Cardiovascular Imaging

OTHER VOLUMES IN THE
EXPERT RADIOLOGY SERIES

Abdominal Imaging

Head and Neck Imaging

Imaging of the Chest

Imaging of the Musculoskeletal System

Imaging of the Spine

Image-Guided Interventions

FORTHCOMING VOLUMES IN THE
EXPERT RADIOLOGY SERIES

Breast Imaging

Gynecologic Imaging

Imaging of the Brain

Pediatric Neuroimaging

Obstetric Imaging

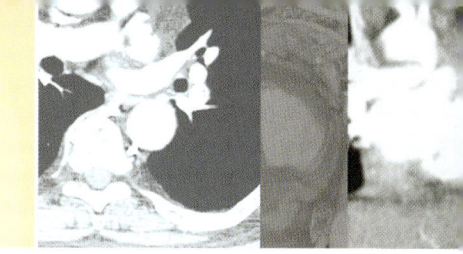

Cardiovascular Imaging
Volume II

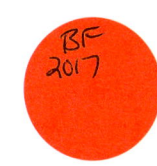

Vincent B. Ho, MD, MBA, FAHA
Fellow, American Heart Association
Professor, Uniformed Services University of the Health Sciences
President, North American Society for Cardiovascular Imaging
Guest Researcher, National Institutes of Health
Editorial Board, *Circulation: Cardiovascular Imaging*
Bethesda, Maryland

Gautham P. Reddy, MD, MPH
Professor of Radiology
Vice Chair for Education
Director of Thoracic Imaging
Department of Radiology
University of Washington School of Medicine
Seattle, Washington

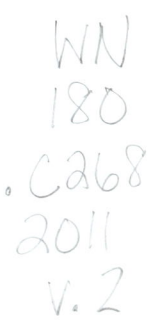

ELSEVIER
SAUNDERS

ELSEVIER
SAUNDERS

3251 Riverport Lane
St. Louis, Missouri 63043

CARDIOVASCULAR IMAGING ISBN: 978-1-4160-5335-4

Copyright © 2011 by Saunders, an imprint of Elsevier Inc.

No part of this publication may be reproduced or transmitted in any form or by any means, electronic or mechanical, including photocopying, recording, or any information storage and retrieval system, without permission in writing from the publisher. Details on how to seek permission, further information about the Publisher's permissions policies and our arrangements with organizations such as the Copyright Clearance Center and the Copyright Licensing Agency, can be found at our website: www.elsevier.com/permissions.

This book and the individual contributions contained in it are protected under copyright by the Publisher (other than as may be noted herein).

Notices

Knowledge and best practice in this field are constantly changing. As new research and experience broaden our understanding, changes in research methods, professional practices, or medical treatment may become necessary.

Practitioners and researchers must always rely on their own experience and knowledge in evaluating and using any information, methods, compounds, or experiments described herein. In using such information or methods they should be mindful of their own safety and the safety of others, including parties for whom they have a professional responsibility.

With respect to any drug or pharmaceutical products identified, readers are advised to check the most current information provided (i) on procedures featured or (ii) by the manufacturer of each product to be administered, to verify the recommended dose or formula, the method and duration of administration, and contraindications. It is the responsibility of practitioners, relying on their own experience and knowledge of their patients, to make diagnoses, to determine dosages and the best treatment for each individual patient, and to take all appropriate safety precautions.

To the fullest extent of the law, neither the Publisher nor the authors, contributors, or editors, assume any liability for any injury and/or damage to persons or property as a matter of products liability, negligence or otherwise, or from any use or operation of any methods, products, instructions, or ideas contained in the material herein.

The opinions or assertions contained herein are the private views of the authors and are not to be construed as official or reflecting the views of the Department of Defense or the Uniformed Services University of the Health Sciences.

Library of Congress Cataloging-in-Publication Data
Cardiovascular imaging / [edited by] Vincent B. Ho, Gautham P. Reddy.—1st ed.
 p. ; cm.
 Includes bibliographical references and index.
 ISBN 978-1-4160-5335-4
 1. Cardiovascular system—Diseases—Diagnosis. 2. Diagnostic imaging. I. Ho, Vincent B.
II. Reddy, Gautham P.
 [DNLM: 1. Cardiovascular Diseases—diagnosis. 2. Diagnostic Imaging—methods. 3. Diagnostic Techniques, Cardiovascular. WG 141 C2686 2010]
 RC670.C364 2010
 616.1′075—dc22
 2010021017

Publishing Director: Linda Duncan
Acquisitions Editor: Rebecca Gaertner
Developmental Editor: Jennifer Shreiner
Publishing Services Manager: Patricia Tannian
Project Manager: Fran Gunning
Project Manager: Carrie Stetz
Design Direction: Steve Stave

Printed in China

Last digit is the print number: 9 8 7 6 5 4 3 2 1

Working together to grow
libraries in developing countries

www.elsevier.com | www.bookaid.org | www.sabre.org

ELSEVIER BOOK AID International Sabre Foundation

*To our families, mentors, colleagues, fellows, residents, and students—
this book is for you.*

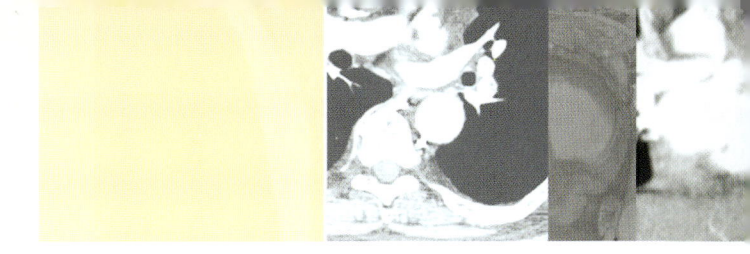

Contributors

Theodore P. Abraham, MD, FACC, FASE
Associate Professor of Medicine
Johns Hopkins University;
Vice-Chief of Cardiology
Co-Director, Echocardiography
Director, Johns Hopkins Hypertrophic
  Cardiomyopathy Clinic
Director, Translational Cardiovascular Ultrasound
  Laboratory
Baltimore, Maryland

Christopher J. Abularrage, MD
Assistant Professor of Surgery
Attending Surgeon
Division of Vascular Surgery and Endovascular
  Therapy
The Johns Hopkins University School of Medicine
Baltimore, Maryland

Mouaz H. Al-Mallah, MD, MSc, FACC, FAHA, FESC
Associate Professor of Medicine
Wayne State University
Detroit, Michigan;
Consultant Cardiologist and Division Head, Cardiac
  Imaging
King Abdul-Aziz Cardiac Center
King Abdul-Aziz Medical City (Riyadh)
National Guard Health Affairs
Saudi Arabia

Mehran Attari, MD
Assistant Professor
Internal Medicine, Cardiology
University of Cincinnati College of Medicine;
Director
Electrophysiology Laboratory
University of Cincinnati Medical Center
Cincinnati, Ohio

Jonathan Balcombe, MD
Radiologist
Imaging On Call
Poughkeepsie, New York

Sanjeev Bhalla, MD
Associate Professor of Radiology
Washington University
Mallinckrodt Institute of Radiology;
Chief, Cardiothoracic Imaging Section
Barnes Jewish Hospital
St. Louis, Missouri

Kostaki G. Bis, MD, FACR
Clinical Professor
Oakland University William Beaumont School of
  Medicine
Rochester Hills, Michigan;
Associate Director, Body Imaging
Department of Radiology
William Beaumont Hospital
Royal Oak, Michigan

Michelle M. Bittle, MD
Assistant Professor
University of Washington
Harborview Medical School
Seattle, Washington

Ron Blankstein, MD
Instructor in Medicine
Harvard Medical School
Brigham and Women's Hospital
Boston, Massachusetts

Thorsten Bley, MD
Assistant Professor
Department of Radiology
University Medical Center Hamburg-Eppendorf
Hamburg, Germany

David A. Bluemke, MD, PhD
Director
Radiology and Imaging Sciences
National Institutes of Health
Bethesda, Maryland

Jamieson M. Bourque, MD, MHS
Fellow in Cardiovascular Disease and Advanced Cardiovascular Imaging
University of Virginia Health System
Charlottesville, Virginia

Lawrence M. Boxt, MD
Professor of Radiology
Albert Einstein College of Medicine;
Director of Cardiac CT and MR Imaging
Division of Cardiology
Montefiore Medical Center
Bronx, New York

Lynn S. Broderick, MD
Professor
Department of Radiology
University of Wisconsin-Madison
Madison, Wisconsin

Thomas G. Brott, MD
Professor, Department of Neurology
Associate Dean for Research
Mayo Clinic
Jacksonville, Florida

Allen Burke, MD
Associate Professor of Pathology
University of Maryland School of Medicine
University of Maryland Medical System
Baltimore, Maryland

Alexander Bustamante, MD
Cardiology Staff
National Naval Medical Center
Bethesda, Maryland

Hugh Calkins, MD
Professor
Medicine and Cardiology
Director, Electrophysiology
Director, ARVD Program
Johns Hopkins Hospital
Baltimore, Maryland

Jeffrey P. Carpenter, MD
Professor and Chief
Department of Surgery
UMDNJ-Robert Wood Johnson Medical School
Camden, New Jersey;
Vice President for Perioperative Services and Chief of Surgery
Cooper Health System
Voorhees, New Jersey

James C. Carr, MD, FFR RCSI
Associate Professor of Radiology and Medicine
Northwestern University Feinberg School of Medicine;
Director of Cardiovascular Imaging
Northwestern Memorial Hospital
Chicago, Illinois

Frandics P. Chan, MD, PhD
Associate Professor of Radiology
Stanford University School of Medicine
Department of Radiology
Stanford, California

Joseph Jen-Sho Chen, MD
Radiology Resident
University of Maryland Medical Center
University of Maryland School of Medicine
Baltimore, Maryland

Bennett Chin, MD
Associate Professor of Radiology
Duke University School of Medicine
Associate Professor of Radiology
Duke University Medical Center
Durham, North Carolina

Jonathan H. Chung, MD
Fellow and Clinical Assistant, Cardiothoracic Imaging
Harvard Medical School
Massachusetts General Hospital
Boston, Massachusetts

William R. Corse, DO
Director of Cardiovascular MRI
Doylestown Hospital
Doylestown, Pennsylvania

Carlos Cuevas, MD
Assistant Professor
Department of Radiology, Body Imaging Section
University of Washington School of Medicine
Assistant Professor
University of Washington Medical Center
Seattle, Washington

Zelmira Curillova, MD
Division of Cardiology
Department of Medicine
VA Boston Healthcare System
West Roxbury, Massachusetts

Ricardo C. Cury, MD
Consulting Radiologist
Massachusetts General Hospital
Harvard Medical School
Boston, Massachusetts;
Director of Cardiac MRI and CT
Baptist Cardiac and Vascular Institute
Miami, Florida

David H. Deaton, MD, FACS
Chief, Endovascular Surgery
Associate Professor of Surgery
Georgetown University Hospital
Washington, DC

Subrato J. Deb, MD, FCCP
Assistant Professor of Surgery
Uniformed Services University
F. Edward Hébert School of Medicine
Bethesda, Maryland;
Cardiovascular and Thoracic Surgeon
Western Maryland Regional Medical Center
Cumberland, Maryland;
Cardiothoracic Surgeon
National Naval Medical Center;
Captain, United States Navy
Naval Reserve, National Naval Medical Center
Bethesda, Maryland

Patrick J.H. de Koning, MSc
Researcher, Image Processing
Leiden University Medical Center
Department of Radiology, Division of Image Processing
Leiden, The Netherlands

J. Kevin DeMarco, MD
Associate Professor
Michigan State University
East Lansing, Michigan;
Attending Radiologist
Lansing, Michigan

Albert de Roos, MD
Professor of Radiology
Leiden University Medical Center
Leiden, The Netherlands

Swati Deshmane, MBBS, DMRD
Research Volunteer
Cardiovascular Imaging
University of California Los Angeles
Los Angeles, California

Lisa M. Dias, MD
Diagnostic Radiology Resident
Department of Radiology
William Beaumont Hospital
Royal Oak, Michigan

Marcelo F. Di Carli, MD, FACC, FAHA
Director, Noninvasive Cardiovascular Imaging Program
Chief, Division of Nuclear Medicine and Molecular Imaging
Brigham and Women's Hospital
Boston, Massachusetts

Manjiri Dighe, MD, DMRE
Assistant Professor
University of Washington Medical Center
Seattle, Washington

Vasken Dilsizian, MD
Professor of Medicine and Radiology
University of Maryland School of Medicine
Chief, Division of Nuclear Medicine
Director, Cardiovascular Nuclear Medicine and PET Imaging
University of Maryland Medical Center
Baltimore, Maryland

Vikram S. Dogra, MD
Professor of Radiology, Urology, and Biomedical Engineering
Director of Ultrasound and Radiology Residency
University of Rochester School of Medicine
Rochester, New York

Jeremy C. Durack, MD
Assistant Professor of Radiology
University of California San Francisco
San Francisco, California

James P. Earls, MD
Medical Director
Cardiovascular CT and MRI
Fairfax Radiological Consultants PC
Fairfax, Virginia

Frederick K. Emge, MD
Departments of Surgery, Radiology, Pediatric Cardiology, and Cardiothoracic and Vascular Surgery
Geisinger Medical Center
Danville, Pennsylvania

A. Sanli Ergun, PhD
Assistant Professor
TOBB-University of Economy and Technology
Ankara, Turkey

Elif Ergun, MD
Instructor in Radiology
Ankara Training and Research Hospital
Ankara, Turkey

Stanford Ewing, MD, FAAP, FRCP(C)
Clinical Assistant Professor
University of Pennsylvania;
Attending Pediatric Cardiologist
Children's Hospital of Philadelphia
Philadelphia, Pennsylvania

Peter Faulhaber, MD, MA
Associate Professor of Radiology
Case Medical Center
Case Western Reserve University;
Director
Clinical PET
University Hospitals Case Medical Center
Cleveland, Ohio

Elliot K. Fishman, MD
Professor of Radiology and Oncology
Johns Hopkins University School of Medicine;
Director, Diagnostic Imaging and Body CT
Johns Hopkins Hospital
Baltimore, Maryland

Mark A. Fogel, MD, FACC, FAHA, FAAP
Associate Professor of Pediatrics and Radiology
Director of Cardiac MRI
University of Pennsylvania School of Medicine;
Children's Hospital of Philadelphia
Philadelphia, Pennsylvania

Thomas K.F. Foo, PhD
Assistant Professor
Department of Radiological Sciences
Uniformed University of the Health Sciences
Bethesda, Maryland;
Manager, MRI Lab
GE Global Research
Niskayuna, New York

Aletta Ann Frazier, MD
Associate Professor of Diagnostic Radiology
University of Maryland School of Medicine
Baltimore, Maryland;
Biomedical Illustrator in Radiologic Pathology
Armed Forces Institute of Pathology
Washington, DC

Tamar Gaspar, MD
Faculty of Medicine
Technion-Israel Institute of Technology;
Head of Cardiovascular Imaging
Carmel Medical Center
Haifa, Israel

Eva Maria Gassner, MD
Department of Radiology
University Hospital Innsbruck
Innsbruck, Austria

Jon C. George, MD
Adjunct Research Instructor
Cardiovascular Research Center
Temple University School of Medicine
Philadelphia, Pennsylvania

Thomas C. Gerber, MD, PhD
Professor of Medicine and Radiology
Mayo Clinic College of Medicine
Rochester, Minnesota;
Consultant in Cardiology
Mayo Clinic
Jacksonville, Florida

Christian L. Gilbert, MD, FACS
Associate Medical Director
The International Children's Heart Foundation
Memphis, Tennessee

Robert C. Gilkeson, MD
Associate Professor
Case Western Reserve University;
Section Chief, Cardiothoracic Imaging
University Hospitals Case Medical Center
Cleveland, Ohio

James F. Glockner, MD, PhD
Assistant Professor
Consultant
Mayo Clinic
Rochester, Minnesota

Michael B. Gotway, MD
Clinical Associate Professor of Diagnostic Radiology
and Biomedical Imaging and Pulmonary/Critical
Care Medicine
University of California
San Francisco, California;
Scottsdale Medical Imaging, Ltd., an affiliate of
Southwest Diagnostic Imaging
Scottsdale, Arizona

Curtis E. Green, MD
Professor of Radiology and Medicine
University of Vermont College of Medicine;
Staff Radiologist
Fletcher Allen Healthcare
Burlington, Vermont

S. Bruce Greenberg, MD
Professor of Radiology
Arkansas Children's Hospital
University of Arkansas for Medical Sciences
Little Rock, Arkansas

Heynric B. Grotenhuis, MD, PhD
Pediatric Cardiologist
Leiden University Medical Center
Leiden, The Netherlands

Martin L. Gunn, MB, ChB, FRANZCR
Assistant Professor
Department of Radiology
University of Washington
Seattle, Washington

Sandra Simon Halliburton, PhD
Adjunct Professor of Chemical and Biomedical
Engineering
Cleveland State University;
Cardiac Imaging Scientist
Cleveland Clinic
Cleveland, Ohio

Ulrike Hamper, MD
Professor of Radiology, Urology, and Pathology
Johns Hopkins University School of Medicine
Baltimore, Maryland

Christopher J. Hardy, PhD
Principal Scientist
GE Global Research
Niskayuna, New York

Jeffrey C. Hellinger, MD
Assistant Professor of Radiology
The Children's Hospital of Philadelphia
Philadelphia, Pennsylvania

Miguel Hernandez-Pampaloni, MD, PhD
Assistant Professor of Radiology
Chief, Nuclear Medicine
University of California San Francisco
San Francisco, California

Charles B. Higgins, MD
Professor of Radiology
University of California San Francisco
San Francisco, California

Vincent B. Ho, MD, MBA, FAHA
Fellow, American Heart Association
Professor, Uniformed Services University of the Health Sciences
President, North American Society for Cardiovascular Imaging
Guest Researcher, National Institutes of Health
Editorial Board, *Circulation: Cardiovascular Imaging*
Bethesda, Maryland

Maureen N. Hood, MS, RN, RT(R)(MR)
Assistant Professor
Department of Radiology and Radiological Sciences
Uniformed Services University of the Health Sciences
F. Edward Hébert School of Medicine
Bethesda, Maryland

Michael D. Hope, MD
Assistant Professor of Radiology
University of California San Francisco
San Francisco, California

Thomas A. Hope, MD
Resident in Radiology
University of California San Francisco
San Francisco, California

Jiang Hsieh, PhD
Adjunct Professor
Medical Physics Department
University of Wisconsin-Madison
Madison, Wisconsin;
Chief Scientist
GE Healthcare
Brookfield, Wisconsin

W. Gregory Hundley, MD
Professor
Wake Forest University School of Medicine
Winston-Salem, North Carolina

John Huston 3d, MD
Professor of Radiology
Mayo Clinic College of Medicine
Rochester, Minnesota

Neil R.A. Isaac, MD
Radiologist
North York General Hospital
Toronto, Ontario

Benjamin M. Jackson, MD, MS
Assistant Professor of Surgery
Division of Vascular Surgery and Endovascular Therapy
University of Pennsylvania
Philadelphia, Pennsylvania

Aditya Jain, MBBS, MPH
Research Fellow
Johns Hopkins Hospital
Baltimore, Maryland

Olga James
Nuclear Medicine Resident
Duke Hospital
Durham, North Carolina

Cylen Javidan-Nejad, MD
Assistant Professor
Mallinckrodt Institute of Radiology
Washington University;
Fellowship Director
Section of Cardiothoracic Imaging
Mallinckrodt Institute of Radiology
St. Louis, Missouri

Jean Jeudy, MD
Assistant Professor
Department of Diagnostic Radiology and Nuclear Medicine
University of Maryland, School of Medicine
Baltimore, Maryland

Saurabh Jha, MBBS, MRCS
Assistant Professor of Radiology
University of Pennsylvania
Philadelphia, Pennsylvania

Pamela T. Johnson, MD
Assistant Professor
Johns Hopkins University School of Medicine
Assistant Professor of Radiology
Johns Hopkins Hospital
Baltimore, Maryland

Praveen Jonnala, MD
Radiologist
Interventional Radiologist and Cardiac Imager
Long Beach Memorial Medical Center
Long Beach, California

Wouter J. Jukema, MD, PhD
Professor, Cardiology
Leiden University Medical Center
Department of Radiology, Division of Image
  Processing
Leiden, The Netherlands

Bobby Kalb, MD
Assistant Professor
Emory University School of Medicine
Atlanta, Georgia

Sanjeeva P. Kalva, MD
Assistant Professor of Radiology
Harvard Medical School
Assistant Radiologist
Massachusetts General Hospital
Boston, Massachusetts

John A. Kaufman, MD, FSIR
Radiologist
Professor of Radiology
Chief, Vascular Interventional Radiology
Dotter Interventional Institute
Oregon Health Sciences University
Portland, Oregon

Aoife N. Keeling, MD, FFR RCSI
Fellow
Cardiovascular and Interventional Radiology
Northwestern Memorial Hospital
Chicago, Illinois

Danny Kim, MSE, MD
Assistant Professor of Radiology
New York University School of Medicine
New York University Langone Medical Center
New York, New York

Sooah Kim, MD
Assistant Professor of Radiology
New York University School of Medicine
New York University Langone Medical Center
New York, New York

TaeHoon Kim, MD
Associate Professor of Radiology
Yunsei University College of Medicine;
Associate Professor
Department of Radiology
Gangnam Serverance Hospital, College of Medicine
Seoul, Korea

Amy Kirby, MD
Medical Director
Ponca City Regional, Logan Medical Center
Kingfisher Regional Medical Center
Oklahoma City, Oklahoma;
Eagle Eye Radiology
Reston, Virginia

Jacobo Kirsch, MD
Section Head
Cardiopulmonary Radiology
Cleveland Clinic Florida
Weston, Florida

Jonathan D. Kirsch, MD
Assistant Professor, Diagnostic Radiology
Associate Chief, Section of Ultrasound
Yale University School of Medicine
Yale-New Haven Hospital
New Haven, Connecticut

Pieter H. Kitslaar, MSc
Researcher, Image Processing
Leiden University Medical Center
Department of Radiology, Division of Image
  Processing
Leiden, The Netherlands

Michael V. Knopp, MD, PhD
Professor of Radiology
Director, Wright Center of Innovation in Biomedical
  Imaging
Novartis Chair of Imaging Research
The Ohio State University
Columbus, Ohio

Marc Kock, MD
Department of Radiology
Albert Schweitzer Hospital
Dordrecht, The Netherlands

Maureen P. Kohi, MD
Clinical Fellow
University of California San Francisco
San Francisco, California

Gerhard Koning, MSc
Researcher, Image Processing
Leiden University Medical Center
Department of Radiology, Division of Image
  Processing
Leiden, The Netherlands

Christopher M. Kramer, MD
Professor
Department of Radiology and Medicine
Director
Cardiovascular Imaging Center
University of Virginia Health System
Charlottesville, Virginia

Mayil S. Krishnam, MD, MRCP, DMRD (UK), FRCR (UK), ABR
Associate Clinical Professor
University of California Irvine
Irvine, California;
Director, Cardiovascular and Thoracic Imaging
UCI Medical Center
Orange, California

Rajesh Krishnamurthy, MBBS
Clinical Assistant Professor of Radiology and Pediatrics
Baylor College of Medicine;
Radiologist
EB Singleton Department of Pediatric Radiology
Texas Children's Hospital
Houston, Texas

Lucia J.M. Kroft, MD, PhD
Radiologist
Leiden University Medical Center
Leiden, The Netherlands

Rahul Kumar, MD
Clinical Cardiology Fellow
Wake Forest Baptist Medical Center
Winston-Salem, North Carolina

Raymond Kwong, MD, MPH, FACC
Assistant Professor of Medicine
Harvard Medical School;
Director, Cardiac Magnetic Resonance Imaging
Brigham and Women's Hospital
Boston, Massachusetts

Brajesh K. Lal, MD, FACS
Associate Professor, Departments of Vascular Surgery,
  Physiology, and Bioengineering
University of Maryland
Baltimore, Maryland

Warren Laskey, MD
Professor of Medicine
Chief, Division of Cardiology
University of New Mexico School of Medicine;
Chief, Division of Cardiology
University of New Mexico Hospital
Albuquerque, New Mexico

Vivian Lee, MBA, MD, PhD
Vice-Dean for Science
Chief Scientific Officer
Professor of Radiology
New York University Medical Center
New York, New York

Christianne Leidecker, PhD
Scientific Collaboration Manager
Siemens Medical Solutions USA, Inc.
Malvern, Pennsylvania

Tim Leiner, MD, PhD
Associate Professor of Radiology
Utrecht University Medical Center
Department of Radiology
Utrecht, The Netherlands

Rachel Booth Lewis, MD
Assistant Professor of Radiology
Uniformed Services University of Health Sciences;
Staff Radiologist
National Naval Medical Center
Bethesda, Maryland;
Chief of Gastrointestinal Radiology
Armed Forces Institute of Pathology
Washington, DC

Jonathan Liaw, MD, MRCP, FRCR
Assistant Professor of Diagnostic and Interventional
  Imaging
University of Texas Houston Medical School;
Assistant Radiologist
Memorial Hermann Hospital
Houston, Texas

Harold Litt, MD, PhD
Assistant Professor of Radiology and Medicine
University of Pennsylvania School of Medicine;
Chief, Cardiovascular Imaging Section
Hospital of the University of Pennsylvania
Philadelphia, Pennsylvania

Derek G. Lohan, MD
Consultant Radiologist
Galway University Hospitals;
Department of Radiology
Hospital Ground, Merlin Park Hospital
Galway, Republic of Ireland

Roi Lotan, MD
Faculty
Robert Wood Johnson University Hospital
New Brunswick, New Jersey

Amit Majmudar, MD
Nuclear Medicine/PET Specialist
Diagnostic Radiology
Radiology, Inc.
Powell, Ohio

Amgad N. Makaryus, MD
Assistant Professor of Clinical Medicine
New York University School of Medicine
New York, New York;
Director of Cardiac CT and MRI
Department of Cardiology
North Shore University Hospital
Manhasset, New York

Jeffrey H. Maki, MD, PhD
Department of Radiology
University of Washington School of Medicine
Puget Sound VA Health Care Service
Seattle, Washington

Neil Mardis, DO
Assistant Professor of Radiology
University of Missouri;
Pediatric Radiologist
The Children's Mercy Hospital and Clinics
Kansas City, Missouri

Henk A. Marquering, PhD
Assistant Professor, Cardiovascular Image Processing
Amsterdam Medical Center
Department of Biomedical Engineering and Physics
Amsterdam, The Netherlands

Diego Martin, MD, PhD
Professor of Radiology
Director of MRI
Emory University School of Medicine
Atlanta, Georgia

Alison Knauth Meadows, MD, PhD
Assistant Professor of Radiology and Pediatrics
University of California San Francisco
San Francisco, California

Lina Mehta, MD
Assistant Professor of Radiology
Associate Dean for Admissions
Case Western Reserve University
University Hospitals Case Medical Center
Cleveland, Ohio

Kristin Mercado, MD
Fellow in Cardiovascular Imaging
Harvard Medical School
Brigham and Women's Hospital
Boston, Massachusetts

Steven A. Messina, MD
Resident
Diagnostic Radiology and Nuclear Medicine
Department of Radiology
University of Florida College of Medicine
Gainesville, Florida

Cristopher A. Meyer, MD
Professor
University of Wisconsin School of Medicine and Public Health
Madison, Wisconsin

Mariana Meyers, MD
Resident
University Hospitals Case Medical Center
Cleveland, Ohio

Donald L. Miller, MD
Professor of Radiology and Radiological Sciences
Uniformed Services University of the Health Sciences;
Interventional Radiologist
Department of Radiology
National Naval Medical Center
Bethesda, Maryland

Edward J. Miller, MD, PhD
Assistant Professor
Uniformed Services University of the Health Sciences;
Staff Cardiologist
National Naval Medical Center
Bethesda, Maryland

Tan-Lucien Mohammed, MD
Residency Program Director, Imaging Institute
Fellowship Program Director, Section of Thoracic Imaging
Staff Radiologist, Section of Thoracic Imaging
Cleveland Clinic
Cleveland, Ohio

Phillip Moore, MD, MBA
Professor of Clinical Pediatrics
University of California San Francisco Medical School;
Director, Pediatric and Adult Congenital Cardiac Catheterization Laboratory
University of California San Francisco
San Francisco, California

Mariam Moshiri, MD
Clinical Assistant Professor
University of Washington
Clinical Assistant Professor
Director of Body Imaging Fellowship
University of Washington Medical Center
Seattle, Washington

Gaku Nakazawa, MD
CV Path Institute
Gaithersburg, Maryland

Gautam Nayak, MD
Department of Cardiology
National Naval Medical Center
Bethesda, Maryland

Kenneth J. Nichols, PhD
Associate Professor of Radiology
Hofstra University
Hempstead, New York;
Senior Medical Physicist
Division of Nuclear Medicine & Molecular Imaging
North Shore-Long Island Jewish Medical Center
Manhasset & New Hyde Park, New York

Jonathan A. Nye, PhD
Assistant Professor
Department of Radiology
Emory University
Atlanta, Georgia

James K. O'Donnell, MD
Professor of Radiology
School of Medicine
Case Western Reserve University;
Director of Nuclear Medicine
Case Medical Center
University Hospitals of Cleveland
Cleveland, Ohio

Karen G. Ordovas, MD
Assistant Professor of Radiology
University of California San Francisco
San Francisco, California

Hideki Ota, MD, PhD
Research Fellow
Michigan State University
East Lansing, Michigan

Jaap Ottenkamp, MD, PhD
Pediatric Cardiologist
Leiden University Medical Center
Leiden, The Netherlands

Maitraya K. Patel, MD
Assistant Professor of Radiology
David Geffen School of Medicine at UCLA
Los Angeles, California

Smita Patel, MBBS, MRCP, FRCR
Associate Professor of Radiology
University of Michigan Medical School
University of Michigan Medical Center
Ann Arbor, Michigan

Aurélio C. Pinheiro, MD, PhD
Post-Doctoral Research Fellow
Adult Echocardiography Laboratory
Johns Hopkins University
Baltimore, Maryland

Benjamin Pomerantz, MD
Instructor of Radiology
Harvard Medical School;
Assistant Radiologist
Massachusetts General Hospital
Boston, Massachusetts

Martin R. Prince, MD, PhD
Professor
Weill Cornell Medical Center;
Professor
Columbia College of Physicians and Surgeons
New York, New York

Joan C. Prowda, MD, JD
Associate Clinical Professor of Radiology
Columbia University College of Physicians and Surgeons;
Associate Attending
New York Presbyterian Hospital
New York, New York

Chirapa Puntawangkoon, MD
Research Fellow
Wake Forest University School of Medicine
Winston-Salem, North Carolina

Steven S. Raman, MD
Associate Professor of Radiology
David Geffen School of Medicine at UCLA
Los Angeles, California

Gautham P. Reddy, MD, MPH
Professor of Radiology
Vice Chair for Education
Director of Thoracic Imaging
Department of Radiology
University of Washington School of Medicine
Seattle, Washington

Johan H.C. Reiber, PhD
Head, Division of Image Processing
Leiden University Medical Center
Department of Radiology, Division of Image Processing
Leiden, The Netherlands

Justus E. Roos, MD
Assistant Professor
Stanford University;
Assistant Professor
Department of Radiology
Medical Center Stanford University
Stanford, California

Stefan G. Ruehm, MD, PhD
Associate Professor and Director, Cardiovascular CT
Director, Cardiovascular Imaging
Santa Monica Hospital
University of California Los Angeles;
Department of Radiology
Medical Center and Orthopedic Hospital
David Geffen School of Medicine at UCLA
Los Angeles, California

Raymond R. Russell, MD, PhD
Associate Professor of Medicine and Diagnostic Radiology
Yale University School of Medicine
New Haven, Connecticut

Marcel Santos, MD, PhD
Attending Radiologist
University Hospital of the School of Medicine of Ribeirao Preto
Sao Paulo, Brazil

U. Joseph Schoepf, MD, FAHA, FSCBT-MR, FSCCT
Professor of Radiology and Medicine
Director of Cardiovascular Imaging
Medical University of South Carolina
Charleston, South Carolina

Leslie M. Scoutt, MD
Professor of Diagnostic Radiology
Yale University School of Medicine;
Chief, Ultrasound Service
Yale-New Haven Hospital
New Haven, Connecticut

Laureen Sena, MD
Clinical Instructor
Harvard Medical School;
Staff Radiologist
Children's Hospital
Boston, Massachusetts

Nidhi Sharma, MD
Fellow, Section of Molecular and Functional Imaging
Cleveland Clinic
Cleveland, Ohio

Rajesh Sharma, MD
Department of Radiodiagnosis
Government Medical College Hospital
Jammu, India

Matthew J. Sharp, MD
Staff Radiologist
Portland Veterans Affairs Medical Center
Adjunct Professor, Oregon Health and Sciences University
Portland, Oregon

John J. Sheehan, MD, MRCSI, FFRRCSI
Assistant Professor of Radiology
The University of Chicago, Pritzker School of Medicine;
Director of Cardiovascular Imaging
NorthShore University Health System
Chicago, Illinois

Mark Sheldon, MD
Assistant Professor of Medicine
University of New Mexico, School of Medicine;
Assistant Professor
University of New Mexico Health Sciences Center
University of New Mexico Hospital
Albuquerque, New Mexico

Marilyn J. Siegel, MD
Professor of Radiology and Pediatrics
Washington University School of Medicine
St. Louis, Missouri

Albert J. Sinusas, MD
Professor of Medicine and Diagnostic Radiology
Director, Animal Research Laboratories, Section of Cardiovascular Medicine
Director, Cardiovascular Nuclear Imaging and Stress Laboratories
Yale University
New Haven, Connecticut

Ting Song, PhD
Assistant Professor
Department of Radiology
Uniformed Services University of the Health Sciences;
Scientist
GE Healthcare
Bethesda, Maryland

Anand Soni, MD
Cardiac Imaging Fellow
Massachusetts General Hospital
Harvard Medical School
Boston, Massachusetts

William Stanford, MD
Professor Emeritus
Roy T. and Lucille A. Carver College of Medicine
The University of Iowa;
Professor Emeritus
Department of Radiology
The University of Iowa Hospitals and Clinics
Iowa City, Iowa

Alexander B. Steever, MD
Assistant Clinical Professor of Radiology
Columbia University Medical Center
Harlem Hospital
New York, New York

Robert M. Steiner, MD
Professor of Radiology and Medicine
Temple University School of Medicine
Philadelphia, Pennsylvania;
Clinical Professor of Radiology
Stanford University School of Medicine
Stanford, California;
Chief, Thoracic Radiology
Temple University Hospital
Philadelphia, Pennsylvania

Jadranka Stojanovska, MD
Clinical Lecturer
Department of Radiology
University of Michigan Medical School
University of Michigan Medical Center
Ann Arbor, Michigan

Harikrishna Tandri, MD
Assistant Professor of Cardiology
Johns Hopkins Hospital
Baltimore, Maryland

Shawn D. Teague, MD
Associate Professor of Clinical Radiology
Indiana University School of Medicine
Indianapolis, Indiana

John S. Thurber, MD
Assistant Professor of Surgery
Uniformed Services University of the Health Sciences
F. Edward Hébert School of Medicine;
Integrated Chief of Cardiothoracic Surgery
Attending Cardiothoracic Surgeon
Captain, Medical Corps
United States Navy
National Naval Medical Center
Bethesda, Maryland;
Walter Reed Army Medical Center
Washington, DC

Ahmet T. Turgut, MD
Associate Professor in Radiology
Ankara Training and Research Hospital
Ankara, Turkey

Rob J. van der Geest, MSc
Assistant Professor, Image Processing
Leiden University Medical Center
Department of Radiology, Division of Image Processing
Leiden, The Netherlands

Ronald van 't Klooster, MSc
Researcher, Image Processing
Leiden University Medical Center
Department of Radiology, Division of Image Processing
Leiden, The Netherlands

Jens Vogel-Claussen, MD
Assistant Professor
Johns Hopkins University;
Department of Radiology
Tübingen University
Tübingen, Germany

John R. Votaw, PhD
Professor and Vice Chair for Research
Department of Radiology
Emory University
Atlanta, Georgia

Thomas G. Vrachliotis, MD, PhD
Director of Interventional Radiology
Henry Dunant Hospital
Athens, Greece

Dharshan Raj Vummidi, MRCP, FRCR
Acting Instructor and Senior Fellow in Cardiothoracic Imaging
University of Washington
Seattle, Washington

Stephen Waite, MD
Assistant Professor of Clinical Radiology and Internal Medicine
Chief of Cardiovascular Radiology
SUNY Downstate
Brooklyn, New York

T. Gregory Walker, MD
Instructor in Radiology
Harvard Medical School
Associate Radiologist
Fellowship Director, Vascular Imaging and Intervention
Massachusetts General Hospital
Boston, Massachusetts

Gaby Weissman, MD
Assistant Professor of Medicine
Georgetown University;
Cardiac Imaging
Washington Hospital Center
Washington, DC

Charles S. White, MD
Professor of Radiology
Director of Thoracic Imaging
Department of Radiology
University of Maryland
Baltimore, Maryland

Kevin K. Whitehead, MD, PhD
Assistant Professor of Pediatrics
University of Pennsylvania School of Medicine;
Noninvasive Imaging
Children's Hospital of Philadelphia
Philadelphia, Pennsylvania

Oliver Wieben, PhD
Assistant Professor
Departments of Medical Physics and Radiology
University of Wisconsin
Madison, Wisconsin

Eric E. Williamson, MD
Assistant Professor, Cardiovascular Radiology
Mayo Clinic Rochester
Rochester, Minnesota

Priscilla A. Winchester, MD
Associate Professor of Clinical Radiology
Weill Cornell Medical College
New York Presbyterian Hospital
New York, New York

Carol C. Wu, MD
Clinical Instructor
Harvard Medical School
Assistant Radiologist
Massachusetts General Hospital
Boston, Massachusetts

Louis Wu, MD, CM
Director, MRI
Department of Radiology
Lakeridge Health Oshawa
Oshawa, Ontario, Canada

Vahid Yaghmai, MD, MS
　Associate Professor
　Northwestern University;
　Medical Director CT
　Northwestern Memorial Hospital
　Chicago, Illinois

Douglas Yim, MD
　Assistant Professor of Radiology and Radiologist
　　Sciences
　Uniformed Services University of the Health Sciences;
　Chief, Interventional Radiology
　National Naval Medical Center
　Bethesda, Maryland

Phillip M. Young, MD
　Assistant Professor of Diagnostic Radiology
　Mayo Clinic College of Medicine;
　Senior Associate Consultant in Diagnostic Radiology
　Mayo Clinic
　Rochester, Minnesota

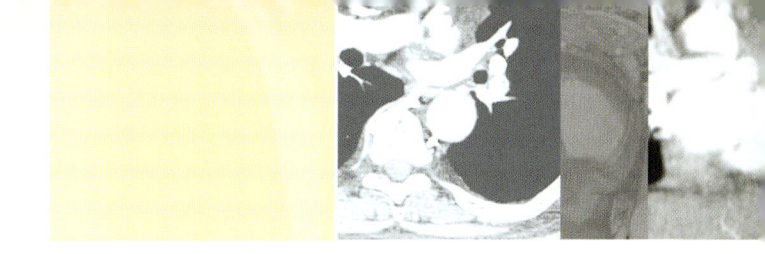

Preface

The ability to image the cardiovascular system has improved exponentially over the past 20 years. This project began rather modestly but quickly ballooned to a two-volume book of 119 chapters as we began to lengthen our list of the most important cardiovascular imaging techniques and common conditions. We were fortunate to have enlisted an excellent group of highly dedicated experts from the best universities and cardiovascular centers in the world.

Our book consists of two volumes: Cardiac Imaging (Volume I) and Vascular Imaging (Volume II). Section 1 of Volume I begins with an introduction to normal cardiac embryology, anatomy, and physiology. Section 2 reviews the physics and technical considerations for the various cardiac imaging techniques ranging from plain film, echocardiography, and invasive catheterization to advanced cardiac CT, MR, SPECT, and PET/CT. This section is supplemented by special discussions on CT dose reduction strategies, CT and MR contrast agents, MR safety, radiopharmaceuticals, and pharmacologic stress agents. Section 3 is dedicated to cardiac interventions, covering both percutaneous as well as open procedures. In Section 4, coronary artery imaging is reviewed with detailed discussions of imaging of coronary artery calcium, congenital coronary anomalies, obstructive coronary disease, coronary artery aneurysms, and coronary revascularization procedures. Section 5 reviews the wide variety of acyanotic and cyanotic congenital heart disease with special mention of coarctation of the aorta as well as vascular rings and slings. In Section 6, the pathologic basis for ischemic heart disease is reviewed and followed by detailed discussions of myocardial perfusion, function, and viability as determined by CT, MR, and radionuclide imaging. Valvular heart disease is reviewed in Section 7. Section 8 details the various forms of cardiomyopathy (i.e., dilated, restrictive, and hypertrophic), including chapters on arrhythmogenic right ventricular dysplasia and myocarditis. Section 9 provides a brilliant pictorial of cardiac tumors. In Section 10, pericardial diseases are discussed.

Volume II is devoted to vascular imaging and begins with Section 11, which reviews normal arterial and venous anatomy in the thorax, abdomen, pelvis, and extremities. Section 12 provides a technical and clinical discussion of vascular ultrasound, CT angiography (CTA), MR angiography (MRA), CTA/MRA image postprocessing, and vascular applications of nuclear medicine. Section 13 provides a review of the various arterial percutaneous and open procedures. Noninvasive imaging of atherosclerotic plaque ("plaque imaging") is reviewed in Section 14. In Section 15, carotid artery disease and imaging using ultrasound, CTA, and MRA are reviewed. Section 16 discusses common vascular thoracic conditions such as thoracic aortic aneurysm, acute aortic syndrome, aortic trauma, aortitis, pulmonary thromboembolism, pulmonary arterial hypertension, pulmonary edema and pulmonary hemorrhage, and vasculitis. This is followed by Section 17, which explores imaging considerations for the various abdominal vascular conditions such as abdominal aortic disease, endograft arterial repair, open surgical arterial repair, renal artery hypertension, renal and central venous conditions, hepatic transplantation, and renal and pancreatic transplantation. In Section 18, peripheral arterial disease and lower extremity imaging are described, with inclusion of newer techniques for peripheral CTA and MRA. In Section 19, upper extremity vascular imaging applications, including hemodialysis fistulas, are discussed.

This project is the culmination of many years of experience from a multitude of contributors with a variety of backgrounds. We hope that readers will enjoy reading the chapters as well as appreciate the expert recommendations provided by our contributors.

In addition to the contributing authors, we would like to thank many people at Elsevier—notably Rebecca Gaertner for entrusting this most important portion of the *Expert Radiology* collection to us, Jennifer Shreiner for providing critical and timely editorial guidance and assistance, and Fran Gunning and Carrie Stetz for providing terrific closure for this project.

VINCENT B. HO, MD, MBA, FAHA
Bethesda, Maryland

GAUTHAM P. REDDY, MD, MPH
Seattle, Washington

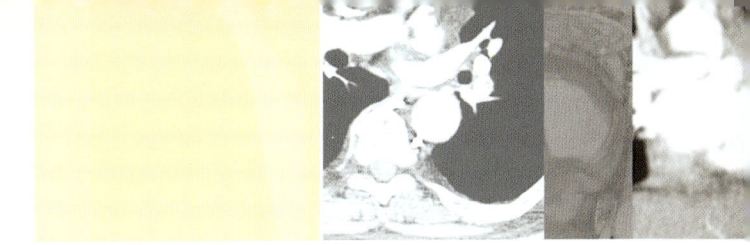

Contents

VOLUME I

PART ONE: AN INTRODUCTION TO THE HEART

CHAPTER 1 **Embryologic Basis and Segmental Approach to Imaging of Congenital Heart Disease** 3
Rajesh Krishnamurthy

CHAPTER 2 **Cardiac Anatomy** 30
Dharshan Raj Vummidi and Gautham P. Reddy

CHAPTER 3 **Coronary Anatomy** 38
Jadranka Stojanovska and Smita Patel

CHAPTER 4 **Physiology of the Heart** 57
Phillip M. Young and Thomas C. Gerber

PART TWO: CARDIAC IMAGING TECHNIQUES

CHAPTER 5 **Radiology of the Heart: Plain Film Imaging and Diagnosis** 71
Robert M. Steiner

CHAPTER 6 **Echocardiography** 98
Theodore P. Abraham and Aurélio C. Pinheiro

CHAPTER 7 **Diagnostic Coronary Angiography** 123
Curtis E. Green

CHAPTER 8 **Physics of Cardiac Computed Tomography** 133
Christianne Leidecker

CHAPTER 9 **Clinical Techniques of Cardiac Computed Tomography** 143
Shawn D. Teague

CHAPTER 10 **Radiation Dose Reduction Strategies in Cardiac Computed Tomography** 150
Sandra Simon Halliburton

CHAPTER 11 **Contrast Agents and Medications in Cardiac Computed Tomography** 156
Justus E. Roos

CHAPTER 12 **Image Postprocessing in Cardiac Computed Tomography** 167
Elliot K. Fishman and Pamela T. Johnson

CHAPTER 13 **Methods for Cardiac Magnetic Resonance Imaging** 180
Thomas K.F. Foo and Christopher J. Hardy

CHAPTER 14 **Clinical Techniques of Cardiac Magnetic Resonance Imaging: Morphology, Perfusion, and Viability** 201
Louis Wu and Gautham P. Reddy

CHAPTER 15 **Clinical Techniques of Cardiac Magnetic Resonance Imaging: Function** 215
Rahul Kumar and W. Gregory Hundley

CHAPTER 16 **Clinical Techniques of Cardiac Magnetic Resonance Imaging: Functional Interpretation and Image Processing** 227
Chirapa Puntawangkoon and W. Gregory Hundley

CHAPTER 17 **Magnetic Resonance Evaluation of Blood Flow** 239
Michael D. Hope, Karen G. Ordovas, Thomas A. Hope, Alison Knauth Meadows, Charles B. Higgins, and Gautham P. Reddy

CHAPTER 18 **Contrast Agents in Magnetic Resonance Imaging** 251
Michael V. Knopp

CHAPTER 19 **Magnetic Resonance Imaging Safety** 261
Maureen N. Hood

CHAPTER 20 **Physics and Instrumentation of Cardiac Single Photon Emission Computed Tomography** 270
Edward J. Miller and Raymond R. Russell

CHAPTER 21 **Clinical Single Photon Emission Computed Tomography Cardiac Protocols** 281
Miguel Hernandez-Pampaloni

CHAPTER 22 **Radiopharmaceutical Single Photon Emission Computed Tomography Imaging Agents** 298
Alexander Bustamante and Gautam Nayak

Contents

CHAPTER 23 Physics and Instrumentation of Cardiac Positron Emission Tomography/Computed Tomography 304
John R. Votaw and Jonathan A. Nye

CHAPTER 24 Clinical Techniques of Positron Emission Tomography and PET/CT 325
Marcelo F. Di Carli and Mouaz H. Al-Mallah

CHAPTER 25 Radiopharmaceuticals and Radiation Dose Considerations in Cardiac Positron Emission Tomography and PET/CT 339
Gaby Weissman and Albert J. Sinusas

CHAPTER 26 Pharmacologic Stress Agents 352
Alexander Bustamante and Gautam Nayak

PART THREE: CARDIAC INTERVENTIONS

CHAPTER 27 Congenital Percutaneous Interventions 363
Phillip Moore

CHAPTER 28 Congenital Cardiac Surgery 383
Frederick K. Emge and Christian L. Gilbert

CHAPTER 29 Percutaneous Catheter-Based Treatment of Coronary and Valvular Heart Disease 393
Mark Sheldon and Warren Laskey

CHAPTER 30 Surgery for Acquired Cardiac Disease 412
John S. Thurber and Subrato J. Deb

CHAPTER 31 Imaging of Atrial Fibrillation Intervention 442
Cristopher A. Meyer and Mehran Attari

PART FOUR: CORONARY ARTERY IMAGING

CHAPTER 32 Coronary Calcium Assessment 457
William Stanford

CHAPTER 33 Congenital Coronary Anomalies 466
James P. Earls

CHAPTER 34 Indications and Patient Selection in Obstructive Coronary Disease 477
Eva Maria Gassner and U. Joseph Schoepf

CHAPTER 35 Interpretation and Reporting in Obstructive Coronary Disease 493
Tamar Gaspar

CHAPTER 36 Coronary Artery Aneurysms 509
Jon C. George, Mariana Meyers, and Robert C. Gilkeson

CHAPTER 37 Imaging of Coronary Revascularization: Coronary Stents and Bypass Grafts 515
Jean Jeudy, Stephen Waite, and Joseph Jen-Sho Chen

PART FIVE: CONGENITAL HEART DISEASE

CHAPTER 38 Coarctation of the Aorta 535
Marilyn J. Siegel

CHAPTER 39 Vascular Rings and Slings 542
Marilyn J. Siegel

CHAPTER 40 Magnetic Resonance Imaging of the Aorta and Left Ventricular Function in Inherited and Congenital Aortic Disease 549
Heynric B. Grotenhuis, Jaap Ottenkamp, Lucia J.M. Kroft, and Albert de Roos

Section One: **Acyanotic Heart Disease with Increased Vascularity**

CHAPTER 41 Atrial Septal Defect 563
Amgad N. Makaryus and Lawrence M. Boxt

CHAPTER 42 Ventricular Septal Defect 572
Amgad N. Makaryus and Lawrence M. Boxt

CHAPTER 43 Patent Ductus Arteriosus 583
Cylen Javidan-Nejad

Section Two: **Cyanotic Heart Disease with Increased Vascularity**

CHAPTER 44 Transposition of the Great Arteries 601
Frandics P. Chan

CHAPTER 45 Truncus Arteriosus 616
Frandics P. Chan

CHAPTER 46 Anomalous Pulmonary Venous Connections and Drainage 625
Laureen Sena and Neil Mardis

CHAPTER 47 Tetralogy of Fallot 640
S. Bruce Greenberg

CHAPTER 48 Ebstein Anomaly 654
Jeffrey C. Hellinger

CHAPTER 49 Complex Congenital Heart Disease 656
Kevin K. Whitehead, Stanford Ewing, and Mark A. Fogel

CHAPTER 50 Magnetic Resonance Imaging in the Postoperative Evaluation of the Patient with Congenital Heart Disease 689
Alison Knauth Meadows, Karen G. Ordovas, Charles B. Higgins, and Gautham P. Reddy

PART SIX: ISCHEMIC HEART DISEASE

CHAPTER 51 Atherosclerotic Coronary Artery Disease 705
Allen Burke, Gaku Nakazawa, and Charles S. White

CHAPTER 52 Acute Coronary Syndrome 715
Joseph Jen-Sho Chen and Charles S. White

CHAPTER 53 Magnetic Resonance and Computed Tomographic Imaging of Myocardial Perfusion 726
Ricardo C. Cury, Anand Soni, and Ron Blankstein

CHAPTER 54 Nuclear Medicine Imaging of Myocardial Perfusion 738
Olga James, Kenneth J. Nichols, and Bennett Chin

CHAPTER 55 Magnetic Resonance and Computed Tomographic Imaging of Myocardial Function 752
Kristin Mercado and Raymond Kwong

CHAPTER 56 Nuclear Medicine Imaging of Ventricular Function 771
Bennett Chin and Kenneth J. Nichols

CHAPTER 57 Magnetic Resonance Imaging of Myocardial Viability 781
Zelmira Curillova and Raymond Kwong

CHAPTER 58 Nuclear Medicine Imaging of Myocardial Viability 790
Steven A. Messina and Vasken Dilsizian

CHAPTER 59 Postoperative Imaging of Ischemic Cardiac Disease 810
Praveen Jonnala, Swati Deshmane, and Mayil S. Krishnam

PART SEVEN: VALVULAR HEART DISEASE

CHAPTER 60 Aortic and Mitral Valvular Disease 827
Roi Lotan and Jens Vogel-Claussen

CHAPTER 61 Tricuspid and Pulmonary Valvular Disease 839
Jeffrey C. Hellinger

PART EIGHT: CARDIOMYOPATHIES AND OTHER MYOCARDIAL DISEASES

CHAPTER 62 Dilated Cardiomyopathy 851
James F. Glockner

CHAPTER 63 Restrictive Cardiomyopathy 861
James F. Glockner

CHAPTER 64 Hypertrophic Cardiomyopathy 874
Gautham P. Reddy, Matthew J. Sharp, and Karen G. Ordovas

CHAPTER 65 Arrhythmogenic Right Ventricular Dysplasia 884
Aditya Jain, Harikrishna Tandri, Hugh Calkins, and David A. Bluemke

CHAPTER 66 Myocarditis 896
Carol C. Wu and Mayil S. Krishnam

PART NINE: TUMORS AND MASSES

CHAPTER 67 Cardiac Tumors 905
Aletta Ann Frazier and Rachel Booth Lewis

PART TEN: PERICARDIAL DISEASE

CHAPTER 68 Pericardial Effusion 941
Lynn S. Broderick

CHAPTER 69 Acute Pericarditis 945
Lynn S. Broderick

CHAPTER 70 Constrictive Pericarditis 949
Lynn S. Broderick

VOLUME II

PART ELEVEN: VASCULAR ANATOMY AND CIRCULATION/ARTERIAL ANATOMY

CHAPTER 71 Arterial Anatomy of the Thorax 955
Amy Kirby, Jacobo Kirsch, and Eric E. Williamson

CHAPTER 72 Arterial Anatomy of the Abdomen 969
Jeremy C. Durack and Maureen P. Kohi

CHAPTER 73 Arterial Anatomy of the Pelvis and Lower Extremities 978
Douglas Yim and Donald L. Miller

CHAPTER 74 Arterial Anatomy of the Upper Extremities 989
Douglas Yim and Donald L. Miller

CHAPTER 75 Venous Anatomy of the Thorax 996
Jacobo Kirsch, Amy Kirby, and Eric E. Williamson

CHAPTER 76 Venous Anatomy of the Abdomen and Pelvis 1005
Jeremy C. Durack and Maureen P. Kohi

CHAPTER 77 Venous Anatomy of the Extremities 1019
Jeffrey C. Hellinger

PART TWELVE: NONINVASIVE VASCULAR IMAGING TECHNIQUES

CHAPTER 78 Vascular Ultrasonography: Physics, Instrumentation, and Clinical Techniques 1033
Elif Ergun, Ahmet T. Turgut, A. Sanli Ergun, and Vikram S. Dogra

CHAPTER 79 Physics of Computed Tomography 1047
Jiang Hsieh

CHAPTER 80 Computed Tomographic Angiography: Clinical Techniques 1055
John J. Sheehan, Aoife N. Keeling, Vahid Yaghmai, and James C. Carr

CHAPTER 81 Magnetic Resonance Angiography: Physics and Instrumentation 1078
Oliver Wieben and Thorsten Bley

CHAPTER 82 **Magnetic Resonance Angiography: Clinical Techniques** 1102
Stefan G. Ruehm and Derek G. Lohan

CHAPTER 83 **Basic Three-Dimensional Postprocessing in Computed Tomographic and Magnetic Resonance Angiography** 1120
Ting Song, William R. Corse, and Vincent B. Ho

CHAPTER 84 **Advanced Three-Dimensional Postprocessing in Computed Tomographic and Magnetic Resonance Angiography** 1128
Rob J. van der Geest, Pieter H. Kitslaar, Patrick J.H. de Koning, Ronald van 't Klooster, Wouter J. Jukema, Gerhard Koning, Henk A. Marquering, and Johan H.C. Reiber

CHAPTER 85 **Nuclear Medicine: Extrathoracic Vascular Imaging** 1144
Amit Majmudar and James K. O'Donnell

PART THIRTEEN: CATHETER ANGIOGRAPHY AND INTERVENTIONS

CHAPTER 86 **Percutaneous Vascular Interventions** 1155
Jonathan Liaw, Benjamin Pomerantz, and Sanjeeva P. Kalva

CHAPTER 87 **Vascular Surgery** 1172
Christopher J. Abularrage and David H. Deaton

PART FOURTEEN: ATHEROSCLEROSIS

CHAPTER 88 **Noninvasive Imaging of Atherosclerosis** 1193
Jamieson M. Bourque and Christopher M. Kramer

PART FIFTEEN: THE CAROTID ARTERIES

CHAPTER 89 **Carotid Artery Disease** 1217
Brajesh K. Lal and Thomas G. Brott

CHAPTER 90 **Ultrasound Evaluation of the Carotid Arteries** 1227
Leslie M. Scoutt, Jonathan D. Kirsch, and Ulrike Hamper

CHAPTER 91 **Magnetic Resonance and Computed Tomographic Angiography of the Extracranial Carotid Arteries** 1251
J. Kevin DeMarco, John Huston 3d, and Hideki Ota

PART SIXTEEN: THE THORACIC VESSELS

CHAPTER 92 **Thoracic Aortic Aneurysms** 1271
Saurabh Jha and Harold Litt

CHAPTER 93 **Acute Aortic Syndrome** 1288
TaeHoon Kim and Harold Litt

CHAPTER 94 **Thoracic Aortic Trauma** 1306
Jonathan Balcombe and Harold Litt

CHAPTER 95 **Thoracic Aortitis** 1314
Neil R.A. Isaac and Harold Litt

CHAPTER 96 **Subclavian Steal Syndrome** 1326
Dharshan Raj Vummidi and Gautham P. Reddy

CHAPTER 97 **Acute Pulmonary Thromboembolic Disease** 1332
Nidhi Sharma and Tan-Lucien Mohammed

CHAPTER 98 **Chronic Pulmonary Embolism** 1344
Sanjeev Bhalla

CHAPTER 99 **Pulmonary Hypertension** 1353
Michael B. Gotway

CHAPTER 100 **Pulmonary Edema** 1373
Michael B. Gotway

CHAPTER 101 **Pulmonary Hemorrhage and Vasculitis** 1383
Michael B. Gotway

PART SEVENTEEN: THE ABDOMINAL VESSELS

CHAPTER 102 **The Abdominal Aorta** 1397
Martin L. Gunn, Jonathan H. Chung, Michelle M. Bittle, and Jeffrey H. Maki

CHAPTER 103 **Postendograft Imaging of the Abdominal Aorta and Iliac Arteries** 1420
Thomas G. Vrachliotis, Kostaki G. Bis, and Lisa M. Dias

CHAPTER 104 **Open Repair of Abdominal Aortic Aneurysms and Postoperative Assessment** 1439
Lisa M. Dias, Kostaki G. Bis, and Thomas G. Vrachliotis

CHAPTER 105 **Magnetic Resonance Imaging of Vascular Disorders of the Abdomen** 1451
Marcel Santos, Bobby Kalb, and Diego Martin

CHAPTER 106 **Renal Artery Hypertension** 1471
Tim Leiner

CHAPTER 107 **Renal Arteries: Computed Tomographic and Magnetic Resonance Angiography** 1483
Danny Kim, Sooah Kim, and Vivian Lee

CHAPTER 108 **Renal Artery Scintigraphy** 1492
Lina Mehta, James K. O'Donnell, and Peter Faulhaber

CHAPTER 109 **Sonography of the Renal Vessels** 1497
Rajesh Sharma and Vikram S. Dogra

CHAPTER 110 **Inferior Vena Cava and Its Main Tributaries** 1524
Carlos Cuevas, Manjiri Dighe, and Mariam Moshiri

CHAPTER 111 **Vascular Imaging of Hepatic Transplantation** 1544
Maitraya K. Patel and Steven S. Raman

CHAPTER 112 **Vascular Imaging of Renal and Pancreatic Transplantation**   1559
Alexander B. Steever, Martin R. Prince, Priscilla A. Winchester, and Joan C. Prowda

PART EIGHTEEN: THE LOWER EXTREMITY VESSELS

CHAPTER 113 **Peripheral Artery Disease**   1573
Benjamin M. Jackson and Jeffrey P. Carpenter

CHAPTER 114 **Lower Extremity Operations and Interventions**   1585
T. Gregory Walker, Sanjeeva P. Kalva, and John A. Kaufman

CHAPTER 115 **Computed Tomographic Angiography of the Lower Extremities**   1610
Saurabh Jha and Harold Litt

CHAPTER 116 **Peripheral Magnetic Resonance Angiography**   1628
Tim Leiner

PART NINETEEN: THE UPPER EXTREMITY VESSELS

CHAPTER 117 **Vascular Diseases of the Upper Extremities**   1643
Tim Leiner and Marc Kock

CHAPTER 118 **Venous Sonography of the Upper Extremities and Thoracic Outlet**   1661
Jonathan D. Kirsch, Ulrike Hamper, and Leslie M. Scoutt

CHAPTER 119 **Hemodialysis Fistulas**   1672
Tim Leiner

Index   I-1

PART ELEVEN

Vascular Anatomy and Circulation/ Arterial Anatomy

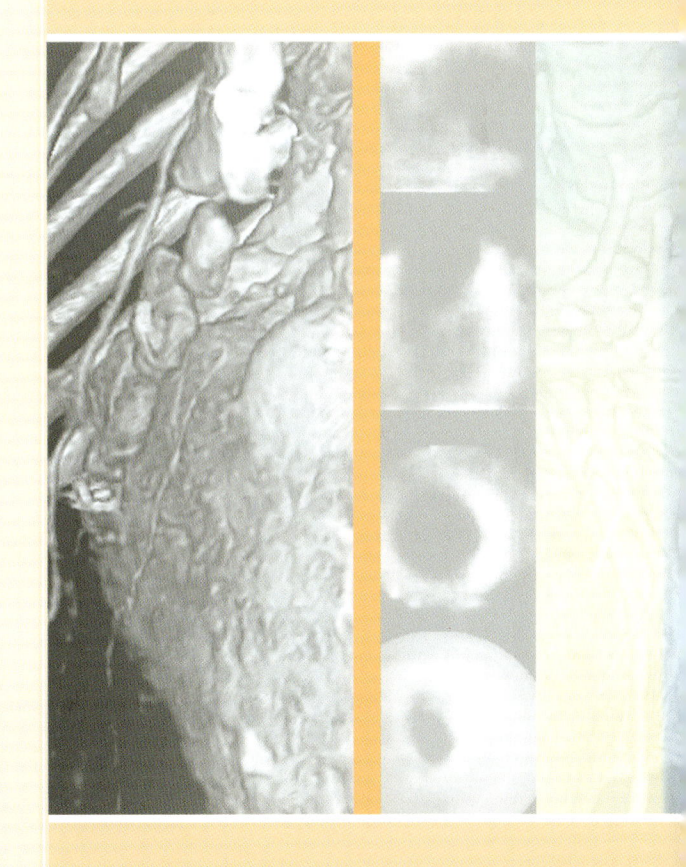

CHAPTER 71

Arterial Anatomy of the Thorax

Amy Kirby, Jacobo Kirsch, and Eric E. Williamson

The arterial anatomy of the chest can be complex, and recognition of normal and variant anatomy is important in everyday practice. Although chest radiography is the modality most commonly performed for initial assessment of the chest and included vasculature, arterial anatomy can be difficult to evaluate by this modality because of the superimposition of structures within the mediastinum and hilar regions. CT and MRI have come to play a key role in the evaluation of the mediastinal structures, including not only the solid organs but the vasculature as well. The imager's role in the recognition of normal and variant vascular anatomy is important for diagnosis and management of the patient as well as for surgical planning.

The arterial systems in the chest can be divided into systemic arteries, which transport the oxygenated blood to the body through the aorta and its branches, and the pulmonary arteries, which deliver blood to the lungs for oxygenation. The systemic arteries consist of the thoracic aorta and its branches, the bronchial arteries, and the chest wall arteries. The systemic and pulmonary arterial anatomy is discussed here, including both normal and variant anatomy.

THORACIC AORTA

Normal Anatomy

The thoracic aorta can be divided into five segments: the aortic root, the ascending aorta, the proximal and posterior aortic arch (or aortic isthmus), and the descending aorta (Fig. 71-1). The aortic root is the short segment of the aorta that arises from the left ventricle to include the aortic valve and the sinuses of Valsalva. The right and left coronary arteries arise from the sinuses of Valsalva (Fig. 71-2). The sinotubular junction delineates this segment from the ascending aorta, which extends from the sinotubular junction to the first branch of the aortic arch. Although the average diameter of the ascending aorta is 3.5 cm, the diameter at which surgical repair is considered is 5.5 cm.[1] The ascending aorta is branchless. It remains enveloped within the uppermost extent of the serous pericardium, and in some cases, in the presence of pericardial fluid, the transverse pericardial recess can be seen surrounding part of the ascending aorta. As the ascending aorta travels cephalad, it curves toward the right just above the right atrium and slightly anterior to the superior vena cava. It conventionally lies to the right of the main pulmonary artery and anterior to the right pulmonary artery, which branches from the main pulmonary artery at a lower level than that of the left pulmonary artery (Figs. 71-3 and 71-4).

The aortic arch is defined from the origin of the right brachiocephalic artery to the insertion of the ductus arteriosus, the ligamentum arteriosum in the adult. The arch courses obliquely through the anterior mediastinum from anterior to posterior and horizontally from right to left. Anterior to the arch lies the prevascular space, which is typically composed of mediastinal fat. The trachea is posterior to the proximal portion of the arch and is located to the right of the distal or posterior arch. The superior vena cava is conventionally to the right of the proximal arch (Fig. 71-5). The proximal aortic arch typically includes three branches in the following order from right to left: the right brachiocephalic, the left common carotid, and the left subclavian artery (Fig. 71-6). The distal segment of the arch, also known as the aortic isthmus, includes the portion extending from the left subclavian artery to the ligamentum arteriosum (Fig. 71-7). The ligamentum arteriosum represents the remnant of fetal circulation that shunts blood from the pulmonary artery to the arch and can often be identified in adults by associated calcification.

The descending aorta is divided into thoracic and abdominal portions. The thoracic segment of the descending aorta extends from the ligamentum arteriosum to the diaphragmatic aortic hiatus, at approximately

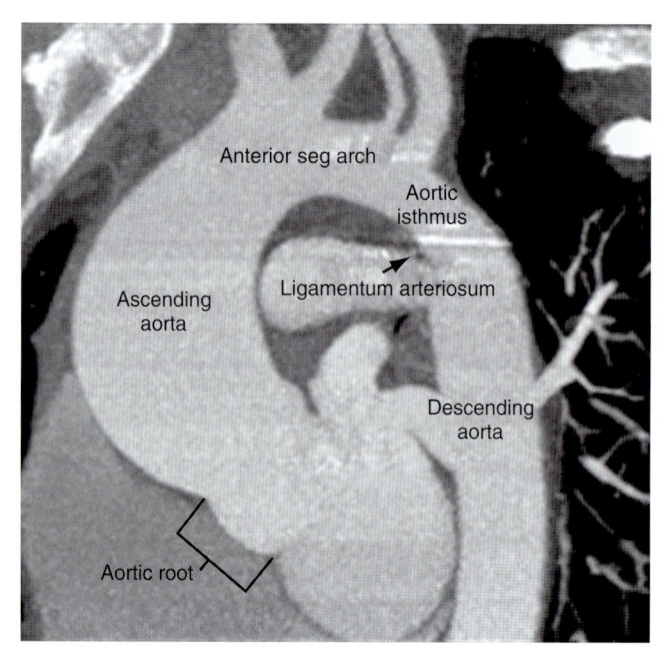

FIGURE 71-1 Oblique sagittal reformatted CT image of the thoracic aorta shows the following aortic segments: aortic root; ascending aorta; aortic arch, including the anterior arch and posterior arch (or aortic isthmus); and descending aorta. Note the ligamentum arteriosum, which demarcates the aortic isthmus from the descending aorta. Anterior Seg Arch, anterior segment of the aortic arch.

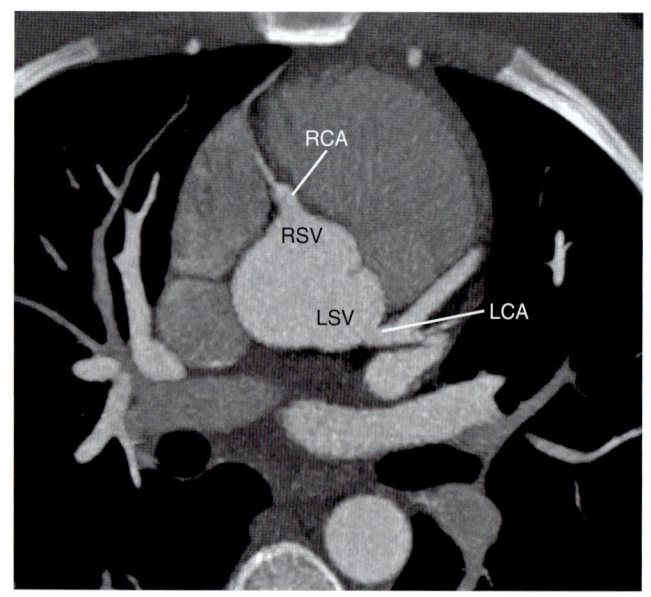

FIGURE 71-2 Axial contrast-enhanced image through the aortic root shows the ostia of the right and left coronary arteries from the right and left sinuses of Valsalva, respectively. RCA, right coronary artery; LCA, left coronary artery; LSV, left sinus of Valsalva; RSV, right sinus of Valsalva.

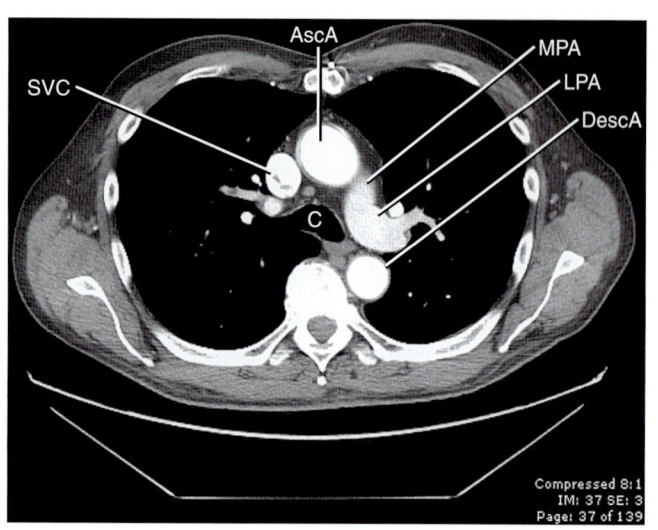

FIGURE 71-3 Contrast-enhanced axial CT image through the middle mediastinum below the level of the arch shows the relationship of the ascending aorta to the surrounding vasculature. It lies anteromedial to the superior vena cava, to the right of the main pulmonary artery (partially shown here) and the left pulmonary artery, which lies directly anterior to the descending aorta. Note that the right pulmonary artery is not seen on this axial slice because it arises from the main pulmonary artery at a level lower than that of the left pulmonary artery. SVC, superior vena cava; AscA, ascending aorta; MPA, main pulmonary artery; LPA, left pulmonary artery; DescA, descending aorta; C, carina.

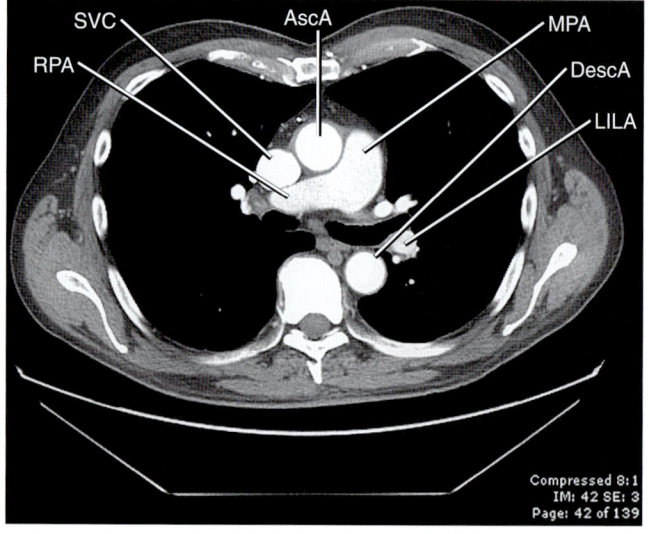

FIGURE 71-4 Contrast-enhanced CT image through the middle mediastinum inferior to Figure 71-3 shows the origin of the right pulmonary artery (RPA) arising from the main pulmonary artery (MPA). The main pulmonary artery lies to the left of the ascending aorta (AscA), and the right pulmonary artery runs posterior to the superior vena cava (SVC). DescA, descending aorta; LILA, left interlobar artery.

T10. The average diameter is 2.48 cm, ranging from 1.6 to 3.7 cm. However, surgical intervention is considered when the diameter is greater than 6.5 cm.[1] The descending thoracic aorta tapers distally and just above the diaphragm has an average diameter of 2.42 cm, with ranges from 1.4 to 3.3 cm.[2] It courses along the left aspect of the spine within the posterior mediastinum. There are several paired branches arising from the descending thoracic aorta, which include the bronchial arteries, the esophageal arteries, and the posterior intercostal arteries. Phrenic branches and pericardial branches are also typically present.

Variant Anatomy

Variant branching patterns of the arch vessels are frequently encountered, particularly within the black population. The term *bovine arch* is a commonly used misnomer that refers to common origin of the brachiocephalic and left common carotid arteries (Fig. 71-8). Cadaveric studies show an overall incidence of 13%, with an incidence of 25% in blacks and 8% in whites.[3] A variant of this, also erroneously referred to as bovine arch, consists of the left common carotid arising as a branch from the brachiocephalic artery, usually between 1 and 2.5 cm from the brachiocephalic origin.[4] The incidence is 9% in the overall population, with 10% seen in blacks and 5% seen in whites.[4]

Anomalies of the aortic arch are rare, with the exception of the left aortic arch with aberrant right subclavian artery, which has an occurrence of 1 : 200.[5] The incidence of the remaining anomalies is reported as less than 1% of all congenital cardiac anomalies; 85% to 95% of the arch anomalies are double aortic arch and right aortic arch with aberrant left subclavian artery.[6] Arch anomalies are characterized by their sidedness as well as by the branching patterns off of the arch. There are five described anomalies: double aortic arch, right-sided aortic arch with mirror-image branching, right-sided aortic arch with abnormal branching, left-sided arch with abnormal branching, and cervical aortic arch.

To understand the origin of these variants, it is necessary to understand the embryology of the aortic arch. There are six paired aortic arches in the fetus as well as two dorsal aortae. The first and second aortic arches contribute to the formation of the stapedial artery. The third arches form the carotid system, including the right and left common, external, and internal carotids. The left fourth arch forms the aortic arch; the right forms a portion of the right subclavian artery. The fifth pair of aortic arches regress in their entirety. The sixth arches contribute to the development of the right and left pulmonary arteries, and the left also forms the ductus arteriosus. The left seventh segmental artery forms the left subclavian artery. The right seventh segmental artery contributes to the distal right subclavian artery. The right subclavian artery also receives contributions from the dorsal aorta.[7] It is the abnormal regression or persistence of these structures that contributes to the anomalies discussed next (Fig. 71-9).[8]

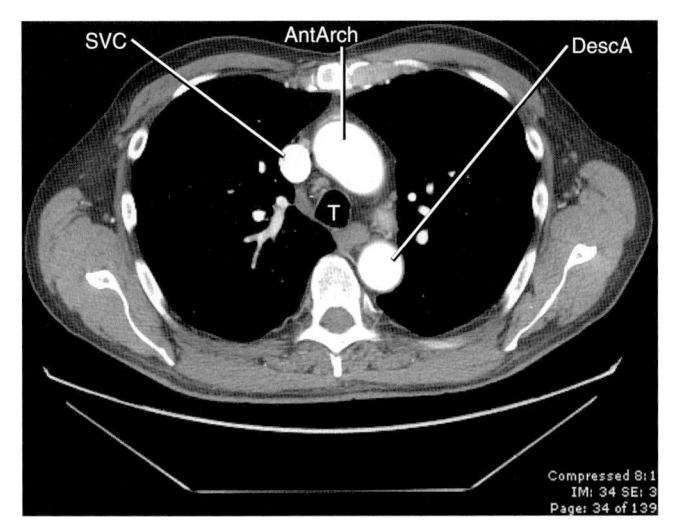

■ **FIGURE 71-5** Contrast-enhanced axial image through the aortic arch shows the anterior segment of the aortic arch (AntArch) directly anterior to the trachea (T) and to the left of the superior vena cava (SVC). DescA, descending aorta.

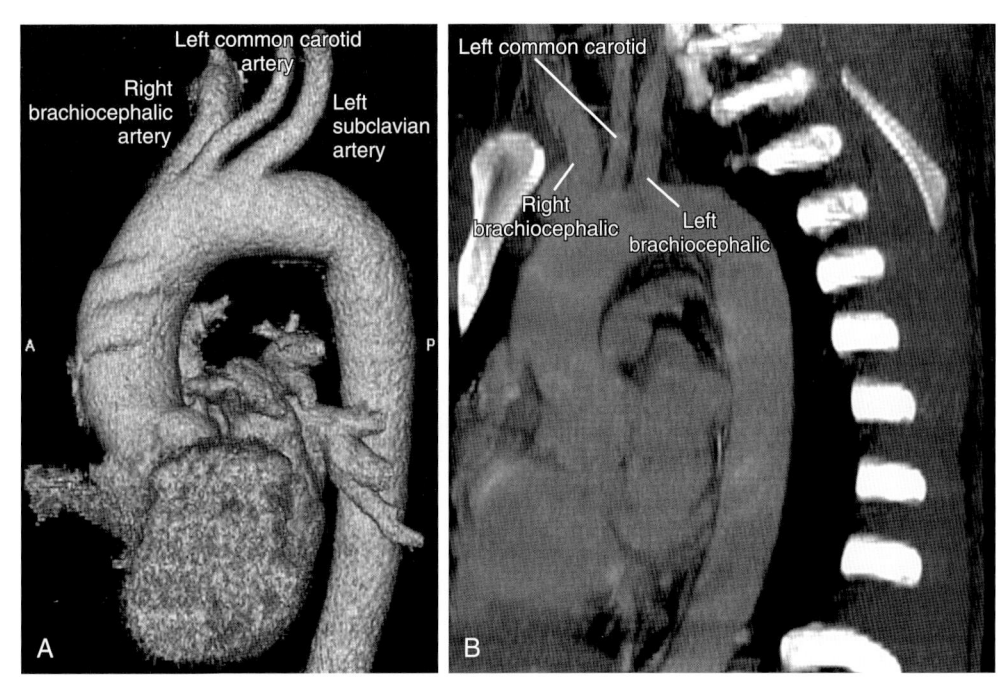

■ **FIGURE 71-6** A, Three-dimensional reconstructed image of the aortic arch and great vessels with conventional anatomy. B, Maximum intensity projection reformatted sagittal oblique image of the thoracic aorta and great vessels with a typical branching pattern.

In the normal development of the arch, the right dorsal aorta as well as a portion of the right sixth aortic arch regresses. In double aortic arch development, both of the paired dorsal aortae persist, with regression or persistence of the sixth arch, which contributes to the formation of the ductus arteriosus. Because there is complete encasement of the trachea and esophagus, patients often present early in life with nonpositional stridor. Double aortic arch can be seen on plain film radiography as a posterior indentation on the trachea by the right arch on lateral view and often on the posteroanterior view as tracheal indentations by the more superior right arch and inferior left arch. However, CT and MRI are the preferred methods for characterization of the anatomy as well as of any associated cardiac anomalies. Axial images demonstrate the "four artery sign," representing paired carotid and subclavian arteries, evenly spaced around the trachea, just cephalad to the aortic arch (Fig. 71-10).[9]

■ **FIGURE 71-7** Oblique sagittal reformatted CT image of the thoracic aorta shows the ligamentum arteriosum, which demarcates the aortic isthmus (AI) from the descending aorta (DA).

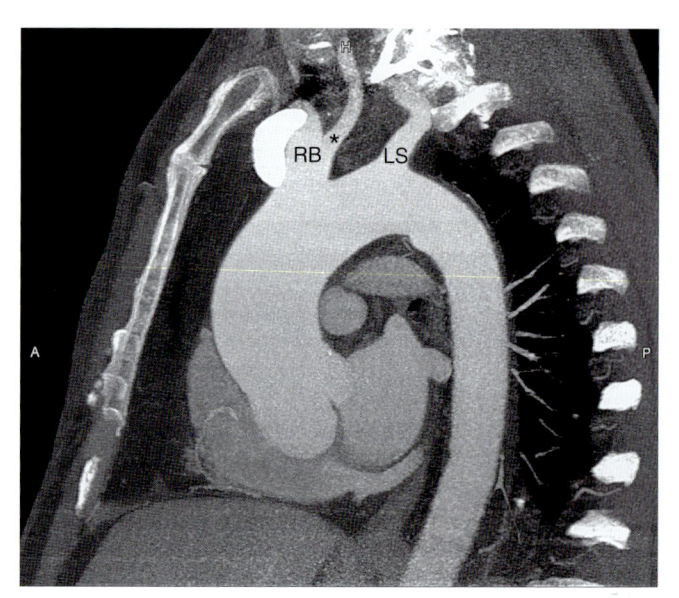

■ **FIGURE 71-8** Sagittal oblique image of the chest through the aortic arch shows a "bovine" arch, with the left common carotid (*asterisk*) originating with the right brachiocephalic artery (RB). LS, left subclavian artery.

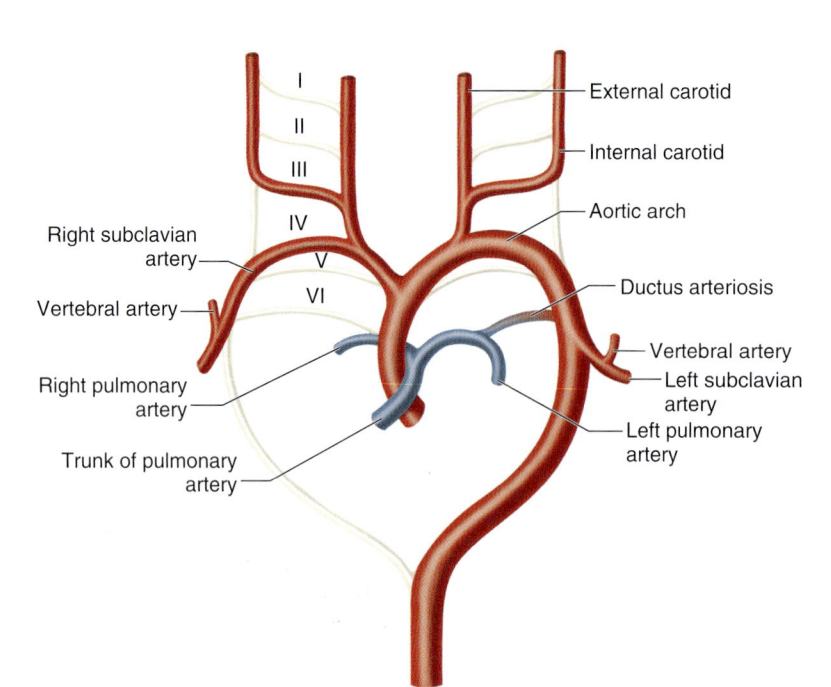

■ **FIGURE 71-9** Embryonic development of the aortic arches. The fully developed form is depicted in red with conventional anatomy. *(Modified from Gray H. Anatomy of the Human Body. Philadelphia, Lea & Febiger, 1918; Bartleby.com, 2000, p 515.)*

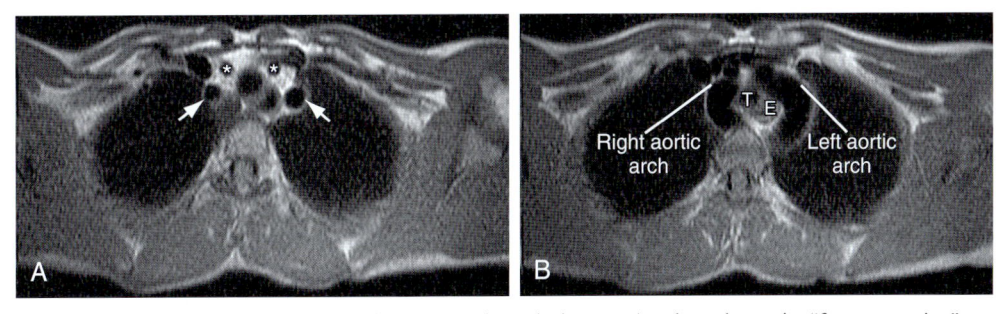

FIGURE 71-10 Double aortic arch. **A,** MR axial black blood image through the superior chest shows the "four artery sign" representing paired carotids (*asterisks*) and paired subclavian arteries (*arrows*), symmetrically oriented in relation to the trachea. **B,** At a slightly lower level, there is both a right aortic arch and left aortic arch encircling both the trachea (T) and esophagus (E), creating a complete vascular ring.

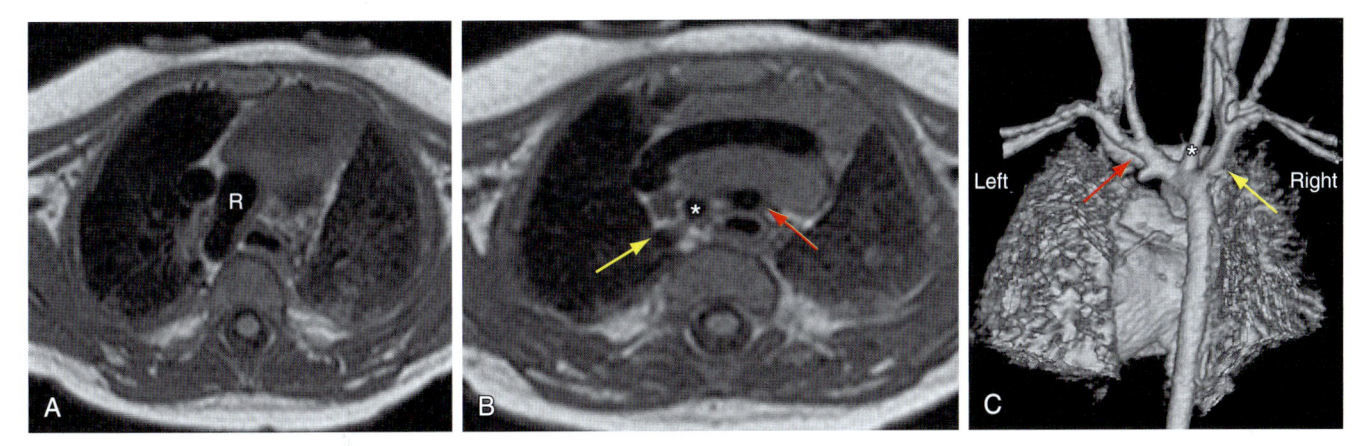

FIGURE 71-11 Right arch with mirror-image branching. **A,** Axial black blood MR image shows a right-sided arch (R). **B,** Caudal to **A,** three vessels are seen in the following order, from left to right: left innominate (*red arrow*), right common carotid (*asterisk*), and right subclavian artery (*yellow arrow*). **C,** Maximum intensity projection image shows the right-sided arch with mirror-image branching of the left innominate (*red arrow*), right common carotid (*asterisk*), and right subclavian artery (*yellow arrow*) arising in mirror-image order from a left arch.

When there is persistence of the right dorsal aorta and the left dorsal aorta regresses, a right-sided arch develops. There are three subtypes of right aortic arch, depending on the branching pattern. Mirror-image branching replicates the order of branching seen with a left-sided aorta, with a left brachiocephalic artery arising first, followed by the right common carotid and then the right subclavian artery (Fig. 71-11). A left-sided ductus arteriosus is typically seen with this entity, passing between the descending aorta and left pulmonary artery. Right aortic arch with mirror-image branching is almost always associated with congenital heart anomalies, most commonly tetralogy of Fallot, reported in 25% of cases.[10]

With right aortic arch with aberrant left subclavian artery, there is abnormal dorsal aortic regression between the origins of the left common and the left subclavian arteries. The left subclavian arises from a retroesophageal diverticulum, which is the remnant of the regressed dorsal segment.[11] The ductus arteriosus arises from this diverticulum and connects to the left pulmonary artery, creating a complete vascular ring (Fig. 71-12). Because this condition forms a complete vascular ring, these patients often present with nonpositional stridor due to airway compression.[11]

Right aortic arch can also be seen with an isolated left subclavian artery, which has no direct communication to the aorta. Instead of originating from the arch, an isolated left subclavian artery arises from the left pulmonary artery through the ductus arteriosus. The embryologic origin of this anomaly is hypothesized to involve regression of the fourth arch as well as a portion of the sixth arch, with migration of the seventh intersegmental artery to the level of the sixth arch, forming the communication between the ductus and the pulmonary artery (which arises from the left sixth arch) and the left subclavian artery (arising from the seventh intersegmental artery).[12] Because of the subclavian's lack of oxygenated blood supply from the arch, this anomaly can present with extremity ischemia and subclavian steal phenomena. Although isolated subclavian artery has been reported on the right, it occurs much more commonly on the left. Right aortic arch with isolated left subclavian artery is almost always associated with congenital heart disease, most commonly with transposition and tetralogy of Fallot. Luetmer[11] described 39 reported cases from 1970 to 1990.

Left-sided aortic arch with aberrant right subclavian artery is the most common aortic arch anomaly, with an occurrence of 1:200.[5] Similar to right arch with aberrant left subclavian, this vascular anomaly results when there is abnormal regression between the right common carotid and right subclavian. The aberrant right subclavian arises from the diverticular remnant of the right aortic arch, also

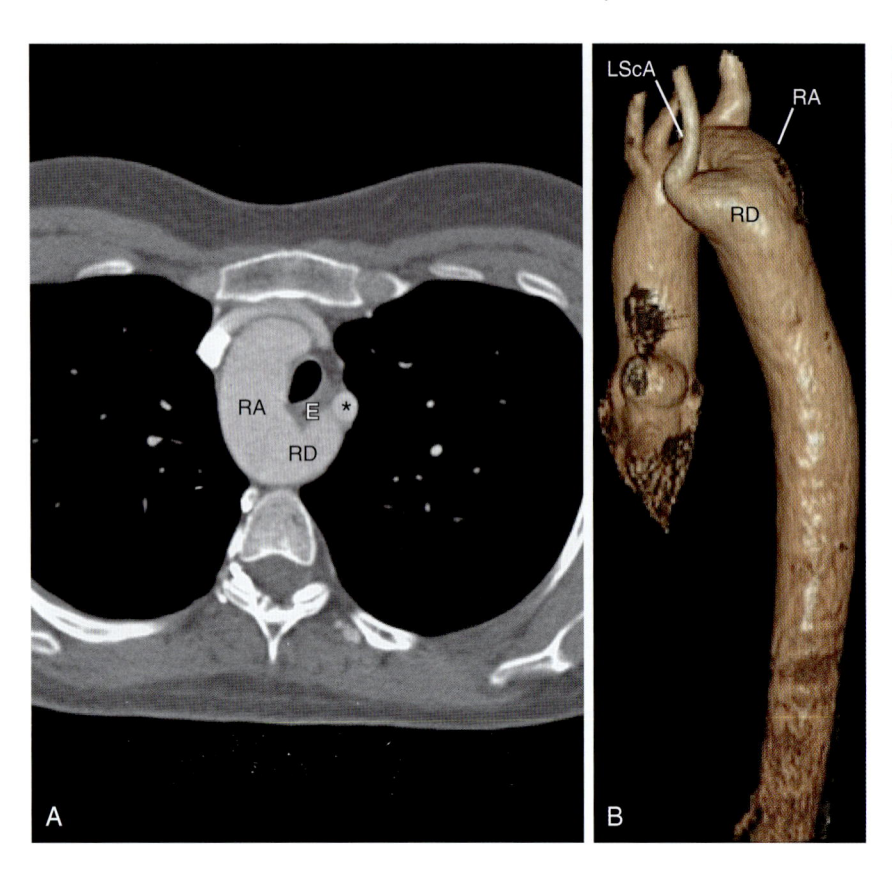

■ **FIGURE 71-12** Right arch with aberrant left subclavian artery. **A,** Axial contrast-enhanced CT image of the chest shows a right-sided aortic arch, with the left subclavian artery (*asterisk*) arising from a retroesophageal diverticulum. **B,** Reconstructed three-dimensional image shows a sagittal oblique view of the right-sided aortic arch with aberrant left subclavian arising from a retroesophageal diverticulum. RA, right-sided arch; RD, retroesophageal diverticulum; E, esophagus; LScA, left subclavian artery.

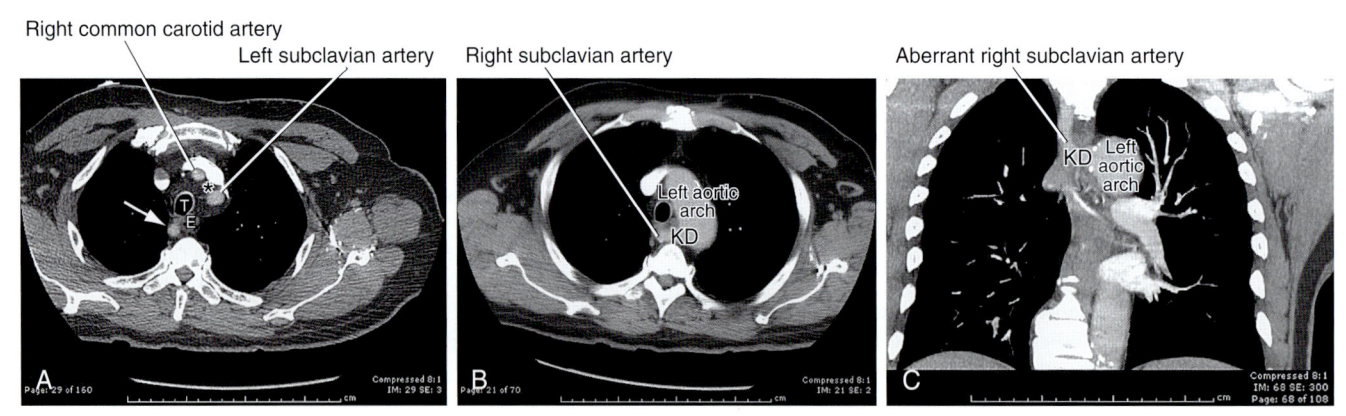

■ **FIGURE 71-13** Left arch with aberrant right subclavian artery. **A,** Contrast-enhanced axial image through the chest shows a vascular structure (*arrow*) posterior and to the right of the trachea (T) and esophagus (E). Note the three vessels in the suspected location of the great vessels on this image. This patient has anomalous origin of the left vertebral artery (*asterisk*) from the arch, accounting for this appearance. **B,** Axial image caudal to A at the level of the arch shows an anomalous right subclavian artery arising from Kommerell diverticulum (KD). In this particular patient, it passes posterior to the esophagus, which is the most common course. **C,** Coronal oblique reformatted image through the arch shows the aberrant right subclavian arising from Kommerell diverticulum and ascending superiorly along the right mediastinum.

called *Kommerell diverticulum*. This aberrant artery most commonly passes posterior to the esophagus, but it can pass between the trachea and esophagus in 18% and anterior to the trachea in 4%.[13] Because this condition does not produce a complete vascular ring, patients are usually asymptomatic (Fig. 71-13).

The aortic arch is typically located between the second costosternal junction on the right and the T4 vertebral body.[14] An anomalous position of the arch, known as the high-riding cervical arch, is variable in position from just above the expected location of the arch to a supraclavicular location, within the soft tissues of the neck. A cervical arch often passes posterior to the esophagus and can be associated with both left and right arches. Although it is controversial, this anomaly is thought to develop as a result of persistent second or third branchial arches,[15] with regression of the normal contributions from the fourth branchial arches. The aortic arch branches can also be anomalous in origin with this entity as well. On plain film radiography, a cervical arch is manifested as a superior mediastinal mass with tracheal deviation. CT shows the arch at or above the thoracic inlet, typically supracla-

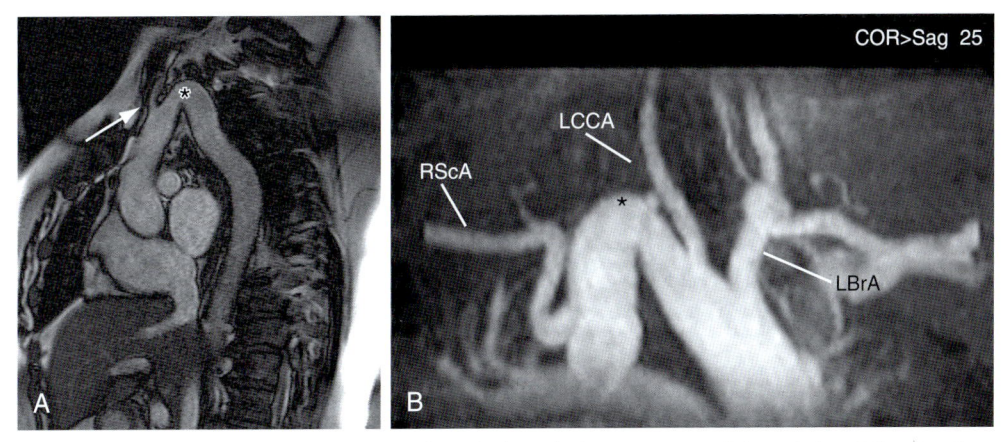

■ **FIGURE 71-14** Cervical arch. **A,** Coronal oblique MR image through the arch shows the apex of the arch (*asterisk*) at the thoracic inlet, with the origin of the right subclavian (*arrow*) coming off inferior to the apex of the arch on this image. **B,** Maximum intensity projection fast spoiled gradient-recalled image of the aortic arch shows the three aortic branches arising from the arch, which extends cranially in relation to the great vessel origins. RScA, right subclavian artery; LCCA, left common carotid artery; LBrA, left brachiocephalic artery.

vicular in location (Fig. 71-14). Clinically, patients can present with a pulsatile neck mass but generally are asymptomatic.

CAROTIDS: COMMON, EXTERNAL, AND INTERNAL

The carotid arteries arise from the third aortic arches embryologically. The right common carotid arises from the right brachiocephalic artery, most commonly at the level of the sternoclavicular joint. In approximately 12% of the population, the origin is above the sternoclavicular joint.[16] The left common carotid can be divided into a thoracic and a cervical portion; the thoracic portion courses from the arch through the superior mediastinum, to the level of the sternoclavicular joint, where it becomes the cervical portion. The common carotid arteries are invested in a carotid sheath, which contains the internal jugular vein and the vagus nerve as well, with the artery medial to the vein and anteromedial to the nerve. The common carotids course obliquely cephalad, passing posterior to the sternoclavicular joints and deep to the sternocleidomastoid muscle, to the level of the thyroid cartilage, approximately C4, where they bifurcate into the internal and external carotid arteries. The bifurcation is the location of the carotid body (also called the carotid glomus or glomus caroticum), which is a cluster of chemoreceptors that can give rise to glomus tumors. In approximately 80% to 85% of patients, the internal carotid artery is posterior or posterolateral to the external carotid (Fig. 71-15).[17]

The external carotid artery supplies the face, scalp, and neck. It courses from the bifurcation at the level of the thyroid cartilage to the posterior aspect of the mandibular neck, where it branches into the superficial temporal and internal maxillary arteries. The external carotid has several branches, which typically arise in the following order: superior thyroid, ascending pharyngeal, lingual, facial, occipital, and posterior auricular arteries, followed by the terminal branches, the maxillary artery and superficial temporal artery (Fig. 71-16).

The internal carotid artery is the primary supply of oxygenated blood to the intracranial structures, including

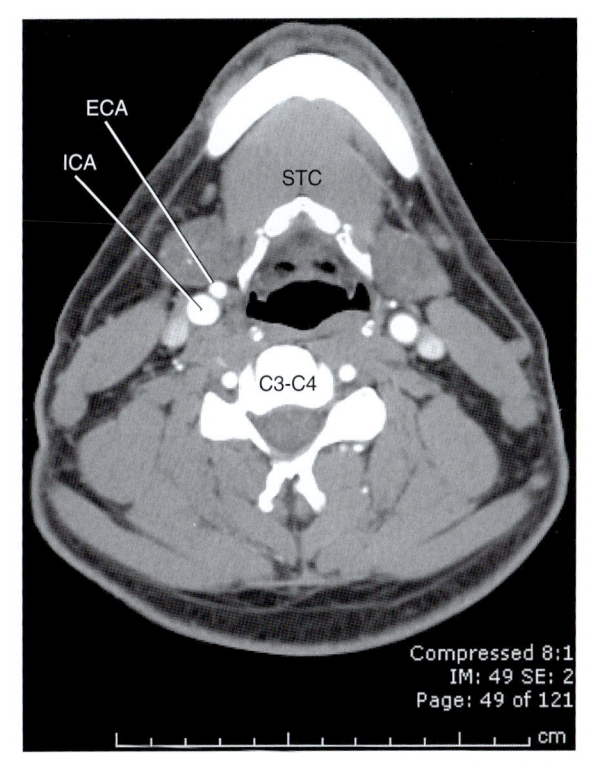

■ **FIGURE 71-15** Contrast-enhanced axial CT image through the neck just above the carotid bifurcation shows the internal carotid artery (ICA) posterolateral to the external carotid artery (ECA). This is at the level of C3-4. Superior thyroid cartilage (STC) is the most stable landmark for the bifurcation.

the anterior brain and the orbits. The internal carotid remains within the carotid sheath and retains the same relationship to the jugular vein and vagus nerve as the common carotid artery. The older classification delineated four segments: the cervical, petrous, cavernous, and cerebral segments. The newer classification system described by Bouthillier[17] divides the internal carotid into the following seven segments: cervical (C1), petrous (C2), lacerum (C3), cavernous (C4), clinoid (C5), ophthalmic (C6), and communicating (C7). The cervical portion extends from the carotid bifurcation to the level of the carotid canal in

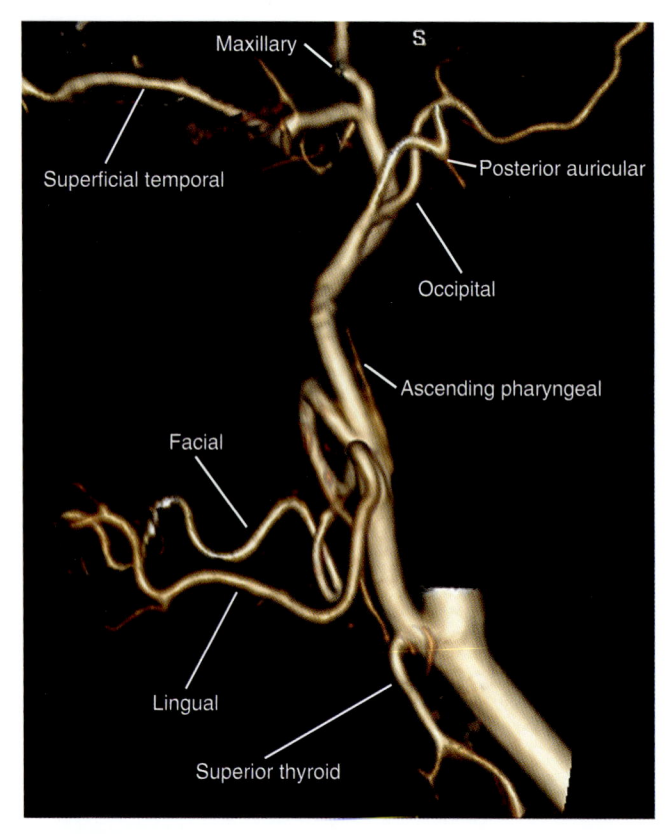

FIGURE 71-16 External carotid branches. Three-dimensional reconstructed image of the external carotid shows its branches in the following order: superior thyroid, lingual, facial, ascending pharyngeal, occipital, posterior auricular (which arises from the occipital in this patient), superficial temporal, and maxillary arteries.

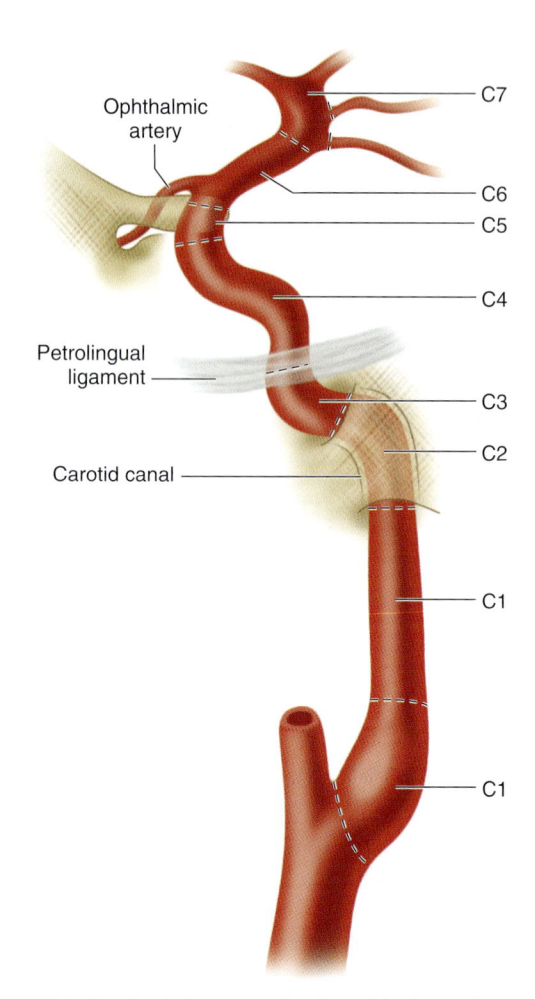

FIGURE 71-17 Cervical segment drawing of the internal carotid. Lateral anatomic diagram depicting the seven internal carotid artery segments: C1, cervical segment (the bulb is indicated by *stippling*, the ascending segment by *horizontal lines*); C2, petrous segment; C3, lacerum segment; C4, cavernous segment; C5, clinoidal segment; C6, ophthalmic segment; C7, communicating segment. (From Osborn AG. Diagnostic Cerebral Angiography, 2nd ed. Philadelphia, Lippincott Williams & Wilkins, 1999, p 58.)

the petrous bone, anterior to the jugular foramen (Fig. 71-17). The carotid bifurcation and the proximal portion of the cervical segment lie within an external anatomic landmark known as the carotid triangle. The triangle is defined anatomically by the sternocleidomastoid muscle posteriorly, the omohyoid muscle anteriorly, and the stylohyoid and digastric muscles superiorly (Fig. 71-18). The petrous segment of the internal carotid artery travels in the carotid canal of the petrous bone, taking a short vertical course before coursing medially and horizontally through the canal. The lacerum segment is a short segment of the internal carotid artery that begins at just above the foramen lacerum (typically filled with fibrocartilage in living patients) and continues to the petrolingual ligament. On exiting the carotid canal, the cavernous segment begins at the petrolingual ligament, ascends to the posterior clinoid process, then passes alongside the body of the sphenoid bone anteriorly, and finally courses vertically on the medial side of the anterior clinoid process, where it perforates the dura and becomes the clinoid segment at the proximal dural ring. The clinoid segment includes the portion of internal carotid artery between the proximal dural ring and the distal dural ring, where it then becomes the ophthalmic segment, which is intradural. The ophthalmic segment extends from the distal dural ring to the posterior communicating artery, with a course that is parallel and posterolateral to the optic nerve. This segment gives off the ophthalmic and superior hypophyseal arteries. The final segment of the internal carotid artery, called the communicating segment, passes between the optic and oculomotor nerves, giving rise to the posterior communicating artery and the anterior choroidal artery before bifurcating into the terminal branches of the internal carotid artery, the anterior cerebral artery and the middle cerebral artery.

Variant Anatomy

The level of the carotid bifurcation can be variable, most commonly above C4 when it occurs. Huber[17a] reported the bifurcation at C4-5 in 48% of 658 bifurcations and at C3-4 in 34%. The most stable anatomic landmark for the bifurcation is the superior thyroid cartilage.[18] The common carotids are most commonly branchless, although sometimes they may give rise to the superior thyroid artery, the inferior thyroid, or, uncommonly, the vertebral artery.

The left common carotid artery most commonly arises from the aortic arch. As previously mentioned, a common

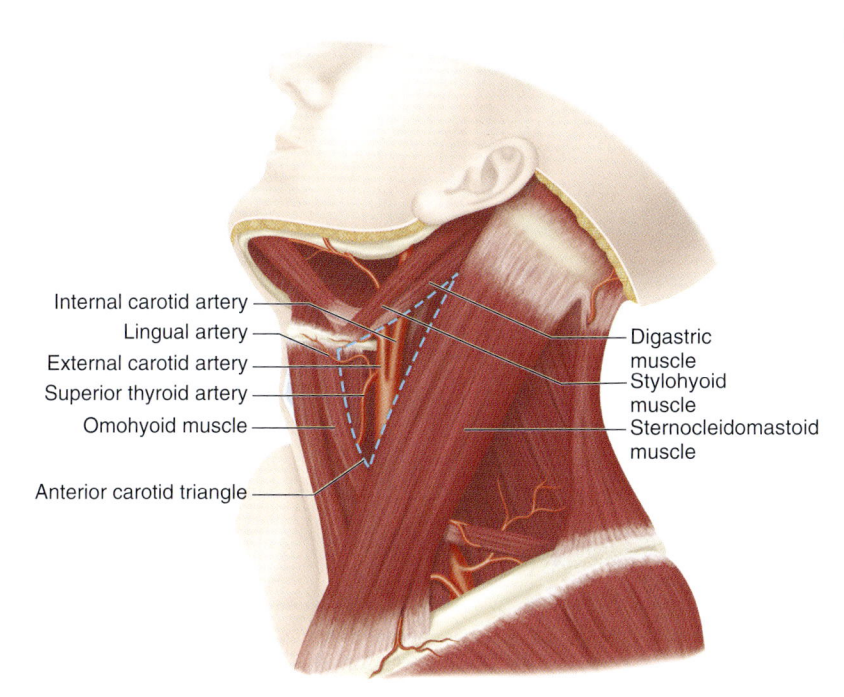

FIGURE 71-18 Carotid triangle. Illustration of the carotid triangle delineates the anterior border by the omohyoid muscle, the posterior border by the sternocleidomastoid muscle, and the superior border by the digastric muscle. The lingual and superior thyroid artery branches from the external carotid are also depicted along with the internal and external carotid arteries.

origin of the left common carotid with the right brachiocephalic is sometimes referred to as a bovine arch, although this can be considered a misnomer because this is not the usual branching pattern in cows. Less common variations include a single trunk giving rise to both carotids and a common origin with the left subclavian, resulting in symmetric bilateral brachiocephalic trunks, occurring in 1.2% to 1.6% of individuals with anomalous branching.[19]

Variations of the external carotid include abnormal course and the absence of one or both of the external carotids. An abnormal position has been reported in 5% of the population by Prendes.[20] Carotid basilar anastomoses are well known, but rare, vascular anomalies in which there is persistence of the primitive segmental arteries, which connect the carotid system to the vertebrobasilar system. Because the segmental arteries are named according to the cranial nerve with which they are associated, the three most common carotid basilar anastomoses arise from persistence of the trigeminal, otic, and hypoglossal arteries (Fig. 71-19). These anastomoses most commonly occur with the internal carotid but have been reported with the common carotid and external carotid arteries as well. A primitive trigeminal artery is the most common of these, with an incidence between 0.1% and 0.6% by angiography.[21] It accounts for 80% to 85% of the persistent carotid basilar anastomoses.[22] In primitive trigeminal artery, the persistent trigeminal artery communicates between the basilar and the internal carotid artery and can be further classified by medial or lateral type (supraclinoid internal carotid artery communication or precavernous internal carotid artery communication, respectively) and the presence or origin of the posterior cerebral artery (Saltzman types I and II). With Saltzman type I, the midbasilar and posterior communicating arteries are usually hypoplastic. With type II, the posterior communicating artery supplies the posterior cerebral artery's territory,

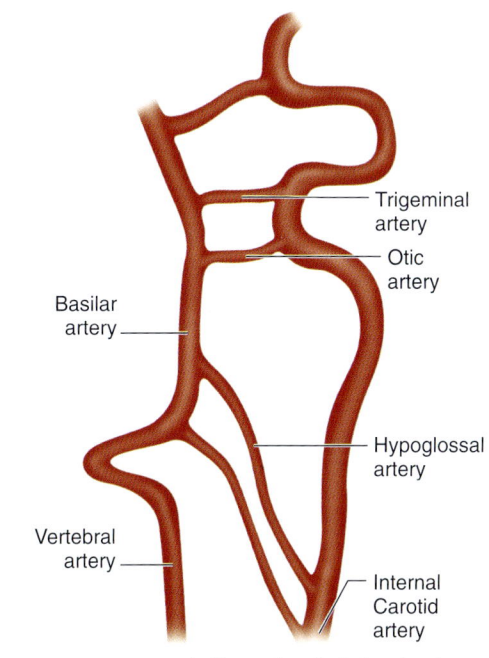

FIGURE 71-19 Anatomic illustration depicting the three most common carotid basilar anastomoses.

and the basilar joins the persistent trigeminal at the level of the superior cerebellar artery (Figs. 71-20 and 71-21).[23] The persistent hypoglossal has a reported incidence between 0.03% and 0.26% on cerebral angiography.[24] Fetal origin of the posterior cerebral artery arising from the supraclinoid portion of the internal carotid artery with no communication with the basilar artery occurs in 10% of the population on the right and left sides individually and in 8% bilaterally (Fig. 71-22).

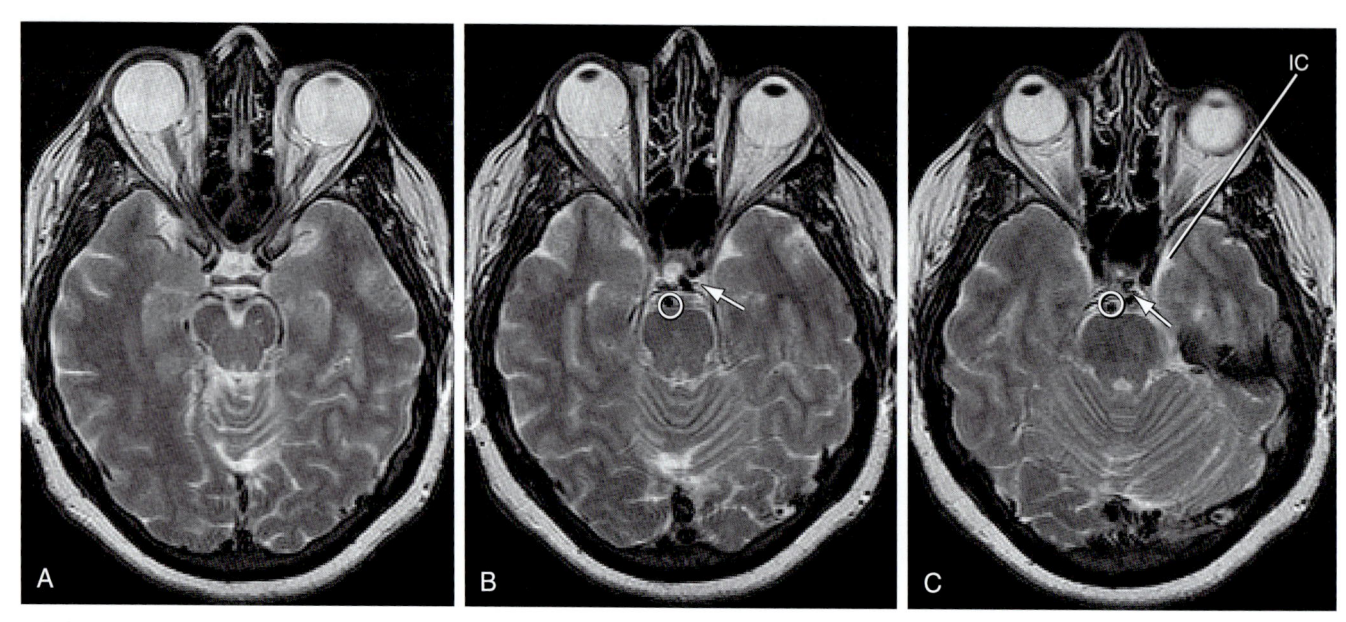

FIGURE 71-20 Persistent trigeminal artery, Saltzman type II. T2-weighted axial MR image of the brain shows a vascular structure (*arrows*) coursing along the dorsal aspect of the left cavernous sinus, between the internal carotid and the basilar artery (*circled*). IC, internal carotid.

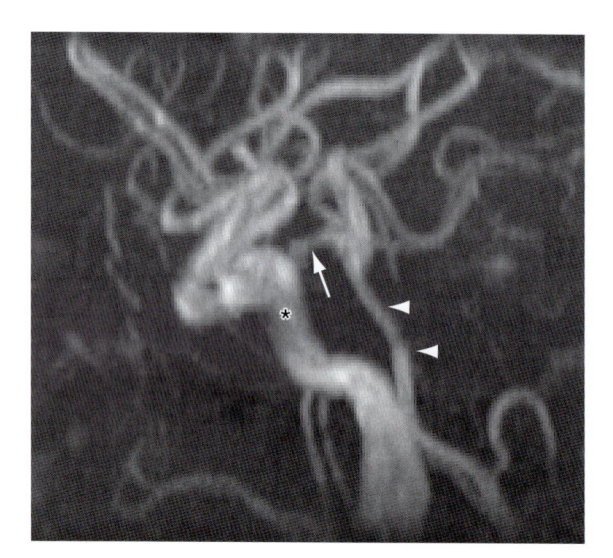

FIGURE 71-21 Persistent trigeminal artery, type II. MR angiography of the brain in a separate patient shows a persistent trigeminal artery (*arrow*) arising from the basilar artery (*asterisk*) and joining the internal carotid (*arrowheads*).

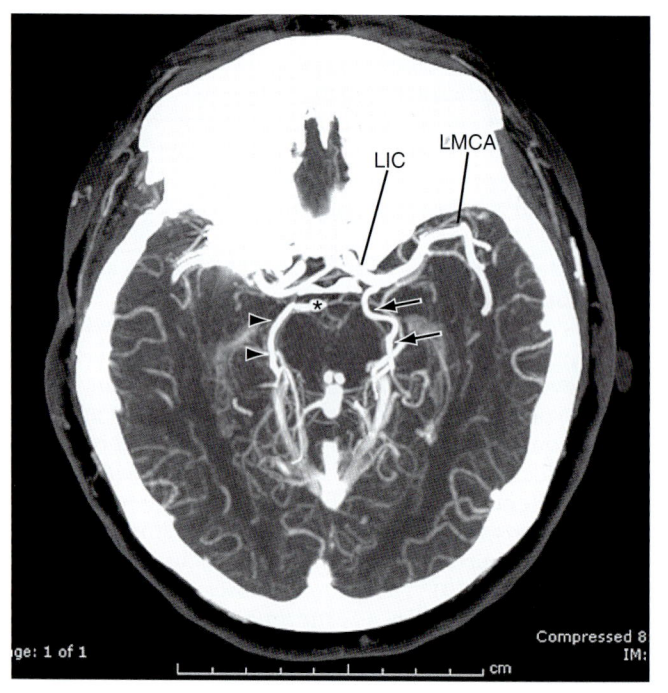

FIGURE 71-22 Left fetal origin of the posterior cerebral artery. CT angiography of the cerebral vasculature shows the left posterior cerebral artery (*arrows*) arising from the left internal carotid near the origin of the left middle cerebral artery. Note the origin of the right posterior cerebral artery (*arrowheads*) from the basilar artery (*asterisk*). LIC, left internal carotid; LMCA, left middle cerebral artery.

CHEST WALL ARTERIES

The chest wall arteries include the internal thoracic arteries and the intercostal arteries, which serve as an important collateral pathway with aortoiliac occlusion or stenosis as well as aortic coarctation.

The internal thoracic arteries are also referred to as the internal mammary arteries and are important for cardiac bypass grafting. They are paired arteries, coursing vertically along the anterior chest wall just posterior to the sternum and medial to the nipple. At approximately the sixth intercostal space, each artery divides into the musculophrenic and the superior epigastric artery. Other branches include the thymic and pericardiophrenic arteries. The internal thoracic arteries give off paired anterior intercostal arteries that continue around the chest wall to anastomose with their correlative posterior intercostal arteries. These intercostal arteries course inferiorly to their corresponding ribs one to six and accompany the intercostal vein (superior to the artery) and nerve (inferior to the artery) in each respective rib space. The first and second posterior intercostal arteries arise from the costocervical trunk, which is the first branch of the subclavian artery. The remaining posterior intercostals arise from the descending thoracic aorta.

BRONCHIAL ARTERIES

The bronchial arteries are the systemic blood supply to their corresponding airways (trachea, extrapulmonary and intrapulmonary airways) and their supporting structures, regional lymph nodes, and esophagus as well as the vasa vasorum of the aorta, pulmonary artery, and pulmonary vein. They terminate at the level of the respiratory bronchioles and form anastomoses with the pulmonary arteries to supply the visceral pleura as well.

The bronchial arteries frequently demonstrate variable origin, branching patterns, and course. The most common configuration includes two bronchial arteries on the left and one on the right. The right bronchial artery most commonly arises from the first aortic intercostal artery. However, most often the left bronchial arteries originate directly from the descending thoracic aorta, between the levels of the T5 and T6 vertebrae. Bronchial arteries that originate outside this area are considered to be anomalous. Hartmann and colleagues[25] found that in symptomatic patients presenting with hemoptysis, 36% had at least one bronchial artery of ectopic origin. Of these, 19% had a common bronchial trunk and 81% had isolated right or left bronchial arteries. The most common locations for ectopic origins of the bronchial arteries include the concavity of the aortic arch (74%), the subclavian artery (10.5%), and the descending aorta (8.5%).

PULMONARY ARTERIES

The pulmonary arteries transport deoxygenated blood to the lungs for oxygenation. The transport of deoxygenated rather than of oxygenated blood is a unique feature of the pulmonary arteries; the remainder of the arterial system transports oxygenated blood. The pulmonary trunk arises from the right ventricle, coursing superiorly and posteriorly, passing anterior to the ascending aorta and then to the left of the ascending aorta, where it bifurcates into the right and left main pulmonary arteries at approximately T5-6 (Fig. 71-23). The pulmonary trunk is completely enveloped in pericardium.

The right main pulmonary artery has a horizontal course, posterior to the ascending aorta and superior vena cava, running anterior to the right main bronchus. At the root of the right lung, the right pulmonary artery gives off two branches; the smaller supplies the upper lobe of the lung, and the larger supplies the middle and lower lobes (Fig. 71-24).

The left main pulmonary artery also courses horizontally and lies anterior to the left bronchus. At the root of the left lung, it also gives off two branches, supplying the upper and lower lobes (Fig. 71-25). The remnant of the ductus arteriosus, the ligamentum arteriosum, runs from the proximal aspect of the left pulmonary artery to the concave surface of the aortic arch, just distal to the origin of the left subclavian artery.

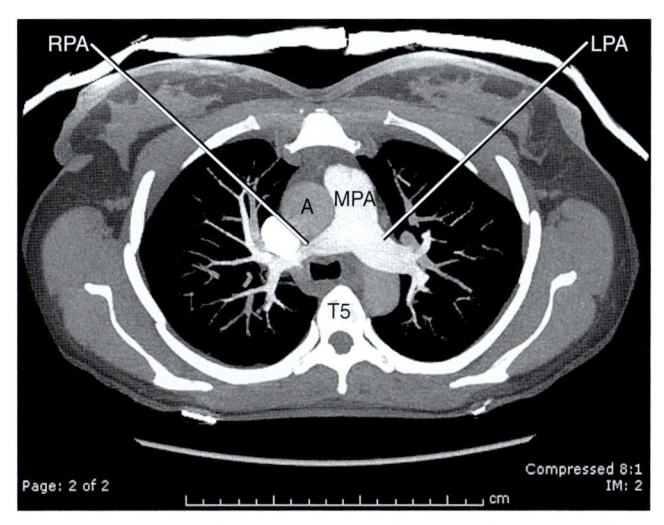

■ **FIGURE 71-23** Pulmonary anatomy. The main pulmonary trunk (MPA) passes anterior and then to the left of the ascending aorta (A), bifurcating at approximately T5-6 into right and left main pulmonary arteries. RPA, right pulmonary artery; LPA, left pulmonary artery.

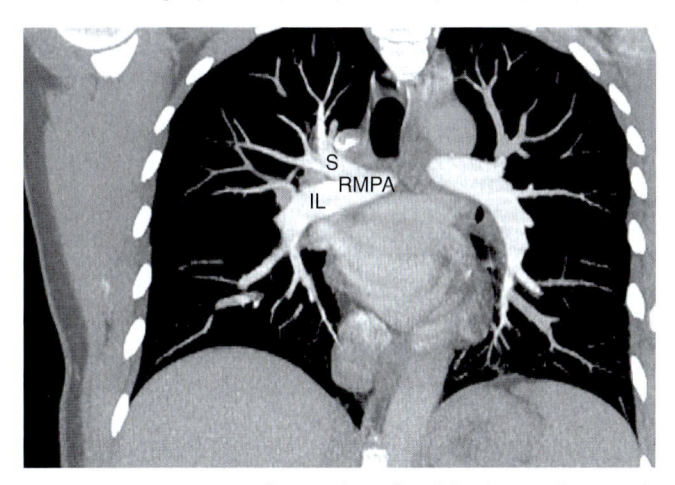

■ **FIGURE 71-24** Coronal CT angiography of the chest at the root of the right lung shows the right main pulmonary artery bifurcating into two branches. The larger (IL, interlobar artery) supplies the middle and lower lobes; the smaller (S, superior lobar artery) supplies the upper lobe. RMPA, right main pulmonary artery.

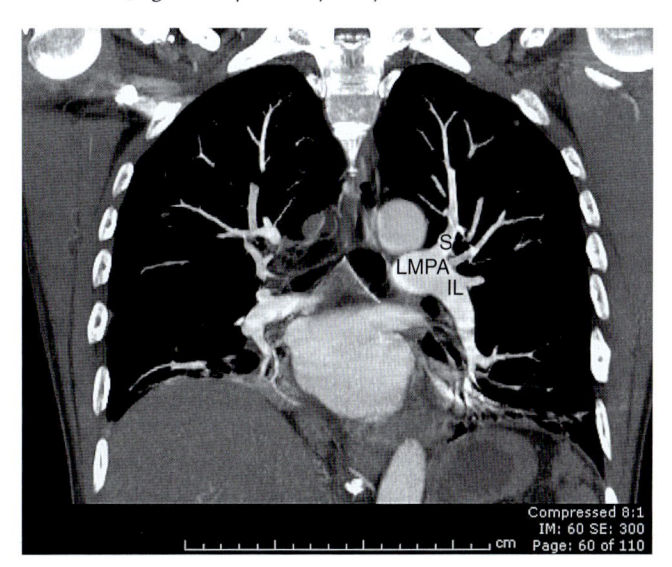

■ **FIGURE 71-25** Coronal CT angiography of the chest through the left hilum shows the bifurcation into the superior lobar artery (S) and inferior lobar artery (IL). LMPA, left main pulmonary artery.

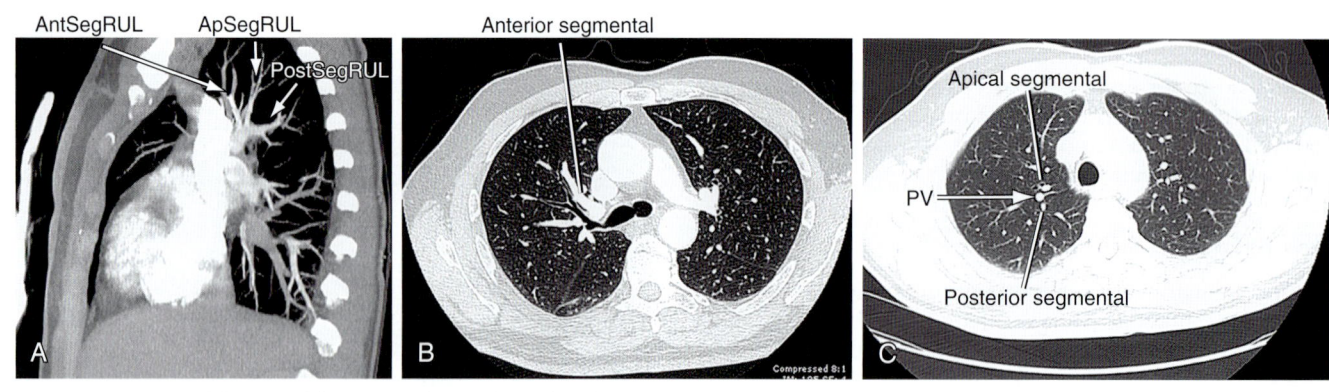

FIGURE 71-26 Right upper lobe segmental anatomy of the pulmonary arteries. **A,** Coronal oblique CT angiography of the pulmonary arteries shows the three segments of the right upper lobe (RUL): anterior segmental artery, posterior segmental artery, and apical segmental artery. **B,** Contrast-enhanced axial image at the level of the carina shows the anterior segmental pulmonary artery. **C,** More cephalad to **B,** the apical and posterior segmental arteries are shown. Note that the arteries run with the bronchi, whereas the pulmonary vein (PV) runs separate from the bronchus.

The pulmonary segmental arteries and their corresponding bronchi are based on segmental anatomy of the lungs, with usually 10 segments on the right and eight on the left. The bronchopulmonary segments include both bronchial and pulmonary arteries and the corresponding bronchus. They are located centrally within each pulmonary segment. The pulmonary veins and lymphatics run between the segments and therefore are separate.

The right upper lobe is supplied by three segmental branches, the anterior, posterior, and apical segmental arteries, which arise from the ascending branch of the right main pulmonary artery (Fig. 71-26). The descending branch, the interlobar artery, which supplies the middle and lower lobes on the right, gives rise to the superior basal segmental artery and the middle lobar artery as the first branches at approximately the same level. The superior basal segmental artery originates from the posterior aspect of the interlobar artery; the middle lobar artery originates from the anterior aspect of the interlobar artery and further bifurcates into medial and lateral segmental arteries (Fig. 71-27). More caudally, the interlobar artery gives off the medial basal segmental and the anterior basal segmental artery, followed inferiorly by the posterior basal segmental artery and the lateral basal segmental artery (Fig. 71-28).

The left pulmonary artery divides into the ascending and descending branches, in similar fashion to the right pulmonary arterial system; however, the upper lobe is supplied by the anterior segmental artery and the apicoposterior segmental artery, which arise from the superior lobar pulmonary artery (Fig. 71-29). The descending branch, the interlobar artery, gives off the superior basal segmental artery and the lingular artery first, with the superior basal segmental artery at a slightly higher level than the lingular arteries, followed by the basal segments: anteromedial basal segment, posterior basal segment, and lateral basal segment (Fig. 71-30).

Variant Anatomy

Variations of the pulmonary artery include the pulmonary arterial sling and aberrant origin from the ductus arteriosus. Pulmonary arterial sling occurs when the left main pulmonary artery arises from the posterior right main pulmonary artery, courses around the right main stem bronchus, and then passes between the esophagus and the trachea, compressing the trachea (Fig. 71-31). Before the advent of cross-sectional imaging, this anomaly was diagnosed by barium studies, which demonstrated anterior indentation of the esophagus and posterior indentation of the trachea. The ligamentum venosum attaches to the main pulmonary artery, passing to the left of the trachea and attaching to the posterior aortic arch, completing the ring.

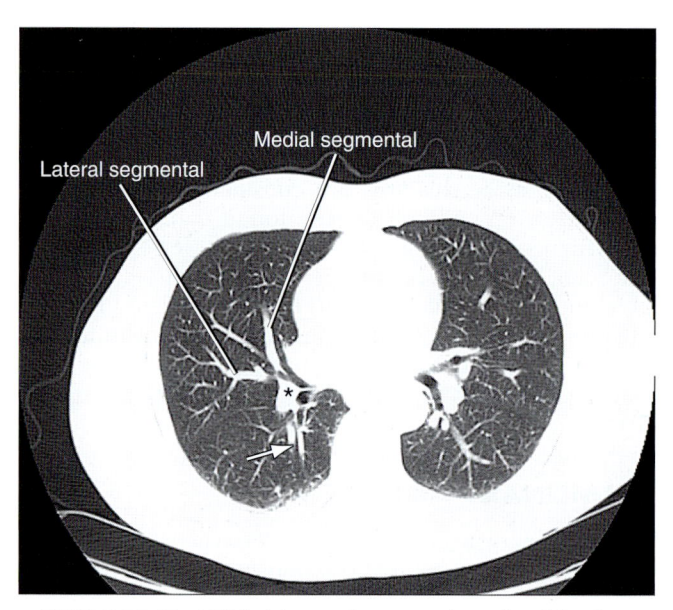

FIGURE 71-27 Middle lobe arteries. CT angiography of the chest shows the medial and lateral segmental branches of the middle lobe on the right, along with their corresponding bronchi. These originate from the anterior aspect of the interlobar artery (*asterisk*); the superior segmental artery arises posteriorly at the same level (*arrow*).

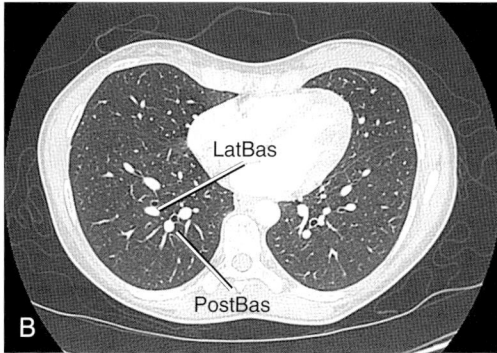

■ **FIGURE 71-28** Right lower lobe pulmonary arterial supply. **A,** CT angiography of the chest shows medial and anterior basal segmental arteries with their corresponding bronchi. **B,** The lateral basal and posterior basal segments arise more inferior to **A**. MedBas, medial basal segmental artery; AntBas, anterior basal segmental artery; LatBas, lateral basal segmental artery; PostBas, posterior basal segmental artery.

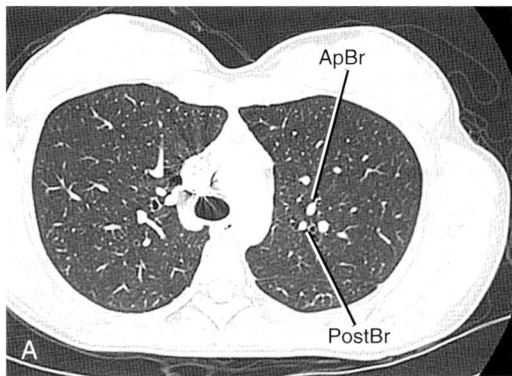

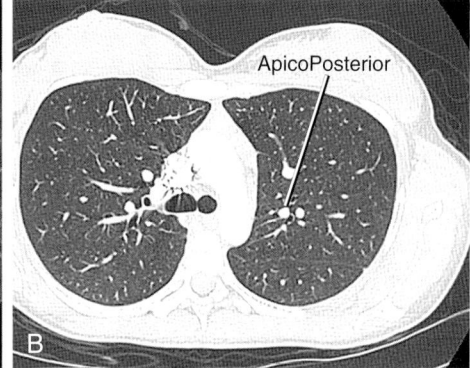

■ **FIGURE 71-29** Left upper lobe pulmonary arteries. **A,** CT angiography of the chest shows the apical and posterior segmental branches of the apicoposterior pulmonary artery of the left upper lobe. **B,** Image caudad to **A** shows the apicoposterior segment before it branches into apical and posterior segments. PostBr, posterior branch of the apicoposterior segmental artery; ApBr, apical branch of the apicoposterior segmental artery.

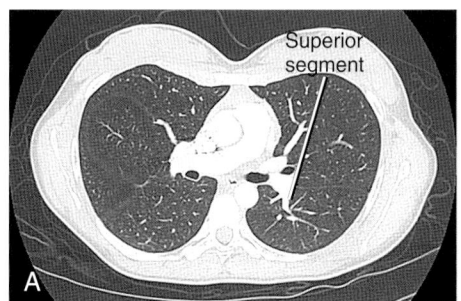

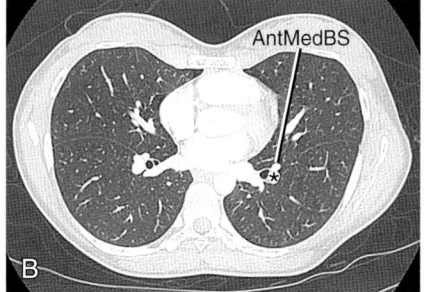

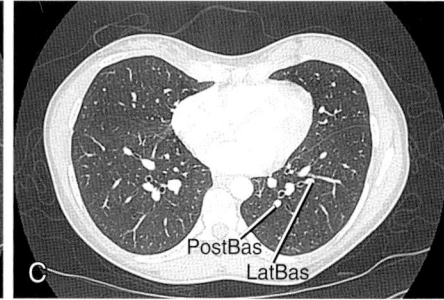

■ **FIGURE 71-30** Left lower lobe pulmonary arterial anatomy. **A,** CT angiography of the chest shows the superior segmental artery arising from the interlobar artery, which is superior to the origin of the lingular artery (not shown). **B,** Caudal to the origin of the superior and lingular arteries, the anteromedial basal segmental artery arises from the anterior aspect of the descending left pulmonary artery (*asterisk*). **C,** The posterior basal and lateral basal segmental arteries originate at a more inferior level and in similar fashion to the right lower lobe anatomy. AntMedBS, anterior medial basal segment; LatBas, lateral basal segment; PostBas, posterior basal segment.

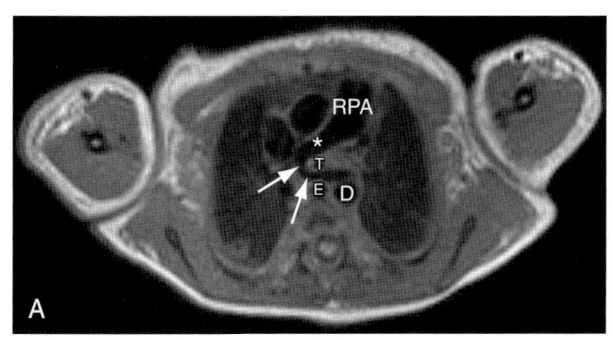

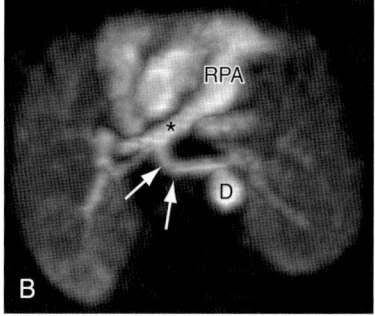

■ **FIGURE 71-31** Axial black blood MR image (**A**) and maximum intensity projection image (**B**) of the pulmonary arteries show the left main pulmonary artery (*arrows*) arising from the right main pulmonary artery (*asterisk*), coursing behind the trachea (T) and anterior to the descending aorta (D) and esophagus (E). RPA, right pulmonary artery.

SUMMARY

Although individually the arterial anomalies of the chest are relatively rare, the variety of anomalies as well as the increasing prevalence of cross-sectional imaging of the chest makes the possibility of encountering a vascular anatomic variant in daily clinical practice very likely. Therefore, the imager should be familiar with normal arterial anatomy and the common anatomic variants.

KEY POINTS

- Knowledge of arterial anatomy is important for the interpretation of imaging examinations.
- It is important to be aware of normal variants.

SUGGESTED READING

Uflacker R. Atlas of Vascular Anatomy: An Angiographic Approach. Philadelphia, Lippincott Williams & Wilkins, 2006, p 135.

REFERENCES

1. Elefteriades JA. Natural history of thoracic aortic aneurysms: indications for surgery, and surgical versus nonsurgical risks. Ann Thorac Surg 2002; 74:S1877-S1880.
2. Aronberg DJ, Glazer HS, Madsen K, Sagel SS. Normal thoracic aortic diameters by computed tomography. J Comput Assist Tomogr 1984; 8:247-250.
3. De Garis CF, Black IB, Riemenschneider EA. Patterns of the aortic arch in American white and Negro stocks, with comparative notes on certain other mammals. J Anat 1933; 67:599-618.
4. Layton KF, Kallmes DF, Cloft HJ, et al. Bovine aortic arch variant in humans: clarification of a common misnomer. AJNR Am J Neuroradiol 2006; 27:1541-1542.
5. Donnelly LF, Fleck RJ, Pacharn P, et al. Aberrant subclavian arteries: cross-sectional imaging findings in infants and children referred for evaluation of extrinsic airway compression. AJR Am J Roentgenol 2002; 178:1269-1274.
6. Kocis KC, Midgley FM, Ruckman RN. Aortic arch complex anomalies: 20-year experience with symptoms, diagnosis, associated cardiac defects, and surgical repair. Pediatr Cardiol 1997; 18:127-132.
7. Congdon ED. Transformation of the aortic-arch system during the development of the human embryo. Contrib Embryol 1992; 68:47-110.
8. Lowe GM, Donaldson JS, Backer CL. Vascular rings: 10-year review of imaging. Radiographics 1991; 11:637-646.
9. Kleinman PK, Spevak MR, Nimkin K. Left-sided esophageal indentation in right aortic arch with aberrant left subclavian artery. Radiology 1990; 191:565-567.
10. Nadas AS. Pediatric Cardiology, 2nd ed. Philadelphia, WB Saunders, 1963, p 430.
11. Luetmer PH, Miller GM. Right aortic arch with isolation of the left subclavian artery: case report and review of the literature. Mayo Clin Proc 1990; 65:407-413.
12. Kalke BR, Magotra R, Doshi SM. A new surgical approach to the management of symptomatic aberrant right subclavian artery. Ann Thorac Surg 1987; 44:86-89.
13. Gray H, Pick TP, Howden R. Gray's Anatomy: The Unabridged Running Press Edition of the American Classic. Philadelphia, Running Press, 1991, p 478.
14. Harley HR. The development and anomalies of the aortic arch and its branches. With the report of a case of right cervical aortic arch and intrathoracic vascular ring. Br J Surg 1959; 46:561-573.
15. Gray H. Anatomy of the Human Body. Philadelphia, Lea & Febiger, 1918; Bartleby.com, 2000, p 551.
16. Trigaux JP, Delchambre F, Van Beers B. Anatomical variations of the carotid bifurcation: implications for digital subtraction angiography and ultrasonography. Br J Radiol 1990; 747:181-185.
17. Bouthillier A, van Loveren H, Keller JT. Segments of the internal carotid artery: a new classification. Neurosurgery 1996; 38:425-433.
17a. Huber P. Cerebral Angiography. 4th ed. Stuttgart, Germany, Thieme, 1982.
18. Ribeiro RA, Ribeiro JA, Rodrigues Filho OA, et al. Common carotid artery bifurcation levels related to clinical relevant anatomical landmarks. Int J Morphol 2006; 24:413-416.
19. Uflacker R. Atlas of Vascular Anatomy: An Angiographic Approach. Philadelphia, Lippincott Williams & Wilkins, 2006, p 135.
20. Prendes JL, McKinney WM, Buonanno FS, Jones AM. Anatomic variations of the carotid bifurcation affecting Doppler scan interpretation. J Clin Ultrasound 1980; 8:147-150.
21. Hahnel S, Hartmann M, Jansen O, Sartor K. Persistent hypoglossal artery: MRI, MRA and digital subtraction angiometry. Neuroradiology 2001; 43:767-769.
22. Caldemeyer KS, Carrico JB, Mathews VP. The radiology and embryology of anomalous arteries of the head and neck. AJR Am J Roentgenol 1998; 170:197-203.
23. Uchino A, Sawada A, Takase Y, et al. MR angiography of anomalous branches of the internal carotid artery. AJR Am J Roentgenol 2003; 181:1409-1414.
24. De Caro R, Parenti A, Munari PF. The persistent primitive hypoglossal artery: a rare anatomic variation with frequent clinical implications. Ann Anat 1995; 177:193-198.
25. Hartmann IJ, Remy-Jardin M, Menchini L. Ectopic origin of bronchial arteries: assessment with multidetector helical CT angiography. Eur Radiol 2007; 17:1943-1953.

CHAPTER 72

Arterial Anatomy of the Abdomen

Jeremy C. Durack and Maureen P. Kohi

The organs and blood vessels of the abdomen and pelvis may be afflicted by a variety of disease processes, including inflammatory, infectious, neoplastic, autoimmune, traumatic, and degenerative. Many of these conditions may be treated with medical or surgical therapies, although sufficient blood supply to the affected region is often the critical factor for prognosis. Pharmacotherapeutic treatment requires distribution through a rich and redundant network of arterial blood flow. For endovascular or surgical procedures in the abdomen and pelvis, an understanding of normal and variant arterial anatomy is vital.

Modern intravascular contrast imaging enables exquisite visualization of the vascular supply to the abdomen and pelvis. More specifically, multiphase CT and MRI, as well as extended-run angiography, display arterial, portal venous, and venous anatomy and may provide valuable information in settings of altered vascular physiology. In this and subsequent chapters, we will demonstrate and highlight interesting and clinically important alterations in blood flow to these regions.

NORMAL ANATOMY
General Anatomic Descriptions

The abdominal aorta and its branches are responsible for the arterial blood supply to the abdominal organs (Figs. 72-1 and 72-2). From the thoracic cavity, the aorta courses through the diaphragm slightly to the left of midline at the aortic hiatus, most commonly anterior to the twelfth thoracic vertebral body.[1] The normal aorta measures 1.5 to 2 cm in diameter and diminishes in caliber until its terminal bifurcation, typically at the level of the fourth lumbar vertebral body. During the process of vasculogenesis, embryonic folding during the fourth week parallels fusion of the paired dorsal aortae into a single median dorsal aorta in the abdomen.[2] Major branches from the dorsal abdominal aorta subsequently develop ventrally, laterally, and posterolaterally and may be divided into four groups (Table 72-1).

Group 1 includes branches formed by the union of vitelline arteries arising from the wall of the yolk sac that supply organs depending on their location in the primitive gut.[2] The developing gastrointestinal tract, or primitive gut, is often divided into the foregut, midgut, and hindgut. The foregut gives rise to the esophagus, stomach, proximal half of the duodenum, liver, and pancreas. The midgut gives rise to the distal half of the duodenum, jejunum, ileum, cecum, appendix, ascending colon, and the right two thirds of the transverse colon. The hindgut gives rise to the left two thirds of the transverse colon, descending colon, sigmoid colon, and rectum. From the dorsal aorta, the three dominant vitelline arteries are further refined into the celiac trunk, superior mesenteric artery, and inferior mesenteric artery, which correspond to the three primitive gut regions, respectively.

Group 2 (renal and adrenal branches) includes branches supplying the kidneys and adrenal glands.

Group 3, the gonadal arteries (testicular and ovarian), supply the testes and ovaries. The gonadal arteries develop from lateral splanchnic branches of the abdominal aorta.

Group 4 (terminal and posterior branches) include the media sacral artery, lumbar arteries, and common iliac arteries. Posterolateral arterial branches develop along the course of the aorta by the end of the third week.

The arterial supply of the pelvic organs and pelvic wall courses through the internal iliac arteries, which originate at the bifurcation of the common iliac artery at the sacroiliac junction. Arterial anatomy of the pelvis is presented in Chapter 73.

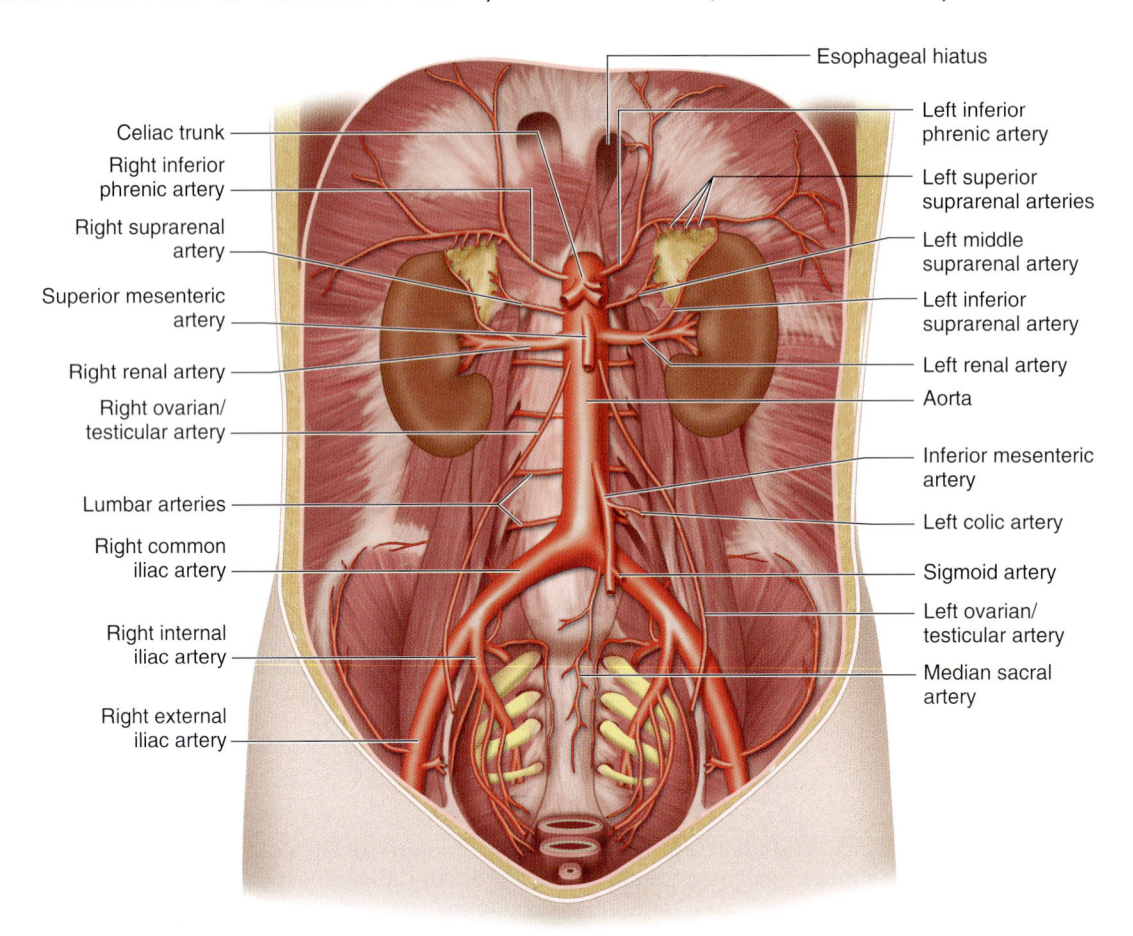

■ **FIGURE 72-1** Arterial anatomy of the abdomen. The major branches of the abdominal aorta are depicted. All abdominal organs have been removed except the kidneys.

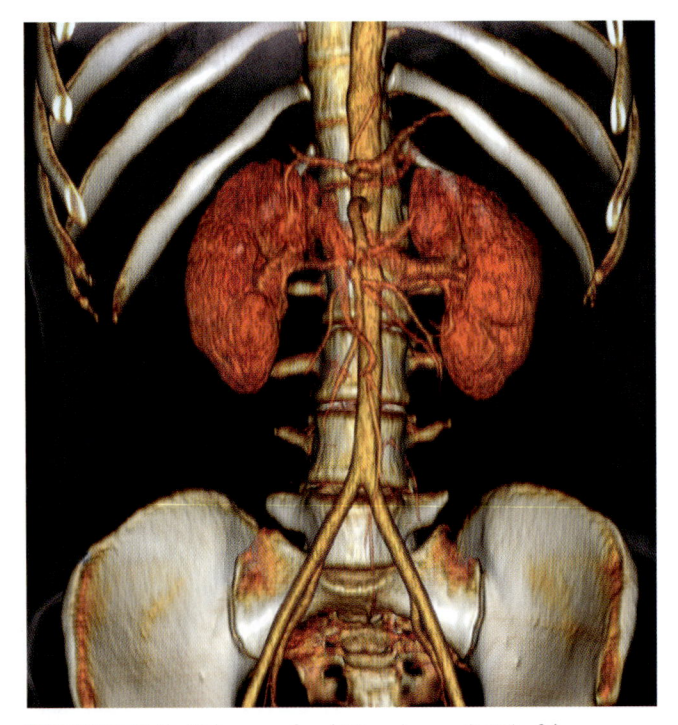

■ **FIGURE 72-2** Volume rendered CT angiogram (CTA) of the abdominal aorta. The celiac trunk, superior mesenteric artery, renal arteries, and inferior mesenteric artery are visible on this CT scan performed with an intravenous contrast agent. CT imaging was timed for optimal opacification of the abdominal aorta and its arterial branches.

Detailed Description of Specific Areas

Normal Variants

Group 1: Celiac Trunk and Mesenteric Arteries

The celiac trunk is a short (1 to 2 cm) ventral branch of the abdominal aorta arising below the aortic hiatus, typically between T12 and L1 (Fig. 72-3).[1,3,4] The foregut organs are supplied by the celiac trunk's trifurcated branches, the left gastric, common hepatic, and splenic arteries, in up to 75% of individuals (Fig. 72-4). Rarely, a common origin of the celiac and superior mesenteric artery develops; however, most variants involve separate origins of one or more of the three main celiac branches. The left gastric artery is ordinarily the first and smallest celiac branch, supplying the distal esophagus and stomach. Coursing along the lesser curvature of the stomach, the left gastric branches unite with the right gastric branches, forming a vascular arcade. Further anastomoses exist between the left gastric artery and the short gastric arteries from the splenic artery as well as the left gastroepiploic (sometimes called gastro-omental) artery.

The splenic artery is the largest and often most tortuous branch of the celiac trunk. Throughout its course superior to the pancreas, it supplies the pancreatic body and tail with multiple small penetrating branches, along with two larger branches, the dorsal pancreatic and greater pancreatic arteries. As previously noted, the splenic artery

TABLE 72-1	Major Branches of the Abdominal Aorta
Group	Arterial Branches
Group 1	
Foregut	Celiac trunk
Esophagus	Left gastric artery
Stomach	Esophageal branches
Proximal half of	Splenic artery
duodenum	Pancreatic branches
Liver	Short gastric branches
Pancreas	Left gastroepiploic artery
	Common hepatic artery
	Hepatic artery proper
	Cystic artery
	Gastroduodenal artery
	Supraduodenal branch
	Right gastroepiploic artery
	Anterior and posterior superior pancreaticoduodenal arteries
	Right gastric artery
Midgut	Superior mesenteric artery
Distal half of duodenum	Inferior pancreaticoduodenal artery
Jejunum	Jejunal arteries
Ileum	Ileal arteries
Cecum	Appendicular artery
Appendix	Ileocolic artery
Ascending colon	Right colic artery
Right two thirds of transverse colon	Middle colic artery
Hindgut	Inferior mesenteric artery
Left two thirds of transverse colon	Left colic artery
Descending colon	Sigmoid artery
Sigmoid colon	Superior rectal artery
Rectum	
Group 2	
Kidney	Renal arteries
Adrenal glands	Inferior phrenic arteries
	Superior adrenal arteries
	Middle adrenal arteries
	Inferior adrenal arteries
Group 3	
Testes and ovaries	Testicular and ovarian arteries
Group 4	
Terminal and posterior branches	Common iliac arteries
	Median sacral artery
	Lumbar arteries

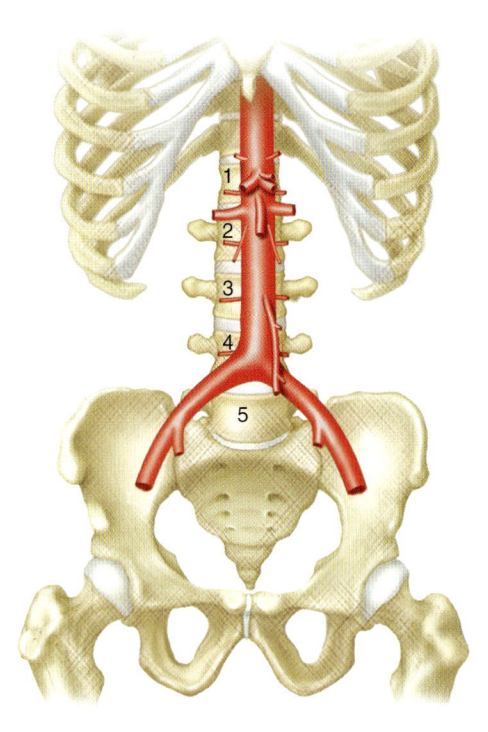

■ **FIGURE 72-3** Location of major abdominal aortic branches relative to the spine. The celiac trunk typically arises anteriorly between the twelfth thoracic (T12) and first lumbar vertebral (L1) bodies. The superior mesenteric artery usually arises anterior to L1 and the inferior mesenteric artery arises anterior to L3. The renal arteries may emerge from T12 to L2, although they most commonly emerge between L1 and L2.

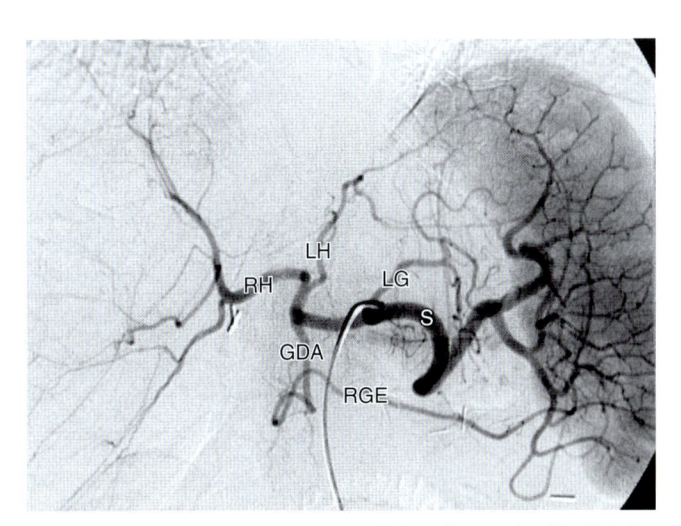

■ **FIGURE 72-4** Selective angiogram of the celiac trunk. This digitally subtracted fluoroscopic image was obtained following injection of contrast through a catheter inserted into the origin of the celiac trunk. GDA, gastroduodenal artery; LG, left gastric artery; LH, left hepatic artery; RGE, right gastroepiploic artery; RH, right hepatic artery; S, splenic artery.

supplies the stomach through the short gastric arteries and left gastroepiploic artery. The left gastroepiploic artery also connects with the right gastroepiploic artery, which feed the stomach and surrounding omentum. Finally, true to its name, the splenic artery's terminal organ is the spleen.

Rounding out the branches of the celiac trunk is the common hepatic artery, an intermediate-sized branch that gives rise to the gastroduodenal artery, right gastric artery and proper hepatic artery. The branching pattern of the proper hepatic artery is frequently variable. Conventionally, the artery divides at the porta hepatis into the right and left hepatic arteries (Fig. 72-5). The described branching pattern of the common hepatic artery into right and left hepatic arteries at the portohepatic artery is seen in only 36% to 50% of patients, according to multiple cadaveric and angiographic studies. In approximately 12% of patients, the right hepatic artery originates from the superior mesenteric artery, a variant described as a replaced right hepatic artery. Furthermore, an accessory right hepatic artery in addition to a conventional right hepatic artery was found in approximately 2.5% of patients in one cadaveric study. The left hepatic artery originates from the left gastric artery, also referred to as a replaced left hepatic artery, in approximately 4.5% to 6% of patients. In about

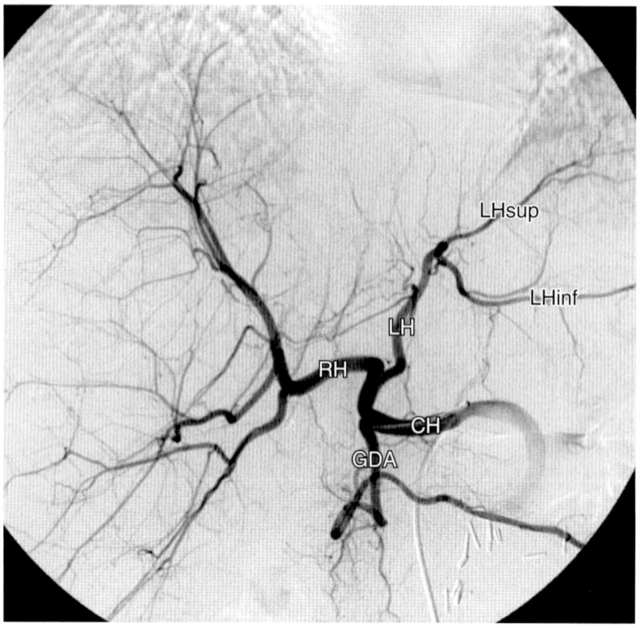

FIGURE 72-5 Selective angiogram of the common hepatic artery. This digitally subtracted fluoroscopic image was obtained following injection of contrast through a catheter inserted into the common hepatic artery. CH, common hepatic artery; GDA, gastroduodenal artery; LH, left hepatic artery; LHinf, inferior branch of the left hepatic artery; LHsup, superior branch of the left hepatic artery; RH, right hepatic artery.

2% of patients, the common hepatic artery arises from the superior mesenteric artery. The right hepatic artery then gives rise to the cystic artery, which furnishes the gallbladder with arterial blood. There is a single cystic artery in about 80% of patients. The cystic artery arises from the right hepatic artery about half the time, followed in decreasing prevalence by the accessory right hepatic, distal common hepatic, left hepatic, proximal common hepatic, proper hepatic, and gastroduodenal arteries. Two cystic arteries, usually both from the right hepatic artery, may be seen in approximately 19% of patients, whereas three cystic arteries have been found in less than 1% of those examined.[5,6]

The gastroduodenal artery is a short, vertically oriented branch of the common hepatic artery that often gives rise to the supraduodenal artery. In a study of 30 patients, the supraduodenal artery was identified in 93%, most frequently originating from the gastroduodenal artery. The supraduodenal artery supplies the distal two thirds of the upper portion of the duodenum and the supraduodenal and retroduodenal portions of the common bile duct. Anastomoses with the right gastric and posterior superior pancreaticoduodenal arteries were discovered in half of cases in a study by Bianchi and Albanese.[7] The gastroduodenal artery then divides further into the anterior superior pancreaticoduodenal artery, posterior superior pancreaticoduodenal artery, and right gastroepiploic artery. The anterior and posterior superior pancreaticoduodenal arteries anastomose with the anterior and posterior branches of the inferior pancreaticoduodenal artery from the superior mesenteric artery, providing blood to the duodenum and surrounding pancreas.

Superior Mesenteric Artery

The superior mesenteric artery is the second large ventral branch of the abdominal aorta, typically emerging 1 cm below the celiac trunk, anterior to the first lumbar vertebral body. It supplies the midgut organs through its main (and largely intuitively named) branches, the inferior pancreaticoduodenal, jejunal, ileal, ileocolic, right colic, and middle colic arteries (Figs. 72-6 to 72-9). The inferior pancreaticoduodenal artery supplies the head of the pancreas and duodenum. The superior mesenteric artery anastomoses with the anterior and posterior superior pancreaticoduodenal arteries originating from the gastroduodenal artery. Jejunal arteries form numerous anastomoses, resulting in extensive vascular arcades and collaterals supplying the jejunum and its mesentery. The ileocolic artery ramifies into multiple small branches, one of which is the appendicular artery supplying the appendix. The right and middle colic arteries deliver blood to the ascending colon and the proximal two thirds of the transverse colon and mesocolon.

Inferior Mesenteric Artery

The inferior mesenteric artery is the most inferior of the visceral arteries from the abdominal aorta, generally located anterior to the L3 vertebral body. It supplies the hindgut through its major branches, the left colic artery, sigmoid artery, and superior rectal artery (Fig. 72-10). The left colic artery supplies the distal third of the transverse colon and descending colon and forms numerous vascular arcades and collaterals. The embryologic division between the midgut and hindgut is an area sensitive to ischemia, sometimes referred to as a watershed area of the transverse colon. The sigmoid arteries supply the distalmost aspect of the descending colon, along with the sigmoid colon. The superior rectal artery flows to the superior aspect of the rectum and forms copious collaterals with the middle and inferior rectal arteries, branches of the internal iliac and internal pudendal arteries, respectively.

Group 2: Renal and Adrenal Arteries

Group 2 includes branches supplying the kidneys and adrenal glands. The kidneys migrate superiorly from a sacral level during development and are progressively but transiently supplied by lateral aortic branches as they move up. Ultimately, the main renal arteries emerge between L1 and L2 in approximately 75% of the population, whereas the remaining 25% of individuals may have renal origins anywhere from the T12 through L2 vertebral levels. Anatomic variants are common, occurring in up to 40% of those studied.[8,9] Accessory or aberrant vessels may arise from iliac, superior and inferior mesenteric, adrenal, inferior phrenic, right hepatic, intercostal, median sacral, lumbar, or right colic arteries. Patients with ectopic or horseshoe kidneys, or other renal anomalies, are more likely to demonstrate aberrant arterial origins. About 30% of individuals have supernumerary renal arteries and, of those, they are unilateral in about 30% and bilateral in about 10% of cases. Renal arteries taking origin from the aorta most frequently arise laterally, although infrequently

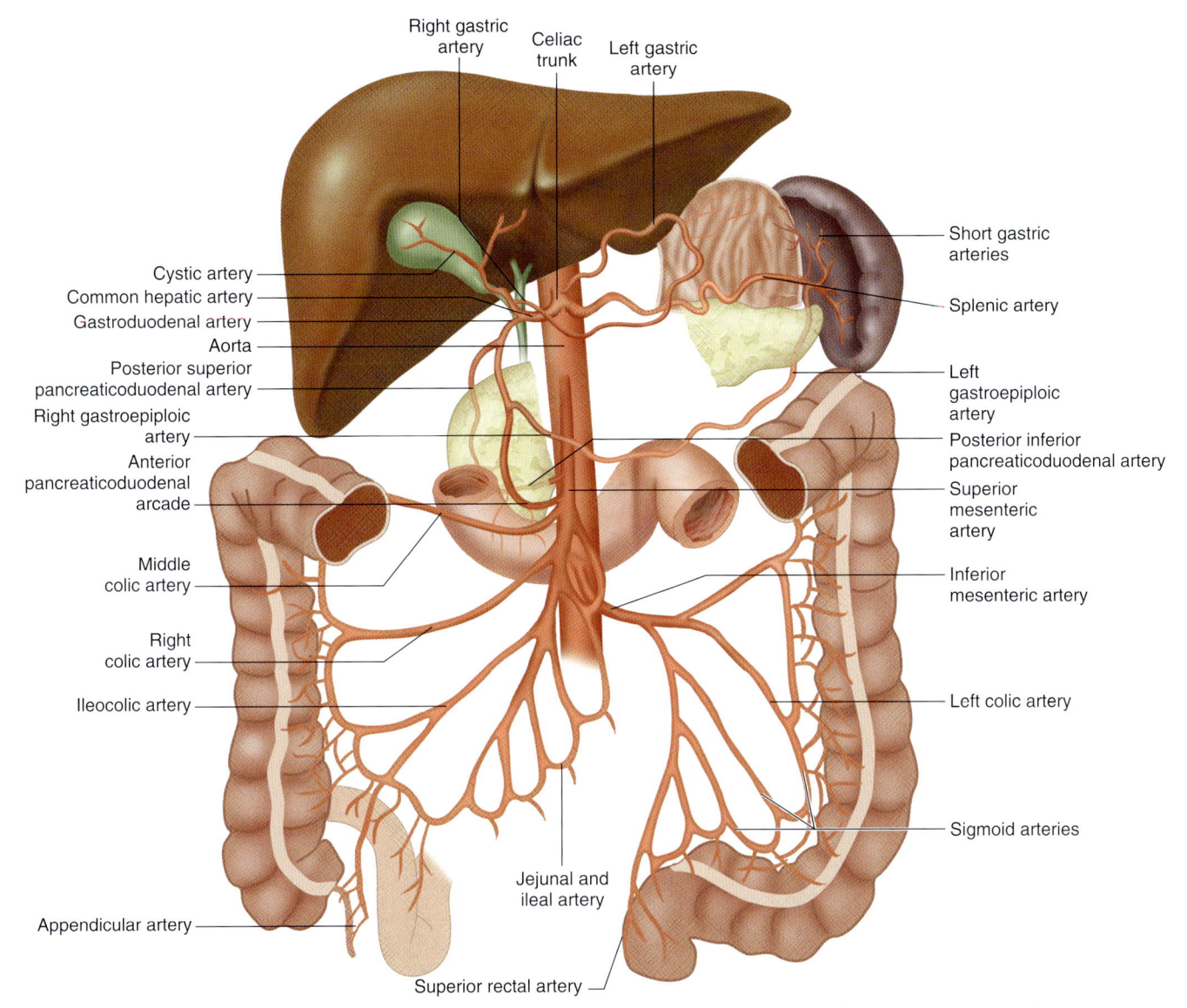

FIGURE 72-6 Arterial supply to the abdominal organs: abdominal aorta, celiac trunk, and superior and inferior mesenteric arteries. The stomach, pancreas, and small and large intestines have been partially removed to highlight arterial vasculature.

the left renal artery arises posterolaterally and the right renal artery arises anterolaterally. Proximal division of the renal artery occurs in approximately 15% of individuals. Additionally, branching proximal to the renal hilum may provide blood supply to the proximal ureter, gonadal arteries, perinephric tissues, renal capsule, and/or adrenal glands. Knowledge of these renal variants is tremendously important for operative planning, and imaging for anatomic delineation is routine for renal donor candidates.

The three adrenal arteries are refined during the process of kidney ascension, which occurs by the sixth week of development. When the kidney has completed its upward migration, the superior adrenal artery begins to supply the maturing diaphragm, forming the inferior phrenic artery. Superior suprarenal artery branches from the inferior phrenic continue to supply the adrenal gland to varying degrees. Supplemental arterial supply comes from the middle suprarenal artery, which typically arises between T12 and L1, most commonly from the lateral aorta, although celiac, superior mesenteric, or lumbar artery origins have been demonstrated. The inferior suprarenal arteries are variable in their origin, in part related to the fact that the main renal arteries develop from the inferior adrenals during renal migration.[10,11] Persistent arterial branches to the adrenal gland from the renal arteries occur in about 80% of individuals from the right and in 60% of individuals from the left. Some studies have shown that those with supernumerary renal arteries possess inferior adrenal branches with greater frequency. Furthermore, inferior suprarenal arteries may stem from renal capsular, inferior phrenic, or interlobar renal arteries.

The inferior phrenic arteries provide blood supply to the abdominal aspect of the diaphragm and originate from the aorta and celiac axis with the highest and almost equal frequency, although numerous variant origins have been reported. The hepatic, superior mesenteric, left gastric, renal, and adrenal arteries have all been demonstrated to give origin to inferior phrenic arteries. If derived from the

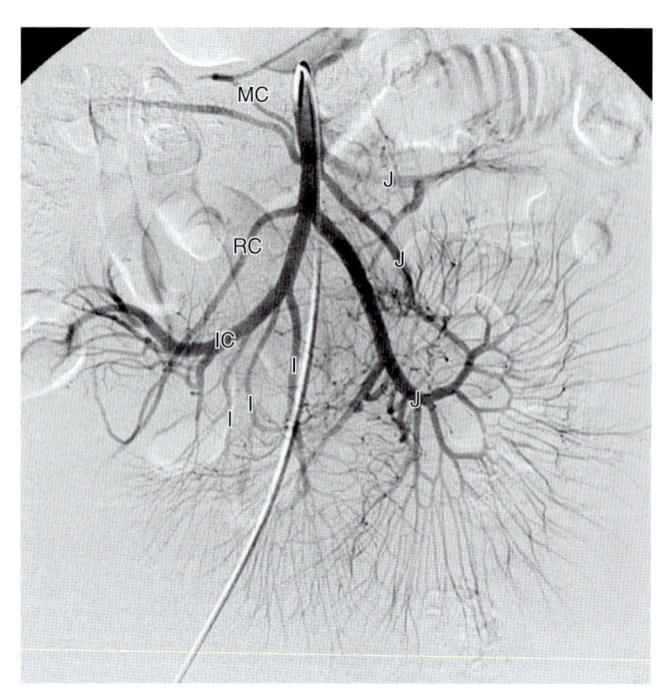

■ **FIGURE 72-7** Selective angiogram of the superior mesenteric artery. This early digitally subtracted fluoroscopic image was obtained following injection of contrast through a catheter inserted into the superior mesenteric artery. I, ileal arterial branches; IC, ileocolic artery; MC, middle colic artery; J, jejunal arterial branches; MC, middle colic artery; RC, right colic artery.

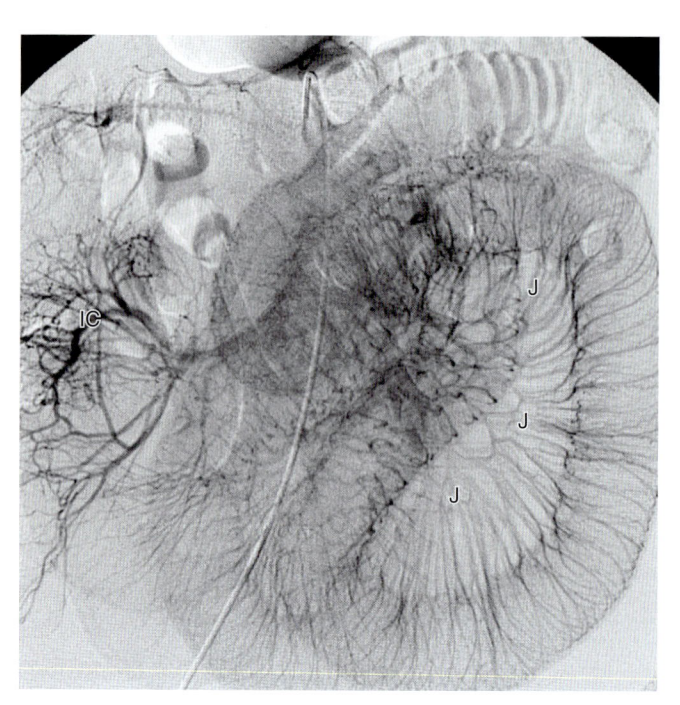

■ **FIGURE 72-9** Later phase digitally subtracted fluoroscopic image acquired after injection of contrast through a superior mesenteric artery catheter, highlighting small arteries supplying the jejunum. IC, ileocolic artery; J, jejunal arterial branches.

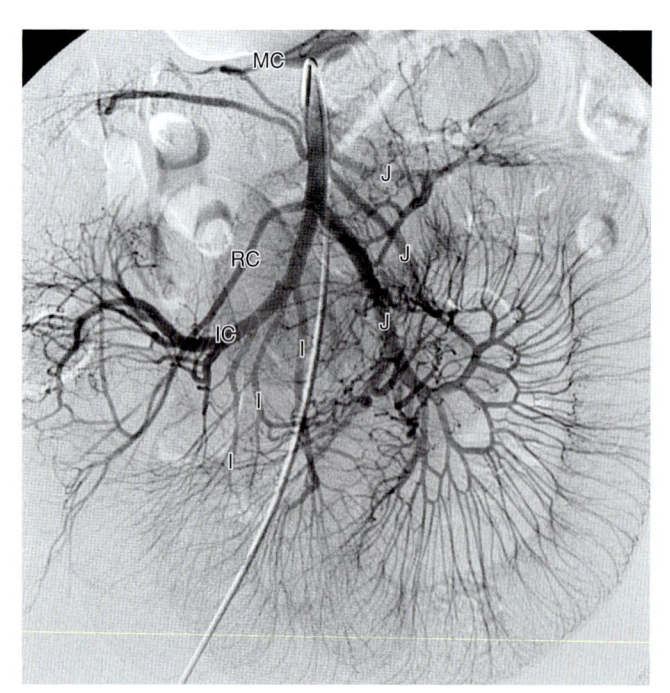

■ **FIGURE 72-8** This digitally subtracted fluoroscopic image was acquired several seconds after injection of contrast through a superior mesenteric artery catheter. I, ileal arterial branches; IC, ileocolic artery; MC, middle colic artery; J, jejunal arterial branches; MC, middle colic artery; RC, right colic artery.

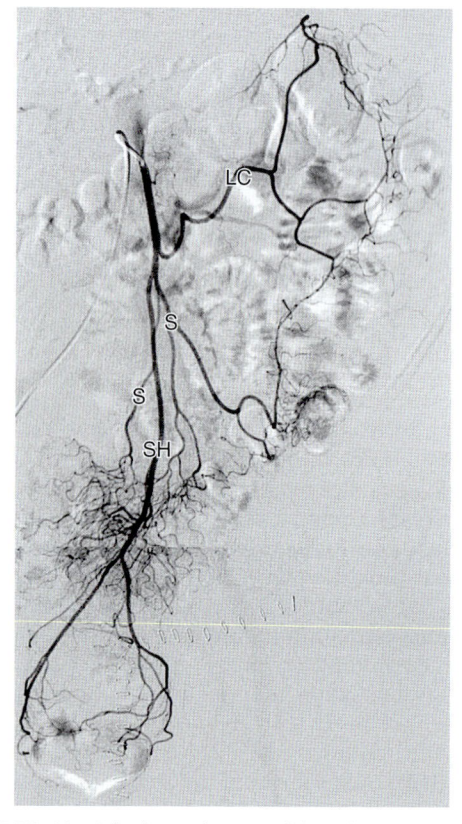

■ **FIGURE 72-10** Selective angiogram of the inferior mesenteric artery. This digitally subtracted fluoroscopic image was obtained following injection of contrast through a catheter inserted into the origin of the inferior mesenteric artery. LC, left colic artery; S, sigmoid arterial branches; SH, superior hemorrhoidal artery.

TABLE 72-2 Inferior Phrenic Artery Origins Studied at Autopsy (%)

Origin	Aorta	Celiac	Left Gastric	Renal
Common trunk	18.6	13.4		
Independent left-right	13.4	18.3		
Right	16.2	7.6		
Left	11.7	18.9		
Total right	48.2	39.3	3.1	7.6
Total left	43.7	50.6	4.1	0.9

Adapted from Kadir S. Atlas of Normal and Variant Angiographic Anatomy. Philadelphia, WB Saunders, 1991.

aorta, they are usually found between T12 and L2, but may be distributed from T9 to L2. The left and right inferior phrenic arteries may begin as a common trunk, or independently. Kadir has combined data from autopsy studies into a single table (Table 72-2).[12]

The inferior phrenic artery is the most common vessel to supply extrahepatic blood to hepatocellular carcinomas in the liver. To prevent bleeding complications during surgical resection or recurrence after endovascular treatment, arterial supply to hepatocellular tumors should be defined.

Group 3: Gonadal Arteries

Group 3 includes the gonadal arteries supplying the testes and ovaries. The gonadal arteries develop from lateral splanchnic branches of the abdominal aorta. Most commonly, gonadal arteries are single bilaterally and arise ventrally near the level of the second lumbar vertebra, taking a horizontal course (anterior to the inferior vena cava on the right) initially before diving caudally. Multiple gonadal arteries are more common on the left and a common origin, although rare, can emerge from either the aorta or renal artery. Approximately 5% to 20% arise superior to L2 and may originate from the main or accessory renal artery in up to 6% of individuals.[13,14] A course posterior to the inferior vena cava may occur in cases of high right gonadal artery origin. Rarely, a gonadal artery arises from an adrenal, lumbar, or iliac artery. Closer to the gonadal arterial origin, branching supply to the ureter, perirenal adipose tissue, and retroperitoneal lymph nodes may be seen. Frequently tortuous distally, the ovarian artery provides tubal and ureteric branches in addition to supplying the ovaries and regions of inguinal skin.

The aberrant origin and course of gonadal arteries may have implications for surgery, particularly urologic or retroperitoneal procedures. Prior knowledge of aberrant anatomy is important for surgical planning. Anatomic variance may be difficult to discern on aortography due to the small size of the gonadal vessels (about 1 mm in diameter) and their visualization in only one-third of cases. Conversely, hypertrophic ovarian arteries may be discovered prior to or following procedures to treat symptomatic uterine fibroids.

Group 4: Terminal and Posterior Branches

Group 4 includes the median sacral artery, lumbar arteries, and common iliac arteries. Posterolateral arterial branches develop along the course of the aorta by the end of the third week. These branches further refine into intercostal arteries in the thoracic region and lumbar arteries more caudally. Most often there are four pairs of lumbar arteries, which anastomose with the lower intercostal, subcostal, iliolumbar, deep iliac circumflex, and inferior epigastric arteries. The medial sacral artery, which runs medially and inferiorly from the aortic bifurcation, represents a continuation of the dorsal aorta. Small lumbar arteries representing a fifth pair sometimes originates from the medial sacral artery. Not surprisingly, the median sacral artery may also sprout from the lowest pair of lumbar arteries. The aorta terminates at its bifurcation into the common iliac arteries, usually at the L4 or L5 level. With age, the aorta and common iliac arteries may become tortuous, so that the aortic bifurcation descends to a more caudal position.

Differential Considerations

A number of eponymous vascular anastomoses can hypertrophy as a result of flow limitations in the abdominal arterial system. Frequently, these anastomoses increase in prominence as atherosclerotic vascular narrowing progresses. For example, multiple collaterals exist between branches of the superior and inferior mesenteric arteries and between the celiac and superior mesenteric arteries. The marginal artery of Drummond is formed by the anastomosis of a transverse branch of the middle colic artery with an ascending branch of the left colic artery.[1,4] This artery is a marginal colonic artery that lies along the mesenteric border of the left colon. The arc of Riolan is a more medial anastomotic connection between the left colic and middle colic arteries (Fig. 72-11). The arc of Buehler is formed by the anastomosis of the celiac artery and superior mesenteric artery.

Fibromuscular disease is a nonatheromatous and noninflammatory process that causes arterial narrowing and aneurysms. While the cause of fibromuscular disease or dysplasia (FMD) is not well understood, the process tends to occur in women between the age of 40 and 60 years, frequently involves the renal arteries, and results in renovascular hypertension in about one-third of patients. Various forms of dysplasia or hyperplasia can involve the media, intima, or adventitia of the vascular wall. The most common type, medial fibroplasia (60% to 70%), produces alternating thick and thin fibromuscular ridges resulting in a string of beads appearance angiographically (Fig. 72-12). The mid to distal renal arteries are typically affected (60% to 75%), although abnormalities in the carotid and intracranial arteries (25% to 30%), mesenteric arteries (9%), and external iliac arteries (5%) may also be seen.

Pertinent Imaging Considerations

Cancers of the liver, whether primary or metastatic, can be treated in a number of ways depending on tumor size, location, origin, and patient comorbid conditions. Radioembolization using yttrium-90 microspheres is an innovative procedure whereby inoperable cancers may be treated endovascularly. The microspheres are delivered intraarterially in the hepatic artery so that the radioactive

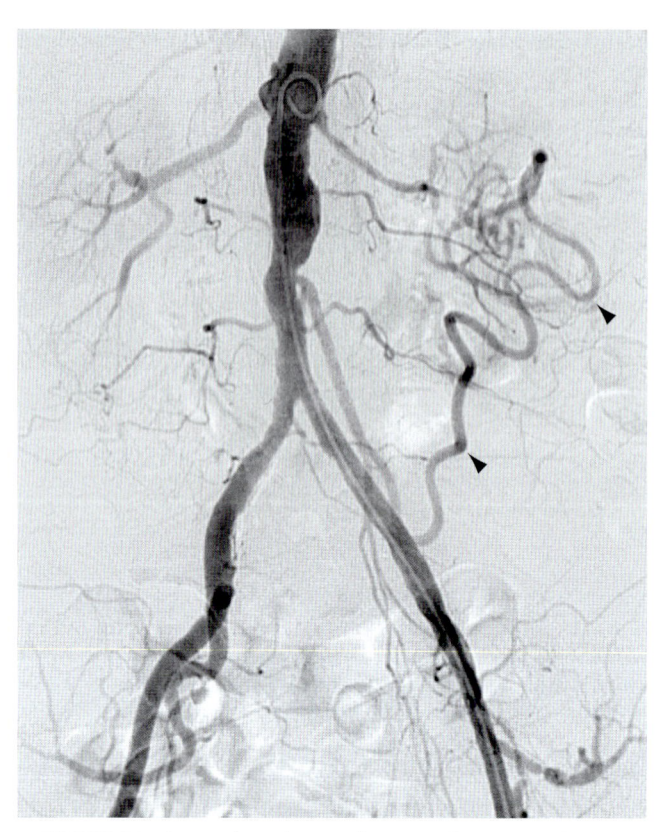

■ FIGURE 72-11 Aortic angiogram demonstrating mesenteric anastomosis. *Arrowheads* point to a prominent arc of Riolan, an anastomosis between the superior and inferior mesenteric arteries, which has enlarged due to severe narrowing of the proximal superior mesenteric artery from atherosclerotic disease.

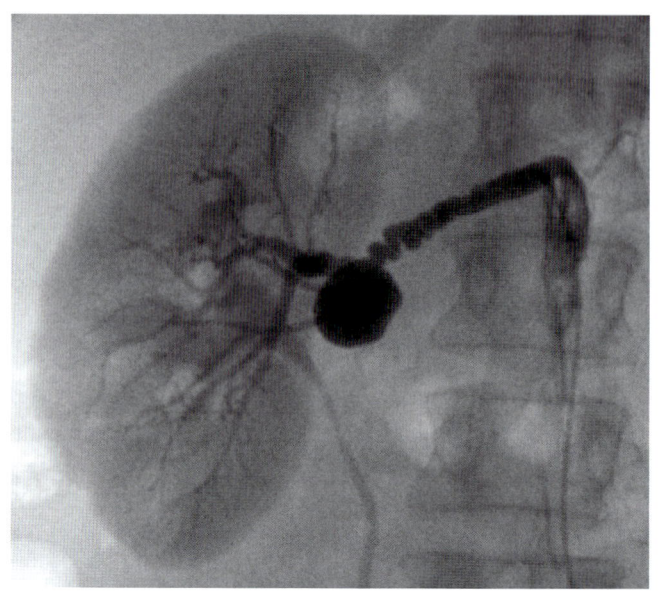

■ FIGURE 72-12 Fibromuscular disease affecting the renal artery. A fluoroscopic image from a selective right renal angiogram demonstrates both a characteristic string of beads appearance to the mid to distal renal artery and a saccular aneurysm.

element yttrium-90 is deposited within tumor blood vessels, radiating and destroying tumor cells. In planning for this procedure, it is critical that all the arterial vasculature of the upper abdomen is visualized, minimizing nontarget embolization of gastrointestinal or other organs. Conventional arteriography of the celiac axis and superior mesenteric artery is fastidiously performed prior to the procedure to visualize the relevant arterial anatomy. Arterial vessels supplying the gastrointestinal tract or other nontarget organs can then be embolized endovascularly prior to radionuclide therapy.

KEY POINTS

- Arterial phase imaging in the abdomen can be acquired by CT or MRI following intravenous injection of contrast agents.
- Direct contrast angiography can be performed by catheterization of the abdominal aorta or selective catheterization of aortic branch vessels.
- Variations in abdominal arterial anatomy are common and may be important for understanding disease processes and treatment options.

SUGGESTED READINGS

Capuñay C, Carrascosa P, Martín López E, et al. Multidetector CT angiography and virtual angioscopy of the abdomen. Abdom Imaging 2009; 34:81-93.

Hazirolan T, Metin Y, Karaosmanoglu AD, et al. Mesenteric arterial variations detected at MDCT angiography of abdominal aorta. Am J Roentgenol 2009; 192:1097-1102.

Iezzi R, Cotroneo AR, Giancristofaro D, et al. Multidetector-row CT angiographic imaging of the celiac trunk: anatomy and normal variants. Surg Radiol Anat 2008; 30:303-310.

Smith CL, Horton KM, Fishman EK. Mesenteric CT angiography: a discussion of techniques and selected applications. Tech Vasc Interv Radiol 2006; 9:150-155.

Zhang H, Zhang W, Juluru K, Prince M. Body magnetic resonance angiography. Semin Roentgenol 2009; 44:84-98.

REFERENCES

1. LaBerge J, Gordon R, Kerlan R, Wilson W. Interventional Radiology Essentials. Philadelphia, Lippincott Williams & Wilkins, 2000.
2. Larsen WJ, Sherman LS, Potter SS, Scott WJ. Development of the vasculature. In Larsen WJ, Sherman LS, Potter SS, Scott WJ (eds): Human Embryology, 3rd ed. Philadelphia, Churchill Livingstone, 2001, pp 195-234.
3. Netter F. Atlas of Human Anatomy, 2nd ed. Altona, Manitoba, Canada, Friesens, 1997.

4. Gray H. Anatomy of the Human Body, 20th ed. Available at: http://www.bartleby.com/107. Accessed September 27, 2009.
5. Covey AM, Brody LA, Maluccio MA, et al. Variant hepatic arterial anatomy revisited: digital subtraction angiography performed in 600 patients. Radiology 2002; 224:542-547.
6. Nelson T, Pollak R, Jonasson O, Abcarian H. Anatomic variants of the celia, superior mesenteric, and inferior mesenteric arteries and their clinical relevance. Clin Anat 1988; 1:75-91.
7. Bianchi HF, Albanese EF. The supraduodenal artery. Surg Radiol Anat 1989 11:37-40.
8. Fine H, Keen EN. The arteries of the human kidney. J Anat 1966; 100:881-894.
9. Harrison LH, Flye MW, Seigler HF. Incidence of anatomical variants in renal vasculature in the presence of normal renal function. Ann Surg 1978; 188:83-89.
10. Gagnon R. The arterial supply of the human adrenal gland. Rev Can Biol 1957; 16:421-433.
11. Toni R, Mosca S, Favero L, et al. Clinical anatomy of the suprarenal arteries: a quantitative approach by aortography. Surg Radiol Anat 1998; 10:297-302.
12. Kadir S. Atlas of Normal and Variant Angiographic Anatomy. Philadelphia, WB Saunders, 1991.
13. Merklin RJ, Michels NA. The variant renal and suprarenal blood supply with data on the inferior phrenic, ureteral and gonadal arteries. J Int Coll Surg 1958; 29:41-76.
14. Asala S, Chaudhary SC, Masumbuko-Kahamba N, Bidmos M. Anatomical variations in the human testicular blood vessels. Ann Anat 2001; 183:545-549.

CHAPTER 73

Arterial Anatomy of the Pelvis and Lower Extremities

Douglas Yim and Donald L. Miller

The major arteries of the pelvis and lower extremities are frequently involved by systemic diseases, especially atherosclerosis and diabetes mellitus. The existence of frequent anatomic variations and complex collateral pathways means that the anatomy as presented in textbooks often does not correspond to the clinical situation. In addition, certain specific arterial abnormalities in the pelvis and popliteal fossa can be symptomatic and clinically important.

NORMAL ANATOMY OF THE PELVIS

General Anatomic Descriptions

The abdominal aorta divides into the common iliac arteries at approximately the level of L4. The middle sacral artery, usually a very small vessel, arises from the posterior surface of the aortic bifurcation and extends inferiorly along the anterior surface of the sacrum, in the midline, to the distal tip of the coccyx. The length of the common iliac artery is variable. Each common iliac artery divides into an external iliac artery and internal iliac artery (Fig. 73-1).

The external iliac artery has only two branches, the deep circumflex iliac and inferior epigastric arteries. Both arise approximately at the point where the inguinal ligament crosses anterior to the external iliac artery, and both serve as markers on arteriograms for the junction of the external iliac artery and common femoral artery. Some experts consider the inferior epigastric artery to arise from the proximal femoral artery. The deep circumflex iliac artery extends superolaterally from its origin on the lateral aspect of the external iliac artery, and supplies the pelvic side wall. It anastomoses with the iliolumbar and superior gluteal arteries, branches of the internal iliac artery, and with the ascending branch of the lateral circumflex femoral artery, a branch of the profunda femoral artery.

The inferior epigastric artery arises from the medial aspect of the external iliac artery and dips inferiorly and medially before turning superiorly to course deep to the rectus abdominis muscle in the anterior abdominal wall (Fig. 73-2). Superiorly, it anastomoses with the superior epigastric artery, a branch of the internal thoracic artery.

The internal iliac artery has anterior and posterior divisions. Branches of the anterior division primarily supply the pelvic viscera, whereas branches of the posterior division supply pelvic bones and muscles (Fig. 73-3A).

Typically, the three branches of the posterior division are the iliolumbar artery, lateral sacral artery, and superior gluteal artery (see Fig. 73-3B). The iliolumbar artery extends laterally and superiorly to divide into two branches that supply the iliacus muscle and ilium (iliac branch) and the psoas major and quadratus lumborum muscles (lumbar branch). The lateral sacral artery extends medially and then superiorly to supply the spinal meninges and the roots of the sacral nerves. The superior gluteal artery, the largest branch of the internal iliac artery, extends laterally, passes above the piriformis muscle through the greater sciatic foramen as it leaves the pelvis posteriorly, and supplies the gluteal muscles, overlying soft tissues and skin. These posterior division branches may, on occasion, arise from the anterior division or from trunks formed by various combinations of internal iliac artery branches (see later).

The anterior division of the internal iliac artery divides into a number of named arteries. As with the posterior division branches, the anterior division vessels may occasionally arise from the posterior division or from trunks formed by various combinations of internal iliac artery branches.

The three principal branches of the anterior division are the obturator artery, inferior gluteal artery, and internal pudendal artery (Fig. 73-4A). The obturator artery courses along the pelvic brim, bifurcates above the obtura-

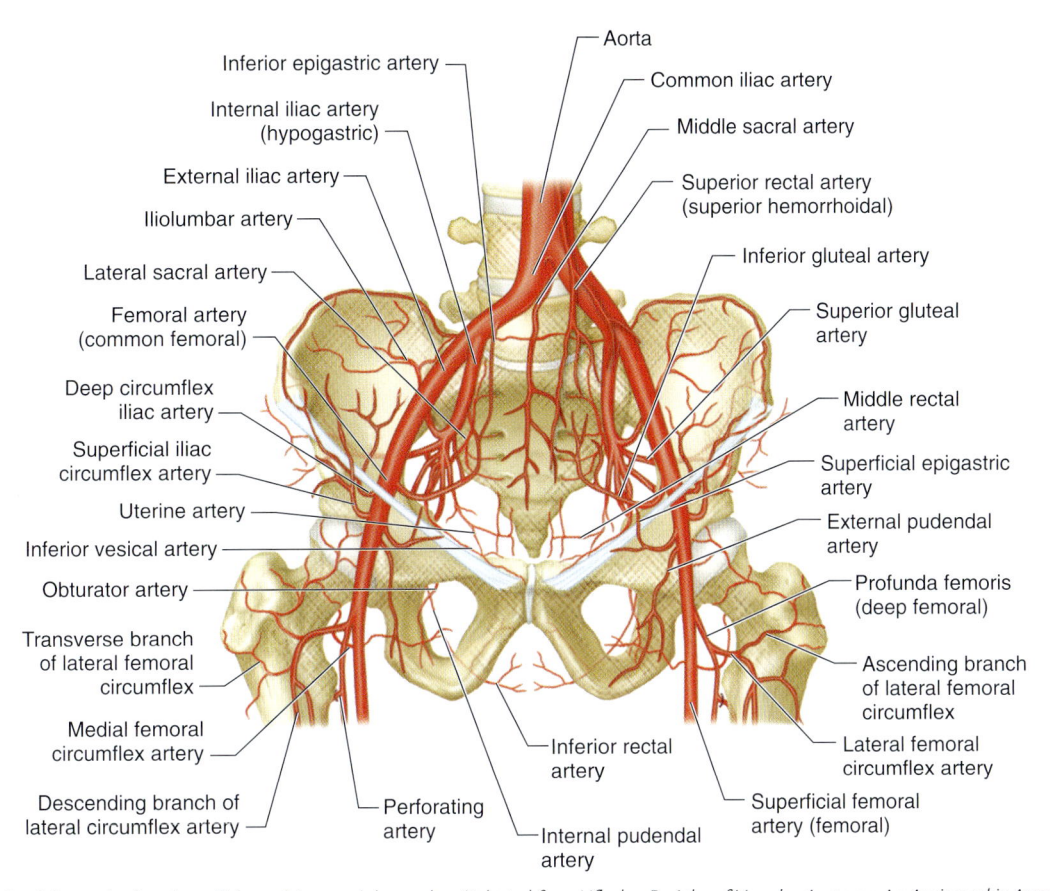

CHAPTER 73 • *Arterial Anatomy of the Pelvis and Lower Extremities* 979

■ **FIGURE 73-1** Schematic drawing of the pelvic arterial vessels. (Adapted from Uflacker R. Atlas of Vascular Anatomy: An Angiographic Approach, 2nd ed. Philadelphia, Lippincott Williams & Wilkins, 2006.)

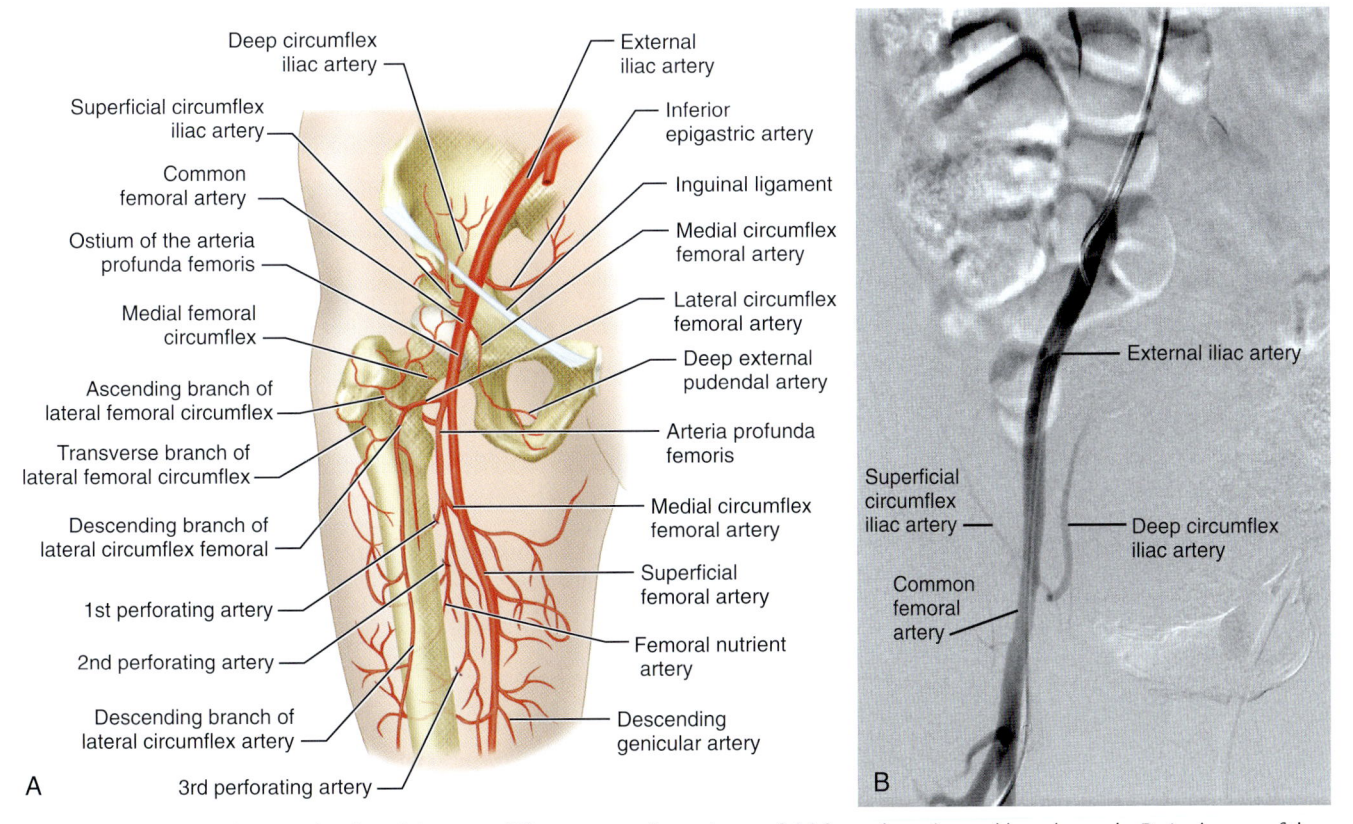

■ **FIGURE 73-2** A, Schematic drawing of the external iliac, common femoral, superficial femoral arteries, and branch vessels. B, Angiogram of the right external and common iliac arteries and branch vessels (contralateral oblique view). (A, adapted from Uflacker R. Anatomy Atlas of Vascular Anatomy: An Angiographic Approach, 2nd ed. Philadelphia, Lippincott Williams & Wilkins, 2006.)

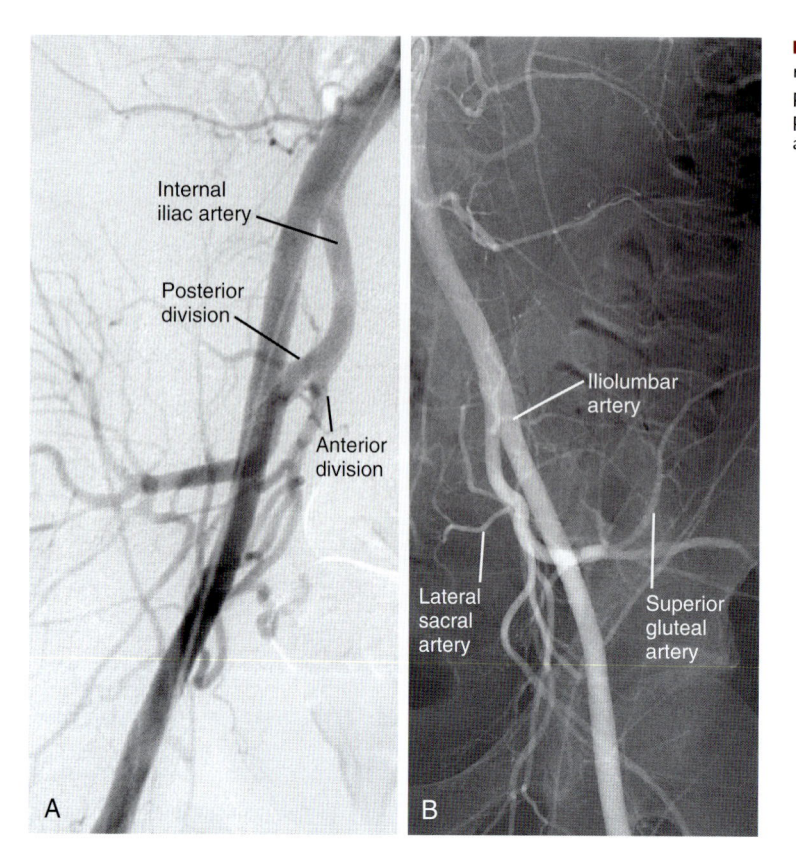

FIGURE 73-3 **A,** Angiogram of the right internal iliac artery, with anterior and posterior divisions. **B,** Angiogram of the posterior division of the left internal iliac artery.

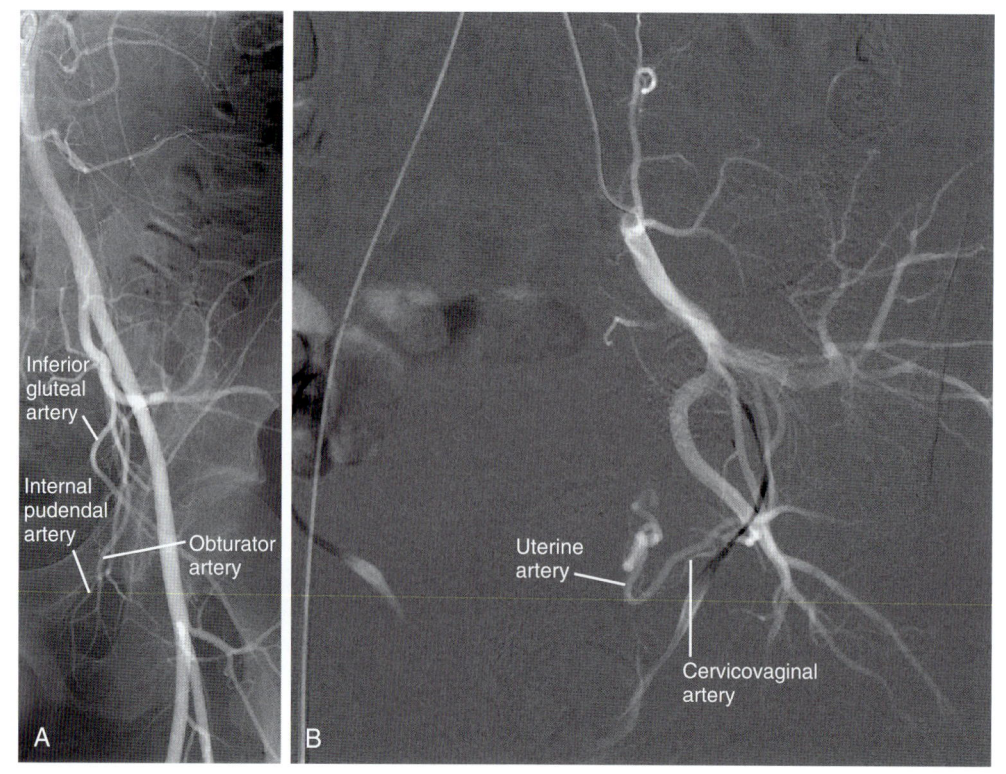

FIGURE 73-4 **A,** Angiogram of the anterior division of the left internal iliac artery. **B,** Angiogram of the left uterine artery, with cervicovaginal branch.

tor notch, and passes laterally through the obturator foramen to supply muscles of the thigh and ligament of the femoral head. It is usually the most lateral of the anterior division branches. A distal branch of the obturator artery anastomoses with the medial circumflex femoral artery, a branch of the profunda femoral artery. The inferior gluteal artery has a variable intrapelvic course, typically concave laterally. It courses inferiorly, anterior to the piriformis muscle and sacral plexus, extends laterally, and exits the bony pelvis via the greater sciatic notch. It supplies the muscles and skin of the buttock and posterior surface of the thigh. In rare cases, it gives rise to a persistent sciatic artery (see later). The internal pudendal artery courses inferiorly along the anterior surface of the piriformis muscle, lateral to the inferior gluteal artery, and enters the ischiorectal fossa through the lesser sciatic foramen. It has numerous small named branches. It supplies the perineum and external genitalia.

The remaining branches of the anterior division are less prominent (see Fig. 73-1). The superior vesical artery has an inferomedial course until it reaches the lateral aspect of the bladder, at which point it courses along the superior surface of the bladder; its position varies depending on the degree of bladder distention. It supplies up to 80% of the bladder, as well as the distal ureters and, in males, the ductus deferens. The inferior vesical artery has an inferomedial course whose position is not dependent on the degree of bladder distention. It is a small vessel, difficult to appreciate angiographically, which supplies the inferolateral surface of the bladder, the trigone and, in males, the seminal vesicles and prostate. In females, the analogous vessel is sometimes termed the *vaginal artery*. It supplies the vagina, posteroinferior portions of the bladder, and pelvic part of the urethra. The vaginal artery may be a single vessel or two or three separate arteries. The inferior vesical artery often forms a common trunk with the middle rectal artery. The middle rectal artery may arise from the anterior division, but is frequently a branch of another artery in the internal iliac artery distribution. This small vessel is the most posterior of the anterior division vessels, and descends inferomedially to the ipsilateral side of the middle portion of the rectum. It anastomoses with the superior and inferior rectal arteries to supply the rectum and sometimes inferior vesical–vaginal artery territory. The uterine artery has a characteristic U-shaped course; it descends, turns medially to course along the broad ligament, and then ascends in the parametrium along the lateral border of the uterus. The cervicovaginal artery, which supplies the cervix and vagina, arises near the junction of the medial and ascending portions. The ascending portion is typically convoluted and gives off numerous convoluted branches that extend medially (see Fig. 73-4B). In postpartum women, the uterine artery may extend superiorly, without demonstrating the U-shaped course typical of the nongravid uterus.

Other arteries arise outside the pelvis but terminate within it. These are the superior rectal artery, which is the continuation of the inferior mesenteric artery in the pelvis, and the gonadal arteries—internal spermatic (testicular) arteries in the male and ovarian arteries in the female. The gonadal arteries arise from the abdominal aorta at the L2 or L3 level and accompany the gonadal veins into the pelvis.

Detailed Description of Specific Areas

Normal Variants

The common iliac arteries are absent in fewer than 1% of individuals. In this case, the aorta divides into four branches, the internal and external iliac arteries bilaterally.

Variations of the internal iliac artery and its branches are common. Typically, the internal iliac artery divides into two branches, as noted earlier. However, this arrangement is seen in approximately 60% of cases, and the remaining 40% demonstrate one (10%), three (20%), or four or more (10%) principal trunks. The sequence of branch origins and trunk formation is extremely variable. The obturator artery may arise from the external iliac artery or the inferior epigastric artery. A persistent sciatic artery, which arises from the inferior gluteal artery, is a rare but clinically important variant (Fig. 73-5). Because it is often symptomatic, it is discussed separately later.

Differential Considerations

Arterial bypass grafts for infrarenal aortic or iliac artery disease originate from the axillary artery or the infrarenal

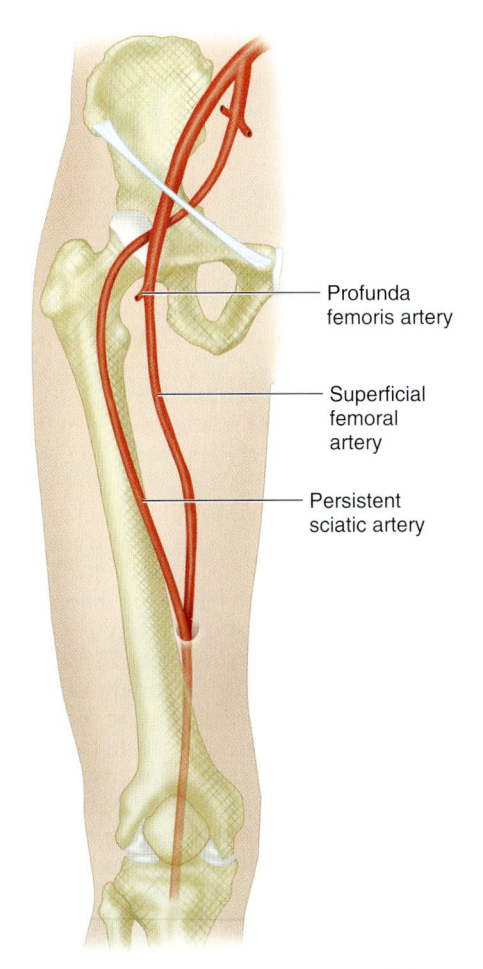

■ **FIGURE 73-5** Schematic drawing of persistent sciatic artery.

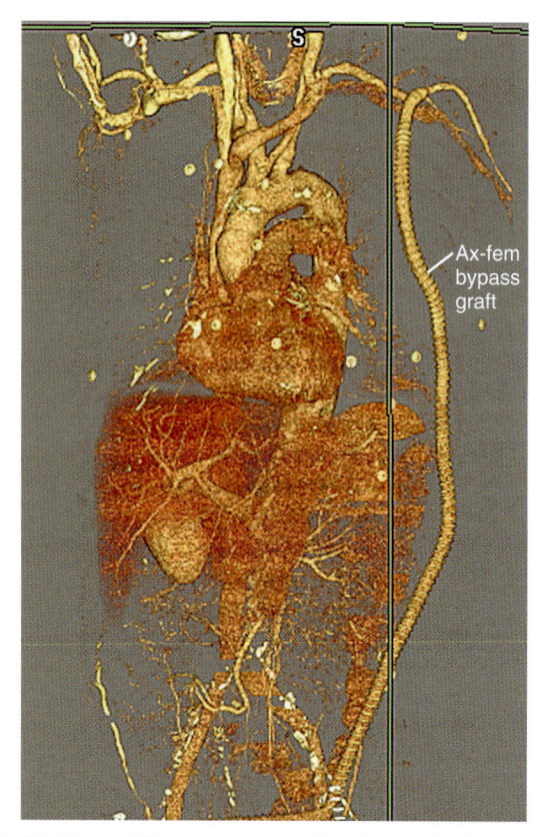

FIGURE 73-6 CTA scan showing axillary-femoral (Ax-fem) bypass graft.

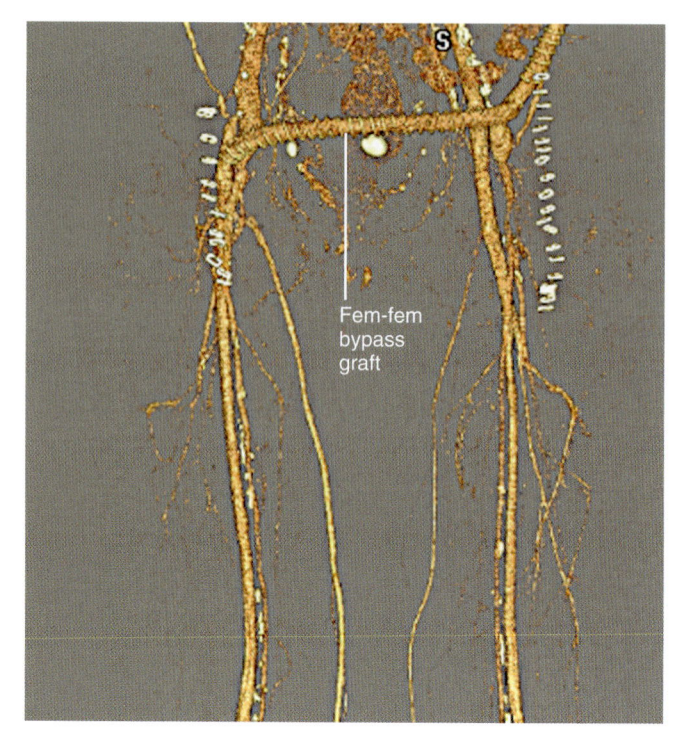

FIGURE 73-7 CTA scan showing femoral-femoral (Fem-fem) bypass graft.

aorta and insert in the external iliac, common femoral, or profunda femoral arteries, depending on the site(s) of disease (Fig. 73-6). Common femoral artery to common femoral artery grafting can be performed for unilateral common iliac or external iliac artery disease (Fig. 73-7). Lower extremity atherosclerosis requiring surgical bypass can be treated with a graft originating at the common femoral artery and terminating at the popliteal artery (ideally, superior to the knee joint), posterior tibial artery, or anterior tibial artery, as required (Fig. 73-8).

In the pelvis, a persistent sciatic artery can be clinically important. The sciatic artery normally involutes by the 22-mm embryo stage, with remnants persisting as the proximal portion of the inferior gluteal artery, popliteal artery, and peroneal artery.[1] Rarely, the sciatic artery persists, either because of failure of development of the superficial femoral artery or failure of regression of the sciatic artery.[2] A persistent sciatic artery is the continuation of the internal iliac artery (see Fig. 73-5), arising from the anterior division distal to the origin of the internal pudendal artery. It follows the course of the inferior gluteal artery through the greater sciatic foramen, where it may accompany the posterior cutaneous nerve or sciatic nerve. It continues inferiorly along the posterior aspect of the adductor magnus and then passes through the popliteal fossa to form the popliteal artery and supply the leg and foot.[1] The reported incidence, based on angiographic series, is 0.01% to 0.05%.[2] Bilateral persistent sciatic arteries are estimated to occur in about 10% of these individuals.[2]

Approximately 60% of individuals with a persistent sciatic artery are symptomatic. The most common symptom is lower extremity ischemia.[3] Approximately 40% of patients with a persistent sciatic artery develop an aneurysm of the vessel at the level of the greater trochanter, believed to be caused by repetitive microtrauma from the sacrospinal ligament and piriformis muscle during hip

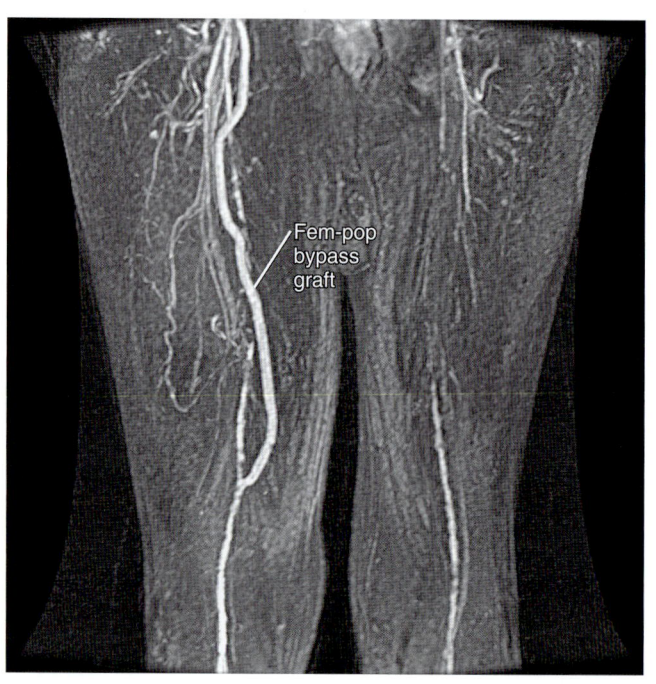

FIGURE 73-8 CTA scan showing femoral-popliteal (Fem-pop) bypass graft.

flexion and extension.⁴ These patients may present with thrombosis, distal embolization, or a buttock mass. Symptomatic patients have a risk of limb loss as high as 25%.

On imaging studies in these individuals, the internal iliac artery is larger than the external iliac artery. The persistent sciatic artery is ectatic and courses laterally at the level of the femoral head before turning inferiorly. On oblique views, it can be appreciated as a posterior structure. The external iliac artery and common femoral artery are in their normal locations, but may be small. The superficial femoral artery tapers in the thigh, may bifurcate on the region of the adductor canal, and then disappears. Persistent sciatic arteries are readily appreciated on CT angiography (CTA), which also permits the determination of aneurysm size, despite the possible presence of luminal thrombus.³

Pertinent Imaging Considerations

Adequate evaluation of the pelvic arteries on CTA or MR angiography (MRA) requires viewing of data in oblique orientations that are easily provided using various postprocessing methods such as maximum intensity projection, multiplanar reformation, and volume-rendered viewing. Conventional angiographic experience has shown that an anterior oblique view usually is best for evaluating the ipsilateral common femoral artery bifurcation and contralateral common iliac artery bifurcation. Evaluation of collateral flow and of specific branches of the internal and external iliac arteries may require individualized views.

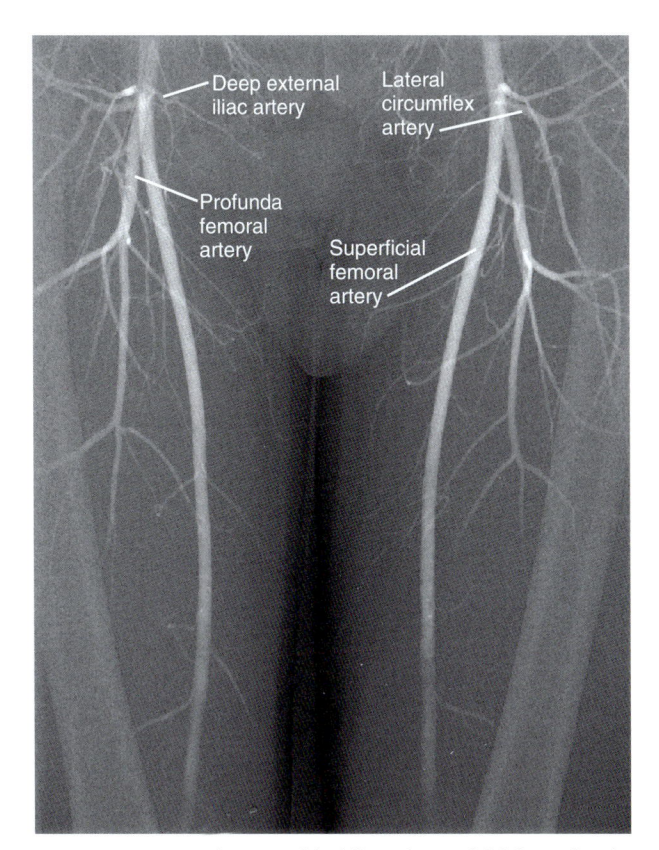

■ **FIGURE 73-9** Angiogram of the bilateral superficial femoral and profunda femoral arteries.

NORMAL ANATOMY OF THE LOWER EXTREMITIES

General Anatomic Descriptions

The femoral artery (usually referred to in clinical practice as the common femoral artery) is the continuation of the external iliac artery distal to the inguinal ligament. It is the usual percutaneous access site for catheter angiography. The femoral artery is variable in length. It divides into the profunda femoral artery posterolaterally and the superficial femoral artery anteromedially (Fig. 73-9) and may also give rise to the superficial circumflex iliac artery, external pudendal arteries, and muscular branches, although this is variable.

The profunda femoral artery (deep femoral artery) is the largest branch of the femoral artery and supplies the thigh muscles anteriorly and posteriorly. It normally gives rise to the medial and lateral circumflex femoral arteries and then continues inferiorly as it gives off several perforating branches (see Fig. 73-9).

The superficial femoral artery extends inferiorly to the inferior end of the adductor canal (Hunter's canal), where it continues as the popliteal artery (Fig. 73-10A). The adductor canal is a fascia-lined compartment bounded by the vastus medialis muscle anteriorly and laterally and the adductor magnus and adductor longus muscles posteriorly, which winds medially and posteriorly around the femur. The junction of the superficial femoral artery and popliteal artery is thus in the distal thigh, and not at the level of the knee joint, as is occasionally—and incorrectly—stated in clinical practice. The superficial femoral artery serves as conduit to the leg and foot. It gives rise to multiple small muscular branches and, just superior to its entrance into the adductor canal, it gives rise to the descending (supreme) genicular artery.

The popliteal artery extends from the inferior aspect of the adductor canal to a point inferior to the knee, where it divides into the tibial and peroneal arteries. Along its course, posterior to the femur and the tibia, it gives off a small medial genicular artery, multiple sural arteries, medial and lateral superior genicular arteries, and medial and lateral inferior genicular arteries (see Fig. 73-10B). The last four genicular arteries wrap around the femur and tibia to form an anastomotic network around the patella. They supply the articular capsule and ligaments of the knee joint. The sural arteries extend inferiorly to supply the calf muscles.

In the leg, the popliteal artery gives off the anterior tibial artery at the level of the inferior edge of the popliteus muscle. The popliteal artery continues as the tibioperoneal trunk, which then divides into the posterior tibial artery and peroneal artery (see Fig. 73-10).

The anterior tibial artery, a major source of supply to the foot, passes anteriorly between the two heads of the tibialis posterior muscle and through the interosseous membrane to the anterior leg. It extends inferiorly, medial to the fibula and continues on to the dorsum of the foot. After it crosses the inferior extensor retinaculum, it becomes the dorsalis pedis artery (Fig. 73-11).

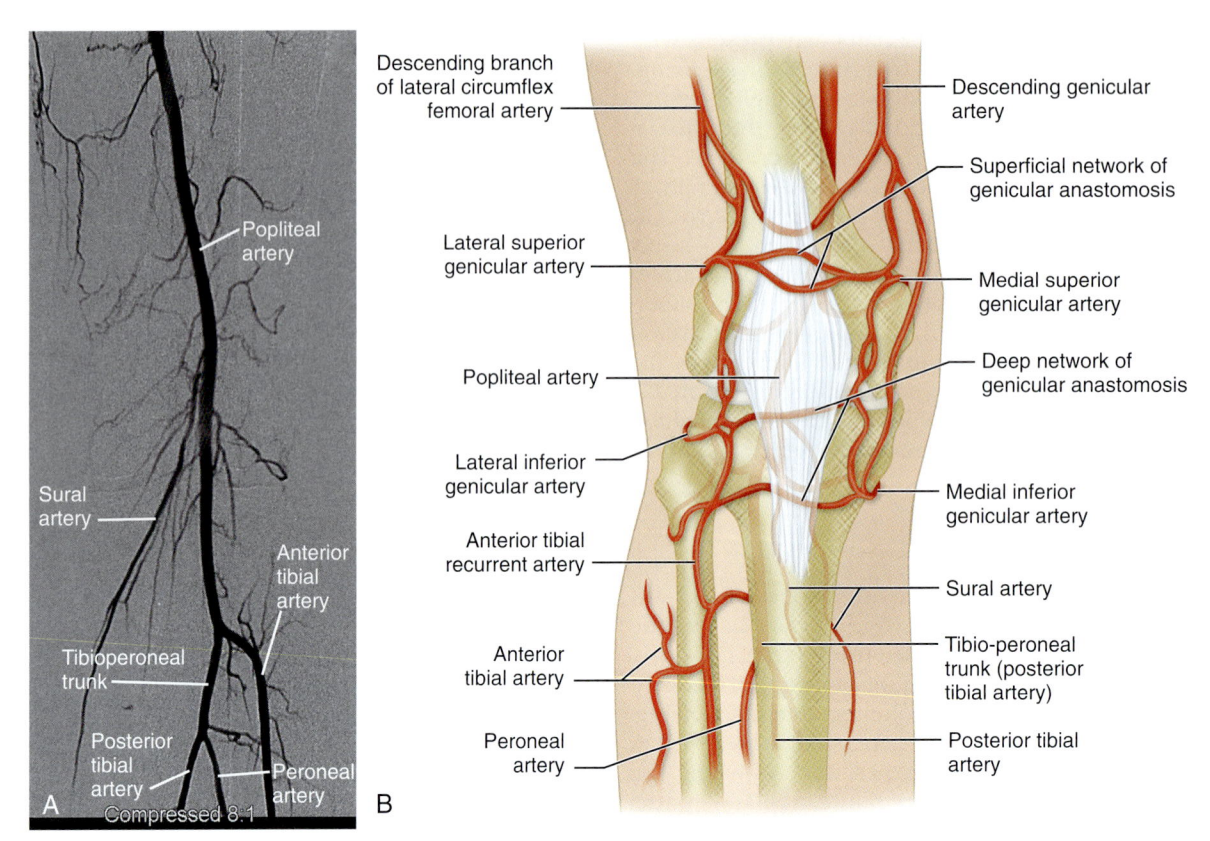

FIGURE 73-10 **A,** Angiogram of the left popliteal artery to trifurcation. **B,** Schematic drawing of the popliteal artery and branch arteries around the knee. (**B,** adapted from Uflacker R. Atlas of Vascular Anatomy: An Angiographic Approach, 2nd ed. Philadelphia, Lippincott Williams & Wilkins, 2006.)

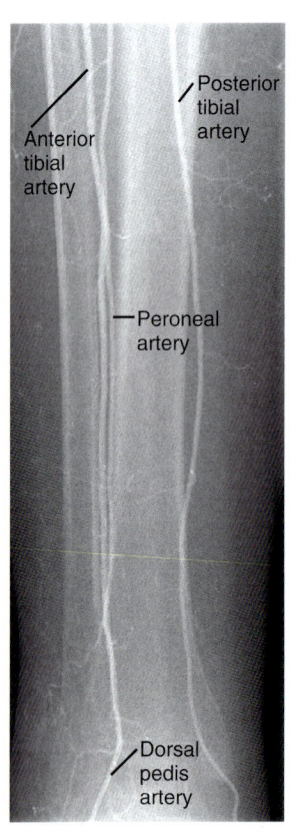

FIGURE 73-11 Angiogram of the right runoff arteries—anterior tibial, peroneal, and posterior tibial arteries.

The posterior tibial artery, also a major source of supply to the foot, extends inferiorly in the posterior leg to reach the ankle behind the medial malleolus and continues on to the foot. In a frontal view, the posterior tibial artery is the most medial of the three major calf vessels (see Fig. 73-11).

The peroneal artery arises from the tibioperoneal trunk and extends inferiorly to a point about 5 cm superior to the lateral malleolus, where it divides into a perforating branch. This anastomoses with a branch of the anterior tibial artery and a communicating branch that anastomoses with a branch of the posterior tibial artery. On both frontal and lateral views, the peroneal artery is projected between the anterior tibial and posterior tibial arteries.

In the foot (Fig. 73-12), the posterior tibial artery divides into a relatively small medial plantar artery, which runs along the first ray, and a larger lateral plantar artery. These vessels run in the plantar aspect of the foot. The lateral plantar artery runs laterally and distally to the base of the fifth metatarsal and then swings medially to form one side of the plantar arch, which supplies plantar metatarsal and common digital arteries to the forefoot.

The dorsalis pedis artery runs in the dorsum of the foot to the level of the metatarsal heads, where it swings laterally as the arcuate artery and gives off a variable number of metatarsal arteries and dorsal digital arteries to supply the forefoot. The arcuate artery anastomoses via a deep plantar branch with the lateral plantar artery to complete the plantar arch. Near its origin, the dorsalis pedis artery

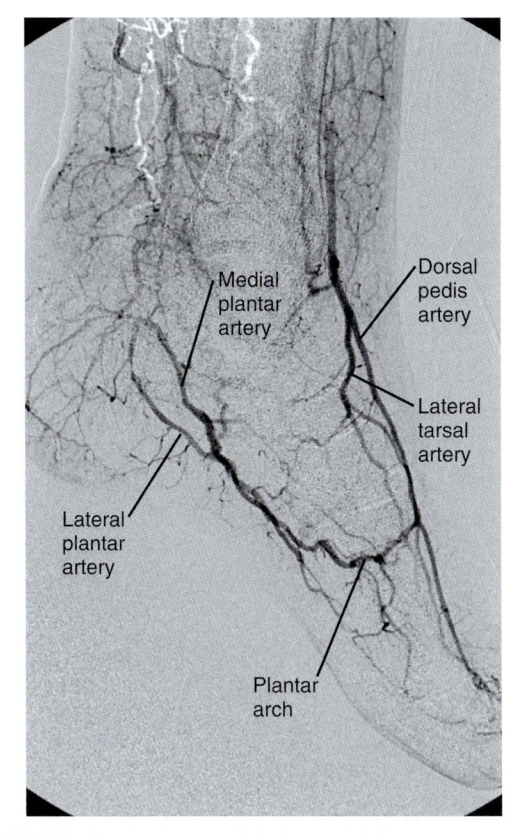

FIGURE 73-12 Angiogram of the lateral left foot.

gives off a lateral tarsal branch, which may anastomose distally with the arcuate artery.

Detailed Description of Specific Areas

Normal Variants

The classic description of profunda femoral artery anatomy is accurate in only about 60% of limbs. In the remainder, one or more of the profunda femoral artery branches arises from the femoral artery. This is important information for the vascular surgeon planning an arterial bypass with an anastomosis to the femoral artery or profunda femoral artery. In fewer than 1% of patients, the origin of the profunda femoral artery is superior to the inguinal ligament. The profunda femoral artery lies lateral or posterolateral to the superficial femoral artery in only 50% of limbs. It is posterior to the superficial femoral artery in 40% of limbs, and medial to the superficial femoral artery in 10% of limbs. This information is valuable to the vascular surgeon and awareness of these variants is essential for the interpreting physician who is performing vascular ultrasound examinations.

The division of the popliteal artery into anterior tibial, posterior tibial, and peroneal arteries (the so-called trifurcation) follows the classic description in approximately 90% of limbs. In approximately 4% of limbs, there is a true trifurcation, with no tibioperoneal trunk. In approximately 1% of limbs, the posterior tibial artery is the continuation of the popliteal artery and the other branch of the popliteal artery is a combined trunk that divides into the anterior tibial and peroneal arteries. In approximately 3% of limbs, the anterior tibial artery arises from the popliteal artery superior to the popliteus muscle (high origin).

In 6% and 5% of limbs, the anterior tibial and posterior tibial arteries, respectively, may be hypoplastic or congenitally absent. In these limbs, the perforating and communicating branch, respectively, of the peroneal artery is enlarged and continues to the foot as the dorsalis pedis or posterior tibial artery. The peroneal artery is congenitally absent in fewer than 0.1% of limbs.

Collateral Pathways

Numerous collateral pathways exist through the pelvic vasculature to mitigate the effects of occlusions or severe stenoses of the infrarenal abdominal aorta, common iliac artery, internal iliac artery, external iliac artery, and common femoral artery. These may be broadly grouped into anterior, central, and posterior pathways.

The anterior pathway extends across the anterior chest wall and anterior abdominal wall via the internal thoracic artery and intercostal arteries, through the superior and inferior epigastric arteries, to the distal external iliac artery (Fig. 73-13). The posterior pathway extends from the posterior chest wall and posterior abdominal wall to the internal iliac artery via intercostal and lumbar arteries, and then through the iliolumbar and superior gluteal arteries. Both anterior and posterior collateral pathways provide alternate routes for ipsilateral arterial flow from the aorta to the pelvis.

There are several central collateral pathways. There is a pathway from the abdominal aorta to the internal iliac artery via the inferior mesenteric artery, through anastomoses between the superior rectal artery and the middle and inferior rectal arteries. There are also multiple ipsilateral-contralateral pathways across the midline in the pelvis via the lateral sacral arteries posteriorly and most of the visceral branches anteriorly.

Finally, there are collateral pathways from the pelvis to the lower extremity—from the internal iliac artery to the ipsilateral femoral artery via the internal pudendal artery through anastomoses with the external pudendal arteries, from the external iliac artery to the ipsilateral profunda femoral artery via the deep circumflex iliac artery through anastomoses with the lateral circumflex femoral artery, and from the internal iliac artery to the ipsilateral profunda femoral artery via the obturator artery and the gluteal arteries through anastomoses with the circumflex femoral arteries and perforating branches.

Collateral formation in the thigh is common in patients with calf claudication, because the superficial femoral artery is a common site of atherosclerosis, especially as it exits the adductor canal. Collateral pathways are from the profunda femoral artery branches to the superficial femoral artery and from the superficial femoral artery proximal to the lesion to the superficial femoral artery distal to the lesion via muscular branches (Fig. 73-14).

There are numerous collateral pathways in the region of the knee. The genicular arteries form a rich anastomotic network, which comes into play when there is stenosis or occlusion of the popliteal artery. Collateral flow via the distal branches of the peroneal artery can supply the foot

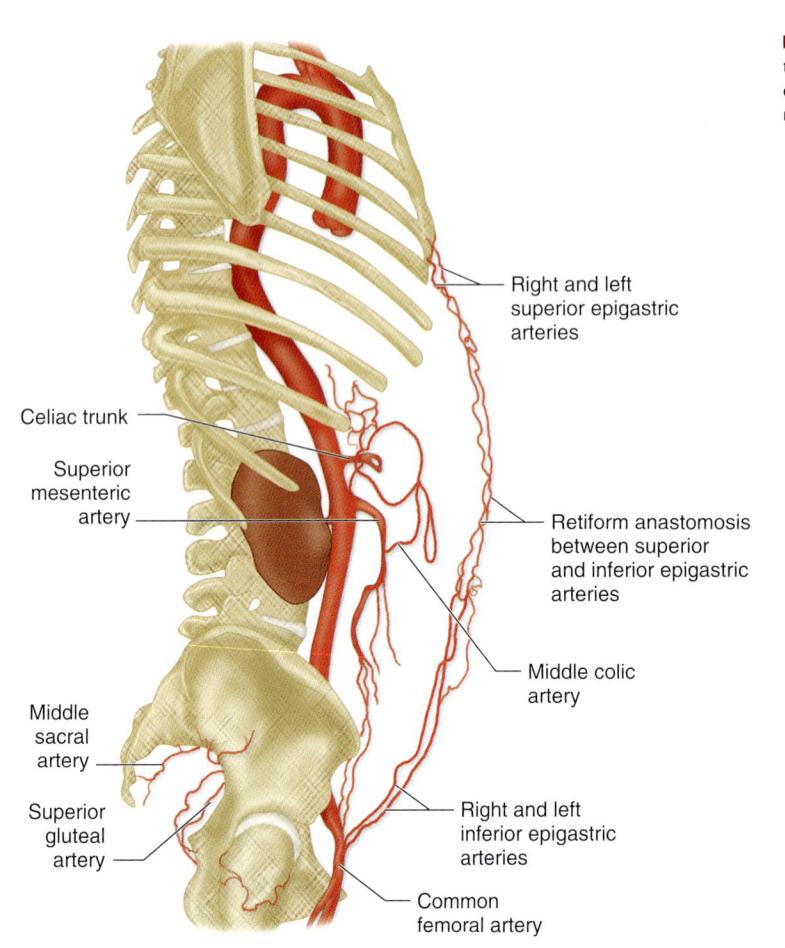

FIGURE 73-13 Schematic drawing of the thoracoabdominal arterial anastomosis through the superior epigastric and inferior epigastric arteries; three-dimensional reconstruction, lateral view.

in patients with occlusion of the anterior tibial or posterior tibial artery (Fig. 73-15).

The plantar arch of the foot is complete in 99% of limbs. The blood supply to each of the metatarsals and toes is extremely variable with respect to the predominant supply from the dorsal or plantar arteries.

Differential Considerations

Pathologies of clinical importance in the knee include popliteal entrapment, adventitial cystic disease, and popliteal artery aneurysms.

Popliteal artery entrapment syndrome (PAES) is caused by a congenital anomaly in the anatomic relationships between the popliteal artery and soft tissue structures of the popliteal fossa, most commonly the medial head of the gastrocnemius. Strenuous athletic activity can cause repetitive compression or microtrauma to the popliteal artery and may result in foot or calf claudication. Symptoms usually develop over time, but acute onset after strenuous exercise has also been described. Ultimately, popliteal artery aneurysm, pseudoaneurysm, atherosclerosis, thrombosis, or thromboembolism may occur. It is a rare disorder, with an estimated prevalence of 0.16%.[5]

Most patients with popliteal artery entrapment syndrome are young men—active individuals, physically fit, and otherwise in good health.[6] Most are athletes or on active military duty. More than 80% are younger than 30 years; fewer than 10% are older than 50 years.[7] One or both lower extremities may be affected.

Numerous classification schemes have been proposed, based on the anatomy of the entrapment. Whelan and colleagues[8] have described four anatomic variations, and Rich and associates[9] added a fifth variant. More recently, the Popliteal Vascular Entrapment Forum has modified the classification to include functional entrapment.[10] In type I anatomy, the popliteal artery passes medially to the normally inserted medial head of the gastrocnemius muscle. In type II anatomy, the popliteal artery is in its normal position but passes medial to an abnormal medial head of the gastrocnemius muscle, which inserts too far laterally on the distal femur. In type III anatomy, a normally positioned popliteal artery is either compressed by an aberrant muscle slip of the medial head of the gastrocnemius muscle or passes through the medial head of the gastrocnemius. In type IV anatomy, the posterior aspect of the popliteal artery is compressed by an anomalous fibrous band or by the popliteus muscle. The artery may or may not pass medially to the medial head of the gastrocnemius.

In the study by Rich and coworkers,[9] patients who had entrapment by branches of the tibial nerve were included in this group. In type V, the popliteal vein is involved, as well as the popliteal artery. Imaging studies typically demonstrate the artery deviated medially at the level of the knee. Type VI is functional entrapment, with normal

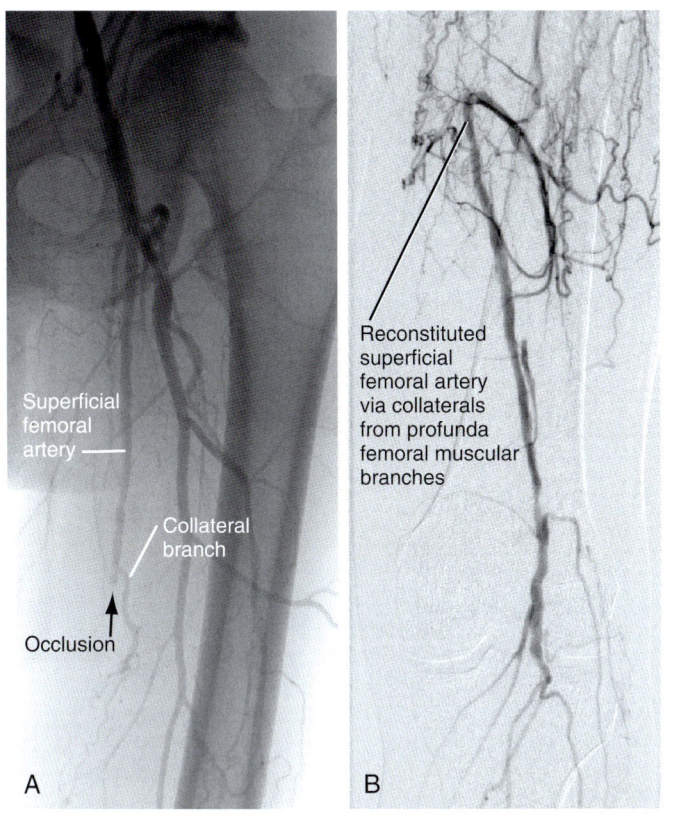

■ **FIGURE 73-14** **A,** Angiogram of the proximal left superficial femoral artery, with a distal occluded segment and reconstitution downstream via collaterals. **B,** Angiogram of the distal left superficial femoral artery via muscular collaterals from the profunda femoral artery.

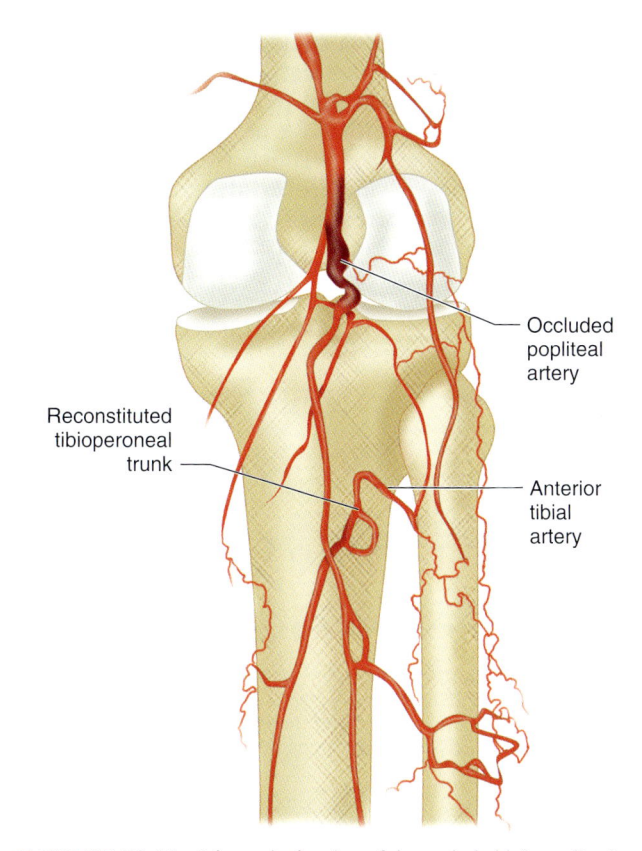

■ **FIGURE 73-15** Schematic drawing of the occluded left popliteal artery, with reconstitution of the anterior tibial artery and tibioperoneal trunk via collaterals.

anatomy and compression caused by hypertrophied muscles. Other unusual anatomic variants also exist.

Adventitial cystic disease (ACD) is a rare disorder of uncertain cause characterized by mucoid cysts in the adventitia of the arterial wall. The incidence has been estimated as 1 in 1200 cases of claudication.[11] The mass effect of the cysts compresses the arterial lumen and compromises flow. ACD has been reported in the popliteal artery in the popliteal fossa, the external iliac artery, and less commonly in the distal brachial, radial and ulnar arteries. It is most commonly seen in men ages 20 to 50 years.[10]

Popliteal artery ACD is a classic although rare cause of lower extremity claudication. Arterial imaging often demonstrates a smooth tapering stenosis (scimitar sign) or smooth concentric or eccentric stenoses.[12] MRI and ultrasound demonstrate mucoid cysts, which are hyperintense on T2-weighted images and of variable intensity on T1-weighted images.[10] Treatment with cyst aspiration under ultrasound guidance has been suggested but is not always successful.[12,13] Surgical unroofing of the cysts and bypass grafting are more commonly performed.

The popliteal artery is considered aneurysmal when its diameter exceeds 7 mm.[14] This vessel is the most common site of aneurysm formation in the peripheral vasculature, accounting for approximately 80% of peripheral arterial aneurysms.[15] Popliteal artery aneurysms are usually at least 20 mm in diameter at diagnosis, are bilateral in 50% of cases, and are associated with an aortic aneurysm in 40% of cases.[15] They are secondary to atherosclerosis in nearly 90% of patients.[16] Other uncommon causes include trauma, infection (mycotic aneurysm), connective tissue disorders (e.g., Marfan syndrome, Ehlers-Danlos syndrome), vasculitis and, rarely, pregnancy.[14] Because most cases are caused by atherosclerosis, the patient population is typically older and predominantly male.

Approximately 25% to 45% of popliteal artery aneurysms are asymptomatic at the time of diagnosis.[14,16] Patients with symptomatic popliteal artery aneurysms typically present with acute or chronic limb ischemia caused by thrombosis of the aneurysm or distal embolization of thrombotic material.[10] These complications will eventually occur in 18% to 75% of patients. Acute limb ischemia has a relatively poor prognosis, with a 15% amputation rate because of occlusion of runoff vessels.[15] By contrast, treatment of asymptomatic popliteal aneurysms yields a 5-year graft patency of 80% and 98% limb salvage. Popliteal artery aneurysm rupture is uncommon. Symptomatic patients are treated surgically with exclusion of the aneurysm, thrombectomy, and bypass grafting. If the patient can tolerate an additional period of ischemia during therapy, thrombolysis is highly successful for recanalizing the distal vessels to provide targets for bypass grafting.

Pertinent Imaging Considerations

The arteries of the thigh and knee usually can be evaluated adequately in a frontal view. Imaging of the popliteal artery in the popliteal fossa sometimes requires a lateral view. A frontal view of the leg often demonstrates the distal anterior tibial artery and peroneal artery superimposed. When imaged with CTA or MRA, these vessels should also be evaluated in a lateral view, as should the vessels of the foot. Specific provocative maneuvers have been described to elicit vascular compression in patients with popliteal entrapment.[10]

> **KEY POINTS**
>
> - Knowledge of the expected and possible variant arterial anatomy of the pelvis and lower extremities is essential for successful CTA and MRA scan prescription and interpretation.
> - Consideration of the clinical indication for a pelvic and/or lower extremity CTA and MRA will assist in the proper selection of imaging parameters (e.g., anatomic coverage, spatial resolution).
> - Evaluation of pelvic and lower extremity by CTA and MRA is optimized by oblique viewing of data using image postprocessing (e.g., maximum intensity projection, multiplanar reconstruction, and volume rendering).

SUGGESTED READINGS

Kadir S. Atlas of Normal and Variant Angiographic Anatomy. Philadelphia, WB Saunders, 1991.

Lippert H, Pabst R. Arterial Variations in Man. Classification and Frequency. Munich, JF Bergmann Verlag, 1985.

Merland J-J, Chiras J. Arteriography of the Pelvis. Diagnostic and Therapeutic Procedures. New York, Springer-Verlag, 1981.

Uflacker R. Atlas of Vascular Anatomy. An Angiographic Approach, 2nd ed. Philadelphia, Lippincott Williams & Wilkins, 2007.

Valentine RJ, Wind GG. Anatomic Exposures in Vascular Surgery. Philadelphia, Lippincott Williams & Wilkins, 2003.

REFERENCES

1. Mandell VS, Jaques PF, Delany DJ, Oberheu V. Persistent sciatic artery: clinical, embryologic, and angiographic features. AJR Am J Roentgenol 1985; 144:245-249.
2. Kurtoglu Z, Uluutku H. Persistent sciatic vessels associated with an arteriovenous malformation. J Anat 2001; 199(Pt 3):349-351.
3. Jung AY, Lee W, Chung JW, et al. Role of computed tomographic angiography in the detection and comprehensive evaluation of persistent sciatic artery. J Vasc Surg 2005; 42:678-683.
4. Kritsch D, Hutter HP, Hirschl M, Katzenschlager R. Persistent sciatic artery: an uncommon cause of intermittent claudication. Int Angiol 2006; 25:327-329.
5. Bouhoutsos J, Daskalakis E. Muscular abnormalities affecting the popliteal vessels. Br J Surg 1981; 68:501-506.
6. Collins PS, McDonald PT, Lim RC. Popliteal artery entrapment: an evolving syndrome. J Vasc Surg 1989; 10:484-489.
7. Rosset E, Hartung O, Brunet C, et al. Popliteal artery entrapment syndrome: anatomic and embryologic bases, diagnostic and therapeutic considerations following a series of 15 cases with a review of the literature. Surg Radiol Anat 1995; 17:161-169.
8. Whelan TJ, Haimovici H. Popliteal artery entrapment syndrome. In Haimovici H (ed). Vascular Surgery: Principles and Techniques, 2nd ed, vol 2. New York, McGraw-Hill, 1984, pp 557-567.
9. Rich NM, Collins GJ Jr, McDonald PT, et al. Popliteal vascular entrapment. Its increasing interest. Arch Surg 1979; 114:1377-1384.
10. Holden A, Merrilees S, Mitchell N, Hill A. Magnetic resonance imaging of popliteal artery pathologies. Eur J Radiol 2008; 67:159-168.
11. Flanigan DP, Burnham SJ, Goodreau JJ, Bergan J. Summary of cases of adventitial cystic disease of the popliteal artery. Ann Surg 1979; 189:165-175.
12. Cassar K, Engeset J. Cystic adventitial disease: a trap for the unwary. Eur J Vasc Endovasc Surg 2005; 29:93-96.
13. Do DD, Braunschweig M, Baumgartner I, et al. Adventitial cystic disease of the popliteal artery: percutaneous US-guided aspiration. Radiology 1997; 203:743-746.
14. Wright LB, Matchett WJ, Cruz CP, et al. Popliteal artery disease: diagnosis and treatment. Radiographics 2004; 24:467-479.
15. Thompson MM, Bell PR. ABC of arterial and venous disease. Arterial aneurysms. BMJ 2000; 320:1193-1196.
16. Davidovic LB, Lotina SI, Kostic DM, et al. Popliteal artery aneurysms. World J Surg 1998; 22:812-817.

CHAPTER 74

Arterial Anatomy of the Upper Extremities

Douglas Yim and Donald L. Miller

The major arteries of the upper extremities are less frequently involved by systemic diseases such as atherosclerosis and diabetes than the vessels of the lower extremity. However, the unique combination of the glenohumeral joint, scapula, and thorax, along with their surrounding muscles and ligaments, form potential spaces for vessel constriction, which may lead to significant obstructive symptoms.

NORMAL ANATOMY OF THE SUBCLAVIAN ARTERY

General Anatomic Descriptions

The subclavian artery arises from the brachiocephalic trunk (innominate artery) on the right and from the aorta on the left. It runs within the thoracic cage to the first rib, where it becomes superficial to the bony thorax and becomes the axillary artery. It gives rise to the vertebral artery, the internal thoracic artery (internal mammary artery), and the thyrocervical and costocervical trunks. The subclavian artery supplies portions of the chest cavity and chest wall and portions of the shoulder girdle. Ascending branches off the subclavian artery supply portions of the anterior neck, spinal cord, and brain (Fig. 74-1).

The vertebral artery is the first branch of the subclavian artery. The thyrocervical trunk and internal thoracic artery arise opposite each other from the anterosuperior and anteroinferior aspect of the subclavian artery. The thyrocervical trunk divides into the inferior thyroid artery with its characteristic looping course, the transverse cervical artery and the suprascapular artery (Fig. 74-2). It supplies the anterior neck, including the thyroid gland and the superior portion of the esophagus, as well as portions of the shoulder. The internal thoracic artery travels slightly anterior and inferiorly, deep to the thorax, to supply the rib cage and portions of the mediastinum. Inferiorly, it continues as the superior epigastric artery and anastomoses with the inferior epigastric artery in the anterior abdominal wall. The costocervical trunk arises distal to the thyrocervical trunk from the posterosuperior aspect of the subclavian artery. It divides into the deep cervical artery and supreme intercostal artery (highest intercostal artery) to supply the first two or three intercostal spaces and the deep structures of the neck (Fig. 74-3).

The axillary artery runs between the thorax and the arm, from the lateral edge of the first rib to the lower border of the tendinous attachment of the teres major muscle. It gives rise to a number of branches that supply the shoulder region and chest wall. The axillary artery is divided into three parts, from medial to lateral.

The first part of the axillary artery, from the first rib to the medial border of the pectoralis minor muscle, gives rise to the superior thoracic artery, also called the highest thoracic artery. It supplies the chest wall (Fig. 74-4).

The second part of the axillary artery, posterior to the pectoralis minor muscle, gives rise to the thoracoacromial artery and lateral thoracic artery, which supply the shoulder, anterior axilla, and chest wall (see Fig. 74-4). The thoracoacromial artery pierces the overlying costocoracoid membrane anteriorly, dividing into pectoral, acromial, clavicular and deltoid branches. The lateral thoracic artery courses inferiorly to anastomose with the internal thoracic, subscapular, and intercostal arteries, along with pectoral branches of the thoracoacromial artery. It supplies lateral mammary branches in women and is also called the external mammary artery.

The third part of the axillary artery extends laterally from the outer border of the pectoralis minor muscle to the lower border of the teres major muscle and gives rise to three branches, the subscapular artery and the anterior and posterior circumflex humeral arteries, which supply the posterior and lateral axilla (see Fig. 74-4). The subscapular artery divides into the circumflex scapular artery, the infrascapular artery (largest branch), and the dorsal thoracic artery. These branches anastomose with the

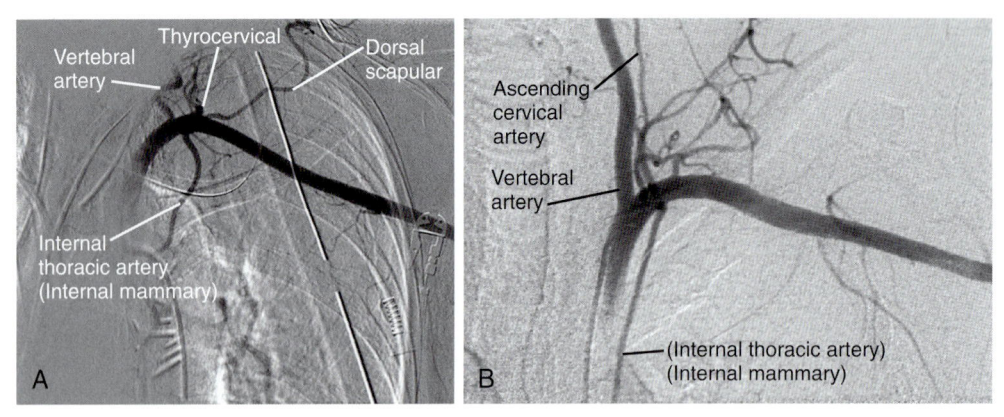

FIGURE 74-1 A, B, Angiogram of the left subclavian artery and branches.

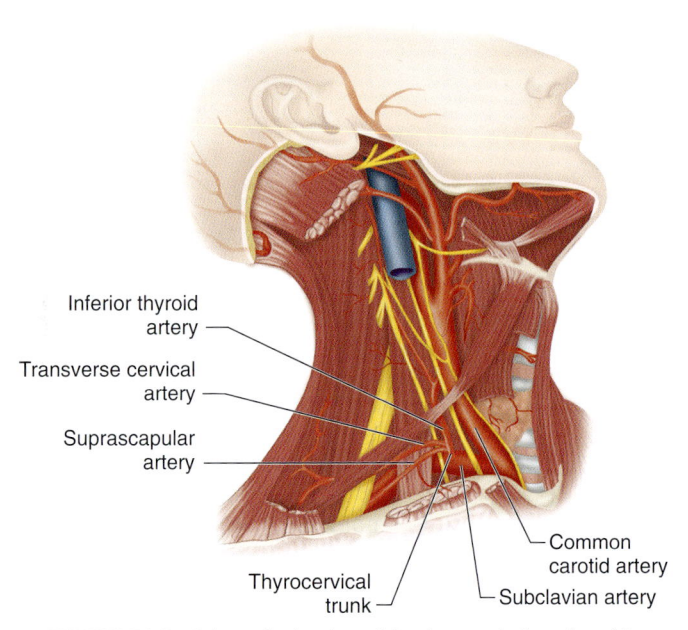

FIGURE 74-2 Schematic drawing of the thyrocervical trunk and its branches.

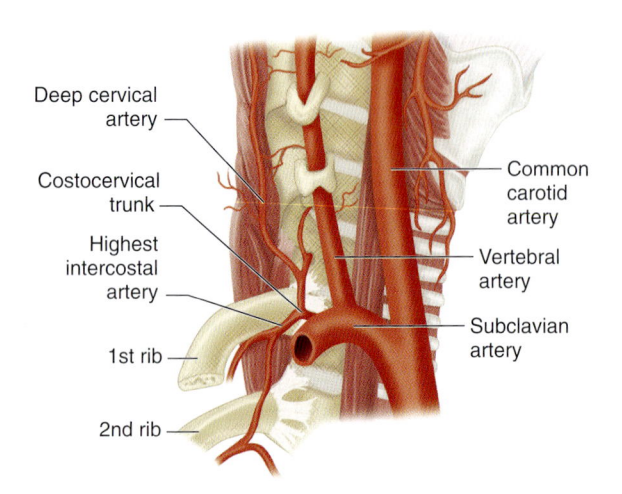

FIGURE 74-3 Schematic drawing of the costocervical trunk and its branches.

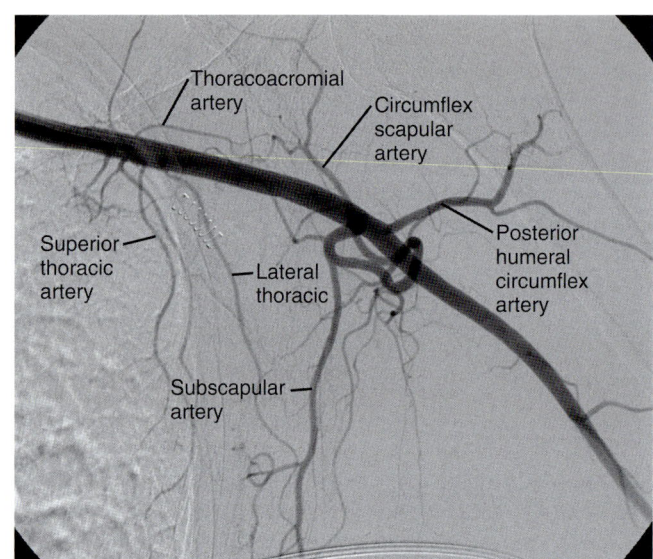

FIGURE 74-4 Angiogram of the left axillary artery and its branches.

lateral thoracic artery, intercostal arteries, and the deep branch of the transverse cervical artery. The anterior and posterior circumflex humeral arteries pass around the surgical neck of the humerus. The posterior circumflex humeral artery is the larger of the two.

Detailed Description of Specific Areas

Normal Variants

Most variations of the subclavian artery are related to the origins of the branches of the thyrocervical trunk and internal thoracic artery. Any or all of these arteries may arise separately from the subclavian artery or may be combined as a common trunk. Less commonly, branches of the costocervical trunk may arise from the thyrocervical trunk, or vice versa. These variations are generally important only to interventionalists who do parathyroid arteriography or who need to treat hemoptysis by embolizing the supreme intercostal artery, superior thoracic artery, or lateral thoracic artery.

Variations in the origins of the axillary artery branches are very common; the "normal" situation as seen in

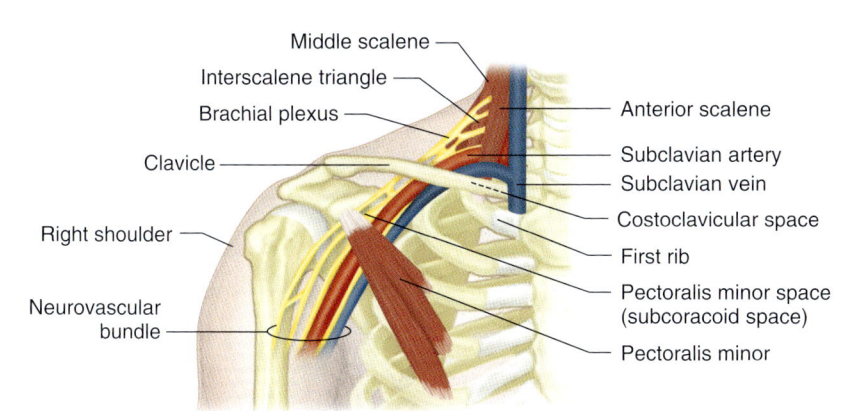

FIGURE 74-5 Schematic drawing of the spaces forming the thoracic outlet.

textbooks occurs in probably fewer than 10% of limbs. Trunk formation of some of the branches of the axillary artery is seen in approximately 50% of all upper extremities. The most common trunk formations are the subscapular artery–posterior circumflex humeral artery and a common origin of both circumflex humeral arteries.

Differential Considerations

Thoracic Outlet Syndrome

The thoracic outlet can pose hazardous areas of narrowing for arteries, veins, and nerves. The subclavian and axillary arteries are subject to compression at several narrow spaces along their course out of the thorax. The most common sites are the interscalene triangle, costoclavicular space, and subcoracoid space (Fig. 74-5). Compression of the neurovascular bundle is the most common form of thoracic outlet syndrome (TOS) causing neurologic symptoms. However, the arterial type, seen in 1% to 2% of cases, is associated with the most serious complication of limb ischemia, which can result in limb loss. This chronic arterial compression is generally made worse with certain arm positions leading to intimal and medial wall injury. Over time, repetitive vessel trauma and flow disturbances promote poststenotic dilation, aneurysm formation, premature atherosclerosis, and/or embolization of platelet-fibrin deposits or thrombus from the diseased wall, leading to complete vessel occlusion. Both duplex ultrasound and CT angiography are used to detect vessel abnormalities in patients with suspected TOS. However, Longley and colleagues[1] have observed an incidence of asymptomatic compression of the subclavian artery on Doppler ultrasound as high as 20% in normal volunteers.

Quadrilateral Space Syndrome

The quadrilateral space is bounded by the humerus, teres major and teres minor muscles, and long head of the triceps muscle (Fig. 74-6). Because the posterior circumflex humeral artery and axillary nerve run through the quadrilateral space, compression of these structures by surrounding fibrous bands can lead to this syndrome. It is most evident in the abducted and externally rotated position. The phenomenon appears to be caused by compression of the axillary nerve rather than arterial compression. Mochizuki and associates[2] have observed occlusion of the posterior circumflex humeral artery in 5 of 6 (80%) of asymptomatic volunteers, suggesting that demonstration of arterial compression is not helpful in establishing the diagnosis.

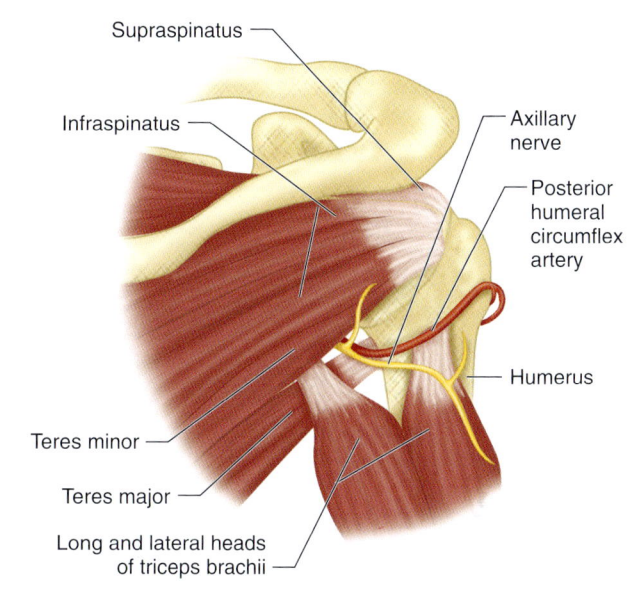

FIGURE 74-6 Schematic drawing of the quadrilateral space.

NORMAL ANATOMY OF THE BRACHIAL ARTERY

General Anatomic Descriptions

The brachial artery is the continuation of the axillary artery from the lower border of the teres major muscle to the level of the radial neck. The artery takes a medial course along the humerus, partially overlapped by the biceps and coracobrachialis muscles. It then takes a gradual turn anteriorly to the antecubital fossa, where it lies between the biceps tendon laterally and the median nerve medially. Here the vessel divides into the radial and ulnar arteries (Fig. 74-7). The brachial artery serves as a potential arterial access site because of its course along

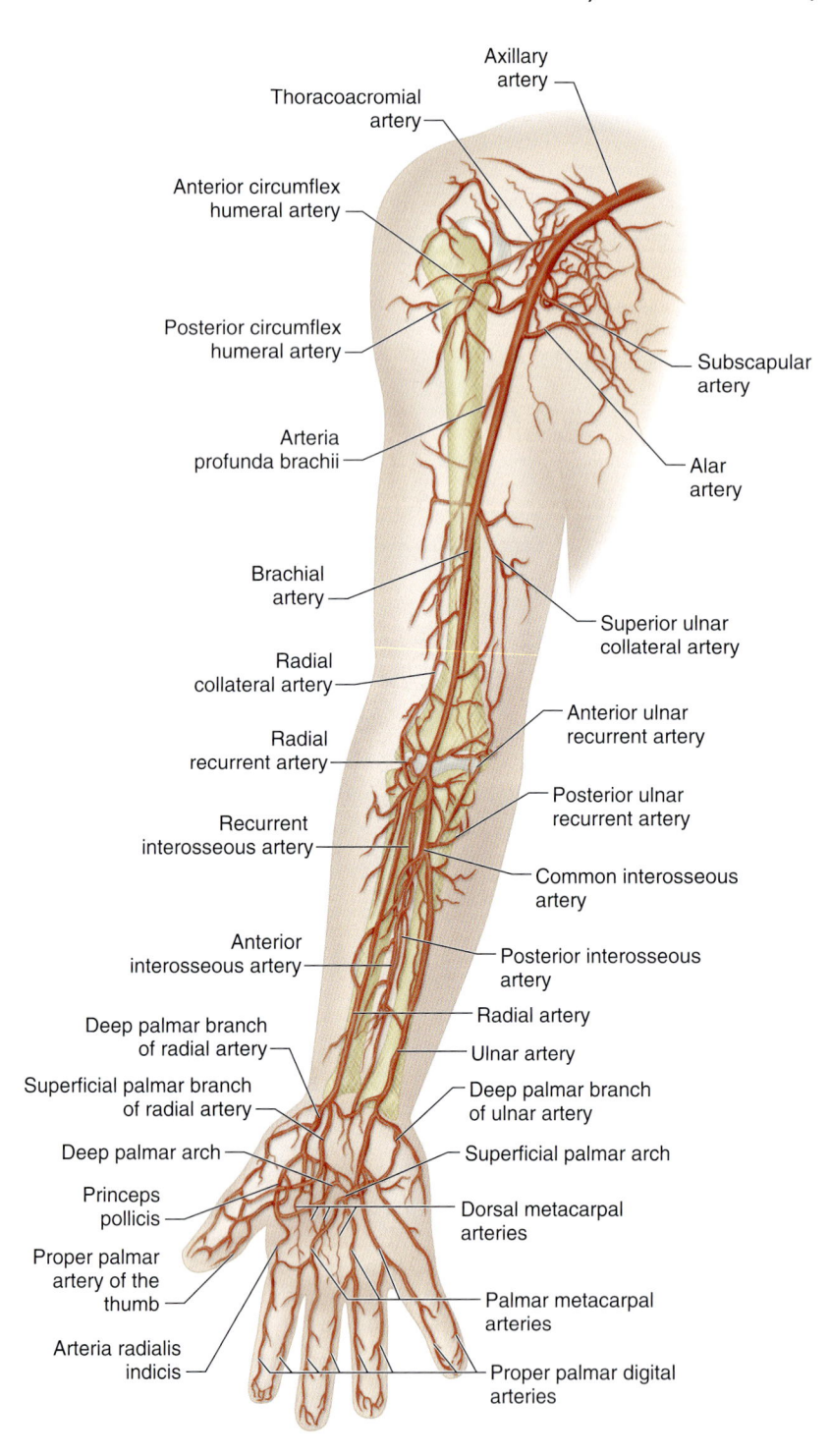

FIGURE 74-7 Schematic drawing of the brachial artery and branches. *(Adapted from Uflacker R. Atlas of Vascular Anatomy: An Angiographic Approach, 2nd ed. Philadelphia, Lippincott, Williams & Wilkins, 2006.)*

the humerus, which allows compressive hemostasis against the underlying bone.

The brachial artery has multiple branches to include smaller muscular and nutrient vessels. However, the main branch arteries are the deep brachial and superior ulnar collateral arteries (Fig. 74-8). The deep brachial artery arises proximally and crosses posterior to the humerus, along with the radial nerve. It then divides into smaller collateral branches along the radial border of the humerus. The deep brachial artery first gives off the deltoid artery, which courses superiorly to collateralize with branches of the posterior humeral circumflex artery. The next branch is the middle collateral artery, which courses distally to anastomose with the interosseous recurrent artery and the rich collaterals about the elbow (see Fig. 74-7). The deep brachial artery then continues as the radial collateral artery to anastomose with the radial recurrent artery and the rich collaterals about the elbow, acting as an important alternative pathway when the brachial artery is occluded at the elbow.

CHAPTER 74 • *Arterial Anatomy of the Upper Extremities*

At the elbow, the brachial artery divides into the radial and ulnar arteries (Fig. 74-9). The radial artery begins in the antecubital fossa about 1 cm below the elbow joint. Although it is smaller than the ulnar artery, it is a more direct continuation of the brachial artery. The radial artery follows the course of the radius toward the lateral wrist, crosses the floor of the anatomic snuffbox formed by the scaphoid and trapezium, and ends by completing the deep palmar arch as it anastomoses with the deep palmar branch of the ulnar artery (Fig. 74-10).

The branches of the radial artery include the radial recurrent artery, muscular perforators, the deep palmar branch of the radial artery, and the superficial palmar branch of the radial artery. In the proximal forearm, the radial recurrent artery (see Fig. 74-9) ascends to anastomose eventually with the terminal portion of the deep brachial artery (radial collateral artery), thus serving as an important collateral in the elbow region. In the distal forearm and wrist, the deep palmar branch of the radial artery arises near the lower border of the pronator quadratus muscle and runs across the palmar aspect of the carpal bones. It anastomoses with the deep branch of the ulnar artery. The superficial palmar branch artery arises

■ **FIGURE 74-8** Angiogram of the left brachial artery and branches.

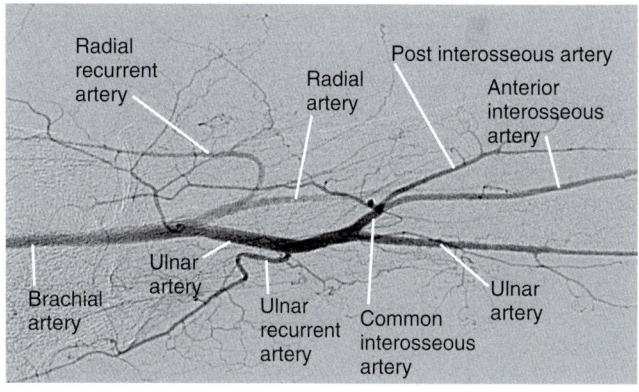

■ **FIGURE 74-9** Angiogram of the brachial artery bifurcation at the antecubital fossa.

■ **FIGURE 74-10** Schematic drawing of the hand. *(Adapted from Uflacker R. Atlas of Vascular Anatomy: An Angiographic Approach, 2nd ed. Philadelphia, Lippincott, Williams & Wilkins, 2006.)*

from the radial artery just proximal to the wrist, coursing forward through the thenar eminence. It normally anastomoses with the terminal portion of the ulnar artery to form the superficial palmar arterial arch (see Fig. 74-10).

The ulnar artery also begins in the antecubital fossa. It is larger than the radial artery and follows the general course of the median nerve. Distally, the continuation of the ulnar artery is the superficial palmar arterial arch, which anastomoses with the superficial palmar branch of the radial artery.

The branches of the ulnar artery include the ulnar recurrent artery, posterior ulnar recurrent artery and common interosseous artery (see Fig. 74-9). The anterior ulnar recurrent artery is an important collateral around the medial aspect of the elbow. This vessel arises immediately inferior to the elbow and ascends to anastomose with the superior and inferior ulnar collateral arteries. The posterior ulnar recurrent artery is also an important collateral around the medial aspect of the elbow. This vessel arises somewhat more distally than the anterior ulnar recurrent artery, ascending posterior to the medial epicondyle of the humerus to anastomose with the superior and inferior ulnar collateral and interosseous recurrent arteries. The common interosseous artery arises immediately inferior to the radial tuberosity and quickly divides into the anterior and posterior interosseous arteries (see Fig. 74-9). The anterior interosseous artery descends along the volar surface of the interosseous membrane in the forearm, giving off muscular branches and the nutrient arteries of the radius and ulna. At the superior border of the pronator quadratus muscle, the anterior interosseous artery pierces the interosseous membrane to reach the dorsum of the forearm and anastomose with the posterior interosseous artery. The posterior interosseous artery descends along the dorsal surface of the interosseous membrane where, at the distal part of the forearm, it anastomoses with the termination of the anterior interosseous artery and with the dorsal carpal network. From the proximal aspect of the posterior interosseous artery, there is a branch (the posterior interosseous recurrent collateral) that ascends to the interval between the lateral epicondyle and olecranon to anastomose with the radial collateral branch of the deep brachial artery, posterior ulnar recurrent artery and inferior ulnar collateral artery.

Detailed Description of Specific Areas

Normal Variants

Approximately 20% of limbs have a high origin of one or more of the arteries to the arm or some other variant of the arteries in the arm. Approximately 4% have a high origin of the superficial brachial artery, 13% have a high origin of the deep brachial artery, and 5% have a deep brachial artery arising from the posterior circumflex humeral artery. An additional 20% of individuals have other, relatively unimportant variants.

With regard to arterial variations in the arm and forearm, the superficial brachial artery can replace the brachial artery (9%) or occur in addition to it (13%). Additionally, the superficial brachial artery can continue as the sole supply to the radial artery (5%) or the sole supply to all

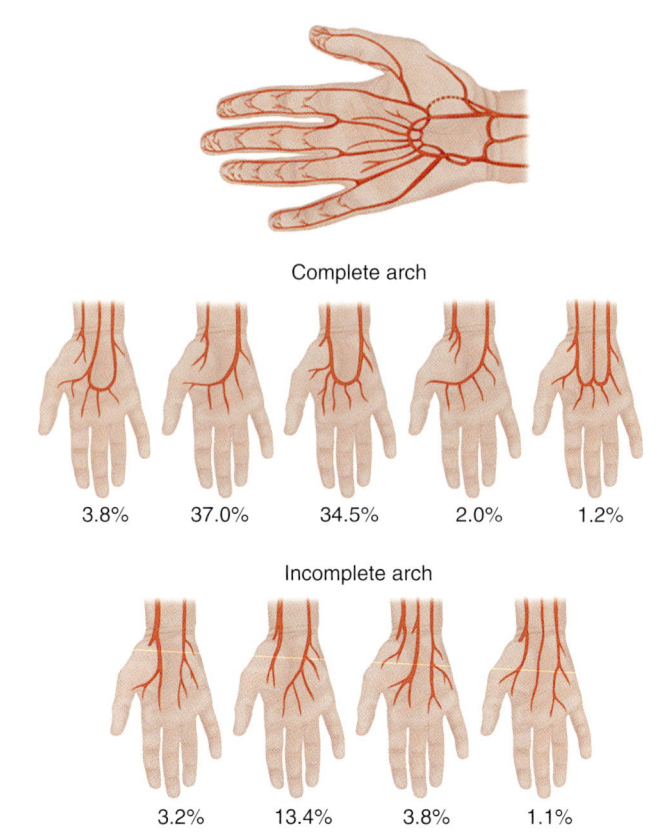

FIGURE 74-11 Schematic drawing of the hand, with arch variations. *(Adapted from Uflacker R. Atlas of Vascular Anatomy: An Angiographic Approach, 2nd ed. Philadelphia, Lippincott, Williams & Wilkins, 2006.)*

forearm arteries (6%). A persistent median artery (8%) arises from the common, anterior, or posterior interosseous artery and runs parallel to the median nerve.

NORMAL ANATOMY OF THE RADIAL AND ULNAR ARTERIES

General Anatomic Descriptions

Both the radial and ulnar arteries supply blood to the hand. The radial artery leaves the forearm by coursing dorsally to enter the anatomic snuffbox, deep to the tendons of the abductor pollicis longus, extensor pollicis longus, and brevis muscles to the proximal space between the metacarpal bones of the thumb and index finger. Finally, it passes forward between the two heads of the first interosseous dorsalis muscles, into the palm of the hand, where it crosses the metacarpal bones. At the ulnar side of the hand, it unites with the deep palmar branch of the ulnar artery to form the deep palmar arch (see Fig. 74-10).

The ulnar artery enters the hand along the ulnar border of the wrist, crossing the transverse carpal ligament along the radial border of the pisiform bone. Immediately distal to the pisiform bone, the ulnar artery divides into two branches, which contribute to the completion of the superficial and deep palmar arches. The deep palmar arch gives rise to three palmar metacarpal arteries that run

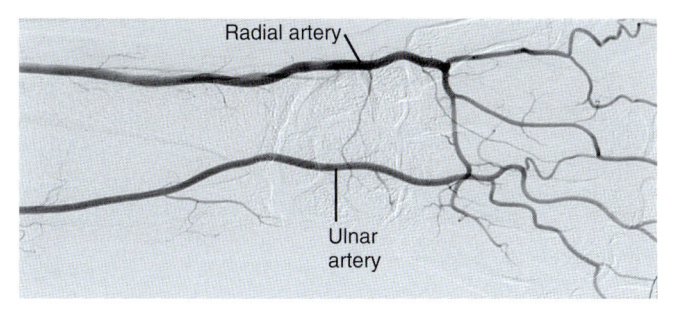

FIGURE 74-12 Angiogram of an incomplete palmar arch.

Detailed Description of Specific Areas

Normal Variants

There are numerous variants of the palmar arches and digital arteries (Fig. 74-11). The superficial palmar arch may be complete (42%) or incomplete (58%) (Fig. 74-12). If the superficial palmar arch is prominent, the deep palmar arch will be small, and vice versa. Both palmar arches supply the fingers in only 40% of limbs.

distally, joining the common palmar digital arteries that arise from the superficial palmar arch. Proper palmar digital arteries arising from the common palmar digital arteries supply the index, middle, ring, and little fingers. The radial artery gives off the princeps policis artery and radialis indicis artery (the digital arteries to the thumb and the lateral side of the index finger).

> **KEY POINTS**
> - Individual institutions may have a preference between CTA and MRA, depending on equipment and expertise. It is best to consult the institution about their preferred imaging modality to obtain the highest quality vascular imaging.
> - Catheter-directed angiography still remains the gold standard.

SUGGESTED READINGS

Kadir S. Atlas of Normal and Variant Angiographic Anatomy. Philadelphia, WB Saunders, 1991.

Lippert H, Pabst R. Arterial Variations in Man. Classification and Frequency. Munich, JF Bergmann Verlag, 1985.

Uflacker R. Atlas of Vascular Anatomy: An Angiographic Approach, 2nd ed. Philadelphia, Lippincott Williams & Wilkins, 2006.

REFERENCES

1. Longley D, Yedlicka J, Molina E, et al. Thoracic outlet syndrome: evaluation of the subclavian vessels by color duplex sonography. AJR Am Roentgenol 1992; 158:623-630.

2. Mochizuki T, Isoda H, Masui T, et al. Occlusion of the posterior humeral circumflex artery: detection with MR angiography in healthy volunteers and in a patient with quadrilateral space syndrome. AJR. Am J Roentgenol 1994; 163:625-627.

CHAPTER 75

Venous Anatomy of the Thorax

Jacobo Kirsch, Amy Kirby, and Eric E. Williamson

Understanding of the normal anatomy of the thoracic venous system is paramount to the effective daily practice of the imager. This understanding is crucial not only in assessing the normal contours and outlines of the vasculature on plain film radiographs but also in recognizing anomalous or aberrant presentations of that anatomy with cross-sectional imaging. It is often these variations in the anatomy that produce symptomatic disease in the patient, rendering the imager a key player in diagnosis. Venous anatomy or variations thereof can also be crucial to surgical colleagues for operative planning and follow-up.

Although plain film radiography was once considered the gold standard for chest evaluation, both multidetector computed tomography and magnetic resonance imaging are becoming indispensable for delineation of the different drainage patterns of the thoracic venous system. This is particularly true with the thoracic veins because they can be highly variable and tend to be tortuous with complex branching patterns, particularly in the setting of collateral development. In this chapter, we aim to depict the conventional anatomy of the thoracic venous system as well as common anatomic variants and their clinical significance.

NORMAL ANATOMY
General Anatomic Description

The thoracic veins can be divided in two groups: those that transport systemic (nonoxygenated) blood from the body to the right side of the heart and those that carry pulmonary (oxygenated) blood from the lungs to the left side of the heart. The systemic veins can be further subdivided into the deep system, which includes the venae cavae and the subclavian, brachiocephalic, and jugular veins; and the superficial system, which includes the chest wall veins and the azygos, hemiazygos, and paraspinal veins. We discuss the systemic veins first, beginning with the deep system followed by the superficial system, and then the pulmonary venous system, describing normal and variant anatomy of each.

THE VENAE CAVAE

The venae cavae are the two largest veins in the thorax. They drain the systemic blood directly into the right atrium. The superior vena cava conveys most of the supradiaphragmatic blood return, and the inferior vena cava drains the blood from the infradiaphragmatic structures.

The Superior Vena Cava

The superior vena cava (SVC) is the primary means of blood return to the heart from the upper extremities, head, and neck. It forms from the convergence of the right and left brachiocephalic veins (also known as the innominate veins) and ends at its entrance into the right atrium. The lower half of the vessel lies within the pericardium.[1] The SVC has a slightly convex vertical course, with its apex to the right, beginning immediately below the first costosternal junction and ending opposite the upper border of the third right costal cartilage. It measures approximately 7 cm in length, with its midpoint near the level of the carina on a frontal chest radiograph.[2]

In cross-sectional imaging, the beginning of the SVC can be recognized at the junction of the brachiocephalic veins in the upper mediastinum, posterior and slightly inferior to the right clavicular head and just above the prevascular space (Fig. 75-1). The course of the SVC lies slightly to the right of midline, adjacent to the ascending aorta, and passes anterior to the right pulmonary artery before entering the heart (Fig. 75-2). When CT imaging of the chest is performed after an upper extremity injection of intravenous contrast material, the SVC can often be recognized as the densely opacified structure draining into the heart and creating some streak artifact in this area.

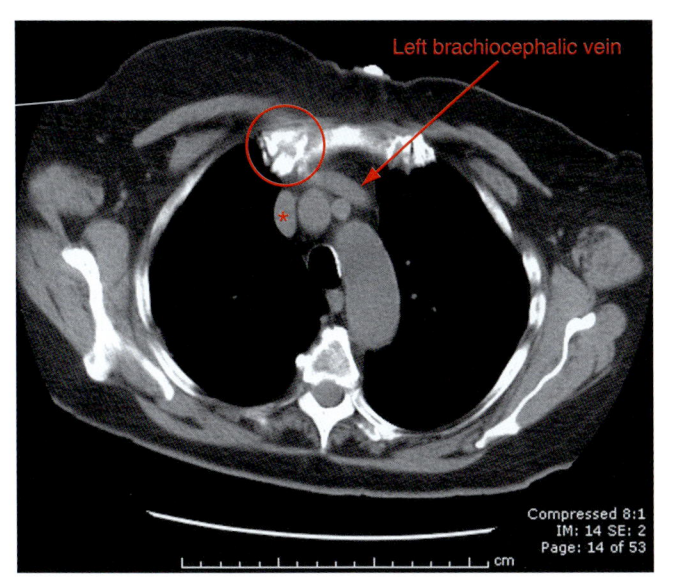

FIGURE 75-1 CT image of the chest without contrast enhancement at the inferior aspect of the right sternoclavicular articulation (*circle*) shows the left brachiocephalic vein crossing anterior to the great vessels to join the right brachiocephalic vein (*asterisk*) and forming the superior vena cava (not shown).

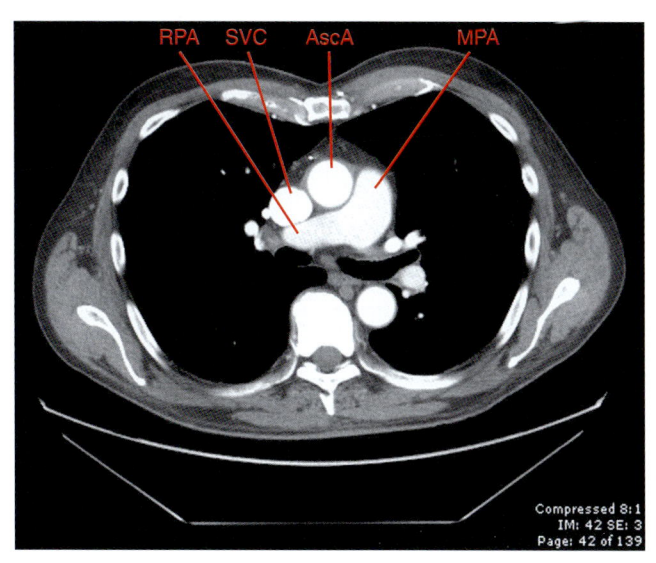

FIGURE 75-2 Contrast-enhanced CT image at the level of the pulmonary trunk shows the superior vena cava (SVC) to the right of the ascending aorta (AscA) and anterior to the right pulmonary artery (RPA). MPA, main pulmonary artery.

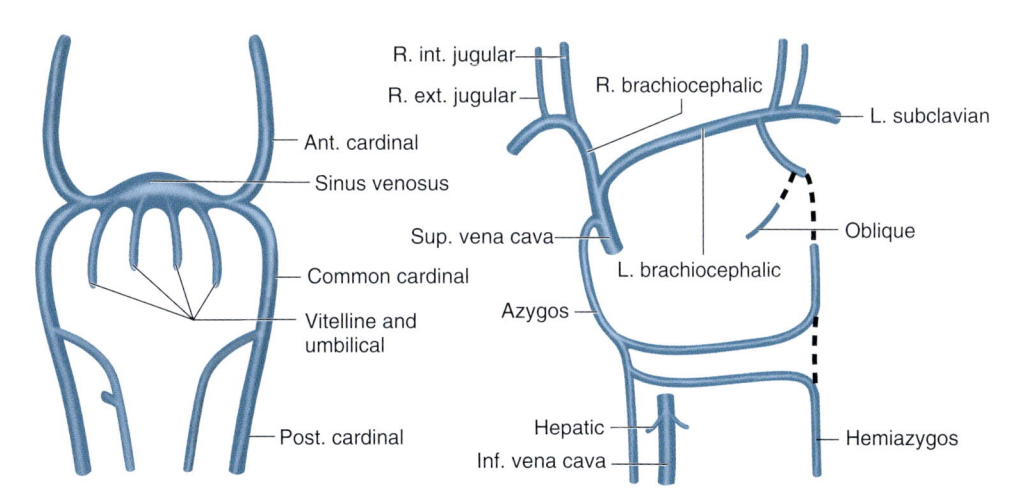

FIGURE 75-3 Embryologic anatomy illustration.

Variant Anatomy

The SVC anomalies can be divided into those associated with a right-sided SVC, a left-sided SVC, or a duplicated SVC. Right-sided SVC anomalies are the rarest of the SVC variants and include variations in the normal junction, with a right-sided SVC draining directly into the left atrium or having a very low insertion into the right atrium.

To understand the duplicated and left-sided SVC variants, one must first understand the venous embryologic development. The venous system begins its development in the earliest stages of intrauterine life as a symmetrical structure of paired cardinal and subcardinal veins. Early in the intrauterine period, the paired cardinal veins run the entire length of the embryo. There is a larger and more developed dorsally positioned caudal tract (the right and left posterior cardinal veins) and a more ventrally located cranial tract (the right and left anterior cardinal veins). The common cardinal veins originate from where the posterior and anterior cardinal veins converge and reach the primitive heart, the sinus venosus, from both the right and left sides. In a normal progression of development, the inferior portion of the left anterior cardinal vein regresses, and an anastomotic channel is formed between the right and left anterior cardinal veins, which becomes the left brachiocephalic vein. This vein allows drainage from the left side to the right. The superior portion of the left anterior cardinal vein becomes the superior intercostal vein, which drains the second and third left intercostal spaces. The normal right-sided SVC forms from the right common cardinal vein and the right anterior cardinal vein.[3] When the left distal anterior cardinal vein persists, a left-sided vena cava forms (Fig.

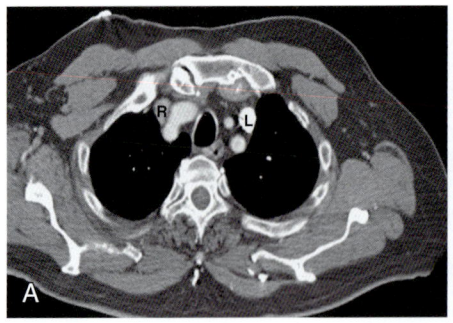

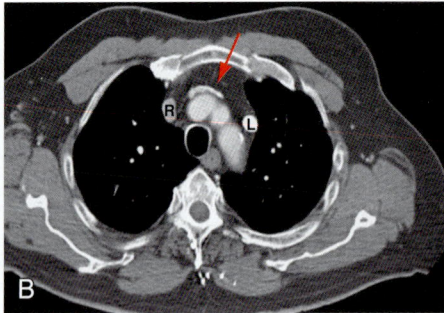

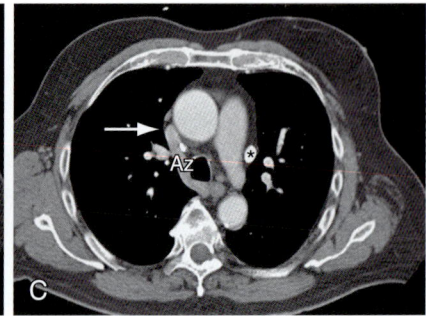

■ **FIGURE 75-4** Duplicated SVC. **A,** There is dense contrast material within a left SVC (L) that courses laterally and to the left of the arch vessels (*asterisk*). **B,** At the level of the arch, it courses laterally along the left aspect of the mediastinum, while the conventional right-sided brachiocephalic (R) vein is also present, receiving the atrophic left brachiocephalic vein (*arrow*) to form the right-sided SVC. **C,** The right SVC (*white arrow*) is in its expected position to the right of the aortic arch and great vessels. It receives the azygos inferiorly (Az) as the left SVC (*asterisk*) is noted to the left of the main pulmonary trunk (P).

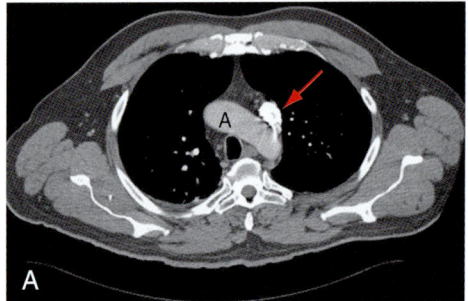

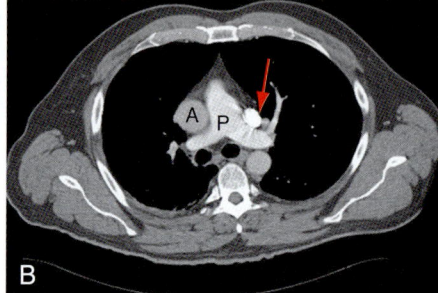

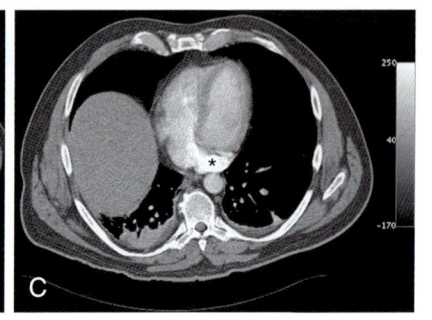

■ **FIGURE 75-5** Left-sided SVC. Contrast material is seen within a left-sided SVC (*red arrow*), coursing to the left of the aortic arch (A) in **A** and to the left of the aorta and main pulmonary artery (P) in **B**. It drains into the coronary sinus (*asterisk*) in **C**. Note the absence of the right-sided SVC in this patient.

75-3). The incidence of a left-sided vena cava is 0.3% to 0.5% in the general population and 4% in patients with congenital heart disease.[4]

A left-sided SVC may or may not be accompanied by regression of the right anterior cardinal vein and the right common cardinal vein, which form the normal right-sided SVC. Without regression, both a right and left SVC develop, resulting in a duplicated SVC system, with an absent left brachiocephalic vein and smaller right SVC in 65% of cases (Fig. 75-4). Duplicated SVC occurs in 0.3% to 0.5% of the population and in approximately 11% of patients with congenital heart disease.[5]

With regression of the cardinal veins that form the right SVC, blood from the right side of the embryo drains from the right brachiocephalic vein to the left SVC, which then drains most commonly into the coronary sinus and on into the right atrium. Cross-sectional imaging of a left-sided SVC shows it coursing caudally to the left of the aortic arch and left main pulmonary artery within the mediastinum, passing medially to the left superior pulmonary vein, before emptying into the coronary sinus (Fig. 75-5). Although it is most commonly asymptomatic, the resultant dilation of the coronary sinus can rarely cause conduction abnormalities. In the absence of other congenital cardiac anomalies, a left-sided SVC with absent right SVC and visceroatrial situs solitus occurs in fewer than 0.1% of the population.[6] Finally, a left-sided SVC can drain directly into the left atrium, producing a right-to-left shunt. This anomaly is rare and is usually associated with congenital cardiac anomalies.

The Inferior Vena Cava

The thoracic segment of the inferior vena cava (IVC), the suprahepatic segment, is very short; it crosses the diaphragm through the caval opening or foramen in the central tendon at approximately the level of T8. Branches of the phrenic nerve that are separated by fibrous pericardium accompany it.[7] The drainage of the IVC into the right atrium is considered to be a reliable marker for determination of the atrial situs because the suprahepatic IVC almost never drains into a different cavity.[8] The normal embryologic precursor to the suprahepatic IVC is the right supracardinal vein.

Variant Anatomy

Developmental anomalies of the IVC are rare, occurring in fewer than 1% of those with congenital heart disease.[9] The embryogenesis of the IVC involves formation of several anastomoses of three paired embryonic veins. Variations in this development result in several important anomalous drainage patterns. The most common variation is absence of the suprahepatic IVC with azygos continuation of the IVC. It results from the involution of a segment of the supracardinal vein, leading to drainage of the infrahepatic IVC into the azygos vein; the hepatic veins continue to drain directly into the right atrium.[8] The prevalence is 0.6%.[10] An enlarged azygos vein will then join the SVC at the normal location in the right paratracheal space. Imaging findings include absence of the suprahepatic

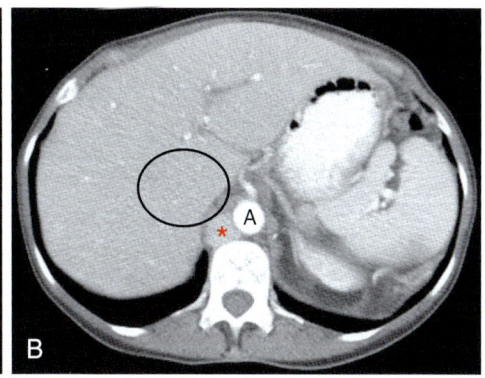

FIGURE 75-6 Azygos continuation of the IVC. **A,** Axial contrast-enhanced image through the chest shows a large vascular structure to the right of the descending aorta (A) that is an enlarged azygos (*asterisk*). Note on image **B** the absence of the intrahepatic portion of the IVC (*circle*) as well as the enlarged azygos to the right of the abdominal aorta.

segment on the lateral view of a chest radiograph and a mass in the right paratracheal space on the anteroposterior view, in the expected region of the azygos vein. Cross-sectional imaging delineates the dilated azygos ascending along its normal course to drain into the SVC (Fig. 75-6).

VEINS THAT DRAIN THE UPPER EXTREMITIES AND HEAD INTO THE CHEST

General Anatomic Description

The subclavian and jugular veins represent the major routes of venous drainage of the head and neck and upper extremities. There is considerable variation in their size and anatomy between sides and between individuals. However, physiologically important abnormalities involving these systems are uncommon.

The venous drainage of the head and neck is provided primarily by a paired triple jugular system composed of both deep and superficial vessels: the internal, external, and anterior jugular veins.[11] The jugular veins converge with the subclavian veins to form the brachiocephalic veins, also referred to as the innominate veins.

The subclavian veins drain the upper extremities, and after receiving the jugular drainage, they continue to the SVC as the brachiocephalic veins. The main tributaries of the brachiocephalic vein include the vertebral, internal mammary, and inferior thyroid veins, in that order from proximal to distal.[7] These are discussed in subsequent sections. The right brachiocephalic vein is the shortest of the two and has an almost vertical course until it forms the SVC at its junction with the left brachiocephalic, which is longer and crosses midline, passing behind the sternal manubrium and anterior to the aortic branches.

Variant anatomy of the brachiocephalic veins is rare and is reported in 0.2% to 1% of all cardiac anomalies.[12] These predominantly involve coursing of the left brachiocephalic vein under the aortic arch, superior to the pulmonary artery, and are associated with other congenital heart anomalies, most commonly tetralogy of Fallot.[12] Cross-sectional imaging can clearly differentiate this from a persistent left-sided SVC or vertical vein and can be important in presurgical planning for congenital heart disease.

VEINS THAT DRAIN THE CHEST WALL

General Anatomic Description

The principal veins on the internal surface of the thorax are the internal thoracic veins, which ascend lateral to the sternum and medial to the internal thoracic (mammary) arteries. They mainly receive blood from the anterior intercostal veins, and they usually vary from one to two on each side. At the approximate level of the sternomanubrial joint, the thoracic veins will join into a common trunk that joins the right and left brachiocephalic veins.[13] It is estimated that approximately half of the population will have two veins on each side of the sternum, 10% will have a single vein on each side, and the remaining population has a combination of one and two on either side.[13] The internal thoracic veins run medial to the internal thoracic arteries.

Each intercostal space has two anterior intercostal veins and one posterior intercostal vein. The drainage of the anterior veins is to the internal and lateral thoracic veins, as previously mentioned.

The posterior veins will drain to different systems, depending on their level; the lower eight drain to the azygos system on the right and the accessory hemiazygos and hemiazygos veins on the left. The first posterior intercostal veins drain into the respective right and left brachiocephalic vein. The second, third, and sometimes fourth intercostal veins will drain into the ipsilateral brachiocephalic vein through one of its tributaries, the superior intercostal vein.[7] The left superior intercostal will form an arch on the left side of the mediastinum that is analogous to the azygos arch on the right, sometimes called the hemiazygos arch, which most of the time is diminutive (Fig. 75-7). About 75% of the time, this vein will connect to the accessory hemiazygos vein.[14] This is the so-called aortic nipple sometimes seen on the frontal chest radiograph.[15]

The Azygos Veins

1-SVC
2-Azygos vein
3-Hemiazygos vein
4-Accessory hemiazygos vein

■ **FIGURE 75-7** Illustration of the posterior venous drainage of the thorax, with the azygos, hemiazygos, and accessory hemiazygos draining the intercostals bilaterally. The superior intercostal vein is also depicted, which conventionally drains the second through the fourth posterior intercostal veins on the left and the second and third posterior intercostal veins on the right.

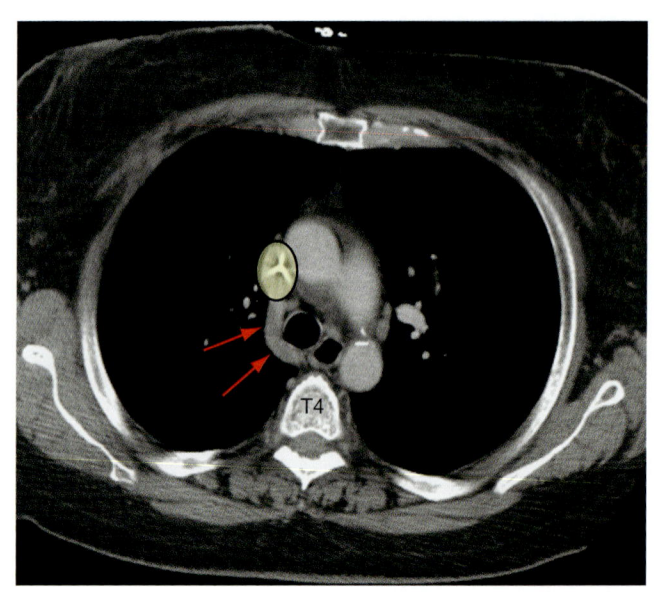

■ **FIGURE 75-8** Azygos vein on axial CT. Axial contrast-enhanced CT image of the chest shows the azygos (*arrows*) with a conventional course along the right mediastinum, draining into the SVC (*depicted in yellow*) at T4. Note the beam hardening artifact from the indwelling catheter.

THE AZYGOS AND HEMIAZYGOS SYSTEMS

General Anatomic Description

The azygos system is a paired paravertebral system. Interestingly, the azygos and hemiazygos veins are the only large veins in the thoracic cavity with valves.[16]

Embryologically, the azygos vein is formed from the right posterior cardinal vein inferiorly and the right supracardinal vein superiorly. It originates as the confluence of the lumbar venous plexus in the abdomen and extends cephalad, entering the thorax through the aortic hiatus or behind the lateral aspect of the right diaphragmatic crus. It continues to the right of the spine, and at the approximate level of T4, it creates the azygos arch where it joins the SVC (Fig. 75-8). This can sometimes be seen with aberrant SVC catheter positioning, with the tip directed over the SVC on the anteroposterior view and directed posteriorly on the lateral radiograph, indicating its position within the azygos vein (Fig. 75-9).

On the left, the hemiazygos and accessory hemiazygos veins are embryologically derived from the left supracardinal vein. Similar to the azygos on the right, the perilumbar veins usually form the hemiazygos vein. The hemiazygos vein ascends to the left of the spine until it reaches the level of T8, where it crosses over the midline to join the azygos vein (Fig. 75-10). From then on, the continuation of the venous system on the left is called the accessory hemiazygos vein, which has a variable amount of branches communicating with the azygos, hemiazygos, or left brachiocephalic vein.[17]

Normal Variants

The azygos lobe, a normal variation, is present in 0.4% to 1.0% of the population. When present, it may alter the shape of the SVC and the location of the azygos arch.[18] This anomaly is formed by the indentation of the right upper lobe by an invagination of the azygos arch, which brings with it four layers of pleura (two layers of visceral pleura and two layers of parietal pleura). On plain film examinations of the chest, an azygos lobe is recognized as a curvilinear density with a distal teardrop shadow arising from the upper right mediastinum, coursing through the medial aspect of the apex of the lung. On cross-sectional examinations, an azygos fissure can be seen as a curved tubular vascular structure at the right upper thorax separated from the mediastinum by interposed lung parenchyma (Fig. 75-11). Embryologically, formation of an azygos lobe results from failure of the posterior cardinal vein to migrate over the apex of the lung, and the vein courses through lung parenchyma.

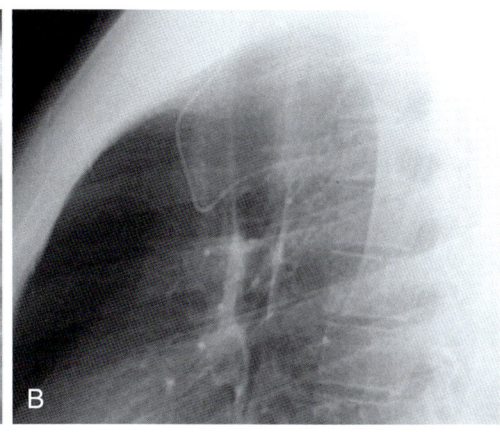

■ **FIGURE 75-9** Posteroanterior and lateral chest radiographs show an azygos lobe (*arrows*) with a left peripherally inserted central catheter line directed laterally and posteriorly, indicating aberrant placement within the azygos vein (*asterisk*).

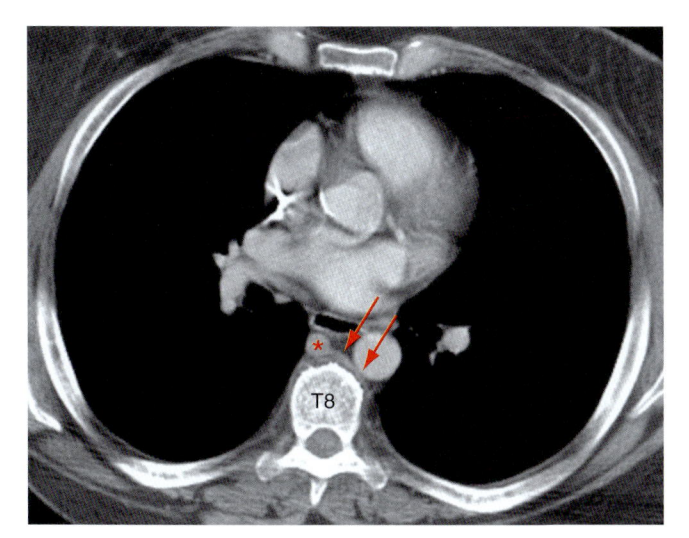

■ **FIGURE 75-10** Axial contrast-enhanced image of the chest shows the hemiazygos (*arrows*) draining into the azygos (*asterisk*) at approximately T8.

THE PULMONARY VEINS

General Anatomic Description

During embryonic development, two pulmonary veins from each lung join to form a common pulmonary vein. These common veins unite with a pulmonary bud from the primitive left atrium, which results, in most people, in four individual pulmonary veins, two for each lung (expected to occur in approximately 66% to 70% of the population). However, significant variations in the embryologic process can lead to variations in the number, site, and branching pattern of pulmonary veins. If there is underincorporation of the pulmonary veins into the left atrium, a common pulmonary vein will result. On the other hand, overincorporation of the common pulmonary vein into the dorsal left atrium results in supernumerary pulmonary veins.[19] Most of the adult left atrium is also derived from this primitive common pulmonary vein, which becomes incorporated into the left atrial wall as it expands in size.[7,20]

Approximately 70% of patients have two separate ostia on the right side for upper and lower lobe pulmonary veins. The majority of the remaining individuals will have three to five pulmonary vein ostia; less than 2% have a common ostium on the right. On the left, it is expected that approximately 85% of patients will have two ostia, for the upper and lower lobe veins; virtually all the remainder have a single common ostium as a less common variant (Fig. 75-12).[21] When present, accessory veins are named for the pulmonary lobe or segment that they drain. The superior pulmonary veins are found in front of the pulmonary arteries. In the left lung root, the superior pulmonary vein is in front of the left main bronchus, and the inferior pulmonary vein is below it. In the right lung root, the pulmonary veins are similarly distributed above and below the right bronchus.[7]

The pulmonary veins do not closely follow the bronchi, and they run in intersegmental septa (Fig. 75-13). These veins drain the lungs and enter the left atrium from superior and inferior to the oblique fissure on each side. The portion of the left atrium defined by the boundaries of the pulmonary veins is the anterior wall of the oblique pericardial sinus, which is separated from the esophagus by the fibrous pericardium.[7]

Detailed Description of Specific Areas

Normal Variants

Anomalous pulmonary venous anatomy occurs when pulmonary veins drain into a structure other than the left atrium. Partial anomalous pulmonary venous return occurs when at least one of the pulmonary veins drains into the left atrium.[20] If no pulmonary veins drain into the left atrium, the resulting condition is total anomalous pulmonary venous return (TAPVR), also known as total anomalous pulmonary venous connection.

Premature atresia of the right or left portion of the primordial pulmonary vein while primitive pulmonary-systemic connections are still present results in a partial anomalous pulmonary venous connection.[22] This anomalous pulmonary venous connection creates a system whereby oxygenated blood is returned to the right atrium

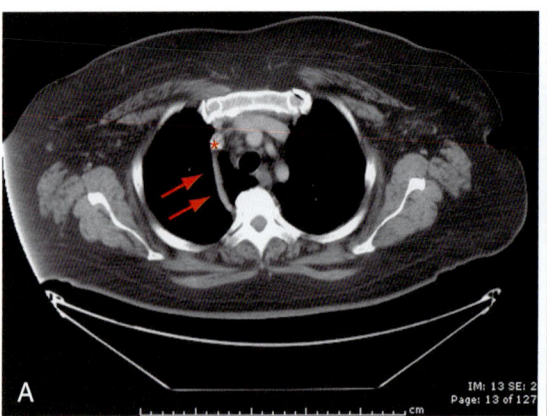

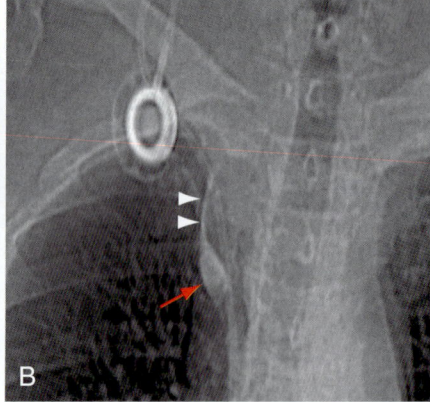

■ **FIGURE 75-11** **A,** Axial contrast-enhanced image of the upper chest shows a vascular structure (*arrows*) coursing through the medial aspect of the right upper lobe, draining into the SVC (*asterisk*). **B,** Correlative scout film of the chest shows the azygos (*arrow*) and the course of the azygos arch (*arrowheads*). Note the catheter within the SVC.

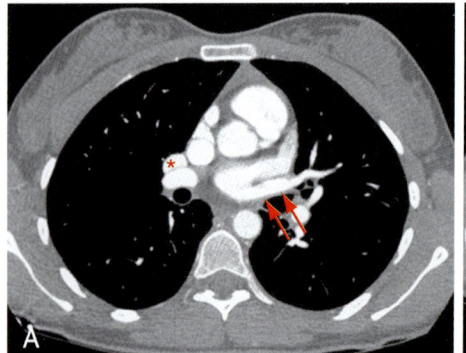

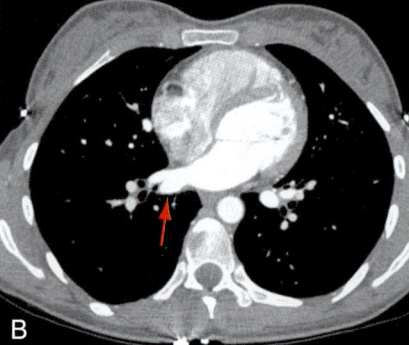

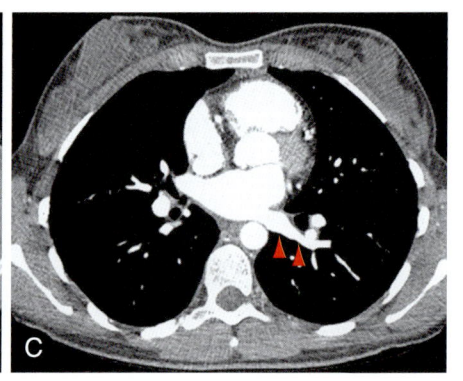

■ **FIGURE 75-12** Pulmonary vein anatomy. **A,** Contrast-enhanced axial CT image shows the right superior pulmonary vein (*asterisk*) anterior to the right main pulmonary artery and the origin of the left superior pulmonary vein (*arrows*) from the left atrium. Note the superior pulmonary vein anterior to the left main bronchus. **B** and **C,** Caudal to image **A,** the right inferior pulmonary vein (*arrow*) and the left inferior pulmonary vein (*arrowheads*) are depicted at their respective origins. This patient has conventional anatomy, with two right and two left pulmonary veins.

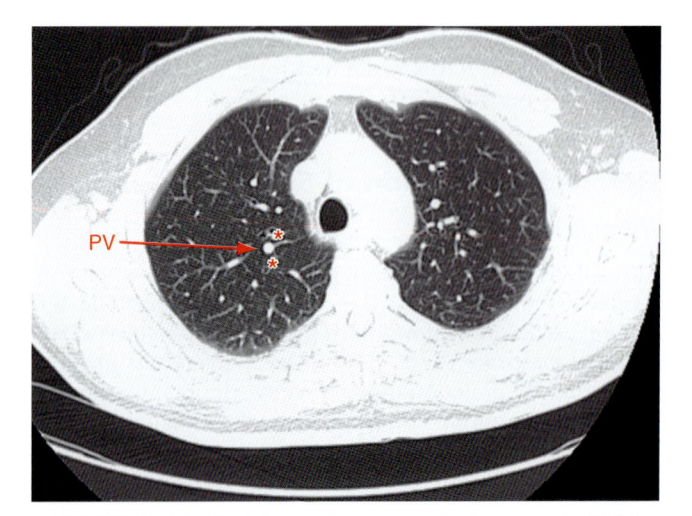

■ **FIGURE 75-13** The left superior segmental pulmonary vein (PV) is shown on this non–contrast-enhanced CT image of the chest coursing by itself in the interlobar septa. Note the segmental pulmonary arteries (*asterisks*) that course adjacent to their corresponding bronchi.

or its tributaries instead of to the left atrium, creating a left-to-right shunt.[23-25] The described prevalence of a partial anomalous pulmonary venous connection is 0.4% to 0.7%, with 90% of them being right sided (Fig. 75-14).[26-28] Between 80% and 90% of patients with this condition will have an associated atrial septal defect of either the sinus venosus or secundum type.[22,29]

TAPVR occurs when all the pulmonary veins fail to connect to the left atrium and instead connect to a systemic vein or veins. The location of this connection is used to categorize this anomaly, and there are four types: above the heart (supracardiac, type I), below the heart (infracardiac, type II; Fig. 75-15), to the right atrium or coronary sinus (cardiac, type III), or some combination of these types (mixed, type IV). Because the anomalous pulmonary venous return results in a left-to-right shunt, with mixing of the systemic venous and pulmonary venous blood, there is resultant cyanosis, necessitating a patent foramen ovale or ductus arteriosus for compatibility with life. Accurate delineation of the different subtypes is crucial in determining the appropriate surgical management.

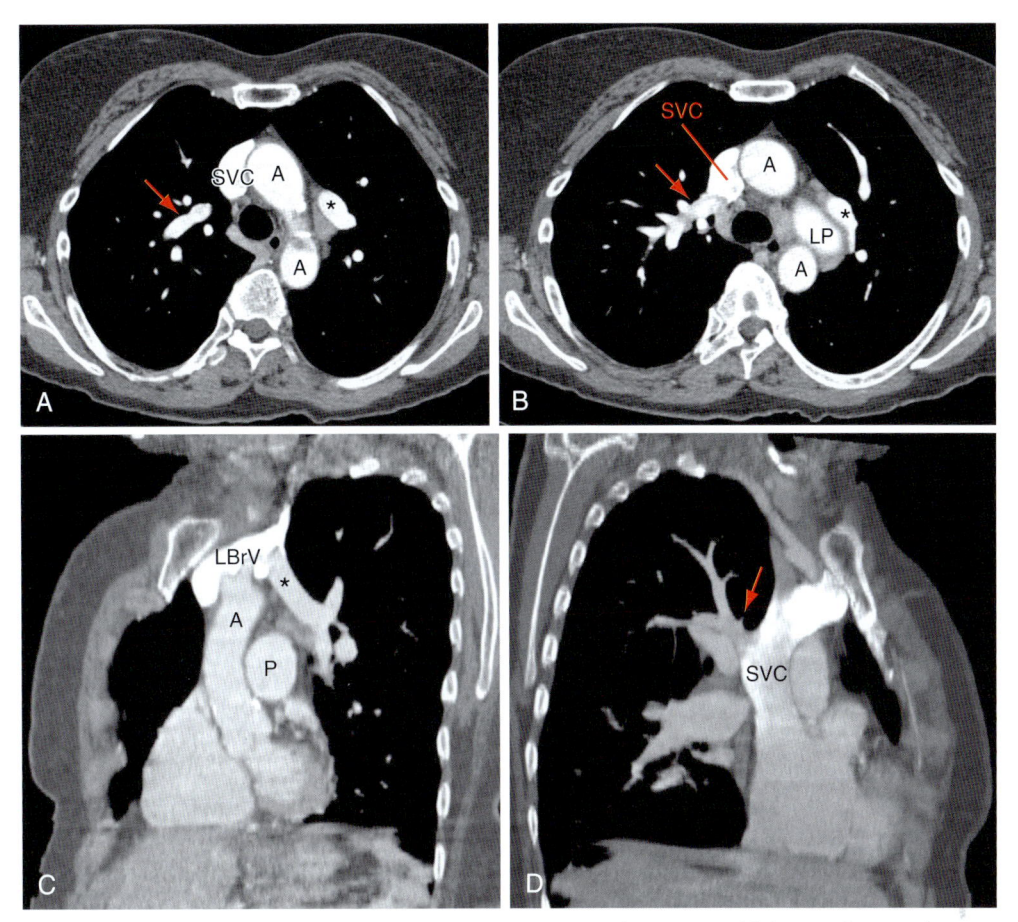

■ **FIGURE 75-14** Partial anomalous pulmonary venous return. **A** and **B,** There are right (*arrow*) and left (*asterisk*) anomalous superior pulmonary veins emptying into the SVC on the right and into the brachiocephalic on the left. **C,** Reformatted sagittal oblique image of the left side of the chest shows anomalous superior pulmonary vein (*asterisk*) draining into the left brachiocephalic vein (LBrV). **D,** Reformatted sagittal oblique image of the right side of the chest shows anomalous superior pulmonary vein (*arrow*) draining into the SVC. A, aorta; P, pulmonary artery; LP, left pulmonary artery.

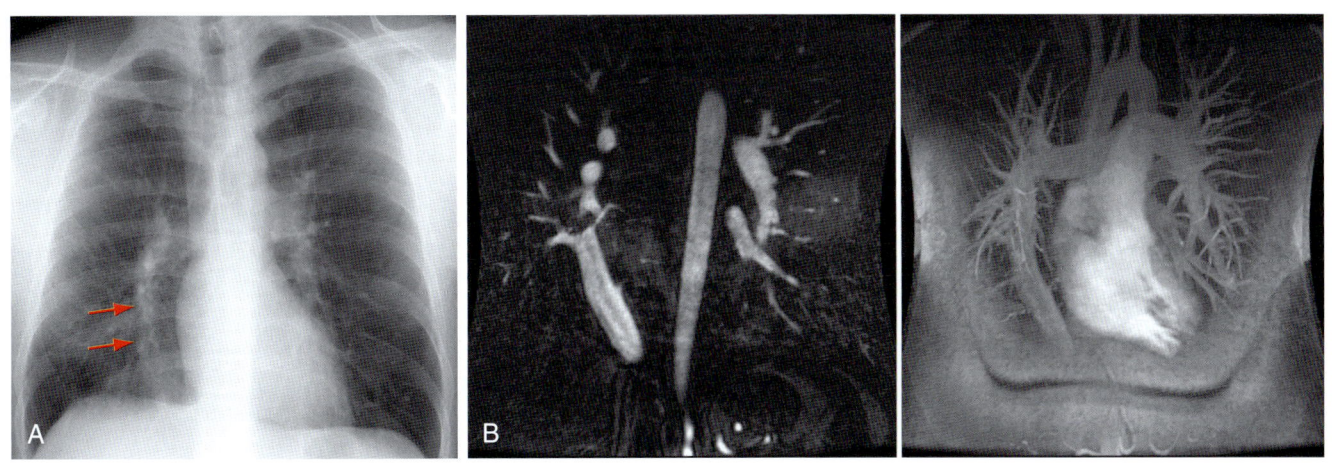

■ **FIGURE 75-15** Total anomalous pulmonary venous return, type II. **A,** Plain film of the chest shows a linear density (*arrows*) extending from the hilum to the diaphragm on the right, representing the "scimitar sign." **B,** Coronal MR angiography and maximum intensity projection images show anomalous drainage of the right pulmonary veins to the level of the diaphragm, with connection to the infradiaphragmatic IVC (not shown).

The incidence of TAPVR is 0.008% in the general population and 2.2% in patients with congenital heart disease.[30] The supracardiac form is the most common, representing 45%.[31] Most commonly, with the supracardiac type of TAPVR, the pulmonary veins empty into the vertical vein, which empties into the left brachiocephalic vein and then into the SVC. The infracardiac form occurs in approximately 26% of patients with TAPVR.[31] Because pulmonary venous obstruction is virtually invariably seen with this form, infracardiac TAPVR is the most severe form, presenting with cyanosis in the first day of life. In this form, the pulmonary veins empty into the portal vein, IVC, or hepatic veins. The cardiac form of TAPVR represents 13%, with the pulmonary veins emptying into the right atrium or coronary sinus. The mixed type is the rarest, representing 5% of this anomaly.[31]

> **KEY POINTS**
>
> - To interpret image examinations, it is necessary to be familiar with normal anatomy and variants.

SUGGESTED READINGS

Godwin JD, Chen JT. Thoracic venous anatomy. AJR Am J Roentgenol 1986; 147:674-684.

REFERENCES

1. Gray H. Anatomy of the Human Body. Philadelphia, Lea & Febiger, 1918; Bartleby.com, 2000, p 666.
2. Mahlon M, Yoon H. CT angiography of the superior vena cava: normative values and implications for central venous catheter position. J Vasc Interv Radiol 2007; 18:1106-1110.
3. Minniti S, Visentini S, Procacci C. Congenital anomalies of the venae cavae: embryological origin, imaging features and report of three new variants. Eur Radiol 2002; 12:2040-2055.
4. Cha EM, Khoury GH. Persistent left superior vena cava: radiologic and clinical significance. Radiology 1972; 103:375-381.
5. Demos TC, Posniak HV, Pierce KL, et al. Venous anomalies of the thorax. AJR Am J Roentgenol 2004; 182:1139-1150.
6. Bartram U, Van Praagh S, Levine JC, et al. Absent right superior vena cava in visceroatrial situs solitus. Am J Cardiol 1997; 80:175-183.
7. Lawler L, Fishman EK. Thoracic venous anatomy multidetector row CT evaluation. Radiol Clin North Am 2003; 41:545-560.
8. Kirsch J, Araoz PA, Breen JF, Chareonthaitawee P. Isolated total anomalous connection of the hepatic veins to the left atrium. J Cardiovasc Comput Tomogr 2007; 1:55-57.
9. Peterson RW. Infrahepatic interruption of the inferior vena cava with azygos continuation (persistent right cardinal vein). Radiology 1965; 84:304-307.
10. Bass JE, Redwine MD, Kramer LA, et al. Spectrum of congenital anomalies of the inferior vena cava: cross-sectional imaging findings. Radiographics 2000; 20:639-652.
11. Schummer W, Schummer C, Bredle D, Fröber R. The anterior jugular venous system: variability and clinical impact. Anesth Analg 2004; 99:1625-1629.
12. Chen SJ, Liu KL, Chen HY, et al. Anomalous brachiocephalic vein: CT, embryology, and clinical implications. AJR Am J Roentgenol 2005; 184:1235-1240.
13. Loukas M, Tobola MS, Tubbs RS, et al. The clinical anatomy of the internal thoracic veins. Folia Morphol (Warsz) 2007; 66:25-32.
14. Godwin JD, Chen JT. Thoracic venous anatomy. AJR Am J Roentgenol 1986; 147:674-684.
15. Ball JB Jr, Proto AV. The variable appearance of the left superior intercostal vein. Radiology 1982; 144:445-452.
16. Yeh BM, Coakley FV, Sanchez HC, et al. Azygos arch valves: prevalence and appearance at contrast-enhanced CT. Radiology 2004; 230:111-115.
17. Dudiak CM, Olson MC, Posniak HV. CT evaluation of congenital and acquired abnormalities of the azygos system. Radiographics 1991; 11:233-246.
18. Smathers RL, Buschi AJ, Pope TL Jr, et al. The azygous arch: normal and pathologic CT appearance. AJR Am J Roentgenol 1982; 139:477-483.
19. Konin GP, Jain VR, Fisher JD, Haramati LB. The ambiguous pulmonary venoatrial junction: a new perspective (review). Int J Cardiovasc Imaging 2008; 24:433-443. Epub 2007 Oct 2.
20. Lacomis JM, Wigginton W, Fuhrman C, et al. Multi-detector row CT of the left atrium and pulmonary veins before radio-frequency catheter ablation for atrial fibrillation. Radiographics 2003; 23(Spec No):S35-S48.
21. Marom EM, Herndon JE, Kim YH, et al. D variations in pulmonary venous drainage to the left atrium: implications for radiofrequency ablation. Radiology 2004; 230:824-829.
22. Senocak F, Ozme S, Bilgic A, et al. Partial anomalous pulmonary venous return. Evaluation of 51 cases. Jpn Heart J 1994; 35:43-50.
23. Herlong JR, Jaggers JJ, Ungerleider RM. Congenital Heart Surgery Nomenclature and Database Project: pulmonary venous anomalies. Ann Thorac Surg 2000; 69(Suppl):S56-S69.
24. Spindola-Franco H, Fish BG. Radiology of the heart. In Radiology of the Heart: Cardiac Imaging in Infants, Children, and Adults. New York, Springer-Verlag, 1985, pp 317-322.
25. White CS, Baffa JM, Haney PJ, et al. MR imaging of congenital anomalies of the thoracic veins. Radiographics 1997; 17:595-608.
26. Brody H. Drainage of the pulmonary veins into the right side of the heart. Arch Pathol 1942; 33:221-240.
27. Healy JE. Anatomic survey of anomalous pulmonary veins: their clinical significance. J Thorac Surg 1952; 23:433-443.
28. Van Meter C Jr, LeBlanc JG, Culpepper WS III, et al. Partial anomalous pulmonary venous return. Circulation 1990; 82:IV195-IV198.
29. Toyoshima M, Sato A, Fukumoto Y, et al. Partial anomalous pulmonary venous return showing anomalous venous return to the azygos vein. Intern Med 1992; 31:1112-1116.
30. Ferencz C, Rubin JD, McCarter RJ, et al. Congenital heart disease: prevalence at livebirth. The Baltimore-Washington Infant Study. Am J Epidemiol 1985; 121:31-36.
31. Delisle G, Ando M, Calder AL, et al. Total anomalous pulmonary venous connection: report of 93 autopsied cases with emphasis on diagnostic and surgical considerations. Am Heart J 1976; 91:99-122.

CHAPTER 76

Venous Anatomy of the Abdomen and Pelvis

Jeremy C. Durack and Maureen P. Kohi

The venous drainage of the abdomen is primarily mediated through the portal venous system and the inferior vena cava (IVC). These two systems are separate from each other in their organ drainage, but unite proximal to the IVC's diaphragmatic hiatus to return blood from the abdomen and pelvis to the right atrium. The venous drainage of the pelvis is largely mediated through the common iliac veins, which unite to form the IVC. It is important to remember that abdominal and pelvic venous vasculature are highly variable; therefore, canonical representations are frequently oversimplifications.

ABDOMEN: PORTAL VENOUS CIRCULATION

General Anatomic Description

The portal venous system is composed of the veins that drain the abdominal viscera, spleen, pancreas, and gallbladder. Nearly 80% of hepatic inflow comes from the portal vein. Visceral blood enters the liver via the portal vein, which ramifies to smaller caliber veins, eventually reaching the hepatic sinusoidal level. From there, postsinusoidal blood drains into the hepatic veins, which route all of the venous outflow from the liver to the IVC and systemic circulation.

Detailed Description of Specific Areas

Portal Vein

The portal vein (PV) is approximately 7 to 8 cm long in adults and is formed by the union of the splenic vein and superior mesenteric vein at the level of the second lumbar vertebra.[1] It lies posterior to the pancreatic head and anterior to the IVC (Figs. 76-1 to 76-3). The PV enters the liver at the porta hepatis, where it runs posterior and medial to the bile duct and posterior and lateral to the hepatic artery. At the porta hepatis, the PV divides into the right and left PVs. Of note, the adult PV and its tributaries are devoid of valves. However, in the fetus and for a brief postpartum period, valves can be found in portal tributaries.

Conventionally, the right PV first receives blood returning from the cystic vein and then enters the right hepatic lobe, where it divides into anterior and posterior trunks, supplying hepatic segments 5 through 8. The left PV, which is longer but typically smaller in caliber, is discussed in terms of a more proximal transverse portion and more distal umbilical portion. The left PV supplies hepatic segments 1 through 4. Along its course, the left PV merges with the paraumbilical veins and ligamentum teres (obliterated left umbilical vein) and is united to the IVC by the ligamentum venosum (obliterated ductus venosus).

Inflow to the PV is supplied by the superior mesenteric, splenic, right gastric, left gastric (coronary), paraumbilical, and cystic veins.

Superior Mesenteric Vein

The superior mesenteric vein (SMV) drains the small intestine, cecum, appendix, and the ascending and transverse portions of the colon (see Fig. 76-1). It courses posterior to the head of the pancreas and horizontal segment of the duodenum, and lies anterior to the IVC. The SMV unites with the splenic vein to form the main PV.

Mesenteric tributaries of the SMV include the jejunal, ileal, ileocolic, right colic, and middle colic veins. The nonmesenteric supply to the SMV comes from the right gastroepiploic and inferior pancreaticoduodenal veins.

The jejunal and ileal veins are named after their respective arteries and conform to the same arcade distribution. They drain the jejunum and ileum into the SMV, typically on the left side.

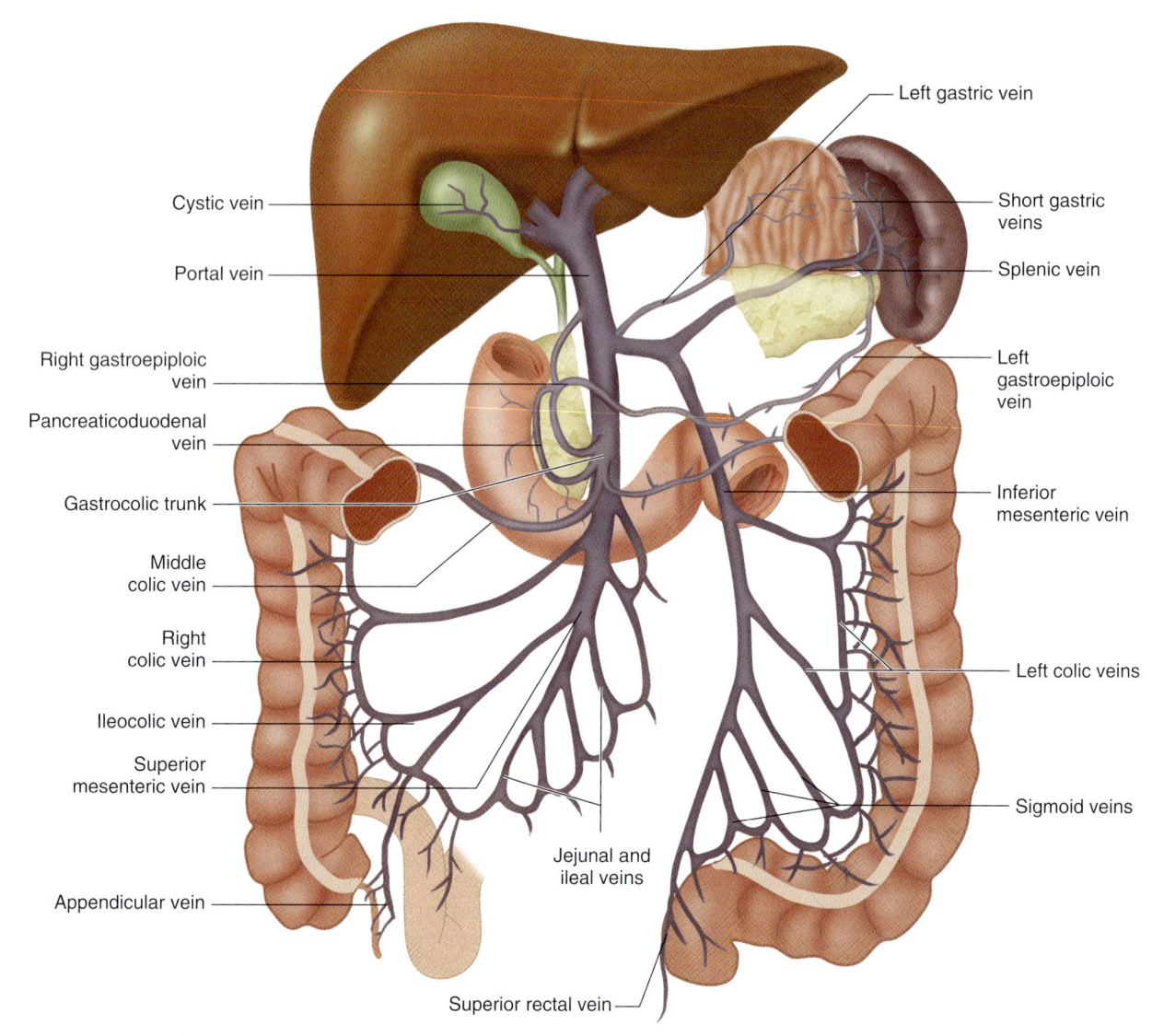

■ **FIGURE 76-1** Portal venous system and systemic drainage of the small and large intestines. The stomach, pancreas, and small and large intestines have been partially removed to highlight portal venous vasculature.

The ileocolic vein is formed by the union of the anterior and posterior cecal veins, appendicular veins, the last ileal vein, and a colic vein. The ileocolic vein can anastomose with the ileal veins and right colic vein and it eventually drains into the SMV on the right.

The right colic vein drains the right colon and can anastomose with the ileocolic and middle colic veins into the SMV. The middle colic vein drains the transverse colon via its left and right branches.

The right gastroepiploic vein courses along the greater curvature of the stomach and drains the greater omentum, distal body, and antrum of the stomach into the SMV. It can form connections with the left gastroepiploic vein and can serve as collateral circulation in the setting of splenic vein thrombosis.

The pancreaticoduodenal veins drain the head of the pancreas and duodenal wall into the SMV. These veins conform to the same anatomy as the pancreaticoduodenal arteries, with anterior and posterior venous arcades between the superior and inferior pancreaticoduodenal veins.

Splenic Vein

The splenic vein (lienal vein) is the second largest tributary of the PV and measures about 1 cm in diameter. The main splenic vein is formed by the union of two (76%), three (20%), or four (4%) inflow veins.[2]

Conventionally the following veins drain into the splenic vein—short gastric, left gastroepiploic, pancreatic, and inferior mesenteric veins. The short gastric veins include four or five veins, which drain the fundus and part of the greater gastric curvature. These veins also communicate with the inferior esophageal veins and can enlarge significantly in the setting of portal hypertension, presenting a risk for esophageal variceal bleeding.

The left gastroepiploic vein courses along the greater curvature of the stomach and drains the walls of the

FIGURE 76-2 Main portal vein and venous drainage of the stomach, spleen, and duodenum. The liver has been retracted to reveal portal venous vasculature.

stomach and greater omentum before joining the splenic vein.

The pancreatic veins include a number of small vessels draining the body and tail of the pancreas into the splenic vein.

The inferior mesenteric vein drains the rectum via the superior rectal vein, the sigmoid colon via the sigmoid vein, and the left colon via the left colic vein into the splenic vein.

Gastric Veins

The right gastric vein courses along the lesser curvature of the stomach, draining the stomach into the PV. The left

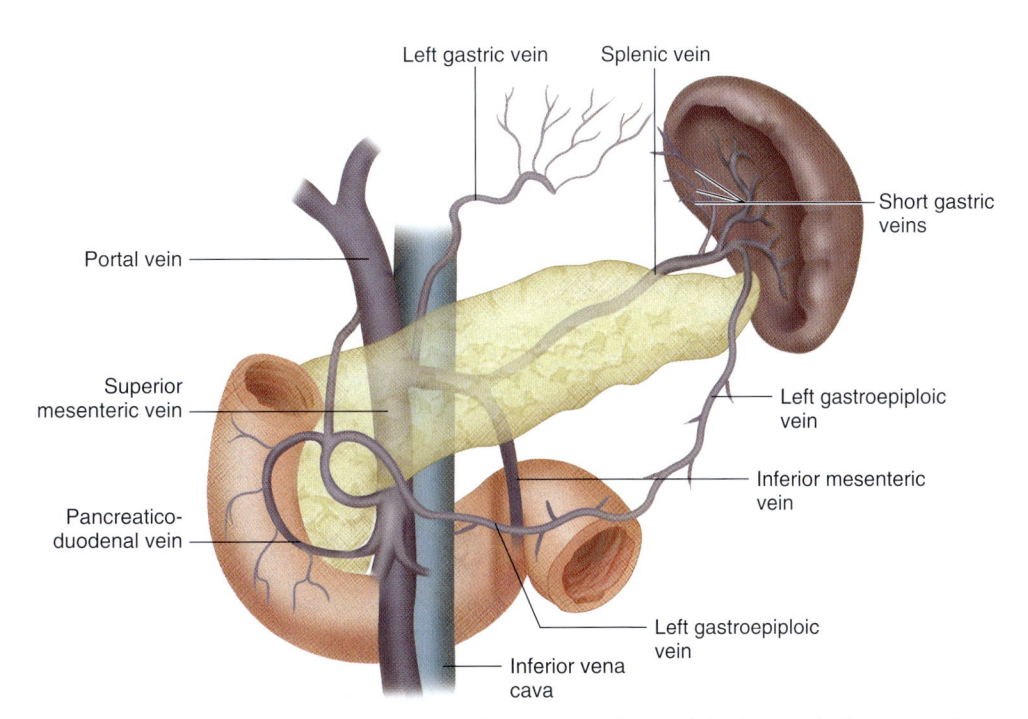

FIGURE 76-3 Main portal vein and venous drainage of the stomach, pancreas, spleen, and duodenum. The liver, stomach, mesentery, and portions of the small intestine have been removed to highlight portal venous vasculature.

gastric vein (coronary vein) drains the gastric walls into the PV. It also connects with the lower esophageal vein through multiple anastomoses.

Paraumbilical Veins

The paraumbilical veins are small in caliber and variable in number and are found extending along the ligamentum teres and median umbilical ligament. These short veins connect the anterior abdominal wall veins to the portal venous system. As such, they can offer collateral venous circulation in the case of portal obstruction.

Cystic Vein

The cystic vein drains the gallbladder into the right PV.

Normal Variants

In a study by Koc and colleagues, a total of 318 branching variants and anomalies of the portal venous system were observed in 307 (27.4%) of 1120 patients[3]; 72.6% of patients demonstrated conventional anatomy. The most frequent variation was trifurcation of the PV, detected in 12.4% of patients. In these individuals, the PV divided into a left portal branch, right anterior portal branch, and right posterior portal branch. The next most common variant was a right posterior portal branch as the first branch of the main portal vein, detected in 9.2% of cases. In 3.6% of patients, there were variants of PV origin in segments IV and VIII of the liver.

Another variant of the PV seen in very rare cases is infracardiac total anomalous pulmonary venous return (TAPVR), in which the pulmonary veins drain into the PV. The incidence of TAPVR is approximately 2% of all congenital heart defects and, in 15% of cases, the pulmonary veins drain into the portal venous system (type III).[3,4]

In most cases, the SMV is formed by its chief tributaries. However, in almost 13% of cases, the main trunk of the SMV is absent and large right and large left mesenteric branches join the splenic vein to form the portal vein.[3,4]

The inferior mesenteric vein demonstrates considerable anatomic variability. In a study by Graf, the inferior mesenteric vein drained into the splenic vein in 56% of patients, but in 18% it drained into the splenoportal angle, and in the remaining 26% drainage was observed into the superior mesenteric vein.[5]

Differential Considerations

Portal Hypertension

The PV normally provides up to 80% of the total hepatic blood flow. Normal pressure in the PV ranges from 5 to 10 mm Hg, although clinically relevant alterations in portal pressures may be best considered in relative terms. The portosystemic gradient (PSG), or pressure difference between the PV and IVC (or the right atrium), is normally 3 to 6 mm Hg. In the setting of portal hypertension, the absolute portal pressure may rise above 11 mm Hg, and the portosystemic gradient may rise above 6 mm Hg.

TABLE 76-1 Causes of Portal Hypertension

Prehepatic	Intrahepatic	Posthepatic
Portal vein thrombosis	Cirrhosis Schistosomiasis Noncirrhotic portal fibrosis	Right-sided heart failure Hepatic outflow obstruction (Budd-Chiari syndrome) Constrictive pericarditis

A number of different factors can result in increased pressure in the portal system. These can be divided into prehepatic, intrahepatic and posthepatic causes (Table 76-1).

The most common causes of portal hypertension include cirrhosis, noncirrhotic portal fibrosis, Budd-Chiari syndrome, and schistosomiasis. The increase in portal venous pressure results in the formation of multiple portosystemic collateral vessels. These vessels function to divert blood away from the region of increased pressure and into the systemic circulation. Four main groups of portosystemic collaterals will be discussed.

1. The first group is represented by collaterals between the left gastric (coronary vein) and short gastric veins of the portal system with the intercostal veins, esophageal vein, and azygos tributaries of the IVC. This group may manifest clinically through sequelae of esophageal and gastric fundal varices (Fig. 76-4).
2. The second group, located in the anterior abdominal wall, is composed of communication between the

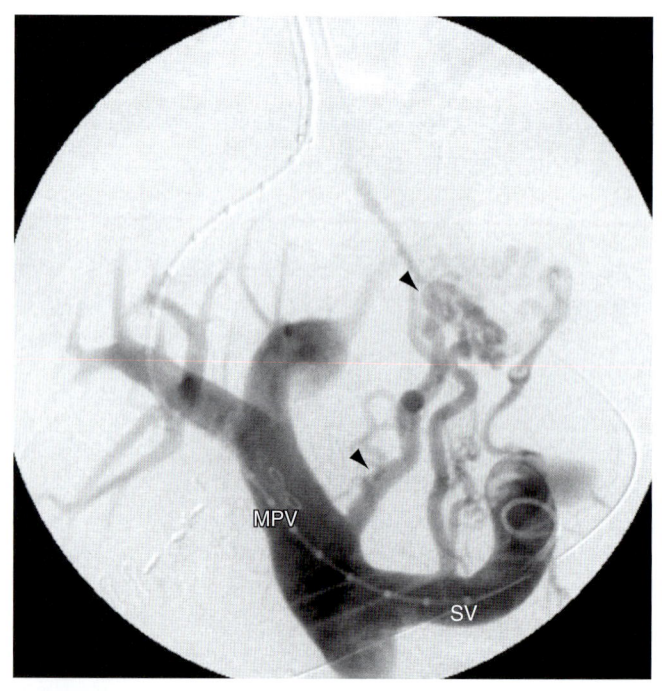

■ **FIGURE 76-4** Esophageal varices from portal hypertension. This digitally subtracted fluoroscopic image was obtained during a transjugular intrahepatic portosystemic shunt (TIPS) procedure following injection of contrast through a catheter inserted into the splenic vein. Large esophageal varices are indicated by arrowheads. MPV, main portal vein; SV, splenic vein.

vestiges of the umbilical circulation of fetal life and veins of the anterior abdominal wall. These collaterals produce varices radiating from the umbilicus, most often referred to as caput medusae.
3. The third group, located in the retroperitoneum, comprises collateral formation between the splenic vein and the left renal vein. These collaterals are often referred to as spontaneous splenorenal shunts.
4. The fourth group is located at the anal canal where the superior rectal vein, tributary of the portal venous system, anastomoses with the middle and inferior rectal veins. These veins may become dilated and pressurized, resulting in symptomatic rectal varices.

Patients with portal hypertension may be asymptomatic, but most manifest with variceal bleeding, ascites, splenomegaly, or encephalopathy. In variceal bleeding, 85% of cases result from variceal hemorrhage at the gastroesophageal junction. Bleeding from gastric and esophageal varices account for 17% of cases of acute massive upper gastrointestinal hemorrhage.[6]

Direct pressure recording of the PV through arterial portography or indirect measurement by wedged hepatic venography can be used to diagnose portal hypertension. However, portal hypertension can also be noted on computed tomography (CT) or ultrasound. CT signs of portal hypertension include dilated portal vein (>13 mm), splenomegaly, ascites, and portosystemic collaterals. Sonographic signs of portal hypertension include ascites, splenomegaly, PV enlargement (>13 mm measured in the anteroposterior direction), portosystemic collaterals, enlarged hepatic arteries, and hepatofugal (reversed) portal flow.

Treatment options for portal hypertension include medical management, surgical devascularization with portosystemic shunt formation, transjugular intrahepatic portosystemic shunt (TIPS), and liver transplantation.[7]

ABDOMEN: SYSTEMIC VENOUS CIRCULATION

General Anatomic Description

The abdominal systemic venous circulation courses through the IVC. Proximal to the right atrium, the systemic and portal venous circulations unite to drain the abdominal and pelvic organs.

Detailed Description of Specific Areas

The IVC is formed by the union of the common iliac veins at the level of the fifth lumbar vertebra (Fig. 76-5).[1] It ascends to the right of the abdominal midline, anterior to the vertebral column, in the retroperitoneal space and traverses the tendinous portion of the diaphragm at the level of the eighth thoracic vertebra, draining into the right atrium. A semilunar valve is present at its atrial orifice (valve of the inferior vena cava), which in fetal life serves to direct blood through the foramen ovale into the left atrium, which becomes rudimentary in the adult.

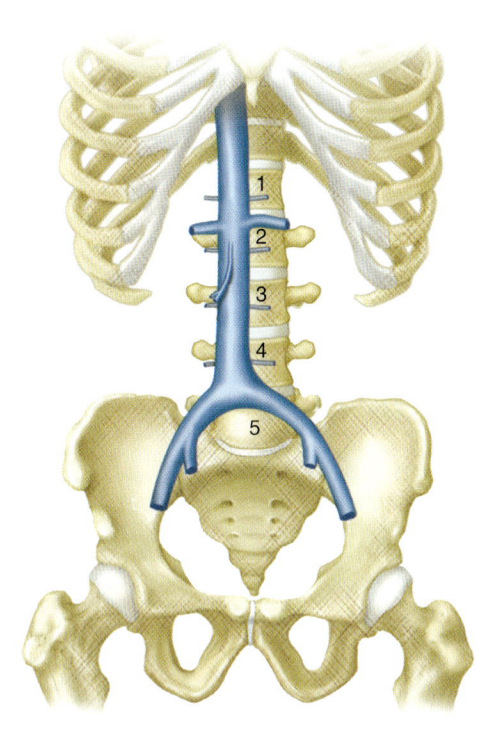

■ **FIGURE 76-5** Location of major vena caval inflow relative to the spine. The renal veins typically join the inferior vena cava between L1 and L2. The convergence of the common iliac veins most often occurs at the L5 vertebral level.

Inflow to the Inferior Vena Cava

Inferior vena caval inflow comes from the lumbar, renal, right inferior phrenic, right testicular or ovarian, right suprarenal, and hepatic veins (Fig. 76-6).

Lumbar Veins

Four paired lumbar veins drain the lumbar musculature and vertebral plexus into the IVC.[2] The lumbar veins are interconnected via longitudinal veins called the ascending lumbar veins, which allow for communication between the common iliac and iliolumbar veins. The ascending lumbar veins join the subcostal veins and form the azygos vein on the right and the hemiazygos vein on the left.

Renal Veins

The renal veins are located anterior to the renal arteries and drain into the IVC. The left renal vein is the longer than the right and courses between the aorta and origin of the SMV. The left renal vein receives blood from the left testicular or ovarian, left inferior phrenic, and left suprarenal veins.

Right Inferior Phrenic Vein

The right inferior phrenic vein follows the course of the inferior phrenic artery and drains into the IVC. Note the different drainage pattern from the left inferior phrenic vein, which drains into the left renal vein.

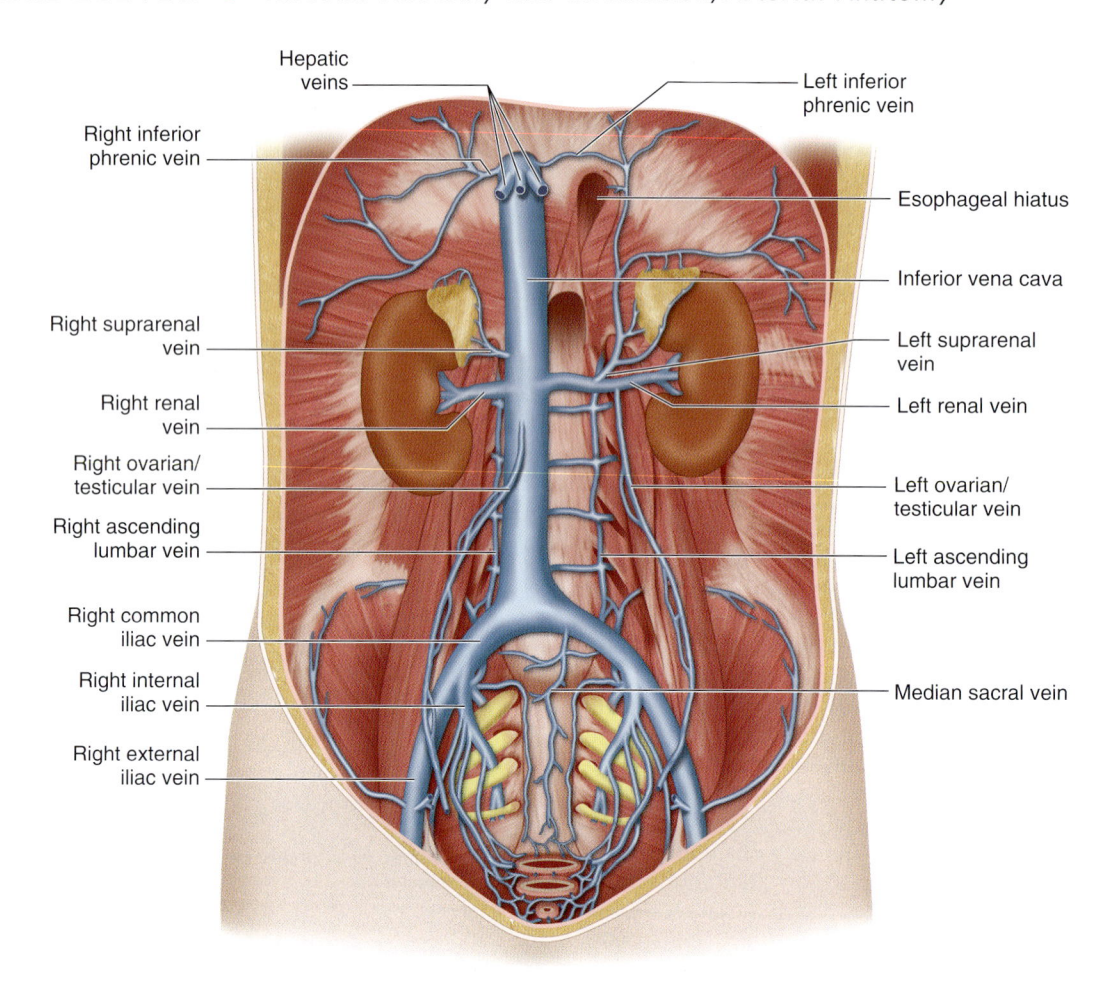

FIGURE 76-6 Abdominal and pelvic venous return to the inferior vena cava. The abdominal and pelvic organs, except for the kidneys, have been removed to reveal the inferior vena cava and inflowing veins.

Right Testicular or Ovarian Vein

The right testicular or ovarian vein drains into the IVC. The left testicular or ovarian vein drains into the left renal vein. Of note, valves are present in the testicular veins and are occasionally present in the ovarian veins. Incompetent valves may account for cases of pelvic congestion syndrome and male infertility (see subsequent discussion).

Right Suprarenal Vein

The right suprarenal vein drains directly into the IVC, superior to the orifice of the right renal vein. The left suprarenal vein drains into the left renal vein.

Hepatic Veins

The hepatic veins drain the liver parenchyma and do not contain valves. Most commonly, three large hepatic veins emerge from the posterior superior surface of the liver—the right, middle, and left hepatic veins. In addition, small accessory veins drain directly into IVC. These additional veins generally drain the caudate lobe or the right hepatic lobe.

The right hepatic vein courses along the right hepatic fissure, dividing the right lobe into anterior (segments V and VIII) and posterior segments (VI and VII).

The middle hepatic vein courses along the middle hepatic fissure and divides the right hepatic lobe from the left hepatic lobe. This vein drains the medial aspect of the left lobe (segment IV) and large portions of the right lobe (segment V). The middle and left hepatic veins typically unite into a common trunk before draining into the IVC.

The left hepatic vein drains the left lateral segments (segments II and III) and also receives tributaries from segment IV. As noted, this vein generally unites with the middle hepatic vein proximal to draining into the IVC.

The caudate lobe vein directly drains the caudate lobe into the IVC.

Normal Variants

In a large study by Koc and associates, 58.2% of patients demonstrated conventional hepatic vein anatomy.[3] The most common hepatic vein variant (prevalence, 69.5% to 86%) is the presence of an inferior right hepatic vein (IRHV), which usually drains segment VI. Knowledge of the number of IRHVs and the distance from each IRHV to the IVC is important for surgical planning prior to liver transplantation. In cases of rare multiple IRHVs, some of these veins drain into the adrenal vein before joining the IVC (prevalence, 0.2%). Another common variant found in 65% to 85% of individuals is a common trunk for the middle and left hepatic veins proximal to their insertion into the IVC.

The presence of multiple renal veins is the most common renal vein variation, with a prevalence of 9% to 30%. A circumaortic renal vein is the most common variation of the left renal vein, with a prevalence of 8.7%. Less commonly, a retroaortic left renal vein is noted, with a prevalence of 2.1%.[3]

In studies of IVC development in the domestic cat, variations of vena caval anatomy were classified based on abnormal regression or persistence of the various embryonic veins.[8] In total, 14 theoretical variations were suggested. We will discuss the most common variations of the IVC.

A left-sided IVC forms when the left supracardinal vein persists, seen in 0.2% to 0.5% of the population. In most cases, a true left IVC unites with the left renal vein, crosses to the right side (anterior to the aorta), and joins the right renal vein, forming a normal right-sided IVC. This variation is important to recognize to prevent misdiagnosis (e.g., adenopathy) and for planning endovascular procedures in the abdomen.

In 0.2% to 0.3% of the population, a double IVC forms when both supracardinal veins persist. The two vessels often demonstrate marked size discrepancy. This anomaly should be suspected in the setting of recurrent pulmonary embolism following single IVC filter placement. In most cases, the left-sided IVC joins the left renal vein, which drains in a conventional fashion into the right-sided IVC. In 0.6% of individuals, there is azygos continuation of the IVC, with absence of the hepatic segments of the IVC.[8]

Differential Considerations

Budd-Chiari Syndrome

First discussed in 1845 by George Budd and then further detailed by Hans Chiari in 1899, the Budd-Chiari syndrome (BCS) is marked by obstruction of the hepatic venous outflow system. Hepatic venous obstruction can occur at any level from the small hepatic veins to the caval-atrial junction. Although BCS is rare, it can be a life-threatening condition that can present relatively acutely or develop gradually. Causes of BCS can be primary (e.g., congenital membranous webs), or secondary (e.g., polycythemia vera, paroxysmal nocturnal hemoglobinuria, hypercoagulable states, oral contraceptive–induced, or pregnancy).[9] In approximately two thirds of cases, no cause can be established.

Classically, BCS manifests with the triad of abdominal pain, ascites, and hepatomegaly. However, patients often present with portal hypertension, variceal bleeding, and jaundice. The clinical presentation varies based on the chronicity of the disease process. In acute BCS, patients may experience sudden onset of right upper quadrant pain. In chronic BCS, hepatomegaly, ascites, and portal hypertension become evident.

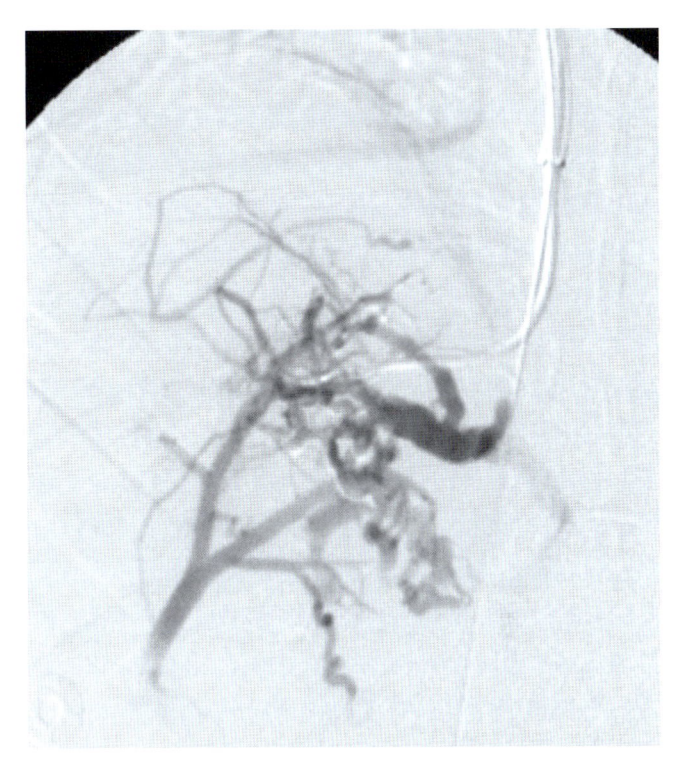

■ **FIGURE 76-7** Hepatic venogram in Budd-Chiari syndrome. This digitally subtracted fluoroscopic image from a right hepatic venogram demonstrates tortuous intrahepatic venous collaterals from hepatic venous outflow obstruction.

Diagnosis may be achieved more invasively through hepatic venography or hepatic biopsy. Other noninvasive modalities such as magnetic resonance imaging (MRI), ultrasound, and CT serve as excellent diagnostic tools.[10-12] With CT and MRI, signs of BCS include ascites, hepatomegaly, nonvisualization of the hepatic veins, and prominent enhancement of the central liver, with enhancement of the periphery only on delayed images. The caudate lobe is usually spared because it drains separately into the inferior vena cava.

Multiple intrahepatic and extrahepatic venous collateral pathways exist in the setting of BCS.[13,14] The intrahepatic collateral veins serve to divert blood away from the occluded hepatic veins, draining into a patent hepatic or systemic vein. These veins usually are curvilinear and tortuous, often resembling a comma—hence, the "comma sign" of BCS (Fig. 76-7).

Treatment options for BCS include medical managements of symptoms, surgery, transjugular intrahepatic portosystemic shunt formation, or liver transplantation.

Nutcracker Syndrome

First described in 1950, the nutcracker syndrome results from compression of the left renal vein between the aorta and the superior mesenteric artery (SMA).[15]

Typically, the space in which the left renal vein courses anterior to the aorta and deep to the SMA is 4 to 5 mm and is maintained by retroperitoneal fat and the third segment of the duodenum. The pathophysiology of this syndrome is not completely understood; however, if the

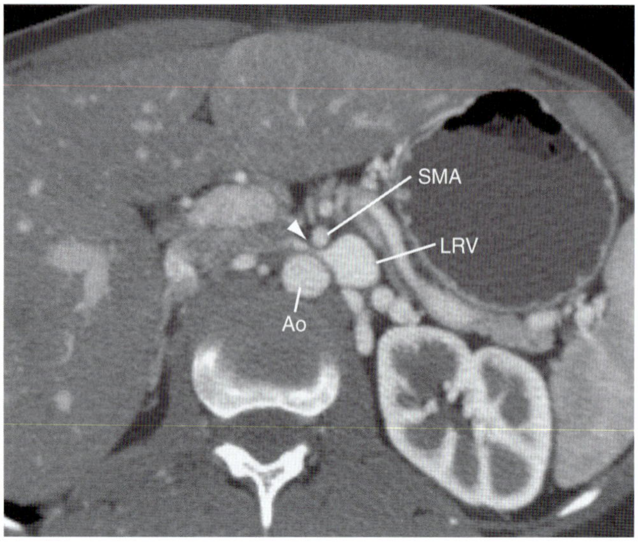

FIGURE 76-8 Nutcracker syndrome. This axial CT image demonstrates severe narrowing of the left renal vein as it passes between the superior mesenteric artery and aorta (*arrowhead*). Ao, aorta; LRV, left renal vein; SMA, superior mesenteric artery.

aortomesenteric angle is narrow (perhaps because of abnormal SMA branching), left renal vein compression occurs (Fig. 76-8). Increased left renal vein pressures and surrounding venous collateral formation may be appreciated.[16] The syndrome typically occurs in young, previously healthy patients. The most common clinical presentation is hematuria in the absence of renal pathology and presence of gonadal varices. Hematuria may be caused by rupture of congested renal vein tributaries into the renal collecting system. Diagnostic modalities include CT, ultrasound, and venography, with pressure gradient measurements obtained between the left renal vein and IVC. Treatment options include surgical intervention or minimally invasive intravascular stent placement.[17]

PELVIS: SYSTEMIC VENOUS CIRCULATION

General Anatomic Descriptions

The systemic venous drainage of the pelvis primarily flows through the common iliac veins and their tributaries. The right and left common iliac veins merge at the level of the fifth lumbar vertebra to form the IVC.

Detailed Description of Specific Areas

Common Iliac Veins

The common iliac veins are formed by the union of the internal (hypogastric) and external iliac veins anterior to the sacroiliac joint.[1,2] Typically, the right common iliac vein is shorter than the left and is positioned posteriorly and laterally to the corresponding artery. The left common iliac vein is positioned at first on the medial aspect of the corresponding artery but then courses posterior to the artery, and can be compressed between the spine and the artery (see later, "May-Thurner Syndrome").

External Iliac Veins

The external iliac vein is the continuation of the common femoral vein at the level of the inguinal ligament. On the right, it is first medial and then posterior to the corresponding artery. On the left, the vein runs medial to the corresponding artery (Fig. 76-9). The tributaries of each external iliac vein include the inferior epigastric, deep circumflex iliac, and pubic veins.

The inferior epigastric vein courses along the corresponding artery, draining into the external iliac vein about 1.25 cm above the inguinal ligament. Marching superiorly, the deep circumflex iliac vein joins the external iliac vein about 2 cm above the ligament, whereas the pubic vein serves as the conduit between the obturator veins and external iliac vein.

Internal Iliac Veins

The internal iliac vein is situated medial to the corresponding artery and, at the pelvic brim, joins the external iliac vein to form the common iliac vein. Tributaries of each internal iliac vein have often been separated into three groups.

The first group includes tributaries that originate outside the pelvis and includes the superior and inferior gluteal, internal pudendal, and obturator veins. The second group includes the lateral sacral veins, which lie anterior to the sacrum. The final group includes tributaries originating in visceral venous plexuses and includes the middle rectal, vesical, uterine, and vaginal veins.

Group 1: Venous Origin Outside the Bony Pelvis

The superior gluteal veins receive tributaries from the buttock and enter the pelvis through the greater sciatic foramen. The inferior gluteal veins drain the upper portion of the posterior thigh and enter the pelvis through the greater sciatic foramen. The internal pudendal veins begin in the deep veins of the penis and prostatic venous plexus in the male and the uterovaginal plexus in the female (Figs. 76-10 and 76-11). These veins course alongside the corresponding artery to form a single vein draining into the internal iliac vein. The internal pudendal veins also receive tributaries from the urethral bulb, perineal, and inferior rectal veins.

The obturator vein enters the pelvis through the superior aspect of the obturator foramen. It is typically positioned between the ureter and the internal iliac artery as it drains into the internal iliac vein.

Group 2: Lateral Sacral Veins

The lateral sacral veins accompany the corresponding arteries on the anterior surface of the sacrum and drain into the paravertebral and internal iliac veins. Note that the median sacral veins run alongside the median sacral artery anterior to the sacrum before merging into a single vein, which usually joins the left common iliac vein.

FIGURE 76-9 Venous drainage of the female pelvis, anterior view. The pelvic organs have been removed to highlight the complex venous drainage of the pelvis.

Group 3: Venous Origin in Visceral Plexuses

The rectal venous plexus is positioned around the rectum and communicates with the vesical plexus (in males) and the uterovaginal plexus (in females; Fig. 76-10). The plexus consists of an internal submucosal portion and external muscular portion. At the anal canal, the plexus is composed of veins with longitudinal orientation, which are prone to become varicose, resulting in internal hemorrhoids. The internal portion of the plexus drains into the superior rectal vein and also communicates with the external portion.

The external portion of the plexus has various drainage sites. The most inferior aspect of the external rectal plexus is drained by the inferior rectal veins into the internal pudendal vein. The middle portion is drained by the middle rectal vein, which itself drains into the internal iliac vein. The most superior portion of the external rectal

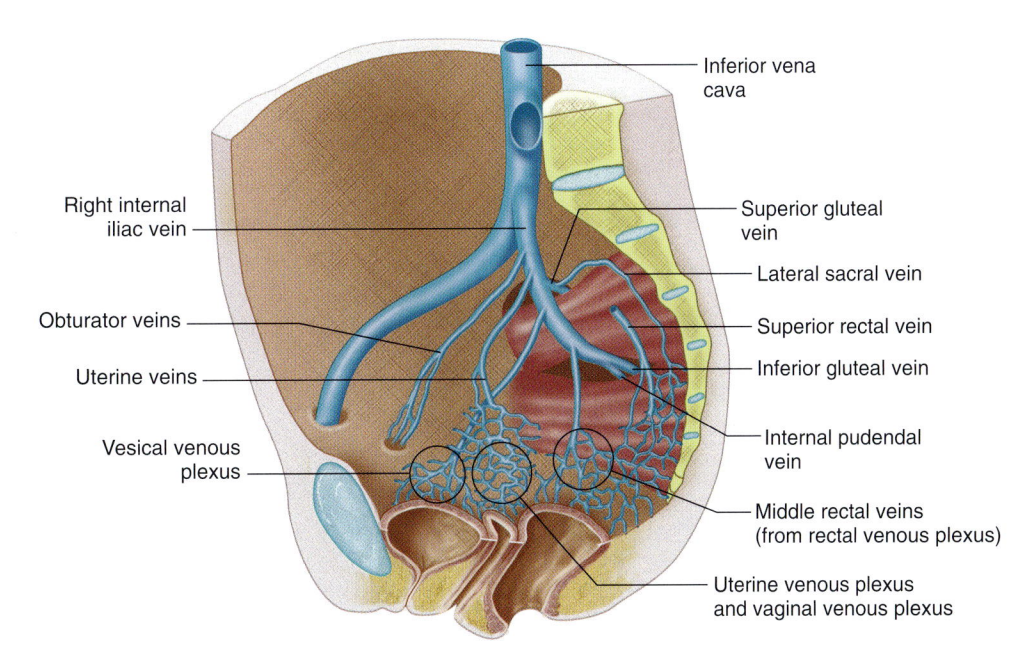

FIGURE 76-10 Lateral view of the venous drainage of the female pelvis. The right pelvic veins are depicted, emphasizing the venous plexuses of the bladder, female genitalia, and rectum.

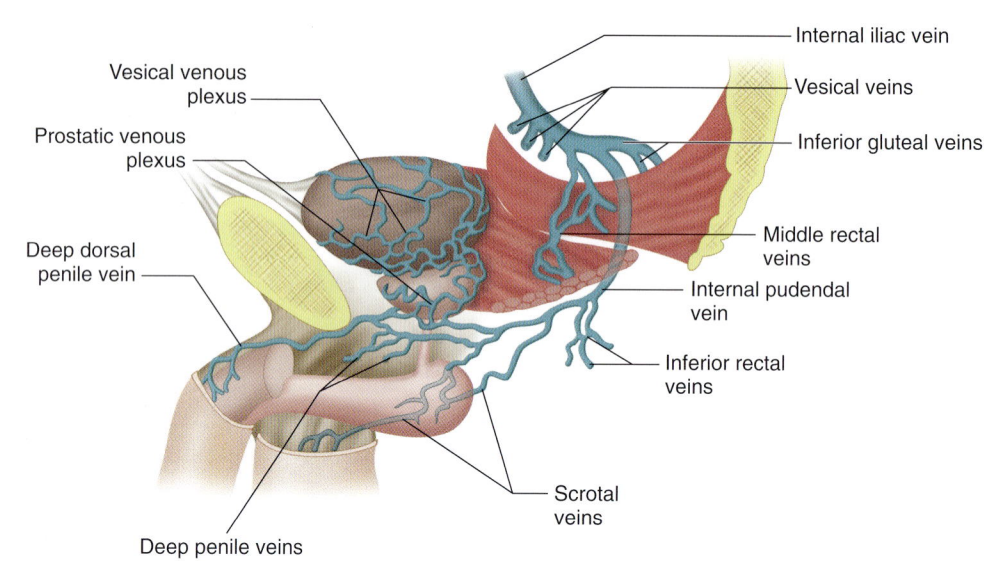

FIGURE 76-11 Lateral view of the venous drainage of the male pelvis. The male venous plexuses for the genitalia, bladder, and rectum are depicted.

plexus drains into the superior rectal vein, which ultimately drains into the inferior mesenteric vein, a tributary of the portal venous system. This communication between the systemic and portal venous systems allows for portosystemic collaterals in the setting of portal hypertension.

The pudendal plexus receives the deep dorsal vein of the penis and branches from the bladder and prostate. This plexus communicates with the vesical plexus and subsequently the internal pudendal vein. There are venous communications between the prostatic plexus and pudendal plexus.

The dorsal veins of the penis are composed of superficial and deep veins. The superficial vein drains the prepuce and skin of the penis into the external pudendal vein. The deep vein drains the glans penis and corpora cavernosa into the prostatic venous plexus and communicates with the internal pudendal veins.

The vesical venous plexus is situated on the inferior aspect of the bladder and at the base of the prostate. It communicates with the prostatic venous plexus in males and the vaginal venous plexus in females.

The uterine plexus communicates with the ovarian and vaginal plexuses and is drained by a pair of uterine veins into the internal iliac vein. The vaginal plexus communicates with the uterine, vesical, and rectal plexus and is drained by the vaginal veins into the internal iliac veins.

Normal Variants

Developmental anomalies of the IVC may result in variability in pelvic venous outflow, although relatively rarely.

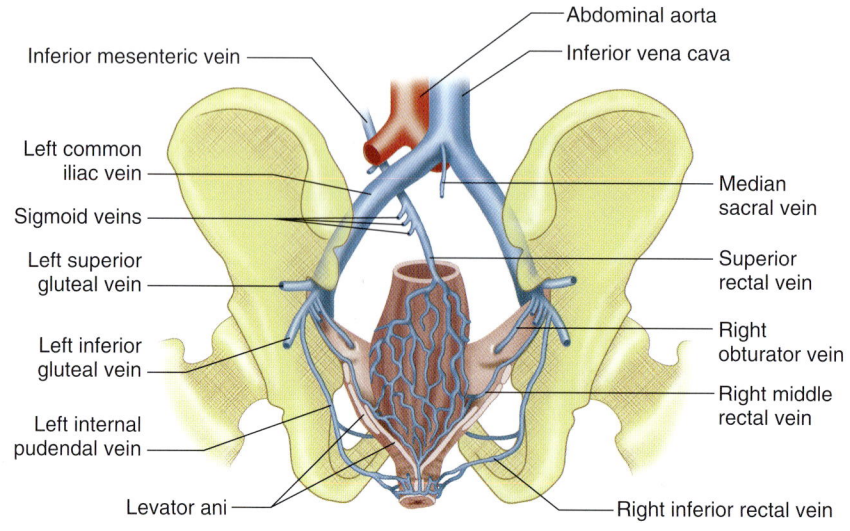

FIGURE 76-12 Posterior view of rectal venous drainage.

On occasion, the left common iliac vein has been seen to ascend into the abdomen, receive the left renal vein, and subsequently cross anterior to the aorta to join the inferior vena cava.[3]

Differential Considerations

May-Thurner Syndrome

May-Thurner syndrome (also known as iliac vein compression syndrome, Cockett syndrome, iliocaval compression syndrome, or pelvic venous spur) is characterized by obstruction of the left common iliac vein related to compression by the overlying right common iliac artery.[1] The mechanism of obstruction is caused by the physical entrapment of the vein between the artery and the spine or by extensive intimal hypertrophy of the vein resulting from the chronic pulsatile force of the anteriorly situated common iliac artery.

Following examination of 430 cadavers in 1957, May and Thurner described iliac compression syndrome and documented decreased venous flow resulting from intimal changes.[18] They theorized that the intimal changes resulted from continual compression of the left common iliac vein by the right common iliac artery. The transmitted arterial pulsation may cause opposing venous walls to contact, resulting in endothelial irritation and subsequent proliferation. This may explain the formation of intraluminal webs or spurs within the iliac vein, sometimes visualized using intravascular ultrasound. Sequelae of venous compression include reduction of venous outflow and deep vein thrombosis of the left iliofemoral system (Fig. 76-13). Other symptoms include leg swelling, varicosities, chronic venous stasis ulcers, and symptomatic pulmonary emboli.

The true prevalence of this disorder is unknown. May-Thurner syndrome is estimated to occur in 2% to 5% of patients undergoing evaluation for lower extremity venous disorders. Approximately 70% to 87% of cases are in females typically around 40 years of age. Early diagnosis of common iliac vein obstruction is important for prognosis. Iliac venography is the optimal diagnostic test because venous compression may be visualized in conjunction with pressure gradient measurements to determine the hemodynamic significance of the compression. Surrounding venous collaterals may be seen on iliac venography, either via conventional angiography or contrast-enhanced CT.

Treatment options for May-Thurner syndrome include endovascular thrombolysis followed by venous dilation and endovascular stent placement at the site of compression. Surgical options, including left common iliac vein bypass, may also be considered.

Pelvic Congestion Syndrome

It is estimated that 30% of all women experience chronic pelvic pain (CPP) during their lifetime. CPP is an enigmatic condition defined as noncyclic pain lasting longer than 6 months. Many different entities can result in CPP, including endometriosis, fibroids, and pelvic congestion syndrome (PCS). The medical literature suggests that 30% of chronic pelvic pain symptoms are caused by PCS.

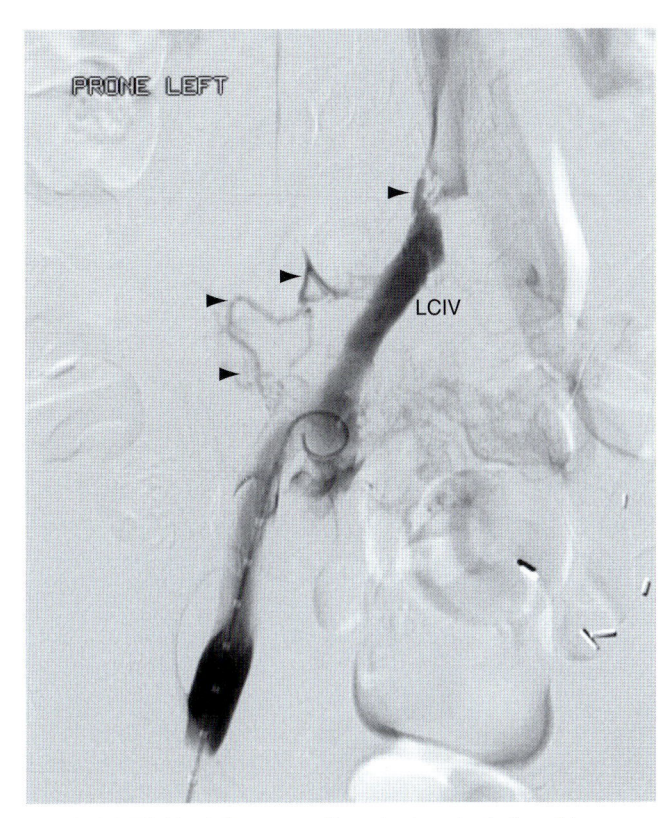

FIGURE 76-13 Left common iliac vein thrombosis from May-Thurner syndrome. This digitally subtracted fluoroscopic image from a selective contrast injection of the left common iliac vein demonstrates a thrombus near the confluence with the inferior vena cava (*large arrowhead*). There are numerous small venous collateral pathways to bypass the obstructed vein (*small arrowheads*).

PCS relates to ovarian and pelvic vein dilation, resulting in blood pooling and pain in the region of the uterus, ovaries, and vulva (Fig. 76-14). This condition is analogous to varicoceles in men.[19] PCS is prevalent in women younger than 45 years of age (child-bearing age). The syndrome is uncommon in nulliparous women. It has been estimated that 15% of women between the ages of 20 and 50 years have pelvic varicose veins, although not all experience noncyclic pain. PCS has also been associated with polycystic ovaries and hormonal dysfunction. Symptoms of PCS include dull pain in the lower abdomen and lower back that increases on standing or with pregnancy, dyspareunia, dysmenorrhea, vaginal discharge, irritable bladder, and varicose veins involving the legs.

The diagnosis of PCS is challenging because other causes of CPP must be excluded. Useful modalities for the diagnosis of PCS include pelvic venography, MRI, ultrasound, and CT.[20] On ultrasound, the ovarian and pelvic varicoceles are dilated and often tortuous, with surrounding dilated pelvic venous plexuses demonstrating reversed (caudal) flow within the ovarian vein. CT may demonstrate varicose veins surrounding the uterus and ovaries, with retrograde filling of dilated ovarian veins from the left renal vein in the arterial phase. Of note, dilated pelvic veins larger than 5 mm in diameter is consistent with varices and larger than 8 mm in diameter is suggestive of PCS, given the appropriate clinical symptomatology.

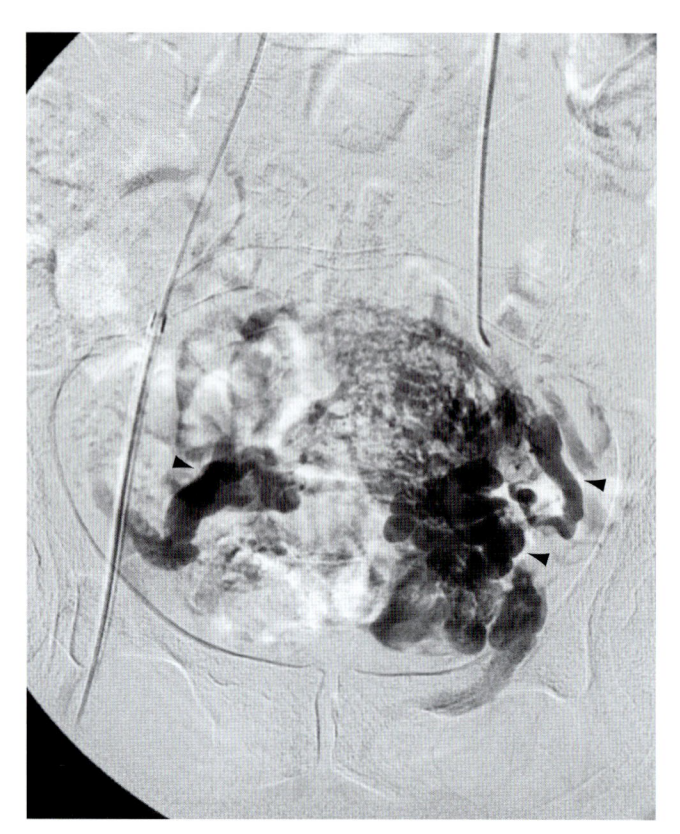

FIGURE 76-14 Dilated pelvic veins in pelvic congestion syndrome. This digitally subtracted fluoroscopic image from contrast injection of pelvic veins in a patient with pelvic pain demonstrates numerous tortuous and dilated varicose veins (*arrowheads*).

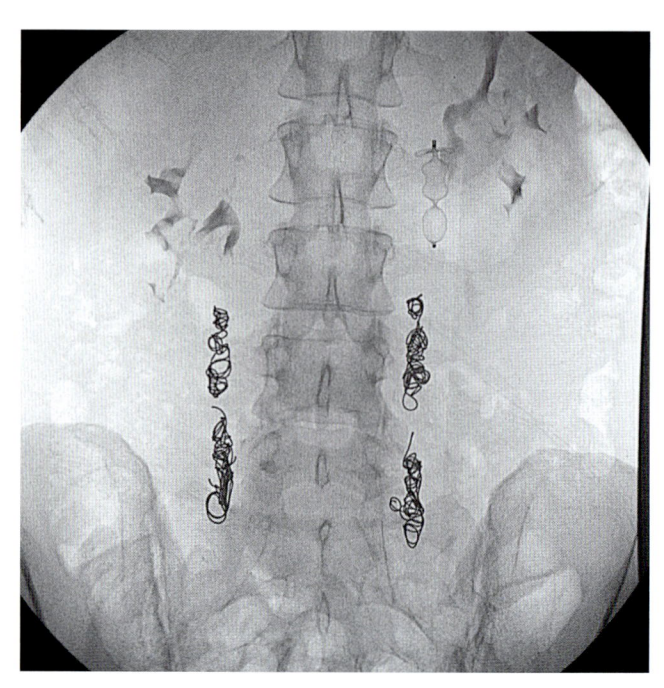

FIGURE 76-15 Coil embolization of bilateral ovarian veins to treat pelvic congestion syndrome. This fluoroscopic image was obtained after coil embolization of the ovarian veins, reducing flow to the previously visualized pelvic varices.

Numerous treatment options are available for PCS.[21] Medical management with analgesics and hormones can be effective, but does not cure the underlying cause of pain. Surgical options including hysterectomy and bilateral salpingo-oophorectomy have been performed. However, minimally invasive options include endovascular embolization of the varicose ovarian veins using metallic coils (Fig. 76-15). This procedure is reportedly successful in terms of symptom relief in approximately 85% to 95% of patients.

Pertinent Imaging Considerations

Portal venous imaging requires attention to the timing of contrast injections for optimal opacification of portal structures, whether via conventional angiography, CT, or MRI.

During catheter angiography, indirect portograms are often well visualized in the late venous phases following injection of the celiac or superior mesenteric arteries. Alternatively, direct portography is possible from several approaches. Catheterization of the portal vein itself can be achieved from a transhepatic or transjugular route. The spleen may be injected with contrast, a technique known as splenoportography, or an umbilical vein may be large enough for direct puncture and subsequent portal imaging.

Cross-sectional portal venous imaging is commonly performed during multiphase CT or MR abdominal studies. The optimal portal venous scan delay from the time of peripheral venous contrast injection is routinely calculated using a timing bolus, in which peak aortic enhancement is determined. When additional scanning parameters such as contrast injection rates are taken into consideration, the results are often spectacular, with minimal contamination from nonportal vascular opacification (Fig. 76-16). CT portography combining catheter angiography with direct superior mesenteric arterial injections has emerged as a superior means to evaluate the portal venous system. In particular, when there is clinical concern for PV thrombosis or portal hypertension, CT portography may be invaluable for surgical planning.

KEY POINTS

- Venous vasculature in the abdomen and pelvis is highly variable.
- Blood returning from the mesenteric, gastroduodenal, pancreatic, splenic, and cystic veins passes through the portal venous system.
- Abdominal systemic drainage is mediated by the inferior vena cava.
- Numerous portosystemic and portoportal anastomoses exist, which can play an important role in the clinical manifestations of portal hypertension.
- Imaging of the portal venous system can be achieved indirectly through arterial portography or directly through transhepatic portography, splenoportography, or catheterization and injection of the umbilical vein.

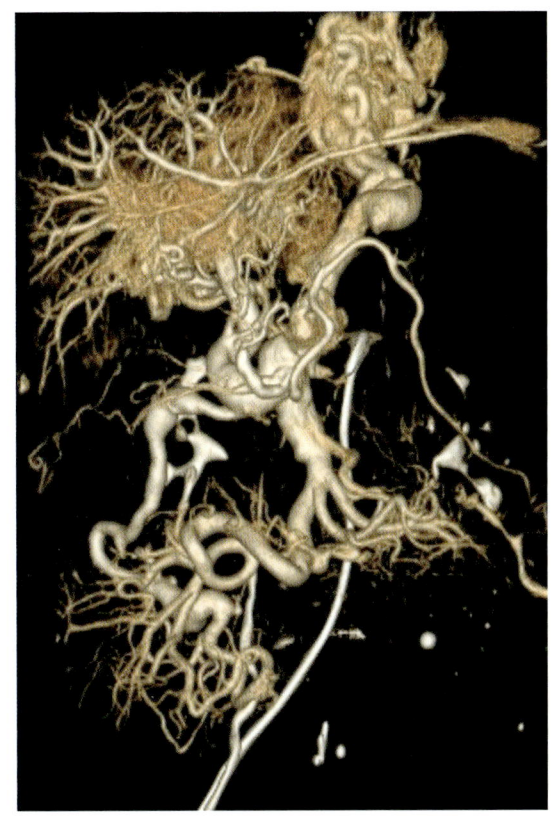

■ **FIGURE 76-16** CT portography. This is a volume-rendered CT image of the portal venous system following injection of contrast agent directly into the superior mesenteric artery. Imaging was delayed until the portal venous system was optimally opacified.

SUGGESTED READINGS

Gallego C, Velasco M, Marcuello P, et al. Congenital and acquired anomalies of the portal venous system. Radiographics 2002; 22:141-159.

Kang HK, Jeong YY, Choi JH, et al. Three-dimensional multi-detector row CT portal venography in the evaluation of portosystemic collateral vessels in liver cirrhosis. Radiographics 2002; 22:1053-1061.

Koc Z, Ulusana S, Oguzkurta L, Tokmaka N. Venous variants and anomalies on routine abdominal multi-detector row CT. Eur J Radiol 2007; 61:267-278.

Minniti S, Visentini S, Procacci C. Congenital anomalies of the venae cavae: embryological origin, imaging features and report of three new variants. Eur Radiol 2002; 12:2040-2055.

REFERENCES

1. LaBerge J, Gordon RL, Kerlan RK Jr, Wilson MW. Interventional Radiology Essentials. Philadelphia, Lippincott Williams & Wilkins, 2000.
2. Uflacker R. Atlas of Vascular Anatomy: An Angiographic Approach. Philadelphia, Lippincott Williams & Wilkins, 1997.
3. Koc Z, Ulusan S, Oguzkurt L, Tokmak N. Venous variants and anomalies on routine abdominal multi-detector row CT. Eur J Radiol. 2007; 61:267-278.
4. Bharati S, Lev M. Congenital anomalies of the pulmonary veins. Cardiovasc Clin 1973; 5:23-41.
5. Graf O, Boland GW, Kaufman JA, et al. Anatomic variants of mesenteric veins: Depiction with helical CT venography. AJR Am J Roentgenol 1997; 168:1209-1213.
6. Gines P, Cardenas A, Arroyo V, Rodes J. Management of cirrhosis and ascites. N Engl J Med 2004; 350:1646-1654.
7. Thompson ABR, Shaffer EA. First Principles of Gastroenterology: The Basis of Disease and an Approach to Management. Mississauga, Ontario, Canada, Astra Pharma 1994.
8. Bass JE, Redwine MD, Kramer LA, et al. Spectrum of congenital anomalies of the inferior vena cava: cross-sectional imaging findings. Radiographics 2000; 20:639-652.
9. Fitzgerald O, Fitzgerald P, Cantwell D, Mehigan JA. Diagnosis and treatment of the Budd-Chiari syndrome in polycythaemia vera. Br Med J 1956; 2: 1343-1345.
10. Vogelzang RL, Anschuetz SL, Gore RM. Budd-Chiari syndrome: CT observations. Radiology 1987; 163:329-333.
11. Erden A, Erden I, Karayalçin S, Yurdaydin C. Budd-Chiari syndrome: evaluation with multiphase contrast-enhanced three-dimensional MR angiography. AJR Am J Roentgenol 2002; 179:1287-1292.
12. Mathieu D, Vasile N, Menu Y, et al. Budd-Chiari syndrome: dynamic CT. Radiology 1987; 165:409-413.
13. Cho O-K, Koo J-H, Kim Y-S, et al. Collateral pathways in Budd-Chiari syndrome: CT and venographic correlation. AJR Am J Roentgenol 1996; 167:1163-1167.
14. Takayasu K, Mizuguchi Y, Muramatsu Y, et al. Neovasculature of benign thrombus of the inferior vena cava demonstrated by

computed tomography during hepatic arteriography, mimicking a small hepatocellular carcinoma. Jpn J Clin Oncol 2003; 33:44-46.
15. Takebayashi S, Ueki T, Ikeda N, Fujikawa A. Diagnosis of the nutcracker syndrome with color Doppler sonography: correlation with flow patterns on retrograde left renal venography. AJR Am J Roentgenol 1999; 172:39-43.
16. Kim SH, Cho SW, Kim HD, et al. Nutcracker syndrome: diagnosis with Doppler US. Radiology 1996; 198:93-97.
17. Park YB, Lim SH, Ahn JH, et al. Nutcracker syndrome: intravascular stenting approach. Nephrol Dial Transplant 2000; 15:99-101.
18. Cil BE, Akpinar E, Karcaaltincaba M, Akinci D. Case 76: May-Thurner syndrome. Radiology 2004; 233:361-365.
19. Koc Z, Ulusan S, Tokmak N, et al. Double retroaortic left renal veins as a possible cause of pelvic congestion syndrome: imaging findings in two patients. Br J Radiol 2006; 79:152-155.
20. Park SJ, Lim JW, Ko YT, et al. Diagnosis of pelvic congestion syndrome using transabdominal and transvaginal sonography. AJR Am J Roentgenol 2004; 182:683-688.
21. Ganeshan A, Upponi S, Hon LQ, et al. Chronic pelvic pain due to pelvic congestion syndrome: the role of diagnostic and interventional radiology. Cardiovasc Intervent Radiol 2007; 30:1105-1111.

CHAPTER 77

Venous Anatomy of the Extremities

Jeffrey C. Hellinger

The upper and lower extremity peripheral venous systems comprise three main types of veins—superficial, deep, and perforating. The superficial and deep subsystems are defined by major and tributary veins linked by the perforating veins as well as venous networks (plexi), with the goal of directing all venous blood return into the deep system in peripheral, mid, or central extremity venous segments. Wide variability is often encountered in this anatomy, with origins for both systems beginning peripherally at the hand or foot for the upper and lower extremities, respectively. The superficial veins are located subcutaneously within the superficial fascia. The deep veins are located intramuscularly, deep to the superficial fascia, accompanying the extremity arteries (venae comitans). Perforating veins cross the muscular fascial layer, typically bridging flow from superficial to deep veins. Valves function in superficial, deep, and perforating veins to keep blood flowing antegrade and prevent blood flowing from the deep to superficial veins. Valves are more prevalent in the deep veins for both the upper and lower extremities.[1-5]

In general, the extremity veins are thin wall structures with little to no elastic lamina, resulting in passive distensible conduits with large compliance. The deep veins, however, inherit strength directly by having a greater degree of elastic lamina and indirectly by way of muscular contractions, countering gravity and central venous filling pressures to propagate blood flow toward the central veins and heart.[5-6] The well-orchestrated anatomic physiology between the deep venous pumps, valves, and perforating veins becomes particularly apparent in the setting of elevated central venous pressures, incompetent valves, immobility, obstructed central or deep extremity veins, or a combination of these conditions.

UPPER EXTREMITY

Veins for the upper extremity direct blood flow from the hand, wrist, forearm, upper arm, and shoulder to the ipsilateral central thorax veins and ultimately the superior vena cava. In the hand, forearm, and upper arm, the superficial system functions as the principal means for venous drainage. As a result, the caliber of the superficial veins is generally larger than the deep veins. The major superficial veins of the hand, forearm, and upper arm exist as single structures and infrequently have accessory veins. The smaller deep veins occur in pairs, alongside the respective arteries. All upper extremity venous drainage transitions to the deep system at the axilla, with a single main venous channel crossing the costoclavicular space into the thoracic central venous system. Within the axillae and thorax, the major deep veins occur as single structures, accompanying the adjacent artery.[7-10]

Superficial Veins of the Upper Extremity

In the hand, veins and their tributaries can be divided into dorsal and palmar (volar) subsystems, with dominant drainage through the dorsal subsystem, enforced through the valves. Communication, however, occurs between both, at the digital, metacarpal, and wrist levels.

The dorsal veins include the dorsal digital veins, dorsal metacarpal veins, and dorsal venous network (plexus). Dorsal digital veins form by coalescence of dorsal distal digital venules and venous arches, and extend bilaterally along the length of dorsum of the fingers. They communicate at multiple levels via small oblique venous connections. The dorsal digital veins from the ulnar aspect of the index finger, radial aspect of the fifth finger, and both sides of the third and fourth fingers, along with intercapitular veins between the digits, drain into three superficial dorsal metacarpal veins. The metacarpal veins, in turn, feed into the dorsal venous network, which is located at the mid and base of the metacarpals (Fig. 77-1).[9]

Along the radial aspect of the hand, the dorsal venous network receives dorsal veins of the thumb and dorsal vein of the radial aspect of the index finger and continues with cephalad drainage, forming the cephalic vein. Along the ulnar aspect of the hand, the dorsal venous plexus

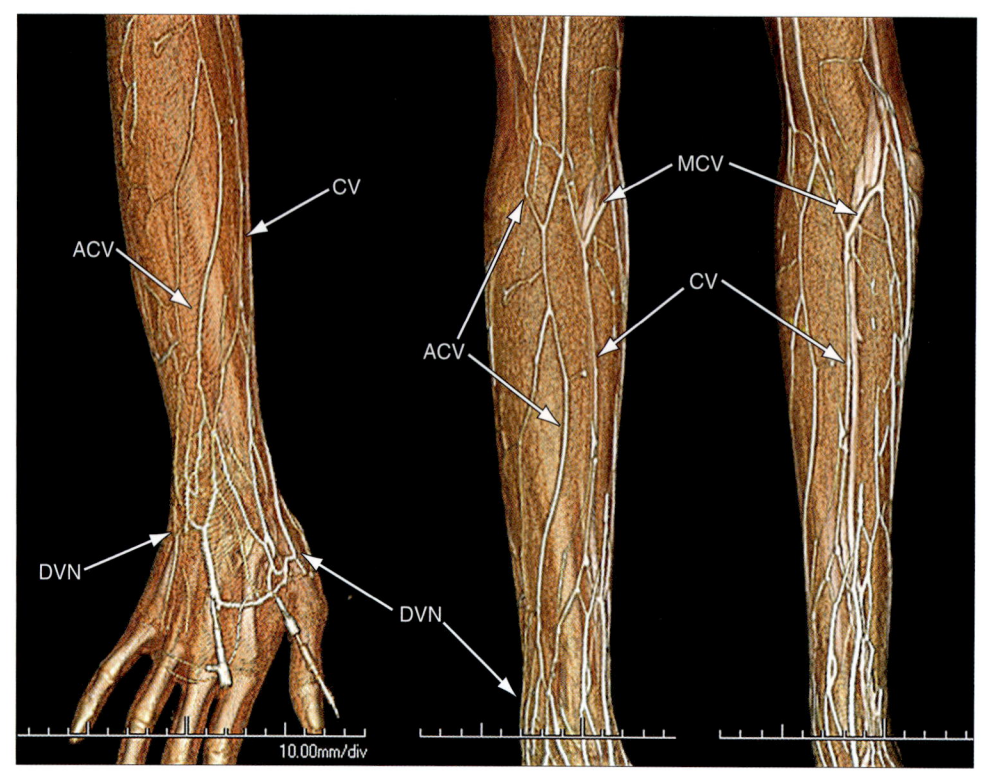

FIGURE 77-1 Direct CT venogram of the right hand forearm. ACV, accessory cephalic vein; CV, cephalic vein; DVN, dorsal venous network; MCV, median cubital vein.

receives the dorsal vein from the ulnar aspect of the fifth finger and continues with cephalad drainage, forming the basilic vein. The median portion of the network variably may drain to the mid-forearm cephalic vein via a communicating (accessory) vein (Fig. 77-2).[8]

The palmar veins of the hand include palmar digital veins and palmar venous plexus. Palmar digital veins parallel the dorsal digital veins, along the palmar surface. There are three routes of drainage for the palmar digital veins. Two are within the superficial system and include the palmar venous network and dorsal digital and metacarpal veins. The palmar venous network lies at the thenar and hypothenar eminences and drains primarily into the median antecubital vein of the forearm. Drainage into the dorsal digital veins and dorsal metacarpal veins occurs by way of intercapitular veins in the digital web spaces at the metacarpal heads. The third route is into the common and metacarpal palmar veins of the palmar deep system.[2,3]

In the forearm, main superficial venous drainage occurs via the cephalic, basilic, and median antecubital veins (Fig. 77-3). The cephalic and basilic veins ascend to the elbow along the radial and ulnar aspects of the forearm, respectively, with continuation into the upper arm. The cephalic vein, basilic vein, or both, may form the dominant drainage route into the upper arm.

The cephalic vein transitions from the dorsal to volar surfaces in the distal third of the forearm. Along its course in the forearm, the cephalic vein receives dorsal and volar tributaries. Just proximal to the elbow, the cephalic vein gives off the median basilic vein, which ascends obliquely over the volar surface, crosses the antecubital fossa, and drains into the basilic vein. The cephalic vein then crosses the ventrolateral aspect of the elbow, in a groove between the brachioradialis and biceps brachii muscles. An accessory cephalic vein is often present, with variable morphology. Most commonly, it arises from the dorsal venous plexus or from a dorsal forearm tributary network and courses along the radial aspect of the forearm, lateral to the cephalic vein. It drains into the cephalic vein below the elbow. Alternatively, the accessory cephalic vein may form a venous bridge between cephalic vein segments below and above the elbow. The accessory cephalic vein often supplies a dorsal oblique branch, forming a second level of communication between the cephalic and basilic veins within the forearm.[8]

The basilic vein in the forearm primarily courses along the dorsal surface, receiving tributary drainage from the respective region. It transitions to the volar surface in the proximal forearm, just below the elbow, where it receives the median cubital vein. The basilic vein crosses the ventromedial antecubital fossa, between the biceps brachii and pronator teres.

The median antecubital vein ascends along the ventromedial surface of the forearm with tributary drainage into the basilic vein or median cubital vein. Alternatively, the median antecubital may divide into two branches, one that drains into the basilic vein (median basilic vein) and the other into the cephalic (median cephalic) vein.

In the upper arm, the basilic and cephalic veins are the major routes for superficial venous drainage, with ultimate runoff into the deep system (Figs. 77-4 and 77-5). The basilic vein is typically larger than the cephalic vein, coursing medial to the biceps brachii. The smaller cephalic vein courses lateral to the biceps brachii. The basilic vein

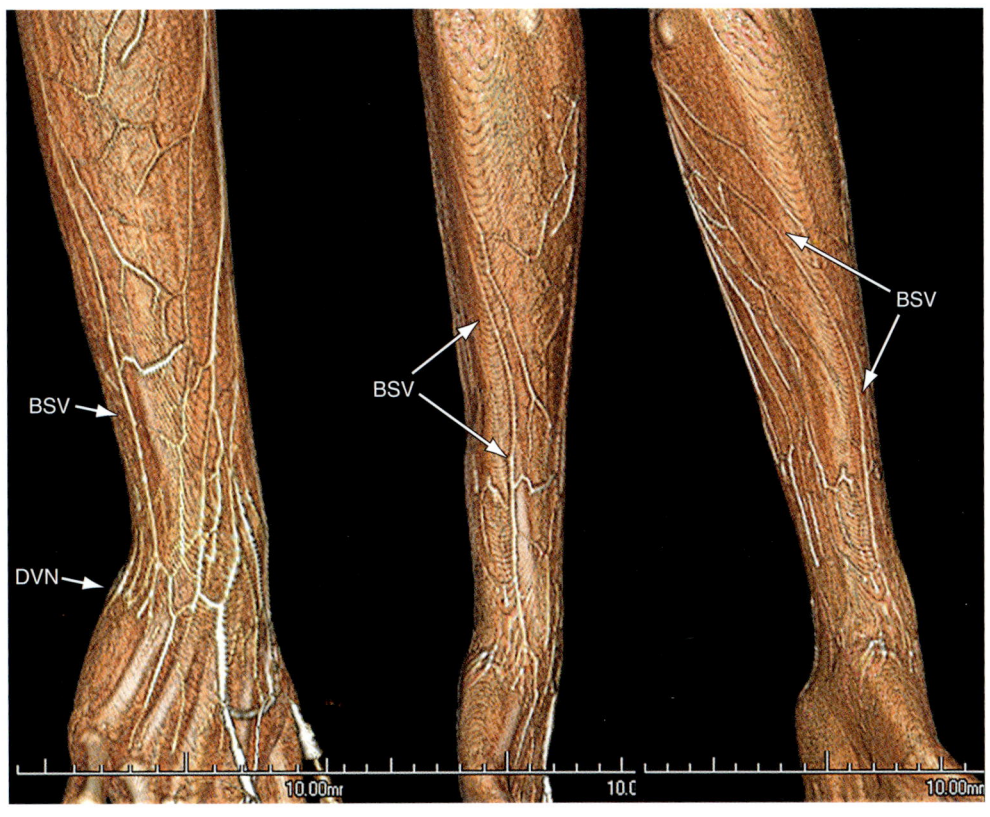

■ **FIGURE 77-2** Direct CT venogram of the right forearm. BSV, basilic vein; DVN, dorsal venous network.

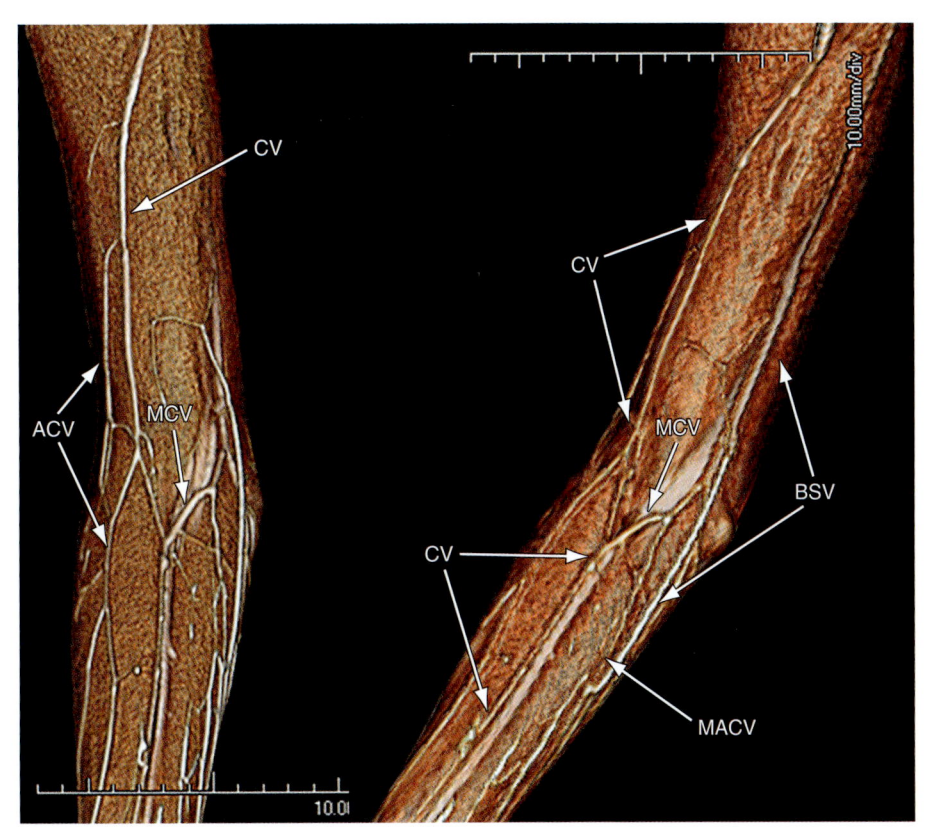

■ **FIGURE 77-3** Direct CT venogram at the right elbow. ACV, accessory cephalic vein; BSV, basilic vein; CV, cephalic vein; MACV, median antecubital vein; MCV median cubital vein.

FIGURE 77-4 Direct CT venogram of the right upper arm and central thorax. AXV, axillary vein; BRV$_L$, brachial vein, lateral; BRV$_M$, brachial vein, medial; BSV, basilic vein; CV, cephalic vein.

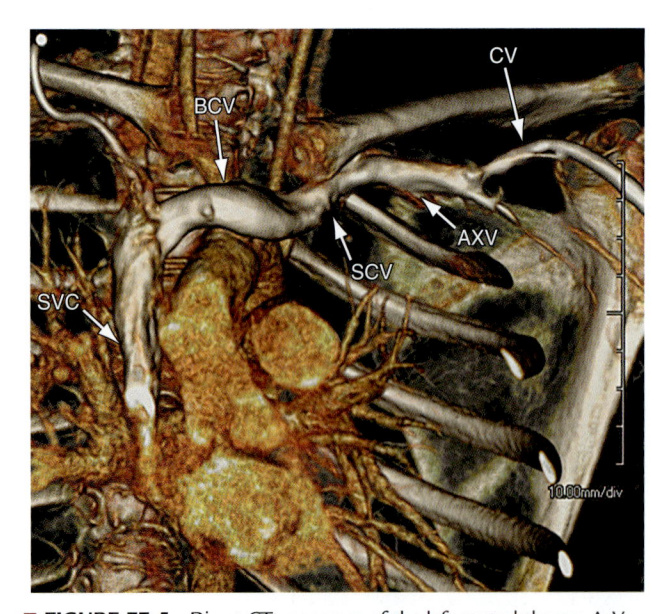

FIGURE 77-5 Direct CT venogram of the left central thorax. AxV, axillary vein; BCV, brachiocephalic vein; CV, cephalic vein; SCV, subclavian vein; SVC, subclavian vein.

ascends initially within the superficial fascia, but then perforates the deep fascia at the midarm level. Subsequent to this, the basilic vein courses along the medial aspect of the brachial artery until the inferior margin of the teres major muscle, at which point it joins the brachial vein (deep system) to form the axillary vein (deep system). The cephalic vein ascends completely within biceps superficial fascia, entering the infraclavicular fossa between the pectoralis major and deltoid muscles.[8] It then courses medial, in the clavipectoral triangle, entering the cranial aspect of the central axillary vein with acute angulation, below the clavicle. The cephalic veins typically have a valve just proximal to its junction with the axillary vein.

Deep Veins of the Upper Extremity

In the hand, the superficial and deep palmar venous arches form the most peripheral major venous conduits of the upper extremity deep system. Usually duplicated with interconnections between each individual pair of arches, the palmar arches parallel the arterial arches and receive drainage corresponding to the respective arterial arch branches. These include common palmar digital veins for the superficial palmar venous arch and palmar metacarpal veins for the deep venous arch. The palmar metacarpal veins also communicate with the dorsal metacarpal veins via perforating veins, forming a means for the deep palmar venous arch to drain the dorsal metacarpal veins as well. The superficial palmar arch courses to the ulnar side of the wrist and drains into ulnar veins, whereas the deep palmar venous arch courses to the radial side of the wrist and drains into radial veins. Branches from the deep palmar arches and the proximal ulnar and radial veins form a carpal venous plexus, which drains into the volar and dorsal interosseous veins.[4]

In the forearm, the radial, ulnar, and interosseous paired deep veins ascend on either side of the respective companion arteries (Fig. 77-6). The ulnar veins are typically larger in caliber because there is more dominant

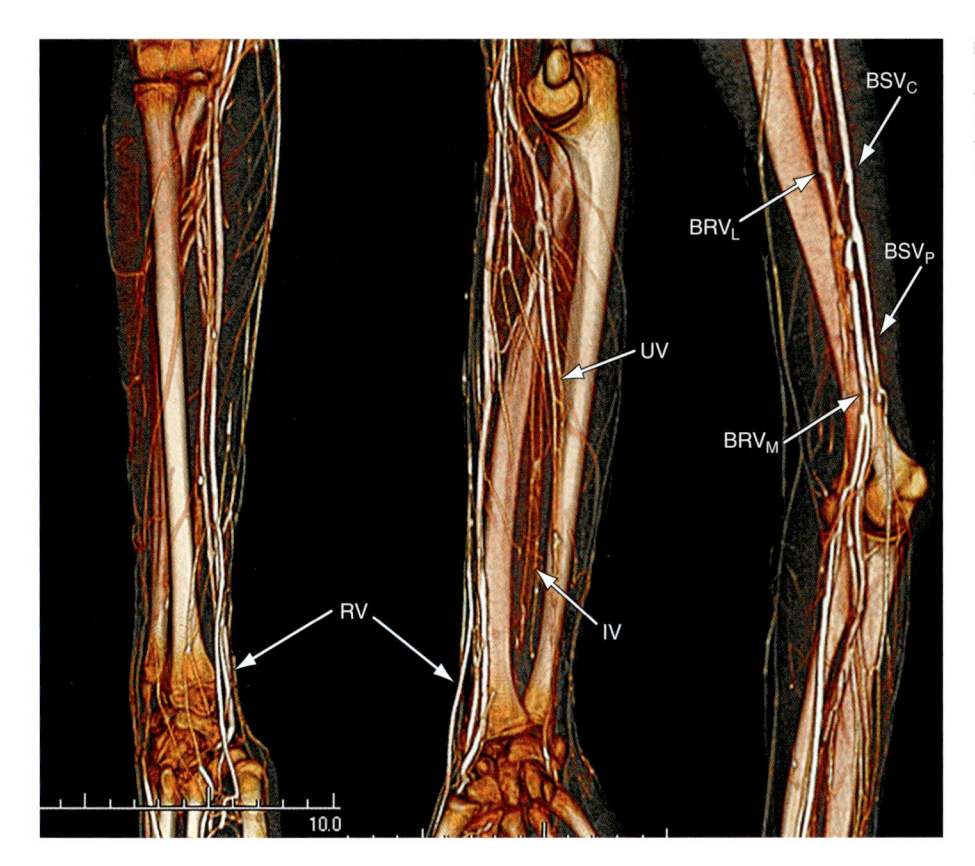

FIGURE 77-6 Direct CT venogram of the left forearm and elbow. BRV_L, brachial vein, lateral; BRV_M, brachial vein, medial; BSV_C, basilic vein, central; BSV_P, basilic vein, peripheral; IV, interosseous vein; RV, radial vein; UV, ulnar vein.

drainage through the superficial palmar venous arch. Proximal to the elbow, the interosseous veins drain into the ulnar veins, which then give off tributary veins to the median cubital vein. At the elbow, the radial and ulnar veins coalesce to form the paired deep brachial veins (see Fig. 77-6).

In the upper arm, the paired brachial veins ascend on either side of the brachial artery, receiving small venous branch tributaries. At the level of the teres major, the brachial veins coalesce with the basilic vein to form the axillary vein. The medial brachial vein may join the basilic vein prior to this junction. The axillary vein courses to the thoracic inlet as a single vein medial and caudad to the axillary artery. It crosses the first rib into the costoclavicular space, transitioning to the subclavian vein. In addition to the cephalic vein, the axillary vein receives venous tributaries corresponding to the axillary branch arteries (see Figs. 77-4 to 77-6).

Centrally in the thorax, deep venous drainage of the upper extremities occurs by way of the subclavian and brachiocephalic veins (see Fig. 77-6). The subclavian vein extends from the first rib to the level of the clavicular head, where it joins with the internal jugular vein to form the brachiocephalic vein. The subclavian vein lies anterior and caudad to the subclavian artery and courses posterior to the scalenus anterior. Important tributaries include the external jugular, anterior jugular, and dorsal scapular veins. The right and left thoracic ducts drain into the ipsilateral subclavian veins at the respective confluences with their internal jugular veins.[7,10]

The right and left brachiocephalic veins join together to form the superior vena cava, which then drains into the right atrium (see Fig. 77-6). The right brachiocephalic vein has a short vertical course and lies anterior and to the right of the brachiocephalic artery. The left brachiocephalic vein has a longer, horizontal oblique course, and lies anterior to the aortic arch branch arteries. Common brachiocephalic vein tributaries include the vertebral, internal mammary, inferior thyroid, and supreme intercostal veins.[7,10]

LOWER EXTREMITY

The lower extremity superficial and deep venous systems in the foot, leg, and thigh direct blood flow to the ipsilateral pelvic veins and ultimately to the inferior vena cava (Figs. 77-7 and 77-8). Similar to the upper extremity, both systems have an integrated relationship, linked by major and minor perforating veins as well as by tributary veins and networks at standard and variable levels.[1,5,11,12] Drainage ultimately transitions to the deep system at the groin. In distinction to the upper extremity, the deep system plays a more dominant role. In part, this is because of the greater dependence on deep intermuscular veins functioning as pumps to expel venous blood against gravity into the central venous system with each muscle contraction. The deep plantar veins of the foot and paired deep veins of the calf serve as the principle physiologic pumps to generate this flow (Figs. 77-9 and 77-10).[5,6] Valves are more numerous in the lower extremity and, overall, have a greater prevalence in the deep veins and in the more peripheral lower extremity venous segments. The lower extremity superficial system draining the subcutaneous tissues is distinguished from upper extremity counterparts

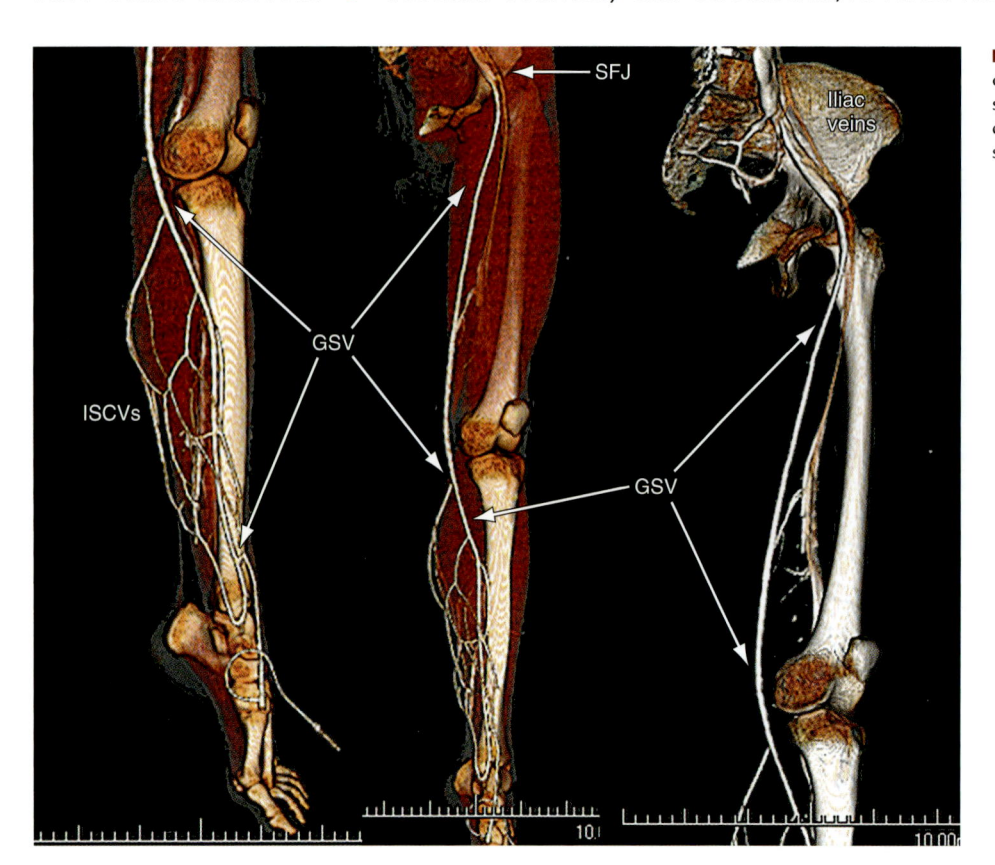

■ **FIGURE 77-7** Direct CT venogram of the left lower extremity. GSV, great saphenous vein; ISCVs, intersaphenous communicating veins; SFJ, saphenofemoral junction.

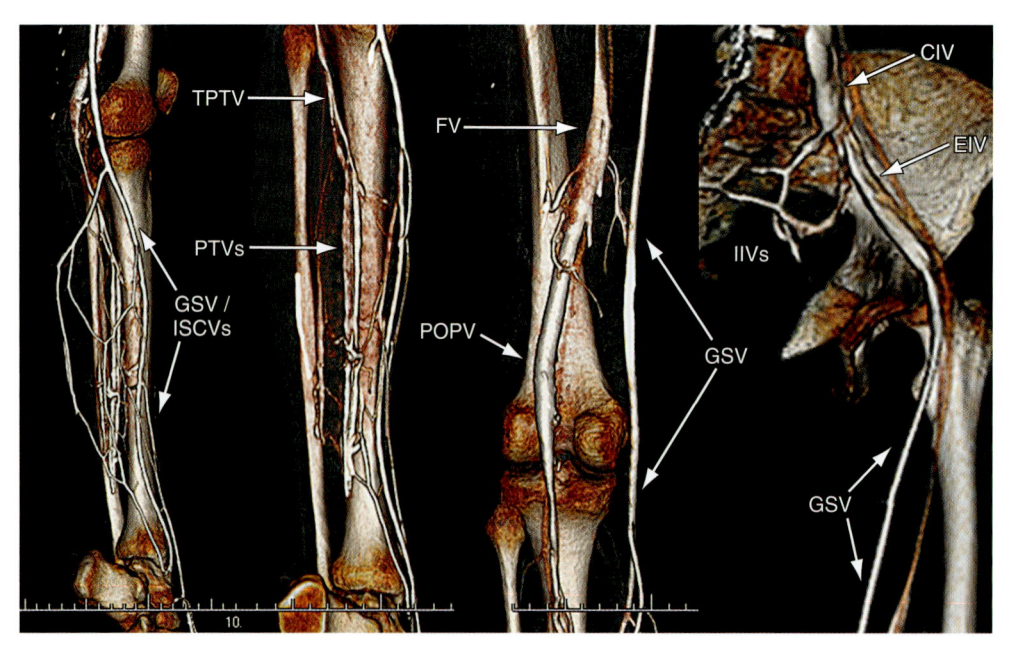

■ **FIGURE 77-8** Direct CT venogram of the left lower extremity. CIV, common iliac vein; EIV, external iliac vein; FV, femoral vein; GSV, great saphenous vein; IIVs, internal iliac veins; ISCVs, intersaphenous communicating veins; POPV, popliteal vein; PTV, posterior tibial vein; TPTV, tibioperoneal trunk vein.

in that the two major superficial veins, the great and small saphenous veins, are enveloped with their own saphenous fascia layer, forming the saphenous compartment. All other superficial tributary veins course between the superficial and muscular fascia layers.[11,12]

Superficial Veins of the Lower Extremity

In the foot, the superficial veins can be divided into two main subsystems, those for the dorsum of the foot and those for the plantar surface. Of the two, the dorsal

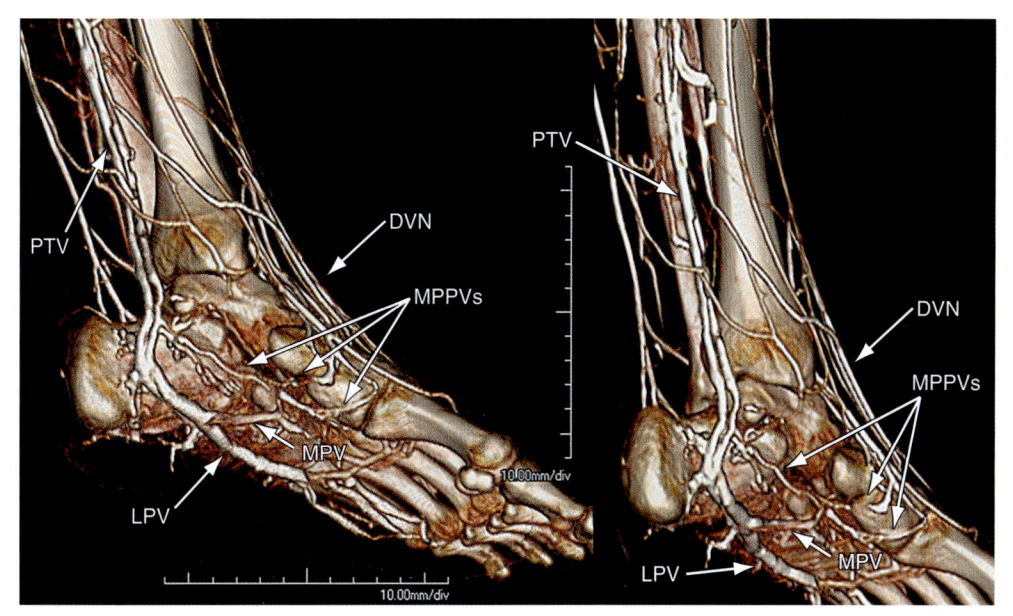

FIGURE 77-9 Direct CT venogram of the left lower extremity. DVN, dorsal venous network; LPV, lateral plantar vein; MPV, medial plantar vein; MPPVs, medial plantar perforating veins.

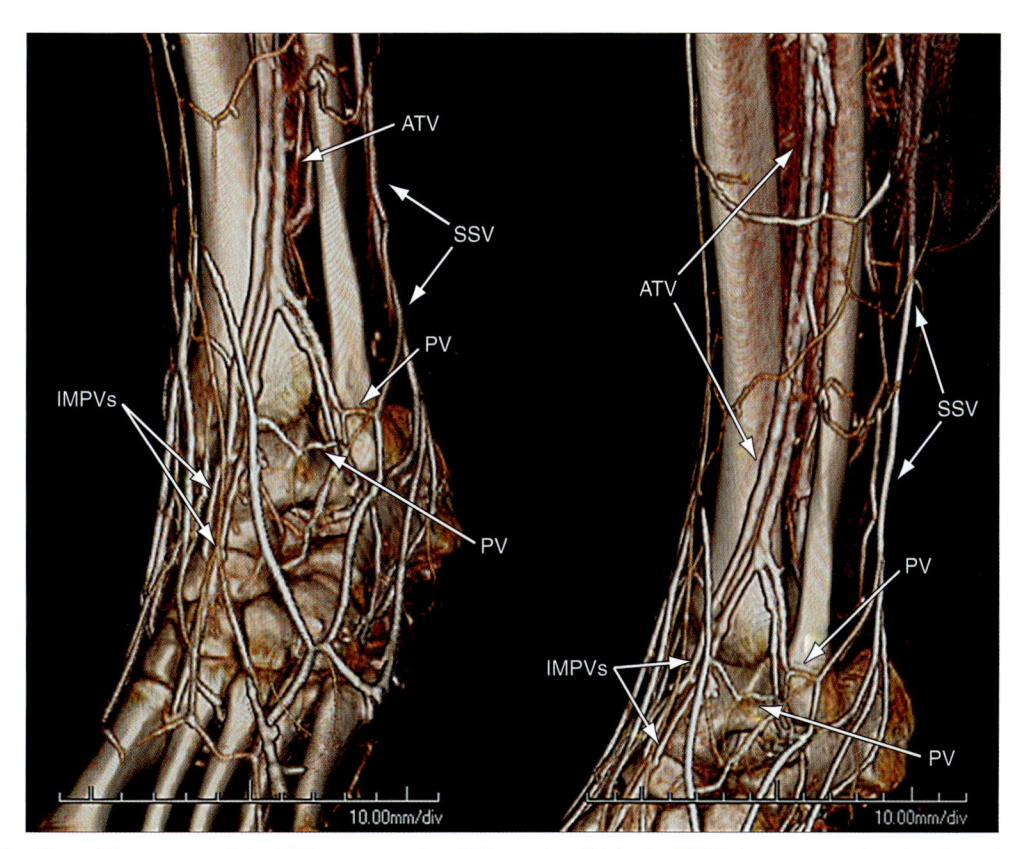

FIGURE 77-10 Direct CT venogram of the left lower extremity. ATV, anterior tibial vein; IMPVs, intermetatarsal perforating veins; PVs, perforating veins; SSV, short saphenous vein.

superficial veins function in a more dominant capacity, giving origin to the great and small saphenous veins. Beginning peripherally at the toes and extending centrally to the ankle, the superficial dorsal veins of the foot include the dorsal digital veins, dorsal metatarsal veins, dorsal venous arch, medial marginal vein, and lateral marginal vein, and dorsal venous network. All lie within the dorsal subcutaneous superficial fascia. The dorsal digital veins course along the lateral dorsal margins of the toes and converge in the webs between the toes to form the dorsal metacarpal veins. The dorsal metacarpal veins, in turn, feed into the dorsal venous arch (Fig. 77-11). The dorsal

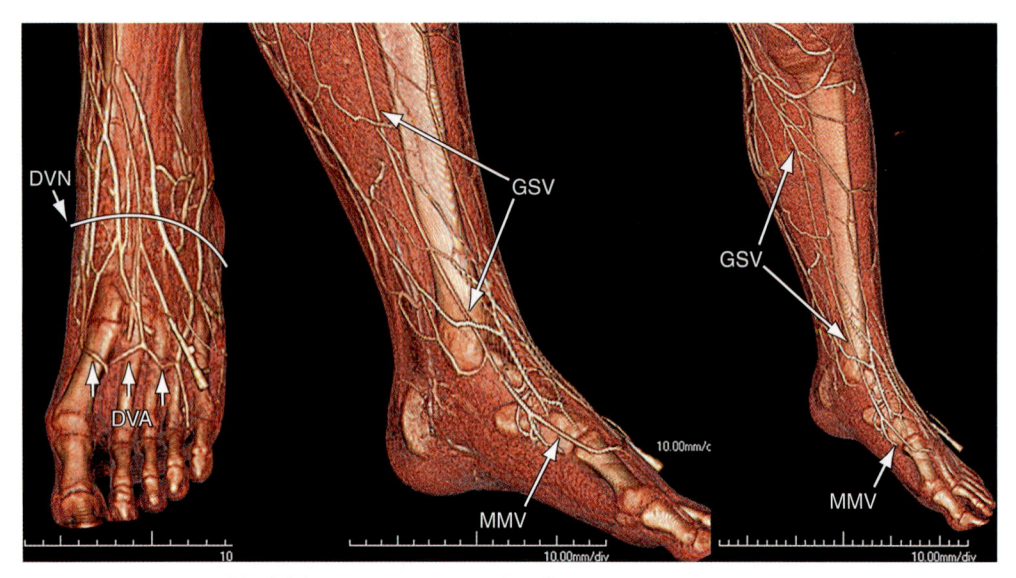

■ **FIGURE 77-11** Direct CT venogram of the left lower extremity. DVA, dorsal venous arch; DVN, dorsal venous network; GSV, great saphenous vein; MMV, medial marginal vein.

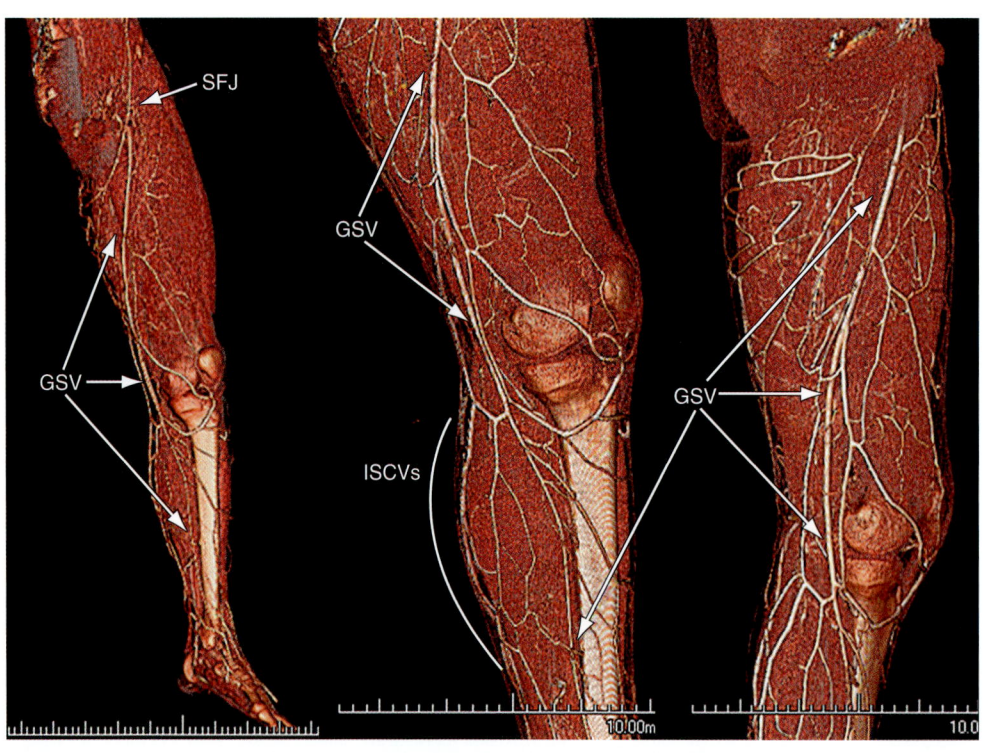

■ **FIGURE 77-12** Direct CT venogram of the left lower extremity. GSV, great saphenous vein; ISCVs, intersaphenous communicating veins; SFJ, saphenofemoral junction.

venous arch extends medially as the medial marginal vein and laterally as the lateral marginal vein. The medial marginal vein courses to the medial ankle, continuing as the great saphenous vein (Figs. 77-11 and 77-12). The lateral marginal vein courses along the lateral border of the foot to the ankle, where it continues as the small saphenous vein (Fig. 77-13). Central to the dorsal venous arch, the dorsal venous network receives small tributaries from the dorsal arch, dorsal superficial veins along the mid and basilar metatarsals and tarsals and, finally, plantar superficial veins (see Figs. 77-11 and 77-13). This network is continuous with the superficial dorsal veins of the lower leg and feeds tributaries into the medial marginal vein and the great saphenous vein.[11,12]

The plantar superficial veins of the foot form an intricate subcutaneous network of fine veins extending from the forefoot to the hind foot. They drain into the deep plantar veins via perforating vertical veins along the intermuscular septa and into the dorsal superficial veins via medial, lateral, and interdigitary communicating veins.[13]

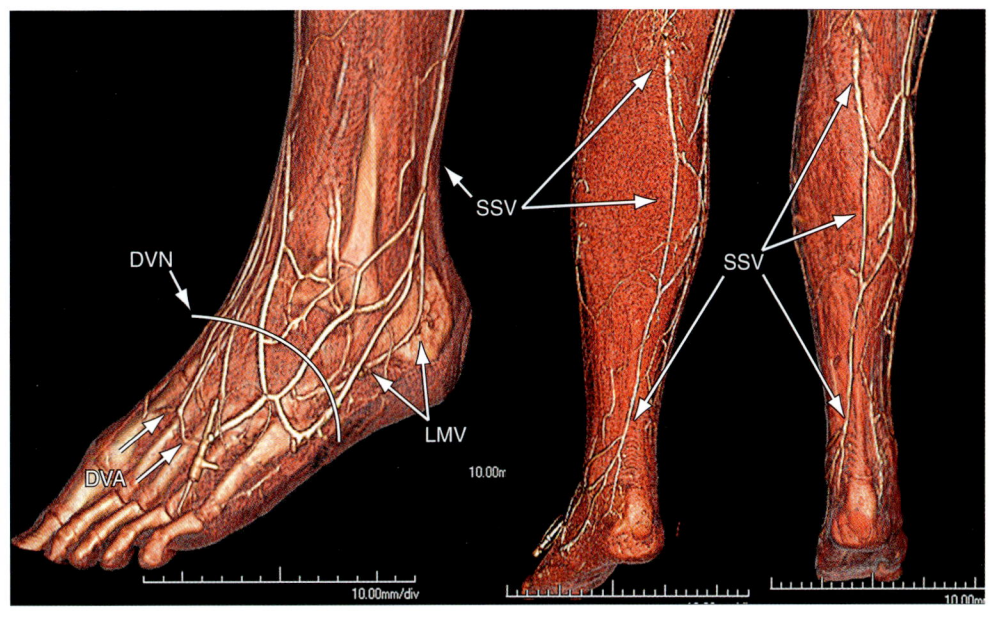

FIGURE 77-13 Direct CT venogram of the left lower extremity. DVA, dorsal venous arch; DVN, dorsal venous network; LMV, lateral marginal vein; SSV, short saphenous vein.

In the leg and thigh, the great and small saphenous veins are the principle, constant superficial veins. The great saphenous vein is present in both the leg and thigh, whereas the small saphenous vein most commonly only drains the calf. Communication between the great and small saphenous veins occurs in the leg via one or more intersaphenous oblique coursing veins.[11,12]

The great saphenous vein, continuing from its medial marginal vein origin, crosses anterior to the medial malleolus and ascends along the anteromedial aspect of the leg with the saphenous nerve (see Figs. 77-7, 77-11, and 77-12). At the knee, the great saphenous vein passes posteromedial to the medial tibial and femoral condyles and enters the thigh. In the thigh, the great saphenous vein courses anteromedially to just below the inguinal ligament, where it crosses the deep fascia at the saphenous vein opening and terminates in the anterior aspect of the femoral vein (saphenofemoral junction). Anterior and posterior accessory veins of the great saphenous vein run parallel to and are located anterior and posterior to the great saphenous vein, respectively. Both have tributary greater saphenous venous drainage in the leg and, ultimately, at the intervalvular great saphenous venous segment, just peripheral to the saphenofemoral junction. In addition to these accessory veins, a superficial accessory great saphenous vein may parallel the great saphenous vein more superficially in the leg and thigh. Tributary drainage at the intervalvular segment also includes the anterior and posterior circumflex veins of the thigh, superficial inferior epigastric veins of the lower abdominal-pelvic wall, superficial circumflex iliac veins of the lateral iliac region, and superficial external pudendal vein of the pubic and perineal regions (Fig. 77-14). The anterior and posterior circumflex veins may arise from the remnant lateral venous system, but the posterior circumflex vein may also arise from the small saphenous vein. Rather than running off into the great saphenous vein, the anterior and posterior circumflex veins may drain into the anterior and posterior accessory veins of the great saphenous vein, respectively.[11,12]

The small saphenous vein, continuing from its lateral marginal vein origin, crosses posterior to the lateral malleolus and ascends with the sural nerve, in the midline of the calf (see Fig. 77-13). Most commonly, the small saphenous vein enters the popliteal fossa, crossing the deep fascia between the heads of the gastrocnemius muscles to terminate in the popliteal vein (saphenopopliteal junction) within 5 cm above the knee joint. Less commonly, the small saphenous veins may drain into the popliteal vein more than 5 cm above the knee joint, may pierce the deep fascia below the fossa, or may terminate in veins other than the popliteal vein, including the great saphenous vein (via the posterior circumflex vein), superficial communicating veins, and deep thigh muscular perforators. Rather than terminating, the small saphenous vein may have axial (deep) extension or postaxial (dorsal) extension into the thigh. A superficial accessory small saphenous vein may be present, ascending parallel to the small saphenous vein, superficial to the saphenous compartment.[11,12]

Deep Veins of the Lower Extremity

In the foot, the deep veins include the plantar digital veins, plantar metatarsal veins, deep plantar arch, medial plantar veins, and lateral plantar veins. Plantar digital veins are located along the plantar surfaces of the digits, receiving drainage from the plantar plexuses of each digit. They converge into four deep plantar metatarsal veins in the intermetatarsal grooves, where there is also communication to the dorsal digital veins. The deep plantar metatarsal veins drain into the plantar venous arch, paralleling the plantar arterial arch. Outflow from the plantar venous arch occurs by way of the medial and lateral deep plantar

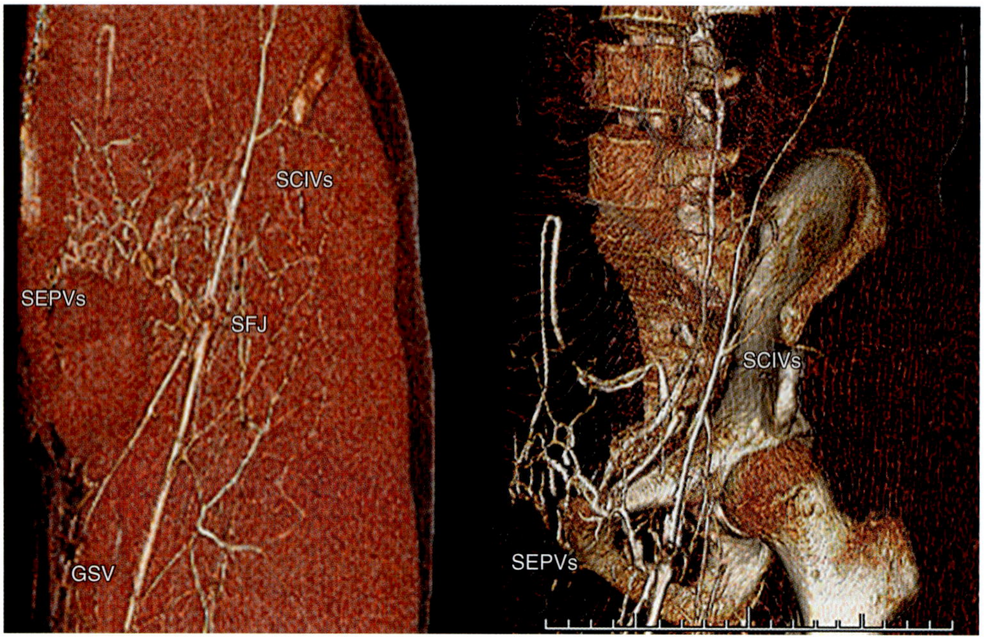

■ **FIGURE 77-14** Direct CT venogram of the left lower extremity. GSV, great saphenous vein; SCIVs, superficial circumflex iliac veins; SEPVs, superficial external pudendal veins; SFJ, saphenofemoral junction.

veins, which course along the medial and lateral inner plantar surfaces, respectively (see Fig. 77-9). The medial and lateral deep plantar veins function as the primary reservoir for the plantar venous pump, converging posterior to the medial malleolus to form the paired posterior tibial veins.[5,6,11]

The deep veins of the leg consist of three pairs of intermuscular veins and numerous intramuscular veins. The six intermuscular veins include the posterior tibial veins, peroneal veins, and anterior tibial veins (see Figs. 77-8 to 77-10). The posterior tibial and peroneal veins are located in the deep posterior compartment of the calf and the anterior tibial veins are located in the anterior compartment. From their plantar vein origins medial to the ankle, the posterior tibial veins course cephalad in the medial aspect of the deep posterior compartment, alongside the posterior tibial artery. The peroneal veins form at and drain the lateral aspect of the ankle and course in the central aspect of the deep posterior compartment, adjacent to the fibula, paired with the peroneal artery. Accessory deep venous drainage from the plantar veins may occur into the peroneal vein. The peroneal veins unite with the posterior tibial veins to form a common tibioperoneal vein. The anterior tibial veins are formed from the dorsal first intermetatarsal perforating veins, which travel with the dorsal pedis artery. Extending cephalad from the dorsal ankle level, the anterior tibial veins course in the anterior compartment lateral to the tibia along the interosseous membrane, with the corresponding anterior tibial artery. These veins drain the dorsum of the foot and anterior compartment muscles. At the inferior margin of the popliteal fossa, they cross the interosseous membrane and unite with the tibioperoneal trunk to form the popliteal vein. The popliteal vein courses cephalad across the knee joint into the thigh, traversing the adductor hiatus to become the femoral vein. In addition to draining the tibial and peroneal veins, the popliteal veins receive the sural veins and, as discussed, the short saphenous vein.[5,11]

Most deep intramuscular veins in the leg are minor tributaries into the paired deep intermuscular veins. The exception to this is the soleus and gastrocnemius deep veins. Both sural veins form from sinusoidal venous networks in the respective muscles of the superficial posterior compartment of the calf. The soleus veins may drain into the popliteal vein or adjacent muscular veins, whereas the gastrocnemius veins (medial gastrocnemius vein, lateral gastrocnemius, and intergemellar vein) may drain into the popliteal vein or short saphenous vein.[5,11]

In the thigh, the femoral and deep femoral veins comprise the major components of the deep system (see Fig. 77-8). Beginning as the continuation of the popliteal vein at the adductor hiatus, the femoral vein extends cephalad through the adductor canal, coursing alongside the femoral artery, initially posterolaterally, becoming medial to the femoral artery as it enters the femoral triangle in the groin. It receives small muscular venous tributaries primarily from the anterior and medial compartments. The deep femoral vein parallels the corresponding femoral profunda artery, coursing posterior and lateral to the femoral vein, between the anterior and medial compartments of the thigh, draining primarily posterior and lateral muscle groups. The medial and lateral circumflex veins typically drain into the femoral vein but, not uncommonly, may also drain into the deep femoral vein. In the proximal thigh, several centimeters below the inguinal ligament, the deep femoral vein joins with the femoral vein posteriorly to form the common femoral vein. After receiving the greater saphenous vein anteriorly, the common femoral vein crosses the inguinal ligament to become the external iliac vein.[5,11]

In the pelvis, the external iliac vein courses cephalad as a single vein, joining with the ipsilateral internal iliac vein to form the common iliac vein (see Fig. 77-8). Bilateral common iliac veins unite to form the inferior vena cava, which then traverses the abdomen and directs blood flow back to the right atrium. The right common iliac vein has a more direct path to the inferior vena cava, whereas the left crosses midline to reach the right-sided inferior vena cava. The right common iliac artery may cross the left common iliac vein, potentially resulting in anterior compression.[5,11]

Perforator Veins of Lower Extremity

The perforating veins in the lower extremity course obliquely across the deep fascia and communicate with unidirectional valves between the superficial and deep veins. Although these veins may have variable morphology and number, there are groups of perforating veins that maintain a consistent location. In the foot, these standard perforating veins include the dorsal foot intercapitular perforator veins and medial, lateral, and plantar foot veins, whereas in the ankle, they include the medial, lateral, and anterior perforating veins. In the leg, there are four main groups of constant perforators, corresponding to the anterior (anterior perforators), lateral (lateral perforators), deep posterior (paratibial and posterior tibial medial perforators), and superficial posterior (medial gastrocnemius, lateral gastrocnemius perforators, and intergemellar perforators) muscle compartments. The standard perforators at the knee include medial, lateral, infrapatellar, suprapatellar, and popliteal fossa perforating veins. In the thigh, the perforators are defined as medial, anterior, lateral, and posterior perforating veins. The medial perforators include the femoral canal and inguinal perforating veins. The anterior and lateral perforators are grouped according to the respective muscle compartments. The posterior perforators are divided into posteromedial thigh perforators (adductor muscles), sciatic perforators (posterior midline thigh), and posterolateral perforators (posterior muscle compartment). Perforating veins also occur in the gluteal muscles and are divided into superior, mid, and lower perforators.[5,11,12]

> **KEY POINTS**
> - The peripheral venous systems in the extremities are composed of three main types of veins: superficial, deep, and perforating.
> - In-depth knowledge of venous anatomy is vital for the interpretation of imaging examinations of peripheral veins.

SUGGESTED READINGS

Hellinger JC, Epelman M, Rubin GD. Upper extremity computed tomographic angiography: state of the art techniques and applications in 2010. Radiol Clin North Am 2010; 48:397-421.

Uhl JF, Gillot C. Embryology and three-dimensional anatomy of the superficial venous system of the lower limbs. Phlebology 2007; 22: 194-206.

REFERENCES

1. Thomson H. The surgical anatomy of the superficial and perforating veins of the lower limb. Ann R Coll Surg Engl 1979; 61:198-205.
2. Nystrom A, Friden J, Lister GD. Superficial venous anatomy of the human palm. Scand J Plast Reconstr Surg Hand Surg 1990; 24:121-127.
3. Nystrom A, von Drasek-Asher G, Lister GD. The palmer digital venous anatomy. Scand J Plast Reconstr Surg Hand Surg 1990; 24:113-119.
4. Nystrom A, Friden J, Lister GD. Deep venous anatomy of the human palm. Scand J Plast Reconstr Surg Hand Surg 1991; 25:233-239.
5. Tretbar LL. Deep veins. Dermatol Surg 1995; 21:47-51.
6. White JV, Katz ML, Cisek P, Kreithen BA. Venous outflow of the leg: anatomy and physiologic mechanism of the plantar venous plexus. J Vasc Surg 1996; 24:19-824.
7. Godwin JD, Chen JTT. Thoracic venous anatomy. Am J Roentgenol 1986; 147:674-684.
8. Hallock GG. The cephalic vein in microsurgery. Microsurgery 1993; 14:482-486.
9. Moss SH, Schwartz KS, von Drasek-Ascher G, et al. Digital venous anatomy. J Hand Surg Am 1985; 10:473-482.
10. Chasen MH, Charnsangavej C. Venous chest anatomy: clinical implications. Eur J Radiol 1998; 27:2-14.
11. Caggiati A, Bergan JJ, Gloviczki P, et al. Nomenclature of the veins of the lower limbs: an international interdisciplinary consensus statement. J Vasc Surg 2002; 36:416-422.
12. Uhl JF, Gillot C. Embryology and three-dimensional anatomy of the superficial venous system of the lower limbs. Phlebology 2007; 22:194-206.
13. Imanishi N, Kish K, Chang H, et al. Anatomical study of cutaneous venous flow of the sole. Plast Reconstr Surg 2007; 120:1906-1910.

PART TWELVE

Noninvasive Vascular Imaging Techniques

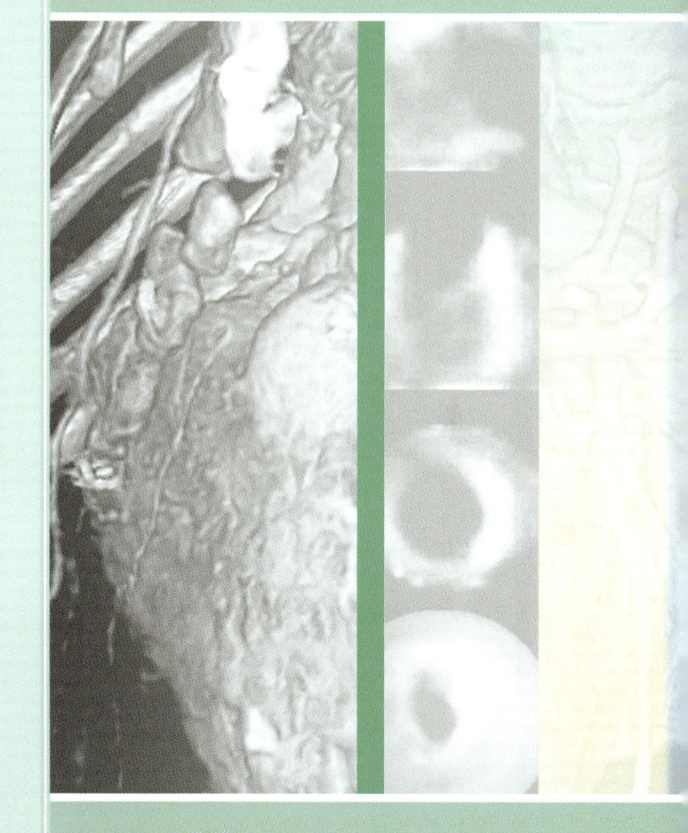

CHAPTER 78

Vascular Ultrasonography: Physics, Instrumentation, and Clinical Techniques

Elif Ergun, Ahmet T. Turgut, A. Sanli Ergun, and Vikram S. Dogra

This chapter reviews the physics of ultrasound imaging and blood flow studies, including the physics of contrast agents. The emphasis is placed on Doppler ultrasonography because it plays a major role in vascular ultrasonography. Technical aspects of Doppler ultrasonography are described, including indications, strategies to optimize the parameter settings to obtain a correct image, accurate image interpretation, Doppler artifacts, pitfalls and their solutions, and postprocessing of the images.

DESCRIPTION OF TECHNICAL REQUIREMENTS

The main technical requirements are familiarity with ultrasound physics, instrumentation, and artifacts.

Physical Principles and Instrumentation in Vascular Ultrasonography

Ultrasound imaging is based on sound propagation in the body and its reflections from scatterers in the tissue and bloodstream, and reflections from interfaces between different tissues (Fig. 78-1). The reason for reflection and scattering is the difference in the mechanical impedances of different tissue and scatterers. The reflected and scattered ultrasound waves are collected with transducer arrays and converted to an image, which reveals the anatomic structures of the body.

Ultrasound transducer arrays are conventionally made of piezoelectric material, which is a special kind of crystal that converts electrical energy into acoustic energy and vice versa. By electronically controlling the hundreds of elements of which the transducer arrays are composed, these arrays can focus, steer, or translate the ultrasound beam. The first step to form an image is to transmit a focused ultrasound beam into the body that travels more or less along a line, and the echoes coming from the reflectors and scatterers along this line are collected by the transducer array. While receiving the echoes, the transducer array is dynamically focused to find the gray-scale value of a pixel on the line—black pixel means there is nothing to reflect ultrasound. This forms an image line. The steps that form an image line are repeated hundreds of times while the beam is translated or steered (or both) from line to line. As shown in Figure 78-2, four basic types of transducers are used in ultrasound imaging, which are classified according to how the image lines are formed: linear sequenced array, curvilinear array, linear phased array, and vector array.[1]

Typically, there are hundreds of pixels along an image line. The number of pixels is chosen so as not to degrade the axial resolution (i.e., resolution along an image line). More pixels do not always mean better resolution, however. The length of the ultrasound pulse (number of cycles × the wavelength) sets the ultimate limit on the axial resolution. The shorter the pulse, the higher is the axial resolution. The number of lines in an image is chosen to avoid losing resolution and important anatomic information (the use of too few lines can lead to missing anatomic structures), and to avoid decreasing the frame rate (too many lines means lower frame rate).

The above-described image formation results in the conventional B-mode image, in which strong reflectors are depicted by white pixels, and weak reflectors are depicted as darker shades of gray. In B-mode images, blood appears dark and is considered anechoic mainly because the scatterers in the blood, predominantly red blood cells, are very small and have very low back-scattering coefficients.

FIGURE 78-1 A and B, Ultrasound beams are reflected from tissue interfaces (**A**) and scattered from particles within the tissue and body fluids (**B**).

Vascular ultrasonography makes use of different techniques that enhance signals coming from the bloodstream to be able to image blood flow. First and most widely used of these is Doppler ultrasonography.[2-5] In the Doppler technique, the signals coming from moving scatterers are enhanced, whereas stationary echoes are suppressed, which effectively displays blood flow information.

A more recently developed modality used for blood flow imaging is B-flow.[6] The appearance of B-flow images is similar to that of B-mode images, and this technique overcomes some of the pitfalls of Doppler ultrasonography. A third modality used for blood flow imaging is contrast-enhanced harmonic imaging. In this modality, contrast agents, which are essentially gas-filled bubbles, are injected into the bloodstream. Contrast agents boost the echogenicity of the blood, and are used to enhance the signal coming from the blood in Doppler ultrasonography and B-flow imaging.

Doppler Ultrasonography

The Doppler effect, named after the Austrian mathematician and physicist Christian A. Doppler (1803-1853) who first hypothesized it, simply states that for a stationary observer, the apparent frequency of a wave emitted from a moving source changes proportional to the relative velocity of the source with respect to the observer (Fig. 78-3 is a conceptual drawing of wave fronts generated by a moving source). In simple terms, *relative velocity* is the rate of change of the distance between the source and the observer. In that sense, it could be the observer that is moving. The Doppler frequency shift solely depends on the relative velocity regardless of who or what is moving.

Although Doppler developed his hypothesis for light waves, he also noted that the same hypothesis applied to sound waves. The Doppler effect is observed most easily with sound waves because, in the audible range, our ears can hear and detect changes in frequency (pitch). Imagine (or rather remember) a vehicle passing by while honking, or an ambulance, fire truck, or police car with sirens blaring. The pitch of the siren is noted to change while passing by: the siren starts with a high pitch; when getting close, the pitch starts to drop; the siren attains the actual pitch right when passing by and continues to drop thereafter. Figure 78-4 shows a simulated example, in which

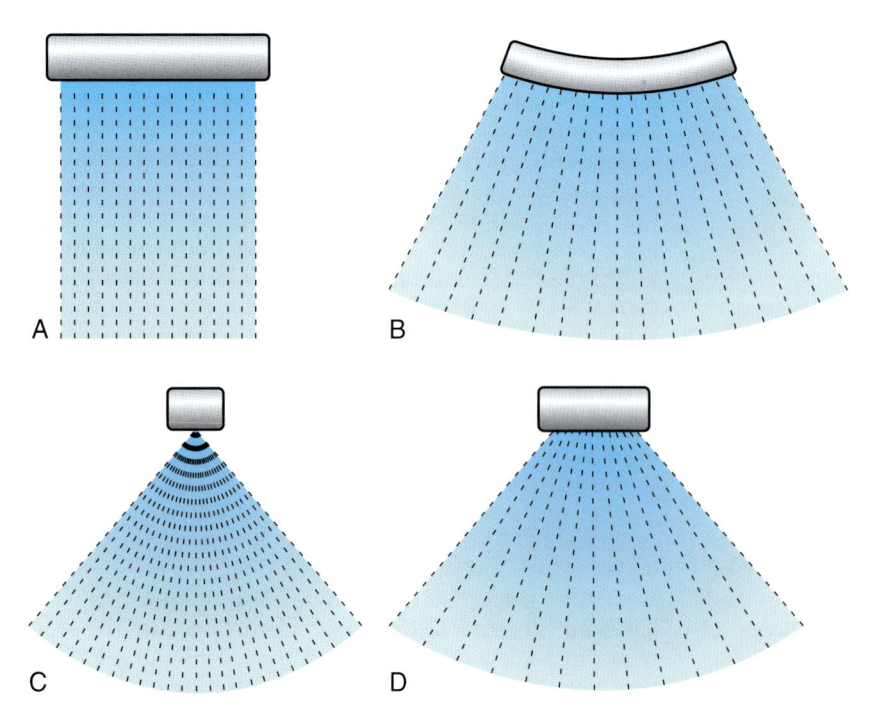

FIGURE 78-2 Types of transducers. **A**, Linear sequenced array. **B**, Curvilinear array. **C**, Linear phase array. **D**, Vector array.

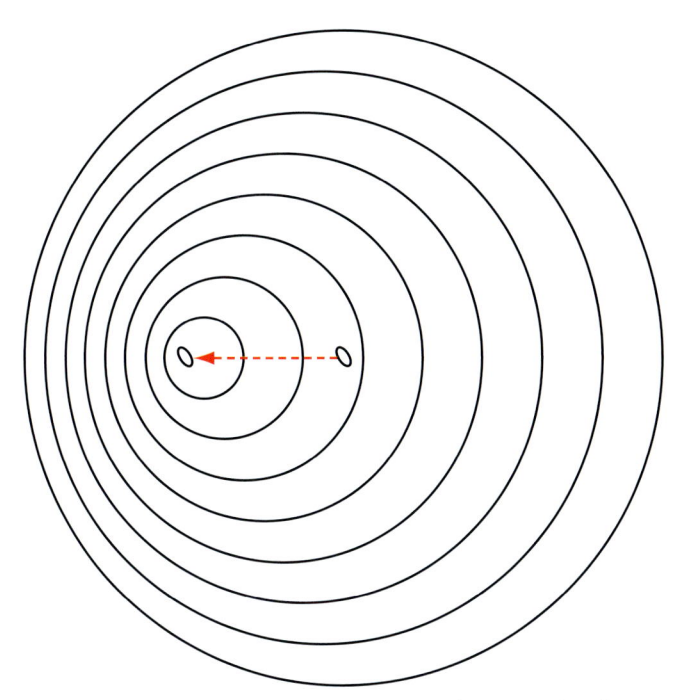

FIGURE 78-3 A moving source generates a shorter wavelength (corresponding to higher frequency) ahead of itself and a longer wavelength (corresponding to lower frequency) behind itself compared with the wavelength it would generate while stationary.

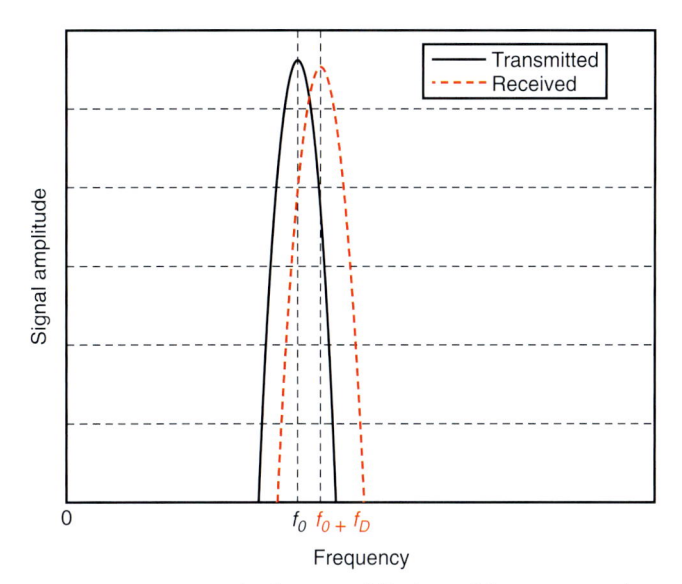

FIGURE 78-4 Doppler frequency shift observed for a target moving toward the observer: The *solid curve* represents the frequency spectrum of the transmitted signal, whereas the *dashed curve* represents the frequency spectrum of the received signal. The difference between these two spectra is a result of the Doppler shift.

the solid and dashed curves show the frequency spectrum of the transmitted and received signals.

In ultrasonography, the Doppler effect is applied to identify tissue motion, blood flow, and vessel structures. The simplest application of Doppler effect in ultrasonography is fetal heart rate monitoring. These devices detect the motion of the fetal heart and convert it into audible sound. More sophisticated Doppler instruments that visualize blood flow and vessel structures are now integrated into most modern ultrasound imaging systems.[1]

In blood flow imaging, the Doppler signal is generated by blood cells that back-scatter the transmitted ultrasound wave. The back-scattering coefficient of the cells is a quadratic function of their relative size with respect to the wavelength.[2] The blood is mostly composed of red and white blood cells and water. In B-mode imaging, blood is almost anechoic because of the very small back-scattering coefficient of blood cells. The echoes coming from the surrounding tissue dominate the image. In Doppler imaging, in which the surrounding tissue is stationary, the moving blood cells generate the Doppler signal. Although white blood cells are larger, red blood cells are more numerous in the blood and generate most of the Doppler flow signal.

The Doppler frequency shift f_D is formulated as:

$$f_D = 2 \cdot f_0 \cdot v_{s,r} \cdot \cos(\theta)/c$$

where f_0 is the frequency of the transmitted ultrasound wave, $v_{s,r}$ is the relative velocity of the moving target with respect to the transducer, and c is the speed of sound in tissue (on average 1540 m/s); θ is the angle of the direction of the moving target with respect to the transducer. This angle is zero when the target is moving head on toward the transducer, and it is 90 degrees when the target is moving parallel to the transducer surface. The factor 2 comes from the fact that the targets (e.g., blood cells in this case) are reflectors, and the transmitted signal is twice subjected to Doppler shift.

The Doppler signal is proportional to this frequency shift f_D. The previous formula captures some of the attributes of Doppler imaging. The Doppler signal is proportional to the transmitted ultrasound frequency, so higher frequencies are preferred. Another reason for preferring higher frequencies is the back-scattering coefficient of blood cells. As mentioned previously, the back-scattering coefficient of cells is a quadratic function of the size of the cells in relation to the wavelength. Because wavelength is inversely proportional to the frequency, using higher ultrasound frequencies (shorter wavelength) increases the back-scattering coefficient significantly. Attenuation in tissue, which is an exponential function of frequency, ultimately limits the frequency and penetration depth, however. Stated in another way, for a target depth, there is always an optimal Doppler frequency dictated by these three factors. The cosine term accounts for the angular dependence of the Doppler signal. It is strongest when the blood flow is parallel to the ultrasound beam, and is zero when the blood flow is at right angles to the ultrasound beam. The Doppler signal is also proportional to the velocity of the blood cells and the number of blood cells in the sample volume interrogated by the ultrasound beam. Because the number of blood cells per unit blood volume is more or less constant, it is the spot volume of the ultrasound beam that determines the strength of the Doppler signal.[3]

Although we have been talking about Doppler frequency shift, in modern ultrasound systems the phase shift, not the frequency shift, is measured. Making true frequency measurements requires the system to use continuous wave ultrasound signals, which means complete loss of axial resolution for an ultrasound image. Because of this, ultrasound systems now use pulsed wave ultrasound techniques, which measure the phase shift in the received signal using a mathematical process called *autocorrelation*. This technique is achieved by interrogating the same sample volume multiple times (at least 3, typically 10 to 20 times), and correlating the echoes.[1] Because measuring the phase shift is essentially equivalent to measuring the Doppler frequency shift within certain limitations, all the arguments we made before about Doppler frequency shift remain the same.

In B-mode imaging, the ultrasound pulse length is typically kept at minimum for best axial resolution. In Doppler imaging, shortest possible pulse length is insufficient to extract phase shift information, however, and several cycle pulses are used. As mentioned before, the Doppler signal strength is proportional to the ultrasound beam volume, which is proportional to the pulse length—more blood cells generate larger signal. In that sense, it is better to use long pulses in Doppler imaging, although at the expense of axial resolution. Two types of Doppler ultrasound equipment are clinically available: continuous wave and pulsed Doppler devices.

Continuous Wave Doppler Imaging

The continuous wave Doppler device, which continuously transmits and receives signals, requires two separate sections mounted in the ultrasound probe; one is the transmitting transducer, and the other is the receiving transducer. This is a simple process and it works well when only the magnitude of the Doppler shift frequency is required.[7] It does not provide directional information about the flow, however, and does not have any axial resolution. The Doppler signal comes from a large sample volume, which is essentially the intersection of the transmit and receive beams. Vascular structures at different depths are sampled simultaneously.[2] The major advantage of this system is that aliasing does not occur, and continuous wave Doppler is more sensitive to slow flow than pulsed Doppler.

Pulsed Wave Doppler Imaging

Most modern ultrasound systems use pulsed Doppler techniques, which provide depth and sample volume control. In contrast to continuous wave Doppler systems, pulsed wave Doppler systems do not generate continuous signals, but transmit pulses of ultrasound and then switch to receive mode. The system has only one transducer, which transmits and receives signal, instead of separate transmitting and receiving transducers as in continuous wave Doppler. Color Doppler and spectral Doppler use pulsed wave ultrasound, but data are processed in different ways to obtain a Doppler sonogram in spectral Doppler and color flow image in color Doppler.

Color Doppler Imaging

Color Doppler images are generated in the same way as conventional B-mode images. After interrogating a scan line multiple times, the phase shift information obtained by autocorrelation is converted to velocity information for every pixel on the scan line—typically hundreds of pixels per scan line. The sign of the velocity information (i.e., the direction of the flow) is coded with two colors—typically blue and copper for positive and negative—and the mean velocity value is coded as levels of these two colors. The same process is repeated for all the scan lines. The color-coded scan lines are compounded to form the color Doppler image. The end image is a representation of the flow velocity in the scan area (depth and width of interest), which is typically set by the user.

Color Doppler imaging has three major limitations: aliasing, angle dependence, and low frame rate. The pulse repetition frequency (PRF) of the pulses that are used to interrogate each scan line is determined by the depth of interest. The system waits for the echoes from deepest locations to fire the next pulse. The PRF sets the maximum velocity that the system can detect without aliasing. Flows faster than the maximum velocity appear as if flowing in the opposite direction with a different velocity (faster flows are displayed under a different alias). Aliasing can be avoided only with high PRF.[1,2]

The Doppler shift is angle-dependent by nature. Around 90 degrees of incidence, there is no Doppler shift, and so there is no velocity information to display. Typically, these regions appear black on the screen with opposite flows on both sides. This appearance can be avoided only by looking at the same vessel from an angle so that 90 degrees of incidence is avoided.[1,2]

The low frame rate of color Doppler imaging is a result of the necessity to interrogate the same scan line multiple times. In contrast to B-mode images, it takes at least 3, and typically 10, times more time to generate a single scan line. The problem with low frame rate for Doppler imaging is that a significant portion of the cardiac cycle appears across the image. That is, by the time the image advances from the first scan line to the last, the body is at a different stage of the cardiac cycle. The color image is not an instantaneous snapshot of blood flow.[1] There is no elegant remedy for this problem. One can only reduce the scan area and scan depth, and increase PRF to improve the frame rate.

Power Doppler Imaging

Power Doppler imaging is a flow imaging modality that has gained great popularity in the last decade. At the expense of loss of flow speed, direction, and character information, power Doppler imaging is able to display flow information free of angle dependence and aliasing effects. In simple terms, power Doppler imaging interrogates the power of the flow signal, not its speed and direction. Rather than displaying the Doppler shift spectrum in which each frequency of the spectrum corresponds to a flow speed component, it displays the integrated power of all these components. Because all the flow components are integrated, power Doppler has significantly more signal-to-noise ratio compared with color Doppler. In addition, power Doppler is not affected much by the cardiac cycle, and it is possible to use low PRF values to detect slow flow and averaging to improve signal-to-noise ratio further.[1,4] With all these advantages, power Doppler is an excellent tool for imaging vessel structures and imaging small low-flow vessels.

Spectral Doppler Imaging

The Doppler signal is generated by the blood cells contained in the volume of the ultrasound beam. At 7.5 MHz with F/2 aperture, the spot size of the ultrasound beam is typically 0.4 mm × 1 mm (wavelength at 7.5 MHz is 0.2 mm). With five cycles of pulsed ultrasound (also called gate length), the ultrasound beam volume is 0.4 mm^3, which contains 105 to 106 blood cells. Each of these cells moves at a different speed and direction, and contributes to a different component of the Doppler shift spectrum. In color Doppler, ensemble average and variance of all the cells within the ultrasound beam are displayed. The spectral content, or equivalently the different velocity content, information is lost in color Doppler. In power Doppler, the loss of information is even greater.

Spectral Doppler is an imaging modality in which Doppler shift spectrum is not lost and displayed. Because of the extent of the information, it is impossible to display the spectral information for a scan area as in color Doppler. Rather, the spectral Doppler information is displayed only for a point in the image area selected by a gate called *range gate*.[1,3] The spectral Doppler display is a two-dimensional display with time on the *x*-axis and frequency on the *y*-axis, so that it displays the Doppler shift spectrum (corresponding to velocity components) as a function of time. Spectral Doppler displays vital information about the type of flow and is used to detect abnormal flow conditions (e.g., caused by plaque or stenoses or punctured vessels).[1]

B-Flow Imaging

In Doppler ultrasonography, long pulses are used to be able to visualize weak flow signals, which compromise axial resolution. Besides, generating an image line typically takes 10 to 20 firings along the same line, which severely limits the frame rate. Finally, Doppler images are overlaid on B-mode images, which sometimes results in the obstruction of vessel walls and important diagnostic information.

B-flow imaging uses coded excitation to enhance the flow signal, and it equalizes the tissue signal to display tissue and flow signals simultaneously.[6] There is no loss of information because of overlaying of images. In addition, coded excitation allows the use of long pulses without degrading the axial resolution, and these pulses are done close to the frame rate of the usual B-mode image.[8] In all, B-flow imaging provides a precise depiction of the blood flow, vessel structures, and surrounding tissue simultaneously at the resolution and frame rate of B-mode images. Because of the ability of B-flow to scan at high frame rates, it is also used to visualize the interaction of blood flow with anatomic structures inside the vessel.[6]

With all the above-mentioned advantages, B-flow imaging allows the depiction of plaque characteristics even better than color Doppler and B-mode imaging, and is useful in carotid imaging. It can also be used to show small venous thrombi as a filling defect of the vessel lumen. It is useful in evaluating complex flow states, such as with bypass grafts, arteriovenous fistulas, pseudoaneurysm, and dialysis fistulas, in which color Doppler artifacts may obscure flow information.[9]

Major disadvantages are that B-flow imaging does not provide velocity information and gives only visual and qualitative information about flow. Ultrasound attenuation is another limitation of the system, which means depiction of flow characteristics in deep vessels such as of the abdomen is not as good as the depiction in superficial vessels, so it is used mainly in superficial vascular imaging.

Contrast-Enhanced Harmonic Imaging

Ultrasound propagation in tissue is nonlinear by nature. Nonlinear wave propagation in tissue generates harmonics of the transmitted signal. If a 5-MHz signal is transmitted, part of the signal is transferred to 10 MHz. The received signal is filtered around 10 MHz to generate the harmonic image. Normally, high-frequency signals are attenuated severely, and this happens in the transmit and receive directions. By harmonic imaging, one can transmit at lower frequency (5 MHz) and receive at the harmonic frequency (10 MHz), and save one-way attenuation.

Aside from having a high back-scattering coefficient, ultrasound contrast agents are also known to have a highly nonlinear response.[10,11] That is, when excited by an ultrasound beam, the back-scattered echo from a contrast agent contains harmonics of the transmitted signal. Because contrast agents are introduced into the bloodstream and perfuse into the vessel structure completely, contrast-enhanced harmonic imaging is a powerful tool for vascular ultrasonography, and it generated great interest in early tumor angiogenesis detection. One of the pitfalls of harmonic imaging is the harmonic signal generated by the tissue itself. Because contrast agents have a unique nonlinear response, using specific complex pulse sequences that suppress tissue harmonics and enhance contrast agent harmonics mitigates this pitfall.[12]

TECHNIQUE OF DOPPLER ULTRASONOGRAPHY

Indications

The most simplistic role of all Doppler systems is determination of blood flow. Flow characteristics, such as flow direction and flow velocity, can also be determined. Doppler ultrasonography has a wide range of indications in diagnostic radiology, including the evaluation of carotid and vertebral artery disease, deep vein thrombosis and venous incompetence, peripheral arterial disease, disease of the portal and hepatic venous system, renal artery disease, and mesenteric ischemia. Doppler ultrasonography also can be used in obstetric and gynecologic applications, including ovarian torsion, ectopic pregnancy, and intrauterine growth retardation. Vascular characterization of tissue and solid masses, to distinguish between testicular torsion and epididymo-orchitis, evaluation of suspected vasculogenic impotence, and evaluation of dialysis fistula function are further indications for Doppler ultrasonography.

Contraindications

There are no contraindications of Doppler ultrasonography. However, because absorption of ultrasound energy increases the body temperature locally, there is a theoretical risk to the fetus during extended use of ultrasonography.[13] In Doppler imaging, the average power sent into the body is significantly larger than typical B-mode. Especially in spectral Doppler, this power is concentrated on a small sample volume. As a rule of thumb, diagnostic Doppler ultrasonography is used in pregnancy only when a medical benefit is expected. The power output of the machine should always be checked, and minimum level of acoustic power and dwell time necessary to obtain the required diagnostic information should be used. This principle is referred as ALARA (as low as reasonably achievable).[14]

Technique

The outcome of Doppler ultrasound examination is strongly influenced by the applied technique, which depends on the precise indication. There are also a variety of technical parameters of Doppler ultrasonography of which the operator should be aware regardless of the application. Changes in these parameters influence color and spectral components of Doppler ultrasound examination. Knowing these operator-dependent parameters and the physical principles underlying them is crucial to obtain a correct diagnostic image. Most modern ultrasound machines have preset parameters that vary according to the region being examined, but it is still required to optimize the parameters for each patient and for the desired diagnostic information.

Choice of Instrumentation

Color Doppler imaging permits rapid assessment of flow over a large region, and highlights gross circulation abnormalities, such as stenosis, aneurysm, and turbulent flow. Analysis of these specific sites by spectral Doppler provides detailed information about flow characteristics and enables quantification of flow. The two modes are complementary to each other, and combined use of them increases the diagnostic information about blood flow.

Choice of Probe and Frequency

The choice of the transducer depends on the clinical application and on the body habitus of the patient. Frequently, more than one transducer is used during an examination. Many factors influence the choice of frequency. The frequency determines the axial resolution and depth of the image. As the insonating frequency increases, attenuation of the ultrasound wave by the tissue increases, and penetration depth decreases. Detecting deep flow requires the use of lower frequencies. Also, low frequencies are less susceptible to aliasing and allow examination of high-velocity flow without aliasing. Sensitivity to flow increases with high frequencies because Doppler shift increases as the insonating frequency increases. Axial resolution is higher with higher frequencies.[2,7] There is a compromise between axial resolution, sensitivity to flow, and depth. The highest frequency that would achieve the best resolution and highest Doppler shift with sufficient penetration should be chosen.

On the basis of this principle, examination of superficially situated vascular structures as in peripheral vasculature is performed by steered linear array transducers with frequencies of 5 MHz or greater. Curvilinear or convex probes in which insonating frequency ranges from 2.5 to 5 MHz are well suited for abdominal scanning.[7,15] Trapezoid field of view convex array is a common configuration for transvaginal and transrectal applications.[7]

Sample Volume

The effective sample volume size in color Doppler is influenced by the size of the color box. The color box or color region of interest defines the volume of tissue in which color processing occurs. The shape, size, and location of the box are adjustable, and image resolution and quality are affected by the box size. In principle, the size of the color box should be kept as small as possible, and the location of it should be as superficial as possible, while still providing the necessary information. The box size is kept small: as the width and depth of the color box increase, more color processing is needed, which reduces the frame rate. A small-sized color box also allows a higher scan line density, which provides better spatial resolution. The color box should be located as superficial as possible because a deeper box demands a low PRF and is more susceptible to aliasing.

In spectral Doppler, sample volume, which is also referred to as the gate size, defines the size and location of the area from which the Doppler information is obtained. Although larger sample volume results in higher signal-to-noise ratio, it may include erroneous signal arising from the adjacent vessels and from the movement of the vessel wall (Fig. 78-5).[7,16] The gate size or sample volume in spectral Doppler should be kept as small as possible. A smaller sample volume also increases the frame rate and the spatial resolution. If it is kept too small, it may give the false impression of reduced or even absent flow.[16]

Choice of Pulse Repetition Frequency/Velocity Scale

The most important factor that has an influence on PRF is the velocity of flow. As a rule of thumb, a low PRF value should be used to look at low velocities, and a high PRF value should be used to look at high velocities. Low PRF in the presence of a high-velocity flow produces aliasing (Figs. 78-6 and 78-7). High PRF reduces the sensitivity to flow, and an examination with high PRF may miss the signals from low-velocity flow (see Figs. 78-6 and 78-7).[14] When searching for signals, examination should be started with the lowest PRF. When the flow signal is detected, PRF can be increased.[7] Depth of the image is another factor affecting PRF. As the depth increases, it takes a longer time for the sound waves to traverse tissue, which increases the time interval between pulsing and sampling. Deeply situated flow should be examined with low PRF values. Using lower PRF values decreases the frame rate.

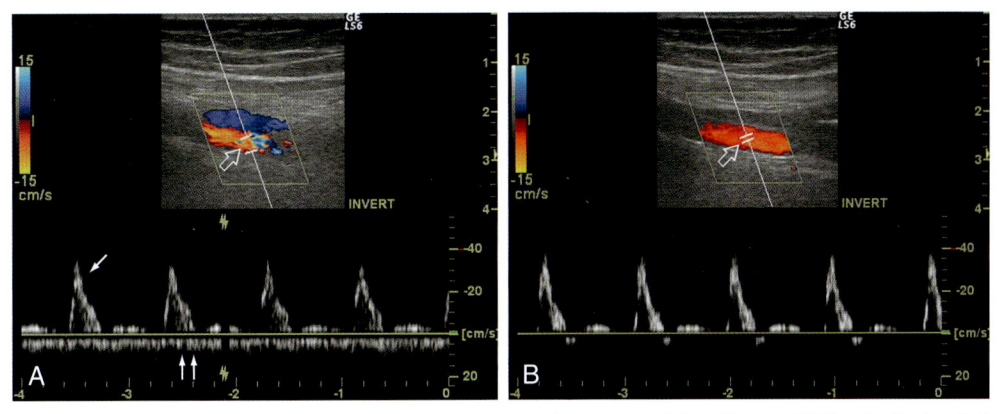

CHAPTER 78 • *Vascular Ultrasonography: Physics, Instrumentation, & Clinical Techniques* 1039

■ **FIGURE 78-5** **A**, Gate or sample volume (*open arrow*) includes signals from the artery and the vein. Arterial flow is displayed above the spectrum (*arrow*); venous flow is displayed below the spectrum. **B**, Sample volume or gate (*open arrow*) size is reduced, and signal only from the artery is included, which is displayed clearly on the spectrum above the baseline.

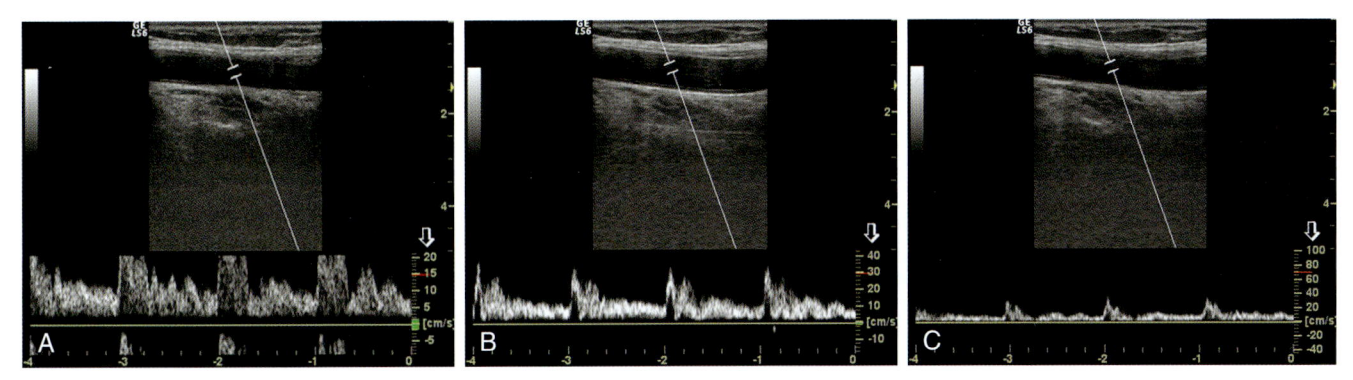

■ **FIGURE 78-6** Effect of PRF/velocity scale setting on spectral Doppler. **A**, Aliasing occurs because of low PRF/velocity scale setting (30 cm/s [*arrow*]). The systolic peak terminates abruptly and wraps around to project below the baseline. **B**, A clear spectrum without aliasing is obtained by increasing PRF/velocity scale to 40 cm/s (*arrow*). **C**, PRF/velocity scale is increased further to 100 cm/s (*arrow*), and the spectrum is compressed along the baseline.

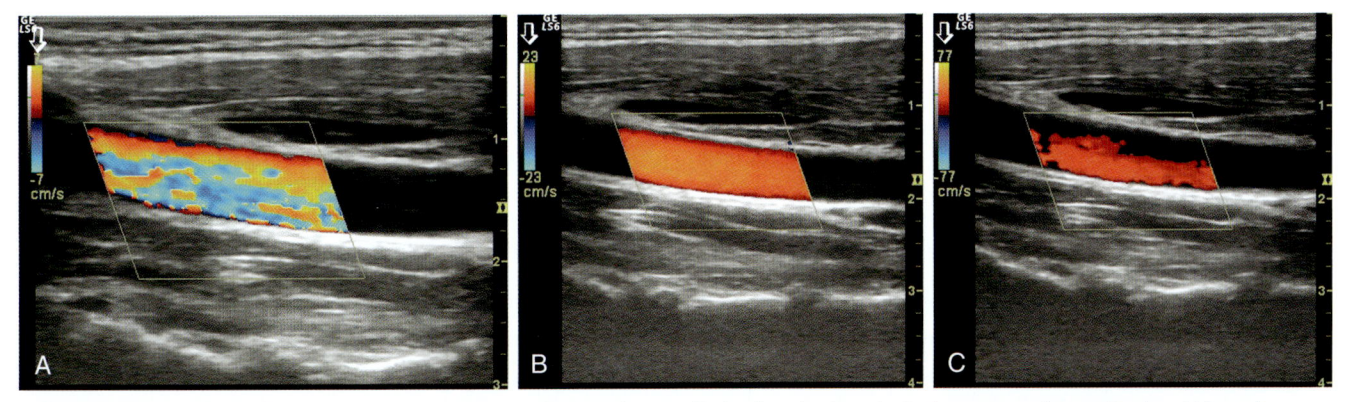

■ **FIGURE 78-7** Effect of PRF/velocity scale setting on color Doppler. **A**, Aliasing in color Doppler is shown as a mixture of red and blue color mimicking the appearance of flow reversal. PRF/velocity scale is 7 cm/s (*arrow*). **B**, With an appropriately set PRF/velocity scale, aliasing disappears, and flow direction is correctly displayed. **C**, PRF/velocity scale is increased further to 77 cm/s (*arrow*). The lumen filling with color is incomplete.

Angle of Insonation and Angle of Correction

The angle of insonation is the angle between the transducer and the vessel being examined. Remember the formulation of Doppler frequency shift f_D, which is:

$$f_D = 2 \cdot f_0 \cdot v_{s,r} \cdot \cos(\theta)/c$$

As easily understood from this equation, Doppler frequency shift is directly proportional to the cosine of the angle θ. As the transducer gets more aligned with the vessel, which means as θ gets smaller, the Doppler shift frequency increases. When the transducer is aligned with a vessel, the largest Doppler shift is obtained, but at such small angles technical difficulties occur in obtaining signal.

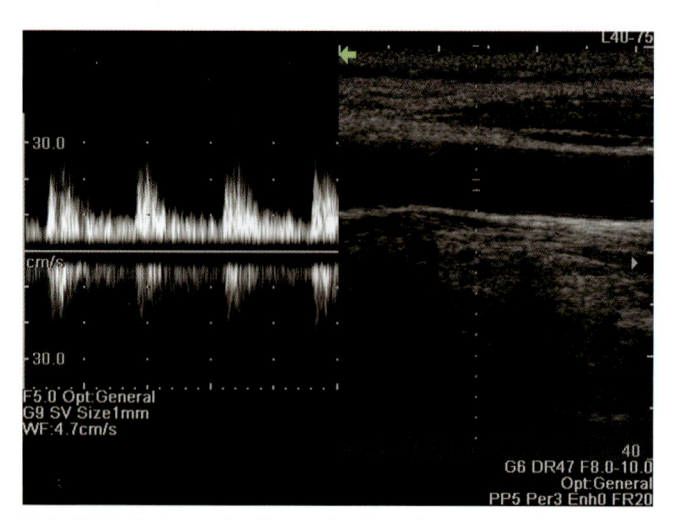

■ **FIGURE 78-8** Angle of insonation is 90 degrees, and the spectrum shows a mirror pattern in which flow appears equally above and below the baseline.

Theoretically, Doppler shift frequency is zero, and no signal can be detected as the angle reaches 90 degrees. At angles approaching 90 degrees, directional knowledge of flow is lost, and flow appears equally above and below the zero line forming the mirror image artifact (Fig. 78-8). The ideal angle of insonation is between 30 degrees and 60 degrees.[2]

Angle correction refers to adjustment of Doppler angle in spectral Doppler. It is used to calculate the velocity of flow as Doppler devices are equipped to calculate flow velocity from the Doppler frequency shift if the angle between the sound beam and the flow direction is measured and indicated to the machine by the operator. For accurate flow measurement, Doppler angle should not be greater than 60 degrees. At angles exceeding 60 degrees, small errors in angle measurement cause large errors in angle-corrected velocity computations.[2,7]

Power and Gain

Acoustic power generated by the Doppler device and transmitted to the tissue is an important factor affecting the sensitivity to flow. Color Doppler and spectral Doppler use higher average power than B-mode ultrasonography. Most devices allow the operator to control the power output according to the specific application. It must be set as low as possible and should be increased only if there is no other way to eliminate noise and detect a Doppler signal.[7] Power output control is crucial, especially in obstetric Doppler applications.

Gain in spectral and color Doppler determines the overall sensitivity to flow. In color Doppler examinations with appropriate gain settings, color should occupy the full anteroposterior diameter of the vessel (Fig. 78-9A). The spectrum should be clearly visible and free of noise with optimal spectral gain; this can be achieved by first increasing receiver gain until noise is displayed, then after a signal is obtained, gain is reduced until noise disappears. Gain settings that are too high cause loss of directional information and produce mirror image artifact in spectral Doppler, whereas aliasing and color noise in the surrounding tissues occur in color Doppler (see Fig. 78-9B). If gain is set too low, slow flow cannot be detected (see Fig. 78-9C).[15]

Appropriately set B-mode gain is also important in color Doppler imaging. If it is set too high, it may suppress color within the vessel. When examining slow flow, decreasing B-mode gain helps to display the vessel in color flow imaging.

High-Pass Filter

Doppler frequency shift is generated also by soft tissue motion, such as the movement of vessel wall and cardiac structures or movement owing to respiration. Such signals have higher amplitude than signals generated by blood flow and may overwhelm the signal of flow.[2,17,18] Doppler equipment compensates for this effect by employing filters that cut out the high-amplitude, low-frequency Doppler signals generated by tissue movement. Because the dominant contribution to this signal is from the vessel wall movement, the filter is referred to as a wall filter. It is actually a high-pass filter. Filtering reduces the background noise and provides a clearer signal.[19] Depending on the flow characteristics and desired clinical application, the operator can vary the cutoff frequency of the wall filter. A high-pass filter limits the minimum velocities that can be measured by the system, and it removes not only high-amplitude, low-frequency soft tissue components, but also slow flow components with frequency shifts below the

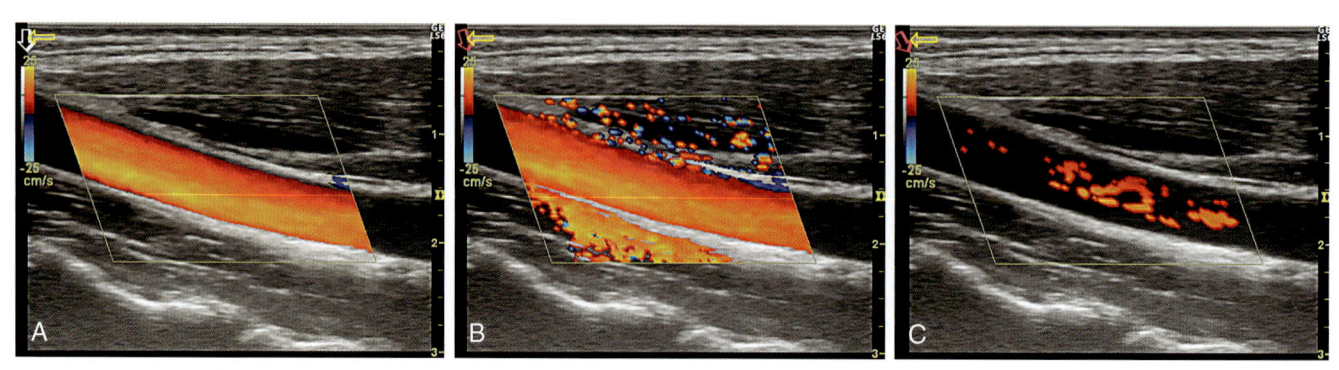

■ **FIGURE 78-9** **A,** Color Doppler image obtained with appropriately set color gain in which color occupies the full anteroposterior diameter of the vessel. **B,** Color noise occurs in the surrounding soft tissues because of high color gain. **C,** Color gain is so low that most of the flow knowledge is lost, and luminal filling with color is incomplete.

cutoff frequency of the filter. If the filtration is set too high, diagnostic velocity information can be lost.[20]

Baseline Shift

Color baseline appears as a horizontal black line on the color bar. Spectral baseline is the time axis of the spectral display. If aliasing occurs, and PRF cannot be increased because of the depth of the investigation, lowering the color or spectral baseline reduces aliasing and optimizes the display of flow.

Color and Spectrum Invert

Flow toward the transducer typically appears red at color Doppler and above the baseline (positive flow) on the spectrum. The Doppler system allows the operator to change the hue assigned to the direction of flow and to invert the spectral display simply by adjusting an inversion button. By this function, it is possible always to display arteries in red and veins in blue in color Doppler, and arterial flow above the baseline in spectral Doppler.

Dwell Time

Dwell time, which is also known as ensemble length or packet size, is a parameter of color Doppler. In color Doppler imaging as mentioned earlier, several pulses are necessary to obtain each line of Doppler information. Number of pulses used for each line is referred to as *packet size* and determines the duration of Doppler sampling for each line. As it increases, sensitivity to flow and color spatial resolution increases. However, the frame rate becomes slower, which may limit the ability of color Doppler to depict rapidly changing hemodynamics.

Focal Zone

In most duplex systems, the focal zone is automatically placed at the depth of the sample volume. In color Doppler systems, the operator determines the location of the focus. Spatial resolution is best at the focal zone, and flow is better detected here.[7]

TABLE 78-1 Color Doppler and Spectral Doppler Artifacts

Artifacts Related to Instrumentation and Settings
Aliasing
Wall filter setting
Gain setting
Directional ambiguity
Grating and side-lobe artifact
Spectral broadening artifact

Artifacts Related to Anatomic Factors
Mirror image artifact
Flow direction artifact

Artifacts Unrelated to Vascular Structures and Blood Flow (Color in Nonvascular Structures)
Edge artifact
Twinkle artifact
Color flash artifact
Pseudoflow artifact

TABLE 78-2 Doppler Signal

Doppler Signal Depends on
Blood velocity—Doppler frequency increases as velocity increases
Ultrasound frequency—higher insonation frequency gives increased Doppler frequency; as in B-mode ultrasound, increased frequency of ultrasound has poorer tissue penetration
Angle of insonation—Doppler frequency increases as ultrasound beam becomes more aligned to flow direction; as the angle of insonation reaches 90 degrees, Doppler signal progressively decreases

TABLE 78-3 Aliasing

To Avoid Aliasing
Decrease insonating frequency
Increase angle of insonation
Increase PRF
Change baseline setting

Artifacts, Pitfalls, and Solutions in Doppler Ultrasonography

Artifacts in spectral and color Doppler imaging may be due to physical limitations of the modality, inappropriate equipment settings, or some anatomic factors (Table 78-1). The operator should be aware of the appearances of typical Doppler artifacts and factors that have an influence on the Doppler signal so as not to make false interpretations. The effects of inappropriate equipment settings on the obtained image are discussed in detail in the previous section. Some of the most important parameters are reviewed here.

Aliasing

Aliasing is a fundamental limitation of pulsed wave Doppler systems. There is no such limitation in continuous wave Doppler. As mentioned earlier, the system transmits a pulse to the target and waits for the received echo to obtain a Doppler signal. The sampling frequency of the Doppler signal is referred to as PRF. The sampling frequency should provide sufficient time for the system to collect all signals from one pulse before the next pulse is generated. PRF limits the maximum Doppler shift that can be measured by the pulsed wave Doppler system. When the frequency of Doppler signal exceeds one half of the PRF (Nyquist sampling rate), this results in the ambiguity of the Doppler signal that is termed *aliasing*.[9,20] In spectral tracing, this ambiguous signal is "wrapped around" and depicted as if flow is in the reversed direction (see Fig. 78-6A). Color aliasing projects the color of reversed flow in the central areas of higher laminar velocity (see Fig. 78-7A).[20] Awareness of some technical and physical issues (Table 78-2) helps to build strategies that avoid aliasing (Table 78-3).

Wall Filter Setting

Diagnostically significant flow information, especially about low-velocity flow, may be lost if wall filter is set too high.[20] When the area of investigation has a low-velocity

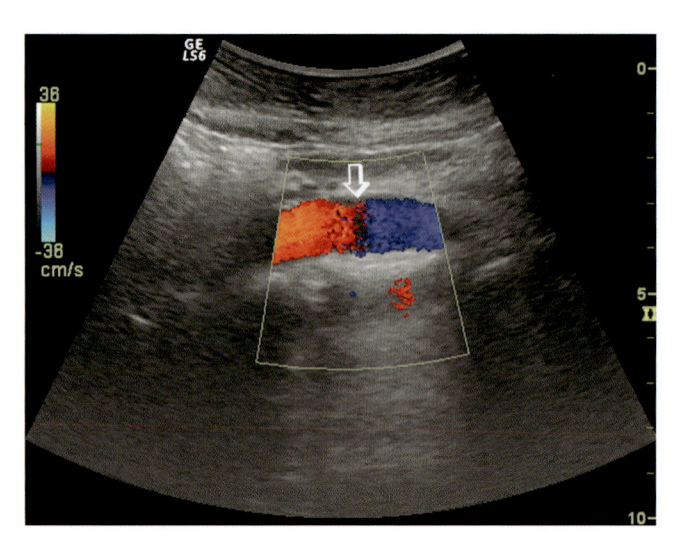

FIGURE 78-10 Color Doppler image of abdominal aorta obtained by a convex probe. The vessel is coded by different colors in different segments. Doppler shift is absent at the small colorless region (*arrow*) where flow is perpendicular to the angle of insonation.

flow pattern, no filtering or little filtering should be used. There are other system parameters such as PRF and frame rate that have an effect on filtering. In some systems, wall filter automatically increases as the PRF is increased.[7,14] The processing time and Doppler sensitivity decrease as the frame rate increases; if high frame rates are used, wall filter should be reduced.

Gain Setting

When color or spectral gain is too low, it gives a false impression of absence of flow. Too high B-mode gain may suppress color in the vessel, especially when the flow velocity is low. While examining vessels with slow flow velocities, color and spectral gain should be high enough so that signal free of noise is detected, and B-mode gain should be as low as possible.

Directional Ambiguity

Directional ambiguity can result when the insonating angle is 90 degrees. It may display absence of flow in color Doppler. With linear transducers, this is a more significant problem, but beam steering can improve the angle and alleviate this problem. With sector transducers, the same artery is coded in different colors in different segments of the vessel, and a small colorless region exists at the point where the flow is perpendicular to the beam (Fig. 78-10).[2,20]

Grating or Side-Lobe Artifact

Electronically focused transducers concentrate the insonating beam toward the sample volume. Because of design of the transducers, weak secondary lobes of focused sound may insonate areas unrelated to the primary beam, and if reflected echoes from these regions are strong enough, they are displayed in the image. Convex probes are more susceptible to this artifact than linear probes. These off-axis lobes can insonate vessels unrelated to Doppler sample volume, and if Doppler signal is strong enough, it can be displayed in the spectrum in regions where no Doppler signal is expected.[20]

Spectral Broadening Artifact

Angle of insonation and velocity of flow are the two factors that may cause spectral broadening. It is mainly observed in stenotic arterial segments, but may also occur in a normal arterial segment owing to the insonating angle approaching 90 degrees.

Mirror Image Artifact

Mirror image artifact, which is commonly observed in B-mode imaging, can also occur in color Doppler and spectral Doppler imaging. In color Doppler imaging, it occurs in a vessel that is adjacent to a highly reflective surface, such as lung.[21] The subdiaphragmatic region of the liver and supraclavicular region are also notorious for this artifact.[20]

In spectral Doppler, mirror image artifact is displayed as a similar time-velocity spectrum appearing below and above the zero line (see Fig. 78-8). It occurs at large angles of insonation especially when large receiver gain is used to detect weak Doppler signals.[2]

Flow Direction Artifact

In color Doppler imaging, flow toward and away from the transducer is encoded in different hues, so the veins and arteries are coded in different colors. The operator assigns the hue to the direction of flow. In some anatomic regions where vessels diverge, the color is not an absolute indicator of the vessel type (artery or vein) (Fig. 78-11). In such regions, the device codes arteries in red and blue. Use of spectral Doppler helps alleviate this problem.

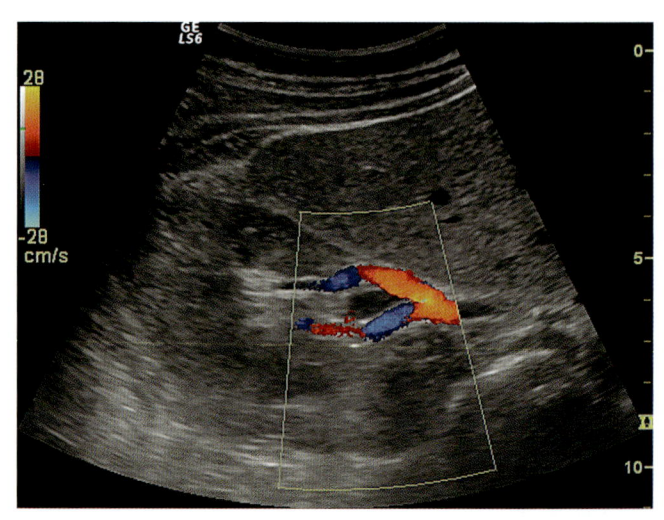

FIGURE 78-11 Color Doppler image of the renal artery. The vessel bifurcates, and branches of the artery diverge and are coded in different colors.

Color in Nonvascular Structures and Color Modulation of Biologic Movement

In color flow devices, any motion of a reflector relative to the transducer produces a Doppler shift and is modulated into color by the device. An artifactual impression of flow is produced and is referred to as the *color flash artifact*.[2,20,22] To compensate for this problem, most color flow devices are equipped with motion discriminators that separate true flow from random motion of soft tissues.

Low level signals arising from hypoechoic areas such as cysts and collections do not trigger the motion discriminators, and color flash artifacts occur in such regions.[20] Artificial color signals may be observed in dilated bile ducts and gallbladder, especially if the color sensitivity settings are high.[23] Transient color flash artifact may also occur because of patient motion (e.g., respiration, cardiac pulsations, and bowel movement) or transducer motion.

Pseudoflow artifact, which is closely related to color flash artifact, occurs secondary to fluid motion. This artifact may be caused by motion of ascites or urine. Spectral analysis of these regions helps to differentiate color flash or pseudoflow artifact from real blood flow because it reveals a spectrum that is very atypical for a vessel.[22]

Twinkle Artifacts

Strongly reflective granular interfaces, such as urinary tract stones or parenchymal calcifications, cause twinkle artifacts, which appear as rapidly fluctuating mixtures of red and blue pixels imitating turbulent flow.[22] Discrimination of this artifact from a real turbulent flow is easy because spectral imaging reveals no flow, and spectrum is flat.

Edge Artifact

Edge artifact is related to strong specular reflectors and occurs as color along the rim of calcified structures, such as bone or gallstones. As in twinkle artifacts, spectral imaging displays a flat spectrum.[22]

Image Interpretation

The image generated by spectral Doppler technique is known as the *Doppler spectrum* (Fig. 78-12). This is a graph that displays different Doppler shift frequencies present in the sample volume over a short time.[9] Three characteristics of the signal—frequency, amplitude, and time—are displayed on the spectrum.

Amplitude illustrates the power of the spectrum and is displayed on the z-axis as brightness of the pixel. Time is displayed on the horizontal axis, which is the baseline. Direction of the flow relative to the transducer is shown relative to the baseline.

The Doppler frequency shift is displayed on the vertical axis. Doppler devices are equipped to calculate the velocity from the frequency shift using the angle that is measured by the operator. The calculated velocity is also displayed on the vertical axis of the spectrum.

The shape of this spectrum is referred to as a *waveform*. Each vessel in the body has an expected flow waveform and color flow properties. Changes in these flow characteristics may indicate disease. Understanding the color Doppler and spectral Doppler features of normal and diseased vessels are crucial for accurate diagnosis.

Blood flow in arteries has a laminar pattern in which blood in the center of the vessel has a higher speed than blood at the periphery. In this pattern, most of the blood cells has a uniform speed. In spectral Doppler, laminar flow pattern is displayed as a thin line outlining a clear space referred as the *spectral window*.[9] Turbulent flow, which is usually observed in pathologic conditions, may be shown in normal arteries in some situations (Table 79-4). Each cardiac cycle induces cyclic changes in arterial flow and causes variations in the velocity ranges during systole and diastole. Arteries have a distinct waveform that begins with systole and ends at the end of diastole. The shape of this wave reveals information about a crucial flow property of arteries, the pulsatility (Fig. 78-13).

Venous flow is slower than arterial flow, and its detection requires low PRF and low wall filtering. Venous flow is continuous, but respiratory and cardiac modulations can be observed in flow, especially in the central veins. The respiratory modulation appears as enhancement of velocities during expiration in the subdiaphragmatic territory veins. This phenomenon exists in the supradiaphragmatic territory during inspiration. Cardiac modulation is

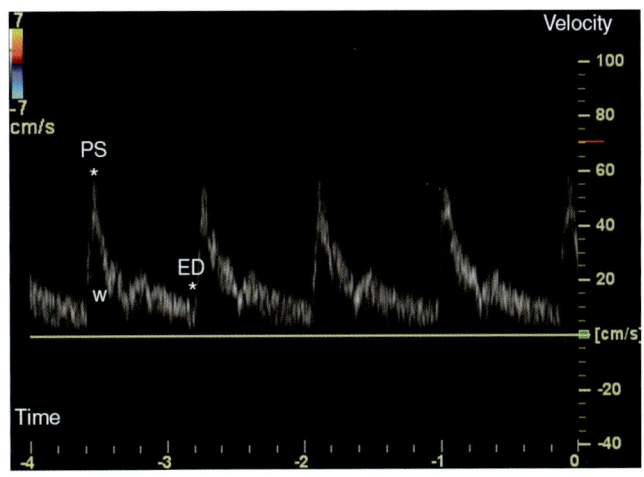

FIGURE 78-12 Doppler spectrum displaying arterial flow with a moderate resistance. Velocity is displayed on the vertical axis, and time is displayed on the horizontal axis. Direction of flow is determined relative to the baseline. This spectrum displays flow toward the transducer above the baseline. Flow toward the transducer is always represented by a positive velocity value. Brightness of the pixel correlates with the number of erythrocytes that have the corresponding velocity. The dark window (w) under the spectral trace represents that the number of erythrocytes having the corresponding velocities at that specific time is zero. ED, end-diastole; PS, peak systole.

TABLE 78-4 Turbulent Flow
Decrease in vessel diameter (stenosis), increase in flow velocity (arteriovenous shunt), and decreased blood viscosity are causes
Can be observed at bifurcation points, and curves and kinks
Flow is disorganized and displayed as spectral broadening, and fill-in of the spectral window in spectral Doppler
Reversed flow is observed in color and spectral Doppler

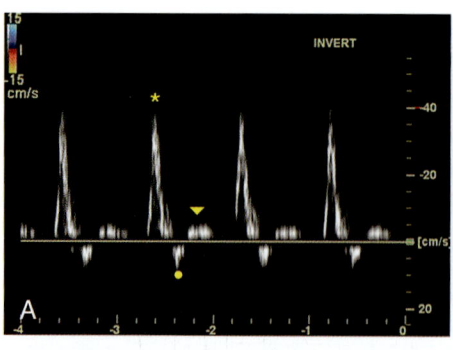

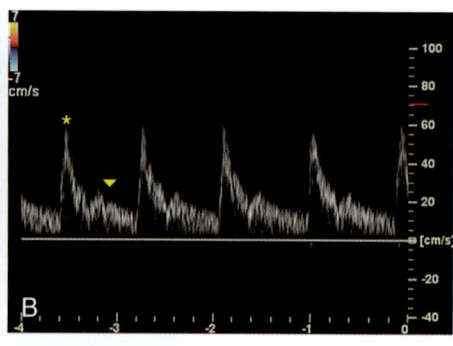

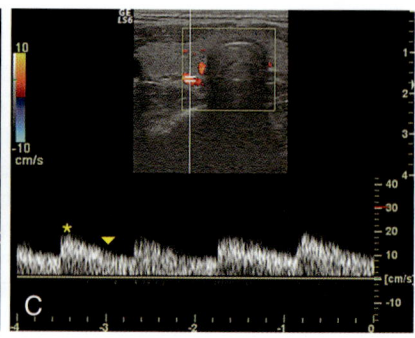

FIGURE 78-13 Spectral displays of various arterial flow patterns. **A,** High-resistance flow pattern, which is typically observed in the extremity arteries. In this triphasic pattern, systolic peak (*asterisk*) is narrow. There is a flow reversal (*bullet*) in early diastole; after a brief forward diastolic flow (*arrowhead*), flow is absent at the late diastole. **B,** Flow with moderate resistance. Systolic peak (*asterisk*) is narrow; forward flow, which is persistent throughout diastole (*arrowhead*), is observed. **C,** Low-resistance arterial flow displayed by broad systolic peak and prominent forward flow throughout diastole.

observed in the abdominal veins that are located close to the heart, such as the inferior vena cava and hepatic veins; this appears as a short reversal of flow during diastole.[24]

Arterial Stenosis

Spectral Doppler Changes

The flow velocity and acceleration are highest at the site of maximum stenosis. Commonly used stenotic zone velocities are peak systolic velocity (PSV) and end-diastolic velocity (EDV). PSV is the first Doppler parameter that becomes abnormal in the stenotic zone, whereas EDV remains normal with less than 50% diameter narrowing. Systolic velocity ratio (PSV in the stenotic zone/PSV in the normal zone proximal to the stenosis) is another important parameter of arterial stenosis and compensates for patient-to-patient hemodynamic variabilities.[9]

In the poststenotic region, flow is disorganized, and turbulent flow with negative frequencies predominating in systole is observed. The resistance to flow increases in the prestenotic region where high-resistance flow pattern is observed. In the region distal to the stenosis, flow resistance decreases, and pulsus parvus et tardus is observed with rounded systolic peak, reduced PSV, slower acceleration, and increased diastolic flow.[24]

Color Doppler Changes

There is a localized aliasing in the region of stenosis where the reduction in caliber can also be visually observed. Reverse flow with color inversion is observed in the immediate poststenotic zone. When narrowing is severe, turbulence in the poststenotic zone becomes so high that an artifact caused by the wall vibrations arises in the perivascular soft tissues. This artifact is displayed as a random color map.[9,25]

Aneurysm and Pseudoaneurysm

Velocities decrease in the aneurysmatic region because of an increase in the vessel diameter. The spectrum is dampened, and color encoding is poor inside the lumen. A helical flow is displayed as a multiphasic spectrum and a mixture of red and blue color. Pseudoaneurysms have a communication with the arterial lumen via a narrow neck in which a to-and-fro flow pattern is observed.[24]

Arteriovenous Shunts (Malformations and Fistulas)

Peripheral resistance is severely decreased in the region of the arteriovenous shunts. The enormous increase in velocities causes a very turbulent flow with transmission of mechanical vibrations to the perivascular tissue. Afferent and efferent vessel diameters increase. The afferent arterial flow is turbulent with high velocities in systole and diastole. The efferent venous flow has a clear cardiac modulation with increased velocities during systole.

Steal Phenomenon

Changes in the flow characteristics first appear at diastole as a decrease in the diastolic velocities. For that reason, the earliest finding is an increase in the resistive index. As the pathology advances, flow is reversed at diastole. Flow is totally reversed in systole and in diastole when the stealing effect increases.

Venous Obstruction and Venous Thrombosis

Flow is decreased, and cardiac or respiratory modulation is lost in the upstream region of venous obstruction. In venous thrombosis, no flow is shown inside the lumen, although the setting parameters of the device are optimal. Compressibility of the vein is lost if the thrombosed vein is superficial. Venous occlusion in the veins draining an organ, such as the renal vein, causes an increase in the arterial resistive index of that organ.

Postprocessing

Flow characteristics can be determined qualitatively by visual analysis of the spectral waveform and color Doppler images. It is also possible to obtain quantitative information about the flow from these images. Many techniques have been proposed for quantifying flow. They are velocity measurements and other parameters derived from

TABLE 78-5 Doppler Indices

Resistive index (RI)[26] = (A − B)/A
Pulsatility index (PI)[27] = (A − B)/mean
Systolic-to-diastolic ratio (A/B ratio)[28] = A/B

A, peak systolic frequency; B, end-diastolic frequency.

these measurements, such as volume blood flow and waveform indices.

Velocity Measurements

When the beam/flow angle is known, measurement of mean velocity, EDV, and maximum flow velocity, which is the PSV for arterial flow, is possible from the spectrum.

Doppler Indices

Further analysis of the spectrum and calculating some indices help to describe the complex waveform in a simple way and to evaluate organ blood flow. Commonly used indices available on most scanners are resistive index, systolic/diastolic ratio, and pulsatility index (see Table 78-5 for calculations). The major advantage of these indices is that they are independent of the transmit frequency and Doppler angle.

Acceleration Time and Acceleration Index

Acceleration time and acceleration index are also important parameters obtained from the Doppler spectrum. They quantify the flow.[9] In systole, the flow velocity accelerates very rapidly in the arteries, and the time needed to reach the maximum systolic velocity is referred as the *acceleration time*.

Volume Blood Flow Measurement

Quantification of flow volume is possible with color Doppler and duplex Doppler instruments. Different techniques are used to calculate flow volume, but it is simply calculated by multiplying luminal area with the mean velocity. This calculation is done automatically by the ultrasound machine. Measurement of flow volume is fraught with difficulties even under ideal conditions. Errors may arise because of many factors, including shape of the vessel, inaccurate estimation of the mean velocity, and variation in the vessel diameter (e.g., artery diameters are smaller during systole).[2] Volume flow measurements have found surprisingly little use in a clinical setting. Parameters such as pulsatility index seem to be more

helpful in defining many physiologic and pathologic conditions.[2,9] Increased resistance to flow may increase cardiac contractility, and flow may be maintained until late in the disease.

In color Doppler imaging, visualization of the stenotic vessel segment with its residual lumen is possible. Most modern instruments are equipped to calculate the percent stenosis of diameter and area from this image.

Reporting

There are general principles in reporting, given the fact that the report depends on the specific clinical application. The report should contain information that describes the qualitative color and spectral flow characteristics. The necessity of obtaining quantitative data from the device by postprocessing of the image depends on the region of examination and the type of vessel being examined. In case such data are obtained, they should be included in the report.

KEY POINTS

- Doppler ultrasonography uses the Doppler effect to image blood flow. The fundamental function of Doppler ultrasonography is the determination of blood flow, but other flow characteristics, such as flow direction and velocity, can also be determined.
- Modern Doppler devices use pulsed Doppler systems and have color Doppler, spectral Doppler, and power Doppler options.
- Color Doppler ultrasonography and spectral Doppler ultrasonography are complementary to each other. Color Doppler ultrasonography enables assessment of blood flow over a large region, but gives qualitative information about the flow. Spectral Doppler ultrasonography provides detailed and quantitative knowledge about the flow, but in a small region.
- Power Doppler ultrasonography is able to display flow information free of angle dependence and aliasing effects. It has significantly more signal-to-noise ratio compared with color Doppler. Power Doppler is an excellent tool for imaging vessel structures and imaging small low-flow vessels.
- Various technical parameters, such as PRF and angle of insonation, have an effect on the image obtained by Doppler ultrasonography. To obtain a correct image and to interpret images correctly, the operator should be aware of these parameters and the physical principles underlying them.
- B-flow imaging and contrast-enhanced harmonic imaging are the other modalities of vascular ultrasonography.

SUGGESTED READINGS

Campbell SC, Cullinan JA, Rubens DJ. Slow flow or no flow? Color and power Doppler US pitfalls in the abdomen and pelvis. RadioGraphics 2004; 24:497-506.

Grenier N, Basseau F, Rey MC, et al. Interpretation of Doppler signals. Eur Radiol 2001; 11:1295-1307.

Nelson TR, Pretorius DH. The Doppler signal: Where does it come from and what does it mean? AJR Am J Roentgenol 1988; 51:439-447.

Pozniak MA, Zagzebski JA, Scanlan KA. Spectral and color Doppler artifacts. RadioGraphics 1992; 12:35-44.

Scoutt LM, Zawin ML, Taylor KJW, et al. Doppler US, part II: clinical applications. Radiology 1990; 174:309-319.

Taylor JWK, Holland S. Doppler US, part I: basic principles, instrumentation, and pitfalls. Radiology 1990; 174:297-307.

Teh J. Applications of Doppler imaging in the musculoskeletal system. Curr Probl Diagn Radiol 2005; 35:22-34.

Wells PN. Ultrasound in vascular pathologies. Eur Radiol 1998; 8:849-857.

REFERENCES

1. Frederick WK. Diagnostic Ultrasound, Principles and Instruments. Philadelphia, Saunders, 2006.
2. Taylor KJW, Holland S. Doppler US, part I: basic principles, instrumentation, and pitfalls. Radiology 1990; 174:297-307.
3. Nelson TR, Pretorius DH. The Doppler signal: where does it come from and what does it mean? AJR Am J Roentgenol 1988; 51:439-447.
4. Martinoli C, Derchi LE, Rizzatto G, et al. Power Doppler sonography: general principles, clinical applications, and future prospects. Eur Radiol 1998; 8:1224-1235.
5. William JZ, Pellerito JS. Introduction to Vascular Ultrasonography. Philadelphia, Saunders, 2004.
6. Chiao RY, Mo LY, Hall AL, et al. B-mode blood flow imaging. In IEE Ultrasonics Symposium, 2000, pp 1469-1472.
7. Burns PN. Interpreting and analysing the Doppler examination. In Taylor JW, Burns PN, Wells PNT (eds). Clinical Applications of Doppler Ultrasound. Philadelphia, Lippincott-Raven, 1995, pp 55-98.
8. O'Donnell M. Coded excitation system for improving the penetration of real-time phased-array imaging systems. IEEE Trans Ultrason Ferroelectr Freq Control 1992; 39:341-351.
9. Zweibel WJ, Pellerito JS. Basic concepts of Doppler frequency spectrum analysis and blood flow imaging. In Zweibel WJ, Pellerio JS (eds). Introduction to Vascular Ultrasonography. Philadelphia, Saunders, 2005, pp 61-89.
10. Simpson DH, Burns PN, Averkiou MA. Techniques for perfusion imaging with microbubble contrast agents. IEEE Trans Ultrason Ferroelectr Freq Control 2001; 48:1483-1494.
11. Chang PH, Shung KK, Wu SJ, et al. Second harmonic imaging and harmonic Doppler measurements with Albunex. IEEE Trans Ultrason Ferroelectr Freq Control 1995; 42:1020-1027.
12. Hope-Simpson D, Chin C, Burns P. Pulse inversion Doppler: a new method for detecting non-linear echoes from microbubble contrast agent. IEEE Trans Ultrason Ferroelectr Freq Control 1999; 46:372-382.
13. Scoutt LM, Zawin ML, Taylor KJW, et al. Doppler US, part II: clinical applications. Radiology 1990; 174:309-319.
14. Maulik D. Biological safety of diagnostic sonography. In Maulik D (ed). Doppler Ultrasound in Obstetrics and Gynecology. Berlin, Springer-Verlag, 2005, pp 95-111.
15. Foley WD, Erickson SJ. Color Doppler flow imaging. AJR Am J Roentgenol 1991; 156:3-13.
16. Kruskal JB, Newman PA, Sammons LG, et al. Optimizing Doppler and color flow US: application to hepatic sonography. RadioGraphics 2004; 24:657-675.
17. Rubin JM. Spectral Doppler US. RadioGraphics 1994; 14:139-150.
18. Powis RL. Color flow imaging. RadioGraphics 1994; 14:415-428.
19. Teh J. Applications of Doppler imaging in the musculoskeletal system. Curr Probl Diagn Radiol 2006; 35:22-34.
20. Pozniak MA, Zagzebski JA, Scanlan KA. Spectral and color Doppler artifacts. RadioGraphics 1992; 12:35-44.
21. Middletoon WD, Melson GL. The carotid ghost: a color Doppler ultrasound duplication artifact. J Ultrasound Med 1990; 9:487-493.
22. Campbell SC, Cullinan JA, Rubens DJ. Slow flow or no flow? Color and power Doppler US pitfalls in the abdomen and pelvis. RadioGraphics 2004; 24:497-506.
23. Mitchell DG, Burns P, Neddleman L. Color Doppler artifacts in anechoic regions. J Ultrasound Med 1990; 9:255-260.
24. Grenier N, Basseau F, Rey MC, et al. Interpretation of Doppler signals. Eur Radiol 2001; 11:1295-1307.
25. Mitchell DG. Color Doppler imaging: principles, limitations and artifacts. Radiology 1990; 177:1-10.
26. Pourcelot L. Applications clinique de l'examen Doppler transcutane. In Peronneau P (ed). Velocitmetric Ultrasonor Doppler. Inserm 1974; 34:213-240.
27. Gosling RG. Extraction of physiological information from spectrum analyzed Doppler-shifted continuous wave ultrasound signals obtained noninvasively from the arterial tree. In Hill DW, Watson BW (eds). I.E.E. Medical Electronic Monographs, 13-22, Peter Peregrinus, London, 1976, pp 73-125.
28. Stuart B, Drumm J, Fitzgerald DE, et al. Fetal blood velocity waveforms in normal pregnancy. Br J Obstet Gynaecol 1980; 876:780-785.

CHAPTER 79

Physics of Computed Tomography

Jiang Hsieh

FUNDAMENTALS OF X-RAY PHYSICS

In the diagnostic x-ray energy range between 20 keV and 140 keV, there are three types of interactions between x-ray photons and the patient: photoelectric effect, Compton scatter, and coherent scatter.[1-3] In photoelectric interaction, the incident x-ray photon energy is greater than the binding energy of a deep shell electron. By giving up its entire energy in liberating the electron, the original x-ray photon no longer exists. When the hole created at the deep shell is filled by an outer shell electron, a characteristic radiation is generated. Because the probability of such interaction is proportional to the cube of the atomic number of the matter, tissues with small differences in atomic numbers result in a greater difference in the x-ray photon absorption and lead to greater contrast between different tissues.

In Compton scatter interaction, the energy of the incident x-ray photon is considerably higher than the binding energy of the electron, and the incident x-ray photon is deflected or scattered with partial loss of its initial energy while freeing up the electron from the atom. The scattered photon may be deflected at any angle ranging from 0 to 180 degrees and consequently provides little information about the location of interaction and the original photon path. The scattered photon may undergo additional collisions before exiting the patient. This type of interaction is the most important interaction mechanism in tissue-like materials.

The third and less important type of interaction is the coherent scattering or Rayleigh scattering. Little energy is lost in such interaction. In medical imaging, all three types of interactions are combined in the measurement, and only the composite effect is observed. Interaction of x-ray photons with matter is governed by Beer's law, which can be described by the following equation for a monoenergetic x-ray beam:

$$I = I_0 e^{-\mu \cdot \Delta x}$$

where I_0 is the intensity of the x-ray beam impinging on a uniform material of thickness Δx, I is the x-ray intensity after passing through the material, and μ is the linear attenuation coefficient of the material; μ changes with the input x-ray energy and varies for different materials. Figure 79-1 shows, on a logarithmic scale, μ as a function of energy for soft tissue (red), cortical bone (green), and iodine (blue). It is clear from the figure that significant difference exists between the attenuation coefficients for the three materials, and iodine is more attenuating to the x-ray photons than the bone, which in turn is more attenuating than the soft tissue. As a result, when iodine-based contrast material is injected intravenously into the patient and imaged under x-ray examination, blood vessels generate stronger attenuating signals and therefore become more visible over the diagnostic x-ray energy range.

The x-ray photons produced by the x-ray tube on all clinical x-ray devices today have a wide energy spectrum. For example, when 120 kVp is prescribed on an x-ray CT scanner, x-ray energies ranging from 20 keV to 120 keV are emitted. Because the amount of attenuation to these x-ray photons varies significantly, even for a single material as demonstrated in Figure 79-1, the measured attenuation of an object is consequently the averaged effects of different energy x-ray photons weighted by their spectrum.

IMPORTANT PERFORMANCE PARAMETERS OF X-RAY COMPUTED TOMOGRAPHY

There are many parameters that define the performance of a CT scanner.[1,4-6] During the system design, conscious decisions have to be made to trade off some performance parameters against others to optimize the overall performance for a particular application. In this section, a few important performance parameters of the CT system are discussed, and it should be understood that this is by no means a complete list.

Spatial resolution defines the ability of a CT scanner to resolve closely spaced high-contrast objects and is often specified in terms of line pairs per centimeter (lp/cm). A pattern of 1 lp/cm is formed by a pair of high- and low-intensity bars, each 5 mm in width, as shown in Figure 79-2A; a pattern of 4 lp/cm contains four such high- and low-intensity bars within each centimeter space, as depicted in Figure 79-2B. It is clear from the figure that as the width of the bars is reduced and the bars are closely packed together, it becomes increasingly difficult for a CT system to resolve or to identify the bars individually. To measure the spatial resolution of a CT system, standard bar phantoms are scanned and reconstructed. An example of such a phantom (Catphan) is shown in Figure 79-3. In this phantom, bar patterns of different frequencies are positioned at a fixed radius from the phantom center, and system response to these frequencies can be evaluated from a single scan.

To quantitatively describe the spatial resolution performance, modulation transfer function (MTF) is typically employed. If we plot the profile of the original 4 lp/cm bar pattern object, we obtain a set of rectangular functions as shown by the upper portion of Figure 79-3C. In a similar fashion, we can plot the profile of the reconstructed image of the same bar pattern and obtain a smoothed version of the original rectangular pattern shown by the lower portion of Figure 79-2C. Because of the limited frequency response of the system, both the sharpness and the peak-to-valley magnitude of the reconstructed bar pattern are reduced compared with the original. In the

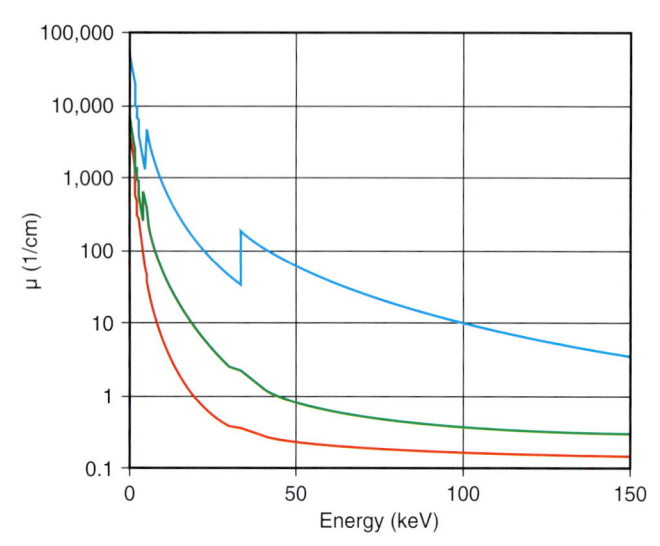

■ **FIGURE 79-1** Linear attenuation coefficients as a function of energy: red, soft tissue; green, bone; blue, iodine.

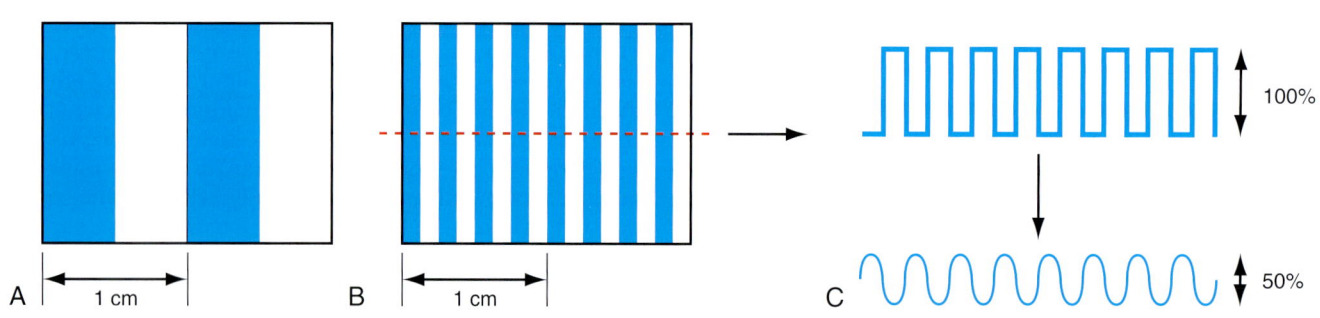

■ **FIGURE 79-2** Illustration of CT resolution testing pattern: **A**, 1 lp/cm; **B**, 4 lp/cm; **C**, profiles of the object and reconstructed image.

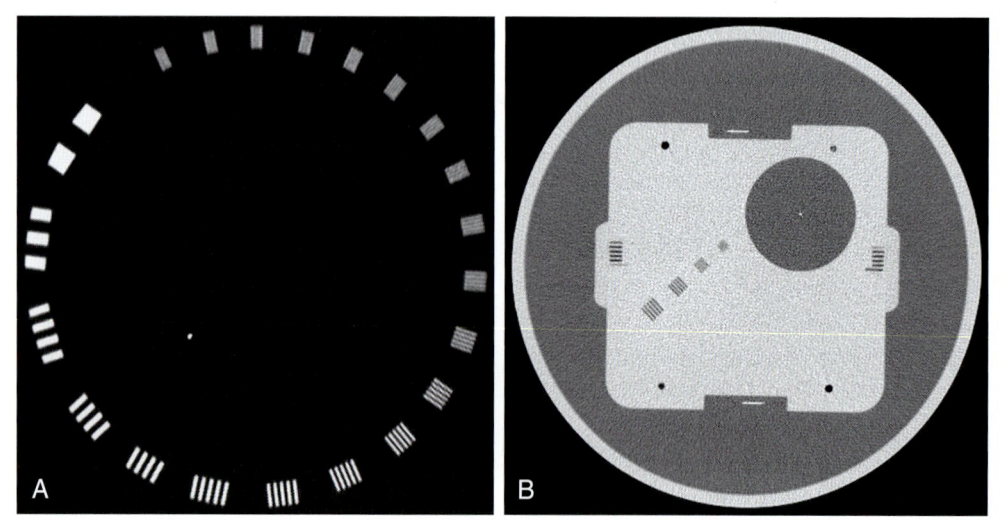

■ **FIGURE 79-3** Reconstructed images of resolution phantoms. **A**, Catphan. **B**, GE Performance phantom. (*B courtesy of GE Healthcare Technologies, Waukesha, Wisc.*)

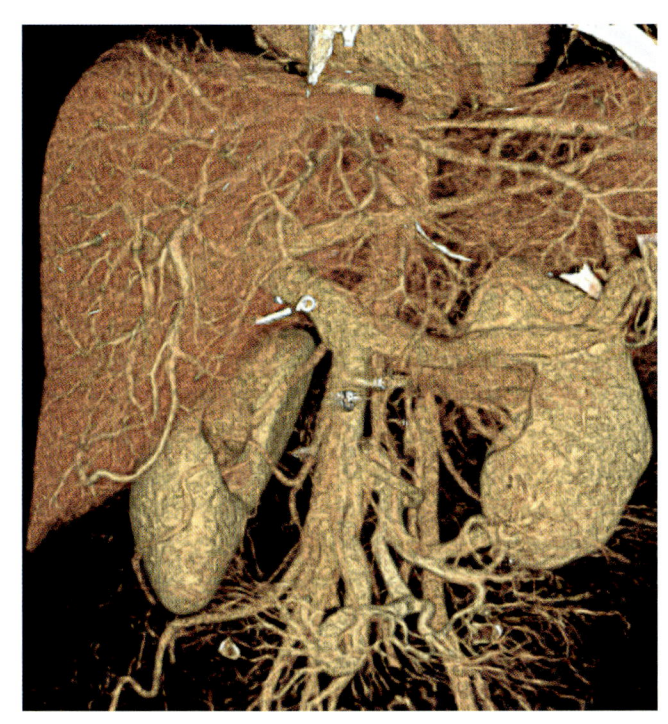

FIGURE 79-4 CT angiography study of a patient performed on a multislice CT scanner.

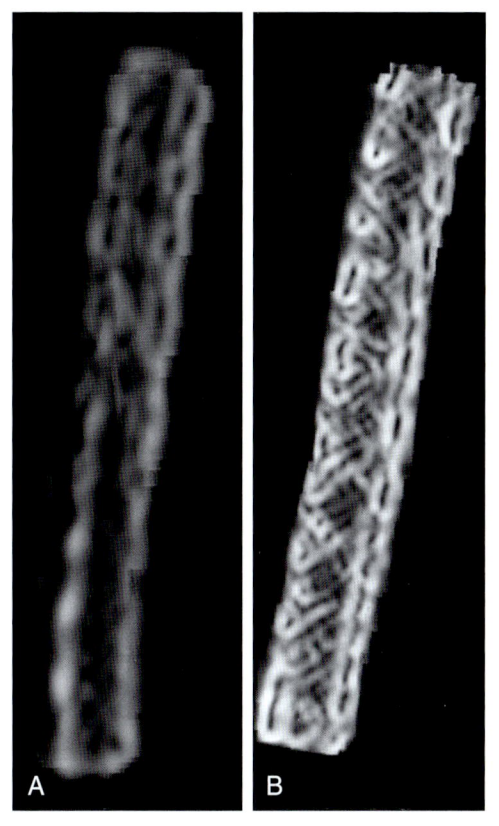

FIGURE 79-5 Volume rendered images of a 3-mm stent. **A,** The multislice CT image. **B,** High-definition image. *(Courtesy of GE Healthcare Technologies, Waukesha, Wisc.)*

example shown, the magnitude of the reconstructed object is only 50% of the original. Therefore, the MTF value at 4 lp/cm for this system is 0.5. By plotting the peak-to-valley magnitude over different frequencies, a complete MTF curve is obtained. The MTF accurately describes a system's frequency response and is a good indicator of the system's ability to resolve small objects. Alternatively, MTF curves can be obtained from the reconstructed phantom image of a thin wire, based on the fact that MTF is the magnitude of the Fourier transform of the point-spread function. Figure 79-3B shows a reconstructed image of a GE Performance phantom, and the wire section of the image is extracted to generate the MTF curve.

The most commonly quoted spatial resolution specifications are the 50% MTF, 10% MTF, and 0% MTF, which represent the frequencies at which the peak-to-valley magnitude of the CT system drops to 50%, 10%, and 0% of the scanned bar pattern. There are many factors that have an impact on the MTF, such as x-ray focal spot size, detector size, sampling frequency, system geometry, and reconstruction algorithm.

The importance of spatial resolution can be easily understood because it is an indicator of how well a small structure can be visualized. For example, Figure 79-4 depicts a volume rendered image of a CT angiography scan collected on a multislice CT scanner. High spatial resolution enables the clear visualization of small vascular structures. Another example is depicted in Figure 79-5 of two volume rendered images of a stent. Clear visualization of the stent allows the evaluation and assessment of its integrity or potential of restenosis in many clinical applications. Figure 79-5A was obtained on a multislice CT scanner; Figure 79-5B was obtained on a high-definition scanner. Because of the increased spatial resolution offered by the high-definition scanner, the stent structure is better visualized.

Another important performance parameter is the CT number uniformity and accuracy. CT number is defined by the following equation:

$$CT = \frac{\mu - \mu_w}{\mu_w} \times 1000$$

where μ is the linear attenuation coefficient of the object of interest and μ_w is the linear attenuation coefficient of water; the quantity is measured in Hounsfield units, honoring the inventor of the x-ray CT scan. On the basis of this definition, water automatically has a value of zero and air has a value of −1000. To ensure the CT number accuracy, water phantoms are often scanned, and the average CT number inside the water phantom is measured to ensure that it is within the tolerance limit of a few Hounsfield units. The selection of water phantoms for quality control is not accidental because the attenuation characteristics of human soft tissues are similar to those of water. Figure 79-6 depicts the reconstructed image of a 20-cm water phantom. For typical tests, several regions of interest are selected across the entire phantom to ensure that the CT number accuracy is maintained in the entire reconstruction field of view.

The CT number accuracy of a CT scanner can be affected by many factors, such as beam hardening, scatter, long-term stability of components, and other calibration issues. Therefore, periodic quality assurance testing is necessary to ensure that a CT scanner is performing within its designed specification. Recent research and development activities of dual-energy CT place an even higher importance on CT number accuracy because good material decomposition relies on the accuracy and reproducibility of the reconstructed CT numbers of different materials.

One of the more complex performance parameters is perhaps the low contrast detectability (LCD). LCD indicates a scanner's ability to identify small objects whose CT number difference to their background is small, and its performance depends not only on the size and contrast of the low-contrast objects to their background but also on the noise level present in the image. Because noise in the image is closely linked to the noise in the projection data, LCD needs to be specified with the specific phantom used in the test and the dose level in the scan. For example, the LCD specification generated with a Catphan of 3 mm, 0.3%, at 18 mGy and 5-mm slice thickness indicates that when the phantom is scanned with a dose level of 18 mGy and reconstructed at 5-mm slice thickness, 3-mm objects with 3 HU difference to their background can be visualized. For illustration, Figure 79-7A shows a reconstructed LCD section of a Catphan. Cylindrical objects of various sizes and contrast levels to the background are contained in the phantom of uniform background. Historically, the LCD specification was generated with human observers. Each observer was asked to identify the smallest cylinder with the lowest contrast in a set of reconstructed images. By incorporation of results generated on multiple images and with multiple observers, the LCD specification was produced. It is clear that such a method is highly subjective, and large variation among observers is expected. To overcome such shortcoming, several image processing–based methodologies were proposed. Given the limited scope of this chapter, any details are not discussed here.

Because image noise plays an important role in LCD, it is important to understand the impact of the reconstruction algorithm on LCD. For illustration, Figure 79-7 depicts the same LCD scan data reconstructed with two different reconstruction algorithms. The image depicted in Figure 79-7A was reconstructed with a filtered back-projection algorithm, which is a class of algorithm used by all vendors on the commercially available clinical scanners. The image depicted in Figure 79-7B, on the other hand, was reconstructed with an advanced statistical reconstruction that accurately models the statistics of the CT system. It is clear that better visualization of the LCD objects is achieved by the advanced statistical reconstruction. The 0.3% disks (shown in the outer ring between the 12- and 2-o'clock positions) that cannot be resolved in Figure 79-7A are now visible in Figure 79-7B. A similar result is also observed in a clinical study performed on a multislice CT scanner, as shown in Figure 79-8A and B. Note that by suppressing the noise in the images generated by filtered back-projection, density variations in the low-contrast tissues can be better visualized in Figure 79-8B.

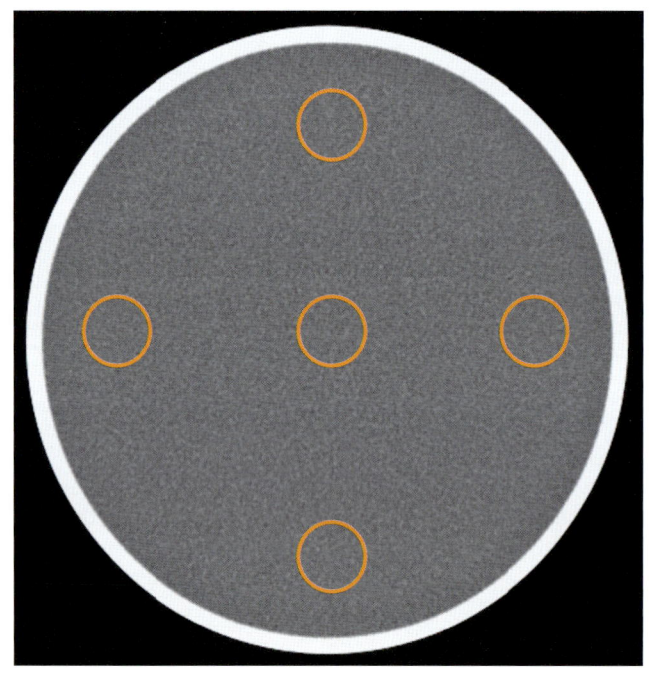

■ **FIGURE 79-6** Reconstructed image of a 20-cm water phantom.

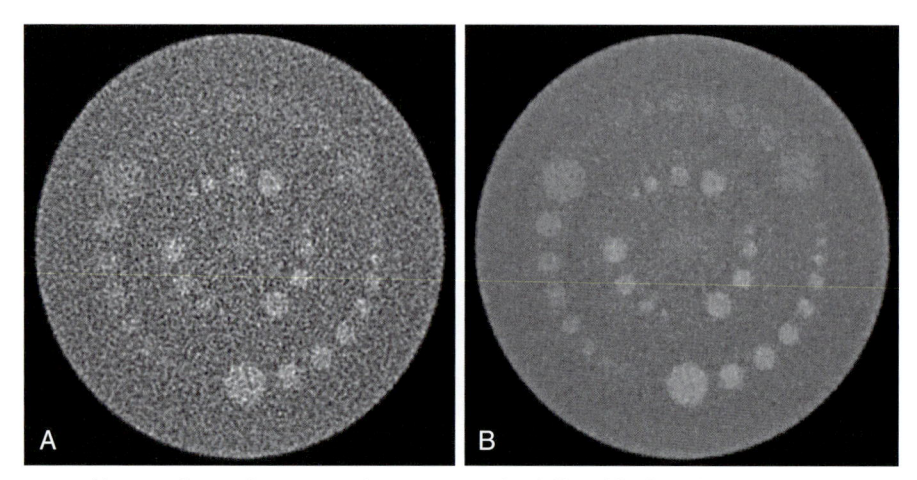

■ **FIGURE 79-7** Reconstructed images of a Catphan LCD section. **A,** Conventional filtered back-projection reconstruction. **B,** Advanced statistical reconstruction.

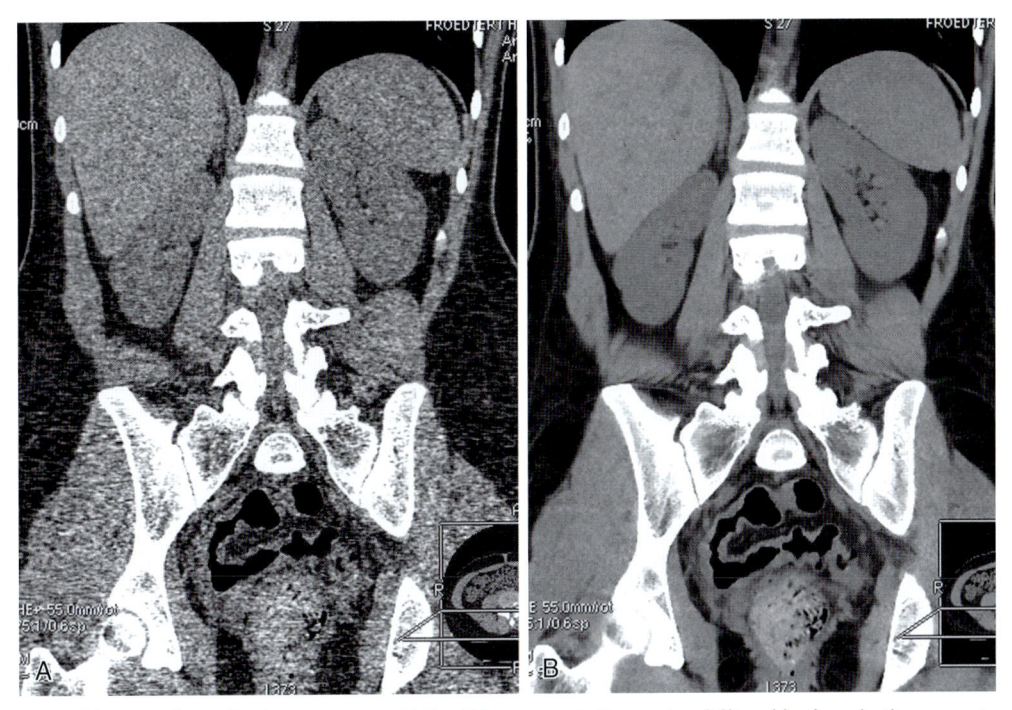

FIGURE 79-8 Coronal images of a patient's scan on a multislice CT scanner. **A,** Conventional filtered back-projection reconstruction. **B,** Advanced statistical reconstruction.

There are other performance parameters important to the specification of a CT scanner, such as temporal resolution, image artifacts, noise uniformity, spatial resolution uniformity, and dose efficiency. Interested readers can find relevant material in reference 1.

STEP-AND-SHOOT VERSUS HELICAL

Helical or spiral CT (HCT) was introduced in the early 1990s to overcome the lengthy delay in the traditional step-and-shoot mode of data acquisition.[7-10] Before the introduction of HCT, the patient and the table remained stationary during the data acquisition. Once the data collection is completed, the table is indexed to the next location for scanning. The table indexing time is typically on the order of a second. When the gantry rotation speed is slow, the amount of time spent on table translation is relatively small and constitutes a small fraction of the total study time. As the gantry speed increases, the table translation time becomes a significant portion of the overall scan time. Considering that the patient is holding his or her breath during CT scans to reduce motion-induced artifacts, a significant portion of the patient breath-hold time is wasted on indexing the patient because no data acquisition takes place during the patient indexing.

In HCT, the patient's table is translated at a constant speed while continuous data acquisition takes place. Relative to a fixed location on the patient, the x-ray source trajectory forms a helix (shown in Fig. 79-9), and the name of HCT is a reflection of such trajectory. In the early days of HCT development, there were lively debates on the naming convention: helical versus spiral. These debates ended without a clear winner, and both names are used interchangeably today.

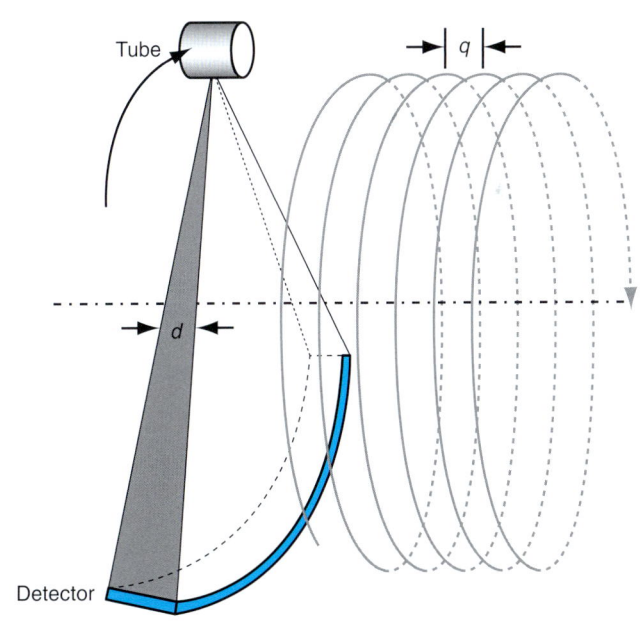

FIGURE 79-9 Illustration of helical data acquisition.

To characterize the nature of the helical trajectory, helical pitch is typically used. Helical pitch, h, is defined as the ratio of the table traveling distance in one gantry rotation, q, over the x-ray beam collimation width at the isocenter, d:

$$h = \frac{q}{d}$$

A higher h value indicates a faster table translation, assuming the gantry rotation speed is kept constant. An added advantage of the HCT mode of acquisition is the uniform sampling pattern along the patient's long axis. Note that in the step-and-shoot mode of data acquisition, the patient is scanned at discrete locations. For example, if a 2.5-mm source collimation is used for data acquisition, the table is typically indexed every 2.5 mm to acquire a consecutive set of slices. In HCT mode, however, the table moves in a continuous fashion, and the data are collected uniformly along the patient's long axis, z. Because the data acquisition is uniform along z, images can be reconstructed at arbitrary locations and spacing. If we use the same 2.5-mm source collimation example, images can be reconstructed at every 1.25 mm or finer to satisfy the Nyquist sampling criteria and to enable improved image quality in reformatted or volume rendered images. For illustration, Figure 79-10A shows a coronal image of a patient's scan reconstructed with 2.5-mm slice thickness at 2.5-mm spacing. Close inspection of the boundaries of the air pockets and contrast-enhanced organs shows discontinuities or stair-stepping artifacts, a clear indication of undersampling along the z-axis. For helical reconstruction, the images are reconstructed with the same slice thickness (2.5 mm) but at 1.0-mm spacing. Stair-stepping artifacts are completely eliminated in the coronal image as shown in Figure 79-10B. These advantages come at the price of increased complexity in reconstruction.

Less than a decade ago, the majority of the commercially available CT scanners were built with single-row detectors, in which the coverage along the patient's long axis is linked directly to the pre-patient collimation and the slice thickness. To scan a large volume in a short time for CT angiography applications (to keep up with the contrast bolus), higher helical pitch (h) was often used. For a single-slice scanner, a higher helical pitch often leads to an increased level of helical artifacts and degraded slice profiles. One often must trade off the coverage speed with the image quality. For illustration, Figure 79-11 shows the reconstructed images of a helical body phantom. The oval high-density objects are ellipsoids placed at an angle with respect to the patient's long axis to simulate ribs. The air pocket at the center is shaped as an ellipsoid. It is clear from the figure that as the helical pitch increases, the distortion and shading artifacts around ribs and air pocket increase. The monotonic behavior of artifacts versus helical pitch is mainly a single-slice scanner behavior. The relationship between artifacts and helical pitch is more complex for the case of a multislice scanner.

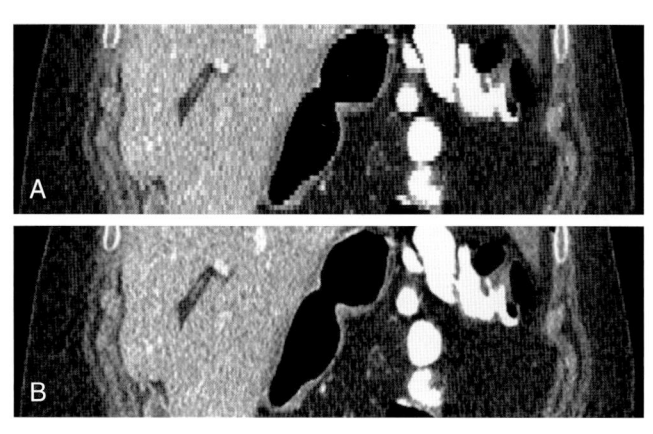

■ **FIGURE 79-10** Coronal images of a clinical study. **A,** A 2.5-mm slice thickness without overlap. **B,** A 2.5-mm slice at 1.0-mm spacing.

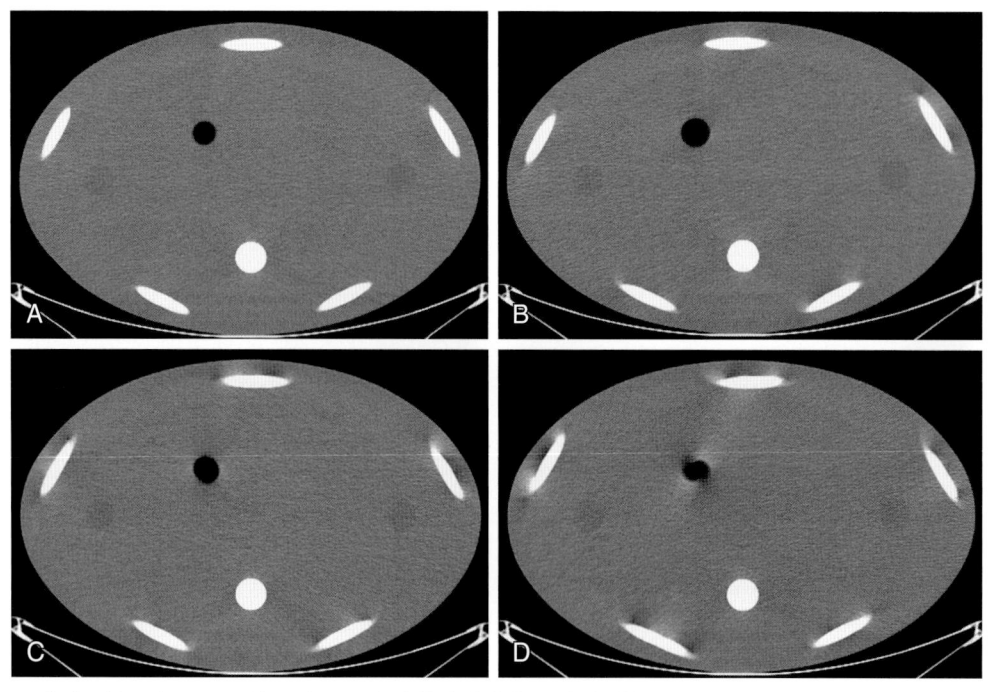

■ **FIGURE 79-11** Helical artifacts increase with an increase in helical pitch for a single slice: **A,** $h = 0$; **B,** $h = 1$; **C,** $h = 1.5$; **D,** $h = 2.0$.

There are other considerations in the selection of the helical pitch as well. One of the considerations is the noise level in the reconstructed images. As a general rule of thumb, the number of projections used to reconstruct an image is roughly inversely proportional to the helical pitch. For example, the number of views used in a 0.5:1 pitch scan is roughly twice as many as the number of views used in the 1:1 pitch. If other scanning parameters are kept constant, the 0.5 pitch image will be generated with nearly twice as much photon flux as the pitch 1 case; thus, the noise in the image should be scaled down by roughly $\sqrt{2}$. This offers additional flexibility in scanning of large patients when the maximum x-ray tube power is limited.

MULTISLICE COMPUTED TOMOGRAPHY

Although the very first CT scanner built more than three decades ago was a multislice CT scanner (dual slice), many people consider the commercial introduction of the four-slice scanner in the late 1990s the turning point of the multislice revolution, a reflection of its clinical impact, not a simple specification or slice count.[11-14] As the name implies, a multislice CT scanner divides each single-row detector cell into multiple detector cells along the gantry rotation axis (z-axis), as shown in Figure 79-12.

The advantage of the multislice CT scanner is its large detector coverage along the patient's long axis without trading off the spatial resolution in z. In a single-slice scanner, the z-coverage and the slice thickness are both controlled by the pre-patient collimator. If a 10-mm z-coverage is desired, the slice thickness of the detector is also 10 mm. Therefore, there is a one-to-one relationship between the coverage and z-resolution. For a multislice scanner, the slice thickness is no longer determined by the pre-patient collimation; it is determined by the size of the finely divided detector cells (if we ignore focal spot size and other factors). A larger coverage in z requires a larger number of detector rows.

There are two different types of detector designs used in the multislice CT scanner: matrix detector and adaptive detector (Fig. 79-13). In the matrix detector configuration, all detector rows are diced into identical sizes, and acquisition slice thickness is solely defined by the detector cell size. Different slice thickness can be obtained by combining several detector rows before or during the reconstruction process. In the adaptive detector scheme, the sizes of detector rows change symmetrically with respect to the detector center, and acquisition slice thickness is defined by the combination of detector cell aperture and pre-patient collimation. Similar to the matrix detector configuration, different slice thickness can be achieved by combining multiple detector rows. There are pros and

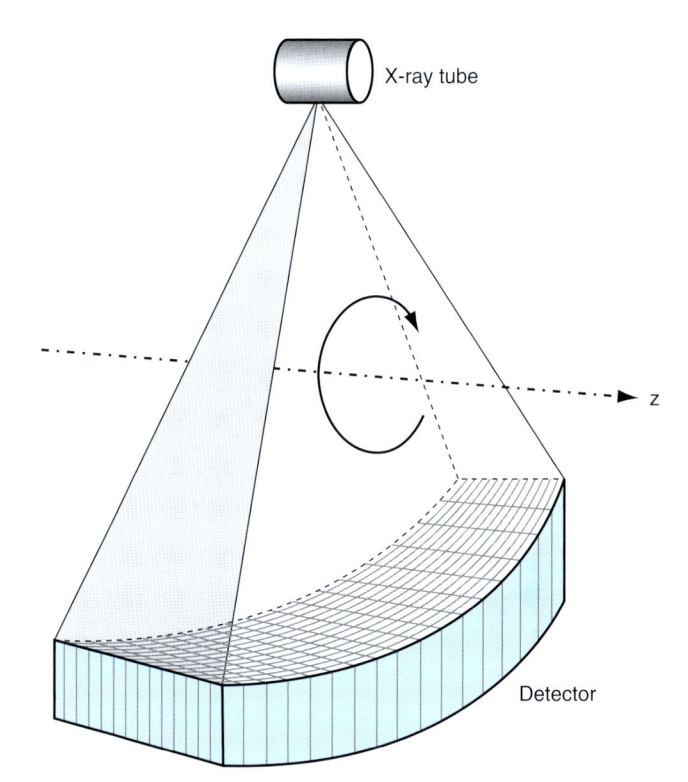

■ **FIGURE 79-12** Illustration of multislice CT configuration.

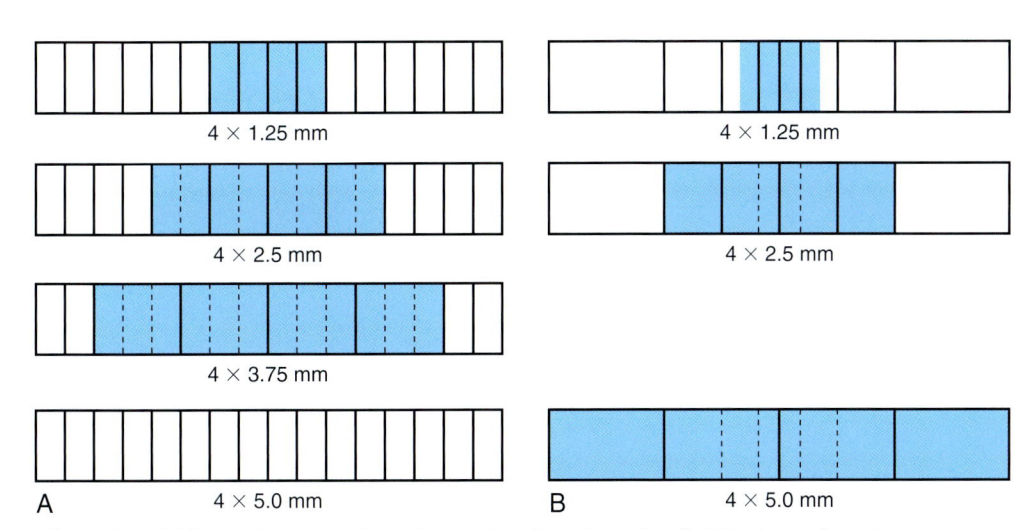

■ **FIGURE 79-13** Illustration of different detector configurations. **A**, Matrix configuration. **B**, Adaptive configuration.

cons with each approach, and given the limited scope of this chapter, detailed discussion is omitted here.

If the introduction of helical CT marks the era of single-organ coverage in a single breath-hold, the realization of the multislice CT marks the era of isotropic spatial resolution anywhere at any time. With the introduction of the 64-slice scanners, the time it takes to scan an anatomy in most cases is no longer limited by the data acquisition speed of the scanner. In fact, in many clinical practices, the scan speed is purposely throttled back to avoid overrunning the contrast agent.

There are many technical challenges facing multislice CT development as the number of slices increases significantly beyond 64-slice configuration. These challenges include the cone-beam artifacts for step-and-shoot mode scans, longitudinal truncation issues, over-beaming issues, increased scatter, degraded heel effect of the x-ray tube, compromised dose efficiency, and reduced effectiveness of the x-ray tube current modulation. Some of the challenges, such as over-beaming, can be addressed by modification of existing CT designs. Other challenges, such as cone-beam artifacts for step-and-shoot mode acquisition, remain difficult, and significant research efforts are continuing to minimize their clinical impact.

KEY POINTS

- Important parameters that define the performance of a CT scanner include spatial resolution, CT number uniformity and accuracy, and low contrast detectability.
- Temporal resolution, image artifacts, noise uniformity, spatial resolution uniformity, and dose efficiency are other parameters of performance.
- Helical CT uses continuous table translation during scanning, which is faster than step-and-shoot scanning and avoids misregistration artifact.
- Multislice CT allow fast scanning of a large volume, which is ideal for vascular imaging.

SUGGESTED READINGS

Boone JM. X-ray production, interaction, and detection in diagnostic imaging. In Beutel J, Kundel HL, VanMetter RL (eds). Handbook of Medical Imaging. Bellingham, Wash, SPIE Press, 2000, pp 3-78.

Hu H. Multi-slice helical CT: scan and reconstruction. Med Phys 1999; 26:1-18.

Hsieh J. CT image reconstruction. In Goldman LW, Fowlkes JB (eds). Categorical Course in Diagnostic Radiology Physics: CT and US Cross-Sectional Imaging. Oakbrook, Ill, Radiological Society of North America, 2000, pp 53-64.

Hsieh J. Computed Tomography: Principles, Design, Artifacts, and Recent Advances. Bellingham, Wash, SPIE Press, 2003.

REFERENCES

1. Hsieh J. Computed Tomography: Principles, Design, Artifacts, and Recent Advances. Bellingham, Wash, SPIE Press, 2003.
2. Boone JM. X-ray production, interaction, and detection in diagnostic imaging. In Beutel J, Kundel HL, VanMetter RL (eds). Handbook of Medical Imaging. Bellingham, Wash, SPIE Press, 2000, pp 3-78.
3. Johns HE, Cunningham JR. The Physics of Radiology. Springfield, Ill, Charles C Thomas, 1983.
4. Judy PF. Evaluating computed tomography image quality. In Goldman LW, Fowlkes JB (eds). Medical CT and Ultrasound: Current Technology and Applications. Madison, Wisc, Advanced Medical Publishing, 1995, pp 359-377.
5. McCollough CH, Zink FE. Performance evaluation of CT systems. In Goldman LW, Fowlkes JB (eds). Categorical Courses in Diagnostic Radiology Physics: CT and US Cross-Sectional Imaging. Oakbrook, Ill, Radiological Society of North America, 2000, pp 189-207.
6. American Association of Physicists in Medicine. Specification and Acceptance Testing of Computed Tomographic Scanners. New York, AAPM, 1993. Report no. 39.
7. Kalender WA, Seissler W, Vock P. Single-breath-hold spiral volumetric CT by continuous patient translation and scanner rotation. Radiology 1989; 173(P):414.
8. Crawford CR, King K. Computed tomography scanning with simultaneous patient translation. Med Phys 1990; 17:967-982.
9. Wang G, Vannier MW. Longitudinal resolution in volumetric x-ray computerized tomography—analytical comparison between conventional and helical computerized tomography. Med Phys 1994; 21:429-433.
10. Hsieh J. A general approach to the reconstruction of x-ray helical computed tomography. Med Phys 1996; 23:221-229.
11. Wang G, Lin TH, Cheng P, Shinozaki DM. A general cone-beam reconstruction algorithm. IEEE Trans Med Imaging 1993; 12:486-496.
12. Taguchi K, Aradate H. Algorithm for image reconstruction in multi-slice helical CT. Med Phys 1998; 25:550-561.
13. Hu H. Multi-slice helical CT: scan and reconstruction. Med Phys 1999; 26:1-18.
14. Hsieh J. CT image reconstruction. In Goldman LW, Fowlkes JB (eds). Categorical Course in Diagnostic Radiology Physics: CT and US Cross-Sectional Imaging. Oakbrook, Ill, Radiological Society of North America, 2000, pp 53-64.

CHAPTER 80

Computed Tomographic Angiography: Clinical Techniques

John J. Sheehan, Aoife N. Keeling, Vahid Yaghmai, and James C. Carr

Since the introduction of multidetector computed tomography (MDCT), one now has the ability to image the entire arterial tree in a noninvasive fashion. Optimal technical considerations for performing MDCT angiography (MDCTA) are essential for accurate diagnosis and atherosclerotic disease stratification. This chapter focuses on the various technical aspects necessary for CT angiography (CTA) acquisition. The different protocols for assessment of the cerebral, carotid, coronary, aortic, and peripheral arteries are outlined. In addition, the issue of radiation dose reduction, optimal bolus delivery of contrast material, and methods of postprocessing are described. Previously, digital subtraction angiography (DSA) was the only established reliable imaging technique to quantify atherosclerotic disease load; however, in this new millennium, MDCTA may now challenge the old gold standard.

DSA remains the gold standard method for evaluation of atherosclerosis within the vasculature; however, this is a minimally invasive technique with the potential for iatrogenic complications. Therefore, noninvasive imaging methods are desirable among patients and physicians alike. With the advent of MDCT, noninvasive angiography has become a viable option as a result of increased speed, spatial resolution, and volume coverage. CTA revolutionized vascular imaging when vessels smaller than 1 mm in diameter were imaged with single-slice spiral CT.[1-5] However, because of the small volume of coverage and limitations in the speed of image processing, CTA did not become widely used until the introduction of MDCT in 1998.[6-8] With the advent of MDCT, temporal and spatial resolution of the scanners significantly improved.[9,10] Gantry rotation times of 0.28 to 0.5 second with slice thickness of 0.33 to 0.75 mm are now available on most MDCT scanners.

With MDCT, there are several parallel detectors along the z-axis, and multiple channels of data (currently up to 320) significantly improve z-axis resolution. This allows isotropic resolution for most vascular applications with images obtained during a single short breath-hold. The result has been elimination of the tradeoff between spatial resolution (z-axis) and scanning range, an important limitation of single-detector spiral CT.[11,12] Hence, a significant benefit has been a paradigm shift from single-slice to volumetric data acquisition. This, in turn, has made imaging of different vascular phases with a single bolus of contrast material a reality.[7] Isotropic data sets allow three-dimensional reconstruction and a variety of postprocessing methods to enable both diagnostic interpretation and eloquent anatomic and pathologic arterial display.

Cardiac imaging was previously confined to plain film, invasive coronary angiography, nuclear medicine, and echocardiography. Noninvasive imaging of the heart with CT and magnetic resonance imaging (MRI) has changed our approach to imaging of cardiac disease. The advent of MDCT with electrocardiographic (ECG) synchronization has established several clinical roles in the evaluation of coronary artery disease, coronary artery anomalies, coronary stent, coronary bypass analysis, and coronary plaque characterization.

The advantages of CTA include lower cost and the ability to potentially reduce the total volume of contrast material administered. With the fastest scanners currently available, abdominal CTA can be performed with as little as 50 mL of contrast material with the use of saline flush.[13,14] This requires meticulous attention to the timing of bolus administration of the contrast material, which is discussed later in this chapter. In evaluation of life-threatening vascular disease, such as traumatic aortic injury or pulmonary embolus, CTA has a clear advantage because of short acquisition times.[15]

An important advantage of CTA over catheter angiography is its ability to examine the vessel wall as well as its lumen. The adjacent organs can also be evaluated (e.g., staging of pancreatic adenocarcinoma). Another advantage of CTA is the ability to evaluate a vessel in projections that cannot be obtained with conventional techniques.

Increased utility of CT has led to significant increase in radiation exposure and concerns about its effect.[16] CT currently accounts for approximately 75% of the total radiation dose delivered by medical imaging.[17] Development of automatic tube current modulation software that is now available on all advanced MDCT systems has been a positive side effect of this awareness. Tube current modulation automatically adjusts the current during scanning to decrease the amount of radiation in anatomic regions that do not require higher current (e.g., lung bases or above the iliac crest) while maintaining image quality.[16] In the appropriate setting, CTA may be performed with a reduced kilovoltage setting to decrease radiation to the patient and to improve signal-to-noise ratio.[18]

TECHNICAL REQUIREMENTS
Technical Components and Design
Image Quality

Factors affecting image quality and characteristics of CTA images include temporal and spatial resolution. Spatial resolution refers to the degree of blurring in the image and the ability to discriminate objects and structures of small size. Axial resolution within the scan plane can be improved by using a small field of view, larger matrix size, smaller focal spot, and smaller detectors. The demand for high spatial resolution to visualize the various coronary segments that course with decreasing diameter to the apex is high. One of the major goals of MDCT technology development has been to obtain similar spatial resolution in all directions, also expressed as *isotropic spatial resolution*.[19] CTA requires high spatial resolution to enable accurate detection and interrogation of small arterial branch vessels. Both in-plane and through-plane spatial resolutions are important indices that require optimization to provide isotropic source data. Isotropic means that the spatial resolution is approximately equal in all planes, which is necessary to enable multiplanar image reconstruction after acquisition. Isotropic data avoid loss of spatial resolution in one plane and reduce partial volume effects after source data reconstruction.[20] The increased scanner detector numbers has allowed increased through-plane spatial resolution as the detector width is reduced with increased numbers (1 to 1.25 mm with 4-detector row CT, 0.5 to 0.625 mm with 64-detector row CT).[21] The new MDCT scanners have not improved in-plane spatial resolution; this is determined by detector geometry and the convolution kernel (reconstruction algorithm).[20] Temporal resolution is defined as the required time for data acquisition per slice. It represents the length of the reconstruction window during each heart cycle, which is determined by the gantry speed.

Noise is the random fluctuation of pixel values in a region that receives the same radiation exposure of another. Noise is an important determinant of CT image quality and limits the visibility of low contrast structures. It is determined primarily by the number of photons used to make an image (quantum mottle). Increasing tube current and voltage can reduce it. It can also be reduced by increasing voxel size (decreasing matrix size, increasing field of view, or increasing slice thickness).

Contrast is the difference of the intensity of one area relative to another. Image contrast is the difference in the intensity of a lesion and that of the surrounding background. CT is superior to conventional radiography for detecting low contrast differences. CT contrast is the difference in the Hounsfield unit (HU) values between tissues. CT contrast increases as tube voltage (kV) decreases and is not affected by tube current (mAs). Adding a contrast medium such as iodine can increase contrast. The displayed image contrast is determined by the CT window (width and level).

Scanner Design

Since the first pencil beam EMI scanner in 1972, there have been numerous generations of CT scanners. The first four generations of scanners all had a single row of detectors (single slice) with evolving x-ray tube and detector configurations. Initially, for these generations, the image data were acquired one slice at a time. This involved scanning a slice and then moving the patient table to the next slice position and scanning again, otherwise known as step-and-shoot. The next advancement was the introduction of helical (spiral) CT, which involved continuous moving of the patient table through the CT gantry, as the tube rotated around the patient. The relationship between the patient and tube motion is called pitch, which is defined as table movement (mm) during each full rotation of the x-ray tube divided by the collimation width (mm). A faster pitch means thicker slices, reduced resolution, but lower scan time and lower patient dose. A pitch of greater than 1 will leave gaps between slabs, and a pitch of less than 1 will allow necessary overlap among slabs.

Electron-beam CT technology, also known as *fifth-generation CT*, provides excellent temporal resolution that allows freezing of cardiac motion through very short acquisition times. In electron-beam CT, the detectors are stationary. The x-ray source is fixed. It consists of a 210-degree ring of tungsten. This is bombarded by an electromagnetically focused beam of electrons fired from an x-ray gun. The patient is placed between the x-ray source and detector, obviating the need for moving any part of the scanner during the examination. Whereas electron-beam CT has better temporal resolution at present (50 ms), the spatial resolution is not nearly as good as that of MDCT because the collimators are too thick.

Detectors

The next major advancement was the development of MDCT. This incorporated the use of multiple rows of detectors to detect wider fan beams. This configuration makes more efficient use of x-ray tube output and covers a larger area in the patient's z-axis (long axis) for every tube rotation. Unlike in conventional CT, the slice thickness of MDCT is determined by detector width and not by collimator thickness. The number of rows has increased at a rapid pace during recent years, covering 2, 4, 8, 16, 32, 64, 128, 256, and now 320 slices. The current driving force behind this rapid evolution is coronary artery disease.

Flying focal spot technology improves spatial resolution without decreasing the size of the detector elements by use of two overlapping x-ray beams without a corresponding increase in dose. Detector elements of 0.6 mm can be used to acquire 0.33-mm spatial resolution images.

Diagnostic performance in coronary CTA is primarily determined by temporal resolution, which is the required time for data acquisition per slice. The determinant of this is the gantry rotational speed. For the typical setup of a single tube and detector, half a gantry rotation is necessary to acquire the data for volume reconstruction, that is, temporal resolution is equal to half gantry rotation. The temporal resolution of a 64-slice CT scanner with a gantry rotation of 330 ms is 166 ms. For motion-free images to be obtained at any phase in the cardiac cycle, a temporal resolution of 10 ms is required. Achievement of such high temporal resolution is impossible with CT. As a result, cardiac CT phase reconstruction is centered on the quiescent or low-motion window in end-diastole. The postulated required temporal resolution for reliable cardiac imaging is in the range of 65 ms.[22] One manufacturer has developed a 256-slice CT scanner (128 × 0.625) with a rotation time of 270 ms and temporal resolution of 135 ms. However, with automatic multisegmental reconstructions with voxel-based optimization, temporal resolutions up to 68 ms are achieved.

Other platforms use dual-source CT technology, which comprises two x-ray tubes and two corresponding detectors. The two acquisition systems are mounted on the rotating gantry, with an angular offset of 90 degrees. For cardiac imaging, a detector configuration of 64 × 0.6 mm is used, whereby two subsequent 64-slice readings with a flying focal spot are combined into two 128-slice projections, with isotropic spatial resolution of 0.33 mm. With the tube rotation time of 280 ms, data can be sampled over only 90 degrees of a gantry rotation (as opposed to 180 degrees with single-source systems), resulting in the industry's fastest temporal resolution of 75 ms. The ultra-fast tube rotation and table feed enable acquisition of the entire heart in 250 ms within a single diastolic phase without a breath-hold, resulting in reduced dose down to an unprecedented 1 mSv or less.

The newly developed 320-slice CT scanner with 0.5-mm detectors (16-cm coverage along the patient's z-axis) images the body in a cylindrical fashion and can scan the entire heart prospectively, in one heartbeat without any table movement. This is expected to reduce the likelihood of both cardiac and respiratory motion artifacts.

Dual Energy

One of the more recent advances in CT has been the introduction of dual energy. In dual-energy mode, the two tubes emit x-ray spectra of different energy levels that are simultaneously registered in their corresponding detector array. At any given time point, this provides synchronous dual-energy image formation for the entire anatomy encompassed by the scan range. This enables differentiation of scanned tissues with different spectral properties, allowing the identification and subtraction of vessel wall calcification.

Image Acquisition and Reconstruction

CTA can be performed with or without ECG gating. The advantage of gating is that it significantly minimizes motion of the aorta or coronary arteries related to cardiac motion and systolic pressure changes. Two types of triggering or ECG gating exist: retrospective and prospective.

Retrospective Gating

Cardiovascular MDCT imaging is currently predominantly performed in the spiral (helical) mode; data are acquired by constant rotation of the x-ray tube/detector system throughout the entire cardiac cycle (continuous scanning). The data acquired are linked to the ECG tracing, allowing retrospective reconstruction of multiple cardiac phases when the study is complete. A specific phase within the R–R interval can be chosen to create a stack of images.

There are two techniques to retrospectively gate the scan to the ECG for image reconstruction. In one technique, the images are collected from one particular point in time in the cardiac cycle, which is defined as a percentage of the R–R interval. Alternatively, this point in time is defined at an absolute fixed time in milliseconds before or after the R–R interval. This latter method is better for irregular heart rhythms.

Retrospective gating allows faster coverage of the heart than does prospective triggering because images are reconstructed at every heartbeat. Continuous spiral acquisition allows overlapping of image sections and therefore permits 20% greater in-plane spatial resolution than that allowed by the collimator itself, resulting in a resolution of 0.6 mm for a 0.75-mm section and 0.4 mm for a 0.6-mm section.

Continuous acquisition throughout the cardiac cycle also allows retrospective reconstruction at different phases of the cardiac cycle. This permits selection of the best phases for each of the coronary arteries and their segments where there is least motion and best image quality. Retrospectively, individual heartbeats may be deleted, or the reconstruction interval for an individual beat can be shifted manually if there are arrhythmias or variable heart rates. Retrospective triggering is the preferred method of triggering for assessment of cardiac function and valve disease.

Prospective Gating

Prospective ECG triggering is a sequential scan in which data acquisition is prospectively triggered by the ECG signal in diastole. Data are collected only at a predefined cardiac phase, established by the operator before the acquisition.

With this technique, tube current is turned on only at a predefined point after the R wave (a constant cardiac phase). At all other times between each R-R interval, no radiation is emitted. This triggering method requires a regular heart rhythm; otherwise, the image created during each heartbeat will occur at a different part of the cardiac phases, resulting in artifacts. Prospective gating is most often used for calcium scoring. Prospective gating reduces the radiation dose by up to 10 times. However, this occurs at the expense of unavailability of systolic phases for additional image reconstruction (which may be needed if diastolic images are suboptimal). In addition, assessment of cardiac function is not possible.

Hsieh and coworkers[23] have developed a new approach for CTA referred to as prospectively gated axial. This technique uses a combined step-and-shoot axial data acquisition and an incrementally moving table with prospective adaptive ECG triggering. This method takes advantage of the large-volume coverage available with the 64-slice MDCT scanner that enables complete coverage of the heart in two or three steps. With this technique, the table is stationary during the image acquisition. It then moves to the next position for another scan initiated by the subsequent cardiac cycle. The result is very little overlap between the scans, significant (50% to 80%) reduction in radiation dose, and more robust and adaptive ECG gating. Earls and associates[24] reported an effective dose for the prospectively gated axial group (mean, 2.8 mSv) that was significantly lower than that for the retrospectively gated helical group (mean, 18.4 mSv). This represents a reduction in mean effective dose to the patient by up to 80% from the retrospectively gated helical to the prospectively gated axial approach.

ECG Dose Modulation

Dose modulation is used to help reduce the radiation exposure. During retrospective scanning, the tube current (mA) is turned on continuously during the examination. The tube current is dialed down by 80% during systole. Although the lower milliamperage may result in a suboptimal quality image, this may not be of clinical consequence. The reduced dose of radiation is therefore applied before 35% and after 80% of the R-R interval, which reduces the radiation dose by up to 40% of the usual dose. With most machines, dose modulation is the default mode and needs to be turned off if it is not desired. With increased heart rates, dose modulation cannot be used.

Reconstruction Techniques

Reconstruction of images for the evaluation of arteries uses thin slices with the smallest field of view (e.g., 18 to 20 cm) that encompasses only the heart. If the entire chest needs to be evaluated, a larger field of view is used with thicker slices. Additional data sets with a larger field of view that includes the entire chest should be reconstructed for the evaluation of extracardiac structures.

Kernel or reconstruction filters determine the balance between image resolution and smoothness (or signal-to-noise ratio). Smooth kernels are used for coronary CTA. Sharper kernels provide better definition of lumen borders and reduce blooming artifacts from high-density structures (e.g., stent) at the expense of higher image noise. The use of smooth kernels provides images with lower noise at the expense of possibly increased blooming of calcium and stents.

Contrast Detection and Administration

With shortened acquisition times of MDCT, optimization and maximization of vascular enhancement have become more challenging.[25,26] CTA requires excellent contrast enhancement of the targeted vessels. A good-quality CT angiogram requires an arterial density value of greater than 200 HU.[27,28] This should be achieved rapidly, and the peak should coincide with the acquisition interval. It is therefore crucial to time the contrast bolus correctly. However, rapid administration of contrast material shortens the plateau phase of contrast enhancement, thus creating further challenge for correct timing of the study.[25,26,29] For most CTA applications, an injection rate of 4 to 5 mL/sec yields optimal vascular enhancement.

Several factors affect time to peak from the start of contrast bolus administration. These include the iodine content of the contrast material, the injection rate, and the patient's cardiac status.[25,26,30,31] A faster injection rate, for example, can achieve a higher density in the targeted vessel and results in a higher quality CT angiogram. It also separates the arterial from the portal venous phase and hence results in excellent image quality without cross-contamination by different phases.[25] Contrast material with higher iodine concentration improves vascular enhancement if all other parameters are held constant.[25,32] An important consideration with the 16- and 64-slice scanners is the possibility of "outrunning" the contrast bolus in patients with low cardiac output or in cases that require long z-axis coverage (e.g., combination of extremity and abdominal CTA); to overcome this issue, one can slow down the scanner by increasing the gantry rotation time and slowing the table speed.[33,34]

Fixed Scan Delay

Few authors currently use the method of setting a standard timed scan delay after the intravenous administration of contrast material to acquire images in the arterial phase.[35,36] By setting the same scan delay for every patient, one is assuming that exactly the same hemodynamic conditions exist in all patients. This method does not accommodate patients with any variation from the normal (i.e., low blood pressure, low cardiac outputs, hypovolemia, high outputs). We would not agree with employing this method of a fixed scan delay time.

Bolus Tracking

To more accurately determine the optimal scan delay after intravenous administration of contrast material in patients with variable hemodynamics, the technique of contrast bolus tracking can be employed. Used by many authors,[37,39] this is an efficient way to optimize arterial opacification. Initially, a single low-dose CT image is obtained, without administration of contrast material, at the level of the common carotid for the carotids, the ascending aorta for the coronary and thoracic aorta, and the celiac axis for the abdominal aorta and runoffs. A 10- to 15-mm^2 circular region of interest is placed inside the middle of the aortic lumen, and this will subsequently measure the Hounsfield units of the aortic lumen on subsequent scanning. At 8 to 10 seconds after intravenous administration of contrast material, serial low-dose monitoring CT scans are obtained at the same table position at 1-second intervals. When the region of interest detects a preset contrast enhancement level (usually 100 to 150 HU value), there is automatic triggering of the scanner to acquire images in the desired scan range. This time-efficient method ensures optimal arterial enhancement within the region of interest, which can be moved to a different arterial location if desired. It enables lower contrast use and reduces scan-to-scan and patient-to-patient variability in arterial opacification.

Test Bolus

Another method to optimize arterial contrast opacification is that of a test bolus or timing bolus acquisition. Described by a number of authors,[38,40] this technique involves intravenous administration of a small bolus (20 to 30 mL) of contrast material followed by serial CT data acquisitions at one table position, usually at the levels described for bolus tracking. Images are acquired, after a scan delay of 8 to 10 seconds, every 1 to 2 seconds for a predetermined number of images (20 to 40) or until the CT technologist chooses to manually stop the acquisition after the contrast peak within the aorta. A time versus Hounsfield unit (attenuation) curve is then generated by placing a region of interest over the contrast-opacified aorta. The time taken to reach peak opacification is then used as the scan delay for the actual CTA and thus corresponds to the time taken for the contrast material to pass from the intravenous injection site of interest. This method is useful as it detects variable transit times between patients with different hemodynamic states and allows individualization of scan delays.

Adaptive Method

The runoff vessels in the symptomatic limb can be problematic with CTA as a result of proximal/in-flow stenosis or, alternatively, distal hyperemia at the site of arterial ulceration; these can cause arterial flow discrepancy between the two lower limbs. Thus, one limb will have a faster flow rate than the other, resulting in good contrast opacification of the arteries ipsilaterally but failed opacification contralaterally. CT fails at eliciting dynamic information. This problem may be somewhat reduced by use of an adaptive method of contrast detection that was described by Qanadli and associates.[41] This method is similar to that of a test bolus technique in that a small 30-mL contrast bolus is administered intravenously, followed by two low-dose (20 mA, 120 kV) CT acquisitions. The first is at the level of the descending thoracic aorta (at vertebra level T12) acquired 20 seconds after the start of intravenous administration of the contrast material for 10 seconds; the second level is the popliteal arteries below the knee acquired 30 seconds after the start of the intravenous bolus (i.e., after the aortic level is finished). Three time-density curves are created, one from the aortic level and one from each of the popliteal artery levels. The time to peak contrast enhancement is then determined for each level (aortic time = T1; popliteal time = T2). If the right and left popliteal times are different, the symptomatic leg or the longer time is taken to be T2. The aortopopliteal transit time (Tt) is determined from T2 − T1. The CT gantry rotation time and table speed are then set to match Tt in order that the popliteal artery will be imaged at peak enhancement. T1 is the delay time between commencement of the usual intravenous contrast bolus and commencement of data acquisition.[41] Laswed and colleagues[42] applied this adaptive method clinically in patients with peripheral arterial disease, with DSA correlation, and determined that MDCTA has a sensitivity and specificity of 100% for arterial lesion detection on a per-patient basis. Analyzed on a per-segment basis, MDCTA had a sensitivity and specificity for lesion detection of 91% and 96%, respectively, in the below-knee arteries and 100% and 90%, respectively, in the distal pedal arteries. This method was found to be reproducible, had high image quality, avoided the problem of venous overlay, and resolved the issue of differential peripheral arterial opacification.[42]

Contrast Media Concentration

A recent review attempted to determine the difference that contrast media iodine concentration makes to image quality of MDCTA in the peripheral vasculature.[43] All of the studies reviewed used iodine concentrations of 300 mg/mL and higher; whereas improved arterial enhancement and visualization were demonstrated with higher iodine concentrations, there was no clear evidence of a significant difference in diagnostic efficacy for the different iodine concentrations.[43] Iezzi and coworkers,[44] comparing iodine concentrations of 300 mg/mL with 400 mg/mL on a 4-detector scanner, also determined no significant differences in diagnostic ability of CTA for peripheral arterial disease. This could perhaps be explained by applying findings from the coronary CTA literature, whereby Becker and colleagues[45] determined that coronary artery attenuation levels of 250 to 300 HU were optimal for the evaluation of coronary artery disease because higher attenuation values may underestimate the amount of atherosclerosis owing to obscuration of vessel wall calcification. In our institution, we use a contrast media iodine concentration of 350 mg/mL.

Dual-Head Power Injectors

To achieve the desired arterial Hounsfield unit, a fast iodinated contrast injection with a tight arterial contrast bolus is necessary. Thus, patients will need to have a well-positioned, large-bore (18-gauge), intravenous cannula within the antecubital fossa. A dual-head power injector permits both contrast material and saline to be administered separately, concurrently, and sequentially. This means that two separate injection phases are possible, the first with 100% iodinated contrast material and the second with a 100% saline flush. The advantages of this method are that the arterial contrast enhancement is improved and prolonged, the contrast dose is reduced because most of the administered contrast material is within the arterial side, and the saline flush at the end clears dense contrast material from the superior vena cava to avoid streak artifact.[14,30,46] The value of a triphasic injection strategy with an extra second phase comprising a contrast-saline mixture could also potentially reduce the requirements for contrast material. The new multislice scanners in combination with dual-head injectors allow marked decrease in the amount of contrast material used for routine CTA. However, the total volume of contrast material administered for a routine abdominal CT study (usually 150 mL of 300 mg/mL concentration of contrast material) should not change if solid organs, such as liver, are evaluated in conjunction with CTA. Lowering of the total volume of contrast material may potentially reduce the sensitivity of lesion detection.[12,32]

Many authors have reported the use of gadolinium chelates for CTA in patients who have diminished renal function.[47-50] Although gadolinium is radiodense and may be used as a contrast agent with radiography, many gadolinium-based products have higher osmolality than iodine-based contrast media and are therefore potentially more nephrotoxic. More important, there have been several reports of nephrogenic systemic fibrosis leading to serious physical disability in patients with end-stage renal disease receiving gadolinium-containing contrast agents.[51,52]

TECHNIQUES

Indications and Technique Description

Scan protocols are highly variable and depend to a large extent on the type of MDCT scanner available (i.e., 4-, 16-, 64-, 128-, or 320-detector or dual energy) and also the manufacturer of the scanner. A suitable protocol should be chosen and programmed into the individual scanner for routine use. For the best CTA, a 16-slice scanner or higher should be used. A summary of the various protocols for the different vascular territories is outlined for a typical 64-slice MDCT scanner (Table 80-1).

Cerebral CTA

Intracranial vascular disease can now be identified and characterized noninvasively by visualization of the blood vessels with contiguous thin slices and creation of isotropic maximum intensity projection (MIP) images and three-dimensional volume rendered reformations. The newer generation of MDCT scanners, such as the 320-slice CT scanner, allows dynamic entire-volume imaging, producing CT-DSA in all dimensions (two-, three-, and four-dimensional). The time-resolved data sets can be used to perform three-dimensional perfusion with quantification. This technique is not likely to completely replace conventional diagnostic DSA as it has inferior spatial and temporal resolution.

The scanning volume of CTA is determined on the basis of the location of vascular lesions or suspected vascular lesions on CT, MRI, or magnetic resonance angiography. If the lesions are suspected in the supratentorial or circle of Willis region, the scan volume begins at the level of the sellar floor and extends cranially. If the lesions are multiple or unknown, the scan volume can be extended caudally to the level of the foramen magnum. If required, the extracranial vasculature (carotids and aortic arch) can be evaluated by extending the scan volume farther caudal to the level of the aortic arch.

Automated bolus tracking is the preferred technique to reliably obtain the optimal arterial phase by placing a region of interest on the internal carotid artery close to the skull base. An injection volume of 75 mL of a contrast agent with high iodine concentration (350 mg/mL) at a flow rate of 5 mL/sec is typically used. Images are acquired in the caudal to cranial direction with a slice thickness of 1 mm, slice interval of 0.5 mm, and 0.6 mm of collimation (Fig. 80-1).

Carotid CTA

In the United States, stroke is the leading cause of adult disability and the third leading cause of death; only heart disease and cancer cause more deaths annually. About 80% of strokes are ischemic strokes. Ischemic cerebrovascular events are often related to atherosclerotic narrowing at the carotid bifurcation. Conventional DSA is the reference standard for the evaluation of carotid artery disease.[53,54] The advantage of noninvasive CTA is the reduction in cost and procedural risks. With conventional DSA, several studies have demonstrated up to a 4% risk of transient ischemic attack or minor stroke, a 1% risk of major stroke, and a small (<1%) risk of death.[55] Plaque composition can be evaluated by CTA, which is an important indicator of plaque stability and helps with the assessment of risk factors for thromboembolic events. Noninvasive CTA provides the necessary information required before carotid endarterectomy and endovascular therapies.

The scanning volume of CTA is determined on the basis of the initial anteroposterior and lateral topograms. The volume should include all the vascular structures from the aortic arch to the intracranial circulation at the level of the external auditory meatus.

Automated bolus tracking or test bolus triggering techniques can reliably obtain the optimal arterial phase by placing a region of interest on the aortic arch. An injection volume of 75 mL of a contrast agent with high iodine concentration (350 mg/mL) at a flow rate of 5 mL/sec is typically used. Images are acquired in the caudal to cranial direction with a slice thickness of 1 mm, slice interval of 0.5 mm, and 0.6 mm of collimation (Fig. 80-2).

Thoracic CTA

The disease processes affecting the aortic root and thoracic aorta include aneurysmal dilation, aortic dissection along with intramural hematoma, and penetrating ulcer. By diagnosis, surveillance, and monitoring, imaging plays an important role in determining the timing and role of endovascular and surgical intervention.

Conventional DSA is regarded as the reference standard for evaluation of the thoracic arterial system. CTA of the thoracic aorta is currently the preferred method, however, for follow-up of patients with thoracic aortic aneurysms.[56]

CHAPTER 80 ● Computed Tomographic Angiography: Clinical Techniques 1061

TABLE 80-1 Summary of the Various Protocol Parameters for the Different Vascular Territories on a Typical 64-Slice MDCT Scanner

	Cerebral	Carotid	Thoracic Aorta	Pulmonary Artery	Coronary	Abdominal Aorta	Lower Extremity
Intravenous contrast agent	Yes	Yes	Yes	Yes	Yes	Yes	Yes
Contrast type	350	350	350	300	350	350	350
Contrast volume (mL)	75	75	100	120	100	100	150
Saline volume (mL)	80 (test 40/chase 40)	70 (test 40/chase 30)	70 (test 40/chase 30)	70 (test 40/chase 30)	70 (test 40/chase 30)	90 (test 40/chase 50)	90 (test 40/chase 50)
Rate (mL/sec)	5	5	5	4	5	5	5
Scan delay	Bolus tracking	Bolus tracking	Bolus tracking	Bolus tracking	Test bolus triggering	Bolus tracking	Bolus tracking
Placement of region of interest for detection of contrast	Internal carotid artery	Aortic arch	Ascending aorta	Pulmonary trunk	Ascending aorta	Aorta at celiac artery	Aorta at celiac artery
Scout views		Anteroposterior and lateral	Anteroposterior	Anteroposterior	Anteroposterior	Anteroposterior	Anteroposterior
Start position	Vertex	Aortic arch	Apices	Apices	Aortic arch	Diaphragm	Above celiac
End position	Head	External auditory canal	Mid kidney	Below lung bases	Apex of heart	Symphysis pubis	Through bottom of feet
Display field of view	Entire head	Entire head	Entire chest	Entire chest	Cone to heart	Entire AP	Entire AP
Slice thickness (mm)	1	1	1.5	1.5	0.75	2	1
Interval (mm)	0.5	0.5	1	1.5	0.5	2	1
Collimator (mm)	0.6	0.6	0.6	0.6	0.6	0.6	0.6
Reconstruction kernel (siemens)	H45f	B20f	B40f	B40f	B40f	B40f	B40f
Rotation time (seconds)	0.5	0.33	0.5	0.33	0.33	0.33	0.33
Direction	Caudal-cranial	Caudal-cranial	Cranial-caudal	Cranial-caudal	Cranial-caudal	Cranial-caudal	Cranial-caudal
kV/mAs	120/340	120/250	120/250	120/240	120/240	120/260	120/175
Breathing instructions	N/A	N/A	Technician inspiration	Technician inspiration	Technician inspiration	Technician inspiration	Technician inspiration
Window level	CTA	CTA	Abdomen	Mediastinum	Mediastinum	Abdomen	Abdomen

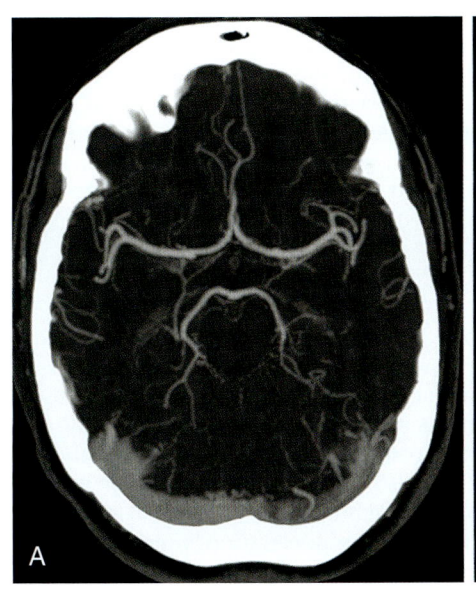

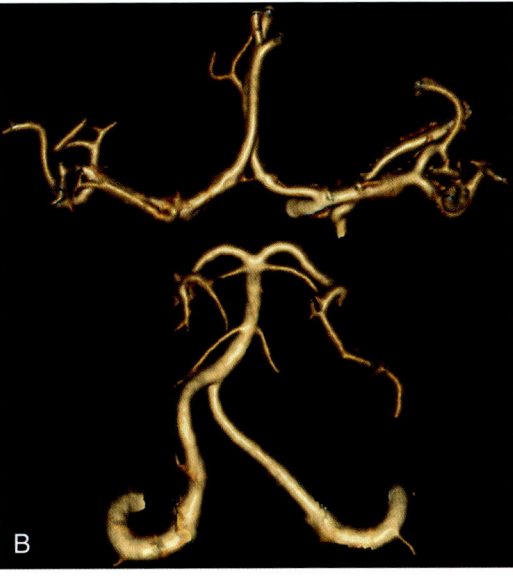

■ FIGURE 80-1 Axial MIP image (A) and volume rendered image (B) of CTA of the intracranial vessels demonstrating normal anatomy.

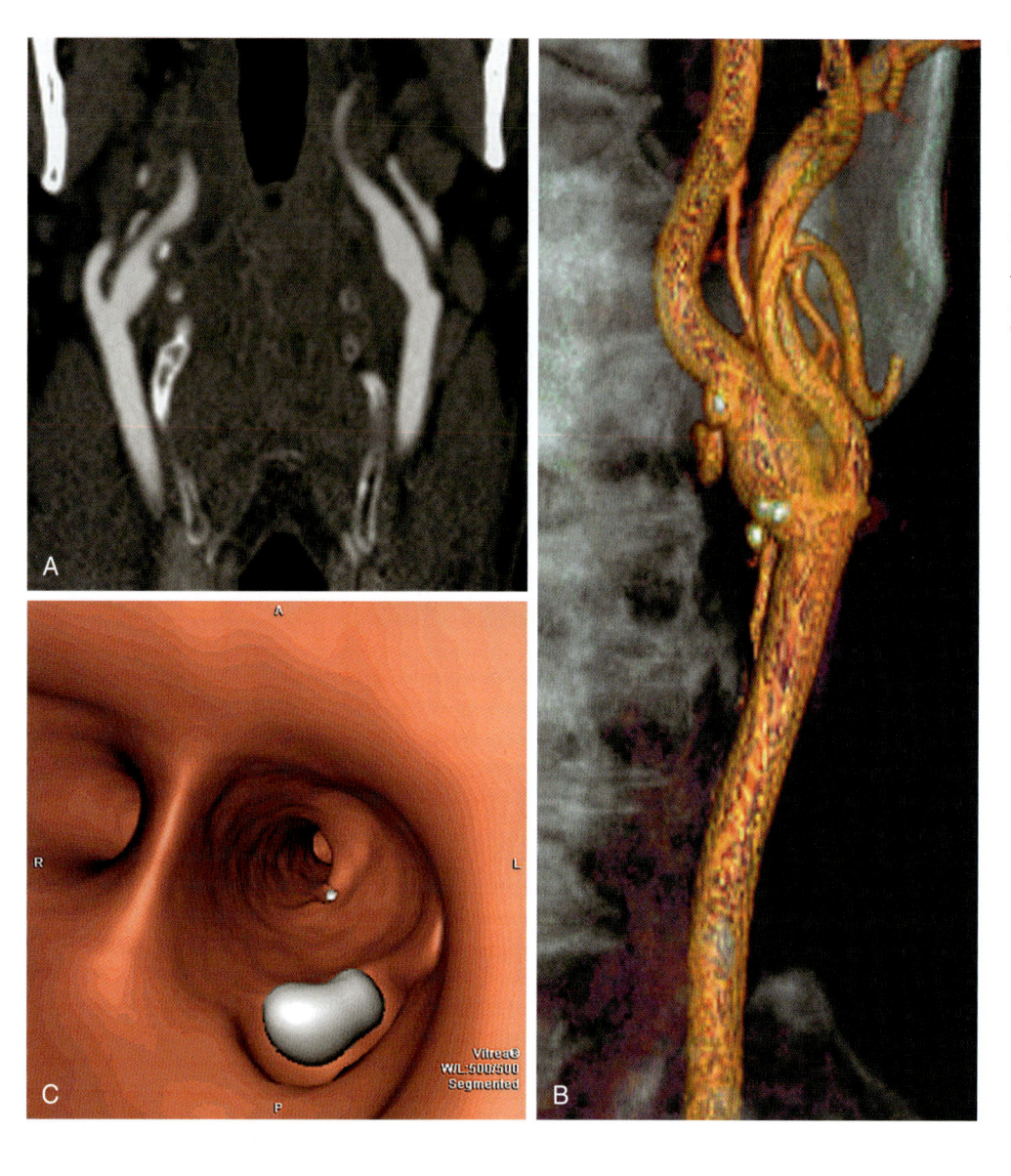

FIGURE 80-2 Coronal MIP image of the carotid vessels (**A**) shows calcified and soft plaque causing moderate stenosis of the right internal carotid artery beyond the bulb. The volume rendered image of the right side (**B**) demonstrates the eccentric calcified plaque causing predominantly positive remodeling. The in-vessel view (**C**) shows the calcified plaque lying within the wall of the carotid bulb.

It can, in addition to evaluating luminal disease, assess the vessel wall for plaque composition, hematoma, and dissections. Three-dimensional images demonstrate the normal anatomic relationship of the branch vessels, the mediastinal structures, and the extent of the disease process.

Faster imaging acquisitions and ECG-triggered gating allow nearly complete suppression of respiratory and cardiac motion. Motion artifact in the region of the aortic root can be misinterpreted as aortic dissection. The main disadvantage of retrospective ECG gating, which is increased patient dose, can be overcome by performing prospective gating instead.

The scanning volume of CTA is determined by the indication. It is typical to start at the lung apices, which provides adequate coverage of the supra-aortic vessels. The end position is typically at the level of the mid-kidney; however, if a dissection is suspected, the coverage can be extended to the groin. ECG gating is usually reserved for the evaluation of aortic dissections along with aortic root and ascending aortic aneurysmal disease.

Automated bolus tracking or test bolus triggering techniques can reliably obtain the optimal arterial phase by placing a region of interest on the ascending aorta. An injection volume of 100 mL of a contrast agent with high iodine concentration (350 mg/mL) at a flow rate of 5 mL/sec is typically used. Images are acquired in the cranial to caudal direction with a slice thickness of 1.5 mm, slice interval of 1.0 mm, and 0.6 mm of collimation (Figs. 80-3 to 80-5).

Pulmonary CTA

The introduction of MDCT has led to CTA being the technique of choice for the evaluation of most known or suspected pulmonary vascular pathologic processes. Spatial resolution has improved significantly, allowing the detection of very small peripheral pulmonary emboli.[57] Pulmonary CTA can also be used to evaluate for pulmonary hypertension, systemic arterialization of the lung parenchyma in pulmonary sequestration, pulmonary arteriovenous malformations, and congenital pulmonary vas-

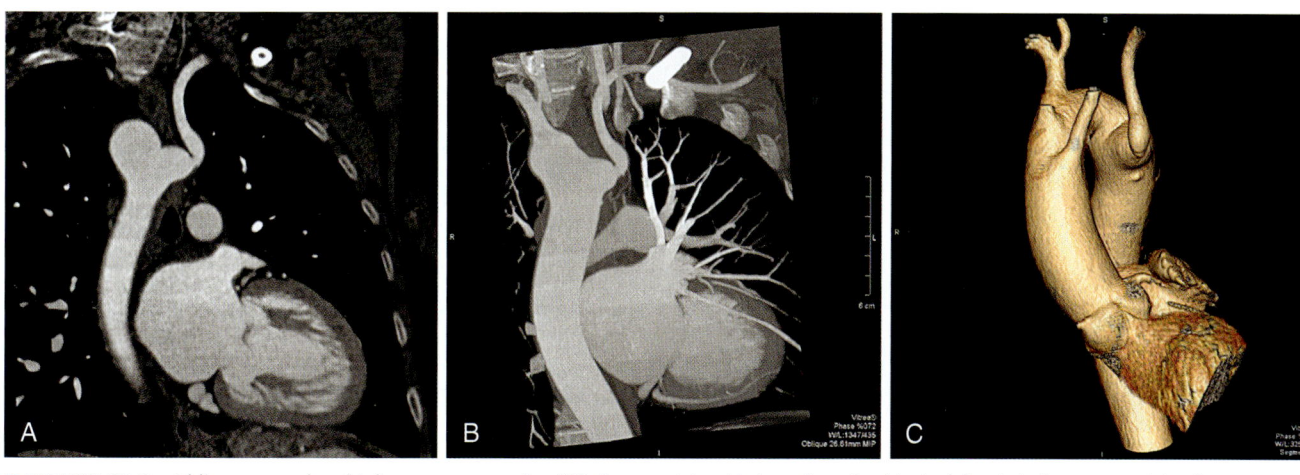

■ **FIGURE 80-3** Oblique coronal multiplanar reconstruction (**A**) shows a right-sided aortic arch with the left subclavian artery arising from a diverticulum of Kommerell. A thick MIP image (**B**) and volume rendered image (**C**) help demonstrate the vascular relationships.

cular anomalies. For the evaluation of pulmonary embolism, conventional DSA is still considered the gold standard, but it is rarely used.[58,59]

The scanning volume starts at the lung and extends caudally to below the lung bases. Automated bolus tracking can reliably obtain the optimal arterial phase by placing a region of interest on the main pulmonary trunk. An injection volume of 120 mL of a contrast agent with high iodine concentration (350 mg/mL) at a flow rate of 4 mL/sec is typically used. Images are acquired in the cranial to caudal direction with a slice thickness of 1.5 mm, slice interval of 1.5 mm, and 0.6 mm of collimation (Figs. 80-6 to 80-9).

Coronary CTA

Invasive coronary angiography remains the gold standard to determine the precise location and degree of stenosis because of its high spatial and temporal resolution (0.13 to 0.30 mm and 20 ms). It also allows therapeutic angioplasty and stenting at the time of the procedure. However, it is an expensive procedure with significant radiation exposure and carries a small risk of serious complications.[60] Furthermore, only one third of these examinations are performed in conjunction with an interventional therapeutic procedure.[61] Twenty percent of patients have normal or minimal coronary artery disease. Thus, a noninvasive assessment of coronary arteries is highly desirable for the diagnosis of coronary artery disease.

Coronary artery disease is a more systemic, diffuse condition, and the treatment is likewise often systemic. Whereas it is important to identify, to quantify, and to treat discrete, significant obstructive lesions, it may also be just as important to determine whether atherosclerotic plaque is present in the coronary arteries so that systemic therapies and lifestyle modifications can be initiated. Until the development of MDCT, CT in the assessment of coronary artery disease was restricted to the detection and quantification of coronary artery calcium. CT has a number of advantages over invasive coronary angiography. It is a noninvasive, three-dimensional technique that can obtain a calcium score, has a high negative predictive value for coronary artery disease, has the potential to characterize plaque components, provides additional anatomic information, and entails no recovery time after the study.

Patients who are not good candidates for CTA include those with unstable acute coronary syndrome who may need percutaneous coronary intervention, patients in atrial fibrillation, those with renal failure, and those with allergy to iodinated contrast material. Obesity limits the ability to obtain diagnostic examinations because of the increased soft tissue attenuation and image noise. With body mass indices above 30, it has been shown that the

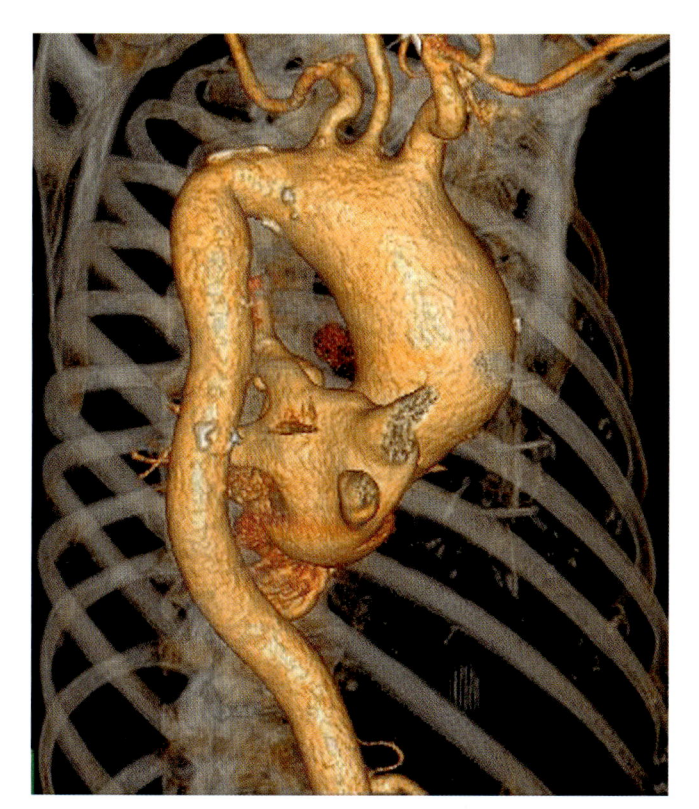

■ **FIGURE 80-4** Volume rendered image of ECG-gated CTA of the thoracic aorta demonstrates a large fusiform aneurysm of the ascending thoracic aorta.

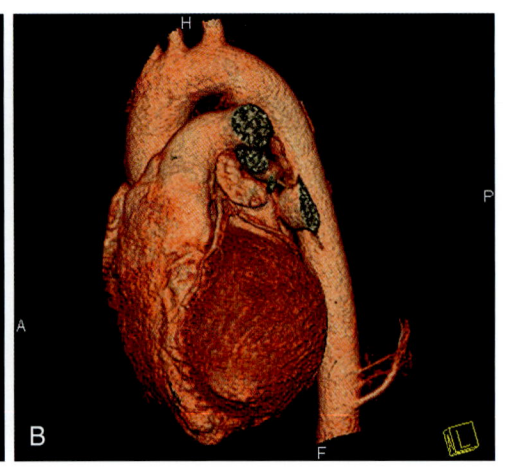

FIGURE 80-5 Oblique MIP image (**A**) and volume rendered image (**B**) of CTA of the thorax demonstrate three arteries arising from the distal descending thoracic aorta to supply the left lower pulmonary lobe, consistent with a sequestration.

accuracy of the test falls below that for patients of normal weight.[62] Coronary artery calcification also reduces the diagnostic accuracy of CTA.

To conduct a coronary CTA examination, intravenous access is obtained, ideally with an 18-gauge antecubital catheter in the right arm. Next, breath-holding is practiced with the patient, and the patient is instructed to avoid swallowing and movement for avoidance of step artifact in the resultant image. β Blockade is used to achieve slower heart rates, either intravenously or orally, depending on the clinical setting. A sample protocol includes intravenous injection of metoprolol (5 mg) repeated up to three times, depending on the heart rate. Alternatively, oral dosing can be administered the night before and the morning of the examination. Slowing of the heart rate is essential for image quality in 16- and 64-slice CT. A study of dual-source CT demonstrated slightly lower per-segment evaluability for high heart rates without β blockade but no decrease in diagnostic accuracy for the detection of coronary artery stenosis.[63] Nitroglycerin (0.4 mg sublingually) is given to vasodilate the coronary arteries and to improve visualization.

The scanning volume starts at the aortic arch and extends caudally to the apex of the heart. Test bolus triggering can reliably obtain the optimal arterial phase by placing a region of interest on the ascending thoracic aorta. An injection volume of 100 mL of a contrast agent with high iodine concentration (350 mg/mL) at a flow rate of 5 mL/sec is typically used. Images are acquired in the cranial to caudal direction with a slice thickness of 0.75 mm, slice interval of 0.6 mm, and 0.6 mm of collimation (Fig. 80-10).

A protocol similar to that used to image the coronary arteries can be applied to assess the pulmonary and cardiac veins. To assess the pulmonary vein ostia, a contrast bolus of more than 100 mL is recommended with gating optional. The time to scan will be slightly earlier than for the coronaries, with a scan duration of only 2 seconds necessary. Bolus tracking technique can be used with the region of interest placed within the left atrium to optimize opacification of the pulmonary vein ostia.

A popular protocol for administration of contrast material uses a triphasic injection; the first phase is contrast material, the second phase is an admixture (70% saline/30% contrast material), and the third phase is a bolus chaser of saline alone. The advantage of this triphasic technique is that it will produce enough contrast in the right ventricle to allow visualization of the septum for left ventricular functional assessment. The rate of infusion of contrast material is a critical determinant of the quality of the image. A minimal flow rate of 5 mL/sec is optimal for the general population. For obese patients, higher rates should be attempted.[64]

Personalized, computerized, patient-based dosing of contrast media delivery protocols are showing promise, helping to produce diagnostic quality images more consistently for coronary CTA. They personalize the scan delay, flow rate, and volume for each of the three phases of injection on the basis of the patient's weight, scan time, time to aorta peak, HU peak number, and concentration of iodine used (300 or 350 mL).

FIGURE 80-6 Volume rendered axial image of CTA of the pulmonary artery demonstrates a pseudoaneurysm of the right lower lobe pulmonary artery.

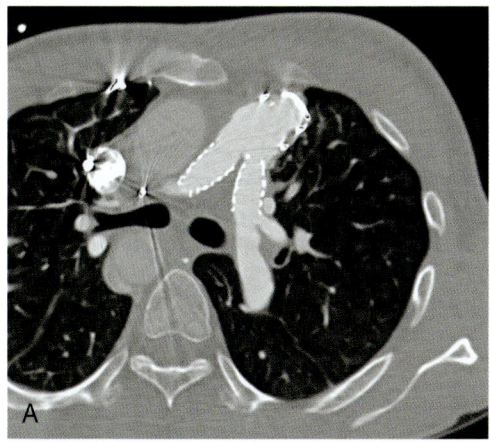

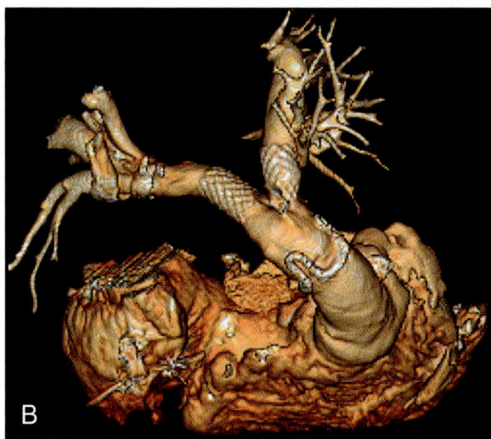

CHAPTER 80 • *Computed Tomographic Angiography: Clinical Techniques* 1065

■ **FIGURE 80-7** Axial thin MIP image (**A**) of CTA of the pulmonary artery shows bilateral pulmonary artery stents. The volume rendered image (**B**) demonstrates the stents and the pulmonary valve prosthesis.

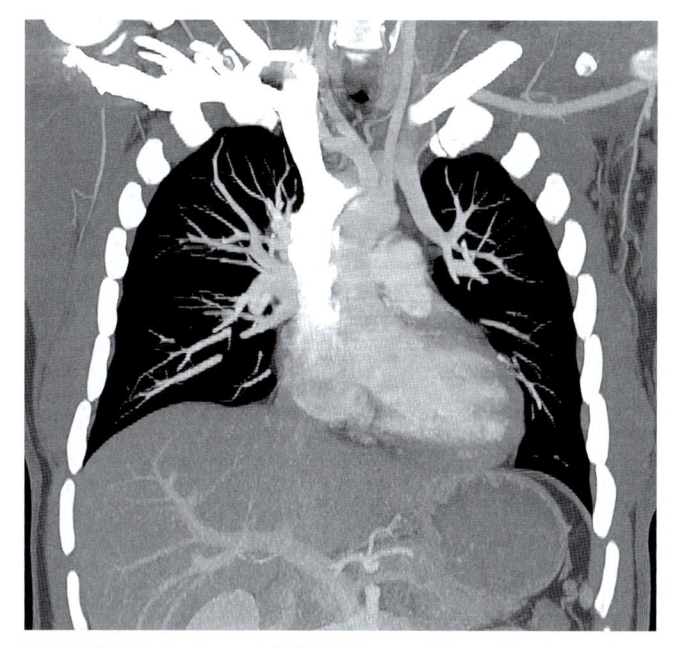

■ **FIGURE 80-8** Coronal thick MIP image of CTA of the thorax shows a left superior pulmonary vein draining vertically into the left brachiocephalic vein, consistent with anomalous pulmonary venous return.

Abdominal CTA

Common abdominal applications of CTA include evaluation of the abdominal aorta, preoperative and postoperative assessment for kidney and liver transplantation, preoperative planning for hepatic segmentectomy and pancreatic surgery, and evaluation of mesenteric ischemia and gastrointestinal hemorrhage. The protocols for each application should be individually tailored to optimize imaging of the targeted vascular structures. For example, planning of a Whipple procedure should include both arterial and portal venous phase images.

Abdominal Aorta

Full assessment of aortic dissection by CTA requires unenhanced CT followed by contrast-enhanced CT. Unenhanced CT is useful for detection of dense intramural hematoma that may be mistaken for chronic thrombus on the enhanced images.

The scanning volume starts at the diaphragm and extends caudally to the symphysis pubis. Bolus tracking triggering can reliably obtain the optimal arterial phase by placing a region of interest on the aorta at the level of the celiac artery. An injection volume of 100 mL of a contrast

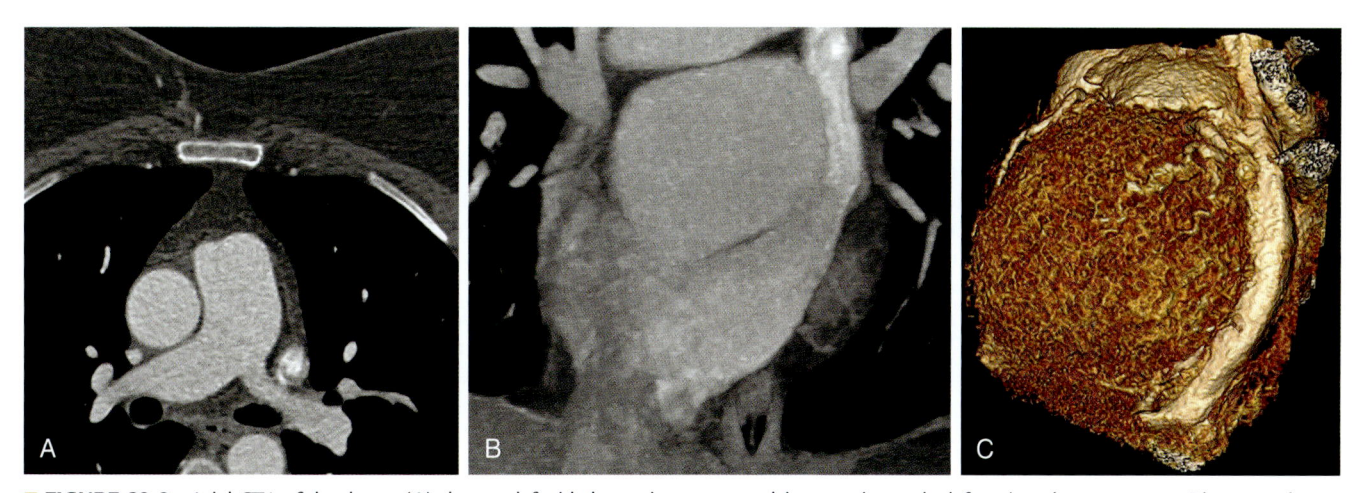

■ **FIGURE 80-9** Axial CTA of the thorax (**A**) shows a left-sided superior vena cava lying anterior to the left main pulmonary artery. The coronal oblique MIP image (**B**) and volume rendered image (**C**) demonstrate the vein draining into the coronary sinus.

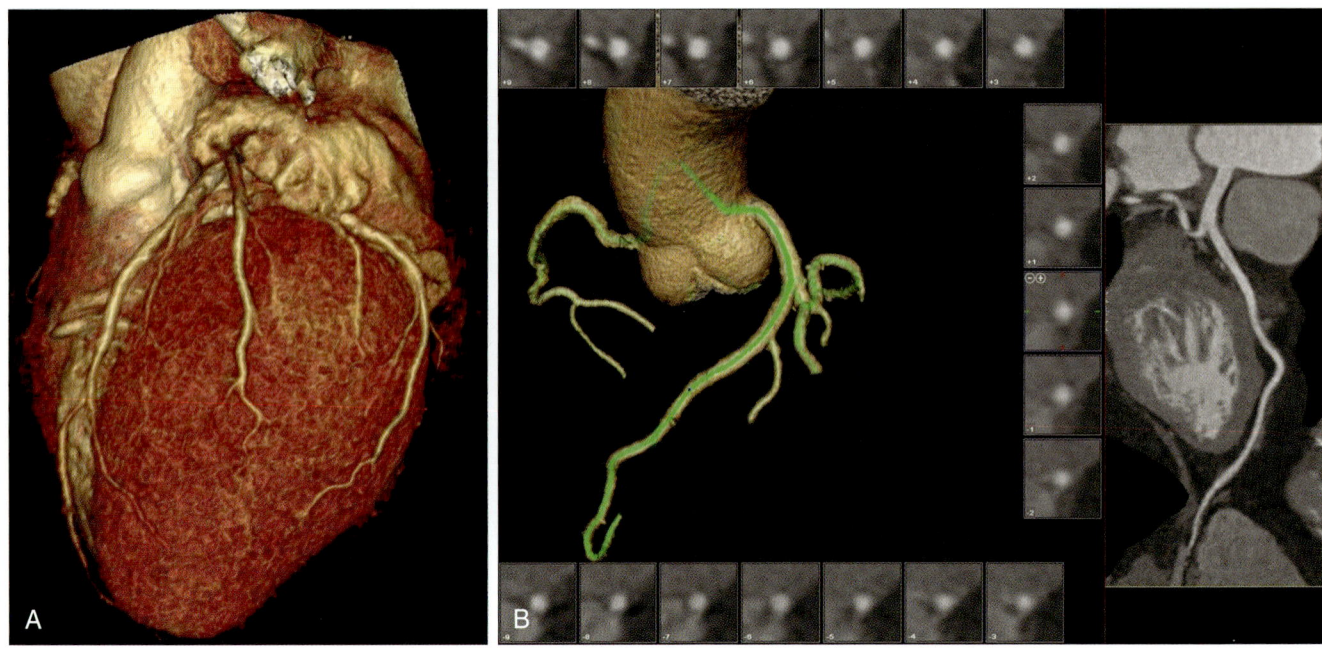

■ **FIGURE 80-10** **A,** Volume rendered technique shows the relationship of the coronary arteries to the cardiac chambers. **B,** The vessel-only view of the left anterior descending artery alongside the curved planar reformat. The blue dot on the distal left anterior descending artery corresponds to the central axial image.

agent with high iodine concentration (350 mg/mL) at a flow rate of 5 mL/sec is typically used. Images are acquired in the cranial to caudal direction with a slice thickness of 2.0 mm, slice interval of 2.0 mm, and 0.6 mm of collimation (Fig. 80-11).

Patients treated with endovascular aneurysm repair undergo frequent imaging by CTA to monitor for endoleak, stent migration, or fracture as well as stability of aneurysm size (Fig. 80-12).[65] Increase in the diameter of an aneurysm is associated with endoleak. Evaluation of an endoleak requires unenhanced CT imaging as well as imaging during arterial and venous phases of contrast enhancement. Unenhanced images are used to detect artifact from calcification or embolization material that may mimic endoleak on the enhanced images. Venous phase images have been shown to enhance the detection rate of endoleaks.

Pancreas

Staging of pancreatic cancer with multiphasic CT is now the standard of care in many institutions.[66] It requires arterial, parenchymal, and portal venous phase images to evaluate the solid organs and the mesentery.[67-69] Addition of a non–contrast phase allows detection of parenchymal and vascular calcifications. Neutral oral contrast agents help distend the bowel and improve visualization of the bowel wall. Positive oral contrast agents (e.g., iodine-based agents) obscure vascular detail and should be avoided in all abdominal CTA.

Although curved multiplanar reformations of the pancreas improve visualization of the parenchyma and pancreatic duct, MIP and volume rendered images are needed for vascular analysis (Fig. 80-13).[70,71] The newest generation of scanners allows rapid multiplanar and maximum intensity projections on the scanner, thus obviating the need for routine data transfer to an independent image processing workstation.

Renal Imaging

A comprehensive examination includes non–contrast-enhanced images to evaluate for renal calculi and vascular calcification, arterial phase to detect vascular anatomic variants and anomalies, nephrographic phase to detect renal parenchymal abnormalities, and excretory phase to evaluate the collecting systems and ureters.[72-75] Coronal thin-slab MIP images are useful for optimal visualization of the renal arteries (Fig. 80-14).[76] However, because MIP images do not provide spatial depth, volume rendered images are also beneficial (Fig. 80-15). It is feasible to scan the renal vasculature with 50 mL of nonionic iodinated contrast material and saline chase using a dual injector on a 16- or 64-slice CT scanner with excellent results.[14] However, to improve opacification of the ureters, saline bolus or diuretics may be beneficial.[77]

Hepatic and Mesenteric Vasculature

CTA allows excellent visualization of the hepatic and mesenteric vasculature (Fig. 80-16). Because of high temporal resolution, it may be necessary to scan the region of interest twice; a "pure" arterial phase does not allow evaluation of the venous structures. This is necessary because incomplete enhancement of the mesenteric venous branches during late arterial phase may mimic thrombosis.

Celiac and mesenteric stenoses are best visualized by sagittal thin-slab MIP or volume rendered images (Fig. 80-17). However, a thin-slab coronal MIP image also provides an excellent overview of the mesenteric vascular structures as well as the bowel loops (Fig. 80-18).[78] The

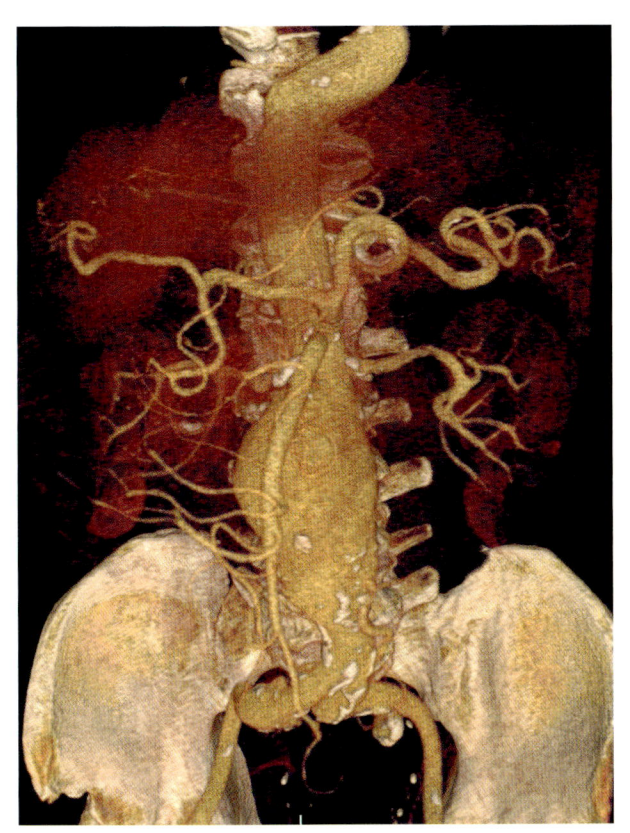

■ **FIGURE 80-11** A volume rendered image of CTA of the abdominal aorta demonstrates a fusiform aneurysm of the infrarenal abdominal aorta.

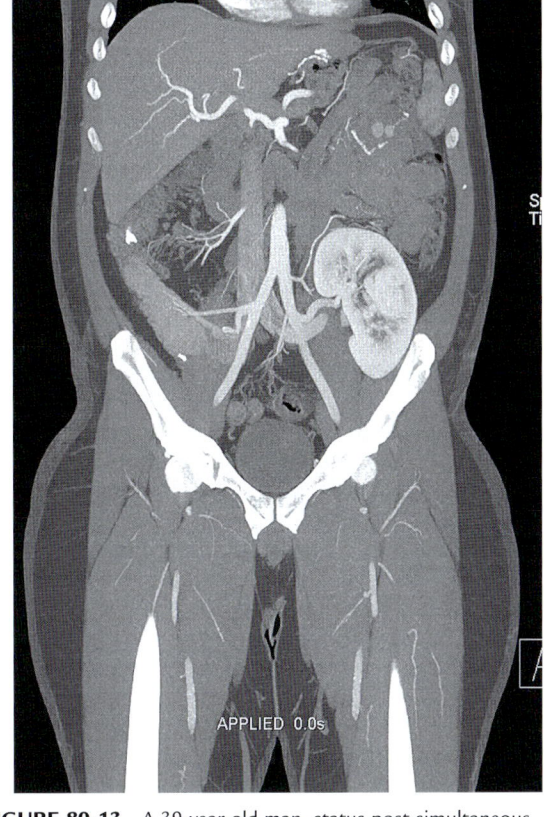

■ **FIGURE 80-13** A 39-year-old man, status post simultaneous pancreas-kidney transplantation. This coronal MIP image from MDCTA demonstrates widely patent renal transplant and pancreatic transplant arteries anastomosing with both native common iliac arteries.

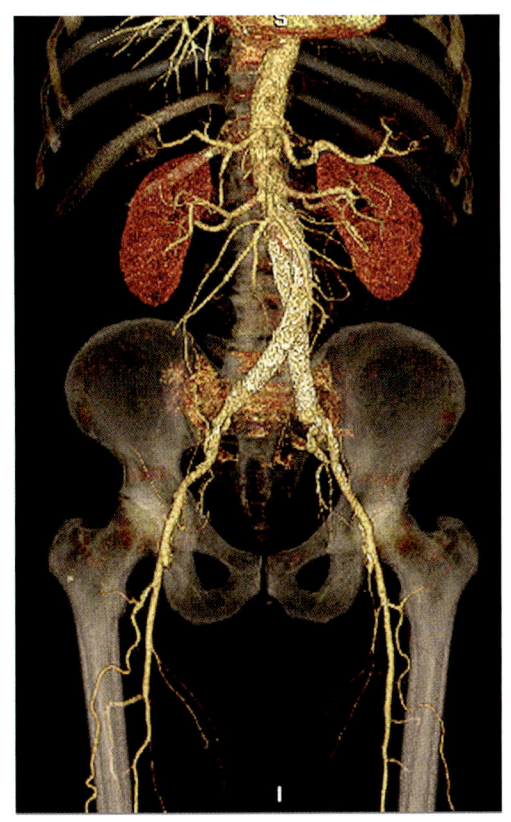

■ **FIGURE 80-12** A volume rendered image of CTA of the abdominal aorta demonstrates bi-limbed endovascular stent grafts within the abdominal aorta, extending into the iliac vessels.

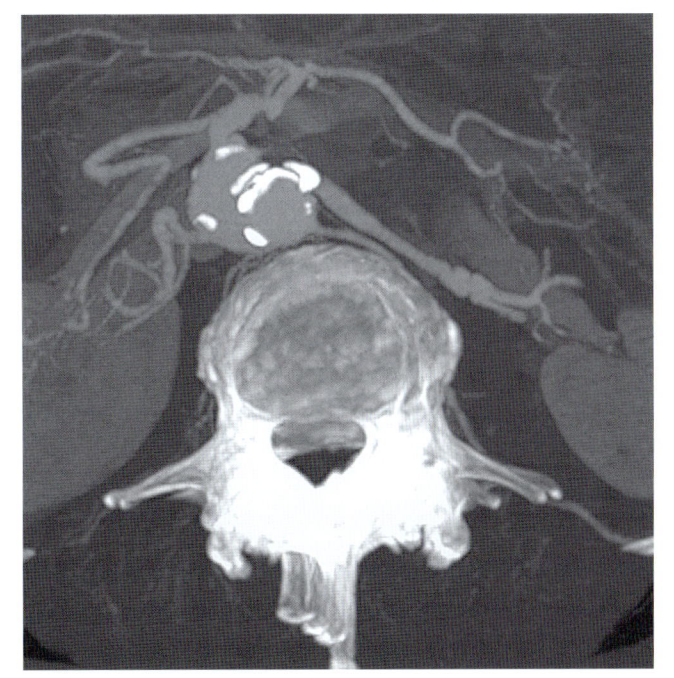

■ **FIGURE 80-14** Axial oblique thick MIP image demonstrates beading of the distal left renal artery, suggestive of fibromuscular dysplasia.

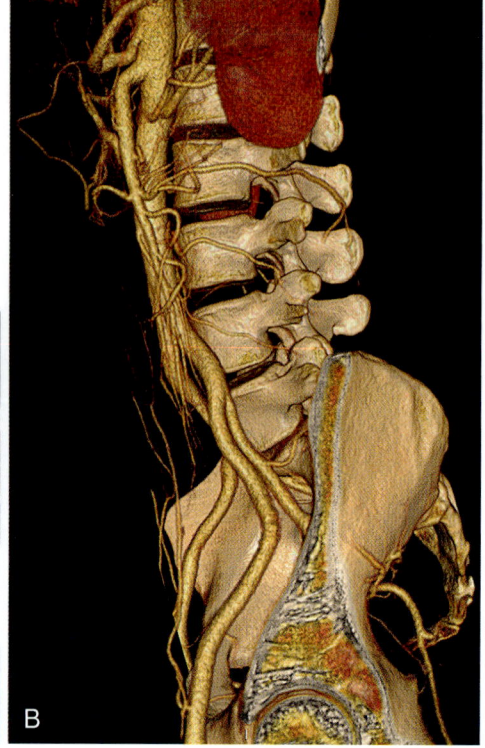

■ FIGURE 80-15 Axial thick MIP image (A) of renal CTA of a healthy renal donor demonstrates an accessory renal artery anterior to the main left renal artery. The volume rendered image (B) helps define the anatomic relationships.

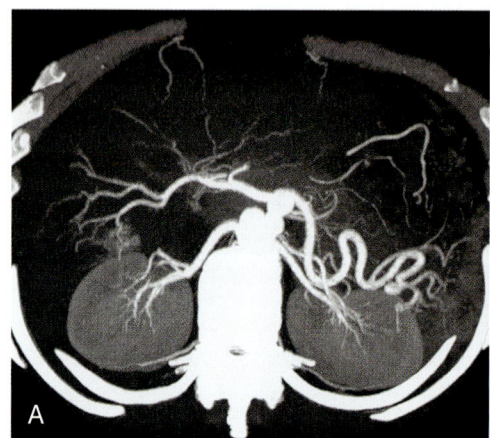

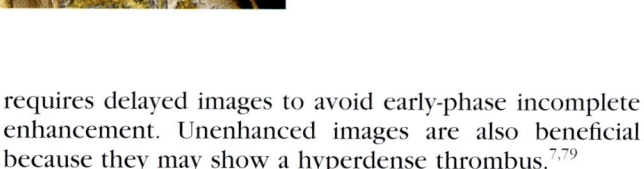

use of neutral oral contrast agents is important in evaluating the mesentery to improve visualization of the bowel mucosa.

Acute mesenteric ischemia is a life-threatening event that may be caused by a variety of factors. These include embolic phenomenon, severe hypoperfusion, thrombosis of stenotic vessels, dissection, hypercoagulable states, and vasculitis. Diagnosis of mesenteric venous thrombosis requires delayed images to avoid early-phase incomplete enhancement. Unenhanced images are also beneficial because they may show a hyperdense thrombus.[7,79]

Lower Extremity CTA

Most institutions will initially perform a scout view, from the diaphragms to the feet; an optional non–contrast-enhanced acquisition from the celiac axis to the feet; and an arterial phase–timed acquisition from the celiac axis to the feet, with the option of a second later limited acquisition from the lower thighs to the feet in the event that the contrast material has a slower transit time on the symptomatic side.

Bolus tracking triggering can reliably obtain the optimal arterial phase by placing a region of interest on the aorta at the level of the celiac artery. An injection volume of 150 mL of a contrast agent with high iodine concentration (350 mg/mL) at a flow rate of 5 mL/sec is typically used. Images are acquired in the cranial to caudal direction with a slice thickness of 1.0 mm, slice interval of 1.0 mm, and 0.6 mm of collimation (Figs. 80-19 to 80-24).

Because most patients who are having peripheral CTA have known peripheral arterial disease, one would expect them to have some arterial stenoses or occlusions; thus, a fast scan time is not always desirable because one does not want to scan ahead of the contrast bolus. Thus, a table pitch of 1.1, gantry rotation of 0.37 second, table increment of 21.1 mm/360-degree rotation, and table speed of 63 mm/sec will all result in a scan time of 23 seconds and will require a fast contrast injection bolus. However, if one suspects more severe atherosclerosis, a slower contrast injection bolus and correspondingly slower/longer scan

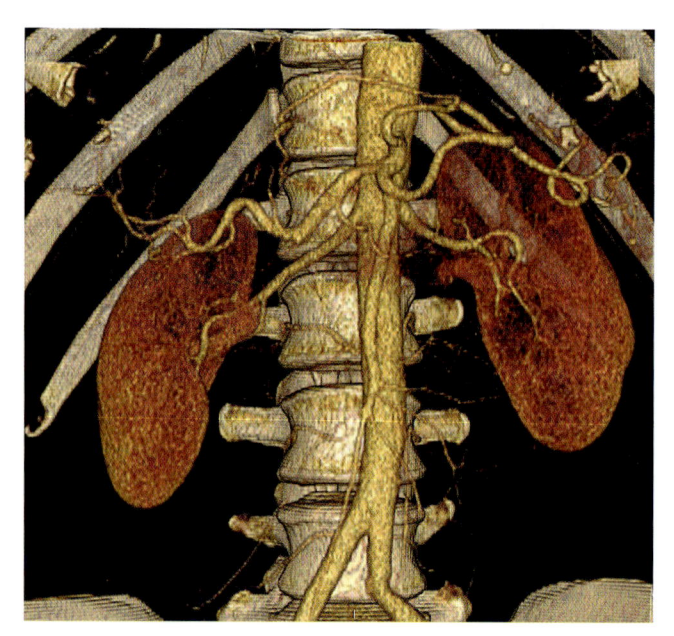

■ FIGURE 80-16 Volume rendered image of the abdominal aorta demonstrates an accessory left hepatic artery arising from the celiac axis.

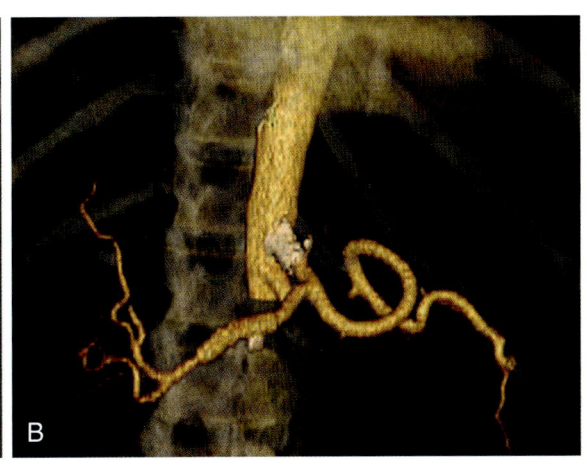

FIGURE 80-17 Sagittal MIP image (**A**) and volume rendered image (**B**) of the abdominal aorta show a metal endovascular stent placed in the proximal celiac artery.

time is desirable. Longer scan time can be achieved by reducing the table speed through the scanner (i.e., the pitch) and by slowing the gantry rotation time. Thus, in this scenario, a table pitch of 0.85, gantry rotation of 0.5 second, table increment of 17 mm/360-degree rotation, and table speed of 32 mm/sec will all result in a scan time of 40 seconds. As mentioned previously, different detector numbers and different manufacturers will require different scan protocols.

Pitfalls and Solutions

Artifacts

Streak artifacts can be noted around high-attenuation structures, such as endovascular stents, pacing wires, and coils, and can obscure adjacent structures. These are difficult to avoid and can be reduced with special artifact reduction software developed by the manufacturers.

High-attenuation structures such as stents and calcified plaques can appear enlarged ("bloomed") because of partial volume averaging effects. This results in overestimation of the size of the calcified plaque. This can obscure the coronary lumen, limiting the estimation of stenosis in the affected segments. Although sharper filters or kernels and thinner slices (0.5 to 0.6 mm) may reduce the artifact with stents, this has little effect on calcification.

FIGURE 80-18 Coronal MIP image of CTA of the mesenteric vessels shows a focal mycotic aneurysm of the distal superior mesenteric artery.

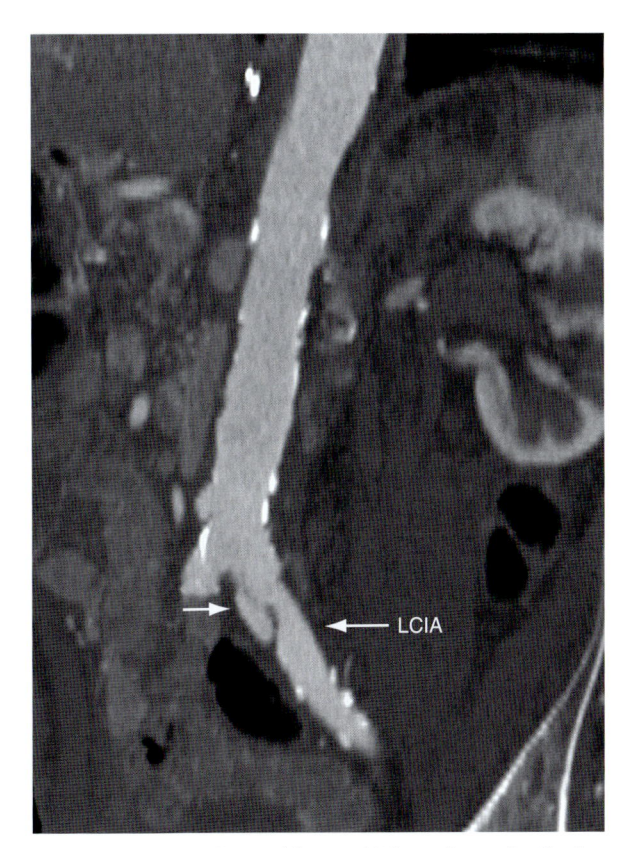

FIGURE 80-19 A 76-year-old man with intermittent claudication at 500 m. Left anterior oblique coronal MDCTA demonstrates a localized dissection flap (*arrow*) with a corresponding moderate stenosis of the left common iliac artery (LCIA).

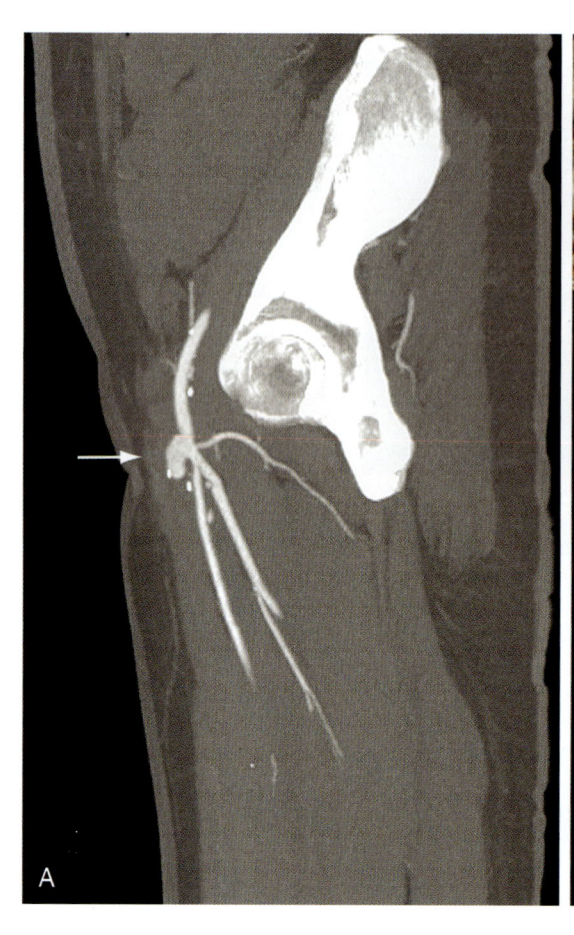

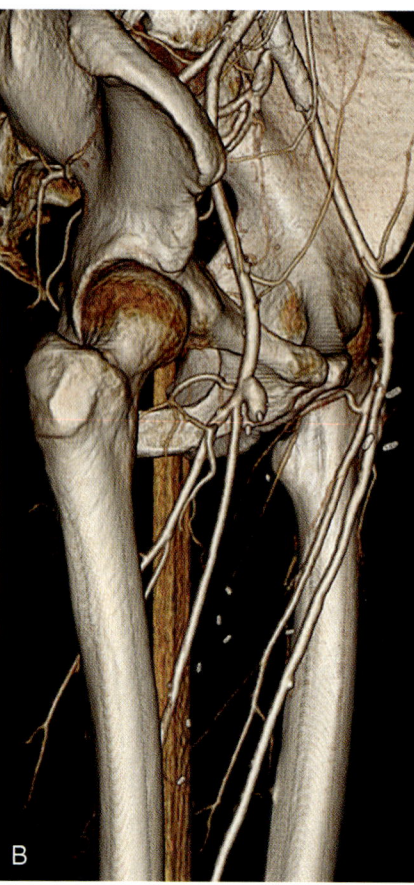

FIGURE 80-20 A 40-year-old man with peripheral arterial disease, status post left common iliac artery and left external iliac artery stenting through the right common femoral artery approach. Sagittal MIP image from MDCTA (**A**) demonstrates a right common femoral arterial pseudoaneurysm (*arrow*). Volume rendered view (**B**) demonstrates the right common femoral arterial pseudoaneurysm; note the left common and external iliac arterial stents in situ.

Beam hardening is important to recognize. This artifact is a low-density focus in a reconstructed image, appearing similar to noncalcified coronary atherosclerotic plaque. It is a result of low-energy photon absorption as the x-ray beam crosses a high-density structure, such as a surgical clip or calcification. In areas neighboring the dense structure, the high-energy beam passes through with little absorption, resulting in a low-density focus. It occurs in one direction of the scan plane.

Other types of artifacts commonly observed in the thorax are due to incomplete breath-holding, observed on sagittal or coronal views. These are seen as "stair-step" artifacts through the entire data set, including nonmoving structures, such as the bones. Adequate instruction to the patient before imaging is essential to avoid such artifacts.[80]

Many unique artifacts can result from imaging of the rapidly moving heart, the most common of which is the result of cardiac pulsation.[19] This produces an image with horizontal slabs of the image in displaced alignment. The second type is banding artifacts, which result from an increased heart rate during the scan. These are similar in appearance to pulsation artifacts. These artifacts especially occur in patients with high heart rates, in patients with heart rate variability, and in the presence of irregular or ectopic heart beats (e.g., premature ventricular contractions and atrial fibrillation). These can be minimized by scanning with higher temporal resolution on the order of 50 ms or by multisecond reconstruction with MDCT. A β blocker should be used to reduce the heart rate to less than 65 beats/min.[81] Recent data support high diagnostic accuracy for the detection of coronary artery stenosis with the use of dual-source CT without β blockade, attributed to the improved temporal resolution (75 to 83 ms) compared with single-source MDCT (166 ms).[82] However, in clinical practice, the exact role of β blockade in dual-source imaging is yet to be determined, especially at high heart rates.

Radiation and Dose

There has been rapid evolution in MDCT technology with increasing temporal and spatial resolution, allowing rapid imaging of a greater population of patients than in previous years. With this evolution, the scientific and public awareness of the radiation risks associated with this technology has been increasing. Therefore, it is essential for operators to understand the effects of the radiation exposure delivered and to implement techniques that reduce this exposure.

Potential biologic effects from ionizing radiation depend on the radiation dose and the biologic sensitivity of the tissue or organ system irradiated. Effective dose (E) is the descriptor that reflects this difference in biologic sensitivity. The units of E are sieverts (Sv), often expressed as millisieverts (mSv). Not all tissues are equally sensitive to the effects of ionizing radiation. Therefore, tissue-weighting factors (Wt) assign a particular organ or tissue the proportion of the risk of stochastic effects (e.g., cancer and genetic effects) resulting from irradiation of that tissue

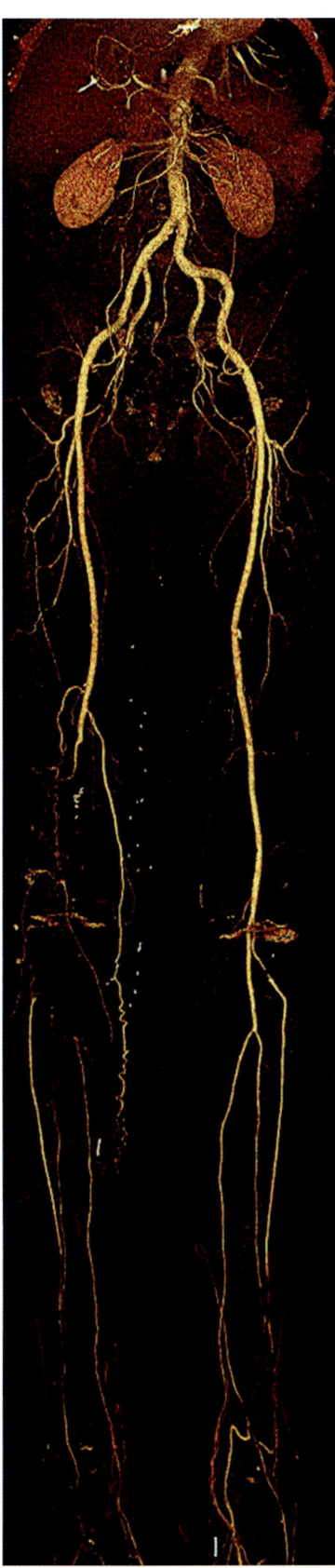

CHAPTER 80 • *Computed Tomographic Angiography: Clinical Techniques* 1071

■ **FIGURE 80-21** A volume rendered view of CTA of the lower extremities shows occlusion of the right distal superficial femoral artery at the level of Hunter's canal.

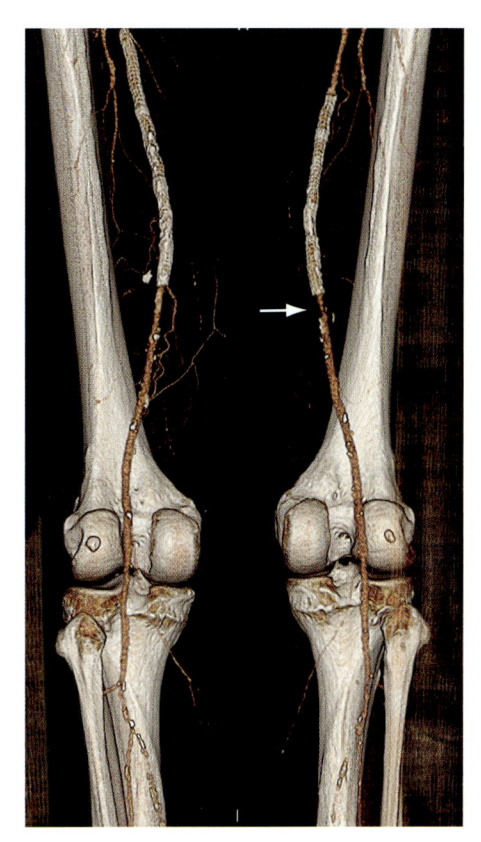

■ **FIGURE 80-22** A 58-year-old woman complaining of intermittent claudication at 200 m. This posterior volume rendered view of MDCTA demonstrates bilateral superficial femoral arterial stents in situ, with evidence of a tight stenosis within the right superficial femoral artery distal to the stent (*arrow*).

compared with uniform whole-body irradiation. The x-ray radiation that everyone is exposed to each year from natural sources amounts to 2 to 5 mSv.

CT contributes to 75% of the total collective dose from ionizing radiation to the public from medical imaging.[17] With the increasing widespread use of CT and individual patients having multiple scans during their lifetime, low-dose techniques are increasingly desired. The goal is to keep doses "as low as reasonably achievable" (ALARA). This represents a practice mandate adhering to the principle of keeping radiation doses to patients and personnel as low as possible. Among the most widely known protocols, such as calcium scoring studies, the effective dose is relatively small, 1 to 3 mSv.[83] The effective radiation dose with retrospectively gated coronary angiography by 64-slice MDCT is estimated to be approximately 11 to 22 mSv.[80]

Clinically, studies performed with higher milliamperage have less noise and higher signal-to-noise ratio and contrast-to-noise ratio, which is visually more appealing and useful in heavily calcified or stented vessels. However, doubling of the tube current doubles the radiation dose. Lowering of the tube voltage allows significant reduction in effective dose as increasing the kilovoltage by 15% has the same effect as doubling of the milliampere-seconds. The tradeoff for lower tube voltage is increased noise; however, use of 100 kV for patients with low body mass index results in increased intensity of iodinated contrast media as 100 kV is closer to the k-edge of iodine.

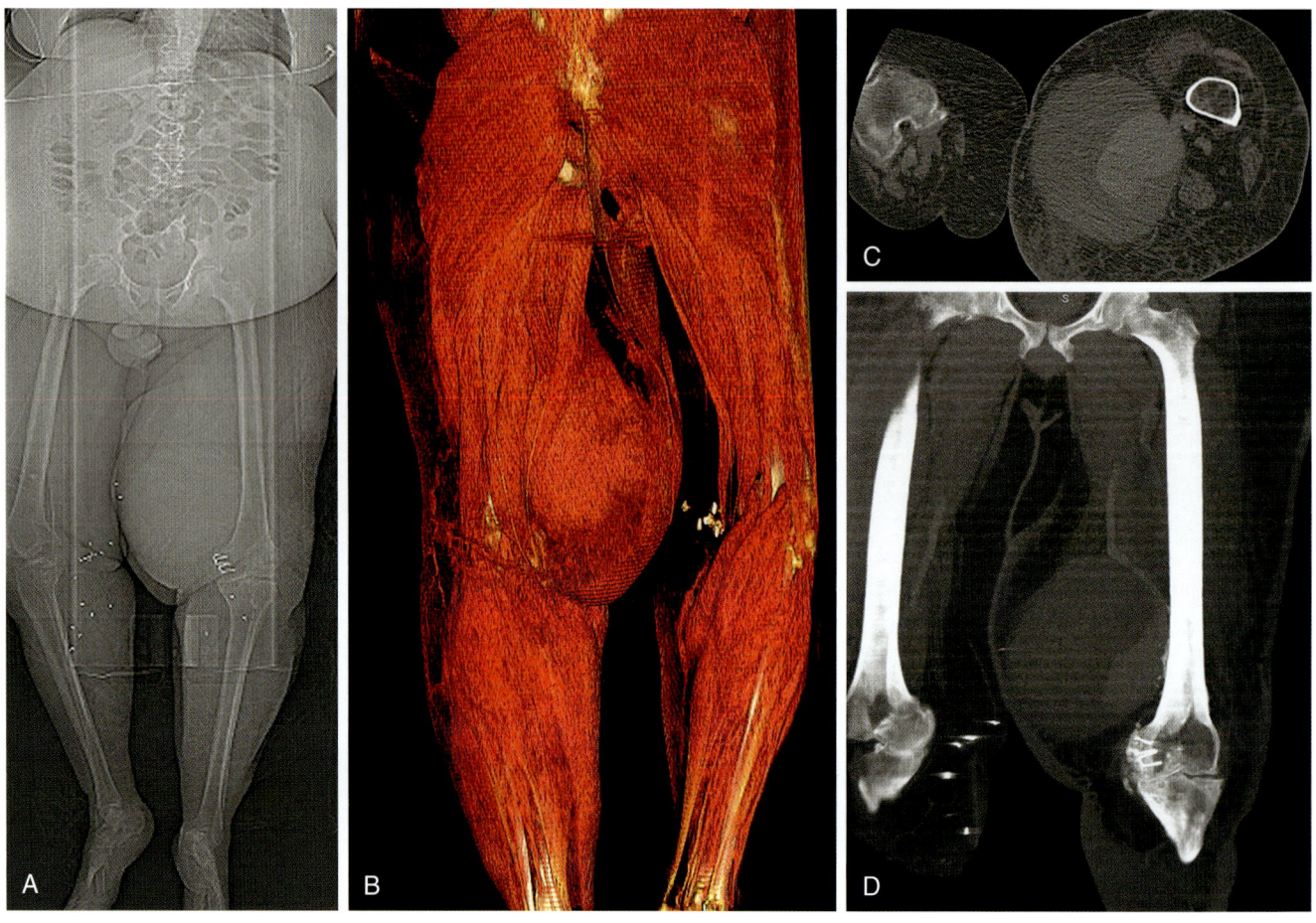

FIGURE 80-23 A 48-year-old man presented to the emergency department after a fall from a stepladder; 5 years previously, he had a posterior left knee dislocation after a road traffic accident. MDCT topogram (**A**) demonstrates a markedly swollen left thigh. The volume rendered image (**B**) demonstrates the large hematoma adjacent to the distal left superficial femoral artery displacing the soft tissues medially. Axial contrast-enhanced CT (**C**) shows a large hematoma medially within the left thigh and a large pseudoaneurysm within the hematoma. Coronal MIP image from MDCTA (**D**) demonstrates the pseudoaneurysm donor artery, which is the superficial femoral artery.

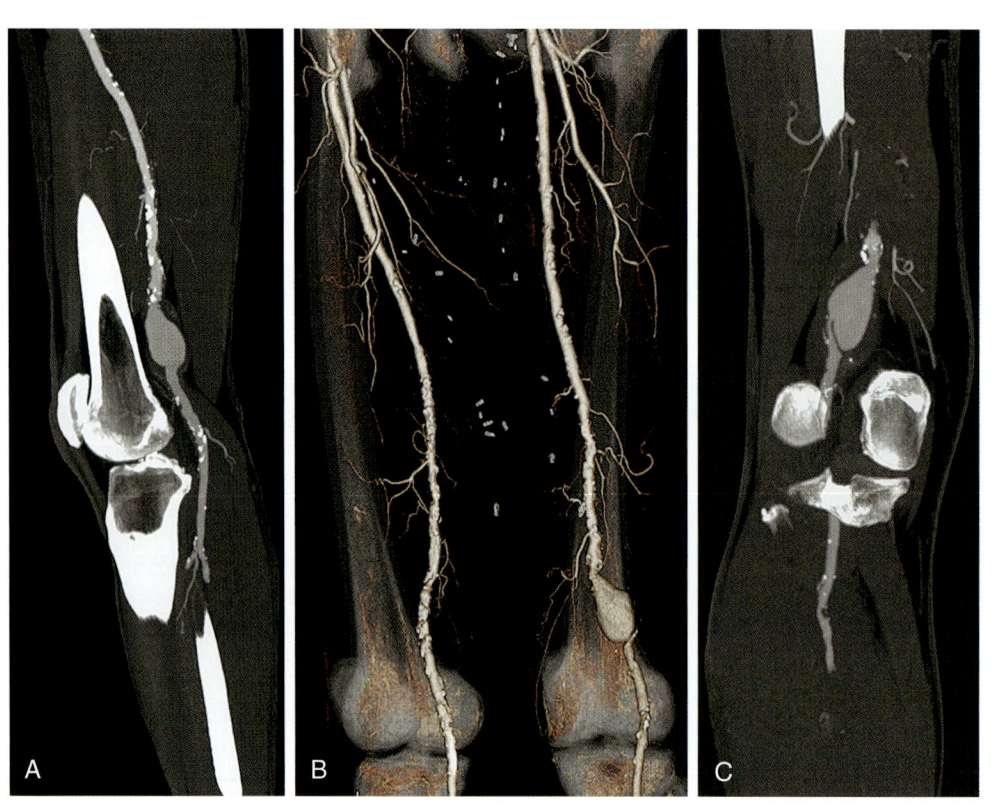

FIGURE 80-24 A 69-year-old man with a swelling behind the right knee. Sagittal MIP image from MDCTA (**A**) demonstrates a fusiform aneurysm of the proximal popliteal artery with minimal mural hematoma. Volume rendered posterior view (**B**) demonstrates the fusiform right popliteal aneurysm. Coronal MIP image from MDCTA (**C**) shows a popliteal tight stenosis inferior to the fusiform aneurysm.

Adaptive scanning reduces the radiation exposure of dose-sensitive anatomic regions, such as the female breast. This is done by switching the x-ray tube assemblies off during the rotation phase in which the anatomic regions concerned are most directly exposed to radiation. In this way, it is possible to reduce the radiation exposure of individual anatomic regions, such as the breasts, by up to 40%. Furthermore, an adaptive dose shield can block irrelevant pre-spiral and post-spiral radiation with dynamic diaphragms, thus ensuring that only a minimum and clinically essential radiation exposure occurs. This enables an additional 25% reduction of the dose required for routine examinations.

Fraioli and colleagues[84] performed peripheral CTA at 50 mAs, 100 mAs, and 130 mAs in three groups of patients with peripheral arterial disease and compared the findings with the gold standard, DSA.[84] No difference in qualitative analysis of arterial segments was determined between the three CTA groups; similar sensitivity and specificity for diagnosis of peripheral arterial disease were achieved with CTA performed at 50 mAs, 100 mAs, and 300 mAs. Thus, optimal image quality with diagnostic accuracy for peripheral arterial disease was achieved with the low-dose technique, allowing a 74% reduction in effective dose to the patient.[84] Similarly, for renal arterial CTA in potential living renal donors, 100 kVp achieved diagnostically acceptable CT images with a significant radiation dose reduction compared with CTA at 120 or 140 kVp.[85] In our institution, Farrelly and colleagues have demonstrated a significant reduction in radiation dose by performing low peak tube voltage, prospectively ECG-gated CTA of thoracic aortas without loss of image quality. The mean radiation dose of the retrospectively gated–120 kVp was 26 mSv compared with 2.94 mSv for the prospectively gated–100 kVp studies. The latest coronary CTA protocols using prospective gating reduce the radiation doses to less than 3 mSv.[24]

Strategies for reduction of radiation dose in cardiac MDCT include the following[86]:

Optimize scan parameters
- Weight-adjusted tube current (mA)
- Reduce kilovoltage to 100 kV in patients with low body mass index
- Limit z-axis coverage
- Reduce field of view

ECG dose modulation
- Up to 40% dose reduction

Prospective gated axial
- Up to 80% dose reduction

Adaptive scanning
- Up to 40% dose reduction to the breast
- Up to 25% reduction by eliminating pre-spiral and post-spiral radiation

Garnet-based gemstone scintillator detectors
- Up to 50% dose reduction

Dual-source detectors
- With temporal resolution of 75 ms, table feed of 43 cm/sec, entire heart scan in 250 ms with <1 mSv

New reconstruction algorithms (automatic statistical iterative reconstruction)

Bismuth breast shields

The implementation of these techniques and other dose reduction strategies evolving industry-wide will greatly minimize the radiation risks associated with CTA.

Image Interpretation

Postprocessing

Thinner slice acquisition with CTA has resulted in a significant increase in the number of images acquired. Hence, "data overload" has been a direct side effect of isotropic and near-isotropic scanning. CTA of the abdominal aorta and its branches on the newest scanners generates more than 1000 images.[87] As the volume of data significantly increases, the processing power of many of the current image processing workstations is pushed to its limits. Because of the large volume of data obtained with CTA, accurate, time-efficient, and reproducible image postprocessing to enable disease interpretation is now a requirement.[88-91] The axial image plane, formerly the plane with highest image quality in a single-detector CT scanner acquisition, is no longer the only plane available for image interpretation[92]; however, it remains mandatory to review these axial planes to ensure detection of extra-arterial disease.[89] For the majority of patients with arterial disease, axial image viewing is time-consuming, inefficient, and often less accurate than viewing of reformatted images.[93] With MDCTA acquisition, near-isotropic data sets can be obtained and thus manipulated in all imaging planes and projections without significant loss of image quality to enable eloquent display of the arterial anatomy and pathology.[94] Therefore, a dedicated three-dimensional workstation to enable a real-time interactive approach to image manipulation and interpretation has now become a necessity. Many authors advocate the use of three-dimensional image display, both for diagnosis by the interpreting physician and for procedure planning by the interventionalist.[91,95-97] Available image postprocessing techniques on the clinical three-dimensional workstations include multiplanar reconstruction (MPR), maximum intensity projection (MIP), volume rendering technique (VRT), and shaded surface display (SSD). Postprocessing of the source data not only improves visualization of the vascular structures and their relationship to the adjacent organs but also decreases the number of slices needed for the review of the data set.[98,99] Images can be processed on the scanner or a freestanding image processing workstation. Thicker slices may be produced for review of the axial images on PACS.[100] When the attenuation of vessels is usually more than or nearly 300 HU, the image quality of MPR, MIP, and VRT is usually satisfactory. Most institutions, including that of the authors, routinely use a combination of the MIP and volume rendered display of data for CTA because these two are complementary. Whereas volume rendering is useful for the display of soft tissues and three-dimensional relationships, MIP provides a more detailed view of the vessels within the slab of data and is less operator dependent.[101]

Multiplanar Reconstruction

The MPR algorithm enables a reordering of specific acquired image voxels along a predefined vascular centerline to provide a two-dimensional image of the vessel of interest (see Fig. 80-5A). As all arteries are curved at some point in their distribution, curved MPR (CMPR) is an extension of the MPR process that enables display of a curved plane prescribed along an individual vessel contour or centerline, thus displaying the entire vessel midline on a single two-dimensional image.[94] CMPRs provide a comprehensive cross-sectional display of arterial luminal sizes over long segments and can be especially useful in review of large vascular territories, such as the peripheral arterial tree.[102] CMPRs are the most equipped postprocessing method to reduce artifact from vessel calcification and arterial stents. However, CMPR is user dependent because it requires manual or semiautomated tracing of each vessel centerline.[95] Also, it is imperative that at least two orthogonal planes for each arterial segment be created to ensure accurate quantification of eccentric atherosclerotic plaque.[89] The orthogonal planes are, in fact, essential for determination of the true cross-sectional diameter of a vessel. Other limitations of CMPRs are that only one arterial segment can be displayed at a time and the limited spatial perception due to the absence of anatomic landmarks, such as vessel bifurcations.[103] A new potential solution for these limitations has been described, that of multipath curved planar reformations (MPCPRs).[104] This MPCPR method permits multiple longitudinal vessel cross sections to be displayed simultaneously and therefore allows branching patterns to be seen without obscuration of vessel wall calcifications and stents, and it enables restoration of spatial perception. Roos and colleagues[105] think that MPCPR is currently the most comprehensive technique to visualize the peripheral arteries in patients with peripheral arterial disease; however, it cannot completely replace MIP and VRT.

Maximum Intensity Projection

The technique of MIP provides images that most closely resemble those obtained with conventional DSA and therefore are often desired by interventionalists to enable a quick overall review of the vasculature for anatomic and significant lesion determination before endovascular or surgical treatment. To obtain the MIP image, a specific algorithm is applied to the source data within the three-dimensional workstation. This algorithm involves applying a threshold attenuation value and selecting out the highest attenuation voxels along lines projected through the given volume data set.[106] These selected high-attenuation voxels are then incorporated into a two-dimensional angiogram-like image, useful for demonstrating vessel opacification and residual vessel lumen (see Figs. 80-1A, 80-3B, 80-14, 80-15A, 80-18, and 80-20A). The limitations of MIP include vessel obscuration by other high-attenuation voxels, such as calcification, stents, or bone, and the inability to display three-dimensional relationships of vessels and adjacent anatomic structures.[107] These limitations become a major problem with heavy arterial wall calcification or arterial stents because the vessel lumen can become obscured.[38] Also, when vessel relationships need to be determined before surgical intervention, this two-dimensional MIP method is limited.[108] However, MIP weaknesses can be reduced by editing adjacent high-density structures (bones, vessel wall calcification, and stents), using alternate planes of projection and setting variable attenuation threshold values.[94]

Volume Rendering Techniques

Again, dedicated computer software on the three-dimensional workstation allows a VRT algorithm to be applied to the source data. The principle of volume rendering involves taking the entire volume of source data, adding the contributions of each voxel along a line from the viewer's eye through the data set, and displaying the resulting composite for each pixel of the display (see Figs. 80-1B, 80-2B, 80-4, 80-7B, 80-10A, 80-12, and 80-20B).[107] VRT preserves three-dimensional anatomic relationships, unlike MIP; however, VRT, like MIP, still has limitations with vessel calcification and arterial stents. Therefore, this fundamental limitation precludes the exclusive use of volume rendering and MIP techniques in a large proportion (approximately 60%) of patients with peripheral arterial disease.[109]

Shaded Surface Display

SSD is a process in which apparent surfaces are determined within the volume of data and an image representing the derived surfaces is displayed.[107] SSD provides an anatomic overview, but like MIP and volume rendering techniques, it has difficulty discriminating calcification, fails to display lumen detail, and can overestimate stenosis; therefore, SSD is generally not recommended for vessel caliber measurements.[94]

Combination of Methods

In clinical practice, combinations of the available three-dimensional reformatting methods are employed to accurately diagnose atherosclerosis (see Fig. 80-10B). Anatomic overview and quick significant disease localization can be achieved with the MIP or the VRT images. If arterial calcification or a stent obscures the arterial lumen, a combination of MPR and CMPR is used. In the event that complete evaluation of all arterial segments is hindered, review of the original axial source images can be performed.

Postprocessing Limitations

Technical limitations to postprocessing may exist, with the main ones being secondary to heavy arterial wall calcification or the presence of an arterial stent, as discussed before. Review of the axial source data can be a simple measure to overcome these problems. Postprocessing artifacts can also occur secondary to inadvertent vessel subtraction, particularly with MIP images, and production of pseudostenosis or occlusions in MPRs (especially curved MPRs) as a result of inaccurate centerline definition. Volume rendered images may not demonstrate aneurysmal dilation of a vessel because of partial luminal thrombosis. Again, the axial source data can act to solve these problems. To date, there are no fully automated algorithms to detect vessel centerlines, to segment out bony structures, or to detect or to subtract vessel wall calcification. However, with constant software updates, these tools are likely to become available in the near future.[80] A new investigational tool is dual-energy CTA that allows automatic subtraction of bone and potentially calcified atherosclerotic plaque, based on differential attenuation of bone, calcium, and iodine on a dual-energy scan.

CONCLUSION

Since the introduction of MDCT, one now has the ability to image the entire arterial tree in a noninvasive fashion. CTA is the byproduct of rapid advances in CT technology and has replaced catheter angiography in many institutions. Both image acquisition and processing techniques can significantly affect diagnostic image quality. A thorough knowledge of the scanner hardware and the ability to optimize the technical and contrast parameters are, therefore, essential for performing CTA to achieve accurate diagnosis and atherosclerotic disease stratification. Care must be taken to maintain radiation dose as low as is reasonably achievable. Several recently developed techniques that allow significant reductions to radiation dose are facilitating the acceptance of this modality as a safe and accurate alternative to currently used conventional diagnostic tests. Previously, DSA was the only established reliable imaging technique to quantify atherosclerotic disease load; however, in this new millennium, CTA may now challenge the old gold standard.

> **KEY POINTS**
>
> - Image acquisition and processing techniques can significantly affect diagnostic image quality.
> - Knowledge of scanner hardware and optimization of techniques and contrast parameters are essential in performing CT.
> - Recently developed techniques allow significant reductions to radiation dose, facilitating acceptance of this modality as a safe and accurate alternative to other conventional diagnostic alternatives.

SUGGESTED READING

1. Yaghami V, Sahani D. Advances in MDCT. Radiol Clin North Am 2009; 47:1-183.

REFERENCES

1. Rubin GD, Dake MD, Napel SA, et al. Three-dimensional spiral CT angiography of the abdomen: initial clinical experience. Radiology 1993; 186:147-152.
2. Adachi H, Ino T, Mizuhara A, et al. Assessment of aortic disease using three-dimensional CT angiography. J Card Surg 1994; 9:673-678.
3. Napel S, Marks MP, Rubin GD, et al. CT angiography with spiral CT and maximum intensity projection. Radiology 1992; 185:607-610.
4. Dillon EH, van Leeuwen MS, Fernandez MA, Mali WP. Spiral CT angiography. AJR Am J Roentgenol 1993; 160:1273-1278.
5. Galanski M, Prokop M, Chavan A, et al. Renal arterial stenoses: spiral CT angiography. Radiology 1993; 189:185-192.
6. Rydberg J, Buckwalter KA, Caldemeyer KS, et al. Multisection CT: Scanning techniques and clinical applications. Radiographics 2000; 20:1787-1806.
7. Fishman EK. From the RSNA Refresher Courses: CT Angiography: clinical applications in the abdomen. Radiographics 2001; 21:3S-S16.
8. Lawler LP, Fishman EK. Three-dimensional CT angiography with multidetector CT data: study optimization, protocol design, and clinical applications in the abdomen. Crit Rev Comput Tomogr 2002; 43:77-141.
9. Rubin GD. MDCT imaging of the aorta and peripheral vessels. Eur J Radiol 2003; 45:S42-S49.
10. Rubin GD, Shiau MC, Leung AN, et al. Aorta and iliac arteries: single versus multiple detector-row helical CT angiography. Radiology 2000; 215:670-676.
11. Vrtiska TJ, Fletcher JG, McCollough CH. State-of-the-art imaging with 64-channel multidetector CT angiography. Perspect Vasc Surg Endovasc Ther 2005; 17:3-8.
12. Saini S. Multi-detector row CT: principles and practice for abdominal applications. Radiology 2004; 233:323-327.
13. Schoellnast H, Tillich M, Deutschmann MJ, et al. Aortoiliac enhancement during computed tomography angiography with reduced contrast material dose and saline solution flush: influence on magnitude and uniformity of the contrast column. Invest Radiol 2004; 39:20-26.
14. Utsunomiya D, Awai K, Tamura Y, et al. 16-MDCT aortography with a low-dose contrast material protocol. AJR Am J Roentgenol 2006; 186:374-378.
15. Anderson SW, Lucey BC, Varghese JC, Soto JA. Sixty-four multidetector row computed tomography in multitrauma patient imaging: early experience. Curr Probl Diagn Radiol 2006; 35:188-198.
16. Kalra MK, Maher MM, Toth TL, et al. Strategies for CT radiation dose optimization. Radiology 2004; 230:619-628.
17. Mettler FA, Wiest PW, Locken JA, Kelsey CA. CT scanning: patterns of use and dose. J Radiol Prot 2000; 20:353-359.
18. Wintersperger B, Jakobs T, Herzog P, et al. Aorto-iliac multidetector-row CT angiography with low kV settings: improved vessel enhancement and simultaneous reduction of radiation dose. Eur Radiol 2005; 15:334-341.
19. Mahesh M, Cody DD. Physics of cardiac imaging with multiple-row detector CT. Radiographics 2007; 27:1495-1509.
20. Lell MM, Anders K, Uder M, et al. New techniques in CT angiography. Radiographics 2006; 26(Suppl 1):S45-S62.
21. Flohr TG, Stierstorfer K, Ulzheimer S, et al. Image reconstruction and image quality evaluation for a 64-slice CT scanner with z-flying focal spot. Med Phys 2005; 32:2536-2547.
22. Jahnke C, Paetsch I, Achenbach S, et al. Coronary MR imaging: breath-hold capability and patterns, coronary artery rest periods, and beta-blocker use. Radiology 2006; 239:71-78.
23. Hsieh J, Londt J, Vass M, et al. Step-and-shoot data acquisition and reconstruction for cardiac x-ray computed tomography. Med Phys 2006; 33:4236-4248.
24. Earls JP, Berman EL, Urban BA, et al. Prospectively gated transverse coronary CT angiography versus retrospectively gated helical technique: improved image quality and reduced radiation dose. Radiology 2008; 246:742-753.

25. Bae KT. Peak contrast enhancement in CT and MR angiography: when does it occur and why? Pharmacokinetic study in a porcine model. Radiology 2003; 227:809-816.
26. Bae KT, Tran HQ, Heiken JP. Uniform vascular contrast enhancement and reduced contrast medium volume achieved by using exponentially decelerated contrast material injection method. Radiology 2004; 231:732-736.
27. Macari M, Israel GM, Berman P, et al. Infrarenal abdominal aortic aneurysms at multi-detector row CT angiography: intravascular enhancement without a timing acquisition. Radiology 2001; 220:519-523.
28. Johnson PT, Fishman EK. IV contrast selection for MDCT: current thoughts and practice. AJR Am J Roentgenol 2006; 186:406-415.
29. Kim M-J, Chung YE, Kim KW, et al. Variation of the time to aortic enhancement of fixed-duration versus fixed-rate injection protocols. AJR Am J Roentgenol 2006; 186:185-192.
30. Fleischmann D. Use of high concentration contrast media: principles and rationale—vascular district. Eur J Radiol 2003; 45(Suppl 1):S88-S93.
31. Fleischmann D, Rubin GD, Bankier AA, Hittmair K. Improved uniformity of aortic enhancement with customized contrast medium injection protocols at CT angiography. Radiology 2000; 214:363-371.
32. Furuta A, Ito K, Fujita T, et al. Hepatic enhancement in multiphasic contrast-enhanced MDCT: comparison of high- and low-iodine-concentration contrast medium in same patients with chronic liver disease. AJR Am J Roentgenol 2004; 183:157-162.
33. Fleischmann D, Hallett RL, Rubin GD. CT angiography of peripheral arterial disease. J Vasc Interv Radiol 2006; 17:3-26.
34. Fleischmann D, Rubin GD. Quantification of intravenously administered contrast medium transit through the peripheral arteries: implications for CT angiography. Radiology 2005; 236:1076-1082.
35. Adriaensen ME, Kock MC, Stijnen T, et al. Peripheral arterial disease: therapeutic confidence of CT versus digital subtraction angiography and effects on additional imaging recommendations. Radiology 2004; 233:385-391.
36. Catalano C, Fraioli F, Laghi A, et al. Infrarenal aortic and lower-extremity arterial disease: diagnostic performance of multi-detector row CT angiography. Radiology 2004; 231:555-563.
37. Martin ML, Tay KH, Flak B, et al. Multidetector CT angiography of the aortoiliac system and lower extremities: a prospective comparison with digital subtraction angiography. AJR Am J Roentgenol 2003; 180:1085-1091.
38. Ofer A, Nitecki SS, Linn S, et al. Multidetector CT angiography of peripheral vascular disease: a prospective comparison with intra-arterial digital subtraction angiography. AJR Am J Roentgenol 2003; 180:719-724.
39. Willmann JK, Mayer D, Banyai M, et al. Evaluation of peripheral arterial bypass grafts with multi-detector row CT angiography: comparison with duplex US and digital subtraction angiography. Radiology 2003; 229:465-474.
40. Rubin GD, Schmidt AJ, Logan LJ, Sofilos MC. Multi-detector row CT angiography of lower extremity arterial inflow and runoff: initial experience. Radiology 2001; 221:146-158.
41. Qanadli SD, Chiappori V, Kelekis A. Multislice computed tomography of peripheral arterial disease: new approach to optimize vascular opacification with 16-row platform. Eur Radiol 2004; 14(Suppl 2):806.
42. Laswed T, Rizzo E, Guntern D, et al. Assessment of occlusive arterial disease of abdominal aorta and lower extremities arteries: value of multidetector CT angiography using an adaptive acquisition method. Eur Radiol 2008; 18:263-272.
43. Johnson PT, Fishman EK. IV contrast selection for MDCT: current thoughts and practice. AJR Am J Roentgenol 2006; 186:406-415.
44. Iezzi R, Cotroneo AR, Filippone A, et al. Four-detector row computed tomographic angiography in the evaluation of infrarenal aorta and peripheral arterial occlusive disease: influence of contrast medium concentration. J Comput Assist Tomogr 2008; 32:690-696.
45. Becker CR, Hong C, Knez A, et al. Optimal contrast application for cardiac 4-detector-row computed tomography. Invest Radiol 2003; 38:690-694.
46. Hittmair K, Fleischmann D. Accuracy of predicting and controlling time-dependent aortic enhancement from a test bolus injection. J Comput Assist Tomogr 2001; 25:287-294.
47. Karcaaltincaba M, Foley WD. Gadolinium-enhanced multidetector CT angiography of the thoracoabdominal aorta. J Comput Assist Tomogr 2002; 26:875-878.
48. Pena CS, Kaufman JA, Geller SC, Waltman AC. Gadopentetate dimeglumine: a possible alternative contrast agent for CT angiography of the aorta. J Comput Assist Tomogr 1999; 23:23-24.
49. Chicoskie C, Tello R. Gadolinium-enhanced MDCT angiography of the abdomen: feasibility and limitations. AJR Am J Roentgenol 2005; 184:1821-1828.
50. Wicky S, Greenfield A, Fan C-M, et al. Aortoiliac gadolinium-enhanced CT angiography: improved results with a 16-detector row scanner compared with a four-detector row scanner. J Vasc Interv Radiol 2004; 15:947-954.
51. Grobner T. Gadolinium—a specific trigger for the development of nephrogenic fibrosing dermopathy and nephrogenic systemic fibrosis? Nephrol Dial Transplant 2006; 21:1104-1108.
52. Thomsen HS. Nephrogenic systemic fibrosis: a serious late adverse reaction to gadodiamide. Eur Radiol 2006; 16:2619-2621.
53. Estol C, Claasen D, Hirsch W, et al. Correlative angiographic and pathologic findings in the diagnosis of ulcerated plaques in the carotid artery. Arch Neurol 1991; 48:692-694.
54. Ricotta JJ, Schenk EA, Ekholm SE, DeWeese JA. Angiographic and pathologic correlates in carotid artery disease. Surgery 1986; 99:284-292.
55. Davies KN, Humphrey PR. Complications of cerebral angiography in patients with symptomatic carotid territory ischaemia screened by carotid ultrasound. J Neurol Neurosurg Psychiatry 1993; 56:967-972.
56. Chiles C, Carr JJ. Vascular diseases of the thorax: evaluation with multidetector CT. Radiol Clin North Am 2005; 43:543-569, viii.
57. Ghaye B, Szapiro D, Mastora I, et al. Peripheral pulmonary arteries: how far in the lung does multi-detector row spiral CT allow analysis? Radiology 2001; 219:629-636.
58. Crawford T, Yoon C, Wolfson K, et al. The effect of imaging modality on patient management in the evaluation of pulmonary thromboembolism. J Thorac Imaging 2001; 16:163-169.
59. Prologo JD, Glauser J. Variable diagnostic approach to suspected pulmonary embolism in the ED of a major academic tertiary care center. Am J Emerg Med 2002; 20:5-9.
60. Scanlon PJ, Faxon DP, Audet AM, et al. ACC/AHA guidelines for coronary angiography. A report of the American College of Cardiology/American Heart Association Task Force on practice guidelines (Committee on Coronary Angiography). Developed in collaboration with the Society for Cardiac Angiography and Interventions. J Am Coll Cardiol 1999; 33:1756-1824.
61. American Heart Association. 2002 Heart and Stroke Statistical Update. Dallas, TX, American Heart Association, 2002.
62. Raff GL, Gallagher MJ, O'Neill WW, Goldstein JA. Diagnostic accuracy of noninvasive coronary angiography using 64-slice spiral computed tomography. J Am Coll Cardiol 2005; 46:552-557.
63. Johnson TR, Nikolaou K, Wintersperger BJ, et al. Dual-source CT cardiac imaging: initial experience. Eur Radiol 2006; 16:1409-1415.
64. Rodriguez-Granillo GA, Rosales MA, Degrossi E, et al. Modified scan protocol using multislice CT coronary angiography allows high quality acquisitions in obese patients: a case report. Int J Cardiovasc Imaging 2007; 23:265-267.
65. Golzarian J, Valenti D. Endoleakage after endovascular treatment of abdominal aortic aneurysms: diagnosis, significance and treatment. Eur Radiol 2006; 16:2849-2857.
66. Brugel M, Link TM, Rummeny EJ, et al. Assessment of vascular invasion in pancreatic head cancer with multislice spiral CT: value of multiplanar reconstructions. Eur Radiol 2004; 14:1188-1195.
67. Foley WD, Mallisee TA, Hohenwalter MD, et al. Multiphase hepatic CT with a multirow detector CT scanner. AJR Am J Roentgenol 2000; 175:679-685.
68. Foley WD. Special focus session: multidetector CT: abdominal visceral imaging. Radiographics 2002; 22:701-719.
69. Fletcher JG, Wiersema MJ, Farrell MA, et al. Pancreatic malignancy: value of arterial, pancreatic, and hepatic phase imaging with multi-detector row CT. Radiology 2003; 229:81-90.
70. Nino-Murcia M, Jeffrey RB Jr, Beaulieu CF, et al. Multidetector CT of the pancreas and bile duct system: value of curved planar reformations. AJR Am J Roentgenol 2001; 176:689-693.
71. Vargas R, Nino-Murcia M, Trueblood W, Jeffrey RB Jr. MDCT in pancreatic adenocarcinoma: prediction of vascular invasion and

resectability using a multiphasic technique with curved planar reformations. AJR Am J Roentgenol 2004; 182:419-425.
72. Urban BA, Ratner LE, Fishman EK. Three-dimensional volume-rendered CT angiography of the renal arteries and veins: normal anatomy, variants, and clinical applications. Radiographics 2001; 21:373-386.
73. Raman SS, Pojchamarnwiputh S, Muangsomboon K, et al. Utility of 16-MDCT angiography for comprehensive preoperative vascular evaluation of laparoscopic renal donors. AJR Am J Roentgenol 2006; 186:1630-1638.
74. Patil UD, Ragavan A, Nadaraj, et al. Helical CT angiography in evaluation of live kidney donors. Nephrol Dial Transplant 2001; 16:1900-1904.
75. Kim J-K, Park S-Y, Kim H-J, et al. Living donor kidneys: usefulness of multi-detector row CT for comprehensive evaluation. Radiology 2003; 229:869-876.
76. Kim JK, Kim JH, Bae S-J, Cho K-S. CT angiography for evaluation of living renal donors: comparison of four reconstruction methods. AJR Am J Roentgenol 2004; 183:471-477.
77. Noroozian M, Cohan RH, Caoili EM, et al. Multislice CT urography: state of the art. Br J Radiol 2004; 77:S74-S86.
78. Kirkpatrick IDC, Kroeker MA, Greenberg HM. Biphasic CT with mesenteric CT angiography in the evaluation of acute mesenteric ischemia: initial experience. Radiology 2003; 229:91-98.
79. Bradbury MS, Kavanagh PV, Bechtold RE, et al. Mesenteric venous thrombosis: diagnosis and noninvasive imaging. Radiographics 2002; 22:527-541.
80. Hoffmann U, Ferencik M, Cury RC, Pena AJ. Coronary CT angiography. J Nucl Med 2006; 47:797-806.
81. Leschka S, Wildermuth S, Boehm T, et al. Noninvasive coronary angiography with 64-section CT: effect of average heart rate and heart rate variability on image quality. Radiology 2006; 241:378-385.
82. Achenbach S, Ropers D, Kuettner A, et al. Contrast-enhanced coronary artery visualization by dual-source computed tomography—initial experience. Eur J Radiol 2006; 57:331-335.
83. Hunold P, Vogt FM, Schmermund A, et al. Radiation exposure during cardiac CT: effective doses at multi-detector row CT and electron-beam CT. Radiology 2003; 226:145-152.
84. Fraioli F, Catalano C, Napoli A, et al. Low-dose multidetector-row CT angiography of the infra-renal aorta and lower extremity vessels: image quality and diagnostic accuracy in comparison with standard DSA. Eur Radiol 2006; 16:137-146.
85. Sahani DV, Kalva SP, Hahn PF, Saini S. 16-MDCT angiography in living kidney donors at various tube potentials: impact on image quality and radiation dose. AJR Am J Roentgenol 2007; 188:115-120.
86. Paul JF, Abada HT. Strategies for reduction of radiation dose in cardiac multislice CT. Eur Radiol 2007; 17:2028-2037.
87. Rubin GD. Data explosion: the challenge of multidetector-row CT. Eur J Radiol 2000; 36:74-80.
88. Fishman EK. High-resolution three-dimensional imaging from sub-second helical CT data sets: applications in vascular imaging. AJR Am J Roentgenol 1997; 169:441-443.
89. Fleischmann D, Hallett RL, Rubin GD. CT angiography of peripheral arterial disease. J Vasc Interv Radiol 2006; 17:3-26.
90. Kirchgeorg MA, Prokop M. Increasing spiral CT benefits with post-processing applications. Eur J Radiol 1998; 28:39-54.
91. Lawler LP, Fishman EK. Multi-detector row CT of thoracic disease with emphasis on 3D volume rendering and CT angiography. Radiographics 2001; 21:1257-1273.
92. Fleischmann D, Rubin GD, Paik DS, et al. Stair-step artifacts with single versus multiple detector-row helical CT. Radiology 2000; 216:185-196.
93. Ota H, Takase K, Igarashi K, et al. MDCT compared with digital subtraction angiography for assessment of lower extremity arterial occlusive disease: importance of reviewing cross-sectional images. AJR Am J Roentgenol 2004; 182:201-209.
94. Lawler LP, Fishman EK. Multidetector row computed tomography of the aorta and peripheral arteries. Cardiol Clin 2003; 21:607-629.
95. Prokesch RW, Coulam CH, Chow LC, et al. CT angiography of the subclavian artery: utility of curved planar reformations. J Comput Assist Tomogr 2002; 26:199-201.
96. Raman R, Napel S, Rubin GD. Curved-slab maximum intensity projection: method and evaluation. Radiology 2003; 229:255-260.
97. Rankin SC. CT angiography. Eur Radiol 1999; 9:297-310.
98. Yaghmai V, Nikolaidis P, Hammond NA, et al. Multidetector-row computed tomography diagnosis of small bowel obstruction: can coronal reformations replace axial images? Emerg Radiol 2006; 13:69-72.
99. Cody DD. AAPM/RSNA Physics Tutorial for Residents: Topics in CT: image processing in CT. Radiographics 2002; 22:1255-1268.
100. Prokop M. General principles of MDCT. Eur J Radiol 2003; 45:S4-S10.
101. Fishman EK, Ney DR, Heath DG, et al. Volume rendering versus maximum intensity projection in CT angiography: what works best, when, and why. Radiographics 2006; 26:905-922.
102. Napoli A, Fleischmann D, Chan FP, et al. Computed tomography angiography: state-of-the-art imaging using multidetector-row technology. J Comput Assist Tomogr 2004; 28(Suppl 1):S32-S45.
103. Raman R, Napel S, Beaulieu CF, et al. Automated generation of curved planar reformations from volume data: method and evaluation. Radiology 2002; 223:275-280.
104. Kanitsar A, Fleischmann D, Wegenkittl R, et al. CPR: curved planar reformation. IEEE Computer Society 2002; 37-44.
105. Roos JE, Fleischmann D, Koechl A, et al. Multipath curved planar reformation of the peripheral arterial tree in CT angiography. Radiology 2007; 244:281-290.
106. van Ooijen PM, Ho KY, Dorgelo J, Oudkerk M. Coronary artery imaging with multidetector CT: visualization issues. Radiographics 2003; 23:e16.
107. Calhoun PS, Kuszyk BS, Heath DG, et al. Three-dimensional volume rendering of spiral CT data: theory and method. Radiographics 1999; 19:745-764.
108. Kim JK, Kim JH, Bae SJ, Cho KS. CT angiography for evaluation of living renal donors: comparison of four reconstruction methods. AJR Am J Roentgenol 2004; 183:471-477.
109. Koechl A, Kanitsar A, Lomoschitz E. Comprehensive assessment of peripheral arteries using multi-path curved planar reformation of CTA datasets. Eur Radiol 2003; 13:268-269.

CHAPTER 81

Magnetic Resonance Angiography: Physics and Instrumentation

Oliver Wieben and Thorsten Bley

Magnetic resonance imaging (MRI) provides several useful approaches for the assessment of vascular disease. Signal properties of flowing blood can be exploited to differentiate the blood pool from stationary tissue with positive (bright blood imaging) or negative (black blood imaging) contrast and to provide functional information in terms of velocity maps and flow measurements. In another technique, contrast-enhanced MR angiography (CE-MRA), a venously injected gadolinium (Gd) chelate contrast agent mixes with blood and alters its signal properties. The major advantage of MR angiography (MRA) is the capability to capture comprehensive information for all voxels within a larger three-dimensional imaging volume, allowing for the display of tortuous vessel paths in various modes and for reformatting of data for viewing in arbitrary planes. MRA is noninvasive, with only a venous puncture in the case of CE-MRA, and provides information about the surrounding soft tissues. Other MRI sequences can be added to extend the scope of the examination (e.g., vessel wall imaging, diffusion and perfusion imaging, functional MRI studies).

The performance of an MRA requires attention to detail because overall scan time must be optimized to provide sufficiently high spatial resolution for diagnosis. Typically, the operator must balance concerns related to anatomic coverage with the constraints placed on proper spatial resolution and overall scan time or temporal resolution. Prolonged MRA scan times increase the acquisition's susceptibility to image blurring artifacts from bulk body motion and physiologic motion related to respiration and cardiac contraction.

There have been dramatic improvements in MR hardware and acquisition approaches over the past decades, many of which have proved beneficial for or were inspired by angiography applications; these now allow for more rapid imaging with improved image contrast and reproducible image quality. This chapter discusses some underlying physical principles of vascular imaging using MRI and the instrumentation and acquisition approaches for typical MRA examinations. In addition, the various mechanisms for vascular bright blood vascular depiction using CE-MRA, time-of-flight MRA (TOF MRA), phase contrast MRA, and steady-state free precession MRA will be discussed. It should be noted that the terminology for MR techniques can sometimes be confusing, not only because there are many variants of related schemes, but also because various vendors usually market these technologies under different trade names.[1]

DATA ACQUISITION AND IMAGE RECONSTRUCTION

MRI is based on the nuclear magnetic resonance phenomenon, which arises in atoms with an odd number of protons and/or an odd number of neutrons. Almost all clinical MRI, including angiography applications, is based on the signal from the hydrogen nucleus, ^1H, a single, positively charged proton that is the most abundant in the body (mainly in H_2O but also in fat and other compounds). From a classic physics perspective, each proton has a magnetic dipole moment and behaves like a tiny bar magnet when interacting with a magnetic field. In the absence of an external magnetic field, the axes of the magnetic dipole moments are randomly arranged so that they in aggregate cancel each other out and result in a net magnetization of zero. However, in the presence of an external magnetic field, or B_0, the magnetic dipole moments of the protons will align parallel or antiparallel with the external field. In thermal equilibrium, slightly more spins are aligned parallel than antiparallel with the

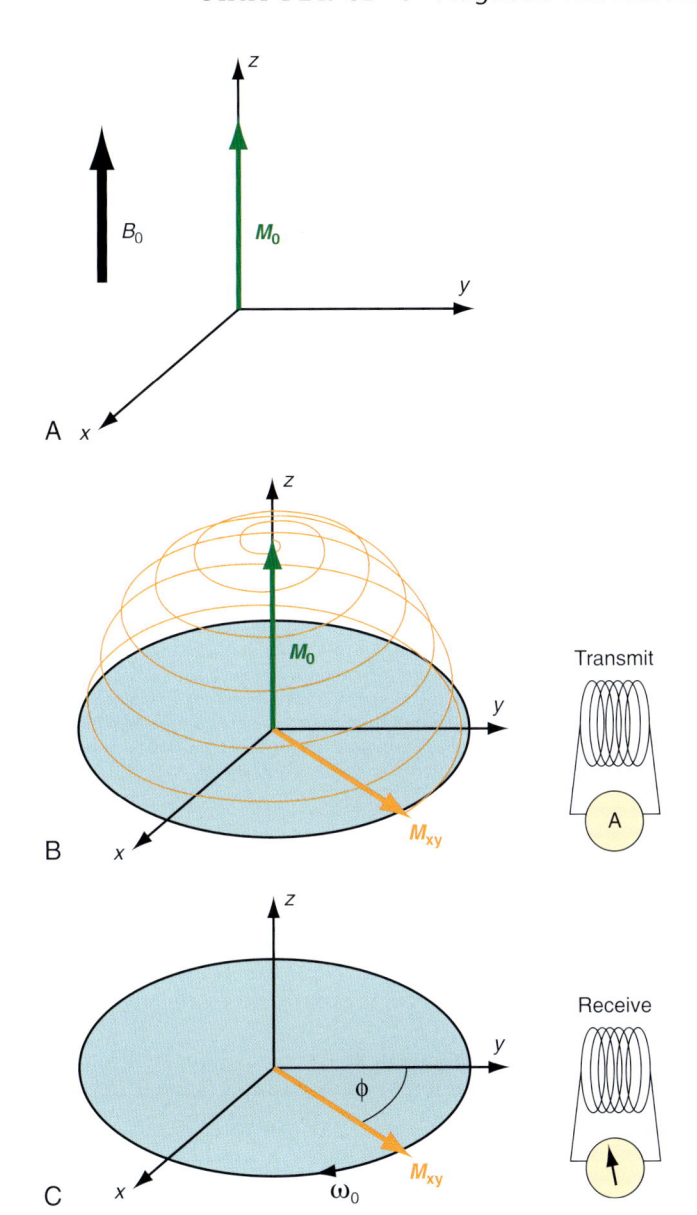

FIGURE 81-1 A, In thermal equilibrium, the net magnetization is aligned with the direction of the main magnetic field, B_0. B, With an RF system that generates an RF field tuned to the resonance frequency of the spin ensemble, the net magnetization (M_0) can be tipped into the transverse plane. C, The transverse magnetization, M_{xy}, precesses at the Larmor frequency, ω_0, thereby creating an oscillating signal that can be measured with a receiver coil.

external magnetic field because it requires less energy. The result is a net magnetization that becomes the signal source in MR experiments. As shown in Figure 81-1A, this vector quantity is aligned with the direction of the main magnetic field. To measure signal from the net magnetization, it has to be "tipped" away from its orientation along the main magnetic field into the transverse plane. Once it is tipped away from the longitudinal axis, the magnetization vector rotates, or precesses, around that axis with a characteristic frequency, as given by the Larmor equation:

$$\omega_0 = -\gamma B_0 \qquad (1)$$

where ω_0 is referred to as the Larmor frequency, γ is the gyromagnetic ratio of protons (42.58 MHz/T) and B_0 is the magnetic field flux of the main field. The precessing transversal magnetization M_{xy} creates a weak radiofrequency (RF) field that can be recorded with a properly tuned coil (e.g., 63.87 MHz at B_0 = 1.5 T) circularly polarized about the axis of precession. As illustrated in Figure 81-1B, the tipping of the net magnetization vector is accomplished with a second RF system that can generate an oscillating magnetic field, B_1, close to the resonance frequency, a concept called RF excitation. In practice, the RF pulse is played out very shortly (in the order of milliseconds) and a remarkably small B_1 field is sufficient for RF excitation (e.g., ~50 mT in comparison to B_0 = 1.5 T).

Once the RF field is turned off, the spin system returns into its thermal equilibrium state. The rate of regrowth for the longitudinal magnetization follows an exponential waveform described by its characteristic time constant, called T1, referred to as the longitudinal relaxation time. The regrowth rate depends on the properties of the nucleus and its interactions with the environment. Meanwhile, the signal decrease in the transversal magnetization component is described by the exponential time constant called T2, the transversal relaxation time, and reflects dephasing caused by interactions between neighboring nuclei; also, it does not depend on the nucleus or chemical compound alone. Additional parameters contribute to the T2 relaxation, so that the T1 and T2 relaxation processes cannot be predicted from one another.

Multiple RF excitations are needed to acquire enough data for a two-dimensional image. The time between successive excitations is controlled by the MRI parameter repetition time (TR). The time between an RF excitation and the recording of the signal is controlled by the MRI parameter echo time (TE). Both of these parameters have an impact on the measured MR signal because they dictate how much time is allowed for the decay of the transversal magnetization (TE) or the regrowth of the longitudinal magnetization (TR). The actual measured MR signal depends on the T1 and T2 relaxation times, proton density, choice of TR and TE, and other imaging parameters, but also on factors such as motion, diffusion, and temperature. In MRA, the goal is to generate high signal differences between blood and surrounding background tissues, which is achieved by incorporating the motion of the blood using noncontrast MRA techniques or T1 shortening of blood by a circulating Gd chelate contrast agent using CE-MRA. Typical relaxation times are T1/T2 = 1200/250 ms for arterial blood and T1/T2 = 1200/220 ms for venous blood at 1.5 T.[2] Whereas T1 increases with field strength for most tissues (1600 ms for arterial blood), the T2 undergoes a small decrease.

Image Encoding

To create an image, the spatial distribution of the protons has to be resolved. Spatial encoding is achieved with the use of spatially and temporally varying magnetic fields. In the first step, the signal-generating volume is reduced to a slice (two-dimensional imaging) or volume (three-dimensional imaging) by selective excitation. A linear magnetic field gradient is superimposed onto the main magnetic field in the slice (or volume) direction simultaneously with the RF excitation. Consequently, the resonance frequency

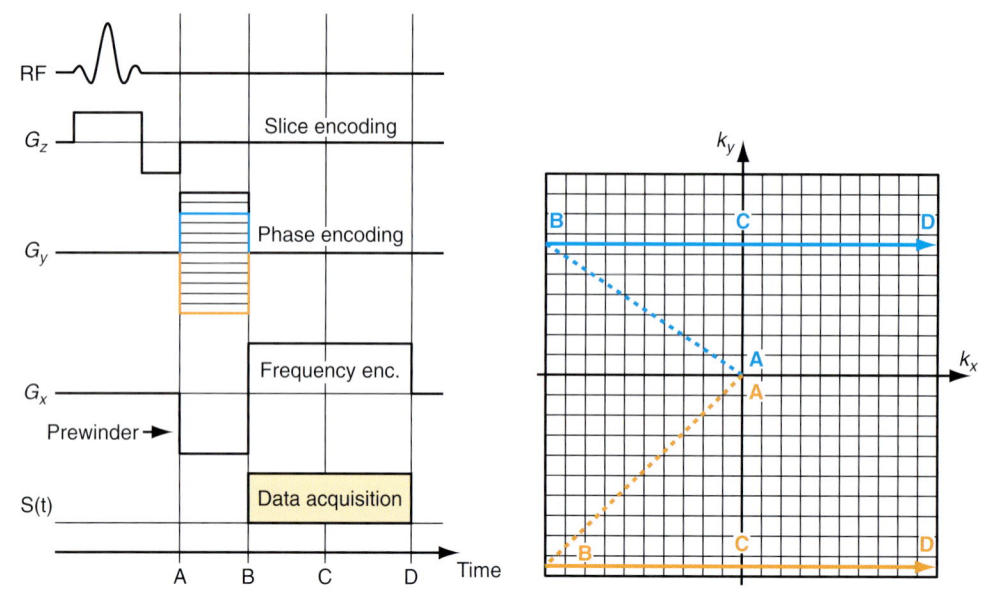

FIGURE 81-2 Basic gradient echo pulse sequence for two-dimensional Fourier transform k-space scanning. An RF pulse and slice-encoding gradient, followed by a refocusing gradient, are played out simultaneously to excite spins in a slice. Frequency encoding is achieved with a linear gradient applied during data acquisition, resulting in the sampling of k-space along the frequency encoding direction k_x. A prewinding gradient is required to start the acquisition with negative spatial frequencies. The measurement is repeated with stepwise changing phase-encoding gradients for sampling along the frequency-encoding direction with different offsets in the phase-encoding direction k_y. The signed area under the gradients steers the sampling path, here shown for two phase-encoding settings (*orange* and *blue*) and their characteristic time points A, B, C, and D.

of the spin system is linearly varying as well. The RF system generates a pulse that excites not only a single precession frequency but all the frequencies contained in the desired slice or volume. Spins located outside the desired volume are not excited because their precession frequency is higher or lower than the frequency band covered by the RF excitation. Theoretically, this concept could be repeated in orthogonal directions ultimately to excite only a single point in the object, and then repeat the measurement until all points in the image are sampled. However, a much more efficient approach is Fourier encoding, whereby each sampled signal contains contributions from all spins in the object, therefore dramatically increasing the SNR of the acquisition. Figure 81-2 shows a basic example for a Fourier-encoded two-dimensional acquisition in the form of a pulse sequence diagram that illustrates the timing for RF excitation, the gradients, and data acquisition.

A second linear field gradient, called the frequency-encoding gradient, is applied during data sampling so that the precession frequency of the net magnetization varies linearly. Thus, the detected signal becomes a summation of all encoded frequencies and its spatial distribution can be derived by a one-dimensional Fourier transform. This encoding scheme makes MRI a spectroscopic imaging method. Unfortunately, the second spatial dimension cannot be encoded simultaneously during readout because this would result in a nonunique allocation of frequency and spatial location. Instead, the gradients are applied sequentially, with the drawback of extended imaging times.

The third gradient, called the phase-encoding gradient, is switched on and off prior to the frequency-encoding gradient. This leads to a linearly varying phase of the net magnetization vectors along the direction of that gradient, providing encoding for a single spatial frequency. In other words, with properly controlled gradients, the time-dependent MR signal actually samples the spatial frequencies of the object in two dimensions. Figure 81-2 shows how the sampling trajectory in the spatial frequency space, also called k-space, is controlled by the area under the gradient waveforms.

If that experiment is repeated several times with varying phase-encoding gradients, then multiple spatial frequencies are sampled in the phase-encoding direction as well and an image can be reconstructed via inverse two-dimensional Fourier transform. Figure 81-3 shows an example of a sagittal head scan. The received signal is digitized by an analog to digital converter and a discrete inverse two-dimensional Fourier transform generates the corresponding image, which contains magnitude (length of the transversal magnetization) and phase information (position in the transverse plain in respect to the coil axis) for each voxel. Most MRI relies on the magnitude image only. However, in some applications, such as phase contrast MRA, the phase information plays an essential role in generating image contrast.

Suppose an acquisition matrix contained 256 data points in the frequency and 256 data points in the phase-encoding direction. The reconstructed image is also described by a 256×256 matrix. For a two-dimensional acquisition, the total scan time is given by the number of phase-encoding steps multiplied by the repetition time (i.e., TR). Volumetric imaging can be accomplished by successive imaging of two-dimensional slices (i.e., two-dimensional MRA), or by excitation of an entire imaging volume (i.e., three-dimensional MRA) and the use of phase encoding in the third dimension for a true three-dimensional data acquisition. Either option prolongs the total scan time proportional to the number of slices (two-

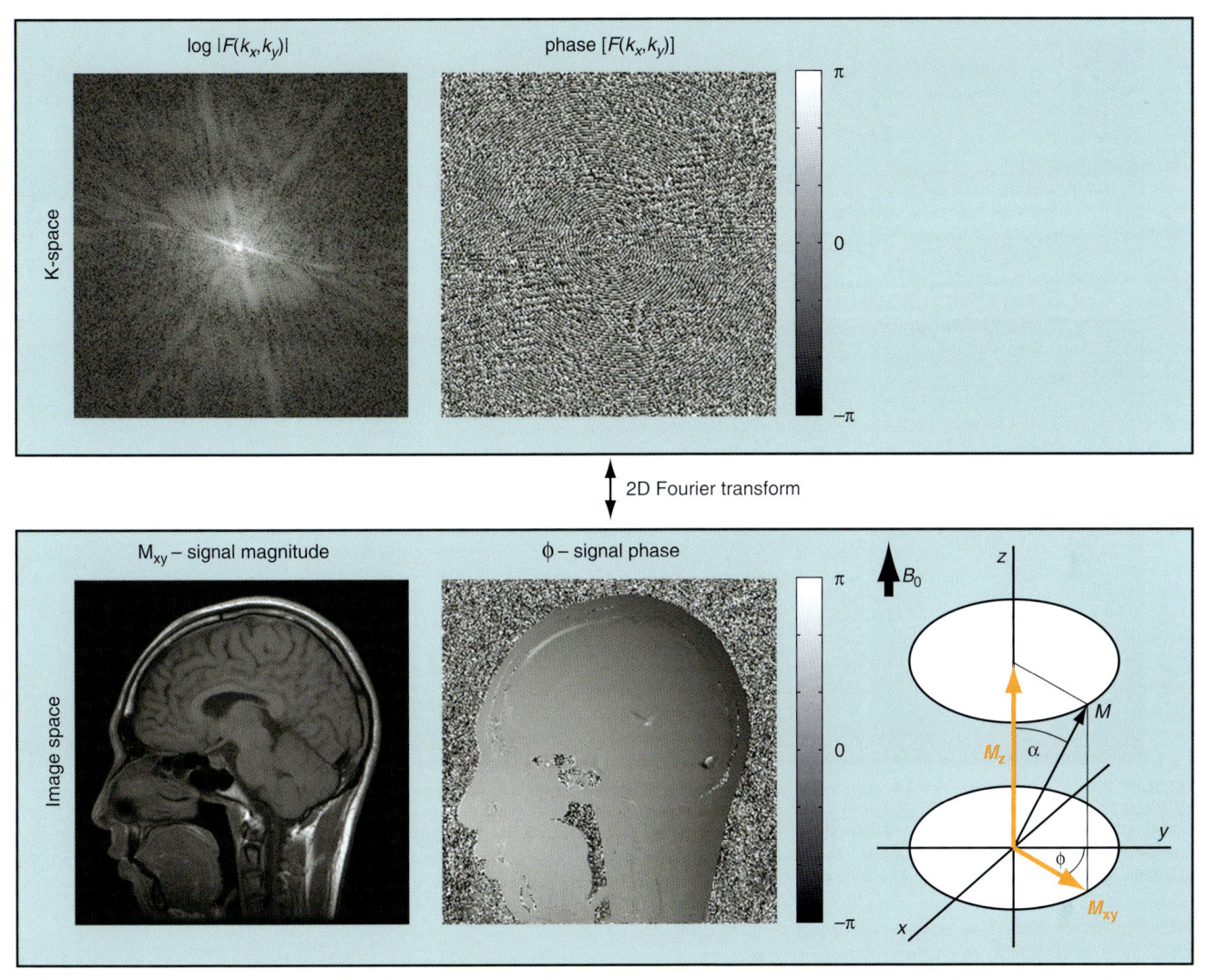

FIGURE 81-3 Two-dimensional (2D) Fourier transform pair. The acquired complex k-space data are reconstructed into image space via a 2D Fourier transform. The resulting signal has a magnitude and a phase component, representing the transversal magnetization M_{xy} and its position ϕ in a unit circle in respect to a receiver axis. The highest signal can be obtained with a flip angle of $\alpha = 90$ degrees, which tips the magnetization vector completely into the transversal plane. Note that the k-space magnitude is shown on a logarithmic scale.

dimensional) or partitions (three-dimensional) in the volume.

Figure 81-4 provides some insight about the signal distribution in k-space. For this image, most of the signal energy is located around the origin of k-space. This area defines the weighting for the low spatial frequencies, which define the coarse outline of the imaged object yet lacks information on edges. The broad pattern of the phantom can be identified even with less than 0.5% of the k-space samples from the full-resolution image. However, all the detail is lost, which is defined in the unsampled higher spatial frequencies. The difference in images between the low-resolution images and the fully sampled image reveals the errors caused by limiting the acquisition to lower spatial frequencies only.

The basic signal-to-noise ratio (SNR) in MR acquisitions is given by

$$\text{SNR} \propto B_0 \times (\text{voxel volume}/\text{noise volume}) \times \sqrt{T_{acq}} \quad (2)$$

where T_{acq} represents the data acquisition time.[3] Based on this relationship, one notes that the desirable properties for MRA, such as small voxel size for higher spatial resolution imaging and short acquisition times for fast scans, are detrimental to the obtainable SNR. Frequently, compromises in scan parameter choices are necessary for optimization of MRA for imaging individual vascular territories, with each offering unique challenges for proper visualization by MRA.

TECHNICAL REQUIREMENTS

The basic components of an MRI system are (1) a magnet that creates a strong static magnetic field, (2) an RF system that excites nuclei with a magnetic moment via RF pulses and detects the electrical signals created by the excited nuclei, and (3) a set of gradient coils that generates secondary static magnetic fields in a controlled fashion to

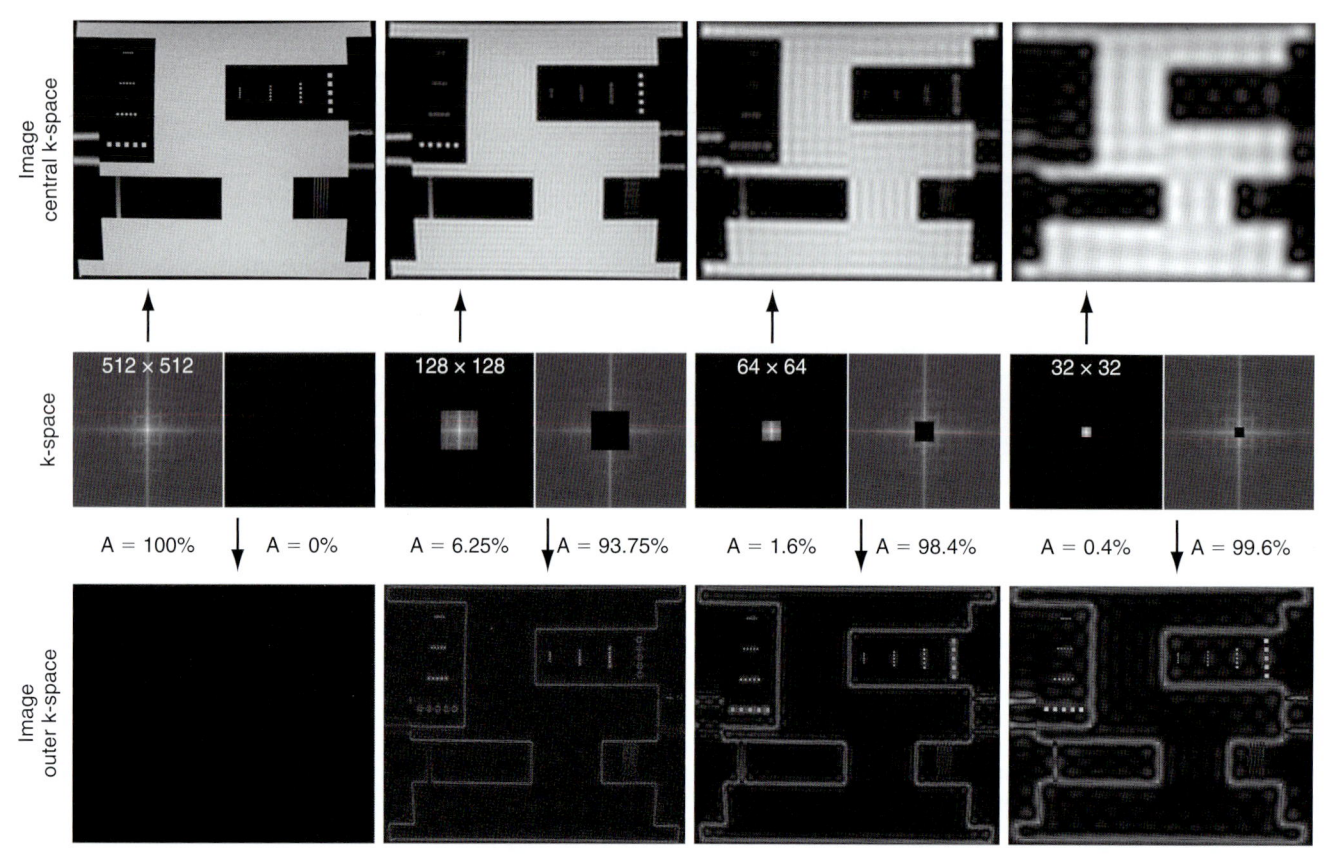

FIGURE 81-4 A high-resolution phantom scan reconstructed from different k-space subregions. The *upper row* is reconstructed when the central 512 × 512 (full resolution), 128 × 128, 64 × 64, and 32 × 32 samples are used for the reconstruction. This is equivalent to using 100%, 6.25%, 1.6%, or 0.4% of all sampled data. The lower row represents reconstruction results when the remaining peripheral k-space data are used for the image reconstruction instead. Whereas the central k-space samples define the low spatial frequencies and most of the image contrast, the peripheral k-space data define the higher spatial frequencies and, therefore, fine structures and edges.

superimpose linear field gradients onto the main field for spatial encoding.

Magnetic Resonance Scanner

Each MR scanner is designed to provide a magnetic field, B_0, that is homogeneous over the imaging volume, stable over time, and against the influence of external sources. The magnetic induction of the field, also frequently referred to as the magnetic field strength, is measured in tesla (T) or gauss (G), where $1 \text{ T} = 10^4$ G. The most common modern MR scanners used in clinical practice are whole-body scanners that rely on a superconducting magnet with a field strength of 1.5 or 3 T. For comparison, the field strength of a 1.5-T MR scanner is about 30,000 times stronger than the earth's magnetic field (~0.5 G). Superconducting MR scanners contain several coils that run in series to form a solenoid and create a cylindrically symmetrical magnetic field, with the main magnetic field aligned with the z-axis of the cylindrical housing (Fig. 81-5). They operate near absolute zero temperature (~4 K, or −270° C) to effectively eliminate electrical resistance in the coil wires, allowing large currents that generate high magnetic fields. Other MR scanner designs include resistive magnetic fields (without superconductivity) that operate at lower magnetic field strengths (<0.15 T), permanent magnetic fields that have intermediate field

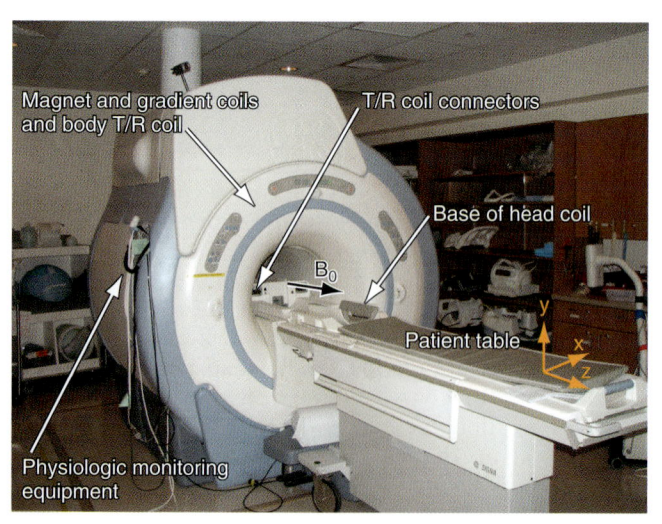

FIGURE 81-5 A 1.5-T MR system with a superconducting magnet, gradient coils, and a body transmit-receive RF system enclosed in the housing. The patient table, connectors for external transmit-receive or receive-only coils, and physiologic monitoring equipment are also shown. The main magnetic field is aligned with the table axis, called the z-axis by convention.

Coils

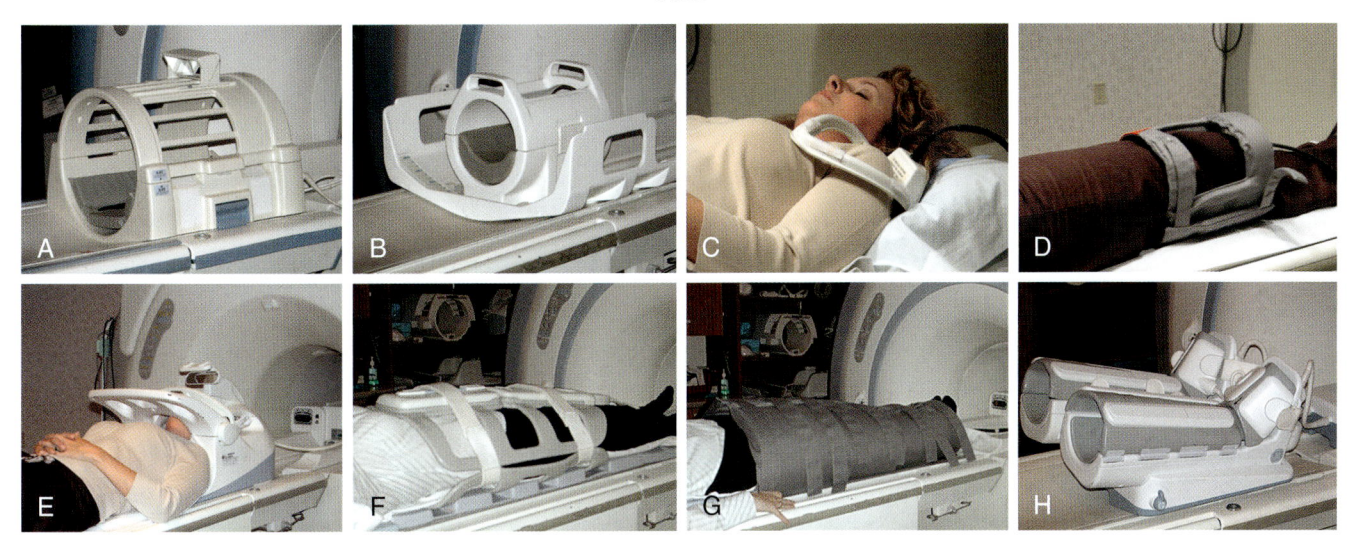

FIGURE 81-6 RF coils used for MR scanning. Bird cage coils for head (**A**) and knee (**B**) imaging are single-coil transmit and receive coils with a very homogeneous B_1 field. Single-channel surface coils such as the shoulder coil (**C**) or general purpose flex coil (**D**) are designed to have a high local sensitivity. Multielement coil arrays can combine the benefits of local sensitivity and larger coverage, here shown for an eight-channel neurovascular coil (**E**), eight-channel body phased-array coil (**F**), four-channel lower extremity coil (**G**), and eight-channel lower leg coil (**H**).

strength (<0.7 T), smaller bore diameter MR scanners for extremity imaging, and open bore designs (usually <0.7 T) to improve patient comfort and reduce claustrophobia. Imaging at lower field strengths reduces some of the problems encountered at higher fields, such as reduced RF penetration and increased energy absorption. However, MRA applications greatly benefit from imaging at higher field strength because the SNR increases linearly with field strength. MR scanners with field strengths of 3 T are becoming more prevalent in clinical settings and favorable results have been reported with these systems[4]; more recently, higher field 7-T research MR systems are being investigated.[5]

Gradient System

The magnetic field gradient system typically consists of three orthogonal gradient coils embedded within the housing of the scanner. Gradient coils are designed to produce a spatially varying magnetic field that can be temporally altered. Although these additional magnetic fields are dramatically smaller than the main magnetic field, they are an essential component for spatial encoding of the signal distribution in the imaging volume of interest. Gradients are rated by their maximum gradient strength (the higher the better) and the time needed to rise to the maximum gradient strength (slew rate—the faster the better). The gradient waveforms in Figure 81-2 are idealized in that they can be switched on and off instantaneously.

Gradient systems have undergone dramatic improvements over the last decade and modern equipment can provide maximum gradient strengths of about 50 mT/m and slew rates of 200 T/m/s. MRA applications greatly benefit from high-performance gradients because they enable faster imaging for higher temporal sampling of data, which can be used to improve spatial or temporal resolution. Faster imaging speeds are particularly helpful to assess the dynamic progression of a contrast bolus using multiphase or time-resolved MRA, or to ensure sufficient spatial resolution during a single breath-hold MRA acquisition. The minimization of imaging parameters such as the echo time, TE, or the repetition time, TR, are facilitated by the availability of high-performance gradients and provide additional benefits for image quality (see later).

Radiofrequency System

The RF system serves the purpose of converting pulsed oscillating currents from a power amplifier into an oscillating magnetic field, also referred to as the B_1 field, for the excitation of the nuclear spin system. This is accomplished by a transmitter coil tuned to the resonance frequency of the spin system under investigation. Such coils are designed to provide a uniform B_1 field over the imaging volume to ensure uniform spin excitation. So-called birdcage coils are well suited for this purpose and exist as whole-body coils built into the scanner housing and as specialty coils, such as for head or knee imaging (Fig. 81-6).

A receiver coil is used to detect the RF field created by the precessing magnetization of the nuclear spins after their excitation. The same coil may be used for transmitting and receiving the RF signals, which are referred to as transmit-receive coils (see Fig. 81-6A and B). However, in many applications, it is advantageous to use special local coils that are sensitive only to the signal from the region close to the coil. Such local coils can have a significantly better SNR, as described by equation 2, especially compared with the whole-body transmit-receive coil that encounters noise contributions from the whole volume within it that is much larger than that of smaller local coils. Figure 81-6 shows examples of such local coils, including a shoulder coil (C) and a multipurpose flex coil (D).

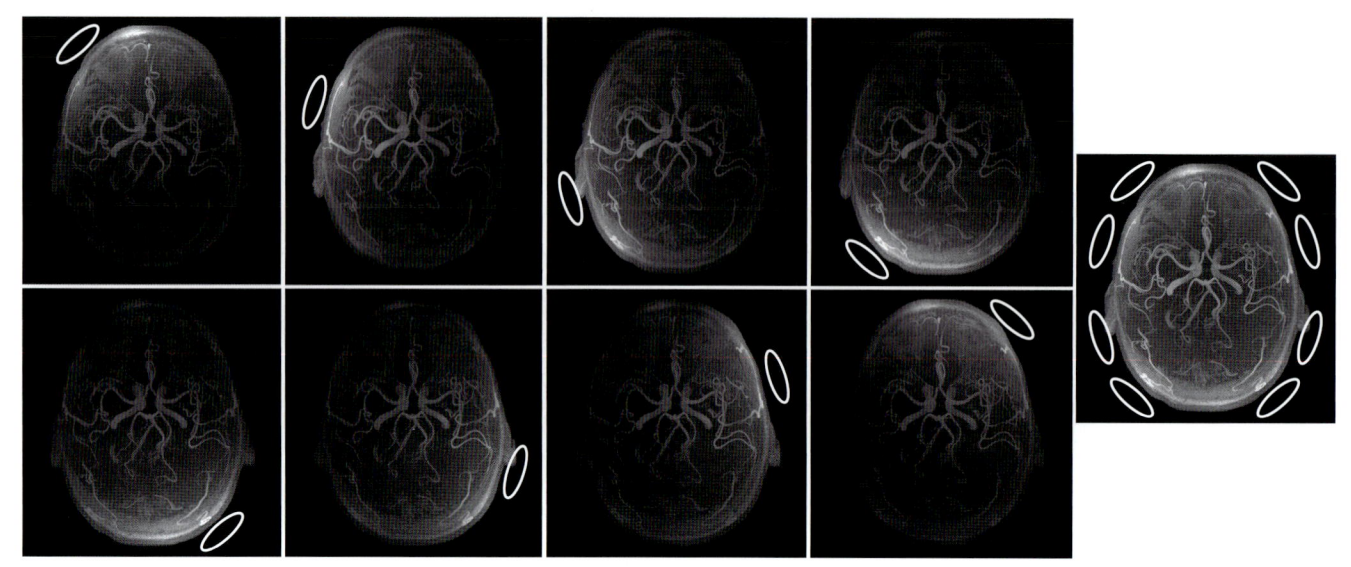

FIGURE 81-7 TOF angiography data set acquired with an eight-channel head coil. Shown are images reconstructed for each individual coil with increased local sensitivity (small images) and after combining all images as the square root of the sum of the squares from all individual coil images. *(Courtesy of Dr. Alexej Samsonov, University of Wisconsin-Madison, Madison, Wis.)*

Coil arrays consist of multiple local receiver coils to provide a larger coverage with the SNR advantage of local coils. These multielement RF coils have become very common and are available for many applications in many body regions (Fig. 81-6E-H). Figure 81-7 demonstrates the local coil sensitivities of an eight-channel head coil in a three-dimensional TOF MRA and the cumulative image obtained from combining all channels. Data from multiple coils cannot be combined during acquisition and must be stored individually. Therefore, the acquired data size increases linearly with the number of coils, and image reconstruction must be completed for each channel before they can be combined. However, current reconstruction engines are prepared to handle the additional workload for 8 to 16 channels without significant delays.

Parallel Imaging

More recently, scan time reduction methods were developed that explore the redundancy in the information contained in multiple receiver coils with partly overlapping sensitivity regions. SMASH (**s**im**u**ltaneous **a**cquisition of **s**patial **h**armonics),[6] SENSE (**sens**itivity **e**ncoding),[7] and GRAPPA[8] are acquisition and reconstruction methods from this group referred to as parallel imaging, which have found rapid commercial adaptation for cardiovascular imaging, especially CE-MRA. With this approach, the equivalent of multiple-phase encoding steps is acquired during a single readout. Although the advantage of accelerated imaging comes at the expense of a reduction in SNR, it can be highly beneficial in situations in which there is sufficient SNR and rapid image acquisition is desired. Basically, all CE-MRA applications fall into this category because faster imaging can improve the frame rate for dynamic acquisitions or reduce breath-hold lengths or other artifacts related to patient motion. As shown in Figure 81-8, attention has to be paid to potential local noise amplifications from the reconstruction process, frequently described as g-factor maps, when using high acceleration factors.

The scan time reduction factor that can be obtained with parallel imaging depends on the number of independent coil elements and their arrangement. Therefore, further increases in the number of coil elements and receiver channels promise even greater reductions in scan time. Consequently, the recent progress in parallel imaging has led to renewed interest in coil design and receiver systems. New MRI platforms provide the ability to connect many coil elements and acquire the signal from as many as 16 to 32 receivers simultaneously and systems with even more channels are being explored. With higher receiver coil counts, the SNR and coverage can be further improved or higher acceleration factors can possibly be obtained. Current design problems, such as with the decoupling of individual coil elements, has limited commercial coil designs to 8 to 32 elements. In research settings, systems with up to 128 receiver channels have been recently evaluated and demonstrated regional SNR benefits and high acceleration factors for cardiovascular applications as compared with lower count coil arrays.[9] However, the lack of penetration for small coils might limit additional benefits for regions of interest that are more distant from the body surface. It remains to be seen at which point additional coil elements are still beneficial, especially when the noise in the MR system becomes dominated by electrical noise from the receiver system, instead of intrinsic noise contributions caused by random motion of electrons in the patient's tissue.

Patient Monitoring

Patient monitoring systems are crucial components for vascular imaging because several approaches require synchronization with the cardiac cycle or feedback on the

Coil sensitivities

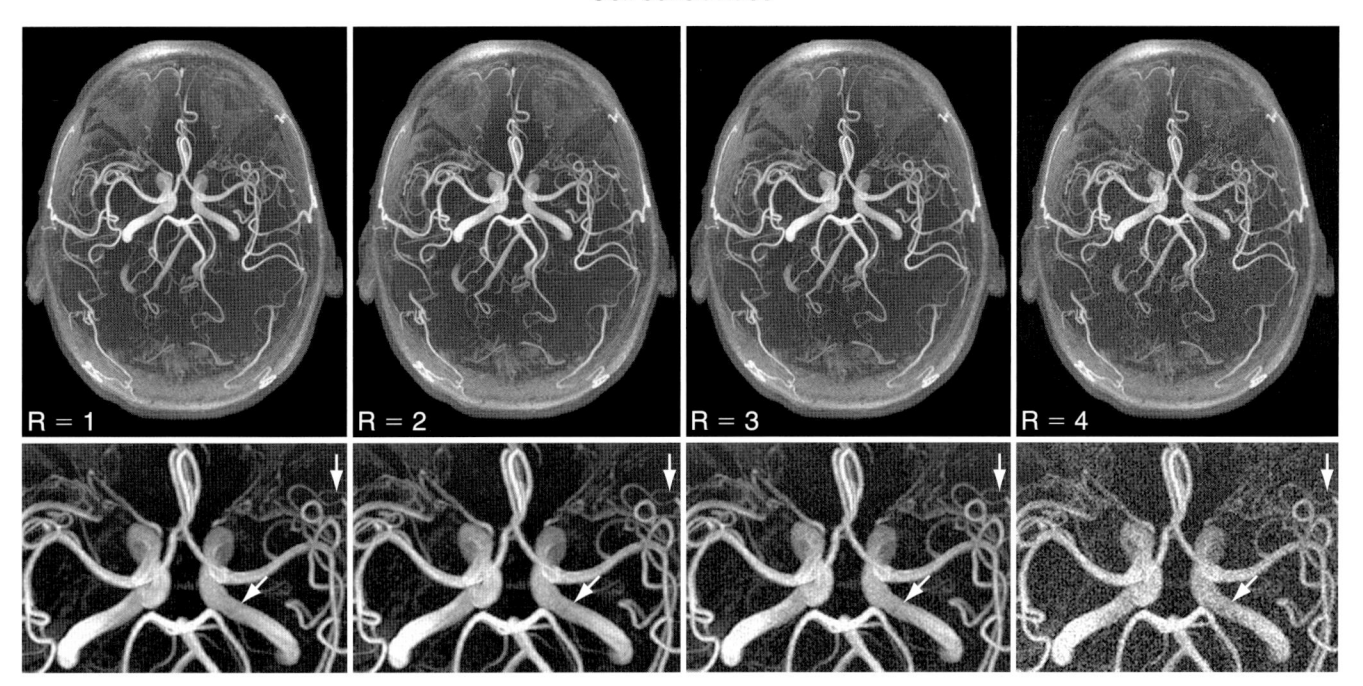

■ **FIGURE 81-8** MRA data reconstructed with a SENSE (1) based parallel imaging reconstruction using all the data from a fully sampled acquisition. The enlargements (*bottom row*) demonstrate good image quality for R = 2 but a decreased SNR and local noise enhancements for R = 3, which renders the images nondiagnostic, for a reduction of R = 4 with dramatic noise enhancements that obscure vessel anatomy. 100% reduction factor R = 1; 50% (R = 2); 33% (R = 3); 25% (R = 4). (*Courtesy of Dr. Alexej Samsonov, University of Wisconsin-Madison, Madison, Wis.*)

respiratory motion for optimized image quality. To accommodate these needs, most MR systems are equipped with a pulse oximeter probe, an electrocardiogram (ECG) gating system, and stress transducer systems worn as a belt around the abdomen to track abdominal distention during respiration.

The most precise synchronization with the cardiac cycle is obtained with R wave detection from an ECG signal. It requires the placement of three or four MR-compatible electrodes on the subject's chest and the connection to an amplifier system. ECG readings from within the MR scanner are often suboptimal for proper diagnostic ECG interpretation because of magnetohydrodynamic effects, which most notably manifest themselves as enlarged T waves. These enlarged T waves can cause problems in gated acquisitions when they are mistaken as the trigger point from the R wave. Vector gating systems that process multiple leads simultaneously, as well as careful electrode placement, can minimize erroneous ECG gating results. Another source for suboptimal gating results can be unwanted signal perturbations into the ECG leads from gradient switching and RF transmission. Heavy shielding or shortening of the ECG cables can minimize these effects. Use of fiberoptic ECG cables for extended connections can also reduce these concerns. An alternative to ECG gating is to use optically based arterial blood oxygen saturation monitors (SaO_2) in the form of finger probes or reflectance probes for cardiac imaging synchronization. The setup for these measurements is simple but the signal has a less distinct peak within the cardiac cycle for gating, making it less desirable for acquisitions that need precise synchronization.

Stress transducer systems provide a similarly simple approach for the tracking of the respiratory cycle. However, they can lack precision because they track the abdominal circumference instead of the targeted image area, can undergo baseline drifts, and can pose difficulties in shallow breathers. A more precise but also more complex approach is the use of navigator echoes that track the position of the lung-liver interface (i.e., hemidiaphragm) and determine the respiratory cycle of the patient, typically during tidal respiration.

Power Injector

For CE-MRA, a Gd-based contrast agent is injected intravenously, usually into an antecubital vein. The injection of the contrast agent is followed by the injection of sterile saline to flush the contrast material out of the delivery system and ensure that the contrast bolus is sufficiently central within the body. Although manual injections are possible, the use of a computer-controlled, MR-compatible power injector is usually preferred. The power injector is more precise in delivering reproducible injection rates and its use omits the need for an operator in the scan room during imaging. Power injectors also provide features to assist in dynamic timed studies and breath-hold maneuvers and allow for multiphase injections. A typical system consists of a delivery component in the scan room and a user console in the operator room (Fig. 81-9). Manual injections have the advantage that the physician is right next to the patient and can better monitor the administration of contrast agent and the status of the patient.

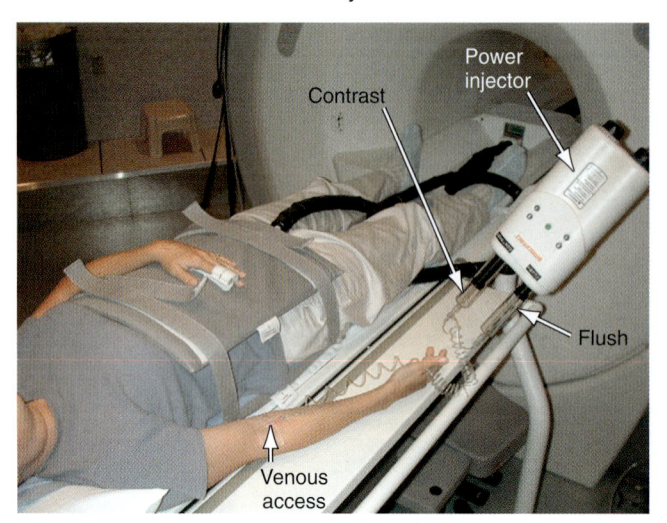

FIGURE 81-9 MR-compatible power injector during patient preparation. A computer-controlled delivery system injects the contrast agent and the saline flush into the antecubital vein through a common line.

TECHNIQUES

Contrast-Enhanced Magnetic Resonance Angiography

CE-MRA[10] has gained widespread clinical acceptance because of its ability to provide diagnostic angiographic data sets very quickly and reliably. In many practices, CE-MRA has replaced conventional x-ray angiography as the preferred method for angiographic depiction of specific anatomic regions such as the aorta, carotid arteries, and peripheral arteries.

The exposure to gadolinium-based contrast material has been associated with the development of nephrogenic systemic fibrosis (NSF).[11] Patients with compromised kidney function are at risk and proper screening (knowledge of the patient's renal function—estimated glomerular filtration rate [GFR] and serum creatinine level) is important to minimize potential risks. A more detailed discussion of NSF can be found in Chapter 18.

CE-MRA typically uses traditional extracellular MR contrast agents based on Gd, which is a paramagnetic metal ion that decreases T1 and T2 relaxation times. Because of the toxicity of Gd in pure form, it is chelated with ligands in formulations used in clinical practice. Basically, all CE-MRA acquisitions take advantage of the T1-shortening effect of the blood signal when it mixes with the Gd chelate contrast agent, resulting in a more rapid regrowth of the longitudinal magnetization. The MR acquisition is typically performed with a T1-weighted three-dimensional spoiled gradient echo pulse sequence with short TRs to maximize the contrast between the blood pool (high signal) and stationary tissue (low signal). The contrast medium bolus is intravenously administered, usually with a power injector at a fixed rate (e.g., 2 mL/sec) for single-station MRA examinations or possibly as a biphasic injection (e.g., 1.5 and 0.5 mL/sec). Both weight-based dosing (e.g., 0.2 mmol/kg Gd chelate contrast agent) and fixed dosing (e.g., 20 mL) of contrast medium can be used for CE-MRA, with the overall intent of reducing the T1 of blood to as low as 50 ms during the first pass. The specifics of the injection protocol should be tailored for the vascular territory, imaging pulse sequence, contrast agent, and specific condition and circulatory time of the patient. A discussion of specific MRA protocol considerations can be found elsewhere in this text in chapters that relate to the vascular territory and/or the underlying suspected pathologic condition.

The MR signal in CE-MRA is dominated more by the T1-shortening effect of the blood signal caused by the presence of the circulating contrast agent and less by signal properties related to flowing blood. CE-MRA, in essence, provides a lumenogram similar to that of conventional x-ray angiography or CTA. T1 weighting is achieved with spoiled gradient echo pulse sequences with small flip angles and short TE and TR values. Short repetition times leave little time for signal regrowth between successive excitations and form the basis for good background suppression. Therefore, only tissues with a short T1 time will generate significant signal contributions (Fig. 81-10). A pitfall of this technique is its application in regions of the body where there is an abundance of fat in the surrounding background tissue. In these cases, the signal of surrounding fat may diminish the apparent contrast-to-noise discrimination of the arterial segments from signal of surrounding fat. Fat suppression or image subtraction of pre-contrast mask data sets can be used to improve the depiction of arteries on CE-MRA in such cases.

Bolus Timing for Contrast-Enhanced Magnetic Resonance Angiography

To optimize image quality, the data acquisition has to be synchronized with the contrast bolus transit through the target vasculature, which is typically arterial. The imaging objective is thus to capture critical image data during the arterial first passage of the bolus prior to contrast bolus progression and signal enhancement of the veins, and prior to significant dilution of the contrast bolus within the arterial tree (Fig. 81-11). Several approaches have been proposed to acquire the data during peak arterial Gd concentration so that a high SNR image without venous contamination is obtained. The simplest way to estimate the arrival time of the bolus is the best guess technique. However, this is also a highly inaccurate technique because the arrival time depends on a variety of parameters, such as the patient's cardiac output, size, and underlying vascular pathology.

Contrast bolus arrival time can be determined for an individual patient by performing a preliminary timing scan with a low dose of contrast agent (e.g., a 1- to 2-mL Gd chelate contrast agent test bolus).[12] With this method, a series of two-dimensional images of the target arterial tree is rapidly acquired (typically about one image/sec) and analyzed for arrival time of the test bolus into the artery under investigation. Based on these images, the arrival time for a full injection is predicted and a suitable delay time for the start of the data acquisition is determined. Disadvantages of the technique include a prolonged examination time for two injections and the use of additional

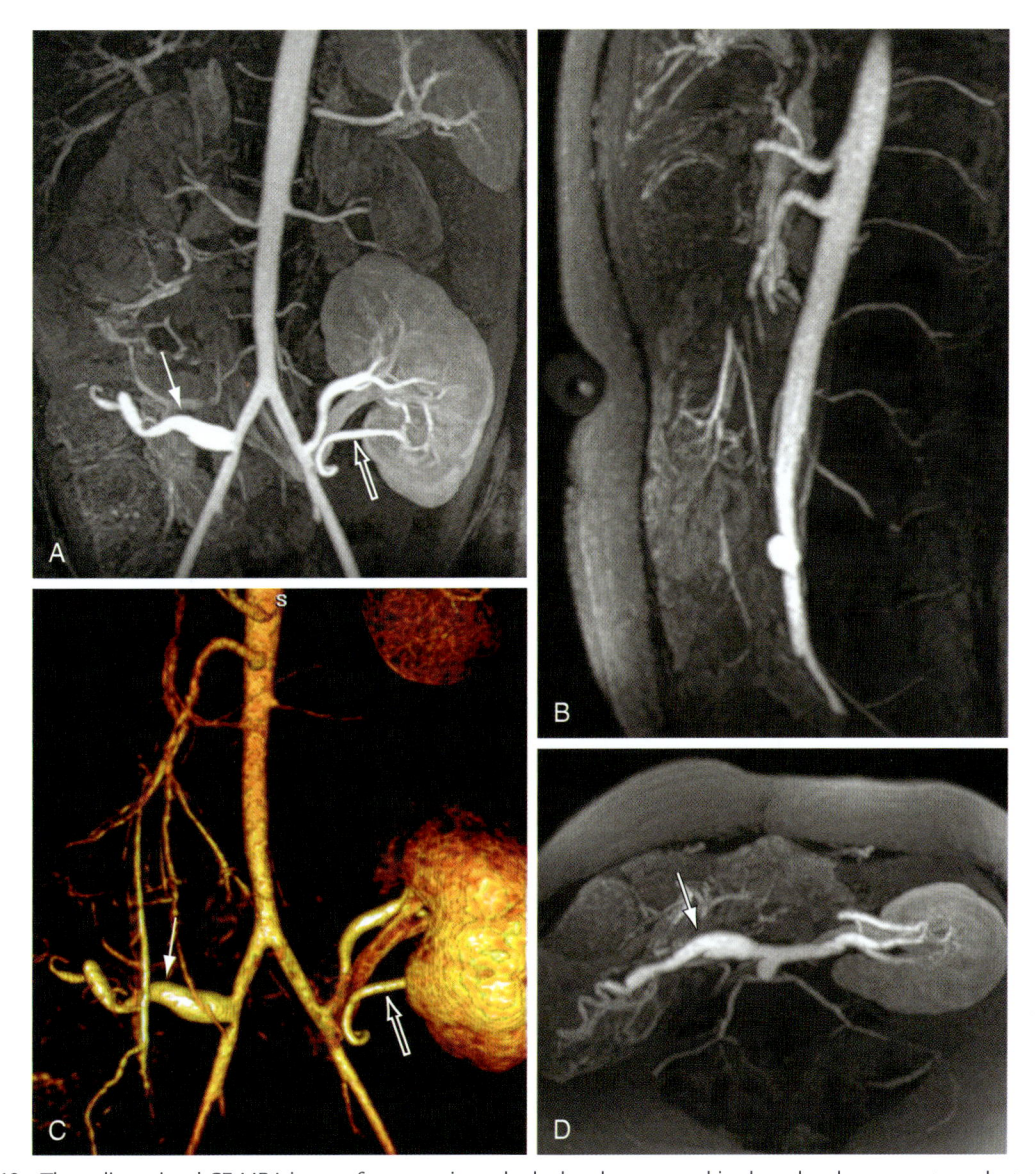

FIGURE 81-10 Three-dimensional CE-MRA images from a patient who had undergone combined renal and pancreas transplantations displayed as coronal (**A**), sagittal (**B**), transversal (**D**) maximum intensity projection (MIP) images, with a volume rendering technique (VRT) (**C**). Note the patent pancreas transplant artery (*arrows*), renal transplant artery, and accessory renal transplant artery (*open arrows*).

contrast agent, which will necessarily increase the signal contributions of adjacent background tissues and the urinary system. Also, the arrival time of the contrast may vary because of differences in breathing or the initiation of a breath-hold.

Another timing method is to integrate an automated detection scheme that can monitor the signal in an arterial voxel[13] or a near–real-time two-dimensional image display (MR fluoroscopy) of the region of interest[14] that can be used to monitor for contrast bolus arrival and initiate the scan on arrival of the contrast bolus. These latter techniques have the advantage of a single injection for the CE-MRA itself and thus improved background signal suppression.

Magnetic Resonance Angiography Scan Time

Another consideration for CE-MRA is overall scan time for image acquisition. As noted, the duration of preferential arterial enhancement by the contrast bolus provides the ideal imaging window for CE-MRA. In some cases, such as with the carotid arteries, this window can be as brief as 5 seconds. Moreover, CE-MRA in the body is often improved if performed during a breath-hold because respiratory motion can result in significant blurring on CE-MRA. These time constraints limit the maximal achievable spatial resolution for a given three-dimensional MRA acquisition. For example, if one wants to acquire a cubic volume with an isotropic spatial resolution of 256 voxels in each dimension (Fig. 81-12A) and a typical TR of 5 ms, then the total scan time would be $T_{scan} = TR \times N_y \times N_{sl} = 328$ sec, where N_y and N_z represent the number of phase encoding steps in y and z. Instead, a reduced data set is sampled to limit the scan duration to 10 to 30 seconds, either with compromised spatial resolution by symmetrical k-space reduction (see Fig. 81-12B), reduced coverage (see Fig. 81-12C), asymmetrical reductions in k-space that maintain the spatial resolution by exploring symmetries in

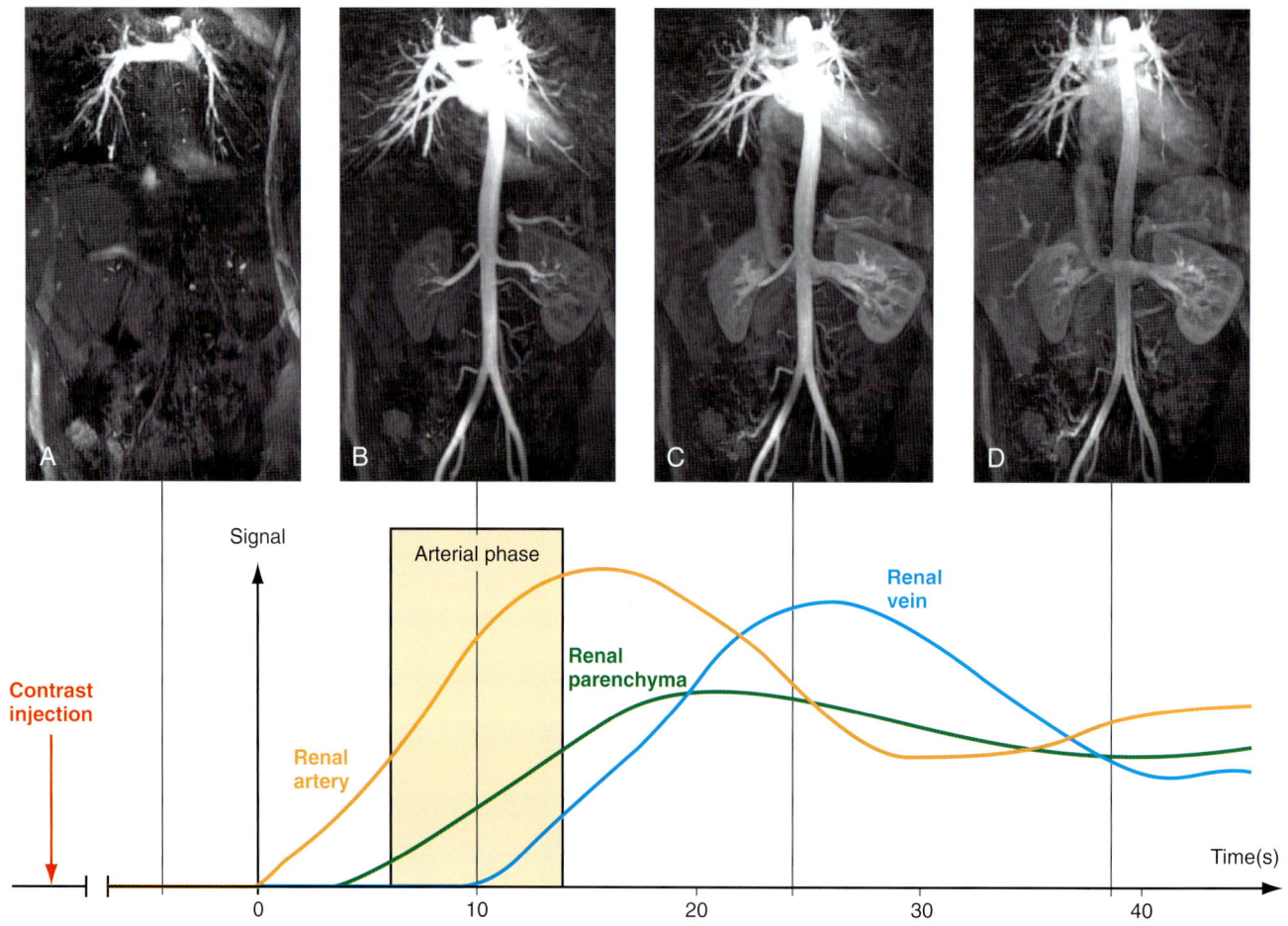

FIGURE 81-11 Bolus passage in CE MRA with an extracellular contrast agent. After venous injection of the contrast agent, the bolus travels through the right ventricle, pulmonary system (**A**), and left ventricle before it enters the systemic vasculature (**B**). It then enters the venous system through the capillary bed (**C**) and transition of the contrast material from the intravascular compartment into interstitial space occurs (**C, D**). Usually, images from the arterial phase (**B**) are desired to visualize arteries with high contrast to the surrounding tissue and veins.

k-space (see Fig. 81-12D),[15] reduction of phase encoding steps with parallel imaging (see Fig. 81-12E),[6-8] or a combination of these techniques in a single- or double-phase encoding direction.

K-Space View Ordering

If it were possible to extend the scan time beyond the period of preferential arterial enhancement (i.e., arterial phase) without signal from the veins, the obtainable spatial resolution could be improved. To this end, sampling schemes have been developed that tailored the temporal order of the phase-encoding steps to optimize image quality. Because the central spatial frequencies (i.e., central k-space data) define the image contrast, it is necessary to acquire these portions of k-space during the peak of the arterial signal intensity, before the bolus arrives in the veins.[16] Higher spatial frequencies that dominate the edge information of an image (i.e., peripheral k-space data) can be acquired even after venous contamination to provide the desired spatial resolution with minimal signal interference from venous structures.

In traditional three-dimensional MR acquisition schemes, sequential phase-encoding schemes are applied (Fig. 81-13A). The first acquired view in such a scheme is the most distant from the origin of k-space. Line after line of k-space is acquired linearly by advancing one phase encode (here, k_z) from its minimum to its maximum, while the other phase encode is kept constant (here, k_y). However, this scheme is not well suited to ensure sampling of the central k-space region during peak arterial enhancement. To this end, centric view-encoding k-space schemes were developed whereby the views near the k-space origin are acquired during the initial period of the scan. Centric view encoding k-space schemes facilitate better synchronization of key central k-space image data acquisition with the arrival of the contrast bolus. One such implementation is linear centric view encoding (see Fig. 81-13B), in which the views are ordered in a double loop; the outer one (here, k_y) is ordered based on its distance from the origin ($+\Delta k_y, -\Delta k_y, +2\Delta k_y, -2\Delta k_y,...$) whereas the inner loop (here, k_z) is still chosen sequentially. A further optimized variation of this scheme is the so-called elliptical centric view ordering.[17] In this approach, the temporal order of the acquisition of k-space lines is determined by their distance in the k_y-k_z plane to the center of k-space, providing a more compact and true centric encoding in both phase-encoding dimensions. The larger the distance between a k-space point and the origin, the later that particular k_x line is sampled (see Fig. 81-13C). When

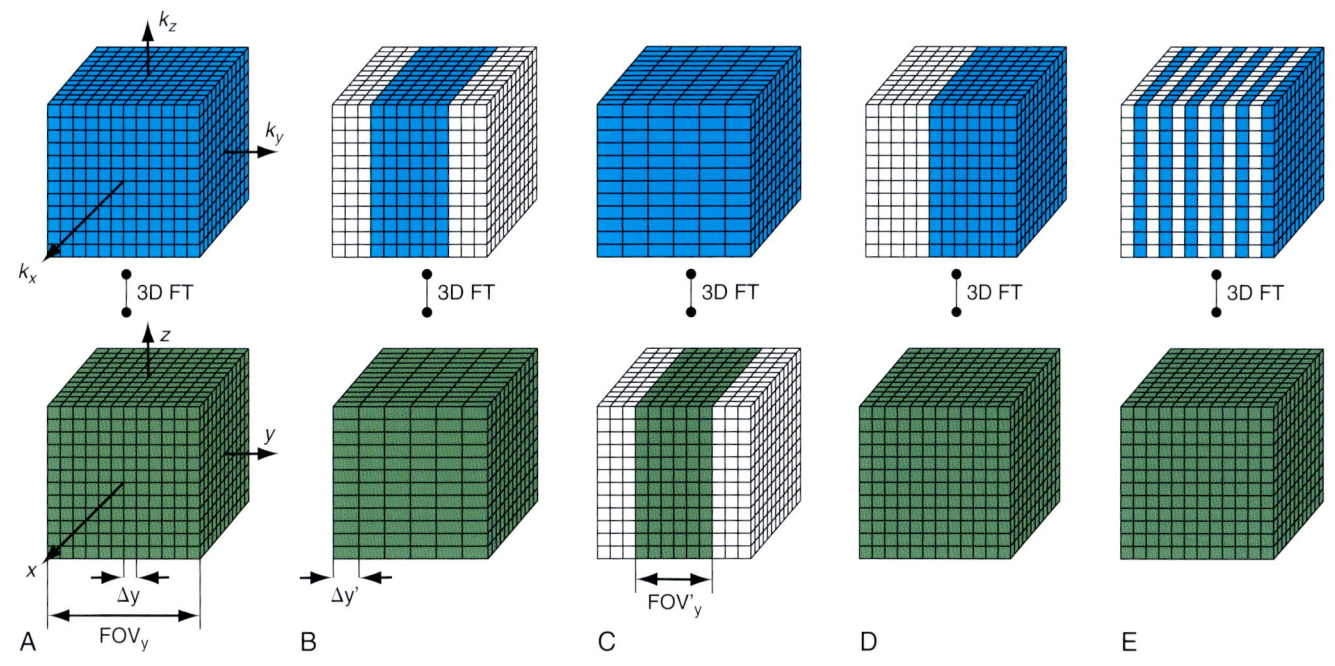

FIGURE 81-12 With three-dimensional MR acquisitions, a volume in k-space is sampled and image volumes are reconstructed via three-dimensional Fourier transforms. High-resolution, large-coverage scans are time-consuming (**A**). Scan time savings can be achieved if a smaller matrix is sampled, such as with compromised spatial resolution in a phase-encoding direction (**B**), reduced coverage in a phase-encoding direction (**C**), partial Fourier acquisitions that assume certain symmetries in k-space (**D**), reduction of phase-encoding steps with parallel imaging (**E**), or a combination of these techniques. Here these schemes are shown for reductions in k_y but, in practice, they can also be used in k_z or in both phase-encoding directions.

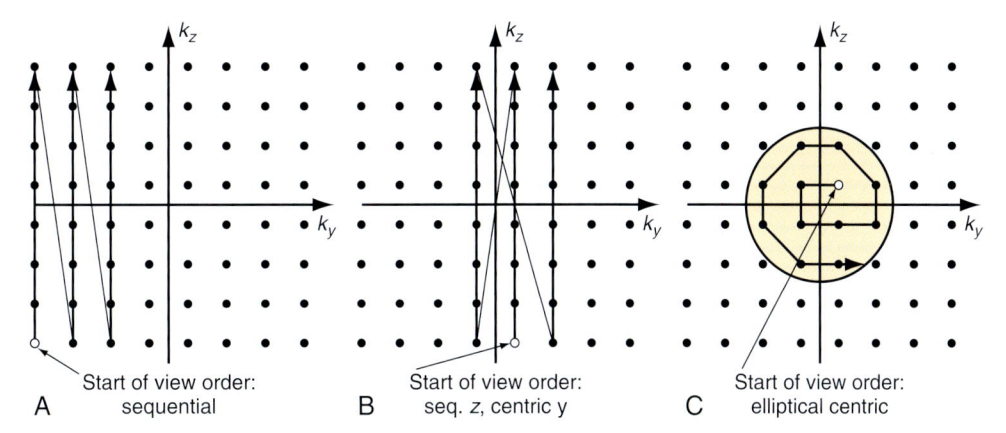

FIGURE 81-13 View-ordering schemes for three-dimensional MRI. Each readout is represented by a dot and the readout direction is perpendicular to the shown k_y-k_z plane. **A,** Sequential phase encoding is well suited to image static objects. In CE-MRA, the limited time available to acquire data from arterial structures is devoted only to the contrast defining central k-space region, either with centric (**B**) or elliptical centric (**C**) view ordering. Only the first encoding steps are displayed in this figure.

properly timed, such ordering allows for the acquisition of the central k-space data during the signal intensity peak in the arteries and the higher spatial frequencies thereafter. It is also more robust to artifacts generated by the modulation of the contrast concentration and suppression of motion artifacts.[18] An example of such an acquisition is shown in Figure 81-10, demonstrating the large coverage, high spatial resolution, and three-dimensional reformatting capabilities of a CE-MRA data set acquired in a single breath-hold. Elliptical centric view ordering is particularly helpful for imaging arterial territories such as the carotid arteries, which can have especially brief periods of preferential arterial enhancement.

Time-Resolved Contrast-Enhanced Magnetic Resonance Angiography

Time-resolved CE-MRA has several advantages over the acquisition of a single time frame. With proper frame rates, arterial-only images are obtained without the need for any synchronization of the acquisition and arrival of the bolus. In addition, this technique provides temporal information related to the bolus progression that may be required to properly discern complex blood flow states, such as late-filling vessels in areas of severe stenoses, slow-filling vascular leaks, or relative filling patterns in complex vascular lesions (e.g., arteriovenous malforma-

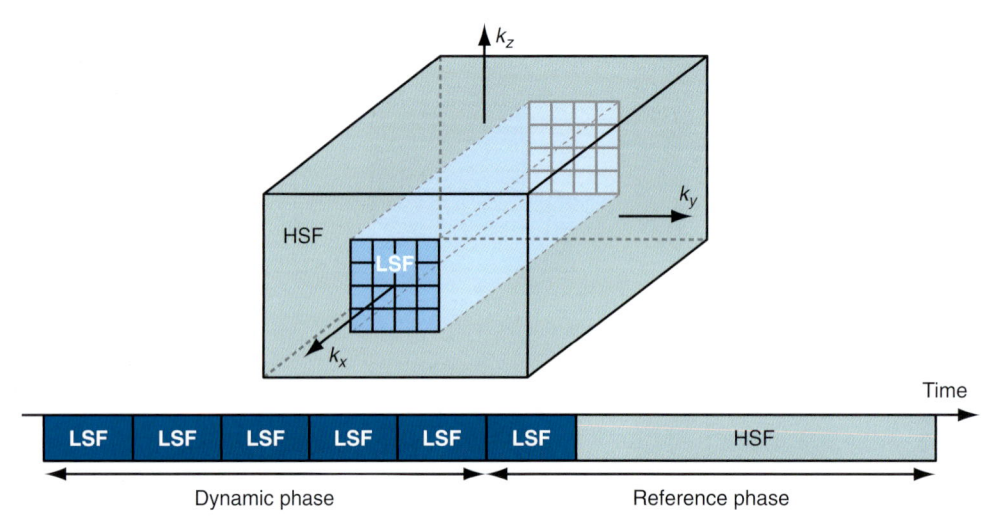

■ **FIGURE 81-14** Dynamic CE-MRA with keyhole imaging. K-space is divided into a central k-space region representing the low spatial frequencies (LSF) and image contrast, and the high spatial frequencies (HSF) representing the image detail. To allow for higher frame rates, only the central region is updated during the dynamic phase, whereas the high spatial frequencies are only acquired once at the end of the scan. Dynamic images are reconstructed by updating the central k-space region.

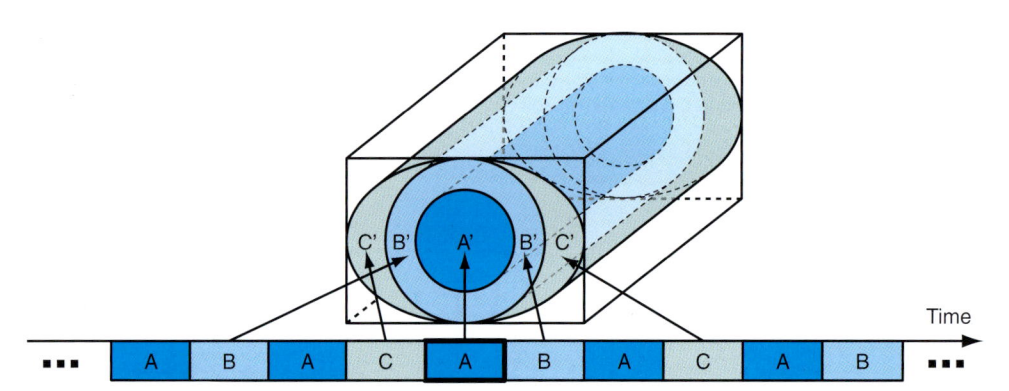

■ **FIGURE 81-15** Scheduling algorithm and data sharing scheme in three-dimensional TRICKS. The k-space regions are scheduled so that the central region, A, is acquired every other time frame, while the outer portions of k-space, B and C, are sampled less frequently. Information from the regions is shared for the reconstruction of image sets. In this example, the central region A′ of the reconstructed time frame is the actually acquired region, A, whereas regions B′ and C′ are linearly interpolated from adjacent regions.

tions). However, decreasing the scan time usually requires undesirable compromises in the spatial resolution. To facilitate dynamic acquisitions with high spatial resolution, data-sharing techniques are now commonly used.

In keyhole imaging, the acquisition process is split into a dynamic phase, in which central k-space data are acquired rapidly but with limited spatial resolution, and a subsequent second phase, whereby the missing high spatial frequency data (i.e., peripheral k-space data) is acquired to provide image detail.[18,19] These two acquisitions are then combined to generate a dynamic series with high spatial and high temporal resolution by updating only the central k-space region (Fig. 81-14). The underlying assumption is that most of the signal changes are reflected in the central k-space region (see Fig. 81-4). The drawback of the approach is the missing dynamic information about high spatial frequencies. Dynamic information is captured only with low spatial resolution whereas the high spatial frequency data, which define finer structures such as smaller vessels, are acquired only once and shared across the acquisition. If the relevant information under investigation contains changes in the outer portions of k-space, then keyhole imaging can produce images with an erroneous time course.[20]

Another commercially available approach, three-dimensional TRICKS, also shares data among time frames but does not update the central region alone. In three-dimensional TRICKS (three-dimensional *t*ime-*r*esolved *i*maging of *c*ontrast *k*inetic*s*) imaging,[21] k-space is divided into subvolumes based on their distance to the center of k-space. Figure 81-15 shows an implementation of TRICKS with an elliptical centric view ordering scheme whereby the phase- and slice-encode ordering is based on their distance in the k_y-k_z plane from the center of k-space. In this figure, the subvolumes consist of a cylinder for the region containing lower spatial frequencies (A) and cylindrical shells of equal volume for the regions representing higher spatial frequencies (B and C). In practice, most examinations are acquired with a decreased spatial resolution in the slice-encoding direction, z, for a decreased imaging time and higher SNR. In this case, the higher spatial frequency regions become incomplete cylindrical shells. The central region, A, contains the low spatial frequency information and is sampled every second time

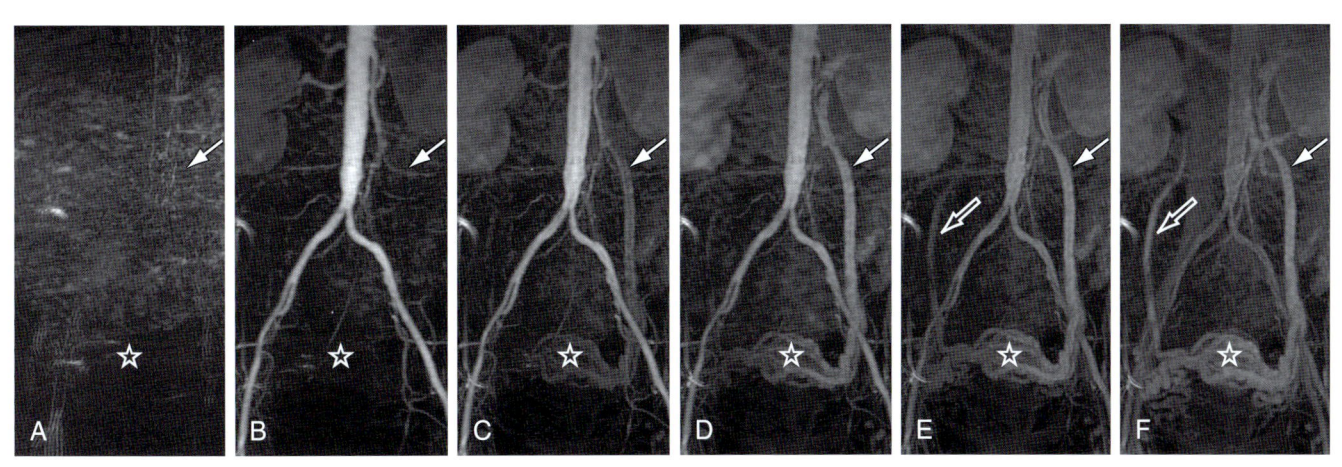

FIGURE 81-16 Abdominal-pelvic three-dimensional CE-MRA with TRICKS. The time shows MIP images prior to the arrival of the bolus (**A**), early arterial enhancement (**B**), an enlarged left gonadal vein (**C-F**, *solid arrows*), and a plexus of parauterine varices (**C-F**, *asterisks*), consistent with pelvic congestion syndrome. The MIP images of several time frames reveal a clear separation of the arterial and venous phase and also show that the right gonadal vein (**E**, **F**, *arrows*) is filled significantly later.

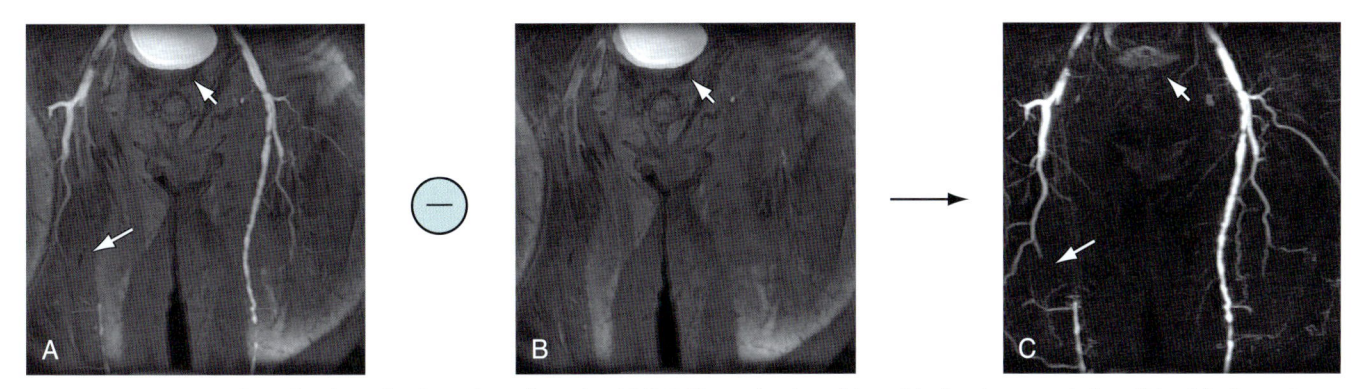

FIGURE 81-17 Mask mode subtraction for a three-dimensional MR DSA examination of the pelvis showing an occlusion of the right femoral artery (*long arrows*). **A**, MIP image of peak arterial enhancement. **B**, MIP image from a precontrast mask. **C**, Obtained by subtracting **B** from **A** on a slice-by-slice basis. As a result, stationary background noise from tissue and accumulation of contrast agent from an earlier injection, such as a signal in the urinary bladder (*short arrows*), is removed. Delineation of the vessels from the background is significantly improved in the subtracted image. (*Courtesy of Dr. Frank R. Korosec, University of Wisconsin-Madison, Madison, Wis.*)

frame, whereas regions B and C are sampled every fourth time frame only. For each newly sampled k-space subvolume, a complete k-space volume is assembled by temporal interpolation of the adjacent subvolumes acquired before, during, and after the current time frame.

This approach continuously acquires data during the passage of the contrast agent and is relatively insensitive to variation in timing and shape of the contrast bolus. An example for an examination of the abdominal and pelvic vasculature is shown in Figure 81-16. The maximum intensity projection (MIP) images represent reformats of three-dimensional volumes reconstructed for each time frame.

Mask Mode Subtraction

CE-MRA examinations usually include the acquisition of a precontrast mask so that techniques similar to those of digital subtraction angiography can be incorporated into the image display. Subtraction of a precontrast mask increases the contrast in the image by suppressing stationary background signals. The images must be subtracted prior to the calculation of the MIP images to reflect the properties in the three-dimensional data set. As a result, smaller vessel details can be identified.

Figure 81-17 shows an example of mask mode subtraction for an examination of the pelvis. Mask mode subtraction is extremely beneficial when using multiple injections of a Gd chelate contrast agent because the accumulated effects of prior contrast administration can be minimized by the use of imaging subtraction. With this method, time-varying background signals caused by patient motion or motion of the gastrointestinal tract are not affected. Although the contrast in the images is improved by mask mode subtraction, the actual SNR is decreased by $\sqrt{2}$, because the noise of the two images is additive.

Time-of-Flight Magnetic Resonance Angiography

Image contrast in TOF MRA relies on the inflow of blood into the imaging slice so that the signal from moving blood is brighter than that from stationary tissue. Because TOF MRA is inflow dependent, it is best suited for vascular territories that allow for slice orientations with pronounced inflow effects, such as the lower extremities or carotid arteries, which have straight vessel paths and little in-plane flow. As a non–CE-MRA technique, TOF MRA provides an alternative to CE-MRA in patients with

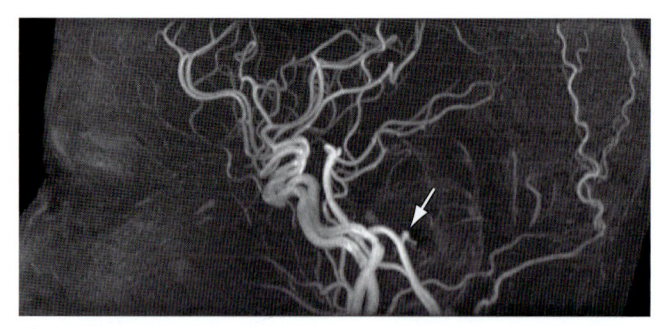

FIGURE 81-18 MIP image of an intracranial TOF examination acquired at 3 T with submillimeter isotropic resolution reveals a 1-mm posterior inferior cerebellar artery (PICA) aneurysm (*arrow*) as an incidental finding in a 38-year-old female volunteer.

contraindications to Gd chelate contrast agents. It is routinely used for cranial MRA, providing spatial resolution and image quality superior to CE-MRA because the scan time is not limited to an arterial-venous window (Fig. 81-18). However, in vessels with more tortuous pathways with in-plane components and slow flow, TOF MRA acquisitions can suffer from disease-mimicking signal voids.

Two-Dimensional Time-of-Flight

The TOF acquisition strategy aims to saturate partially the longitudinal magnetization of nonmoving spins so that unaffected moving spins appear bright in comparison.[22] Similar to CE-MRA, a spoiled gradient echo sequence is used to achieve this goal. With this acquisition, the repeated RF pulses used for excitation in the beginning of each TR diminish the available longitudinal magnetization until an equilibrium between signal regrowth from relaxation and signal decrease from the RF excitation is reached (Fig. 81-19). The actual signal depends on the TR, the T1 of the tissue, and the flip angle. In two-dimensional TOF imaging, the imaging slice is oriented perpendicular to the flow direction. Stationary tissue experiences all RF pulses and will only have small signal contributions in the resulting image. However, only a few RF excitations will affect flowing blood as it enters the imaging slice, resulting in a relatively high signal contribution in the angiogram. The longer the blood stays in the imaging slice, the more the signal differences diminish. Consequently, the vessel to background contrast decreases as the slice thickness increases or the velocity of blood flow decreases. A longer TR will increase the vascular signal but will also increase the signal from background tissues and lengthen the scan time. Therefore, intermediate TR times are usually chosen. An increased flip angle will decrease the signal contribution from stationary tissues, but signal from blood that undergoes multiple RF excitations will also decrease (see Fig. 81-19). Therefore, intermediate flip angles are used for most clinical applications.

Without any further modifications, arterial and venous blood flow will cause a bright signal in TOF angiograms. In most applications, it is desirable to image selectively the arteries or veins only. This can be easily achieved with the use of saturation bands in vascular regions with arterial and venous flow in opposing directions.[23] With this approach, a saturation pulse is applied parallel to the imaging slice to eliminate unwanted inflow signal from a particular direction. Figure 81-20 demonstrates an example of arterial and venous suppression in an axial slice through the neck with the use of superior and inferior saturation slabs.

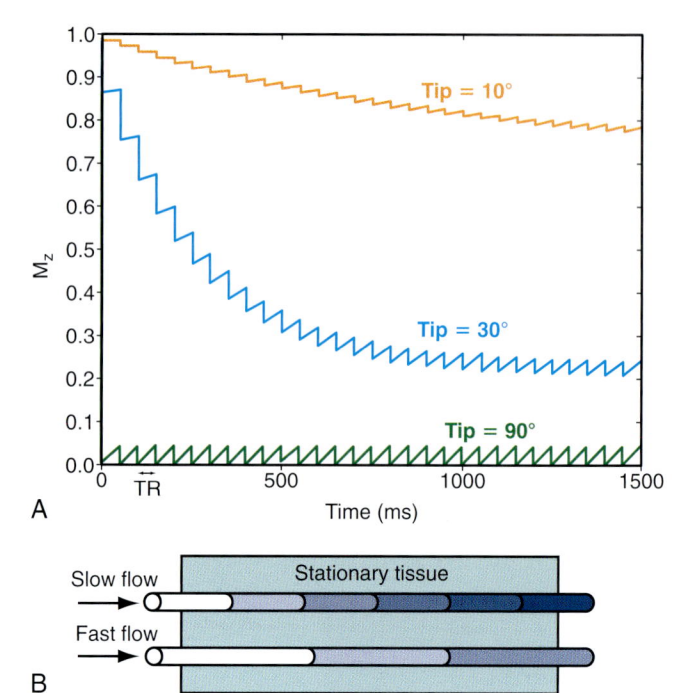

FIGURE 81-19 Contrast mechanism in TOF MRA. **A,** Repeated RF excitations decrease the longitudinal magnetization (M_z) until the regrowth during each TR equals the decrease from the excitation pulse. The signal behavior depends on the T1 (here, 1200 ms), flip angle (varied from 10 to 30 degrees and 90 degrees), and TR time (here, 50 ms). **B,** Higher contrast for fast-flowing blood that experiences fewer RF excitations in the imaging slice or volume as compared with slower flowing blood that can suffer from partial saturation effects.

Volume data can be achieved with two-dimensional TOF MRA whereby a series of contiguous two-dimensional slices are acquired sequentially over the vascular territory of interest. In most cases, two-dimensional TOF MRA is accompanied by a saturation band (e.g., inferior saturation band for lower extremity arterial imaging) that is applied sequentially with each two-dimensional slice, a feature also known as a walking saturation band. This approach is commonly used in TOF examination of the lower extremities in which coverage of the vessels from the pelvis to the feet is achieved with sets of axial slices that are acquired over multiple stations (Fig. 81-21). TOF examinations in the abdomen, pelvis, and lower extremities typically must be cardiac gated because of the flow pulsatility that can result in significant fluctuations in arterial signal and artifacts. The acquisition of central k-space data during systole optimizes arterial inflow signal on TOF MRA.

Disadvantages of two-dimensional TOF acquisitions include the relatively long acquisition times, which reduce patient comfort and increase the likelihood for bulk patient motion artifacts. Because temporary motion might affect only a single slice, this could result in a focal decreased signal and mimic the appearance of vascular disease, such as stenosis. Moreover, the relatively thick

CHAPTER 81 ● *Magnetic Resonance Angiography: Physics and Instrumentation* **1093**

■ **FIGURE 81-20** Inflow effect and the use of saturation slabs in TOF MRA to tailor the image characteristics to the desired anatomic information. **A,** With no saturation slab, venous and arterial inflow, such as from the carotid artery (*open arrow*) and jugular vein (*solid arrow*) contribute to the signal in the axial slice through the neck. **B,** When placing a saturation slab superior to the imaging slice, the magnetization of the inflowing venous blood will be saturated and the arterial signal will dominate the image. **C,** A saturation slab placed inferior to the imaging slide causes the opposite effect, with suppression of the arterial signal and a bright venous signal.

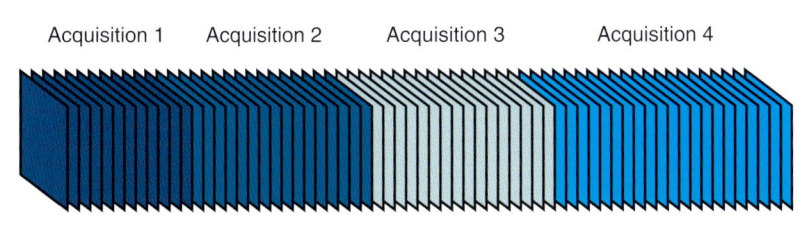

■ **FIGURE 81-21** Sequential two-dimensional TOF examination of the lower extremities. The scan is completed in four separate acquisitions because of the limited field of view for an MR image free of geometric distortions. Multiple axial slices are acquired at each of the four stations and displayed as a coronal MIP image.

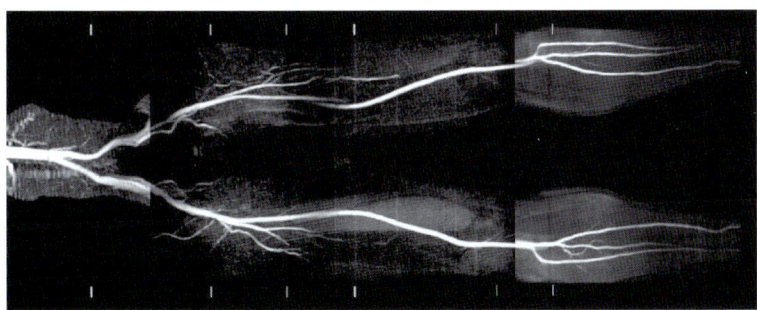

slices and longer TE associated with two-dimensional TOF imaging can further contribute to signal loss in areas of complex flow, such as downstream of a stenosis, or areas of irregular luminal geometry, such as with atherosclerotic plaque. All these lead to a tendency to underestimate luminal diameter and to possible overestimation of a stenosis to the point of even simulating an arterial occlusion. However, two-dimensional TOF may serve as a good screening method for the presence of vascular disease in vascular territories such as the carotid arteries.

Three-Dimensional Time-of-Flight

In three-dimensional TOF MRA,[24] the SNR is improved compared with sequential two-dimensional TOF because all the magnetization in the excited volume contributes to the signal of each sampled data point. In addition, the slice encoding for thin slices less than 1 mm thick, with reasonable echo times for artifact suppression, poses major challenges to two-dimensional TOF but can easily be achieved with three-dimensional TOF. The phase-encoding steps and not the slice-encoding gradient determine the slice thickness in three-dimensional TOF. The increased spatial resolution reduces intravoxel dephasing and permits the visualization of smaller vessels that otherwise might be obscured by partial voluming effects.

The drawback of three-dimensional TOF is the reduction in the inflow effect because the moving blood remains longer in the imaging volume and experiences more RF excitations. The flip angle is reduced (<30 degrees) to preserve signal contributions from slower moving blood. However, signal from stationary tissue is also increased and leads to diminished vessel contrast.

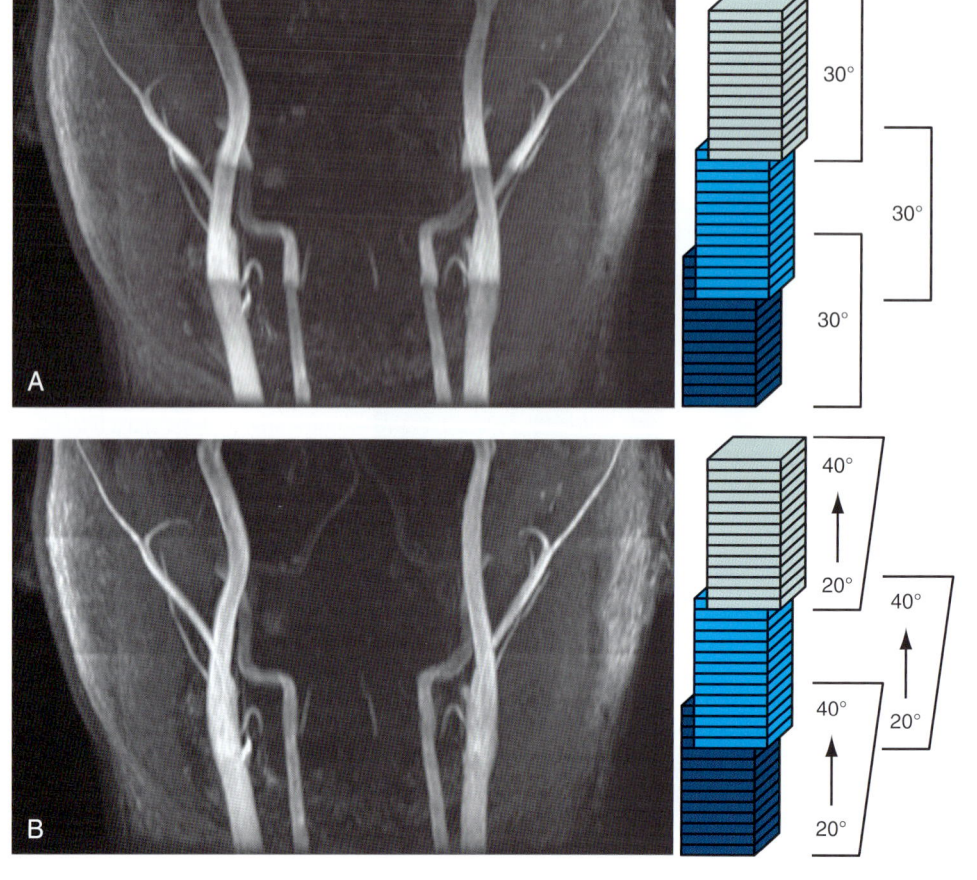

FIGURE 81-22 Volumetric TOF acquisition with MOTSA (multiple overlapping thin slab angiography).[24] This neck examination was acquired with three partially overlapping thin slabs to provide large coverage with thin slices, high SNR, and good vessel contrast. **A,** When a constant flip angle of 30 degrees is used, the vessel signal decreases as the arterial blood travels supine and experiences additional RF pulses (*arrows*). **B,** The homogeneity of the vessel signal can be further improved with ramped flip angles to counteract this effect. *(Courtesy of Dr. Frank R. Korosec, University of Wisconsin-Madison, Madison, Wis.)*

Sequential Three-Dimensional Time-of-Flight

The signal loss of flowing blood from saturation in a thick three-dimensional volume can be reduced by exciting smaller volumes. The use of MOTSA (multiple overlapping thin slab angiography)[25] provides large coverage with thin slabs (i.e., thin volumes), thereby combining benefits from two-dimensional (reduced blood saturation) and three-dimensional TOF (small voxels, high SNR, and short TE). Overlapping of the thin slabs reduces artifacts from slab profiles and partial saturation, making this approach the method of choice for cranial and carotid MRA, in which high spatial resolution is essential (Fig. 81-22A; see Figs. 81-7 and 81-18). Such volumetric acquisitions benefit from ramped flip angles designed to counteract the signal loss from partial saturation effects when blood moves through the imaging volume. A lower flip angle, in which the arterial blood enters the imaging volume, and a higher flip angle, in which the arterial blood leaves the imaging slice, provide a homogeneous vessel signal across the imaging volume (see Fig. 81-22B). The linearly varying flip angle reduces saturation effects for the blood entering the volume and increases the signal for the blood leaving the volume. The amplified saturation of blood exiting the volume is inconsequential because it will not be used for signal generation once it has left the imaging volume.

Phase Contrast Magnetic Resonance Angiography

Phase contrast MRA (PC MRA) provides quantitative velocity and flow measurements in vascular territories throughout the body and, like TOF, can be acquired in two-dimensional or three-dimensional modes. Two-dimensional PC MRA is commonly used in an ECG-gated cine mode for the dynamic assessment of cardiac valve function, pulmonary and systemic flow, and unusual shunt determinations in patients with congenital heart disease. In addition, MR angiograms can be derived from the acquired data, making this approach another alternative to CE-MRA in patients who cannot be given Gd chelate contrast agents. PC MRA works well for two-dimensional projections through thick sections and, compared with TOF methods, smaller vessels with low blood velocities can be identified. PC MRA is also particularly good when performed following the administration of Gd chelate contrast agents and is a good alternative when the initial CE-MRA scan is nondiagnostic.[26]

Whereas the imaging contrast between blood and surrounding tissues in all other MRA techniques is based on the magnitude of the magnetization, PC MRA uses bipolar gradients for phase manipulation of the magnetization.[27] Figure 81-23 demonstrates how the gradient pair causes the phase of stationary spins to accumulate to zero,

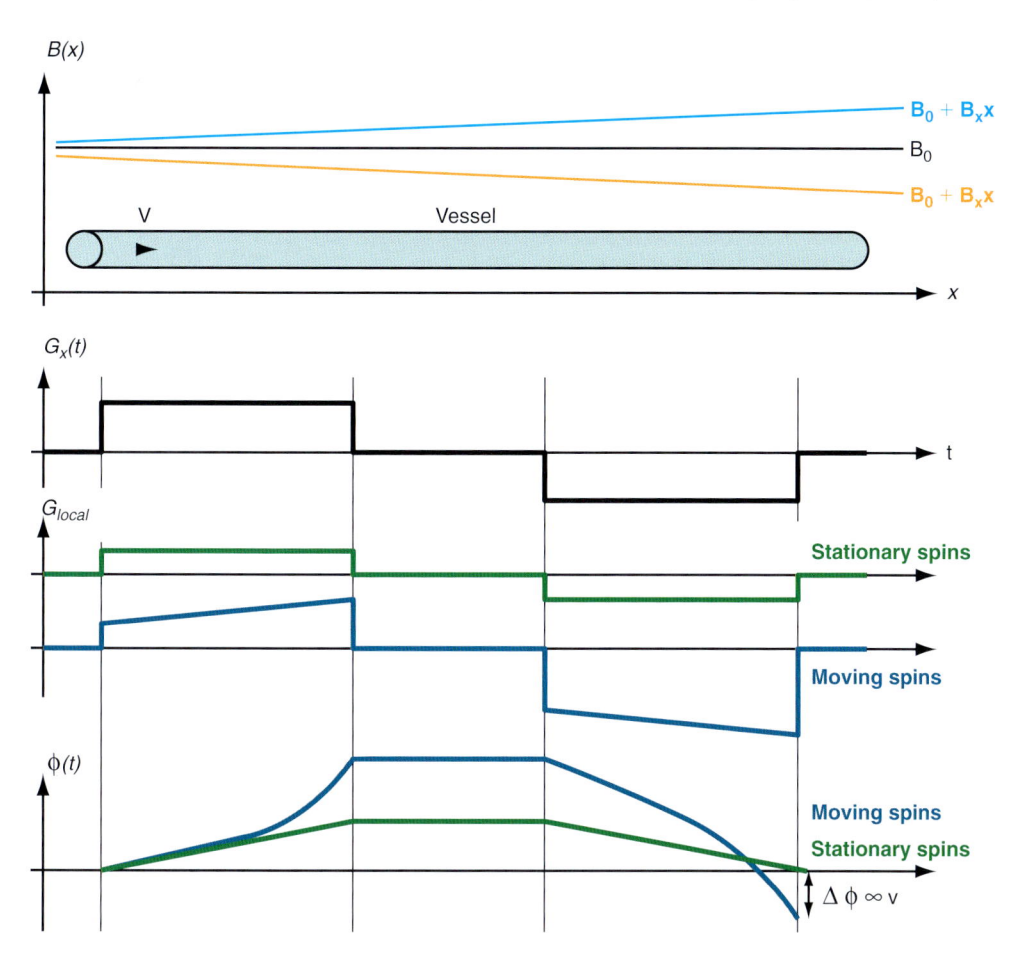

FIGURE 81-23 Velocity encoding in PC MRI. A field gradient, G_x, is applied along a direction, here shown for the x-axis. The gradient is switched on and off in the shape of a bipolar gradient with a positive and negative lobe, $G_x(t)$. Stationary tissue experiences a positive and negative magnetic field superimposed to the stationary field B_0, resulting in a zero phase from a faster and slower precession at the end of the bipolar gradient. Blood that moves along the direction of the gradient experiences a varying field while the bipolar gradient is switched on. The resulting net phase, $\Delta\varphi$, is proportional to the velocity, v.

whereas spins that move along the axis of the gradient accumulate a net phase proportional to their velocity. Because MR images contain unpredictable phase contributions from magnetic susceptibilities, eddy currents, measurement imperfections, and other sources, a reference image without velocity encoding has to be acquired. On subtraction of the reference phase from the velocity-encoded image, these local phase offsets are removed. Therefore, one-directional velocity encoding requires the acquisition of two images, thereby doubling the scan time. In the phase difference image, the signal in each voxel is linearly proportional to its velocity. Blood moving along one direction of the gradient axis is assigned a bright (white) signal and blood moving along the opposite direction is assigned a dark (black) signal. PC acquisitions, therefore, can provide directional information of blood flow. A magnitude image is also reconstructed as the average of the two acquisitions to provide anatomic information. The velocity-encoding direction can be perpendicular to the imaging plane (through-plane flow) or in plane in the phase or frequency direction. For pulsatile flow measurements, cine PC imaging with ECG gating[28] is performed to capture the flow dynamics for multiple time points within the cardiac cycle. Because of the slower acquisition speed of MRI, data sampling for cine series stretches over multiple heartbeats. Reductions in scan time because of high-performing gradients (shorter TR) and parallel imaging can improve the temporal and spatial resolution achievable for cine PC imaging within a patient-friendly breath-hold duration. Figure 81-24 shows a magnitude image and several phase difference images at peak systolic flow for an oblique imaging plane in a chest that was oriented perpendicularly to the path of the ascending aorta with through-plane velocity encoding.

The application of bipolar gradients along a second and third gradient axis extends the technique to two-dimensional and three-dimensional flow encoding. The same reference image can be used for calculating the directional phase differences, yet the total scan time is prolonged to three or four acquisitions, respectively. Figure 81-25 shows an example of three-directional velocity encoding for a slice covering the aortic arch. The different in-plane and through-plane components of the velocity vector can be appreciated as three gray-scale images. The concept can be further extended to volumetric cine imaging,[29] thereby providing comprehensive information on the anatomy and velocity fields over a vascular territory.

One important parameter in PC MR is the proper choice of the velocity-encoding setting. The velocity of a voxel is determined by its phase accumulation, whereas the bipolar gradient waveform is played out. Because the phase is a cyclic entity, there is a maximum and a minimum phase indistinguishable from a wrapped phase. For example, a precession of +190 and −270 degrees results in the same final position on the unit circle. Because the precession path to the final position is unknown in PC

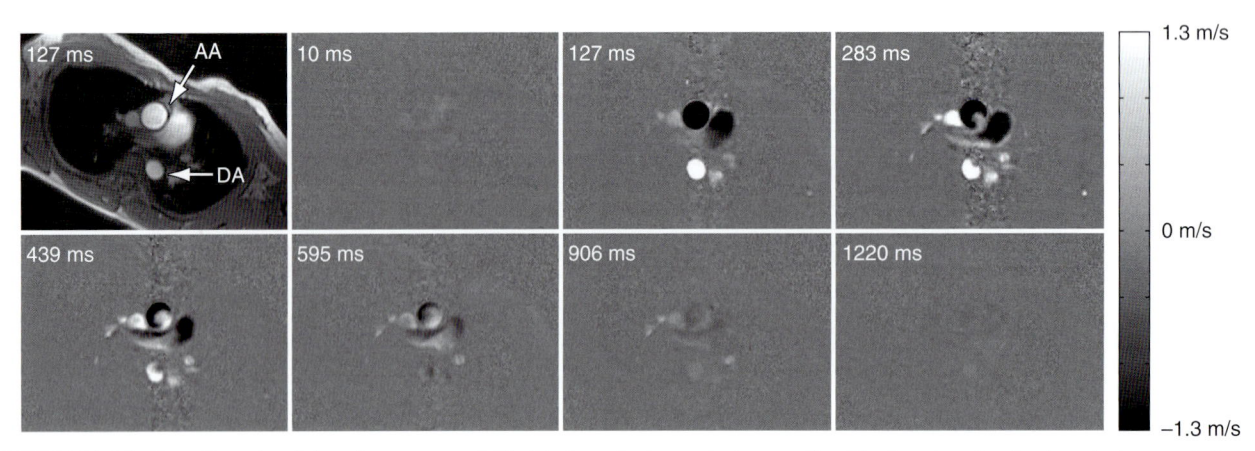

■ **FIGURE 81-24** Two-dimensional cine phase contrast MR with through-plane velocity encoding. The imaging slice for the velocity-encoded acquisition was placed perpendicular to the orientation of the ascending aorta (AA). The magnitude image and the selected seven cine frames from the velocity-encoded images show the ascending and descending aorta (DA). The gray-scale intensity is proportional to the velocity in each voxel, with dark values indicating flow in the inferior to superior direction and bright voxels indicating flow in the opposite direction.

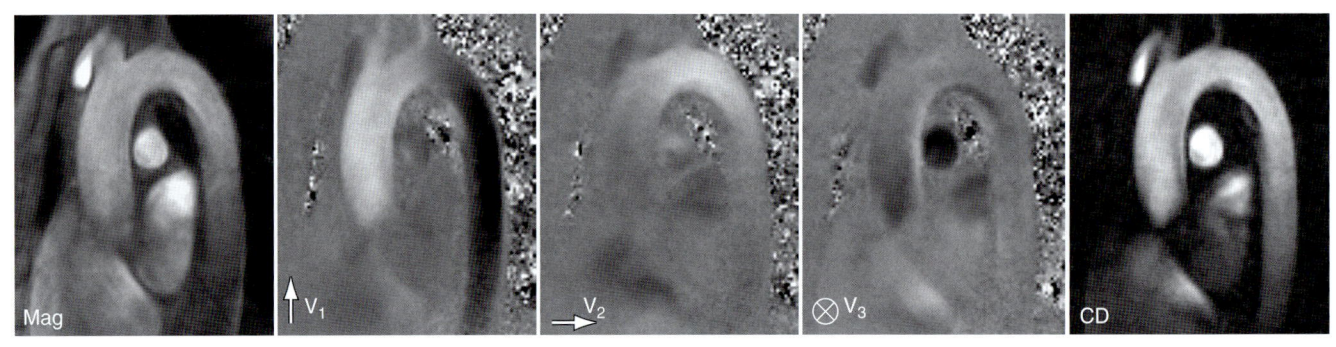

■ **FIGURE 81-25** PC MRA with three-directional flow encoding. The imaging slice was oriented along the orientation of the aortic arch and shows a single time frame of a three-directional cine acquisition. CD, complex difference image as an angiogram that shows vessel anatomy only based on the three velocity components, but without quantitative information; Mag, magnitude image; v_1, velocity component in the inferior to superior in-plane direction; v_2, velocity component in the anterior to posterior in-plane direction; v_3, velocity component in the left to right direction (through-plane).

MR, only phase precessions less than +180 or −80 degrees can be uniquely identified with the proper velocity. The velocity corresponding to a 180-degree phase is referred to as the velocity-encoding parameter (Venc) of the acquisition and must be carefully adjusted to the imaging task. If chosen too low, velocity aliasing from phase wrap will occur, which can result in a heterogeneous signal within the vessel (and inaccurate flow measurements if flow quantification is performed). If chosen too high, the phase difference data will have a small signal range and a decreased velocity-to-noise-ratio (VNR), secondary to a higher noise floor. Venc is determined by the shape of the bipolar gradient waveform.

Figure 81-26 shows an example of an axial imaging slice in the neck with optimized Venc settings for arterial flow analysis (50 cm/sec) and cerebrospinal fluid (CSF) flow analysis (5 cm/sec) and an intermittent Venc of 30 cm/sec. In practice, the bipolar gradient waveform is automatically calculated from a user input on the desired Venc based on reference velocities for normal vessels or expected velocity ranges. Ideally, the Venc is set slightly above the peak velocity within the vessel of interest. However, peak velocity, especially in diseased vessels, may be difficult to predict, and the PC acquisition may need to be repeated at a more appropriate Venc setting if the initial Venc setting is suboptimal.

Several factors lead to an increased susceptibility of PC MR to intravoxel dephasing:

1. The presence of velocity-encoding gradients increases the minimum TE, which in turn allows more intravoxel dephasing from all sources, including magnetic susceptibility.
2. Voxels that contain heterogeneous velocity components will have a decreased net phase. This is a common occurrence in areas of disturbed flow. Again, the longer the TE, the more pronounced the effects become. The artifacts can be reduced by minimizing the TE (e.g., by using fractional echo acquisitions and high-performance gradients) and by decreasing the voxel size.
3. The imaging gradients themselves cause intravoxel dephasing while spins move during their application. Gradient moment nulling[30] is used to reduce these effects but also further lengthens the TE.

Postprocessing

In addition to the magnitude and phase image, complex difference (CD) images can be derived from PC acquisitions. The complex difference image is obtained as the length of the vector obtained by complex subtraction of the velocity-encoded data from the reference data, thereby

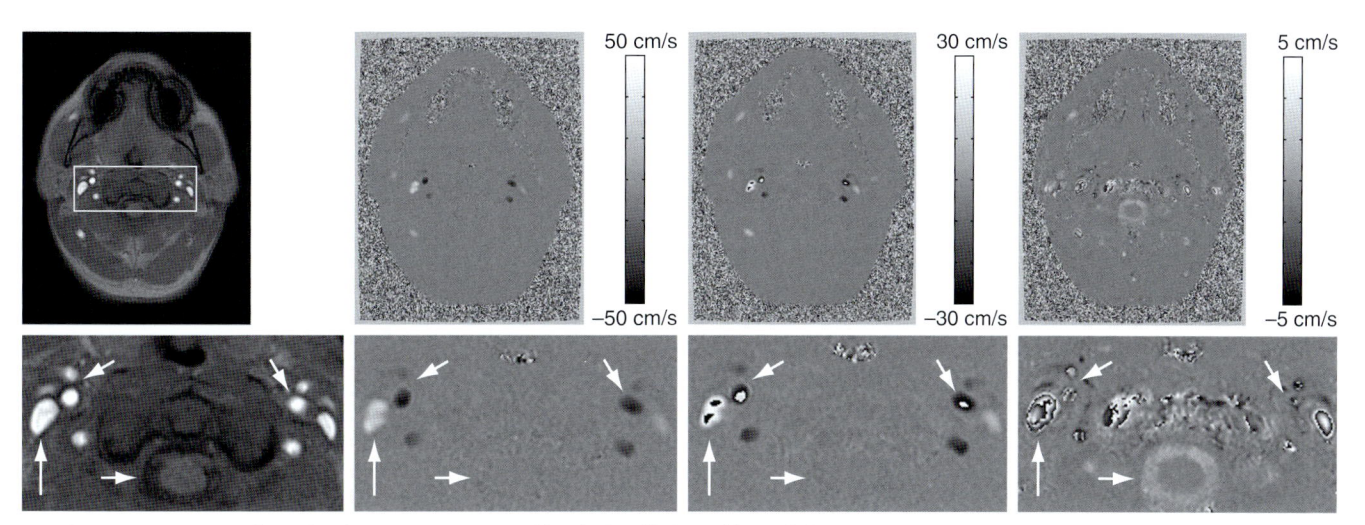

FIGURE 81-26 Two-dimensional PC measurements with velocity aliasing. This axial cine PC series was acquired at the neck of a healthy volunteer with Venc settings of ±50, ±30, and ±5 cm/s. With a Venc of ±50 cm/s, the flow through the carotid artery (*small arrows*) and the jugular vein (*long arrows*) remains artifact free because all velocities in the imaging slice are within the encoded velocity range. If the Venc is reduced to 30 cm/s, then velocity aliasing occurs in the carotid arteries and the right jugular vein during peak systolic flow. If the Venc is reduced further, severe aliasing occurs in almost all vessels, but the velocities of the slow-flowing CSF (*bold arrows*) can be quantified while it is hidden in the noise level with the higher Venc acquisitions.

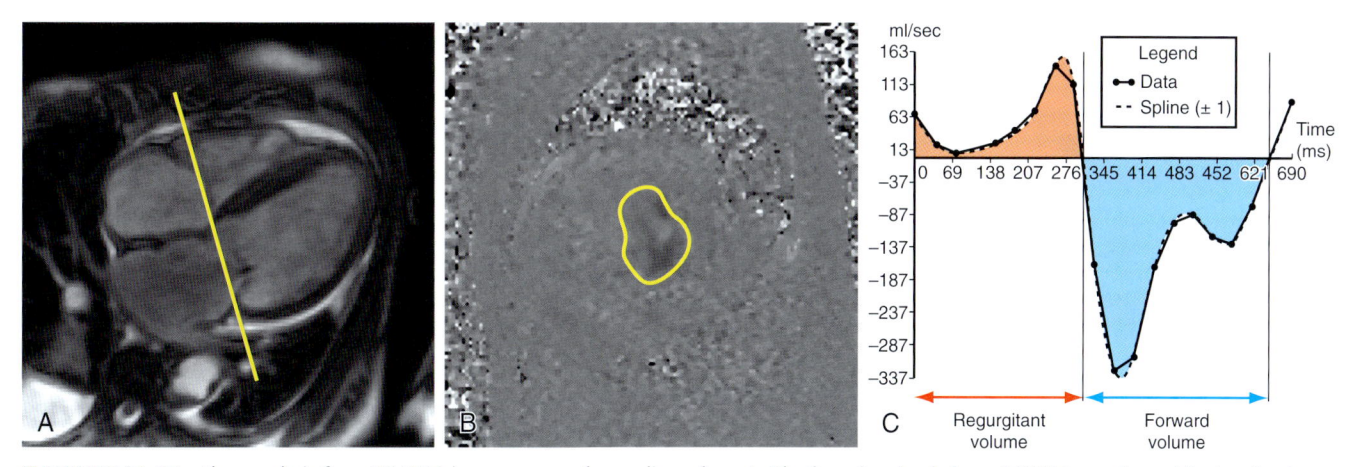

FIGURE 81-27 Flow analysis from PC MRA images across the cardiac valves. **A,** The four-chamber balanced SSFP image is used for localization of the valve plane (*yellow line*). **B,** The regurgitant jet is used to prescribe the phase contrast acquisition perpendicular to the jet. A manually drawn region of interest delineates the area from which the desired flow information is obtained. **C,** The areas over and under the flow curve as a function of time determine the regurgitant volume (*red area*) and forward volume (*blue area*). *(Courtesy of Dr. C. Francois, University of Wisconsin-Madison, Madison, Wis.)*

incorporating phase and magnitude into the calculation. As opposed to phase difference images, complex difference images are non-negative and do not suffer from discontinuities from velocity aliasing. As shown in Figure 81-25, they are well suited for the display of vessel paths with good background suppression, but do not provide quantitative or directional flow information.

Flow quantification is performed with software packages that allow for the interactive definition of regions of interests (ROIs). In a two-dimensional image with through-plane velocity encoding, the volume flow rate through a voxel is calculated as

$$Q_{voxel} = \text{velocity} \times \text{area}$$

where Q_{voxel} is given in mL/min, velocity is determined using the phase map images (cm/sec), and area is given by the spatial resolution of the phase map (cm^2). The flow rate through a vessel is simply determined by integration over a manually or semiautomatically defined cross-sectional ROI that encompasses the vessel circumference. Flow volumes throughout the cardiac cycle can be calculated by integration over the sampled time points, as shown in the valve analysis in Figure 81-27.

Flow analysis and visualization for cine three-directional volumetric velocity mapping has gained significant interest but is currently limited to research applications, partly because of the lack of intuitive analysis platforms. Advanced visualization techniques such as particle tracers, streamlines, and velocity vectors are limited to specialized software platforms (Fig. 81-28). However, the availability of comprehensive information on cardiovascular anatomy and function from a single examination is appealing and possibly allows for the derivation of additional hemodynamic parameters, such as trans-stenotic pressure gradi-

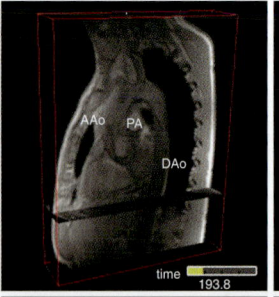

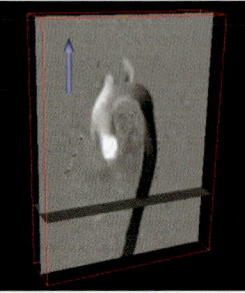

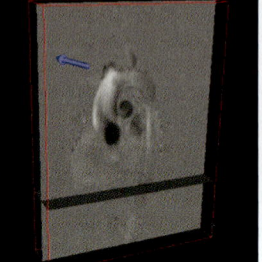

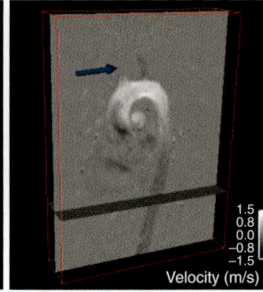

Data acquisition: Flow-sensitive 4D MRI
- ECG gating
- Adaptive navigator respiration control
- Three-directional velocity encoding

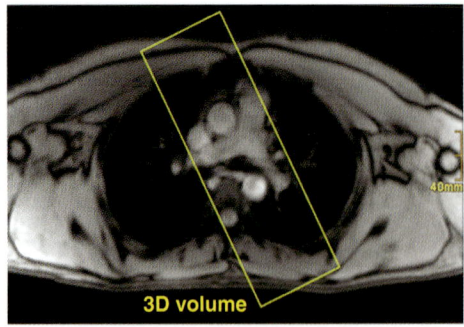

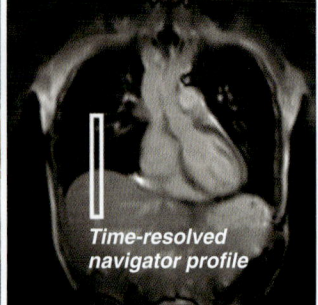

Raw Data
Three-spatial dimensions
Three-velocity directions
Time, cardiac cycle

3-D Visualization

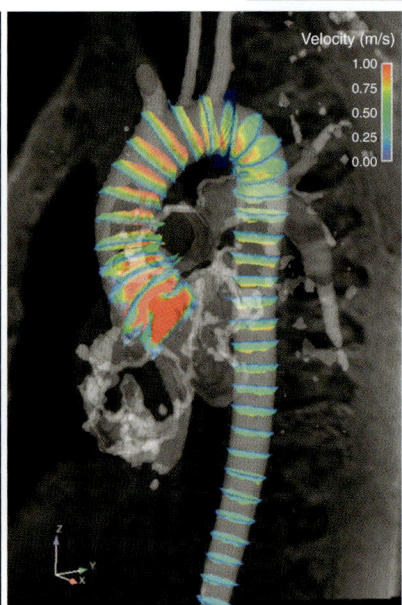

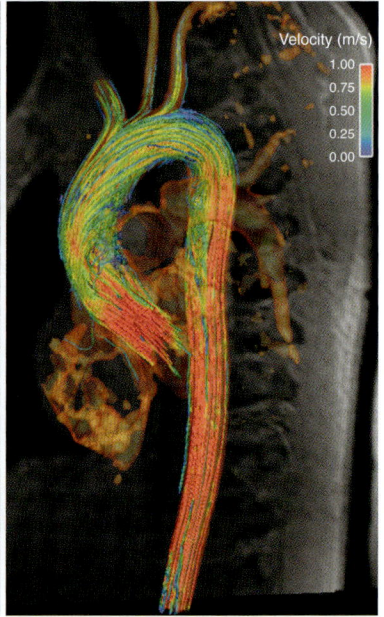

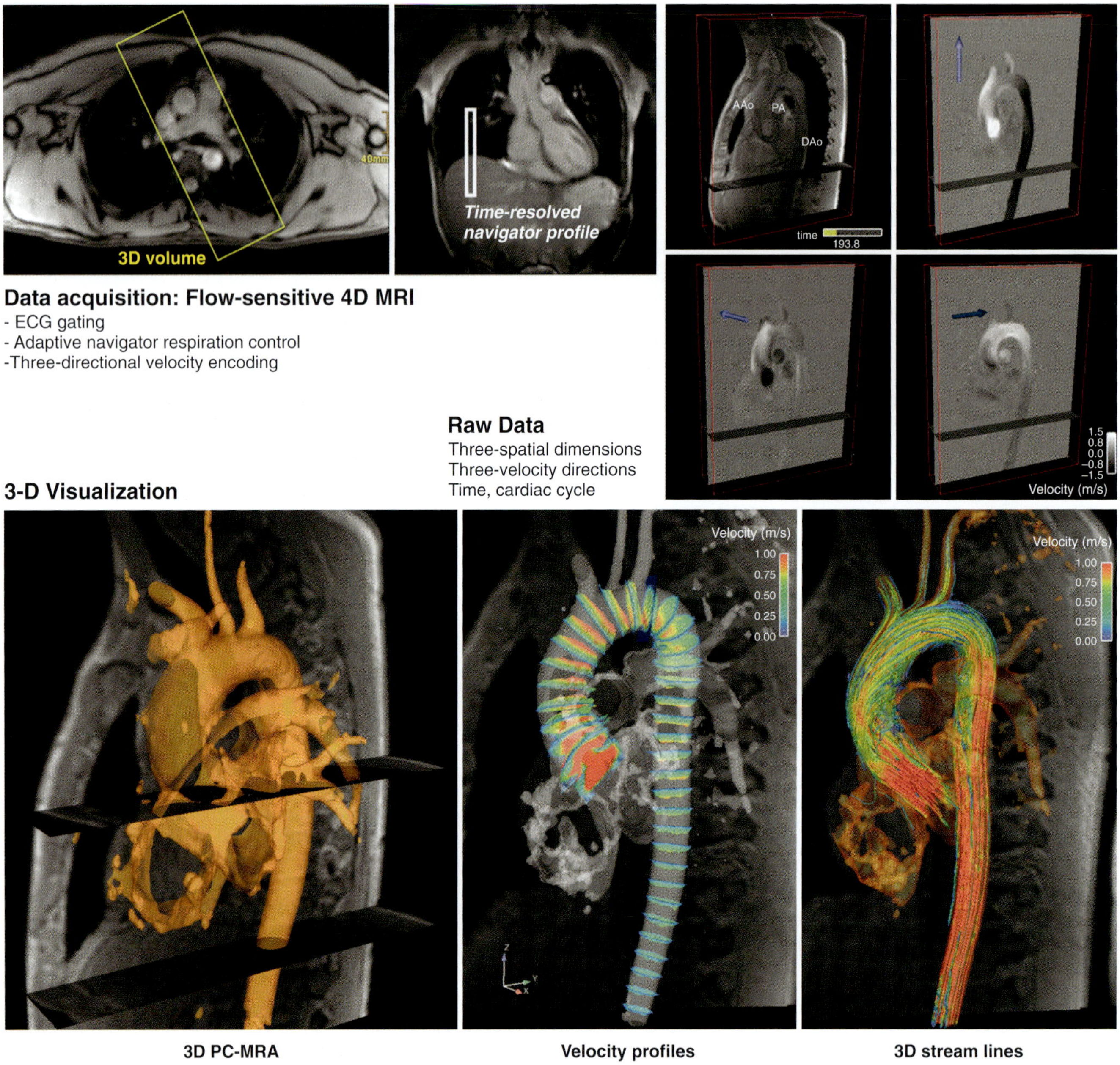

3D PC-MRA Velocity profiles 3D stream lines

FIGURE 81-28 Flow-sensitive four-dimensional (4D) MRI provides volumetric, three-directional, cine PC measurements. The acquisition allows for the capture of complex hemodynamic and postprocessing with advanced visualization software and the derivation of additional hemodynamic parameters. This acquisition uses a navigator signal for respiratory gating of the lung/liver tissue interface. *(Courtesy of Dr. Michael Markl, University Hospital. Freiburg, Germany.)*

ents and wall shear stress within the limits of the spatial resolution of the acquisition. Without taking advantage of accelerated imaging methods, the total scan time for such measurements, T_{scan}, becomes prohibitively long:

$$T_{scan} = (N_{FD} + 1) \times N_{PE} \times N_{SE} \times T_R \times T_{cp}$$

where N_{FD} = no. of flow-encoding directions, N_{PE} = no. of phase-encoding directions, N_{SE} = no. of slice-encoding directions, T_R = repetition time, and T_R = no. of cardiac phases. Similar to CE-MRA, accelerated PC imaging approaches include partial Fourier acquisitions, view sharing and temporal interpolation schemes, and use of parallel imaging techniques.

Steady-State Free Precession Magnetic Resonance Angiography

In balanced steady-state free precession (SSFP) imaging, the magnetization is manipulated so that both the transverse and the longitudinal components reach a steady state and contribute to the MR signal. The clinical adaptation of this imaging approach, also known as true fast imaging with steady-state precession (trueFISP), fast imaging employing steady-state acquisition (FIESTA), and balanced fast field echo (bFFE), had been delayed until recent hardware improvements, particularly in gradient performance and field shimming, minimized, image-degrading artifacts. This sequence is extensively used for the evaluation of cardiac function.[31]

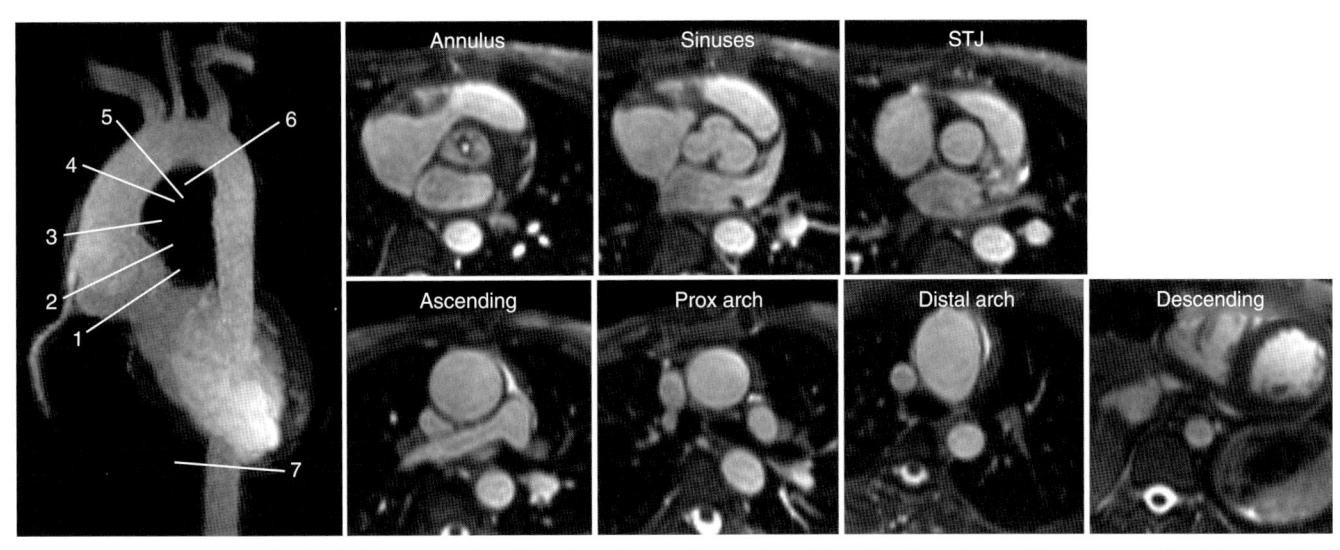

■ **FIGURE 81-29** Images obtained with bSSFP MRA of the thoracic aorta in a patient with a dilated aortic root. The volume-rendered image (*left*) demonstrates the large coverage of the acquisition. Multiplanar reformats of the source images are shown at seven levels (1-7) and provide high signal from blood because of the T2 over T1 contrast. Fat suppression was used in the ECG-gated sequence. (*Courtesy of Dr. C. Francois, University of Wisconsin-Madison, Madison, Wis.*)

Whereas the image contrast in the rapid spoiled gradient echo sequence depends mostly on T1-dependent and inflow effects for a high blood signal, SSFP provides an inherently high steady-state signal for species with a large T2/T1 ratio, such as in blood. This property explains its extensive use in the evaluation of cardiac function, with striking contrast between the blood pool and the myocardium. However, not only blood has a large T2/T1 ratio, and the challenge for SSFP MRA applications becomes the suppression of unwanted signals, particularly from fat and veins. Fat suppression is usually accomplished with water-selective excitation pulses or repeated spectral fat saturation pulses. Figure 81-29 shows MRA scans of the thoracic aorta acquired with an SSFP sequence and fat suppression.

In SSFP MRA, data are acquired with very short TR times (~3 ms), allowing for breath-held ECG-gated acquisitions. This approach is becoming a promising alternative for patients with contraindications to CE-MRA with Gd chelate contrast agents. Several modified acquisition schemes have been suggested to improve signal suppression from fat and veins, including the use of arterial spin labeling or saturation bands similar to the ones used in TOF imaging for the suppression of venous signal and slab-selective spin inversions.[2] Future clinical evaluations are needed to assess their reliability over a broad patient base. It must also be noted that signal on SSFP MRA is good after the administration of Gd chelate contrast agents and provides an additional imaging option following CE-MRA if specific regions need reassessment.[32]

Black Blood Imaging

One final technique, black blood imaging, requires specific mention, because it also can be used for the depiction of blood vessels. With black blood imaging techniques, the stationary tissue produces a signal with high amplitude, whereas the signal from moving spins is nulled.[33] This is the reverse of all other MRA techniques described here, which result in bright vascular signals. Black blood methods are based on spin-echo sequences with long TR times. The most common approach for generating this contrast is by the use of a black blood pulse consisting of two consecutive 180-degree excitation pulses (double-inversion recovery fast spin echo [DIR FSE]). The first pulse is a non–slice-selective pulse that effectively inverts the magnetization in the excitation volume of the transmit coil. As a result, the initial value of the normalized longitudinal magnetization is not 0, as is the case for a 90-degree excitation, but −1. The second pulse is selective to the magnetization of protons in the imaging slice, basically reversing the previous inversion. However, the protons outside the imaging slice are not affected by the second inversion pulse. Therefore, they undergo T1 relaxation to return to their equilibrium state (Fig. 81-30). The magnetization of blood entering the imaging slice will undergo the same relaxation and its image signal can be nulled when the data acquisition is synchronized with the zero crossing of the longitudinal magnetization. The acquisitions are usually based on fast spin-echo sequences with cardiac gating to allow for imaging with long TRs, ensuring the proper regrowth of the longitudinal magnetization prior to the next excitation.

Black blood imaging is of value whenever high contrast between the vessel lumen and vessel wall is desired and is typically performed as a two-dimensional acquisition. This technique is particularly useful for imaging atherosclerotic plaque, vasculitis, coronary arteries, and cardiac and intravascular masses and clots (see Fig. 81-30). Furthermore, non–contrast-enhanced MRA sequences that rely on bright blood signal can suffer from signal dephasing in areas of complex flow, resulting in the overestimation of stenoses. Black blood sequences do not suffer from this artifact because the acquisition is designed to provide no signal from within the lumen and can serve as a good adjunct to bright blood MRA for vascular diagnosis. However, drawbacks of this approach include insufficient contrast in regions with low signal intensity background, such as air and bone, and persistent signals in vessels with slow or recirculating blood.

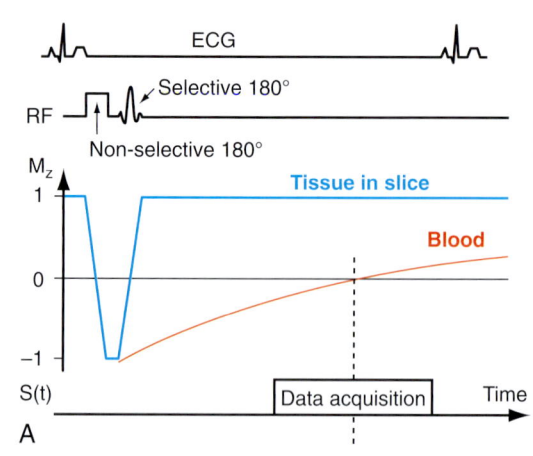

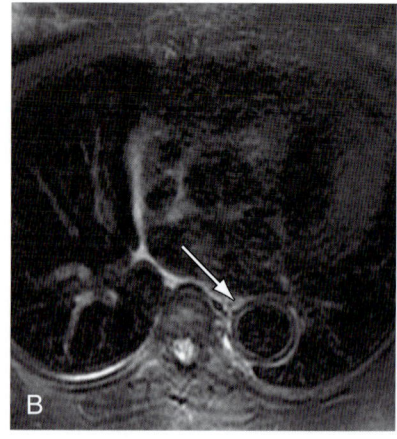

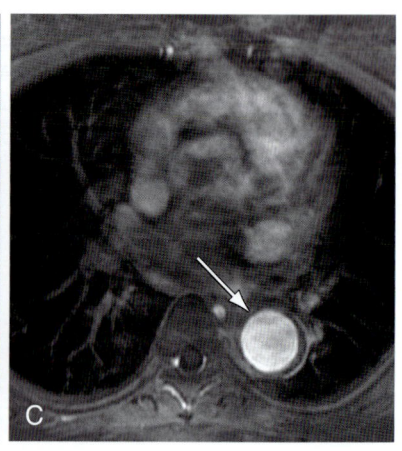

FIGURE 81-30 Black blood MRA with double inversion pulse. **A,** The first 180-degree pulse is nonselective and excites all protons inside and outside the imaged slice. The second 180-degree pulse is slice-selective and inverts only the magnetization of protons within the slice. The protons in blood entering the imaging slice have undergone only the nonselective excitation and their longitudinal magnetization, M_z, undergoes T1 relaxation. The data acquisition is centered around the zero crossing of the blood magnetization to null the signal from blood in the resulting image. **B,** This is demonstrated in a patient with Takayasu arteritis in whom the aortic wall is thickened (*arrow*) and displays increased signal intensity in T2-weighted black blood images resembling those in aortitis. The hypointense signal of the blood provides a clear separation of the vessel wall and aortic lumen. **C,** For comparison, the corresponding T1-weighted image with fat saturation obtained after IV contrast injection is displayed (*arrow*).

KEY POINTS

- Various MR techniques (e.g., contrast enhancement, time-of-flight, phase contrast, black blood, steady-state free precession) that can provide illustration of blood vessels are available.
- Hardware developments, such as more rapid and stronger gradients systems and the availability of multicoil receiver systems, together with novel acquisition schemes such as parallel imaging, have led to significantly accelerated MRA scans.
- Optimized MRA protocol development requires an understanding of the tradeoffs regarding anatomic coverage, spatial and temporal resolution, and signal-to-noise ratio.
- Contrast-enhanced MRA is a widely used clinical technique that requires synchronization of the MRA image acquisition (notably the central k-space views) with the arrival of the contrast bolus into the target vascular bed.
- TOF MRA relies on the inflow effect of flowing blood and is best suited for vessels with relatively straight trajectories, such as the carotid arteries or peripheral arteries.
- Phase contrast MRA can provide quantitative flow measurements and directional information.

SUGGESTED READINGS

Larkman DJ, Nunes RG. Parallel magnetic resonance imaging. Phys Med Biol 2007; 52:R15-R55.

Lotz J, Meier C, Leppert A, Galanski M. Cardiovascular flow measurement with phase-contrast MR imaging: basic facts and implementation. Radiographics 2002; 22:651-671.

Montgomery ML, Case RS. Magnetic resonance imaging of the vascular system: a practical approach for the radiologist. Top Magn Reson Imaging 2003; 14:376-385.

Paschal CB, Morris HD. K-space in the clinic. J Magn Reson Imaging 2004; 19:145-159.

Rohrer M, Geerts-Ossevoort L, Laub G. Technical requirements, biophysical considerations and protocol optimization with magnetic resonance angiography using blood-pool agents. Eur Radiol 2007; 17(Suppl 2):B7-B12.

Shetty AN, Bis KG, Shirkhoda A. Body vascular MR angiography: using two-dimensional and three-dimensional time-of-flight techniques. Concepts Magn Reson 2000; 12:230-255.

Willinek WA, Schild HH. Clinical advantages of 3.0 T MRI over 1.5 T. Eur J Radiol 2008; 65:2-14.

Wilson GJ, Hoogeveen RM, Willinek WA, et al. Parallel imaging in MR angiography. Top Magn Reson Imaging 2004; 15:169-185.

Wright GW. Magnetic resonance imaging. IEEE Signal Process 1997; 14:56-66.

Zhang H, Maki JH, Prince MR. three-dimensional contrast-enhanced MR angiography. J Magn Reson Imaging 2007; 25:13-25.

REFERENCES

1. WR Nitz, MR imaging: acronyms and clinical applications. Eur Radiol 1999; 9:979-997.
2. Miyazaki M, Lee VS. Nonenhanced MR angiography. Radiology 2008; 248:20-43.
3. Macovski A. Noise in MRI. Magn Reson Med 1996; 36:494-497.
4. Gibbs GF, Huston J 3rd, Bernstein MA, et al. Improved image quality of intracranial aneurysms: 3.0-T versus 1.5-T time-of-flight MR angiography. Am J Neuroradiol 2004; 25:84-87.

5. von Morze C, Xu D, Purcell DD, et al. Intracranial time-of-flight MR angiography at 7T with comparison to 3T. J Magn Reson Imaging 2007; 26:900-904.
6. Sodickson DK, Manning WJ. Simultaneous acquisition of spatial harmonics (SMASH): fast imaging with radiofrequency coil arrays. Magn Reson Med 1997; 38:591-603.
7. Pruessmann KP, Weiger M, Scheidegger MB, et al. SENSE: sensitivity encoding for fast MRI. Magn Reson Med 1999; 42:952-962.
8. Griswold MA, Jakob PM, Heidemann RM, et al. Generalized autocalibrating partially parallel acquisitions (GRAPPA). Magn Reson Med 2002; 47:1202-1210.
9. Schmitt M, Potthast A, Sosnovik DE, et al. A 128-channel receive-only cardiac coil for highly accelerated cardiac MRI at 3 Tesla. Magn Reson Med 2008; 59:1431-1439.
10. Prince MR, Yucel EK, Kaufman JA, et al. Dynamic gadolinium-enhanced three-dimensional abdominal MR arteriography. J Magn Reson Imaging 1993; 3:877-881.
11. Thomsen HS, Morcos SK, Dawson P. Is there a causal relation between the administration of gadolinium based contrast media and the development of nephrogenic systemic fibrosis (NSF)? Clin Radiol 2006; 61:905-906.
12. Earls JP, Rofsky NM, DeCorato DR, et al. Breath-hold single-dose gadolinium-enhanced three-dimensional MR aortography: usefulness of a timing examination and MR power injector. Radiology 1996; 201:705-710.
13. Foo TKF, Saranathan M, Prince MR, Chenevert TL. Automated detection of bolus arrival and initiation of data acquisition in fast, three-dimensional, gadolinium-enhanced MR angiography. Radiology 1997; 203:275-280.
14. Wilman AH, Riederer SJ, Huston J, et al. Arterial phase carotid and vertebral artery imaging in three-dimensional contrast-enhanced MR angiography by combining fluoroscopic triggering with an elliptical centric acquisition order. Magn Reson Med 1998; 40:24-35.
15. McGibney G, Smith MR, Nichols ST, Crawley A. Quantitative evaluation of several partial Fourier reconstruction algorithms used in MRI. Magn Reson Med 1993; 30:51-59.
16. Maki JH, Prince MR, Londy FJ, Chenevert TL. The effects of time varying intravascular signal intensity and K-space acquisition order on three-dimensional MR angiography image quality. J Magn Reson Imaging 1996; 6:642-651.
17. Wilman AH. Riederer SJ. Performance of an elliptical centric view order for signal enhancement and motion artifact suppression in breath-hold three-dimensional gradient echo imaging. Magn Reson Med 1997; 38:793-802.
18. Jones RA, Haraldseth O, Muller TB, et al. K-space substitution: a novel dynamic imaging technique, Magn Reson Med 1993; 29:830-834.
19. van Vaals JJ, Brummer ME, Dixon WT, et al. Keyhole method for accelerating imaging of contrast agent uptake. J Magn Reson Imaging 1993; 3:671-675.
20. Bishop JE, Santyr GE, Kelcz F, Plewes DB Limitations of the keyhole technique for quantitative dynamic contrast-enhanced breast MRI. J Magn Reson Imaging 1997; 7:716-723.
21. Korosec FR, Frayne R, Grist TM, Mistretta CA Time-resolved contrast-enhanced three-dimensional MR angiography. Magn Reson Med 1996; 36:345-351.
22. Wehrli FW, Shimakawa A, Gullberg GT, MacFall JR. Time-of-flight MR flow imaging: selective saturation recovery with gradient refocusing. Radiology 1986; 160:781-785.
23. Felmlee JP, Ehman RL. Spatial presaturation: a method for suppressing flow artifacts and improving depiction of vascular anatomy in MR imaging. Radiology 1987; 164:559-564.
24. Dumoulin CL, Souza SP, Walker MF, Wagle W. Three-dimensional phase contrast angiography. Magn Reson Med 1989; 9:139-149.
25. Parker DL, Yuan C, Blatter DD. MR angiography by multiple thin slab three-dimensional acquisition. Magn Reson Med 1991; 17:434-451.
26. Hood MN, Ho VB, Corse WR. Three-dimensional phase-contrast magnetic resonance angiography: A useful clinical adjunct to gadolinium-enhanced three-dimensional renal magnetic resonance angiography? Milit Med 2002; 167:343-349.
27. Moran PR. A flow velocity zeugmatographic interlace for NMRI in humans. Magn Reson Imaging 1982; 1:197-203.
28. Nayler GL, Firmin DN, Longmore DB. Blood flow imaging by cine magnetic resonance. J Comput Assist Tomogr 1986; 10:715-722.
29. Wigstrom L, Sjoqvist L, Wranne B. Temporally resolved three-dimensional phase-contrast imaging. Magn Reson Med 1996; 36:800-803.
30. Haacke EM, Lenz GW. Improving MR image quality in the presence of motion by using rephasing gradients. AJR Am J Roentgenol 1987; 148:1251-1258.
31. Carr JC, Simonetti O, Bundy J, et al. Cine MR angiography of the heart with segmented true fast imaging with steady-state precession. Radiology 2001; 219:828-834.
32. Foo TK, Ho VB, Marcos HB, et al. MR angiography using steady-state free precession. Magn Reson Med 2002; 48:699-706.
33. Jara H, Barish MA. Black-blood MR angiography. Techniques, clinical applications. Magn Reson Imaging Clin North Am 1999; 7:303-317.

CHAPTER 82

Magnetic Resonance Angiography: Clinical Techniques

Stefan G. Ruehm and Derek G. Lohan

Since its inception slightly more than 2 decades ago, MR angiography has become a preferred noninvasive imaging technique for a wide range of clinical indications. Concomitant technical developments in CT angiography have challenged the potential dominance of MR angiography, most notably during the recent era of multidetector CT. MR angiography permits comprehensive multiplanar endoluminal and vascular mural evaluation with exquisite soft tissue contrast, however, in the absence of ionizing radiation exposure or the requirement for iodine-based contrast medium administration. This chapter reviews the spectrum of unenhanced and gadolinium contrast-enhanced MR angiography techniques, highlighting the current and potential future roles of each in contemporary medical imaging.

DESCRIPTION OF TECHNICAL REQUIREMENTS

Consistent achievement of high-quality diagnostic MR angiography examinations depends on a synergy between appropriate MRI hardware and software and technologist-patient communication. Compromise in any of these components is certain to have a detrimental effect on image quality. Although detailed consideration of the wide range of currently available technical components is beyond the scope of this chapter, many key considerations do exist, each of which is briefly considered.

Field Strength

It has been established that signal-to-noise ratio (SNR) increases in an approximately linear fashion with magnetic field strength, which provides the opportunity for immensely superior vascular depiction with imaging at 3.0 T compared with 1.5 T. High field strength imaging is associated with a realm of potential challenges, however, which are relatively less significant at 1.5 T, including specific absorption rate considerations, $T2^*$ and dielectric resonance effects, and a greater incidence of clinically appreciable peripheral nerve stimulation.[1] Use of a 3.0 T system demands familiarity with methods of avoiding and addressing these challenges such that compromised patient safety or image quality is not acceptable. Although higher field strength has advantages for MR angiography, it is not essential, and high-quality diagnostic examinations are routinely produced on 1.5 T MRI systems.

Gradient Coils

More recent developments in MRI hardware design have facilitated further improvements in gradient coil performance.[2] High-performance gradient coils enable optimization of vascular SNR. These SNR improvements incur a penalty, however, in the form of energy deposition and increases in specific absorption rate. In practical terms, limitations in specific absorption rate often necessitate a compromise in attainable slice coverage for a particular repetition time (TR).

Phased-Array Surface Coils and Parallel Imaging Techniques

Comprising multiple integrated receiver coils, phased-array coils combine the advantages of high SNR achieved by smaller coils with the benefits of improved volume coverage, previously afforded only by large coil elements. Parallel imaging techniques (e.g., sensitivity encoding, or

SENSE),[3] whereby incomplete k-space sampling is tolerated by coil sensitivity profile calculation of the missing data, allow for significant improvements in temporal resolution, spatial resolution, or volume coverage. Parallel imaging depends on phased-array surface coils for its application. Parallel imaging improvements are attained at the expense, however, of reduced SNR. Such SNR loss may be offset, and even reversed, by imaging at higher field strengths (e.g., 3.0 T), allowing the benefit of ever-increasing acceleration factors to be realized without compromise in field of view (FOV) or spatial resolution.[4]

ECG Gating

Cardiac gating is typically unnecessary for most body MR angiography applications. During contrast-enhanced MR angiography, implementation of ECG gating would markedly prolong the already relatively protracted data acquisition times currently achievable (approximately 20 seconds), beyond the restrictions allowed by first-pass of the contrast bolus. In certain situations, availability of cardiac gating is desirable, however; these include vascular flow quantification using phase contrast flow-sensitive techniques and three-dimensional steady-state free precession (SSFP) coronary and thoracic aortic MR angiography, both of which are considered in greater detail later.

Careful Patient Preparation

High-quality MR angiography depends on a combination of adequate MRI scanner technology, experienced staff capable of exploiting this technology and modifying the imaging protocol when necessary, and an informed patient capable of adhering to the operator instructions. The impact of this last prerequisite on image quality cannot be overstated. Careful patient preparation results in improved patient cooperation with breath-hold instructions and a reduction of motion artifacts. This level of patient cooperation can be achieved only by complete and detailed explanation of the MRI experience to the patient in a comforting environment before the examination, while addressing the patient's concerns in a considerate manner.

TIME OF FLIGHT MAGNETIC RESONANCE ANGIOGRAPHY

Repetitive successive radiofrequency pulses, if applied at a magnitude and rate sufficient to prevent interval T1 recovery, results in saturation of signal from tissue within the imaged volume.[5] Time of flight (TOF) MR angiography exploits this saturation effect, providing untainted visualization of the signal produced by unsaturated entry of blood (i.e., through-plane blood flow) without the requirement for contrast agent administration. Unidirectional flow may be imaged through the use of presaturation pulses (also known as saturation bands) to eliminate signal from spins traveling in the opposite direction, with the effect of providing pure angiographic or venographic depiction, as desired. These attributes have made TOF MR angiography the most established MR angiography technique currently available, particularly with regard to the carotid, vertebral, and intracranial vascular territories.

Numerous potential implementations of this technique are available. Each varies in its degree of suitability, depending on the clinical indication. Two-dimensional TOF MR angiography involves the excitation of a single anatomic section and has proven useful for the evaluation of anatomic regions where respiratory or cardiac motion precludes useful volumetric evaluation (e.g., chest or abdomen). Multiple breath-holds and sequential, independent two-dimensional TOF MR angiography acquisitions may be used in this instance to provide diagnostic quality examinations, even in dyspneic patients (Fig. 82-1). Three-dimensional TOF MR angiography is preferred for intracranial evaluation in particular, permitting detailed volumetric data acquisition at submillimeter voxel resolution and the potential for subsequent postprocessing (Fig. 82-2). Multiple overlapping thin slab acquisition (MOTSA) represents a compromise in two-dimensional and three-dimensional techniques, integrating the advantages of three-dimensional imaging with the relatively fewer limitations of the two-dimensional approach. MOTSA combines multiple, relatively thin three-dimensional slabs to provide clinically useful volume coverage.[6]

Indications

Before the widespread introduction of contrast-enhanced MR angiography techniques for comprehensive large-volume anatomic vascular coverage, TOF MR angiography represented the cornerstone of MR angiography throughout the body. Contrast-enhanced MR angiography, however, required revision of many diagnostic algorithms in favor of this faster and typically higher quality method. Nonetheless, TOF MR angiography remains the technique of choice for intracranial vascular depiction, a reflection of its superb spatial and contrast resolution and its patient acceptability.[7] Advances in MRI hardware, including the introduction of dedicated head and neck coils and resultant implementation of parallel imaging techniques, have enhanced the value of this approach in clinical practice further.

TOF MR angiography also remains a common means of extracranial carotid arterial evaluation. Artifact relating to patient motion or swallowing often produces less adequate results compared with intracranial imaging. The superb quality of vascular depiction obtained on supra-aortic contrast-enhanced MR angiography studies suggests that TOF MR angiography may soon be superseded by this contrast-enhanced technique for routine extracranial carotid MR evaluation. In the presence of contraindications to contrast administration, TOF MR angiography may also be valuable in head and neck venous imaging, particularly imaging of the intracranial venous sinuses.

Contraindications

No contraindications particular to TOF MR angiography exist, such that it may be safely performed in any patient

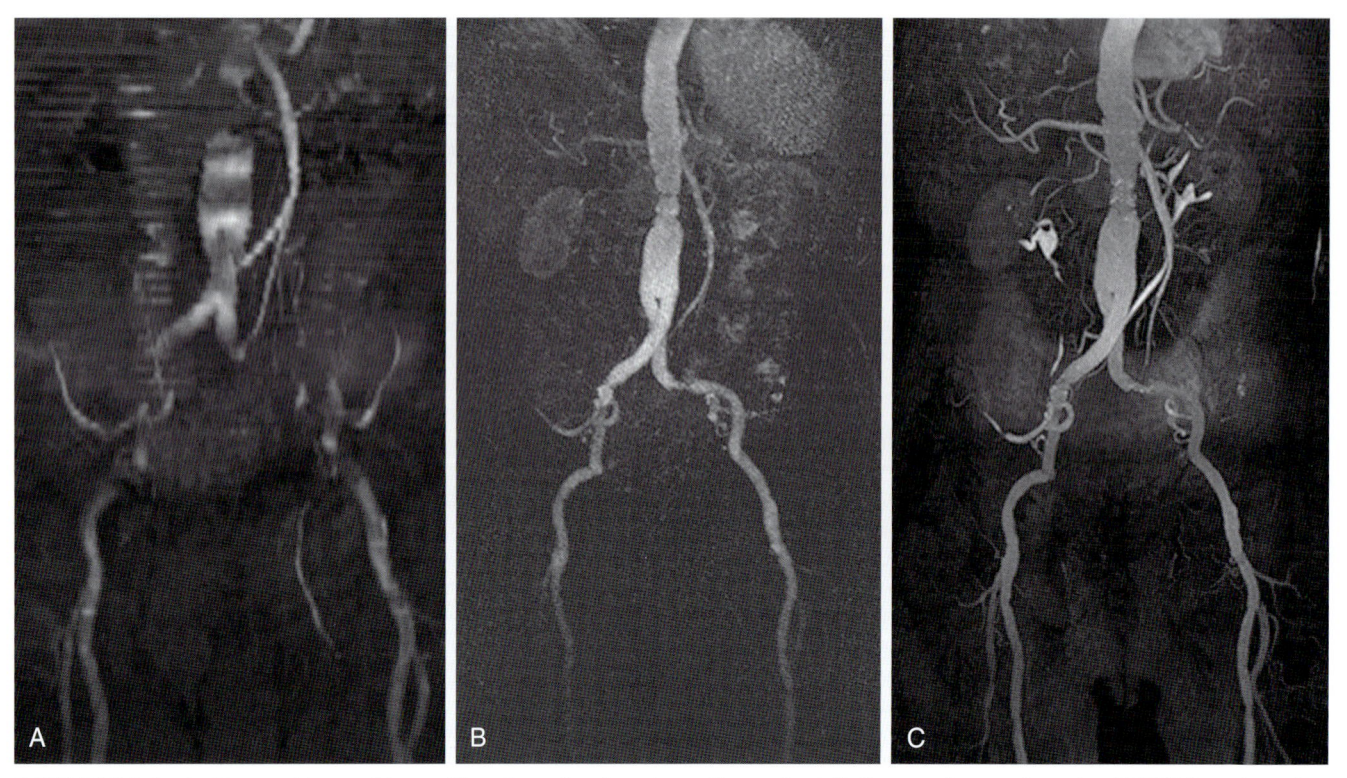

■ **FIGURE 82-1** An 88-year-old man with aortoiliac atherosclerosis and aortoiliac grafts. **A-C,** Comparative two-dimensional TOF MR angiography (**A**), arterial phase TR MR angiography frame (**B**), and full-thickness three-dimensional contrast-enhanced MR angiography (**C**) coronal images illustrate the typical image quality of each technique when imaging this anatomic region. Performed properly, three-dimensional contrast-enhanced MR angiography provides the highest spatial resolution image.

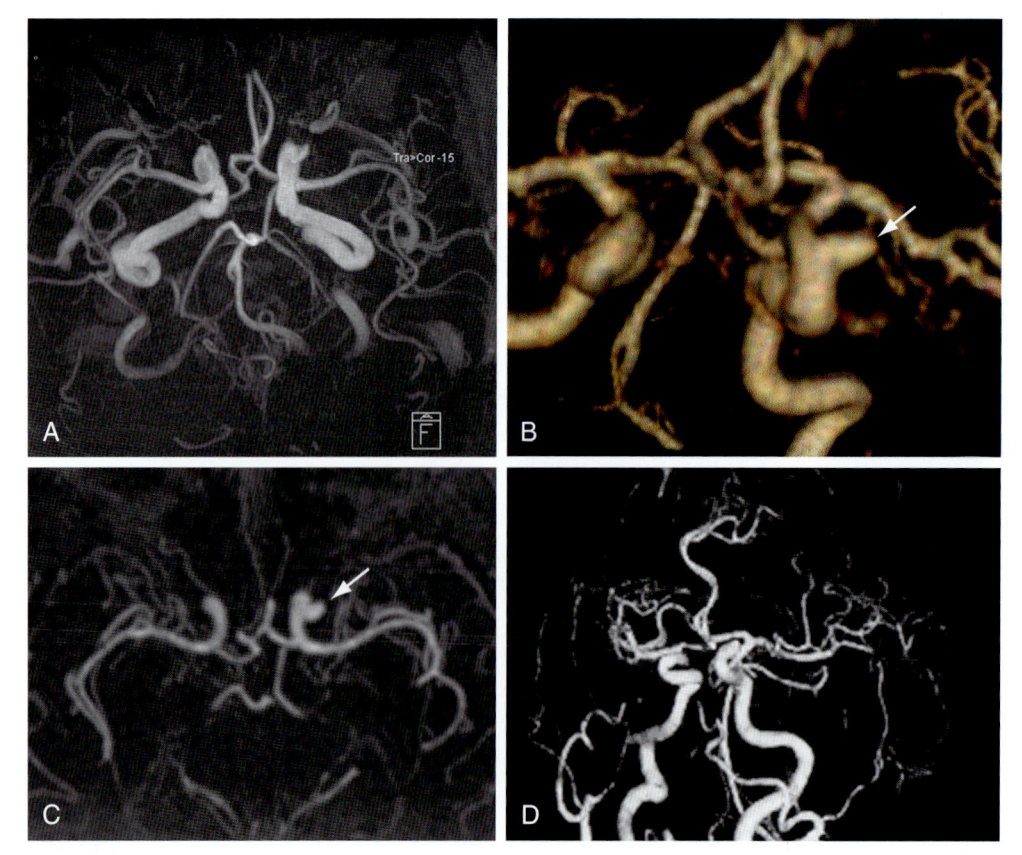

■ **FIGURE 82-2** Periophthalmic intracranial aneurysm. **A-D,** Full-thickness MIP (**A**) and volume-rendered reconstructions (**B**) from TOF MR angiography examination, and axial thin-section MIP (**C**) and coronal oblique full-thickness volume rendered (**D**) reconstructions from contrast-enhanced MR angiography provide comparable information regarding aneurysm morphology and location (*arrow* in **B** and **C**).

undergoing an MRI examination. This attribute has undoubtedly contributed to the popularity of this technique and helped maintain its position as a significant part of the diagnostic algorithm.

Pitfalls and Solutions

Despite its popularity and widespread implementation, TOF MR angiography may be extremely challenging to implement and interpret because of its numerous potential pitfalls.[8]

Saturation

As explained, successful TOF MR angiography depends on saturation of signal from static tissue, such that "fresh" through-plane vascular spins produce an appreciable signal. Saturation of blood signal occurs if blood flow is slow or persists within the imaging field (e.g., vessel coursing in-plane) and can result in suboptimal vascular visualization, to the point of potentially mimicking a vascular occlusion. This situation is of particular significance with regard to the use of three-dimensional TOF MR angiography, owing to the more extensive volume coverage required for most body applications. Numerous potential solutions to this dilemma exist, including optimization of TR and imaging plane, reduction of flip angle and echo time (TE), and use of thinner slices. Three-dimensional TOF MOTSA provides the advantages of three-dimensional TOF MR angiography, but by using thinner three-dimensional slabs, minimizes the saturation effects over that of a single large three-dimensional volume. If saturation effects persist in small, slow-flow vessels, administration of a small amount of T1-shortening paramagnetic contrast agent may prove effective, although at the risk of inducing adjacent soft tissue enhancement and venous contamination.[9]

Prolonged Imaging Times

Data acquisition is directly related to TR, which must be maintained sufficiently brief to achieve tissue saturation. Too brief a TR fails to allow sufficient time for "fresh" unsaturated spins to enter the imaging section, however, resulting in suboptimal vascular signal.

Intravoxel Dephasing

Intravoxel dephasing is an undesirable effect that manifests as vascular signal loss and results from complex or turbulent flow patterns that result in loss of the phase coherence of moving spins. Complex and turbulent flow patterns are seen in the presence of tortuous or stenotic vessels. Intravoxel dephasing can result in the overestimation of a stenosis on MR angiography. The identification of intravoxel dephasing can be beneficial, however, as a tool for the detection of a hemodynamic stenosis (e.g., coarctation of the aorta) or valvular dysfunction (e.g., aortic stenosis or insufficiency) on cine bright blood MRI. Appropriate remedies include use of smaller voxel sizes, thinner slices, and reducing the TE.

Image Interpretation

Postprocessing

A TOF MR angiography data set is volumetric and comprises voxels, acquired in slices (two-dimensional TOF) or in the form of digital sections known as partitions (three-dimensional TOF). Selection of isotropic voxel dimensions minimizes the image distortions seen on multiplanar off-axis reconstruction. TOF MR angiography data are most often presented in the form of a full-thickness maximum intensity projection (MIP), rotated through 360 degrees in anteroposterior (somersault) and transverse planes. As a result, small aneurysms or luminal surface irregularities (e.g., intimal flap or ulceration) may not be as well appreciated or may be missed. It is recommended that the partition "source data" are also reviewed so that subtle abnormalities are not concealed by overlapping vessels in areas of complex vascularity.

Reporting

Confident, accurate reporting of TOF MR angiography examinations necessitates that the potential pitfalls referred to earlier and their imaging manifestations are recognized and correctly interpreted. Because there is a tendency for each of these unwanted effects to result in intraluminal signal loss, either focal or widespread, failing to recognize them may result in considerable overestimation in the degree of vascular steno-occlusive disease and prompt unnecessary invasive investigation.

PHASE CONTRAST MAGNETIC RESONANCE ANGIOGRAPHY

Phase contrast MR angiography is an unenhanced approach to imaging that employs bipolar phase-encoding gradient pairs to encode flow velocity in the gradient direction. Stationary background tissue accumulates a net phase shift of zero. Moving spins experience a net phase shift that produces signal and the image contrast necessary to distinguish between moving and stationary tissue (i.e., angiography).[10] Phase contrast MR angiography requires the operator selection of a velocity encoding (VENC) in cm/s, which is responsible for determination of the flow sensitivity of the acquisition. Because assignment of phase shift is limited to a range of −180 degrees to +180 degrees, the VENC represents a flow velocity that would cause a maximal phase shift of 180 degrees. For optimal sensitivity, this VENC should be selected to correspond with or slightly exceed the highest velocity present within the vessel in question. For intracranial applications, a VENC of 70 to 80 cm/s is often sufficient for arterial imaging, whereas a factor of 20 to 30 cm/s should be applied for venous imaging.[11] If the flow velocity exceeds the chosen VENC, aliasing results with the effect of apparent flow reversal.

In addition to providing a visual representation of flowing blood, phase contrast MR angiography allows quantitative evaluation of flow velocity, typically acquired in cine mode (i.e., cine phase contrast). This evaluation reflects the direct relationship between the phase shift experienced by flowing spins and their velocity. This technique is being increasingly recognized regarding its potential utility throughout the vascular system, particularly in regard to estimation of pressure gradients or flow quantification.

Indications

Before the widespread availability of contrast-enhanced and increasingly impressive TOF techniques, phase contrast MR angiography was relatively successful in the evaluation of various vascular territories. In recent times, this approach has been relegated in importance to that of a "last resort," should the other angiographic techniques discussed in this chapter be unsuccessful or contraindicated. Phase contrast MR angiography has regained some of its former popularity more recently because of its flow quantification capabilities. Our experience suggests that phase contrast flow quantification is a valuable, versatile tool in the noninvasive evaluation of flow characteristics within almost any vascular bed.[12] Although this technique has not yet been incorporated into widespread clinical practice, its future potential remains encouraging.

Contraindications

Absolute contraindications to phase contrast MR angiography are those of MRI in general; any patient in whom MRI is deemed safe may potentially undergo this angiographic technique. The relatively long data acquisition times involved (often >20 minutes) may render phase contrast MR angiography as a relative contraindication in patients with unstable or rapidly declining clinical condition.

Pitfalls and Solutions

The limitations of phase contrast MR angiography are similar to those of TOF MR angiography, including in-plane saturation, velocity aliasing, voxel dephasing, and long acquisition times. The flip angle may be increased in the presence of intravoxel dephasing or decreased if spin saturation is experienced. VENC may also be increased or decreased to prevent aliasing and poor image contrast. Administration of the contrast agent gadolinium-chelate improves vascular depiction on phase contrast MR angiography and may be considered for further augmentation of luminal vascular image contrast. Nonetheless, despite the presence of potential solutions to many phase contrast MR angiography pitfalls, this technique remains inferior to alternative angiographic approaches, and has been excluded from routine clinical practice for the purpose of vascular depiction.

THREE-DIMENSIONAL STEADY-STATE FREE PRECESSION MAGNETIC RESONANCE ANGIOGRAPHY

SSFP is a low flip angle gradient-recalled-echo (GRE) technique that induces a persistent level of tissue magnetization by means of a TR that is significantly shorter than the T2 of tissue. As a result, this approach permits bright blood vascular imaging, the signal from which is a reflection of the inherent T2/T1 ratio of blood, while precluding gadolinium-chelate contrast agent administration.[13] Owing to a very short TR and large flip angle, two-dimensional SSFP techniques allow rapid subsecond image acquisition that does not require respiratory suspension, even when imaging the chest. These attributes have resulted in the adoption of SSFP as a cornerstone imaging technique in many aspects of cardiac imaging, including two-dimensional single-shot multiplanar morphologic and ECG gated cine functional myocardial assessment.

Many three-dimensional implementations of SSFP have been successfully evaluated for the purpose of vascular imaging, most notably with regard to the coronary and renal arteries.[14,15] In exploiting the intrinsic T2/T1 signal of blood, three-dimensional SSFP MR angiography allows large FOV vascular coverage, while avoiding the data acquisition constraints because of the contrast bolus imposed during contrast-enhanced MR angiography. Combining three-dimensional SSFP MR angiography with navigator gating allows free-breathing nonenhanced chest and abdominal vascular depiction. Further addition of ECG gating has allowed the realization of free-breathing coronary MR angiography, although at the expense of often prolonged acquisition times (≥10 minutes) (Fig. 82-3). The potential of parallel imaging techniques to aid in reduction of these acquisition times has been evaluated, providing encouraging results to date. Implementation of this data-sharing technique does incur penalties with regard to SNR, however, with the effect of image degradation that may be poorly tolerated.

Indications

Physicians have seemed reluctant to integrate three-dimensional SSFP MR angiography into routine clinical practice; this is a reflection of the long imaging durations required for its successful implementation. In many cases, this technique is used because of necessity rather than desire, with a typical scenario involving a patient with contraindications to CT angiography or conventional catheter angiography or both, in whom confirmation of vascular patency is required. Nonetheless, the potential value of this approach has gradually achieved acknowledgment in recent times with its successful application to aortic, renal, carotid, and peripheral arterial imaging. The current environment of heightened sensitivity toward the administration of intravenous gadolinium-chelate contrast agents, discussed in greater detail subsequently, may also serve to broaden the spectrum and availability of this versatile technique.

Contraindications

After general contraindications to MRI have been excluded, all patients may be considered candidates for three-dimensional SSFP MR angiography. This technique may play a significant role in the future with increasing acceptance of this technique into routine imaging practice.

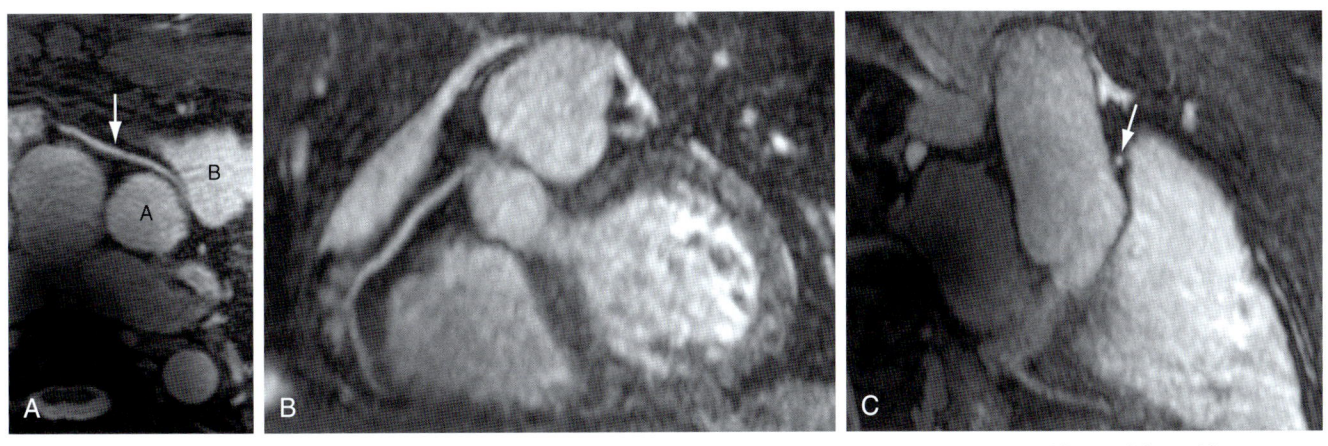

■ **FIGURE 82-3** Navigator-gated coronary three-dimensional SSFP MR angiography. **A-C,** MPR reconstructions (**A,** oblique axial; **B,** oblique coronal; **C,** oblique sagittal) from the same data set illustrating an aberrant origin of the right coronary artery (*arrow*). This vessel may be confidently visualized throughout much of its length, passing proximally between the ascending aorta (A) and pulmonary trunk, following an interarterial course. Motion artifacts were minimized by the use of respiratory and ECG gating.

Pitfalls and Solutions

SSFP techniques are sensitive to off-resonance artifacts, manifesting as dark bands traversing the images acquired. These potentially detrimental regions may prove particularly difficult to avoid when imaging at 3.0 T. Preventive methods have been described, including small volume frequency scouting to select the optimal frequency at which the bands are eradicated.[16]

Whole heart coronary MR angiography using three-dimensional SSFP may represent a source of considerable frustration owing to its occasional production of poor-quality studies despite its apparently adequate implementation. In many cases, these suboptimal studies stem from poor delineation of the luminal and mural margins, with resultant blurring of the images obtained. Because successful three-dimensional SSFP demands careful coordination of numerous key components, knowledge of each is necessary so that the offending factor may be addressed.[17]

Heart Rate and Rhythm

ECG gated studies involve data acquisition during a predefined interval of the cardiac cycle. Erratic cardiac rhythms serve to deprive each cycle of this portion of the R-R interval, prolonging data acquisition times. Tachycardia also has a detrimental effect on three-dimensional SSFP imaging, increasing the degree of cardiac motion experienced during a single image acquisition window.

Respiratory Rhythm

Ideal conditions for respiratory-navigated MR angiography studies involve a patient with a slow, consistent respiratory pattern, such that its predictability may be employed in selecting a window during which data acquisition occurs. In the absence of such conditions, rapid or varying respiratory rates and depths prolong study times and predispose toward degradation of image quality.

Respiratory Acceptance Window

High-quality free-breathing SSFP MR angiography requires that k-space filling occurs during a specific phase of respiration. This requirement has the effect of ensuring that the structures within the imaging FOV maintain a near-exact position throughout data acquisition. Definition of an acceptance window (the volume within which the diaphragm must be located for data collection to occur) for respiratory navigation represents a compromise between image quality and duration of the examination. When acceptance windows are narrow, k-space filling occurs for a diminutive proportion of each respiratory cycle, and study times are prolonged, although less respiratory motion artifact results. Conversely, loosening of acceptance window constraints expedites study durations through an increase in the respiratory phase during which data collection occurs, although at the expense of compromised image quality.

Navigator Band Location

Triggering of k-space filling depends on identification of a soft tissue interface within a predefined acceptance window. Commonly employed interfaces include interfaces between the lung and liver or mediastinum. Adequate selection of navigator band location is central to the successful implementation of this technique. Sharply defined interfaces allow confident automated detection of the tissue margin, whereas ill-defined margins (e.g., between liver and atelectatic lung) make identification of the interface difficult.

Patient Motion

A perpetual source of image degradation during MRI, patient motion is of particular relevance to three-dimensional SSFP MR angiography because of the relatively long imaging durations involved. The long duration has the effect of introducing motion artifact and degradation of image quality. Although shortening of the duration of the

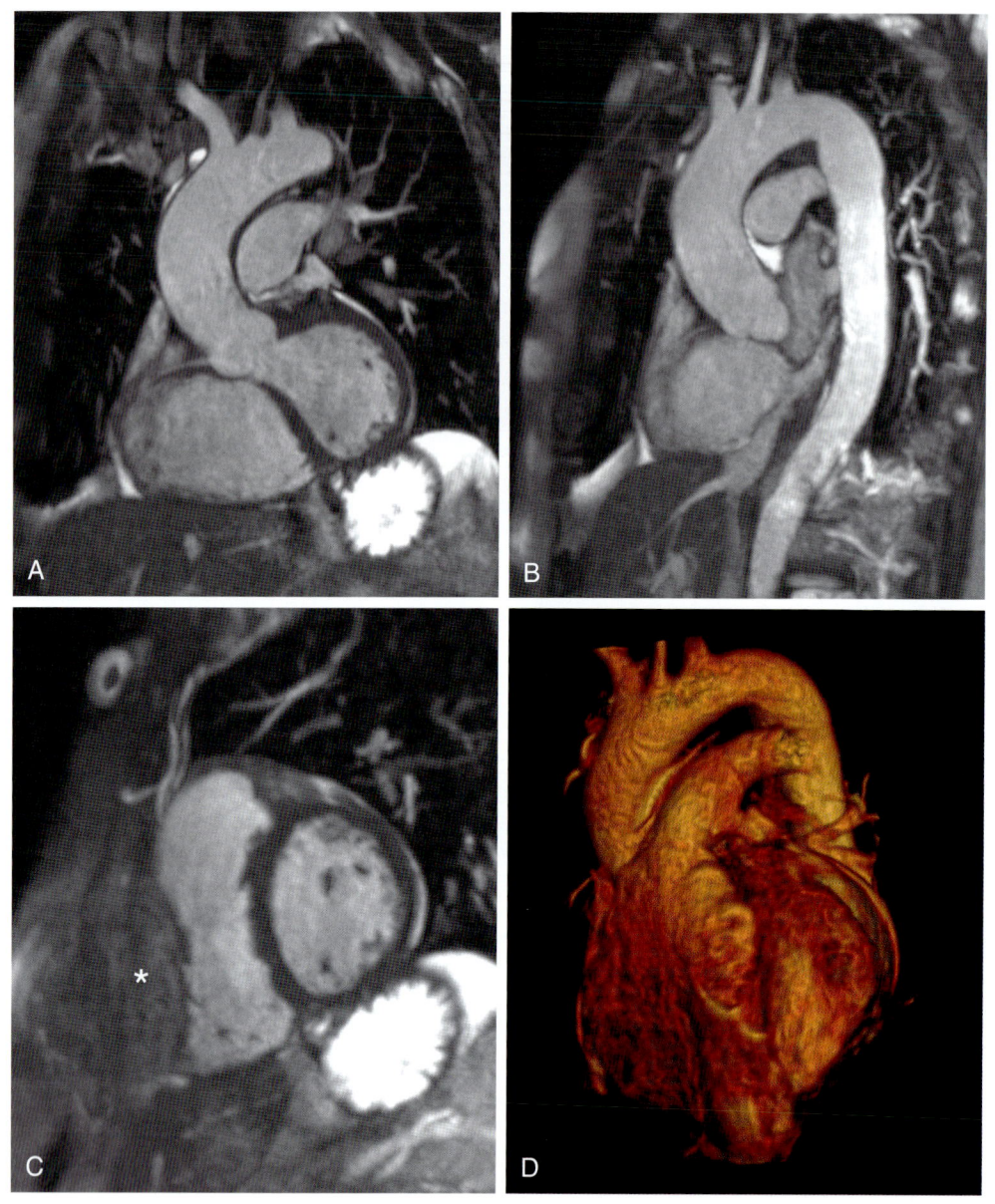

■ **FIGURE 82-4** Thoracic three-dimensional SSFP MR angiography. Acquisition of an isotropic three-dimensional data set allows reconstruction in any desired plane without loss of in-plane resolution. **A** and **B**, Coronal (**A**) and sagittal oblique (**B**) images show the thoracic aorta without motion artifact. **C**, There is a metastatic lesion (*asterisk*) in the sternum, its effect on the right ventricle being readily appreciable in this sagittal image. **D**, Volume-rendered three-dimensional reconstruction.

examination (by widening the respiratory navigation acceptance window or removal of ECG gating) may reduce the probability of significant patient motion, these adjustments also have the effect of compromising image integrity.

Image Interpretation

Postprocessing

The volumetric nature of three-dimensional SSFP MR angiography with near-isotropic voxel dimensions permits data reconstruction in any desired plane without incurring penalties with regard to image distortion (Fig. 82-4). Comprehensive multiplanar vascular evaluation is typically feasible on the basis of a single acquisition. Coronary artery assessment generally involves curved multiplanar reconstruction (MPR) processing, allowing visualization of the arterial lumen throughout its length, despite its tortuous course. Short-axis reconstructions (perpendicular to the vascular lumen) at sites of suspected pathology may also be derived from this data set. Renal artery evaluations generally involve coronal oblique and axial reconstructions.

Reporting

As explained previously, free-breathing, ECG gated three-dimensional SSFP MR angiography exploits the T2/T1 signal ratio of blood for signal generation. In contrast to the other angiographic techniques discussed, SSFP MR angiography provides concomitant arterial and venous

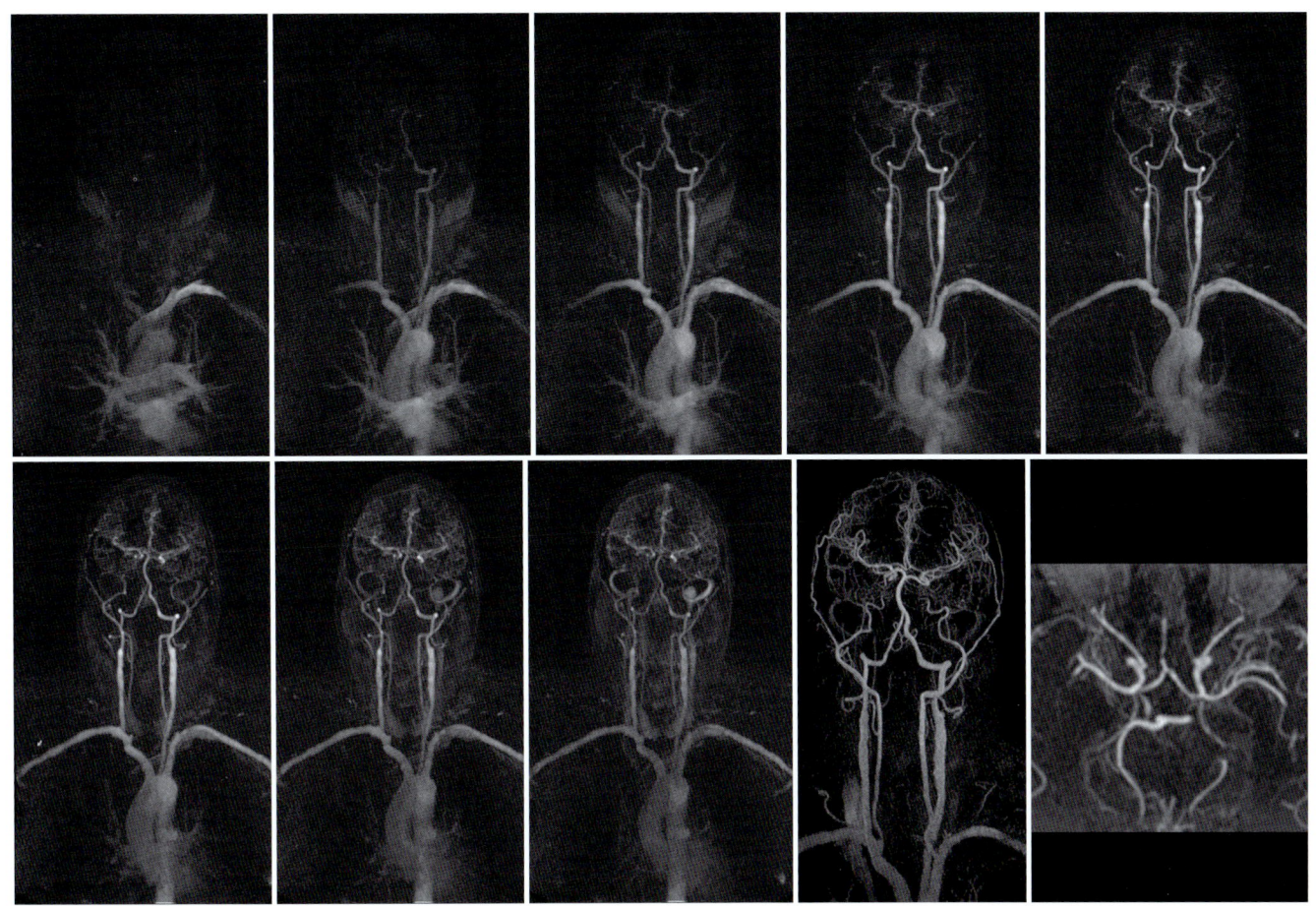

FIGURE 82-5 Bilateral internal carotid arterial bulb occlusions. Sequential time resolved MR angiography frames and full-thickness MIP from contrast-enhanced MR angiography (*bottom right two frames,* coronal and axial MIPs) examination fail to show opacification of the internal carotid arteries from their origins. The vertebral arteries, collateral pathway, and external carotid circulation are prominent, including ophthalmic branches.

luminal depiction. This wealth of information should be evaluated carefully for the presence of incidental or subclinical vascular abnormalities, within the arterial and the venous territories.

TIME RESOLVED MAGNETIC RESONANCE ANGIOGRAPHY

Time resolved MR angiography is a dynamic approach to contrast-enhanced angiography that involves rapid sequential imaging of an anatomic volume during the luminal transit of a contrast bolus (Fig. 82-5). Although most commonly implemented as a two-dimensional technique for the purpose of "bolus timing" in preparation for subsequent high-resolution contrast-enhanced MR angiography, more recent three-dimensional applications of TR MR angiography have shown considerable promise with regard to functional vascular imaging and evaluation of visceral perfusion.

Regardless of the approach used, time resolved MR angiography involves the use of a T1-weighted GRE sequence with sufficiently short TR to allow repeated imaging at temporal resolutions of 1 to 2 seconds per frame. Achievement of such ultrashort temporal resolutions demands that compromises are made, however, most commonly with respect to spatial resolution. One approach is to allow concessions in the slice-select direction, as described by Finn and colleagues.[18] Although this method precludes off-axis reconstruction of the volumetric data obtained, this is rarely of sufficient impact to limit the diagnostic utility of the studies performed. Alternatively, through-plane resolution comparable to that of the in-plane direction may be employed, although at the expense of less frequent data refreshment.[19]

Enthusiasm regarding the potential value of time resolved MR angiography in clinical practice stems from its ability to permit starting imaging before the arrival of the contrast bolus and continuation of imaging throughout the arterial and venous phases of luminal opacification. As a result, TR MR angiography is free from the bolus-timing constraints of contrast-enhanced MR angiography and the ever-present threat of venous contamination occasionally experienced during contrast-enhanced MR angiography.

Indications

Widespread appreciation of the potential utility of time resolved MR angiography has resulted in its successful application across a wide range of disciplines (Figs. 82-6 and 82-7). Our experience with this technique has been considerable and similarly encouraging. Table 82-1 sum-

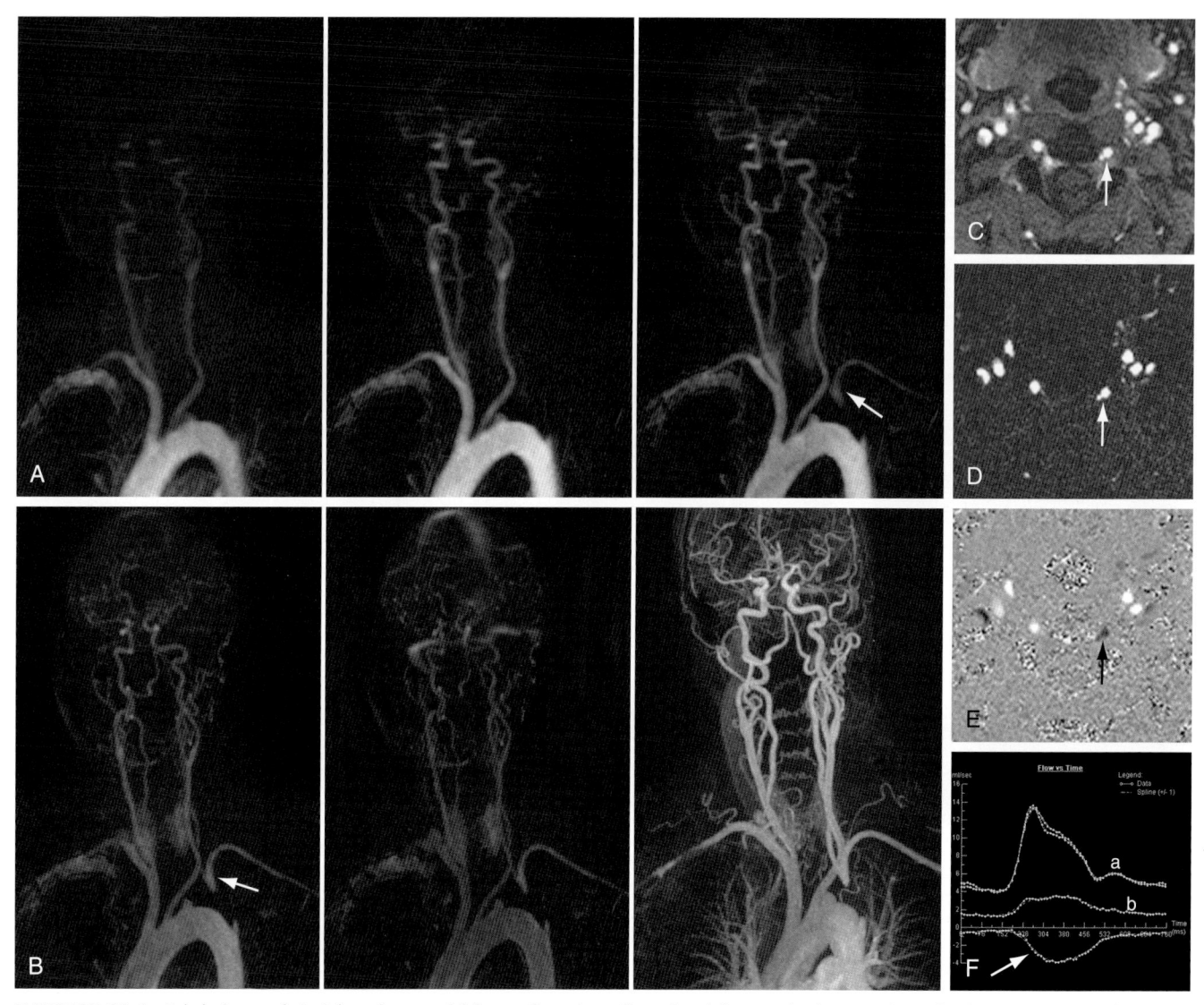

■ FIGURE 82-6 Subclavian steal. A, Selected sequential frames from three-dimensional time resolved MR angiography shows proximal occlusion of the left subclavian artery with collateral circulation via retrograde flow in the left vertebral artery (*arrow*). B, This pathway is eloquently depicted by three-dimensional contrast-enhanced MR angiography (*arrow*). C-E, Cine axial phase contrast imaging at the level of the mid-common carotid arteries confirms the presence of retrograde left vertebral arterial flow (*arrow* in C-E; C, magnitude image; D, speed or angiographic image (all flow bright); E, phase map image (ascending flow is bright and descending flow is black). On phase map images (E), retrograde flow within the left vertebral artery is confirmed by its black signal. On the phase map image, flow is bright in the right vertebral and carotid arteries. F, On flow analysis, there is negative flow or descending flow (*arrow*) measured within the left vertebral artery compared with the positive flow or ascending flow within the carotid arteries (a) and the right vertebral artery (b).

marizes proven indications for the use of time resolved MR angiography, including suggested applications that are based on our personal experience to date.

Contraindications

A significant proportion of current interest in time resolved MR angiography has been generated as a result of its relative lack of specific contraindications: it may be performed in any patient in whom contrast-enhanced MR angiography is planned. When general contraindications to MRI (e.g., severe claustrophobia, presence of certain implanted metallic devices such as cardiac pacemaker leads) and previous severe reactions to gadolinium-chelate contrast agents have been excluded, time resolved MR angiography can be considered in all patients.

The potential role of time resolved MR angiography in clinical practice has been readdressed in recent times as a result of the emergence of a potential link between administration of gadolinium-chelate contrast agents and development of the potentially fatal condition nephrogenic systemic fibrosis in patients with severe, end-stage renal failure.[20] Although some authors have questioned the justification for contrast-enhanced MR angiography and time resolved MR angiography in these patients, others have focused on the potential of time resolved MR angiography to replace its high-resolution three-dimensional counterpart in certain instances. Such preclusion of the requirement for contrast-enhanced MR angiography is wholly desirable, a reflection of the ability of time resolved MR angiography to provide highly diagnostic studies with the injection of only 0.01 to 0.02 mmol

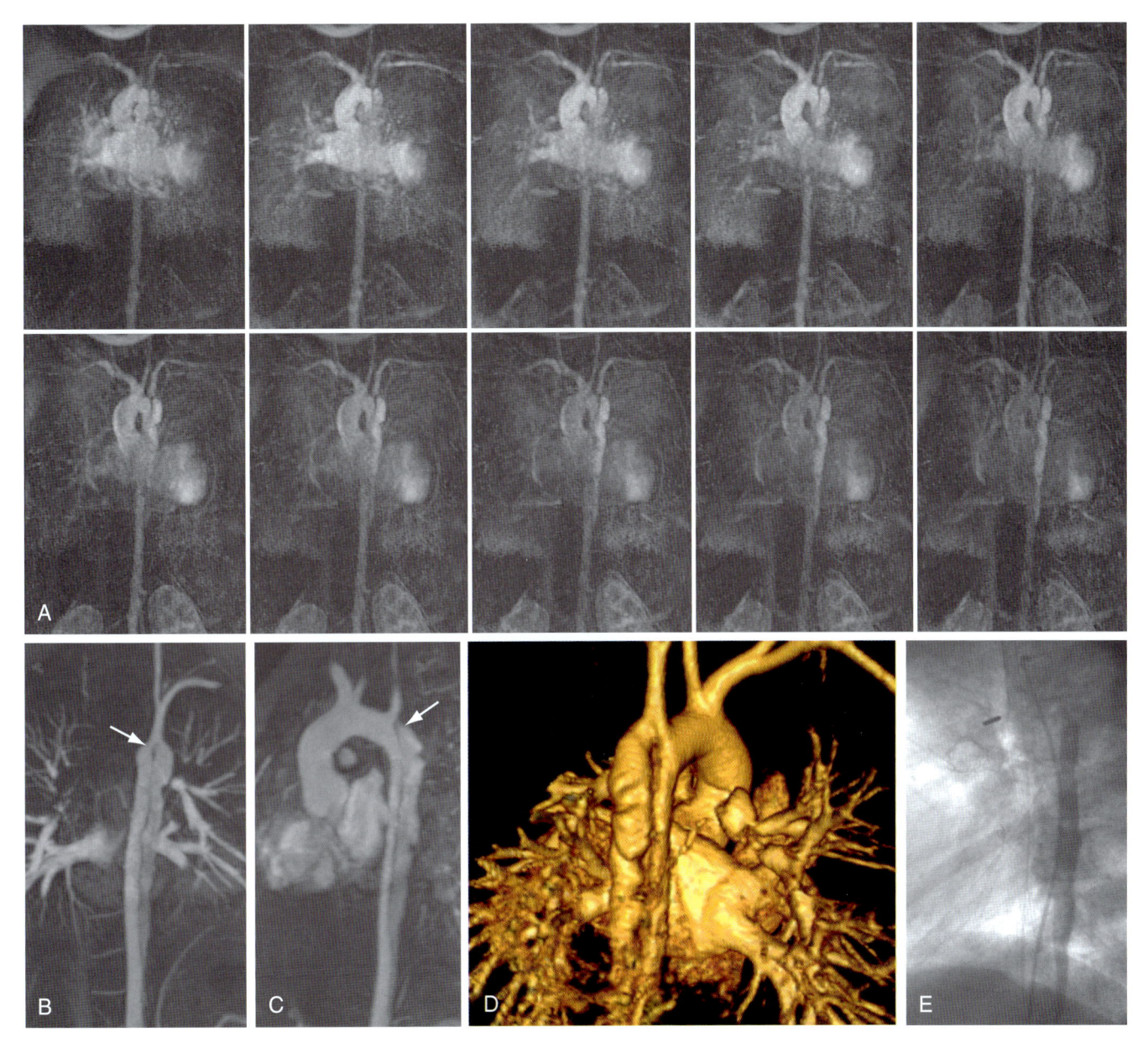

CHAPTER 82 ● *Magnetic Resonance Angiography: Clinical Techniques* 1111

■ **FIGURE 82-7** Iatrogenic type B aortic dissection in a 10-year-old boy. **A,** Disparity between true and false luminal flow is seen on time resolved MR angiography frames (these frames are of diagnostic quality despite respiratory motion). **B-D,** The intimal flap is clearly visible on direct coronal (**B**) and sagittal oblique (**C**) three-dimensional contrast-enhanced MR angiography MIP and volume-rendered (**D**) reconstructions, obtained with suspended respiration. **E,** This dissection was subsequently confirmed at conventional catheter angiography.

of gadolinium-chelate contrast agent per kilogram of patient body weight compared with 0.1 to 0.2 mmol/kg for contrast-enhanced MR angiography.[21]

Pitfalls and Solutions

Time resolved MR angiography represents a balance between in-plane spatial resolution, through-plane spatial resolution, FOV, and rate of temporal data refreshment. Because the equilibrium between these factors is often quite tenuous, improvement in one parameter often incurs penalties with respect to one or more of the others. Many of the pitfalls of time resolved MR angiography occur as a result of this complex relationship, such as exclusion of a vital vascular structure owing to FOV constraints, inability to produce suitable off-axis MIPs as a result of limited through-plane resolution, or failure of detection of a transient vascular phenomenon because of suboptimal temporal resolution. Avoidance of such adversities involves careful preemptive tailoring of the imaging plane, three-axis spatial resolution, and temporal resolution to suit the clinical indication. In many cases, technical restrictions prevent avoidance of all of these pitfalls during a single time resolved MR angiography acquisition. As a result, a low threshold should be maintained for consideration of multiple time resolved MR angiography acquisitions using complementary parameters so that a comprehensive morphologic and dynamic evaluation is obtained.

TABLE 82-1 Indications for the Use of Time Resolved Magnetic Resonance Angiography

Discipline	Application
Neurovascular	Cerebral and spinal vascular malformations
	Spinal arteriovenous shunts
	Subclavian steal syndrome
	Dural arteriovenous fistulas
	Carotid bifurcation imaging
	Postoperative assessment of extracranial to intracranial arterial bypass
	Intracranial venous sinus evaluation
	Assessment of bilateral symmetric cerebral parenchymal perfusion in the presence of internal carotid or vertebrobasilar steno-occlusive disease
Cardiac	Work-up of complex pediatric and adult congenital heart disease
	Evaluation of patency of intracardiac and extracardiac surgical shunts (e.g., Fontan, Glenn shunt)
	Detection of right-to-left intracardiac shunts
Pulmonary	Assessment of pulmonary perfusion
	Differentiation between idiopathic and thromboembolic pulmonary hypertension
	Evaluation of pulmonary arteriovenous malformations
	Primary screening of patients with suspected pulmonary embolism
	Pulmonary venous ostial evaluation for stenosis
	Pulmonary venous assessment for anomalous drainage
Chest/abdomen	Assessment of differential flow in true and false lumens after aortic dissection
	Evaluation for endoleaks after endograft repair of abdominal aortic aneurysm
	Preoperative evaluation of hepatic arterial and portal venous anatomy in potential liver donors
	Determination of adequacy of renal parenchymal perfusion in the presence of renal artery stenosis
Extremity	Evaluation of the hemodynamic significance of infrageniculate arterial occlusive disease
	Assessment of soft tissue enhancement in the presence of cellulitis
	Determination of degree of arteriovenous shunting in peripheral arteriovenous malformations
Venous	Confirmation of venous patency
	Determination of dominant venous collaterals in the presence of venous occlusion
General (incidental detection)	Hypervascular thyroid nodules
	Unknown arterial abnormalities (e.g., splenic/renal artery aneurysms)

Image Interpretation

Postprocessing

Generally, time resolved MR angiography is postprocessed inline on the MRI console, involving subtraction of the initial unenhanced data set from all subsequent data sets and presentation of the subtracted temporal volumes in a full-thickness MIP format for immediate review. Certain situations may require that off-axis reconstruction of one or more of the volumetric data sets be obtained, the diagnostic quality of which largely depends on the through-plane resolution and relative magnitudes of in-plane and through-plane resolutions. In cases in which these postprocessed images are inadequate for diagnostic interpretation, repeat time resolved MR angiography at a different projection or imaging parameters or both should be considered in view of the relatively small contrast dose involved.

Reporting

A single time resolved MR angiography acquisition, often of duration of no longer than 20 seconds, provides a considerable amount of morphologic and dynamic information that should be alluded to in the ensuing report. Arterial luminal patency, directional flow, parenchymal perfusion, venous drainage, and a wide variety of site-specific considerations, including degree of arteriovenous shunting within vascular malformations and differential perfusion with regard to symmetric viscera, must be carefully evaluated to detect subtle derangements. Because other MR angiography techniques provide little if any dynamic vascular information, particular reference should be made to this parameter when considering any time resolved MR angiography examination.

THREE-DIMENSIONAL CONTRAST-ENHANCED MAGNETIC RESONANCE ANGIOGRAPHY

High-resolution three-dimensional contrast-enhanced MR angiography has become one of the most powerful diagnostic tools in diagnostic imaging. This is due in large part to the introduction of high field MRI systems with rapid high-performance gradient coils and the development of phased array coils and, subsequently, parallel imaging techniques.[22] These advances have conspired to make large FOV high-resolution three-dimensional contrast-enhanced MR angiography during comfortable breath-hold times and in the absence of venous contamination a clinical reality.

Contrast-enhanced MR angiography depends on the ability of intravenously administered gadolinium-chelate contrast agents to shorten the T1 time of the target vascular bed. Properly timed, the T1 signal from the target vascular territory far exceeds that of adjacent nonenhanced extravascular background soft tissue, allowing confident detailed evaluation of luminal patency or mural irregularity. Using a three-dimensional T1-weighted spoiled GRE sequence similar to that described for time

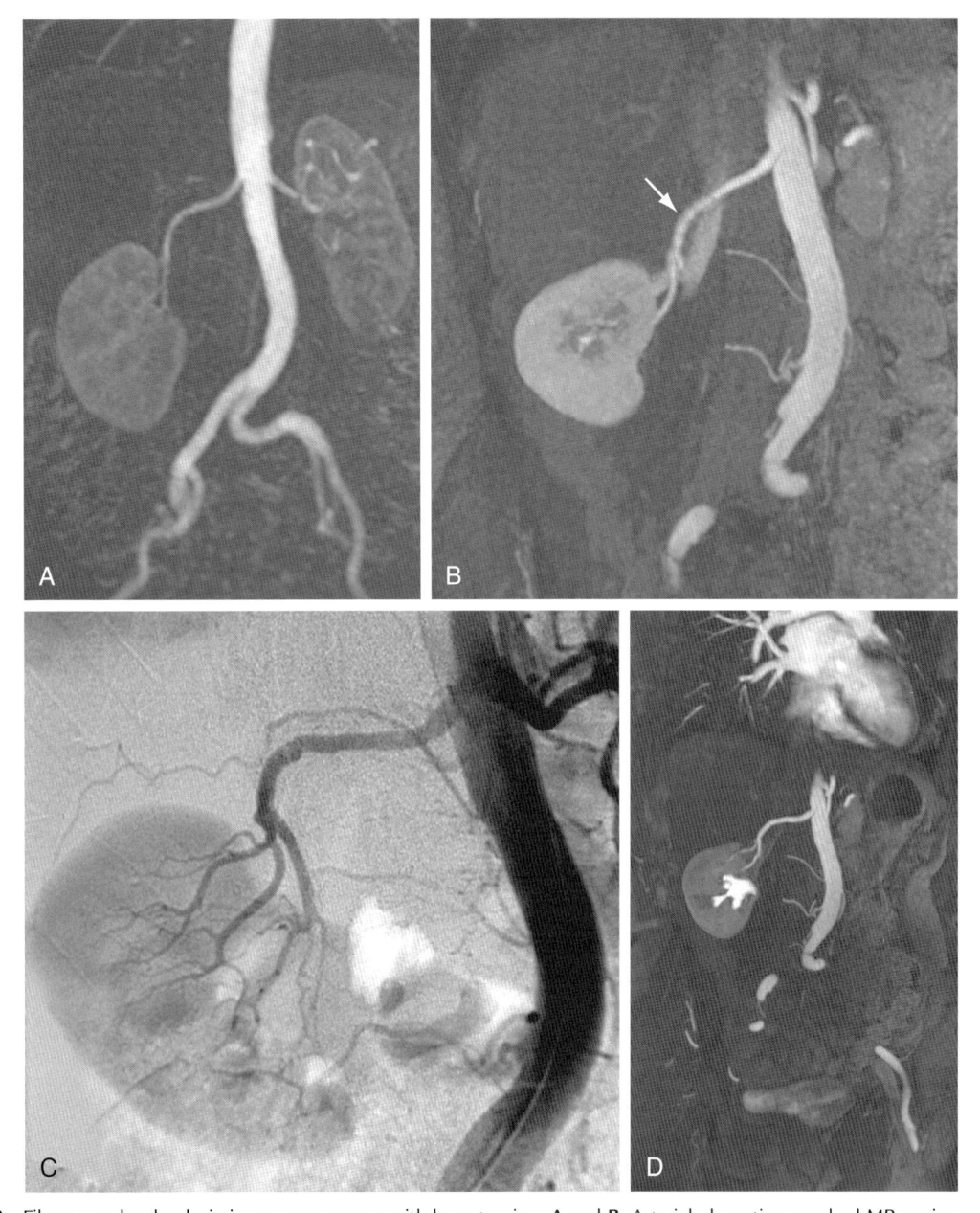

■ **FIGURE 82-8** Fibromuscular dysplasia in a young woman with hypertension. **A** and **B,** Arterial phase time resolved MR angiography reconstruction (**A**) and coronal oblique contrast-enhanced MR angiography MIP (**B**) show characteristic renal arterial "beading" of the right renal artery (*arrow*) of fibromuscular dysplasia. **C,** This was confirmed on conventional x-ray angiography and treated using percutaneous balloon angioplasty, with satisfactory clinical improvement. **D,** A good therapeutic result is also noted on postoperative contrast-enhanced MR angiography.

resolved MR angiography, the presence of an ultrashort TR results in saturation of signal from background soft tissues, enhancing the conspicuity of contrast-enhanced blood. The illustration of vessels may be augmented further by acquisition of an unenhanced data set before administration of contrast agent for use in subsequent "mask" subtraction.

Indications

The efficacy of three-dimensional contrast-enhanced MR angiography has been proven for almost every vascular territory, with the result that it has now replaced conventional diagnostic angiography as the imaging modality of choice for various clinical applications. The most common indication for contrast-enhanced MR angiography is the investigation of suspected atherosclerotic steno-occlusive disease.[23] This approach allows comprehensive, large-volume, detailed evaluation for the presence of mural irregularity, stenosis, dissection, or aneurysmal dilation, and permits accurate assessment of their effect on the adjacent vessel lumen. The most common territories routinely evaluated using this technique are extracranial carotid, supra-aortic, thoracic and abdominal aortic, renal, mesenteric, and peripheral extremity vessels (Figs. 82-8, 82-9, and 82-10).

Pulmonary vascular imaging has also benefited significantly from developments in contrast-enhanced MR angiography; this technique allows depiction of branch vessels of calibers of 1 to 2 mm. Contrast-enhanced MR angiogra-

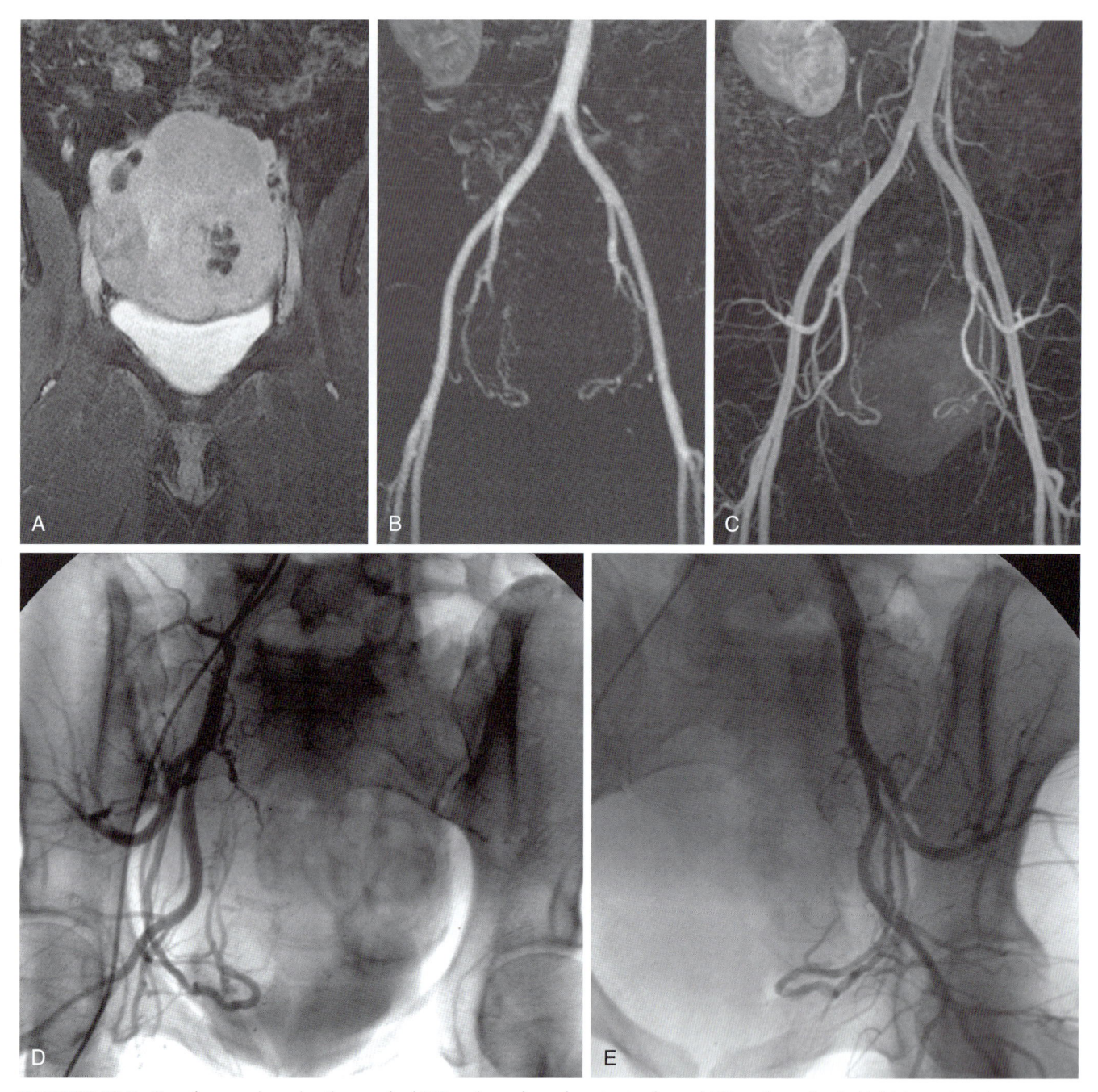

FIGURE 82-9 Vascular mapping using time resolved MR angiography and contrast-enhanced MR angiography. **A,** Multiple uterine leiomyomas seen on postcontrast fat-saturated T1-weighted GRE imaging. **B** and **C,** Isolated arterial phase TR MR angiography (**B**) and full-thickness contrast-enhanced MR angiography MIP (**C**), performed as a prelude to interventional therapy, allow high-quality depiction of the internal iliac arteries and branch vessels in the absence of venous contamination. **D** and **E,** Conventional catheter angiography, obtained at the time of fibroid embolization, are provided for comparison.

phy has now become a valuable tool in the evaluation of suspected pulmonary hypertension and determination of its potential etiology, such as chronic thromboembolic disease. The efficacy of this technique in diagnosis of acute pulmonary embolism has also been shown, and this may be of particular value in patients in whom iodinated contrast media are undesirable or contraindicated.[24]

The reproducibility of contrast-enhanced MR angiography has also led to its widespread adoption in the follow-up of patients who have undergone open surgical intervention for atherosclerotic occlusive disease, most often in the form of bypass grafts, especially extra-anatomic bypass grafts. Although the presence of anastomotic hemostatic clips occasionally may preclude visualization of such conduits throughout their length owing to metallic susceptibility artifact, this is rarely of such severity as to limit diagnostic interpretation.[25] Three-dimensional contrast-enhanced MR angiography has also proven to be of high diagnostic utility in the diagnosis of acute aortic events, such as dissection or intramural hematoma, vascular inflammatory conditions (e.g., Takayasu and giant cell arteritis), evaluation of coronary arterial

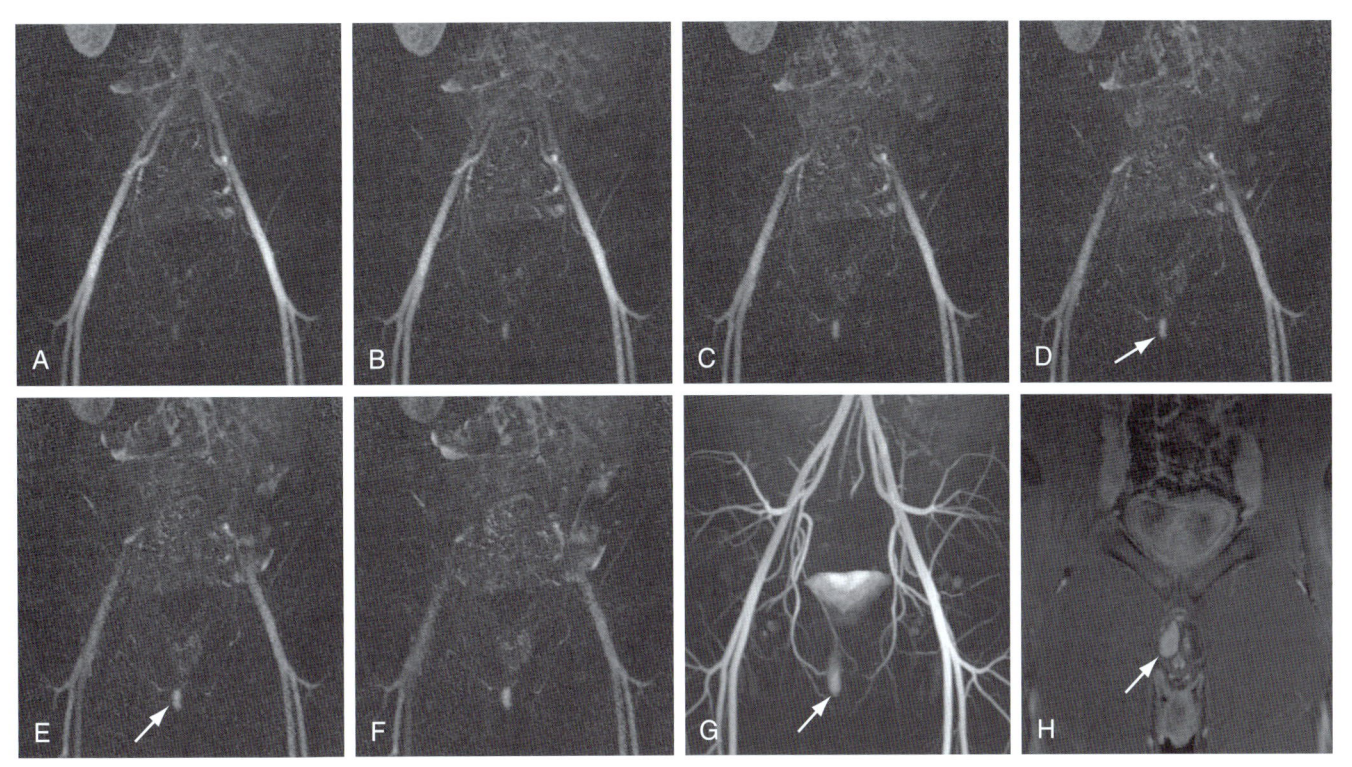

FIGURE 82-10 Traumatic arteriocavernosal fistula. **A-G,** Opacification of the right corpus cavernosum (*arrows* in **D, E,** and **G**) is seen on late arterial phase time resolved MR angiography images (**A-F**) and first-pass contrast-enhanced MR angiography (**G**). **H,** Disparity between right (*arrow*) and left cavernosal opacification is seen on postcontrast two-dimensional coronal fat-saturated T1-weighted imaging.

course and patency, and pediatric vascular abnormalities, including aortic coarctation (Figs. 82-11 and 82-12) and truncus arteriosus (Fig. 82-13), among many other conditions (Fig. 82-14).

Contraindications

As considered previously with regard to time resolved MR angiography, after general contraindications to MRI and previous reactions to gadolinium-chelate contrast agents have been excluded, contraindications specific to contrast-enhanced MR angiography relate to more recently developed concerns regarding the potential induction of nephrogenic systemic fibrosis. Contrast-enhanced MR angiography does differ from time resolved MR angiography, however, because the dose of contrast agent required is considerably larger. The larger dose is needed because of the longer acquisition times involved, demanding protracted bolus infusions at rates sufficient to reduce adequately the T1 of blood in which the contrast agent resides at a level sufficient for diagnostic interpretation. Although little is known at present regarding the relationship between gadolinium-chelate contrast agents and nephrogenic systemic fibrosis, current U.S. Food and Drug Administration recommendations are that these agents should be avoided, if possible, in high-risk individuals. In this situation, dose reduction using TR MR angiography or obviation of the need for contrast administration by use of one of the alternative MR angiography techniques described earlier may be considered, depending on the clinical indication.

Pitfalls and Solutions

Successful high-resolution contrast-enhanced MR angiography may be a challenging feat even with a cooperative subject, unless one possesses knowledge of the numerous grounds for potential error during this technique. Important prerequisites for diagnostic contrast-enhanced MR angiography include the following:

1. Timing data acquisition such that it corresponds with the arrival of the contrast bolus within the vessels in question. Specifically, filling of the center of k-space should be synchronized with peak luminal enhancement of the target vascular territory.
2. Maintenance of a compact contrast bolus with the effect of optimizing the T1 difference between enhanced blood and adjacent soft tissues.
3. Complete data acquisition during a period sufficient for avoidance of venous contamination.
4. Optimization of signal reception after the contrast medium is within the vascular territory of interest.
5. Prevention of patient motion artifact, in particular artifact related to respiratory suspension when imaging the chest and abdomen.

Compromise in any of these prerequisites may result in suboptimal contrast-enhanced MR angiography. Premature central k-space filling relative to the peak of the contrast bolus may result in intraluminal "pseudofilling defects" owing to inappropriate filling of the low spatial frequency data in this region of k-space. Failure of coordination of the contrast bolus and data acquisition such that

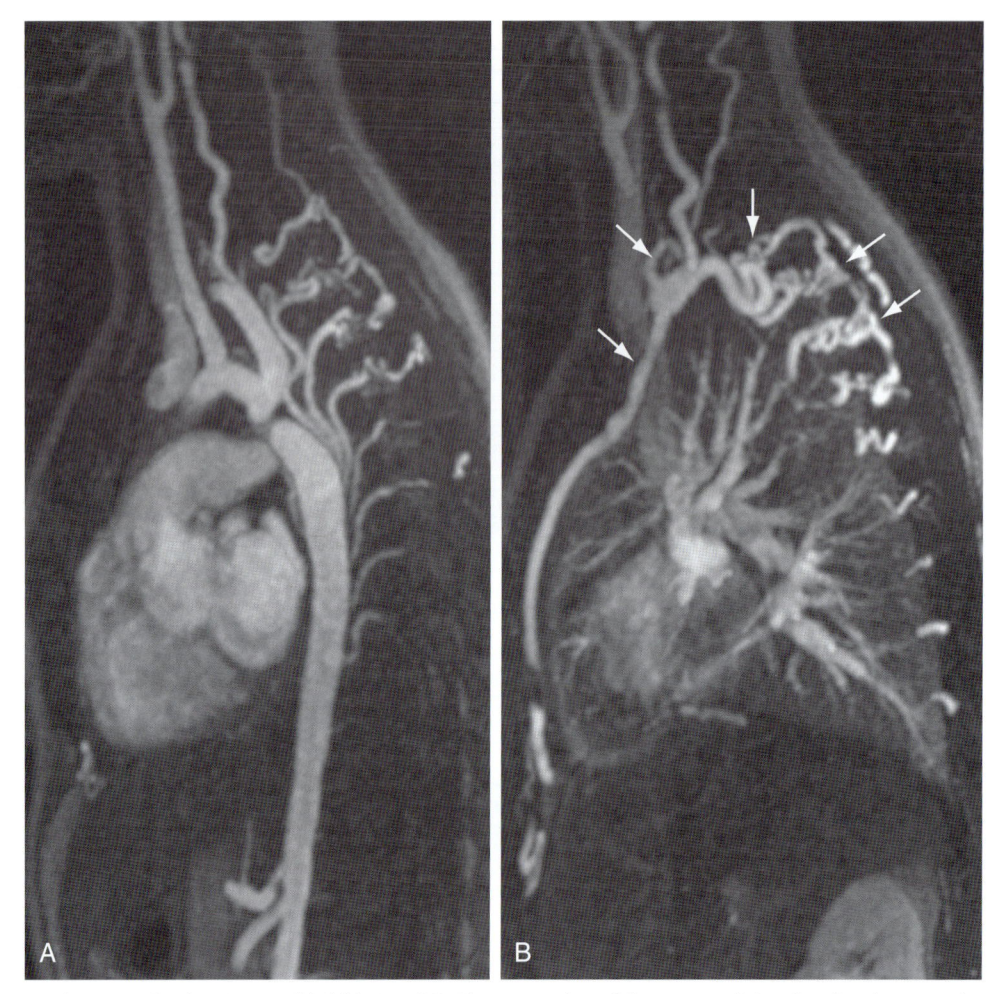

FIGURE 82-11 Aortic coarctation in a 2-year-old child. **A** and **B**, The coarctation of the aorta and the abundant intercostal, parascapular and internal mammary collateral vessels (*arrows* on **B**) are well illustrated on contrast-enhanced MR angiography sagittal oblique MIPs.

the arterial phase has passed and venous contamination is present may also obscure vascular detail, which is a particular disadvantage when imaging the lower extremities. Dispersion of the contrast bolus or poor signal reception may result in inadequate luminal enhancement, making identification of subtle vascular abnormalities impossible. Motion artifact also may have a significantly detrimental effect on image quality, owing to the production of blurring of vessel margins.[26]

Preemptive avoidance of many of these potential adversities is often readily achievable, however. Numerous methods have been developed to aid in bolus timing, including use of a test bolus, "fluoroscopic" or automated bolus detection of contrast arrival, incorporation of a fixed delay between contrast injection and start of data acquisition, and repetitive scanning so that different phases of opacification are obtained.[27] Although some methods (e.g., test bolus, real-time "fluoroscopy," and automated bolus detection algorithm) may be expected to produce more consistent results than others (e.g., fixed delay and multiphase imaging), familiarity with more than one technique is recommended so that timing issues in uncharacteristic cases may be addressed. Optimization of intravascular signal should involve a combination of MRI-compatible power injector and appropriate surface receiver coils, such that image contrast between the lumen and extravascular soft tissues is maximal. Motion artifact may be difficult, or occasionally impossible, to address—particularly in dyspneic patients because of the relatively long breath-hold times required for chest and abdominal contrast-enhanced MR angiography (approximately 20 seconds). Nonetheless, preprocedural coaching of patient respiratory suspension and attention to patient fears should represent a routine part of any contrast-enhanced MR angiography examination.

Image Interpretation

Postprocessing

Three-dimensional contrast-enhanced MR angiography provides a complete volumetric data set amenable to a wide variety of image post-processing.[28] MPRs are of significant practical value in the assessment of vascular patency, particularly in regions where overlapping vascular structures with tortuous courses are present (e.g., chest MR angiography). This holds particularly true when isotropic or near-isotropic voxels have been acquired because MPR allows reconstruction at any conceivable projection without the risk of image distortion or elongation. In certain instances, curved MPRs (whereby the axis of the reconstruction deviates from a single plane) may

CHAPTER 82 ● *Magnetic Resonance Angiography: Clinical Techniques*

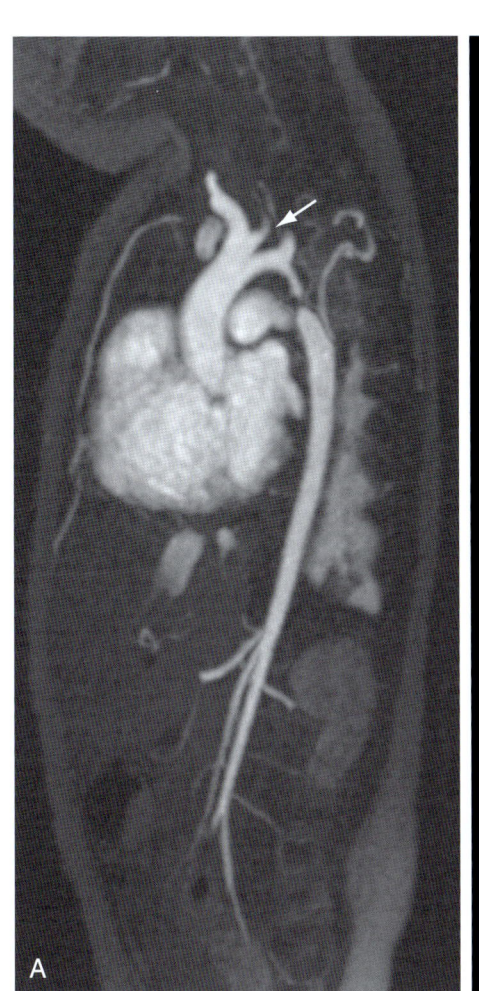

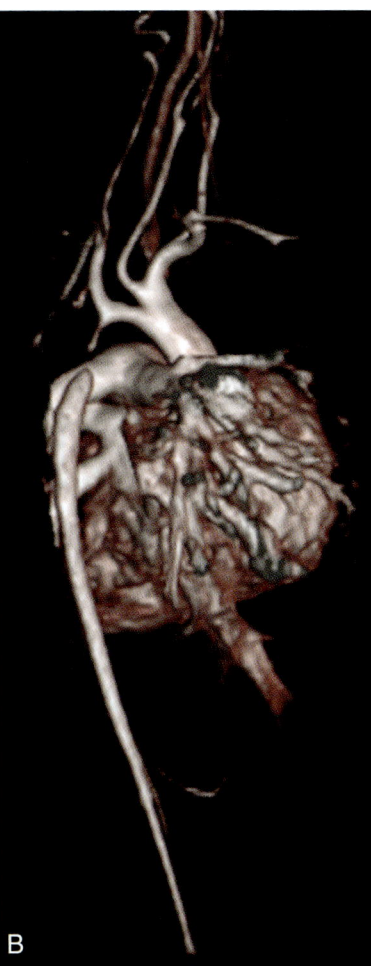

■ FIGURE 82-12 Newborn girl with preductal interruption of the aortic arch. **A** and **B**, On contrast-enhanced MR angiography (**A**, oblique sagittal MIP; **B**, opposite oblique sagittal volume rendered), hypoplasia of the aortic arch distal to the left subclavian origin is seen, followed by a short segment of occlusion (*arrow* on **A**). The distal thoracic aorta is perfused by a large patent ductus arteriosus.

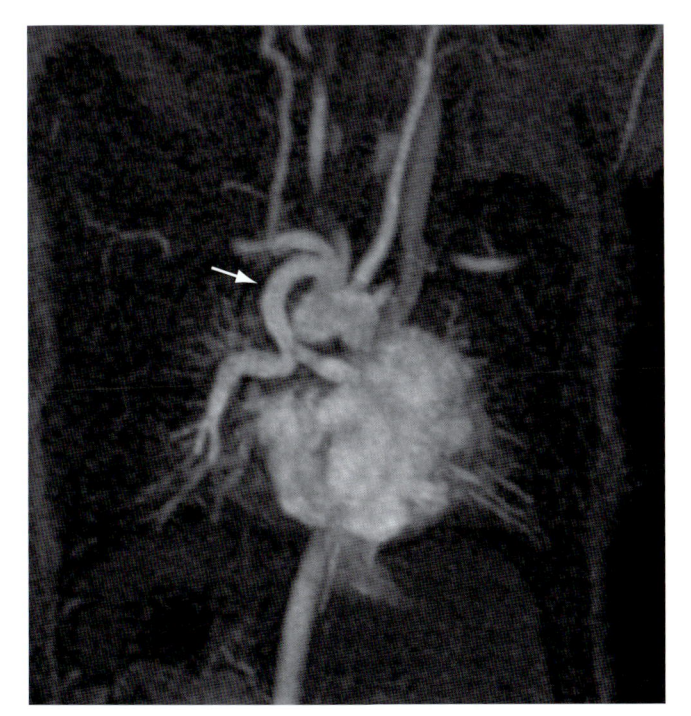

■ FIGURE 82-13 Newborn with a variant of truncus arteriosus type 1. On contrast-enhanced MR angiography, the pulmonary trunk (*arrow*) arises directly from the innominate artery, subsequently branching into normal-sized pulmonary arteries.

also be considerably valuable, most commonly in the determination of changes in caliber of long, tortuous vessels, such as the coronary arteries and thoracic aorta.

MIP reconstructions increase the conspicuity of the contrast-enhanced lumen by mapping the maximum signal intensity value at each location within a desired plane. Thin-section MIPs are popular in the evaluation of vascular patency, although they are known to result in overestimation of the significance of luminal stenoses, when present. Specific rotational full-thickness MIPs are routinely used at many institutions because they provide a quick means for demonstration of overall luminal integrity and vascular patency in a series of fixed projections.

Volume rendered techniques are among the most versatile for reconstructing three-dimensional contrast-enhanced MR angiography data. Volume rendering makes use of the information within each voxel to provide a two-dimensional projection of the three-dimensional data set, without compromise in through-plane attributes, and retains depth perception, a distinct advantage over MIP that provides a two-dimensional projection without depth information.

Reporting

Reporting of contrast-enhanced MR angiography examination requires that numerous key considerations are taken into account, including the following:

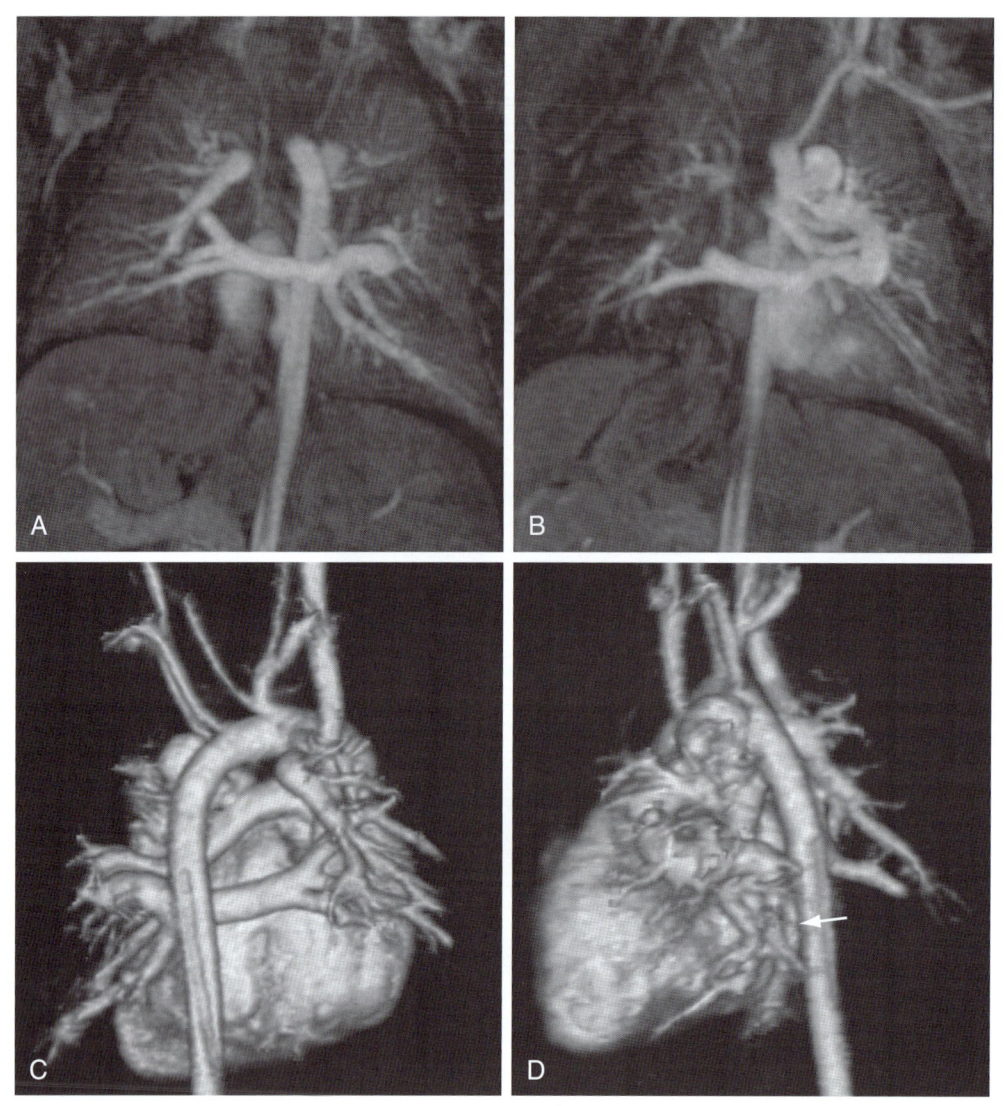

FIGURE 82-14 Total anomalous pulmonary venous return in a 2-month-old girl. **A-D,** Coronal contrast-enhanced MR angiography MIP reconstructions (**A** and **B**) and volume rendered reconstructions (**C** and **D**) illustrate confluence of the pulmonary veins bilaterally to form a horizontal vein with a vertical component (*arrow*) on the left side that subsequently drains to the coronary sinus. Volume rendered reconstructions are often valuable in preoperative assessment.

1. Location and morphology of vessel origins
2. Mural irregularity and, if present, the distribution and likely etiology of this irregularity (e.g., atherosclerosis, arteritis)
3. Focal mural pathology, in the form of plaque ulceration, dissection, or intramural hematoma
4. Location of stenoses and degree of associated luminal compromise
5. Presence, location, and extent of collateral circulatory pathways
6. Asymmetry in visceral enhancement and perfusion
7. Presence of vascular mural enhancement
8. Abnormal communication between two vascular territories or arteriovenous shunting

Because of its ability to provide high-resolution submillimeter-voxel data acquisition over large FOVs, careful analysis of a contrast-enhanced MR angiography examination and each of the vessels imaged is an arduous task. For this reason, initial analysis of the full-thickness MIP is preferred by some interpreting physicians, providing the physician with a "short list" of regions warranting further attention on MPR, subvolume MIP, or individual contrast-enhanced MR angiography partitions.

KEY POINTS

- The term *MR angiography* encompasses a variety of imaging techniques (e.g., TOF MR angiography, phase contrast MR angiography, SSFP MR angiography, time resolved MR angiography, contrast-enhanced MR angiography), each unique in design, implementation, and clinical applicability.
- An understanding of each technique, including common pitfalls and solutions, facilitates investigational versatility and improvements in image quality.
- Full exploitation of the promise of MR angiography techniques necessitates familiarity with appropriate hardware and data postprocessing tools.

SUGGESTED READINGS

Grobner T, Prischl FC. Gadolinium and nephrogenic systemic fibrosis. Kidney Int 2007; 72:260-264.

Ho VB, Foo TK, Czum JM, et al. Contrast-enhanced magnetic resonance angiography: technical considerations for optimized clinical implementation. Top Magn Reson Imaging 2001; 12:283-299.

Kramer H, Michaely HJ, Reiser MF, et al. Peripheral magnetic resonance angiography at 3.0 T. Top Magn Reson Imaging 2007; 18:135-138.

Meaney JF, Goyen M. Recent advances in contrast-enhanced magnetic resonance angiography. Eur Radiol 2007;17(Suppl 2):B2-B6.

Michaely HJ, Dietrich O, Nael K, et al. MRA of abdominal vessels: technical advances. Eur Radiol 2006; 16:1637-1650.

Ozsarlak O, Van Goethem JW, Maes M, et al. MR angiography of the intracranial vessels: technical aspects and clinical applications. Neuroradiology 2004; 46:955-972.

Stuber M, Weiss RG. Coronary magnetic resonance angiography. J Magn Reson Imaging 2007; 26:219-234.

Yucel EK, Anderson CM, Edelman RR, et al. AHA scientific statement. Magnetic resonance angiography: update on applications for extracranial arteries. Circulation 1999; 100:2284-2301.

Zhang H, Maki JH, Prince MR. 3D contrast-enhanced MR angiography. J Magn Reson Imaging 2007; 25:13-25.

REFERENCES

1. Bernstein MA, Huston J 3rd, Ward HA. Imaging artifacts at 3.0 T. J Magn Reson Imaging 2006; 24:735-746.
2. Rohrer M, Geerts-Ossevoort L, Laub G. Technical requirements, biophysical considerations and protocol optimization with magnetic resonance angiography using blood-pool agents. Eur Radiol 2007; 17(Suppl 2):B7-B12.
3. Pruessmann KP, Weiger M, Scheidegger MB, et al. SENSE: sensitivity encoding for fast MRI. Magn Reson Med 1999; 42:952-962.
4. Frydrychowicz A, Bley TA, Winterer JT, et al. Accelerated time-resolved 3D contrast-enhanced MR angiography at 3T: clinical experience in 31 patients. MAGMA 2006; 19:187-195.
5. Bosmans H, Marchal G, Lukito G, et al. Time-of-flight MR angiography of the brain: comparison of acquisition techniques in healthy volunteers. AJR Am J Roentgenol 1995; 164:161-167.
6. Davis WL, Blatter DD, Harnsberger HR, et al. Intracranial MR angiography: comparison of single-volume three-dimensional time-of-flight and multiple overlapping thin slab acquisition techniques. AJR Am J Roentgenol 1994; 163:915-920.
7. Sadikin C, Teng MM, Chen TY, et al. The current role of 1.5T non-contrast 3D time-of-flight magnetic resonance angiography to detect intracranial steno-occlusive disease. J Formos Med Assoc 2007; 106:691-699.
8. Wilcock DJ, Jaspan T, Worthington BS. Problems and pitfalls of 3D TOF magnetic resonance angiography of the intracranial circulation. Clin Radiol 1996; 50:526-532.
9. Ishimaru H, Ochi M, Morikawa M, et al. Accuracy of pre- and post-contrast 3D time-of-flight MR angiography in patients with acute ischemic stroke: correlation with catheter angiography. AJNR Am J Neuroradiol 2007; 28:923-926.
10. Dumoulin CL, Souza SP, Walker MF, et al. Three-dimensional phase contrast angiography. Magn Reson Med 1989; 9:139-149.
11. Marks MP, Pelc MJ, Ross MR, et al. Determination of cerebral blood flow with a phase-contrast cine MR imaging technique: evaluation of normal subjects and patients with arteriovenous malformation. Radiology 1992; 182:467-476.
12. Baledent O, Gondry-Jouet C, Stoquart-Elsankari S, et al. Value of phase contrast magnetic resonance imaging for investigation of cerebral hydrodynamics. J Neuroradiol 2006; 33:292-303.
13. Reeder SB, Herzka DA, McVeigh ER. Signal-to-noise ratio behavior of steady-state free precession. Magn Reson Med 2004; 52:123-130.
14. Zagrosek A, Noeske R, Abdel-Aty H, et al. MR coronary angiography using 3D-SSFP with and without contrast application. J Cardiovasc Magn Reson 2005; 7:809-814.
15. Maki JH, Wilson GJ, Eubank WB, et al. Steady-state free precession MRA of the renal arteries: breath-hold and navigator-gated techniques vs CE-MRA. J Magn Reson Imaging 2007; 26:966-973.
16. Wansapura J, Fleck R, Crotty E, et al. Frequency scouting for cardiac imaging with SSFP at 3 Tesla. Pediatr Radiol 2006; 36:1082-1085.
17. Stuber M, Weiss RG. Coronary magnetic resonance angiography. J Magn Reson Imaging 2007; 26:219-234.
18. Finn JP, Baskaran V, Carr JC, et al. Thorax: low-dose contrast-enhanced three-dimensional MR angiography with subsecond temporal resolution—initial results. Radiology 2002; 224:896-904.
19. Korosec FR, Frayne R, Grist TM, et al. Time-resolved contrast-enhanced 3D MR angiography. Magn Reson Med 1996; 36:345-351.
20. Sieber MA, Peitsch H, Walter J, et al. A preclinical study to investigate the development of nephrogenic systemic fibrosis: a possible role for gadolinium-based contrast media. Invest Radiol 2008; 43:65-75.
21. Michaely HJ, Nael K, Schoenberg SO, et al. Renal perfusion: comparison of saturation-recovery TurboFLASH measurements at 1.5T with saturation-recovery TurboFLASH and time-resolved echo-shared angiographic technique (TREAT) at 3.0T. J Magn Reson Imaging 2006; 24:1413-1419.
22. Michaely HJ, Herrmann KA, Kramer H, et al. High-resolution renal MRA: comparison of image quality and vessel depiction with different parallel imaging acceleration factors. J Magn Reson Imaging 2006; 24:95-100.
23. Hansen T, Ahlstrom H, Johansson L. Whole-body screening of atherosclerosis with magnetic resonance angiography. Top Magn Reson Imaging 2007; 18:329-337.
24. Pleszewski B, Chartrand-Lefebvre C, Qanadli SD, et al. Gadolinium-enhanced pulmonary magnetic resonance angiography in the diagnosis of acute pulmonary embolism: a prospective study on 48 patients. Clin Imaging 2006; 30:166-172.
25. Loewe C, Cejna M, Schoder M, et al. Contrast material-enhanced, moving-table MR angiography versus digital subtraction angiography for surveillance of peripheral arterial bypass grafts. J Vasc Interv Radiol 2003; 14(9 Pt 1):1129-1137.
26. Spincemaille P, Hai ZX, Cheng L, et al. Motion artifact suppression in breath hold 3D contrast enhanced magnetic resonance angiography using ECG ordering. Conf Proc IEEE Eng Med Biol Soc 2006; 1:739-742.
27. Shetty AN, Bis KG, Kirsch M, et al. Contrast-enhanced breath-hold three-dimensional magnetic resonance angiography in the evaluation of renal arteries: optimization of technique and pitfalls. J Magn Reson Imaging 2000; 12:912-923.
28. Lell M, Fellner C, Baum U, et al. Evaluation of carotid artery stenosis with multisection CT and MR imaging: influence of imaging modality and postprocessing. AJNR Am J Neuroradiol 2007; 28:104-110.

CHAPTER 83

Basic Three-Dimensional Postprocessing in Computed Tomographic and Magnetic Resonance Angiography

Ting Song, William R. Corse, and Vincent B. Ho*

The three-dimensional data acquired by computed tomography angiography (CTA) or magnetic resonance angiography (MRA) can be processed off-line using a variety of commercially available techniques that enable isolation and improved viewing of specific vascular segments and their anatomic relationships. The most popular and widely available postprocessing tools for CTA and MRA data are multiplanar reformation (MPR), maximum intensity projection (MIP), and volume rendering (VR).[1-5] This chapter reviews these basic methods for postprocessing of CTA and MRA data, highlighting their strengths and pitfalls. For different clinical applications, the specific methods of highest value will vary. Individual techniques for various anatomic regions are covered elsewhere in this text.

MULTIPLANAR REFORMATION

MPR refers to the reconstruction of three-dimensional data into a new orientation. For example, a volumetric CTA data set acquired in the axial plane can be reconstructed for viewing in a coronal plane or a plane of any obliquity using MPR. MPR images can be reconstructed into linear (e.g., coronal, sagittal, axial, oblique; Figs. 83-1 and 83-2) or curved plane images (Fig. 83-3). The process does not change the original data or voxels. In the MPR process, interpolation is needed to rearrange data into a different coordinate system. Curved reformatting is useful for viewing tortuous vessels such as the coronary arteries on CTA because it unravels the tortuous segments for linear viewing of the vessel (i.e., straightens out the vessel in length). It is particularly useful for showing vascular detail in cross-sectional profile along the vessel length, facilitating characterization of stenoses or other intraluminal abnormalities. The pitfall is that manual definition of curved planes may not be accurate for actual measurements and is potentially a time-consuming process because operator interaction is often required. Automated curve detection methods can expedite processing but fail if there are image artifacts within the data (e.g., motion blurring or high-value nonvascular structures such as calcium on CTA). These may be erroneously labeled as vessel lumen, thereby introducing inaccurate curved vascular lumen reformation.

Nearest Neighbor Interpolation

Interpolation is an important concept in the context of image reconstruction. As demonstrated in Figure 83-4, a slice of an original acquired image is composed of known data points. In this example, the circles are known data grids. Triangles are points that need to be interpolated because of MPR needs. The left known data signal inten-

---

*The opinions or assertions contained herein are the private views of the authors and are not to be construed as official or reflecting the views of the Department of Defense or the Uniformed Services University of the Health Sciences.

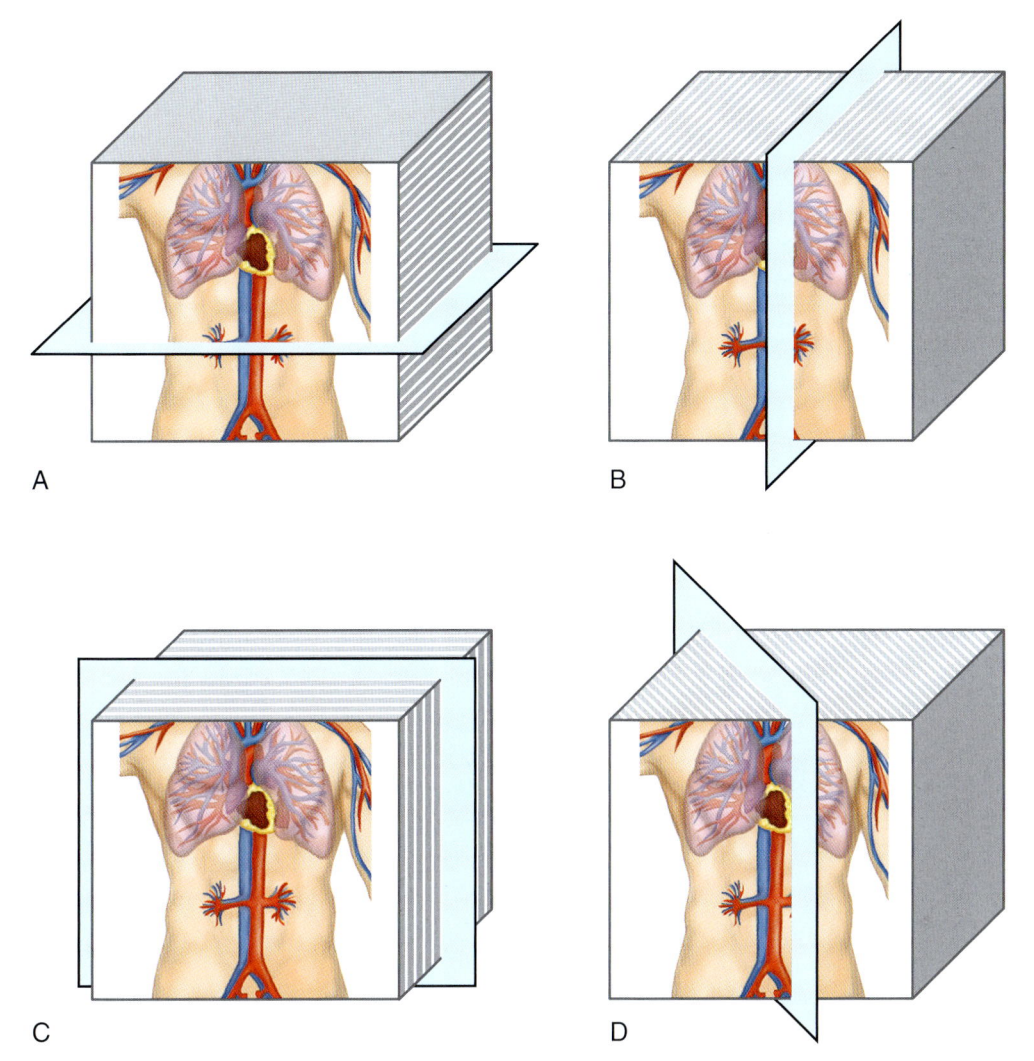

FIGURE 83-1 Multiplanar reformation (MPR). **A,** The diagram represents a stack of axial images that can be reconstructed and interpolated to a three-dimensional volume. Sagittal (**B**) and coronal (**C**) MPR views can be sampled and generated from it. **D,** It can also be sampled in an arbitrary oblique MPR view, which can be used for improved visualization of specific vascular segments.

sity (SI) value is $SI_a = 100$, and right known signal intensity value is $SI_b = 100$. The simplest interpolation is the nearest neighbor. In nearest neighbor interpolation, the new interpolated data point (i.e., triangle) is closer to the right data point, where SI_b is, so the unknown interpolated signal intensity (SI_i) is set to be the same as SI_b, that is, SI_i.

Linear Interpolation

Another simple method is linear interpolation. Using the same example as in Figure 83-4, the distance for the points are $x_a = 1$, $x_i = 3$, and $x_b = 4$. The signal intensities for known points are $SI_a = 10$ and $SI_b = 100$. The interpolated value SI_i for the triangle is linear interpolation as given by equation (1):

$$SI_i = SI_a + ([x_i - x_a][SI_b - SI_a])/(x_b - x_a). \quad (1)$$

Therefore $SI_i = 70$. This example is a one-dimensional demonstration. Three-dimensional (3D) interpolation is used in 3D data processing. Furthermore, additional, more sophisticated interpolation such as the cubic spline approach is sometimes used. The basic concept behind MPR is to use acquired known image data from CTA or MRA data sets to generate new or "unknown" data for viewing of the data in different views by interpolation.

MAXIMUM INTENSITY PROJECTION

MIP is another common method for two-dimensional projectional viewing CTA and MRA three-dimensional data. In MIP, the highest signal intensity values are projected from the data encountered by a ray cast through an object to the viewer's eye (Fig. 83-5). MIP is not averaging the average signal intensities from slice to slice along the projected axis (mean value); instead, it finds the highest value along a projection line and assigns that value to the pixel represented on the two-dimensional projected image. For CTA, the pixel values are in density or Hounsfield units; for MRA, the pixel values are in signal intensity. In this way, three-dimensional data can be collapsed into a two-dimensional projection image (see Fig. 83-2). MIP can be generated using the whole three-dimensional volume or a smaller subvolume (slab, or subvolume MIP; Figs. 83-6 and 83-7).

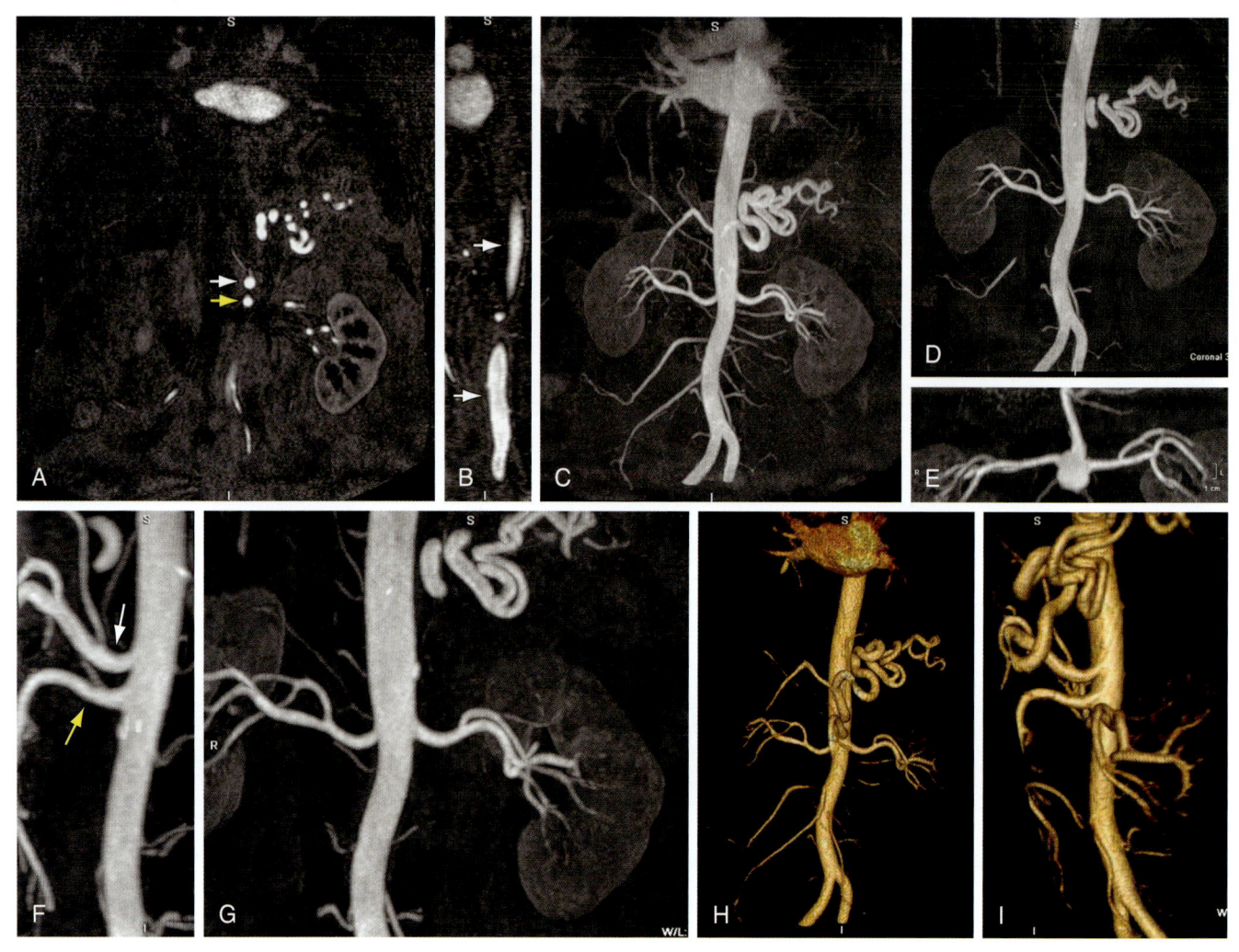

■ **FIGURE 83-2** Normal renal contrast-enhanced three-dimensional MPR. With MPR, a single-voxel view of the three-dimensional data set can be individually visualized. **A,** On the coronal MPR, the celiac trunk (*white arrow*) and superior mesenteric artery (*yellow arrow*) are seen but their relationship to the renal arteries and aorta is not evident because the coronal MPR does not include these structures. **B,** Similarly, on a sagittal MPR, only a portion of the abdominal aorta (*arrows*) is included on this coronal MPR obtained at the edge of the abdominal aorta. **C,** On a whole-volume coronal MIP, the renal arteries and their origin from the abdominal aorta are much more clearly viewed than on the thin single-voxel MPR. On subvolume MIP (**D,** coronal; **E,** axial; **F,** sagittal; **G,** oblique coronal), overlapping structures can be excluded from the slab to visualize the renal arteries preferentially. **F,** On the sagittal subvolume MIP, the origins of the celiac trunk (*white arrow*) and superior mesenteric artery (*yellow arrow*) can be clearly seen arising anteriorly from the abdominal aorta. On VR (**H,** coronal; **I,** oblique sagittal), the observer is provided with improved depth perception of the abdominal aorta and renal arteries compared with MIP images (compare **H** with **C**).

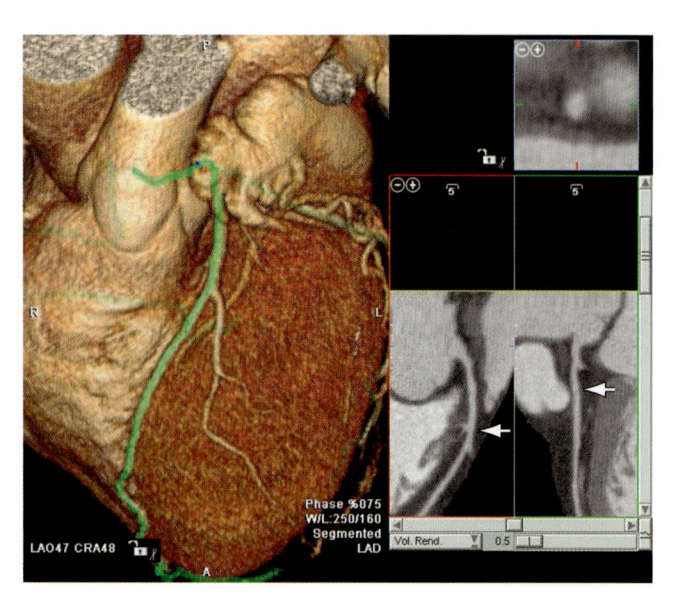

■ **FIGURE 83-3** Normal coronary CTA. *Lower right images,* The proximal left anterior descending (LAD) coronary artery (*arrows*) is well seen on curved MPR. *Top right image,* Cross section of the proximal LAD is shown. *Left,* Actual green line tracing used to predict the curved MPR on a VR projection of the coronary CTA. Ao, aortic root.

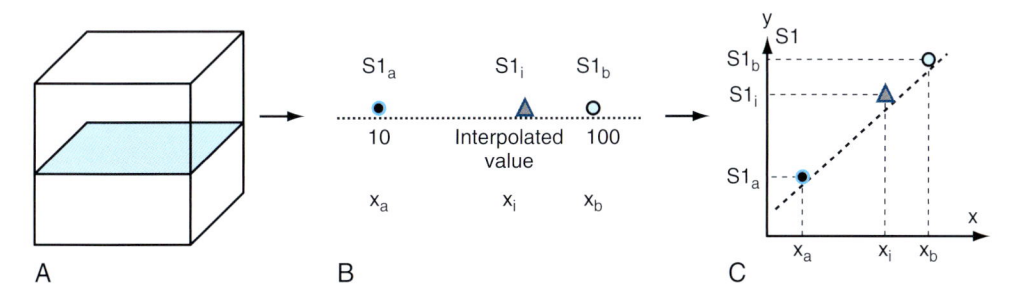

CHAPTER 83 • Basic Three-Dimensional Postprocessing in CT and MR Angiography 1123

■ **FIGURE 83-4** Multiplanar reformation. **A,** A slice of the original acquired image composed of known data points. **B,** Example of two known grids with an oblique line that are defined by oblique MPR. Circles are data grids that are known. Triangles are points that need to be interpolated because of MPR needs. **C,** Explanation in SI − x coordinate.

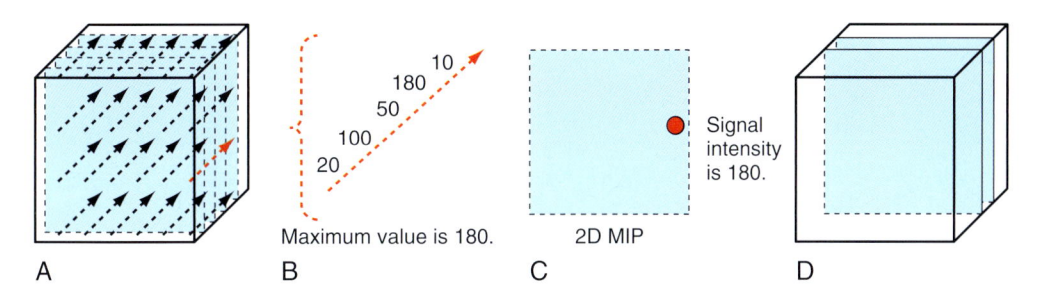

■ **FIGURE 83-5** Maximum intensity projection. **A,** Three-dimensional MRA data set. The viewer's eye cast ray projections from front to back into the page. **B,** One of the projection rays is zoomed in, with signal intensities of 20, 100, 50, 180, and 10. The highest intensity is 180. **C,** Corresponding projected point on two-dimensional MIP image. A signal intensity of 180 is assigned to that pixel. **D,** Subvolume MIP that is projected through limited volume, or slab, of the entire three-dimensional data set.

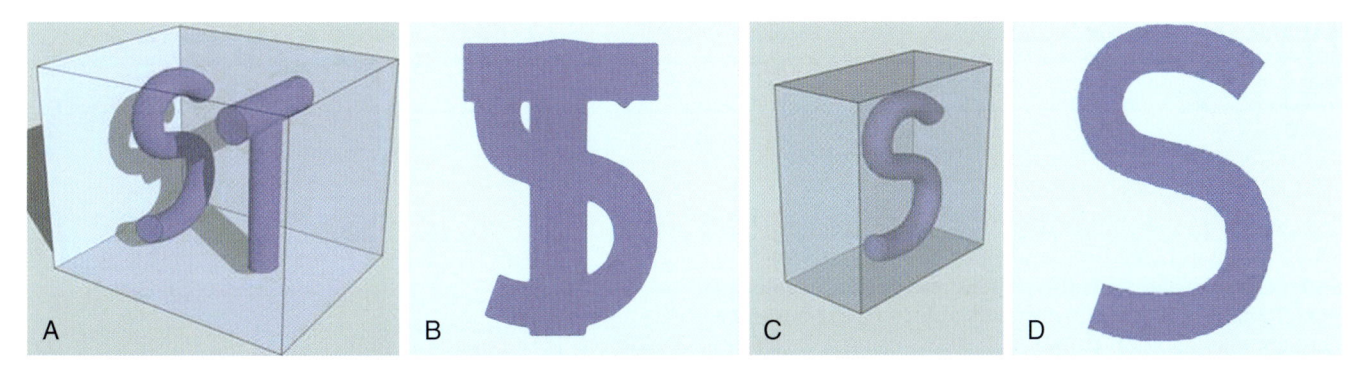

■ **FIGURE 83-6** Subvolume MIP. **A,** Two parallel three-dimensional objects (letters S and T) will overlap each other on a frontal MIP projection **(B)** such that the margins of the individual letters overlap and are not distinct. **C,** On a subvolume MIP, one object (S) can be isolated from the other object (T) and reconstructed so that only the target object will be seen on the subvolume MIP **(D)**.

MIP is useful for projected viewing of CTA and MRA in views similar to conventional x-ray angiograms. MIP images provide the big picture but are often suboptimal for viewing specific segments that are tortuous, such as near vessel origins or bifurcations, where subvolume MIP may be more helpful, especially if there are overlapping vessels such as the celiac artery (Fig. 83-8). Furthermore, because it projects simply brightest value, full-volume or thick MIP processing does not provide depth perception because the three-dimensional data are collapsed for viewing of only the brightest values. Subvolume MIP provides planar viewing of thinner volumes versus single-voxel viewing using MPR but may also mask luminal abnormalities. With MIP, the pitfall is that of a loss in depth information. Therefore, MIP misrepresents anatomic spatial relationships in depth directions. Moreover, MIP shows only the highest intensity along the projected ray. A high-intensity mass such as calcification will obscure information from intravascular contrast material. Vessels with low signal intensity values may be partially or completely imperceptible on MIP images. Alternatively, the bright signal of the lumen may mask subtle detail such as an intimal tear in an arterial dissection.

VOLUME RENDERING

Volume rendering (VR) is a visualization technique that represents a three-dimensional CTA or MRA data set (see Figs. 83-2, 83-7, and 83-8) as an opaque or translucent fashion but preserves the depth information of the data

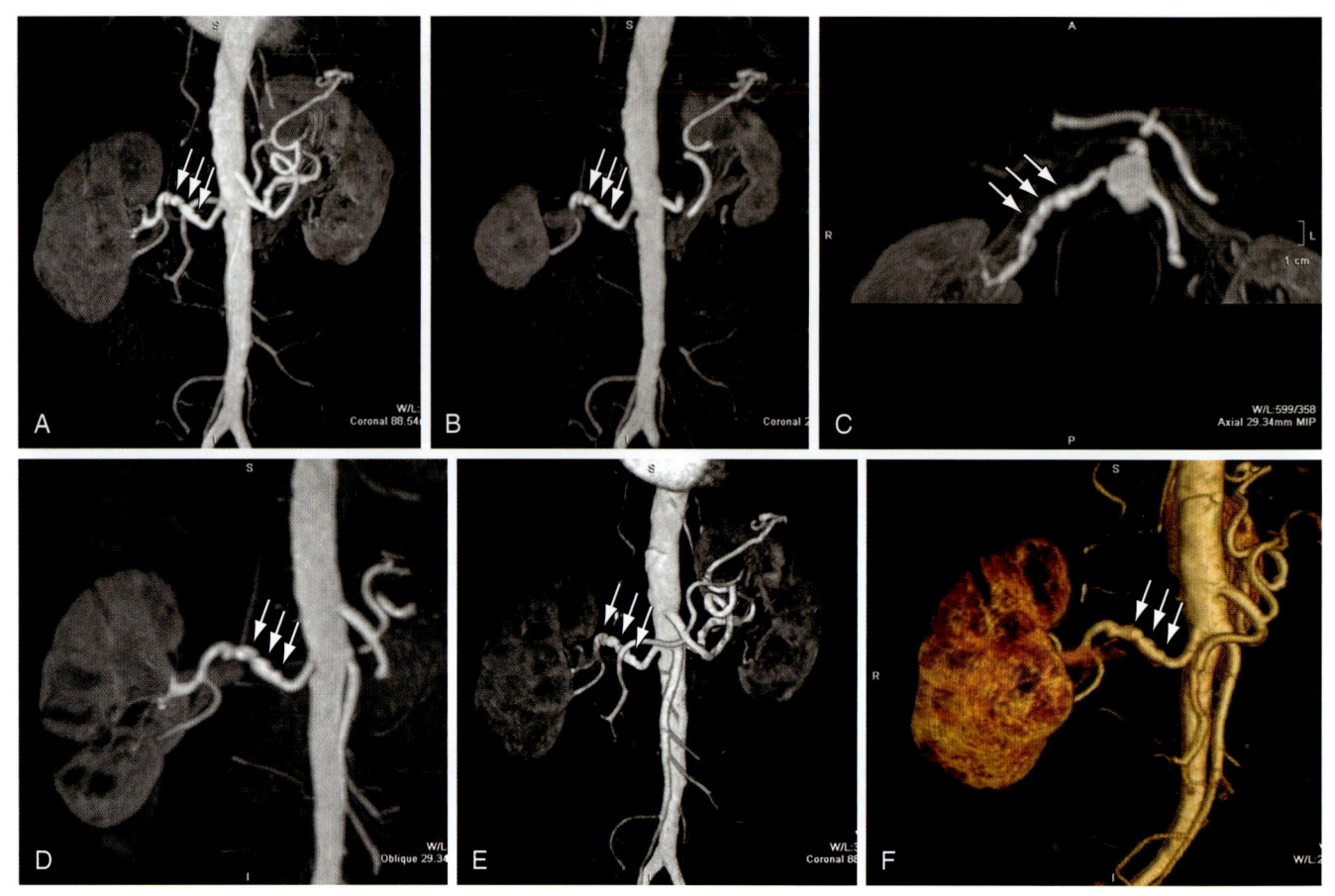

FIGURE 83-7 Renal fibromuscular dysplasia (FMD) on contrast-enhanced three-dimensional MRA. On MIP (**A**, coronal thick slab; **B**, coronal thin slab; **C**, thin slab axial; **D**, thin slab oblique coronal), the typical string of beads appearance of FMD (*arrows*) is seen in the mid–right renal artery. Minimizing the target volume on a subvolume MIP allows improved viewing of the three-dimensional data so that overlapping structures can be removed (compare **A** with **B**). This is seen also on VR (**E**, coronal; **F**, oblique coronal). The improved depth perception is evident on VR (compare **F** with **D**).

set, which is not afforded by MIP reconstruction (Fig. 83-9). It has replaced most imaging applications such as surface rendering, with the notable exception of interior vessel analysis. VR assigns opacity values based on a percentage classification from 0% to 100% using a variety of computational techniques. It uses all acquired data, so it needs greater processing power than the other applications discussed. Once the data have been assigned percentages, each tissue is assigned a color and degree of transparency. Then, by casting simulated rays of light through the volume, VR generates a three-dimensional image. The color used in volume rendering is a pseudocolor, which does not represent the true optical color of the tissues. However, color enhances the human eyes' ability to perceive depth relationships (see Fig. 83-3). On VR reconstruction, the three-dimensional data can be visualized using various degrees of opacity and transparency, which afford different viewing perspectives of the image data (Fig. 83-10).

The basic idea of volume rendering is to find the best approximation of the low-albedo volume rendering optical model that represents the relation between the volume intensity and opacity function and the intensity in the image plane. A common theoretical model on which VR algorithms are based is described in equation (2)[6]:

$$I_\lambda(x, r) = \sum_{k=1}^{M} C_\lambda(s_k)\alpha(s_k) \cdot \prod_{i=1}^{k-1}(1-\alpha(s_i)) \qquad (2)$$

where α is the opacity samples along the ray and C is the local color values derived from the illumination model. All algorithms obtain colors and opacities in discrete intervals along a linear path and composite them in front to back order. The raw volume densities are used to index the transfer functions for color and opacity; thus, the fine details of the volume data can be expressed in the final image using different transfer functions.

Therefore, there are many adjustable parameters in volume rendering, such as window center, window width, color, transparency, degree of opacity, and shading. Different vendors have different standards for parameters as well as core algorithms for volume rendering, so the appearance of rendered images may vary slightly among vendors.

In the volume rendering process, geometric structures from volume data and render volumes are based on fuzzy or percentage classification and are different from, and generally more useful than, images generated using surface rendering. VR is actually a direct volume-rendering (DVR) method. DVR techniques include ray casting, splatting,

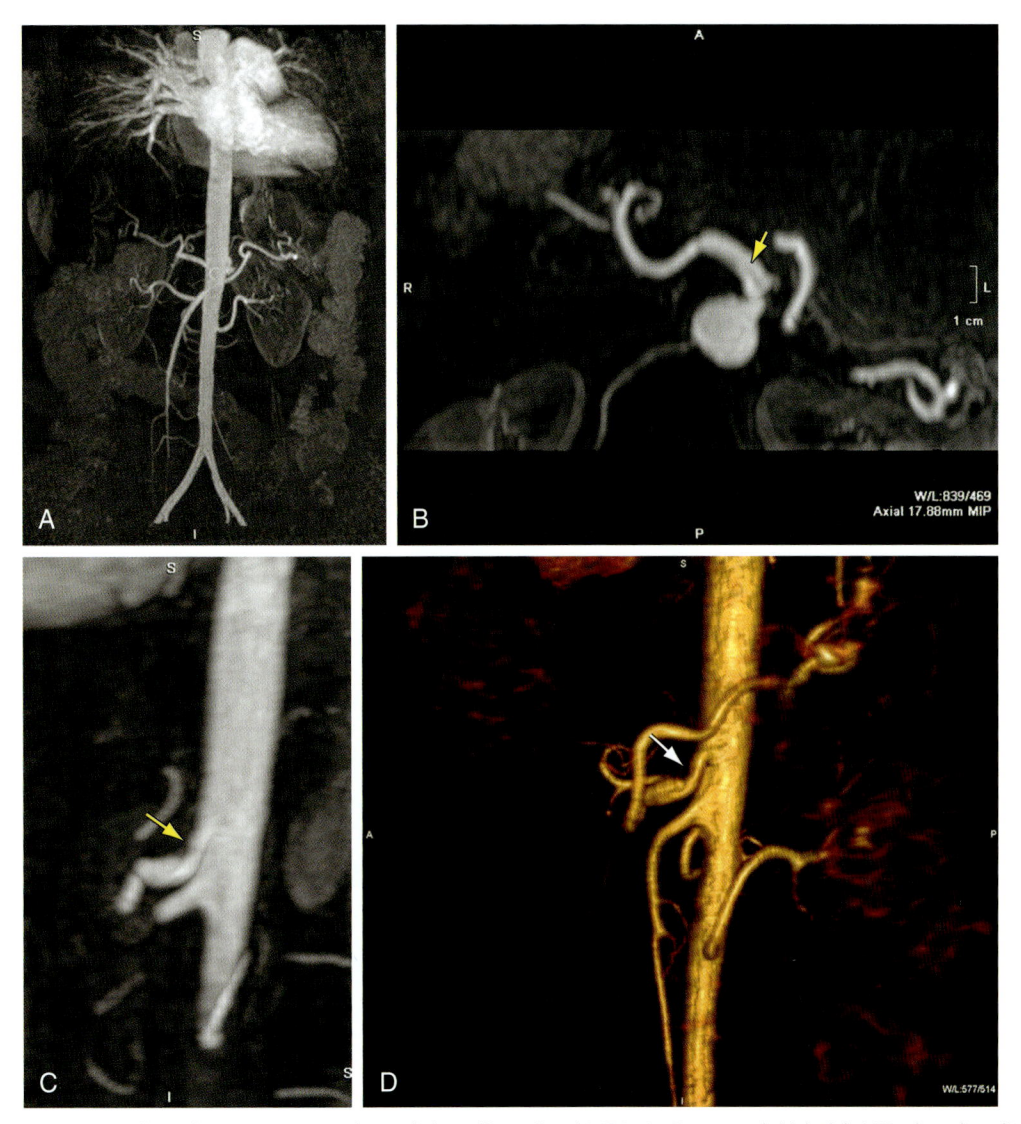

■ FIGURE 83-8 Celiac artery dissection on contrast-enhanced three-dimensional MRA. **A,** On coronal thick slab MIP, the celiac dissection is not clearly seen. **B,** However, on axial subvolume MIP, an intimal flap (*arrow*) is noted in the proximal celiac artery. **C,** Sagittal subvolume MIP shows the celiac artery dissection (*arrow*) as a spiral indentation to the superior surface of the proximal true lumen of the proximal celiac artery. Note that on contrast-enhanced MRA, gadolinium chelate contrast medium fills both the true and false lumen, if patent. In these images, the true lumen (inferior channel) is well seen but there is incomplete filling of the superiorly located false lumen, which results in the appearance of a superior spiral indentation to the proximal celiac artery. **D,** On oblique sagittal VR, the spiral indentation of the unopacified false channel (*arrow*) and the intimal flap just distal to the indentation are more clearly demonstrated.

shear warp, texture mapping, and hardware-driven volume rendering. Each approach has its own advantages and disadvantages. Shear warp and three-dimensional texture mapping volume rendering are devised to maximize frame rates at the expense of image quality and are used for the assessment of dynamic three-dimensional data sets. Image-aligned splatting and ray casting are devised to achieve high image quality at the expense of performance. A combination of these techniques is possible based on specific applications. However, this discussion is beyond the scope of this basic introductory chapter on three-dimensional postprocessing.

KEY POINTS

- Three-dimensional data sets from CTA and MRA can be viewed using a variety of postprocessing tools, most commonly, multiplanar reformation, maximum intensity projection, and volume rendering.
- MPR provides reconstructed viewing of three-dimensional data in an arbitrary plane that can be linear (e.g., axial, coronal, sagittal, oblique) or curved.
- MIP generates two-dimensional projectional views of the three-dimensional data set and can be performed as a thick full data or thinner slab subvolume reconstruction. Subvolume MIP provides improved ability to isolate and view specific vascular segments.
- VR retains image depth information for improved viewing of vascular structures compared with MIP.

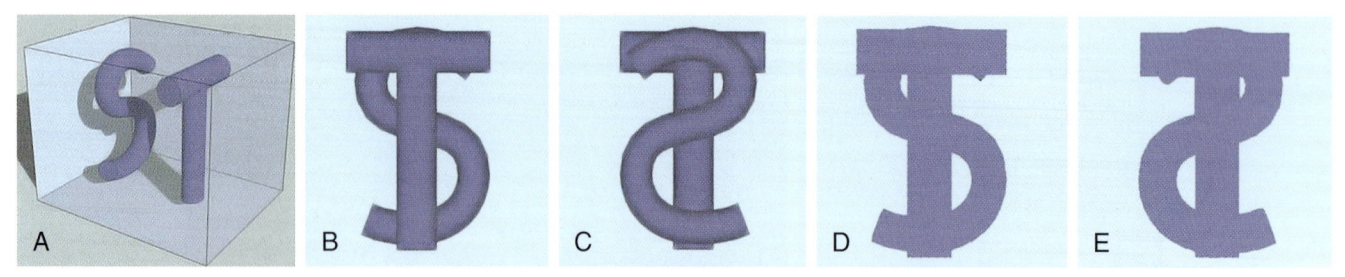

■ **FIGURE 83-9** Volume rendering versus maximum intensity projection reconstruction. **A**, Two three-dimensional objects are shown. If volume rendering is used, the depth information is preserved, thereby showing the relationship between the two objects in a front view (**B**) or back view (**C**). However, on MIP reconstruction, separation of the objects (S and T) is not evident because the contours of the objects overlap and blend, making visual separation difficult. On the MIP images (**D**, front view; **E**, back view), the contours of both objects blend and it is hard to see the spatial depth relationship (i.e., which is in the foreground versus which is in the background).

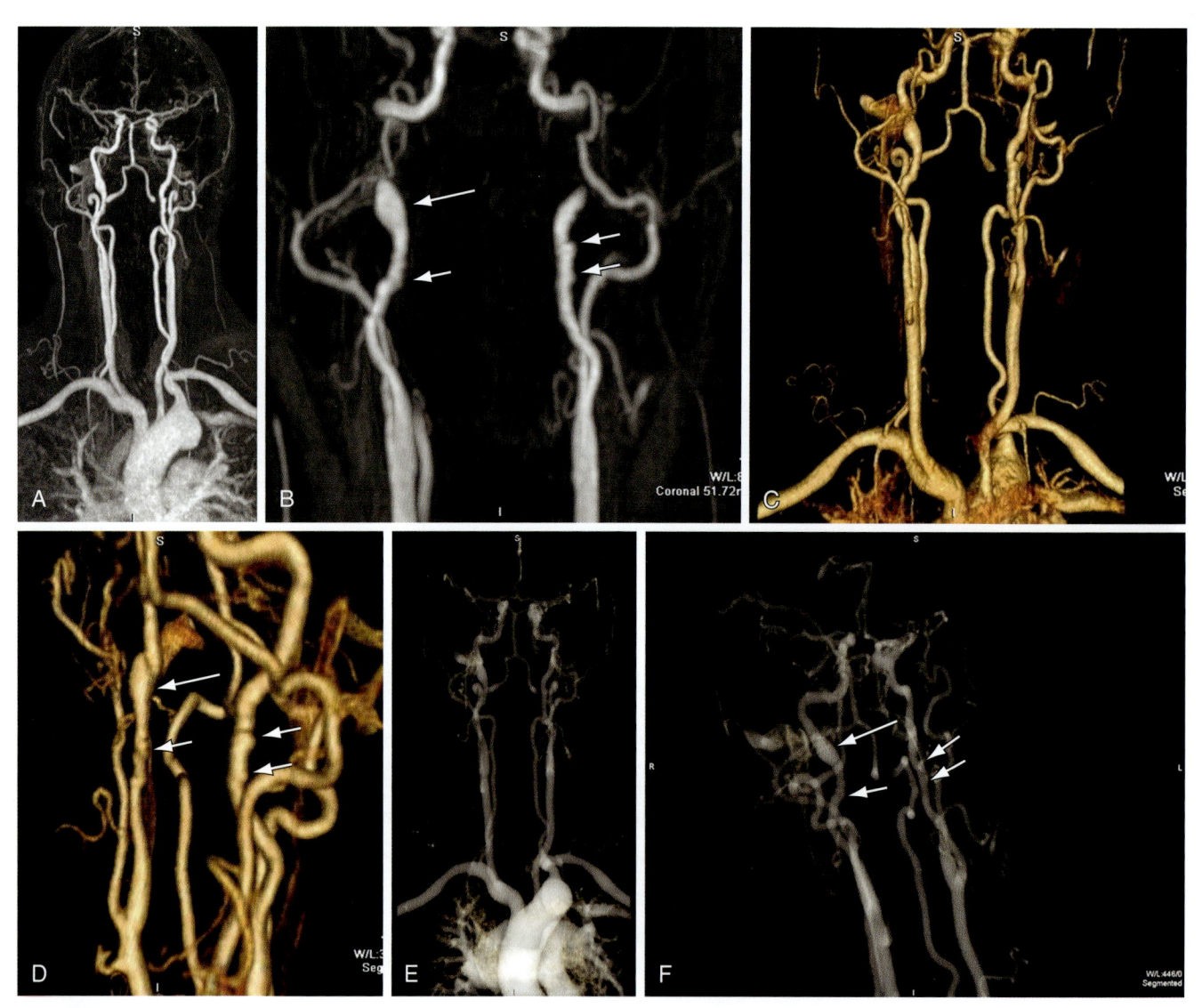

■ **FIGURE 83-10** Bilateral internal carotid artery fibromuscular dysplasia (FMD). **A**, On thick slab MIP, the string of beads appearance characteristic for FMD is not immediately evident. **B**, However, on thinner subvolume MIP, the string of beads appearance is seen in both internal carotid arteries (*arrows*), with an aneurysm (*large arrow*) in the distal right internal carotid artery. On opaque volume rendered (VR) (**C**, coronal; **D**, oblique sagittal), the string of beads (**D**, *arrows*) and distal right aneurysm (**D**, *large arrow*) is again noted. Similarly on translucent VR views (**E**, coronal; **F**, oblique sagittal), the same findings are noted. On translucent VR views, one can see through the vascular structures.

SUGGESTED READINGS

Cody DD. AAPM/RSNA physics tutorial for residents: topics in CT. Image processing in CT. Radiographics 2002; 22:1255-1268.

Fishman EK, Ney DR, Heath DG, et al. Volume rendering versus maximum intensity projection in CT angiography: what works best, when and why. Radiographics 2006; 26:905-922.

Calhoun PS, Kuszyk BS, Heath DG, et al. Three-dimensional volume rendering of spiral CT data: theory and method. Radiographics 1999; 19:745-764.

REFERENCES

1. Lell MM, Anders K, Uder M, et al. New techniques in CT angriography. Radiographics 2006; 26:S45-S62.
2. Dalrymple NC, Prasad SR, Freckleton MW, Chintapalli KN. Informatics in radiology (infoRAD): introduction to the language of three-dimensional imaging with multidetector CT. Radiographics 2005; 25:1409-1428.
3. Cody DD. AAPM/RSNA physics tutorial for residents: topics in CT. Image processing in CT. Radiographics 2002; 22:1255-1268.
4. Fishman EK, Ney DR, Heath DG, et al. Volume rendering versus maximum intensity projection in CT angiography: what works best, when and why. Radiographics 2006; 26:905-922.
5. Calhoun PS, Kuszyk BS, Heath DG, et al. Three-dimensional volume rendering of spiral CT data: theory and method. Radiographics 1999; 19:745-764.
6. Levoy M. Efficient ray tracing of volume data. ACM Trans Graphics 1990; 9:245-261.

CHAPTER 84

Advanced Three-Dimensional Postprocessing in Computed Tomographic and Magnetic Resonance Angiography

Rob J. van der Geest, Pieter H. Kitslaar, Patrick J.H. de Koning,
Ronald van 't Klooster, Wouter J. Jukema, Gerhard Koning,
Henk A. Marquering, and Johan H.C. Reiber

INTRODUCTION

Over the past several years, the research and developments in visualization and quantitative analysis, as well as the clinical usage of cardiovascular MRI and, in particular, of multidetector computed tomography (MDCT) have made major progress. Both acquisition techniques have in common that enormous amounts of data are being generated that need to be visualized in a proper manner for interpretation purposes. It has been clear for many years that cardiovascular MRI has all the ingredients for the "one-stop-shop" approach, allowing the assessment of anatomy, function, perfusion, infarct imaging, flow, as well as spectroscopy, although imaging time has been a major limitation. These possibilities led to a data explosion, making it difficult to visualize, interpret all the data, and come to a diagnosis by the cardiologist/interpreting physician. Given these developments, it has been clear that quantitation of all these data sets becomes an imperative for various reasons. It has been documented that the variability in the quantitative analyses has been much smaller than by visual interpretation, leading to smaller population sizes in clinical trials with all the subsequent advantages, such as lower costs of the trials, results available earlier, and so on. In addition, quantitation will lead to an efficiency improvement in the clinical setting: less dependency on the experience of the interpreter, the analyses can be preprocessed for the final approval by the cardiologist/interpreting physician, and all the results can be stored right away in the hospital picture archiving and communication system (PACS) system. Given all the high expectations of molecular imaging and the hope to better understand the atherosclerotic process, MR vessel wall imaging appears to be an excellent means to study the changes in the vessel wall and the composition of the atheroma.

With the enormous technical developments in multislice CT now with 256 and 320 slice scanners, the depiction of anatomy in particular has become astonishing. An enormous advantage of CT is the very short acquisition times from one to a few cardiac cycles; greatest disadvantage is the radiation dose, although great efforts are underway to diminish that as much as possible. There has been a growing clinical interest in the use of the MDCT system for noninvasive coronary angiography. Visualization of the data sets is commonly done by 3D workstations, which increasingly provide some quantitation results as well, although the variabilities in the analyses have been enormous and clinically often not acceptable, even raising questions by the Food and Drug Administration (FDA). It has been evident that more complex segmentation techniques are necessary, and that validation of the results is a must. Also, MDCT is developing toward the assessment of function, perfusion, and viability, and the analysis of heart valves. In this chapter, we will describe and illustrate segmentation and quantitation approaches for both CT angiography (CTA) and MR angiography (MRA).

3D Postprocessing in Computed Tomographic Angiography

For the analysis of vessel structures in CTA data a number of postprocessing (image processing) steps are required. The first step is the (automated) extraction of the vessel centerline, which forms the foundation for a number of subsequent postprocessing steps. For stenosis quantification in the vessel, lumen contours are detected in a stretched vessel image based on the extracted centerline. In the next section these steps will be discussed in more detail.

Automated Vessel Extraction

Segmentation and analysis of vessels in 3D image data has been an area of research for many years. In general, the definition of the vessel centerline is a first major step in the process of segmentation and analysis of vessels. Existing methods for the determination of vessel centerlines can roughly be grouped into two categories: a minimal cost path calculation;[1] and methods based on first obtaining the whole set of image pixels containing the vessel (segmentation) and next gradually reducing these sets of pixels to a single centerline (skeletonization).[2] The first type is typically computationally faster and avoids the error-sensitive segmentation step. However, the minimal cost path may deviate from the true lumen center at strong curvatures of the vessels. Furthermore, the intermediate result of the second type does provide some advantages such as the visual evaluation of the presegmentation of the vessel (tree).

The presented method consists of the following steps: (1) the presegmentation of the coronary vessels; (2) the extraction of the vessel's centerline; (3) a reformatting of the image volume to produce a stack of cross-sectional images perpendicular to the centerline; (4) a combination of longitudinal and transversal contour detection approaches; and (5) the quantification of vessel morphologic parameters. These five steps will be described in more detail in the following paragraphs.

Coronary Vessel Presegmentation

The first step in the segmentation and analysis process is a presegmentation step based on the so-called *fast-marching level* set method (called WaveProp for short).[3] The WaveProp algorithm simulates the propagation of a wave through a medium starting from a user-selected source point, in this case the ostium of a vessel. The wave propagates through the volume set with a propagation speed given by the so-called *speed function*; this speed function can be designed based on image intensities in such a way that the wave propagates fast in the structures of interest (high intensities in a blood vessel) and slow in the remaining structures (low image intensities). By this image-based approach, the propagation automatically provides an initial segmentation of the vessel lumen.

For a complete analysis of a segment of a single vessel, the user places a proximal point at the beginning of the vessel and a distal point at the end of the vessel of interest. The expansion or propagation process stops when the wave propagation reaches the end point.

Centerline Detection

The fastest path, which is the path connecting the start and end point, can be obtained using a so-called *steepest-descent* approach by backtracking the path of an accepted voxel in the wave propagation to the source (starting point) following the minimal travel time (highest speed). However, the fastest path tends to deviate from the center of the lumen by taking the inside curve at bending vessels. To correct the fastest path such that it follows the center of the lumen, a modified distance transformation is used.[4] This distance map defines for each voxel the minimal distance to a nonaccepted voxel, and as a result, the highest values represent the center of the segmented vessels. An example is given in Figure 84-1.

Curved Multiplanar Reformatting

Because of its tortuous course and the presence of other structures such as the heart chamber, the visual evaluation of the segmented vessels may still be cumbersome. When the vessel's centerline is known, a curved multiplanar reformatted (CMPR) image along the vessel's course can be constructed (Fig. 84-2). The goal of CMPR visualization is to make a vessel visible in one single image over its entire length. Traditionally, two separate approaches have been used in the construction: stretched CMPR or straightened CMPR. The stretched CMPR displays a tubular structure in one 2-D plane without overlap, whereas the straightened CMPR produces a linear representation of the vessel that simulates the vessel as if it has been pulled straight. To optimize the image for contour detection, we follow the latter approach. The reformatted image contains a stack of 2D images that are perpendicular to the centerline. The third dimension, Z, in this image represents the distance to the source point along the centerline, such that the centerline is transformed into a straight line running through the X-Y center of the stack of images.

Contour Detection

For the quantitative results to be insensitive to image noise, the contour detection needs to be relatively insensitive and robust to image distortions. Straight-forward contour detection methods based on thresholds of image intensities solely, second-order derivatives or the full-width half maximum method[5] are sensitive to image noise, and as a result limit the algorithm to adapt to variations in the dosage or distribution of contrast agent.[5] Commonly, contour detection for the determination of vessel dimensions is carried out solely on the 2D cross-sectional planes perpendicular to the vessel's centerline. To minimize the sensitivity to image noise, we use information of the complete 3D shape of the vessel. The reformatted CMPR image enables the use of multiple 2D contour detections. For that reason, we suggest the following approach, which has been successful in IVUS applications.[6]

Through the stack of images, a number of longitudinal cut planes (typically 4 to 6) can be defined, which are perpendicular to the transversal planes and pass through the center of the CMPR image, and thus through the cen-

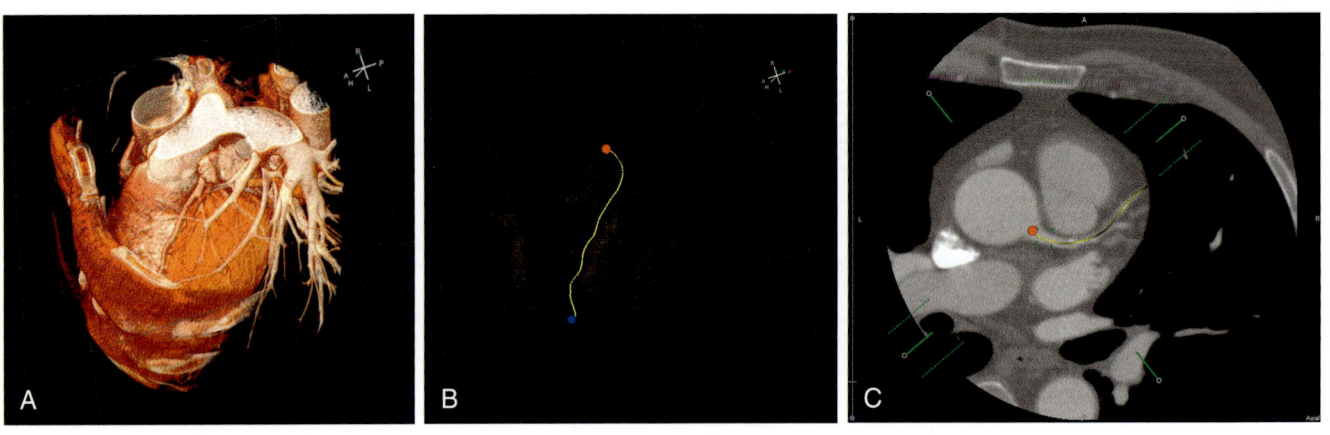

■ **FIGURE 84-1** **A,** Volume rendering of CTA volume of the heart. **B,** Centerline obtained from the start (*red*) and end (*blue*) points. **C,** Centerline overlayed in the axial slice.

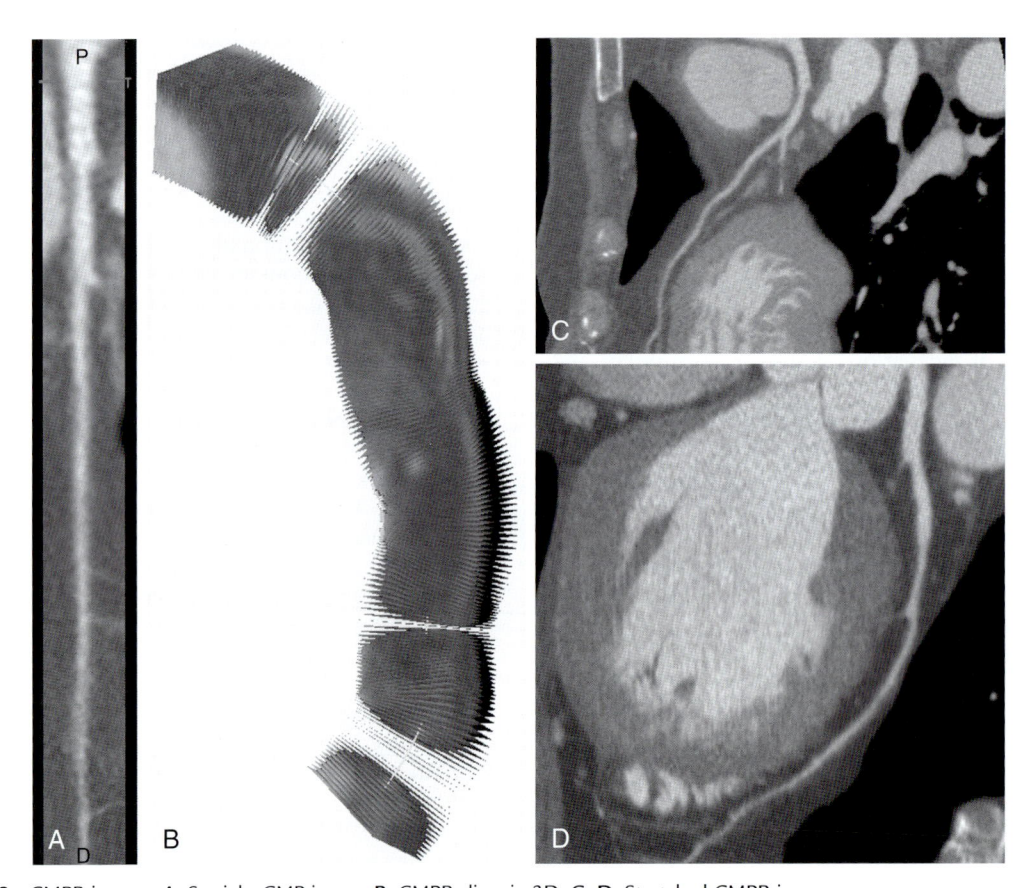

■ **FIGURE 84-2** CMPR images. **A,** Straight CMP image. **B,** CMPR slices in 3D. **C, D,** Stretched CMPR images.

terline of the vessel (Fig. 84-3). These cut planes are subsequently used for the contour detection along the course of the vessel.[7] Experiments have demonstrated that the construction of four cut planes is sufficient for the longitudinal contour detection.

The longitudinal vessel borders are detected using the model-guided minimum cost approach (MCA)[8]. The cost function is based on a combination of spatial first-, and second-derivative gradient filters in combination with knowledge of the expected CT values, and curvature of the coronary vessels. Because the 3D shape of the vessel resembles a smoothly curved tube, the two vessel boundaries in a longitudinal cut plane are detected simultaneously.[9] This means that a well-defined vessel border at one side can support the detection of the vessel border at the other side. This mutual guidance by the simultaneous detection of the vessel boundaries is especially helpful at locations with strong partial volume effects or close to bifurcations. In these cases, the shape of the opposite contour follows the shape of the well-defined edge.

Next, the four longitudinal cut planes displaying its associated contours are presented for visual inspection (Fig. 84-4A). In some cases, such as at the presence of strong calcifications or odd branchings, manual correction

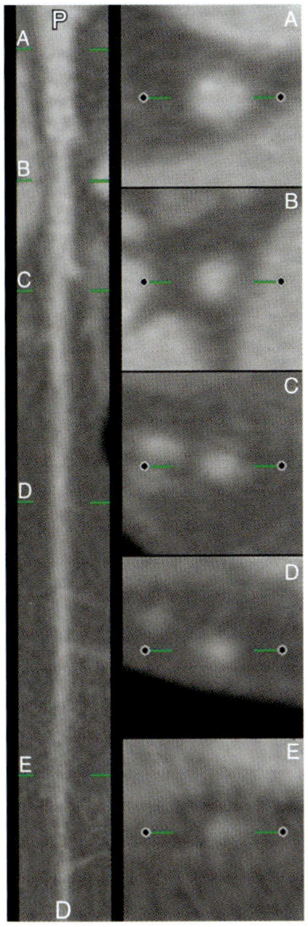

FIGURE 84-3 A single longitudinal cut slice (*left*) and four transversal slices at the corresponding positions (*right*) in the CMPR image.

of the contours may be necessary, and can easily be carried out. The longitudinal detected vessel contours produce a series of intersection points with the transversal slices. These points have two functions: (1) they are used to specify the region of interest for the MCA contour detection in the transversal images; and (2) they function as attraction points with an adjustable strength to attract the contour detection to areas close to these points. The advantage of using attraction points instead of forcing contours to run through the intersection points is that small deviations in the longitudinal contours do not force the transversal contour to follow this point and makes the transversal contour detection less sensitive to small variations in the longitudinal contours. The contours in single transversal images can also be manually corrected by adjusting a part of the contour or by moving an attraction point (see Fig. 84-4B).

Stenosis Quantification

When the contours in the stack of transversal images have been detected, possibly corrected and approved, vessel-related parameters such as the lumen cross-sectional area and diameter are calculated for each individual image (cross-section). Based on this series of measurements, the area function along the vessel and the corresponding minimum and maximum values are determined. The cross-sectional area is directly related to the hemodynamic properties of vessels and is, therefore, expected to be more significant than the vessel diameter measurements.

However, because of the historical popularity of projection angiography, the vessel diameter is still commonly used for the quantification of vessel stenosis. We propose using both. Following van Bemmel and colleagues, an average radius of the lumen is derived by comparing the measured area with the area of a circle with a given radius.[10] From the actual area function from the beginning to the end of a vessel, a reference area (or diameter function) can be derived, representing to the best of our knowledge the size of the vessel before the obstructions became apparent. This reference function is determined by a repeated linear regression fit of the lumen area as a function of the longitudinal distance.[11] The user may flag areas that are suspicious and may cause an erroneous determination of the trend. For example, it is difficult to produce accurate reference contours of a vessel in the vicinity of large bifurcations, or ectatic areas. For such cases, it is justified to remove (flag) these parts from the calculation of the reference function.

In the vessel, three segments are automatically detected: (1) the diseased part or obstructed segment, (2) the proximal, and (3) the distal normal segment, in which the lumen area is representative for the nondiseased state of the vessel. The degree of stenosis is given by the ratio of either the radius or area of the most narrowed segment of the vessel and its corresponding reference radius or area, respectively.

Application for X-Ray Angiographic Planning Purposes

Motivated by the growing number of MDCT scans that are available prior to an invasive cardiac catheterization procedure, we have investigated the possible use of such data for the planning of a coronary interventional procedure. More specifically, there has been a need for the determination of optimal angiographic views for coronary bifurcations, and we believe that MDCT can support such procedures.

Principle

The optimal angiographic view is defined as the angle that minimizes the amount of foreshortening and vessel overlap in resulting x-ray angiograms. A three-dimensional representation of the coronary tree can be used to simulate all possible angiographic views with the computer. For each simulated angiographic view, the resulting amount of foreshortening and vessel overlap can be assessed, and from such data the optimal viewing angle can be derived. In our system, the amount of foreshortening is determined from a representation of the centerlines of the coronary arteries. For the calculation of the amount of vessel overlap, a surface representation of the coronary tree is used.

Segmentation Steps

To obtain the centerline and surface model representation of the coronary trees from the CTA data set, a method similar to the approach described earlier can be used. The only difference is that some presegmentation steps are

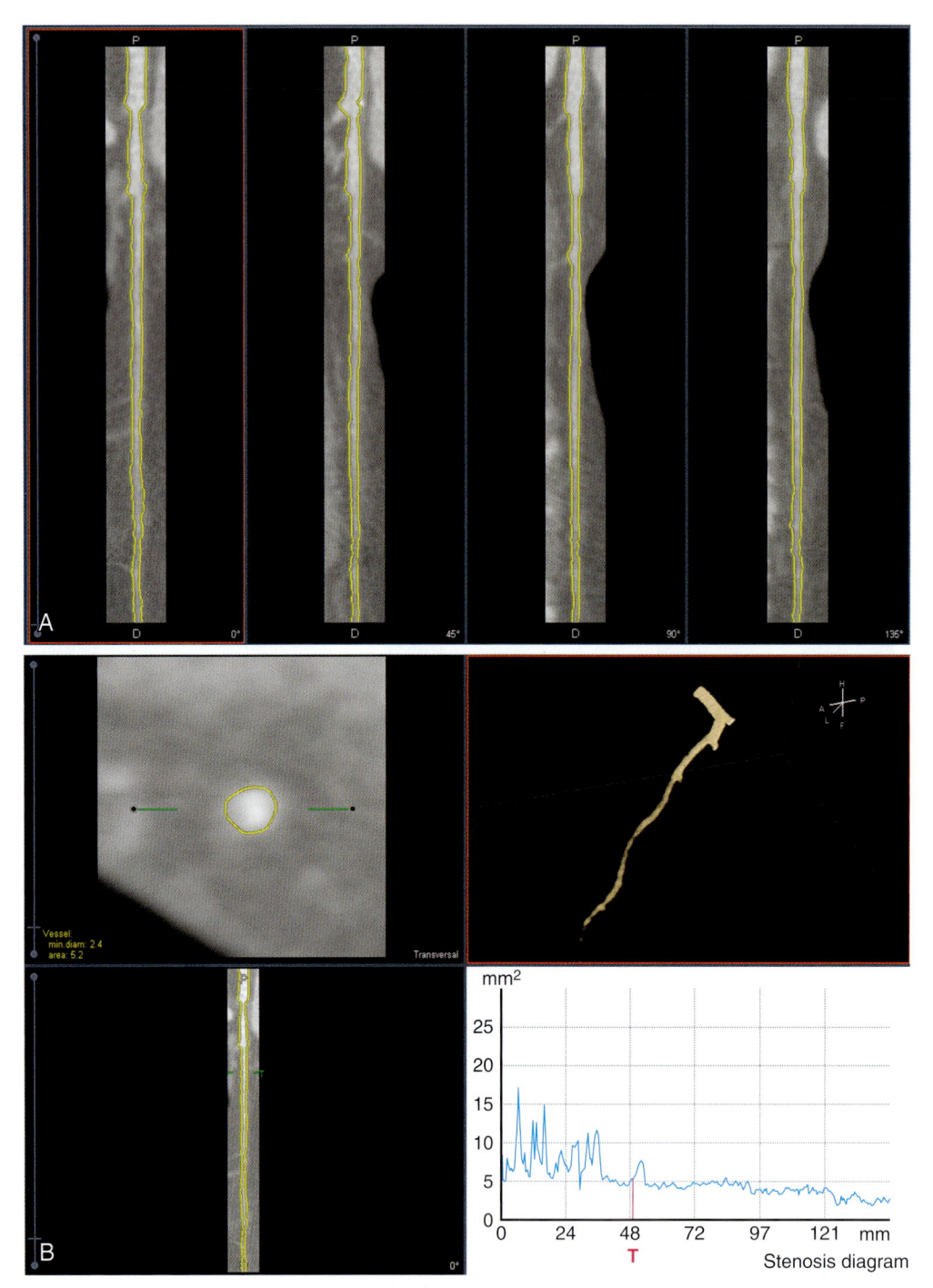

FIGURE 84-4 **A,** Four longitudinal cut planes with the detected contours. **B,** Overview of the vessel analysis results.

applied before extracting the vessels. Also, the end points for the centerlines within the coronary tree are now automatically found, so that only a single user-defined start point is needed.[12]

The before-mentioned presegmentation step removes large contrast-filled structures in the image. The removal (or masking) of the large contrast-filled regions, like the heart chambers and the aorta, prevents the WaveProp algorithm from leaking. Starting from a user-defined seed point in the ostium of the coronary tree, the propagation method will result in a complete segmentation of the arteries in the tree. From this user-defined point, the "root" point, the extremities of the coronary tree, called the "leaf points", can be determined automatically. Next, the centerlines of the coronary tree are detected as described earlier. An example of the outcome of these segmentation steps is presented in Figure 84-5.

Region of Interest

To obtain the optimal angiographic viewing angle for a specific bifurcation, a region of interest for that bifurcation is defined at 10 mm distance from the bifurcation point (D_{region} in Fig. 84-6A).

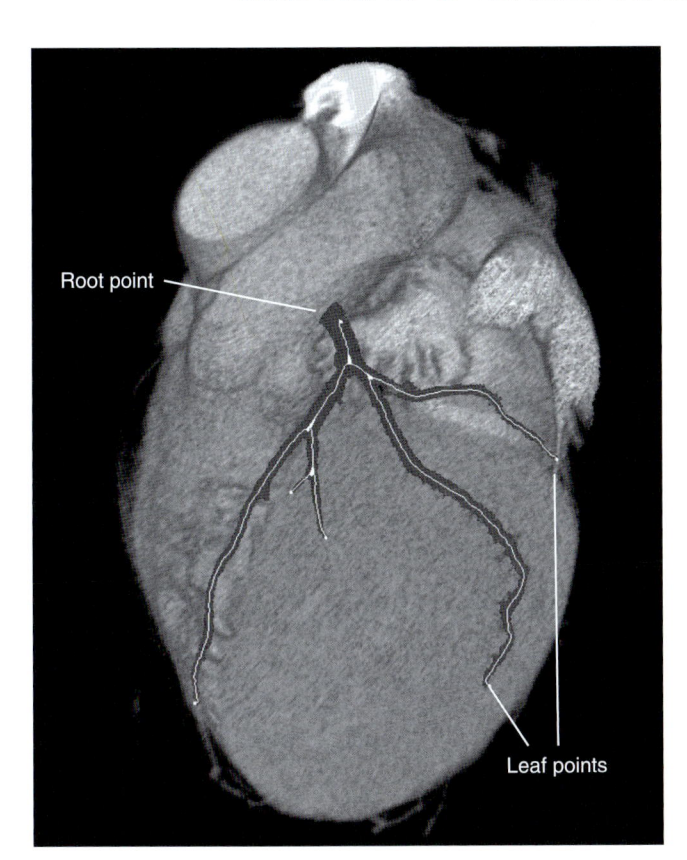

FIGURE 84-5 Volume rendering of the heart with a segmented left coronary tree. The "leaf" and "root" points are indicated, as well as the extracted centerlines.

Projection Overlap

To determine the projection overlap for a bifurcation, the projected image of only the bifurcation region is calculated first, followed by the calculation of the projection of the remainder of the coronary tree (without the bifurcation). The projection overlap for the bifurcation is defined by the number of pixels that appear in both the projection of the bifurcation and the projection of the whole coronary tree. Figure 84-6 shows examples of the projection overlap of a bifurcation for different angles. To distinguish between the examples a and c, which have similar overlap and foreshortening values, a second overlap measure is defined, which is denoted by the internal overlap. This internal overlap determines the overlap that individual branches of the bifurcation have with each other. For this, the three branches of the bifurcation are separated from each other (see Fig. 84-6A) and the overlap between each branch pair is calculated. The internal overlap for the whole bifurcation is defined by the maximum value of these pair-wise overlap values.

Simulating Angiographic Views

The percentage of foreshortening, overlap, and internal overlap for a bifurcation are calculated for a range of rotation and angulation angles. In this study, we limited the rotations between RAO 40 and LAO 60; the minimum and maximum angulations were set to caudal 35 and cranial 30, respectively. These values are in agreement with the ranges used in clinical practice. Figure 84-7 shows an example of two x-ray angiograms and two simulated views from the same projection angle.

Optimal Angiographic View

A convenient representation for the measurements is a two dimensional map. The horizontal axis in this map represents the rotation angle and the vertical axis represents the angulation angle (Fig. 84-8). The optimal viewing angle is determined by combining the results of the foreshortening, overlap, and internal overlap calculations. In terms of the map representations, this comes down to creating a new combined viewing map. For this combined map, the overlap and internal overlap map are used to create a mask map that excludes regions in the foreshortening map as optimal angle candidates. This mask is constructed by allowing only angles that result in less than 20% overlap and less than 10% internal overlap. To prevent the algorithm from choosing angles too close to regions of high overlap, an additional border at 10 degrees' distance from these regions is added to the mask as a "safety zone." The optimal angle is automatically determined as the angle with the minimum amount of foreshortening in the combined map.

3D Postprocessing in MRA

The accurate assessment of the presence and extent of vascular disease and planning of vascular interventions based on MRA also require accurate determination of vessel dimensions. MRA data sets are generally evaluated on 2D maximum intensity projections (MIP) using either visual inspection or caliper measurements. However, MIP renderings suffer from a decreased SNR and may lead to an underestimation of the vessel width. It may also lead to a misinterpretation of the actual vascular morphology because an MIP presents only a 2D representation of the actual 3D anatomy. Reviewing the original source images is, therefore, considered mandatory to come to a reliable assessment.

Although MRA provides accurate 3D visualization of the vascular lumen, additional MR vessel wall imaging phase sequences may be employed for a detailed evaluation of the arterial wall. Currently the degree of lumen stenosis is used as a marker for high-risk plaques. However, lumen narrowing is not a good estimator of plaque size and probably underestimates the atherosclerotic burden. For instance, Glagov and colleagues demonstrated that, because of compensatory enlargement of the adventitial boundary, vessels can suffer a large increase in atherosclerotic plaque mass without luminal narrowing.[13] The North American Symptomatic Carotid Endarterectomy Trial (NASCET) and the Asymptomatic Carotid Atherosclerosis Study (ACAS) supported this hypothesis by demonstrating that lumen narrowing is a poor predictor of plaque vulnerability.[14,15] High resolution MR has emerged as the potential leading noninvasive imaging modality for characterizing atherosclerotic plaque in vivo. Recent literature has documented MR capabilities of identifying atherosclerotic plaque components,[16,17] plaque areas and volumes, and its

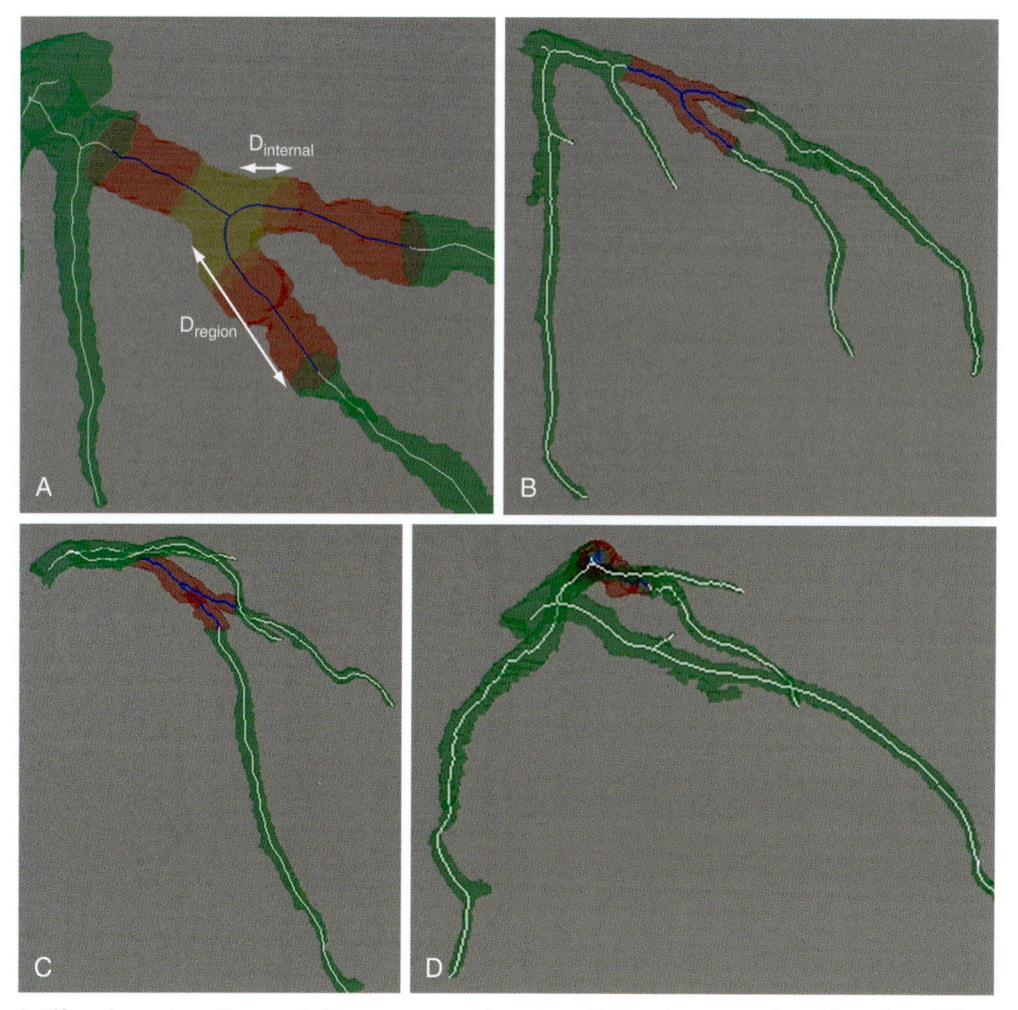

■ **FIGURE 84-6** *A,* Bifurcation region of interest. Left coronary tree with a selected bifurcation area projected from three different angles. *B,* RAO 35, CAUD 40 projection with 27% foreshortening and 14% overlap. *C,* LAO 60, CAUD 18 projection with 86% foreshortening and 75% overlap. *D,* LAO 1, CRAN 30 projection with 26% foreshortening and 13% overlap. CAUD, caudal; CRAN, cranial; LAO, left anterior oblique; RAO, right anterior oblique.

potential for monitoring the progression and regression of plaque lesions.[18,19]

The combination of MRA and vessel wall imaging (VWI) in a single imaging session makes MR imaging a unique imaging modality to study the vascular system. Accurate and reproducible measurements are of extreme importance for routine clinical application. Techniques for computerized quantitative analysis of MRA and MR VWI studies are described in the following sections.

Automated Vessel Lumen Analysis from MRA Studies

To improve the conventional analysis of MRA imaging studies, it is desirable to obtain quantitative morphologic information directly from the 3D images and not to rely on MIP projections. Hence, accurate 3D segmentation tools are required. Vessel segmentation of 3D images has been investigated by many researchers. However, the majority of this research focused on enhancing the 3D visualization of the vascular structures in the image, and not on accurate quantification of these structures. More research is required on automated quantification of the luminal dimensions to grade the severity of stenoses or other vascular abnormalities. A description of select developed techniques and the results of various validation studies are presented subsequently.

User Interaction

Before performing the automated 3D pathline detection, the first step in the analysis process is to select the vessel segment of interest. This is necessary because an MRA data set typically encompasses a large volume containing multiple arteries. To simplify the selection, the user needs to define a proximal (start) and a distal (end) point inside the vessel of interest in the 3D data space. Placing a point in 3D space requires the definition of three coordinates. However, an MIP is a 2D projection image which can provide only two coordinates (either xy, xz, or yz). Therefore, at least two MIP views are needed to obtain all three coordinates (the third MIP image can be used for verification purposes). The third coordinate from an MIP can be calculated using a depth buffer or Z-buffer, which stores

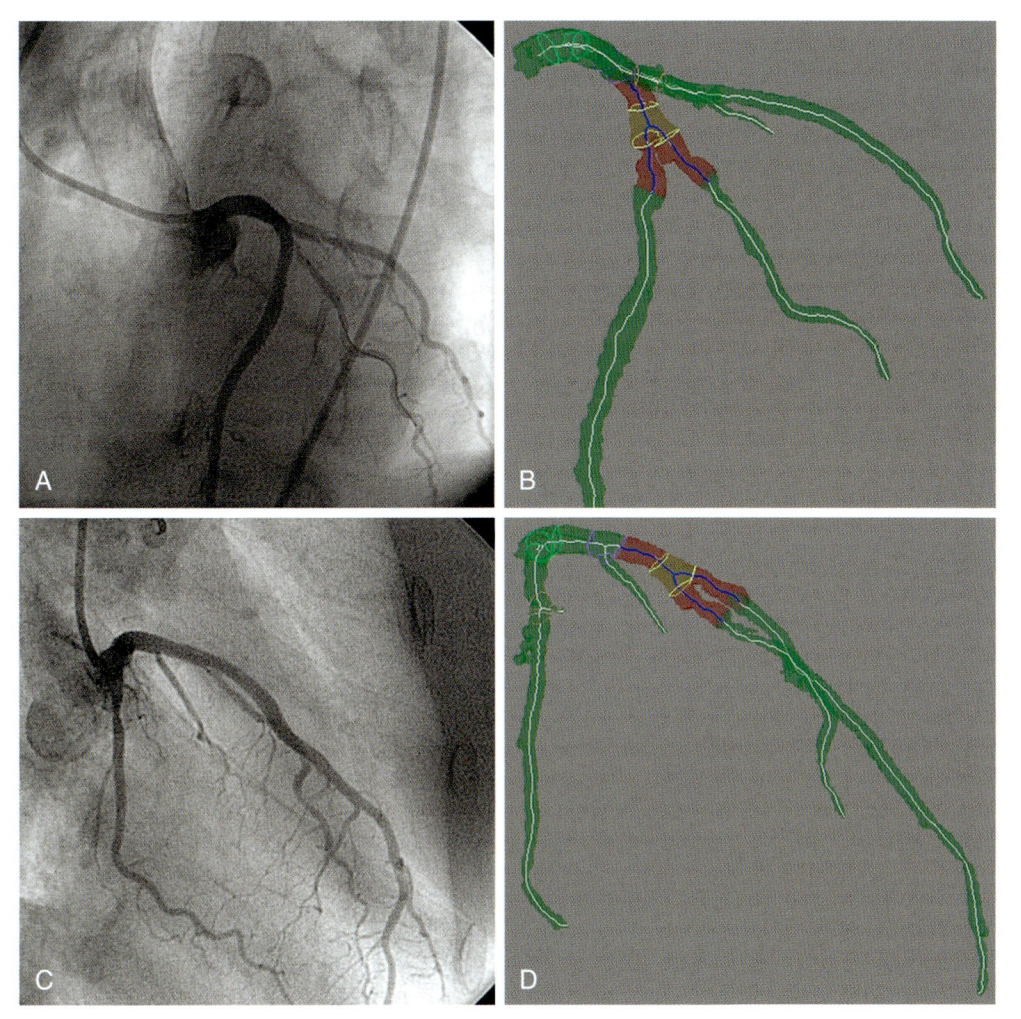

FIGURE 84-7 Comparison of x-ray angiograms and projections of segmented coronary arteries from CTA. Angiogram (**A**) and simulated projection (**B**) for LAO 42, CRAN 28. Angiogram (**C**) and simulated projection (**D**) for RAO 37, CAUD 18.

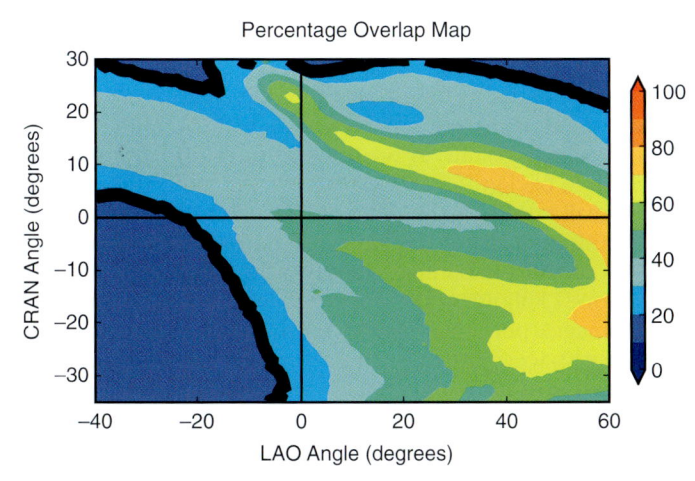

FIGURE 84-8 Example of a map demonstrating the amount of overlap for a bifurcation for all possible rotation and angulation angles. The *bold lines* indicate the threshold values for 20% overlap.

the location at which the maximum intensity is found. To avoid additional computational costs, the Z-buffer can be calculated simultaneously during the MIP construction. After the proximal and the distal points are defined, a 3D pathline is automatically detected through the vessel segment. The detected pathline can be visualized by projecting it onto the MIP images for the visual verification purposes by the user. In case the pathline is not valid, the user may reposition the proximal and distal points or place one or more intermediate points on the vessel segment and run the pathline detection again.

Automated Vessel Pathline Detection

The automated 3D pathline detection is based on the fast marching level set method (FMLSM), as discussed previously in the section on CTA postprocessing. The FMLSM numerically approximates the propagation of a wave through a medium and computes the arrival time of the wave at each image element. The wave propagation speed is set to be higher in regions of high signal intensity (i.e.,

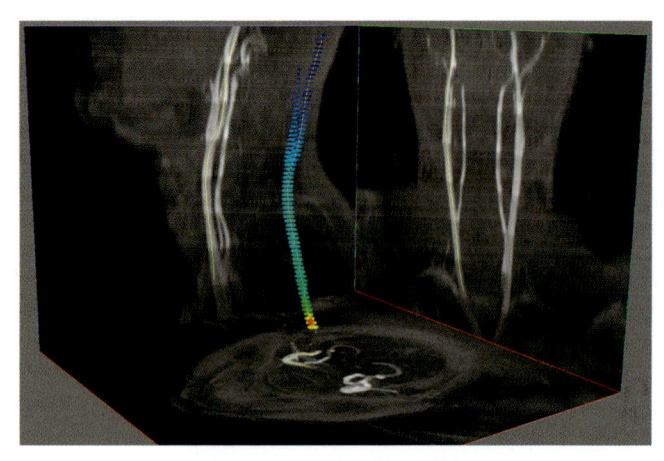

■ **FIGURE 84-9** Intermediate result of the pathline detection algorithm. Proximal point (*in red*) and distal point (*in blue*) represent the user-defined start and end point of the vessel segment of the right carotid artery. Colorized voxels in the vessel indicate the arrival times obtained by applying the wavefront propagation algorithm. The three background images show MIP reformats of the volume data in three orthogonal directions.

TABLE 84-1		Results of Pathline Detection	
Observer	Segments	Classified Correctly	Success (%)
A	43	40	93
B	43	40	93

the vessel lumen) and lower in regions of low intensity. The propagation starts at the indicated proximal point and continues until the wavefront reaches the distal point (Fig. 84-9). Using a steepest-descent approach, the optimal trajectory from the distal to the proximal point can be calculated. However, the pathline found using this approach will not be at the desired center of the lumen at every location. Especially in curved segments, the pathline usually follows the inside curve. Therefore, a postprocessing step based on a distance transform is performed to relocate the pathline toward the center of the lumen.

Validation of the MRA Pathline Detection

Validation of the automated pathline detection approach has been performed on in-vivo data sets of peripheral arteries of seven patients.[2] Three studies were acquired for each patient, covering the abdomen and the upper and lower parts of the legs, respectively. This resulted in a total of 20 CE-MRA studies (1 study of the lower legs had to be rejected due to severe motion artifacts). Two sequences were used in this study. Sequence 1 used a breath-hold, T1-weighted turbo field echo (TFE) sequence with the following imaging parameters: TR/TE/α = 4.1/1.3/50 degrees, field of view (FOV) 345 × 345 mm^2, 81% rectangular, and scan matrix 256 × 126. This resulted in a spatial resolution of 1.4 × 2.7 mm^2. Using a 512 × 512 reconstruction matrix, the pixel size was 0.7 × 0.7 mm^2. The slice thickness was 2.8 mm with a 50% overlap. A total of 55 slices were acquired with a total acquisition time of 25 s. Sequence 2 used a T1-weighted 3D spoiled gradient-echo sequence with the following imaging parameters: TR/TE/α = 10/4.8/50 degrees, FOV 450 × 450 mm^2, 80% rectangular, and scan matrix 256 × 182. This resulted in a spatial resolution of 1.8 × 2.5 mm^2. Using a 256 × 256 reconstruction matrix, the pixel size was 1.8 × 1.8 mm^2. The slice thickness was 2.4 mm with a 50% overlap. A total of 60 slices were acquired with a total acquisition time of 60 s. The abdominal section was acquired using sequence 1, whereas both peripheral sections were acquired using sequence 2.

Two independent observers analyzed the studies by specifying the proximal and distal points of the vessel segments. Only the major vessels were studied, which were the aorta and the common iliac, external iliac, femoral, and popliteal arteries. The observers were instructed to analyze the two longest segments in each study. In the abdominal study, three vessels (the aorta and the left and the right common iliac arteries) had to be analyzed. The total number vessel segment to analyze was 49 segments, 6 of which had to be rejected because no vessel was visible owing to an occlusion of the vessel. After the analysis was completed, the observers visually inspected the detected centerline and classified the result as correct or incorrect. A centerline was classified as correct if the projection of the centerline onto each of the MIP images was within the vessel. Additionally, the 3D path could be examined together with a volume rendering of the original image if the projections were not clear enough. The results of the validation are provided in Table 84-1. It shows that in all but three cases, a correct centerline was detected by both observers. The three failures were caused by brighter vessels running close and parallel to the vessel of interest and were identical for both observers. Placing an additional support point in the vessel segment of interest was sufficient to obtain a correct pathline in these cases.

Vessel Lumen Segmentation in MRA

Based on the detected pathline the lumen boundaries are detected using either an edge-based or intensity-based approach. For smaller diameter vessels, detection of the vessel boundaries based on the edges can be inaccurate due to the relatively poor resolution of the MRA acquisition, which results in an unclear transition from vessel lumen to background. Alternatively, the lumen boundaries for small vessel can be detected based on the observation that the intensity at the vessel boundary is approximately 30% of the maximum intensity in the vessel cross-section.[20] Following this approach, a series of reformatted 2D images perpendicular to the pathline is generated at evenly spaced intervals. In each of these 2D images the luminal contour is detected by applying the proper threshold. Figure 84-10 illustrates the lumen contour detection technique. Subsequently, the series of contours in the 2D cross-sectional images is transformed back to 3D space resulting in a triangulated mesh, which can be used to derive various quantitative parameters describing the lumen dimensions of the analyzed vessel segment. Figure 84-11 shows an example of an automatically analyzed vessel segment and its derived quantitative parameters.

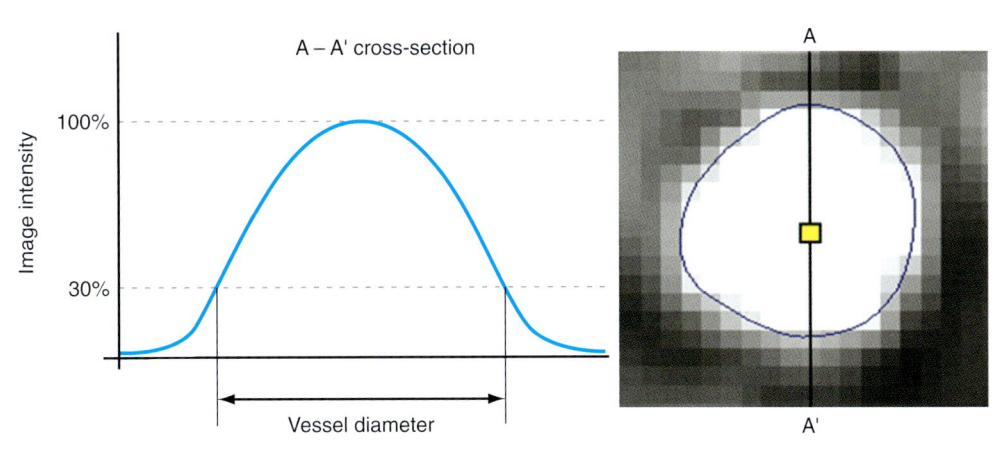

FIGURE 84-10 Vessel lumen boundary detection using the full width 30% maximum criterion. Based on the maximum intensity in the vessel lumen, close to the lumen center, the vessel boundary is defined at the location where the intensity is equal to 30% of the maximum value.

A drawback of the threshold-based approach applied in the sequence of cross-sectional 2D images is that it may result in an unrealistic, irregular, 3D segmentation. In the presence of other vessel running close to the vessel segment of interest or stenotic areas where the maximum intensity at the location of the pathline is low, overestimation of the lumen contour may occur in individual slices. A potential solution to this problem is the use of a 3D tubular model that is fit to the actual image data. The tubular model fitting to the cross-sectional images is based on a threshold approach or image gradient features. By constraining the allowed deformation of the tubular model, such an approach is much less sensitive to image artifacts at particular locations. Promising results of the 3D tubular model fitting has been presented by Makowski and associates.[21] Figure 84-12 shows an example of a vessel segment detected using the tube fitting approach.

Validation of the Automated MRA Lumen Segmentation

To validate the lumen segmentation algorithm against a true gold standard, MRA acquisitions were obtained from five phantoms having an identical reference diameter of 6.8 mm and different obstruction diameters simulating varying degrees of stenosis severity. The results of reference and obstruction diameter assessment by MRA are listed in Table 84-2. For each of the phantoms, the obstruction diameter was accurately assessed using the automated method with an error of $1.0 \pm 3.7\%$. For the regions with an obstruction, however, overestimation of the diameter occurred for the more severe stenoses. This result can be explained by the relatively poor resolution of the MRA acquisition. Given the actual spatial resolution in the order of $2 \times 2 \times 2$ mm^3, the diameter values in the stenotic region of the phantoms with the most severe stenosis correspond to either 1.5 or 1 voxel. The results indicate that for accurate diameter measurements, the spatial resolution should be such that at least three voxel elements along the vessel diameter are present.

De Vries and colleagues evaluated the described MRA contour detection technique for the automated detection of aortoiliac stenoses in 3D contrast-enhanced MRA in patients with peripheral arterial disease.[22] In this study, 25 patients were included in which intra-arterial digital subtraction angiography (IA-DSA) was available and used as a standard of reference. Three blinded observers independently evaluated the CE-MRA data sets for stenoses using semiautomated analyses. In addition, three other observers independently evaluated the data sets using conventional measurements of stenosis severity. For computerized analysis, a stenosis was considered significant if the reduction in luminal area exceeded 50% of a chosen reference segment. An example of such analysis is given in Figure 84-13. During conventional analysis, linear dimensions were measured using a 3D workstation in MIP reformats and original source images. In total, 125 vessel segments were evaluated using both approaches. On IA-DSA, 28 significant lesions were identified in 20 patients. Agreement between MRA and IA-DSA (as expressed using the kappa values) was $\kappa = 0.78$ for semiautomated MRA analysis and $\kappa = 0.70$ for conventional MR analysis (p = NS). This indicates that the automated analysis performs similarly to conventional analysis.

Automated Assessment of Vessel Wall Morphology

A typical MR vessel wall imaging protocol consists of multiple acquisitions using different contrast weightings to allow accurate quantification of vessel wall morphology and characterization of plaque components. However, if only morphologic information is required about the vessel wall, a single high-resolution vessel wall imaging (VWI) series may be sufficient, providing good depiction of the luminal and outer wall boundaries.

The initial step for vessel wall analysis is the automated detection of the luminal and outer wall boundaries in the 2D VW images. Adame and coworkers have described a model-based contour detection technique that can be applied for various arteries and has been validated on carotid and aortic MR studies.[23,24] Starting with a manually identified point in the lumen center, an edge-based segmentation technique is applied based on ellipse fitting and dynamic programming. For the detection of the lumen

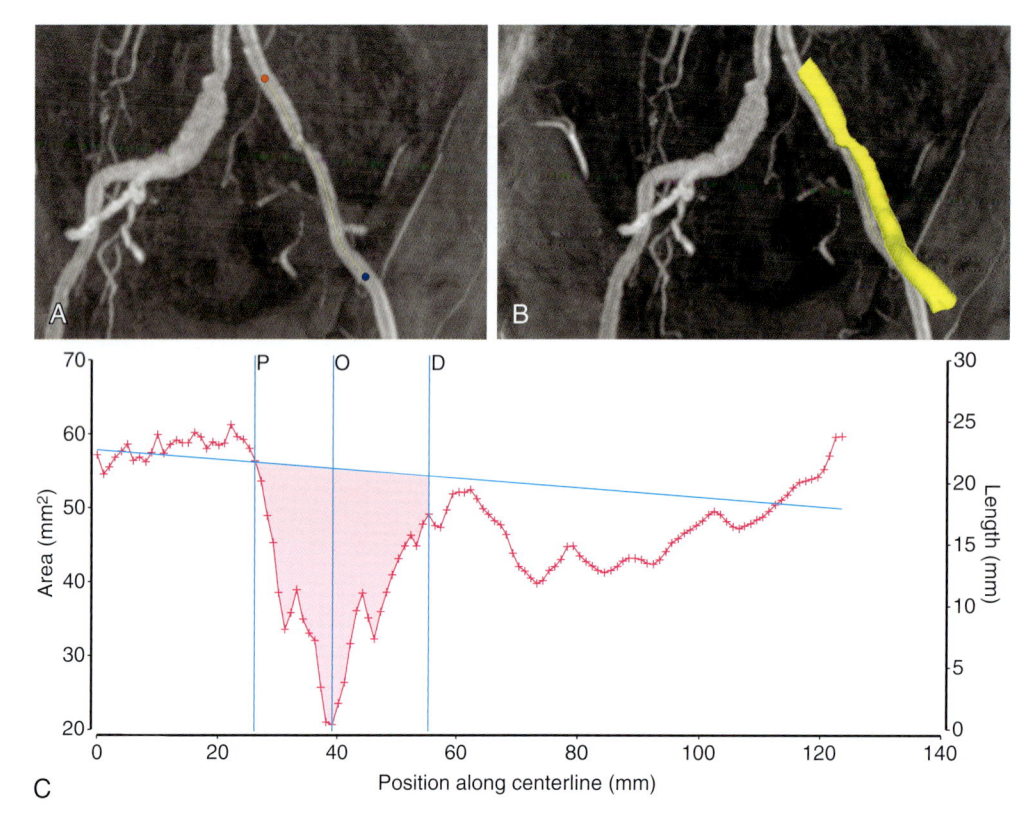

■ **FIGURE 84-11** Example of an automated stenosis analysis for a lesion in the left iliac artery. **A,** The *red and blue dots* represent the user-defined start and end point of the segment to be analyzed. The detected lumen pathline is shown in *yellow*. **B,** Detected luminal surface. **C,** Graph illustrating the vessel's cross-sectional area as a function of the position along the pathline (in *red*). The *blue line* indicates the reference area, which is an approximation of the lumen area as it would be in the nondiseased state. The percent stenosis is derived by dividing the actual cross-sectional area by the reference area at the corresponding location. As an alternative, the reference area can also be derived from a normal segment distal or proximal to the actual lesion.

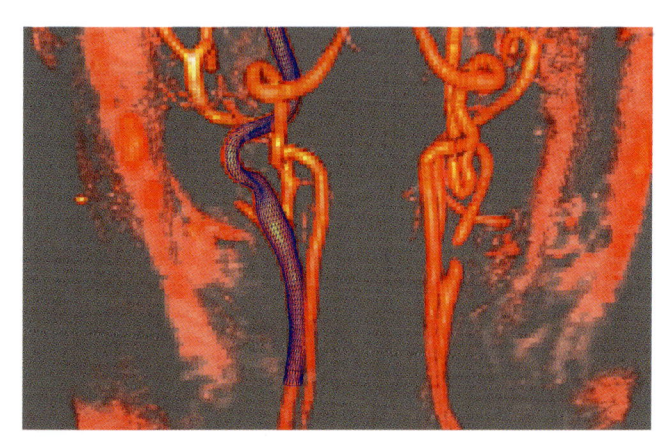

■ **FIGURE 84-12** Result of 3D lumen segmentation using a tube fitting approach. A major advantage is the use of the 3D spatial coherency of the lumen surface. This makes this approach less sensitive to local image artifacts.

boundaries, information about the approximate size and shape is incorporated in the algorithm, as well as the fact that the lumen area has lower signal intensity than the vessel wall. Accurate detection of the outer wall is, in general, more challenging because the intensities of surrounding tissue may be lower, higher, or have a similar intensity as the vessel wall. Alternatively, because the shape of the outer wall boundary can be approximated by an ellipse, reliable edge information at a local level is less important. Therefore, for the detection of the outer wall, the first step is to fit an ellipse around the available lumen contour on the image edges. The resulting ellipse is then slightly deformed locally based on a subsequent dynamic programming step.

In carotid studies of 17 patients,[23] an excellent agreement was observed between contour areas obtained by automated contour detection and contour areas derived from manual tracings (mean difference for lumen areas: 9.1% ± 21.7% and for outer contour areas: 5.4% ± 19.1%). The contour detection approach was also validated for aortic vessel wall dimensions based on MR VW studies of 28 patients.[24] Mean difference for automated versus manually derived contour areas was 0.97% ± 3.4% for lumen and 1.3% ± 6.7% for outer contour areas, respectively. In addition, in the same study, it was observed that the agreement of wall thickness measurements between automated detection and manual contour tracing was higher than the agreement between two manual observers. Figure 84-14 shows an example of automatically detected contours and derived wall thickness measurements in the thoracic aorta following this approach. Figure 84-15 provides an example of a vessel wall analysis of a segment of the common carotid artery.

CHAPTER 84 • Advanced Three-Dimensional Postprocessing in CT and MRA 1139

TABLE 84-2 Results of Measurements of the Reference and Obstruction Diameters Using Automated MRA Analysis

Phantom Number	True Reference Diameter [mm]	MRA-Derived Reference Diameter [mm]	True Obstruction Diameter [mm]	MRA-Derived Obstruction Diameter [mm]
1	6.80	7.25 ± 0.09	5.58	5.54
2	6.80	6.96 ± 0.08	4.69	5.09
3	6.80	6.66 ± 0.11	3.47	4.68
4	6.80	6.87 ± 0.12	2.92	5.18
5	6.80	6.65 ± 0.11	1.97	5.02

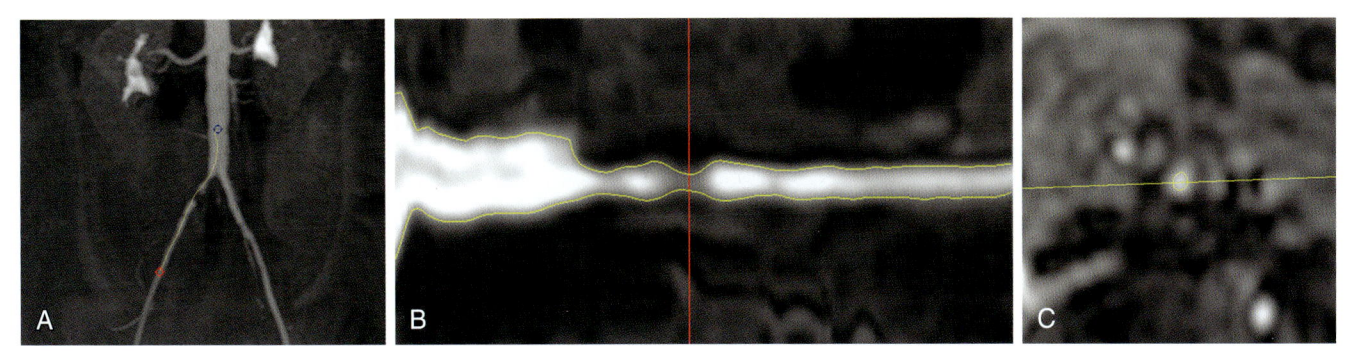

■ **FIGURE 84-13** MRA analysis of a lesion in the right iliac artery. **A,** Detected pathline. **B,** Longitudinal reformat view showing the detected luminal boundaries in a stretched view. **C,** Cross-sectional view at the location of the minimal luminal area.

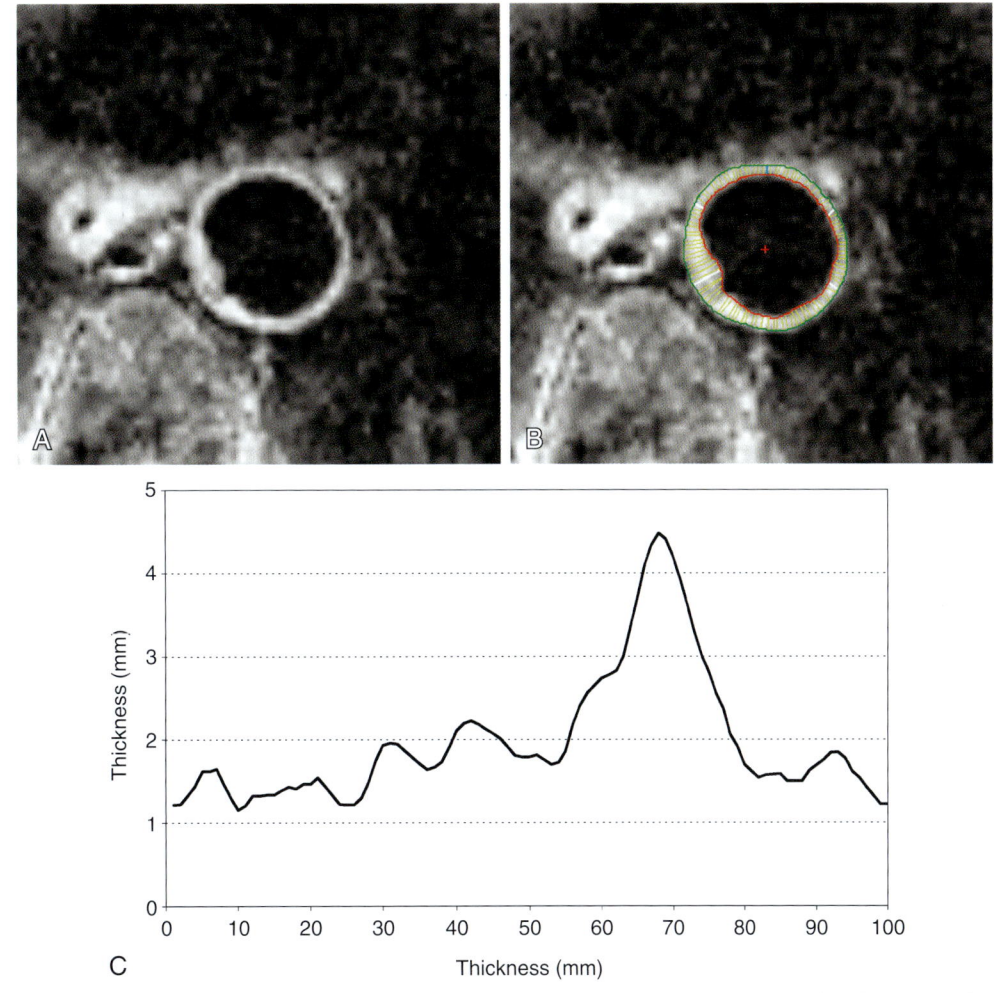

■ **FIGURE 84-14** Result of wall thickness analysis of the thoracic aorta. **A,** MR vessel wall images at the level of the thoracic descending aorta. **B,** Automatically detected luminal (*red*) and outer contours (*green*) and wall thickness measurements using the centerline method. Wall thickness chords (*yellow*) are generated at 100 positions along the vessel circumference starting at the 12 o'clock position (*blue tick mark*). **C,** Graph showing local wall thickness along the vessel wall circumference.

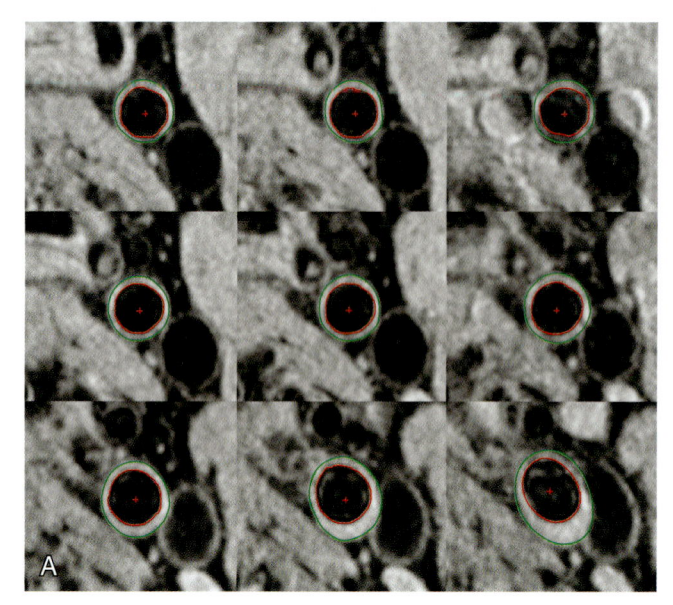

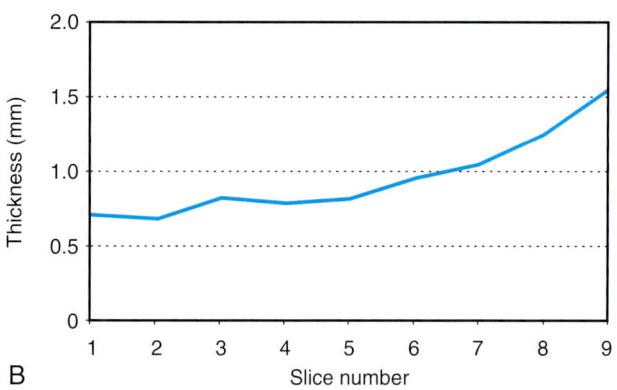

FIGURE 84-15 Result of wall thickness analysis of the common carotid artery. **A,** Automatically detected luminal and outer wall contours in nine consecutive slices. **B,** Graph showing mean wall thickness for each slice level.

TABLE 84-3	Plaque Characterization Using Multispectral MRI*		
	T1W	**PDW**	**T2W**
Calcium	Hypointense	Hypointense	Hypointense
Lipid	Hyperintense	Hyperintense	Hypointense
Fibrous tissue	Isointense	Hyperintense	Isointense to hypointense

*Classification of MR signal intensity is relative to the signal of the sternocleidomastoid muscle in the same image.

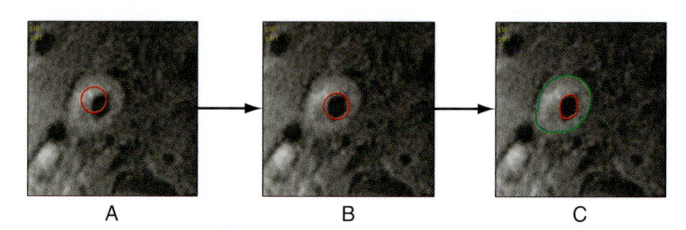

FIGURE 84-16 Automated contour detection in T1w vessel wall image based on available lumen segmentation in CE-MRA sequence. **A,** The result of the MRA lumen segmentation is transferred to the T1w image. **B,** T1w image after lumen registration. **C,** Lumen refinement and outer wall contour detection.

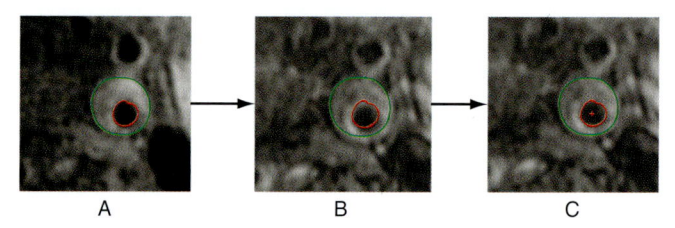

FIGURE 84-17 Automated registration of vessel lumen and outer contours of T1w image to T2w image. **A,** Detected lumen and outer contour in a T1w image. **B,** Transfer of both contours to the T2w image. **C,** Resulting T2w image after the application of automatic registration.

Plaque Assessment

For detailed characterization of the plaque composition, multiple VWI series need to be acquired using different contrast-weightings (e.g., T1, T2, proton density). Each contrast-weighting can be optimized in such a way that it targets a specific tissue type causing a high or low signal excitation of this tissue compared to surrounding tissues. For visual plaque assessment, a decision scheme can be used like the one provided in Table 84-3, taking into account the signal intensities in the vessel wall as seen in the various sequences. Quantitative analysis of such extensive vessel wall examinations requires: (1) registration of the multiple series to correct for patient motion that occurs between the series; (2) detection of luminal and outer boundaries in the vessel segment of interest; (3) detection and classification of relevant plaque components; and (4) assessment of parameters accurately describing the vascular pathology. This analysis approach can be integrated into a single system.[25]

The first step in the analysis is the identification of the vessel segment of interest by indicating a proximal and distal point in the 3D MRA data set as described earlier.

The resulting 3D segmentation is transferred to the images of the T1-weighted (T1w) series using an automated registration procedure (Fig. 84-16). Because the in-plane resolution of the T1w series is higher than that of the MRA series, the lumen contours in the T1w images are further refined using a dynamic programming approach based on the edges in the T1w images. Subsequently, the outer contours are detected in the T1w images based on ellipse fitting followed by dynamic programming. When lumen and outer contours are available for the T1w series, these contours are transferred to the other available VWI series. During this step, another registration step needs to be performed to correct for patient motion between imaging series (Fig. 84-17).

In the previous steps all available image information was aligned and for each location inside the vessel wall signal intensities from multiple contrast weightings are known. In order to compare these intensities amongst multiple patients, the MR signal intensities need to be normalized. In the process of conventional manual plaque assessment, the expert manually segments the vessel wall by deciding whether a region of interest is hypointense

FIGURE 84-18 Image of a T1w sequence showing outlines of the left and right sternocleidomastoid muscles.

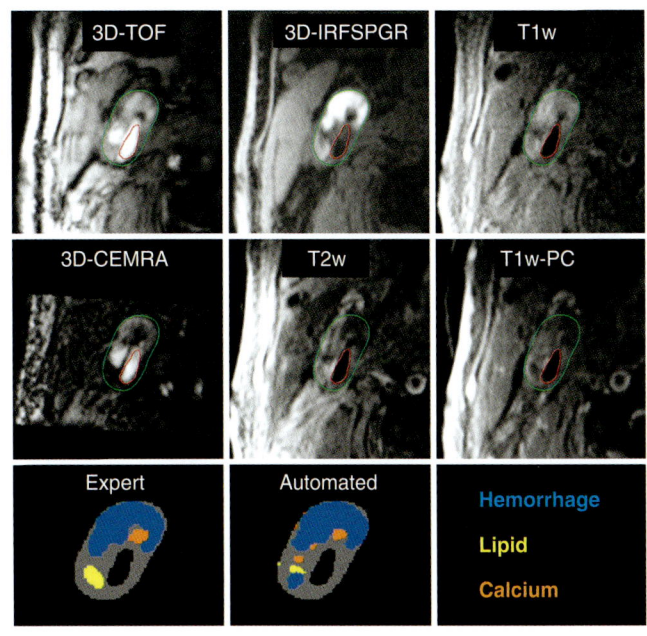

FIGURE 84-19 *Top two rows*: Cross-sectional images at the bifurcation level of a carotid artery with extensive disease using a multi-sequence in-vivo 3T MR protocol with lumen and outer contours defined. Good agreement is observed between expert segmentation of plaque components and result of automated plaque segmentation. TOF, time of flight, IRFSPGR, inversion recovery fast spoiled gradient recalled, T1w, T1-weighted, CE-MRA, contrast-enhanced MRA, T2w, T2-weighted, T1w-PC, T1-weighted postcontrast. *(Images courtesy of JK DeMarco, MD.)*

or hyperintense compared to the sternocleidomastoid muscle, the anterior muscle in the neck (Fig. 84-18). In our automated approach, the signal intensity of the sternocleidomastoid muscle is determined by selecting a region of interest around the vessel and the median value of that region is assumed to resemble the signal intensity of the sternocleidomastoid. The signal intensities of each slice and MR sequence are divided by the found median value, resulting in a normalized image set.

The last step of the automated vessel wall analysis is the classification of the plaque content inside the vessel wall. A statistical pattern recognition system is employed to automatically classify the contents of the vessel wall. Pattern recognition aims to classify data (patterns) based on either a priori knowledge or on statistical information extracted from the patterns. The former is called *supervised classification*; the latter *unsupervised classification*. The patterns to be classified are usually groups of measurements or observations, defining points in an appropriate multidimensional space. The output classes of the classifier are in this case labels of different tissues, for example, fibrous tissue, lipid, hemorrhage, and calcium. The first step of the pattern recognition system is the collection of measurements and observations. For each location inside the vessel wall, that is, for each pixel in the MR images, characteristics such as image intensities from multiple sequences, edge information and morphologic properties (e.g., the thickness of the vessel wall) can be obtained. The aim of this step is to collect as much relevant information as possible about that certain location. The more information that can be incorporated into the system, the better a decision can be made about that location in the vessel wall. In the second step, a supervised classifier is trained using a priori knowledge. Representative example data sets containing image information and expert segmentation are used to obtain the a priori knowledge. This is accomplished by extracting patterns from the image information as well as by corresponding output classes as assigned by the expert segmentation. The classifier is then trained by determining the boundaries in the multidimensional space between patterns of different classes extracted from the example data. Different methods exist to define these boundaries resulting in different types of classifiers. When the boundaries are known, an unseen pattern (i.e., a pixel inside the vessel wall) is tested by assigning probabilities of the target classes to it using the boundaries obtained during training. The class with the highest probability determines the class of the unseen pattern. An example of an automatic classification based on six MR sequences is shown in Figure 84-19. Different classifiers were evaluated for this kind of classification problem. It has been shown by Hoffman and colleagues that more complex classifiers do not have major advantages over more basic classifiers.[26]

Although the classification is normally applied to single pixels, the result of the classification is usually interpreted in plaque lesions. In a typical classification result, lesions are already visible but also scattering of pixels is apparent. Postprocessing can be applied to the classification result to remove scattered pixels and create smooth lesions. Postprocessing can be performed on the output of the classifier or a level set approach can be used where the classification output serves as an initial segmentation result. Another approach is to use a classifier that takes the neighborhood of a pixel into account during the classification, thereby reducing the amount of scattered pixels in the end result.[26]

The performance of a pattern recognition system is generally evaluated by looking at the amount of correctly classified patterns, whereas plaque is generally assessed by counting plaque lesions; the exact plaque boundaries are of less importance. The number of correctly classified lesions is an essential measure used to evaluate the automatic system. A lesion is said to be correctly classified when it has an overlap of at least 50% with the gold standard lesion. Other interesting measures are the area of the total found plaque and the amount of overlap between the gold standard and automated segmentation. Quantification of the plaque volume allows for longitudinal studies because plaques can be followed over time and the change in plaque volume can be evaluated.

> **KEY POINTS**
> - Quantitative analysis based on automated contour detection techniques provides objective and reproducible data about vessel sizes in CTA and MRA.
> - Coronary CTA has developed into a readily available noninvasive imaging modality to detect the presence or absence of coronary obstructions; radiation dose is still an issue of concern.
> - MRA allows the noninvasive depiction of peripheral vessels; there is no radiation hazard, but the spatial resolution is limited.
> - MR vessel wall imaging allows an excellent depiction of the plaque burden in the wall, and potentially about the plaque composition.

SUGGESTED READINGS

Achenbach S. Computed tomography coronary angiography J Am Coll Cardiol 2006; 48:1919-1928.

Briley-Saebo KC, Mulder WJM, Mani V, et al. Magnetic resonance imaging of vulnerable atherosclerotic plaques: current imaging strategies and molecular imaging probes. J Magn Reson Imaging 26:460-479, 2007.

Finn JP, Nael K, Deshpande V, et al. Cardiac MR imaging: state of the technology. Radiology 2006; 241:3354.

Fuster V, Fayad ZA, Moreno PR, et al. Atherothrombosis and high-risk plaque. Part II: Approaches by noninvasive computed tomographic/magnetic resonance imaging. J Am Coll Cardiol 2005; 46:1209-1218.

Jacobs MA, Ibrahim TS, Ouwerkerk R. MR imaging: brief overview and emerging applications. Radiographics 2007; 27:1213-1229.

Lindsay AC, Choudhury RP. Form to function: current and future roles for atherosclerosis imaging in drug development. Nature Reviews 2008; 7:517-529.

Mahesh M, Cody DD. Physics of cardiac imaging with multiple-row detector CT. Radiographics 2007; 27:1495-1509.

Pooley RA. Fundamental physics of MR imaging. Radiographics 2005; 25:1087-1099.

Schroeder S, Achenbach S, Bengel F, et al. Cardiac computed tomography: indications, applications, limitations and training requirements. Eur Heart J 2008; 29:531-556.

REFERENCES

1. Frangi AF, Niessen WJ, Hoogeveen RM, et al. Model-based quantitation of 3D magnetic resonance angiographic images. IEEE Trans Med Imaging 1999; 18:946-956.
2. de Koning PJH, Schaap JA, Janssen JP, et al. Automated segmentation and analysis of vascular structures in magnetic resonance angiographic images. Magn Reson Med 2003; 50:1189-1198.
3. Janssen JP, Koning G, de Koning PJH, et al. A novel approach for the detection of pathlines in x-ray angiograms: the wavefront propagation algorithm. Int J Cardiovasc Imaging 2002; 18:317-324.
4. Schirmacher H, Zockler M, Stalling D, Hege HC. Boundary surface shrinking—a continuous approach to 3D center line extraction. Proc. IMDSP 1998; 1:25-28.
5. D'Souze ND, Reinhardt JM, Hoffmann EA. ASAP: Interactive quantification of 2D airway geometry. Physiology and function from multidimensional images. Proc. SPIE Medical Imaging. 1996; 2809:180-196.
6. Dijkstra J, Koning G, Reiber JHC. Quantitative measurements in IVUS images. Int J Card Imaging. 1999; 15:513-522.
7. Koning G, Dijkstra J, von Birgelen C, et al. Advanced contour detection for three-dimensional intracoronary ultrasound: a validation—in vitro and in vivo. Int J Cardiovasc Imaging 2002; 18:235-248.
8. Sonka M, Hlavac V, Boyle R. Image Processing, Analysis, and Machine Vision. Pacific Grove, Calif., PWS Publishing, 1999.
9. Sonka M, Winniford MD, Collins SM. Robust simultaneous detection of coronary borders in complex images. IEEE Trans Med Imag 14:151-161, 1995.
10. van Bemmel CM, Spreeuwers LJ, Viergever MA, Niessen WA. Medical image computing and computer-assisted intervention. In Dohi T, Kikinis R (eds). Lecture Notes in Computer Science. Berlin, Springer, 2002, pp 36-43.
11. Reiber JHC, Koning G, Tuinenburg JC, et al. Quantitative coronary arteriography. In Oudkerk M (ed). Coronary Radiology. Berlin, Springer Verlag, 2004, pp 41-58.
12. Kitslaar PH, Marquering HA, Koning G, et al. CTA derived optimal angiographic viewing angles for coronary x-ray angiography. Proc SPIE Medical Imaging 2008; 6918:68181J-1-69181J-10.
13. Glagov S, Weisenberg E, Zarins DK, et al. Compensatory enlargement of human atherosclerotic coronary arteries. N Engl J Med 1987; 316:1371-1375.
14. North American Symptomatic Carotid Endarterectomy Trial Collaborators. Beneficial effect of carotid endarterectomy in symptomatic patients with high-grade carotid stenosis. N Eng J Med 1991; 325:445-453.
15. ACAS Clinical advisory: carotid endarterectomy for patients with asymptomatic internal carotid artery stenosis. Stroke 1994; 25:2523-2524.
16. Ingersleben GV, Schmiedl UP, Hatsukami TS, et al. Characterization of atherosclerotic plaques at the carotid bifurcation: correlation of high resolution MR with histology. RadioGraphics 1997; 17:1417-1423.
17. Toussaint JF, LaMuraglia GM, Southern JR, et al. Magnetic resonance images lipid, fibrous, calcified, hemorrhagic, and thrombotic components of human atherosclerosis in vivo. Circulation 94:932-938, 1996.
18. Skinner MP, Yuan C, Mitsumori LM, et al. Serial magnetic resonance imaging of experimental atherosclerosis detects lesions, fine structures, progression, and complications in vivo. Nat Med 1995; 1:69-73.
19. Yuan C, Mitsumori LM, Skinner MP, et al. Magnetic resonance imaging techniques for monitoring the progression of advanced

20. Hoogeveen RM, Bakker CJ, Viergever MA. Limits to the accuracy of vessel diameter measurement in MR angiography. J Magn Reson Imaging 1998; 8:1228-1235.
21. Makowski P, deKoning PJH, Angelié E, et al. 3D cylindrical B-spline segmentation of carotid arteries from MRI Images. In Lecture Notes in Computer Science, Biomedical Simulation. Berlin/Heidelberg, Springer, 2006, pp188-196.
22. de Vries M, de Koning PJ, de Haan MW, et al. Accuracy of semiautomated analysis of 3D contrast-enhanced magnetic resonance angiography for detection and quantification of aortoiliac stenoses. Invest Radiol 2005; 40:495-503.
23. Adame IM, van der Geest RJ, Wasserman BA, et al. Automatic segmentation and plaque characterization in atherosclerotic carotid artery MR images. MAGMA 2004; 16: 227-234.

lesions of atherosclerosis in rabbit aorta. Magn Reson Imaging 1996; 14:93-102.

24. Adame IM, van der Geest RJ, Bluemke DA, et al. Automatic vessel wall contour detection and quantification of wall thickness in in-vivo MR images of the human aorta. J Magn Reson Imaging 2006; 24:595-602.
25. Adame IM, de Koning PJH, Lelieveldt BPF, et al. An integrated automated analysis method for quantifying vessel stenosis and plaque burden from carotid MRI images: Combined postprocessing of MRA and vessel wall MR. Stroke 2006; 37:2162-2164.
26. Hofman JM, Branderhorst WJ, ten Eikelder HM, et al. Quantification of atherosclerotic plaque components using in vivo MRI and supervised classifiers. Magn Reson Med 2006; 55:790-799.

CHAPTER 85

Nuclear Medicine: Extrathoracic Vascular Imaging

Amit Majmudar and James K. O'Donnell

Compared with catheter angiography, CT angiography, and MR angiography, nuclear medicine is a small component of extrathoracic vascular imaging. This component is crucial, however; the specific questions answered safely and efficiently by nuclear medicine cannot be answered by any other modality. Historically, radioisotope techniques have been used widely to answer research and clinical vascular questions. Some early nuclear angiographic procedures contributed greatly to our knowledge of cardiac and vascular physiology and diagnosis of various peripheral vascular disorders.[1] These techniques capitalize on the ability of noninvasive radioisotope imaging to depict existing physiologic parameters accurately without changing the physiology being interrogated.

Three specific studies occupy pivotal, indispensable roles in contemporary clinical algorithms: Tc 99m–radiolabeled erythrocyte scanning for acute gastrointestinal bleeding, Tc 99m pertechnetate imaging for the detection and management of Meckel diverticulum causing intermittent gastrointestinal bleeding, and brain perfusion tomographic single photon emission computed tomography (SPECT) imaging before and after administration of acetazolamide (Diamox) for the assessment of cerebrovascular reserve. Modern dynamic imaging techniques, image display, and improvements in erythrocyte labeling efficiency have optimized these studies. Reliable, definitive information is delivered to angiographers, neurointerventionalists, and surgeons to assist in patient management decisions.

Bleeding studies benefit from dynamic cine sequences, which show in rapid succession multiple images acquired at short intervals (Fig. 85-1). This sequence of images gives the interpreting physician greater confidence in localizing a bleeding site or visualizing the progressive accumulation of activity in a Meckel diverticulum (Fig. 85-2). Brain SPECT studies have benefited from advances in software allowing digital image fusion of the radioisotope study with CT or MRI anatomic sectional images, further computer comparison with probabilistic brain atlases, and three-dimensional volume rendering.

Nuclear medicine continues to refine its preexisting role in extrathoracic cardiac imaging even as it expands to assess atherosclerosis with positron emission tomography with ^{18}FDG. This study is still in its experimental phase, but shows great promise as an imaging adjunct.[2]

TECHNICAL REQUIREMENTS

Gastrointestinal bleeding studies including Tc 99m–radiolabeled erythrocyte scans and Tc 99m pertechnetate scans require a standard gamma camera with a large field of view. A low-energy, high-resolution, parallel hole collimator should be used, and a 20% window should be centered at 140 keV. An identical energy window should be used for the acetazolamide brain perfusion SPECT scan, but the gamma camera must have its one or more detector heads mounted on a rotating gantry programmable to rotate in a 360-degree arc around the head of the patient.

GASTROINTESTINAL BLEED LOCALIZATION SCAN

Indications and Contraindications

A Tc 99m–radiolabeled erythrocyte scan should be performed to help localize the vascular origin of acute gastrointestinal bleeding involving the colon. The technique is less accurate in the assessment of upper gastrointestinal

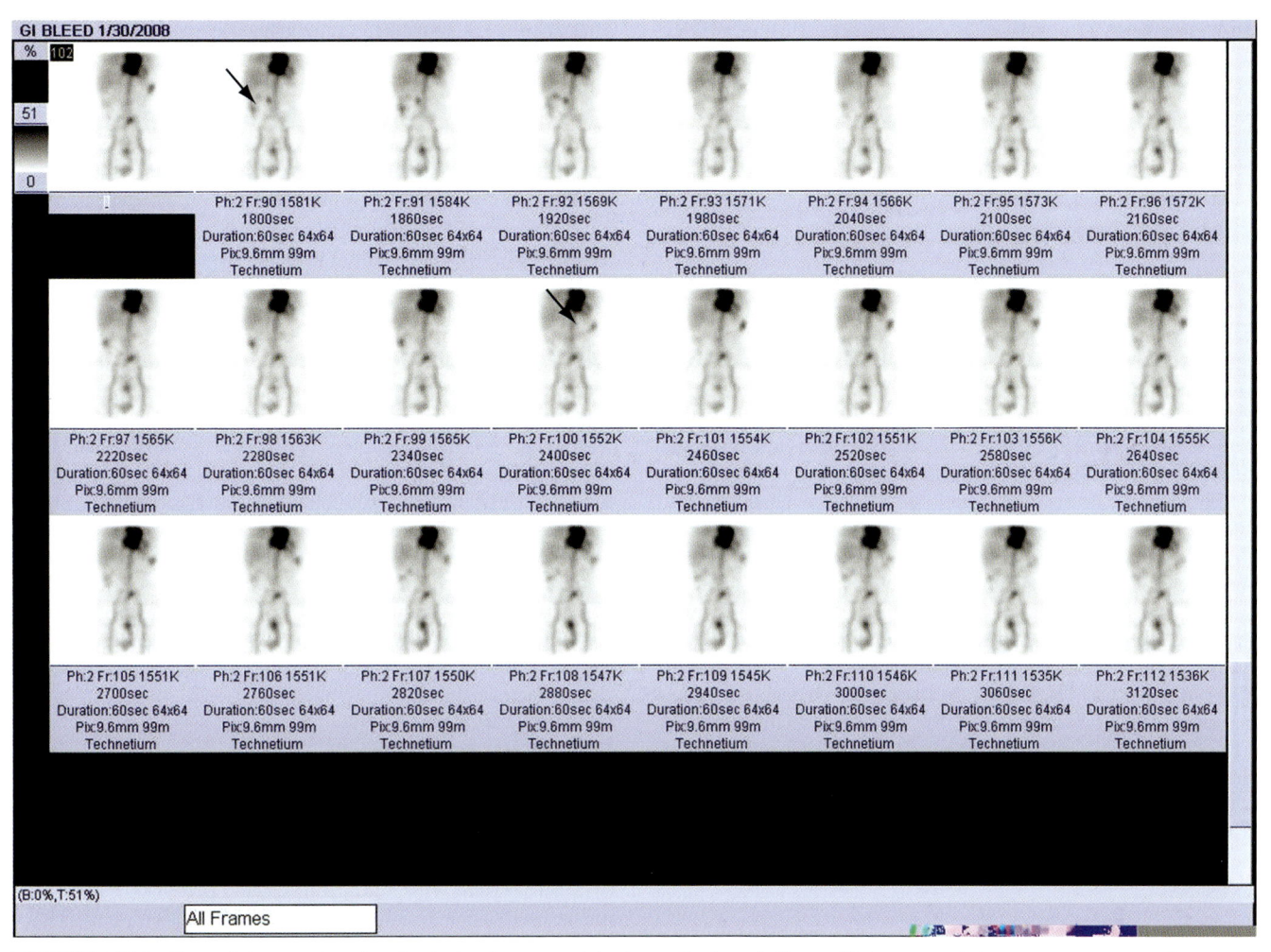

■ **FIGURE 85-1** Dynamic images show intraluminal radiotracer originating at the hepatic flexure (*first row, arrow*) that progresses antegrade, crossing midline along the course of the transverse colon (*second row, arrow*). The *upper left corner image* is a single image from the dynamic cine presentation.

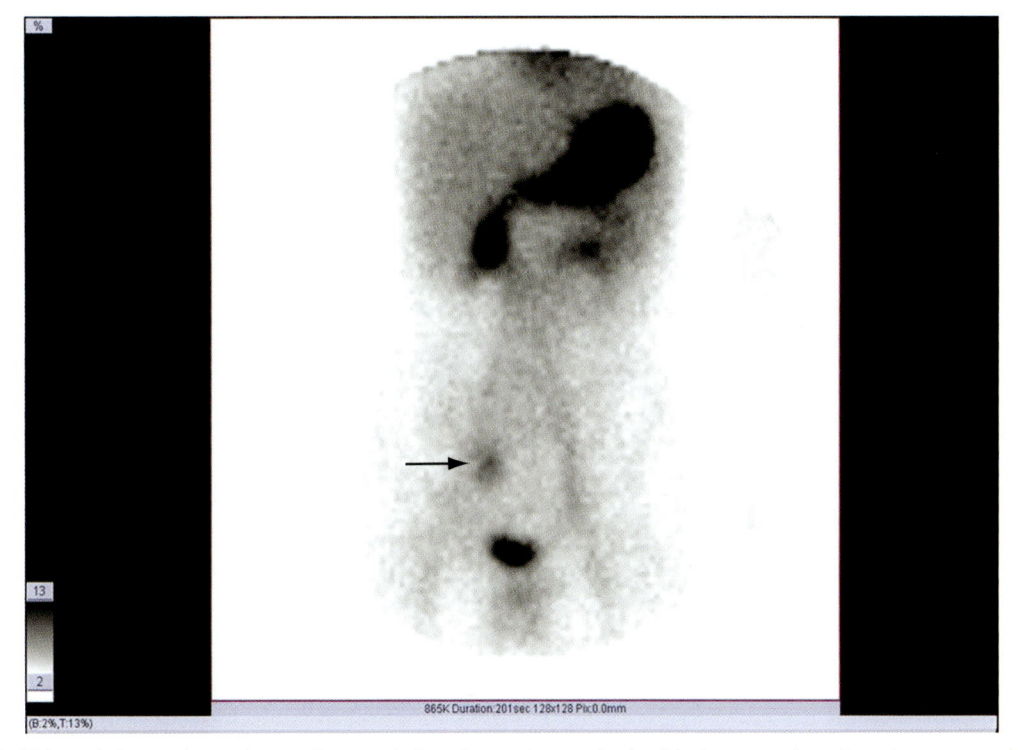

■ **FIGURE 85-2** This static image shows abnormal accumulation of pertechnetate in the right lower quadrant (*arrow*), a common location for a Meckel diverticulum. The intense activity in the upper abdomen conforms to the stomach.

tract bleeding. The only major contraindication is a bleed so rapid that it is best spared scintigraphic interrogation in favor of immediate contrast angiography. The bleeding localization study may require too much radiolabeling preparation and imaging time to be performed on an acutely unstable patient.

Technique Description

No specific patient preparation is required for a Tc 99m–radiolabeled erythrocyte scan. This is an advantage because studies for gastrointestinal bleeding are usually requested emergently. Various labeling methods and kits are available to label the red blood cell, including an in vitro method, an in vivo method, and a hybrid method. The in vitro method using widely available kits typically provides very high labeling efficiency (e.g., Ultratag kit [Mallinckrodt, Inc., St. Louis]) provides a labeling efficiency of 98.5%).[3] What the methods have in common is the use of stannous ion as a reducing agent and the Tc 99m label.

The patient is positioned supine with the camera located anteriorly. On initial intravenous injection of the radiolabeled erythrocytes, initial flow images are obtained at 1 s/frame for 60 frames. Subsequent dynamic images are obtained at 1 min/frame for 60 additional frames. A 128×128 image matrix is normally used for both acquisitions.[4] Additional imaging may be repeated at intervals up to 24 hours, but all acquisitions should be in a dynamic series to enable detection of subtle bleeding sites and peristaltic transit through the bowel.

Pitfalls and Solutions

The most common technical pitfall of the Tc 99m–radiolabeled erythrocyte scan relates to an imperfect tagging of the blood cells, leaving free Tc 99m pertechnetate in the bloodstream. As described earlier, tagging efficiency is typically very high, especially with the in vitro technique. Common drugs such as heparin, penicillin, and iodinated contrast media interfere with the entry of the reducing agent (Sn^{++}) through the red blood cell membrane, however, causing an increased amount of free pertechnetate in the blood.[5] Also, alternative in vivo labeling techniques may allow a certain amount of free pertechnetate to circulate.

Free pertechnetate appears in the stomach where it is physiologically secreted by the gastric parietal cells (see Fig. 85-2). This activity has an intraluminal configuration and moves antegrade over time. This movement can simulate an upper gastrointestinal bleed. In some instances, an upper gastrointestinal bleed may have been ruled out from a recent endoscopy, or the clinical presentation may not be consistent with one. A static image of the neck also reveals physiologic uptake of pertechnetate in the thyroid gland. After confirmation of the presence of free pertechnetate, the best solution is to allow for it in the interpretation. A brisk lower gastrointestinal bleed should be differentiated easily on dynamic imaging.

Another pitfall, related to the physiology of gastrointestinal bleeding itself, is intermittent bleeding. In Tc 99m sulfur colloid scanning (no longer commonly performed), after an initial 20-minute window, the study ceases to be diagnostic because of rapid radiopharmaceutical clearance by the liver. With Tc 99m–radiolabeled erythrocyte scans, however, delayed imaging up to 24 hours is possible. Delayed imaging can solve the problem of bleeding that has stopped temporarily during the initial imaging session.

Several factors must be accounted for to maximize the diagnostic utility of delayed scanning. First, the patient should be rescanned as soon as possible after the repeat bleed comes to clinical attention. The images obtained should be dynamic; this is the only way to localize the bleed. Localization is often impaired because the intraluminal blood, a strong peristaltic stimulant, has progressed distal to the actual bleeding site.

Interpretive pitfalls consist of confounding patterns of activity. The only solution for these interpretive pitfalls is for the interpreter to be aware of their appearance. Physiologic penile blood flow may be mistaken for rectal bleeding, or mesenteric vascular activity may overlie the expected location of the bowel. What these confounding patterns have in common is their lack of intraluminal configuration and the absence of antegrade or retrograde movement over time. Table 85-1 presents examples of these patterns.

Image Interpretation

Postprocessing

For Tc 99m–radiolabeled erythrocyte scan, postprocessing is minimal. The images are simply presented in a dynamic series, with static frames also provided for review individually.

Reporting

A Tc 99m–radiolabeled erythrocyte scan report should describe the presence or absence of extravascular activity, where it appears to originate, and whether this activity shows the movement that would be consistent with extravasated blood. Localizing the segment of bowel where the bleed originates helps guide selective angiography and intervention. The quality of the tag, if suboptimal, also warrants comment. If penile blood flow is seen, a mention of its presence avoids confusion among surgeons and other clinicians who may review the scan independently. Communication with collaborating angiographers is also essential to ensure optimization of the subsequent angiographic approach for diagnosis and possible therapeutic intervention.

MECKEL DIVERTICULUM SCAN

Indications and Contraindications

The Tc 99m–pertechnetate scan is useful in detecting a Meckel diverticulum, which contains ectopic gastric mucosa whose acid production ulcerates the small bowel mucosa. These congenital abnormalities are almost always located in the right lower quadrant of the abdomen and manifest with symptomatic gastrointestinal bleeding (see Fig. 85-2). In 50% of cases, diverticula manifest before 2

TABLE 85-1 Confounding Patterns of Activity

Appearance	Description	Etiology
	Focal, rounded, gradually intensifying suprapubic focus without movement (*arrow*)	Physiologic bladder activity
	Focal, rounded area of accumulation along the course of a major vessel (*arrow*) that appears early and shows no peristaltic movement	Vascular aneurysm
	Faint, hazy localization over the abdomen (*arrows*) without peristaltic movement, in a configuration not conforming to bowel lumen	Omental vascular blush
	Linear activity (*arrow*) in a male patient, well below the aortic bifurcation, that shows no movement and appears early. Not to be confused with rectosigmoid bleeding	Penile blood flow

years of age. The pertechnetate administered crosses the placenta,[6] and women of reproductive age should be questioned regarding the possibility of pregnancy.

Technique Description

Scanning for the gastric mucosa in a Meckel diverticulum (also known as Meckel scan) should be obtained with the patient fasting for 4 hours before the scan. The camera is placed in the anterior position relative to the patient, who is positioned semisupine with left side down and right side up; this maneuver minimizes antegrade passage of physiologically secreted gastric pertechnetate activity from the stomach to the proximal small bowel. The field of view is kept with the xiphoid process superiorly and the pubic bone inferiorly, although more of the torso and extremities is inevitably included with very young pediatric patients.

After appropriate positioning, 5 to 10 mCi of Tc 99m pertechnetate is injected intravenously. The dose may be administered by weight for pediatric patients. A standard protocol includes flow images, obtained at 1 s/frame for 60 frames. Dynamic images are obtained at 30 s/frame for 60 additional frames. A 128×128 matrix is used.[4]

Pitfalls and Solutions

Technical pitfalls in Meckel scanning are rare because the radiotracer is simple to prepare. Because pertechnetate is secreted by the gastric mucosa in a Meckel diverticulum, most Meckel diverticula that do not contain gastric mucosa are not detected by the scan. Symptomatic small bowel bleeding is caused by only a few Meckel diverticula that do contain gastric mucosa, however. The physiology of radiotracer localization ensures that the scan detects only symptomatic diverticula—a limitation that is, from the surgeon's standpoint, an advantage.

The most common interpretive pitfall relates to the physiologic excretion of pertechnetate through the renal system. Renal collecting system activity can be present in the expected location of a Meckel diverticulum. A lateral view reliably distinguishes the retroperitoneal structure.

Image Interpretation

Postprocessing

For Tc 99m pertechnetate scans, postprocessing is minimal. The images are simply presented in a dynamic series, with static frames also provided for review individually.

Reporting

The most important information in a Meckel diverticulum scan report is the presence or absence of ectopic gastric mucosa suggestive of a symptomatic Meckel diverticulum. Also important for documentation are the time the activity first appeared, the persistence or intensification of activity, and any other incidental findings. The abnormality usually appears very early in the scan, essentially at the same time as the stomach activity is seen. A delayed appearance may represent urinary collecting system activity, and the location of this activity should be confirmed with additional images (e.g., lateral views).

The wording of a normal pertechnetate scan report is also important. An appropriate normal report states that there is no evidence for ectopic gastric mucosa, not that there is "no Meckel diverticulum." This is because a patient may have a Meckel diverticulum but have a negative scan because the diverticulum contains no gastric mucosa.

BRAIN PERFUSION TOMOGRAPHY

Indications and Contraindications

Acetazolamide-augmented brain perfusion SPECT scans are obtained in patients with compromised carotid circulation who must be evaluated for external-to-internal carotid arterial bypass. If there is appropriate augmentation of cerebral blood flow from baseline after administration of the vasodilator, the cerebrovascular reserve is intact. If there is a failure of perfusion augmentation, this implies a critically stenotic vessel with compromised ability to increase regional blood flow to the brain parenchyma it supplies (Fig. 85-3).

The main contraindication to this study is a sulfa drug allergy. As with any drug allergy, a full investigation into the nature and severity of a past reaction should be obtained. Isolated reports of "steal phenomenon" leading to ischemia exist in the literature,[7] but there are no data to suggest a significant risk of stroke after administration of this carbonic anhydrase inhibitor. Patients should be advised regarding side effects such as nausea, numbness around the mouth or fingers, lightheadedness, or facial flushing.

Technique Description

The patient should be placed in a dark, quiet room for 20 minutes before injection of radiotracer. The patient should not read or speak. Approximately 20 minutes after intravenous injection of 10 mCi of a Tc 99m–radiolabeled lipophilic amine compound—Tc99m HMPAO (Ceretec) or Tc 99m ECD (Neurolite)—a baseline SPECT scan should be acquired. Subsequently, 1 g of acetazolamide is infused intravenously over 5 minutes. Ten minutes after this, a higher dose (30 mCi) of the same Tc 99m radiotracer is administered. Another 20-minute delay precedes the second SPECT image acquisition.[8]

Pitfalls and Solutions

Patient motion is a common technical pitfall with brain SPECT imaging. Postprocessing software is often able to correct for a certain degree of patient motion. If patient stimulation is not minimized before the injection of radiotracer for the baseline and postacetazolamide studies, cortical activation can lead to spurious radiotracer localization. Brain SPECT with a lipophilic amine tracer detects brain perfusion, and brain ^{18}FDG-PET detects metabolism; these are intimately related physiologic processes that can be artifactually altered if the patient is not kept in a dark room with minimal auditory stimuli.

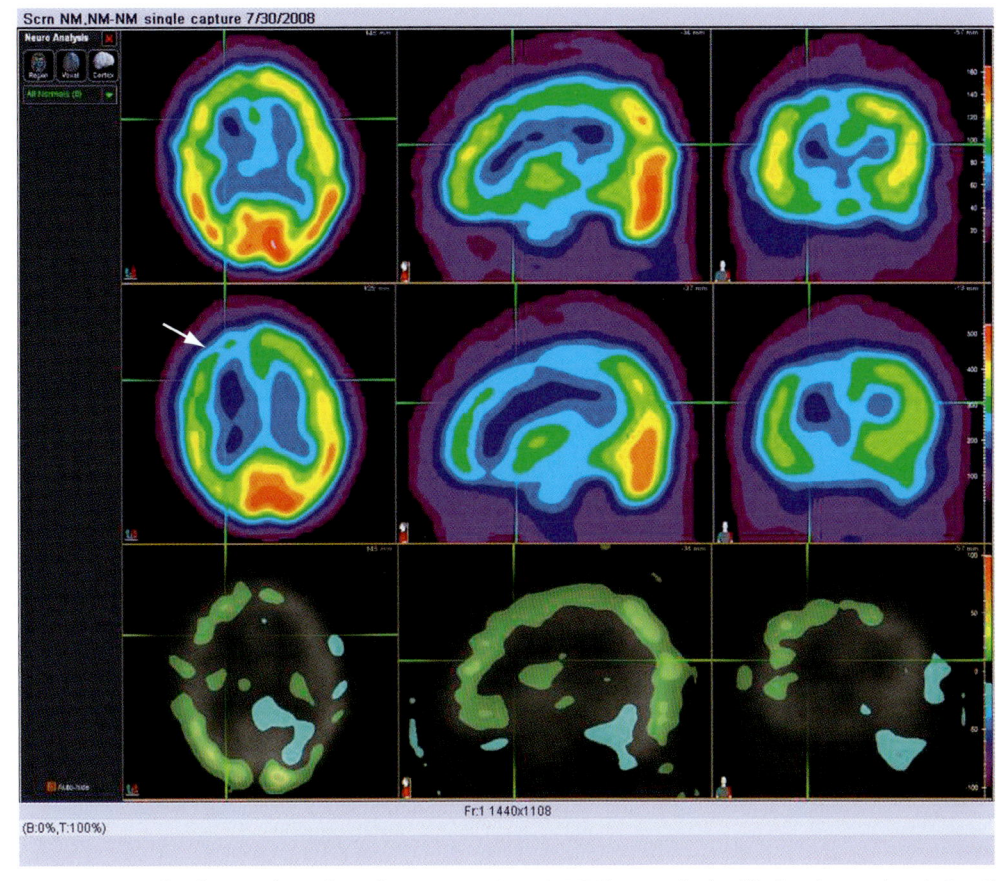

■ **FIGURE 85-3** Juxtaposition and software subtraction of Tc 99m HMPAO SPECT images obtained before (*top row*) and after (*bottom row*) administration of acetazolamide shows failure of augmentation in the right frontal lobe on the study obtained after acetazolamide administration (*arrow, second row*), indicating impaired cerebrovascular reserve.

Postprocessing errors can confound the interpretation as well. Many software programs compare the acquired data with a probabilistic brain atlas.[9] Any results obtained through these means should be verified with direct visual inspection and used at best as an adjunct corroborating the interpreter's own impression.

Interpretive pitfalls are rare with brain SPECT imaging. The vascular changes visualized are often significant ones, in contrast to the more subtle alterations in perfusion seen with interictal and ictal SPECT scans for epilepsy evaluation.

Image Interpretation

Postprocessing

Interpretation involves evaluation of regional brain perfusion in the baseline state and with vasodilator augmentation. Correlation with any anatomic imaging studies, usually MRI of the brain, is helpful and highly advised in elderly patients likely to have cerebrovascular disease. Some software allows digital fusion of the brain SPECT slices with correlative MRI or CT.

Brain SPECT involves more elaborate postprocessing than gastrointestinal bleeding studies. A longer acquisition time per frame on the lower dose baseline scan results in image quality similar to the higher dose postvasodilator scan.

Standard SPECT reconstruction software allows comparison of baseline and postvasodilator images. More quantitative techniques are being developed to enhance diagnostic accuracy. These use iterative reconstruction using ordered subset expectation maximization (OSEM), the technical details of which are beyond the scope of this text. Essentially, the baseline and postacetazolamide data sets are subjected to the same number of reconstruction iterations, followed by three-dimensional processing. This latter step uses either a previously acquired CT scan as an attenuation correction map or preexisting logarithms based on standardized attenuation maps, part of the reconstruction software (e.g., ASTONISH [Phillips Healthcare, Andover, MA]). The images are displayed separately for initial evaluation, with parallel-row, three-dimensional projection and digital subtraction presentations performed at the discretion of the interpreting physician (often using an image processing and presentation software, such as MIM Vista 2.0, Cleveland, OH).

Reporting

Areas of absent or severely limited cerebrovascular reserve appear as areas of decreased perfusion compared with baseline after vasodilator administration (Fig. 85-4). The report should list these areas, ideally taking advantage of digital image fusion or coregistration with correlative anatomic studies, such as MRI or CT.

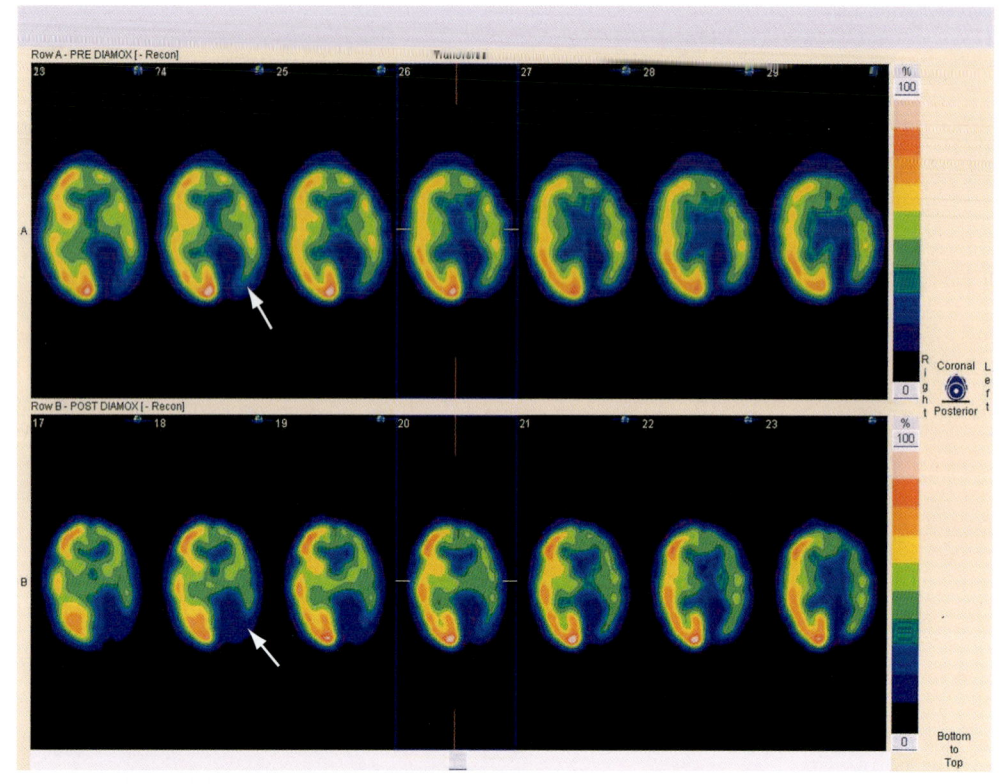

FIGURE 85-4 Tc 99m HMPAO SPECT shows severely impaired perfusion to the left cerebral hemisphere, especially the left parieto-occipital lobe and frontal lobe (*arrows*). The absence of change between studies before and after acetazolamide administration indicates an absence of cerebrovascular reserve.

KEY POINTS

- Tc 99m–radiolabeled erythrocyte scans guide selective angiographic intervention in the setting of acute lower gastrointestinal tract bleeding.
- Tc 99m pertechnetate scanning detects the ectopic gastric mucosa that is present in symptomatic Meckel diverticula.
- Patients undergoing vasodilator-augmented brain SPECT imaging for assessment of cerebrovascular reserve benefit from advanced software analysis for comparison of baseline versus augmented scans and comparison with an atlas of established normals.
- As with all functional imaging studies, an understanding of the physiology to be interrogated, image data acquisition, and postprocessing techniques optimizes the final interpretation.

SUGGESTED READINGS

Grant K, Umphrey H, Liu HG, et al. Clinical use of Diamox brain SPECT: comparison of protocols, evaluation of interpretive findings, and use correlative imaging. J Nucl Med 2007; 48(Suppl 2):214P.

Gutierrez C, et al. The use of technetium-labeled erythrocyte scintigraphy in the evaluation and treatment of lower gastrointestinal hemorrhage. Am Surg 1998; 64:989-992.

Leonidas JC, Germann DR. Technetium-99m pertechnetate imaging in diagnosis of Meckel's diverticulum. Arch Dis Child 1974; 49: 21-26.

Ozgur HT, et al. Correlation of cerebrovascular reserve as measured by acetazolamide-challenged SPECT with angiographic flow patterns and intra- or extracranial arterial stenosis. AJNR Am J Neuroradiol 2001; 22:928-936.

Parkman HP, Maurer AH. Update on gastrointestinal scintigraphy. Semin Nucl Med Volume 2006; 36:110.

REFERENCES

1. MacIntyre WJ, Storaasli JP, Krieger H, et al: I-131-labeled serum albumin: its use in the study of cardiac output and peripheral vascular flow. Radiology 1952; 59:849-857.
2. Rudd JH, Myers KS, Bansilal S, et al. Atherosclerosis inflammation imaging with ^{18}F-FDG PET: carotid, iliac, and femoral uptake reproducibility, quantification methods, and recommendations. J Nucl Med 2008; 49:871-878.
3. Patrick ST, Glowniak JV, Turner FE, et al. Comparison of in vitro RBC labeling with the UltraTag RBC kit versus in vivo labeling. J Nucl Med 1991; 32:242-244.
4. Klingensmith W, Eshima D, Goddard J. Nuclear Medicine Procedure Manual, 2000-2002 edition. Englewood, CO, Wick Publishing, 2002.
5. Saha GB. Characteristics of specific radiopharmaceuticals. In Fundamentals of Nuclear Pharmacy. Berlin, Springer-Verlag, 1992, p 117.

PART
THIRTEEN

Catheter Angiography and Interventions

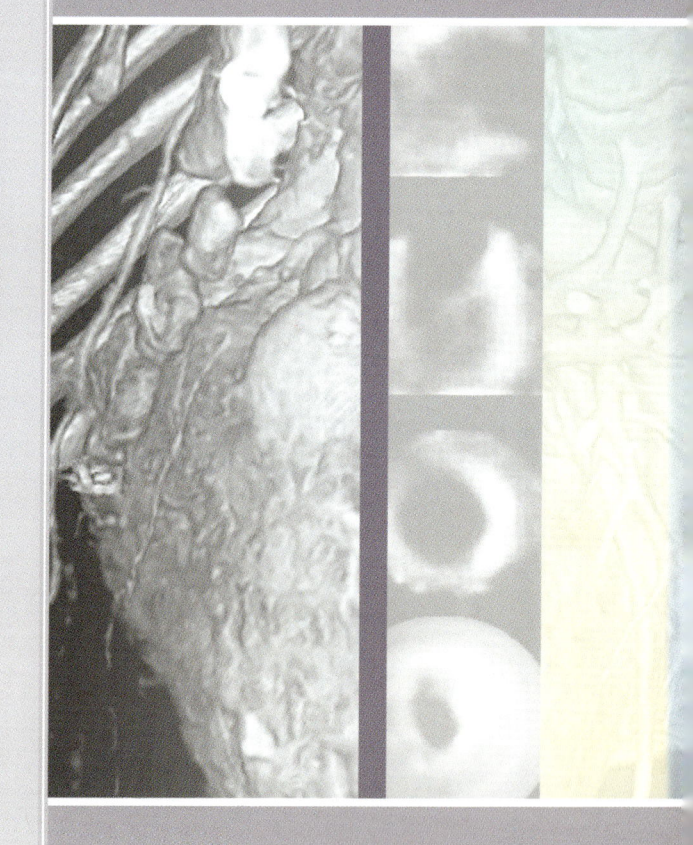

6. Husak V, Wiedermann M. Radiation absorbed dose estimates to the embryo from some nuclear medicine procedures. Eur J Nucl Med 1980; 5:205-207.
7. Komiyama M, Nishikawa M, Yasui T, et al. Reversible pontine ischemia caused by acetazolamide challenge. AJNR Am J Neuroradiol 1997; 18:1782-1784.
8. Juni JE, Waxman AD, Devous MD, et al. Society of Nuclear medicine procedure guideline for brain perfusion single photon emission computed tomography (SPECT) using Tc-99m radiopharmaceuticals. Version 2.0 (approved February 7, 1999).
9. Lee HY, Paeng JC, Lee DS, et al. Efficacy assessment of cerebral arterial bypass surgery using statistical parametric mapping and probabilistic brain atlas on basal/acetazolamide brain perfusion SPECT. J Nucl Med 2004; 45:202-206.

CHAPTER 86

Percutaneous Vascular Interventions

Jonathan Liaw, Benjamin Pomerantz, and Sanjeeva P. Kalva

The first known use of angiography was performed on a cadaver hand in 1896, a year after Roentgen developed the first x-ray. The progress of angiography was initially slow because of the lack of a suitable in vivo contrast medium. Eventually, a contrast agent was developed based on linking iodine to carbon, a formula fundamental to all current iodinated agents. Vascular access remained a problem until 1954, when Seldinger described the technique for percutaneous vascular access.[1] This allowed safe vascular cannulation and resulted in the rapid development of techniques for diagnostic percutaneous angiography.

Percutaneous vascular therapeutic interventions evolved from the successes of diagnostic angiography. The first case of percutaneous revascularization was performed by Dotter and Judkins,[2] who successfully dilated a superficial femoral artery stenosis in 1964 using serial dilation over a percutaneously inserted guide wire. Since then, many technologic innovations in hardware materials, such as balloons, metallic stents and guide wires, have led to the rapid progression of percutaneous vascular interventions. Advances in contrast media and imaging technology, such as digital subtraction angiography, CT, and MRI, have also ushered in new approaches and methods to identify and treat a wide array of vascular diseases through the percutaneous approach. One such example of great clinical usefulness is the use of carbon dioxide (CO_2) as a contrast material for arteriography in digital subtraction angiography system.[3] The knowledge gained through such arterial interventions has been applied for cancer therapy to achieve temporary tumor devascularization in preparation for surgery or to treat the tumor through a combination of chemotherapy and vascular occlusion materials.

In this chapter, we will briefly discuss the tools, principles, and methods of diagnostic arteriography and percutaneous arterial interventions. We have broadly divided arterial interventions into revascularization procedures and vascular exclusion procedures. Our intention is not to provide detailed descriptions of procedures but to provide an overview of the indications, principles, complications, and results. For detailed descriptions of these procedures, refer to the subsequent specialized chapters in this book.

EQUIPMENT AND TOOLS

The essential tools for diagnostic arteriography are catheters, vascular sheaths, and guide wires. In addition to these, revascularization procedures use various types of balloons, metallic stents, and aspiration and infusion catheters. Vascular occlusion and exclusion procedures use particulate materials, metallic coils, detachable balloons, liquid embolic agents, and stent grafts.

Catheters

A catheter commonly serves as a delivery conduit for contrast materials, drugs and embolic devices. Catheters are long hollow tubes made of various materials, usually polyethylene or polyurethane. The size (diameter) refers to the outer diameter of a catheter, with typical sizes varying from 4F to 9F. The inner lumen of a diagnostic catheter is constant, and allows a 0.038-inch diameter guide wire. Within the shaft of a catheter, there is a layer of fine braided wire, resulting in a flexible, kink resistant, torqueable structure. The luminal surface is coated with Teflon or other low-friction substances to provide a low-friction surface for passage of the guide wire and other devices used for peripheral arterial interventions. The tip of the catheter is soft and often tapered. Some catheters have a preformed shape. This may help manipulate the catheter across a vessel or allow selective cannulation of a vessel. Various tip configurations are currently available. Catheter selection depends on the angle at which the target vessel arises from the parent vessel. Several catheters have a reverse curve (e.g., Simmons, SOS omni), which require reformation in a larger vessel to return to the original curve of the catheter.[4] Other catheters have multiple side holes at the tip and allow injection of a large volume of contrast material at a high flow rate.

Microcatheters are generally 3F or smaller in diameter and can be passed through a diagnostic catheter. A microcatheter allows superselective cannulation of a small or tortuous vessel.

Vascular Sheaths and Dilators

Vascular sheaths are generally larger catheters of varying lengths, with a hemostatic valve on the proximal end of the sheath. A side arm is connected to the hemostatic valve. These catheters are inserted over a wire following needle cannulation of the vessel. An inner dilator is present and removed following cannulation of the vessel with the sheath. After removing the dilator, the vascular sheath provides hemostatic access to the vascular system, greatly reducing trauma to the vessel associated with repetitive catheter insertion and manipulation. Most procedures require the use and manipulation of multiple catheters that can be introduced atraumatically to the vessel lumen via the sheath. In addition, sheaths provide support for catheter manipulation and interventions. Sheaths are available in varying sizes, shapes, and lengths. The size (diameter) of sheaths is described in a similar fashion as catheters but, in the case of sheaths, the inner diameter of a vascular sheath is used as the metric, which therefore corresponds to the largest catheter diameter that the sheath will accommodate.

Dilators are short, stiff catheters with a smoothly tapered end. They are passed over a guide wire into the vessel and are used to create a smooth, minimally traumatic tract from the skin surface to the vessel lumen. These are particularly useful for scarred tissue and serial dilations can be performed to enlarge a soft tissue tract to accommodate larger catheters and sheaths. The dilator shape and size are closely matched to the sheath to facilitate nontraumatic introduction of the sheath to the vessel.

Guide Wires

Guide wires are crucial in supporting and steering catheters to the target vessels. They consist of an inner core of stainless steel, wrapped with a smaller wire mandrel. There are multiple guide wire diameters, lengths, stiffnesses, and coatings. The tip of the wire can be angled, flexible, or J-shaped. The length of the flexible tip varies from 1 to 6 cm. A J tip can have a 3-, 5-, 10-, or 15-mm curved radius. Guide wires are typically coated to reduce friction. Some guide wires have a hydrophilic coating, which when wet develop low friction coefficients, thus facilitating advancement in tortuous vessels. Guide wire selection is based on the catheter being used, location of the target vessel, and intervention being performed.

Balloons

Although the first percutaneous angioplasty was described by Dotter and Judkins[2] in 1964, Gruentzig devised the first successful balloon angioplasty in 1976, and this method became widely accepted.[5] The primary mechanism of balloon angioplasty is controlled tear and shearing of the atheromatous plaque, the intima, and the media beneath the plaque.

The characteristics of a balloon depend on the material and its construction. There are essentially two types of balloons, compliant and noncompliant. All balloons have a nominal diameter at a given pressure as well as a predetermined burst pressure.

Compliant and Noncompliant Angioplasty Balloons

Compliant balloons are made of latex, silicone, or polyurethane. These balloons elongate and conform to the vessel rather than dilate as pressure is applied. They are particularly useful for temporary vascular occlusion, embolectomy, or the molding of a stent graft.

Noncompliant balloons are made of noncompliant polymers with high tensile strength. The balloon reaches a nominal predetermined diameter during inflation. These balloons are useful for angioplasty.

Cutting Balloons

The Peripheral Cutting Balloon (Boston Scientific; Natick, Mass) features a noncompliant balloon with three or four small longitudinal blades. These blades lie in balloon recesses when the balloon is deflated. The balloon is introduced via a sheath. Once it reaches the target lesion, the sheath is retracted to expose the cutting balloon. On inflation, the cutting blades incise and fracture the plaque more readily than conventional angioplasty balloons. As a result, this technique may reduce trauma to the vessel. It is critical to retract the cutting balloon into the sheath after angioplasty to avoid trauma to the adjacent nondiseased portion of the vessel.

Cryoplasty Balloons

The PolarCath angioplasty system (Boston Scientific) simultaneously dilates and cools the plaque and vessel wall. Nitrous oxide gas is instilled into the balloon and chills the vessel wall to −10° C over a depth of 500 μm. It is believed that cooling to −10° C can induce cell apoptosis rather than necrosis in smooth muscle cells, resulting in decreased elastic recoil and reduced neointimal hyperplasia. This device is relatively new and more clinical studies are required to provide a robust evidence of the efficacy of this mode of treatment.[6]

Atherectomy Devices

Atherectomy devices (e.g., SilverHawk Plaque Excision System; U.S. Peripheral Products, Plymouth, MN) use a small rotating blade to cut and remove vessel wall atheroma. Theoretically, atherectomy offers the following advantages over conventional percutaneous transluminal angioplasty. It reduces focally and selectively the degree of stenosis by debulking the atheromatous mass, which increases immediate technical success, given the absence of subintimal dissection and local trauma. Although short-term results show a favorable trend toward decreased restenosis rates, long-term efficacy data of this technique is not yet available.[7]

Stents

The first endovascular stent (endovascular splint) was used by Dotter in 1969.[8] Since then, stent technology has grown significantly and revolutionized the percutaneous management of vascular disease. Currently, there are two basic devices, balloon-mounted and self-expanding stents.

Balloon-Mounted Stents

Balloon-mounted stents (e.g., Palmaz, Cordis, Warren, NJ; WaveMax, Abbott, Santa Clara, Calif; Omni-Flex, AngioDynamics, Queensbury, NY;, Express, Boston Scientific; LifeStent, Bard Peripheral Vascular, Tempe, Ariz) are made of stainless steel and require balloon dilation to expand the stent to its working dimension. These stents have high radial strength but are less flexible. If deformed, these stents will undergo permanent plastic deformation and thus should not be placed in locations subject to flexing or compression. When deployed, balloon-mounted stents undergo minimal foreshortening, which allows precise placement; this is particularly useful for the treatment of lesions adjacent to an ostium, bifurcation, or side branch. These stents are not contained within a delivery system, and thus the delivery sheath should be long enough to cover the balloon and stent until deployment. During deployment of these stents, the final length of the deployed stent is inversely related to the final diameter of the deployed stent. The stent used needs to be large enough to prevent stent migration with minimal coverage of the normal adjacent vessel.

Self-Expanding Stents

Self-expanding stents (e.g., Wallstents, Boston Scientific; SMART stents, Cordis) are made from an alloy of nickel and titanium (Nitinol) or stainless steel. Nitinol stents have a thermal memory, which allows them to expand to a predetermined diameter at body temperature. Self-expanding stents will not undergo permanent plastic deformation and therefore are ideal for placement across flexing or compressing regions. They should also be used when relatively longer coverage is needed or in the presence of an associated dissection at the target vessel.

Nitinol stents are somewhat radiolucent, requiring the use of radiopaque markers, which are strategically placed on the stent to allow visualization of the proximal and distal aspects of the stent. In general, a self-expanding stent needs to be 1 to 2 mm larger in diameter than the target vessel. Often, after deployment, an angioplasty balloon is needed to expand the stent fully. Following deployment, self-expanding stents undergo minimal foreshortening, generally less than 7%.

Drug-Eluting Stents

Following angioplasty and stent placement, smooth muscle cells in the arterial wall may undergo hyperplasia, resulting in neointimal hyperplasia and subsequent stenosis within the stent. Drug-eluting stents are designed to decrease stent restenosis rates. Drug-eluting stents contain three components, a metallic stent, a slow-release chemical coating, and a drug. The drug acts locally on the vascular smooth muscle cells, theoretically reducing neointimal hyperplasia that results in decreased stent restenosis. To date, the most promising drugs include sirolimus, zotorolimus, everolimus, and paclitaxel. Long-term data are lacking but multiple studies are underway to assess the efficacy of drug-eluting stents.[9]

Stent Grafts

Stent grafts are covered stents that serve as a vascular conduit. The covering material is generally a synthetic textile such as Dacron, extruded polytetrafluoroethylene (ePTFE), or polyethylene terephthalate (PET). Stent grafts may be balloon-mounted (e.g., Fluency stent, Bard Peripheral) or self-expanding (e.g., Viabahn, W.L. Gore, Flagstaff, Ariz). Common indications for stent grafts are treatment of ruptured or unruptured aneurysm, repair of an inadvertently ruptured vessel during angioplasty, and helping prevent restenosis.[10]

PERCUTANEOUS ARTERIOGRAPHY

High spatial resolution catheter-based angiography is crucial for diagnostic and interventional procedures. It is necessary to provide fine anatomic detail of the target lumen. It is important to optimize the technique to obtain temporal and spatial resolution.

Percutaneous Vascular Access

Vascular access techniques have evolved little since Seldinger described the technique of percutaneous access using a removable core or hollow needle, which allows the insertion of a guide wire.[1] The choice of the vascular access site is based on the procedure being performed, the location of the target vessel, and the degree of focal atherosclerotic disease in the affected vascular region. The access vessel should be readily free of disease. Access may be performed using a single-wall or double-wall technique. Regardless of the technique, once the vessel is accessed, a nontraumatic wire is passed through the lumen of the needle into the vessel. The entrance site to the vessel should be located over a bone whenever possible. This provides a stable object against which to compress the vessel following completion of the procedure and removal of the catheters and sheaths.

Common Femoral Artery Access

The common femoral artery (CFA) is the most common access site used for peripheral diagnostic angiography and intervention. The CFA is a large-caliber artery that can accommodate a large sheath size with minimal trauma to the vessel. The entire vascular system can be accessed from this site.

The CFA may be punctured in a retrograde (toward the head) or an antegrade (toward the foot) direction. In the retrograde direction, the access needle's tip should be aimed at the level of the mid-femoral head. The bifurcation of the CFA is commonly just distal to the mid-femoral head. Fluoroscopic guidance may be used to help identify the appropriate access location.

An antegrade puncture is generally more difficult and the risk of bleeding is increased, particularly in obese patients. To puncture the CFA, the skin entrance site must be higher; the needle needs to be angled at 60 degrees toward the feet, aiming at the mid-femoral head. A combination of fluoroscopic and ultrasound guidance can be used to ensure accurate cannulation.

Brachial and Radial Artery Access

Brachial and radial artery access offers a lower risk of bleeding complications. However, the vessels are small, limiting the usable sheath sizes. In addition, there is an increased risk of distal ischemia if the sheath obliterates the vessel lumen. Also, if instrumentation crosses the origins of the great vessels from this approach, there is an increased risk of embolization to the cerebral and contralateral limb circulation.

Micropuncture access sets are normally used for brachial and radial punctures. Brachial artery puncture is performed with the patient's arm and forearm supinated and slightly abducted. The artery is punctured near the medial antecubital fossa, with care taken to avoid puncturing the artery near the radial nerve. Radial artery puncture is performed with the wrist extended and the forearm supinated.

The brachial and radial arteries are more prone to vascular spasm and thrombosis, particularly during catheter manipulation. Administration of a vasodilator, such as nitroglycerin, or heparin is often given intra-arterially to reduce the incidence of these complications.

Popliteal Artery

Popliteal artery access is usually reserved for revascularization procedures involving the superficial femoral artery (SFA). It is performed with the patient in the prone position. In general, ultrasound-guided arterial puncture is recommended to avoid puncturing the popliteal vein, which may lie superficial to the artery.

Choice of Contrast Agent

The best tolerated and least nephrotoxic iodinated contrast material is nonionic iso-osmolar contrast. Many different brands are available, all of which are generally equal in efficacy.

For patients with renal impairment, the best strategy is to prevent further renal deterioration by avoiding the procedure unless absolutely necessary. Other diagnostic procedures such as magnetic resonance angiography (MRA) or color Doppler sonography may be performed for vascular diagnosis. However, if an endovascular therapeutic intervention is essential for management, catheter angiography can be safely performed if the patient is well hydrated prior to the procedure; the amount of contrast material used during the procedure should be minimized.

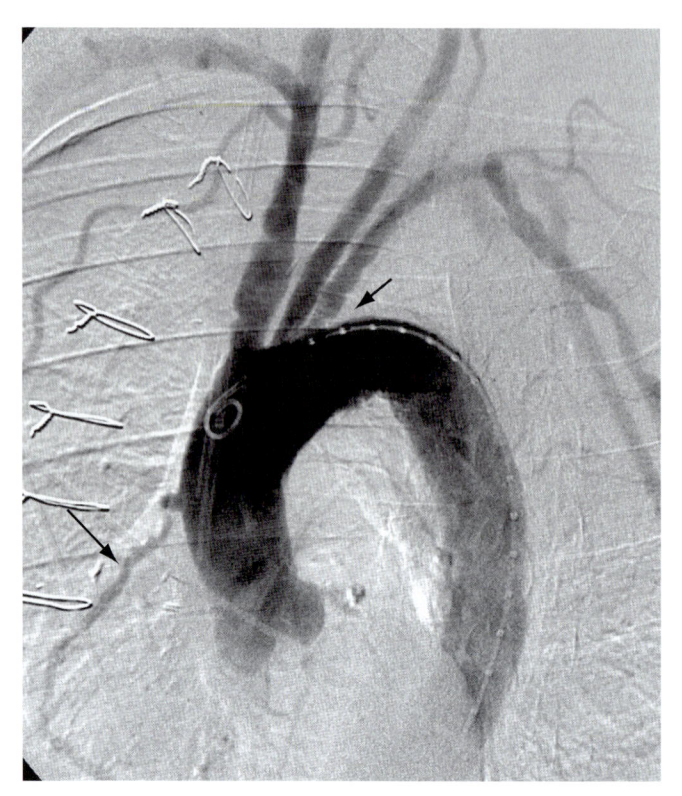

FIGURE 86-1 Arch aortography in a patient suspected of left subclavian stenosis. A pigtail catheter is placed in the ascending aorta and angiography is performed. There is mild stenosis (*short arrow*) of the left subclavian artery. The *long arrow* points to a patent coronary bypass graft.

In addition, oral N-acetylcysteine may be beneficial to reduce the risk for contrast-induced renal impairment.

Gadolinium chelate contrast agents and CO_2 are alternative contrast materials for catheter angiography in renal function–impaired patients. The disadvantage of these contrast agents is that vascular imaging is often suboptimal. In addition, gadolinium chelate contrast materials are associated with increased risk, albeit small, for nephrogenic systemic fibrosis in patients with severe renal impairment.

Specific Regions of Interest

Arch Aortography

Arch aortography is commonly performed for the assessment of atherosclerotic vascular disease, such as stenosis of the origin of the great vessels—the innominate, carotid, and subclavian arteries (Fig. 86-1). It is also used in the evaluation of thoracic aortic aneurysms and dissections, post-traumatic vascular injuries and, in some cases, congenital anomalies of the aorta and/or great vessels, especially if therapeutic intervention is desired.

Abdominal Aortography

Abdominal aortography is commonly performed to evaluate abdominal aortic aneurysms and atherosclerotic vascular disease causing stenosis or occlusion in the aorta, mesenteric, or renal arteries. Additionally, abdominal aortography is routinely performed as the initial step for endovascular procedures involving the mesenteric, renal, and pelvic vasculature.

Pelvic Angiography

Pelvic arteriography is indicated for the diagnosis and management of suspected iliac artery occlusive disease, pelvic trauma, hematuria from the bladder, and arteriovenous malformations in the pelvis.

Carotid and Cerebral Angiography

Carotid and cerebral angiography is indicated for diagnosis and endovascular therapy of steno-occlusive disease, aneurysms, and arteriovenous malformations. Preoperative embolization of intracranial tumors may also be performed. Another less common indication is to assess cross-cerebral perfusion before sacrificing the ipsilateral carotid artery in cases of large inoperable carotid artery aneurysms and during resection of head and neck tumors.

Upper Limb Angiography

Arteriography of the upper limb is commonly performed to investigate vascular compression by bone or ligament (thoracic outlet syndrome), Raynaud's syndrome, subclavian aneurysm, and ischemia (often secondary to embolic occlusion, Buerger disease, or iatrogenic trauma). Atherosclerotic disease is usually focal and located at the origin of the great vessels.

Lower Limb Angiography

Lower extremity arteriography is indicated for the diagnosis and endovascular management of limb ischemia (Fig. 86-2), trauma, vascular malformation, and tumors. Vascular access may be gained through a femoral, brachial, or radial route.

Pulmonary Angiography

Historically, pulmonary angiography had been extensively used for the diagnosis of pulmonary embolism. Currently, its role is limited to interventional procedures for the treatment of massive pulmonary embolism with pharmacomechanical thrombolysis and for pulmonary arteriovenous malformations and aneurysms. With the advent of noninvasive imaging alternatives, notably pulmonary CT angiography, pulmonary angiography is rarely performed for surgical planning in patients with chronic pulmonary thromboembolism. Relative contraindications for pulmonary angiography are the presence of left bundle branch block and severe pulmonary arterial hypertension.

Renal Angiography

Renal angiography is indicated for the diagnosis and management of suspected renovascular hypertension (Fig. 86-3), hematuria of unknown origin, trauma, preoperative assessment of a donor kidney, and postoperative evaluation of a transplanted kidney. It may also be performed for the devascularization of renal tumors prior to surgery or as a palliative therapy.

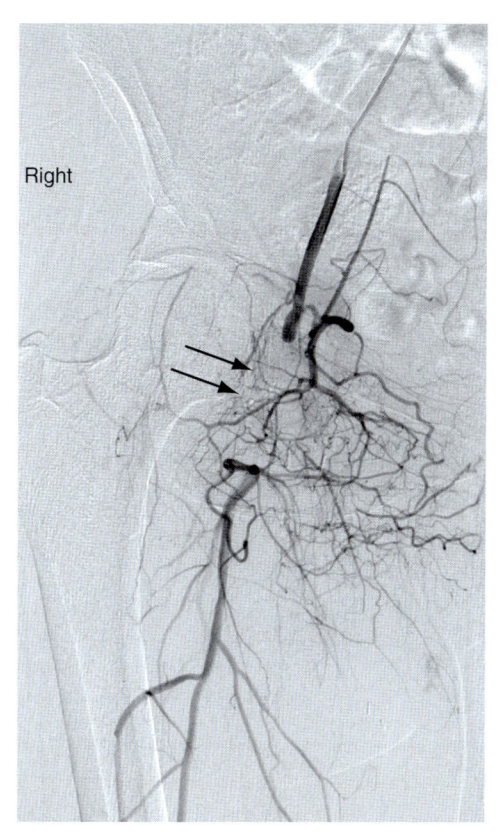

■ **FIGURE 86-2** Right femoral angiography in a patient with rest pain. The catheter is in the right external artery. There is complete occlusion (*arrows*) of the right common femoral artery. The profunda femoris artery is seen in the leg being reformed through collaterals. The superficial femoral artery is also occluded.

Hepatic and Mesenteric Angiography

Hepatic and mesenteric arteriography is indicated for suspected mesenteric ischemia, gastrointestinal bleeding, and vasculitides and for the assessment of variant anatomy prior to catheter-based and colonic interposition procedures. Mesenteric arteriography is also performed as part of an endoleak repair if the inferior mesenteric artery is the source of the endoleak. Other indications of mesenteric arteriography include diagnosis of vascular tumors such as islet cell tumors of the pancreas and assessment of portal venous anatomy through indirect portography.

Indications and Contraindications

Indications for percutaneous arteriography are as follows:

1. Diagnosis and treatment of primary vascular disease—vascular occlusive disease, aneurysm, and arteriovenous malformations
2. Diagnosis, localization, and delineation of highly vascular tumors, such as pancreatic islet cell tumors

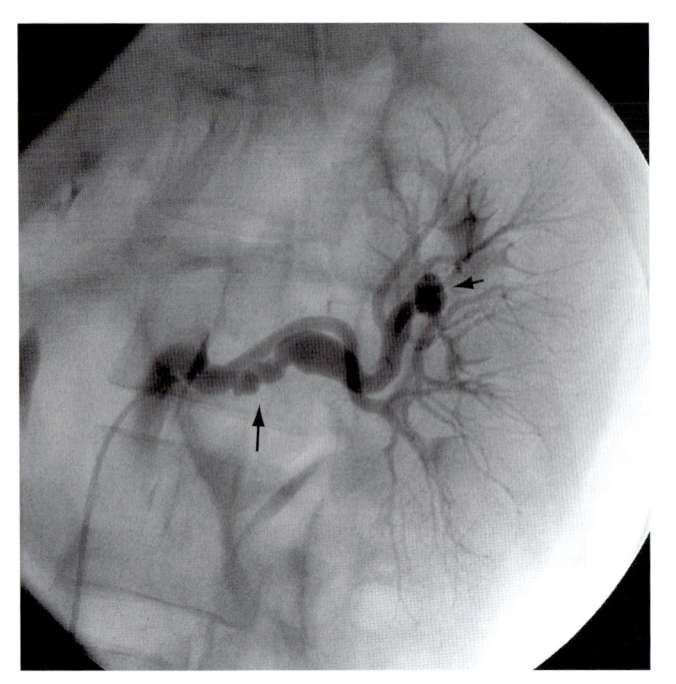

FIGURE 86-3 Left renal angiography in a 24-year-old woman with hypertension and neurofibromatosis. The angiogram shows a dysplastic left renal artery (*long arrow*) with mild stenosis. There is also an intrarenal aneuyrsm (*short arrow*).

3. Evaluation of percutaneous endoluminal therapies such as angioplasty, stenting, atherectomy, embolization, and thrombolysis
4. Diagnosis and treatment of vascular complications in various disease states (e.g., trauma, malignancy)

Contraindications

Few contraindications exist for diagnostic arteriography. Renal insufficiency or renal failure is a relative contraindication for the use of nephrotoxic contrast material. However, iodinated contrast material is cleared by conventional hemodialysis and postprocedural dialysis can reduce the toxicity concerns of iodinated contrast agents. In some cases, CO_2 may be a better alternate contrast material, but its use necessitates digital subtraction angiography. Other relative contraindications for catheter angiography are the presence of septicemia, active vasculitis, or infection at the vascular access site. Patients with an allergy to iodinated contrast material often require premedication or the use of a noniodinated contrast material such as CO_2 or a gadolinium (Gd) chelate contrast agent. Often, the amount of contrast agent used for diagnostic procedures may be less than that required for a diagnostic CT scan.

In pregnant patients, the risks to the fetus also need to be considered in addition to those to the mother relative to the benefits of catheter angiography. In pregnant patients, a noninvasive imaging study such as ultrasound or MRA, without the use of a Gd chelate contrast agent, may be able to provide sufficient diagnostic vascular information for appropriate management of the patient or at least to minimize the extent of catheter intervention, if required.

Outcomes and Complications

Complications of angiography are generally related to the arterial puncture site and nephrotoxic effects of the contrast material.[11,12] The most common puncture site complication is local hemorrhage, which occurs in fewer than 3% of patients. Large hematomas may require transfusion or vascular surgical repair. The risk of hemorrhage is increased with large-caliber catheters, multiple sheath or catheter changes, and patients with bleeding diathesis, local aneurysmal or atherosclerotic arterial disease, or inadequate compression of the puncture artery. In addition to hematoma, false aneurysms (less than 0.5%) and, rarely, arteriovenous fistula formation (less than 0.1%) may occur.

Arterial thrombosis at the puncture site is a rare complication. Arterial spasm, the use of large-caliber sheaths, multiple punctures, polycythemia, hypercoagulable states, and excessive compression of the puncture site also increase the risk of thrombosis.

Subintimal dissection may occur secondary to wire, dilator, or catheter malpositioning. This complication occurs more commonly in the femoral or iliac artery during initial puncture. Frank perforation of the arterial wall is rare.

Embolization into the distal arterial tree occurs most frequently in the lower limbs, given the overwhelming predominance of femoral arterial access. Embolization is caused by thrombus stripping off the guide wire or catheter or by dislodgment of an atheroma (cholesterol emboli) during catheter manipulation. The administration of systemic anticoagulation during the procedure helps reduce the incidence of distal embolization. The use of embolic protection devices during lower extremity interventions also may reduce the incidence of clinically significant distal embolization.[13]

Complications with the use of iodinated contrast material include allergic reactions, renal failure and, rarely, cardiac failure. Premedication with prednisone or diphenhydramine is recommended for patients with a history of minor allergic reactions to contrast materials. As noted, the nephrotoxic effects of contrast can be minimized by preprocedural hydration and possibly the use of N-acetylcysteine. Cardiotoxicity is related to the high osmolarity of the contrast material, largely a historical complication given the widespread current use of low iso-osmolar, nonionic iodinated contrast agents.

Imaging Findings

Preprocedural Planning

Although cross-sectional imaging is often unnecessary for planning angiography, noninvasive imaging with CT angiography (CTA) and MRA is increasingly being used for screening and/or primary diagnosis. CTA and MRA often provide important information concerning the extent of the disease and aid in optimal planning for endovascular interventions. This information may also enable limiting the extent of catheter angiography, thereby decreasing the overall ionizing radiation dose to the patient and potentially the contrast material dose requirement. In

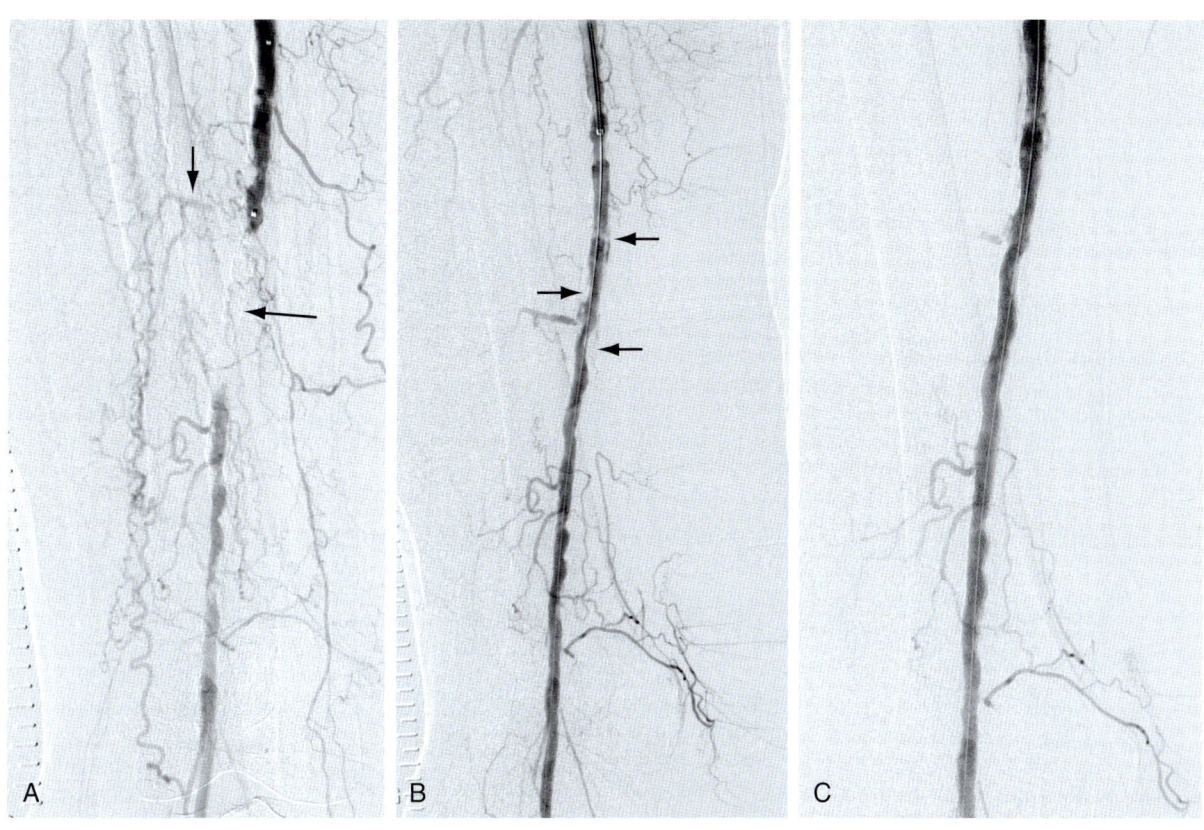

■ **FIGURE 86-4** 62-year-old man with right leg claudication. **A,** Right femoral angiogram shows a short-segment occlusion (*large arrow*) of the distal superficial femoral artery. The popliteal artery is patent and is reconstituted by collaterals (*small arrow*). The occluded segment was treated by balloon angioplasty. **B,** Postangioplasty femoral angiogram shows areas of residual stenosis (*arrows*). This was subsequently treated by placing a self-expanding stent. **C,** Poststent, the femoral angiogram shows no residual stenosis and disappearance of collaterals.

addition, CTA and MRA can provide information regarding the presence and extent of arterial disease at the access site or intervening anatomy that may affect the choice of percutaneous approach or even the preference of therapeutic intervention.

Three-dimensional reformations of CTA or MRA data provide spatial representation of vascular anatomy that often enables improved appreciation of vascular origins and complex geometries of vascular segments. This information aids in the proper selection of angiographic catheters, wires, and therapeutic devices. Radiographic image acquisition during catheter angiography is also optimized if preprocedural knowledge of vessel orientation, course, and branching pattern is obtained on CTA or MRA.

Postprocedural Surveillance

Following diagnostic catheter angiography, all patients are observed for arterial access site complications and distal hypoperfusion. Catheter angiography is generally an outpatient procedure and patients are discharged within 6 hours of the angiographic procedure.

ANGIOPLASTY

Angioplasty was initially described by Dotter and Judkins,[2] who successfully carried out angioplasty of a superficial femoral arterial stenosis using serial dilation. Later, balloon technology was developed by Gruentzig in 1976. Since then, balloon angioplasty has become the standard for revascularization procedures. Successful angioplasty requires careful attention to patient work-up, high-quality angiography, selection of proper hardware, and careful postprocedure management. In general, short-segment stenoses and occlusions respond well to angioplasty.

In addition to routine laboratory work-up and noninvasive vascular studies prior to a planned revascularization procedure, patients should ideally be treated with antiplatelet drugs (e.g., clopidogrel and/or aspirin). Depending on the location of the stenosis or occlusion, an antegrade or retrograde approach is undertaken. In general, a guide catheter or large sheath is placed at the arterial access site to allow angiography of the segment being treated and a balloon catheter to be used. Heparin (70 to 100 U/kg) is administered intravenously prior to crossing the stenosis. The stenosis or occlusion is crossed first with a hydrophilic wire and then with a catheter. The intravascular location of the catheter distal to the stenotic segment is confirmed by contrast material administration and then a stiff working wire (e.g., Rosen or Amplatz wire) is positioned across the stenosis. The catheter is exchanged for a properly sized balloon. The diameter of the balloon is determined by the vascular segment being treated and the size of the normal adjacent vessel. The balloon is inflated, deflated, and removed. Inflation devices are helpful to treat the lesion adequately. A postangioplasty diagnostic arteriogram is obtained (Fig. 86-4) to confirm the therapeutic result. A successful angioplasty is revealed by the absence of any significant residual stenosis (i.e., residual stenosis less than 30%), normalization of intravascular pressures across the stenosis (pressure gradient less than 10 mm Hg), and disappearance of collaterals. Postprocedure, heparin may be infused intravenously for 24 hours.

Special Considerations

Severe or Tight Calcified Stenosis

Wire negotiation through a tight or very severe high-grade stenosis can be challenging. The use of the roadmap feature with digital subtraction angiography is often helpful. A curved guide wire and catheter can be helpful for negotiating across a complex stenosis. In some cases, a subintimal channel with re-entry distal to the lesion may be made (subintimal angioplasty). A very tight or calcified lesion may require progressive dilation with sequentially larger balloons.

Chronic Occlusions

Crossing chronic occlusions presents a particular challenge. New hardware, simultaneous antegrade and retrograde access, and subintimal angioplasty are often useful in such cases. Recently developed tools to help cross chronic occlusions include catheters (e.g., CTO catheter, Cordis), re-entry devices (e.g. Outback, Cordis), an ultrasound-guided re-entry needle for subintimal angioplasty, thermal ablation devices such as a radiofrequency ablation wire (e.g., Safe-Cross wire, IntraLuminal Therapeutics, Menlo Park, Calif), and laser wires (e.g., Excimer laser wire, Spectranetics, Colorado Springs, Colo).

Acute Dissection

Acute dissection during angioplasty may be asymptomatic or may lead to vessel occlusion and/or thrombosis. It may be treated with prolonged balloon inflation across the dissection or with the placement of an intravascular stent.

Acute Thrombosis

Acute thrombosis during the procedure is typically treated with local thrombolytic infusion and/or mechanical thrombectomy or thrombosuction.

Restenosis and Elastic Recoil

Unsuccessful angioplasty caused by recoiling of the vessel may be treated with placement of an intravascular stent. The incidence of postangioplasty neointimal hyperplasia may be reduced with the use of cryoplasty balloons, but data are still lacking concerning their efficacy.

Indications and Contraindications

The main indications for angioplasty vary based on the specific arterial region. They include life-limiting claudication and chronic critical limb or organ ischemia (e.g., rest pain, ulcer, gangrene), bypass graft stenosis, and clinically significant arterial stenoses in the renal artery, mesenteric circulation, and other arterial territories. Angioplasty may also be performed to treat in-stent stenosis (Fig. 86-5). Specific indications for each vascular territory are discussed in subsequent chapters.

Absolute contraindications for angioplasty include a hemodynamically unstable patient and the presence of an ulcerative plaque secondary to its high risk for distal embolization. Multifocal long-segment stenoses and calcified eccentric stenoses respond poorly with angioplasty. Relative contraindications include allergy to contrast material and the presence of renal dysfunction. Pregnant patients present additional considerations related to risks to the fetus. In all cases, discussion and careful assessment of the risks and benefits related to catheter intervention are essential.

Outcomes and Complications

The optimal clinical outcome is a durable improvement of the patient's symptoms. Many early failures of angioplasty were caused by technical problems encountered at the time of the procedure, such as an occlusive dissection adjacent to the intervention site, elastic recoil of a fibrotic lesion, or perhaps an unrecognized lesion that continued to impair flow. Delayed failure occurs when there is restenosis of the treated segment. This is typically seen from 3 months onward and is predominantly caused by neointimal hyperplasia. Late failure occurs as the disease progresses in the inflow and outflow tracts. Vessel patency rates following angioplasty vary significantly, depending on the vascular territory, length of the stenotic lesion, complications during the procedure, and preexisting or unaltered patient factors such as smoking, lifestyle, and the use of antiplatelet medications.

As noted, access site complications include hematoma, pseudoaneurysm, arteriovenous (AV) fistula, and thrombosis. Atheroemboli causing blue toe syndrome occur in less than 1% of patients; dissection and occlusion of the branch vessels occur at a rate of 0.5%. Another rare complication is rupture of the vessel during angioplasty. Predisposing factors for arterial rupture include long-term therapy with corticosteroids and underlying vascular abnormalities such as Marfan syndrome and Ehler-Danlos syndrome. Immediate reinflation of the balloon across the rupture or proximal to the lesion can be a lifesaving maneuver. Urgent surgical repair or endovascular therapy with a stent graft is usually required to stop bleeding. Systemic complications are relatively uncommon and include sepsis (0.2%) and transient acute tubular necrosis (0.3% to 1%).

Imaging Findings

Preprocedural Planning

It is paramount to review previous noninvasive studies (e.g., CTA, MRA, Doppler, ankle-brachial index [ABI] testing) and any prior arteriograms. These are reviewed to assess the extent of the steno-occlusive disease, disease at the access site, anatomy, and disease affecting the distal arterial bed. Imaging studies such as Doppler provide hemodynamic information about the severity of the steno-

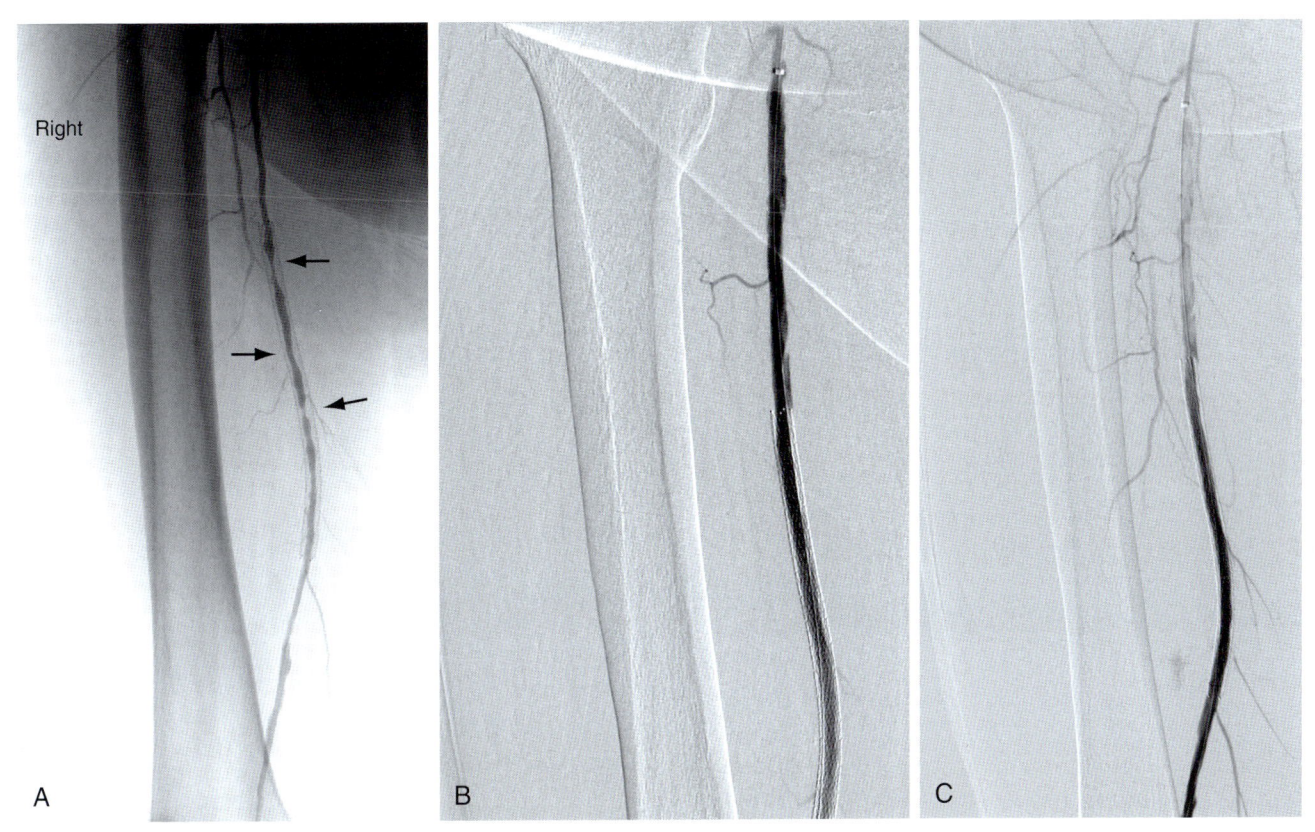

FIGURE 86-5 In-stent stenosis treated with angioplasty. **A,** Right femoral angiogram shows multiple areas of severe stenosis (*black arrows*) within a stent. The stenoses were crossed with a wire and angioplasty was performed. **B, C,** Postangioplasty, there is restoration of the vessel lumen, with no residual stenosis within the stent.

sis. Careful clinical evaluation and recent clinical laboratory studies, in particular renal function, are essential. Administration of antiplatelet medications prior to a planned angioplasty may also improve clinical outcome.[14]

Postprocedural Surveillance

Antiplatelet therapy with aspirin and/or clopidogrel is generally recommended following angioplasty.[14] The duration of antiplatelet therapy is debatable and many interventional interpreting physicians prefer to treat the patient for at least 6 months following angioplasty. It is essential to carry out a postprocedure assessment such as a Doppler ultrasound examination or ABI testing at 24 to 48 hours postangioplasty. Long-term follow-up (e.g., at 1, 3, 6, and 12 months) is also important to monitor patient outcome. Imaging studies such as Doppler or CTA may be performed if there is suspicion of residual or recurrent disease. Secondary interventions with repeat angioplasty or stent placement may be performed to increase the assisted patency following angioplasty.

REVASCULARIZATION WITH STENTS AND STENT GRAFTS

When angioplasty alone is ineffective for treating a stenosis or occlusion, stents and stent grafts provide an alternative solution. It is necessary to have a normal vessel both proximally and distally to allow internal fixation of the device and prevent disease recurrence. Today, many designs are approved by the U.S. Food and Drug Administration (FDA) and numerous devices are being used commercially or in clinical investigations. Stent grafts can also be used to treat aneurysmal disease.

In general, self-expanding stents are preferable for revascularization. However, the design and nature of the delivery system do not allow a precise deployment of the stent in complex locations. As such, balloon-expandable stents are used when location of the stent deployment is complex, as in the treatment of osteal stenosis of the subclavian and renal arteries and intracranial arterial disease.

Primary stenting—direct placement of a stent without prior angioplasty—is often practiced for the treatment of iliac, renal, and subclavian artery disease when the stenosis affects the ostium or is a result of an eccentric ulcerated plaque (Fig. 86-6). Secondary stenting following failed angioplasty or a complication of angioplasty is more commonly done.

The procedure involves the same steps as angioplasty. The stenosis or occlusion is crossed with a wire. The extent, location, and size of the diseased artery are measured and an optimal stent is chosen. The stent is deployed across the disease segment as per the manufacturer's guidelines. Angioplasty of the stent is often performed to bring the stent to the optimal size. If multiple stents are required, deployment of the distal stent should be performed first and adequate overlap of the stents achieved. The deployment of a stent graft for steno-occlusive disease is similar to that used for regular stents. However, when

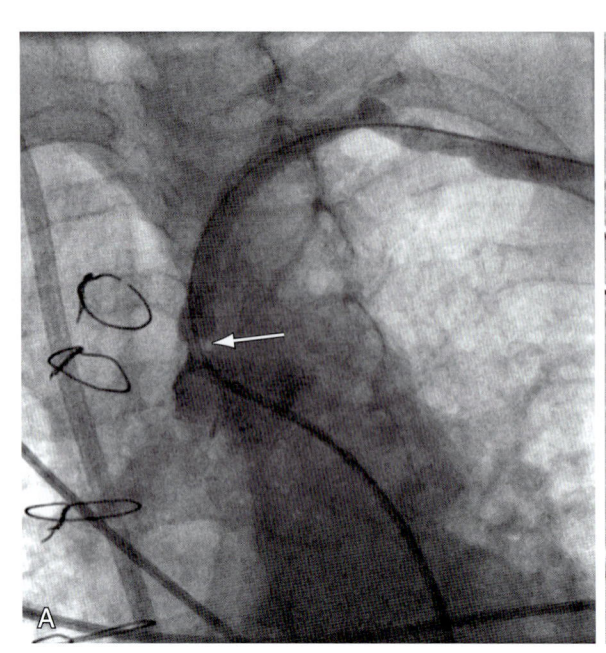

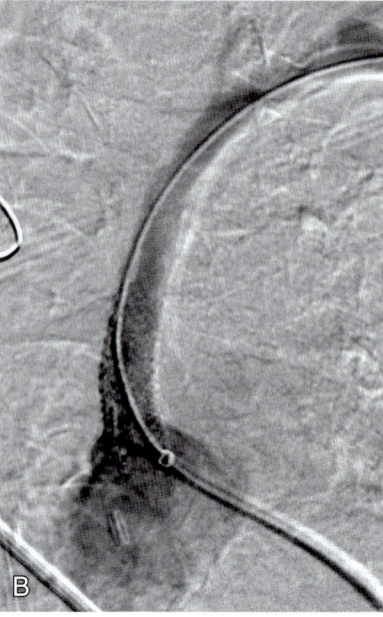

FIGURE 86-6 Left subclavian stenosis treated with primary stenting. **A,** Left subclavian angiogram shows a severe stenosis (*arrow*) at the origin of the vessel. Mild poststenotic dilation is also seen. The stenosis was treated with a balloon-expandable stent. **B,** Poststent, there is no residual stenosis.

stent grafts are chosen to treat an aneurysmal disease, proper planning with regard to the size of the proximal and distal arteries is essential to prevent residual perfusion of the aneurysm.

Indications and Contraindications

Indications for arterial stenting are residual stenosis after angioplasty, postangioplasty dissection, restenosis, eccentric ulcerated plaque with risk of distal embolization, and ostial stenosis of the renal or subclavian arteries. Stent grafts are often used for steno-occlusive disease with an intent to reduce in-stent restenosis. Indications for stent grafts include the treatment of abdominal or thoracic aortic aneurysm, iliac aneurysm, ruptured aneurysm, pseudoaneurysm, ruptured vessel during angioplasty or arterial trauma, and aortic dissection.

The main contraindications for stent grafts include the presence of active infection, bacteremia, or a mycotic aneurysm. Other contraindications for stents include those listed earlier ("Angioplasty").

Outcomes and Complications

In general, stents provide better patency rates compared with angioplasty in the treatment of renal artery disease, subclavian stenosis, and iliac artery disease. The role of stenting has been debated for the treatment of femoropopliteal and infrapopliteal disease. It appears that stents provide better short-term patency rates in the treatment of superficial femoral artery disease.[15] The role of stent grafts in the treatment of aneurysms is now well established for abdominal aortic and iliac artery aneurysms.

The complications of stenting are similar to those for angioplasty. However, stenting carries the risk of stent migration, stent fractures, thrombosis, and restenosis.

Imaging Findings

Preprocedural Planning

Preprocedural planning for stenting is similar to that for angioplasty. It is important to understand the location, extent, and size of the diseased segment and characteristics of the plaque. The distal and proximal normal arterial segments should be assessed for patency, size, and branch vessel origin. In general, stenting across a joint is not preferred because this may increase fracture or crushing of the stent. Similarly, when stent grafts are used for the treatment of steno-occlusive disease, the covering of branch vessels may jeopardize the blood supply to distal organs. Furthermore, covering patent vessels may prevent the formation of collateral pathways in case of stent occlusion.

Postprocedural Surveillance

Surveillance following stent placement for steno-occlusive disease is similar to that for angioplasty. When stent grafts are used for the treatment of aneurysmal disease, imaging surveillance to assess aneurysm size and reperfusion is mandatory at 1 to 3 months and then every year thereafter.

THROMBOLYSIS

Thromboses in the peripheral vascular system are a major cause of morbidity and mortality. An arterial or venous thrombosis can lead to ischemia and tissue infarction. The aim of thrombolysis is to restore blood flow to the ischemic limb or organ and to identify the underlying lesion for treatment via an endovascular approach or surgery.

Several pharmacologic agents are available for thrombolysis, including streptokinase, urokinase and recombinant tissue plasminogen activator (rt-PA). Each has a slightly different mechanism of action but they generally exert their effects by converting plasminogen to plasmin. Plasmin is an enzyme that degrades multiple blood plasma proteins, most notably fibrin (fibrinolysis), the predominant component of fibrin clots. At present, rt-PA has emerged as the most commonly used agent.

During vascular access, care is taken to ensure a single wall puncture to the artery. A diagnostic arteriogram is obtained to assess whether the event is secondary to in situ thrombosis or embolization. Angiography may also provide information about the chronicity of the problem. The arterial inflow, extent of thrombosis, and patency of distal arterial bed are assessed. The thrombus is crossed using a wire and an infusion catheter with multiple side holes is placed within the thrombus. The tip of the infusion catheter should be advanced beyond the thrombus, if possible, and the side holes within the thrombus.

There are multiple regimens for thrombolytic infusion. The most common is a bolus infusion of the thrombolytic agent followed by a continuous infusion for 24 to 48 hours. The catheter may be repositioned during thrombolysis to provide a more even distribution of the thrombolytic agent. Repeat angiograms are obtained at regular intervals to evaluate the progression of thrombolysis. Concomitant low-dose heparin therapy is administered through the arterial sheath or an intravenous route. The patient's activated partial thromboplastin time (aPTT) and hematocrit should be followed during thrombolysis. In addition, serum fibrinogen levels are determined to assess the degree of fibrinolysis, which may correlate with the risk of hemorrhagic complications.

During thrombolysis, there may be a distal embolization as the thrombus fragments. Continued upstream thrombolytic infusion is usually sufficient to lyse any distal thromboemboli. If no improvement occurs within several hours, the infusion catheter can be repositioned within the distal emboli.

Thrombolytic therapy is terminated once antegrade blood flow is established and no significant thrombus remains. In general, thrombolytic therapy is stopped after 48 hours if there is no significant clinical improvement. Thrombolysis is terminated sooner if hemorrhagic complications arise.

After a successful thrombolysis, the patient should be evaluated for any underlying vascular lesion or clotting disorder. If identified, these lesions should be treated to prevent further recurrence.

Special Considerations

Thrombosuction

This technique is done as an adjunct to pharmacologic thrombolysis when there is a large thrombus burden, or in a situation in which chemical thrombolysis alone has failed to clear the thrombus adequately. A large-lumen, nontapered straight catheter is placed into the thrombus. The thrombus is aspirated and suction is maintained while withdrawing the catheter in a smooth motion. These steps are typically repeated several times. This method may also be used when pharmacologic thrombolysis is contraindicated.

Mechanical Thrombolysis

Mechanical thrombectomy devices are used as an adjunct to pharmacologic thrombolysis. These devices excel in the treatment of acute limb ischemia caused by thrombotic occlusion. In addition, there is increasing interest in the use of these devices for the treatment of acute deep venous thrombosis (DVT). Also, these devices allow thrombectomy when pharmacologic thrombolysis is contraindicated or has failed. Several mechanical thrombectomy devices are available.

AngioJet (Possis Medical, Minneapolis) uses retrograde fluid jets to create a negative pressure gradient directed toward the catheter lumen (Bernoulli principle). The thrombus is drawn into the catheter, where it is fragmented by the jets and evacuated from the body. The device consists of a catheter, disposable pump bag and nondisposable motorized drive unit. The catheters have two lumens. The larger lumen allows debris evacuation and guide wire passage while a small profile inner lumen allows the pressurized perfusate to be removed. The pump set pressurizes the saline that energizes the catheter and creates the vacuum. The drive unit activates the pump, monitors safety, and ensures balanced flow and volume of the saline solution. This monitoring and control allow the system to theoretically remain iso-volumetric.

The Arrow Trerotola device (Arrow International, Reading, Pa) is a direct contact mechanical fragmentation device that uses a spinning wire to macerate the thrombus. The device consists of a motor-driven fragmentation cage attached to a drive cable. The cage and drive cable are housed in a 5F catheter containing a self-expanding cage, with a soft rubber distal tip. Once the cage is unsheathed, the cage expands to a predetermined diameter (9 mm). The open cage is rotated within the graft at a fixed speed (3000 rpm) using a separate handheld rotator unit. This device has FDA approval for declotting dialysis access in patients with arteriovenous fistulas and synthetic grafts.

As its name suggests, the ultrasound thrombolytic infusion catheter (EKOS, Bothell, Wash) combines the use of catheter-directed pharmacologic thrombolysis with ultrasound. Ultrasound functions to alter the structure of the thrombus by temporarily increasing its permeability while providing an acoustic pressure gradient that helps move the drug into the thrombus to speed its dissolution (Fig. 86-7).

Indications and Contraindications

Indications for thrombolysis are as follows:

1. Acute thrombotic events with viable extremities and organs. Therapy should be initiated within 4 to 6 hours.
2. Acute thromboses occurring during diagnostic angiography or transcatheter therapy
3. Thrombosis of a mature bypass graft in the presence of demonstrable run-off vessels. However, if it occurs within 4 weeks of bypass graft surgery, it is unlikely to be successful. Surgical thrombectomy with graft revision is often necessary.

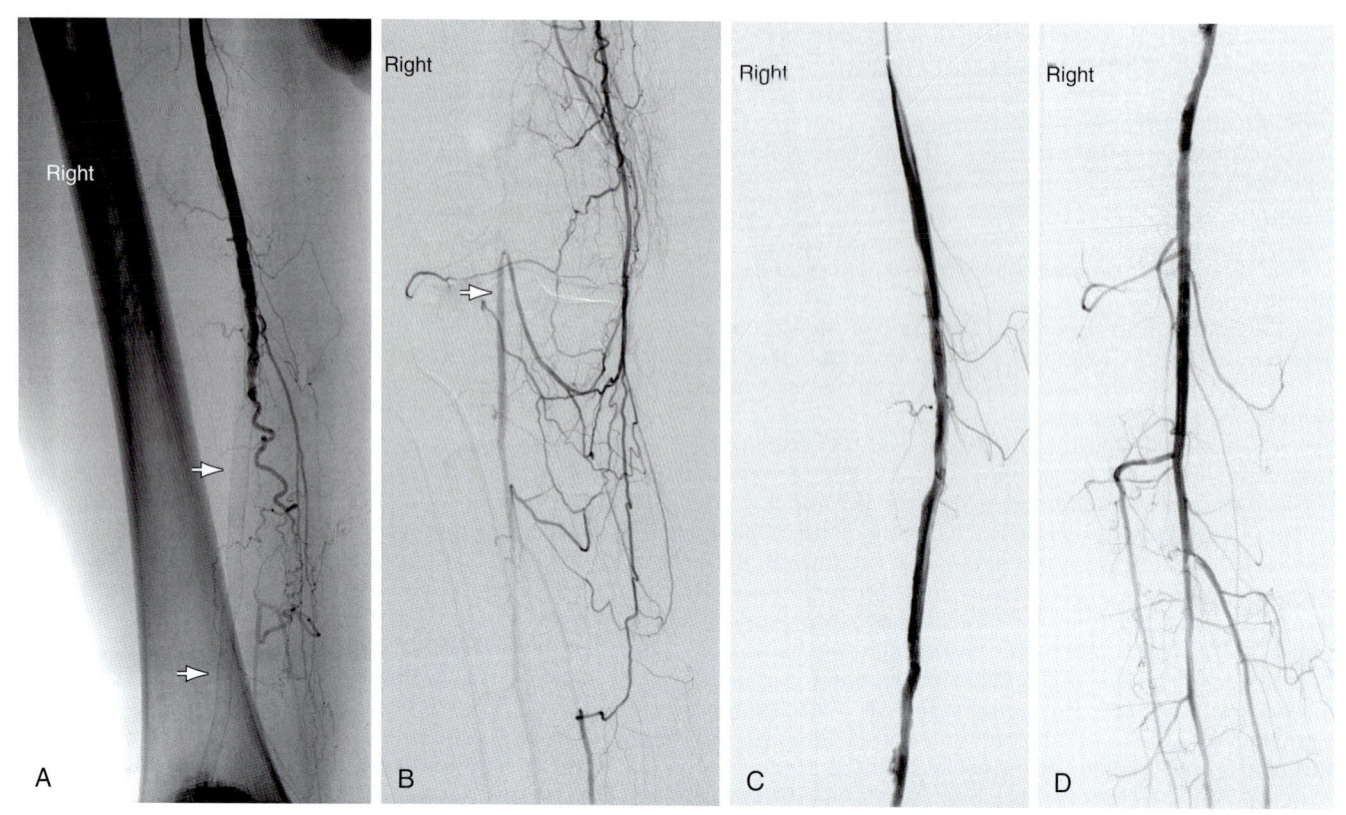

FIGURE 86-7 Acute thrombotic occlusion of femoropopliteal stent. **A,** Right femoral angiogram demonstrates complete occlusion (*arrows*) of femoropopliteal stent. **B,** Distally, there is reconstitution of the below-knee popliteal artery (*arrow*) through collaterals. An EKOS catheter was placed in the thrombus and thrombolysis was performed with rt-PA for 12 hours. **C, D,** Following thrombolysis, there is complete restoration of flow through the stent, with patent run-off vessels.

4. Thrombosis of dialysis related to arteriovenous graft or fistula
5. Acute thrombotic stroke (anterior circulation, less than 6 hours; posterior circulation, 12 to 24 hours)
6. Intracranial venous sinus thrombosis
7. Massive pulmonary embolism with impending cardiorespiratory collapse
8. Central venous access catheter occlusion
9. Extensive peripheral deep vein thrombosis

Thrombolytic therapy is absolutely contraindicated in patients with bleeding diatheses, cerebrovascular accident within 6 months, intracranial surgery within 6 months, gastrointestinal hemorrhage within 10 days, major surgical procedure, and trauma within 10 days. Other absolute contraindications include uncontrolled blood pressure (higher than 180/110 mm Hg), intracranial neoplasm, and arteriovenous malformation. Relative contraindications include renal impairment, hepatic impairment, recent transient ischemic attack, diabetic retinopathy, pregnancy, thrombocytopenia, and coagulopathy.

Outcomes and Complications

The technical success rate is around 80% with urokinases or rt-PA for acute thrombotic occlusions.[16] The success rate decreases with the age of the occlusion. In general, infusion duration is much shorter with rt-PA.

Complications include the following:

1. Transient distal embolization is common in up to 20% of patients and manifests as a transient increase in rest pain. This resolves in a few hours in most patients.
2. Bleeding complications include hematoma at the vascular puncture site (incidence, 15%), gastrointestinal bleeding (10%) and, less frequently, hematuria. The most significant complication is hemorrhagic stroke. The reported risk is up to 2%, with an apparently higher risk with rt-PA. The risk continues for at least 12 to 24 hours following termination of therapy.
3. Systemic complications include acute renal failure (0.3%) and acute myocardial infarction (0.2%).

Imaging Findings

Preprocedural Planning

Careful clinical and laboratory work-up, including a review of all previous angiograms and noninvasive vascular studies, is essential to plan the access site, route to the location of the thrombus, and potential postprocedural issues, such as the placement of indwelling sheaths for ongoing thrombolytic therapy. It is important to assess the extent of thrombus, involvement of branch vessels, and patency of distal arterial flow. Previous imaging studies may provide information about preexisting stenosis or occlusion. It is also important to assess the heart for atrial fibrillation and left atrial thrombus.

Postprocedural Surveillance

Immediate success of thrombolysis is determined by angiography along with noninvasive assessment using ultrasound. Long-term patency rates are improved if the underlying lesions are treated promptly by surgery or percutaneous techniques.

ATHERECTOMY

The concept of removing an obstructive plaque by a catheter-based excision technique was first introduced by Höfling and colleagues.[17] There are several different types of atherectomy devices available, including directional atherectomy devices (e.g., SilverHawk), orbital atherectomy devices (e.g., Diamondback 360, Cardiovascular Systems, Minneapolis), rotational atherectomy devices (e.g., Pathway Jetstream, Pathway Medical Technologies, Kirkland, Wash; Rotablator, Boston Scientific), and laser atherectomy devices (e.g., Excimer laser wire).[18] At present, no specific recommendations have been established for the treatment of lower limb disease with atherectomy devices and there are no long-term results of peripheral application of atherectomy. The procedure involves crossing of a stenotic lesion with a wire and repeatedly passing the atherectomy catheter over the wire to remove the plaque. The size of the atherectomy device depends on the target vessel diameter.

Indications and Contraindications

Currently, no specific recommendations exist for performing atherectomy in the peripheral vascular system. As experience increases, the indications and applications will become more apparent. Certainly, a focal subtotal occlusion, complex stenotic lesion, or discrete lesion within a previously bypassed vessel or stented vessel would be a candidate for atherectomy.

It is clear that atherectomy is contraindicated in certain situations, such as limb-threatening ischemia, total occlusion, occlusion secondary to thrombotic emboli, and multifocal disease in heavily calcified vessels.

Outcomes and Complications

Few large studies exist evaluating the efficacy of atherectomy compared with balloon angioplasty.[19,20] However, there are several theoretic advantages. Physical debulking of the atheromatous plaque compared with fracturing of the media would seem to provide better long-term patency. However, studies have demonstrated that the long-term patency obtained with atherectomy catheters is no better than that achieved with traditional balloon angioplasty.[20,21]

Complications associated with atherectomy are similar to those seen when procedures necessitate the use of large sheaths, including hematoma, dissection, pseudoaneurysm, and complications related to emboli. Additionally, complications from the atherectomy device itself may be encountered, including dissection, tissue emboli or atheroemboli, thrombosis, and vessel damage or perforation.

Imaging Findings
Preprocedural Planning

All patients undergoing atherectomy should be started on antiplatelet therapy with aspirin and clopidogrel prior to the procedure. Evaluation of previous imaging studies is mandatory to assess the lesion of interest as well as any other concomitant peripheral vascular disease. The use of distal embolic protection devices may be indicated, depending on the complexity of the lesion, the device being used, and the operator's preference.

Postprocedure Surveillance

Patients should be maintained on antiplatelet therapy for at least 6 months. Routine postprocedural evaluation with physical examination, ABI tests, and noninvasive vascular studies should be carried out. If there is any suspicion of disease progression, a definitive imaging study should be obtained.

EMBOLIZATION

Embolization refers to the percutaneous therapeutic blockage of blood vessels to stop or prevent hemorrhage, devitalize an organ or tumor, reduce blood flow through a vascular malformation, or redistribute blood flow.

Embolic Agents and Devices

A variety of embolic agents are available, including the following:

1. Particulate agents—gelfoam, polyvinyl alcohol (PVA) particles, trisacryl gelatin microspheres
2. Mechanical occlusion devices—coils, balloons, Amplatz vascular plug
3. Liquid agents—alcohol, n-butyl cyanoacrylate, ethylene–vinyl alcohol copolymers, sodium tetradecyl, sodium morrhuate

Particulate Agents

Gelfoam

Gelfoam is composed of sterile gelatin and is the oldest embolization agent currently used. Because it is biodegradable, it is a temporary embolization agent. Gelfoam is absorbed completely and allows vessel recanalization within days to weeks. Gelfoam is available as a powder or sheet. The powder consists of small particles (40 to 60 μm) and is used for small vessel occlusions. The use of gelfoam powder is associated with a high risk of tissue ischemia and is generally not recommended. Gelfoam sheets are cut to the size required by the operator and are used to occlude larger vessels.

Polyvinyl Alcohol

Currently available particles range from 150 to 1000 μm in size and are homogeneous in size, calibrated by the manufacturer. They are not absorbable and cause near-permanent occlusion. The particles lodge at the arteriolar and capillary level, leading to luminal thrombosis. PVA particles have been extensively used for renal, liver, spleen, and uterine artery embolization.

PVA is usually administered in a mixture of contrast medium under fluoroscopy. Some PVA suspensions have a tendency to clump or float in a suspension. Frequent mixing is therefore required, otherwise clumping of the particles in the catheter or blood vessel may result in a false angiographic end point. Also, during administration, especially when there is slow flow, frequent evaluation for reflux is crucial to avoid nontarget embolization.

Trisacryl Gelatin Microspheres

These particles are hydrophilic, compressible, nonabsorbable, and precisely calibrated. They are available in various sizes, ranging from 40 to 1200 mm. They cause permanent embolization. Similar to PVA particles, they are mixed with contrast material and injected under fluoroscopic guidance. These microspheres can tolerate temporary compression of 20% to 30% to facilitate their passage through the delivery catheter.

Mechanical Occlusion Devices

Coils

Most coils are made of platinum or stainless steel. They are permanent embolic agents used to occlude a vessel or pack an aneurysm sac. Occlusion is a result of coil-induced thrombosis rather than mechanical occlusion. The thrombogenic effect is further improved by Dacron fibers attached to the coils. Coils have three variables—size of the formed coil, length of the coil wire, and diameter of the coil wire. Coils are slightly oversized to pack tightly in the vessel and help reduce the chance of coil migration. Coils are precisely positioned under fluoroscopic guidance. After placement of the first coil, additional coils are deployed until total cessation of blood flow occurs. Mechanical and electrically detachable coils are currently available that allow precise coil placement in more difficult locations.

Balloons

These are permanent embolic agents used to occlude large, high-flow blood vessels. Currently, balloons are rarely used. They have the risk of deflation and migration.

Amplatz Vascular Plug

This plug is made of thin Nitinol wire mesh formed into a plug shape. The Nitinol mesh is radiolucent and it has a platinum band on each side to serve as a marker. The device is secured to the delivery system by a single steel microscrew and is deployed by unscrewing the device from the delivery wire. The delivery system allows precise placement of the plug in the target vessel. The manufacturer recommends oversizing the devices by 30% to 50% to occlude the vessels and prevent risk of distal malposition. The plug occludes the vessel and thrombosis ensues distally because of stasis of blood flow. Often, a single plug can effectively block a blood vessel that would have required many pushable coils, which makes it a very efficient and cost-effective alternative to coils or surgery.

Liquid Embolic Agents

These agents include sclerosants, glue, and thrombin. Common sclerosant agents are absolute ethanol and sodium tetradecyl (STD). Common glue agents are cyanoacrylate and an ethylene–vinyl alcohol copolymer (Onyx Liquid Embolic System, Micro Therapeutics, Irvine, Calif).

Alcohol

This is a permanent embolic agent and is the most commonly used. It causes cell death by dehydration and is highly toxic. Ethanol is administered with contrast material and frequent check angiograms are obtained to assess thrombosis and reflux. Total occlusion of the lumen occurs within minutes. Extravasation should be avoided because this can result in soft tissue swelling and tissue necrosis. Similarly, central nervous system depression, hemolysis, and cardiac arrest can occur if a large amount of absolute alcohol enters the systemic circulation. Balloon-assisted injection of alcohol is often practiced to prevent the systemic spread of alcohol.

n-Butyl Cyanoacrylate

n-Butyl cyanoacrylate (NBCA, glue) is an adhesive that quickly polymerizes when it comes into contact with ionic solutions, blood, or intima of a vessel. Because of the rapid polymerization, coaxial catheterization, precise positioning of the delivery catheter, and considerable skill are required when NBCA is used for embolization. The polymerization can be delayed by adding lipiodol, which allows more distal embolization. When a target location is reached by using a microcatheter, the catheter is flushed with 5% dextrose to clear it of any blood or contrast medium. Under real-time fluoroscopic control, a mixture of NBCA and lipiodol is delivered. As soon as a cast of the vascular tree is seen fluoroscopically, the delivery microcatheter is quickly removed so that the catheter tip does not adhere to the vessel. Again, the catheter is flushed quickly with 50% dextrose so that it can be reused during the same procedure. A foreign body inflammatory reaction is the primary disadvantage of the use of this embolic material.

Sodium Tetradecyl

STD (Sotradecol) is less painful and less toxic than absolute alcohol. It is commonly used for vascular malformations, varices, and varicoceles.

Ethylene–Vinyl Alcohol Copolymer

Onyx is an ethylene–vinyl alcohol (EVOH) copolymer dissolved in an organic solvent and dimethyl sulfoxide

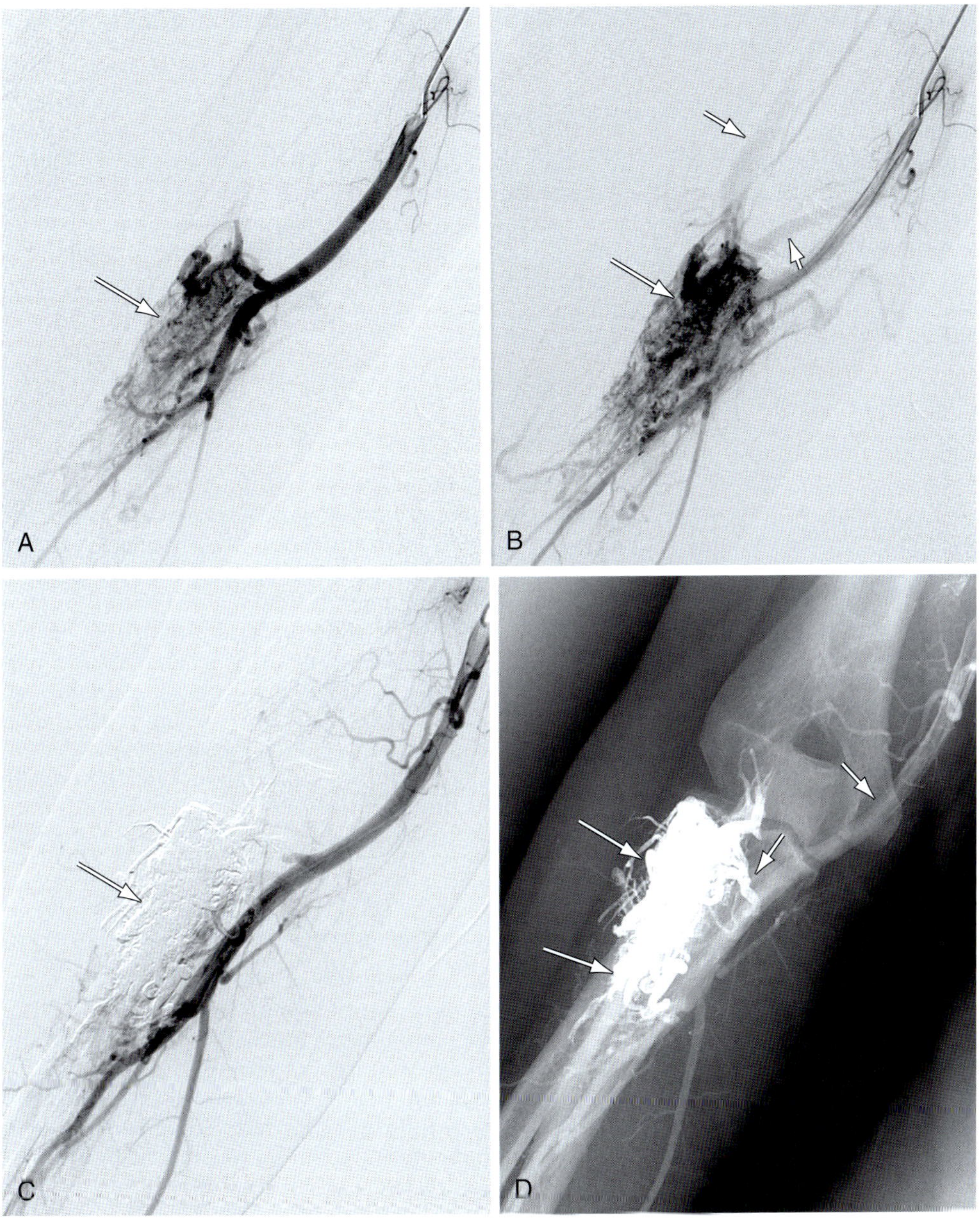

FIGURE 86-8 Right forearm arteriovenous malformation embolized with Onyx. **A,** Right brachial arteriogram shows an AVM (*arrow*) bed through branches of the radial artery. **B,** There is early opacification of the veins (*short arrows*; AVM, *long arrow*). **C, D,** This was treated with Onyx, with a favorable result.

(DMSO). Micronized tantalum powder is added to this mixture to make it radiopaque. When Onyx comes into contact with blood, the DMSO rapidly diffuses, leaving the EVOH to precipitate and solidify at the tip of the catheter in a shape that conforms to a lesion (e.g., an aneurysm). Unlike other liquid embolic agents, Onyx is a nonadhesive material; after it solidifies, it does not adhere to the endothelial wall, and no cases of catheter tip adherence have been documented. The disadvantage of this agent is severe vasospasm precipitated by the rapid injection of DMSO.

Onyx has been used since 1996 in the treatment of cerebral aneurysms and cerebral and peripheral arteriovenous malformations (AVMs; Fig. 86-8).

Thrombin

Thrombin is a topical agent that induces rapid thrombosis when injected intravenously. It is commonly use to treat pseudoaneurysms. Thrombin is reconstituted in saline and contrast material may be added before instillation. Thrombosis is usually achieved within minutes and thus it is important to prevent reflux into the systemic circulation. Gentle injection of contrast material helps monitor the progress of thrombosis to ensure no washout to non-target locations. Lesions with rapid blood flow should not be treated with thrombin.

Principles of Embolization

A detailed description of various embolization procedures is beyond the scope of this chapter. Here we will briefly discuss the principles of embolization.[22] When distal arteriolar or capillary embolization (as in tumor embolization) is desired, particulate or liquid embolizing agents are used. It is important to occlude all collateral supply to the tissue to achieve complete devascularization. When a distal arterial bed needs to be reperfused through collaterals (as in splenic artery embolization for splenic trauma), proximal embolization with mechanical devices is carried out. During therapy of aneurysms and pseudoaneurysms, the arterial inflow and outflow should be occluded to prevent persistent perfusion of the aneurysm. Another option is to completely pack the aneurysm sac with mechanical coils. In the treatment of arteriovenous malformations, all the branch vessels supplying the nidus or the entire nidus should be completely embolized. Arteriovenous fistulas can be treated with coil embolization of the communication or by excluding the communication with a stent graft.

Indications and Contraindications

There are three main therapeutic indications for embolization:

1. In an adjunctive role, embolization is applied to devascularize a tumor prior to surgery or to administer cancer therapy through chemoembolization.
2. In a curative role, embolization is used for the treatment of aneurysms, arteriovenous fistulas (AVFs), AVMs, and treatment of hemorrhage from traumatic or non-traumatic vascular lesions.
3. In a palliative role, embolization is used to relieve symptoms, such as of a large AVM, which cannot be cured by using embolization alone.

Few contraindications exist for embolization. Inability to reach the desired arterial territory because of technical reasons and the risk of nontarget embolization to vital organs remain the most common contraindications.

Outcomes and Complications

Results of embolization vary depending on the disease process and territory involved. Success is high in stopping active bleeding from a ruptured vessel or a tumor.

Complications

Postembolization Syndrome

This syndrome may occur following the embolization of solid organs such as the liver or kidney. It is thought to be caused by the release of vasoactive substances and inflammatory mediators following cellular ischemia and necrosis. Several days after embolization, the patient may develop mild flulike symptoms, including fever, nausea, vomiting, myalgia, arthralgia, and generalized malaise. These symptoms are relatively mild and generally self-limiting; support with oral or, rarely, intravenous hydration and oral analgesics is usually sufficient. The symptoms generally subside after 3 to 5 days.

Nontarget Embolization

The consequences of nontarget embolization obviously depend on the vascular region and tissue being embolized. Additionally, coils may migrate from their intended location if they are improperly sized.

Abscess Formation

Ischemic and necrotic tissue is an excellent culture medium. Depending on the tissue being treated, prophylactic antibiotics may be warranted. Certain patient subsets, such as those with biliary enteric anastamoses, may benefit from several days of pre- and postprocedural antibiotics.

Imaging Findings

Preprocedural Planning

Embolization is almost always performed based on imaging findings or following a previous procedure such as surgery or endoscopy. Detailed evaluation of all available studies must be performed. In addition, the purpose and ultimate goal of the embolization must be discussed with the referring physician. A thorough physical evaluation of the patient and all available laboratory tests must be performed. Numerous variables involved in planning an embolization procedure, including the approach, additional diagnostic imaging, embolic agent(s) being used, and degree of subselective embolization, must be considered prior to beginning the procedure. Each embolization procedure must be custom-tailored to the clinical situation at hand.

Postprocedural Surveillance

The success of any given embolization procedure can usually be ascertained at the time of the procedure. The end point of the embolization is usually determined by the indication of the procedure. Physical examination, laboratory values, and noninvasive studies are used to evaluate the patient following the procedure. Surveillance is performed on a patient by patient basis and can be tailored to the disease process.

KEY POINTS

- Angiography remains the gold standard for the diagnosis of vascular disorders and surveillance of various endovascular therapies.
- Percutaneous vascular interventions are performed primarily to re-establish the arterial supply (e.g., angioplasty, stenting, thrombolysis) or exclusion of blood vessels (e.g., embolization, exclusion with stent grafts).
- Angiography and clinical surveillance are critical for pharmacologic and mechanical thrombolysis.

SUGGESTED READINGS

Allaqaband S, Solis J, Kazemi S, Bajwa T. Endovascular treatment of peripheral vascular disease. Curr Probl Cardiol 2006; 31, 711-760.

Aronow H. Peripheral arterial disease in the elderly: recognition and management. Am J Cardiovasc Drugs 2008; 8, 353-364.

Beard JD. Which is the best revascularization for critical limb ischemia: endovascular or open surgery? J Vasc Surg 2008; 48, 11S-16S.

Mannava K, Money SR. Current management of peripheral arterial occlusive disease: a review of pharmacologic agents and other interventions. Am J Cardiovasc Drugs 2007; 7:59-66.

Stoyioglou A, Jaff MR. Medical treatment of peripheral arterial disease: a comprehensive review. J Vasc Interv Radiol 2004; 15:1197-1207.

REFERENCES

1. Berneus B, Carlsten A, Holmgren A, Seldinger SI. Percutaneous catheterization of peripheral arteries as a method for blood sampling. Scand J Clin Lab Invest 1954; 6:217-221.
2. Dotter CT, Judkins MP. Transluminal treatment of arteriosclerotic obstruction. Description of a new technic and a preliminary report of its application. Circulation 1964; 30:654-670.
3. Hawkins IF. Carbon dioxide digital subtraction arteriography. AJR Am J Roentgenol 1982; 139:19-24.
4. Berman HL, Cornell TJ. A technique for reforming the Simmons curved cerebral catheters. AJR Am J Roentgenol 1982; 139: 824.
5. Jerie P. [Thirty years of the balloon catheter—A. Gruentzig and percutaneous balloon angioplasty.] Cas Lek Cesk 2004; 143: 866-871.
6. Fava M, Loyola S, Polydorou A, et al. Cryoplasty for femoropopliteal arterial disease: late angiographic results of initial human experience. J Vasc Interv Radiol 2004; 15:1239-1243.
7. Zeller T, Rastan A, Schwarzwalder U, et al. Percutaneous peripheral atherectomy of femoropopliteal stenoses using a new-generation device: six-month results from a single-center experience. J Endovasc Ther 2004; 11:676-685.
8. Dotter CT. Transluminally-placed coilspring endarterial tube grafts. Long-term patency in canine popliteal artery. Invest Radiol 1969; 4:329-332.
9. Schmehl J, Tepe G. Current status of bare and drug-eluting stents in infrainguinal peripheral vascular disease. Expert Rev Cardiovasc Ther 2008; 6:531-538.
10. Marin ML, Hollier LH. Endovascular grafts. Semin Vasc Surg 1999; 12:64-73.
11. Halpern M. Percutaneous transfemoral arteriography: an analysis of the complications in 1,000 consecutive cases. Am J Roentgenol Radium Ther Nucl Med 1964; 92:918-934.
12. Nunn DB. Complications of peripheral arteriography. Am Surg 1978; 44:664-669.
13. Lam RC, Shah S, Faries PL, et al. Incidence and clinical significance of distal embolization during percutaneous interventions involving the superficial femoral artery. J Vasc Surg 2007; 46:1155-1159.
14. Dorffler-Melly J, Koopman MM, Prins MH, Buller HR. Antiplatelet and anticoagulant drugs for prevention of restenosis/reocclusion following peripheral endovascular treatment. Cochrane Database Syst Rev 2005; (1):CD002071.
15. Ruef J, Hofmann M, Haase J. Endovascular interventions in iliac and infrainguinal occlusive artery disease. J Interv Cardiol 2004; 17: 427-435.
16. Ouriel K, Veith FJ, Sasahara AA. A comparison of recombinant urokinase with vascular surgery as initial treatment for acute arterial occlusion of the legs. Thrombolysis or Peripheral Arterial Surgery (TOPAS) Investigators. N Engl J Med 1998; 338:1105-1111.
17. Höfling B, Pölnitz AV, Backa D, et al. Percutaneous removal of atheromatous plaques in peripheral arteries. Lancet 1988; 1:384-386.
18. Shrikhande GV, McKinsey JF. Use and abuse of atherectomy: where should it be used? Semin Vasc Surg 2008; 21:204-209.
19. McKinsey JF, Goldstein L, Khan HU, et al. Novel treatment of patients with lower extremity ischemia: use of percutaneous atherectomy in 579 lesions. Ann Surg 2008; 248:519-528.
20. Biskup NI, Ihnat DM, Leon LR, et al. Infrainguinal atherectomy: a retrospective review of a single-center experience. Ann Vasc Surg 2008; 22:776-782.
21. Chung SW, Sharafuddin MJ, Chigurupati R, Hoballah JJ. Midterm patency following atherectomy for infrainguinal occlusive disease: a word of caution. Ann Vasc Surg 2008; 22:358-365.
22. Osuga K, Mikami K, Higashihara H, et al. Principles and techniques of transcatheter embolotherapy for peripheral vascular lesions. Radiat Med 2006; 24:309-314.

CHAPTER 87

Vascular Surgery

Christopher J. Abularrage and David H. Deaton

Vascular disease is typically a longitudinal process that affects patients throughout their life span. The role of the vascular surgeon in managing vascular disease is threefold: identification and monitoring of disease, surgical correction when indicated, and follow-up of surgical results and disease progression. The key to this role is deciding when a patient should undergo surgical correction; this must take into account the risks and benefits of the surgical procedure as well as the durability of the results.

Imaging of the cardiovascular system is a key component of each step in the care of the vascular surgical patient in that it provides the only objective information of the status of the arterial tree in question. Different imaging modalities are relevant at different points during the course of disease management. Whereas one modality may be pertinent in the decision of whether to undergo surgery, another may be more appropriate for preoperative planning or postoperative surveillance. An understanding of their utility at different points in the decision-making process is key to the care of the vascular surgical patient.

CAROTID ENDARTERECTOMY

Description

Carotid endarterectomy is performed through a neck incision along the medial aspect of the sternocleidomastoid muscle. The carotid bifurcation is the most common location of carotid occlusive disease, and control of the common, internal, and external carotid arteries must be obtained. An incision is made along the common carotid extending through the plaque to an area of nondiseased internal carotid artery. The plaque is then elevated from the adventitia along with the intima. Finally, the arteriotomy is closed with a synthetic or autologous patch, which decreases the risk of restenosis compared with primary closure.

Indications

Vascular surgeons are particularly stringent about the indications for carotid endarterectomy because this is one of the few prophylactic operations. Indications for carotid endarterectomy are based on two large, multicenter, randomized trials comparing best medical therapy (antiplatelet) and surgical therapy for carotid stenosis. The North American Symptomatic Carotid Endarterectomy Trial (NASCET) examined patients with a previous history of stroke, transient ischemic attack, or amaurosis fugax within 3 months of enrollment.[1] During 2 years, the risk of stroke in patients with a 70% to 99% stenosis was reduced from 26% to 9% with carotid endarterectomy. The risk of stroke in patients with a 50% to 69% stenosis was reduced from 22% to 16% during 5 years. Given the less substantial benefit seen with the moderate-grade lesions, most vascular surgeons would recommend carotid endarterectomy to symptomatic patients with 50% to 69% stenosis only if they have a substantial life expectancy and low risk of complications related to the surgical intervention. Finally, subgroup analysis revealed an increased risk of stroke in medically treated patients with contralateral carotid occlusions and ulcerated plaques.

The Asymptomatic Carotid Atherosclerosis Study (ACAS) randomized asymptomatic patients to medical and surgical therapy.[2] Carotid endarterectomy reduced the 5-year risk of stroke from 11% to 5% in patients with 60% to 99% stenosis compared with medical therapy. Given an absolute stroke risk reduction of 6% during 5 years, further studies have shown that surgical therapy is most beneficial in patients with 80% to 99% stenosis and in men compared with women. This equates to changing the outcome of approximately 1 in 20 to 30 patients, making the safety and risk reduction in the conduct of intervention for asymptomatic patients of paramount importance. This fact significantly affects the decision-making process regarding carotid imaging for either carotid endarterectomy or carotid stenting. In the ACAS trial, there was a 1.5% risk of stroke from diagnostic angiography alone.

Contraindications

Cardiopulmonary comorbidities preventing surgical intervention and total occlusion of the internal carotid artery are the only absolute contraindications to carotid endarterectomy. The risks related to cardiopulmonary comorbidity may be reduced by the use of local or regional anesthesia, thus limiting the systemic effects of general anesthesia. Carotid endarterectomy is not performed on patients with occlusion of the internal carotid artery as the thrombus typically extends to the ophthalmic artery. Relative contraindications to surgery are based on the exclusion criteria of the NASCET and ACAS trials, including, among others, patients with recent myocardial infarction (symptomatic coronary artery disease), uncontrolled diabetes mellitus, and advanced age. Anatomic risk factors include previous neck irradiation or dissection, tracheal stoma, carotid lesions at or above the second cervical vertebra, contralateral vocal cord paralysis, and previous carotid surgery.

Further studies examined carotid endarterectomy and found that it can be safely performed in patients deemed at high risk, including those 80 years or older and others with significant comorbid conditions, with combined stroke and mortality rates comparable to those found in the NASCET and ACAS studies. Contralateral occlusion was the only predictor for moderately increased perioperative risk of stroke and reduced long-term survival.[3]

Overall, outcomes are based on the surgeon's experience, and decisions about intervention are largely based on the track record of the team performing the procedure.

Outcomes and Complications

Outcomes related to surgical therapy are discussed earlier. The majority of patients do well after carotid endarterectomy and are discharged home by the first postoperative day.

The major complications related to carotid endarterectomy include perioperative stroke, cranial nerve injuries, cardiopulmonary complications, and restenosis. Recurrent stenosis can be in the form of three types occurring at different time stages: (1) residual disease from an incomplete endarterectomy usually can be seen immediately on postoperative imaging; (2) intimal hyperplasia frequently occurs between 2 months and 2 years; and (3) recurrent atherosclerotic disease most often occurs beyond 2 years. Open surgical repair of recurrence in any of these forms carries a higher risk of intraoperative complications, including cranial nerve damage secondary to postoperative scar formation. For this reason, carotid stent angioplasty is frequently used to treat recurrent disease.

One rare complication is hyperperfusion syndrome, which is characterized by a severe, unilateral headache occurring 3 to 7 days after endarterectomy. This has been attributed to the sudden restoration of normal arterial pressures in a vascular bed that has not seen pulsatility and normal pressures for a long period, thus leading to atrophy of the arteriolar restrictive mechanisms and impaired ability of the cerebrovascular circulation to autoregulate after the reestablishment of cranial blood flow. MRI may show reversible vasogenic edema similar to that observed in the posterior leukoencephalopathy syndrome.[4] Treatment includes control of the hypertension that is frequently associated with this phenomenon to prevent cerebral hemorrhage until cerebral autoregulation is reestablished, typically for a few days to 1 week.

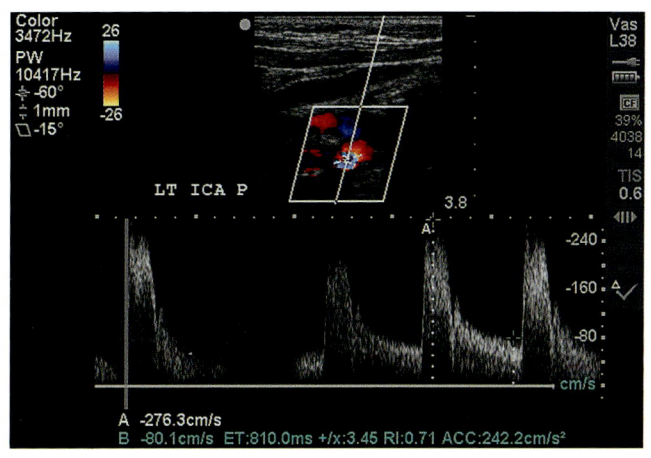

■ **FIGURE 87-1** Duplex ultrasound examination of a patient with left internal carotid artery stenosis. Note the gray-scale lesion on the B-mode image and elevated Doppler velocity measurements across the stenosis.

Imaging Findings

Preoperative Assessment

Duplex ultrasonography is the most common technique used to assess patients suspected of having extracranial cerebrovascular disease. B-mode ultrasonography is used to define location of the stenotic lesion, and Doppler examination is used to measure velocities across the stenosis (Fig. 87-1). B-mode ultrasonography not only delineates the location of a stenosis but also describes the characteristics of the plaque itself. Plaque ulceration as well as plaque calcification or hemorrhage may be seen. B-mode ultrasonography can also evaluate plaque echogenicity and the presence of thrombus. Soft, friable plaques on ultrasound examination are typically less stable than echoic plaques are. Mobile thrombus on ultrasound examination has been associated with an increased risk of stroke.

Velocity measurements across a stenosis are the most important aspect of the preoperative assessment for the vascular surgeon because these measurements are directly correlated with degree of stenosis. Strandness[5] first reported a sensitivity of 99% and a specificity of 84% with duplex ultrasound criteria for the evaluation of carotid disease compared with conventional angiography (Table 87-1). More recently, it has been observed that diagnostic criteria must be altered in the setting of a contralateral severe stenosis or complete occlusion of the internal carotid artery because of a compensatory increase in carotid blood flow. By use of the criteria of AbuRahma,[6] the accuracy of duplex ultrasound measurements can be increased to 96%. No matter which criteria are used, they must be validated by individual vascular laboratories as this technique may be operator and instrument dependent.

Many surgeons will rely on duplex ultrasonography alone in making the decision to perform a carotid endarterectomy. Additional imaging is required in any

TABLE 87-1 Duplex Ultrasound Criteria for Diagnosis of Internal Carotid Artery Stenosis

Stenosis	Criteria	
	Strandness	**AbuRahma**
Normal	PSV < 125 cm/sec No SB Flow reversal in bulb	PSV < 125 cm/sec No SB
1%-15%	PSV < 125 cm/sec No or minimal SB Flow reversal in bulb absent	PSV < 125 cm/sec Minimal SB
16%-49%	PSV > 125 cm/sec Marked SB	PSV < 140 cm/sec EDV < 140 cm/sec
50%-79%	PSV > 125 cm/sec EDV < 140 cm/sec	PSV ≥ 140 cm/sec EDV < 140 cm/sec
80%-99%	PSV < 125 cm/sec EDV > 140 cm/sec	PSV > 140 cm/sec EDV < 140 cm/sec
Occlusion	No flow	No flow

EDV, end-diastolic velocity; PSV, peak systolic velocity; SB, spectral broadening.
Modified from Strandness DE Jr. Extracranial arterial disease. In Strandness DE Jr (ed). Duplex Scanning in Vascular Disorders, 2nd ed. New York, Raven Press, 1993, pp 113-158; and AbuRahma AF, Richmond BK, Robinson PA, et al. Effect of contralateral severe stenosis or carotid occlusion on duplex criteria of ipsilateral stenoses: comparative study of various duplex parameters. J Vasc Surg 1995; 22:751-761.

case in which anatomic factors preclude a complete assessment by ultrasound examination. These include extreme tortuosity, inability to see normal distal internal carotid, or any factor that does not allow complete characterization of the carotid bifurcation and confirmation of a normal distal extracranial internal carotid artery. Furthermore, additional testing should be performed in the presence of the so-called string sign. String sign may occur in two scenarios that are treated differently. In the first, there is slow flow through a high-grade stenosis with an underfilled but normal internal carotid artery. In this case, carotid endarterectomy is beneficial. In the second case, there is a long-segment high-grade stenosis extending into the distal internal carotid artery. These types of lesions are more difficult to treat surgically and are associated with a higher perioperative stroke rate. Combining duplex ultrasonography with either computed tomographic angiography (CTA) or magnetic resonance angiography (MRA) increases the overall accuracy of determining degree of stenosis.

CTA has been used to delineate extracranial cerebrovascular and carotid arch anatomy and has the advantages of minimal discomfort for the patient, relatively low radiation doses, and demarcation of calcific plaques in both the carotid arteries and the aortic arch. Recent three-dimensional reconstructions provide the surgeon with a greater ability in preoperative planning (Fig. 87-2).

MRA is another tool of the vascular surgeon and can be particularly useful in patients with an allergy to intravenous contrast material. Time-of-flight MRA has a tendency to overestimate the degree of stenosis because of local blood flow turbulence. Overestimation of time-of-flight MRA can be reconciled with the performance of gadolinium-enhanced three-dimensional MRA.[7] Both techniques also demonstrate intracranial vessel anatomy along with patency of the communicating arteries.

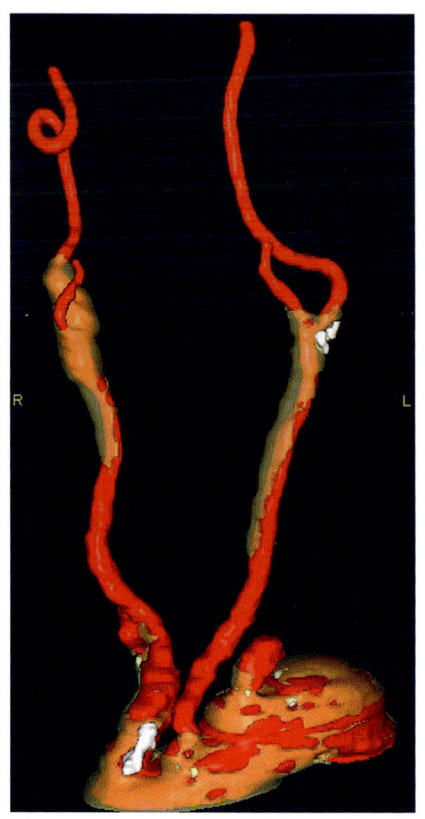

■ **FIGURE 87-2** Postprocessed view of three-dimensional CTA shows a left carotid stenosis with calcification (white) and plaque (yellow).

Catheter angiography (Fig. 87-3), previously considered the gold standard for the assessment of extracranial cerebrovascular disease, has been used less frequently in uncomplicated patients because of the approximately 1.5% risk of stroke. Catheter angiography is now typically reserved for evaluation of patients in whom results from duplex ultrasonography and either CTA or MRA are discordant.

Preoperative Planning

Preoperative planning uses the same techniques discussed before, including duplex ultrasonography, CTA, and MRA. These studies should alert the surgeon of abnormal anatomy, such as an unusually high or low bifurcation or excessive tortuosity, in an effort to avoid injury to important surrounding structures.

Postoperative Surveillance

Postoperative surveillance is accomplished with duplex ultrasonography. This provides an inexpensive, efficient method of monitoring not only the durability of the surgical result but also the progression of disease on the contralateral side. As discussed earlier, recurrent stenosis occurs in three forms and is typically time related. Residual disease can be manifested in the form of postoperative symptoms of amaurosis fugax, transient ischemic attack, or stroke. These patients are brought immediately back to the operating room for re-exploration. If residual disease is identified at the first postoperative duplex scan, patients

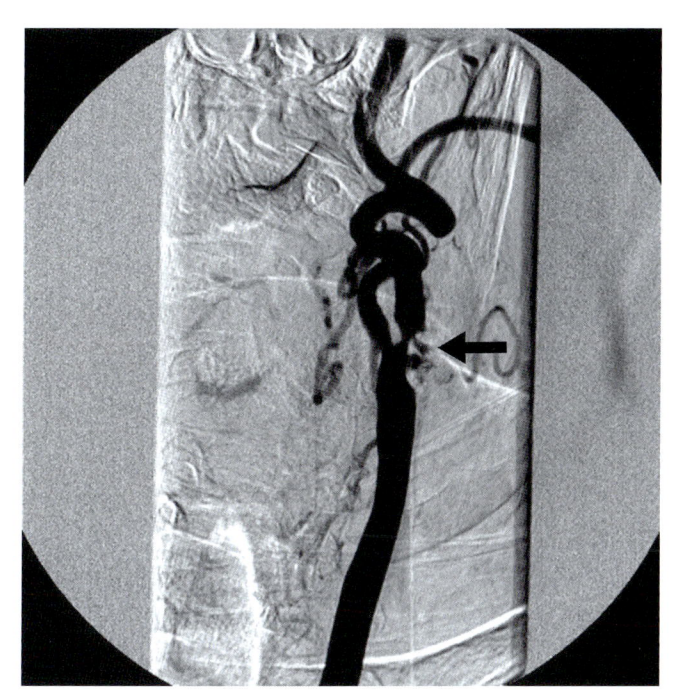

FIGURE 87-3 Digital subtraction angiography showing high-grade stenosis of the internal carotid artery (*arrow*).

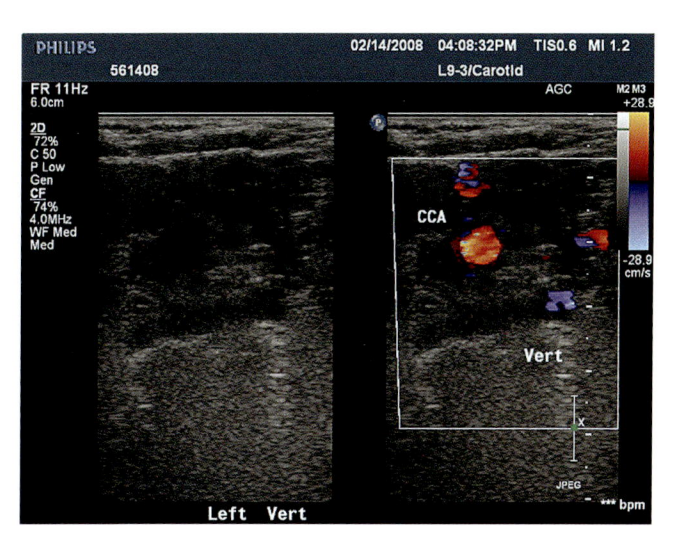

FIGURE 87-4 Duplex ultrasonography of common carotid and vertebral arteries showing reversal of flow within vertebral artery in a patient with subclavian steal syndrome. Note the opposite color of the vertebral artery (blue) compared with the common carotid artery (red).

can be observed if they are asymptomatic or re-explored if the plaque looks unstable. Patients with intimal hyperplasia are most often asymptomatic because these lesions have a very low embolic potential. Therefore, patients with intimal hyperplasia are typically observed until there is progression to a high-grade stenosis or the rare development of symptoms. Recurrent atherosclerotic disease is treated in a manner similar to the primary development of occlusive disease as these lesions are inherently more unstable than their intimal hyperplastic counterparts.

CAROTID-SUBCLAVIAN BYPASS

Description

Carotid-subclavian bypass may be performed through a remote cervical incision just lateral to the sternocleidomastoid muscle. The jugular vein is reflected medially to expose the common carotid artery. The anterior scalene muscle is then divided to expose the subclavian artery. Once proximal and distal control of each artery is obtained, bypass is typically performed with a prosthetic graft as patency is superior to autogenous conduit in this position.[8] On occasion, concomitant disease of the ipsilateral common carotid artery precludes its use as an inflow vessel. In these cases, the contralateral common carotid may be used. The prosthetic graft would then be tunneled across the midline through the retropharyngeal space; this is a more direct path and avoids erosion of the overlying skin or interference with possible subsequent sternotomy or tracheostomy.

Indications

Indications for repair of subclavian stenosis include upper extremity disabling claudication, rest pain, and tissue loss. Patients with subclavian steal syndrome are also candidates for repair. Subclavian steal occurs when there is a stenosis of the first portion of the subclavian artery causing distal pressure to drop below that at the vertebrobasilar junction, with subsequent reversal of flow through the basilar and ipsilateral vertebral arteries. This can lead to vertebrobasilar symptoms of presyncope, syncope, or drop attacks. Finally, carotid-subclavian bypass should be performed in those patients with asymptomatic proximal subclavian stenotic lesions who are undergoing coronary revascularization through the internal mammary artery, as well as in patients with symptomatic coronary steal syndrome from a patent internal mammary artery coronary bypass graft.

Contraindications

Severe cardiopulmonary comorbidity is the only absolute contraindication to carotid-subclavian bypass. As described before, this procedure may be performed through a small incision, and local regional anesthesia may have fewer cardiovascular effects than standard general anesthetic techniques.

Outcomes and Complications

Outcomes from carotid-subclavian bypass are excellent, with 10-year patency rates of 84%.[9] Complications range from a 0% to 1% stroke rate to a 0% mortality rate.[10,11]

Imaging Findings

Preoperative Assessment

Duplex ultrasonography may be used to screen for subclavian stenosis but is limited by the bony structures of the mediastinum. Its usefulness lies in its ability to assess for reversal of blood flow in the vertebral artery with upper extremity exercise (Fig. 87-4) and the adequacy of the common carotid artery for inflow.

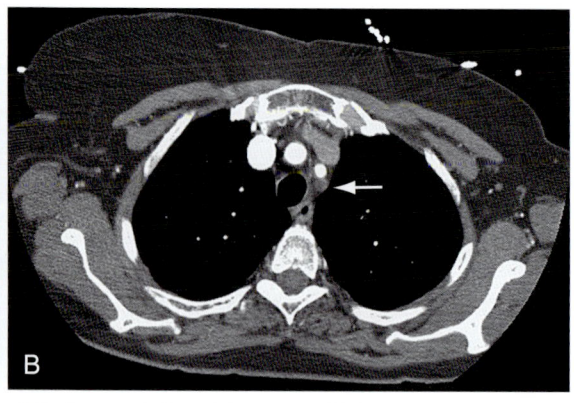

FIGURE 87-5 Coronal reformat (**A**) and axial (**B**) images from CTA show occlusion of the proximal left subclavian artery (*arrows*) in a patient with subclavian steal syndrome.

CTA and MRA are useful tools to assess for lesions of the proximal subclavian artery. As a screening tool, CTA may be more practical because the examination is more widely available and generally quicker to perform.

In cases in which the diagnosis is questionable, digital subtraction angiography may be helpful to demonstrate reversal of flow through the vertebral artery.

Preoperative Planning

Once a subclavian stenosis has been identified, preoperative planning may be accomplished with CTA or MRA (Fig. 87-5). Both evaluate the exact location of the lesion as well as assess possible inflow and outflow vessels. Full appraisal of the aortic arch, its branches, and neck extracranial cerebrovascular vessels is necessary to rule out other pathologic processes. Resolution of the aortic arch and these large-caliber vessels with CTA and MRA is excellent, and they may replace standard angiography.

Digital subtraction angiography may be a useful adjunct for preoperative planning before carotid subclavian bypass. Angiography can identify major inflow and outflow vessels as well as important collaterals (Fig. 87-6).

In cases in which it is necessary to use the contralateral common carotid artery as inflow, CT scanning should be performed to evaluate the retropharyngeal soft tissues.

Postoperative Surveillance

The location of the bypass graft in the neck makes duplex ultrasonography the modality of choice for postoperative graft surveillance. Duplex ultrasonography can identify lesions of the proximal and distal anastomoses along with changes of velocities within the graft.

Once a threatened bypass has been identified with duplex ultrasonography, angiography may be used to further examine the anastomoses and to delineate intragraft stenoses. Endovascular intervention to save the bypass may be performed at this time.

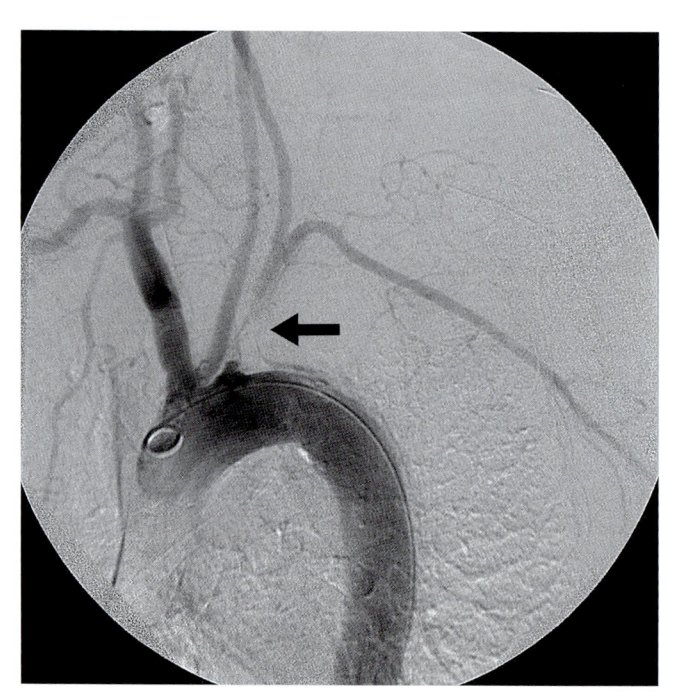

FIGURE 87-6 Digital subtraction angiography showing occlusion of the proximal left subclavian artery (*arrow*) with reconstitution of left vertebral and distal left subclavian arteries. Real-time angiography showed retrograde filling of left vertebral artery.

THORACOABDOMINAL AORTIC ANEURYSM REPAIR

Description

Thoracoabdominal aortic aneurysm (TAAA) repair is performed through a retroperitoneal approach combined with thoracotomy. Intraoperative management of patients with thoracoabdominal aneurysms is dependent on the extent of the aneurysmal degeneration of the aorta. Patients with Crawford extent I and II TAAAs generally require either continuous distal perfusion or left-sided heart bypass; these types of aneurysms are associated with the greatest risk of paraplegia (Fig. 87-7). In the thorax, the recurrent laryngeal and vagus nerves are gently retracted off from the aorta. After cross-clamping of the

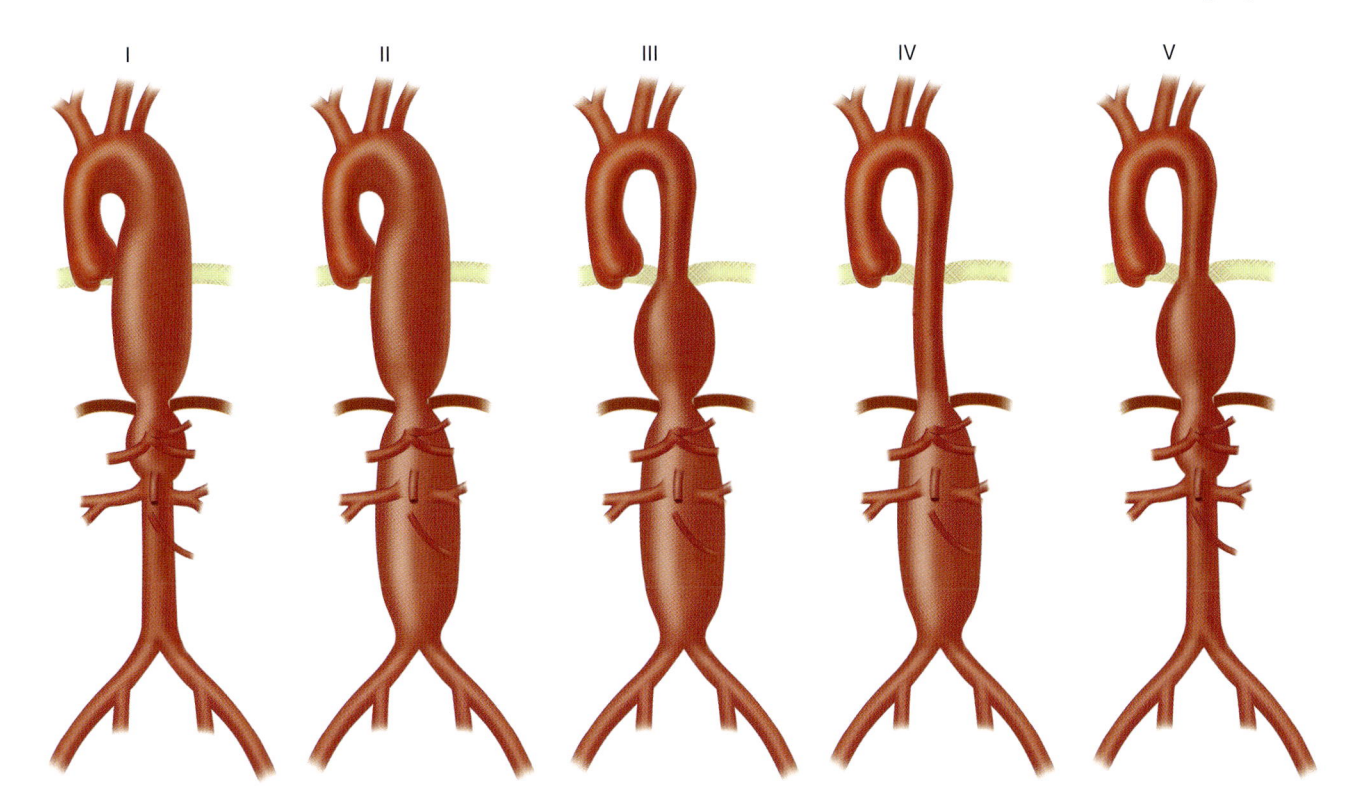

FIGURE 87-7 Crawford classification of thoracoabdominal aneurysms. Extent I, distal to the left subclavian artery to above the renal arteries. Extent II, distal to the left subclavian artery to below the renal arteries. Extent III, from the sixth intercostal space to below the renal arteries. Extent IV, from the 12th intercostal space to the iliac bifurcation (total abdominal aortic aneurysm). Extent V, below the sixth intercostal space to just above the renal arteries.

aorta, the proximal anastomosis is sewn in an endoaneurysmal fashion (end-to-end within the aneurysm sac). All large intercostal arteries from T7 to L2 are reimplanted into the graft, followed by the visceral vessels. If stenoses at the origin of these arteries are encountered, an endarterectomy may be performed. Finally, the distal anastomosis is performed in endoaneurysmal fashion to an uninvolved portion of the distal aorta.

Indications

Asymptomatic TAAAs are repaired if the diameter exceeds 6 cm or if the rate of expansion exceeds 0.5 cm during a 6-month period. TAAAs presenting with abdominal or back pain are repaired immediately as there is an associated higher risk of rupture, especially in the setting of hypotension. Finally, aneurysms producing distal embolization may also be considered for repair regardless of size.

Contraindications

TAAA repair represents one of the most morbid vascular surgical procedures not only because of the risk of paraplegia (up to 13% electively) but also because of a mortality rate of 8%.[12] Patients with prohibitive cardiopulmonary risk are not candidates for this procedure. These patients are typically identified on preoperative cardiac stress testing as well as on preoperative pulmonary function testing. Relative contraindications include decreased life expectancy related to other medical issues.

Outcomes and Complications

The 30-day survival after TAAA repair is approximately 95%. Late survival rates are 55% at 5 years, 29% at 10 years, and 21% at 15 years.[12] Complications related to the surgery are typically pulmonary (32%), cardiac (8%), renal (6%), and spinal (4% to 13%) in nature. Spinal cord ischemia is significantly increased in Crawford extent I and II aneurysms.

Imaging Findings

Preoperative Assessment

Unlike for abdominal aortic aneurysms, no good screening test exists for TAAA. Chest radiography may reveal aortic dilation in the presence of calcification, but the films are frequently normal. The mainstay of preoperative TAAA evaluation is CTA or MRA. Either of these can be used to observe TAAA diameters.

Preoperative Planning

CTA is typically the preferred diagnostic modality for preoperative planning before TAAA repair. CTA identifies the extent of the aneurysm, calcification, thrombus, and accessory vessels. Three-dimensional image postprocessing of CTA data is particularly helpful for elucidating branch vessel anatomy.

Proper synchronization (i.e., timing) of CTA with the contrast bolus for TAAA evaluation may be difficult in

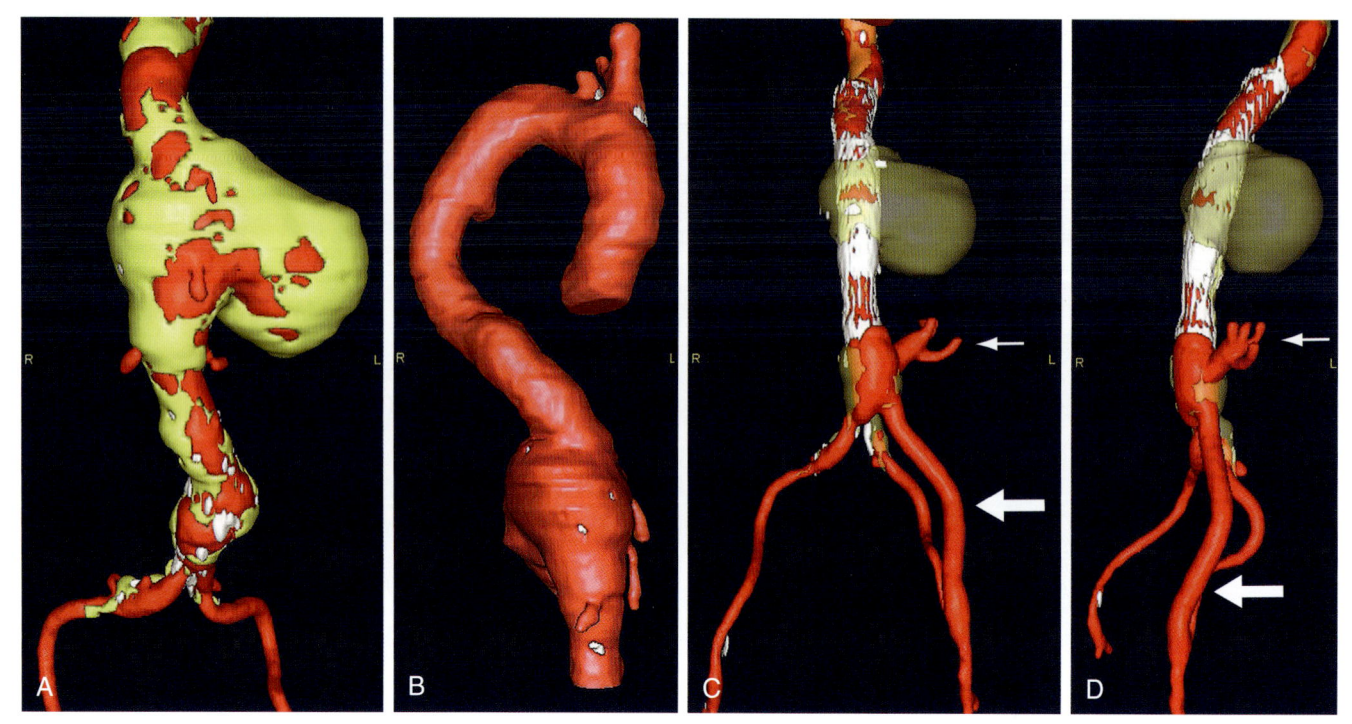

FIGURE 87-8 Preoperative three-dimensional postprocessed views from CTA of a patient with an abdominal aortic aneurysm (**A**) and thoracoabdominal aortic aneurysm (**B**). The patient underwent open debranching of the celiac, superior mesenteric, and bilateral renal arteries with a branched graft from the distal aorta (**C** and **D,** *small arrow*). A distal aorto–left femoral graft was also placed that was used for access in the subsequent endovascular repair (**C** and **D,** *large arrow*).

Crawford extent II aneurysms as these frequently extend the entire length of the aorta. MRI, although not as commonly used as CTA because of a more time-consuming process, may also be used for preoperative planning, especially in patients with an allergy to iodinated contrast agents.

Postoperative Surveillance

Postoperative surveillance of TAAA repair is performed typically with CTA. CTA assesses the durability of the repair, further aneurysmal degeneration of abdominal aorta and its branches, and development of anastomotic pseudoaneurysms.

THORACIC AORTIC ANEURYSM HYBRID PROCEDURES

Description

Thoracic aortic aneurysm (TAA) repair is a morbid procedure because of the necessity for a median sternotomy or posterolateral thoracotomy. Whereas endovascular TAA repair avoids the need for these approaches, anatomic factors such as small access vessels may preclude this. In these cases, hybrid TAA repair may be performed by creating open vascular surgical access to the aorta either distally or proximally. In the case of distal open access, an aortofemoral bypass may be performed either alone or in conjunction with concomitant debranching or repair of an aortic aneurysm (Fig. 87-8). The common iliac artery is oversewn, allowing retrograde blood flow through the aortofemoral limb to the internal iliac artery through the external iliac artery. In the case of proximal access, the arch vessels are debranched from the aorta and reanastomosed to a four-branched prosthetic graft that is anastomosed directly to the ascending aorta (Fig. 87-9). The sheath is then advanced through one of the limbs of the graft, and the TAA is repaired in standard endovascular fashion. At the conclusion of the case, the access limb of the graft is oversewn.

Indications

Endovascular repair of thoracic aneurysms may be limited by device sheath diameter that exceeds the diameter of the access arteries or heavy calcification and tortuosity of the access arteries. In these circumstances, hybrid repair of TAA may be useful. Patients must have TAA morphology that is suitable to endovascular repair.

Contraindications

Contraindications to hybrid TAA repair include cardiopulmonary risk factors as well as anatomic factors of the thoracic aneurysm. Currently, only three devices have been approved by the Food and Drug Administration for endovascular TAA repair (Cook TX, Gore TAG, and Medtronic Talent devices). Anatomic requirements include 20 mm or more of proximal and distal neck length and distal neck diameters of 20 to 42 mm. In cases in which the left subclavian artery needs to be covered with the endovascular stent graft for proximal fixation, contraindications to covering the left subclavian artery with the

CHAPTER 87 • Vascular Surgery 1179

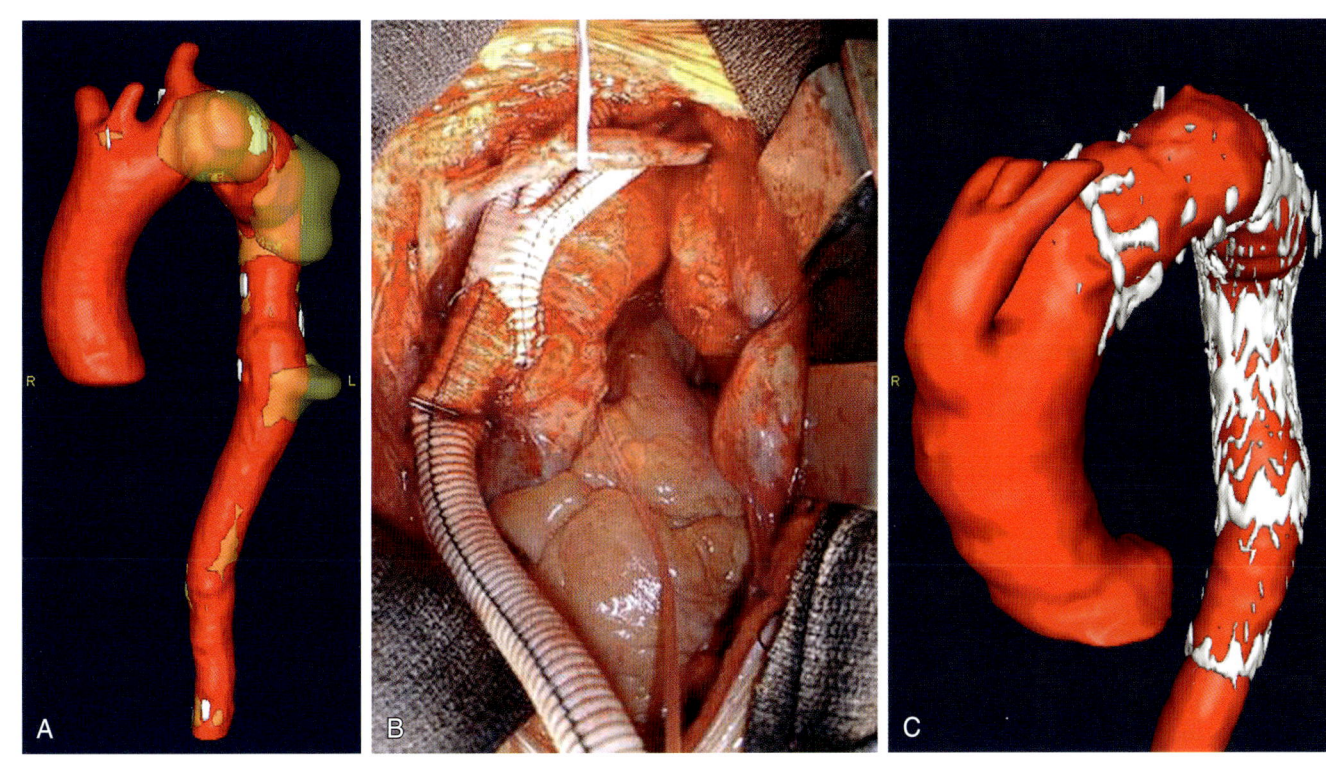

FIGURE 87-9 Preoperative CTA (**A**, oblique sagittal three-dimensional view) of a patient with a thoracic aortic artery aneurysm whose iliac arteries were smaller than the device diameter. A four-limbed bypass was anastomosed to the ascending aorta for device access as well as for debranching of the arch vessels (**B**). Postoperative CTA reveals endovascular exclusion of the aneurysm as well as the three-limbed bypass (**C**, oblique coronal three-dimensional view).

endograft include a patent left internal mammary artery to left anterior descending coronary artery bypass, incomplete circle of Willis, and dominant left vertebral artery. These factors increase the risk of myocardial infarction and stroke.[13] Otherwise, most patients have enough collateral circulation to prevent left upper extremity ischemia, with claudication developing in approximately 16% and rest pain in 5%.[14] In patients with upper extremity rest pain or tissue loss, a left carotid–subclavian bypass may be performed.

Outcomes and Complications

Outcomes of hybrid TAA repairs are similar to those of standard endovascular TAA repair. In the perioperative period, 10% of patients require reintervention; freedom from reintervention approaches 81% by 48 months.[15] Spinal cord ischemic complications, which may occasionally be transient, are experienced by 7% of patients. The perioperative mortality rate is approximately 10% and is half that of an open repair.

Imaging Findings
Preoperative Assessment

Preoperative assessment is similar to that of standard TAA repair. Evaluation of the entire aorta and its branch vessels may be performed with CTA or MRA.

Preoperative Planning

CTA with three-dimensional image postprocessing is key to preoperative planning for hybrid TAA repair. CTA elucidates thrombus, calcification, diameters, landing zones, pathologic changes of the aortic arch and its branches, and iliac or access vessel disease (Fig. 87-9A).

Postoperative Surveillance

Postoperative surveillance of hybrid TAA repair is similar to that of standard TAA repair and is usually adequately accomplished with CTA (Fig. 87-9C).

ABDOMINAL AORTIC ANEURYSM REPAIR
Description

Open repair of abdominal aortic aneurysm (AAA) can be carried out through a midline or retroperitoneal approach; the choice of approach depends on factors related to aneurysm anatomy, involvement of the distal right iliac system, and previous abdominal surgeries. With either procedure, proximal and distal control of the aorta and iliac arteries is obtained. The proximal aortic clamp must be placed on a portion of aorta free from disease. In the case of juxtarenal and suprarenal aneurysms, a supraceliac clamp must be placed. An infrarenal artery clamp is placed just distal to the left renal vein in the case of an infrarenal aneurysm. The aneurysm sac is then opened longitudinally. If a supraceliac clamp is in place, the renal arteries are often flushed with iced heparinized saline to prevent ischemic damage. The proximal anastomosis is sewn in an endoaneurysmal fashion. The visceral vessels may be reimplanted on the graft if that portion of the aorta is aneurysmal. The proximal clamp is then removed and placed on the proximal graft, reestablishing blood flow to the kidneys in the case of supraceliac clamping. All backbleeding lumbar arteries are suture ligated. The inferior mesenteric artery, if patent, may be ligated in the presence of strong backbleeding or reimplanted in the presence of poor backbleeding. The distal anastomoses are then performed in a similar endoaneurysmal fashion. All clamps are removed, and blood flow is reestablished to the lower extremities. Finally, the aneurysm sac is closed over the graft to prevent contact with and possibly erosion into surrounding structures postoperatively.

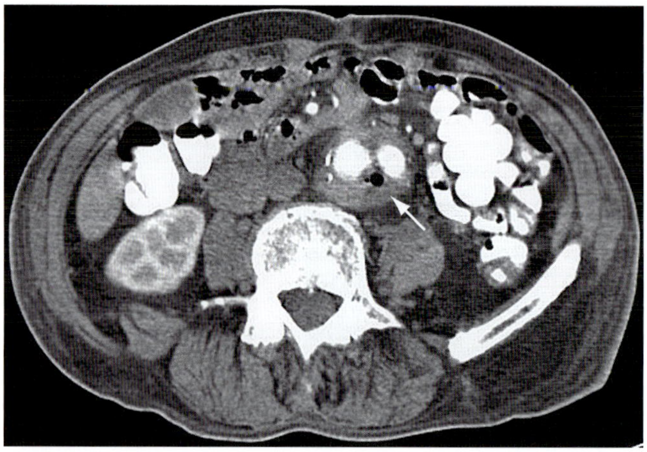

FIGURE 87-10 Postoperative CT scan of a patient who underwent abdominal aortic aneurysm repair showing air within the aneurysm sac (*arrow*), consistent with graft infection.

Indications

The size at which asymptomatic AAA repair is indicated is determined by a composite of the morphology and anatomy of the aneurysm, the medical comorbidities of the patient, and the morbidity and mortality demonstrated by the surgeon. Broadly speaking, 5.5 cm is the size at which the risk of death from the surgical procedure (1% to 5%) is outweighed by the annual risk of rupture (5% to 10%). Other patient groups who may be repaired before this include women with 5-cm AAAs, who have a higher risk of rupture with smaller aneurysm size, and patients with a rapidly expanding AAA (>1 cm per year). According to the Aneurysm Detection and Management (ADAM) study[16] and the U.K. Small Aneurysm Trial,[17] AAAs between 4.5 and 5.5 cm can be safely observed in compliant patients as the risk of open surgery outweighs the risk of rupture. Symptomatic AAAs presenting with abdominal or back pain are repaired immediately as discussed previously for thoracoabdominal aneurysms.

Contraindications

Absolute contraindications to repair of AAA include prohibitive cardiopulmonary risk of surgery; a relative contraindication is decreased life expectancy related to other medical issues. Operative risk is increased in patients with chronic renal insufficiency, chronic obstructive pulmonary disease, congestive heart failure, moderate to severe coronary artery disease, and advanced age.

Outcomes and Complications

Long-term durability of open repair of AAA is excellent, and frequent surveillance is unnecessary. The 30-day mortality of patients undergoing open AAA repair is approximately 5% or less, and the 5-year survival is approximately 70%.

Complications related to AAA repair can be divided into early and late categories. Early complications include, but are not limited to, cardiopulmonary complications, renal failure, distal embolization of thrombus, hemorrhage, and colonic ischemia.

Late complications of AAA repair occur in approximately 7% of patients within 5 years. Aortic graft infection is a dreaded complication. Patients frequently present with fever, bacteremia, or failure to thrive. CT findings include air or fluid around the graft and inflammatory changes in normal tissue planes (Fig. 87-10). Patients undergoing AAA repair may normally have perigraft fluid up to 6 months postoperatively. Differentiation between a graft infection and normal postoperative fluid collections can be accomplished with CT-guided aspiration or indium In 111–tagged white blood cell nuclear scintigraphy.

Anastomotic pseudoaneurysms occur in 0.2% of aortic anastomoses, 1.2% of iliac anastomoses, and 3% of femoral anastomoses.[18] This incidence increases over time, which stresses the importance of follow-up in young patients undergoing AAA repair.

Aortoduodenal fistulas occur approximately 0.9% of the time after AAA repair. Whereas these frequently present as a gastrointestinal bleed, the finding of intravenous contrast agent in the bowel lumen on an intravenous contrast–enhanced only CT scan (no oral contrast agent administered) should alert to this possibility. Emergent upper endoscopy for confirmation of the diagnosis, followed by extra-anatomic bypass and resection of the graft, is warranted.

Imaging Findings

Preoperative Assessment

Ultrasonography is the primary modality for the identification of abdominal aortic aneurysmal disease because of its low cost and ease of detection. Studies have shown that it is helpful not only in patients with pulsatile abdominal masses but also in generalized screening of men older than 60 years[19] or those with a family history of AAA. CT provides more accurate assessment of the diameter as well as extent of aneurysmal degeneration of the aorta and is particularly helpful in aneurysms approaching 4.5 cm.

Preoperative Planning

Similar to preoperative TAAA planning, CTA is often the preferred modality for preoperative planning before AAA repair. Not only does it provide a more accurate diameter measurement than ultrasonography, but it assesses the entire aorta for pathologic changes (Fig. 87-11A). CTA can identify heavy calcification, accessory renal vessels, and retroaortic left renal veins, all of which have implications for intraoperative clamp placement. The recent improvements in three-dimensional image postprocessing and reconstruction of CTA data have enhanced the ability of the vascular surgeon to assess aortic disease and to plan open repair by longitudinally distinguishing intraluminal thrombus from calcification as well as noncircumferential dilation of the aortic wall that might not be as easily seen on standard axial CT images.

MRA, although not as commonly used as CTA, may also be used for preoperative planning, especially in patients with an allergy to iodinated contrast agents. Angiography is useful when there is suspicion of concomitant renal occlusive disease, renovascular hypertension, or other small-vessel anatomy that is often not well delineated by CT.

Postoperative Surveillance

Postoperative assessment of AAA repair is accomplished almost exclusively with CTA (Fig. 87-11B). Open AAA repairs are typically scanned once at 6 to 12 months after surgery, if there are no anatomic concerns. Further scanning is indicated for the development of late symptoms. CTA is helpful not only in assessing the durability of the repair but also for identifying aneurysmal degeneration of the remaining abdominal aorta and its branches, especially the iliac arteries (Fig. 87-12). This becomes clinically relevant beyond 3 mm of dilation and is seen in approximately 13% of patients.[20]

ABDOMINAL AORTIC ANEURYSM HYBRID PROCEDURES

Description

Open access of the iliac arteries may be necessary for endovascular abdominal aortic aneurysm repair (EVAR). This is accomplished through a flank retroperitoneal incision. Vessels are palpated to identify an area that is not heavily calcified. Proximal and distal control of the vessels

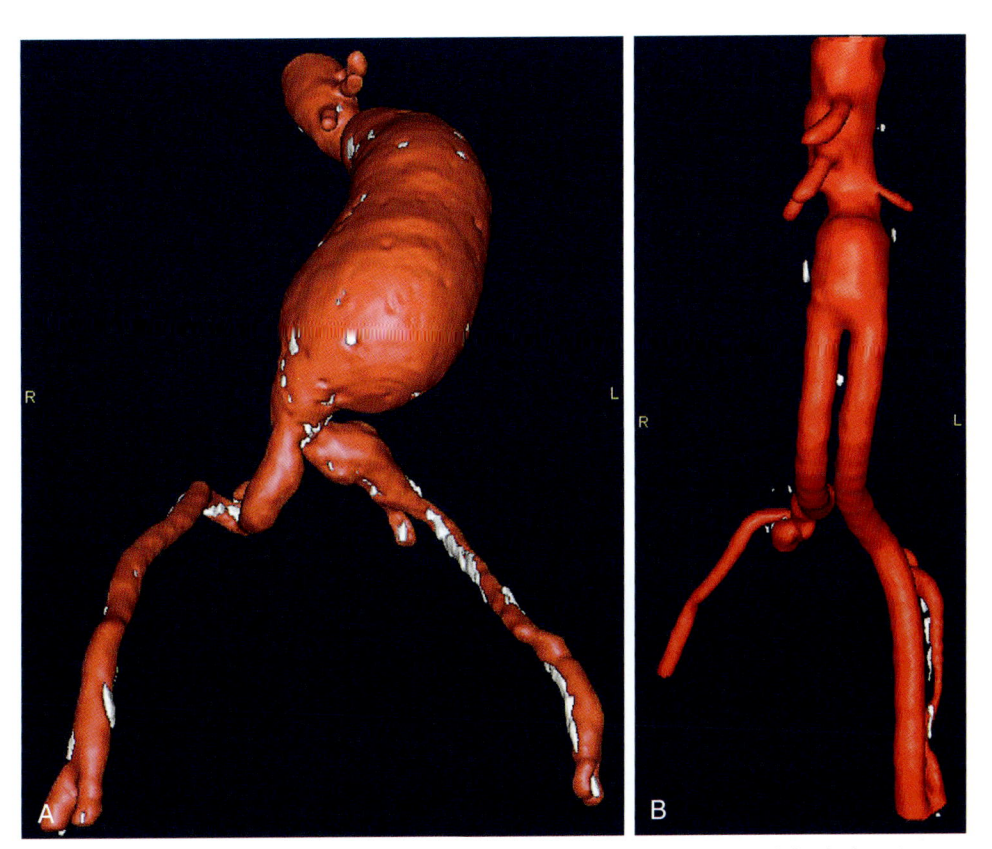

■ **FIGURE 87-11** **A,** Preoperative three-dimensional oblique frontal view from CTA in a patient with an abdominal aortic aneurysm. The patient underwent open aneurysm repair with ligation of the distal left common iliac artery, endarterectomy of the proximal left external iliac artery due to heavy calcification precluding standard anastomosis, and femoral anastomosis of the left graft limb. **B,** Postoperative image shows the aneurysm repair with retrograde flow through the left external iliac artery into the left internal iliac artery.

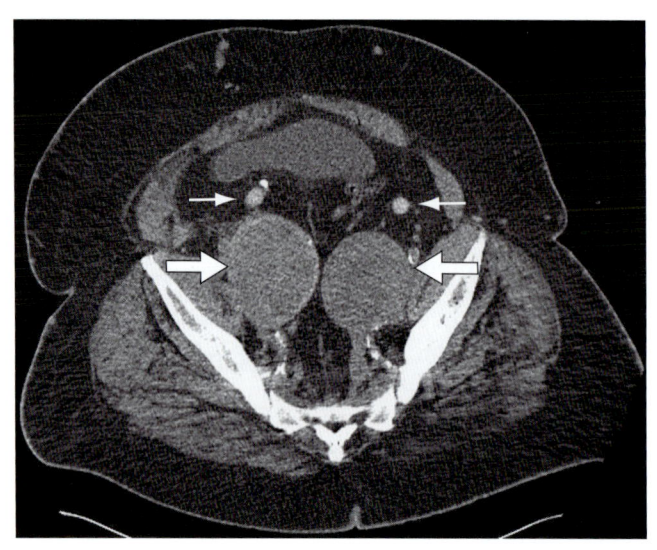

FIGURE 87-12 Postoperative contrast-enhanced CT scan of a patient who 8 years previously underwent an abdominal aortic aneurysm repair with ligation of both internal iliac arteries and anastomosis of the graft limbs to the femoral arteries (*small arrows*). The patient was found to have expansion of the internal iliac artery aneurysms (*large arrows*) due to retrograde flow from pelvic collateral circulation.

is then obtained for introduction of the device in a manner similar to that for standard EVAR.

In patients with AAA and bilateral common iliac artery aneurysms, hybrid repair may be performed by a femorofemoral bypass, followed by an aorto–uni-iliac endograft and then either a contralateral external to internal iliac covered stent or ligation of the contralateral common iliac artery (Fig. 87-13).

Indications

Hybrid procedures for AAA repair may be performed for technical issues when the femoral or iliac access vessels are smaller than the EVAR device diameter, heavily calcified, or tortuous. Hybrid AAA repair may also be performed in patients with concomitant bilateral common iliac artery aneurysms and inadequate distal landing zones (Fig. 87-13A and B). In these patients, standard EVAR covering both internal iliac arteries with the endograft limbs would lead to a high likelihood of pelvic ischemia. Hybrid repair is useful in these situations to avoid the morbidity of an open repair.

Hybrid repairs may also be necessary when there is abnormally low takeoff of a renal vessel or a dominant accessory renal artery (Fig. 87-14). In these situations, an aortorenal or iliorenal bypass may be necessary before the placement of the endograft.

Contraindications

Contraindications to EVAR with hybrid techniques are similar to those of standard AAA repair, although clamping of the iliac arteries is not associated with as high a morbidity as is clamping of the abdominal aorta.

Outcomes and Complications

Outcomes of hybrid AAA repairs are similar to those of standard EVAR.

Imaging Findings

Preoperative Assessment

Preoperative assessment is similar to that of standard AAA repair. Ultrasonography is the customary screening tool. CTA and MRA are useful for precise diameter measurements.

Preoperative Planning

CTA with three-dimensional image postprocessing is key to preoperative planning for hybrid AAA repair. CTA elucidates thrombus, calcification, diameters, landing zones, and iliac artery disease.

Postoperative Surveillance

Postoperative surveillance of hybrid AAA repair is similar to that of standard AAA repair and is typically well accomplished with CTA.

AORTOBIFEMORAL BYPASS

Description

The aorta is accessed through a transperitoneal approach, and the femoral arteries are controlled by bilateral femoral cutdowns. Preoperative planning and the surgeon's preference determine the nature of the proximal anastomosis: end to end or end to side. End-to-side proximal anastomoses preserve pelvic blood flow; end-to-end proximal anastomoses may be preferred to maximize blood flow to the lower extremities in patients with complete occlusion of the aorta and internal iliac arteries. Once the proximal anastomosis is complete, the limbs of the bifurcated graft are tunneled just anterior to the native common and external iliac arteries, posterior to the ureters, and then under the inguinal ligament. The femoral limbs are then anastomosed to the common femoral arteries.

Indications

Aortobifemoral bypass is performed in patients with disabling or lifestyle-limiting claudication, rest pain, or tissue loss and TransAtlantic Intersociety Consensus (TASC) D aortoiliac occlusive disease. In younger patients or those without prohibitive operative risk, aortobifemoral bypass may be more appropriate than endovascular revascularization because of improved long-term patency for TASC C disease.

Contraindications

Aortobifemoral bypass is associated with significant cardiopulmonary morbidity. Patients with cardiopulmonary comorbidities prohibitive of general anesthesia are not

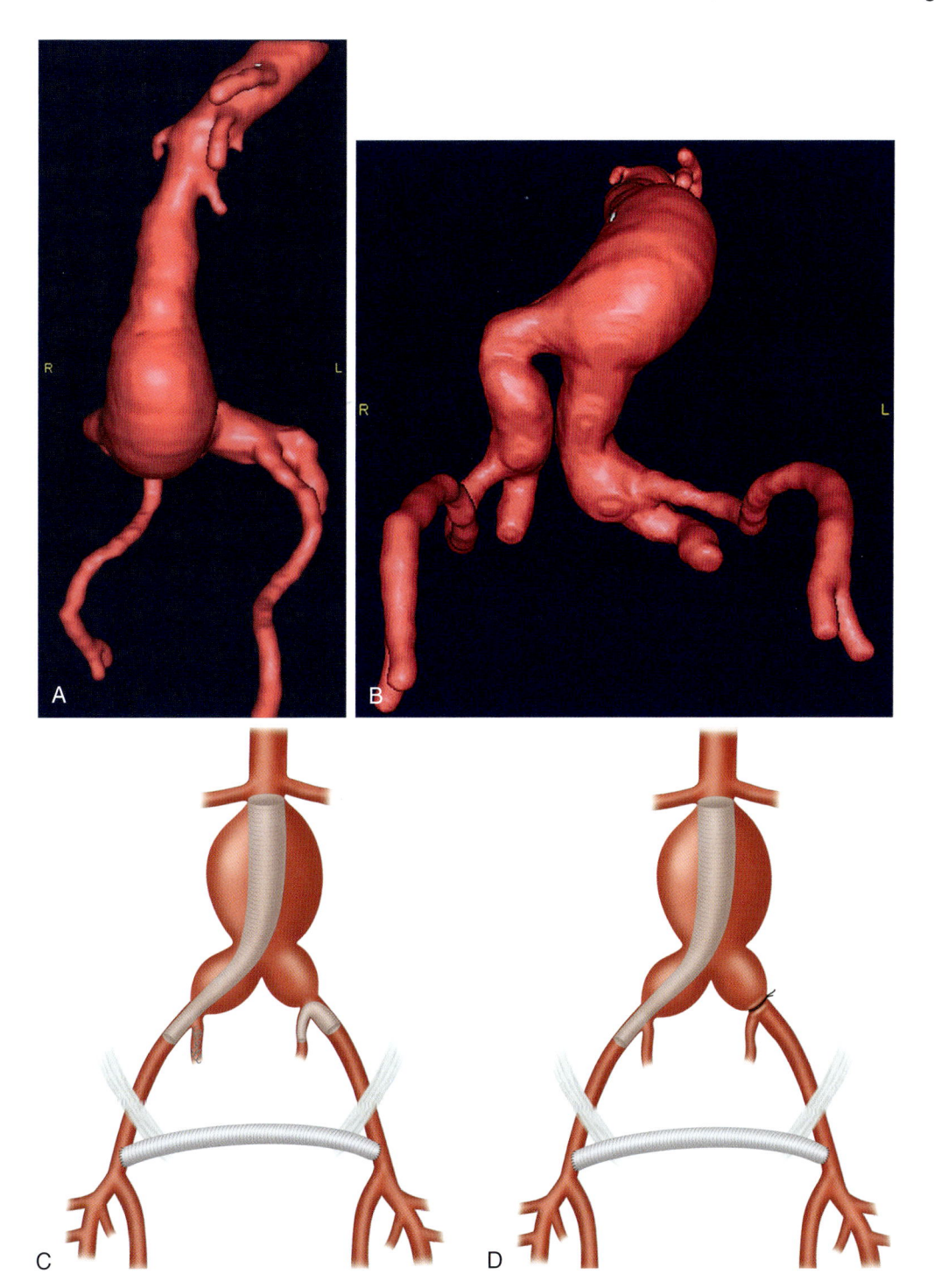

■ **FIGURE 87-13** Preoperative three-dimensional view of CTA (**A,** frontal view; **B,** caudocranial view) in a patient with concomitant abdominal aortic and bilateral common iliac artery aneurysms. The patient underwent a hybrid AAA repair with a femorofemoral bypass, open ligation of the left common iliac artery, and aorto–right external iliac unibody endografting (**C**). Other options for this patient would have included a hybrid AAA repair with a femorofemoral bypass, aorto–right external iliac unibody endograft, and right external–internal iliac artery covered stent (**D**).

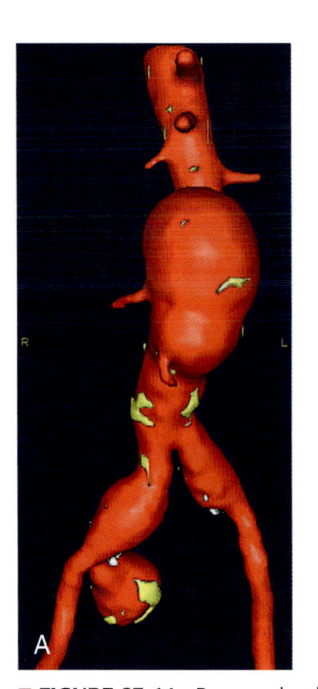

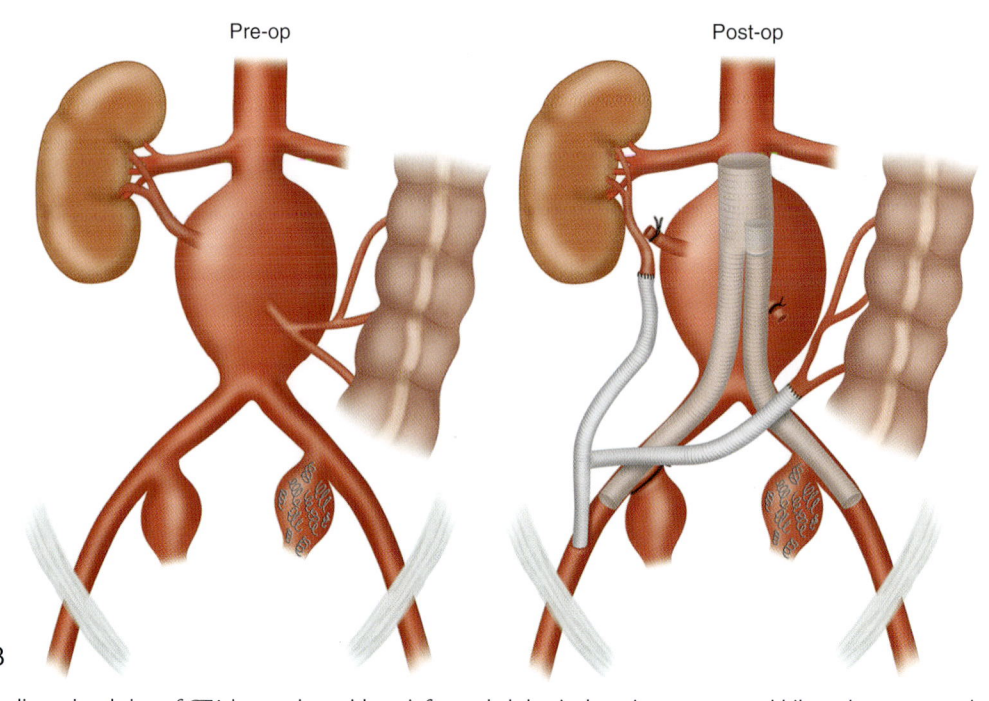

FIGURE 87-14 Preoperative three-dimensional view of CTA in a patient with an infrarenal abdominal aortic aneurysm and bilateral common and internal iliac artery aneurysms with an accessory right renal artery originating from the aneurysm sac (**A**). The left internal iliac artery aneurysm had been previously coil embolized. The patient underwent a hybrid AAA repair (**B**). A bypass from the right external iliac artery to the accessory right renal and inferior mesenteric arteries was performed before endografting to preserve blood flow to the right kidney and pelvis. The aneurysm was then repaired with a standard endograft whose distal limbs covered both internal iliac arteries.

candidates for this procedure. Such patients are better served with extra-anatomic bypass despite the decreased patency rates of these procedures.

Outcomes and Complications

Outcomes of aortobifemoral bypass are excellent, with 5-year patency rates ranging from 85% to 95%. Complications occur infrequently and are typically cardiopulmonary and renal in nature. One unique complication related to this procedure is the development of thigh and buttock claudication in up to 30% of patients undergoing aortobifemoral bypass.[21] This occurs because of a lack of blood flow in the hypogastric system and may be increased in patients with an end-to-end proximal anastomosis. Operative mortality rates range from 2% to 3%.

Imaging Findings

Preoperative Assessment

Preoperative assessment of patients with aortoiliac occlusive disease begins with noninvasive vascular laboratory testing. This may include ankle-brachial indices and segmental pressures (discussed later). Segmental pressures in patients with aortoiliac occlusive disease frequently show blunted waveforms throughout the lower extremities signifying more proximal disease.

Preoperative Planning

Angiography is the gold standard for preoperative planning because it can show the precise pattern of disease

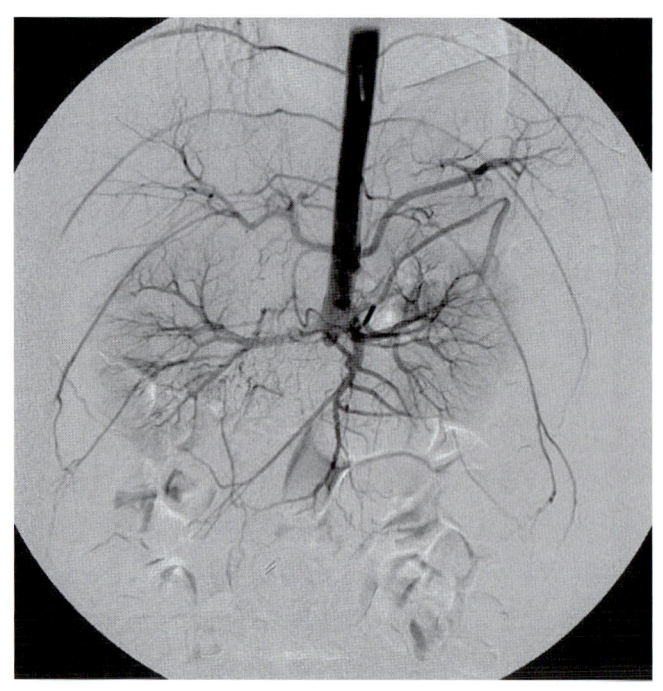

FIGURE 87-15 Digital subtraction angiography demonstrating complete aortic occlusion.

and may assess the patency of the internal iliac arteries. In cases of complete aortic or bilateral iliac artery occlusion, brachial access may be necessary to evaluate the aorta proximal to the occlusion (Fig. 87-15).

Ultrasonography may be used to evaluate femoral anatomy when there is uncertainty of distal external iliac

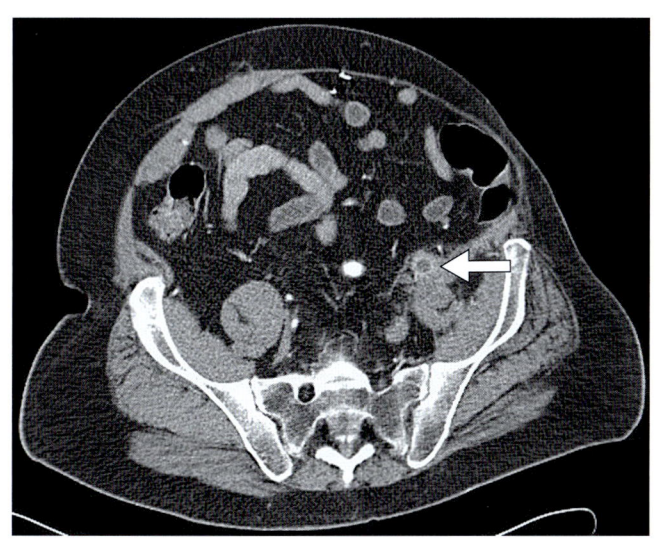

FIGURE 87-16 Postoperative contrast-enhanced CT image shows an occluded left aortobifemoral bypass limb (*arrow*). The patient subsequently underwent left above-knee amputation.

patency or poor imaging of femoral area based on poor delivery of contrast material.

MRA or CTA can be useful for the assessment of patients who have complete occlusion of the bilateral iliac arteries, which would prevent catheter angiographic assessment of the proximal abdominal aorta. CTA can also help delineate aortic thrombus and calcification, both of which have implications in intraoperative aortic clamp placement. MRA provides a viable option for patients in whom the administration of iodinated contrast agents is not desired.

Postoperative Surveillance

Postoperative surveillance may be performed with noninvasive vascular laboratory testing. Duplex ultrasonography can be used to assess graft patency, although this may be limited by bowel gas. More detailed information about graft patency is typically obtained with CTA or MRA. In patients without an iodinated contrast agent allergy, CTA has the advantage of being performed typically in a timelier manner. Compromise of graft patency requires angiographic assessment for anastomotic or intraluminal narrowing amenable to open or endovascular therapies. Finally, more distal peripheral vascular disease may lead to increased resistance within a graft limb and subsequent thrombosis (Fig. 87-16). Evaluation of lower extremity blood flow may be prudent in patients at risk for graft failure.

LOWER EXTREMITY BYPASS
Description

Lower extremity bypass is performed in a variety of manners and is beyond the scope of this chapter. Factors common to all lower extremity bypasses are determination of inflow and outflow vessels, determination of adequacy of the runoff, and choice of conduit. An inflow vessel is defined as the blood vessel of the proximal anastomosis and generally refers to the adequacy of blood flow to the level of the inguinal ligament. Inflow vessels should not have any proximal stenoses that may compromise the blood flow into the conduit. The common femoral artery is most frequently used as inflow, but any artery with in-line flow from the aorta may be used. More distal vessels should be considered to decrease the length of the bypass, a factor associated with increased vein bypass thrombosis. The outflow vessel is defined as the blood vessel of the distal anastomosis. This is generally the most proximal vessel with in-line flow to the foot. Runoff may be defined as continuity of the outflow vessel with the foot or, for the peroneal artery, a direct communication between the delta branches and a pedal vessel. Finally, conduits may be autogenous or nonautogenous. Autogenous conduits include the greater and lesser saphenous veins as well as the basilic and cephalic veins of the arm. Nonautogenous conduits are typically made of polytetrafluoroethylene (PTFE) or polyester.

Once these factors have been determined, the inflow and outflow arteries are controlled both proximally and distally. An arteriotomy is made in the inflow artery, and the conduit is sutured to the artery in continuous fashion. Attention is then turned to the distal anastomosis, where the conduit is sutured in a similar manner. Adequacy of the bypass may be determined with intraoperative arteriography or Doppler ultrasound augmentation with graft compression.

Indications

Indications for lower extremity bypass are disabling or lifestyle-limiting claudication, rest pain, and tissue loss. Bypasses are not typically performed on patients with intermittent claudication; only 20% of these patients will progress to critical limb ischemia during a 10-year period. For these patients, lifestyle modification and exercise are the mainstays of therapy. Endovascular revascularization may also be considered for claudicants, depending on the anatomy and other clinical circumstances.

Contraindications

Contraindications to lower extremity bypass are rare and include cardiopulmonary disease prohibiting anesthesia and untreated hypercoagulable states.

Outcomes and Complications

Outcomes of lower extremity bypass are summarized in Table 87-2. The patency rates of this meta-analysis show that vein bypasses are the conduit of choice.

Complications of lower extremity bypass can be divided into graft-related and non–graft-related categories. Graft thrombosis is the most common complication and a major reason for postoperative graft surveillance (Fig. 87-17). Early graft thrombosis (0 to 30 days) is most likely due to technical error in either performance of the bypass or determination of adequacy of the runoff. Mid graft thrombosis (30 days to 2 years) is typically due to intimal hyperplasia. Late graft thrombosis is usually due to progression of atherosclerosis. Graft infection is another graft-related complication. Infections of autogenous grafts may be treated with antibiotic therapy. Attempts at salvage of

TABLE 87-2 Summary of Patency Rates in Patients Undergoing Lower Extremity Bypass	
Type of Bypass	Primary 5-Year Patency (%)
Above-knee vein bypass	80
Above-knee prosthetic bypass	66
Below-knee vein bypass	72
Below-knee prosthetic bypass	38

TABLE 87-3 Ankle-Brachial Indices and Correlation to Symptoms	
Symptom	Ankle-Brachial Index
Normal	0.80-1.0
Claudication	0.50-0.60
Critical ischemia	<0.30

■ FIGURE 87-17 Digital subtraction angiography showing thrombosis of a prosthetic popliteal dorsalis pedis bypass (*arrow*).

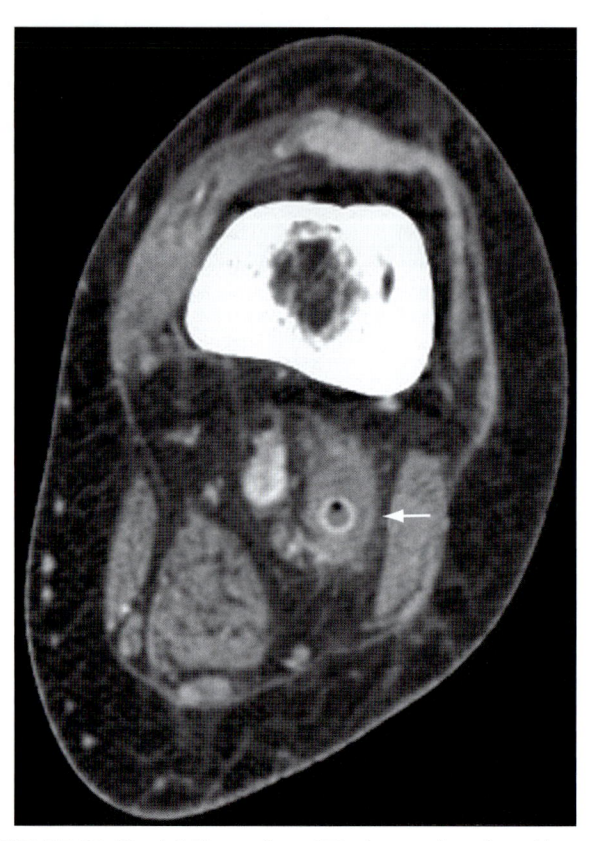

■ FIGURE 87-18 Axial image from CTA shows a thrombosed lower extremity bypass with intraluminal air and surrounding fluid collection (*arrow*) consistent with graft infection.

infected prosthetic grafts can be made, although these frequently need to be excised, especially with involvement of an anastomosis. Fluid collections surrounding a graft on duplex ultrasonography or CTA may be suggestive of graft infection (Fig. 87-18). Non–graft-related complications are typically cardiopulmonary or renal in nature.

Imaging Findings

Preoperative Assessment

Doppler ankle pressure measurements are the most commonly used noninvasive vascular laboratory tests to assess for peripheral vascular disease. The ankle-brachial index is determined by dividing the systolic blood pressure in the brachial artery by the systolic blood pressure at the ankle (the higher of the two values for the dorsalis pedis artery and the posterior tibial artery). The ankle-brachial index has been correlated to degree of symptoms (Table 87-3). The ankle-brachial index may be falsely elevated in heavily calcified arteries, as is typically seen in diabetic patients. Finally, in patients with claudication, the ankle-brachial index may be normal at rest but decreased with exercise. An abnormal exercise response is defined as a 20% decrease from baseline or more than 3 minutes to recover to baseline.

Measurement of pulse volume recordings in the lower extremity is a useful technique to identify significant stenosis in the lower extremity (Fig. 87-19). Blunting of the normal cardiac cycle waveform is typically seen distal to a hemodynamically significant stenosis.

Transcutaneous oxygen tension ($TcPO_2$) measurements are particularly helpful in determining the ability of a wound to heal (Table 87-4). $TcPO_2$ quantifies oxygen molecules transferred to the skin after it is heated with a transducer above 40°C. $TcPO_2$ can be in the form of absolute oxygen tension or regional index, the $TcPO_2$ of the leg divided by the $TcPO_2$ measured at a reference point (chest). This technique has also been shown to be useful in diabetic patients, in whom the ankle-brachial index is unreliable.[22]

Preoperative Planning

Preoperative planning for a lower extremity bypass is typically performed by use of catheter angiography, but CTA and MRA have emerged as suitable preoperative planning

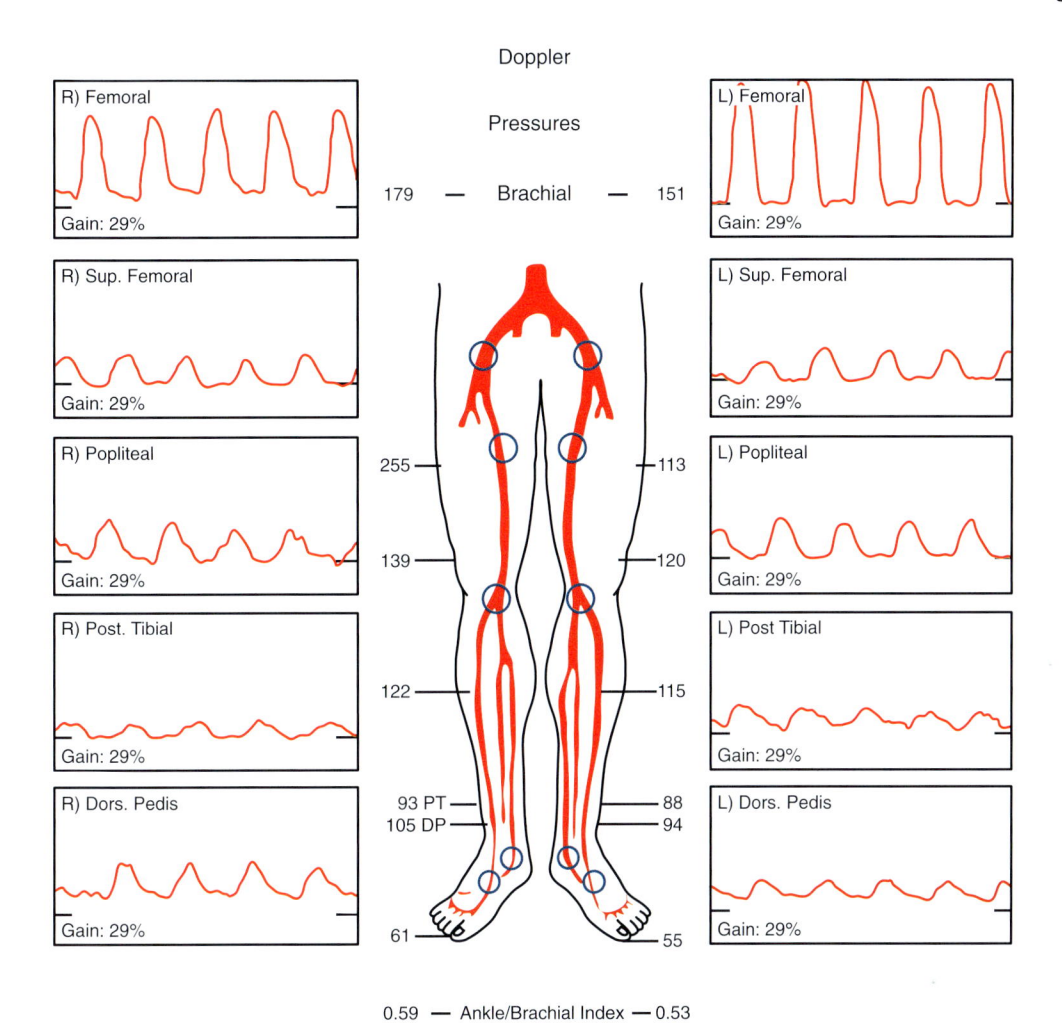

FIGURE 87-19 Pulse volume recordings in a patient with lower extremity disease. Note the failure to augment between the brachial and femoral pressures, signifying aortoiliac disease on the left, and blunting of the waveform below the femoral artery, signifying left superficial femoral artery disease.

TABLE 87-4 Transcutaneous Oxygen Measurements and Correlation to Symptoms

Symptom	Transcutaneous Oxygen Tension (absolute)	Transcutaneous Oxygen Tension (regional index)
Likely to heal	35-40 mm Hg	>0.6
Borderline or delayed healing	25-35 mm Hg	0.4-0.6
Unlikely to heal	<20-25 mm Hg	<0.4

examinations at some sites. Preoperative planning requires the vascular surgeon to identify the exact location of stenoses but also to assess the inflow (site of proximal anastomosis), outflow (site of distal anastomosis), and runoff vessels (arterial tree beyond the distal anastomosis) (Fig. 87-20). Runoff scores have been shown to be one of the strongest predictors for bypass patency and are a key consideration during angiography.[23]

Preoperative vein mapping with duplex ultrasonography can provide detailed information about the quality of a potential vein graft. It can detect constriction of veins secondary to sclerosis, previous manipulation, or thrombophlebitis. It can also assess length and diameter of the vein. These measurements can be particularly important in performing a tibial bypass for which a long segment may be necessary. Diameters of more than 3 mm for reverse[24] and 2 mm for in situ[25] saphenous vein grafts have been recommended to obtain adequate long-term patency.

Postoperative Surveillance

Long-term follow-up of lower extremity bypasses is aimed at early identification of a failing graft and is critical to the long-term success of all lower extremity bypasses as restenosis is frequent. Duplex ultrasonography is frequently used to interrogate a bypass and to identify areas of stenosis with increased velocities (Fig. 87-21). Duplex ultrasonography may also show significantly decreased velocities throughout the graft that may be related to a distal anastomotic stenosis or worsening of the runoff arterial bed. Once a failing graft is identified, angiography must be performed to more accurately delineate the problem. Revision may be performed with both open and endovascular techniques.

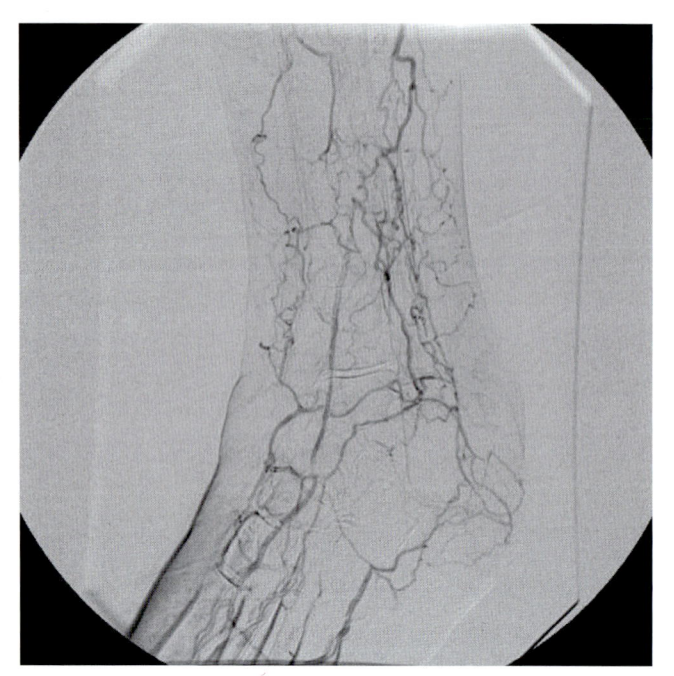

■ **FIGURE 87-20** Digital subtraction angiography showing poor runoff in a patient with toe gangrene. The patient underwent femoral-distal bypass to the dorsalis pedis artery augmented with a distal arteriovenous fistula to improve flow through the bypass.

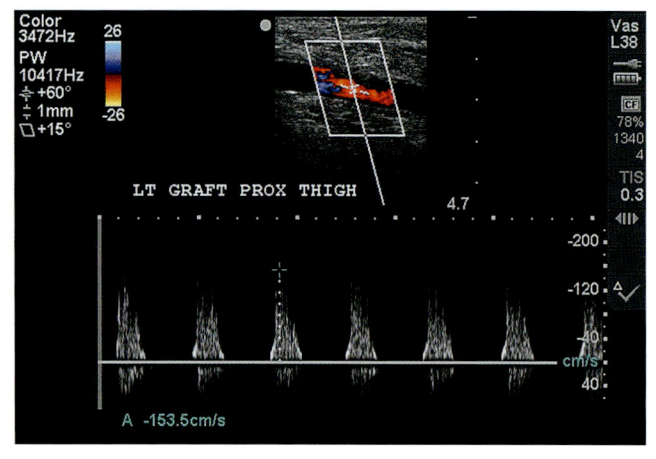

■ **FIGURE 87-21** Duplex ultrasonography of a lower extremity bypass graft stenosis. Note the elevated velocities across the stenosis.

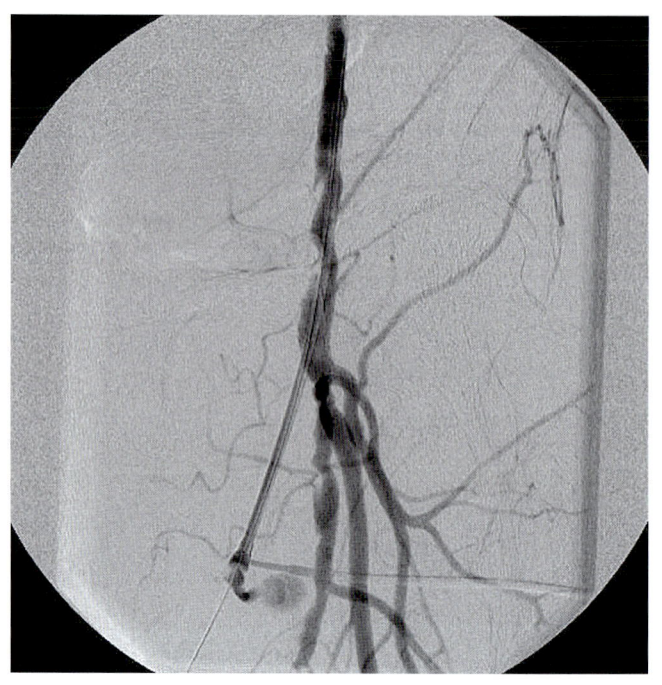

■ **FIGURE 87-22** Digital subtraction angiography showing heavy calcification of the common femoral artery. Open angioplasty allows the surgeon to perform an iliofemoral endarterectomy at the conclusion of the case and thus to improve inflow.

AORTOILIAC AND LOWER EXTREMITY OCCLUSIVE DISEASE HYBRID PROCEDURES

Description

Hybrid procedures for aortoiliac and lower extremity peripheral vascular disease typically involve open access to the femoral arteries for subsequent endovascular intervention either proximally or distally. Open access of the femoral arteries is performed through a standard cutdown technique. Proximal and distal control of the vessel is obtained with vessel loops. This technique allows direct palpation of the artery and identification of an area that is not heavily calcified, and thus it is more appropriate for control with a vascular clamp. At the end of the procedure, the femoral plaque endarterectomy is performed and the vessel is closed with patch angioplasty.

Indications

Patients with heavily calcified femoral arteries are at higher risk of plaque dissection or embolization with percutaneous endovascular interventions. These patients are candidates for open angioplasty. At the conclusion of the procedure, a femoral thromboendarterectomy may serve to increase inflow into the lower extremity.

Contraindications

Open angioplasty can be safely performed with sedation and local anesthesia and thus has few contraindications.

Outcomes and Complications

Outcomes and complications of hybrid procedures are identical to those of their percutaneous counterparts.

Imaging Findings

Preoperative Assessment

Preoperative assessment is similar to that discussed for aortobifemoral bypass and lower extremity bypass.

Preoperative Planning

Duplex ultrasonography or arteriography of the femoral arteries typically shows heavy calcification (Fig. 87-22).

Postoperative Surveillance

Postoperative surveillance is similar to that for endovascular interventions and is discussed in a separate chapter.

KEY POINTS

- Different imaging modalities are relevant at different points during the course of vascular surgical disease management. An understanding of their utility at each point is key to the care of the vascular surgical patient.
- Duplex ultrasonography is useful in the preoperative and postoperative care of patients with carotid artery disease as well as in the follow-up of lower extremity bypass.
- Three-dimensional CT angiography is becoming the preferred modality for preoperative planning of aortic aneurysmal disease because of its ability to provide accurate diameter measurements as well as to assess for other aortic disease.
- Magnetic resonance angiography is a useful adjunct, especially in cases of chronic renal insufficiency.
- Catheter angiography remains the gold standard for the evaluation of lower extremity occlusive disease. Angiography is also useful in cases in which the results of noninvasive imaging studies are discordant.

SUGGESTED READINGS

Ascher E, Marks N. Preprocedural imaging: new options to reduce need for contrast angiography. Semin Vasc Surg 2007; 20:15-28.

Beebe HG, Kritpracha B. Imaging of abdominal aortic aneurysm: current status. Ann Vasc Surg 2003; 17:111-118.

Chiles C, Carr JJ. Vascular diseases of the thorax: evaluation with multidetector CT. Radiol Clin North Am 2005; 43:543-569.

Collins R, Burch J, Cranny G, et al. Duplex ultrasonography, magnetic resonance angiography, and computed tomography angiography for diagnosis and assessment of symptomatic, lower limb peripheral arterial disease: systematic review. BMJ 2007; 334:1257.

Fillinger MF. New imaging techniques in endovascular surgery. Surg Clin North Am 1999; 79:451-475.

Hiatt MD, Fleischmann D, Hellinger JC, Rubin GD. Angiographic imaging of the lower extremities with multidetector CT. Radiol Clin North Am 2005; 43:1119-1127.

Ho VB, Corse WR. MR angiography of the abdominal aorta and peripheral vessels. Radiol Clin North Am 2003; 41:115-144.

Martin ML, Tay KH, Flak B, et al. Multidetector CT angiography of the aortoiliac system and lower extremities: a prospective comparison with digital subtraction angiography. AJR Am J Roentgenol 2003; 180:1085-1091.

Nederkoorn PJ, van der Graaf Y, Hunink MG. Duplex ultrasound and magnetic resonance angiography compared with digital subtraction angiography in carotid artery stenosis: a systematic review. Stroke 2003; 34:1324-1332.

Seifert B, Struwe A, Heilmaier C, et al. Assessment of aortoiliac and renal arteries: MR angiography with parallel acquisition versus conventional MR angiography and digital subtraction angiography. Radiology 2007; 245:276-284.

REFERENCES

1. North American Symptomatic Carotid Endarterectomy Trial Collaborators. Beneficial effect of carotid endarterectomy in symptomatic patients with high-grade carotid stenosis. N Engl J Med 1991; 325:445-453.
2. Executive Committee for the Asymptomatic Carotid Atherosclerosis Study. Endarterectomy for asymptomatic carotid artery stenosis. JAMA 1995; 273:1421-1428.
3. Reed AB, Gaccione P, Belkin M, et al. Preoperative risk factors for carotid endarterectomy: defining the patient at high risk. J Vasc Surg 2003; 37:1191-1199.
4. Karapanayiotides T, Meuli R, Devuyst G, et al. Postcarotid endarterectomy hyperperfusion or reperfusion syndrome. Stroke 2005; 36:21-26.
5. Strandness DE Jr. Extracranial arterial disease. In Strandness DE Jr (ed). Duplex Scanning in Vascular Disorders, 2nd ed. New York, Raven Press, 1993, pp 113-158.
6. AbuRahma AF, Richmond BK, Robinson PA, et al. Effect of contralateral severe stenosis or carotid occlusion on duplex criteria of ipsilateral stenoses: comparative study of various duplex parameters. J Vasc Surg 1995; 22:751-761.
7. Remonda L, Senn P, Barth A, et al. Contrast-enhanced 3D MR angiography of the carotid artery: comparison with conventional digital subtraction angiography. AJNR Am J Neuroradiol 2002; 23:213-219.
8. Ziomek S, Quiñones-Baldrich WJ, Busuttil RW, et al. The superiority of synthetic arterial grafts over autologous veins in carotid-subclavian bypass. J Vasc Surg 1986; 3:140-145.
9. Kline RA, Kazmers A, Friedland MS. Cervical reconstruction of the supra-aortic trunks: a 16-year experience. J Vasc Surg 1999; 29:239-246.
10. AbuRahma AF, Bates MC, Stone PA, et al. Angioplasty and stenting versus carotid-subclavian bypass for the treatment of isolated subclavian artery disease. J Endovasc Ther 2007; 14:698-704.
11. AbuRahma AF, Robinson PA, Jennings TG. Carotid-subclavian bypass grafting with polytetrafluoroethylene grafts for symptomatic subclavian artery stenosis or occlusion: a 20-year experience. J Vasc Surg 2000; 32:411-418.
12. Conrad MF, Crawford RS, Davison JK, Cambria RP. Thoracoabdominal aneurysm repair: a 20-year perspective. Ann Thorac Surg 2007; 83:S856-S861.
13. Feezor RJ, Martin TD, Hess PJ, et al. Risk factors for perioperative stroke during thoracic endovascular aortic repairs (TEVAR). J Endovasc Ther 2007; 14:568-573.
14. Riesenman PJ, Farber MA, Mendes RR, et al. Coverage of the left subclavian artery during thoracic endovascular aortic repair. J Vasc Surg 2007; 45:90-94.
15. Stone DH, Brewster DC, Kwolek CJ, et al. Stent-graft versus open-surgical repair of the thoracic aorta: mid-term results. J Vasc Surg 2006; 44:1188-1197.
16. Aneurysm Detection and Management Veterans Affairs Cooperative Study Group. Immediate repair compared with surveillance of small abdominal aortic aneurysms. N Engl J Med 2002; 346:1437-1444.
17. United Kingdom Small Aneurysm Trial Participants. Long-term outcomes of immediate repair compared with surveillance of small abdominal aortic aneurysms. N Engl J Med 2002; 346:1445-1452.
18. Szilagyi DE, Smith RF, Elliott JP, et al. Anastomotic aneurysms after vascular reconstruction: problems of incidence, etiology, and treatment. Surgery 1975; 78:800-816.
19. Multicentre Aneurysm Screening Study Group. The Multicentre Aneurysm Screening Study (MASS) into the effect of abdominal aortic aneurysm screening on mortality in men: a randomised controlled trial. Lancet 2002; 360:1531-1539.
20. Falkensammer J, Oldenburg WA, Biebl M, et al. Abdominal aortic aneurysm neck remodeling after open aneurysm repair. J Vasc Surg 2007; 45:900-905.

21. Jaquinandi V, Picquet J, Bouyé P, et al. High prevalence of proximal claudication among patients with patent aortobifemoral bypasses. J Vasc Surg 2007; 45:312-318.
22. Williams DT, Price P, Harding KG. The influence of diabetes and lower limb arterial disease on cutaneous foot perfusion. J Vasc Surg 2006; 44:770-775.
23. Seeger JM, Pretus HA, Carlton LC, et al. Potential predictors of outcome in patients with tissue loss who undergo infrainguinal vein bypass grafting. J Vasc Surg 1999; 30:427-435.
24. Wengerter KR, Veith FJ, Gupta SK, et al. Influence of vein size (diameter) on infrapopliteal reversed vein graft patency. J Vasc Surg 1990; 11:525-531.
25. Bergamini TM, Towne JB, Bandyk DF, et al. Experience with in situ saphenous vein bypasses during 1981 to 1989: determinant factors of long-term patency. J Vasc Surg 1991; 13:137-147.

PART
FOURTEEN

Atherosclerosis

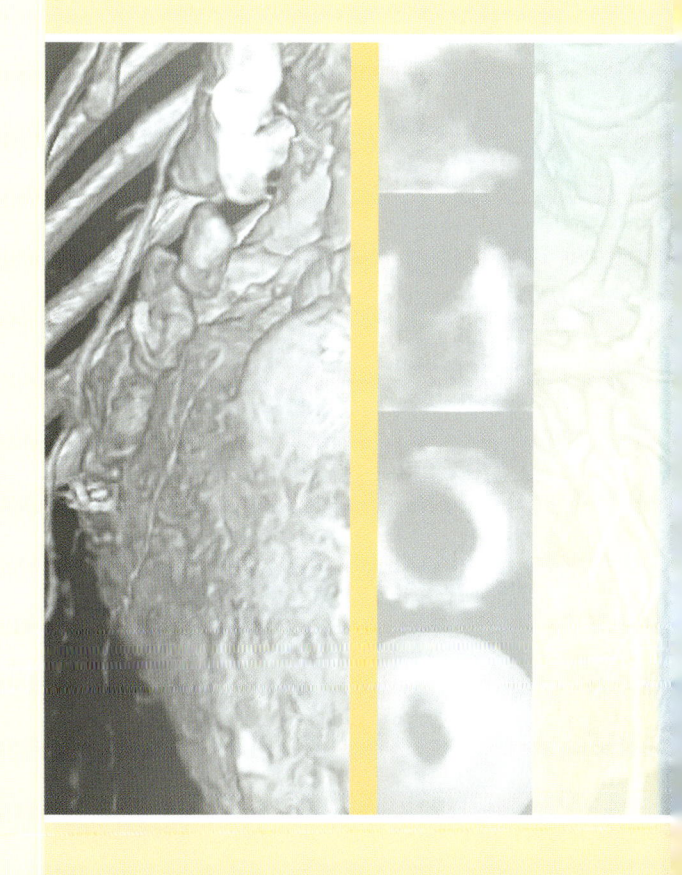

CHAPTER 88

Noninvasive Imaging of Atherosclerosis

Jamieson M. Bourque and Christopher M. Kramer

Atherosclerosis is a disease process in which fatty infiltration and inflammation of the wall of medium to large arteries lead to plaque formation and multiple adverse sequelae including rupture, obstruction, and embolism. It is a major source of morbidity and mortality, with 25 million people in the United States demonstrating at least one clinical manifestation of atherosclerosis.[1] It has been the number one cause of death in the United States since 1900 except for 1918, the year of the influenza epidemic.[2] Atherosclerosis also leads to significant losses in functional capacity and quality of life.

Atherosclerosis should be considered a systemic disease. The primary clinical and research focus has been coronary atherosclerosis; disease in this vascular area affects the most people and is typically the cause of death, even among those with complications of noncoronary vascular disease. It involves almost all arterial beds but most importantly the cerebrovascular, renal, lower extremity, aortic, and mesenteric territories. Although the effects of atherosclerosis vary in each regional circulation, the epidemiology, pathophysiology, presentation, and general treatment strategies are similar and highly linked. The presence of disease and complications in any arterial bed greatly increases the risk of comorbid atherosclerosis and its adverse events in the others.

Noninvasive imaging of the arterial system plays a pivotal role in the diagnosis of atherosclerosis. This disease can often be asymptomatic or with atypical presentation, and the physical examination is imperative but often insufficient. Early diagnosis is of paramount importance as prompt, aggressive therapy significantly reduces atherosclerotic morbidity and mortality.

In this chapter, we focus on noncoronary atherosclerosis, reviewing the epidemiology, pathophysiology, treatment, and noninvasive imaging and other diagnostic strategies available. An understanding of the underlying disease processes and potential therapeutic options is essential to increase the utility and appropriateness of noninvasive evaluation.

ATHEROSCLEROSIS

Definition

Atherosclerosis is a form of arteriosclerosis characterized by the deposition of plaques containing cholesterol and lipids on the innermost layer of the walls of large and medium-sized arteries.[3] The atheroma is a complex of lipids and fibrous tissue with surrounding hypertrophied smooth muscle and inflammatory cells that leads to progressive vessel luminal narrowing and obstruction of blood flow, directly causing or indirectly mediating the many clinical manifestations of atherosclerotic disease.

Prevalence and Epidemiology

The exact overall prevalence of atherosclerosis is not known because of the numerous arterial beds it encompasses and because it is often silent and found only through screening, which is not universally performed. Moreover, atherosclerotic disease often coexists in multiple vascular systems, making the individual disease prevalence not additive. Atherosclerosis does account for almost three quarters of all deaths from cardiovascular disease.[2] The majority of these are from coronary atherosclerosis. Although the mortality from coronary heart disease is decreasing, that from noncoronary atherosclerotic disease is increasing, partly owing to the overall aging of the population. Information on the prevalence of noncoronary atherosclerotic disease and the resultant complications is available for the individual arterial systems affected.

Cerebrovascular Atherosclerotic Disease

Cerebrovascular atherosclerosis has the highest impact of noncoronary disease processes. Stroke is the third leading cause of death in the United States, with an annual incidence of 700,000 events. It is associated with high morbidity and mortality, with a 50% 5-year survival and 15% to 30% risk of permanent disability. Sixty percent of new or recurrent strokes are the result of atherothrombotic disease. One third of these are due to carotid atherosclerosis. At the age of 75 years, 53% of women and 63% of men have carotid stenoses of more than 10%.[4] The presence of carotid bruits approximately doubles the expected stroke risk, but the disease is often in a different cerebral vascular territory and not related to the initial lesion auscultated. Despite the high morbidity and mortality from stroke, individuals with carotid artery disease are more likely to die of cardiovascular causes than of cerebrovascular disease, underscoring the close relationship between noncoronary atherosclerosis and cardiovascular risk.

Peripheral Atherosclerotic Disease

Defining peripheral arterial disease (PAD) as a noninvasive ankle-brachial index (ABI) below 0.90, its prevalence in the lower extremities is 2.5% for those younger than 60 years and increases markedly with age to 18.8% for those 70 years of age or older.[5] Claudication is associated with significant disability and is present in as many as 6% to 7% of the general population 65 years of age and older. The prevalence also varies significantly by risk factor profile. The PAD Awareness, Risk, and Treatment: New Resources for Survival (PARTNERS) study examined PAD prevalence in the American primary care setting and found that the prevalence was as high as 29% in older Americans or those with significant risk factors (especially tobacco use and diabetes). The disease has high morbidity from both peripheral and cardiovascular events. The annual mortality for those with PAD is 4% to 6% and is as high as 25% for the 1% to 2% of patients with critical limb ischemia.[5] Individuals with PAD have a 60% to 80% prevalence of significant coronary artery disease (CAD), with a twofold to sixfold increase in cardiovascular death and a 40% increase in the risk of stroke. PAD is often undetected without careful exercise tolerance questioning and judicious screening, going undiagnosed in as many as 55% of affected individuals.

Aortic Atherosclerotic Disease

Atherosclerosis of the aorta rarely leads to occlusion but causes abdominal aortic aneurysms (AAAs), peripheral embolization of aortic atheromatous material, penetrating aortic ulcers, and intramural hematomas. The prevalences of these entities are difficult to discern as aneurysms have wide variations in definition and the other aortic manifestations are under-reported. The Veterans Affairs Aneurysm Detection and Management (ADAM) study of 125,000 veterans revealed a prevalence of 4.3% and 1.0% for AAAs of 3.0 cm or larger in men and women, respectively, aged 50 to 79 years but only 1.3% and 0.1%, respectively, for AAAs of 4.0 cm or larger.[4] The prevalence increases markedly with age; one Scandinavian study showed a peak of 5.9% for men aged 80 to 85 years and 4.5% for women older than 90 years. This disease is almost always asymptomatic because the clinical manifestations are typically catastrophic. The risk of AAA rupture is amplified with increasing diameter; AAAs larger than 6 cm have a 25% yearly risk of rupture.[4] Despite the focus on rupture, approximately 60% of patients with AAAs die of other cardiovascular complications.

Renal Atherosclerotic Disease

Renal atherosclerotic disease causes 90% of the cases of renal artery stenosis, an uncommon but highly morbid cause of secondary refractory hypertension and renal failure. The prevalence of renal artery stenosis in the population older than 65 years is 6.8%, but it is much higher in high-risk populations. Patients undergoing cardiac catheterization have a 30% prevalence, whereas renal artery stenosis is present in 22% to 59% of those with PAD.[5]

Renal arterial disease has a high rate of progression; occlusion occurs in up to 39% of cases by 5 years. Significant renal impairment in individuals with two functional kidneys typically occurs only with bilateral renal artery stenosis, but 44% of patients have bilateral disease. Almost half of individuals with renal artery stenosis have increased creatinine concentration, and 29% have a 25% to 50% decline in glomerular filtration rate. Despite these factors, patients with renal artery stenosis have a 2-year dialysis-free survival of 97.3% and 82.4% for unilateral and bilateral disease, respectively. The risk of cardiovascular events in this population (more than fourfold increase) far exceeds that of significant renal impairment.[6] Nevertheless, the mortality rate is high with renal artery stenosis and end-stage renal disease, with a mean life expectancy of only 2.7 years.[5]

Mesenteric Atherosclerotic Disease

Because of its vague symptoms and infrequent diagnosis, there are no good studies outlining the true prevalence or natural history of mesenteric arterial disease. Individuals with this condition almost always have concomitant cardiovascular atherosclerotic disease. The majority are older women, with a mean age of 70 years, although biases in testing and symptom presentation limit these observations.

Mesenteric arterial disease causes high morbidity and mortality, with a mortality above 70% for patients with acute mesenteric ischemia, of which 15% is directly attributable to atherosclerotic thrombosis (typically in the superior mesenteric artery). Nonocclusive mesenteric ischemia occurs in approximately 50% of patients, typically from low-flow states such as sepsis or heart failure. Partial atherosclerotic obstruction can certainly play a role in this setting. Chronic mesenteric ischemia also occurs, almost always secondary to atherosclerotic disease, but the clinical presentation of this is nonspecific and therefore underdiagnosed.

Etiology and Pathophysiology

Insight into the pathogenesis of atherosclerosis is essential so that novel imaging techniques can be used and effective therapies can be devised and implemented. Atherosclerosis development represents much more than simply accumulation of lipid. It stems from a series of complex cellular and molecular processes that are initiated as a result of the many known atherosclerotic risk factors and comorbid conditions that cause the initial stages of atherosclerosis to progress in a predictable fashion. The pathophysiologic process of atherosclerosis remains predominantly uniform across the spectrum of affected arterial beds, although there are some key regional differences.

Atherosclerosis is a disease primarily of the large and medium-sized arteries and is increasingly considered primarily an inflammatory process in response to endothelial injury and lipid oxidation. The primary stages of atherosclerosis are

1. accumulation of inflammatory cells, such as macrophages and smooth muscle cells;
2. accumulation and necrosis of a lipid core; and
3. formation of extracellular matrix, which creates a fibrous cap over the enlarging lipid core and accumulating inflammatory cells.

Positive feedback leads to repeated cycles of this process, and progressive arterial dilation (Glagov phenomenon) and eventually luminal encroachment occur. Severe luminal narrowing can result in myocardial ischemia and symptoms. Alternatively, rupture of the fibrous cap can occur, leading to rapid platelet aggregation, thrombosis, rapid vessel obstruction, and clinical events. Several hypothetical frameworks have been developed to help explain this complex process.

Response to Injury Hypothesis

The primary step in the formation of atherosclerosis is the development of vessel wall endothelial dysfunction, which occurs as a response to injury from risk factors such as elevations and alterations in low-density lipoprotein (LDL), genetic abnormalities, and toxic free radicals stemming from tobacco use.[7]

These adverse processes stimulate the production of cytokines, growth factors, and vasoconstrictive agents. They also lead to inflammatory cell and platelet adhesion, amplified endothelial permeability, smooth muscle cell proliferation, and loss of activity of vasodilatory and fibrinolytic agents such as nitric oxide, causing increased endothelial procoagulancy. Endothelial damage also leads to platelet deposition and resultant monocytic and T-cell infiltration. Cumulatively, these factors lead to increased oxidative stress, which facilitates the next step in the atherosclerotic process.

Oxidation Hypothesis

Oxidation of LDL is required for its uptake by macrophages and accumulation within the vessel wall.[8] Arterial LDL is progressively oxidized by oxygen free radicals and internalized by macrophages, forming lipoperoxides, a reactive species that triggers further LDL oxidation and plasma membrane destruction. Oxidized LDL is also a potent chemoattractant for macrophages, inducing the expression of vascular cell adhesion molecules and inhibiting macrophage mobility, thereby furthering macrophage and lipid accumulation within the vessel wall. These lipid-laden macrophages are known as foam cells because of their histologic appearance.[7] As these foam cells accumulate, they undergo apoptosis and necrosis from increased proteolytic activity, forming a necrotic lipid core.

Extracellular Matrix Formation and the Fibrous Cap

Progressive inflammation leads to activation of the infiltrating T lymphocytes and macrophages. These then secrete a variety of cytokines, chemokines, lytic enzymes, and growth factors that stimulate the formation of an extracellular matrix. Continued development of this matrix induces the creation of a fibrous cap over the proliferating smooth muscle cells and necrotic lipid core.

Progression to Clinical Significance

During the initial stages of atherosclerosis, the blood vessel dilates to maintain lumen size, a process known as the Glagov phenomenon (Fig. 88-1). However, the repeated cycles of inflammation, smooth muscle cell and fibrous tissue proliferation, and expansion of the lipid core eventually overwhelm the compensatory response, leading to progressive luminal obstruction. Decreased luminal blood flow from the increasing vessel blockage will eventually lead to insufficient supply to meet oxygen demand, and ischemia will ensue.

More rapid vessel occlusion can also occur, leading to ischemia and potentially infarction, depending on the vascular bed. The activated T lymphocytes present can secrete matrix metalloproteinases and other lytic molecules that can degrade the fibrous cap, leading to cap rupture and the uncovering of the prothrombotic elements underneath. This exposure, along with other pro-

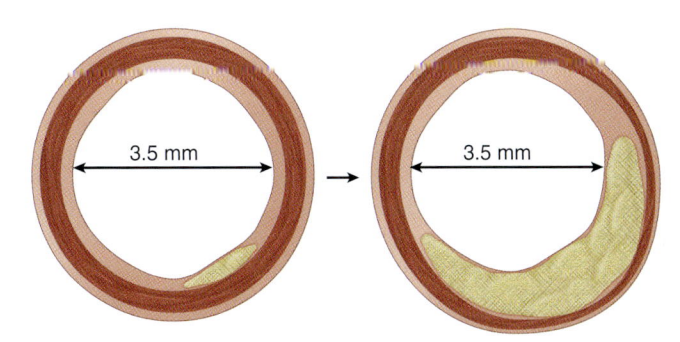

■ **FIGURE 88-1** Glagov phenomenon. The artery on the left has early atherosclerotic findings, including a small lipid core. As the atherosclerosis progresses, the lipid core enlarges, but the artery dilates eccentrically to maintain the original lumen size. Eventually, the lesion progression is sufficient to overload the compensatory dilation, and lumen encroachment occurs (not shown). *(Modified from trackyourplaque.com. Copyright 2006.)*

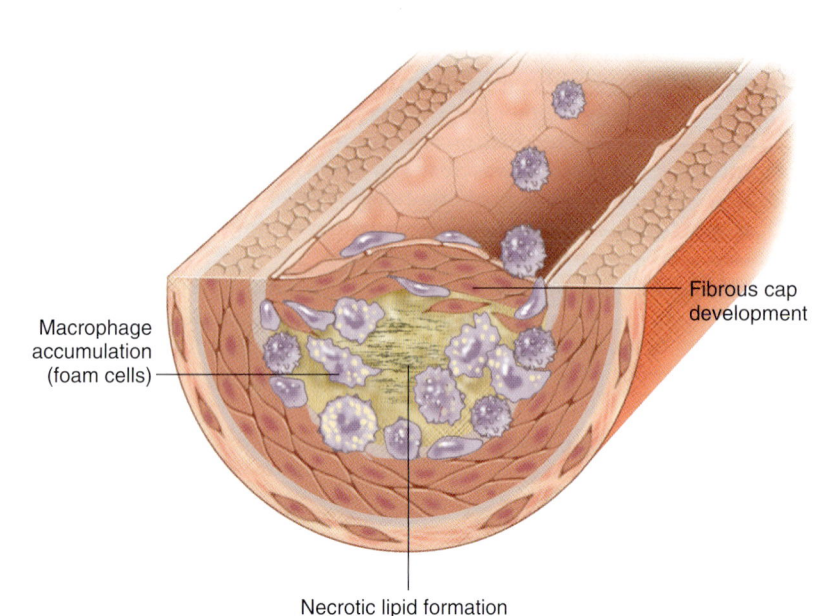

FIGURE 88-2 Atherosclerotic lesion progression. This illustration shows an advanced atherosclerotic plaque with uptake of oxidized LDL by macrophages, which become foam cells. Reactive oxygen species induce necrosis and apoptosis, leading to a necrotic core. Inflammatory cells promote cytokine and growth factor release that stimulates fibrous cap formation. *(Modified from Ross R. Atherosclerosis—an inflammatory disease. N Engl J Med 1999; 340:115.)*

coagulant factors released by activated inflammatory cells, can induce platelet aggregation and ultimately thrombosis and rapid vessel occlusion (Fig. 88-2).

Risk Factors

The risk factors for atherosclerosis are similar across the multiple arterial beds affected, regardless of the end-organ perfused. They fall into two categories: those that are modifiable and those beyond our control. Modifiable risk factors can be further broken down into those that are predominantly a result of lifestyle indiscretions and those that are primarily manifestations of clinical disease that can be treated (Table 88-1).

Risk Factors (Not Modifiable)

Increasing age is the most powerful risk factor for noncoronary atherosclerotic vascular disease (AVD). The atherosclerotic process occurs in a stepwise fashion over time, and those with advanced age are more likely to have a higher burden and greater complexity of disease. Data from the Framingham study show that 7% to 9% of individuals 75 years of age or older have carotid stenoses of 50% or more. In contrast, less than 1% had that degree of obstruction at 50 years of age.[4]

Gender also plays a significant role in the prevalence of atherosclerosis. However, with the increasing number of female smokers and disproportionate prevalence and rate of increase in obesity, these gender differences are narrowing.[2] Race also has a significant impact on the likelihood of atherosclerotic disease. For instance, black populations have a 38% higher incidence than do white populations of ischemic stroke and stroke mortality adjusted for risk factors.[4]

Genetics also plays a significant role in the development of atherosclerosis. This is evident from studies of common carotid artery wall thickness and abdominal calcification, in which familial factors contribute 64% to 92% and 50% of the variation, respectively. Genetically increased risk does not follow a mendelian pattern but is rather the result of changes in multiple genes that have varying effects on the cardiovascular system. The majority of isolated risk-associated genes to date modulate other known cardiovascular risk factors rather than the atherosclerotic process itself. Genes that work independently of known comorbid conditions are the subject of intense ongoing research.

Known genes that promote lipid abnormalities include apolipoprotein E (*APOE*) and cholesteryl ester transfer protein (*CETP*). Mutations in the LDL receptor gene are particularly damaging, leading to familial hypercholesterolemia in its homozygous form and significant lipid abnormalities even when heterozygous, which occurs in approximately 1 in 500 persons.[8] Contributors to the inflammatory process include peroxisome proliferator–activated receptor γ, vascular cell adhesion molecule, and tumor necrosis factor α.[9] Significant research is necessary to identify new genes and to determine the full impact of known genetic abnormalities, their response to environmental conditions, and the subsequent therapeutic implications.

Proinflammatory conditions such as systemic lupus erythematosus and rheumatoid arthritis have up to a 50-fold increase in the risk of AVD, with the largest differences appreciated in younger patients. The proposed mediators of this increased risk include immune complex deposition; increased fibrinogen, von Willebrand factor, and other procoagulants; higher lipoprotein levels from glucocorticoid therapy; and direct vascular injury with endothelial cell progenitor cell depletion. Rarely, vasculitis is the inciting factor. Systemic lupus erythematosus specifically can cause dyslipidemia through lipoprotein lipase autoantibodies and increased oxidized LDL uptake through anti–$β_2$-glycoprotein 1 autoantibodies.

Modifiable Risk Factors

Many of the known modifiable risk factors have well-established interactions with the pathophysiologic processes of noncoronary atherosclerosis. For example,

TABLE 88-1 Risk Factors for the Development of Atherosclerosis

Modifiable Risk Factors
Lifestyle indiscretions
    Obesity
    Tobacco use
    Physical inactivity
Clinical comorbid conditions
    Lipid abnormalities*
        Elevated low-density lipoprotein or total cholesterol level
        Low high-density lipoprotein level
        Elevated triglyceride levels
    Diabetes mellitus
    Metabolic syndrome, insulin resistance
    Hypertension (both systolic and diastolic are independently associated)

Risk Factors (Not Modifiable)
Advanced age
Male gender
Race†
Genetic predisposition (positive family history)
Prothrombotic and proinflammatory comorbid conditions (such as systemic lupus erythematosus, rheumatoid arthritis)

New/Under Investigation
Increased lipoprotein(a)
High-sensitivity C-reactive protein elevation
Homocysteine elevation
Increased fibrinogen

*Each of these lipid abnormalities provides independent incremental risk.
†The black population has a higher rate of atherosclerosis than the white population does.

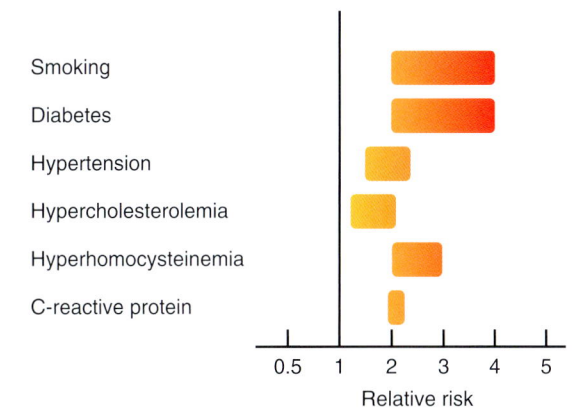

FIGURE 88-3 Relative risk of peripheral arterial disease by risk factor. Tobacco use and diabetes confer the greatest risk of peripheral arterial disease.

hypertension causes increased levels of angiotensin II, which stimulates smooth muscle growth and lipoxygenase activity, a contributor to LDL oxidation and inflammation. Lipoxygenase also increases free radical production and subsequently reduces nitric oxide formation. Homocysteine decreases nitric oxide availability in addition to its direct toxicity to the endothelium and its prothrombotic effects.[7]

Tobacco use and diabetes mellitus appear to confer the greatest risk of noncoronary AVD (Fig. 88-3).[9] Tobacco use doubles the risk of ischemic stroke. Smoking also increases the risk of PAD by twofold to sixfold, and more than 80% of those with PAD have smoked or continue to do so. This effect occurs in a dose-dependent manner.[5] In the Edinburgh Artery Study, the odds ratio (OR) for PAD with tobacco use (OR, 1.8-5.6) was approximately twofold to threefold higher than for CAD (OR, 1.1-1.6).

The proposed pathophysiologic mechanisms for the increased risk of disease in PAD versus CAD are (1) increased endothelial dysfunction (measured through von Willebrand and tissue plasminogen activator antigens), (2) reduced circulating antioxidants, (3) increased plasma fibrinogen levels, and (4) altered lipoprotein profiles. The Edinburgh Artery Study specifically addressed the differential odds ratios by measuring risk factors and analyzing the prevalence of these two conditions in 1592 subjects both with and without a history of tobacco use.[10] This study confirmed increased levels of von Willebrand and tissue plasminogen activator antigens (markers of endothelial disruption), reduced antioxidant levels, and increased fibrinogen levels. However, correction for these variables decreased the PAD odds ratio to only 2.7 from 3.9, with little change in the CAD odds ratio. Although the differential effect of tobacco use was partly mitigated by adjusting for these potential contributors, it is clear that other unknown mechanisms still predominate.[10]

Diabetes mellitus is the other of the two most significant modifiable risk factors, increasing the risk of PAD by 2- to 4-fold and ischemic stroke by 1.8- to 6-fold.[5,11] The risks of critical limb ischemia and major amputation are also higher with diabetes. The pathophysiologic mechanism underlying this increased risk is multifactorial. Increased levels of C-reactive protein promote apoptosis and stimulate procoagulant tissue factors, leukocyte adhesion molecules, and inhibitors of fibrinolysis. The hyperglycemia, insulin resistance, and fatty acid production associated with diabetes reduce the bioavailability of nitric oxide, decreasing vasodilation and allowing increased smooth muscle cell proliferation and platelet activation. Finally, diabetes increases procoagulant tissue factor and fibrinogen production, leading to a hypercoagulable state.[12] Unlike tobacco use, diabetes does not appear to increase the risk of noncoronary AVD disproportionately to the risk of CAD.

Unlike with coronary vascular disease, the lipid abnormality most strongly associated with noncoronary AVD is the combination of high triglyceride and low high-density lipoprotein (HDL) levels, which are also highly linked with diabetes. These lipid abnormalities are closely involved in the noncoronary atherosclerotic process along with increased LDL. Triglyceride-rich lipoproteins stimulate smooth muscle cell proliferation and extracellular matrix deposition. Low levels of HDL increase atherosclerotic risk through a relative decrease in its beneficial processes, including reverse cholesterol transport for its excretion, endothelial protection, and anti-inflammatory effects.[8]

The metabolic syndrome includes these cholesterol derangements as well as abdominal obesity, hypertension, and insulin resistance. This risk factor complex leads to a low-grade inflammatory state with increased levels of C-reactive protein, tumor necrosis factor α, and fibrinogen. Although LDL levels may remain within normal ranges, the particles are smaller and more dense, which renders them prone to detrimental oxidation. Moreover, each component of the metabolic syndrome independently increases atherosclerotic risk. Adipose tissue worsens insulin sensitivity and causes a system-wide pro-inflammatory state. Persistent hyperglycemia from insulin resistance and the high coprevalence of diabetes mellitus lead to advanced glycation end-products that trigger additional arterial inflammation.

Both physical inactivity and obesity have been shown to increase C-reactive protein levels and to cause endothelial dysfunction. They also worsen many other disease states that independently increase the risk of disease. Decreased exercise promotes the formation of proatherogenic cytokines. All of these changes lead to an increased risk of noncoronary AVD.

Novel Risk Factors

Greater understanding of the most common risk factors associated with noncoronary AVD have led to the development of risk scores for stroke and claudication based on the Framingham data. However, novel contributors of risk, especially those estimating inflammation, such as high-sensitivity C-reactive protein, lipoprotein(a), and homocysteine, are challenging these existing paradigms.[9] Lipoprotein(a), for instance, self-aggregates and increases inflammation by impairing fibrinolysis through regulation of fibrinogen activator inhibitor 1 and by inducing smooth muscle cell proliferation.

These novel factors may have additional predictive value only in patients with premature or rapidly progressive disease. Moreover, treatment of these comorbid conditions, such as vitamin supplementation for elevated homocysteine levels, does not necessarily decrease subsequent risk.

There is some variation in risk factors based on the anatomic localization of disease. For instance, in aortic disease, tobacco use continues to play a significant role (partly because of elastin degradation). It and male sex confer the highest risk for AAAs, whereas those of Asian descent rarely develop this disorder. A family history of AAA is especially important. In PAD, however, diabetes plays a larger role, especially for the female gender. PAD appears to have a higher incidence in African-American and Hispanic subgroups. Other than these examples, few data are available on gender- and ethnicity-based risk differences.[9]

Manifestations of Disease

Clinical Presentation

History

The presenting symptoms of noncoronary AVD in the different arterial beds can be found in Table 88-2, which can also be used as a comprehensive vascular review of systems.

The symptoms of noncoronary AVD can be vague and are often mistaken by patients and even clinicians for unrelated conditions with high prevalence in the aging population. It is easy to confuse arthritis and spinal stenosis for claudication, dyspepsia or irritable bowel syndrome for AAA or mesenteric vascular disease, and sinus or migraine headaches and age-related visual changes for the symptoms of cerebrovascular ischemia. The changes in exercise capacity with lower extremity PAD are frequently mistaken for "general deconditioning associated with aging." For this reason, any symptoms that could be related to noncoronary AVD should prompt thorough additional history taking and trigger a full vascular physical examination.

Moreover, patients with risk factors for noncoronary AVD should have a careful vascular review of systems even in the absence of presenting symptoms. This includes all patients older than 70 years, those aged 50 years or older with diabetes or a history of tobacco use, and younger patients with diabetes and any additional atherosclerotic risk factors. Patients with convincing histories

TABLE 88-2 Common Presenting Clinical Findings and Vascular Review of Systems

Condition	Clinical Symptoms and Review of Systems
Cerebrovascular disease	Altered mental status Headaches Vision changes (diplopia, blurred vision, visual field defects) Dysphagia Word-finding or speech articulation difficulties Peripheral motor and sensory deficits

Peripheral arterial disease	Critical limb ischemia
	   Severe, often unremitting resting leg pain
	   Painful arterial insufficiency ulcers on the lower legs and feet
	Chronic ischemia
	   Intermittent claudication (leg fatigue or discomfort during exercise relieved with rest)
	   Poorly healing leg wounds or ulcers

Abdominal aortic disease	Abdominal pain, hypotension, shock in the setting of acute rupture Family history of first-degree relative with AAA Chronic abdominal pain, weight loss, and elevated ESR in patients with an inflammatory AAA
Renal artery stenosis	Accelerating, resistant, or severe hypertension, despite aggressive management with ≥3 drugs Recurrent, unexplained flash pulmonary edema Renal azotemia after ACE inhibitor or ARB

Mesenteric arterial disease	Acute ischemia
	   Abdominal pain out of proportion to physical findings, especially in patients with any known atherosclerotic disease or multiple risk factors
	   Nausea, diarrhea, and lower gastrointestinal blood loss
	Chronic ischemia
	   Chronic, otherwise unexplained, typically postprandial abdominal pain in high-risk individuals
	   Unexplained anorexia and weight loss in high-risk patients with chronic abdominal pain of unknown origin
	   History of atherosclerotic disease and prior revascularization (30%-50% of patients)

AAA, abdominal aortic aneurysm; ACE, angiotensin-converting enzyme; ARB, angiotensin receptor blocker; ESR, erythrocyte sedimentation rate.

should undergo additional vascular assessment irrespective of the vascular physical examination.

Patients with PAD are asymptomatic 20% to 50% of the time. Classic intermittent claudication involves leg fatigue or discomfort, typically in the calf, that occurs only with exertion and is relieved after no more than 10 minutes of rest. This syndrome occurs in only 10% to 35% of patients with PAD. Resting pain and frank gangrene occur with critical limb ischemia, which is present in 1% to 2% of patients with PAD. A large proportion of PAD patients (40% to 50%) have atypical symptoms. This makes a careful physical examination and targeted noninvasive imaging even more important.

AAAs are almost always asymptomatic, although they can be picked up on a careful physical examination. An essential part of a general review of systems is a history of aortic aneurysmal disease in a first-degree relative. Up to 28% of patients with an AAA have a first-degree relative with disease, and the relative risk for male relatives of affected men is as high as 18.[5] Individuals with a family history may have onset of disease at a younger age, although the rate of progression and location do not appear to differ. Inflammatory AAA is one subset that does often have symptoms with no significant differences in risk factor makeup.

Mesenteric arterial disease is poorly studied because of its vague clinical presentation but carries a very poor prognosis and is typically associated with other atherosclerotic disease. The presentation of chronic mesenteric ischemia is fairly uncommon until it has progressed to a high level of severity. The association of abdominal pain with food is not always readily apparent. A high index of suspicion must be maintained in individuals at increased risk, especially those with prior revascularization for atherosclerotic disease, who make up almost half of all patients with this disorder.

Physical Examination

A careful physical examination focusing on the arterial vascular system is essential, especially given the nonspecific nature of much of the history in noncoronary AVD. Given the high coprevalence of coronary vascular disease, a careful cardiac examination should be performed, including assessment of the neck veins, cardiac auscultation, palpation for heaves and thrills and for the point of maximal impulse, and pulmonary auscultation.

The key aspects of the peripheral vascular examination include the following[5]:

- Bilateral brachial blood pressure measurement and comparison for asymmetry.
- Carotid pulse palpation for upstroke, amplitude, and duration, followed by auscultation of the carotids bilaterally and in the suprasternal notch for subclavian bruits.
- Palpation of the abdomen for pulsatile masses and estimated aortic diameter and auscultation for abdominal aortic or renal bruits.
- Evaluation of the presence and intensity of the brachial, radial, ulnar, femoral, popliteal, posterior tibial, and dorsalis pedis pulses by palpation.
- Auscultation of the femoral arteries for bruits bilaterally as well as of other arterial beds as clinically indicated.
- Assessment of the lower extremities, including the feet, for color, temperature, skin integrity, hair loss, and nail hypertrophy.

Hypertension that is resistant to multiple medications, especially in younger patients, can be due to renal artery stenosis. Asymmetric blood pressures in the upper extremities can suggest subclavian or more distal atherosclerosis. Relatively diminished blood pressure in the lower extremities bilaterally suggests aortic narrowing; unilateral decreases suggest iliac atherosclerosis. Patients with cerebrovascular disease and carotid stenosis will often have a delayed carotid pulse with diminished amplitude with or without carotid bruits (which can be absent with severe enough obstruction). AAAs can be manifested with large pulsatile abdominal masses and increased aortic diameter. Femoral or more distal bruits and diminished pulses suggest lower extremity PAD, which is also suggested by cool and pale skin with poorly healing arterial ulcers, shiny and thin skin without hair, and hypertrophic nail beds.

Given the limited sensitivity and specificity of the history and physical examination for noncoronary AVD, any concerning findings should be evaluated further through noninvasive vascular testing.[5]

Imaging Indications and Algorithm

A common theme in the indications for evaluation of atherosclerosis in the various arterial beds is the presence of particularly high-risk or multiple atherosclerotic risk factors. Symptoms of exertional calf pain are much more concerning for atherosclerosis in a 70-year-old patient with diabetes and ongoing tobacco use than in a 20-year-old patient without risk factors and the same symptoms, whose chance for an atherosclerotic etiology is comparatively low.

The algorithm for evaluation of noncoronary atherosclerotic disease typically focuses initially on low-cost, low-risk, noninvasive approaches, followed by more expensive, possibly higher risk modalities for a more robust assessment if the findings on initial examination are abnormal or equivocal.

Screening for atherosclerotic cerebrovascular disease in asymptomatic individuals is not currently recommended because there is a low risk of stroke in asymptomatic patients and surgical outcomes are variable. Several studies have shown that screening leads to more strokes than it prevents and would prevent only approximately 100 strokes for every 10,000 high-risk patients screened. Symptoms are often evaluated with carotid ultrasonography first, followed by magnetic resonance angiography (MRA) or an alternative high-resolution modality for presurgical evaluation or definitive diagnosis as necessary after an abnormal ultrasound study.

Carotid intimal-medial thickness (CIMT) measurement by ultrasonography, on the other hand, is primarily used to evaluate cardiovascular risk and is typically performed in asymptomatic individuals. It is best used in patients with an intermediate risk of cardiovascular disease or with

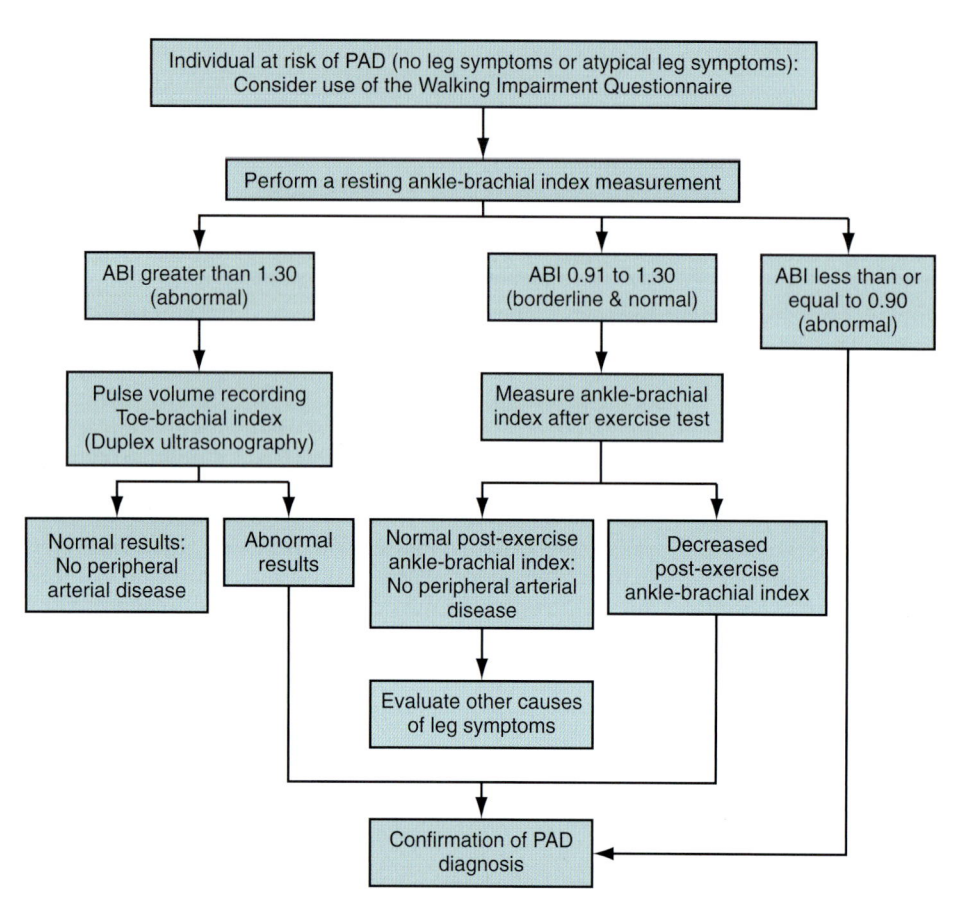

FIGURE 88-4 Diagnostic algorithm for peripheral arterial disease (PAD). (Modified from Hirsch AT, Haskal ZJ, Hertzer NR, et al. ACC/AHA 2005 guidelines for the management of patients with peripheral arterial disease [lower extremity, renal, mesenteric, and abdominal aortic]: executive summary a collaborative report from the American Association for Vascular Surgery/Society for Vascular Surgery, Society for Cardiovascular Angiography and Interventions, Society for Vascular Medicine and Biology, Society of Interventional Radiology, and the ACC/AHA Task Force on Practice Guidelines [Writing Committee to Develop Guidelines for the Management of Patients With Peripheral Arterial Disease] endorsed by the American Association of Cardiovascular and Pulmonary Rehabilitation; National Heart, Lung, and Blood Institute; Society for Vascular Nursing; TransAtlantic Inter-Society Consensus; and Vascular Disease Foundation. J Am Coll Cardiol 2006; 47:1239.)

a strong family history, an especially severe risk factor, or other reason for which the optimal aggressiveness of medical therapy in an individual is unknown. More than 1000 asymptomatic patients in nine studies have shown a strong association between an abnormal CIMT and increased risk of cardiovascular death, nonfatal myocardial infarction (MI), stroke, or a combination of these. The presence of carotid plaque or a CIMT greater than the 75th age- and gender-matched percentile indicates the need for more aggressive medical therapy.[13]

Noninvasive evaluation of PAD almost always starts with ABI ascertainment as a high-risk asymptomatic screening method or to evaluate symptoms in the absence of arterial insufficiency ulcers or critical limb ischemia (Fig. 88-4). ABIs correlate highly with the site and severity of peripheral arterial obstruction as well as with overall cardiovascular risk. Subsequent further studies typically involve high-resolution MRA, computed tomographic angiography (CTA), or digital subtraction angiography.

There are no inexpensive, low-risk screening options to evaluate renal artery stenosis, and symptoms are limited. For this reason, physical examination and laboratory findings prompt further noninvasive evaluation. The two primary clinical findings are hypertension refractory to multiple medications and otherwise unexplained renal insufficiency. Screening should not be undertaken unless intervention is planned for a positive result. In patients at very high risk, invasive angiography can be performed directly, but noninvasive methods such as CTA, MRA, and duplex Doppler ultrasonography carry less risk. MRA has been the modality of choice because of its lack of ionizing radiation and use of a contrast agent without traditional nephrotoxicity. However, patients with a creatinine clearance below 30 mL/min should not be given gadolinium because of the risk of nephrogenic systemic fibrosis, and alternative testing should be chosen.

AAAs are typically discovered as incidental findings or during screening. AAA rupture is catastrophic, and leakage is manifested like other nonatherosclerotic conditions, such that a high index of suspicion must be maintained for those at high risk. As a result of in-depth prevalence data, the guidelines of several major societies, including those of the American College of Cardiology/American Heart Association (ACC/AHA), recommend screening of men aged 65 to 75 years with any past tobacco use history by a physical examination and one-time ultrasound study. Some suggest screening those with a family history of AAA as well. Because of a lower prevalence of disease, they recommend against screening of women (or screening only women with multiple cardiovascular risk factors) or younger or nonsmoking men.

As with renal artery stenosis, there are no good noninvasive screening studies for mesenteric ischemia. Acute ischemia typically requires emergent laparotomy or invasive angiography; noninvasive studies are less commonly used except in equivocal situations. Chronic mesenteric ischemia from arterial disease is more commonly assessed with noninvasive methods such as MRA and CTA, with neither technique having complete dominance.

TABLE 88-3 Sensitivities and Specificities of Noninvasive, Noncoronary Atherosclerosis Assessment Techniques

Arterial Bed and Modality	Sensitivity (%)	Specificity (%)	Finding
Carotid Artery Disease			
Ultrasonography	86	87	70%-99% stenosis[14]
CT	77	95	70%-99% stenosis[15]
MRA	97-100	90-92	70%-99% stenosis[14]
Lower Extremity Arterial Disease			
Ankle-brachial index (ultrasonography)	90	98	≥50% stenosis[16]
Ultrasonography (duplex)	86/80	97/98	≥50% stenosis aortoiliac/femoropopliteal[15]
CT	89-100	92-100	≥50% stenosis
MRA	98	96	
Abdominal Aortic Aneurysm			
Ultrasonography	92-99	100	Various aneurysm diameters
CT	100/100	94	Proximal/distal aneurysm extent (relationship to renals/aortic bifurcation)[17]
MRA	87		Proximal aneurysm extent (relationship to renals)[18]
Angiography	50/89	100/50	Proximal/distal aneurysm extent (relationship to renals/aortic bifurcation)[17]
Renal Atherosclerotic Disease			
Ultrasonography	98	99	60%-99% stenosis (aortic/renal Doppler ratio ≥ 3.5 or peak velocity >200 cm/s)[15]
CT	91-92	99	≥50% stenosis[5]
MRA	90-100	76-94	>50% stenosis[19]
Mesenteric Arterial Disease			
Ultrasonography	90/93	91/100	≥50% superior mesenteric arterial/celiac stenosis (end-diastolic velocity >45/55 cm/s)[15,20]
CT	92	100	Acute occlusion[21]
MRA	100	95-100	Celiac, superior mesenteric arterial, inferior mesenteric arterial stenosis ≥75%[22]

CT, computed tomography; MRA, magnetic resonance angiography.

Imaging Techniques and Findings

The sensitivities and specificities of the multiple imaging modalities that are used to assess noncoronary atherosclerotic disease are presented in Table 88-3.

Radiography

Because of its inability to assess vascular structures, radiography has limited ability to assist in the assessment of atherosclerotic disease. Calcification is well visualized with general radiography, especially diffuse calcification of the aorta on chest radiography or calcification of carotid plaques on dental panoramic radiography. Any such findings can trigger further evaluation and potentially additional noninvasive assessment. Other than as a spurious finding on radiographs performed for other clinical indications, atherosclerosis should not be assessed by radiography.

Ultrasonography

Ultrasonography of the peripheral or cerebrovascular arterial system has well-established utility in the diagnosis and management of atherosclerotic disease. It is easy to perform, carries minimal risk (with no ionizing radiation), and is fairly reproducible.

Two-dimensional images are obtained in real time by use of B-mode (brightness) technology with transducers of varying frequencies. High-frequency transducers provide excellent resolution but have poor depth of penetration. Lower frequency probes provide improved depth for imaging structures, such as the abdominal aorta and renal and mesenteric vasculature, at the sacrifice of resolution. Concurrent Doppler analysis of blood flow is typically performed.

Ultrasonography has demonstrated utility in all of the noncoronary arterial beds. In the cerebrovascular arterial system, carotid ultrasound examination is performed in patients with symptoms of cerebrovascular ischemia or an asymptomatic bruit to assess for focal atherosclerotic plaques quantified through Doppler analysis. An increase in velocity typically does not occur until a stenosis of 50% or more is present. The plaque thickness can be assessed (with discrete plaques defined as a 50% increase in wall thickness), but this typically correlates poorly with the overall plaque size and volume because it is one two-dimensional measurement.[23] Despite these limitations, this technique remains a primary tool to investigate for significant cerebrovascular atherosclerotic disease.

An assessment of the overall atherosclerotic burden can also be obtained for epidemiologic or risk stratification purposes through measurement of the CIMT (Fig. 88-5).[23] An absolute cutoff is difficult to ascertain because age has a large effect on the CIMT. Moreover, because of the frequent inability to separate the intima from the media, diseases such as hypertension that cause medial hypertrophy increase the CIMT in the absence of atherosclerosis. However, increasing CIMT has been shown to correlate well with cardiovascular morbidity, with an age- and

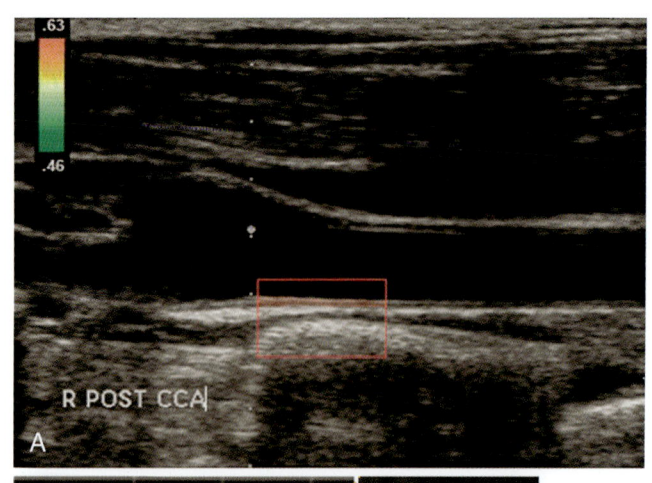

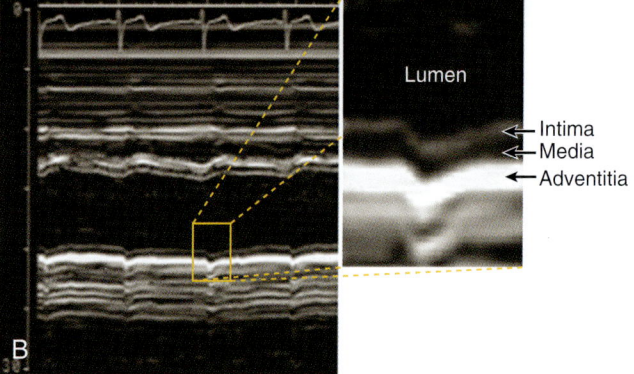

FIGURE 88-5 Carotid intima-media thickness evaluation by ultrasonography. **A,** Right common carotid artery of a 39-year-old man with a prominent family history of premature coronary artery disease and hyperlipidemia with the posterior wall highlighted. The increased intima-media thickness is consistent with advanced atherosclerosis despite a low Framingham risk score. **B,** Carotid artery with vascular wall highlighted. All three layers (intimal, medial, and adventitial) are clearly visualized. *(Reprinted with permission from Hurst RT, Ng DW, Kendall C, Khandheria B. Clinical use of carotid intima-media thickness: review of the literature. J Am Soc Echocardiogr 2007; 20:907.)*

sex-adjusted 15% and 18% increase in risk of MI and stroke, respectively, with each 0.1-mm increase in CIMT.[24] Interobserver variability is good, averaging approximately 0.4 mm with a 3.1% coefficient of variation for experienced readers. Although it has significant value as a predictor of adverse outcome in large populations, CIMT has extensive variability not directly related to atherosclerosis that limits its ability to provide sufficient prognostic information at the level of the individual patient at this time. A consensus statement of the American Society of Echocardiography recommends against CIMT in patients with established atherosclerosis or use in serial fashion to assess progression.[13]

In the peripheral arterial system, ultrasonography has utility in the measurement of ABIs, in the evaluation of brachial artery reactivity, and for arterial duplex scanning. ABI assessment uses hand-held Doppler ultrasound, although this is not an imaging study. The ratio of the ankle to the higher of the brachial systolic blood pressures is obtained; a ratio below 0.90 indicates moderate to significant upstream peripheral arterial obstruction. This technique has fair test-retest reliability (±10% to 16%) and a sensitivity and specificity of 90% and 98%, respectively, for a peripheral arterial stenosis of 50% or more. An ABI below 0.40 is consistent with severe ischemia. Symptomatic patients with normal ABIs can often have dysfunction unmasked with exercise (treadmill or active, repeated pedal plantar flexion). Abnormal ABIs correlate with claudication and functional status (walking distance, overall physical activity) and indicate a higher risk of overall mortality and likelihood of CAD (relative risks at 4 years of 3.1 and 3.7, respectively) and stroke.[16]

Brachial artery reactivity testing assesses the endothelial dysfunction that typically precedes the clinical manifestations of atherosclerosis, making it potentially effective for screening the early stages of disease. Forearm ischemia is created with blood pressure cuff inflation for more than 5 minutes, and the percentage increase in brachial artery diameter is compared with baseline. Functional endothelium releases nitric oxide and should induce reactive hyperemia, increasing the vessel diameter. Flow-mediated dilation of less than 10% was associated in one study with an increased risk of MI and revascularization.[25] The major limitation of this technique is the large variation between patients in the vasodilator response to forearm ischemia, and its clinical use is minimal.

Arterial duplex ultrasonography is performed in stepwise fashion along the entire vessel in the extremity of interest. Color Doppler study is used to identify stenoses, which are then quantified by pulse- and continuous-wave velocities. This technique was evaluated in a meta-analysis of 14 studies that showed sensitivities and specificities of 86% and 97% for aortoiliac disease (≥50% stenosis) and 80% and 98% for femoropopliteal disease.[15] In many instances, ultrasonographic evaluation can avoid invasive diagnostic angiography for patients before intervention, with a 97% accuracy compared with arteriography. It can also be used for serial surveillance of grafts and native vessels after stent placement.

Arterial duplex ultrasonography is also very useful in the assessment of renal and mesenteric atherosclerotic disease. An aortic–renal artery Doppler ratio of 3.5 or higher or a peak systolic velocity above 200 cm/sec corresponds to a stenosis of 60% to 99% with a sensitivity of 98%, specificity of 99%, positive predictive value of 99%, and negative predictive value of 97%.[15] This technique may also predict blood pressure and renal function improvement with revascularization through the resistive index; a value above 80 is associated with a small chance of improvement. Limitations include the need for deep penetration, which is difficult in obese patients, and a relatively poor sensitivity (approximately 60%) for identifying accessory renal arteries.

Mesenteric duplex ultrasonography is contraindicated in the evaluation of acute intestinal ischemia because of the deep location, lack of fasting and optimal timing in the early morning to avoid excessive bowel gas, increased time required for ultrasound examination, and abdominal distention and fluid often present with this condition.[5] Ultrasonography is a good screening modality for chronic mesenteric arterial obstruction, on the other hand, with a sensitivity exceeding 90% for 50% celiac or superior mesenteric arterial stenoses and a 99% negative predictive value. Thus, a normal study should induce work-up of nonatherosclerotic causes of abdominal pain. Mesenteric evaluation is also limited by large body habitus, examiner experience, gas pattern, and prior abdominal surgery.

Ultrasonography is an ideal method for screening abdominal and peripheral arterial aneurysms, with 95% sensitivity and nearly 100% specificity. Aortic wall thrombus and calcification are also assessed. Ultrasonography also evaluates invasive arteriographic complications such as pseudoaneurysms, hematomas, and arteriovenous fistulas. Thrombin injection of pseudoaneurysms was successful in one cohort 94% of the time with no complications noted.

Future advancements in ultrasonography for the assessment of atherosclerotic disease include increased use of three-dimensional probes, hand-held ultrasound machines with increased portability, and additional clinical applications of brachial artery reactivity and CIMT measurement.

Computed Tomography

Multidetector CTA provides rapid, high-resolution assessment of arterial patency. Because of its three-dimensional volumetric acquisition, the anatomy of interest can be assessed in multiple planes with multiple angles after a single acquisition. Moreover, as opposed to conventional angiography, CTA provides good visualization of adjacent anatomic structures and can visualize vessel diameter independent of the lumen. Compared with MRA, CTA has minimal flow-related distortion and improved visualization of calcification and metallic implants such as stents. However, CTA does require ionizing radiation and nephrotoxic iodinated contrast material.

Recent improvements in CTA have markedly shortened image acquisition times that enabled broader anatomic coverage such that a full lower extremity arterial study can now be performed. Moreover, the improved speed allows more detailed visualization of smaller vessels with thinner sections, greater detail, and more uniform vascular enhancement, often with lower doses of contrast agents.[5,15] A single breath-hold (if necessary) image is obtained with multiple contiguous or overlapping axial cross sections of the region of interest. These images have the highest diagnostic utility and less chance for artifacts related to postprocessing. However, the more typical angiographic appearance is created with digital smoothing to reduce stair step artifacts and multiple techniques, such as multiplanar reformation, maximum intensity projection, and volumetric rendering.

CTA provides a high-resolution image of the carotid artery lumen, and lumen diameter can be determined with high accuracy from the three-dimensional reconstructed images (Fig. 88-6). A meta-analysis comparing CTA with invasive cerebral angiography has shown CTA to identify 70% to 99% stenoses with good sensitivity (77%) and excellent specificity (95%). It is especially important to differentiate near from total occlusions, as a benefit has not been shown for revascularization in patients with total occlusions. CTA is 97% to 100% sensitive and 99% to 100% specific for this differentiation.[15] Like MRA and ultrasonography, CTA has a significantly lower sensitivity and specificity for the identification of 50% to 69% stenoses.

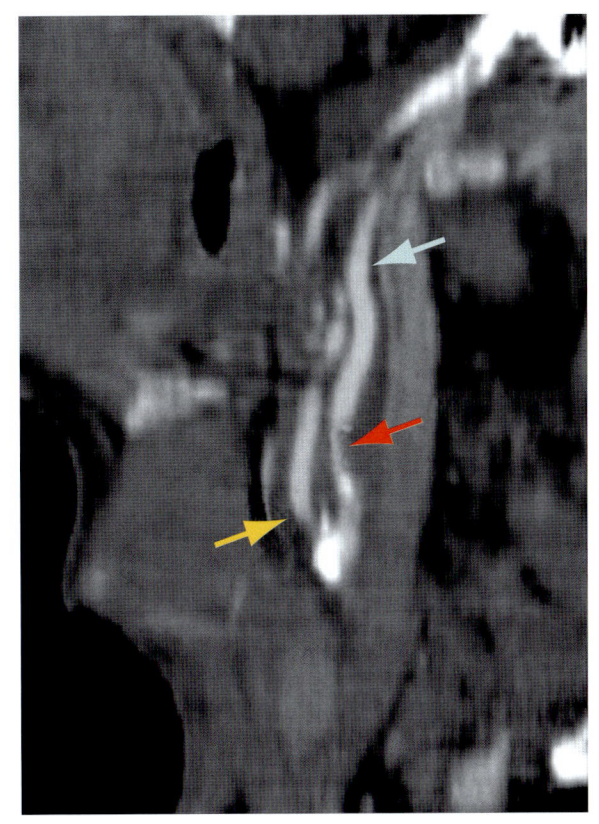

■ **FIGURE 88-6** CTA of the right carotid system in a 79-year-old patient with a history of transient ischemic attack. Severe right carotid bulb stenosis can be clearly visualized (red arrow). The blue arrow represents the right internal carotid artery, and the yellow arrow shows the right external carotid artery. (Reprinted with permission from Saba L, Sanfilippo R, Pirisi R, et al. Multidetector-row CT angiography in the study of atherosclerotic carotid arteries. Neuroradiology 2007; 49:623.)

Given the exposure to ionizing radiation and nephrotoxic contrast agents, CTA is considered a third-line test compared with ultrasonography and MRA for carotid evaluation. It is often used when ultrasonography and MRA disagree or when the patient has a contraindication to MRA.

CTA has an increasing role in peripheral arterial evaluation of the location and extent of significant stenoses as full peripheral "runoff" studies can now be performed. It has been found to have a concordance of 100% with conventional angiography. In addition, 26 additional segments were identified on CTA that were not assessable during angiography because of insufficient opacification distal to significant occlusions. Analyses with multidetector CT have found sensitivity to range from 89% to 100% for stenoses of more than 50%, with specificity of 92% to 100%. Evaluation of grafts and stents after revascularization as routine surveillance has not yet been studied. Assessment of distal calf and foot vessels was previously problematic, but the increasing number of slices obtained (64-slice with 256-slice scanners under development) may eliminate this issue.

The renal and mesenteric arteries can be imaged with high resolution by CTA. With use of multidetector CT to assess renal atherosclerosis, the sensitivity is 91% to 92%, with specificity of 99% compared with MRA.[5] The interobserver and intermodality agreements between CTA and MRA are excellent (κ, 0.88-0.90). The need for 100 to 150 mL of contrast material limits the use of CTA in renal insufficiency, but this amount is expected to decrease with further technologic advancement.

CTA of the mesenteric arterial system shares the same beneficial attributes. Intestinal obstruction is common in higher risk groups but not diagnostic of ischemia because acute intestinal ischemia is uncommon. Diagnosis relies on the combination of diagnostic findings and a compatible history and physical examination and laboratory results. Abdominal CT scanning is often performed before mesenteric ischemia is suspected, and the following findings should suggest this condition: intestinal distention, increased intestinal wall thickness, intestinal perforation, pneumatosis intestinalis, and portal venous air. None of these findings is specific, however, for mesenteric ischemia.

Irrespective of the arterial bed analyzed, CTA has the benefits of high spatial resolution and the ability to image extravascular structures, nonocclusive vessel wall abnormalities, and stents and vessels near to other metallic structures. It is an appropriate test for those with claustrophobia and contraindications to MRA, such as implantable defibrillators and pacemakers. However, it is typically used only if ultrasonography and MRA are contraindicated or conflicting because it requires ionizing radiation (thought to be one fourth of the median dose for digital subtraction angiography) and potentially nephrotoxic iodinated contrast material. However, in patients presenting with nonspecific signs or symptoms, CT is a valuable screening tool that can provide excellent evaluation for nonvascular sources of the patient's complaints.

Future advances in computed tomography include reduced radiation and contrast burden to allow whole-body CT for plaque distribution, vascular road mapping, calcium burden, and guided intervention.

Magnetic Resonance

MRA is an imaging method widely used to assess the effects of noncoronary atherosclerosis in a rapid fashion with high image quality. Unlike comparable techniques such as CTA and invasive angiography, MR uses contrast agents (gadolinium based) that lack nephrotoxic effects and avoids the use of ionizing radiation. Recently, however, a new, highly morbid condition, nephrogenic systemic fibrosis, has been discovered that is linked to use of gadolinium in patients on hemodialysis. This observation prevents the use of gadolinium-enhanced MRA in patients with significant renal dysfunction (use of renal replacement therapy or glomerular filtration rate ≤30 mL/min/1.73 m^2). Other disadvantages include the contraindication to MRI with pacemakers and defibrillators, the potential for claustrophobia, and the difficulty with access for unstable patients.

In patients with advanced renal dysfunction, non–contrast-enhanced MRA can be performed by time-of-flight imaging with suppression of background tissue and bright in-flowing blood. This method is time-consuming and has significant flow-related signal loss. Moreover, it may overestimate the degree of stenoses because of retrograde collateral flow. Its current limitations relegate this technique to a supplementary role only in patients with intact renal function, and other imaging methods should be considered in those with significant renal dysfunction. More recently, three-dimensional steady-state free precession has been found to be a promising non-contrast alternative for diagnostic arterial illustration.

The primary clinical use of MRA in the evaluation of atherosclerosis remains assessment of the vascular lumen. Significant technologic improvements have led to new sequences, such as contrast-enhanced time-resolved three-dimensional MRA, in which the images are presented in a fashion similar to angiograms. They provide extensive clinical information but require relatively long scanning times, and multiple acquisitions may be necessary, especially for aortic and peripheral vascular runoff. Other than to assess asymptomatic vascular aneurysms, the remaining MRA indications to evaluate the peripheral circulation are in symptomatic patients.

An exciting new frontier in MR assessment of atherosclerosis is vessel wall imaging with plaque assessment and resolution of individual plaque components.[26] Other imaging techniques primarily focus on the arterial lumen. However, because of positive arterial remodeling (the Glagov effect; see Fig. 88-1), luminal obstruction does not occur until 40% of the intima is occupied by plaque. This phenomenon allows significant underestimation of the burden of disease by currently used imaging modalities. Moreover, the majority of clinical events are initiated at sites with nonsignificant obstruction. Vessel wall imaging with MR uses special sequences that can provide an estimate of fibrous cap thickness and lipid core volume, which are critical determinants of plaque stability or lack thereof.[26] Vessel wall imaging can assess earlier atherosclerotic changes than are visible with traditional techniques. It is not widely used in clinical practice, and further research is necessary before its routine adoption. It remains an exciting, ongoing new direction.

Contrast-enhanced MRA remains a method of choice to evaluate the carotid arteries (ACC/AHA class I recommendation).[5] This technique was formerly thought to overestimate plaque burden. However, it is more likely that digital subtraction angiography underestimated asymmetric stenoses because of the limited number of carotid artery projections available. It remains highly sensitive and specific for the diagnosis of high-grade carotid stenoses. In a 2006 meta-analysis, the sensitivity and specificity for diagnosis of a 70% to 99% carotid stenosis were 94% and 93%, respectively, compared with invasive angiography. It is critical to separate high-grade stenoses from complete occlusions, and the sensitivity and specificity of MRA compared with invasive angiography for this difference ranges from 97% to 98% and 99% to 100%, respectively.

Contrast-enhanced MRA can also be combined with other imaging modalities to ensure a definitive diagnosis. It is commonly used in tandem with carotid duplex ultrasonography. Ultrasonography can overestimate near-occlusions, which can preclude beneficial surgical therapy if the lesion is misclassified as a total occlusion. MRA can provide important additional information to avoid misdiagnosis in these circumstances.

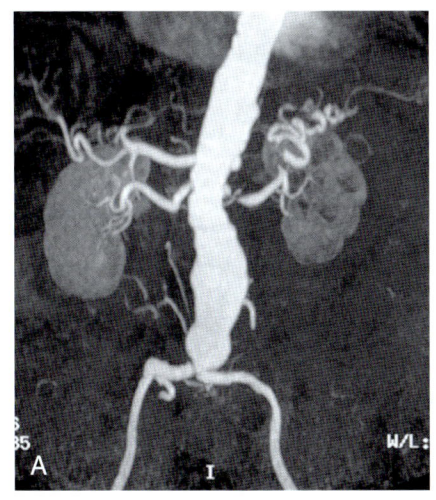

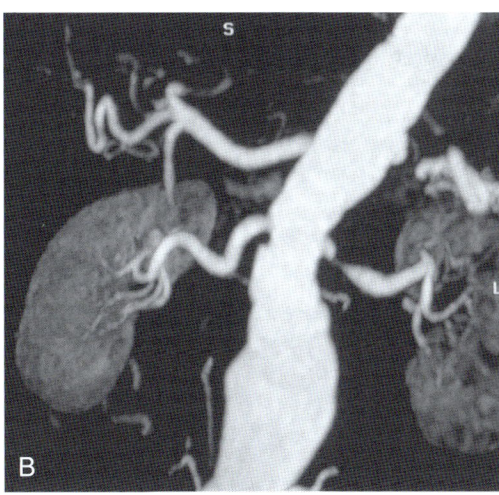

■ **FIGURE 88-7** Severe left renal artery stenosis on contrast-enhanced three-dimensional MRA (**A**, coronal maximum intensity projection; **B**, oblique coronal subvolume maximum intensity projection). The diffuse irregularity and fusiform aneurysm of the abdominal aorta reflect extensive atherosclerosis. *(Reprinted with permission from Ho VB, Corse WR. MR angiography of the abdominal aorta and peripheral vessels. Radiol Clin North Am 2003; 41:115-144.)*

MRA of the peripheral arterial circulation can be achieved through multiple techniques, such as time-resolved three-dimensional MRA and bolus chase three-dimensional MRA. It performs well in determining the location and degree of atherosclerotic stenosis and has rendered invasive diagnostic angiography almost unnecessary. With use of intraoperative angiography as the gold standard, MRA has accuracy similar to that of invasive catheter angiography; both have accuracies of 91% to 99% for a stenosis of 50% or more and close agreement (91% to 97%), which makes MRA a good technique for preoperative evaluation.[5] Compared with ultrasonography, the sensitivity is improved with MRA (98% versus 88%), with similar specificity (96% and 95%, respectively). It can overestimate stenoses because of turbulent flow.

MRA can be used to evaluate patients after bypass with excellent sensitivity and specificity (both 90% to 100%), especially with gadolinium enhancement. Care should be taken, however, as metal clip or metallic stent artifacts can appear similar to stenosis or mimic arterial occlusion.

A previous limitation of MRA was assessment of the small runoff vessels, and these are now adequately visualized at least as well as with invasive techniques. In fact, in one study of patients with diabetes and chronic limb ischemia, 38% of patients had pedal vessels identified by MRA that were not visualized by conventional angiography. The superiority of MRA in this circumstance is not well established, however.

MRA had previously been used extensively in patients with significant renal dysfunction to evaluate for renal artery stenosis and is increasingly regarded as the first-line study (Fig. 88-7). Unfortunately, more caution must be taken given the recently discovered risk of nephrogenic systemic fibrosis. Compared with catheter-based contrast angiography, MRA can identify renal artery stenosis secondary to atherosclerotic disease with sensitivities ranging from 90% to 100%, specificities of 76% to 100%, and accuracy approaching 100%. The interobserver agreement was high, as was that between modalities (κ, 0.88-0.90).[5] MRA can also evaluate the surrounding vasculature and the renal parenchyma, and it may even assess renal function. It has a more limited role in the evaluation of patients with renal stents because of artifact that limits intra-stent analysis of stenosis.

Use of MRA in mesenteric ischemia is less well established. In acute mesenteric ischemia, there are few data evaluating the use of MRA. It is unclear if MRA can assess the distal vasculature adequately for microthromboemboli and areas of nonocclusive ischemia. Angiography can evaluate for these entities and is still the test of choice. In addition, vascular access in these patients who are often severely ill is limited. CT is generally preferred in this setting as it allows improved access to the patient, is lower in cost, and has high sensitivity for detection of mesenteric venous thrombosis.[27]

MRA in chronic mesenteric ischemia is still experimental but likely plays a larger role than in acute ischemia. Compared with angiography, three-dimensional, gadolinium-enhanced MRA has been found to have 100% sensitivity, specificity of 95% to 100%, and accuracy approaching 100% for the diagnosis of celiac, superior mesenteric arterial, and inferior mesenteric arterial proximal stenoses. Specificity is limited by occasional inability to analyze the inferior mesenteric artery. There are few data on more distal disease. As in other vascular beds, MRA should not be used to evaluate disease in deployed stents in the mesenteric arterial system.

MRA provides an excellent assessment of AAAs. It is typically used in the chronic setting, with acute evaluation done predominantly by CT because of its rapidity. Although diagnostic images can be obtained with two-dimensional time-of-flight methods, these have been largely replaced by three-dimensional contrast-enhanced MRA. This technique can identify the diameter and extent of aneurysms as well as branch vessel involvement in a fashion similar to catheter angiography and CT. Phase contrast MR can be used to identify and to quantitate flow in false channels if present.

MRA has been used increasingly in the preoperative assessment before AAA repair. One study of 28 preoperative patients found MRA to correctly predict the proximal extent of the aneurysm and thereby appropriate proximal cross-clamp sites in 87% of patients. Proximal anastomotic sites were identified with similar high accuracy in both

MRA and catheter angiography (95% to 97%). Moreover, MRA was able to assess for iliac or femoral aneurysms, which complicate bypass, with sensitivity of 79% and specificity of 86%.[10]

The future is bright for MR assessment of peripheral atherosclerotic disease. In addition to the direct visualization of the vessel wall and its components, which will likely soon be available in mainstream clinical practice, MR will increasingly be evaluated with use of metabolic and molecular tracers to assess this disease process at its earlier stages. Once disease is present, MR guidance for interventions will be an exciting development, providing a road map for the highly variant vessel anatomy without the need for ionizing radiation.

Nuclear Medicine/Positron Emission Tomography

Radionuclide techniques to evaluate noncoronary atherosclerotic disease currently have very limited clinical value. Positron emission tomography and single photon emission computed tomography can image both perfusion and metabolic abnormalities and provide a functional assessment of their disease in quantifiable fashion. Current research focuses on anatomic correlation with symptoms and outcomes. Muscle perfusion can be difficult to differentiate from skin perfusion.[28]

MRA, ultrasonography, and CTA can provide an assessment of localization and extent of disease with far more precision. They also have more background research to validate their findings and are often less expensive and faster. There are currently no clinical applications of metabolic imaging in noncoronary atherosclerosis, and promising agents, such as radiolabeled platelets and lipoproteins, have ongoing technical limitations. Ongoing research and technical advancement may identify relevant metabolic tracers and increase the role of these imaging modalities in the future.[28]

Angiography

Invasive catheter angiography has been widely available for a long time. It has been considered the gold standard for defining vascular anatomy and pathology. Digital subtraction angiography has intrinsic high resolution, and individual vessels can be selectively evaluated. Moreover, hemodynamic information can be captured to evaluate physiology, whereas it can be estimated only indirectly with noninvasive techniques. Bolus chasing, rapid acquisition of images, three-dimensional reconstruction, and smaller catheters have further improved the utility of digital subtraction angiography, which decreases the dose of contrast material, improves visualization of the vascular tree, and speeds acquisition time compared with conventional angiography.[15]

Although the safety profile has improved with further technologic refinements, this technique remains invasive with inherent risk of bleeding, vascular dissection, downstream thrombosis, and other complications. Moreover, it requires ionizing radiation and nephrotoxic contrast agents, which are avoided in many noninvasive techniques such as ultrasonography and MRI. For these reasons, other noninvasive techniques have been improved and have replaced angiography as the first-line diagnostic test for many indications. Angiography is now typically reserved for resolution of conflicting or inadequate noninvasive results and for therapeutic intervention.

Conventional cerebral angiography has been the gold standard to evaluate for carotid stenoses. It evaluates the entire carotid system and can provide important ancillary information, such as collateral flow. However, up to 77% of those evaluated for ischemic symptoms, even in the setting of stroke or transient ischemic attack, have absent disease, and angiography is associated with a small but significant risk of serious neurologic complications (up to 6%) and even death, especially in those at highest risk for cerebrovascular symptoms, such as those with hypertension, diabetes, PAD, and renal dysfunction. Moreover, because of the limited number of projections attainable, digital subtraction angiography can underestimate the degree of stenosis when eccentric plaques are present. For these reasons, angiography is considered only for patients with conflicting results or scheduled for therapeutic intervention. It also has advantages in the evaluation of suspected non-AVD, such as vasculitis. In the remainder of patients, ultrasonography, MRA, and CTA are preferentially used.

Likewise, in PAD, invasive angiography is typically reserved for those with conflicting or inconclusive noninvasive results, although it retains an ACC/AHA class I indication, especially in the setting of planned revascularization. Smaller catheters, improved access site choice (such as radial access), and closure device use have improved the safety of this procedure. It is important that suspected vessels be selectively imaged; this improves the overall accuracy and reduces the burden of contrast material. A complete study should include assessment of the major bifurcations in profile without vessel overlap (iliac, femoral, and tibial), and indeterminate lesions should have translesional pressure gradients measured (Fig. 88-8).[5] Although digital subtraction angiography has been traditionally used for preoperative evaluation, it has several important limitations, such as poor identification of distal vessels in the setting of critical limb ischemia and underestimation of eccentric lesions.

Conventional angiography is still frequently used in the assessment of renal artery stenosis because it can be performed as an adjunct assessment at the time of coronary or peripheral angiography. This is performed either through direct renal artery cannulation or "flush" aortography. In other settings, noninvasive testing is typically the first-line investigation, especially in patients at higher risk of complications, such as those with diabetes or renal disease. Contrast-induced renal failure occurs less than 3% of the time in patients without significant risk factors, 5% to 10% of the time in patients with diabetes or renal dysfunction, and in 10% to 50% of those with both comorbid conditions. Preprocedural oral administration of *N*-acetylcysteine may lower this risk to a small degree.

Invasive angiography is controversial in the setting of acute intestinal ischemia because it takes extra time that may be critical in determining the patient's outcome. In many instances, proceeding directly to exploratory laparotomy is the appropriate course. However, angiography detects arterial occlusion with high sensitivity (>90%) and

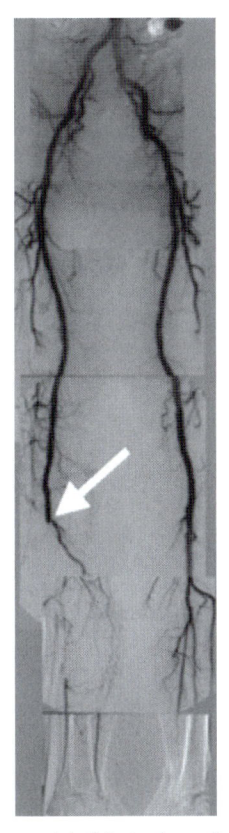

■ **FIGURE 88-8** Intra-arterial digital subtraction angiogram of a 65-year-old man with known peripheral arterial disease and pain-free walking distance of less than 200 m. Bilateral atherosclerotic changes and occlusion of the right tibioperoneal trunk (*arrow*) are apparent. (Reprinted with permission from Herborn CU, Goyen M, Quick HH, et al. Whole-body 3D MR angiography of patients with peripheral arterial occlusive disease. AJR Am J Roentgenol 2004; 182:1427.)

TABLE 88-4 Differential Diagnosis of Noncoronary Atherosclerotic Disease

Affected Arterial Bed	Differential Diagnosis*
Cerebrovascular arterial disease	Seizures (Todd paralysis) Migraine headaches Intracerebral hemorrhage Brain tumors Nonatherosclerotic syncope Multiple sclerosis Vestibulopathy Conversion disorder Metabolic disarray (hypoglycemia, acute renal failure)
Peripheral arterial disease	Nerve root compression Spinal stenosis Hip arthritis Arthritic or inflammatory foot processes Venous claudication
Renal arterial disease	Fibromuscular dysplasia Renal parenchymal disease Aortic coarctation Primary hyperaldosteronism Pheochromocytoma Medication effects
Abdominal aortic aneurysm and mesenteric arterial disease	Aortic dissection Vasculitis Peritonitis Mesenteric venous thrombosis Intestinal obstruction Pancreatitis Diverticulitis Biliary disease Inferior myocardial ischemia or infarction

*This list represents the most common alternative diagnoses. It is not exhaustive.

can assist in differentiating occlusive from nonocclusive disease and in presurgical planning.[29] Moreover, therapy in the form of intra-arterial vasodilators or thrombolytic therapy can be given, or thrombectomy devices can be deployed. This approach is best for patients who present long after symptom onset, with an unclear diagnosis, or with a high likelihood of nonocclusive disease. Angiography should not be used in those with concurrent hypotension or in the setting of vasopressors because these can falsely mimic nonocclusive disease. Moreover, beneficial vasodilators cannot be given in this circumstance.[29]

In chronic mesenteric ischemia, catheter angiography can display arterial obstruction in a fashion similar to that in the other arterial beds. An important caveat is that the majority of chronic mesenteric disease occurs at the origin of the major mesenteric arteries, such as the superior and inferior mesenteric arteries. Angiography may miss these lesions if the catheter is selectively engaged into the partially obstructed vessel. Lateral aortography can help display the origin of disease. In complete superior mesenteric artery origin occlusion, the entire vessel may not be seen, the "naked aorta" sign. A prominent meandering artery can represent an enlarged marginal artery of Drummond rather than chronic atherosclerotic disease.[29] As with invasive angiography in other arterial distributions, the limited projections of the mesenteric arteries obtained can lead to underestimation of eccentric vessels.

Differential Diagnosis

Clinical Presentation

The differential diagnosis for noncoronary atherosclerosis is broad and specific to the arterial bed affected (Table 88-4). Consideration of any possible alternative diagnoses is essential before further invasive testing or therapy is undertaken.

The key to differentiating cerebrovascular arterial disease from other intracranial processes is to determine the presence of positive symptoms (such as head jerking) and negative symptoms (such as motor or sensory deficits), their time at onset and duration, chronicity of spells occurring, and whether associated symptoms are present. This is often difficult, and further noninvasive imaging to define atherosclerotic disease combined with other tests, such as electroencephalography, is essential for a definitive diagnosis. For instance, seizures and migraine headaches often have associated positive symptoms that are rare with transient ischemic attacks or strokes from carotid or vertebrobasilar atherosclerotic disease.

Many disease processes involving the spinal cord or musculoskeletal system can have manifestations similar to claudication from PAD. The important differentiators are the location of the discomfort, the onset relative to exercise, and how the discomfort is ameliorated. Nerve root compression typically is manifested with sharp pain radiating down the leg. Spinal stenosis can occur just with standing and is relieved with leaning forward, hip arthritic pain can be present at rest, and venous claudication is usually associated with venous congestion and edema. Claudication rarely involves the foot, so processes isolated to this area usually represent another disease process.

Other forms of secondary hypertension can lead to the same refractory hypertensive state as with renal artery stenosis. Persistent high blood pressure eventually causes renal dysfunction, as do other forms of renal parenchymal disease. Fibromuscular dysplasia causes similar narrowing (although with a characteristic "beads on a string" appearance). However, patients with this disorder are typically younger with fewer cardiovascular risk factors.

AAAs and mesenteric ischemia both cause acute abdominal pain (during AAA rupture and acute mesenteric arterial occlusion) and chronic pain (AAA leakage and chronic mesenteric ischemia) that can have multiple potential causes, as listed in Table 88-2. Noninvasive imaging is essential to help narrow the differential and should be considered in those with a high risk of noncoronary atherosclerotic disease, as in those with multiple cardiovascular risk factors, especially advanced age, male gender, and ongoing tobacco use.

Imaging Findings

Obstructive lesions appreciated on ultrasonography, CTA, MRA, and invasive angiography typically represent atherosclerosis, especially with concurrent cardiovascular risk factors. Notable exceptions include fibromuscular dysplasia, although this typically affects the renal arteries throughout their course and has a unique appearance, and stenoses seen during assessment of the mesenteric arterial vasculature in the setting of pressor or peripheral vasoconstrictor use. These lesions may represent nonatherosclerotic vasoconstriction. Some noninvasive findings may be true but unrelated. A 4.5-cm AAA with no evidence of rupture or leakage is not likely to be the cause of severe, unremitting abdominal pain, and alternative diagnoses should be pursued.

Synopsis of Treatment Options
Medical

The treatment of noncoronary atherosclerosis varies by the vascular bed affected, but the general treatment principles remain the same: aggressive risk factor control to reduce the risk of cardiovascular events and those specific to the involved vessel territory, and specific therapy to address symptoms and functional status.

Cerebrovascular Atherosclerotic Disease

The primary medical therapy for cerebrovascular atherosclerotic disease (primarily carotid and vertebrobasilar disease) involves antihypertensive, lipid-lowering, and antiplatelet medications.

Blood pressure–lowering agents have been shown to dramatically reduce the risk of stroke in both primary and secondary prevention settings. A meta-analysis of randomized controlled trials showed that antihypertensives, including diuretics and β blockers, reduced stroke risk by approximately 40%. The Heart Outcomes Prevention Evaluation (HOPE) and Perindopril Protection Against Recurrent Stroke Study (PROGRESS) trials showed that angiotensin-converting enzyme inhibitors reduce the risk of stroke by 32% to 43% because of both the blood pressure–lowering effect and possibly an independent pathway.

Lipid-lowering therapy is also essential to slow the rate of progression of atherosclerosis and potentially to stabilize plaques. Pravastatin has been shown to reduce stroke risk by 32% and 19% in the Cholesterol and Recurrent Events (CARE) and Long-Term Intervention with Pravastatin in Ischemic Disease (LIPID) trials, respectively. Simvastatin lowered stroke risk by 23% and 25% in the Scandinavian Simvastatin Survival Study (4S) and Heart Protection Study (a study of high-risk patients with atherosclerosis or diabetes), respectively. The remaining statins are thought to have similar benefits through a class effect.

Antiplatelet medications form the third mainstay of therapy. A meta-analysis of 287 trials with 135,000 high-risk patients showed a 22% reduction in stroke with an antiplatelet regimen. Aspirin reduces adverse cardiovascular risk 23% irrespective of its dose. Thienopyridines have an incremental benefit over aspirin (12% odds reduction) as shown in the Ticlopidine Aspirin Stroke Study (TASS) and Clopidogrel versus Aspirin in Patients at Risk of Ischemic Events (CAPRIE) trials with ticlopidine and clopidogrel. Aspirin plus extended-release dipyridamole is just as effective as aspirin alone for reducing death and nonfatal stroke, but a clear benefit over aspirin is debatable after studies with conflicting findings. There is no benefit to warfarin and increased bleeding risk in this clinical situation.

Peripheral Atherosclerotic Disease

The medical management of PAD revolves around two primary goals: (1) risk reduction targeting both cardiac complications and those of the peripheral arterial bed; and (2) management of symptoms and functional status.

PAD is considered a cardiovascular disease risk equivalent, and treatment targets the same medication classes as for other noncoronary atherosclerotic disease: lipid-lowering, antihypertensive, and antiplatelet medications. Patients with PAD should meet the current Joint National Commission hypertension guidelines, which suggest a goal of below 140/90 mm Hg for all patients and below 130/80 mm Hg for those with diabetes or advanced renal disease. Certain classes have been shown to have beneficial effects in addition to their blood pressure–lowering effect. β Blockers reduce MI and death for patients with CAD and prior MI and should be used because they do not reduce walking capacity as previously thought. Angiotensin-converting enzyme inhibitors are also recommended (class IIa); ramipril was studied in the HOPE trial in 4000 patients with PAD and reduced cardiovascular death, nonfatal MI, and stroke by 22%.[5,30] Additional antihypertensives can be added as necessary to achieve goal blood pressure.

Lipid-lowering therapy is another essential component to retard the progression of atherosclerosis. Statins are the definitive first-line therapy and should be used in all patients with PAD unless an allergy or other contraindication exists. The Heart Protection Study included patients with atherosclerosis, many of whom had PAD, and showed a 25% reduction in cardiac events and overall mortality with titration of simvastatin to achieve the National Cholesterol Eduction Program goal LDL of less than 100 mg/dL.[30] Use of statins to attain this goal has an ACC/AHA class I indication; a goal of less than 70 mg/dL is appropriate, especially in patients with multiple or poorly controlled risk factors (class IIa).[5] Patients who require additional LDL lowering despite maximum-tolerated statin use can benefit from niacin therapy, although flushing and sweats can limit the tolerability of this medication. Niacin also assists in raising the HDL level, low values of which are a known independent risk factor for cardiac events. Finally, fibric acid derivatives are beneficial for those with high triglyceride levels, especially in the setting of low HDL level. One study of patients with low HDL levels and CAD showed a 22% reduction in cardiovascular death and nonfatal MI.

Antiplatelet therapy is the third essential drug class that lowers cardiac and vascular events; a meta-analysis of 9716 patients in 42 trials showed a 23% odds reduction. Low- and high-dose aspirin decreases the risk of events. Clopidogrel, an ADP receptor antagonist, is even more effective, leading to a 24% reduction in risk of MI, stroke, or vascular death in patients with PAD compared with aspirin therapy. Both of these therapies have ACC/AHA class I indications for use in PAD. Combination therapy is under further investigation. Oral anticoagulants have minimal increased benefit and an increased bleeding risk and are contraindicated without an additional appropriate indication.

Intensive control of other significant comorbid conditions, such as renal disease and diabetes, can markedly reduce events. The U. K. Prospective Diabetes Study (UKPDS) trial showed a 42% reduction in the risk of cardiac events with a goal A_{1c} of 7% or less. An unpowered secondary analysis showed a nonsignificant 35% reduction in the risk of amputation or death in patients with PAD. Foot care is especially important in patients with PAD, with frequent professional assessment, prompt care for skin breaks, and frequent washing and complete drying.

Lifestyle changes have an essential role in PAD therapy, the most important of which is tobacco cessation. Physician counseling is effective, leading to a 50-fold increase in 1-year cessation rates (increase from 0.1% to 5%). The addition of nicotine replacement therapy increases the 1-year success rate to 16% and of bupropion to 30%.[5] Weight reduction, especially waist circumference, and regular exercise are also critical.

The second key to PAD medical therapy is symptom control and preservation of and improvement in functional status. Exercise is especially important for these two goals. A meta-analysis of supervised exercise rehabilitation showed a more than 180% increase in walking time with just 30 minutes three times weekly. Exercise outside of structured programs does not have well-established benefit but is certainly expected to improve symptoms and function.

Cilostazol is a phosphodiesterase type 3 inhibitor that improves treadmill time and quality of life. A meta-analysis of six trials showed an improved pain-free walking distance of 30% to 60%. Cilostazol is contraindicated in heart failure. Pentoxifylline (a methylxanthine derivative), L-arginine, propionyl-L-carnitine, and gingko biloba are less effective and not used as frequently. Chelation therapy, vitamin E, and prostaglandins such as iloprost have class III indications.[5] Critical limb ischemia is a surgical condition. There is no clear benefit to the parenteral administration of pentoxifylline or prostaglandins.

Aortic Atherosclerotic Disease

Aneurysms are the primary manifestation of aortic atherosclerotic disease, most commonly in the descending aorta. Close surveillance and surgical intervention when the aneurysms reach the appropriate size are the primary treatment options. However, medical therapy is essential to slow the progression and to reduce the risk of rupture. Despite its importance, no specific therapy has been shown to reduce the rate of aneurysm growth.

The greatest risk factors for rupture include tobacco use and uncontrolled hypertension. Ongoing tobacco use increases the aneurysm growth rate by 20% to 25% and significantly increases the risk of rupture. Cessation advice and assistance with psychotropic medication, nicotine replacement, and adjunctive pharmacotherapy are given a class I indication in this setting per the ACC/AHA 2005 guidelines.[5]

Although the effects of dyslipidemia and less severe hypertension are not fully known, the ACC/AHA guidelines suggest treatment of aortic atherosclerotic disease as a CAD risk equivalent. Although there is debate about whether statins retard aneurysm progression, these guidelines suggest that all such patients should be receiving a statin regardless. β Blockers are also recommended under these guidelines; they also may slow aneurysm progression, although a randomized controlled trial did not show significant benefit.

Renal Atherosclerotic Disease

The medical treatment of renal atherosclerotic disease involves both control of the disease process itself and treatment of the resultant complications. Aggressive atherosclerotic risk factor control is necessary to attempt to slow the progression of renal atherosclerosis as for other arterial beds.

Resistant, severe hypertension and progressive renal function decline are the two primary complications of renal atherosclerotic disease and stem from renal artery stenosis. Angiotensin-converting enzyme inhibitors, angiotensin receptor blockers, calcium channel blockers, and β blockers have all been shown to have some effect on renal artery stenosis–associated hypertension. Both angiotensin-converting enzyme inhibitors and angiotension receptor blockers have been shown to slow the decline in renal function.[5]

Mesenteric Atherosclerotic Disease

Acute mesenteric ischemia and infarction require prompt surgical intervention. Medical therapy is often supportive, involving gastric decompression, hemodynamic support, aggressive intravenous antibiotics, and correction of metabolic acidosis.

Thrombolytic therapy is rarely given and can be used only within 8 hours of abdominal pain onset with no clinical evidence of bowel necrosis or other lytic contraindications. In rare circumstances, intravenous heparin and continuous papaverine infusion (a potent vasodilator) can be used with close monitoring. In this situation, the risks of bleeding versus the antiplatelet benefits of aspirin should be carefully considered. Long-term aspirin use can reduce the risk of recurrent ischemia in the setting of acute or chronic ischemia.

Surgical/Interventional

Because of the high rates of cardiovascular comorbidity in patients with noncoronary atherosclerosis, medical therapy is preferred if symptoms and future events can be adequately controlled. In some cases, revascularization is necessary. Given surgical risks and improving technique and technology, there has been a shift toward percutaneous approaches. Choices of revascularization therapy vary by vascular bed affected.

Cerebrovascular Atherosclerotic Disease

Carotid endarterectomy (CEA) is the primary surgical technique for carotid stenoses. It is currently the primary option for revascularization but remains imperfect, with a 3% to 7.4% surgical complication rate. Individuals with symptoms and carotid stenoses of 70% to 99% were found to have a 2.9 relative risk reduction in ipsilateral stroke with CEA compared with medical therapy at 2 years in the North American Symptomatic Carotid Endarterectomy Trial (NASCET). A Department of Veterans Affairs Cooperative Studies trial likewise showed a 3.4 relative risk reduction.[31]

The role of CEA in patients with asymptomatic significant carotid stenoses is controversial. One randomized controlled trial (Asymptomatic Carotid Artery Stenosis [ACAS] trial) found a 53% relative risk reduction in ipsilateral stroke or periprocedural stroke or death for CEA plus optimal medical therapy versus optimal medical therapy alone. The Asymptomatic Carotid Surgery Trial (ACST) showed a similar 46% relative risk reduction in stroke or periprocedural death at 5 years. However, optimal medical therapy at this time did not include statins and the goals of therapy were less aggressive. Careful selection of patients is imperative in this group.

Because of the high risk of CEA, percutaneous revascularization options are undergoing intensive investigation, but their use remains in a state of evolution. Stenting has supplanted angioplasty alone because this technique is not as effective as CEA. The multiple trials examining percutaneous stenting versus CEA have conflicting noninferiority data, and there is no evidence of long-term efficacy with stenting. Small studies with short-term follow-up have shown benefit comparable to that with CEA, with a marginally higher restenosis rate (3% to 4% versus 1%, respectively). Whereas percutaneous revascularization techniques and outcomes data are improved, the American Heart Association/American Stroke Association 2006 guidelines recommend this approach only in patients at high operative risk for CEA, especially those with early post-CEA restenosis or radiation-induced stenosis.[32] Aggressive antiplatelet therapy is especially important in those receiving carotid stents.

Peripheral Atherosclerotic Disease

Revascularization is an important adjunctive therapy in patients with PAD and can be accomplished by endovascular techniques including percutaneous transluminal angioplasty (PTA) and surgical bypass. Unlike with coronary obstruction, revascularization is indicated only in patients with symptoms that induce significant lifestyle or vocational disability and have a reasonable likelihood of improvement with restoration of blood flow. Moreover, intermediate lesions should be evaluated with translesional pressure gradients with and without vasodilation.

Revascularization in patients without symptoms to prevent critical limb ischemia and intervention on lesions without significant pressure gradients are both contraindicated (class III in the ACC/AHA guidelines).[5] Claudication does not often progress to critical limb ischemia. There are limited randomized trial data comparing revascularization to medical therapy.

The location of obstructive atherosclerotic disease and lesion characteristics dictate the form of revascularization. The type of revascularization determines the operative mortality and patency rates (Table 88-5). Focal aortic disease may be treated with surgery or PTA with or without stenting; surgery is recommended for aortic

TABLE 88-5 Vascular Surgical and Percutaneous Transluminal Angioplasty Revascularization Procedure Success and Mortality Rates

Surgical Procedure	Operative Mortality Rate (%)	Expected Patency Rate (%)
Aortobifemoral bypass	3.3	87.5 (5 years)
Aortoiliac or aortofemoral bypass	1-2	85-90 (5 years)
Iliac endarterectomy	0	79-90 (5 years)
Femorofemoral bypass	6	71 (5 years)
Axillofemoral bypass	6	49-80 (3 years)
Axillofemoral-femoral bypass	4.9	63-67.7 (5 years)
Percutaneous transluminal angioplasty or stenting		
Iliac focal stenosis or occlusion	1	60-80 (4-5 years)
With stent placed	—	74 (4 years)
Venous bypass graft stenosis	—	60 (1-3 years)
Femoral-popliteal stenosis	<1	70 (4-5 years)
With stent placed	—	43 (3 years)

Modified from Kandarpa K, Becker GJ, Hunink MG, et al. Transcatheter interventions for the treatment of peripheral atherosclerotic lesions: part I. J Vasc Interv Radiol 2001; 12:683.

disease that extends into the iliac arteries. In the iliac system, surgery is the preferred treatment of long or irregular stenoses or occlusions. PTA has an ACC/AHA class I indication for shorter stenoses or focal occlusions. The patency is 60% to 80% at 4 to 5 years. Patency rates are slightly higher with surgery, but the increased cost and perioperative risk of surgery make PTA safer and less expensive even if repeated revascularization is required. PTA has 1- to 3-year patency rates of 60% for single venous bypass graft stenoses, but this drops to 6% with multigraft involvement.[31] There are limited data suggesting that stenting may be better in the iliac system, and stenting is preferred for lesions of 2.0 cm or larger. The use of drug-eluting stents is not well studied. Stents are recommended in all vessel distributions for salvage therapy.

In the femoral-popliteal area, surgery has good outcomes data. The use of PTA is controversial, but patency rates are as high as 70% at 4 to 5 years. Stents are likely to worsen prognosis, especially in patients with poor distal runoff, probably because of distal embolization, and are contraindicated under the current ACC/AHA guidelines.[5]

There are insufficient data to recommend PTA versus surgical bypass for disease inferior to the popliteal arteries, including the tibial and peroneal arteries. More research is necessary for these sorts of lesions. Comorbid conditions such as diabetes, renal failure, and ongoing tobacco use decrease the benefit of percutaneous approaches and can influence decision-making. PTA is relatively contraindicated for lesions with dense calcification because there is a significant risk of downstream embolization. On the other hand, surgery should generally be avoided in those younger than 50 years who present with aggressive atherosclerotic occlusive disease; surgery has limited durable response in this population.

Aortic Atherosclerotic Disease

Medical therapy is essential to help slow the progression of aortic atherosclerotic disease. However, surgical repair remains the mainstay of therapy for the major complications of aortic atherosclerotic disease, aortic aneurysms and dissections.

Although adjustments for age, gender, and body surface area are necessary, an anteroposterior diameter of 3.0 cm or more is considered diagnostic of an AAA; this exceeds the 95th percentile for size regardless of these variables.

Aortic aneurysms can lead to thromboembolic ischemic events and impinge on neighboring structures, but the primary concern is the risk for rupture. Properly timed, elective intervention is critical for AAAs; repair in this setting has an improving mortality rate of approximately 5% compared with up to 50% during aortic leakage or rupture. Given this dramatic increase in mortality, all symptomatic patients should undergo repair immediately, regardless of aneurysm diameter. For asymptomatic patients, surgical decision-making is based on the risk/benefit ratio of procedural morbidity versus likelihood of rupture, which is directly related to the maximal diameter, rate of expansion, and gender of the patient.[5]

Aneurysm diameter is the primary determinant of appropriate surgical timing. The risk of rupture for aneurysms smaller than 4 cm is quite low, and surgery can be avoided as these patients often die of the complications of comorbid cardiopulmonary disease. However, an analysis of 10 major studies shows an eventual rupture risk for larger aneurysms that increases from 20% for aneurysm diameter of more than 5 cm to 50% for those of more than 7 cm. Monitoring with serial ultrasound studies or computed tomography is recommended every 2 to 3 years for aneurysms smaller than 4 cm and every 6 to 12 months for those 4.0 to 5.4 cm.

Two major trials show no benefit to surgery for aneurysms with a diameter of less than 5.5 cm. Thus, the current recommendation is to repair those with a diameter of 5.5 cm or more (class I indication).[5] AAAs located above the renal arteries have a slightly higher rate of complications, such as acute renal failure and death, and may either be repaired or watched between 5.5 and 6.0 cm. Growth rates above 7 to 8 mm yearly or a diameter two times the size of the largest normal segment should prompt consideration of repair. Given the higher rate of rupture in women (up to four times greater), the American Association for Vascular Surgery recommends consideration of elective repair for aneurysms with diameters as small as 4.5 cm in women.[33]

Percutaneous endograft placement has become a viable alternative to open repair. The morbidity and mortality with this procedure are currently equivalent to those of open repair. There is an acceptably low risk of rupture but no cost savings because the need for reintervention remains high. Moreover, long-term outcomes with endografts are not known. However, endografting may be beneficial for those with excessive risk of complications during open surgical repair. Thus, open repair is currently recommended unless a high risk for complications is present.

Repair of thoracic aortic aneurysms has a higher risk of morbidity and mortality, which makes medical and percutaneous therapy preferential. Endografts are not currently available for this clinical scenario.

Renal Atherosclerotic Disease

Revascularization of renal artery stenosis secondary to atherosclerotic disease can be attained with both percutaneous and surgical approaches. Revascularization is not currently recommended for asymptomatic renal artery stenosis with no evidence of end-organ dysfunction. The ACC/AHA 2005 guidelines give revascularization a class I indication for recurrent unexplained congestive heart failure or flash pulmonary edema.[5] The goal of intervention in this instance is to reverse the persistent activation of the renin-angiotensin system and progressive renal functional deterioration that lead to volume expansion and intolerance to angiotensin-converting enzyme inhibitors and angiotension receptor blockers.

Revascularization receives class IIa indications for control of resistant, rapidly accelerating, or malignant hypertension and for preservation of renal function in patients with bilateral renal artery stenosis or a solitary affected kidney. In the seven studies addressing hypertension in renal artery stenosis, there was a 50% to 75% improvement in hypertension control rate with a resultant decrease in the number of medications required and their doses. However, cure is rare, occurring in only 1% to 19%

of patients, and up to 40% receive no clinical benefit. Moreover, restenosis is a common problem.

Several trials document improvement or stabilization of renal function with percutaneous or surgical correction of renal artery stenosis. However, a significant change in glomerular filtration rate is not typically seen in those with unilateral renal artery stenosis after revascularization, and more research is needed to further define its role in the preservation of renal function.

Surgical or percutaneous intervention may be considered (class IIb indication) for those with unilateral renal artery stenosis and worsening renal function or angina. Correction of renal artery stenosis has been shown to control angina in 88% of patients, presumably because of the decrease in peripheral vasoconstriction and resultant myocardial oxygen demand. With these specific exceptions, aggressive medical therapy remains the primary approach for renal atherosclerotic disease.

Mesenteric Atherosclerotic Disease

The therapy for mesenteric ischemia depends on the acuity of the presentation. Acute mesenteric ischemia frequently leads to sepsis, bowel infarction, and death, making early diagnosis and treatment imperative. Patients with suspected perforation or gangrene should go directly to surgery. Surgical arterial reconstruction involves bypass grafting, local or transaortic endarterectomy, and resection of nonviable bowel segments. These approaches have a 79% 5-year symptom-free survival but very high surgical mortality rate (approximately 70%).[5,34] Repeated laparotomy at 24 to 48 hours can be beneficial to ensure that no infarcted bowel remains.

Given the high surgical mortality, percutaneous approaches can be considered (class IIb in the 2005 ACC/AHA guidelines).[5] However, most patients still require laparotomy because of infarcted bowel, and percutaneous approaches are difficult because the most common site of involvement is at the origin of the major splanchnic vessels and often involves more than one artery. Moreover, in patients with a high degree of damage, restoration of flow can release dangerous endotoxins that can be controlled with surgery but not with percutaneous therapy. However, a percutaneous approach may reduce the magnitude of a dangerous surgery and should thus be considered.

For chronic mesenteric ischemia, either surgical or percutaneous therapy with angioplasty with or without stenting can be considered. There are limited data to compare the two modalities, and the availability and expertise of local vascular surgeons or interventional radiologists influence therapeutic decision-making. Because of the high coprevalence of significant cardiopulmonary conditions, percutaneous approaches are generally preferred except in younger patients with fewer comorbid conditions or in the setting of multiple obstructed vessels or limited vascular access. Given the high operative mortality (up to 11%), surgical therapy is not appropriate for patients with asymptomatic intestinal arterial obstructions unless aortic or renal artery surgery is planned for other indications.

Angioplasty has an 80% technical success rate, with an 80% rate of clinical remission at 2 to 3 years. Although there is a high rate of restenosis (27% to 46% during 1 to 3 years), recurrent obstruction can generally be resolved with additional percutaneous therapy. Although there has been little formal evaluation of stenting, use of stents appears to be at least as effective as primary angioplasty and may reduce the high recurrence rate.[5]

Surgical approaches include bypass grafting (most commonly used), endarterectomy, and reimplantation. The choice of procedure should be guided by the expertise of the individual surgeon as trials have not shown clear superiority of any technique. Revascularization is successful in 98% to 100% of patients, with lower 1- to 3-year recurrence rates of 19% to 24% compared with percutaneous therapy.[5] Regardless of the choice of revascularization technique, close follow-up is essential.

Reporting: Information for the Referring Physician

A full discussion of the specific recommendations for reporting lesions in each arterial bed is beyond the scope of this chapter. However, in screening for or evaluating the symptoms of atherosclerosis, there are several key factors that should be considered. A critical focus should be on the overall presence or absence of atherosclerotic disease, not only to screen for or assess the symptoms of disease in the specific arterial territory but also as a reflection of disease in the coronary system. The presence of noncoronary atherosclerotic disease increases the risk of comorbid CAD by many times, and CAD leads to high morbidity and mortality. Moreover, the presence of atherosclerosis in any arterial bed leads to significant increases in the intensity of risk factor reduction required, especially when other atherosclerotic disease has not previously been identified. The amount of atherosclerosis present is also important to characterize, even if it is not in the form of significant obstructive lesions because a higher burden of disease further increases cardiovascular event rates.

KEY POINTS

- Noncoronary atherosclerotic disease carries a high morbidity and mortality, both from the arterial bed affected and from comorbid coronary artery disease.
- A careful, detailed history and physical examination and a high degree of suspicion are the only ways to adequately assess these often silent or misclassified disease processes.
- Noninvasive modalities have become sufficient for initial and often definitive evaluation of noncoronary atherosclerotic disease without the need for invasive testing.
- CTA provides exquisite resolution but has ionizing radiation and exposure to nephrotoxic contrast agents. MRA avoids these issues but has limited, non–contrast-enhanced use for those with significant renal dysfunction because of the risk of nephrogenic systemic fibrosis with gadolinium.
- Highly effective surgical and percutaneous techniques are available for revascularization, but the key to the treatment of noncoronary atherosclerotic disease is aggressive secondary risk factor reduction with tight blood pressure and lipid control and antiplatelet therapy.

SUGGESTED READINGS

Faxon DP, Creager MA, Smith SC Jr, et al. Atherosclerotic Vascular Disease Conference: Executive summary: Atherosclerotic Vascular Disease Conference proceeding for healthcare professionals from a special writing group of the American Heart Association. Circulation 2004; 109:2595.

Kim AY, Ha HK. Evaluation of suspected mesenteric ischemia: efficacy of radiologic studies. Radiol Clin North Am 2003; 41:327.

Kramer CM, Anderson JD. MRI of atherosclerosis: diagnosis and monitoring therapy. Expert Rev Cardiovasc Ther 2007; 5:69.

Redberg RF, Vogel RA, Criqui MH, et al. 34th Bethesda Conference: Task force #3—What is the spectrum of current and emerging techniques for the noninvasive measurement of atherosclerosis? J Am Coll Cardiol 2003; 41:1886.

Ross R. Atherosclerosis—an inflammatory disease. N Engl J Med 1999; 340:115.

Stein JH, Korcarz CE, Hurst RT, et al. Use of carotid ultrasound to identify subclinical vascular disease and evaluate cardiovascular disease risk: a consensus statement from the American Society of Echocardiography Carotid Intima-Media Thickness Task Force. Endorsed by the Society for Vascular Medicine. J Am Soc Echocardiogr 2008; 21:93.

REFERENCES

1. Faxon DP, Creager MA, Smith SC Jr, et al. Atherosclerotic Vascular Disease Conference: Executive summary: Atherosclerotic Vascular Disease Conference proceeding for healthcare professionals from a special writing group of the American Heart Association. Circulation 2004; 109:2595.
2. Rosamond W, Flegal K, Friday G, et al. Heart disease and stroke statistics—2007 update: a report from the American Heart Association Statistics Committee and Stroke Statistics Subcommittee. Circulation 2007; 115:e69.
3. Atherosclerosis. The American Heritage Dictionary of the English Language, 4th ed. Boston, Houghton Mifflin, 2004.
4. Pasternak RC, Criqui MH, Benjamin EJ, et al. Atherosclerotic Vascular Disease Conference: Writing Group I: epidemiology. Circulation 2004; 109:2605.
5. Hirsch AT, Haskal ZJ, Hertzer NR, et al. ACC/AHA 2005 guidelines for the management of patients with peripheral arterial disease (lower extremity, renal, mesenteric, and abdominal aortic): executive summary a collaborative report from the American Association for Vascular Surgery/Society for Vascular Surgery, Society for Cardiovascular Angiography and Interventions, Society for Vascular Medicine and Biology, Society of Interventional Radiology, and the ACC/AHA Task Force on Practice Guidelines (Writing Committee to Develop Guidelines for the Management of Patients With Peripheral Arterial Disease) endorsed by the American Association of Cardiovascular and Pulmonary Rehabilitation; National Heart, Lung, and Blood Institute; Society for Vascular Nursing; TransAtlantic Inter-Society Consensus; and Vascular Disease Foundation. J Am Coll Cardiol 2006; 47:1239.
6. Kalra PA, Guo H, Kausz AT, et al. Atherosclerotic renovascular disease in United States patients aged 67 years or older: risk factors, revascularization, and prognosis. Kidney Int 2005; 68:293.
7. Ross R. Atherosclerosis—an inflammatory disease. N Engl J Med 1999; 340:115.
8. Mallika V, Goswami B, Rajappa M. Atherosclerosis pathophysiology and the role of novel risk factors: a clinicobiochemical perspective. Angiology 2007; 58:513.
9. Smith SC Jr, Milani RV, Arnett DK, et al. Atherosclerotic Vascular Disease Conference: Writing Group II: risk factors. Circulation 2004; 109:2613.
10. Price JF, Mowbray PI, Lee AJ, et al. Relationship between smoking and cardiovascular risk factors in the development of peripheral arterial disease and coronary artery disease: Edinburgh Artery Study. Eur Heart J 1999; 20:344.
11. Goldstein LB, Adams R, Alberts MJ, et al. Primary prevention of ischemic stroke: a guideline from the American Heart Association/American Stroke Association Stroke Council: cosponsored by the Atherosclerotic Peripheral Vascular Disease Interdisciplinary Working Group; Cardiovascular Nursing Council; Clinical Cardiology Council; Nutrition, Physical Activity, and Metabolism Council; and the Quality of Care and Outcomes Research Interdisciplinary Working Group. Circulation 2006; 113:e873.
12. Peripheral arterial disease in people with diabetes. Diabetes Care 2003; 26:3333.
13. Stein JH, Korcarz CE, Hurst RT, et al. Use of carotid ultrasound to identify subclinical vascular disease and evaluate cardiovascular disease risk: a consensus statement from the American Society of Echocardiography Carotid Intima-Media Thickness Task Force. Endorsed by the Society for Vascular Medicine. J Am Soc Echocardiogr 2008; 21:93.
14. Auerbach EG, Martin ET. Magnetic resonance imaging of the peripheral vasculature. Am Heart J 2004; 148:755.
15. Olin JW, Kaufman JA, Bluemke DA, et al. Atherosclerotic Vascular Disease Conference: Writing Group IV: imaging. Circulation 2004; 109:2626.
16. Vogt MT, Cauley JA, Newman AB, et al. Decreased ankle/arm blood pressure index and mortality in elderly women. JAMA 1993; 270:465.
17. Errington ML, Ferguson JM, Gillespie IN, et al. Complete pre-operative imaging assessment of abdominal aortic aneurysm with spiral CT angiography. Clin Radiol 1997; 52:369.
18. Petersen MJ, Cambria RP, Kaufman JA, et al. Magnetic resonance angiography in the preoperative evaluation of abdominal aortic aneurysms. J Vasc Surg 1995; 21:891.
19. Tan KT, van Beek EJ, Brown PW, et al. Magnetic resonance angiography for the diagnosis of renal artery stenosis: a meta-analysis. Clin Radiol 2002; 57:617.
20. Zwolak RM, Fillinger MF, Walsh DB, et al. Mesenteric and celiac duplex scanning: a validation study. J Vasc Surg 1998; 27:1078.
21. Zandrino F, Musante F, Gallesio I, et al. Assessment of patients with acute mesenteric ischemia: multislice computed tomography signs and clinical performance in a group of patients with surgical correlation. Minerva Gastroenterol Dietol 2006; 52:317.
22. Meaney JF, Prince MR, Nostrant TT, et al. Gadolinium-enhanced MR angiography of visceral arteries in patients with suspected chronic mesenteric ischemia. J Magn Reson Imaging 1997; 7:171.
23. Redberg RF, Vogel RA, Criqui MH, et al. 34th Bethesda Conference: Task force #3—What is the spectrum of current and emerging techniques for the noninvasive measurement of atherosclerosis? J Am Coll Cardiol 2003; 41:1886.
24. Lorenz MW, Markus HS, Bots ML, et al. Prediction of clinical cardiovascular events with carotid intima-media thickness: a systematic review and meta-analysis. Circulation 2007; 115:459.
25. Neunteufl T, Heher S, Katzenschlager R, et al. Late prognostic value of flow-mediated dilation in the brachial artery of patients with chest pain. Am J Cardiol 2000; 86:207.
26. Kramer CM, Anderson JD. MRI of atherosclerosis: diagnosis and monitoring therapy. Expert Rev Cardiovasc Ther 2007; 5:69.
27. Kim AY, Ha HK. Evaluation of suspected mesenteric ischemia: efficacy of radiologic studies. Radiol Clin North Am 2003; 41:327.
28. Wolfram RM, Budinsky AC, Sinzinger H. Assessment of peripheral arterial vascular disease with radionuclide techniques. Semin Nucl Med 2001; 31:129.
29. Martinez JP, Hogan GJ. Mesenteric ischemia. Emerg Med Clin North Am 2004; 22:909.
30. Creager MA, Jones DW, Easton JD, et al. Atherosclerotic Vascular Disease Conference: Writing Group V: medical decision making and therapy. Circulation 2004; 109:2634.
31. Bettmann MA, Dake MD, Hopkins LN, et al. Atherosclerotic Vascular Disease Conference: Writing Group VI: revascularization. Circulation 2004; 109:2643.

32. Sacco RL, Adams R, Albers G, et al. Guidelines for prevention of stroke in patients with ischemic stroke or transient ischemic attack: a statement for healthcare professionals from the American Heart Association/American Stroke Association Council on Stroke: cosponsored by the Council on Cardiovascular Radiology and Intervention: the American Academy of Neurology affirms the value of this guideline. Stroke 2006; 37:577.

33. Brewster DC, Cronenwett JL, Hallett JW Jr, et al. Guidelines for the treatment of abdominal aortic aneurysms. Report of a subcommittee of the Joint Council of the American Association for Vascular Surgery and Society for Vascular Surgery. J Vasc Surg 2003; 37:1106.

34. Cho JS, Carr JA, Jacobsen G, et al. Long-term outcome after mesenteric artery reconstruction: a 37-year experience. J Vasc Surg 2002; 35:453.

PART FIFTEEN

The Carotid Arteries

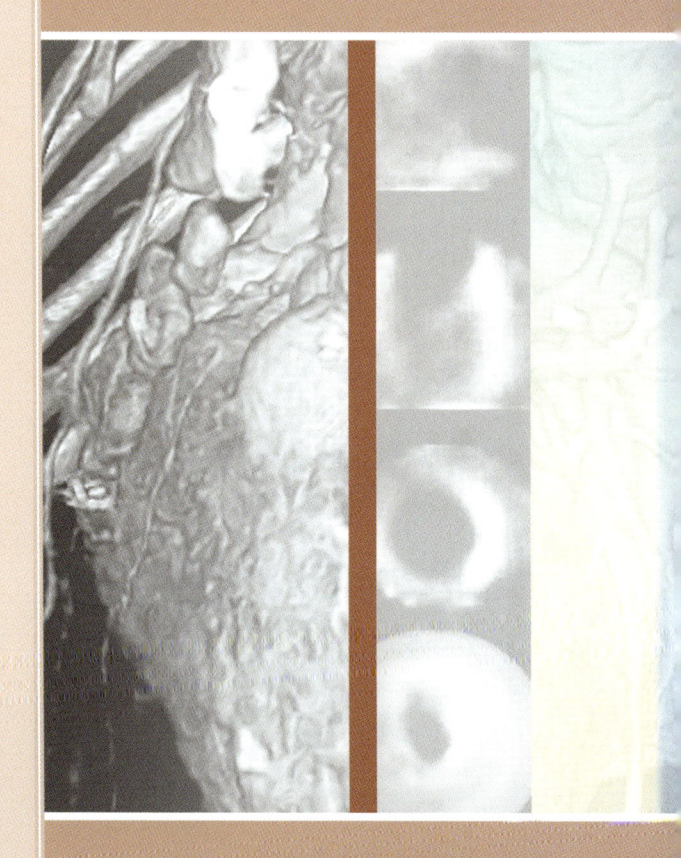

CHAPTER 89

Carotid Artery Disease

Brajesh K. Lal and Thomas G. Brott

The ancient Greeks believed that compression of the carotid artery caused sudden sleep (*karoo,* "to stupefy"). Ambroise Paré later named these arteries "the right and left carotides or sleepy vessels" in the 16th century.[1] In 1914, J. Ramsay Hunt noted that partial or complete occlusion of the carotid artery could be responsible for "cerebral intermittent claudication."[1] In 1935, Aring clarified the differences between brain hemorrhages and infarctions in autopsy cases. The notion that carotid artery occlusive disease can produce a dementia state was proposed soon thereafter.[1] It was postulated that restoration of blood supply could reverse the condition. This inspired the first carotid reconstruction (1951) by Carrea, Molins, and Murphy in Argentina.[1] They performed an anastomosis of the distal internal carotid artery to the external carotid artery after partial resection of a stenosed internal carotid artery. Although DeBakey is credited with performing the first carotid endarterectomy (CEA), the report in 1954 by Eastcott, Pickering, and Rob of a successful carotid reconstruction in a woman after acute stroke provided a major impetus for operative intervention in carotid occlusive disease and introduced CEA as an important procedure in the management of stroke.[1] In the ensuing decades, atherosclerotic carotid occlusive disease has been recognized as, by far, the most common disorder affecting the extracranial carotid artery and has become one of the most intensively studied of vascular diseases. Treatment decisions are appropriately guided by several randomized trials and additional well-designed large cohort studies.

CAROTID ARTERY STENOSIS

Definition

The principal arterial blood supply to the head and neck is from the right common carotid artery originating from the innominate artery, the left common carotid artery arising from the aortic arch, and the two vertebral arteries with origins at the subclavian arteries. Intracranial collateralization between the carotid and vertebral systems is based on the circle of Willis, which becomes an important route of collateral blood flow when the internal carotid artery is occluded. The "classic" complete circle of Willis, however, is present in only about 60% of the population. When the internal carotid artery is occluded, alternative collaterals through the external carotid artery and ophthalmic artery may fill the distal intracranial internal carotid artery. The obvious other collateral is the contralateral internal carotid artery, which supplies the circle of Willis and, through it, the opposite internal carotid artery. The adequacy of collateralization is a major determinant of the occurrence and severity of stroke in the presence of unilateral internal carotid artery occlusion.

Prevalence and Epidemiology

Stroke is the third leading cause of death in the United States. Each year, 600,000 patients suffer a new stroke, and 170,000 deaths per year are attributable to cerebrovascular disease.[2] Stroke is also the leading cause of disability among elderly Americans. Although there has been a 50% reduction in mortality during the last two decades, 21% of survivors will still have a second stroke and 7% a third stroke. Forty percent will require special nursing home care; 10% will require institutionalization involving an expenditure of billions of dollars of the health care budget.[2]

About one third of strokes are thromboembolic in etiology, and atherosclerotic carotid occlusive disease is the most common single cause. The extent to which carotid stenosis or occlusion can be attributed to stroke has been difficult to determine from population studies. Between 1993 and 1997, the Northern Manhattan Study identified cerebral infarction attributable to carotid stenosis in 17 (95% CI, 8 to 26) per 100,000 blacks, 9 (5 to 13) per 100,000 Hispanics, and 5 per 100,000 (2 to 8) whites.[3] Approximately 7% of all first ischemic strokes occurred in the presence of extracranial carotid artery stenosis of 60% or more. Between 1985 and 1989, in the Mayo Clinic study conducted among the population of Rochester, Minnesota, 18% of all first ischemic strokes occurred in the presence of significant extracranial or intracranial carotid artery stenosis.[4]

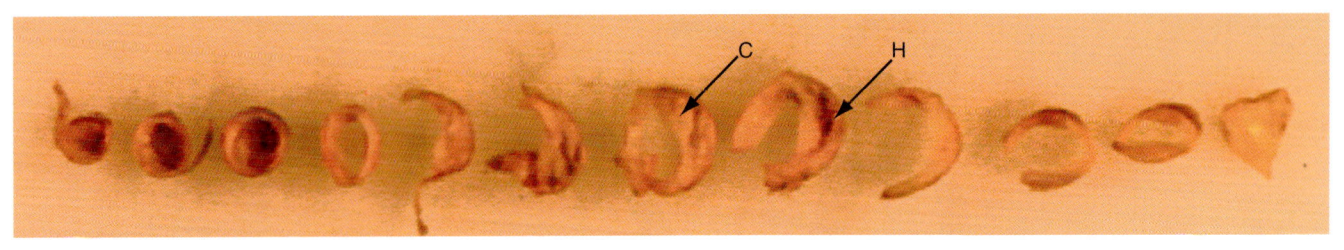

FIGURE 89-1 Serial sections of an explanted carotid atherosclerotic plaque demonstrating an eccentrically located lipid core (C) and intraplaque hemorrhage (H).

A variety of risk factors contribute to an increased risk of stroke. The Framingham study[5] confirmed that there was no difference in incidence related to gender. However, increasing age, systolic and diastolic blood pressure, diabetes, smoking, and cardiovascular diseases were associated with an increased risk for stroke. The age-adjusted relative risk for stroke among hypertensive patients (>160/95 mm Hg) in contrast to normotensive persons (<140/90 mm Hg) is 3.0 in men and 2.9 in women. Smokers may have a 50% increase in risk of atheroembolic stroke compared with nonsmokers.

Etiology and Pathophysiology

The unique hemodynamics at the carotid bifurcation predisposes this area to atherosclerosis. Along the inner wall of the carotid bulb, blood flow remains laminar, with high velocity and high shear stress. Conversely, along the outer wall, there are areas of flow separation, stasis, turbulent flow, and a complex oscillating shear stress pattern that predisposes to atherosclerotic plaque deposition.[6] Although neurologic events have been attributed to progressive stenosis and decreased blood flow from enlarging atherosclerotic plaques, most such events are usually secondary to plaque disruption and atheroembolization from the lesion. Loss of the fibrous cap with exposure of atherosclerotic debris to the flow lumen appears to be responsible for these embolic complications. Additional factors, such as adequacy of collateralization, plaque ulceration or hemorrhage, hypotension, and low cardiac output, also play a contributory role.

Histologic evaluation of atherosclerotic plaques has demonstrated that they originate from fatty streaks that, over time, accumulate into a lipid core.[7] The fatty streak becomes a fibroatheroma as fibrous tissue accumulates over the core and forms a fibrous cap (Fig. 89-1). Through unknown mechanisms, some plaques become unstable, resulting in an enlarging lipid core, intraplaque hemorrhage, plaque enlargement, fibrous cap rupture, ulceration, and luminal thrombosis. These histomorphologic features have been associated with the production of atheroemboli and neurologic symptoms. Specifically, large lipid cores located close to the flow lumen, intraplaque hemorrhage, and fibrous cap disruption with ulceration have frequently been observed in CEA specimens obtained from patients with symptomatic plaques (Fig. 89-2A).[8] Conversely, small lipid cores located deep within the plaque with a thick fibrous cap have been observed in CEA specimens from patients with asymptomatic carotid stenosis (see Fig. 89-2B).[8]

Manifestations of Disease

Clinical Presentation

Because one of the major goals in the management of carotid stenosis is to prevent stroke, the identification of individuals with asymptomatic stenosis becomes an important objective. The incidence of asymptomatic carotid stenosis in the general population is difficult to estimate. In one study of 2000 asymptomatic patients screened by duplex ultrasonography, significant carotid stenosis was found in 32.8% of patients with peripheral vascular disease, 6.8% of patients with coronary artery disease, and 5.9% of patients with significant risk factors.[9] Perhaps the most frequent reason for suspecting a carotid stenosis is a cervical bruit in a high-risk patient. However, bruit is nonspecific and is associated with significant stenosis in only 47% of patients. Conversely, only 60% of significant carotid stenoses will be manifested as a bruit.[10]

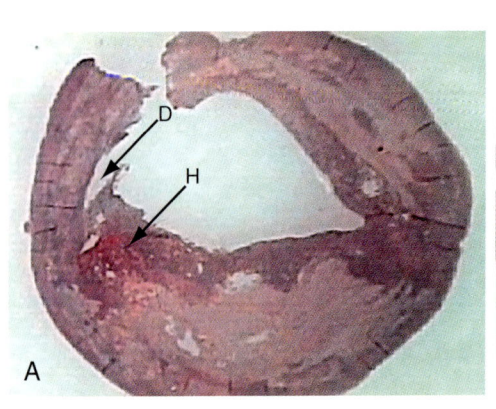

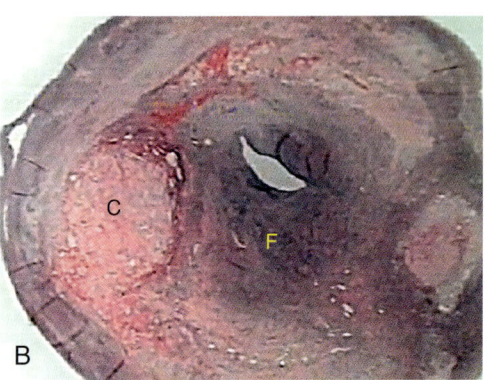

FIGURE 89-2 Photomicrographs of a ruptured carotid atherosclerotic plaque from a patient with a recent nondisabling stroke (A) and an intact plaque from an asymptomatic patient (B). Note the cap disruption (D) and intraplaque hemorrhage (H) in the symptomatic plaque and the deep-seated lipid core (C) with a thick overlying fibrous cap (F) in the asymptomatic plaque.

Although auscultation of a bruit is not a sensitive or specific predictor of carotid stenosis, it remains an important clinical sign in an otherwise asymptomatic patient and must prompt a duplex ultrasound evaluation. Of additional interest is the association of cervical bruit with coronary artery disease. Its presence should also prompt a clinical evaluation for coronary artery disease because the bruit may actually be a more accurate predictor of myocardial infarction than stroke.[10]

Alternatively, patients may first present with a variety of symptoms related to atheroembolic ischemic events. Eye symptoms can result from embolization to the retinal, ophthalmic, or cerebral circulation and include one or more of the following: amaurosis fugax (blurring or loss of vision in the ipsilateral eye, typically described as a curtain or shade falling over the eye), homonymous hemianopia (resulting from emboli to optic radiation), intermittent retinal blindness (loss of vision on exposure to bright light), neovascularization of iris (resulting from ophthalmic artery ischemia), and, rarely, complete blindness (resulting from ischemic optic neuropathy). More commonly, atheroemboli travel to the intracranial circulation and result in lateralizing deficits that may follow several patterns. A transient ischemic attack tends to be a stereotypic and temporary loss of sensory, motor, or visual function that usually lasts for less than 15 minutes. Per definition, patients always return to baseline within 24 hours. Alternatively, patients may have recurring attacks of deficits similar to a transient ischemic attack without an interval allowing complete recovery. The deficit is often the same with each attack, and there is no deterioration in function. These symptoms are associated with a worse outcome and are referred to as crescendo transient ischemic attacks. Patients may also present with recurring attacks of focal neurologic deficits with progressive deterioration in neurologic function. This is termed a stroke in evolution and generally lasts longer than 24 hours. Finally, a completed stroke occurs when a deficit has stabilized beyond 24 hours. The definitions of transient ischemic attack and stroke are evolving. Studies of patients with diffusion-weighted MRI demonstrate that many patients with transient ischemic attacks lasting only hours will actually be shown to have sustained cerebral infarction.[11]

All patients with suspected or confirmed carotid stenosis must undergo a complete neurologic examination to identify potential neurologic deficits and to establish a clinical baseline with which to compare outcomes of future therapeutics. No single outcome measure can describe or predict all dimensions of recovery and disability after acute stroke. Several scales have proved reliability and validity in stroke trials, including the National Institutes of Health Stroke Scale (NIHSS), the modified Rankin Scale, the Barthel Index, the Glasgow Outcome Scale, and the Stroke Impact Scale. The NIHSS comprises 15 items that enable standardized application and measurement of a simple neurologic examination.[12] The scale assesses the level of consciousness, extraocular movements, visual fields, facial muscle function, extremity strength, sensory function, coordination, language, speech, and hemi-inattention. It has undergone extensive validation and is the preferred method of quantification of neurologic deficits in a clinical trial setting.[13-16]

Imaging Indications and Algorithm

A clinically detected carotid bruit, or neurologic symptoms attributable to the carotid artery territory as outlined before, should prompt a noninvasive assessment of the carotid arteries. The most commonly performed study is an ultrasonographic evaluation. Alternative approaches include evaluation with a CT scan or MRI, which have the advantage of being able to incorporate intracranial views to assess for infarctions. However, these studies are more expensive, and the yield for intracranial disease is low. Noninvasive studies typically yield information about the lesion that is reliable enough to plan further management.[17] In cases in which the stenosis is determined to be borderline significant, a second noninvasive study provides complementary information. Exceptional circumstances, such as the inability to differentiate between an occluded and a very tight stenosis, warrant an invasive study such as angiography.

Imaging Techniques and Findings

Angiography

The degree of carotid stenosis generally correlates with risk of stroke in symptomatic extracranial carotid occlusive disease. Cerebral angiography (Fig. 89-3) was the first definitive investigative tool used to visualize and to

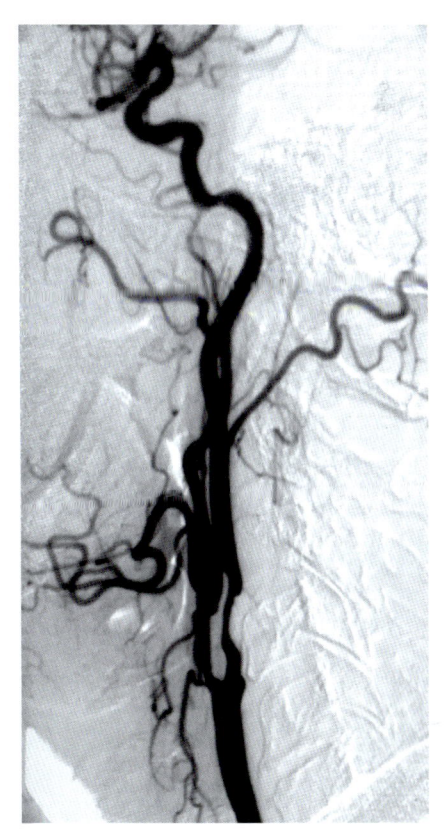

■ **FIGURE 89-3** Selective extracranial carotid circulation angiogram demonstrating a high-grade stenosis in the proximal internal carotid artery. Also note atherosclerotic narrowing of the origin of the external carotid artery.

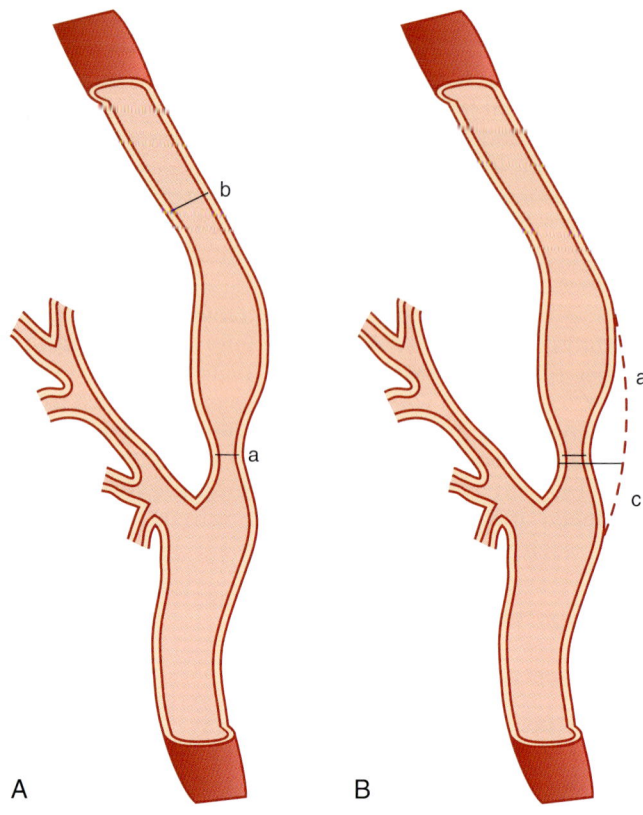

FIGURE 89-4 Two methods of quantifying the degree of internal carotid artery stenosis. **A,** (a/b) × 100 represents the more common method used in the large randomized trials originating in North America. **B,** (a/c) × 100 yields a higher grade of stenosis for a similar amount of luminal loss and is more commonly used in Europe.

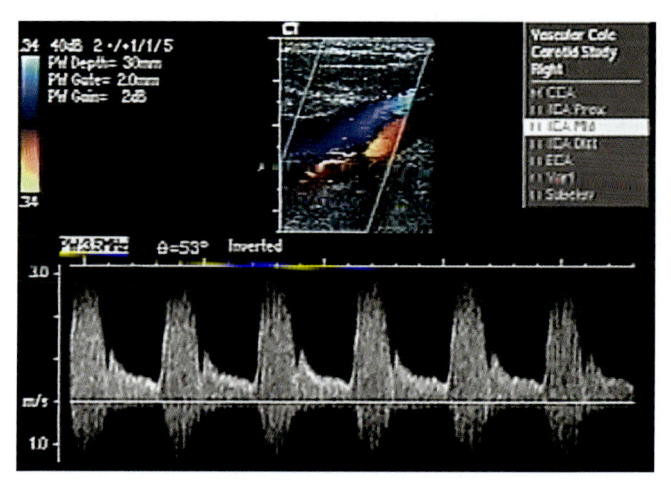

FIGURE 89-5 Duplex ultrasonography of a high-grade internal carotid artery stenosis. Note the high peak systolic and end-diastolic velocities obtained at the stenosis.

quantify carotid stenosis. Multiplanar angiography still remains the gold standard for preoperative delineation of extracranial carotid occlusive disease. Complete details of diagnostic procedures have been included in other chapters in this book. The definition of a significant carotid stenosis has been conventionally accepted as a 50% decrease in the luminal diameter, which translates into a 75% reduction in cross-sectional area. On cerebral angiography, the maximal stenosis is determined on the anteroposterior, lateral, or oblique view. Two methods to estimate the percentage of diameter reduction are in common use (Fig. 89-4). The first (North American) method compares the least transverse diameter at the stenosis with the luminal diameter of the distal internal carotid artery once its walls become parallel. This technique has been used by the majority of carotid atherosclerosis trials.[13-15] The second method compares it with the presumed normal luminal diameter at the stenosis and has been used in Europe.[18] The percentage stenosis measured by the North American method will be lower than the European measurement; for example, North American measurements of 30%, 40%, 50%, 60%, 70%, 80%, and 90% stenosis will correspond to 65%, 70%, 75%, 80%, 85%, 91%, and 97% stenosis, respectively, in Europe. It is therefore important to specify the method used for estimation of percentage stenosis for purposes of comparison with published data.

Ultrasonography

Duplex ultrasonography (Fig. 89-5) emerged about 2 decades ago as a reliable, inexpensive, and safe method of assessing carotid occlusive disease. It is ideal for screening, for observing disease progression or postoperative status, and for intraoperative assessment of CEA. It is being used increasingly as the sole preoperative test before CEA.[17] On a scan, the percentage stenosis is estimated on the basis of peak systolic and end-diastolic velocities. Although the modified University of Washington criteria define this relationship,[19] the Intersocietal Commission for the Accreditation of Vascular Laboratories has recommended that each vascular laboratory generate its own estimates based on the performance of individual devices and technologists.

Computed Tomography and Magnetic Resonance

Magnetic resonance angiography (MRA) and computed tomographic angiography (CTA) are both noninvasive and safe. They are much less operator dependent and can assess intracranial arteries as well as arch origins. Neither MRA nor CTA has the advantage of portability that duplex ultrasonography offers, which still remains by far the least expensive test. Because the limitations of duplex ultrasonography are different from those of MRA and CTA, some centers use these investigations in place of angiography when the results of duplex ultrasonography are equivocal. The use of these two modalities in the diagnostic algorithm is a matter of continuing debate. However, continued use of duplex ultrasonography coupled with improving accuracy of both MRA and CTA has resulted in a decreased reliance on conventional angiography.

Plaque Morphology

A subset analysis of patients randomized in the North American Symptomatic Carotid Endarterectomy Trial (NASCET) showed that for symptomatic patients with no carotid plaque ulceration, the risk of stroke remained constant for all degrees of stenosis of 75% or more.[20]

FIGURE 89-6 Computerized assessment of pixel brightness on B-mode imaging can provide information on the histologic nature of plaque constituents. An intact plaque from an asymptomatic patient (**A**) demonstrates calcification (blue), increased fibrous tissue (green), but a smaller lipid/necrotic core (yellow) and minimal hemorrhage (red). Conversely, a ruptured plaque from a symptomatic patient (**B**) demonstrates minimal calcification and a comparatively larger lipid core with more intraplaque hemorrhage.

Therefore, it is possible that other factors may add to the risk of stroke, such as the histologic composition of the plaque, the plaque surface characteristics (ulceration, hemorrhage), the presence of prior silent but CT-confirmed cerebral infarction, and the status of collateral cerebral circulation. Currently, the most commonly employed clinical predictor for risk of stroke is the severity of stenosis of the carotid arterial plaque. However, the presence of ulceration on carotid plaques is also a marker for stroke risk.[20] Plaques that appear hypoechoic or heterogeneous on duplex ultrasound B-mode imaging may have a high content of lipid or intraplaque hemorrhage that may produce plaque ulceration and a greater embolic potential.[8] Duplex ultrasound examination of the plaque followed by computer-assisted image analysis has recently been suggested as an effective method of objectively characterizing plaque morphology (Fig. 89-6).[21] These morphologic features may also influence the neurologic complication rate associated with revascularization procedures such as carotid artery stenting. MRI also provides excellent soft tissue contrast, offering delineation of important plaque composition features such as the fibrous cap, necrotic core, intraplaque hemorrhage, and calcification (Fig. 89-7). MRI methods that use black blood are effective in delineating the flow lumen and the inner and outer walls of the plaque while eliminating the flow signal. In this protocol, signal heterogeneity has been shown to reflect the complexity of the plaque, consisting of admixtures of necrotic tissue, calcific shards, and intraplaque hematoma. These plaques are probably a greater source of microemboli than is homogeneous fibrous tissue. Significant effort continues to be focused on the identification of noninvasive tissue signatures that may portend future stroke, but additional work is required to identify a definitive marker.

Differential Diagnosis

From Clinical Presentation

A bruit heard over the neck can also be caused by a murmur radiating from a stenosed aortic valve, external carotid artery disease, intraluminal turbulence in the internal carotid artery (dissection), carotid artery aneurysms, external compression from thoracic outlet syndrome, previous scarring due to neck surgery, and a carotid body tumor.

From Imaging Findings

On duplex ultrasonography, other causes of elevated blood flow velocities include hyperdynamic states, aortic valvular lesions, cardiac arrhythmias, and shunting from a contralateral stenosis.

Synopsis of Treatment Options

The first randomized controlled trial comparing pharmacologic with surgical treatment of carotid occlusive disease appeared in 1970.[22] The study reported that the patients undergoing CEA had a lower incidence of stroke and death during long-term follow-up. However, the procedure resulted in a prohibitively high incidence of perioperative stroke rate in that study. With improved surgical technique and selection of patients for operation, a significant decrease in the complication rate of this procedure was noted during the ensuing decade. The ensuing

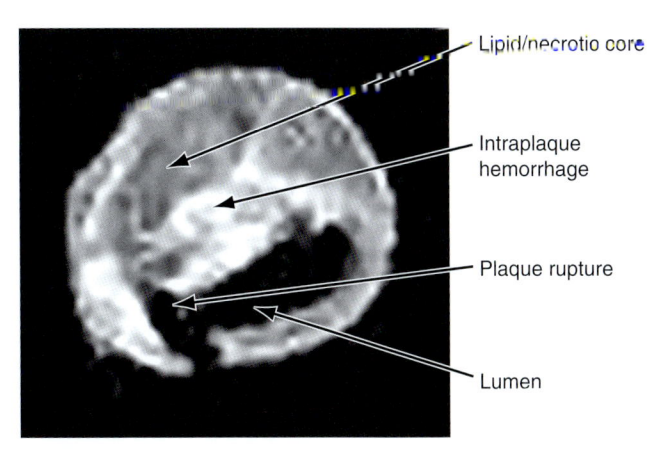

FIGURE 89-7 T1-weighted magnetic resonance image through the area of maximum stenosis of an explanted carotid atherosclerotic plaque.

controversy about the appropriate management of carotid stenosis prompted several randomized controlled multi-institutional trials that have provided statistically reliable results that form the basis for current treatment guidelines.

Symptomatic Carotid Stenosis

Several centers in North America and internationally participated in NASCET,[13] which studied patients with recent hemispheric and retinal transient ischemic attacks or nondisabling strokes and ipsilateral high-grade stenosis (70% to 99%) of the internal carotid artery. The results, published in 1991, showed that the risk of an ipsilateral stroke at 2 years was 26% in medically treated patients and 9% in the surgical patients—an absolute risk reduction of 17%. The European Carotid Surgery Trial[18] published a confirmatory report demonstrating significant benefit of CEA and optimal medical therapy versus best medical care alone. Finally, the Veterans Affairs trial of symptomatic carotid stenosis[23] also confirmed benefit of CEA in a small number of patients; the trial was closed after initial announcement of the NASCET data. Subsequently, the NASCET trialists[15] reported benefit from CEA in patients with 50% to 69% stenosis. The 5-year rate of ipsilateral stroke was 15.7% among patients treated surgically and 22.2% in those treated medically. On the basis of these clinical trials, the Society for Vascular Surgery[24] and the American Heart Association[25] have recommended that symptomatic patients with 50% or more carotid artery stenosis are best treated with CEA and medical therapy.

Asymptomatic Carotid Stenosis

The Veterans Affairs Cooperative Study Group[16] enrolled men with asymptomatic carotid stenosis with diameter reduction of 50% or more. Whereas the combined rate of transient neurologic events and stroke was reduced after CEA, the Asymptomatic Carotid Atherosclerosis Study investigators[14] were the first to report reduction in stroke alone after CEA. In patients with 60% or more diameter-reducing stenosis, the projected 5-year ipsilateral stroke rate for surgically treated patients was 5.1%, whereas it was 11.0% for the medically treated group. These results were mirrored in a larger European trial, in which the benefit of CEA was proved to extend to women also.[26] These trials established the beneficial role of carotid revascularization in reducing the risk of neurologic sequelae in patients with asymptomatic carotid stenosis. On the basis of these results, the Society for Vascular Surgery[24] and the American Heart Association[25] have recommended that asymptomatic patients with 60% or more carotid artery stenosis are best treated with CEA and medical therapy, provided periprocedural morbidity and mortality are less than 3%.

Medical

The major randomized trials addressing management of carotid stenosis have demonstrated the benefit of pharmacologic (antiplatelet) therapy over surgery in a selected subgroup of patients. Furthermore, low periprocedural morbidity in the surgical arm of these studies was achieved in the presence of simultaneous pharmacologic therapy. The Society for Vascular Surgery[24] and the American Heart Association[25] have therefore recommended optimal medical management for all patients with carotid stenosis. Medical therapy should be targeted to achieve a blood pressure below 120/80 mm Hg by lifestyle interventions and antihypertensive treatment, glucose control to hemoglobin A_{1c} below 7% by dietary modifications and hypoglycemic agents, and low-density lipoprotein cholesterol level to 100 mg/dL or even lower for high-risk patients by lifestyle modification and statin therapy. Patients who have smoked in the last year should be counseled to quit. Antiplatelet agents are recommended for patients with ischemic stroke or transient ischemic attack and include aspirin (50 to 325 mg/day), the combination of aspirin, or clopidogrel (75 mg/day).

Surgical

Carotid Endarterectomy

We routinely use general anesthesia for the procedure, although some surgeons perform CEA under cervical block anesthesia. Along with routine monitoring, invasive arterial blood pressure monitoring is recommended during and immediately after the procedure. The operation is accomplished through a longitudinal incision along the anterior border of the sternocleidomastoid muscle. The dissection to expose the internal, external, and common carotid arteries must avoid damage to the superior laryngeal, hypoglossal, glossopharyngeal, marginal mandibular, and vagus nerves. Manipulation of the carotid body must be minimized to prevent bradycardia or hypotension. Systemic heparin is given, and vascular clamps are applied on the proximal uninvolved common carotid artery and the distal nondiseased internal carotid artery and external carotid artery. Many surgeons recommend placement of a temporary shunt from the common carotid artery to the distal internal carotid artery to maintain prograde flow to the brain during the endarterectomy. Others use shunting selectively, based on variables such as internal carotid artery backpressure measurements, operative electroencephalography, sensory evoked potentials, or observation for neurologic events during regional anesthesia. The artery is then incised longitudinally, and the plaque is separated from the common carotid artery and the internal carotid artery. Great care is taken to leave behind a smooth luminal surface with no debris or intimal flaps. The arteriotomy is usually closed with a synthetic or vein patch to prevent restenosis and to reduce perioperative stroke risk. A closed suction drain may also be placed (Fig. 89-8).

Emerging Therapy: Carotid Artery Stenting

During the recent decade, carotid artery stenting (CAS) has been advocated as an alternative treatment to CEA for patients who have carotid stenosis. Several case series, single institutional trials, or registries have reported

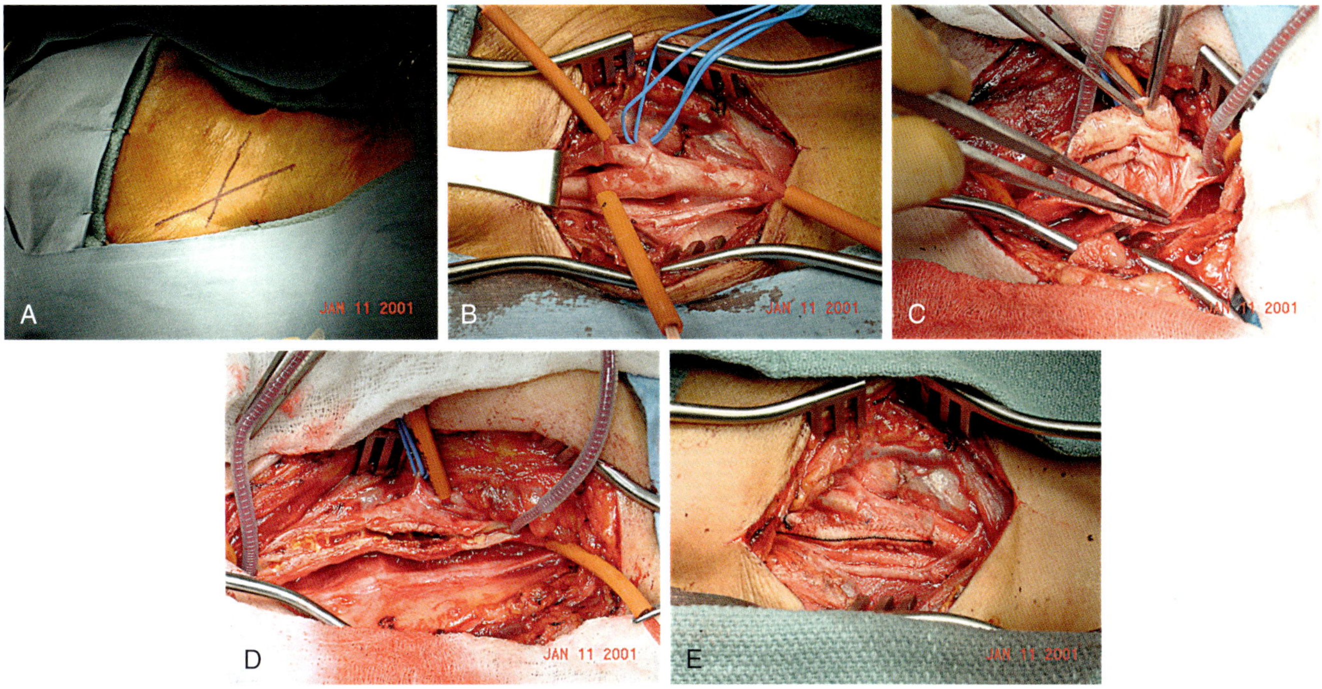

FIGURE 89-8 Carotid endarterectomy. The procedure can be performed through a 2- to 3-inch-long vertical or transverse cervical incision (**A**). Vessel loops are used to control the common, internal, and external carotid arteries after careful dissection (**B**). A shunt can be used to maintain cerebral perfusion, after which the plaque is dissected free through a vertical arteriotomy (**C** and **D**). The arteriotomy is closed with a patch (**E**).

support for this approach.[24] One randomized trial reported potential equivalence of outcomes after CAS versus CEA in high-risk patients.[27] In response to this early enthusiasm, the U. S. Food and Drug Administration approved the use of CAS in selected high-risk patients with symptomatic carotid stenosis in 2004. However, two subsequent randomized trials have shown equivocal results.

The Endarterectomy Versus Angioplasty in Patients with Symptomatic Severe Carotid Stenosis (EVA-3S) trial[28] randomized symptomatic patients with at least 60% carotid stenosis into CAS and CEA. The primary outcome measured was the composite of stroke or death within 30 days of the procedure. As a prerequisite to participation, surgeons had to have successfully performed at least 25 CEA procedures in the previous year, and CAS operators had to have performed at least 12 CAS procedures or 35 stenting procedures in any other artery. Importantly, stent operators with no previous CAS experience could still participate if they were proctored by another qualified operator. The use of an embolic protection device was not mandatory. Enrollment to EVA-3S was stopped in 2005 after 520 patients had been randomized because of a higher stroke and other adverse event rate in patients randomized to CAS. The 30-day stroke and death rate was 9.6% for CAS compared with 3.9% for CEA. Whereas the results provided important information, this study had some limitations that precluded a definitive answer. The experience of the surgeons and CAS operators participating in the trial was unequal, the use of an embolic protection device during CAS was not uniform, the study did not complete enrollment, and more patients assigned to CAS had occlusions of the contralateral carotid artery (5.0% vs.

1.2%), a high-risk anatomic feature limiting the success of CEA.

The Stent-Protected Angioplasty versus Carotid Endarterectomy (SPACE) trial[29] was designed to test whether CAS would be noninferior to CEA in symptomatic patients with carotid artery stenosis of 70% or more. Between 2001 and 2006, 1200 patients were randomized to CEA ($n = 595$) or CAS ($n = 605$). The primary outcome was composite 30-day stroke or death. The prerequisites for participation in the trial were that surgeons should have performed at least 25 CEAs and physicians performing stenting should have carried out at least 25 endovascular interventions, not necessarily involving the carotid arteries. Shunting during CEA and embolic protection during CAS were optional. The study had aimed to randomize 1900 patients but had to be terminated because of inadequate enrollment. Of the patients enrolled, demographics and lesion characteristics were similar in the two treatment groups. At 30 days, there was no significant difference in outcomes between CAS and CEA (30-day stroke and death, 6.8% vs. 6.3%; absolute difference, 0.51% [95% CI, −1.89%-2.91%]. The SPACE study suffered from limitations similar to those observed in the EVA-3S trial, namely, an uneven experience of surgeons versus CAS operators, nonuniform use of embolic protection during CAS, and reduced power due to the inability to complete enrollment.

The safety and efficacy of any new therapy must be clearly established in a controlled, appropriately powered, adequately monitored clinical trial, with appropriately credentialed operators, under Institutional Review Board and U.S. Food and Drug Administration guidelines. In the

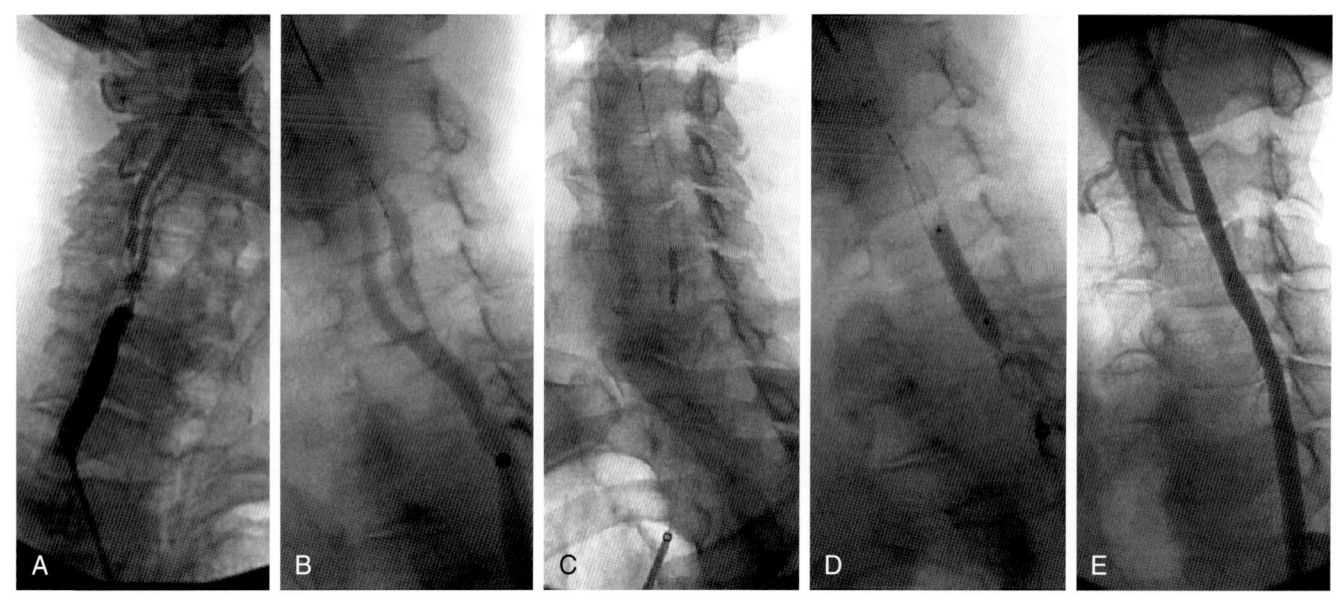

FIGURE 89-9 Carotid artery stenting. The common carotid artery is cannulated most commonly through a transfemoral approach, and the lesion is visualized (**A**). The sheath is advanced to within a few centimeters proximal to the lesion, and an embolic protection device (in this case a filter device) is deployed distal to the lesion (**B**). Protected balloon angioplasty is performed to enable safe passage of the stent (**C**), after which the stent is deployed (**D**, in this case, a nitinol tapered stent). Completion angiography confirms resolution of the stenosis (**E**). Note that caging of the external carotid artery is often necessary to cover the entire lesion and most often does not result in occlusion of that artery.

tradition of the two previous National Institutes of Health–sponsored carotid trials,[13,14] the Carotid Revascularization Endarterectomy versus Stent Trial (CREST)[30] was funded by the National Institute of Neurological Disorders and Stroke. It completed enrollment of more than 2500 asymptomatic and symptomatic patients who were randomized to undergo CAS or CEA in July 2008, and results are anticipated in late 2009. Until the safety and efficacy of CAS can be proved, the widespread clinical application of this technology is not justified. Such procedures must be performed only by properly credentialed physicians in a monitored trial setting.

Procedure

Routinely, two preprocedural antiplatelet agents (aspirin and clopidogrel) are used. Access is generally gained by a transfemoral 6F introducer sheath. Transbrachial or direct carotid exploration and cannulation can be undertaken in selected patients with severe aortoiliac disease. The patient is heparinized to an activated clotting time of 250 to 300 seconds. A 6F long sheath is positioned within the common carotid artery proximal to the lesion. A 0.014-inch guidewire is used to cross the carotid stenosis, over which an embolic protection device (filter or balloon) is passed and deployed distal to the lesion. The lesion is then dilated with a 4-mm low-profile balloon. The same wire is used to deploy a stent across the lesion. Post-stent dilation is accomplished with 5- or 6-mm balloons. Intermittent hand-injection angiography is performed during the entire procedure to confirm appropriate balloon and stent placements; bone landmarks are used for the same purpose. Clopidogrel is discontinued 4 weeks after CAS; aspirin is continued indefinitely (Fig. 89-9).

Current Indications

We have recommended the preferential use of CAS for treatment of patients with neointimal restenosis after CEA and patients with high medical comorbid conditions. Patients with carotid stenosis in whom CEA may be associated with a high incidence of complications may be considered for CAS. These possible indications include carotid stenosis in the presence of prior cervical irradiation, anatomically inaccessible lesions (generally above the C2 vertebra), and severe medical comorbid conditions.

Because of the success of stenting in other vascular beds, particularly in the coronary arteries, patients and their physicians frequently state strong preference for CAS over CEA. In those instances, sufficient evidence now exists to justify CAS as a patient-directed alternative to CEA. However, elderly patients should be cautioned. Because of the findings from the SPACE trial and the CREST lead-in registry, CAS may be proportionally inferior to CEA in patients older than 75 years. Carotid calcification and tortuosity are more prevalent in that group and have been postulated as the causes for the relatively increased 30-day morbidity and mortality in these elderly patients undergoing CAS.

Reporting: Information for the Referring Physician

A clinically detected carotid bruit or neurologic symptoms attributable to the carotid artery territory (stroke, transient ischemic attack, amaurosis fugax) should prompt a noninvasive assessment of the carotid arteries and referral for evaluation of possible carotid artery stenosis.

KEY POINTS

- Randomized trial data confirm that carotid artery revascularization in patients with carotid stenosis reduces the incidences of stroke and death beyond that which can be achieved by optimal medical therapy.
- Because patients must survive several years to derive a benefit from revascularization, the risks of offering the procedure to high-risk individuals must be carefully considered.
- There is Level 1 evidence that revascularization with CEA in carefully selected patients offers an advantage over medical therapy.
- Current information also indicates that revascularization with CAS is technically feasible and can be performed with low periprocedural morbidity, thereby offering a reasonable alternative to CEA.
- Current information, however, does not offer unequivocal evidence to support generalized use of CAS in symptomatic or asymptomatic patients.
- Certain subgroups of high-risk individuals may benefit from CAS, such as patients with surgically inaccessible lesions or difficult surgical dissections. CAS must be recommended with caution in elderly patients.

SUGGESTED READINGS

Barrett KM, Brott TG. Carotid artery stenting versus carotid endarterectomy: current status. Neurosurg Clin North Am 2008; 19:447-458.

Hobson RW 2nd. Randomized clinical trials: how will results influence clinical practice in the management of symptomatic and asymptomatic extracranial carotid occlusive disease? J Vasc Surg 2007; 45(Suppl A):A158-A163.

Hobson RW 2nd, Mackey WC, Ascher E, et al. Management of atherosclerotic carotid artery disease: clinical practice guidelines of the Society for Vascular Surgery. J Vasc Surg 2008; 48:480-486.

Lal BK, Hobson RW 2nd. Treatment of carotid artery disease: stenting or surgery. Curr Neurol Neurosci Rep 2007; 7:49-53.

REFERENCES

1. Thompson J. Carotid artery surgery—historical review In Greenhalgh R, Hollier L (eds). Surgery for Stroke. Philadelphia, WB Saunders, 1993, pp 3-10.
2. Elkins JS, Johnston SC. Thirty-year projections for deaths from ischemic stroke in the United States. Stroke 2003; 34:2109-2112.
3. White H, Boden-Albala B, Wang C, et al. Ischemic stroke subtype incidence among whites, blacks, and Hispanics: the Northern Manhattan Study. Circulation 2005; 111:1327-1331.
4. Petty GW, Brown RD Jr, Whisnant JP, et al. Ischemic stroke subtypes: a population-based study of incidence and risk factors. Stroke 1999; 30:2513-2516.
5. Sacco RL, Wolf PA, Kannel WB, McNamara PM. Survival and recurrence following stroke. The Framingham study. Stroke 1982; 13:290-295.
6. Zarins CK, Giddens DP, Bharadvaj BK, et al. Carotid bifurcation atherosclerosis. Quantitative correlation of plaque localization with flow velocity profiles and wall shear stress. Circ Res 1983; 53:502-514.
7. Stary HC. Natural history and histological classification of atherosclerotic lesions: an update. Arterioscler Thromb Vasc Biol 2000; 20:1177-1178.
8. Lal BK, Hobson RW 2nd, Hameed M, et al. Noninvasive identification of the unstable carotid plaque. Ann Vasc Surg 2006; 20:167-174.
9. Hobson RW. Carotid artery occlusive disease. In Dean RH, Yao JST, Brewster DC (eds). Current Diagnosis and Treatment in Vascular Surgery. New York, Appleton & Lange 1995, pp 80-104.
10. Wolf PA, Kannel WB, Sorlie P, McNamara P. Asymptomatic carotid bruit and risk of stroke. The Framingham study. JAMA 1981; 245:1442-1445.
11. Mlynash M, Olivot JM, Tong DC, et al. Yield of combined perfusion and diffusion MR imaging in hemispheric TIA. Neurology 2009; 72:1127-1133.
12. Brott T, Adams HP Jr, Olinger CP, et al. Measurements of acute cerebral infarction: a clinical examination scale. Stroke 1989; 20:864-870.
13. Beneficial effect of carotid endarterectomy in symptomatic patients with high-grade carotid stenosis. North American Symptomatic Carotid Endarterectomy Trial Collaborators. N Engl J Med 1991; 325:445-453.
14. Endarterectomy for asymptomatic carotid artery stenosis. Executive Committee for the Asymptomatic Carotid Atherosclerosis Study. JAMA 1995; 273:1421-1428.
15. Barnett HJ, Taylor DW, Eliasziw M, et al. Benefit of carotid endarterectomy in patients with symptomatic moderate or severe stenosis. North American Symptomatic Carotid Endarterectomy Trial Collaborators. N Engl J Med 1998; 339:1415-1425.
16. Hobson RW 2nd, Weiss DG, Fields WS, et al. Efficacy of carotid endarterectomy for asymptomatic carotid stenosis. The Veterans Affairs Cooperative Study Group. N Engl J Med 1993; 328:221-227.
17. Kuntz KM, Skillman JJ, Whittemore AD, Kent KC. Carotid endarterectomy in asymptomatic patients—is contrast angiography necessary? A morbidity analysis. J Vasc Surg 1995; 22:706-714; discussion 714-706.
18. Randomised trial of endarterectomy for recently symptomatic carotid stenosis: final results of the MRC European Carotid Surgery Trial (ECST). Lancet 1998; 351:1379-1387.
19. Faught WE, Mattos MA, van Bemmelen PS, et al. Color-flow duplex scanning of carotid arteries: new velocity criteria based on receiver operator characteristic analysis for threshold stenoses used in the symptomatic and asymptomatic carotid trials. J Vasc Surg 1994; 19:818-827; discussion 827-818.
20. Eliasziw M, Streifler JY, Fox AJ, et al. Significance of plaque ulceration in symptomatic patients with high-grade carotid stenosis. North American Symptomatic Carotid Endarterectomy Trial. Stroke 1994; 25:304-308.
21. Lal BK, Hobson RW. Pixel distribution analysis to improve patient selection for CEA and CAS. Endovascular Today 2006; 5:23-26.
22. Fields WS, Maslenikov V, Meyer JS, et al. Joint study of extracranial arterial occlusion. V. Progress report of prognosis following surgery or nonsurgical treatment for transient cerebral ischemic attacks and cervical carotid artery lesions. JAMA 1970; 211:1993-2003.
23. Mayberg MR, Wilson SE, Yatsu F, et al. Carotid endarterectomy and prevention of cerebral ischemia in symptomatic carotid stenosis. Veterans Affairs Cooperative Studies Program 309 Trialist Group. JAMA 1991; 266:3289-3294.
24. Hobson RW 2nd, Mackey WC, Ascher E, et al. Management of atherosclerotic carotid artery disease: clinical practice guidelines of the Society for Vascular Surgery. J Vasc Surg 2008; 48:480-486.
25. Moore WS, Barnett HJ, Beebe HG, et al. Guidelines for carotid endarterectomy. A multidisciplinary consensus statement from the Ad Hoc Committee, American Heart Association. Circulation 1995; 91:566-579.
26. Halliday A, Mansfield A, Marro J, et al. MRC Asymptomatic Carotid Surgery Trial (ACST) Collaborative Group. Prevention of disabling

and fatal strokes by successful carotid endarterectomy in patients without recent neurological symptoms: randomised controlled trial. Lancet 2004; 363:1491-1502.
27. Yadav JS, Wholey MH, Kuntz RE, et al. Protected carotid-artery stenting versus endarterectomy in high-risk patients. N Engl J Med 2004; 351:1493-1501.
28. Mas JL, Chatellier G, Beyssen B, et al. Endarterectomy versus stenting in patients with symptomatic severe carotid stenosis. N Engl J Med 2006; 355:1660-1671.
29. Eckstein H-H, Ringleb P, Allenberg J-R, et al. Results of the Stent-Protected Angioplasty versus Carotid Endarterectomy (SPACE) study to treat symptomatic stenoses at 2 years: a multinational, prospective, randomised trial. Lancet Neurol 2008; 7:893-902.
30. Hobson RW 2nd. CREST (Carotid Revascularization Endarterectomy versus Stent Trial): background, design, and current status. Semin Vasc Surg 2000; 13:139-143.

CHAPTER 90

Ultrasound Evaluation of the Carotid Arteries

Leslie M. Scoutt, Jonathan D. Kirsch, and Ulrike Hamper

Stroke remains the third leading cause of death and is a major cause of morbidity in the United States.[1] Most strokes are due to thromboembolic events rather than to ischemia or reduced perfusion. Whereas the heart is the number one source, 20% to 30% of strokes are believed to be secondary to embolus from plaque or thrombus at the carotid bifurcation.[2] Carotid endarterectomy has been convincingly shown in several prospective multicentered, randomized, double-blind trials to significantly reduce the risk of stroke and death in patients with stenoses of the internal carotid artery (ICA) of more than 60% to 70% compared with optimized medical therapy.[3-6] However, at the time these trials were published in the 1990s, statin therapy was not a part of the standard medical regimen, and double-blind trials comparing carotid endarterectomy with medical management including statin therapy are currently ongoing.

Thus, the identification of patients with ICA stenoses of 60% to 70% is clearly important for patient management, allowing appropriate referral for carotid endarterectomy. Risk factors for disease at the carotid bifurcation include atherosclerosis, hypertension, diabetes mellitus, hyperlipidemia, hypercholesterolemia, obesity, and smoking. Patients with risk factors for carotid plaque, carotid bruits, and symptoms of stroke or transient ischemic attacks are typically referred for evaluation of the carotid arteries, which can be performed with ultrasonography, computed tomographic angiography, magnetic resonance angiography, or conventional angiography. Of these potential screening modalities, carotid ultrasound examination is the most readily available, least invasive, and least expensive. Numerous studies have shown that when it is performed appropriately, ultrasound examination of the carotid arteries is highly accurate for detection of surgical lesions (i.e., ICA stenoses ≥70%),[7-10] and additional confirmatory studies such as CT angiography, magnetic resonance angiography, and conventional angiography are usually unnecessary except in complex cases with discordant findings or poor visualization. The precise method of grading stenoses of the ICA changed with the publication of the North American Symptomatic Carotid Endarterectomy Trial (NASCET).[3] Before the NASCET, the percentage stenosis of the ICA was typically calculated by comparing the width of the residual lumen with the estimated diameter (outer wall to outer wall) of the ICA at the site of the stenosis (Fig. 90-1A). However, because the outer wall of the ICA can be seen on an angiogram only if it is calcified, angiographic measurements of ICA diameter are only estimates in many cases. Hence, this method has significant interobserver and intraobserver variability as well as poor reproducibility. Thus, when the NASCET was designed, the measurement of percentage ICA stenosis was standardized angiographically by comparing the width of the residual lumen at its narrowest point with the diameter of the lumen of the distal normal ICA (beyond any post-stenotic dilation; Fig. 90-1B) because the vessel lumen can be accurately and reproducibly measured on angiographic images. For a given residual lumen, the percentage stenosis is generally higher with the pre-NASCET method of calculating an ICA stenosis.

TECHNICAL REQUIREMENTS

Doppler ultrasound examination of the carotid arteries requires an ultrasound machine with high-resolution gray-scale imaging as well as color Doppler and spectral Doppler capability. A high-frequency 5- to 7.5-MHz linear array transducer should be used to optimize spatial resolution. However, if the carotid arteries are too deep to visualize with the linear array transducer in a patient with a short, thick neck, a lower frequency curved array transducer may be necessary for adequate penetration.

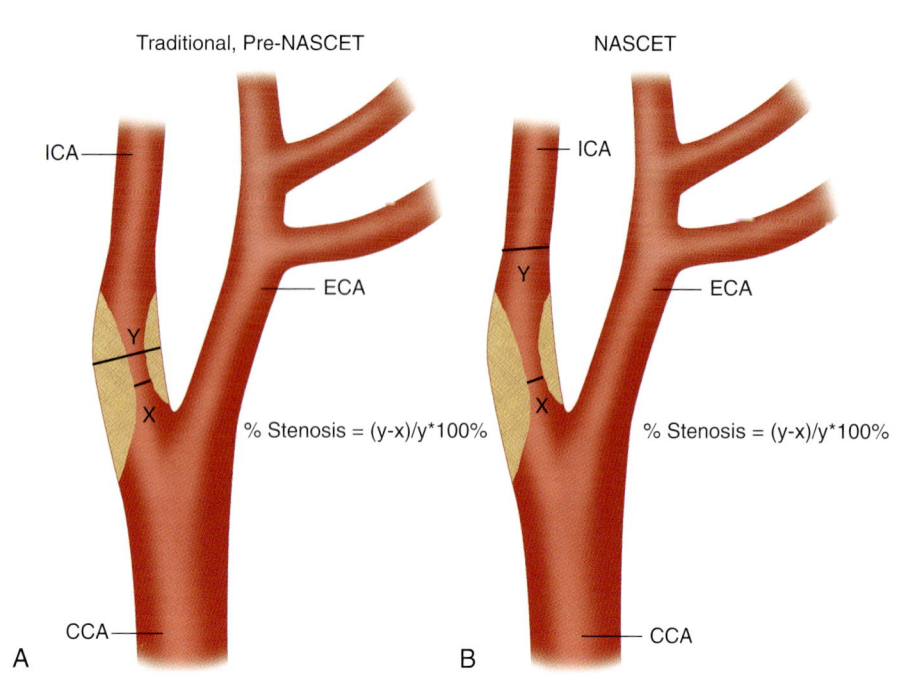

■ **FIGURE 90-1** Schematic diagrams demonstrating the methods of calculating percentage internal carotid artery stenosis. **A,** The pre-NASCET or traditional formula for calculation of an ICA stenosis compares the diameter of the residual lumen with the distance between the outer walls of the ICA at the site of stenosis. On angiograms, this method is less accurate than the NASCET method because of difficulty in identifying the outer wall of the ICA. **B,** Percentage ICA stenosis in the NASCET trial was calculated by comparing the diameter of the residual lumen with the luminal diameter of the distal normal ICA beyond any post-stenotic dilation. This is the currently accepted method of calculating percentage stenosis of the ICA. In general, percentage stenosis is greater when it is calculated by the pre-NASCET or traditional formula than by the NASCET method. CCA, common carotid artery; ECA, external carotid artery; ICA, internal carotid artery.

Technique

Indications

Indications for a carotid ultrasound examination include carotid bruit, stroke, transient ischemic attack, syncope, risk factors for atherosclerosis, preoperative evaluation before major surgery, follow-up for carotid endarterectomy or carotid stent placement, and trauma.

Contraindications

There are no contraindications to an ultrasound examination of the carotid arteries, although the examination may be limited in patients with internal jugular lines or cervical collars.

Technique Description

A complete ultrasound evaluation of the carotid arteries has three components: (1) evaluation of plaque, (2) estimation of ICA stenosis by velocity criteria, and (3) waveform analysis. In evaluation of the ICA for stenosis, velocity criteria should always be correlated with the gray-scale and color estimation of the amount of plaque as well as with the proximal and distal waveforms in the ICA and common carotid artery (CCA). Discrepancies between the different velocity criteria as well as with the gray-scale or color Doppler estimation of percentage stenosis and the waveform pattern should be explained.

The patient is examined in the supine position with the neck extended and slightly turned to the contralateral side. Either a posterior or an anterior approach may be used.

The examination begins with evaluation of plaque burden. Plaque echotexture should be characterized as hypoechoic, heterogeneous, or echogenic (Fig. 90-2). The surface contour of the plaque should be described as smooth or irregular (Fig. 90-3), and the percentage reduction of the arterial diameter by the plaque should be estimated.

Optimal evaluation of plaque requires both gray-scale and color or power Doppler imaging in the longitudinal and transverse planes of the entire CCA and ICA as well as the origin of the external carotid artery (ECA). The focal zone should be set at the level of the far wall of the vessel. The use of spatial compounding and harmonic imaging will also improve gray-scale resolution. The gray-scale gain should be adjusted such that plaque and the vessel wall are easily depicted but artifactual echoes are not present within the vessel lumen. If the gain is set too low, plaque will look artifactually hypoechoic. The color gain should be optimized by slowly increasing the gain until color speckles are noted in the surrounding soft tissues. The gain is then decreased until the color pixels are visible only within the vessel lumen. If the gain is set too high, the color pixels will overwrite or "bleed" over plaque, obscuring visualization of the true extent of plaque burden, particularly during systole, and stenoses may be overlooked (Fig. 90-4). If the gain is too low, sensitivity to blood flow will be decreased, and false-positive diagnoses of occlusion or stenosis will be made. The color velocity scale should be adjusted such that color fills the lumen reaching to the vessel wall. Therefore, the color velocity scale may have to be changed slightly as one interrogates the different vessels in the neck. If the scale is set too low, aliasing will occur, making it more difficult to detect flow disturbances at the site of a stenosis. In addition, color motion artifact, which may obscure visualization of the vessel, is more prominent when the velocity scale or pulse repetition frequency is set too low. The wall filter should

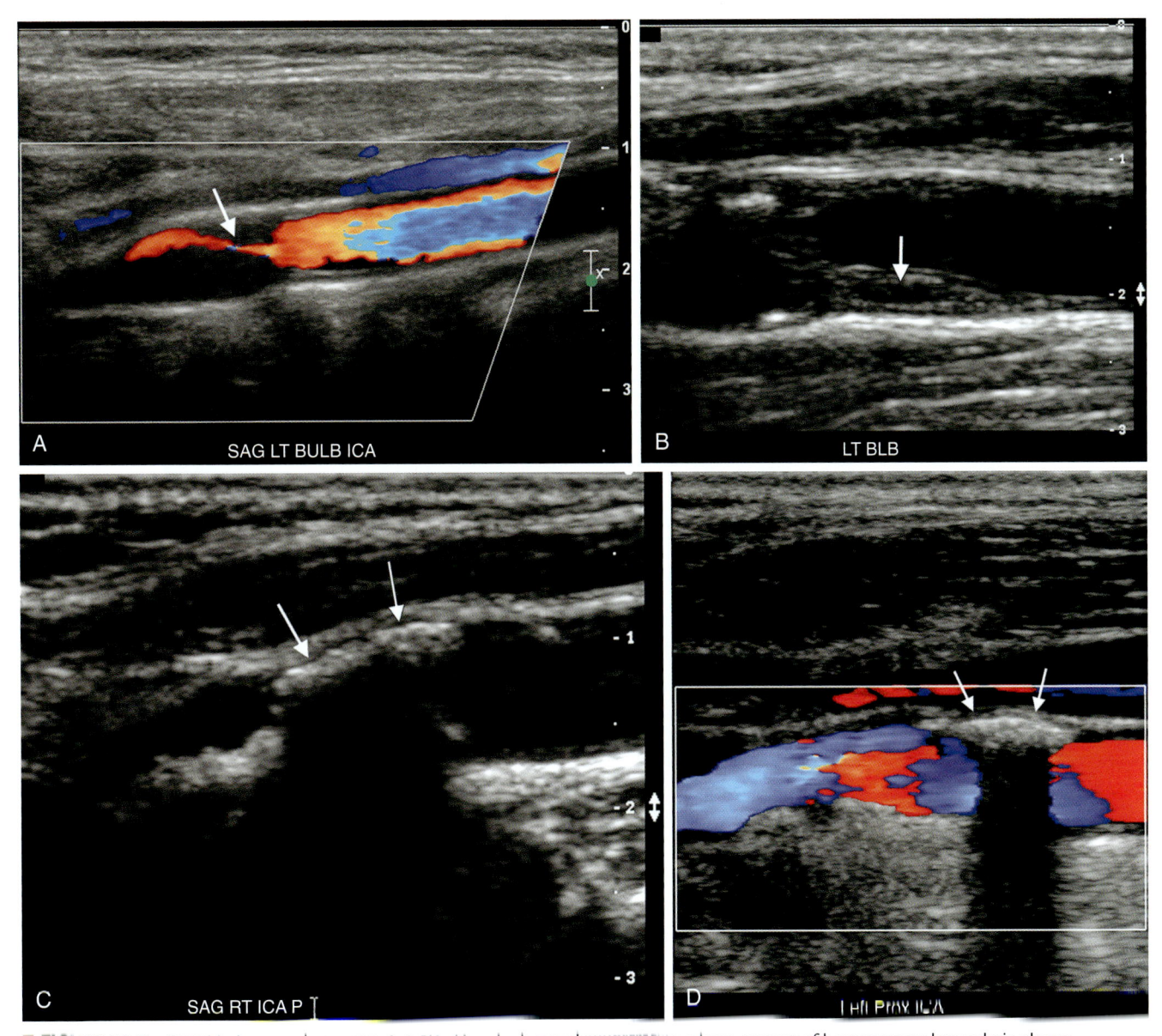

CHAPTER 90 • Ultrasound Evaluation of the Carotid Arteries 1229

FIGURE 90-7 Carotid plaque. **A,** Color Doppler image demonstrating a large amount of homogeneous hypoechoic plaque causing a "string sign" (*arrow*) in the left ICA. **B,** Note focal hypoechoic area (*arrow*) within a heterogeneous plaque in the left carotid bulb. **C,** Note homogeneous echogenic shadowing plaque (*arrows*) in the proximal right ICA. **D,** Color Doppler image demonstrating homogeneous echogenic shadowing plaque (*arrows*) in the left proximal ICA.

be set as low as possible without degradation of the image by motion artifact. Angling of the color box will facilitate evaluation of the direction of blood flow, and a straight, small color box will increase sensitivity to flow. If the vessel lumen cannot be visualized because of shadowing from plaque, an approach to the vessel from different angles (including the transverse plane) or use of a curved array transducer may be helpful.

Once the gray-scale and color or power Doppler images have been obtained, the sonographer should be able to describe the amount and type of plaque in the carotid arteries as well as the relationship of the ICA and ECA to the carotid bulb. Whereas the degree of stenosis can often be estimated on the gray-scale or color Doppler images, precise quantification of stenosis requires accurate measurement of peak systolic velocity (PSV) in the ICA and CCA on the spectral Doppler tracing.

Spectral Doppler tracings are obtained from longitudinal images with the sample volume placed centrally within the vessel lumen or at the brightest spot in any area of focal color aliasing. To optimize the spectral Doppler tracing, the velocity scale and baseline should be adjusted such that the tracing fills the velocity spectrum or scale. If the scale is too high, the waveform will be too small to easily measure or analyze. However, if the scale is too low, the tracing will be too large, and wraparound or aliasing of the systolic velocity peak will occur, making it impossible to accurately measure PSV. The angle of spectral Doppler insonation should be kept between 45 and 60 degrees to minimize error in the calculation of velocity

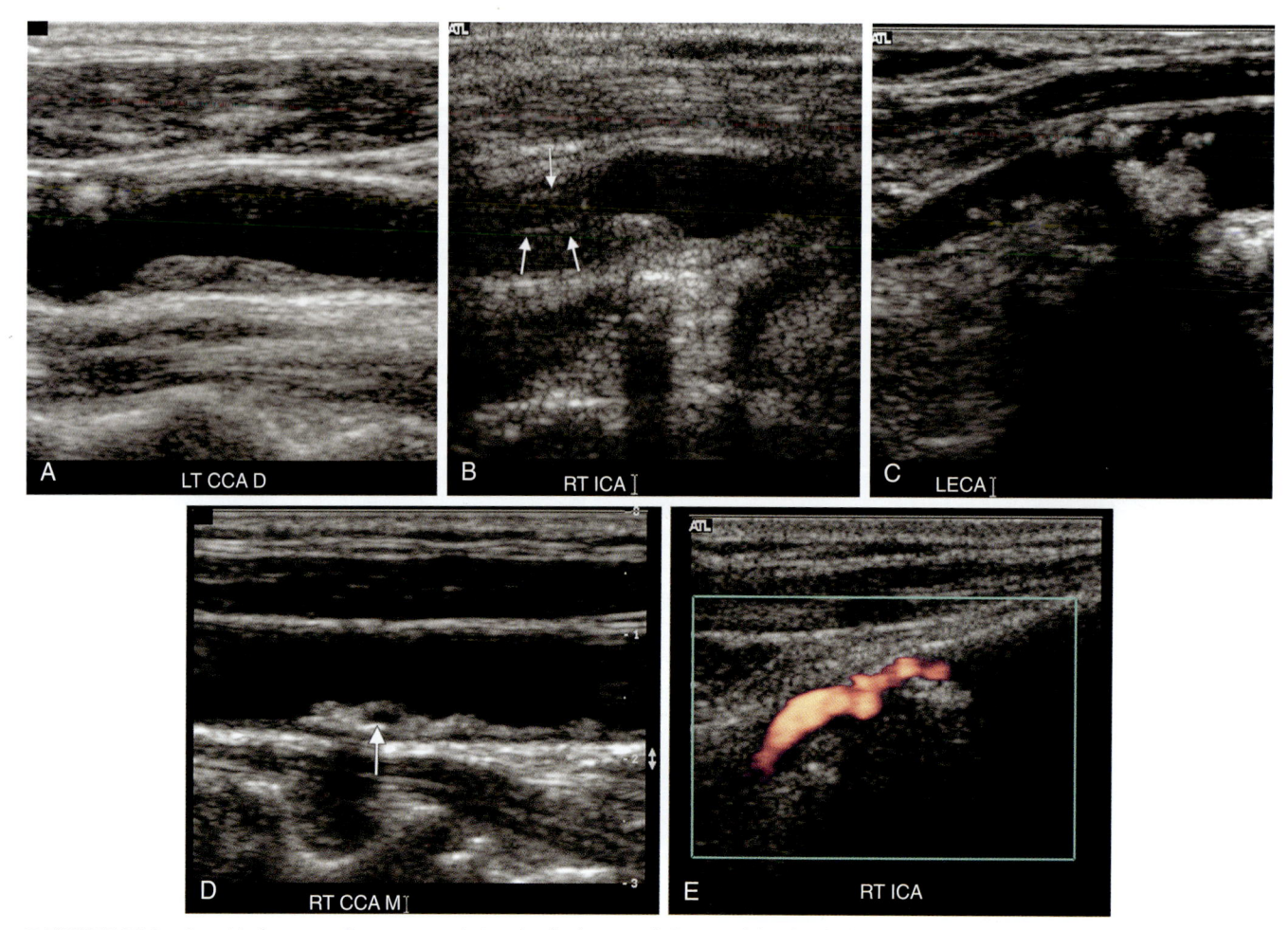

■ **FIGURE 90-3** Carotid plaque: surface contour. **A,** Longitudinal gray-scale image of the distal left CCA demonstrating plaque with a smooth surface contour and heterogeneous echotexture. **B,** Longitudinal gray-scale image reveals a large amount of hypoechoic plaque with a smooth surface contour (*arrows*) along the posterior and anterior walls of the right ICA and bulb. **C** and **D,** Longitudinal gray-scale images of plaque with irregular surface contour from two different patients. Note hypoechoic area within the plaque (*arrow* in **D**). **E,** Longitudinal power Doppler image of the right ICA reveals an irregular residual lumen, indicative of irregular plaque surface.

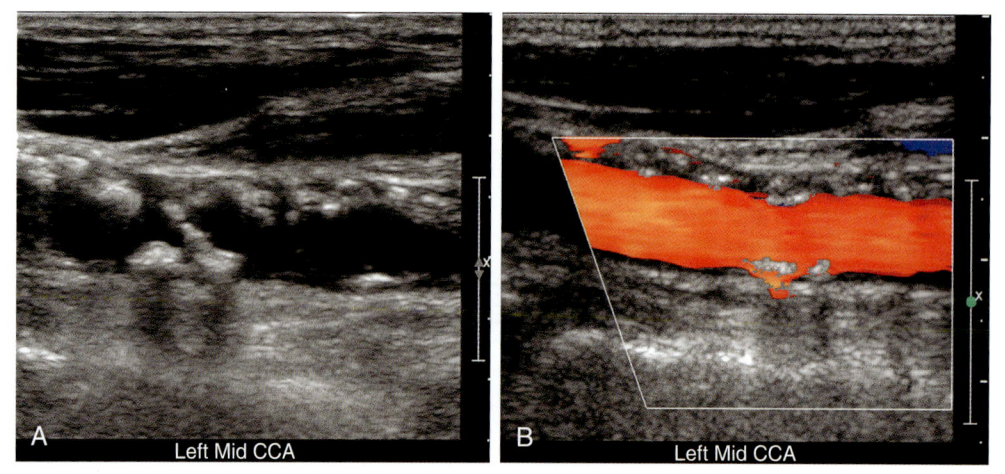

■ **FIGURE 90-4** Color "blooming" artifact. **A,** Note extensive echogenic, irregularly surfaced plaque in the mid left CCA on a longitudinal gray-scale image. **B,** On the color Doppler image, however, the color overwrites and obscures the plaque.

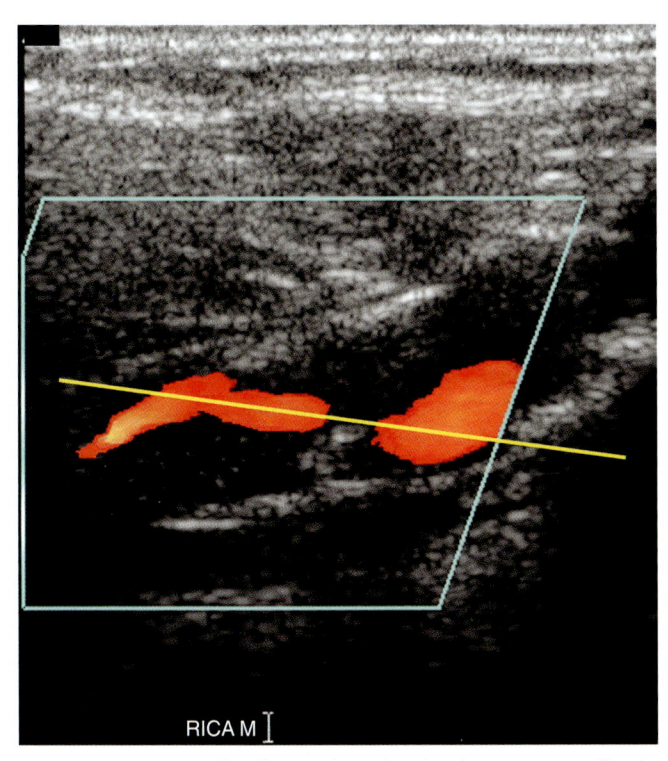

FIGURE 90-5 Angle of insonation. There is a large amount of both hypoechoic and echogenic plaque in the right ICA causing tortuosity and angulation of the vessel lumen in this patient who presented with a carotid bruit. The Doppler angle should be calculated in reference to a vector parallel to the direction of blood flow in the residual lumen (*yellow line*) rather than parallel to the vessel wall.

Protocol

- Longitudinal gray-scale and color or power Doppler images of the proximal and distal CCA, bifurcation, bulb extending into the ICA, and bulb extending into the ECA
- Transverse gray-scale and color or power Doppler images of the proximal and distal CCA, bulb, bifurcation, proximal ICA, and proximal ECA
- Spectral Doppler tracings from the proximal CCA, distal CCA, proximal ICA, mid ICA, distal ICA, proximal ECA, and mid vertebral artery. PSV is recorded for each segment, and end-diastolic velocity (EDV) is noted if it is more than 100 cm/sec. The PSVR is calculated by dividing the highest PSV in the proximal ICA or area of stenosis by the PSV in the distal CCA. PSV in the distal CCA should always be measured 2 to 3 cm proximal to the level of the carotid bulb. Several measurements, optimally three, of PSV should be obtained and the highest velocity recorded.

Additional gray-scale and color or power Doppler images as well as spectral Doppler tracings should be obtained as necessary wherever extensive plaque burden, vessel narrowing, or color aliasing is seen.

Normal Findings

The normal carotid arteries have a thin, regular echogenic wall without focal areas of calcification, intraluminal plaque, or thrombus. Color should fill the vessel lumen homogeneously with a slight central increase in color intensity consistent with normal parabolic or laminar flow. Where the carotid bulb widens, a helical blood flow pattern or reversal of peripheral flow is a normal finding, particularly in younger patients, and is believed to be due to boundary layer separation.

Normal PSV in the CCA is variable and depends on numerous factors, including cardiac output or stroke volume, heart rate, systolic blood pressure, and age. In general, however, PSV in the normal CCA ranges from 70 to 100 cm/sec and decreases gradually as one samples distally.

The CCA, ICA, and ECA demonstrate distinct characteristic waveform patterns. Whereas all segments of the extracranial carotid arteries normally demonstrate a sharp systolic upstroke and thin spectral envelope, the amount of diastolic flow varies in each vessel, reflecting the oxygen consumption and peripheral vascular resistance of the vascular bed supplied. The ECA, which supplies the muscular bed of the scalp, typically demonstrates completely absent or very low velocity end-diastolic flow. Although the amount of diastolic flow in the ECA may vary from patient to patient, it should be symmetric right to left and less than the diastolic flow in the ICA or CCA (Fig. 90-6). An early diastolic notch followed by a short reversal of flow in early diastole is often seen in the ECA. The ICA, which supplies blood to the brain (high oxygen consumption), has a low-resistance waveform pattern with continuous forward, relatively high velocity diastolic flow (Fig. 90-7). The waveform of the CCA demonstrates an intermediate amount of diastolic flow and often demonstrates

from the Doppler frequency shift. If at all possible, the angle should be kept constant on follow-up studies. The angle cursor should be placed parallel to the direction of blood flow in the color jet or vessel lumen rather than parallel to the vessel wall. The direction of blood flow will, in fact, parallel to the vessel wall in most cases, but the jet of blood may travel tangentially or obliquely in relationship to the vessel wall if plaque is irregular or asymmetric (Fig. 90-5). In such cases, the angle correction cursor should be placed parallel to the jet of blood as seen on color Doppler imaging. The sample gate should be kept small, between 1.5 and 2.5 mm in width, and placed in the center of the vessel because PSV will be lower near the vessel wall owing to the geometry of laminar flow and drag from the vessel wall. If the sample gate is too wide, a wider range of velocities will be depicted, and there is the potential risk of falsely creating the appearance of spectral broadening and turbulent flow. Finally, the spectral Doppler gain should be optimized; the gain should be increased until background speckles appear on the spectral tracing and then readjusted downward until the background is homogeneously black. Although incorrect spectral Doppler gain settings rarely cause shifts in PSV of more than 20 cm/sec, such variation in the distal CCA can be important when the PSV in the distal CCA is used as the denominator in calculation of the peak systolic velocity ratio (PSVR). Apparent spectral broadening with "fill in" of the spectral envelope can also be spuriously created if the spectral Doppler gain is set too high.

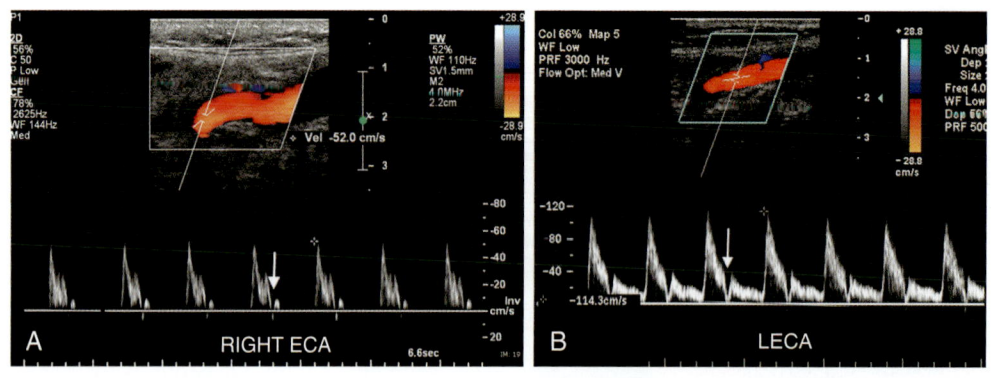

■ **FIGURE 90-6** Normal spectral Doppler tracing of the external carotid artery. The ECA has a higher resistance waveform with less diastolic flow than the ICA. Whereas the amount of diastolic flow may vary from patient to patient, it should be symmetric right to left in a given individual. **A,** This patient has no diastolic flow in the ECA. **B,** In another patient, a small amount of diastolic flow is present. Reversal of flow in early diastole or an early diastolic notch (*arrows*) is a normal finding in the ECA. Note sharp systolic upstroke and thin spectral envelope in the spectral tracings of both ECAs.

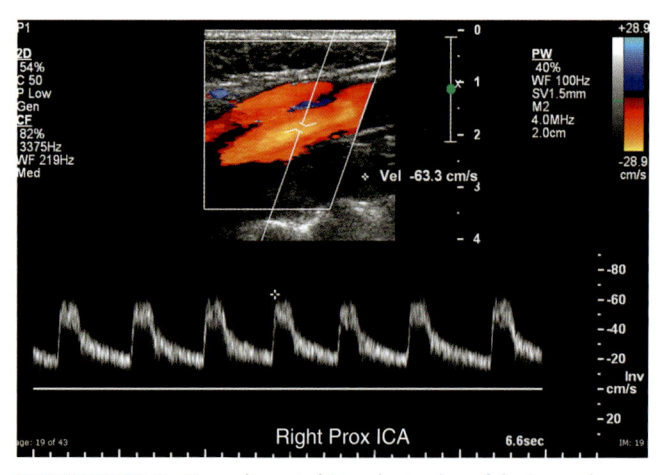

■ **FIGURE 90-7** Normal spectral Doppler tracing of the internal carotid artery. Note that in comparison to the ECA, there is increased diastolic flow, the systolic peak is slightly blunted, and the spectral envelope is slightly widened in the ICA. The systolic upstroke is sharp, and velocity gradually tapers during diastole.

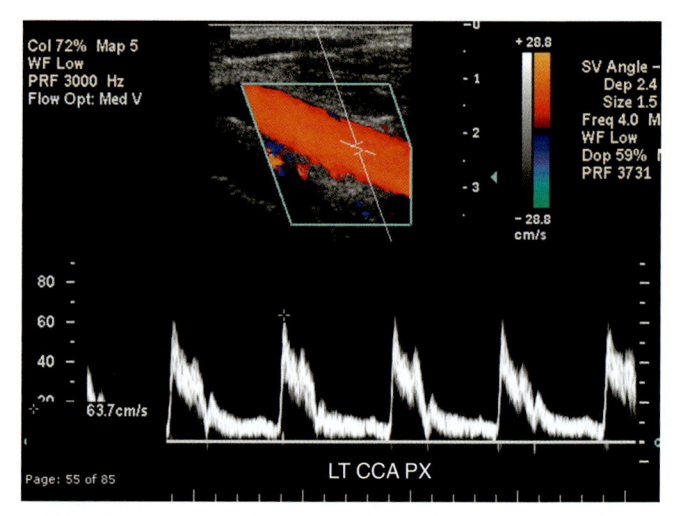

■ **FIGURE 90-8** Normal spectral tracing of the common carotid artery. The systolic upstroke is sharp in the CCA, and there is an intermediate amount of diastolic flow in comparison to the ICA and ECA. An early diastolic notch may be present, but it is less pronounced than in the ECA.

a brief reversal of flow in early diastole (Fig. 90-8). The vertebral artery has a waveform pattern similar to that of the ICA, characterized by a sharp systolic upstroke and continuous forward diastolic flow (Fig. 90-9).

Differentiation of the ICA from the ECA is critically important to avoid misinterpretation of a stenosis in the ECA as a more clinically significant ICA stenosis. The best method of identifying the ECA is by visualization of branches arising from the vessel (Fig. 90-10A). The ICA virtually never gives rise to branch vessels in the neck. Temporal tapping over the ophthalmic artery will generate sharp, spike-like deflections in the waveform of the ECA during diastole (Fig. 90-10B). However, on occasion, transmitted pulsations to the ICA will be observed after temporal tapping, although the deflections are typically blunted in comparison to the deflections observed in the ECA.[7,8] In general, the ECA is smaller, is more medial, and has a higher resistance waveform pattern than the larger posterolateral ICA. However, location and vessel size are not reliable criteria for differentiation of the ICA from the ECA in all patients.

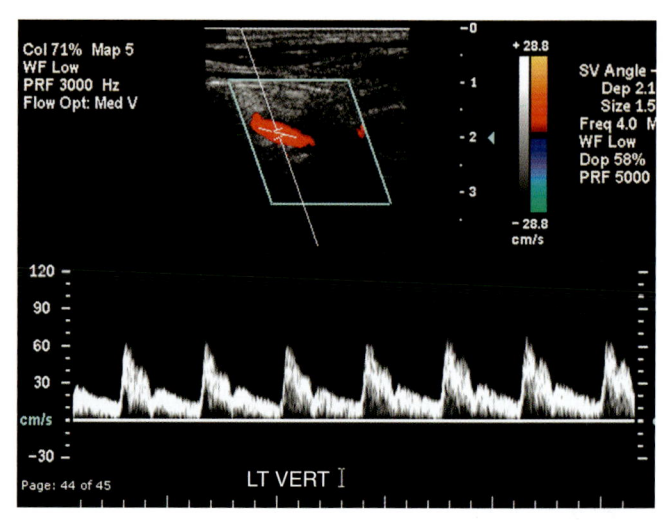

■ **FIGURE 90-9** Normal spectral tracing of the vertebral artery. The waveform of the normal vertebral artery is similar to the waveform of the ICA.

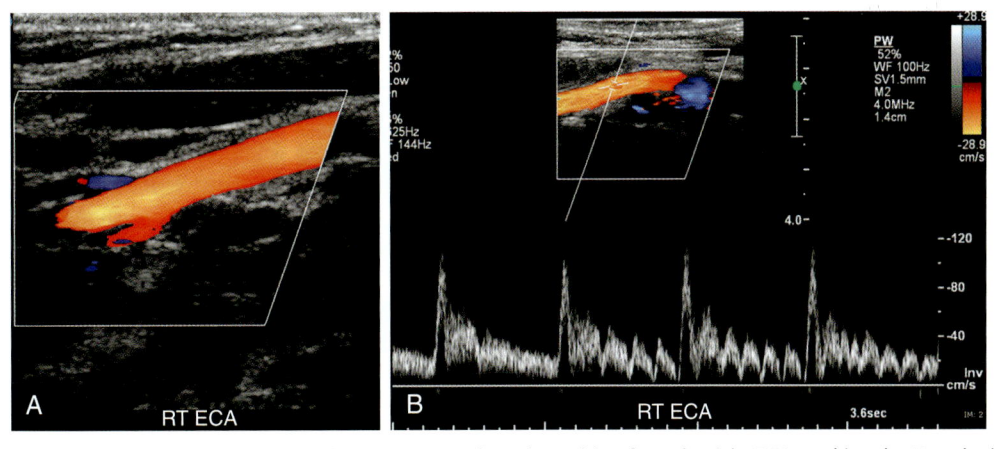

FIGURE 90-10 Identification of the external carotid artery. **A,** Note branches arising from the right ECA on this color Doppler image. Branches almost never arise from the ICA below the skull base. **B,** Note deflections in the spectral tracing from the right ECA due to temporal tapping. These deflections are most easily seen during diastole. Whereas temporal tapping may occasionally cause similar deflections in the ICA or CCA, they will be smaller and less sharply defined than in the ECA.

Grading Stenoses in the Internal Carotid Artery

Grading of stenosis in the ICA by Doppler velocity criteria is based on the simple precept that flow volume is equal to vessel area multiplied by PSV. Because flow volume is a relative constant, PSV is inversely related to vessel lumen diameter. Therefore, if the vessel diameter decreases, PSV must increase to maintain flow volume. As demonstrated by the Spencer diagram, once the vessel diameter decreases by more than 50%, PSV at the site of the stenosis rises exponentially, and this compensatory increase in PSV maintains flow volume until the stenosis reaches approximately 70%.[9] When a stenosis exceeds 70%, flow volume will begin to drop despite continued exponential increase in PSV. Once a stenosis in the ICA becomes greater than approximately 96%, the gradient across the stenosis becomes too high for the pressure generated by the combination of myocardial contractility and vessel elasticity to force blood through the residual lumen, and PSV begins to drop until the vessel occludes and velocity is zero.[9]

Numerous studies have attempted to correlate Doppler measurements of PSV, PSVR, and EDV criteria with angiographically calculated percentage stenosis. Widely variable results have been reported.[10-14] In general, velocity criteria have a higher accuracy and positive predictive value for high-grade stenoses (>70%) and are less reliable for accurate grading of more moderate stenoses (<50%).[12,14] Criteria are probably both machine (possibly even transducer) and laboratory specific and therefore should be validated for each laboratory and machine upgrade if possible. Studies have also demonstrated that vascular laboratories cannot reliably differentiate stenoses in the ICA by 10% increments.[12,14] Accuracy is best achieved by focusing on whether a stenosis is greater than or less than a specific percentage stenosis. In most institutions, carotid endarterectomy is recommended in patients with ICA stenosis of more than 70%. Hence, most vascular laboratories categorize ICA stenoses as less than 50%, 50% to 69%, 70% to 96%, and more than 96%.

A meta-analysis published by Grant and colleagues[12] found that accuracy varied little over a wide range of threshold values for PSV and PSVR, although the sensitivity and specificity were inversely proportional. Hence, the authors recommend that if the Doppler examination is to be used as a screening test, lower thresholds with higher sensitivity should be used. However, if the Doppler examination is intended as a diagnostic test without anticipating confirmation by some angiographic imaging modality, then specificity should be emphasized and higher thresholds are recommended.[12]

In 2002, the Society of Radiologists in Ultrasound (SRU) convened a multidisciplinary panel of experts, including both radiologists and vascular surgeons, to develop a consensus for grading of ICA stenoses by Doppler ultrasonography. The published recommendations of this consensus conference are as follows[13]:

PSV < 125 cm/sec and PSVR < 2.0 suggest a stenosis < 50%
PSV between 125 and 230 cm/sec and PSVR between 2.0 and 4.0 are most consistent with a stenosis of 50% to 69% (Fig. 90-11)
PSV > 230 cm/sec, PSVR > 4.0, and EDV > 100 cm/sec indicate a stenosis of ≥70% to 96% (Figs. 90-12 and 90-13)

Once an ICA stenosis becomes greater than an approximately 96% diameter reduction, PSV velocity begins to drop (Fig. 90-14) until the vessel occludes and the velocity reaches zero.[9] Hence, the panel also recommended that the estimation of diameter reduction by plaque on gray-scale and color Doppler imaging be correlated with the velocity-based estimate of percentage stenosis.[13]

Pitfalls: Technique

Incorrect Choice of Doppler Angle

An incorrect Doppler angle or a Doppler angle that is too high will introduce error into the calculation of PSV. An angle above 60 degrees will result in a falsely elevated PSV (Fig. 90-15). The correct Doppler angle should be calculated in reference to a vector parallel to the vessel lumen or direction of blood flow, which will not necessarily be

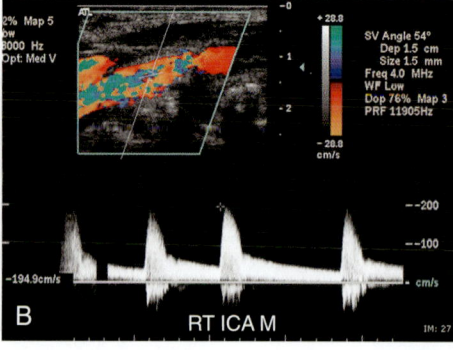

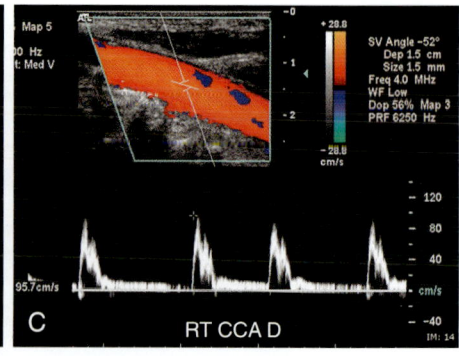

■ **FIGURE 90-11** ICA stenosis, 50% to 69%. **A,** Longitudinal color Doppler image of the right ICA in a patient with a right carotid bruit reveals echogenic plaque and a stenosis at the origin of the right ICA. Note color mosaic just distal to the narrowing of the vessel lumen indicative of increased velocity of flow in the post-stenotic jet. **B,** Spectral tracing reveals a PSV of 195 cm/sec just distal to the stenosis. **C,** PSV in the right CCA is 96 cm/sec. PSVR is approximately 2:1. By SRU criteria, this corresponds to a moderate stenosis of 50% to 69%.

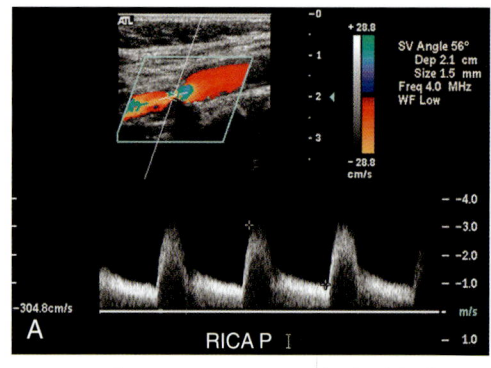

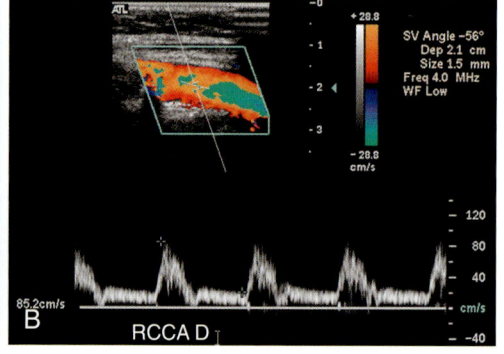

■ **FIGURE 90-12** ICA stenosis, 70% to 96%. **A,** Longitudinal duplex Doppler image of the right ICA in a 73-year-old man presenting with a transient ischemic attack demonstrates that the diameter of the proximal right ICA is narrowed approximately 80%. PSV is 305 cm/sec at the site of the stenosis. **B,** Spectral tracing of the distal right CCA demonstrates a PSV of 85 cm/sec, yielding a PSVR close to 4:1. By SRU criteria, these velocity measurements are consistent with a stenosis of the right ICA of more than 70%, which was confirmed by a CT angiogram.

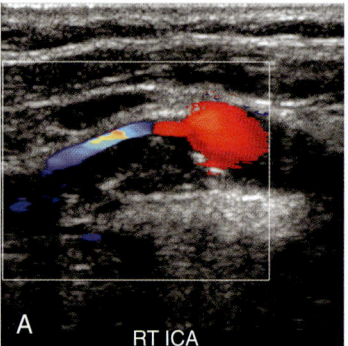

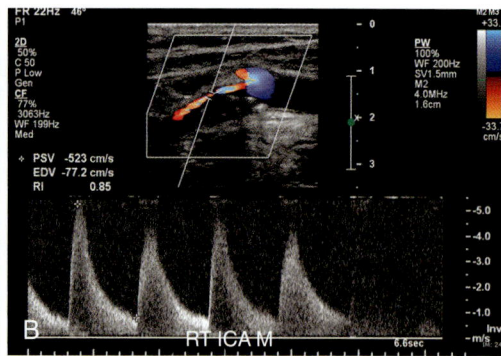

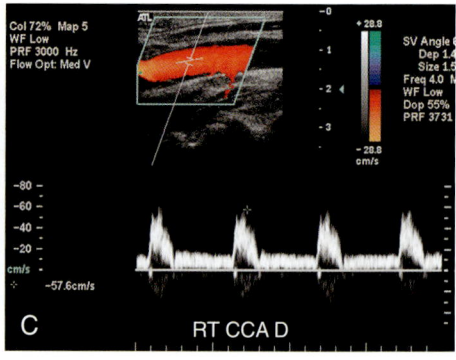

■ **FIGURE 90-13** ICA stenosis, 70% to 96%. Longitudinal color Doppler image of the proximal right ICA (**A**) demonstrates a marked degree of narrowing over a long segment from heterogeneous, largely hypoechoic plaque in a 68-year-old woman presenting with a stroke. By visual inspection, the percentage diameter reduction is estimated at nearly 90%. Spectral Doppler tracing reveals a PSV of 523 cm/sec in the stenosis (**B**), with a PSV of 58 cm/sec in the distal CCA (**C**). PSVR is 9:1. Although it is not possible to accurately classify stenoses at 10% increments by Doppler velocity criteria, these measurements are well above the SRU threshold for a stenosis of 70% or more, and therefore the degree of stenosis is likely in the higher range, approximately 90% diameter reduction, as suggested by the color Doppler image.

parallel to the vessel wall in the case of extensive, irregular plaque (see Fig. 90-5).

Incorrect Gain

If the color gain is set too high, the color will bleed over the vessel wall, obscuring plaque and stenosis (see Fig. 90-4). If the color gain is set too low, the color will not reach the vessel wall and will falsely create the appearance of hypoechoic plaque. If the gray-scale gain is set too low, plaque will appear falsely hypoechoic. Incorrect spectral Doppler gain can also cause slight increase or decrease in measurement of PSV (see earlier).

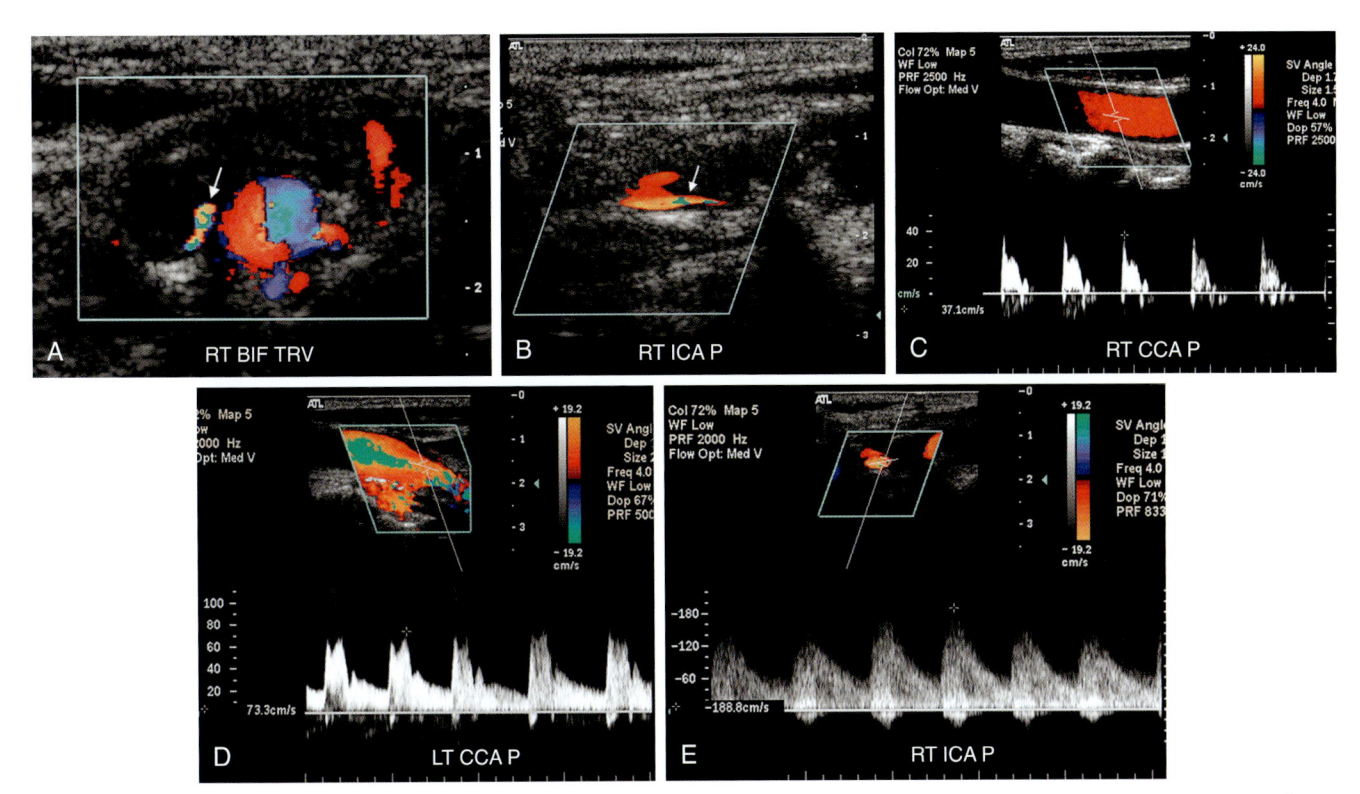

CHAPTER 90 ● *Ultrasound Evaluation of the Carotid Arteries* 1235

■ **FIGURE 90-14** ICA stenosis, greater than 96%. Transverse (**A**) and longitudinal (**B**) color Doppler images reveal a tight stenosis (*arrow*) at the origin of the right ICA. Spectral Doppler tracing of the right CCA (**C**) demonstrates a high-resistance waveform with absent diastolic flow and reduced PSV (37 cm/sec) in comparison to the left CCA (**D**), which has a PSV of 73 cm/sec and a normal amount of diastolic flow. A high-resistance waveform in the CCA suggests a distal high-grade stenosis or occlusion. However, maximum PSV in the right ICA is only 189 cm/sec (**E**). By SRU criteria, this PSV corresponds to only a 50% to 69% stenosis. However, once the percentage diameter reduction exceeds approximately 96%, PSV at the site of a stenosis will drop. Furthermore, PSVR in this patient is more than 5:1, which indicates a stenosis of more than 70% by SRU criteria, confirming a tighter stenosis. Color Doppler images and careful waveform analysis of the proximal and distal vessels are required to differentiate between a high-grade (nearly occlusive) and a more moderate stenosis that may have the same PSV.

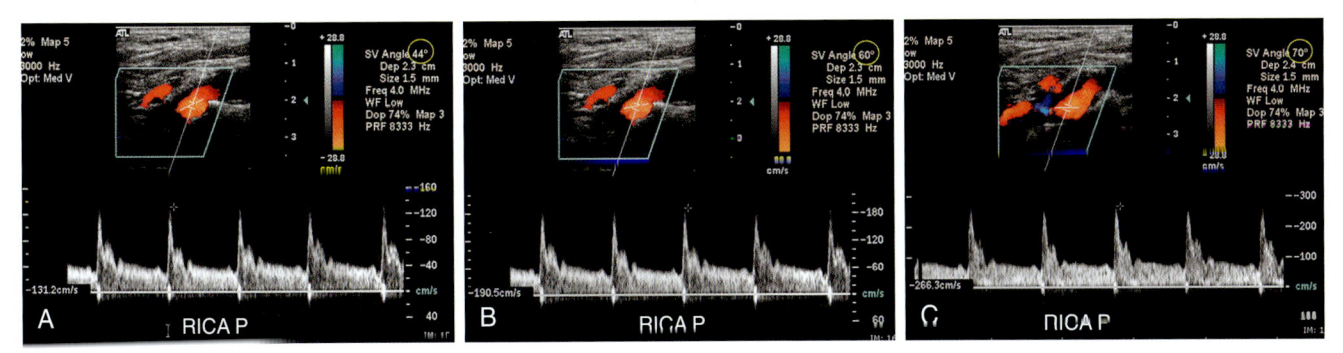

■ **FIGURE 90-15** Effect of Doppler angle on calculated PSV. Three duplex Doppler images are presented of the right ICA at the same location. When the Doppler angle (*yellow circles*) is 44 degrees (**A**), PSV is calculated at 131 cm/sec. However, with a Doppler angle of 60 degrees (**B**), PSV is 190 cm/sec; and when the Doppler angle is 70 degrees (**C**), PSV is calculated at 266 cm/sec. Thus, an incorrect Doppler angle or variations in Doppler angle from examination to examination can introduce significant error into the measurement of PSV.

Pitfalls: Pathology

Tortuous Carotid Artery

When the carotid arteries are tortuous, most commonly in elderly patients, PSV can be elevated without an underlying stenosis (Fig. 90-16). This is due in part to a true increase in PSV as the blood accelerates around the curves but is also likely due to difficulty in assigning a correct Doppler angle along the curved vessel, which results in an overestimation of PSV due to incorrect Doppler angle.

Hence, the sonographer should use caution before diagnosing a carotid stenosis solely on the basis of elevation of PSV in a tortuous vessel without evidence of plaque or vessel narrowing. A true stenosis should cause poststenotic turbulence in addition to an increase in PSV.

Heart Rate

Heart rate affects both PSV and EDV. PSV will be relatively elevated and EDV will be artificially low in patients with

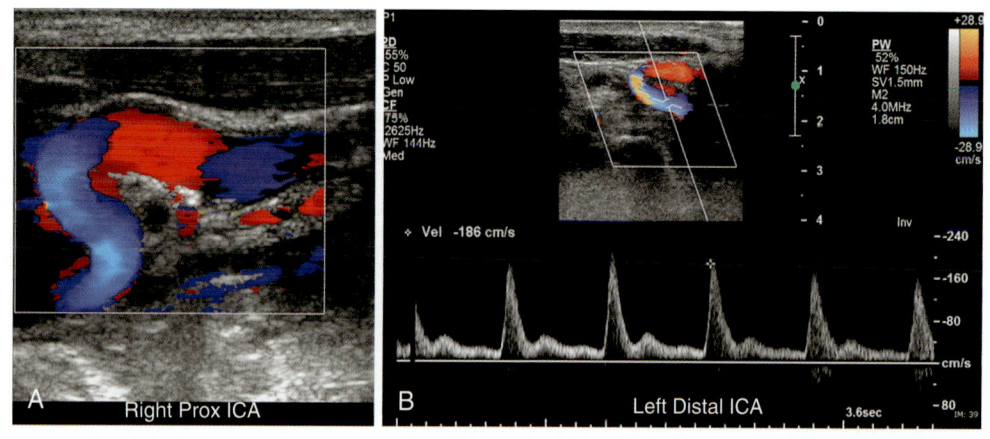

■ **FIGURE 90-16** Tortuous ICA. **A,** Color Doppler image demonstrates a tortuous right ICA. **B,** Duplex Doppler tracing demonstrates a PSV of 186 cm/sec. By SRU criteria, this corresponds to a 50% to 69% stenosis. However, no stenosis was noted on gray-scale or color Doppler imaging. Increased PSV is due to tortuosity of the vessel.

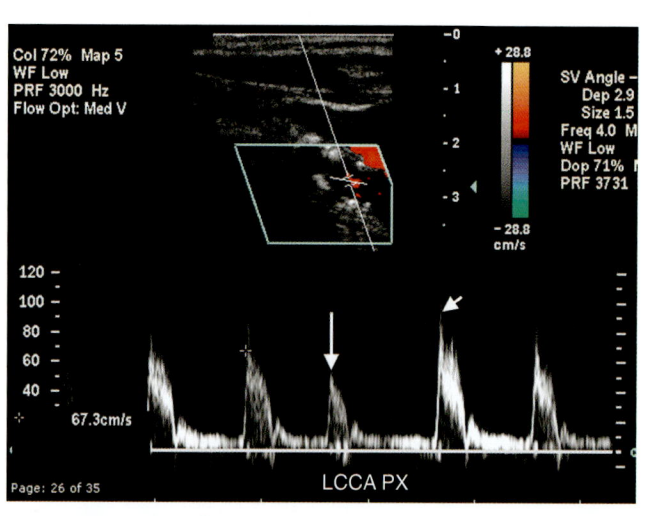

■ **FIGURE 90-17** Effect of heart rate and arrhythmia on PSV. Note variability of PSV in a patient with a premature ventricular contraction and compensatory pause. PSV is decreased during the premature ventricular contraction (*long arrow,* relative tachycardia) and increased in the beat that follows the compensatory pause (*short arrow,* relative bradycardia).

bradycardia. Conversely, in patients with fast heart rates, PSV will be relatively low because of decrease in stroke volume. However, because velocity normally decreases during diastole, EDV will be artificially elevated in patients with tachycardia because of shortening of diastole. Common causes of tachycardia include stress, medications, and thyrotoxicosis. Ventricular conduction defects, medications (including common cardiac drugs such as afterload reducers like propranolol), and hypothyroidism may result in brachycardia. Hence, measurement of PSV and grading of ICA stenoses in patients with cardiac arrhythmias may be problematic. For example, PSV will be increased in the beat after a compensatory pause as a result of relative bradycardia and decreased during a premature ventricular contraction as a result of relative tachycardia (Fig. 90-17). Recommended general guidelines for measurement of PSV in patients with cardiac arrhythmias include the following:

1. Avoid measurement of PSV in a premature ventricular contraction or after a compensatory pause.
2. Measurements should be made at a similar point during the arrhythmia in each vessel segment if the arrhythmia is regular.
3. In the case of an extremely irregular heartbeat, consistently measuring either the most normal appearing cardiac cycle or choosing the highest or lowest PSV in each vessel segment is reasonable. However, a markedly irregular heartbeat does introduce a measure of unreliability to the Doppler criteria.

Long-Segment or Synchronous Involvement

Coexistent disease in the carotid arteries will also make PSV Doppler criteria less reliable. Synchronous disease in the CCA, or tandem lesions, will result in a decrease in PSV for a given percentage stenosis in the ICA. Hence, the entire CCA and ICA must be evaluated, not just the carotid bifurcation. Most ICA stenoses are less than 2 cm in length. However, if a stenosis is unusually long (>2 cm), PSV often drops (possibly because of increased in-flow resistance), although diastolic velocity may remain high (Fig. 90-18). Prior radiation therapy, carotid dissection, arteritis, or fibromuscular dysplasia should be considered when a long-segment stenosis is noted, although diffuse atherosclerosis may also be the cause.

Contralateral Carotid Disease

A high-grade carotid stenosis or occlusion will increase PSV in the contralateral side, especially at the site of a stenosis. Hence, if the PSV seems more elevated than one would expect given the amount of visualized plaque and if the vessel is not tortuous, one should be suspicious of contralateral disease (Fig. 90-19). The degree of increase in velocity is unpredictable and may differ in the CCA and ICA in a given patient. Hence, the use of PSVR may not adequately compensate.[15,16]

Measurements of PSV remain the basis for grading of stenoses of the ICA on Doppler ultrasound examination. However, given the pitfalls in measuring PSV as well as

CHAPTER 90 • *Ultrasound Evaluation of the Carotid Arteries* 1237

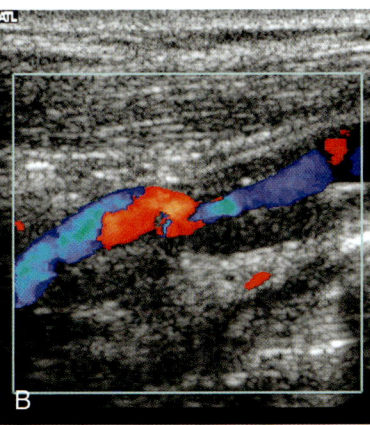

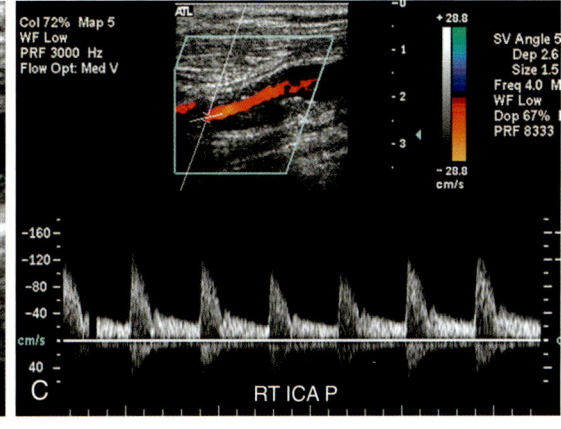

■ **FIGURE 90-18** Long-segment stenosis. Gray-scale (**A**) and color Doppler (**B**) longitudinal images of the right ICA reveal a long-segment high-grade stenosis and extensive hypoechoic plaque (*short arrows*, residual lumen in **A**). However, spectral Doppler tracing (**C**) reveals a maximum PSV of only 120 cm/sec. By SRU criteria, this corresponds to a less than 50% stenosis. However, PSV is artifactually reduced because of the length of the stenosis.

limitations in the applicability of PSV criteria in all patients, the final assessment of an ICA stenosis should always correlate velocity criteria with both gray-scale and color Doppler estimation of plaque burden and waveform analysis of the CCA and ICA. In addition to confirming the presence of a stenosis, abnormalities of the CCA and ICA waveforms can reflect distal or proximal cardiovascular disease not directly assessable by Doppler interrogation.

ULTRASOUND ASSESSMENT OF PLAQUE

Ultrasound evaluation of plaque requires gray-scale and color Doppler imaging in both longitudinal and transverse planes. Such images can be used to estimate percentage diameter reduction by plaque and correlated with PSV measurements. In addition, the echotexture and surface contour of the plaque should be assessed. Plaque should be characterized as hypoechoic or echogenic (see Fig. 90-2) with either a smooth or irregular surface (see Fig. 90-3). Prospective studies have shown that hypoechoic, irregular plaque is associated with an increased risk of neurologic events and increased rate of plaque progression.[17,18]

Whereas echogenic plaque is readily depicted on gray-scale imaging, hypoechoic plaque may not be visible. However, on color Doppler imaging, hypoechoic plaque is readily observed as a signal void (Fig. 90-20). Similarly, surface irregularities are often best seen when outlined by color Doppler flow (Fig. 90-21). Although a pit deeper than 2 mm in a plaque raises concern for ulceration (Fig. 90-22), Doppler ultrasonography is not highly accurate in identifying plaque ulceration. Indentations or divots in plaque identified on color Doppler imaging can, in fact, be endothelialized and therefore not be true ulcers. The same limitation is true for angiography, and plaque ulceration remains primarily a histologic diagnosis. Color Doppler imaging, although necessary for the depiction of hypoechoic plaque, does not eliminate the need for gray-scale evaluation as color blooming, particularly during systole, may overwrite and obscure plaque, thereby causing an underestimation of plaque burden (see Fig. 90-4). Gain settings are important also on gray-scale imaging. If the gain is set too low, plaque will appear falsely hypoechoic, raising unnecessary concern. The percentage diameter reduction is usually best depicted on longitudinal images. However, if the plaque is irregular or eccentric, if there are numerous foci of plaque, or if the vessel lumen is tortuous, transverse images can be extremely helpful, ensuring that the longitudinal image is truly midline and not too lateral or off axis. If the longitudinal image is obtained over an eccentric focus of plaque or too close to the vessel wall, the degree of stenosis will be overestimated. If the vessel lumen is obscured by shadowing from calcified, echogenic plaque, imaging from different planes (i.e., anteriorly or posteriorly), power Doppler imaging, or use of a lower frequency transducer may help visualize the vessel lumen. On occasion, transverse images will eliminate or avoid shadowing from plaque. If the shadowing from plaque obscures the vessel lumen for less than 1 cm, standard PSV criteria can still be used to estimate percentage stenosis because the high-velocity jet caused by a stenosis will persist for approximately 1 cm. However, if more than 1 cm of the vessel length is obscured by shadowing from plaque, the maximal focal elevation of PSV in the post-stenotic jet may be missed, and therefore the use of Doppler velocity criteria to assess carotid stenosis is limited. In such cases, follow-up with CT angiography, magnetic resonance angiography, or conventional angiography is appropriate.

The length of the stenosis should also be considered. Most ICA stenoses are relatively short. If a long-segment stenosis is observed, PSV will be less than expected, although diastolic velocity will remain high (see Fig. 90-18). The relative decrease in PSV is likely due to in-flow resistance. Causes of long-segment stenosis include radiation therapy, carotid dissection, and arteritis (including fibromuscular dysplasia).

Thickening of the wall of the CCA, termed *fibrointimal thickening*, has recently been described as a risk factor for cardiovascular disease (Fig. 90-23).[19,20] Normal wall thickness is likely to be related to race and gender. Measurements should be obtained from the far wall of the CCA or ICA on a magnified image. However, there are

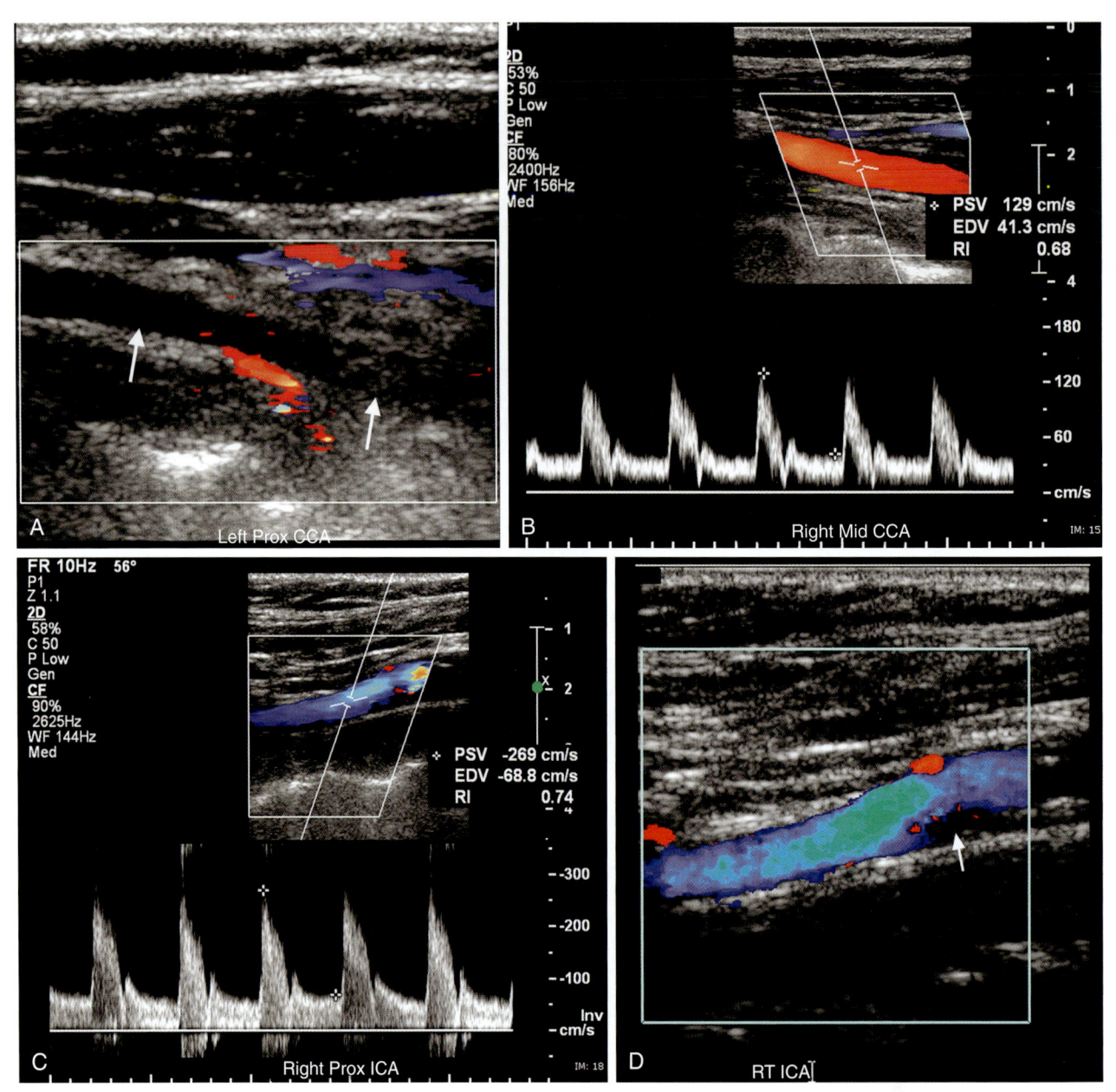

■ **FIGURE 90-19** Effect of contralateral occlusion on PSV. **A,** Longitudinal color Doppler image reveals that the left proximal CCA (*arrows*) is occluded. **B,** PSV is elevated in the mid right CCA (129 cm/sec) and was even more elevated proximally (160 cm/sec; not shown). **C,** PSV is 269 cm/sec in the right ICA. By SRU criteria, this corresponds to a stenosis of more than 70%. However, on color Doppler imaging (**D**), there is only a small amount of plaque noted (*arrow*) in the right ICA consistent with a stenosis of less than 50%. Furthermore, PSVR is approximately 2:1, which corresponds to a stenosis of only 50%. PSV is artificially elevated in the right CCA and ICA because of the occlusion of the left CCA.

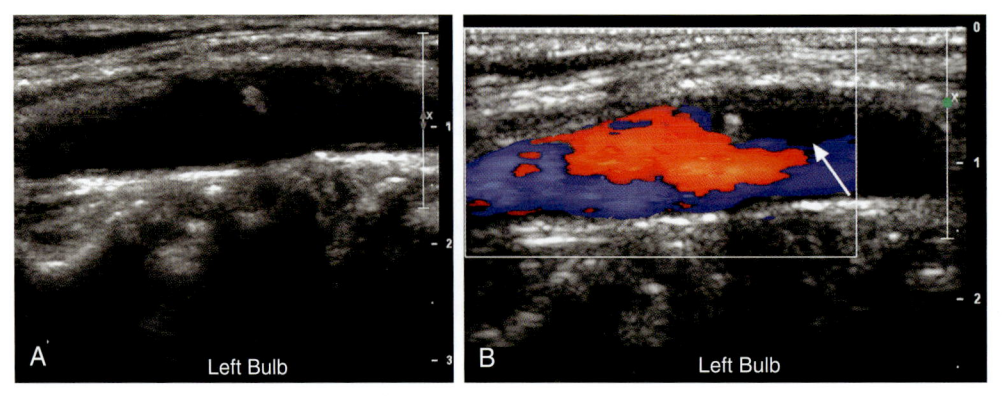

■ **FIGURE 90-20** Hypoechoic plaque. **A,** Longitudinal gray-scale image does not demonstrate the hypoechoic plaque in the left carotid bulb. **B,** However, the hypoechoic plaque (*arrow*) is clearly outlined by color flow on the color Doppler image.

CHAPTER 90 ● *Ultrasound Evaluation of the Carotid Arteries* 1239

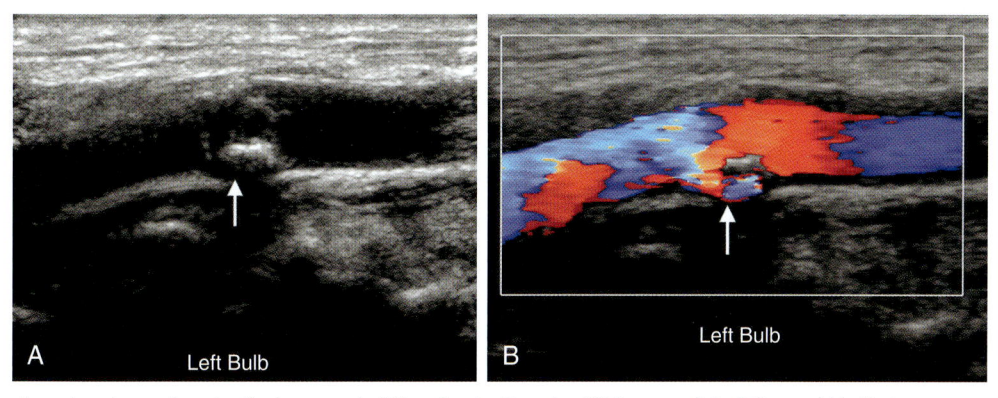

■ **FIGURE 90-21** Irregular plaque. Longitudinal gray-scale (**A**) and color Doppler (**B**) images of the left carotid bulb demonstrate flow (*arrow*) undermining a focus of echogenic, shadowing plaque.

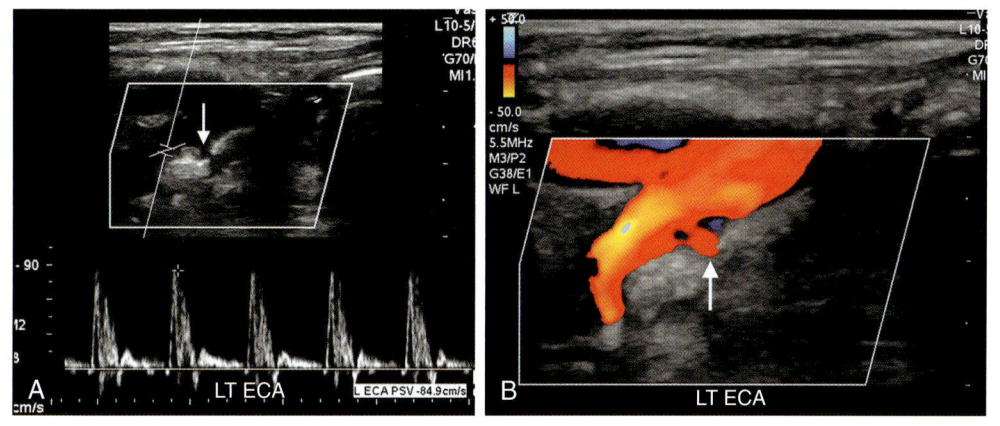

■ **FIGURE 90-22** Ulcerated plaque. Gray-scale (**A**) and color Doppler (**B**) images demonstrating a divot or pit (*arrow*) within a large area of echogenic plaque with an irregular surface. This probably represents an ulcer.

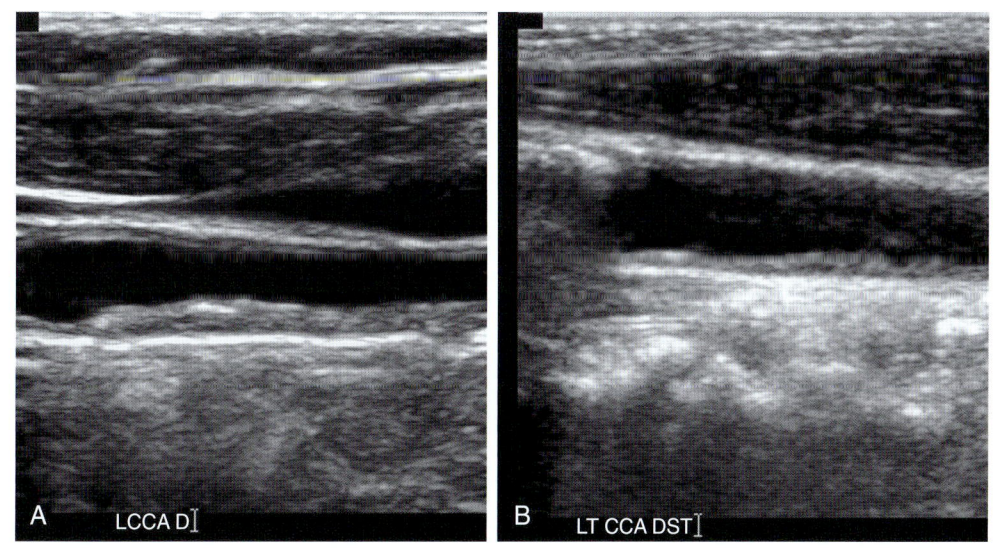

■ **FIGURE 90-23** Fibrointimal thickening. **A** and **B,** Longitudinal gray-scale images demonstrate diffuse hypoechoic, somewhat irregular thickening of the posterior wall of the CCA in two patients with fibrointimal thickening.

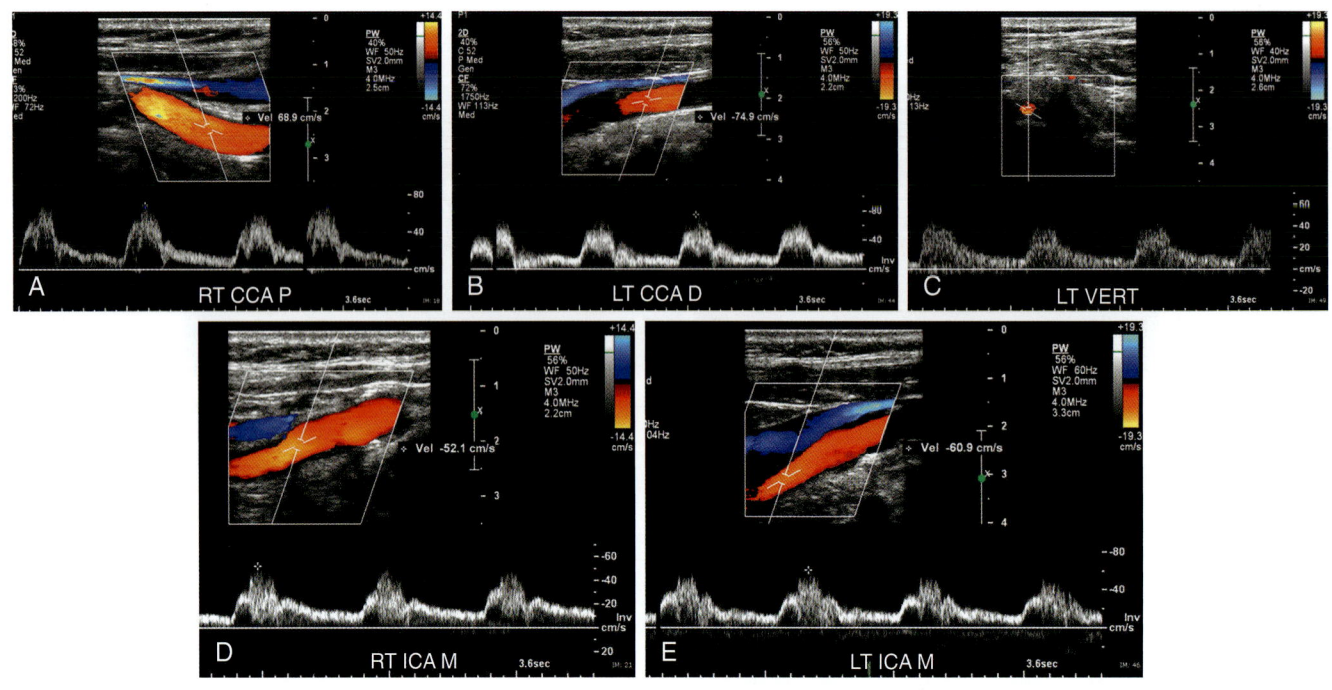

FIGURE 90-24 Aortic stenosis. Note tardus parvus waveform on spectral tracings of the right CCA (**A**), left CCA (**B**), and left vertebral artery (**C**). The delay in systolic acceleration is even more pronounced in the right (**D**) and left (**E**) ICAs. This 79-year-old woman has severe aortic stenosis with a mean aortic valve gradient of 58 mm Hg and valve area of 0.73 cm^2.

technical limitations to accurate measurement and reproducibility of such a thin structure as the vessel wall, and further research in this area continues.

WAVEFORM ANALYSIS OF THE CAROTID ARTERIES

The spectral Doppler waveform of the carotid arteries provides more information than merely a measure of PSV. Analysis of the contour or morphology of the waveform will reveal physiologic information concerning the distal cerebral circulation as well as the heart and more proximal vessels, which cannot be directly visualized on ultrasound examination. The presence of proximal or distal cardiovascular disease can thus be deduced. In addition, changes in the Doppler waveform may also provide clues to uncommon iatrogenic disease in the neck, such as carotid dissections, pseudoaneurysms, and arteriovenous fistulas. Albeit somewhat arbitrarily, abnormalities of the Doppler waveform can be subdivided for the purpose of analysis and description into changes that primarily affect systole, diastole, or the entire cardiac cycle.

Abnormalities of the Systolic Peak

Stenoses in the carotid vessels are the most common cause of changes in the configuration of the systolic peak. Although the focus of the carotid ultrasound examination is generally on the increase in PSV and EDV in an ICA stenosis, broadening of the spectral envelope, fill-in of the spectral window, and turbulence (random forward and backward flow) also occur. However, the outer contour of the systolic peak remains normal with a sharp systolic upstroke. The presence of such changes can help differentiate elevation of PSV due to a stenosis from an increase in PSV due to tortuosity of the vessel or systemic cause of increased PSV, such as hypertension, thyrotoxicosis, bradycardia, or aortic regurgitation (the water-hammer pulse; see later). Conversely, a global decrease in PSV can be seen in patients with hypotension, shock, tachycardia, thoracic aortic aneurysm, or decreased cardiac output (stroke volume) due, for example, to myocardial ischemia, poor myocardial contractility, cardiomyopathy, left ventricular aneurysm, or pericardial effusion.

Parvus Tardus Waveform

A parvus (diminished) tardus (delayed) waveform occurs distal to a severe proximal stenosis.[21,22] The parvus tardus waveform is characterized by decreased PSV and a delayed, more horizontal systolic upstroke with rounding or blunting of the systolic peak. The parvus tardus waveform phenomenon becomes more pronounced the more distal to the stenosis that the vessel is sampled. Hence, it is important to sample the ICA as distally as possible. In addition, the pattern of distribution of the parvus tardus waveform within the vessels in the neck helps pinpoint the location of the proximal stenosis. For example, if only the left CCA, ECA, and ICA have a parvus tardus waveform and if a sharp systolic upstroke is present in the right CCA, right ICA, and both vertebral arteries, the stenosis is likely to be at the level of the origin of the left CCA from the aortic arch. However, involvement of the bilateral CCAs, ICAs, and vertebral arteries is most likely indicative of a stenosis at the level of the aortic valve (Fig. 90-24).[23]

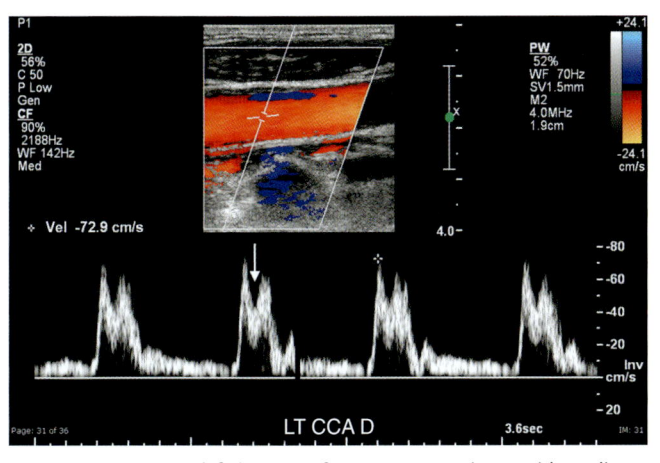

FIGURE 90-25 Bisferiens waveform. Note prominent midsystolic retraction (*arrow*) and two systolic peaks. This young patient has neither aortic regurgitation nor known cardiomyopathy. The bisferiens waveform may not be visualized in all vessels and may be visualized only intermittently in some patients.

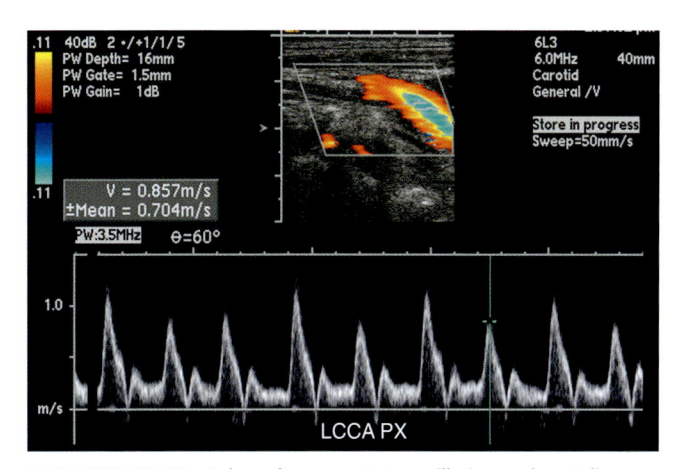

FIGURE 90-26 Pulsus alternans. Note oscillating peak systolic velocities in this 69-year-old man with history of atrial fibrillation, global hypokinesis, and ejection fraction of 30%. The patient had a middle cerebral artery infarct.

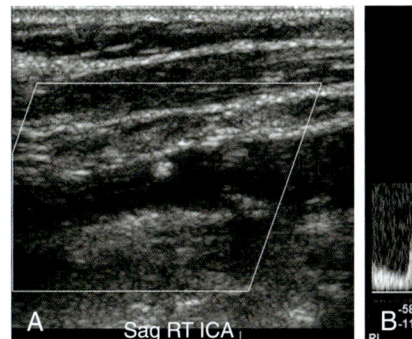

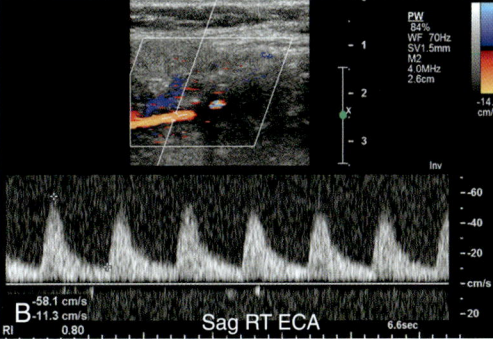

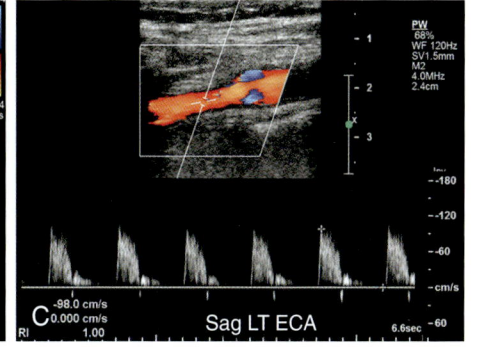

FIGURE 90-27 Internalization of the ECA. Color Doppler image (**A**) from an 83-year-old woman presenting with a stroke demonstrates no evidence of blood flow in the right ICA. Spectral Doppler tracing of the right ECA (**B**) demonstrates increased diastolic flow in comparison to the left ECA (**C**). This phenomenon is termed internalization of the ECA.

Pulsus Bisferiens Waveform

Rarely, two systolic peaks of similar velocity with an interposed midsystolic retraction or deceleration may be observed (Fig. 90-25). This has been termed pulsus bisferiens (Latin, "beat twice"). Whereas this has been described in the literature as most commonly associated with aortic regurgitation (particularly if it coexists with aortic stenosis) and hypertrophic cardiomyopathy,[24] it may more likely be a result of changes in compliance of the vessel wall. In our experience, a bifid systolic peak may be seen in healthy, athletic young individuals or in elderly patients without known underlying heart disease.

Pulsus Alternans Waveform

Alternating systolic velocity peaks, pulsus alternans, may be very rarely observed (Fig. 90-26). The cause of this phenomenon is not known. However, intrinsic myocardial disease, hypocalcemia, and impairment of venous return have been postulated as possible causes.[25]

Abnormalities of Diastolic Flow

The normal ECA demonstrates a characteristic high-resistance waveform pattern with little or no diastolic flow and an early diastolic notch. Although the amount of diastolic flow may vary from individual to individual, the diastolic flow pattern should be symmetric right to left in the same individual. When the ipsilateral ICA is occluded, "internalization" of the ECA may occur, and a lower resistance waveform pattern with increased diastolic flow and asymmetric to the contralateral ECA may be observed (Fig. 90-27).[22,26] This phenomenon is incompletely understood but probably reflects the development of low-resistance collateral pathways. Occlusion of the ipsilateral CCA may sometimes result in a similar waveform pattern in the ECA but with reversed flow if the ICA is reconstituted at the level of the carotid bulb by retrograde flow from the ECA (Fig. 90-28). In such cases, the ECA and ICA waveforms may also demonstrate a delay in systolic upstroke.

A high-resistance waveform pattern with diminished, absent, or reversed diastolic flow is an abnormal finding in the CCA or ICA suggestive of increased peripheral vascular resistance or a distal vascular occlusion or high-grade

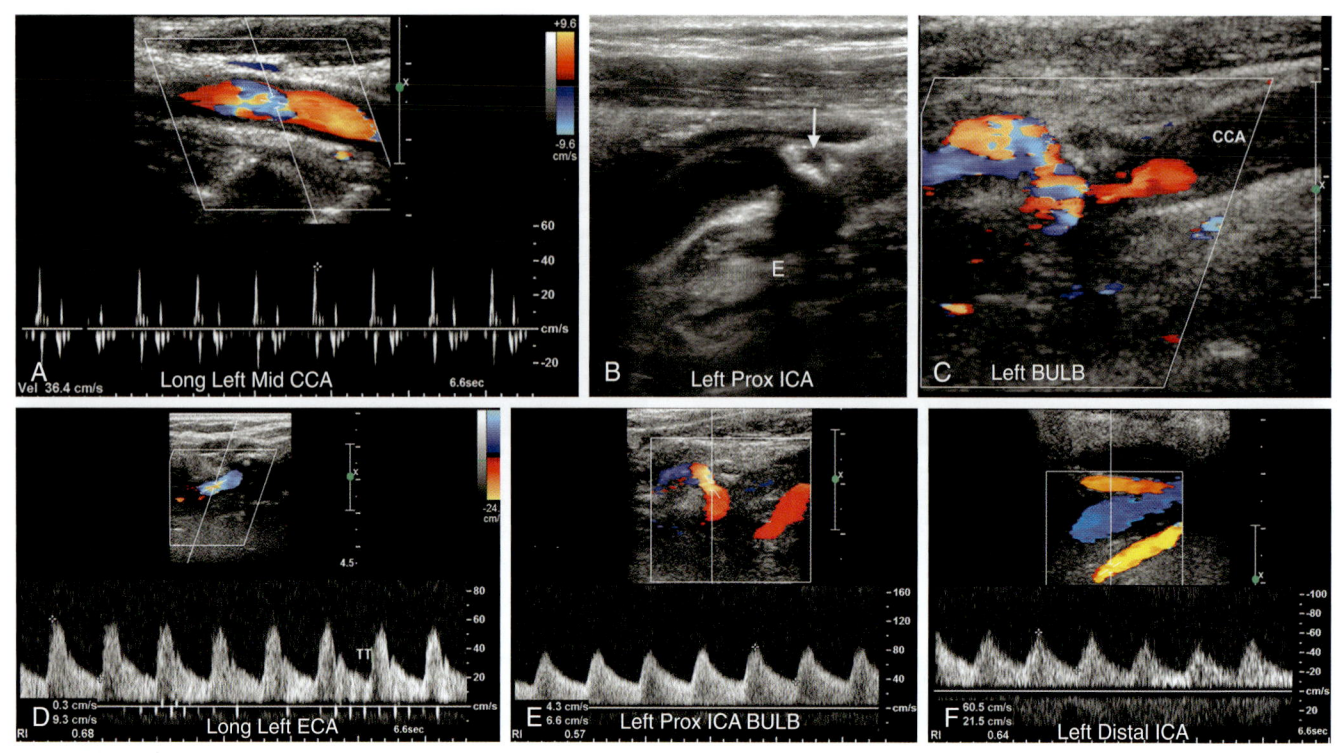

FIGURE 90-28 Occlusion of the common carotid artery. **A**, Spectral tracing of the proximal left CCA from an 81-year-old woman with history of left CCA occlusion demonstrates a high-resistance waveform pattern with absent end-diastolic flow, reversed early diastolic flow, and reduced PSV. **B**, Gray-scale image demonstrates plaque (*arrow*) in the left bulb and distal CCA. E, external carotid artery. **C**, Color flow image demonstrates occlusion of the distal left CCA. Flow is present in the ICA and ECA. There is also a small amount of regurgitant retrograde flow into the distal left CCA below the carotid bulb above the occlusive plaque or thrombus. **D**, Spectral Doppler tracing of the left ECA reveals reversed flow toward the transducer away from the head with increased diastolic flow. Spectral Doppler tracings of the proximal (**E**) and distal (**F**) left ICA reveal that the ICA is reconstituted from reversed flow in the left ECA and demonstrates flow toward the head with a slight delay in systolic upstroke and prominent diastolic flow.

stenosis. When PSV is significantly reduced, this appearance has been described as a "knocking" waveform pattern.[22] A unilateral knocking waveform pattern in the CCA is most commonly observed proximal to a distal high-grade stenosis or occlusion of the ICA or intracerebral vasculature (Figs. 90-28 and 90-29). The reversal of diastolic flow and decrease in PSV become more pronounced the closer to the obstructing lesion that the vessel is sampled. On occasion, a unilateral knocking waveform can be seen in the setting of distal vasospasm, arteritis, or carotid dissection. However, in the case of a carotid dissection, the sampled vessel will typically appear quite narrow over a long segment, and the echogenic dissection flap may also be seen on gray-scale images (see later). Bilateral high-resistance waveform patterns in the ICAs may indicate increased intracranial pressure, diffuse intracerebral vasospasm, or arteritis (Fig. 90-30).

When a high-resistance waveform pattern is noted in the proximal CCAs bilaterally and PSV is increased, aortic regurgitation is the usual cause. The precise diastolic flow pattern depends on the severity of the aortic regurgitation: diastolic flow may be reversed only in early diastole and associated with normal end-diastolic flow; early reversal of diastolic flow may be noted with absent end-diastolic flow; or in severe cases, reversed flow may be seen throughout diastole (Fig. 90-31).[22] This waveform pattern is the Doppler equivalent of the water-hammer pulse detected on physical examination in patients with severe aortic regurgitation. Typically, only moderate to severe aortic regurgitation will disturb the common carotid arterial waveform. The change in diastolic flow pattern and increase in PSV are more pronounced the more proximally one samples the CCA. The waveform pattern in the ICA or even distal CCA will normalize, depending on the severity of the aortic regurgitation. This is a bilateral phenomenon.

Abnormal Waveform Patterns Involving the Entire Cardiac Cycle

Diffusely complex carotid artery waveform patterns affecting the entire cardiac cycle are typically the result of iatrogenic or traumatic conditions. Although uncommon, carotid dissections, pseudoaneurysms, arteriovenous fistulas, and the presence of an intra-aortic balloon pump may be diagnosed by a combination of gray-scale appearance and characteristic waveform.

Dissections of the internal carotid arteries occur most commonly in the setting of trauma from compression of the ICA on the spine. However, spontaneous dissections may occur, particularly in patients with predisposing risk factors, such as Marfan syndrome, Ehlers-Danlos syndrome, fibromuscular dysplasia, cystic medial necrosis, hypertension, and drug abuse. Dissections may also extend

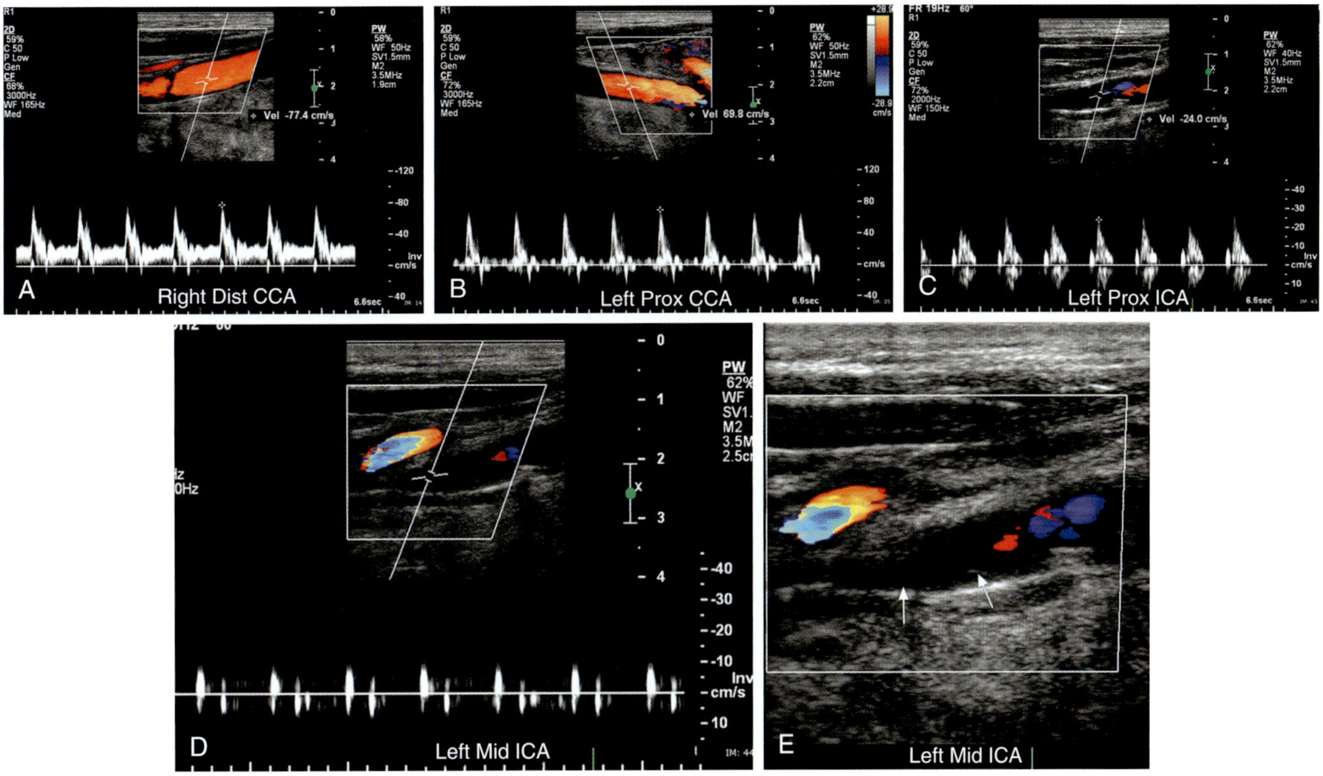

FIGURE 90-29 Knocking waveform pattern. Note asymmetry in the spectral waveforms of the normal right CCA (**A**) and left CCA (**B**). The left ICA has a high-resistance waveform with reduced or absent diastolic flow. PSV, however, is normal. Duplex Doppler interrogation of the proximal left ICA (**C**) and mid left ICA (**D**) reveals a classic knocking waveform pattern with extremely low PSV and absent diastolic flow. PSV is 24 cm/sec in the proximal left ICA and 10 cm/sec in the mid left ICA. PSV decreases as one samples more distally in the left ICA. This is due to complete occlusion of the distal left ICA demonstrated on the sagittal color Doppler image (**E,** *arrows*).

into the CCAs from an aortic dissection. Dissection of the ICA is the most common cause of stroke in young patients, exclusive of cardiac disease. Additional presenting symptoms of carotid dissection include acute onset of headache and Horner syndrome.

Carotid Dissection

In patients with carotid dissection, an echogenic intraluminal flap may be observed on longitudinal or transverse gray-scale images (Fig. 90-32A,B). Flow in both the true and false lumens may be detected on Doppler imaging, albeit with different velocities and waveform patterns (Fig. 90-32C). The spectral Doppler waveform pattern is highly variable, probably related to the length of the dissection, diameter of the lumen, fenestration of the dissection flap, coexisting involvement of aortic dissection, and whether the true or false lumen is sampled (Fig. 90-32D,E). The waveform may be irregular with low-velocity spikes and flutters, making it difficult to distinguish systole from diastole. If the false lumen is thrombosed or if only intramural hematoma is present, gray-scale and color flow imaging will simply reveal a long, smoothly marginated stenosis. The thickening of the arterial wall is typically hypoechoic and may spiral or smoothly taper the distal arterial lumen (Fig. 90-33).[27] A long-segment tapering intraluminal hematoma may create an extremely narrowed lumen with a string sign on color Doppler imaging. In such cases, the waveform may be indistinguishable from a carotid stenosis; the clues to dissection are the length and smoothness of the stenosis, absence of coexistent plaque, and clinical setting. A high-resistance pulsatile but dampened waveform with little or no diastolic flow may be noted proximally in such cases.[27-29]

Carotid Pseudoaneurysm

Pseudoaneurysms arising from the carotid arteries occur most commonly in the CCAs as a result of inadvertent needle sticks during attempts to place an internal jugular central line. However, pseudoaneurysms may also occur in the setting of other forms of penetrating trauma (including drug abuse), blunt trauma, infection, cystic medial necrosis, invasion of the carotid artery by malignant neoplasm, and after carotid endarterectomy. On gray-scale and color Doppler imaging, pseudoaneurysms are easily recognized as an outpouching from the carotid artery. The degree of color fill-in will depend on the amount of intraluminal thrombus (Fig. 90-34A,B). Spectral Doppler interrogation will reveal a "to-and-fro" pattern within the neck, if it is narrow, with flow toward the pseudoaneurysm in systole and back toward the carotid artery during diastole (Fig. 90-34C). If the neck is wide, the waveform will be randomly irregular and turbulent.

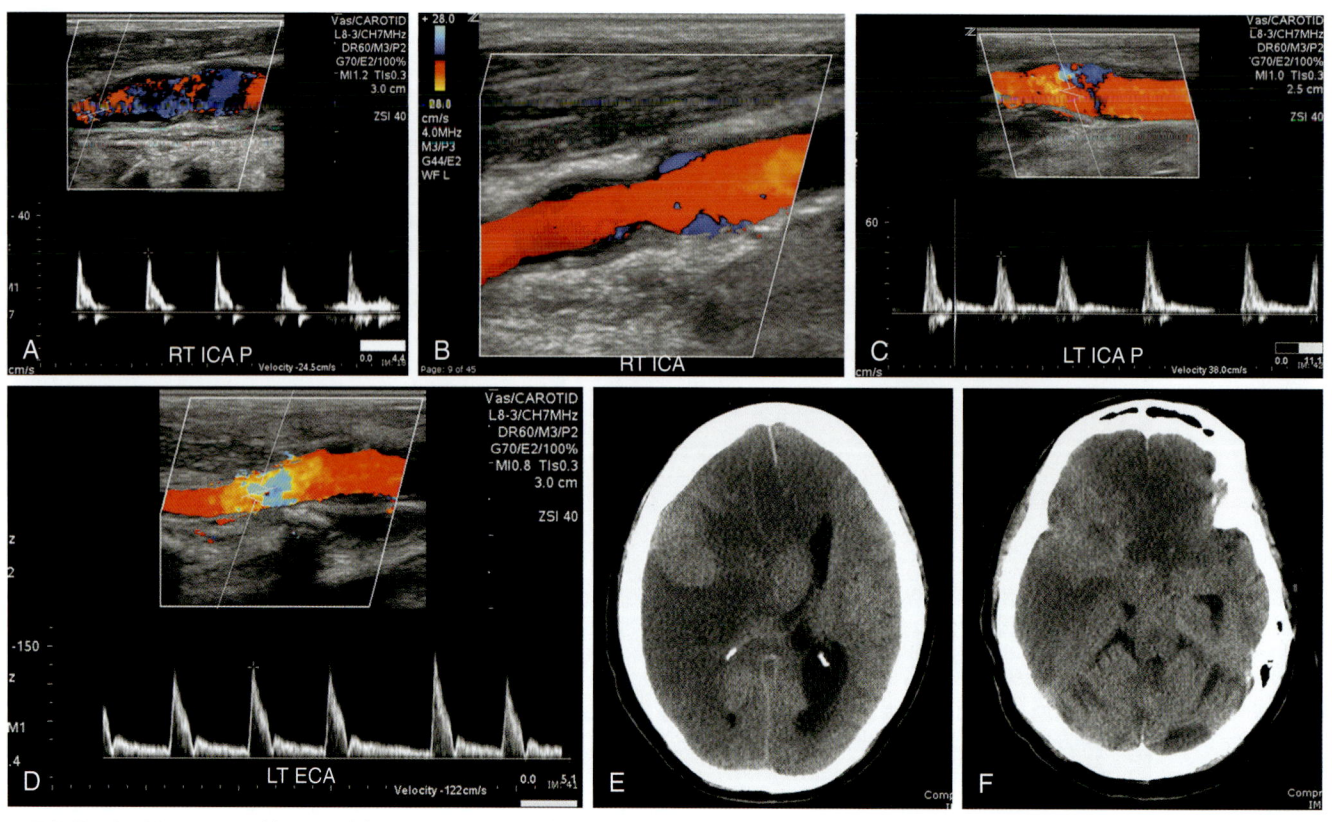

■ **FIGURE 90-30** Increased intracranial pressure. **A,** Spectral tracing of the right ICA from a 75-year-old woman with a large right hemispheric stroke reveals a knocking waveform with decreased PSV (24 cm/sec) and absent end-diastolic flow. **B,** Longitudinal color Doppler image demonstrates that the right ICA is widely patent. Magnetic resonance angiography (not shown) demonstrated occlusion of the right middle cerebral artery. Duplex Doppler interrogation reveals markedly reduced flow, both systolic and diastolic, in the left ICA (**C**), which was widely patent. Note that there is actually more diastolic flow in the left ECA (**D**) than in the ICA. These findings are due to increased intracranial pressure from the large right middle cerebral artery stroke. Axial CT images of the brain reveal both transtentorial (**E**) and uncal (**F**) herniation as well as the large middle cerebral artery stroke. Note midline shift and compression of the left lateral ventricle as well as obliteration of the right lateral ventricle (**E**).

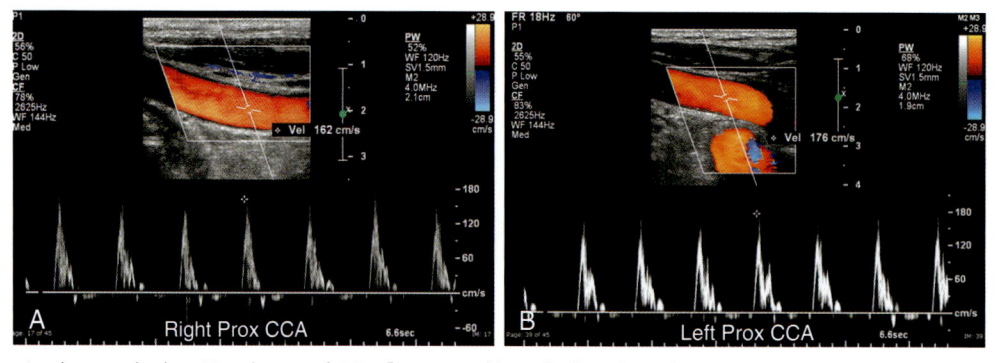

■ **FIGURE 90-31** Aortic regurgitation. Note increased PSV, flow reversal in early diastole, and absent diastolic flow in the right (**A**) and left (**B**) CCAs in a patient with severe aortic regurgitation. Waveforms in the distal ICAs were normal bilaterally.

Arteriovenous Fistula

Arteriovenous fistulas involving the carotid arteries typically occur secondary to trauma or malignant invasion. Color Doppler interrogation may demonstrate the connection between the artery and the vein (Fig. 90-35A,B). Color aliasing due to high-velocity flow within the arteriovenous fistula may be observed, and a color bruit due to tissue reverberation secondary to the high-velocity flow may be seen in the surrounding soft tissues. Spectral Doppler interrogation will reveal a low-resistance waveform pattern characterized by an increase in both peak systolic and end-diastolic flow in the feeding artery. However, the carotid artery distal to the arteriovenous fistula will have a normal waveform pattern. Pulsatile high-velocity flow will be observed in the draining vein (Fig. 90-35C).

Intra-aortic Balloon Pump

Placement of an intra-aortic balloon pump results in a characteristic waveform in the carotid arteries with

CHAPTER 90 • Ultrasound Evaluation of the Carotid Arteries   1245

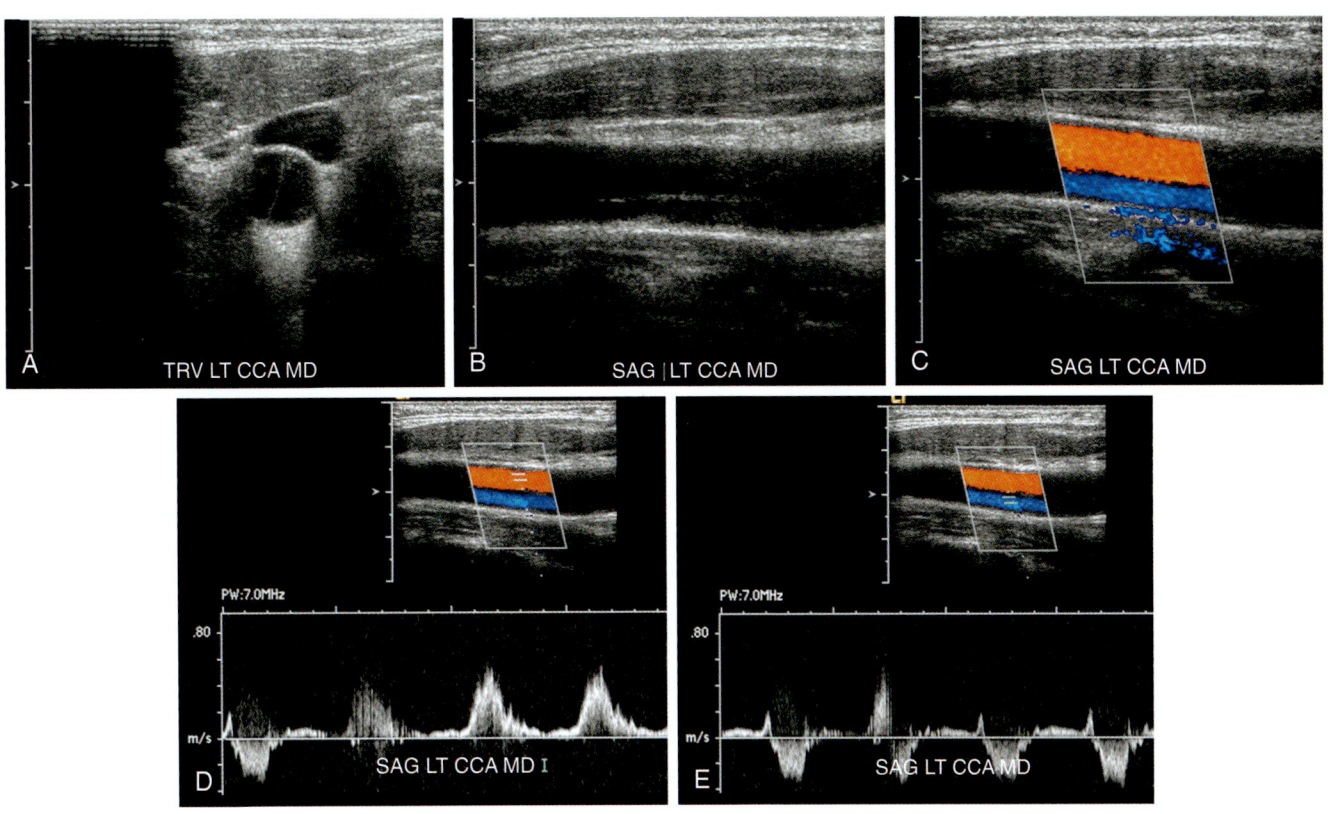

FIGURE 90-32 Carotid dissection. Transverse (**A**) and longitudinal (**B**) gray-scale images of the left mid CCA from a 36-year-old man with Marfan syndrome and a type A aortic dissection reveal a thin dissection flap. **C,** Longitudinal color Doppler image reveals flow in the true lumen (red) and reversed flow in the false lumen (blue). **D,** Spectral Doppler tracing from the true lumen demonstrates a slight delay in systolic upstroke and reduced diastolic flow. **E,** The waveform in the false lumen is extremely irregular, and flow direction is reversed.

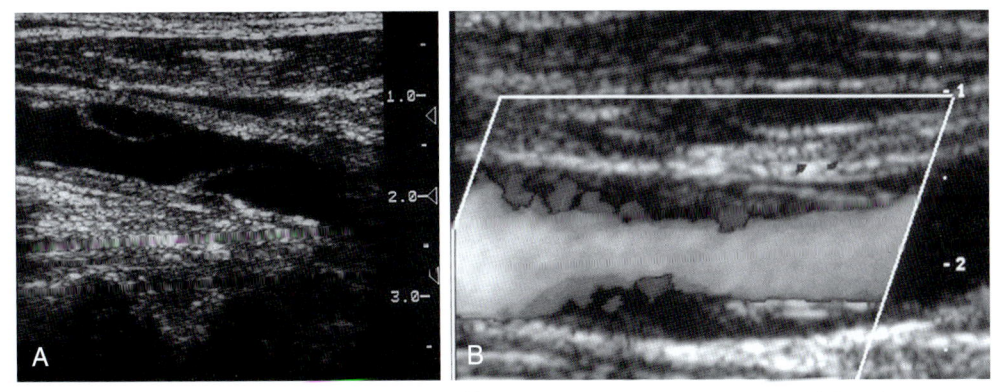

FIGURE 90-33 Intramural hematoma due to carotid dissection. This 22-year-old patient presented with a left neck hematoma and pain after a motor vehicle accident. Color Doppler image demonstrates markedly hypoechoic circumferential "thickening" of the wall of the CCA consistent with an intramural hematoma or thrombosed false lumen. Note that the vessel lumen is narrowed over a long segment. *(From Scoutt LM, Lin FL, Kliewer M. Waveform analysis of the carotid arteries. Ultrasound Clin 2006; 1:133-159.)*

"double systolic peaks." Inflation of the balloon during early diastole causes a second peak of forward flow, increasing flow to the coronary arteries—an intended effect of the balloon pump. Deflation of the balloon at the end of diastole results in a short flow reversal (Fig. 90-36). The intra-aortic balloon pump may be set at different ratios. If it is set at a 1:1 ratio, the pump is activated during every cardiac cycle. When the pump is set at a 1:2 ratio, the balloon pump is triggered to inflate only every second cardiac cycle. Whereas placement of an intra-aortic balloon pump results in an increase of total volume of forward blood flow during systole, PSV is normally decreased. Therefore, carotid stenoses cannot be graded by only using absolute PSV criteria in patients with intra-aortic balloon pumps, and more reliance must be placed on the color Doppler and gray-scale images.

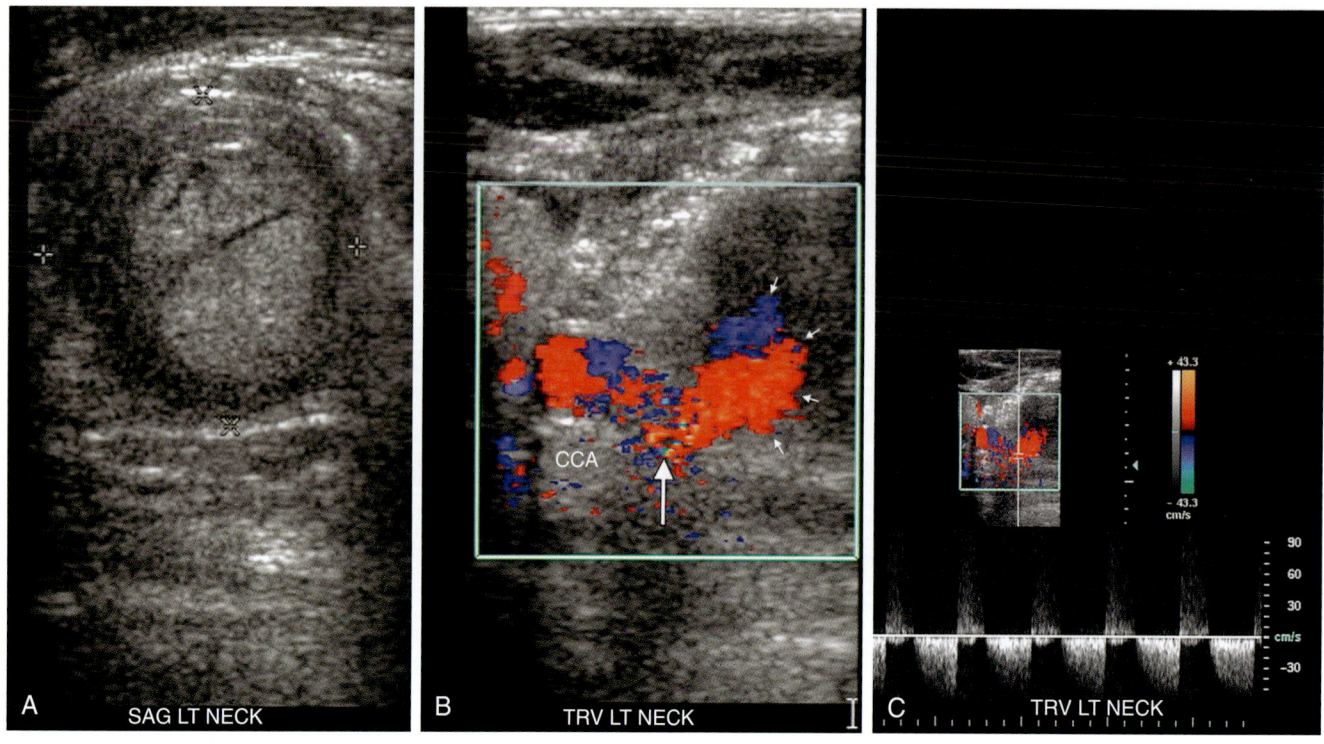

■ **FIGURE 90-34** Pseudoaneurysm of the common carotid artery. **A,** Gray-scale image of the left neck from a 50-year-old man with neck swelling after placement of a central line reveals a mass (*cursors*) representing a largely thrombosed pseudoaneurysm. **B,** Color Doppler image demonstrates the neck arising from the CCA with a small focus of color aliasing (*long arrow*) indicating increased velocity. There is a small amount of flow (*short arrows*) with a yin-yang pattern at the base of the pseudoaneurysm. **C,** Spectral tracing from the neck of the pseudoaneurysm reveals a classic to-and-fro waveform pattern above the baseline in systole and below the baseline in diastole.

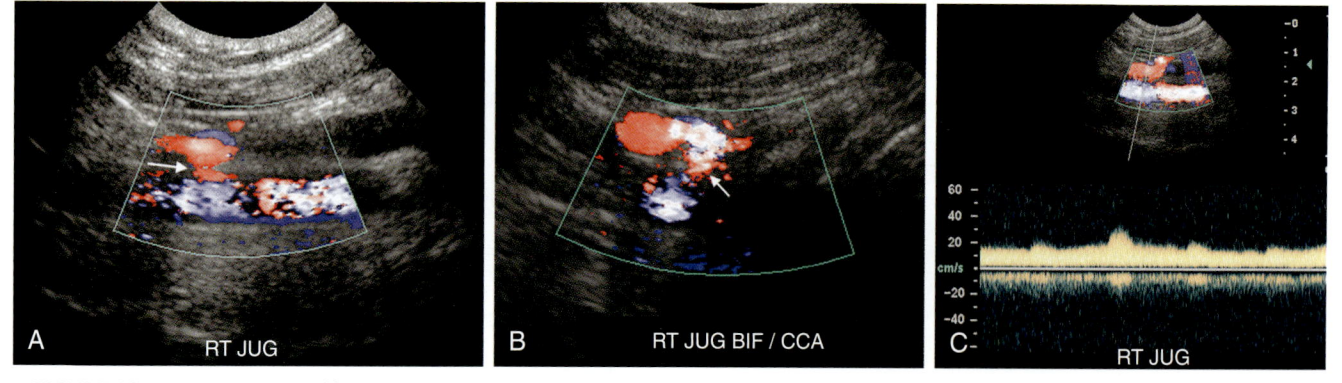

■ **FIGURE 90-35** Common carotid artery to internal jugular fistula. Sagittal (**A**) and transverse (**B**) color Doppler images from a 46-year-old woman with right upper extremity swelling after attempted central line placement demonstrate a connection (arteriovenous fistula, *arrow*) between the right internal jugular vein (red) and CCA (blue). **C,** Spectral Doppler tracing from the right internal jugular vein reveals pulsatile flow.

THE VERTEBRAL ARTERY

In most patients, only the midportion of the vertebral artery in the neck can be directly examined with Doppler ultrasound. However, the presence of distal or proximal disease can occasionally be deduced by analysis of the spectral waveform of the vertebral artery.[30] The normal vertebral artery waveform is symmetric right to left and similar to the waveform of the ICA with a sharp systolic upstroke and continuous forward diastolic flow (see Fig. 90-9).

Asymmetrically increased PSV in a vertebral artery may indicate a proximal stenosis. However, the vertebral arteries are often asymmetric in size, and hence an increase in PSV in one vertebral artery may be simply due to compensatory flow. Increased flow in the vertebral artery may also be noted in the setting of an ipsilateral ICA occlusion. Proximal stenosis of the vertebral artery may also cause a unilateral tardus parvus waveform in the upper to mid vertebral artery. Bilateral tardus parvus waveforms in the vertebral arteries associated with tardus parvus waveforms in the carotid arteries suggest aortic stenosis. A high-resistance waveform pattern with low PSV and absent diastolic flow may indicate a distal stenosis or occlusion of the basilar artery or increased intracranial pressure.[30]

Subclavian Steal Syndrome

Patients with subclavian steal due to a proximal stenosis in the subclavian artery may present with vertigo, syncope, headaches, transient ischemic attacks, visual disturbances, and hearing loss. However, patients may be completely asymptomatic.[31] In patients with complete subclavian steal, reversed flow will be noted in the vertebral artery on Doppler interrogation (Fig. 90-37A). Doppler interrogation of the ipsilateral subclavian artery will demonstrate increased PSV medially and a tardus parvus waveform distally in the axillary and brachial arteries (Fig. 90-37B,C). A "pre-steal" waveform characterized by a sharp midsystolic retraction or deceleration has been described by Kliewer and associates[32] (Fig. 90-38). The depth of the midsystolic retraction depends on the severity of the proximal subclavian stenosis. However, all pre-steal waveforms will demonstrate two systolic peaks. The first is narrow with a sharp upstroke and sharply pointed peak. The second systolic peak is usually of lower velocity and broader as well as rounder in contour. With deeper midsystolic retractions, it may be more difficult to

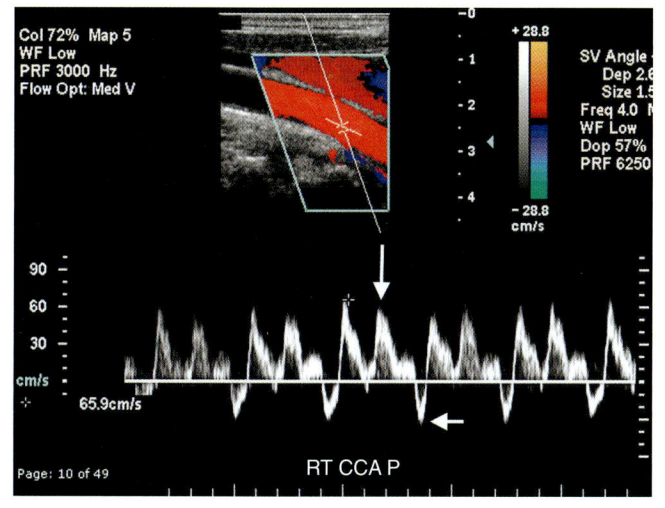

FIGURE 90-36 Intra-aortic balloon pump. Note second peak of forward flow (*long arrow*) resulting from inflation of the intra-aortic balloon pump in early diastole in this patient with ischemic cardiomyopathy. Deflation of the balloon results in a transient reversal of flow (*short arrow*) at the end of diastole.

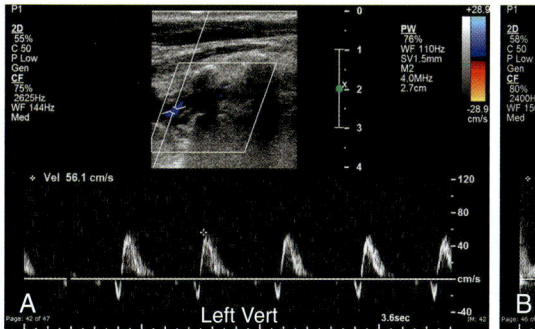

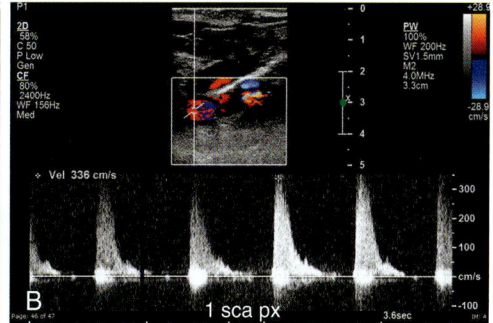

FIGURE 90-37 Subclavian steal. **A**, Spectral Doppler tracing of the left vertebral artery reveals reversed flow heading toward the transducer away from the head. **B**, Note increased PSV of 336 cm/sec in the proximal left subclavian artery in a patient with a left subclavian artery stenosis causing a subclavian steal phenomenon.

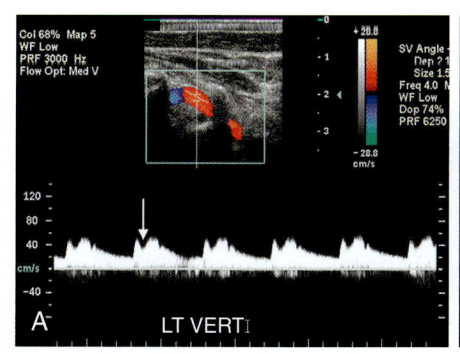

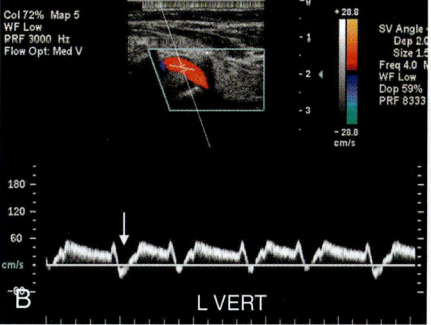

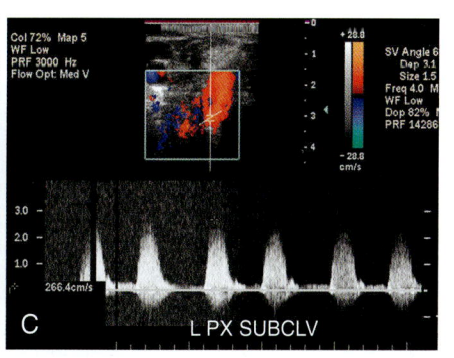

FIGURE 90-38 Pre-steal vertebral artery waveform. **A**, Note midsystolic retraction (*arrow*) in the left vertebral artery in a patient with a moderate left subclavian stenosis on October 6, 2006. **B**, By June 9, 2008, the midsystolic retraction (*arrow*) had deepened, and there was transient flow reversal. **C**, Spectral Doppler tracing of the origin of the left subclavian artery at that time demonstrated a PSV of 266 cm/sec, consistent with a high-grade stenosis.

1248 PART FIFTEEN • *The Carotid Arteries*

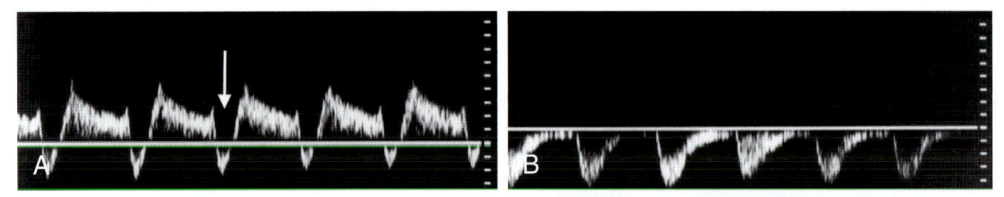

■ **FIGURE 90-39** Subclavian steal—provocative maneuvers. In some cases, provocative maneuvers will deepen the midsystolic retraction in a pre-steal waveform, causing a transient reversal of midsystolic flow or complete flow reversal in the vertebral artery. **A,** Left vertebral artery waveform obtained at rest in an 83-year-old woman who has a known left subclavian stenosis demonstrates a prominent midsystolic retraction with transient reversal of flow (*arrow*). This is a pre-steal waveform, type 4. **B,** After inflation of blood pressure cuff on the left arm and subsequent rapid deflation, there is conversion of the pre-steal waveform to a complete steal, with reversal of blood flow throughout the cardiac cycle. Inflation of the blood pressure cuff causes mild hypoxia in the distal arm. Deflation of the cuff induces relative hyperemia in the distal arm and increases blood flow across the subclavian stenosis, resulting in a complementary pressure drop and change in direction of blood flow in the ipsilateral vertebral artery toward the now lower pressure subclavian artery. (*From Kliewer MA, Hertzberg BS, Kim DH, et al. Vertebral artery Doppler waveform changes indicating subclavian steal physiology. AJR Am J Roentgenol 2000; 174:816-819. Reprinted with permission from the American Journal of Roentgenology.*)

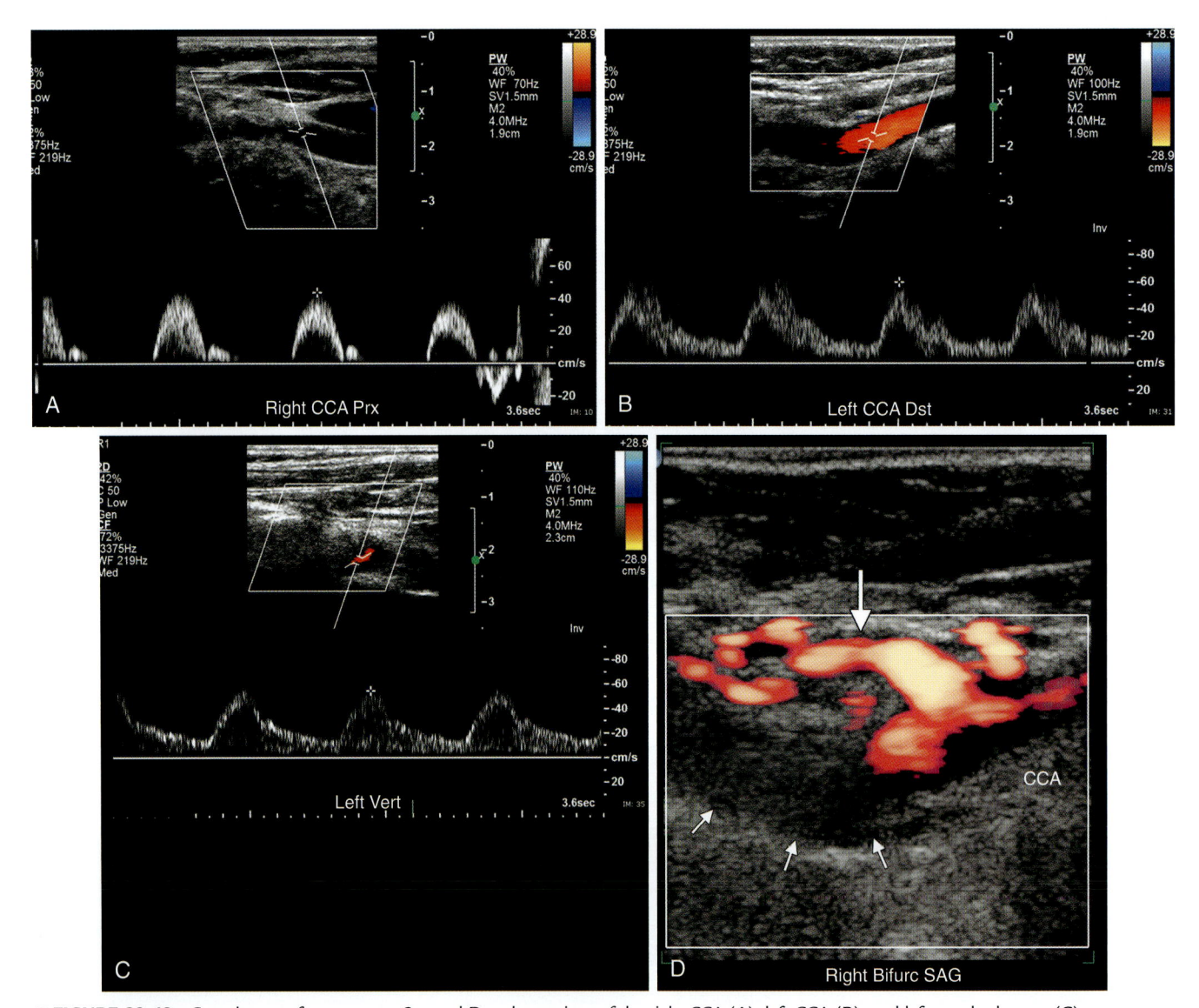

■ **FIGURE 90-40** Complex waveform pattern. Spectral Doppler tracings of the right CCA (**A**), left CCA (**B**), and left vertebral artery (**C**) demonstrate bilateral tardus parvus waveforms with a delay in systolic upstroke and rounding of the systolic peak. However, the amount of diastolic flow is asymmetric right to left, with complete absence of diastolic flow in the right CCA. In addition, PSV is reduced, only 44 cm/sec in the right CCA in comparison to 60 cm/sec in the left CCA. **D,** Power Doppler image demonstrating absence of flow in the right ICA (*short arrows*). Note flow in ECA and branches (*long arrow*) and CCA. This patient has aortic stenosis resulting in bilateral tardus parvus waveforms as well as a complete occlusion of the right ICA resulting in a high-resistance waveform (absent diastolic flow) in the right CCA.

differentiate the second peak from diastole. Provocative maneuvers, such as exercising the hand or inflating a blood pressure cuff above systolic arterial pressure until the hand is mildly symptomatic (usually 3 to 5 minutes), then releasing the cuff and immediately re-evaluating the vertebral artery waveform, can convert a pre-steal waveform into a complete steal or deepen the midsystolic retraction (Fig. 90-39).[32] Grant and colleagues[33] have described a similar waveform pattern in the right common carotid and internal carotid arteries in patients with high-grade stenoses of the innominate artery.

CONCLUSION

Doppler interrogation of the carotid arteries is a highly accurate, readily accessible, inexpensive, and noninvasive method of diagnosis of high-grade (>70%) stenosis of the ICA. With careful attention to technique, longitudinal color and power Doppler images provide morphologic information similar to an angiogram unless the image is degraded by shadowing from calcified plaque. Gray-scale and color Doppler images are important for identification of hypoechoic or irregular plaque, which is believed to progress more rapidly and to pose an increased risk of thromboembolic events. Spectral Doppler interrogation provides not only PSV measurements to used grade stenoses of the ICA but also physiologic information that can provide clues to more proximal or distal cardiovascular disease, which in complex cases may be multifactorial (Fig. 90-40). To avoid pitfalls in the estimation of ICA stenoses, PSV criteria should always be correlated with the gray-scale images and analysis of the spectral waveforms. Similarly, an increase in the PSV of the vertebral artery may indicate a proximal stenosis, and changes in the waveform pattern of the vertebral artery may indicate proximal or distal cardiovascular disease, such as a subclavian steal.

KEY POINTS

- Carotid ultrasound examination is highly accurate for detection of stenoses of the ICA of more than 70%.
- Velocity criteria for grading of ICA stenoses should be validated in individual laboratories and can be chosen to maximize sensitivity or specificity.
- The Society of Radiologists in Ultrasound consensus conference[13] has proposed that a PSV of more than 230 cm/sec and an ICA/CCA PSV ratio above 4.0 are highly accurate criteria for diagnosis of ICA stenoses of more than 70%.
- Velocity criteria should always be correlated with the amount of plaque visualized on gray-scale and color flow imaging as well as waveform analysis.
- Hypoechoic plaque and plaque with an irregular surface are associated with a higher risk of thromboembolic events and more rapid progression.
- Waveforms in the carotid arteries should be symmetric right to left.
- A high-resistance waveform with diminished diastolic flow suggests a distal occlusion, high-grade stenosis, or increased peripheral vascular resistance.
- A tardus parvus waveform with delayed systolic upstroke suggests a proximal stenosis.

SUGGESTED READINGS

Bluth EI. Evaluation and characterization of carotid plaque. Semin Ultrasound CT MR 1997; 18:57-65.
Grant EG, Benson CB, Moneta GL, et al. Carotid artery stenosis: gray-scale and Doppler US diagnosis—Society of Radiologists in Ultrasound Consensus Conference. Radiology 2003; 229:340-346.
Horrow MM, Stassi J. Sonography of the vertebral arteries: a window to disease of the proximal great vessels. AJR Am J Roentgenol 2001; 177:53-59.
Polak JF. Carotid ultrasound. Radiol Clin North Am 2001; 39:569-589.
Robbin ML, Lockhart ME. Carotid artery ultrasound interpretation using a pattern recognition approach. Ultrasound Clin 2006; 1:111-131.
Rohren EM, Kliewer MA, Carroll BA, Hertzberg BS. A spectrum of Doppler waveforms in the carotid and vertebral arteries. AJR Am J Roentgenol 2003; 181:1695-1704.
Scoutt LM, Lin FL, Kliewer M. Waveform analysis of the carotid arteries. Ultrasound Clin 2006; 1:133-159.
Zwiebel WJ, Pellerito JS. Tricky and interesting carotid cases. Ultrasound Q 2005; 21:113-122.
Zwiebel WJ, Pellerito JS. Uncommon but important carotid pathology. Ultrasound Q 2005; 21:131-140.

REFERENCES

1. American Heart Association. Heart Disease and Stroke Statistics—2005 Update. Dallas, TX, American Heart Association, 2005.
2. Timsit SG, Sacco RL, Mohr JP, et al. Early clinical differentiation of cerebral infarction from severe atherosclerotic stenosis and cardioembolism. Stroke 1992; 23:486-491.
3. North American Symptomatic Carotid Endarterectomy Trial Collaborators. Beneficial effect of carotid endarterectomy in symptomatic patients with high grade stenosis. N Engl J Med 1991; 325:445-453.
4. Barnett H, Taylor D, Eliasaw M, et al. Benefit of carotid endarterectomy in patients with symptomatic moderate or severe stenosis. N Engl J Med 1998; 339:1415-1425.
5. Executive Committee for Asymptomatic Carotid Atherosclerosis Study. Endarterectomy for asymptomatic carotid artery stenosis. JAMA 1995; 273:1421-1428.
6. European Carotid Surgery Trialists' Collaborative Group. MRC European Carotid Surgery Trial: interim results for symptomatic patients with severe (70-99%) or with mild (0-29%) carotid stenosis. Lancet 1991; 337:1235-1243.
7. Kliewer MA, Freed KS, Hertzberg BS, et al. Temporal artery tap: usefulness and limitations in carotid sonography. Radiology 1996; 201:481-484.
8. Budorick NE, Rojratanakiat W, O'Boyel MK, et al. Digital tapping of the superficial temporal artery: significance on carotid duplex sonography. J Ultrasound Med 1996; 15:459-464.
9. Spencer MP, Reid JM. Quantitation of carotid stenosis with continuous wave (CW) Doppler ultrasound. Stroke 1979; 10:326-330.
10. Moneta GL, Edwards JM, Chitwood RW, et al. Correlation of North American Symptomatic Carotid Endarterectomy Trial (NASCET) angiographic definition of 70% to 99% internal carotid artery

stenosis with duplex scanning. J Vasc Surg 1993; 17:152-157; discussion 157-159.
11. Carpenter JP, Lexa FJ, Davis JT. Determination of duplex Doppler ultrasound criteria appropriate to the North American Symptomatic Carotid Endarterectomy Trial. Stroke 1996; 27:695-699.
12. Grant EG, Duerinckx AJ, El Saden S, et al. Doppler sonographic parameters for grading of carotid stenosis: is there an optimum method for their selection? AJR Am J Roentgenol 1999; 172:1123-1129.
13. Grant EG, Benson CB, Moneta GL, et al. Carotid artery stenosis: gray-scale and Doppler US diagnosis—Society of Radiologists in Ultrasound Consensus Conference. Radiology 2003; 229:340-346.
14. Sabeti S, Schillinger M, Mlekusch W, et al. Quantification of internal carotid artery stenosis with duplex US: comparative analysis of different flow velocity criteria. Radiology 2004; 232:431-439.
15. AbuRahma AF, Richmond BK, Robinson PA, et al. Effect of contralateral severe stenosis or carotid occlusion on duplex criteria of ipsilateral stenoses: comparative study of various duplex parameters. J Vasc Surg 1995; 22:751-762.
16. Busuttil SJ, Franklin DJ, Youkey JR, Elmore JR. Carotid duplex overestimation of stenosis due to severe contralateral disease. Am J Surg 1996; 172:144-148.
17. Polak JF, Shemanski L, O'Leary DH, et al. Hypoechoic plaque at US of the carotid artery: an independent risk factor for incident stroke in adults aged 65 years or older. Cardiovascular Healthy Study. Radiology 1998; 208:649-654.
18. Bluth EI. Evaluation and characterization of carotid plaque. Semin Ultrasound CT MR 1997; 18:57-65.
19. O'Leary DH, Polak JF, Kronmal RA, et al. Carotid artery intima and media thickness as a risk factor for myocardial infarction and stroke in older adults. Cardiovascular Health Study Collaborative Research Group. N Engl J Med 1999; 340:14-22.
20. O'Leary DH, Polak JF. Intima-media thickness: a tool for atherosclerosis imaging and event prediction. Am J Cardiol 2002; 90:18L-21L.
21. Kotval PS. Doppler waveform parvus and tardus: a sign of proximal flow obstruction. J Ultrasound Med 1989; 8:435-440.
22. Rohren EM, Kliewer MA, Carroll BA, Hertzberg BS. A spectrum of Doppler waveforms in the carotid and vertebral Arteries. AJR Am J Roentgenol 2003; 181:1695-1704.
23. O'Boyle MK, Vibhakar N, Chung J, et al. Duplex sonography of the carotid arteries in patients with isolated aortic stenosis: imaging findings and relation to severity of stenosis. AJR Am J Roentgenol 1996; 166:197-202.
24. Kallman CE, Gosink BB, Gardner DJ. Carotid duplex sonography: bisferious pulse contour in patients with aortic valvular disease. AJR Am J Roentgenol 1991; 157:403-407.
25. Cohn KE, Sandler H, Hancock EW. Mechanisms of pulsus alternans. Circulation 1967; 36:372-380.
26. AbuRahma AF, Pollack JA, Robinson PA, Mullins D. The reliability of color duplex ultrasound in diagnosing total carotid artery occlusion. Am J Surg 1997; 174:185-187.
27. Khaw KT, Griffiths PD. Non-invasive imaging of the cervical carotid and vertebral arteries. Imaging 2001; 13:376-390.
28. Gardner DJ, Gosink BB, Kallman CE. Internal carotid artery dissections: duplex US imaging. J Ultrasound Med 1991; 10:607-614.
29. Hennerici M, Steinke W, Rautonberg W. High-resistance Doppler flow pattern in extracranial carotid dissection. Arch Neurol 1989; 46:670-672.
30. Horrow MM, Stassi J. Sonography of the vertebral arteries: a window to disease of the proximal great vessels. AJR Am J Roentgenol 2001; 177:53-59.
31. Gosselin G, Walker PM. Subclavian steal syndrome: existence, clinical features, diagnosis and management. Semin Vasc Surg 1996; 9:93-97.
32. Kliewer MA, Hertzberg BS, Kim DH, et al. Vertebral artery Doppler waveform changes indicating subclavian steal physiology. AJR Am J Roentgenol 2000; 174:815-819.
33. Grant EG, Elsaden S, Modrazo B, et al. Innominate artery occlusive disease: sonographic findings. AJR Am J Roentgenol 2006; 186:394-400.

CHAPTER 91

Magnetic Resonance and Computed Tomographic Angiography of the Extracranial Carotid Arteries

J. Kevin DeMarco, John Huston 3d, and Hideki Ota

There is clear evidence from multiple carotid trials, including a recent pooled data analysis, that surgical intervention with carotid endarterectomy (CEA) has significant benefits compared with medical therapy in symptomatic patients with severe carotid stenosis.[1-3] Conventional catheter-based invasive angiography with cut film or intra-arterial digital subtraction angiography (DSA) has been the gold standard for measuring the carotid stenosis in these trials. The improved efficacy of noninvasive imaging techniques and the attendant risk of stroke during DSA has led many practices to adopt noninvasive modalities, such as Doppler ultrasound, magnetic resonance angiography (MRA), and/or computed tomography angiography (CTA) to replace this invasive study.

To understand how and when to apply these noninvasive modalities, we need to be able to balance our knowledge of the sensitivity and specificity of ultrasound, CTA, and MRA to identify a severe stenosis with the attendant risks of DSA as well as the risk of CEA. We can borrow a technique called decision analysis to help understand these various factors. Decision analysis takes the sensitivity and specificity of a noninvasive study, risk of stroke with DSA, risk of thromboembolic disease after CEA, risk of withholding CEA in patients with severe symptomatic stenosis, and risk of undergoing CEA with only moderate symptomatic carotid stenosis, as well as the costs of the noninvasive studies DSA, and CEA, into account.[4] The results of this decision analysis allow us to test the risks or costs of various noninvasive carotid stenosis imaging strategies. Decision analysis demonstrates these various tradeoffs, which may not otherwise be apparent. Using DSA alone, all patients face the risk of procedural stroke. With MRA strategy, a few patients with false-positive results face an increased risk associated with CEA and a few patients with false-negative results face an increased risk because of the missed benefits of surgery. As Kuntz and colleagues[4] have illustrated with decision analysis, it is better to have a false-positive result (and perform a CEA in patients with moderate stenosis, with its added slight morbidity per patient) than to have a false-negative result (and allow patients with severe stenosis not to undergo CEA, with a much higher morbidity per patient). Put another way, it is better to send a few extra patients for CEA who may not meet DSA requirements of severe stenosis than to miss patients with severe stenosis and withhold the important benefits of surgery.

Thus, choosing among the noninvasive tests, the option that yields the highest accuracy may not necessarily be better. One must consider the local sensitivity and specificity of a particular noninvasive imaging modality to detect a severe stenosis compared with DSA as well as the angiographic stroke risk and CEA stroke risk when deciding whether the locally acquired ultrasound, CTA, or MRA study can replace DSA in the preoperative evaluation of carotid stenosis (Fig. 91-1). Even when assuming a low angiographic stroke risk of 0.4%, as seen in the Veterans Affairs Cooperative Study, decision analysis has demonstrated that a noninvasive test with a sensitivity of 93% and specificity of 85% resulted in less morbidity than the DSA imaging strategy. This same analysis allows imagers and referring clinicians to compare the relative value of ultrasound, CTA, and MRA to replace DSA using site-specific data instead of relying on published results from outside facilities.

We hope that decision analysis will allow the reader to compare the value of their own ultrasound, CTA, and MRA

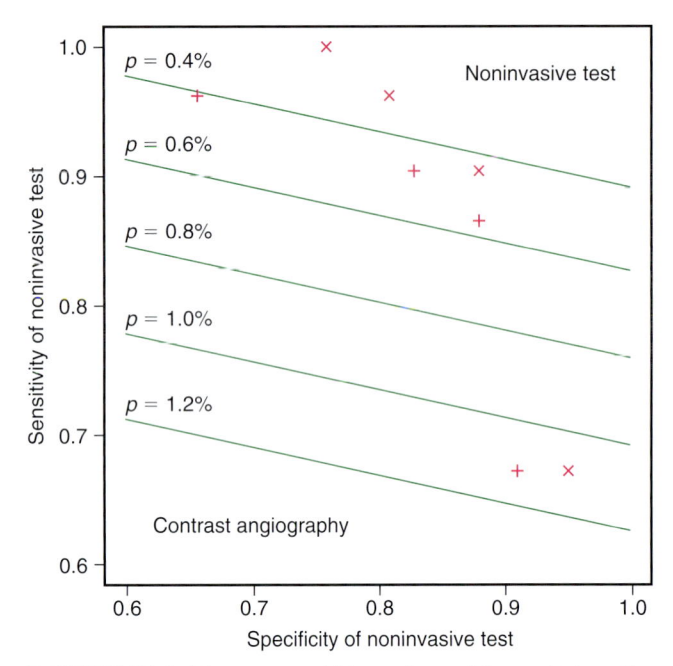

FIGURE 91-1 Three-way sensitivity analyses of the sensitivity and specificity of a noninvasive test and the probability of stroke from catheter angiography ($p = 0.4\%, 0.6\%, 0.8\%, 1.0\%$, and 1.2%). For each line described by angiographic stroke risk (p), the area above the line indicates the region where the noninvasive test is optimal and the area below the line indicates the region where contrast angiography is optimal. Four possible operating points considered for MRA (×) and duplex ultrasound (+) are shown. *(From Kuntz KM, Skillman JJ, Whittemore AD, Kent KC. Carotid endarterectomy in asymptomatic patients—is contrast angiography necessary? A morbidity analysis. J Vasc Surg 1995; 22:706-716.)*

imaging techniques objectively in the depiction of extracranial carotid stenosis. In this chapter, we will discuss the benefits and pitfalls of modern MRA and CTA techniques, as well as recommended protocols for each.

MAGNETIC RESONANCE ANGIOGRAPHY

Technical Requirements

A 1.5- or 3.0-T MR scanner with radiofrequency (RF) coils capable of imaging from the aortic arch through the circle of Willis is required for high-quality carotid MRA. Commercially available eight-channel neurovascular array coils with multiple elements distributed over the head and neck region to support parallel imaging are optimal, although good-quality carotid MRA can be obtained with neurovascular coils not optimized for parallel imaging. Modern gradient systems with a peak gradient amplitude of 30 to 40 mT/m and a slew rate up to 200 mT/m/ms) can support elliptical-centric contrast-enhanced (CE) MRA sequences with minimum repetition times (TRs) on the order of 3 to 5 ms. For CE MRA, a power injector optimizes consistent intravenous gadolinium (Gd)-chelate contrast medium injection rates and allows for accurate timing of the contrast arrival in the carotid arteries.

Techniques

Indications

Despite the availability of high-quality ultrasound, CTA, and MRA, no consensus exists regarding the optimal noninvasive imaging strategy for preoperative evaluation of carotid stenosis. This is particularly true for individual MRA techniques as well. In the 1990s, time-of-flight (TOF) MRA was reported to have good sensitivity and specificity in detecting internal carotid artery stenosis greater than 70% using North American Symptomatic Carotid Endarterectomy Trial (NASCET) criteria identified on DSA.[5-7] However, carotid MRA became more clinically viable with the introduction of CE MRA, which offered the opportunity to cover more of the carotid artery distribution in a fraction of the scan time requirements of TOF MRA. With the advent of elliptical-centric phase reordering and effective timing of the gadolinium contrast bolus, first-pass CE MRA moved from research into routine clinical practice.

Some authors still insist that despite the ability to perform reliable CE MRA, TOF MRA remains the most accurate technique.[8] For those who prefer CE MRA, three competing techniques have evolved. One approach uses multiple time points during the gadolinium bolus arrival with multiple, rapid, three-dimensional acquisitions with relatively low spatial resolution. To achieve a higher spatial resolution and improved temporal resolution, three-dimensional acquisitions reconstructed with a novel oversampling of the center of k-space are possible. This technique is termed *time-resolved imaging of contrast kinetics* (TRICKS).

Contrast-Enhanced Magnetic Resonance Angiography

As experience with gadolinium bolus arrival timing improved, many authors abandoned the time-resolved approach to carotid CE MRA in favor of a higher spatial resolution three-dimensional MRA technique at a single time point (Fig. 91-2). Carotid CE MRA benefits from a large residual carotid retention of the initial bolus of contrast injection and relative lack of motion concerns, which enables the acquisition of longer duration, high spatial resolution three-dimensional MRA. A difficulty with carotid CE MRA, however, has been the relatively brief arteriovenous enhancement window. Jugular venous enhancement can be seen as quickly as 5 seconds following carotid artery enhancement secondary to the lack of Gd-chelate contrast agent penetration of an intact blood-brain barrier and the rapid return of gadolinium contrast through the brain parenchyma to the jugular veins. By modeling the elliptical-centric k-space phase-ordering scheme, which provides a very efficient and compact central k-space sampling, Fain and associates[9] have demonstrated that there is sufficient image contrast for preferential arterial high spatial resolution with the longer acquisition times necessary for high spatial resolution carotid CE MRA. The use of elliptical-centric three-dimensional MRA, in combination with an accurate bolus arrival scan or fluoroscopic triggering, allows for high spatial resolution carotid CE MRA with a voxel size of 1 mm³ or smaller, with reliable and high intra-arterial contrast and very little venous contamination.[10] Use of a neurovascular coil ensures proper coverage of the carotid arteries from the aortic arch through the circle of Willis.

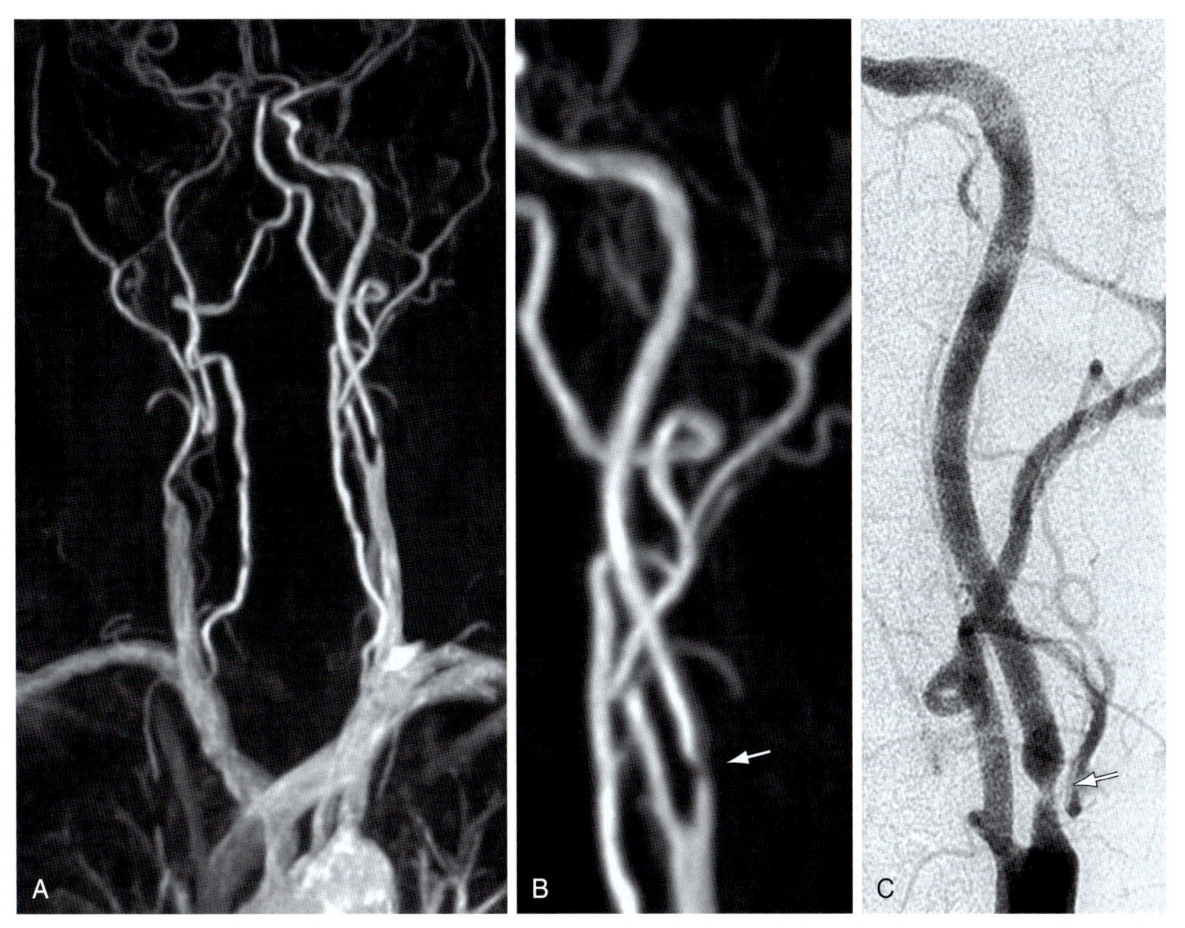

■ **FIGURE 91-2** Comparison of high spatial resolution CE MRA and DSA. **A,** Global MIP of the 0.64-mm^3 resolution CE MRA, with voxel dimensions of 0.81 × 0.81 × 1.0 mm. **B,** Magnified view of the left carotid bifurcation from CE MRA demonstrates a severe stenosis (*arrow*). **C,** Subsequent DSA confirms high-grade stenosis (*arrow*). *(Courtesy of Dr. Winfried. A. Willinek, Department of Radiology, University of Bonn, Bonn, Germany.)*

Spatial Resolution

Hinatiuk and coworkers[11] have reviewed the effect of increased spatial resolution in depicting carotid stenosis as seen on CE MRA at 1.5T. In their patients with carotid artery stenosis, decreasing the voxel volume from 0.9 to 0.53 mm^3 by increasing the scan matrix while keeping the FOV constant caused the scan time to increase from 21 to 40 seconds. The resulting CE MRA with improved resolution from the 0.53 mm^3 resulted in the sharpest depiction of the carotid stenosis. With modern gradient systems, TRs for elliptical-centric acquisitions are roughly half what they were during the early work on carotid CE MRA. The authors made use of the 50% reduction in TR to almost double the spatial resolution of elliptical-centric carotid CE MRA compared with the initial 0.8 to 1.0 mm^3 voxel size while maintaining an imaging time of 40 seconds. This reduction in voxel volume to 0.53 mm^3 resulted in a much better depiction of the carotid stenosis. A total of 30 mL of Gd-chelate contrast medium was used to achieve adequate signal-to-noise ratio (SNR). Further decreases in voxel volume, by extending the acquisition time to 50 to 60 seconds, did not improve the vessel depiction because of both a drop in SNR and sharpness losses, possibly from motion. Nael and colleagues[12] have extended the resolution of elliptical-centric carotid CE MRA to 0.44 mm^3 by making use of the extra SNR at 3.0T.

Parallel Imaging

Parallel imaging is another technique to shorten the acquisition time of first-pass elliptical-centric carotid CE MRA and/or support higher spatial resolution. In general, the efficacious use of parallel imaging allows one to maintain the recommended 1.0 mm or less in plane spatial resolution with a voxel volume of 0.8 mm^3 or less while maintaining adequate SNR to achieve a good image quality. Most authors have recommended using a twofold (i.e., 2×) acceleration factor at 1.5 T. The imaging volume is then increased by 50% in the z direction of the coronal CE MRA acquisition (anteroposterior direction). This simplifies the prescription of the imaging volume. The resulting CE MRA sequence is 25% faster compared with a smaller nonaccelerated prescription. By traversing the center of k-space faster with parallel imaging, the SNR benefits from the gadolinium bolus can be maximized. This helps offset the loss of SNR from the parallel imaging technique. Fourfold acceleration of 3.0-T carotid CE MRA using parallel imaging in phase- and detector row–encoding directions is also possible. Almost isotropic 0.7- × 0.7- × 0.9-mm resolution (0.44 mm^3 voxel volume) CE MRA from the aortic arch through the circle of Willis have been reported with this 3.0-T MR technique.[12] This study demonstrated some of the highest spatial resolution carotid CE MRA examinations ever achieved with a large FOV (Fig. 91-3).

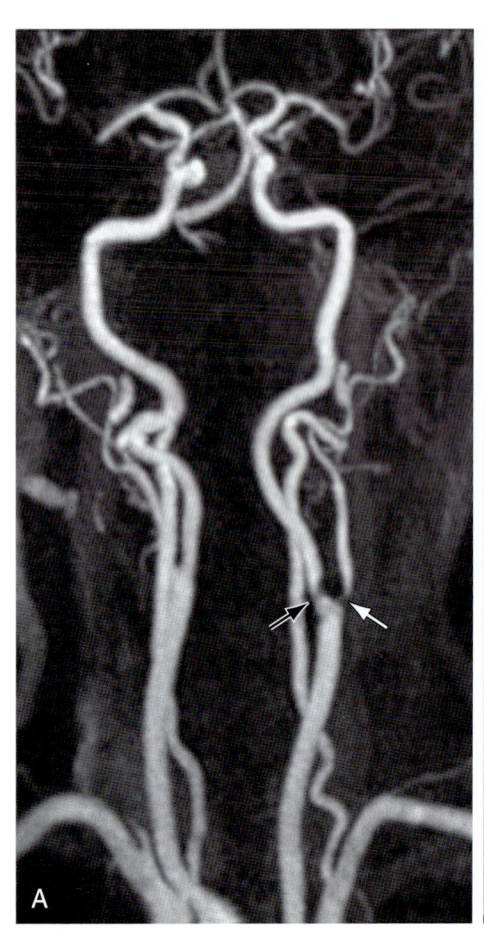

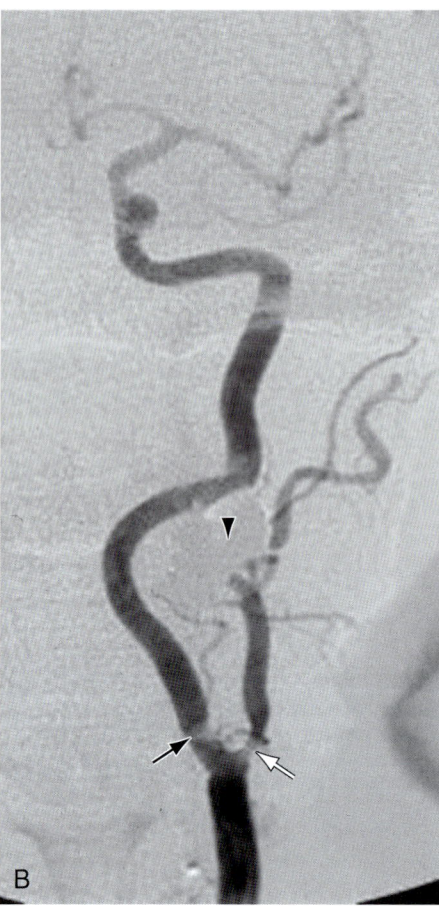

■ **FIGURE 91-3** 3.0-T carotid CE MRA. **A,** 83-year-old woman with history of transient ischemic attack demonstrates a mild stenosis (grade 2, 10% to 50%) at the origins of the left internal carotid artery (*black arrow*) and significant stenosis (grade 3, 51% to 99%) at the origin of the left external carotid artery (*white arrow*) on 3.0-T CE MRA. **B,** Oblique view from DSA confirms the CE MRA findings (*black arrow* and *white arrow*). There is also a small subtraction artifact (*arrowhead*). (From Nael K, Villablanca JP, Pope WB, et al. Supra-aortic arteries: contrast-enhanced MR angiography at 3.0 T—highly accelerated parallel acquisition for improved spatial resolution over an extended field of view. Radiology 2007; 242:600-609.)

Dedicated Carotid Coils

A dedicated neurovascular phased array coil is used in most cases because it not only provides an optimized SNR for carotid imaging and the ability to implement parallel imaging techniques, but also extends carotid artery coverage from its origin at the aortic arch through the circle of Willis. More recently, dedicated carotid surface coils that cover 14 to 18 cm of the midneck have become commercially available at 3.0 T. These dedicated surface coils provide another factor of improvement in SNR compared with the larger FOV clamshell design neurovascular coils that extend from the aortic arch through the circle of Willis. These dedicated carotid surface coils support even higher spatial resolution carotid CE MRA with a voxel size of $0.59 \times 0.59 \times 0.80$ mm without zero filling. This corresponds to a voxel volume of 0.27 mm^3 with dedicated carotid surface coils at 3.0 T compared with 0.44 mm^3 as used by Nael and associates[12] at 3.0 T using a large FOV clamshell neurovascular coil and 0.53 to 0.66 mm^3 as used by Hnatiuk and coworkers[11] and Willinek and colleagues[13] at 1.5 T with a large FOV clamshell neurovascular coil. Carotid CE MRA at 3.0 T using dedicated surface coils results in the highest resolution study achieved to date with CE MRA, and competes favorably with the spatial resolution of the 64-detector CTA.

Field of View

Raw resolution alone may not fully explain the ability to dedicate the carotid lumen stenosis on the CE MRA. According to the study by Fain and associates,[9] one key factor in improving the performance of elliptical-centric phase-reordered CE MRA as measured by the point spread function (PSF) is to minimize the phase FOV in both the *y*- and *z*-axes. By focusing on just the middle 14 to 18 cm of the neck, we can limit the phase FOV in both directions while generating substantially higher spatial resolution CE MRA compared with using a larger FOV and an eight-channel neurovascular coil. At 3.0 T, there is a sufficient carotid SNR to realize improved spatial resolution benefits using a small FOV and dedicated carotid surface coils. The improved PSF provided by the smaller phase FOV should result in a sharper depiction of the arterial lumen boundary compared with a similarly prescribed spatial resolution using a larger FOV. Stated another way, the same spatial resolution prescribed using a large FOV would result in inferior CE MRA compared with a small FOV because of the effect of the smaller phase FOV on the PSF. The arterial lumen boundaries would not be as sharp, despite the same prescribed resolution. This discussion assumes that we somehow generate enough SNR using the larger neurovascular coil, too. In addition to small FOV in the *xy*

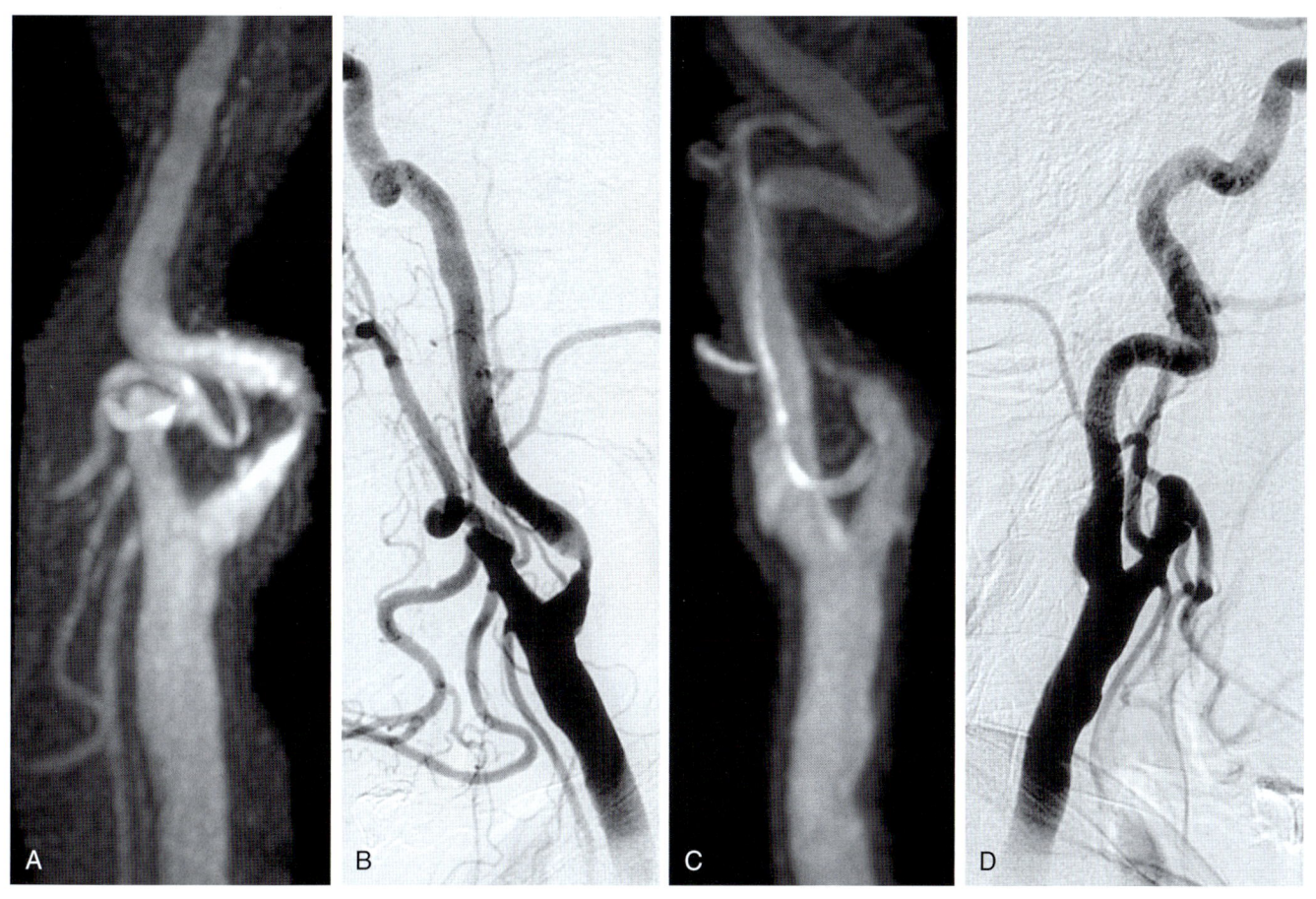

FIGURE 91-4 580-μm, in-plane resolution, 3.0-T carotid CE MRA compared with selective DSA. **A,** Maximum intensity projection of 3.0-T CE MRA demonstrates a severe narrowing of the proximal left internal carotid artery measuring 78% diameter stenosis. **B,** Corresponding selective DSA of the left carotid bifurcation confirms the severe (80%) stenosis. **C,** Plaque at the right carotid bifurcation is causing less than a 30% diameter stenosis, as seen on this maximum intensity projection of 3.0-T CE MRA. **D,** This finding is confirmed on the selective right carotid bifurcation DSA. *(From DeMarco JK, Huston J 3rd, Nash AK. Extracranial carotid MR imaging at 3 T. Magn Reson Imaging Clin North Am 2006; 14:109-121.)*

direction, we can acquire less coverage in the z direction by covering only the middle portion of the neck. Larger phase FOV in the z direction is required to cover the entire course of the carotid artery from the arch through the circle of Willis. If we desire the highest resolution carotid CE MRA, Fain[9] would predict that a small phase FOV of approximately 18 cm in both the y and z direction would be optimal.

Initial results of dedicated carotid coil limited FOV carotid CE MRA have confirmed excellent correlation with DSA (Fig. 91-4).[14] In patients for whom coverage of the carotid arteries that is limited to a 15 to 18 cm FOV in the neck is sufficient, dedicated carotid coil 3.0-T CE MRA represents the highest resolution noninvasive study possible today. This method is particularly well suited for clinical practices in which the decision to proceed to CEA is based on ultrasound without the need of the noninvasive testing to visualize the remainder of the carotid artery directly. If there is a carotid CTA that is limited because of extensive calcifications, the dedicated carotid coil 3.0-T CE MRA can depict the carotid stenosis without artifacts from the calcifications with similar or higher spatial resolution than CTA (Fig. 91-5). The use of such high SNR dedicated carotid surface coils at 3.0 T also makes carotid plaque imaging possible. Although this is still experimental, there is great potential to depict not only carotid ste-

nosis but the underlying plaque causing the narrowing (Fig. 91-6). There is a strong possibility that carotid plaque characteristics as depicted by MRI may be a predictor of which patients with moderate asymptomatic carotid stenosis are at risk to proceed on to stroke or a transient ischemic attack (TIA).[15]

Summary of Using Carotid Contrast-Enhanced Magnetic Resonance Angiography to Depict Carotid Stenosis

This analysis supports the use of first pass elliptical centric carotid CE MRA for the evaluation of carotid stenosis. Attention to technical details such as prescribed matrix size, FOV, use of parallel imaging, MR field strength, and carotid coils will all affect the final image quality of the carotid CE MRA. The optimal combination of these technical factors in various clinical MR configurations will be discussed later in this chapter.

Contraindications: MR Angiography Safety Issues

Nephrogenic Systemic Fibrosis

The concern of nephrogenic systemic fibrosis (NSF) in connection with gadolinium-based contrast agent (GBCA)

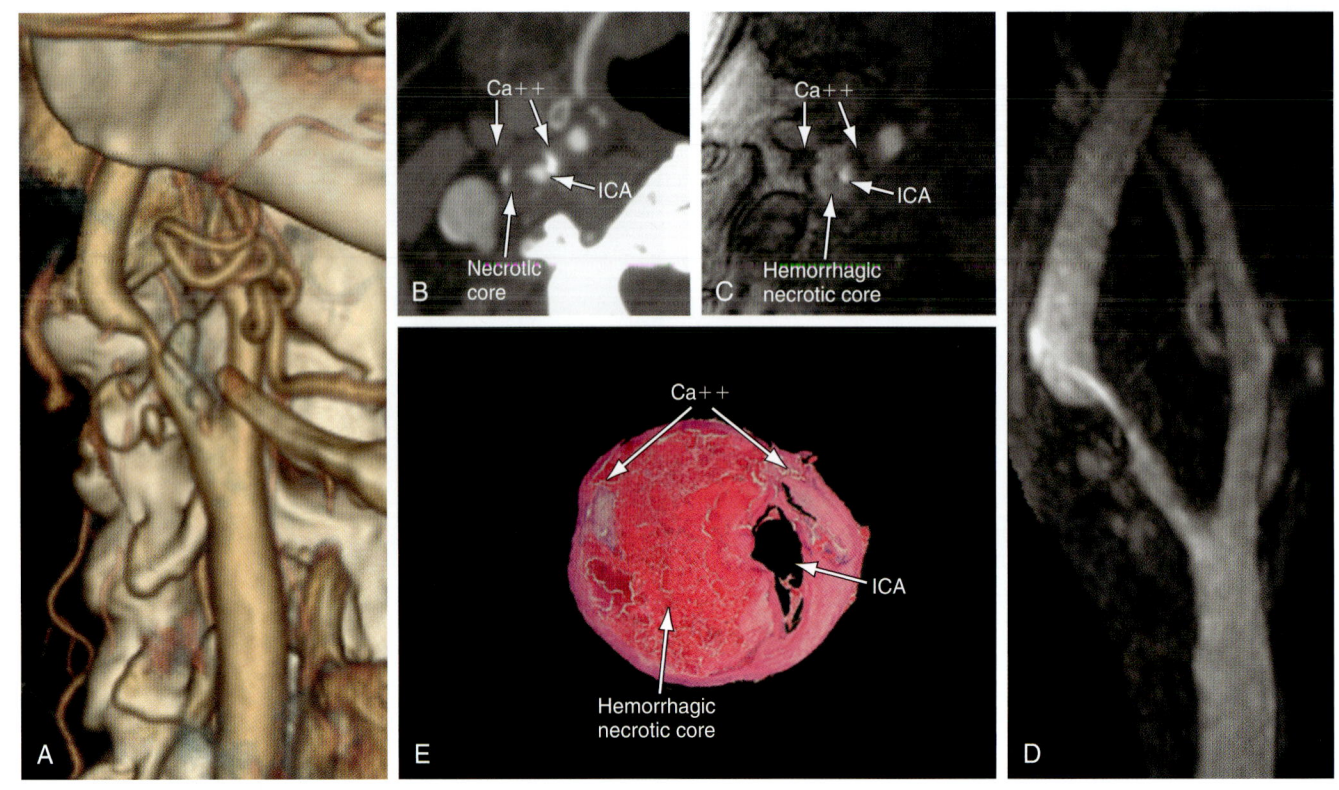

FIGURE 91-5 Comparison of 64-detector CTA and carotid surface coil 3.0-T MRA. **A,** CTA demonstrates a focal severe stenosis of the right internal carotid artery. **B,** Source axial image from CTA reveals a necrotic core as a region darker than muscle, as well as calcifications. **C,** Source axial image from 3.0-T time-of-flight MR angiogram demonstrates high signal intensity in the carotid plaque, indicating that the necrotic core is hemorrhagic. The calcifications are also seen as very dark regions within the carotid plaque. **D,** Maximum intensity projection for the contrast-enhanced carotid 3.0-T MRA confirms a severe stenosis within the proximal right internal carotid artery. **E,** Histologic specimen from the subsequent carotid endarterectomy 2 weeks later confirms the presence of a large hemorrhagic necrotic core and small carotid plaque calcifications.

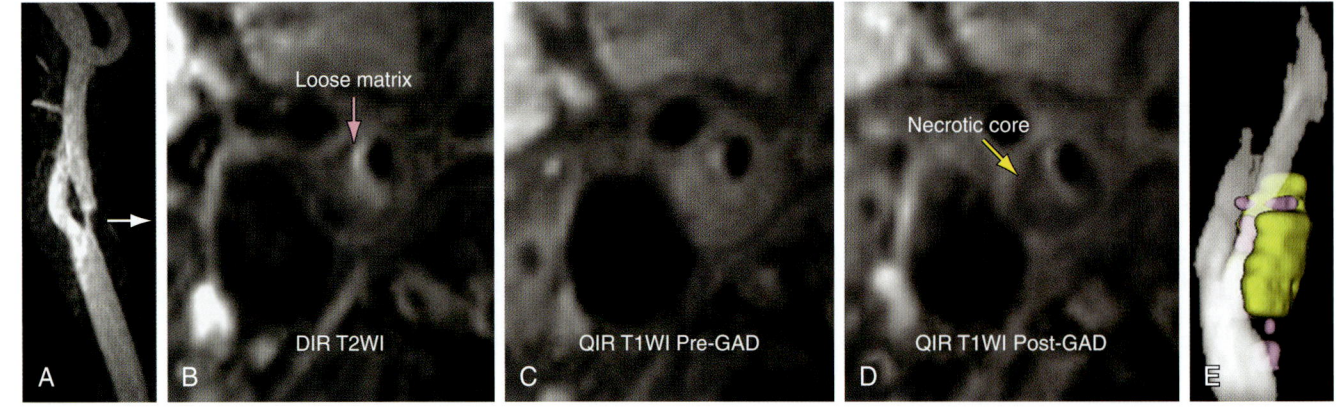

FIGURE 91-6 Carotid surface coil 3.0-T MRA and in vivo carotid plaque imaging in a symptomatic 70-year-old man. **A,** Maximum-intensity-projection of 3.0-T CE MRA demonstrates a severe narrowing of the proximal left internal carotid artery measuring 71% diameter stenosis. **B,** Black blood T2-weighted image along the superior aspect of the severe stenosis demonstrates a region next to the internal carotid artery lumen that is hyperintense to surrounding muscle, compatible with loose matrix involving the fibrous cap (*pink arrow*). Most of the remainder of the plaque is hypointense to muscle, suggesting a large, lipid-rich necrotic core. By comparing the black blood T1-weighted images precontrast (**C**) and postcontrast (**D**), a large nonenhancing region occupying more than 50% of the cross-sectional area of the carotid plaque can be appreciated. This corresponds to a large, lipid-rich necrotic core (*yellow arrow*). **E,** Three-dimensional volume reformatting of the carotid plaque data helps demonstrate the relationship of the large necrotic core (*yellow region*) to the severe carotid stenosis. The visualization is similar to how the plaque looks at surgery. Also, note the depth information in the three-dimensional VR images, which allows the reviewer to see how the necrotic core wraps posterior to the internal carotid artery. These three-dimensional VR images demonstrate complex plaque anatomy in a way that greatly facilitates understanding by the interpreting physician. *(From DeMarco JK, Huston J 3rd, Nash AK. Extracranial carotid MR imaging at 3T. Magn Reson Imaging Clin North Am 2006; 14:109-121.)*

TABLE 91-1 Sample Imaging Parameters for Contrast-Enhanced MRA of the Extracranial Carotid Arteries: Various MR Scanner Platforms

Parameter	1.5 T				3.0 T	
	Mayo[10] (General Electric)	Sonata[11] (Siemens)	Intera[13] (Phillips)	HDx[14] (General Electric)	Trio[12] (Siemens)	HDx[14] (General Electric)
TR (msec)	6.5	3.6	4.8	3.8	3.0	5.6
TE (msec)	1.5	1.2	1.5	1.4	1.2	1.7
Flip angle	45	25	40	35	20	30
Bandwidth (BW)	±32 kHz	440 Hz/pixel	434 Hz/pixel	±83.3 kHz	720 Hz/pixel	±32.5 kHz
FOV (cm)	22	30	35	28	39	15*
Matrix	256 × 224	512 × 410	432 × 432	384 × 256	576 × 561	256 × 256
RFOV	0.7	0.75	0.50	1.0	0.72	1.0
Actual FOV (mm)	220 × 154	300 × 225	350 × 175	280 × 280	390 × 282	150 × 150
Rx matrix	256 × 157	512 × 308	432 × 216	384 × 256	576 × 404	256 × 256
Slab thickness	62	65	60	124	100	36
Number of detector rows	44	54	60	124	112	46
Pixel size	0.86 × 0.98	0.59 × 0.73	0.81 × 0.81	0.73 × 1.09	0.68 × 0.70	0.59 × 0.59
Detector collimation (mm)	1.2	1.2	1.0	1.0	0.9	0.8
Voxel volume (mm)	1.18	0.53	0.66	0.80	0.44	0.28
Parallel image	0	0	0	2x	4x	0
Partial K_y	1.0	0.75	1.0	1.0	0.75	1.0
Partial K_z	1.0	0.75	1.0.	0.8	0.75	1.0
K-space filter	No	No	80%	80%	no	80%
Scan time (sec)	49	40	59	43	20	58

*Dedicated carotid coil.
FOV, field of view; K_y, phase encoding in the y or right-left direction; K_z, phase encoding in the z or anterior-posterior direction; RFOV, rectangular field of view; TE, echo time; TR, repetition time.

injections also needs to be taken in account. Current U.S. Food and Drug Administration (FDA) guidelines recommend caution when injecting GBCA in patients with severe or end-stage chronic kidney disease (glomerular filtration rate < 30 mL/min/1.73 m²) and in patients with acute hepatorenal failure. This occurs uncommonly in outpatients presenting with carotid stenosis. The risk-benefit ratio of GBCA in outpatients with moderate chronic kidney disease (glomerular filtration rate [GFR] from 30 to 59 mL/min/1.73 m²) is less clear. In our experience, the use of high T1-weighted relativity GBCA such as gadobenate dimeglumine (Multihance, Bracco Diagnostics, Milan, Italy) helps minimize the total dose of GBCA administration while supporting a sufficient SNR to produce high image quality carotid CE MRA. Typically, 20 mL of gadobenate dimeglumine is sufficient to maintain a high SNR and image quality of 0.8 mm³ or less resolution carotid CE MRA at 1.5 T. The risk-benefit ratio of carotid CE MRA versus three-dimensional TOF MRA will depend on the local experience and previously determined sensitivity and specificity of each technique to identify a severe carotid stenosis.

Metallic Implants

With increasing use of metallic stents and other implantable devices to treat patients with atherosclerosis, care must be taken to screen patients properly prior to performance of an MRI study. This is especially problematic at 3.0 T, because many manufacturers only certify their metallic stents and devices as safe at 1.5 T. Conditional approval of metallic stents has been increasing, where limitation on gradient amplitude may preclude patients from undergoing carotid MRA.

Summary of Recommended MRA Techniques

Based on published data, it is reasonable to conclude that CE MRA studies using 1.0 mm or less in-plane spatial resolution combined with 0.8- to 1.2-mm-thick partition thickness (≤0.8 mm³ voxel size) can result in accurate MRA examinations that compare favorably with DSA. The specific protocols will vary depending on the available MR field strength, available RF coils and channels, availability of parallel imaging techniques, and available gradient strength and minimum TR for elliptical-centric carotid CE MRA. This is in keeping with the initial simulations of first-pass elliptical-centric phase-reordered CE MRA that predicted the best performance with high resolution while maintaining a minimum-phase FOV in the y and z directions.[9]

A three-way prospective study of a submillimeter spatial resolution first-pass CE MRA, with a time-resolved CE MRA and a noncontrast TOF MRA, in comparison with the gold standard of rotational DSA for the preoperative evaluation of carotid stenosis, would determine which technique is superior if the study included a sufficiently large number of patients. In the absence of such a study, the aforementioned analysis suggests that 1 mm or less in-plane spatial resolution first-pass CE MRA, with a voxel size of 0.8 mm³ or less, perhaps combined with three-dimensional TOF MRA, is the best technique to depict carotid stenosis at the carotid bifurcation. Select recommended protocols are listed in Table 91-1.

The original elliptical-centric carotid CE MRA protocol, as recommended by its developers at the Mayo Clinic in the late 1990s, is listed in the first column of Table 91-1. This carotid CE MRA technique has been shown to provide excellent sensitivity and specificity to detect more than 70% diameter stenosis as compared with DSA. It is critical to note that these high levels of sensitivity and specificity occurred only when maintaining submillimeter in-plane resolution and when measuring stenosis on multiplanar reformation (MPR) and not maximum intensity projections.

With recent improvements in gradient hardware and parallel imaging, further improvements on the original resolution of elliptical-centric carotid CE MRA are possible at 1.5 T. The middle three columns of Table 91-1 illustrate examples from three of the major MRA manufacturers. All imaging parameters listed in Table 91-1 are optimized for high spatial resolution carotid CE MRA using roughly a double dose of a traditional extracellular GBCAs (e.g., 0.2 mmol/kg or roughly 30 mL in most adult patients).

The last two columns highlight the potential for the future. The group at UCLA has combined 3.0 T MR with a dedicated 12-element neurovascular clamshell-style coil and parallel imaging in two directions to achieve higher resolution elliptical-centric carotid CE MRA compared with the results at 1.5 T. (0.44 versus 0.65 mm^3).[12] We have been using research carotid coils (see Table 91-1, far left column) that can image a 15- to 18-cm FOV and cover from the carotid bifurcation to the skull base; combined with 3.0 T MR imaging, this can achieve very high spatial resolution carotid CE MRA (0.28 mm^3 resolution). Most of the major MR manufacturers now or will soon offer similar dedicated clinical carotid surface coils. The first generation of these FDA-approved clinical carotid coils covers the midneck region and are capable of imaging from the carotid bifurcation to near the skull base. Second-generation coils should be able to combine coverage of the midneck with brain imaging at 3.0 T to offer unprecedented resolution with carotid MRA.

Pitfalls and Solutions

Adequate Signal- and Contrast-to-Noise Ratios

In general, properly performed CE MRA will provide a high vascular SNR and CNR. Pushing spatial resolution to the recommended 1.0 mm or less in-plane resolution with a voxel size of 0.8 mm^3 or less requires much attention to technique, equipment selection, and timing of imaging with the transit of the contrast media bolus arrival. All the major MRA manufactures now offer eight-channel or higher neurovascular coils for 1.5- and 3.0-T MRA systems. In addition, many authors now use a 0.2-mmol/kg dose of GBCA or weight-independent dosing of 20 to 30 mL. This is usually injected at 2 to 3 mL/sec followed by a saline flush at a similar rate. This provides a sufficient arterial SNR/CNR to support the recommended higher spatial resolution required for proper first-pass carotid CE MRA in most patients imaged at 1.5 T. It may be possible to use only a single dose of GBCA in combination with 3.0 T to achieve 0.5 mm^3 or lower resolution and still maintain a good SNR/CNR.[16]

Adequate Spatial Resolution While Minimizing Imaging Time and Motion Artifact

It is clear from the work of Hoogeveen and colleagues[17] that at least three pixels are needed across a vessel to define the degree of stenosis. This would suggest that using in-plane resolution on the order of 0.5 to 0.7 mm would improve depiction of relevant stenotic carotid arteries with diameters in the range of 1.5 to 2.5 mm. This assumes that there is a sufficiently high arterial SNR and the examination is not so long as to result in patient motion artifacts.

Image Interpretation

Postprocessing

Use of Direct Caliper Measurements

Subjective visual inspection alone is not recommended for the evaluation of carotid artery stenosis on carotid CE MRA. Subjective inspection may be acceptable as an initial screening tool to exclude the presence of a 70% to 99% stenosis, but caliper measurements are warranted to confirm the presence of such stenosis.[18] As shown Figure 91-7, the maximum intensity projection (MIP) image can strongly suggest a severe stenosis. MPR oblique axial images through the level of maximum stenosis clearly demonstrate only a moderate stenosis, as was confirmed on subsequent DSA. All MRA manufacturers and picture archival and communication system (PACS) vendors now offer simple postprocessing tools to generate MPR in any arbitrary oblique plane. This greatly simplifies the work flow and makes it possible to include a review of MPR images of suspected regions of carotid stenosis in the routine clinical setting.

Use of Multiplanar Reformations in Caliper Measurements of Carotid Stenosis

The MIP algorithm results in decreased noise by decreasing the projected variance of the background compared with that in the source axial images. This leads to increased CNR in the MIP images. However, in the case of a projection through an area with minimal flow-related enhancement, as occurs in regions of carotid stenosis, the MIP algorithm can decrease the CNR so that the vessel is less apparent in the final MIP image. MPR images display the original source axial images in an arbitrary oblique plane. The weighted sum average used to reformat the data leads to an improvement in CNR because of the averaging effect. This improvement in CNR is not dependent on background suppression and vessel contrast is maintained, even in regions of carotid stenosis.[19] MPR of three-dimensional TOF MRA was shown to be highly correlated with DSA for two observers. No statistically significant difference between three-dimensional TOF MPR and DSA was seen. By contrast, the same three-dimensional TOF MRA sequence now analyzed by measurements of carotid stenosis on MIP images did show a significant difference compared with DSA (Fig. 91-8). The MIP images overestimated stenosis by approximately 10%. Lell and associates[20] have also demonstrated the highest concordance of carotid stenosis measurements on carotid MRA using MPR images. Thus, caliper measurements of carotid stenosis as seen on MRA are best performed using MPR and not MIP images.

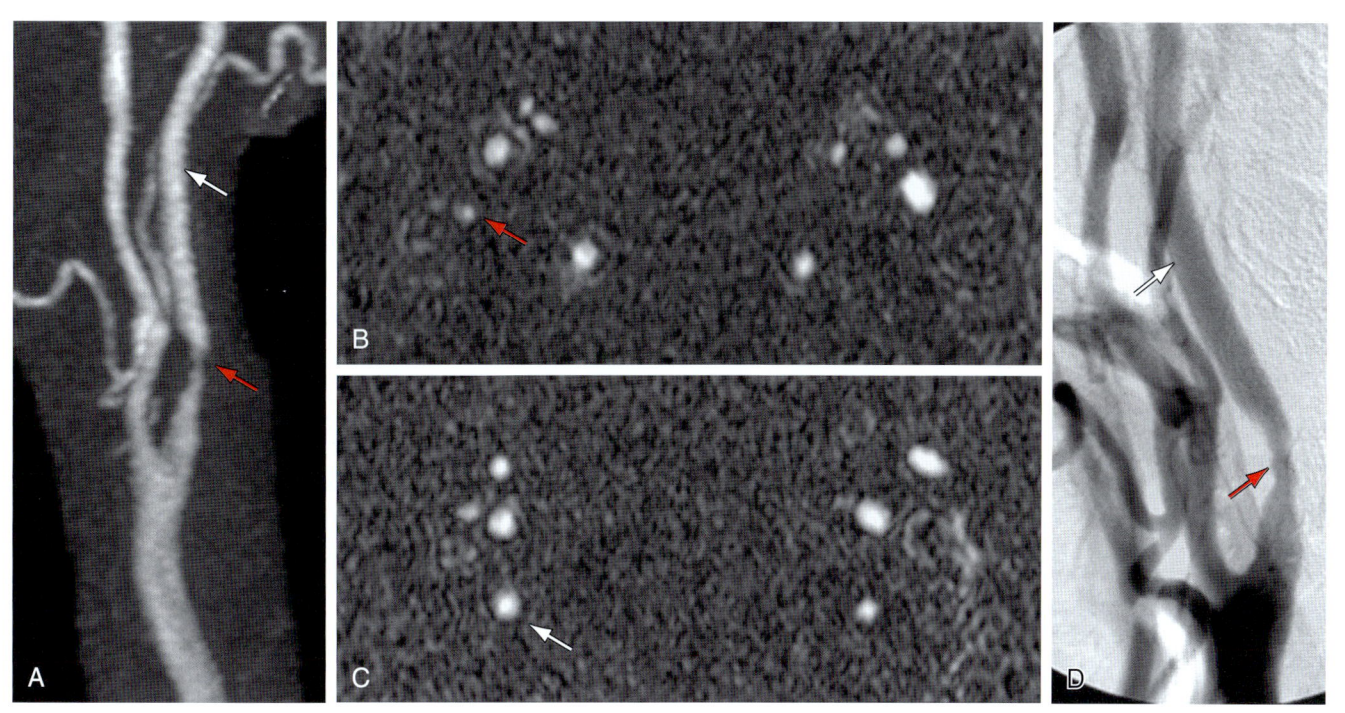

■ **FIGURE 91-7** MPRs of 1.5-T CE MRA correlate better with DSA than MIPs. **A,** Prospective review of the MIP from CE MRA demonstrates a 76% diameter stenosis by NASCET criteria. **B, C,** Axial reformations of the coronal CE MRA at the level of maximum stenosis (*red arrow*) and distal nontapering internal carotid artery (*white arrow*) reveal a less significant stenosis measured as 57%. **D,** DSA confirms only a moderate stenosis measured in a blinded fashion as 58%, which correlated much better with MPR than MIP images.

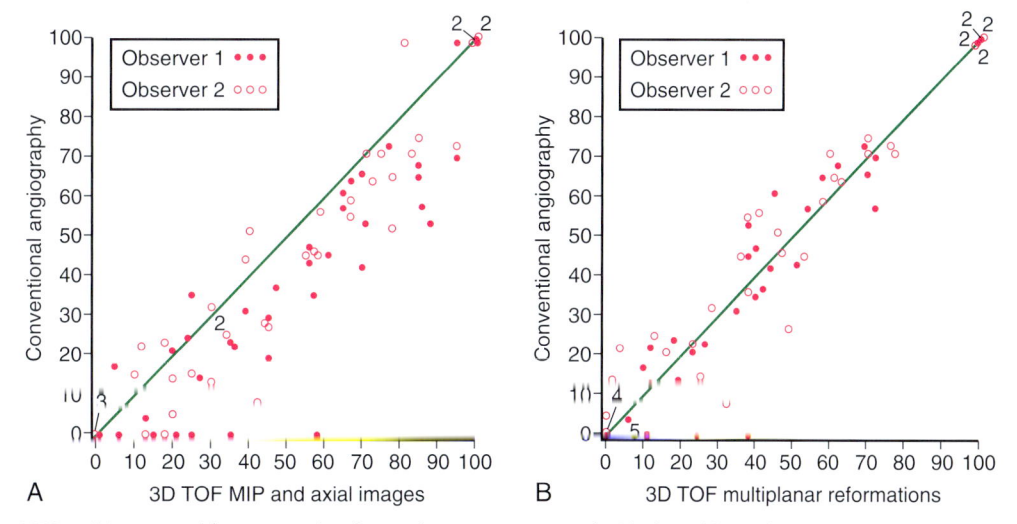

■ **FIGURE 91-8** MPRs of 1.5-T carotid MRA correlate better than MIPs compared with the gold standard DSA. **A,** Two observers measured carotid stenosis on three-dimensional time-of-flight MRA from MIP. Note the consistent overestimation of carotid stenosis on MIP images from MRA compared to DSA. The line represents region of complete agreement between MRA and DSA. **B,** Using MPR, the same two observers in a separate blinded reading session achieved much better correlation between MRA and DSA, with overestimation of stenosis on MRA, as seen when measuring the same sequence on MIP images. (From DeMarco JK, Nesbit GM, Wesbey GE, Richardson D. Prospective evaluation of extracranial carotid stenosis: MR angiography with maximum-intensity projections and multiplanar reformations compared with conventional angiography. AJR Am J Roentgenol 1994; 163:1205-1212.)

Reporting

Criteria for Measuring and Reporting Internal Carotid Artery Stenosis

There are three different methods for quantifying diameter stenosis on CE MRA when using DSA as the gold standard. These include the NASCET, European Carotid Surgery Trial (ECST), and common carotid (CC) methods. NASCET reports the ratio of the stenotic internal carotid artery (ICA) compared with the distal nontapering ICA. ECST uses the estimated diameter of the carotid bulb in the denominator. The CC method uses the distal CC artery (CCA) free of obvious disease as the denominator. When U-King-Im and colleagues[21] evaluated 284 carotid arteries on both CE MRA and DSA, all three methods were adequate for evaluation of DSA. With CE MRA, however, this study supported the use of the NASCET method because of improved sensitivity for the detection of severe stenosis.

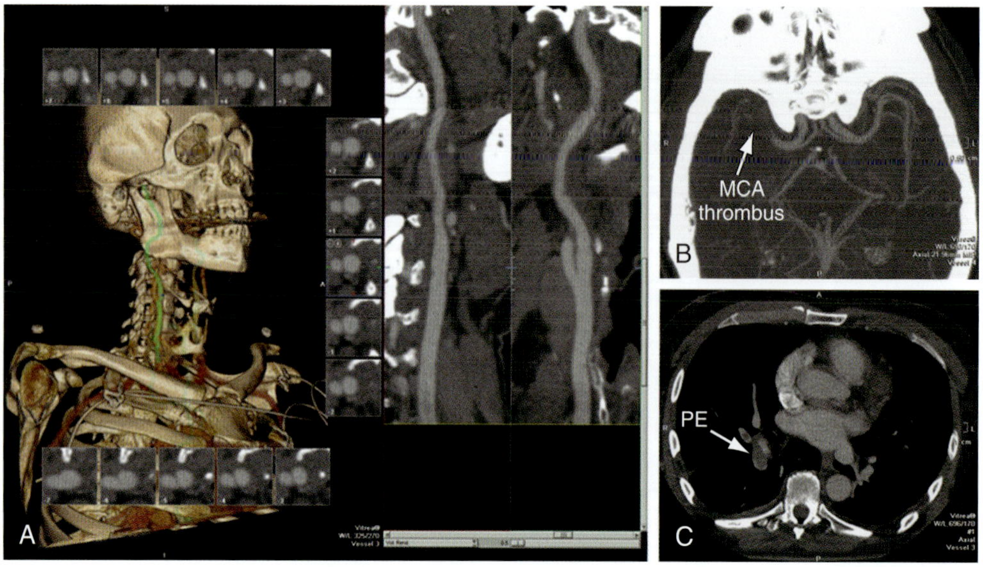

FIGURE 91-9 Acute right middle cerebral artery (MCA) stroke evaluated with CTA. **A,** Isotropic MPRs are possible with 64-slice CTA. Modern workstations can detect the carotid lumen quickly with minimal interaction from the interpreting physician and rapidly generate curved coronal-sagittal MPRs as well as oblique axial images, which represent true cross-sectional views through the carotid artery. There is no significant stenosis. **B,** On the same data set, axial MPR through the brain demonstrates a large right MCA thrombus that is causing the left body stroke symptoms. **C,** Axial MPRs from the same data set through the upper lung demonstrate clinically unsuspected pulmonary embolus. Based on this study, the patient subsequently underwent vascular ultrasound that confirmed a patent foramen ovale (PFO). The patient's PFO allowed lower extremity deep venous thrombosis to embolize to the right MCA. *(Courtesy of Dr. Peter Janick, Lansing Radiology Associates, Lansing, Mich.)*

CAROTID COMPUTED TOMOGRAPHIC ANGIOGRAPHY

Technical Requirements

Detailed protocols including collimation, table speed, and gantry speed are different among scanners provided by multiple vendors. Advances in multidetector CT (MDCT) technology have permitted higher quality CTA with thinner collimation (up to 0.5 mm) and faster gantry speed (up to 0.33 sec/rotation).[22]

In general, four- and eight-detector CT scanners are limited to a slice thickness of 1 mm. More advanced CT designs with 16- and 64- detectors can achieve slice thicknesses as little as 0.5 mm. CT tube rotation speeds have also improved over time. Although vendor specific, in general a four- or eight-detector scanner uses a rotation rate of 0.7 sec/rotation, a 16-detector scanner uses a 0.5 to 0.6 sec/rotation, and a 64-detector scanner uses 0.4 sec/rotation. Advances in CT tube design and heat dissipation has also led to an improvement in carotid CTA quality. Newer MDCT scanners have automatic milliamperage adjustments that are based on in-plane and z-axis attenuation. Synchronizing carotid CTA scanning with peak arterial contrast opacification remains a significant challenge. Faster 64-detector CT may allow the use of smaller amounts of iodinated contrast, but timing becomes even more important. The use of high-concentration contrast medium provides higher peak enhancement and may improve CTA image quality.

Techniques

Indications

Advances in CT scanner technology have resulted in the development of CTA that allows less invasive vascular imaging technique to be used widely in clinical environment. Although earlier studies to evaluate extracranial carotid artery stenosis using single-detector helical CT have shown a certain level of concordance with DSA as the gold standard,[23] single-detector helical CT had tradeoffs of limited scan volume and z-axis resolution. Newer generation MDCT and subsecond rotation capabilities have led to quantum leaps that provide excellent coverage from the aorta arch through the circle of Willis, with z-axis resolutions of 0.5 to 0.625 mm. Using these volume data sets with isotropic submillimeter voxel dimensions, CTA images in every plane of reformation can be generated without losing resolution (Fig. 91-9). Faster gantry rotation speed and increased table speed support higher temporal resolution. Improved spatial and temporal resolution, as well as the development of postprocessing techniques, has allowed multidetector CTA to become a clinically and relevant less invasive technique to evaluate carotid artery disease and has the potential to replace DSA for the evaluation of carotid artery stenosis.

The most common indication for a carotid CTA is evaluation of suspected atherosclerotic ICA stenosis based on a screening duplex ultrasound study. Neurologists and neurosurgeons tend to prefer MRI or MRA evaluation of carotid stenosis, especially if detailed imaging of the brain is required clinically. Vascular surgeons and interventionalists tend to prefer CTA, especially with the familiar depiction of adjacent soft tissues from CT studies (Fig. 91-10). Routine diagnostic invasive DSA to assess carotid stenosis has essentially been replaced by noninvasive methods. As with MRA, there have been significant improvements in CTA technology. Although we will summarize the current peer-reviewed literature, it is important to remember that reported CTA accuracy from single center studies may be difficult to duplicate in clinical

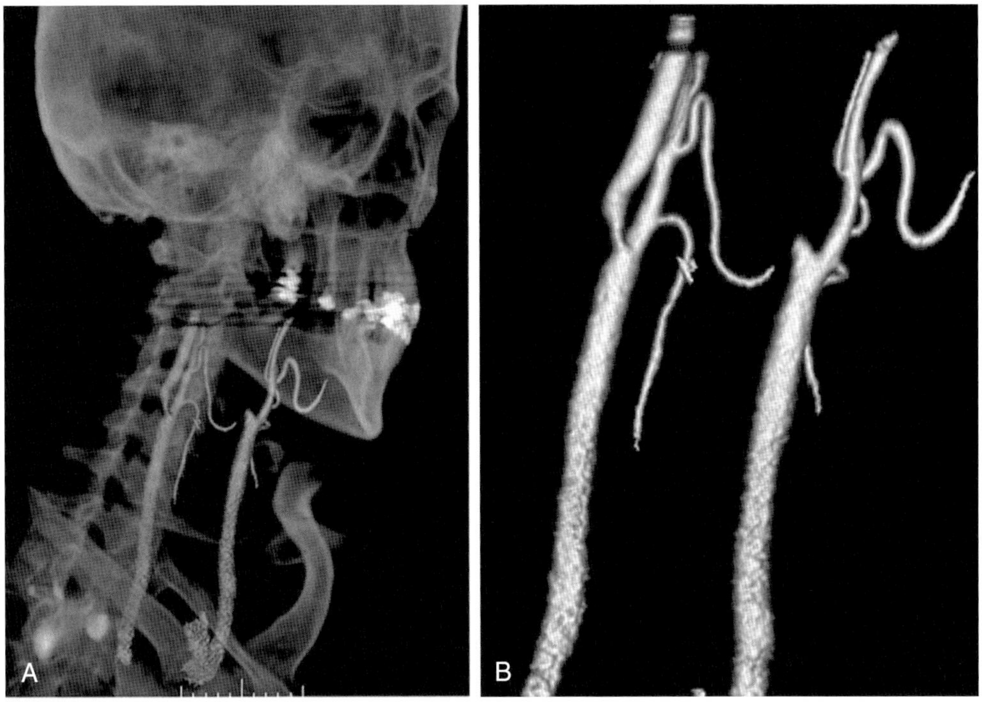

■ **FIGURE 91-10** CTA can present data in a format with which referring vascular surgeons and interventionalists are familiar. **A,** Volume reformations (VR) of a high-resolution carotid CTA data set can be rendered to look strikingly similar to a conventional catheter angiogram, including easy recognition of important anatomic landmarks, such as the angle of the mandible. **B,** The same CTA data set can be segmented to display just the carotid arteries without any overlying bone or soft tissue in a way similar to digital subtraction angiography. *(Courtesy of Dr. Larry Tanenbaum, Department of Radiology, Mount Sinai School of Medicine, New York.)*

practice. As with MRA, we recommend direct comparison of the accuracy of CTA with DSA locally. Local expertise may be a deciding factor in choosing which noninvasive study to use to evaluate suspected carotid stenosis.

In a meta-analysis of 864 patients in 28 studies using a single-detector row CTA technique, Koelemay and coworkers[23] have reported a pooled sensitivity and specificity for detection of a 70% to 99% stenosis that were 85% (95% confidence index [CI], 79 to 89) and 93% (95% CI, 89 to 96). For detection of an occlusion, the sensitivity and specificity were 97% (95% CI, 93 to 99) and 99% (95% CI, 98 to 100). They concluded that CTA is an accurate modality for the detection of severe carotid stenosis, especially for detection of occlusions. Most early experience with single- or four-detector CTA demonstrated a tendency to underestimate carotid stenosis compared with DSA. This leads to high specificity but lower sensitivity with CTA estimation of carotid stenosis. As noted, decision analysis tells us that we need a noninvasive study with high sensitivity to optimize noninvasive imaging strategies and minimize costs and/or morbidity.

Even when limited to four- and eight-detector CTA, limiting collimation to 1 mm may improve correlation of CTA with DSA. Berg and colleagues[24] have reported a 91% accuracy of four-detector CTA with 1-mm collimation compared with rotational DSA, although there was still a tendency to underestimate stenosis on CTA. Bucek and associates[25] have reported 97% sensitivity and 66% specificity in the detection of severe carotid stenosis using four-detector CTA with 1-mm collimation when reviewed by an experienced interpreting physician and using dedicated postprocessing techniques to allow visualization of oblique axial images through the level of maximum stenosis. The accuracy was decreased with a second, less experienced observer. The administration of high-concentration contrast medium and/or the availability of 64-detector CT scanners are expected to reverse the lower sensitivity of single- or four-detector CTA compared with DSA.[26] Again, the role of CTA versus MRA in the evaluation of carotid stenosis identified on screening duplex ultrasound will depend heavily on the local interpreting physician's expertise with each noninvasive technique as well as the referral patterns and preferences of the requesting physicians.

Studies have reported 100% sensitivity and specificity in differentiating complete ICA occlusion from near-occlusion.[25,27] In the largest of these, Chen and coworkers[27] evaluated 57 ICAs with total and near-occlusions with DSA and four-detector CTA. CTA correctly depicted all total and near-occlusions. In total occlusions, the length of the stump and retrograde flow were all accurately described by CTA. In near-occlusions, the sites of tight stenoses were also correctly identified by CTA. It was concluded that CTA may be considered a substitute for DSA in confirming the ultrasound results in diagnosing total versus near-occlusion of an ICA.

The use of stents to treat carotid stenosis has been increasing. CTA, especially with 64-detector CT scanners, can evaluate the status and patency of the carotid artery previously treated with stenting. The success rate in depicting the carotid lumen in the presence of a stent is higher than for the evaluation of coronary stents, given both the larger size of the carotid artery and the decrease

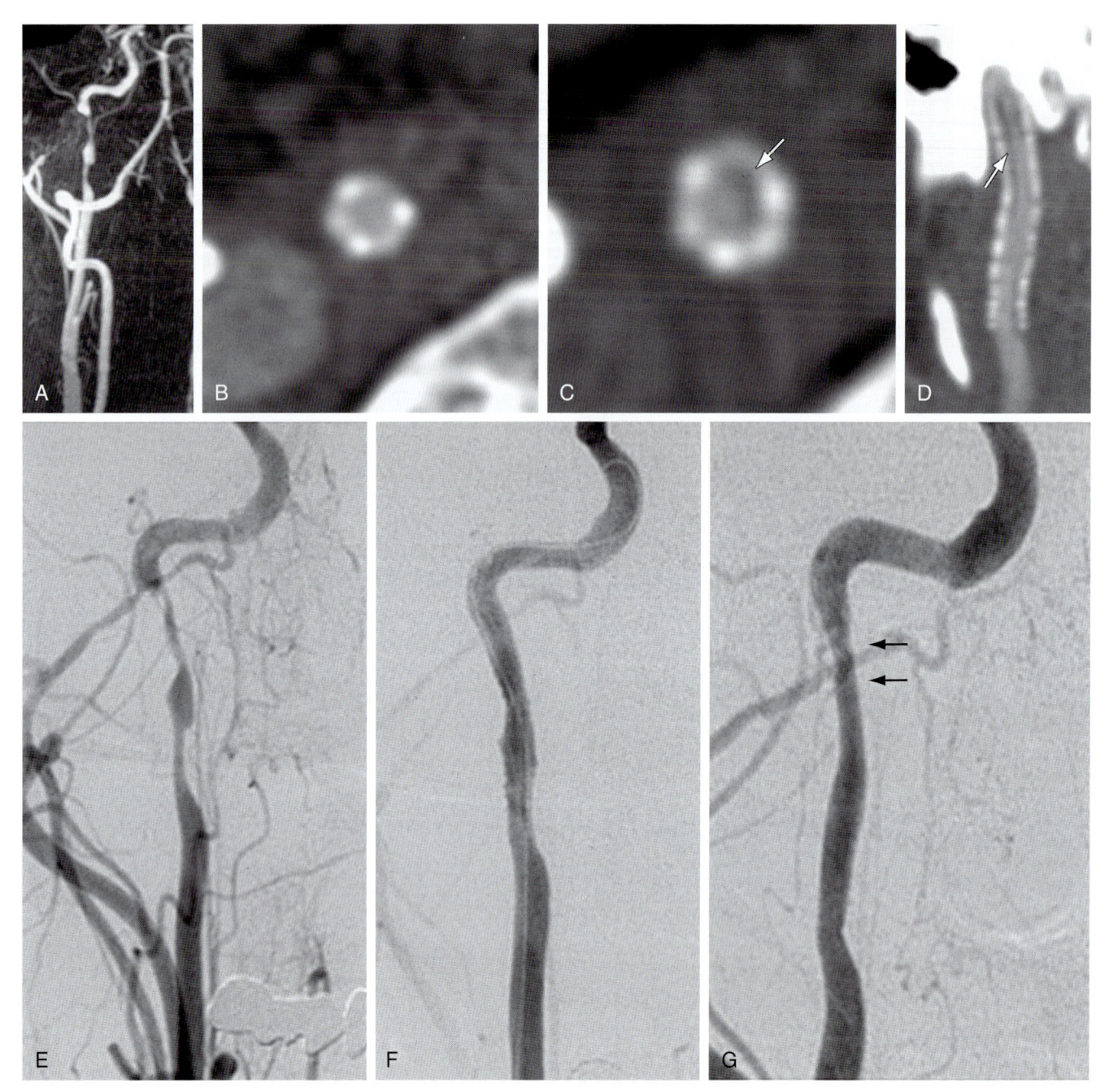

FIGURE 91-11 Restenosis after distal ICA stenting. **A,** Initial contrast-enhanced carotid MRA demonstrated irregular severe distal stenosis. **B,** Source axial image from 64-detector CTA after carotid stenting demonstrates a widely patent distal ICA. **C,** Source axial image from a follow-up 64-detector CTA reveals restenosis within the carotid stent (*arrow*). **D,** The restenosis is better appreciated on the coronal multiplanar reformations (*arrow*). **E,** Initial DSA confirms the irregular high-grade distal ICA stenosis. **F,** Immediate post-stenting DSA shows successful deployment and a widely patent distal ICA. **G,** Follow-up DSA performed because of the results of the CTA confirm restenosis with the previously placed ICA stent (*arrows*). (Courtesy of Dr. Sid Roychowdury, University Radiology Group, New Brunswick, NJ.)

in motion artifact compared with coronary CTA (Fig. 91-11).

Carotid artery dissection is a possible cause of stroke, especially in young patients and patients reporting pain, headache, Horner's syndrome, or neck trauma. Carotid artery dissections typically occur in the distal cervical portion of the ICA and extend into the skull base. CTA may demonstrate long irregular ICA stenosis or tapered occlusion. There may be an intimal flap. Care needs to be taken to evaluate the ICA, especially at the skull base of axial images if there is a clinical concern of carotid dissection. In patients with head and neck trauma, CTA is the fastest and most comprehensive method for evaluating for vascular injury, soft tissue abnormality, and fracture (Fig. 91-12).

Contraindications

Renal Failure

The development of contrast medium–induced nephropathy (CIN) is low in people with normal renal function,

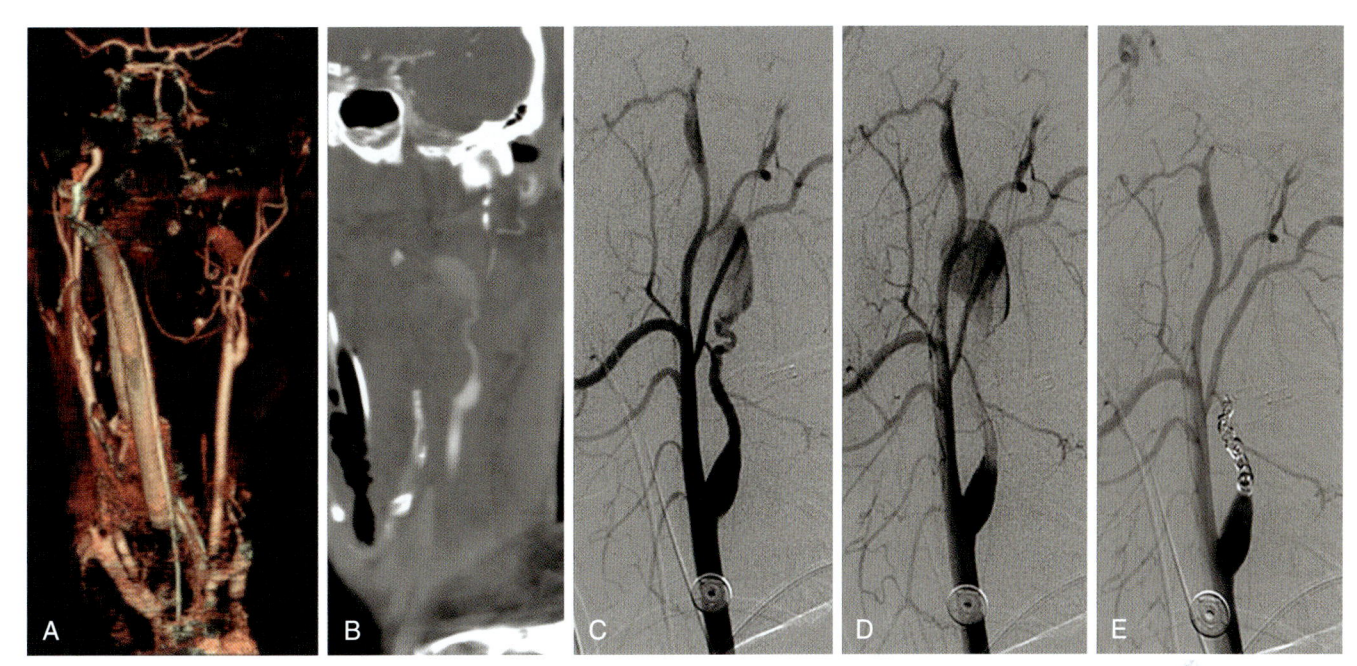

■ **FIGURE 91-12** Traumatic dissection with pseudoaneurysm of left ICA after penetrating knife injury. **A,** Three-dimensional volume reformations with 64-detector CTA demonstrate a post-traumatic pseudoaneurysm of the left ICA. **B,** Oblique coronal multiplanar reformations confirm the presence of the pseudoaneurysm. **C,** Subsequent DSA performed because of the CTA results confirms a traumatic dissection of the left ICA with pseudoaneurysm best appreciated on late images **(D). E,** Postcoiling DSA confirms complete occlusion of the left ICA, with further filling of the traumatic pseudoaneurysm. *(Courtesy of Dr. Sid Roychowdury, University Radiology Group, New Brunswick, NJ.)*

varying from 0% to 5%.[2] Preexisting renal impairment increases the frequency of this complication, ranging from 12% to 27%. Consideration of alternative imaging techniques that do not require administration of a nephrotoxic contrast agent is important. If CTA is necessary clinically in patients with renal impairment, there are several options for pretreatment prior to the CTA to minimize the risk of CIN. Those include volume expansion, use of low- or iso-osmolar contrast media, and stopping nephrotoxic drugs such as nonsteroidal anti-inflammatory drugs.[28] Volume expansion can be achieved with the intravenous injection of 100 mL/hr of 0.9% saline starting 4 hours prior to contrast medium administration and continuing for 24 hours if a patient does not have congestive heart failure. If there is no contraindication to oral administration, free fluid intake should be encouraged. Also, 64-detector CTA has a potential advantage of decreasing the likelihood of CIN by reducing the amount of iodinated contrast material required for good-quality CTA because of the faster scan time. A saline bolus chase is also effective to reduce iodinated contrast material without significantly reducing contrast enhancement in the arterial phase.[29]

Technique Description

CT parameters to obtain optimal image quality on carotid CTA depends on the type of MDCT scanner that is available. In general, the use of the thinnest possible slice thickness is recommended. Although vendor-specific, a detector row thickness of 1 mm is possible with four- or eight-detector CT scanners and slice thicknesses of 0.5 to 0.6 mm are possible with 16- and 64-detector CT scanners. Rotation speed also varies from 0.3 to 0.7 sec/rotation, depending on the number of detectors and the vendor.

Some vendors also allow variable gantry speeds during the acquisition. In these cases, faster acquisition in the neck, where the vessels are larger, and slower acquisition in the head, where the circle of Willis arteries are smaller, is possible. There have also been significant improvements in CT tube design and heat dissipation. In an average-sized patient, with a tube voltage of 120 kVP, milliamperage in the range of 200 to 240 mAs is required for carotid CTA. Modern 16- and 64-detector CT scanners also provide automatic mAs adjustments, with higher mAs through the shoulders to decrease streak artifact. A mAs range of 200 to 800 at 0.4 second with a noise index of 10 provides a good balance of quality and radiation exposure.[30]

Scanning during the peak arterial phase of the intravenous contrast bolus will optimize the carotid CTA image quality. Peak carotid artery opacification depends on a number of factors, such as patient weight, cardiac output, and recirculation of blood pool. With the relatively long scan times necessary with earlier single- and four-detector CT scanners, the variability of peak carotid artery enhancement was not a factor. A standard fixed delay between bolus injection and CTA image acquisition was possible. With the advent of faster carotid CTA scanning possible with 16- and 64-detector scanners, timing becomes critical. Numerous bolus tracking devices with automatic triggering methods are now provided by the CT manufacturers. In addition, a small test bolus method can also be used to time the larger bolus carotid CTA study.

Attention to the type, volume, and site of intravenous injection of iodinated contrast material will affect the final carotid CTA image quality. A large-bore intravenous catheter of at least 20 gauge in the right antecubital fossa is best. Arterial enhancement is provided by the intravenous injection of 80 to 120 mL of nonionic iodinated contrast

TABLE 91-2 Sample Imaging Parameters for CTA with Varying Number of Multiple Detector CT Scanners

Parameter	Number of Detector Rows in CT Scanner		
	4	16	64
Collimation (mm)	1-1.25	0.625-0.75	0.5-0.625
Rotation speed (sec)	0.5	0.5	0.33
Pitch	1.5	1.375	0.9
Coverage in z direction (cm)	25	25	25
Scan time (sec)	21	9	4
Volume of contrast (mL)	120	100	60
Flow rate (mL/sec)	6	5	5

material at a variable rate, from 3 to 6 mL/sec. The volume and rate of injection vary widely, depending on the number of detectors available (Table 91-2). Recently, high-concentration contrast material of 370 to 400 mg I/mL has been shown to provide earlier and higher peak enhancement with lower injection rates of approximately 4 mL/sec. The use of a saline flush after injection of the iodinated contrast can maintain good CTA image quality while minimizing the total dose of contrast injected. The saline flush also minimizes the artifact of highly concentrated contrast in the subclavian vein, which can cause streak artifacts near the aortic arch and takeoff of the great vessels. Schuknecht and colleagues[26] have recently reported their initial experience in 37 patients scanned with a modern 64-detector CT. In their study, a relatively small volume (25 mL) of high-concentration iodinated contrast agent—400 mg I/mL of iomeprol 400 (Bracco Diagnostics)—was injected by a power injector at a flow rate of 4 mL/sec, followed by a 40-mL flush of saline at the same injection rate, which resulted in good-quality carotid CTA in all cases. An automated contrast bolus detection and triggering algorithm provided by the manufacturer were used to time the beginning of the carotid CTA. In older MDCT scanners, in which a short, compact contrast bolus with a saline flush to minimize streak artifact in the subclavian vein was not possible, de Monye and associates[31] demonstrated that the use of a craniocaudal scan direction results in slightly lower attenuation of the carotid arteries and much lower attenuation of the subclavian veins and superior vena cava, with a resulting decrease in streak artifacts near the aortic arch and great vessel takeoff.

Pitfalls and Solutions

Densely calcified plaque, especially at the carotid bifurcation, can lead to an overestimation of the stenosis on CTA because of the blooming artifact. The window level settings are critical to the accurate interpretation of carotid stenosis. The optimal evaluation of carotid stenosis may be from multiplanar reformatted images perpendicular to the longitudinal axis of the ICA at the level of maximum stenosis and the distal nontapering portion of the ICA (oblique axial MPR). Images should be displayed with a window level setting of 700/200 HU unless there are dense calcifications, in which case wider settings (1100/200 HU) are recommended.[20] Calcifications may obscure the true residual carotid lumen on MIPs and volume rendered (VR) images. They are useful for global screening of the large data set from carotid CTA, but accurate assessment of the carotid stenosis requires review of the source axial and oblique axial MPR images.

Artifact from overlapping bone, especially the sternum, can also obscure the aortic arch and the takeoff of the great vessels on MIP or VR images. Curved MPR, thin-section MIP, and bone subtraction algorithms can help in the depiction of stenosis involving the takeoff of the great vessels from the aortic arch. Although still in the development stage, bone subtraction algorithms with motion compensation can provide higher quality CTA than purely rigid registration methods.[32] When there is little swallowing artifact, there is even the potential to remove plaque calcifications at the carotid bifurcation. Others have studied dual-energy CT to automate the segmentation of bone from contrast-enhanced carotid lumen. Initial experience with dual-source MDCT did improve coronary artery depiction from improved temporal resolution, but it is more difficult to segment and subtract bone and calcium from the enhanced arterial lumen. Research in this area is continuing and looks promising.

Another pitfall of carotid CTA is the sheer volume of data to review. Dedicated CTA review workstations greatly improve the work flow. Newer workstations have improved segmentation algorithms that allow rapid generation of curved MPR, VR, and thin-section MIP images, which minimize the time it takes to interrogate visually the entire course of both carotid arteries.

PACSs can also be overwhelmed by the sheer volume of data generated by modern 64-detector MDCT studies. Some centers are choosing to send all CTA data to a separate CTA workstation. Only selected images from the CTA workstation, including 3- to 5-mm-thick axial MPRs to demonstrate the entire region imaged during the carotid CTA are sent for final archiving to the PACS.

Image Interpretation

Postprocessing

To evaluate carotid CTA, both original axial and reformatted images can be used. Current commercially available workstations can generate reconstructed images, including MPR, curved planar reconstruction (CPR), MIP, and VR images. To obtain optimum interpretation of the carotid CTA, the experienced user will use some combination of these images.

Any desired two-dimensional section, which is longitudinal or cross sectional to the vessel axis, can be generated from a stack of CT data with MPR. Cross-sectional MPR images can visualize luminal shape accurately, even if it is eccentric or concentric, and results in good interobserver variability for grading of the degree of stenosis.[4] It is recommended to use cross-sectional MPR images to measure the luminal dimension.[5] Some current workstations can automatically generate consecutive cross-sectional MPR images perpendicular to the vascular axis, with occasional manual correction, which is not a time-consuming method (Fig. 91-13). The drawback of cross-sectional MPR images

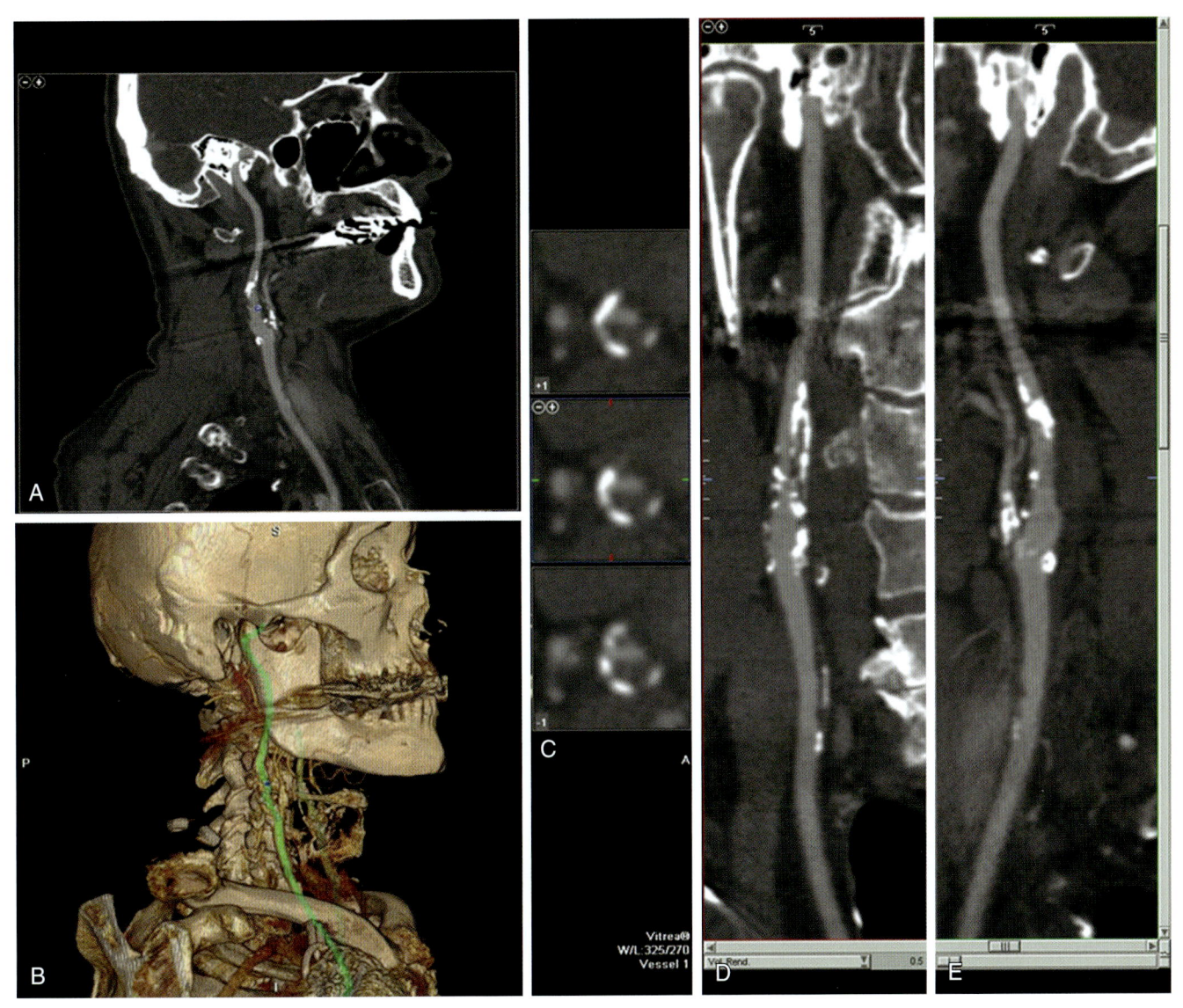

CHAPTER 91 • MR and CT Angiography of the Extracranial Carotid Arteries

■ **FIGURE 91-13** Modern workstations help steamline work flow in the evaluation of complex carotid stenosis. **A,** With minimal interaction by the interpreting physician, workstations can determine the course of the carotid artery with a high-resolution 64-detector CTA data set and display the results as a curved MPR. **B,** The center line of the carotid artery is displayed on volume reformations of the CTA data set. **C,** Oblique axial images at the level of maximum stenosis are automatically generated based on the center line demonstrated in B. **D,** Curved MPRs in the frontal and lateral views (**E**) are presented to allow the interpreting physician to generate true cross-sectional views (oblique axial images) interactively anywhere along the course of the carotid artery. *(Courtesy of Dr. Peter Janick, Lansing Radiology Associates, Lansing, Mich.)*

is that it is difficult to get an overview of the target arteries, which can be overcome by using other imaging technique, such as CPR, MIP, and VR methods. Attention should be paid not to miss multiple lesions at the target artery because tandem lesions are a common feature in atherosclerosis.

CPR in vascular imaging is generated by selecting a curved plane along the central axis of the target vessel. Most vendors provide an automated or semiautomated CPR capability in which the vessel is traced based on Hounsfield units. The automated tracking may not work consistently near contrast-filled veins or bone. The user is usually provided with a tool to quickly correct this target pathway back into the carotid lumen. Although CPR is appropriate to visualize the distribution of disease, including stenosis and plaque components, a drawback is that the images obtained depend on the selected curved plane with the possibility of erroneous appearance of the lesions. Thus, CPR is a quick method to review carotid artery anatomy, especially adjacent to bone or opacified veins, but the user must supplement the CPR with an additional MPR in a second plane, usually perpendicular to the original CPR plane.

An MIP can be generated by extracting the voxels with the highest attenuation value along the projection from any viewing ray, resulting in DSA-like images. Although the MIP images are suitable for viewing the carotid arteries, overlying high-density structures such as bone and calcification can hinder the visualization of the carotid lumen. Unlike volume rendering, MIP images do not provide in-depth information in the image. The plaque calcifications appear overlapped into the opacified carotid artery lumen on the MIP images, making stenosis determination impossible. Bone elimination technique or thin

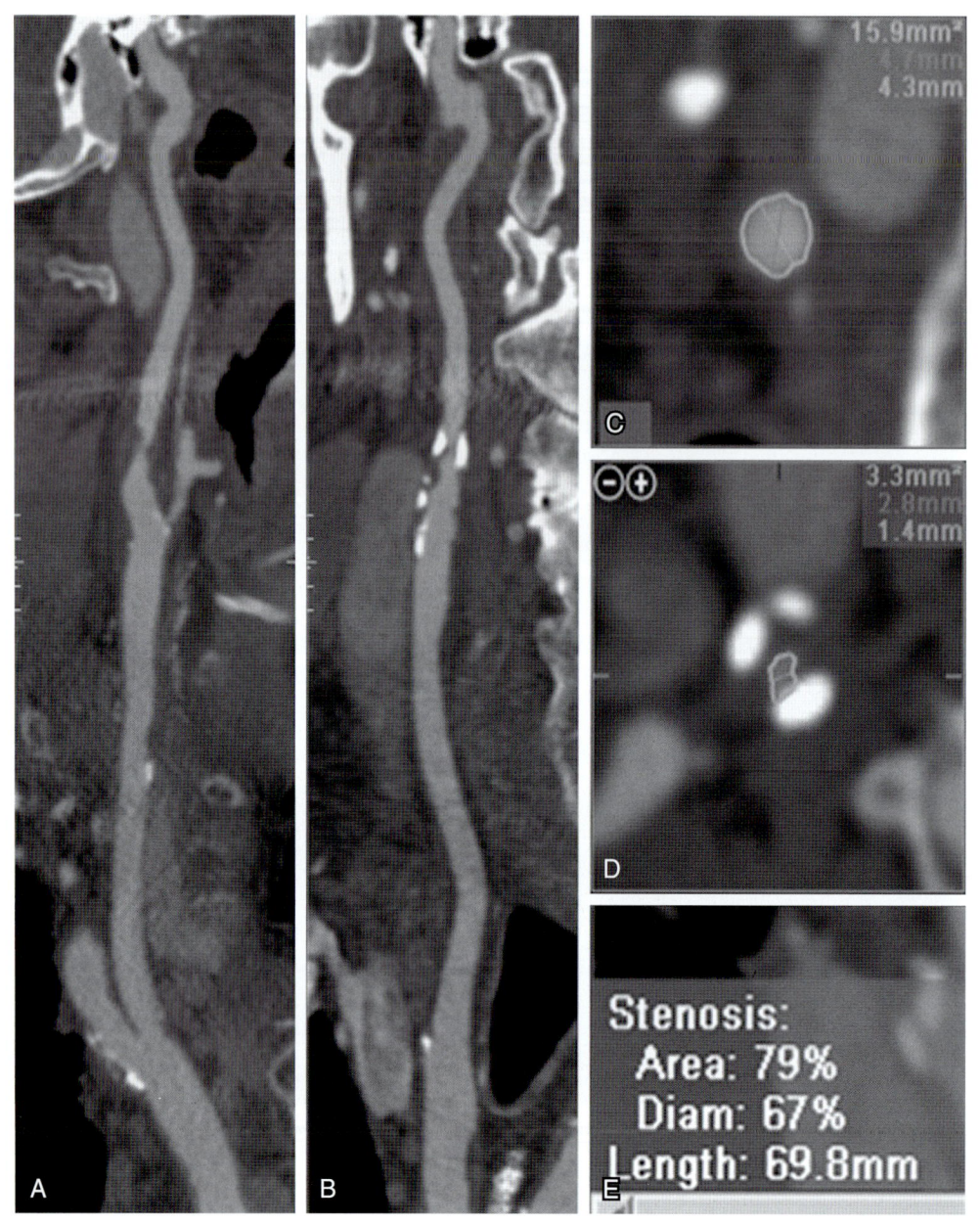

■ **FIGURE 91-14** Automated carotid stenosis. **A, B,** Curved lateral and frontal multiplanar reformations demonstrate ICA stenosis caused by calcified and soft plaque. **C,** Oblique axial MPR demonstrating cross-sectional area of the normal distal ICA is generated based on interpreting physician interaction. **D,** At the level of maximum stenosis, the oblique axial image reveals both soft plaque and calcifications in the carotid plaque. The ICA lumen boundary is automatically detected after a seed point has been placed in the ICA. **E,** Automated percentage diameter and area stenosis are calculated based on minimal interpreting physician interaction. *(Courtesy of Dr. Larry Tanenbaum, Department of Radiology, Mount Sinai School of Medicine, New York.)*

section MIP imaging, where the width is equal to the diameter of the carotid artery to help exclude adjacent bone or enhanced vein, is indispensable to generate MIP images of carotid arteries.

Volume rendering uses all the pixels and can provide a realistic three-dimensional visualization by using different coloring and opacities based on the CT values of voxels. It is an appropriate technique for a quick overview of the carotid arteries on CTA. The drawback in VR images is that the appearance of the target vessel may differ based on the threshold value. Inappropriate window settings can create a pseudostenosis. Overlying dense calcification cannot be differentiated easily from the opacified carotid artery lumen.

In summary, cross-sectional MPR imaging should be used to measure the degree of stenosis accurately with the supplemental use of VR, MIP, or CPR images for the overview of the vascular structure and for planning surgical or interventional radiologic procedures.

Carotid Artery Ulceration

MDCT angiography is helpful for the detection of ulceration. Wintermark and coworkers[33] have demonstrated that CTA performs well in detecting ulcerations ($\kappa <$ 0.855) when compared with histologic examination. Saba and colleagues[34] have demonstrated that MDCT angiography for the detection of carotid ulceration confirmed by surgical specimens reveals 93.9% sensitivity (95% CI, 0.858 to 1.021), and a 98.7% specificity (95% CI, 0.961 to 1.012). They described the usefulness of cross-sectional images and VR to detect ulceration.

Reporting

With the advent of cross-sectional imaging of carotid stenosis by CTA and MRA, direct measurement of both the carotid artery diameter and area stenosis are now possible (Fig. 91-14). Poiseuille's law states that the amount of blood flow in a tubular structure is proportional to the cross-sectional area. This would imply that area stenosis and not diameter stenosis would correlate best with flow in the ICA. Bucek and associates have shown that measurements of the narrowest ICA stenosis on CTA in 178 vessels are a reasonable predictor of the cross-sectional area.[25] This probably explains why the original diameter stenosis measurements from NASCET worked in the first place. When new multicenter trials evaluating CTA and/or MRA to guide medical versus surgical treatments are planned, it would be reasonable to look at direct area stenosis measurements instead of the original indirect NASCET diameter stenosis measurements. Until those studies are available, it is most helpful to report ICA stenosis based on the NASCET criteria. The actual linear measurement of minimal ICA diameter and distal ICA diameter should be reported. The status of the lumen as smooth, irregular, or ulcerated should also be reported. Any tandem stenoses elsewhere in the carotid artery, as well as the status of the circle of Willis, are important to describe. Finally, any significant adjacent soft tissue or bony abnormalities should be reported.

KEY POINTS FOR EXTRACRANIAL CAROTID MR ANGIOGRAPHY

- Contrast agent dose and imaging for high spatial resolution CE MRA are optimized.
- Increasing use of carotid stents may limit MR angiography.
- MRA has several advantages over CTA
  - Has no difficulties imaging calcified carotid artery stenoses
  - Does not require use of ionizing radiation
  - Provides potential for plaque characterization during same examination period
- Near-term improvements with 3.0-T MRA are expected.

KEY POINTS FOR EXTRACRANIAL CAROTID CT ANGIOGRAPHY

- CTA is a fast and readily available technique.
- CTA generally provides higher spatial resolution than MRA.
- Surgeons are typically more comfortable with how the anatomy is displayed.
- CTA can "see through" carotid stents.
- CTA is problematic in patients at risk for CIN and/or who are allergic to iodinated contrast agents.
- There is increasing concern about radiation milliamperage exposure in future CTA units.
- Near-term improvements with increased CT detectors and dual-energy source CT are expected.

SUGGESTED READINGS

Briley-Saebo KC, Mulder WJ, Mani V, et al. Magnetic resonance imaging of vulnerable atherosclerotic plaques: current imaging strategies and molecular imaging probes. J Magn Reson Imaging 2007; 26:460-479.

Enterline DS, Kapoor G. A practical approach to CT angiography of the neck and brain. Tech Vasc Interv Radiol 2006; 9:192-204.

Jewells V, Castillo M. MR angiography of the extracranial circulation. Magn Reson Imaging Clin North Am 2003; 11:585-597.

Kaufmann TJ, Kallmes DF. Utility of MRA and CTA in the evaluation of carotid occlusive disease. Semin Vasc Surg 2005; 18:75-82.

Koelemay MJ, Nederkoorn PJ, Reitsma JB, Majoie CB. Systematic review of computed tomographic angiography for assessment of carotid artery disease. Stroke 2004; 35:2306-2312.

Maldonado TS. What are current preprocedure imaging requirements for carotid artery stenting and carotid endarterectomy? Have magnetic resonance angiography and computed tomographic angiography made a difference? Semin Vasc Surg 2007; 20:205-215.

Nederkoorn PJ, van der Graaf Y, Hunink MG. Duplex ultrasound and magnetic resonance angiography compared with digital subtraction angiography in carotid artery stenosis: a systematic review. Stroke 2003; 34:1324-1332.

Saam T, Hatsukami TS, Takaya N, et al. The vulnerable, or high-risk, atherosclerotic plaque: Noninvasive MR imaging for characterization and assessment. Radiology 2007; 244:64-77.

Takhtani D. CT neuroangiography: a glance at the common pitfalls and their prevention. AJR 2005; 185:772-783.

Wardlaw JM, Chappell FM, Stevenson M, et al. Accurate, practical and cost-effective assessment of carotid stenosis in the UK. Health Technol Assess 2006; 10:1-182.

REFERENCES

1. North American Symptomatic Carotid Endarterectomy Trial Collaborators. Beneficial effect of carotid endarterectomy in symptomatic patients with high-grade carotid stenosis. N Engl J Med 1991; 325:445-453.
2. Randomised trial of endarterectomy for recently symptomatic carotid stenosis: final results of the MRC European Carotid Surgery Trial (ECST). Lancet 1998; 351:1379-1387.
3. Rothwell PM, Eliasziw M, Gutnikov SA, et al. Analysis of pooled data from the randomised controlled trials of endarterectomy for symptomatic carotid stenosis. Lancet 2003; 361:107-116.
4. Kuntz KM, Skillman JJ, Whittemore AD, Kent KC. Carotid endarterectomy in asymptomatic patients—is contrast angiography necessary? A morbidity analysis. J Vasc Surg 1995; 22:706-716.

5. Anderson CM, Lee RE, Levin DL, et al. Measurement of internal carotid artery stenosis from source MR angiograms. Radiology 1994; 193:219-226.
6. Kent KC, Kuntz KM, Patel MR, et al. Perioperative imaging strategies for carotid endarterectomy. An analysis of morbidity and cost-effectiveness in symptomatic patients. JAMA 1995; 274:888-893.
7. Patel MR, Kuntz KM, Klufas RA, et al. Preoperative assessment of the carotid bifurcation. Can magnetic resonance angiography and duplex ultrasonography replace contrast arteriography? Stroke 1995; 26:1753-1758.
8. Townsend TC, Saloner D, Pan XM, Rapp JH. Contrast material-enhanced MRA overestimates severity of carotid stenosis, compared with three-dimensional time-of-flight MRA. J Vasc Surg 2003; 38: 36-40.
9. Fain SB, Riederer SJ, Bernstein MA, Huston J 3rd. Theoretical limits of spatial resolution in elliptical-centric contrast-enhanced three-dimensional-MRA. Magn Reson Med 1999; 42:1106-1116.
10. Huston J 3rd, Fain SB, Wald JT, et al. Carotid artery: elliptical centric contrast-enhanced MR angiography compared with conventional angiography. Radiology 2001; 218:138-143.
11. Hnatiuk B, Emery DJ, Wilman AH. Effects of doubling and tripling the spatial resolution in standard three-dimensional contrast-enhanced magnetic resonance angiography of carotid artery disease. J Magn Reson Imaging 2008; 27:71-77.
12. Nael K, Villablanca JP, Pope WB, et al. Supra-aortic arteries: contrast-enhanced MR angiography at 3.0 T—highly accelerated parallel acquisition for improved spatial resolution over an extended field of view. Radiology 2007; 242:600-609.
13. Willinek WA, von Falkenhausen M, Born M, et al. Noninvasive detection of steno-occlusive disease of the supra-aortic arteries with three-dimensional contrast-enhanced magnetic resonance angiography: a prospective, intra-individual comparative analysis with digital subtraction angiography. Stroke 2005; 36:38-43.
14. DeMarco JK, Huston J 3rd, Nash AK. Extracranial carotid MR imaging at 3 T. Magn Reson Imaging Clin North Am 2006; 14:109-121.
15. Takaya N, Yuan C, Chu B, et al. Association between carotid plaque characteristics and subsequent ischemic cerebrovascular events: a prospective assessment with MRI—initial results. Stroke 2006; 37:818-823.
16. Tomasian A, Salamon N, Lohan DG, et al. A contrast dose reduction study for three-dimensional high spatial resolution contrast-enhanced magnetic resonance angiography of supraaortic arteries at 3.0 Tesla. Annual Meeting of the Society of Cardiovascular MR, Los Angeles, 2008, p 158.
17. Hoogeveen RM, Bakker CJ, Viergever MA. Limits to the accuracy of vessel diameter measurements in MR angiography. J Magn Reson Imaging 1998; 8:1228-1235.
18. U-King-Im J, Graves MJ, Cross JJ, et al. Internal carotid artery stenosis: accuracy of subjective visual impression for evaluation with digital subtraction angiography and contrast-enhanced MR angiography. Radiology 2007; 244:213-222.
19. De Marco JK, Nesbit GM, Wesbey GE, Richardson D. Prospective evaluation of extracranial carotid stenosis: MR angiography with maximum-intensity projections and multiplanar reformation compared with conventional angiography. AJR Am J Roentgenol 1994; 163:1205-1212.
20. Lell M, Fellner C, Baum U, et al. Evaluation of carotid artery stenosis with multisection CT and MR imaging: influence of imaging modality and postprocessing. AJNR Am J Neuroradiol 2007; 28:104-110.
21. U-King-Im JM, Trivedi RA, Cross JJ, et al. Measuring carotid stenosis on contrast-enhanced magnetic resonance angiography: diagnostic performance and reproducibility of 3 different methods. Stroke 2004; 35:2083-2088.
22. Saba L, Sanfilippo R, Phisl R, et al. Multidetector-row CT angiography in the study of atherosclerotic carotid arteries. Neuroradiology 2007; 49:623-637.
23. Koelemay MJ, Nederkoorn PJ, Reitsma JB, Majoic CB. Systematic review of computed tomographic angiography for assessment of carotid artery disease. Stroke 2004; 35:2306-2312.
24. Berg M, Zhang Z, Ikonen A, et al. Multi-detector row CT angiography in the assessment of carotid artery disease in symptomatic patients: comparison with rotational angiography and digital subtraction angiography. AJNR Am J Neuroradiol 2005; 26:1022-1034.
25. Bucek RA, Puchner S, Haumer M, et al. CTA quantification of internal carotid artery stenosis: application of luminal area vs. luminal diameter measurements and assessment of inter-observer variability. J Neuroimaging 2007; 17:219-226.
26. Schuknecht B. High-concentration contrast media (HCCM) in CT angiography of the carotid system: impact on therapeutic decision making. Neuroradiology 2007; 49(Suppl 1):S15-S26.
27. Chen CJ, Lee TH, Hsu HL, et al. Multi-slice CT angiography in diagnosing total versus near occlusions of the internal carotid artery: comparison with catheter angiography. Stroke 2004; 35:83-85.
28. Thomsen HS, Morcos SK. Contrast media and the kidney: European Society of Urogenital Radiology (ESUR) guidelines. Br J Radiol 2003; 76:513-518.
29. Yoon DY, Lim KJ, Choi CS, et al. Sixteen-detector row CT angiography of the brain: comparison of 3 different volumes of the contrast material. J Comput Assist Tomogr 2007; 31:671-676.
30. Enterline DS, Kapoor G. A practical approach to CT angiography of the neck and brain. Tech Vasc Interv Radiol 2006; 9:192-204.
31. de Monye C, de Weert TT, Zaalberg W, et al. Optimization of CT angiography of the carotid artery with a 16-MDCT scanner: craniocaudal scan direction reduces contrast material-related perivenous artifacts. AJR 2006; 186:1737-1745.
32. Lell MM, Ditt H, Panknin C, et al. Bone-subtraction CT angiography: evaluation of two different fully automated image-registration procedures for interscan motion compensation. AJNR Am J Neuroradiol 2007; 28:1362-1368.
33. Wintermark M, Jawadi SS, Rapp JH, et al. High-resolution CT imaging of carotid artery atherosclerotic plaques. AJNR Am J Neuroradiol 2008; 29:875-882.
34. Saba L, Caddeo G, Sanfilippo R, et al. Efficacy and sensitivity of axial scans and different reconstruction methods in the study of the ulcerated carotid plaque using multidetector-row CT angiography: comparison with surgical results. AJNR Am J Neuroradiol 2007; 28: 716-723.

PART SIXTEEN

The Thoracic Vessels

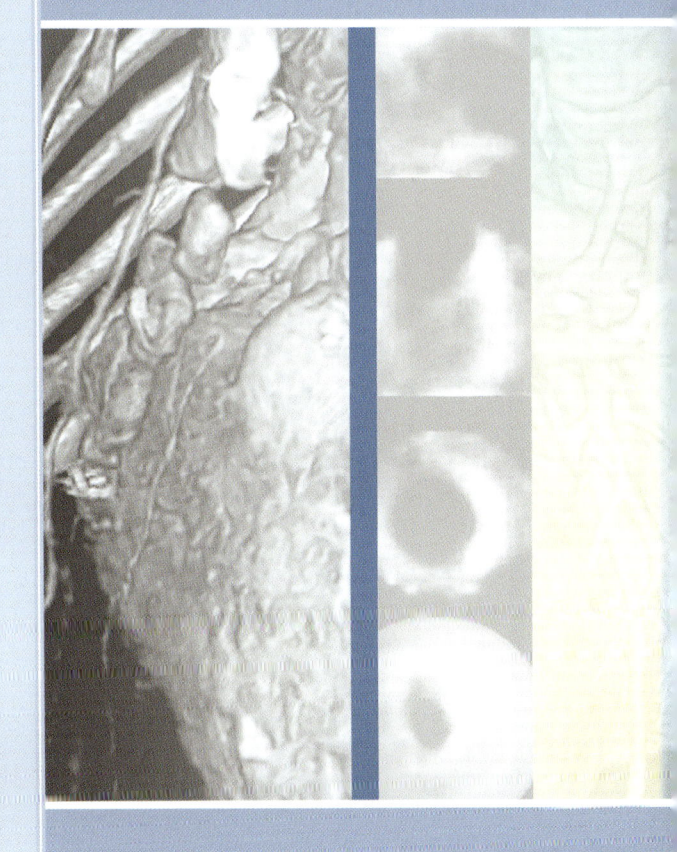

CHAPTER 92

Thoracic Aortic Aneurysms

Saurabh Jha and Harold Litt

Thoracic aortic aneurysms can result from a variety of causes. The underlying cause of a thoracic aortic aneurysm can typically be predicted by its location and morphologic features and by the age of the patient.[1] Whereas the overarching goal of therapy remains similar (i.e., to prevent complications, notably aortic rupture), the nature, timing, and associated operative interventions can differ significantly according to the location and cause of the aneurysm. An example is that of the ascending aortic aneurysm, which by its location is associated with the additional considerations of whether to replace the aortic valve, to reimplant the coronary arteries, and to repair the arch vessels. In addition, assessment of global cardiovascular function is paramount in directing appropriate treatment strategy.

Thoracic aortic aneurysms are less common than their abdominal counterpart.[2] Imaging plays a critical role in diagnosis, treatment planning (i.e., assessment of the need for intervention, urgency of intervention, and type of intervention), and postsurgical surveillance. Moreover, some complications, such as spinal cord ischemia, are germane to surgical repair of thoracic aortic aneurysms, and imaging can provide a road map that may allow prospective modification of surgical technique to reduce the chances of such complications.

THORACIC AORTIC ANEURYSM

Definition

The traditional definition of an aneurysm is dilation of a blood vessel wall so that the resulting caliber is 50% greater.[3] This size-based definition does not account for morphologic characteristics such as focal saccular dilation of the aorta due to trauma, penetrating atherosclerotic ulcer, and infection. These scenarios require an "aneurysm mentality" because saccular aortic dilations are at particular risk for rupture and are thus also classified as aneurysms.

In true aneurysms, the dilation involves all layers of the blood vessel wall. False aneurysms (also known as pseudoaneurysms or saccular aneurysms) occur from disruption of one or more layers of the aortic wall.[4]

Prevalence and Epidemiology

Thoracic aortic aneurysms are less common than abdominal aneurysms, and the prevalence depends on the etiology (Fig. 92-1). Of note, aneurysms due to systemic arterial disease have less male preponderance and a more advanced age at presentation than abdominal aneurysms do, resulting in greater comorbid disease.[2]

The population incidence of detected descending thoracic and thoracoabdominal aortic aneurysms is estimated to be 5.9 new aneurysms per 100,000 person-years. The lifetime probability of rupture in these aneurysms is 75% to 80%.[5]

Etiology and Pathophysiology

The following paragraphs classify aneurysms by underlying etiology and pathogenesis, location, and whether they are true or false. The purpose of such a classification affects the search for associated vascular lesions, the surgical approach, and the potential complications.

Etiology and Pathogenesis

Atherosclerosis

Atherosclerosis affects the aortic wall in many ways, such as through erosion of the internal elastic lamina and subsequent exposure of the medial layer of the aortic wall to the pulse pressure or through ischemia of the media from reduced blood supply due to disease in the vasa vasorum. Another mechanism of aneurysm formation is through progression of atherosclerotic plaque ulceration to a penetrating atherosclerotic ulcer with breakage of the intimal layer. Penetrating atherosclerotic ulcer may result in a saccular aneurysm (Fig. 92-2). Atherosclerotic aneurysms are associated with hypertension, coronary artery disease, and abdominal aortic aneurysms.[4]

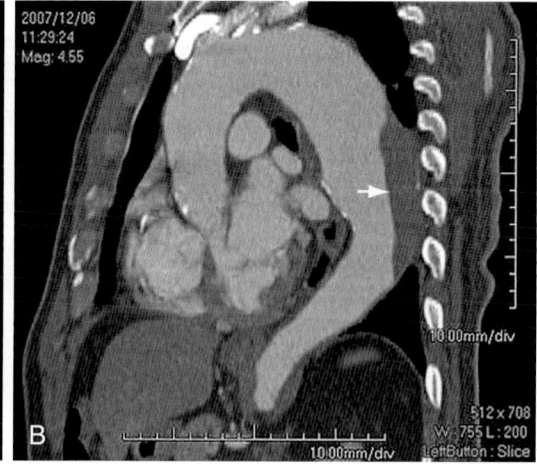

FIGURE 92-1 Atherosclerosis is the most common cause of aneurysms of the descending thoracic aorta. Oblique axial (**A**) and oblique sagittal (**B**) maximum intensity projection CT angiographic images show an aneurysmal descending thoracic aorta with considerable mural thrombus (*arrow*) and atherosclerotic calcifications.

Cystic Medial Necrosis

As the name implies, cystic medial necrosis affects the medial layer of the arterial wall; degeneration of the smooth muscle creates "cystic spaces," resulting in a fusiform aneurysm.[4] This is the most common cause of aneurysms of the ascending aorta. The pathophysiologic process involves the aortic root, resulting in dilation of the annulus of the aortic valve. Associated aortic regurgitation may require concomitant replacement of the aortic valve.[6] Cystic medial necrosis is the hallmark of the pathologic changes in Marfan syndrome (Figs. 92-3 to 92-6). Other connective tissue disorders, such as Ehlers-Danlos and Loeys-Dietz (Fig. 92-7) syndromes, also affect the medial layer of the aorta.[4] These entities are both familial and have an identifiable gene leading to the abnormal biochemistry.

Marfan syndrome is the most common of the connective tissue processes, with an incidence of 1:10,000.[7] Marfan syndrome is an autosomal dominant condition that results in a mutation in the gene encoding fibrillin 1,[8] an essential protein for elastic properties, causing cardiovascular and musculoskeletal abnormalities. The elastin-depleted aorta is stiffer and more prone to dilation as it incurs higher pulse pressure than the normally distensible aorta does. The dilation starts in the root and extends to the mid-ascending aorta.[9] Aortic rupture and dissection are the leading causes of death in patients with Marfan syndrome.[7] Repair in patients with Marfan syndrome is recommended in the asymptomatic patient when the aortic root or ascending aorta exceeds 5 cm in diameter because of the high risk of aortic rupture and aortic dissection.[10] Associated cardiovascular abnormalities include aortic insufficiency and mitral valve prolapse,

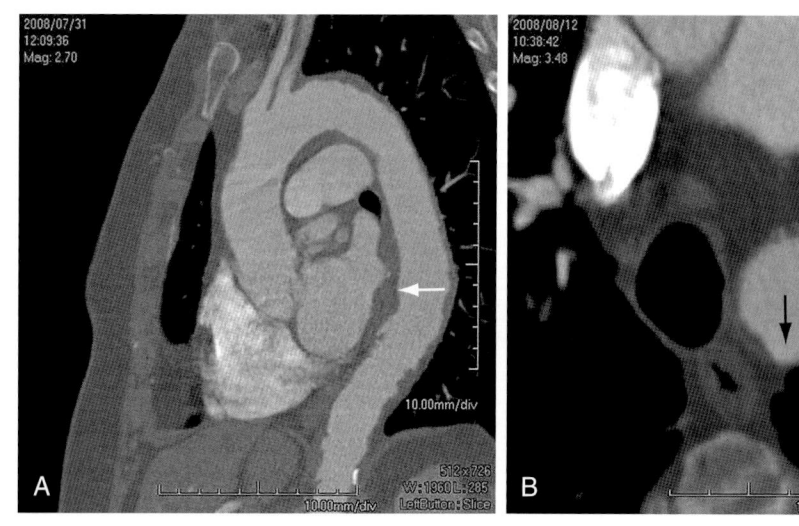

FIGURE 92-2 Ulceration of the atherosclerotic plaque leads to a penetrating atherosclerotic ulcer, which can cause dilation of the aorta (*arrows*). Sagittal oblique maximum intensity projection CT angiographic image (**A**) demonstrates extensive atherosclerotic plaque in the descending thoracic aorta. Plaque ulceration eventually breaks through the intimal layer, causing a penetrating atherosclerotic ulcer, which can result in an aneurysm with a focal bulge or saccular configuration (**B**).

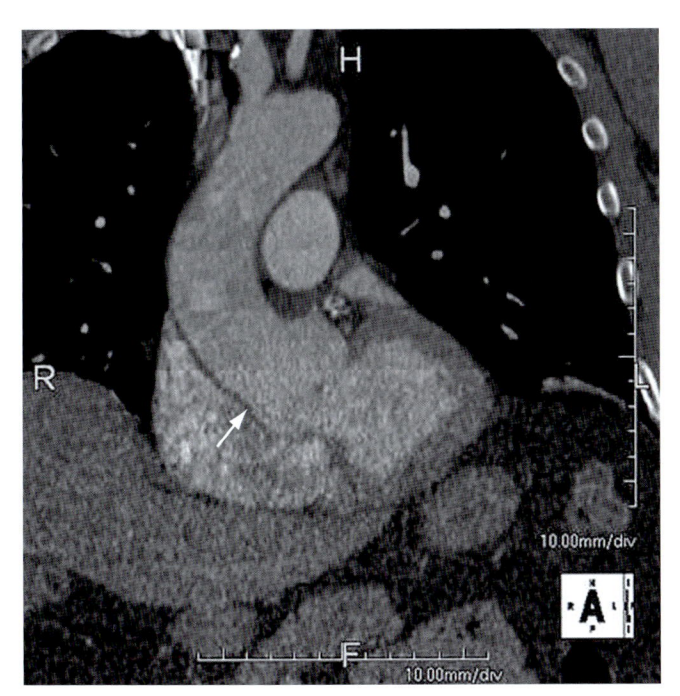

FIGURE 92-3 Oblique coronal reformatted contrast-enhanced CT image shows dilation of the aortic root (*arrow*) and typical effacement of the sinotubular junction in Marfan syndrome.

which frequently necessitate valve repair, and pulmonary artery aneurysms.[9]

Loeys-Dietz syndrome has only recently been characterized as a distinct phenotype that is caused by mutations in genes encoding type 1 or type 2 transforming growth factor β.[11] Aneurysms form at an earlier age than in other connective tissue disorders and tend to rupture at a smaller size, with a greater propensity for dissection. The arteriopathy tends to be more systemic than in Marfan syndrome, and the postoperative surveillance must factor both the repaired artery and the remote arteries including the intracranial circulation.

Vascular Ehlers-Danlos syndrome is an autosomal dominant disorder caused by heterozygous mutations of the *COL3A1* gene. The syndrome is characterized by fragile arterial tissue that not only is prone to aneurysm, dissection, and rupture but can also make surgical repair difficult. Noninvasive imaging, such as computed tomographic angiography (CTA) and magnetic resonance angiography (MRA), is preferred because of the risk of dissection and rupture with arterial access. Unlike Marfan and Loeys-Dietz syndromes, which have a predilection for the aortic root, Ehlers-Danlos syndrome more often affects the visceral arteries.[12]

Dissection

Aortic dissection is different enough in pathogenesis and management to be considered separately from thoracic aortic aneurysms. The term *dissecting aneurysm* is discouraged. Nonetheless, a dissected aorta may become aneurysmal (Fig. 92-8), and an aneurysm may dissect; both scenarios alter the management and approach. Of note, any cause of an acute aortic syndrome can result in aneurysm formation.

Trauma

Blunt thoracic trauma with a sudden deceleration mechanism injures the aorta at its points of relative fixation (due to shear), which includes the aortic isthmus (in the region of the ligamentum arteriosum), the hiatus, and the aortic root, in descending frequency. Injury may cause transection or intimal disruption and, if unrecognized, may be manifested as a saccular aneurysm that may involve disruption of the intima and media (pseudoaneurysm or false aneurysm).[13]

Mild bulging of the proximal descending aorta at the attachment of the ligamentum arteriosum (ductus bump) is a common normal finding and should not be confused with aneurysms in that region, particularly those due to trauma (Fig. 92-9).

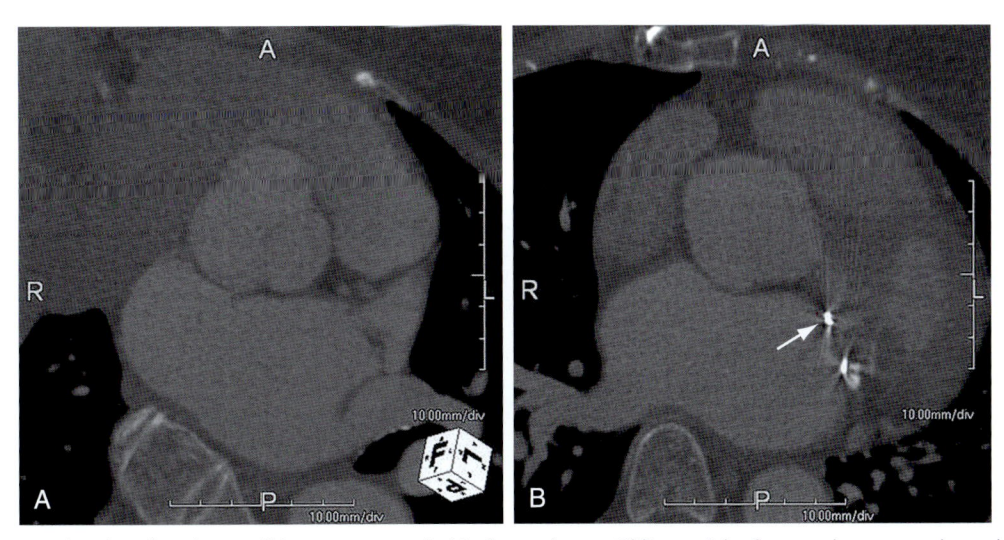

FIGURE 92-4 Associated cardiac abnormalities are common in Marfan syndrome. Oblique axial reformatted contrast-enhanced CT images show a dilated aortic root and mitral valve ring (*arrow*, **B**). The mitral valve was dysfunctional because of associated mitral valve prolapse.

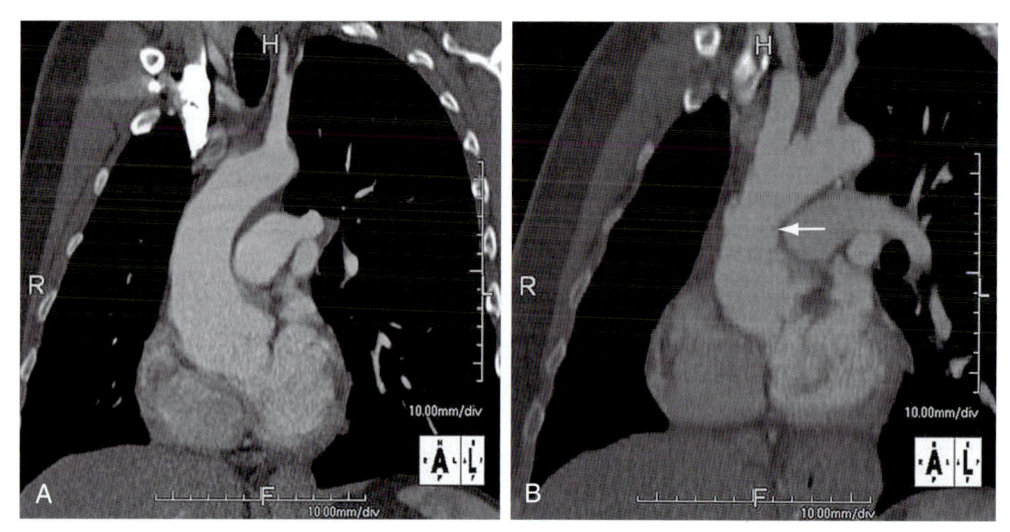

FIGURE 92-5 In Marfan syndrome, the proximal aorta is affected, with the disease commencing at the aortic root. The descending aorta and abdominal aorta are rarely affected. The sinotubular junction can be effaced, resulting in a "spring onion" appearance to the aortic root and ascending aorta. Oblique coronal multiplanar reformatted image before (**A**) and 2 years after (**B**) uncomplicated repair of dilated aortic root. Note the typical appearance of a repaired aorta with kinking at the anastomosis (*arrow*).

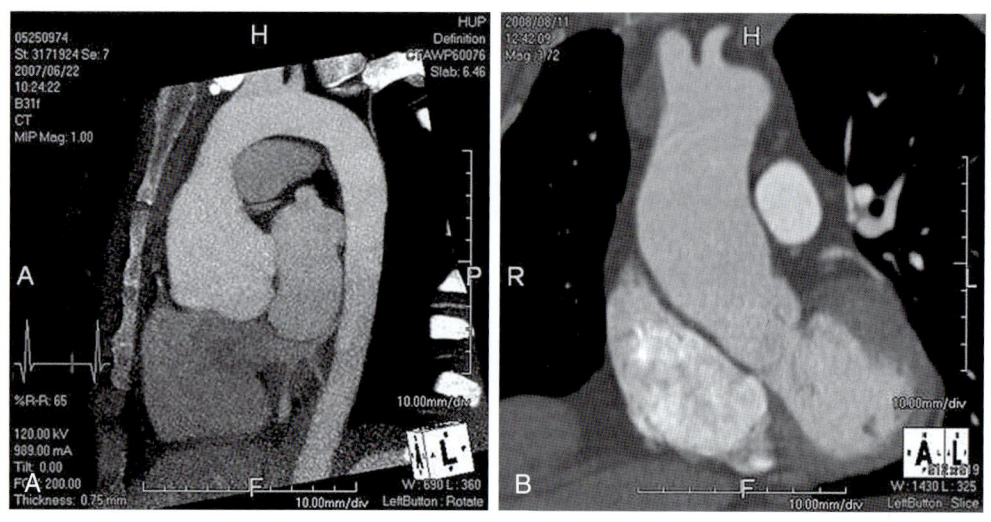

FIGURE 92-6 The dilated root and effaced sinotubular junction (**A**) in Marfan syndrome is of a distinctive configuration. Note the difference in appearance of an ascending aortic aneurysm that spares the root (**B**).

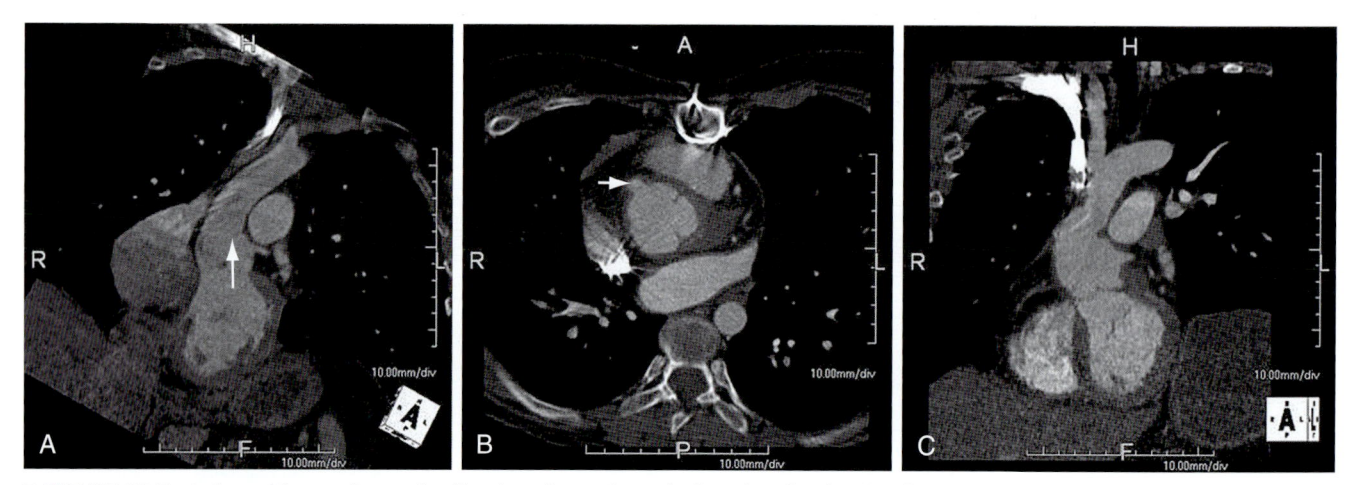

FIGURE 92-7 In Loeys-Dietz syndrome, the dilated aortic root is repaired much earlier than in other connective tissue diseases. Oblique coronal reformatted contrast-enhanced CT image shows a mildly dilated aortic root (*arrow*, **A**), which resulted in a valve-sparing aortic root repair with coronary artery reimplantation (*arrow*, **B**), the modified David procedure (**B** and **C**).

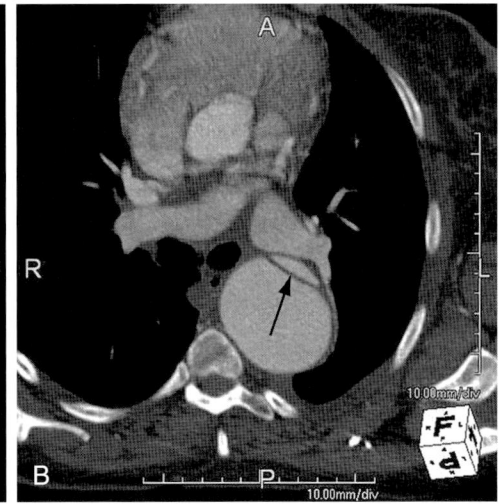

■ **FIGURE 92-8** Sagittal reformatted (**A**) and axial (**B**) contrast-enhanced CT images show a type B dissection (*arrow*) and aneurysm of the descending aorta.

Inflammation and Infection

Infection may primarily involve the artery and secondarily lead to aneurysm, or an aneurysm may become infected. The most common site of infection is the ascending aorta near the sinus of Valsalva (Fig. 92-10).[14] Infected aortic aneurysms, despite the pseudonym mycotic aneurysms, are rarely due to fungal agents and mostly caused by bacteria in an acute or chronic setting, classically due to syphilis.

Infected aortitis leading to aneurysms may occur by direct extension from endocarditis or seeding of the vasa vasorum with infected complexes from remote septic foci. These remote foci may not be clinically evident, and *Salmonella* and *Staphylococcus* are the most common etiologic agents in this situation. Predisposing factors include intravenous drug abuse and immunocompromised state.[15]

Vasculitides such as Takayasu arteritis and giant cell arteritis may lead to aneurysmal dilation, but mural thickening is the predominant finding in such inflammatory conditions. The mural thickening may lead to reduction in luminal caliber even if the adventitia-adventitia measurement indicates arterial enlargement.[16]

Post-stenotic Dilation

Aortic stenosis can cause dilation of the ascending aorta, usually the right lateral and posterior wall, from the post-stenotic jet. This is commonly seen in those with a bicuspid aortic valve (Fig. 92-11), although the dilation may be partly due to a systemic arteriopathy because this condition is also associated with coarctation of the aorta.[17] Coarctation can also lead to post-stenotic dilation.

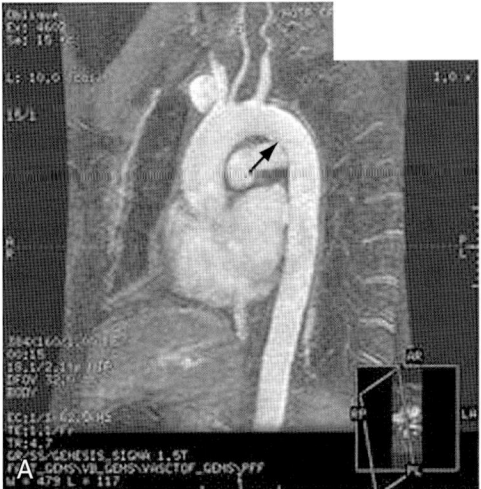

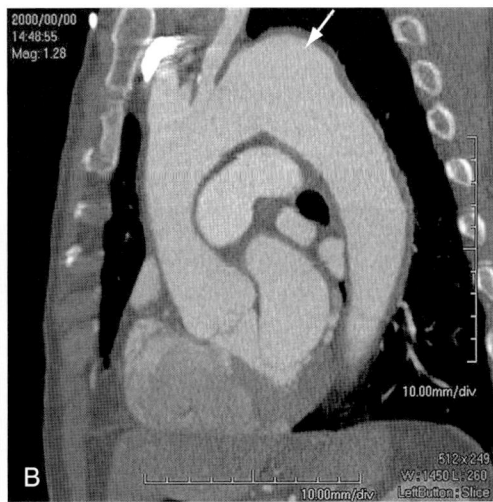

■ **FIGURE 92-9** **A,** Sagittal oblique maximum intensity projection from contrast-enhanced MRA shows mild dilation of the inferior wall of the proximal descending aorta (*arrow*), a common finding known as the ductus bump. **B,** In another patient, an aneurysm (*arrow*) of the proximal descending aorta is shown for comparison.

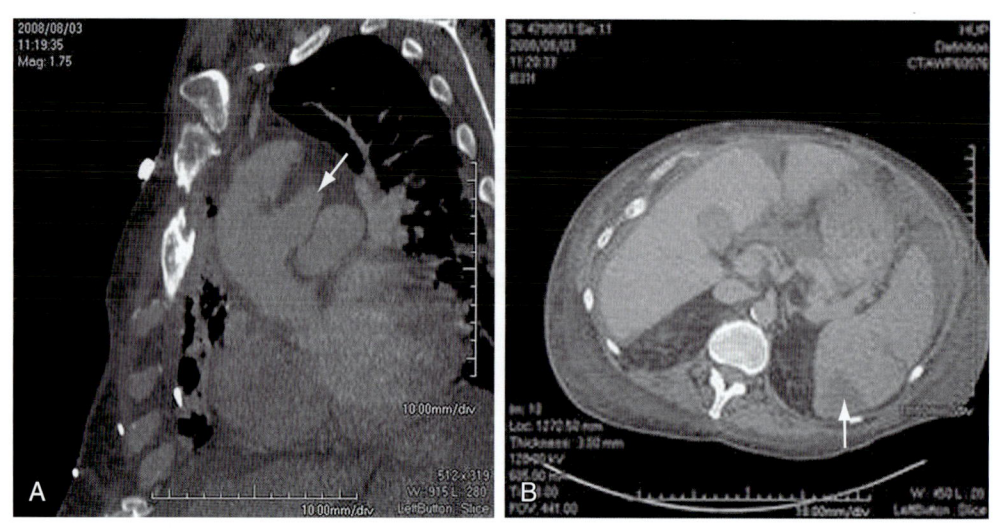

FIGURE 92-10 **A,** Sagittal reformatted contrast-enhanced CT image shows a tubular outpouching (*arrow*) inferior to the aortic arch with a thick rind of surrounding soft tissue. This is an infected aneurysm. **B,** Axial contrast-enhanced CT image shows infarcts (*arrow*) in the spleen due to emboli from the infected complex.

Increased Aortic Flow

The increased stroke volume from aortic regurgitation or from a patent ductus arteriosus can dilate the ascending aorta. Treatment is aimed at treating these entities.

Location

1. Ascending aorta
2. Aortic arch
3. Descending thoracic aorta
4. Thoracoabdominal aortic aneurysms
5. Diffusely aneurysmal aorta

In general, ascending aortic aneurysms are due to cystic medial necrosis. The more common descending thoracic aortic/thoracoabdominal aortic aneurysms are caused by atherosclerosis.

Ascending aortic aneurysms may involve only the supracoronary aorta and spare the aortic root, involve the aortic root only or as well, or result in diffuse tubular dilation.

Thoracoabdominal aortic aneurysms are further divided by the Crawford classification (Fig. 92-12), which is used to determine the operative approach and to counsel the patient about postoperative complications. Crawford I and II start distal to the origin of the left subclavian artery, with Crawford II extending below the renal artery origin. Crawford III starts more distal than Crawford I in the descending thoracic aorta. Crawford IV is essentially an aneurysm of the abdominal aorta that extends to the diaphragmatic hiatus.[18]

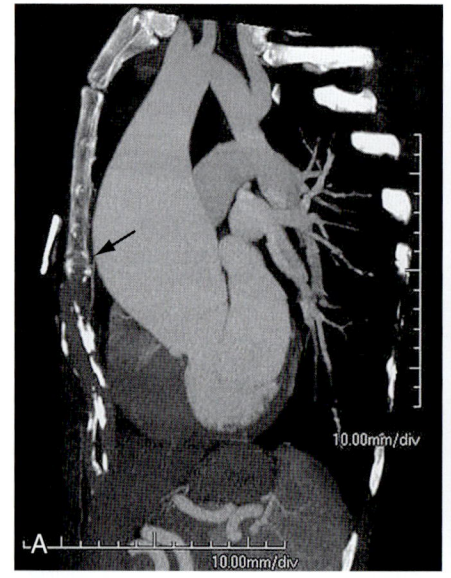

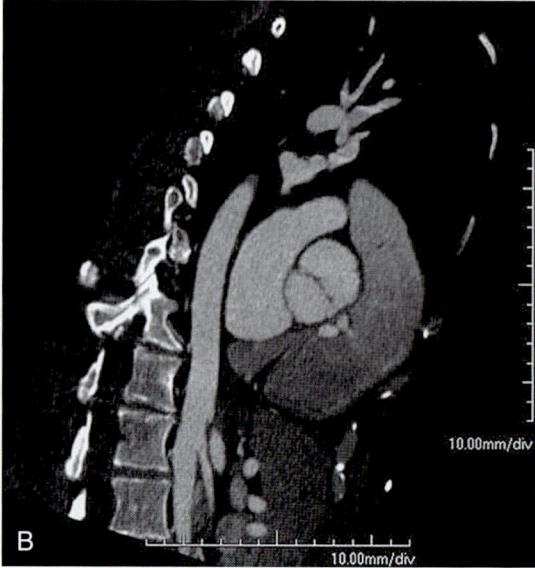

FIGURE 92-11 Sagittal oblique (**A**) and oblique axial (**B**) maximum intensity projection images from contrast-enhanced CT show post-stenotic dilation (*arrow*) of the ascending aorta enlarging the right lateral and posterior wall from bicuspid aortic valve.

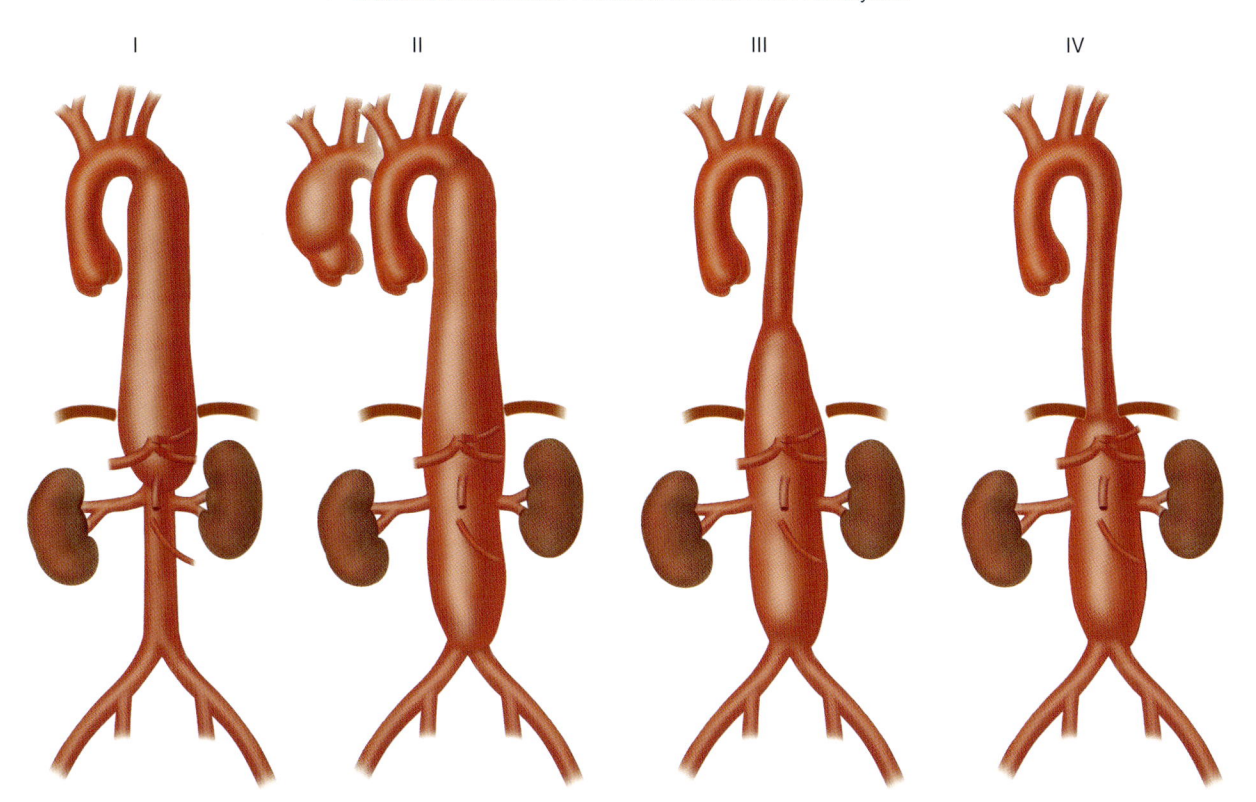

FIGURE 92-12 The Crawford classification of thoracoabdominal aortic aneurysms. *(Reproduced with permission from Coselli J, Lemaire S. Descending and thoraco-abdominal aortic aneurysms. In Kohn LH. Cardiac Surgery in the Adult, 3rd ed. New York, McGraw-Hill, 2007.)*

True and False Aneurysms

All causes of arteriopathy can cause true aneurysms. The causes of false aneurysms, on the other hand, are more typically trauma, infection (i.e., mycotic aneurysm), and penetrating atherosclerotic ulcer. False aneurysms have a saccular morphology, that is, an eccentric bulge, and can be considered a contained rupture (Fig. 92-13). They occur from the disruption of layers of the blood vessel wall and are often contained only by the adventitia and fibrous tissue. This makes them more likely than true aneurysms to rupture for any given size.[1]

Manifestations of Disease

Clinical Presentation

Aneurysms may be detected incidentally, be manifested through local mass effect or systemic symptoms, or cause symptoms from acute rupture.[1,19]

Asymptomatic

Nearly half of thoracoabdominal aortic aneurysms are discovered incidentally, some in the context of vascular disease elsewhere and others on chest radiography or echocardiography. Patients with known phenotype or family history of connective tissue disease should have routine work-up to search for aneurysm.

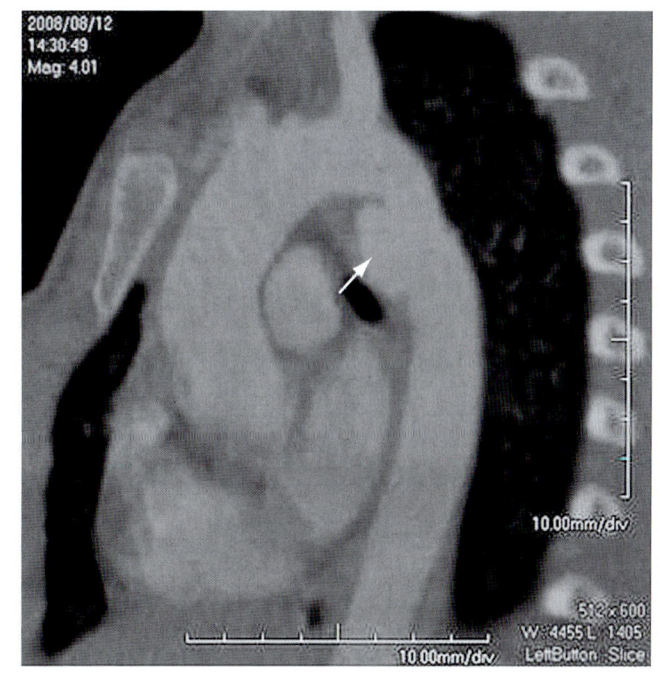

FIGURE 92-13 Sagittal reformatted contrast-enhanced CT image shows a traumatic pseudoaneurysm (*arrow*) in the proximal descending thoracic aorta. Note the typical saccular configuration of the aneurysm.

Local Mass Effect

Symptoms depend on the structure being compressed, such as the airway (breathing difficulty, recurrent pneumonia, and cough), esophagus (dysphagia), pulmonary vein (focal pulmonary edema, varix), systemic veins (limb and facial swelling), and vertebral body (backache). In the event of fistula formation, the patient may present with hemoptysis (airway) or hematemesis (esophagus).

Systemic Symptoms

Inflammatory and infected aneurysms or prosthetic grafts may present with constitutional symptoms such as fever and weight loss.

Embolism of the atherosclerotic plaque or thrombus will cause clinical signs of distal ischemia, such as blue toe syndrome.

Rupture

Chest pain in the context of a known aneurysm signifies increase in size, development of a dissection, or rupture. With rupture, chest pain is accompanied by diaphoresis and hypotension, and the patient may be in extremis. The signs and symptoms may point to end-organ ischemia, such as abdominal pain disproportionate to physical examination findings (mesenteric ischemia), paraplegia (spinal cord ischemia), and angina pectoris (myocardial ischemia).

The strongest predictor of rupture is the initial size of the aneurysm. Also, the etiology of the aneurysm must be taken into consideration as certain connective tissue disorders are associated with rupture at a smaller aneurysm size. For thoracoabdominal aortic aneurysms due to atherosclerosis, the rupture rate is 18% at 2 years for aneurysms greater than 5 cm. Another risk factor for rupture is aneurysm growth of more than 5 mm in 6 months. Aneurysm growth correlates with smoking, forced expiratory volume in 1 second (FEV_1) of less than 1.5 L/min, female sex, and advancing age.[20] The diameter at which elective surgery on the ascending aorta is recommended is considered to be 5.5 cm.[10] Ascending aortic aneurysms grow faster in association with a bicuspid aortic valve (0.19 cm/yr) than with a non–bicuspid valve (0.13 cm/yr).[21]

Imaging Indications and Algorithm

Broadly speaking, imaging aims to define the aneurysm and to determine its extent, to seek associated abnormalities, and to offer surveillance in the postoperative period.

Aneurysm and Its Extent

The questions that need to be answered are

- Does the aneurysm require intervention?
- Is it amenable to endovascular stent placement or does it require a prosthetic graft?

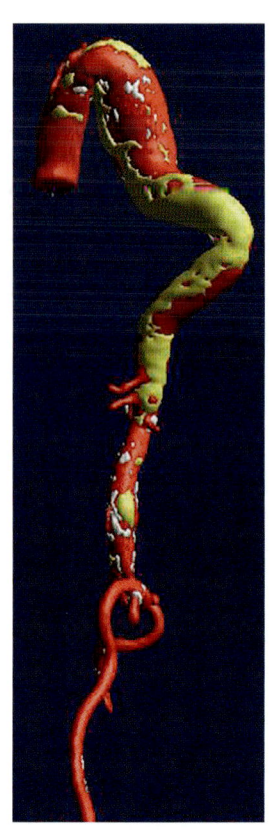

FIGURE 92-14 Color-coded oblique sagittal volume rendered image of the aorta. There are extensive calcifications in the aorta. The calcifications have a green shade. Stent graft placement for the aneurysmal descending thoracic aorta will be difficult because of the severe angulation and tortuosity of the aorta. *(Image courtesy of Dr. Ron Fairman, Chief, Division of Vascular Surgery and Endovascular Therapy, Hospital of the University of Pennsylvania.)*

The following information concerning the aneurysm and vascular tree needs to be determined:

- the size, shape, angulation, and proximal and distal extent of the aneurysm;
- the involvement of the aortic root and arch branch vessels;
- the amount and eccentricity of the mural thrombus;
- the amount and ulceration of the plaque;
- the presence or absence of a dissection;
- the diameter and angulation of the neck of the aneurysm (Fig. 92-14);
- the minimal diameter, tortuosity, and calcification of the iliac arteries; and
- the state of the axillary and subclavian arteries and the intercostal arteries that give rise to the artery of Adamkiewicz.

The state of the axillary and iliofemoral arteries is important to note for many reasons. The iliofemoral arteries provide stent graft access and must be of a certain minimal diameter to allow the sheath to enter without complication. Bypass may use the axillary arteries. In addition, an axillary-femoral bypass may achieve distal aortic perfusion that is critical to reducing visceral ischemia during the cross-clamp period.[1]

Associated Abnormalities

Vascular

Vascular disease is systemic, and assessment of other vascular territories may predict postoperative complications such as renal insufficiency. Assessment of the renal arteries, arch branches, and mesenteric arteries is important in anticipating which vascular beds may be affected by a low-flow/hypotensive state that may be encountered during aneurysm repair. As mentioned, assessment of the arch branches and iliac arteries is also important to plan access.

Cardiac

The major cause of perioperative death and morbidity in patients undergoing vascular surgery for atherosclerotic arterial disease is ischemic heart disease; only 8% of such patients have normal coronary arteries.[22] It is important to identify patients with reduced contractile and perfusion reserve. Concomitant or prophylactic revascularization has not been shown to reduce postoperative outcomes from the cardiac viewpoint, but medical therapy does reduce adverse events in high-risk patients and may influence the surgical approach to reduce operating time.

In the patient with an ascending aortic aneurysm, the state of the aortic root and aortic valve requires evaluation. The degree of aortic regurgitation may be mild and might not merit a concomitant aortic valve replacement during ascending aortic aneurysm repair, but it affects the decision with regard to cross-clamping.[1]

Respiratory

Some of the risk factors for atherosclerotic aneurysms are also those for obstructive lung disease, the diagnosis of which can direct early attention to respiratory support in the perioperative period or favor the use of an endovascular stent graft rather than the open surgical approach. In addition, reduced FEV$_1$ is an independent determinant of growth of an aneurysm.[20]

Postoperative Surveillance

Surveillance in the postoperative period is performed to detect complications that are inherent to the procedure (e.g., endoleaks for stent grafts), to observe for complications due to the hemodynamic alteration consequent to the procedure (e.g., dissection), and to monitor the effects of the causative arteriopathy on the nontreated vasculature.

Imaging Algorithm

No imaging study is all-encompassing, although some studies offer more information than others do. Assessment of the aneurysm extent is best determined by CTA or MRA. Both modalities have inherent advantages and disadvantages, but both can generate diagnostic "luminograms" similar to those of conventional x-ray catheter angiography, and both have the advantage of being able to evaluate the aortic wall and presence of atherosclerotic plaque. Cardiac function is usually assessed by echocardiography, which can be combined with dobutamine stress for contractile reserve. The functional consequence of coronary stenosis is traditionally assessed by stress nuclear medicine (adenosine or dipyridamole), which quantifies perfusion reserve.

The baseline cross-sectional investigation (CTA or MRA) should be chosen to match the one that will be used for follow-up. For example, if the patient is likely to have a stent that is MRI incompatible, the baseline investigation should be CTA. Conversely, if the patient developed anaphylaxis to iodinated contrast medium, MRA should be used for the baseline investigation and follow-up, and an MRI-compatible stent is chosen.

A suggested algorithm:

1. CTA or MRA
2. Echocardiography
3. Carotid duplex ultrasonography
4. Nuclear medicine scan
5. Catheter aortic or coronary angiography (if required)

For surveillance, cross-sectional imaging is performed for uncomplicated cases at 3 months, 6 months, 1 year, and annually thereafter.

Imaging Technique and Findings

Radiography

Chest radiography can suggest the presence of an aneurysm and its complications. Aneurysms often present incidentally on chest radiography. Findings on chest radiography include dilation of the aortic contour (Fig. 92-15) and calcification. Associated cardiac abnormalities will lead to an abnormal cardiac size and configuration.[23]

Dilation of the aortic contour may be focal, segmental, or diffuse. Ascending aortic dilation can be inferred by a right convex contour above the right atrial border. Dilation of the proximal descending aorta, the aortic knob, will cause an indentation on the trachea.

Long-standing aneurysms due to atherosclerosis or syphilis are likely to calcify. Calcification is usually of the intimal layer. Less commonly, the medial layer calcifies, and the calcification has a "railroad" configuration. Diabetes and renal impairment are known causes of medial calcification. Displacement of the intimal calcification, meaning that the calcification is no longer peripheral in location, suggests a dissection or intramural hematoma. Calcification of the mural thrombus or plaque, also known as neointimal calcification, can simulate the displaced calcifications.

Aneurysms of the sinus of Valsalva may mimic a mass on chest radiography. Sinus of Valsalva aneurysms are symmetric or asymmetric. Connective tissue disease typically causes symmetric dilation of the sinuses. The location of the contour abnormality or "mass" on chest radiography can predict the involved sinus. Aneurysms of the right sinus project anteriorly (best seen on the lateral view) and can erode the sternum. Aneurysms from the anterior portion of the noncoronary sinus project over the

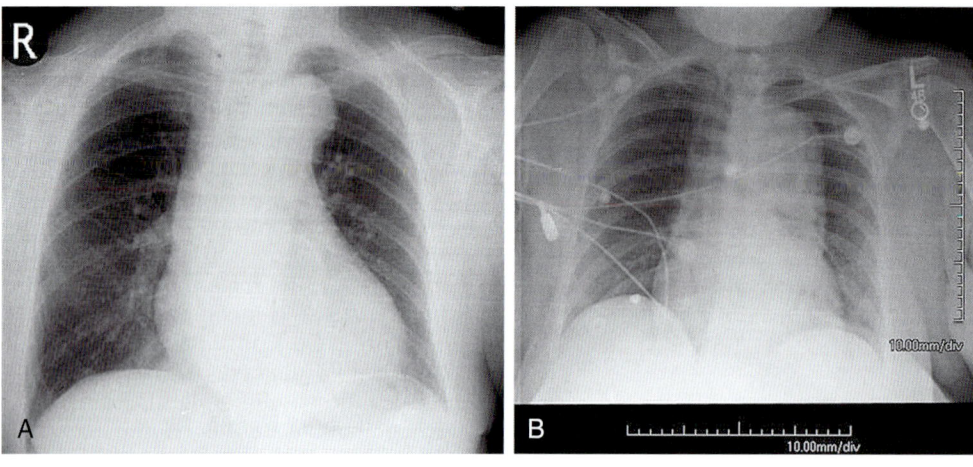

■ **FIGURE 92-15** In two different patients, aneurysms of the ascending (**A**) and descending (**B**) aorta can be seen on plain radiography as enlargement of the aortic contour.

right atrium, and those from the posterior portion of this sinus project over the left atrium.[24]

Rupture of an aneurysm and the presence of a mediastinal hematoma are suggested by the following[1]: displacement of the esophagus, obscuration of the aortic contour, pleural effusion (left), and apical cap (left).

Ultrasonography

Two-dimensional echocardiography (either transthoracic or transesophageal) is not primarily used for the characterization of the aneurysm or the arterial tree. However, the transesophageal approach can provide useful information about the presence of plaque and a dissection flap. The one area not usually visualized by the more invasive but more sensitive transesophageal approach is that part of the ascending aorta overlapped by the trachea because of loss of the acoustic window.[25]

Echocardiography is performed for assessment of valvular function, particularly that of the aortic valve. As mentioned, aortic regurgitation may influence the decision to operate on the aortic valve concurrently. Also, in the presence of aortic regurgitation, cross-clamping should be done with caution, possibly with bypass of the left side of the heart.[1] The intra-aortic balloon pump, a frequent intensive care unit support device, is contraindicated in patients with significant aortic regurgitation.

Carotid duplex ultrasonography is helpful in detecting concomitant carotid artery stenosis and assessing the risk of postoperative complications, such as stroke and subclavian steal phenomenon.

Computed Tomography

With the advent of multidetector CTA and novel contrast injection mechanisms and protocols, CTA has become the most accessible, used, and important modality for the assessment of patients with thoracic aortic aneurysms. Although the risk of radiation exposure and the nephrotoxicity of iodinated contrast medium cannot be discounted, CTA gives excellent spatial and vascular information enabling improved computer postprocessing, such as multiplanar reformation, maximum intensity projection, and volume rendering. Postprocessed viewing of data provides a surgeon or interventionalist with a valuable three-dimensional perspective of the aneurysm, its location, and its position relative to its branch vessels and adjacent structures. The combination of fast acquisition and spatial resolution enables evaluation of the arch to the femoral arteries (and even the toes, if necessary) with the administration of one contrast media bolus ("run") and with only one breath-hold requirement. In addition, ECG-gated cardiac CT can provide information on cardiac function and the coronary arteries. CT of the aortic valve, however, does not provide direct measurement of blood flow, as can be achieved with MRI. Nonetheless, planimetry of CT data can detect and to some extent quantify aortic stenosis (e.g., aortic valve area) or aortic regurgitation (e.g., comparison of right and left ventricular volumes). CTA will assess nonvascular organs, notably the lungs, and may direct the need for pulmonary function tests.[26]

Pre-contrast and arterial phase images are obtained routinely. Delayed (venous phase) images are often beneficial. Venous phase images help in the assessment of solid organs and in the characterization of masses that are incidentally found. Very large aneurysms may not uniformly opacify in the arterial phase, thereby overestimating the size of the thrombus, and only in the venous phase may the true luminal diameter be reflected. Venous phase imaging is routinely obtained in surveillance CT after stent graft placement to detect endoleaks.

Images should be inspected before the administration of contrast material for signs of aortic rupture and for intramural hematoma (Fig. 92-16). Signs of aortic rupture (Fig. 92-17) include irregular aortic wall with broken intimal calcifications, periaortic and mediastinal hematoma, hemothorax (left sided for rupture of aneurysms of the descending aorta), hemopericardium (rupture of ascending aortic aneurysms), and soft tissue "stranding" in the mediastinal fat. Intramural hematoma is indicated by a crescentic high attenuation (50 to 80 HU) along the aortic wall. High attenuation within the mural thrombus is important to identify because this sign is associated with instability and subsequent rupture of aneurysms. Adjacent atelectatic lung should be distinguished from periaortic hematoma.

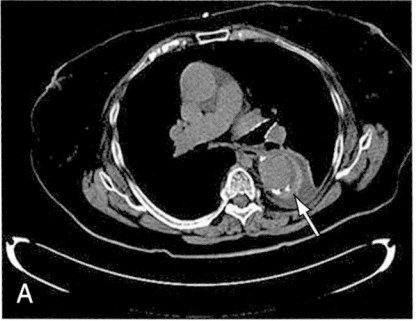

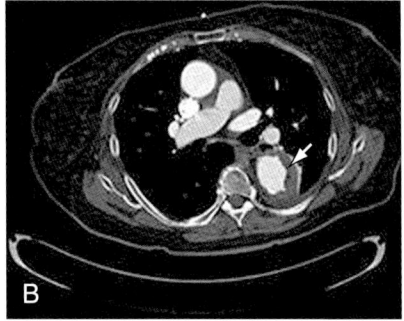

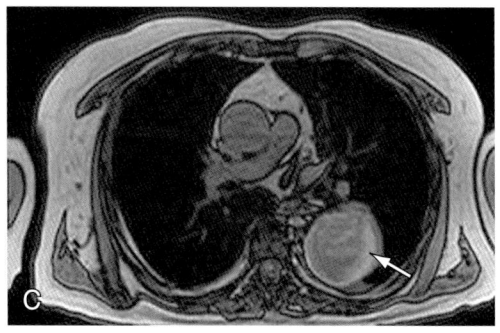

■ **FIGURE 92-16** Intramural hematoma (*arrow*) before (**A**) and after (**B**) contrast-enhanced CT. Subacute blood products are of high attenuation. Note that the intramural hematoma is peripheral to the intimal calcifications. On MRI, the T1-weighted image (**C**) displays the high signal from subacute blood. The intramural hematoma does not enhance (**B**).

A distinction must be made between high attenuation within a mural thrombus and an intramural hematoma. Intramural hematoma is due to bleeding within the medial layer of the aorta and has a smooth margin and a partially circumferential and somewhat helical configuration. Intimal calcifications, if present, are displaced by the intramural hematoma toward the lumen, that is, the hematoma is peripheral to the calcification. Mural thrombus is usually chronic and adherent to the arterial wall. This has an irregular border. The intima is at the periphery of the mural thrombus, that is, the thrombus is internal to the wall of the aorta. Thrombus may calcify, giving the appearance of a displaced intima. However, the distinction can be made by the irregular edge of the thrombus.[27]

Wall thickening of the aorta may be due to an intramural hematoma, a mural thrombus, or an inflammatory process such as vasculitis. Inflammatory wall thickening is distinguishable by the presence of peri-inflammatory fibrosis and wall enhancement.

The aneurysm is best defined on the arterial phase images. A sense of the degree of mural thrombus and atherosclerotic plaque is obtained with the high contrast between lumen and wall. In the setting of an acute rupture, extravasation of contrast material indicates active bleeding and is a sign that must be communicated urgently to the surgeon. However, the absence of extravasated contrast material into the periaortic tissue is not reassuring. To emphasize, the definitive sign of rupture is the periaortic hematoma.

It is critical to ensure that the periaortic process thought to be a hematoma from acute rupture does not enhance in either the arterial or venous phase; mediastinal soft tissue processes such as lymphoma and extramedullary hematopoiesis may have similar imaging features. Similarly, any area questioned in the arterial or venous phase to represent contrast should be correlated with the images obtained before the administration of contrast medium. Calcium and surgical material may not be distinguishable from iodinated contrast media.

Infected aneurysms present as a saccular structure eccentrically from the aortic wall with rapid enlargement, periaortic gas, and erosion of the adjacent osseous structures such as the vertebral body or sternum. Associated reactive adenopathy is frequent.[15]

Magnetic Resonance

MRI can provide much of the same information that CT can, with no radiation and without the complications of iodinated contrast media.[28] However, the use of gadolinium-based contrast agents in patients with severe renal impairment may be a problem secondary to their increased risk for nephrogenic systemic fibrosis.[29] MRI is not as readily available, takes longer to perform than CTA, and may be demanding for the unstable patient. Importantly, MRI does not assess the lungs and cannot detect calcium reliably.

MRI provides flow information and quantifies valvular heart disease with hemodynamic as well as planimetric parameters. MRI also can provide a complete evaluation

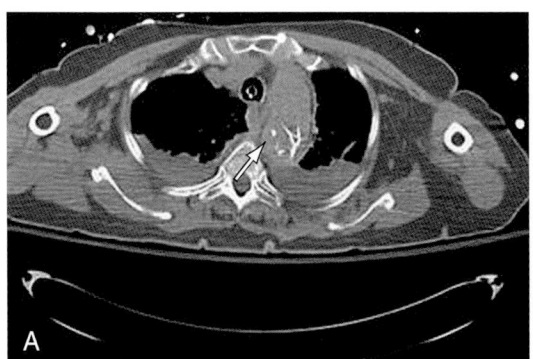

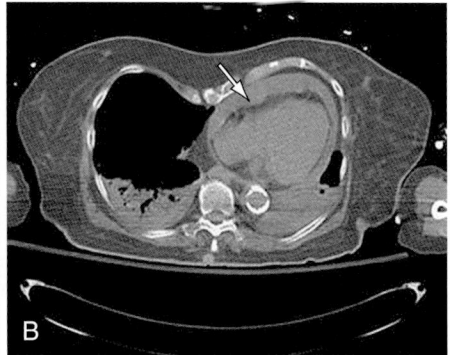

■ **FIGURE 92-17** Non–contrast-enhanced images are crucial in detecting aortic rupture on CT. This patient with a ruptured intramural hematoma (**A**, *arrow*) has hemopericardium (**B**, *arrow*) and bilateral pleural effusions.

of the heart, including function, viability, and contractile or perfusion reserve. Assessment of the coronary arteries by MRI remains an evolving indication.

Multiplanar single-shot fast spin-echo may be used for localizers and overview of anatomy. At least one T1-weighted pulse sequence (e.g., T1-weighted gradient-echo, dual-echo, or fast spin-echo) should be obtained in the axial plane to assess for the presence of hemorrhage in the aortic wall (i.e., intramural hematoma). The post-gadolinium sequence is a three-dimensional spoiled gradient-echo with acquisition parameters optimized for an acquisition that is within the breath-hold capacity of the patient. An axial delayed two-dimensional post-gadolinium pulse sequence, preferably with fat suppression, completes the evaluation. Subtraction images are obtained with use of the pre-gadolinium three-dimensional acquisition as the mask. The angiographic part of MRI is much more amenable to three-dimensional postprocessing, such as maximum intensity projection and volume rendering, than are angiographic images in CT. This is because the nonarterial structures have little contribution to signal, particularly after accurate subtraction.

Although, in general, MRA does not typically require ECG synchronization, the use of prospectively triggered double inversion recovery fast spin-echo black blood imaging allows a better distinction between the aortic wall and lumen, especially near the base of the heart. The addition of inversion recovery fat suppression picks up mural edema, a feature of inflammatory aneurysms.

Cine bright blood images through the thoracic aorta can be useful. In patients with connective tissue disease such as Marfan syndrome, the reduced distensibility of the aorta can be picked up by measuring the change in aortic diameter between end-diastole and end-systole in relation to the pulse pressure.

The morphologic findings of aneurysms are similar to those described with CTA. Subacute blood is of high signal on T1-weighted images, and the signal of the aortic wall and pleural and pericardial effusions should be assessed on this sequence. In the absence of fat suppression, mediastinal hematoma can be difficult to distinguish from fat. Active extravasation of contrast material may be picked up on the multiphase three-dimensional acquisitions or on the delayed venous images.

MRI is more sensitive than is CT in detecting marrow changes due to osteomyelitis that may be associated with infected aortic aneurysms.

Nuclear Medicine/Positron Emission Tomography

Inflammatory aneurysms, infected aneurysms, and infected grafts take up radiotracers indicative of inflammation. Nuclear medicine has a clear role in the evaluation of patients with suspected prosthetic graft infection and equivocal CTA or MRA findings. Leukocytes labeled with technetium Tc 99m exametazime offer the highest sensitivity, although cross-labeling of platelets reduces its usefulness in the early postoperative period. Leukocytes may be labeled with indium 111. The use of gallium requires delayed as well as early imaging. Nuclear medicine lacks spatial sensitivity, and more accurate localization of infection may require CT/PET or CT/SPECT.

Angiography

The use of angiography is declining with the availability of CTA and MRA. Certain indications remain, notably the evaluation of the coronary arteries. Aortography will show the dilated aorta, although it is only a luminogram and does not provide information about the aortic wall, thus underestimating aneurysm size.[30]

In connective tissue disease such as Marfan syndrome, there is effacement of the sinotubular junction, which provides a "spring onion" appearance to the aortic root. Furthermore, aortic root dilation may be symmetric or asymmetric; symmetry is a feature of cystic medial necrosis.

Aneurysms involving the sinus of Valsalva typically have a windsock morphology. A regurgitant jet in diastole signifies aortic incompetence. The sequence of chamber opacification is important to note. For example, early opacification of the right-sided chamber points to a rupture of a sinus of Valsalva aneurysm and fistula or the concomitant presence of aortic insufficiency and a ventricular septal defect.

Differential Diagnosis

From Clinical Presentation

The acute presentation of thoracic aortic aneurysm is typically ominous as it suggests aortic rupture. Patients may have chest pain that can be confused with any number of also dire thoracic conditions, such as myocardial infarction, pulmonary embolism, and aortic dissection.[1] This clinical spectrum is that of acute aortic syndrome and is further discussed in Chapter 93. In most cases, however, the presentation of aortic aneurysms is often asymptomatic, detected incidentally on routine chest radiography or on echocardiography.

From Imaging Findings

The assessment of aneurysms is fairly unequivocal on cross-sectional imaging. On contrast-enhanced CT, paravertebral processes such as lymphoma and extramedullary hematopoiesis can simulate aortic rupture. Evaluation of the images obtained before the administration of contrast material should make the distinction between an inherently high-attenuation process (hematoma) and an enhancing process (malignant neoplasm).[29]

Enlargement of the aorta on plain radiography simulates mediastinal, pulmonary, and paracardiac masses requiring broader differential diagnostic considerations.[23,24] Saccular aneurysms in particular may simulate a mediastinal mass.

Synopsis of Treatment Options

Medical

Medical treatment depends on the cause. Vasculitides such as Takayasu arteritis are treated with steroids. Appropriate antibiotics are used for infected aortic aneurysms and syphilitic aneurysms.[19]

Medical treatment in atherosclerotic aneurysms addresses the treatable risk factors for cardiovascular disease, regardless of whether the patient will have surgical treatment. This might include statins for abnormal lipid profile, antihypertensives, and medications to reduce cardiac workload. For example, the perioperative use of β blockers and statins has been shown to result in fewer adverse cardiac events in the postsurgical period. The use of β blockers can theoretically reduce the wall tension in an aneurysm and thus the risk of rupture.

Medical therapy is not sufficient for the treatment of most causes of thoracic aortic aneurysm, and surgery is the only definitive treatment. Nonetheless, patients with aneurysms due to connective tissue disease are advised to avoid strenuous exercise such as weightlifting. This group of patients requires greater vigilance during pregnancy, including elective cesarean section and peripartum β blockade.

Surgical/Interventional

Open surgery or endovascular stent grafting may be used, depending on aneurysm location, extent, etiology, and characteristics of the patient.

Stent Graft

Stent grafts can be used for aneurysms in the descending thoracic aorta in both the emergent and elective scenario.[31] Not all aneurysms are suitable for treatment by stents. The proximal and distal neck of the aneurysm must be long enough to provide a suitable cuff for proper deployment of a stent. The neck should not exceed 36 mm in diameter, be relatively free of plaque or thrombus, and not be excessively angulated or calcified. The proximal landing zone should be at least 15 mm and may be defined from the origin of either the left subclavian artery or left common carotid artery; if the latter is chosen, the left subclavian artery is necessarily occluded. In that situation, an ipsilateral carotid-subclavian bypass graft is performed to avoid the steal phenomenon and vertebrobasilar insufficiency. Saccular aneurysms due to trauma (including iatrogenic trauma) or penetrating ulcer, because of their focality and relative absence of disease in the proximal and distal landing zones, have the best response rate to stent graft treatment.

The stent is composed of a metallic framework and fabric and is usually self-expanding. The proximal and distal parts of the stent are composed of the metal strut only and not the fabric. The uncovered part of the stent results in better fixation with the arterial wall and allows one to cross an arterial origin without occlusion of flow.

Cross-sectional imaging plays an important role in the pre–stent graft evaluation for accurate sizing of the stent graft. If desired, CTA can also provide comprehensive angiographic information to include the iliac arteries if the surgeon or interventionalist desires evaluation for suitability of the iliac arteries for access. The least tortuous and widest iliac artery is used for access by a femoral arterial surgical cutdown. Alternatively, the iliac arteries can be reached through an extraperitoneal approach, or the stent graft apparatus can be manipulated through a combination of upper extremity and lower extremity vascular access.

Complications of stent grafts include endoleak, stent kinking, migration and fracture, and graft thrombosis and occlusion. Detection of complications warrants surveillance with CTA and MRA.

The stent material determines MR compatibility. Ferromagnetic stents distort the local magnetic field, causing $T2^*$ susceptibility artifacts that may render images nondiagnostic, and safety issues have been raised with one stainless steel stent used for abdominal aortic aneurysms. Nitinol and Elgiloy stents cause relatively little artifact at MRA, with good visualization of the lumen and aneurysm sac. The likely stent choice may be operator specific and, if known prospectively, should influence the baseline imaging test.

Stent migration is more likely to occur in those with atherosclerotic aneurysms whose aorta is more tortuous. Strategies to reduce the chances for or complications of stent migration include a longer proximal landing zone (20 mm) and the use of overlapping stents.[31]

An endoleak is diagnosed by the identification of contrast agent opacification of the excluded aneurysms (Fig. 92-18). Endoleaks due to failure of proximal and distal attachment (type 1) may occur immediately in the period after intervention or after a delay. Delayed type 1 endoleaks suggest graft migration. A proximal landing zone that is short, wide, angulated, ulcerated, or of reverse tapering or trapezoidal morphology predisposes to type 1 endoleak. Retrograde flow through a collateral artery such as the intercostal artery is a type 2 endoleak, which is less common after stent placement in the thoracic aorta than in the abdominal aorta. Type 3 and type 4 endoleaks (due to graft disruption or separation of components in a modular stent graft or porosity, respectively) are less common than type 1 and type 2. In the absence of a visualized endoleak, the continued expansion of the sac is classified as a type 5 endoleak or endotension.

Visualization of the direction of flow characterizes the type of endoleak definitively. This may be possible in high temporal resolution MRA (time-resolved MRA) but usually requires catheter angiography. In the absence of information of the directionality of flow, the type of endoleak can be inferred by the location, configuration, and timing of the appearance of the endoleak. For example, type 1 endoleaks are closer to the stent than the periphery of the sac and tend to be visible in the arterial phase of imaging. Type 2 endoleaks have a peripheral location closest to the feeding artery, have a tubular configuration, and may be visible only in the venous phase.

The CTA protocol for surveillance includes images obtained before the administration of contrast medium and acquisition in both the arterial and venous phases of the examination. The MRA protocol involves the T1-weighted spin-echo sequence to look for subacute blood products and a three-dimensional dynamic arterial phase acquisition, usually with two phases. Delayed two-dimensional gradient-echo acquisitions complete the assessment.

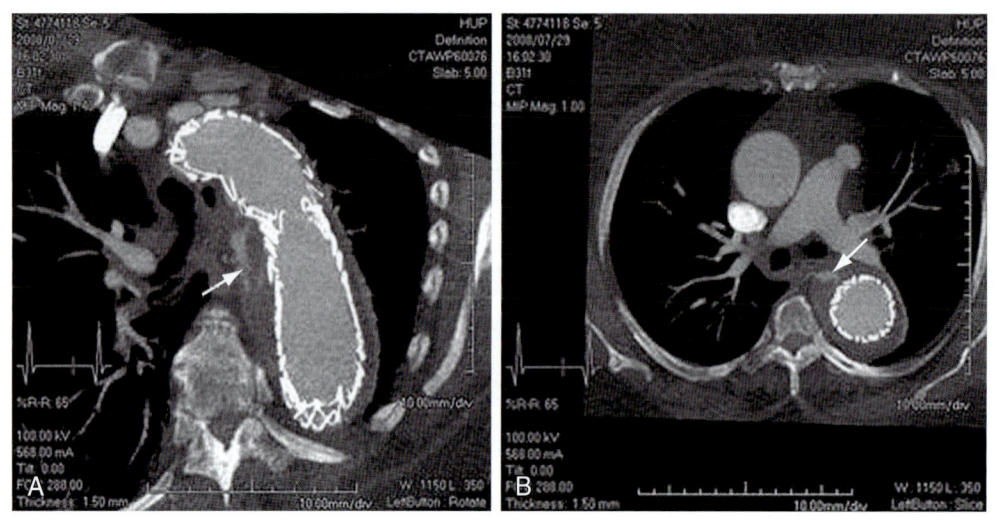

FIGURE 92-18 Oblique maximum intensity projection (**A**) and axial (**B**) contrast-enhanced CT images show a stent in the descending thoracic aorta and an endoleak (*arrow*). The endoleak, located peripherally, appears to connect to an intercostal artery and was presumed to be type 2.

Prosthetic Graft

A description of open surgery for thoracic aortic aneurysms is beyond the scope of this chapter. A brief description is made of the surgical principles. Imagers must be familiar with the surgery to detect complications and to avoid the misinterpretation of expected surgical findings for pathologic changes (Fig. 92-19).

The placement of a prosthetic graft may be without disruption of vascular continuity (interposition graft) or with disruption of vascular continuity (extra-anatomic bypass graft). Interposition grafts may be placed within the native artery (inclusion repair), that is, the aneurysm sac is not repaired and is peripheral to the graft. Alternatively, the aneurysm sac is resected (total repair). Repair of the ascending aorta is accompanied by root repair if the root exceeds 4.5 cm. Surgery of the aortic root may be accompanied by valve repair or coronary artery reimplantation. Surgery may involve the arch in a partial or complete manner, with or without reimplantation of the great arteries. In those with aneurysms of both the ascending and descending aorta, one strategy is a prosthetic graft repair of the ascending aorta and a stent graft repair of the descending aorta.[32]

Complications of Prosthetic Grafts

Imaging has a role to play in the diagnosis or prediction and prevention of complications. These include infection, anastomotic aneurysms and dehiscence, rupture, and paraplegia.

Infection of the graft can have serious consequences locally and systemically, with a high mortality. Local complications can involve the repaired aorta (anastomotic dehiscence, pseudoaneurysm, and rupture) and neighboring nonvascular structures (osteomyelitis). The clinical presentation can be remarkably nonspecific, requiring a high index of suspicion.

CTA and MRA offer effective assessment for graft infection; CTA is more often used. The key to suspicion of infection is the timing of surgery as many of the signs of infection are also expected findings in the early postsurgical period.

CTA signs of infection of prosthetic grafts in the thoracic aorta are perigraft soft tissue rind; fluid in the operative bed (persistence of fluid beyond 3 months of surgery should not be considered normal); air in the vicinity of the graft (this may be normal in the first 10 postoperative days); anastomotic dehiscence and rupture; pseudoaneurysm—2% of patients with graft infection develop pseudoaneurysm, whereas the majority of those with a

FIGURE 92-19 Sagittal oblique reformatted image from contrast-enhanced CT shows the appearance of an ascending aortic prosthetic graft.

CHAPTER 92 • Thoracic Aortic Aneurysms 1285

The most devastating postoperative complication is paraplegia. Despite progress in perioperative care, the incidence of paraplegia has not been reduced to acceptable levels. Risk factors include cross-clamp time of more than 30 minutes, hypotension, and mesenteric ischemia. Operative maneuvers such as sequential reperfusion of the intercostal arteries could be of benefit (Fig. 92-20). Preoperative localization of the artery of Adamkiewicz may be of value, and both CTA and MRA have been used for this purpose (Fig. 92-21). This artery arises from the anterior branch of the radiculomedullary artery, which is a branch of the left posterior intercostal artery (usually 9th to 12th). The diameter of the artery is 0.8 to 1.3 mm, and it has a characteristic hairpin course. Owing to its small diameter and tortuous course, high spatial resolution acquisition with the ability to render three-dimensional reformations is critical.[33]

Reporting: Information for the Referring Physician

A standard report of CTA or MRA should contain a comprehensive report of the aneurysm and the rest of the vascular tree. The report should provide a proper sense of the need for and type of surgery and vascular access as well as insights as to potential procedural complications.

The report can be thought of as having the following components: aneurysm, vascular access, remainder of the arterial tree, and nonvascular findings.

Aneurysm

Are there any signs of rupture? The presence or absence of intramural hematoma or dissection should be commented on. Aneurysm size, shape, extent, proximal neck diameter, distal neck diameter, distance from the left subclavian artery, distance from the celiac artery, and presence and extent of mural thrombus and atherosclerotic plaque are documented.

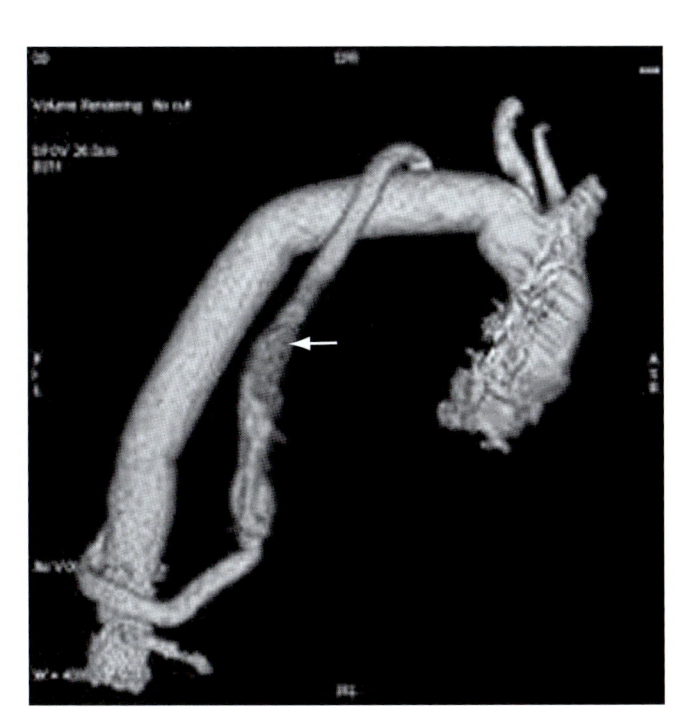

■ **FIGURE 92-20** Volume rendered sagittal oblique image from contrast-enhanced CT shows prosthetic repair of a descending thoracic aortic aneurysm. There is an aorto-aortic extra-anatomic bypass graft (*arrow*) created intraoperatively to ensure perfusion of the intercostal arteries, a mechanism to reduce the risk of paraplegia.

pseudoaneurysm do not have graft infection; fistula; unexplained sternal wound infection or mediastinitis; and tethering of the esophagus.

On MRI, the low signal of air can be difficult to distinguish from calcium, which may also have low signal on all pulse sequences. Nuclear medicine studies help in equivocal cases.

Aneurysms in the repaired aorta may be due to infection or occur at the surgical anastomosis or sites of cannulation for bypass.

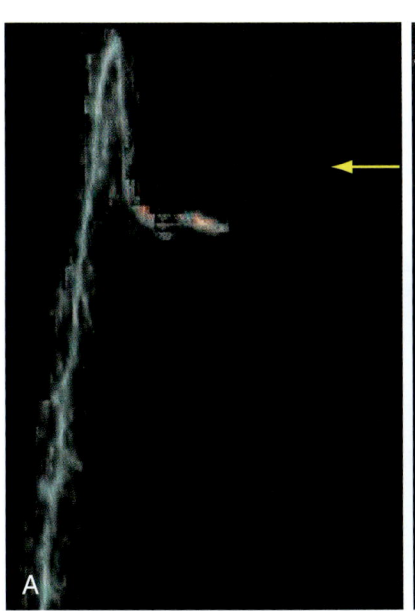

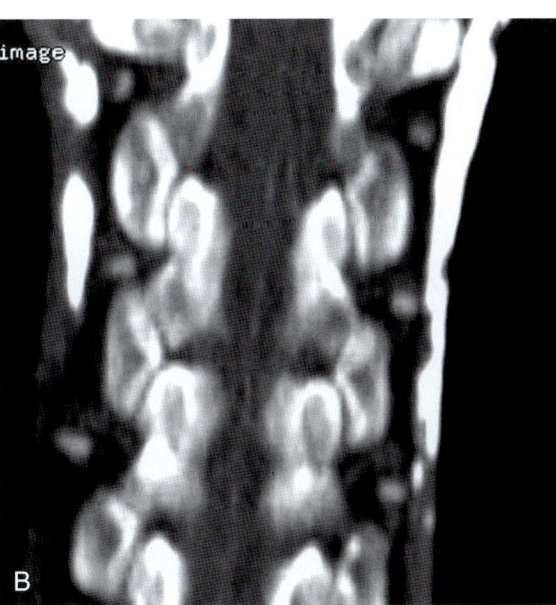

■ **FIGURE 92-21** Volume rendered (**A**) and maximum intensity projection (**B**) images from CE CT show the artery of Adamkiewicz with its characteristic hairpin turn as it enters the spinal cord. (*Images courtesy of Scott Steingall, Chief Technologist, 3 D Lab, University of Pennsylvania.*)

Vascular Access

The state of the iliac arteries and axillary arteries is described. If stent graft placement is planned, the degree of calcification in the iliac and femoral arteries, the tortuosity of the iliac arteries, and their minimal diameters are reported.

Remainder of the Arterial Tree

The patency of branch vessels is reported, particularly of the renal, carotid, subclavian, and vertebral arteries. It is important to describe the origin and path of the artery of Adamkiewicz if surgery on the descending aorta is planned.

Nonvascular Findings

Nonvascular findings are described, such as the lungs and solid abdominal viscera. For lung nodule follow-up, the guidelines of the Fleischner Society are used.[34]

After endovascular stent graft or prosthetic graft placement, surveillance imaging must comment on the presence of complications such as endoleaks and prosthetic graft infection. The size of the aneurysm is measured and compared with the baseline examination finding, which is measured again in the same manner. The vascular access is assessed for complications of access, such as dissection or pseudoaneurysm. The remainder of the arterial tree is assessed for complications of the arteriopathy.

KEY POINTS

- The etiology of thoracic aortic aneurysms can be predicted by the location of the aneurysm.
- Aneurysms of the ascending aorta are usually caused by connective tissue disease such as Marfan syndrome and involve the aortic root.
- Aortic root dilation is accompanied by aortic regurgitation, which may require concomitant valve repair.
- Atherosclerotic aneurysms most often involve the descending aorta.
- Aneurysms of the descending thoracic aorta are amenable to endovascular stent graft placement, particularly those caused by penetrating atherosclerotic ulcer or trauma.
- The baseline imaging modality (CTA or MRA) should be similar to the modality used for postoperative surveillance.
- Description of the artery of Adamkiewicz is of value in patients undergoing open repair of a descending thoracic aortic aneurysm.
- Familiarity with surgical technique is critical for those interpreting postoperative surveillance examinations.
- An index of suspicion is required for prosthetic graft infection.
- The most crucial information in diagnosis of graft infection is the timing of surgery.

SUGGESTED READINGS

Isselbacher EM. Thoracic and abdominal aortic aneurysms. Circulation 2005; 111:816-828.

Johnson PT, Chen J, Loeys B, et al. Loeys-Dietz syndrome: MDCT angiography findings. Am J Radiol 2007; 189:W29-W35.

Macedo TA, Stanson AW, Oderich GS, et al. Infected aortic aneurysms: imaging findings. Radiology 2004; 231:250-257.

Patel HJ, Deeb GM. Ascending and arch aorta: pathology, natural history, and treatment. Circulation 2008; 118:188-195.

Pyeritz RE. The Marfan syndrome. Annu Rev Med 2000; 51:481-510.

Zilocchi M, Macedo TA, Oderich GS, et al. Vascular Ehlers-Danlos syndrome: imaging findings. AJR Am J Roentgenol 2007; 189:712-719.

REFERENCES

1. Curci, JA. Arterial aneurysms—etiologic considerations. In Rutherford RB (ed). Vascular Surgery, 6th ed. Philadelphia, WB Saunders, 2005, pp 475-492.
2. Bickerstaff LK, Pairolero PC, Hollier LH, et al. Thoracic aortic aneurysms: a population-based study. Surgery 1982; 92:1103-1108.
3. Aronberg DJ, Glazer HS, Madsen K, Sagel SS. Normal thoracic aortic diameters by computed tomography. J Comput Assist Tomogr 1984; 8:247-250.
4. Schoen FJ. Blood vessels. In Robbins SL, Cotran RS (eds). Pathologic Basis of Disease, 7th ed. Philadelphia, WB Saunders, 2004, pp 511-555.
5. Davies RR, Goldstein LJ, Coady MA, et al. Yearly rupture or dissection rates for thoracic aortic aneurysms: simple prediction based on size. Ann Thorac Surg 2002; 73:17-27.
6. Brinster DR, Rizzo RJ, Bolman RM III. Ascending aortic aneurysms. In Kohn LH. Cardiac Surgery in the Adult, 3rd ed. New York, McGraw-Hill, 2007, pp 1223-1250.
7. Pyeritz RE, Dietz HC. The Marfan syndrome and other microfibrillar disorders. In Royce PM, Steinman B (eds). Connective Tissue and Its Heritable Disorders, 2nd ed. New York, Wiley-Liss, 2002, pp 585-626.
8. Dietz HC, Pyeritz RE, Hall BD, et al. The Marfan syndrome locus: confirmation of assignment to chromosome 15 and identification of tightly linked markers at 15q15-q21.3. Genomics 1991; 9:355.
9. Marsalese DL, Moodie DS, Vacante M, et al. Marfan's syndrome: natural history and long-term follow-up of cardiovascular involvement. J Am Coll Cardiol 1989; 14:422.
10. Elefteriades JA. Natural history of thoracic aortic aneurysms: indications for surgery, and surgical versus nonsurgical risks. Ann Thorac Surg 2002; 74:S1877-S1880; discussion S1892-S1898.
11. Loeys BL, Schwarze U, Holm T, et al. Aneurysm syndromes caused by mutations in the TGF-ß receptor. N Engl J Med 2006; 355:788-798.
12. Germain DP. Clinical and genetic features of vascular Ehlers-Danlos syndrome. Ann Vasc Surg 2002; 16:391-397.
13. Mirvis SE, Shanmuganathan K, Miller BH, et al. Traumatic aortic injury: diagnosis with contrast-enhanced thoracic CT—five-year experience at a major trauma center. Radiology 1996; 200:413-422.

14. Feigl D, Feigl A, Edwards JE. Mycotic aneurysms of the aortic root: a pathologic study of 20 cases. Chest 1986; 90:553.
15. Hsu RB, Lin FY. Infected aneurysm of the thoracic aorta. J Vasc Surg 2008; 47:270-276.
16. Procter CD, Hollier LH. Takayasu's arteritis and temporal arteritis. Ann Vasc Surg 1992; 6:195-198.
17. Bonderman D, Gharehbaghi-Schnell E, Wollenek G, et al. Mechanisms underlying aortic dilatation in congenital aortic valve malformation. Circulation 1999; 99:2138.
18. Crawford ES, Crawford JL, Safi HJ, et al. Thoracoabdominal aortic aneurysms: preoperative and intraoperative factors determining immediate and long-term results of operations in 605 patients. J Vasc Surg 1986; 3:389-404.
19. Isselbacher EM. Thoracic and abdominal aortic aneurysms. Circulation 2005; 111:816-828.
20. Cambria RA, Gloviczki P, Stanson AW, Cherry KJ Jr. Outcome and expansion rate of 57 thoracoabdominal aortic aneurysms managed nonoperatively. Am J Surg 1995; 170:213-217.
21. Davies RR, Kaple RK, Mandapati D, et al. Natural history of ascending aortic aneurysms in the setting of an unreplaced bicuspid aortic valve. Ann Thorac Surg 2007; 83:1338-1344.
22. Hertzer NR, Beven EG, Young JR, et al. Coronary artery disease in peripheral vascular patients: a classification of 1000 coronary angiograms and results of surgical management. Ann Surg 1984; 199:223-233.
23. Miller WT. Thoracic aortic aneurysms: plain film findings. Semin Roentgenol 2001; 36:288-294.
24. Ominsky SH, Kricun ME. Roentgenology of sinus of Valsalva aneurysms. AJR Am J Roentgenol 1975; 125:571-581.
25. Scott CH, Keane MG, Ferrari VA. Echocardiographic evaluation of the thoracic aorta. Semin Roentgenol 2001; 36:325-333.
26. Nguyen BT. Computed tomography diagnosis of thoracic aortic aneurysms. Semin Roentgenol 2001; 36:309-324.
27. Macura KJ, Corl FM, Fishman EK, Bluemke DA. Pathogenesis in acute aortic syndromes: aortic dissection, intramural hematoma, and penetrating atherosclerotic aortic ulcer. AJR Am J Roentgenol 2003; 181:309-316.
28. Roberts DA. Magnetic resonance imaging of thoracic aortic aneurysm and dissection. Semin Roentgenol 2001; 36:295-308.
29. http://www.fda.gov/cder/drug/infopage/gcca/default.htm.
30. Angiography of the aorta and peripheral arteries. In Baim DS. Grossman's Cardiac Catheterization, Angiography, and Intervention. Philadelphia, Lippincott Williams & Wilkins, 2005, pp 254-281.
31. Garzón G, Fernández-Velilla M, Martí M, et al. Endovascular stent-graft treatment of thoracic aortic disease. Radiographics 2005; 25:S229-S244.
32. Sundaram B, Quint LE, Patel HJ, Deeb GM. CT findings following thoracic aortic surgery. Radiographics 2007; 27:1583-1594.
33. Yoshioka K, Niinuma H, Ohira A, et al. MR angiography and CT angiography of the artery of Adamkiewicz: noninvasive preoperative assessment of thoracoabdominal aortic aneurysm. Radiographics 2003; 23:1215-1225.
34. MacMahon H, Austin JH, Gamsu G, et al; Fleischner Society. Guidelines for management of small pulmonary nodules detected on CT scans: a statement from the Fleischner Society. Radiology 2005; 237:395-400.

CHAPTER 93

Acute Aortic Syndrome

TaeHoon Kim and Harold Litt

Acute aortic syndrome describes a variety of potentially life-threatening aortic pathologic processes. These lesions include aortic dissection, intramural hematoma, penetrating atherosclerotic ulcer, aortic aneurysm leak and rupture, and traumatic aortic transection.[1,2] The clinical presentation is often characterized by acute chest pain in patients with a history of hypertension. Chest pain is variously described as severe, tearing, or migratory. Symptoms can sometimes be confused with acute myocardial infarction or pulmonary embolism. Furthermore, the various types of acute aortic syndromes cannot be reliably differentiated by their clinical presentations.

Acute aortic syndrome is a clinical emergency. Accurate diagnosis and rapid treatment are essential to improve prognosis. Therefore, the aorta must be fully assessed by imaging when the syndrome is suspected. During the last 20 years, new imaging modalities have been developed that dramatically improve assessment of aortic disease. Computed tomography (CT), magnetic resonance imaging (MRI), and ultrasonography allow examination of aortic disease, providing more detail than that of chest radiography or catheter angiography.[3]

The management of acute aortic syndrome remains a therapeutic challenge, and diverse medical, surgical, and percutaneous strategies are continually evolving. As a result of increasing knowledge and better management strategies in this area, the outcomes of patients treated for acute aortic syndromes have improved considerably.

AORTIC DISSECTION

Prevalence and Epidemiology

Aortic dissection is the most common form of acute aortic syndrome. Incidence in the general population is reported from 2.9 to 3.5 cases per 100,000 person-years.[4,5] Two thirds of patients are male. In women, aortic dissection typically presents at an older age (67 years versus 63 years in men).[6]

Etiology and Pathophysiology

The pathology of aortic dissection is a primary intimal tear that allows blood to enter the aortic media, extending proximally and distally into the aortic wall and displacing the intima inward. This entry tear typically occurs at sites of greatest wall tension, notably within a few centimeters of the aortic valve or close to the attachment site of the ligamentum arteriosum.[2,7] The intima and inner part of the aortic media form the intimomedial flap, and the outer part of the aortic media and adventitia form the outer boundary of the false lumen (also known as a false channel; Fig. 93-1). The true lumen is directly connected to the lumen of the unaffected aorta and usually experiences high-velocity flow. The false lumen communicates with the true lumen through the intimal tear and experiences slower, turbulent blood flow. Re-entry tears are usually present in the intima, creating additional communication between the true and false lumens in the distal aorta.[2]

Most patients with aortic dissection have a history of systemic hypertension, which adds to the mechanical strains and shearing forces along the aortic wall. Long-standing hypertension is also associated with increased stiffness of the aortic media, which may introduce additional interlaminar shearing stresses and further contribute to the development of aortic dissection.[2]

Atherosclerotic disease may also be associated with aortic dissection, namely, through the development of a penetrating atherosclerotic ulcer. However, atherosclerosis is not a typical cause of aortic dissection. Dissection in patients with severe atherosclerosis tends to be limited by fibrosis and calcification, but the relationship between an atheroma and the location of aortic dissection is not clear in most patients.[8] Other predisposing factors for aortic

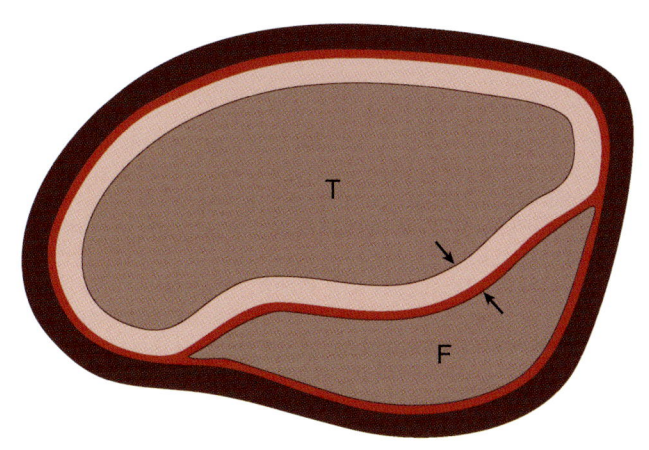

FIGURE 93-1 Schematic diagram of aortic dissection pathology. The aortic media (in red) is partitioned in two parts: one forms part of the dissection flap (*arrows*), the other forms the outer wall of the false lumen. T, true lumen; F, false lumen.

dissection include connective tissue disorders such as Marfan syndrome, Ehlers-Danlos syndrome, bicuspid aortic valve, aortitis, and aortic coarctation. Aortic dissection can also be caused iatrogenically by aortic surgery or percutaneous procedures such as catheterization and placement of intra-aortic balloon pumps.[9,10]

Manifestations of Disease

Clinical Presentation

Aortic dissection often presents as excruciating chest pain in a patient with a history of hypertension. The pain is usually described as severely intense, acute, searing or tearing, throbbing, and occasionally migratory. Involvement of the ascending aorta can cause anterior chest, neck, throat, and even jaw pain, whereas involvement of the descending aorta may cause back and abdominal pain.[11] Ischemic symptoms usually are due to obstruction of the aortic branches by the dissection flap.

Aortic dissection is divided into acute and chronic forms according to the duration of symptoms. An acute form refers to dissection when the diagnosis is made within 2 weeks of symptom onset; in a chronic form, symptoms persist for more than 2 weeks. More than 60% of dissection-related mortality occurs in the first week of disease evolution and 74% within 2 weeks.[12]

Two classifications of aortic dissection are widely used according to the location and extent of involvement of the thoracic aorta. The DeBakey classification system uses three types (Fig. 93-2).[13] Type I dissection involves the ascending aorta, the arch, and a variable length of the descending thoracic and abdominal aorta. Type II dissection is confined to the ascending aorta, and type III dissection may be confined to the descending thoracic aorta (type IIIa) or extend into the abdominal aorta and iliac arteries (type IIIb). The Stanford classification system divides aortic dissection into two types (see Fig. 93-2).[14] Type A involves the ascending aorta, with or without involvement of the arch or the descending thoracic aorta. Type B dissection involves the descending thoracic aorta distal to the origin of the left subclavian artery.

Imaging Indications and Algorithm

Diagnostic imaging is essential for proper evaluation of patients with suspected aortic dissection. The primary goals of imaging are to depict the intimal flap and to

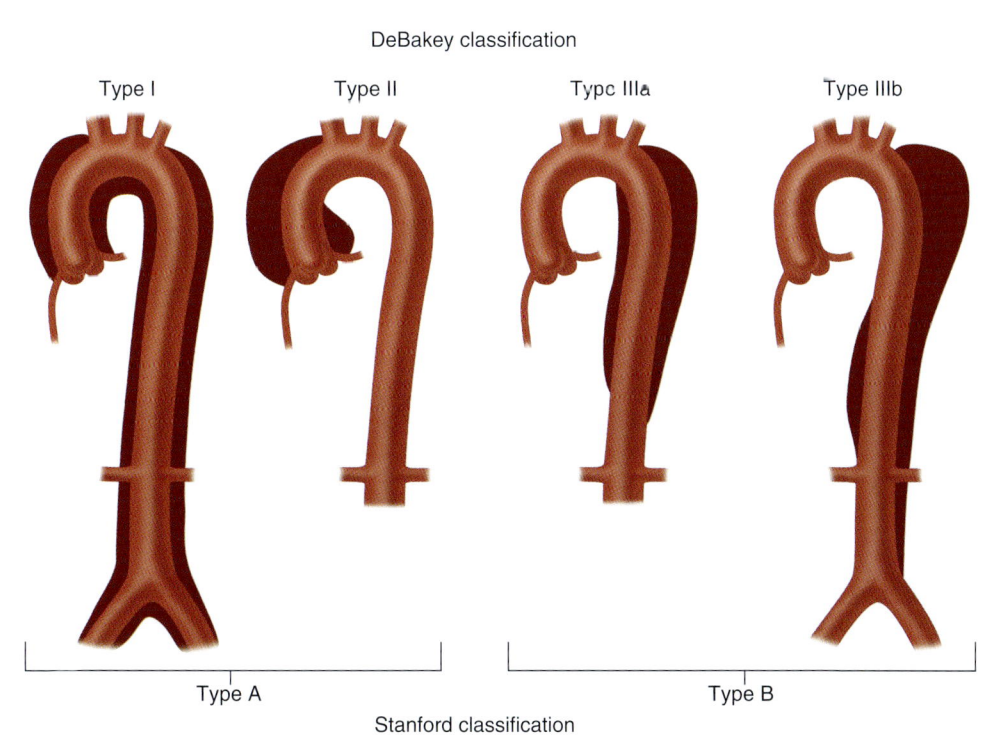

FIGURE 93-2 The two most widely used classifications of aortic dissection. The DeBakey classification includes three types.[14] Type I: the intimal tear usually originates in the proximal ascending aorta; the dissection propagates to the aortic arch and often beyond it distally. Type II: the dissection originates in and is confined to the ascending aorta. Type III: the dissection originates in the descending thoracic aorta (type IIIa) or extends distally down the aorta and iliac arteries (type IIIb); the dissection rarely extends proximally into the aortic arch and ascending aorta. The Stanford classification has two types.[15] Type A: dissection involves the ascending aorta, with or without involvement of the aortic arch or the descending aorta. Type B: dissection does not involve the ascending aorta.

Imaging Techniques and Findings

Radiography

Chest radiography is commonly performed as an initial study in patients with chest pain but is less sensitive for the diagnosis of aortic dissection. Chest radiography, however, does remain important because it may suggest an underlying aortic pathologic process, and it is performed routinely in patients with suspected aortic disease.[15] The most common chest radiographic findings in patients with aortic dissection are widening of the mediastinum and aortic contour, disparity in the size of the ascending and descending aorta, changes in aortic configuration on serial studies, and displacement of a calcified plaque by more than 10 mm (Fig. 93-3).[17] Other findings may include tracheal deviation, inferior displacement of the left main bronchus and opacification of the aorta-pulmonary window, and widening of the left paraspinal line.

In practice, mediastinal widening is often difficult to evaluate on initial chest radiographs because patients are often examined in the supine position with portable radiography and are unable to hold the breath in full inspiration. Individual features suggestive of aortic dissection, such as displacement of aortic calcification, may be misdiagnosed because of the variable positions of the calcified plaque and the lateral aortic border.[17] Proximal dissection is especially difficult to diagnose on chest radiographs. Serial studies can be helpful in identifying the changes between the prior and current studies.

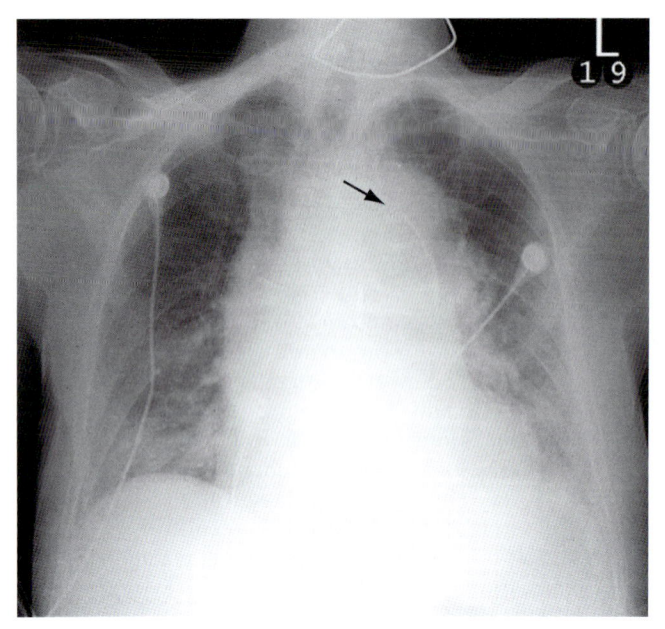

■ **FIGURE 93-3** Anteroposterior chest radiograph shows mediastinal widening and irregular aortic contour. Intimal calcification is displaced near the aortic knob (*arrow*). *(From Kapustin AJ, Litt HI. Diagnostic imaging for aortic dissection. Semin Thorac Cardiovasc Surg 2005; 17:214-223.)*

delineate the extent of aortic involvement and extension into the arch vessels and coronary arteries. It is also important to recognize associated complications, including pericardial hemorrhage, which can lead to life-threatening cardiac tamponade, periaortic or mediastinal hematoma, and pleural hemorrhage.[15]

Imaging techniques for dissection, consisting primarily of radiography and catheter angiography in the past, have changed rapidly in recent years. Multidetector CT (MDCT) and, to a lesser extent, ultrasonography and MRI have taken precedence and relegated catheter angiography to the occasional instance in which noninvasive imaging is not definitive or therapeutic intervention is desired.[15] A meta-analysis found the diagnostic accuracy of CT, transesophageal echocardiography, and MRI to be virtually the same (95% to 100%) for the diagnosis of thoracic aortic dissection.[16]

Ultrasonography

Ultrasound techniques available for evaluation of aortic dissection include transthoracic echocardiography (TTE), transesophageal echocardiography (TEE), and intravascular ultrasound (IVUS).[15] TTE is readily available, noninvasive, and portable but limited by a narrow acoustic window. It can be useful for evaluation of the aortic root, including aortic valve complications or cardiac and aortic wall motion abnormalities. TEE is a relatively invasive diagnostic procedure, but it can be performed at bedside and demonstrate true and false lumens, direction of blood flow, and complications such as aortic regurgitation on Doppler examination (Fig. 93-4). TEE typically provides

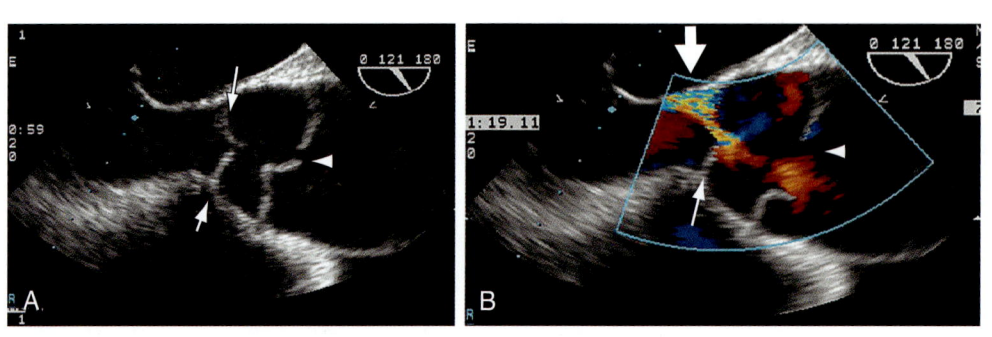

■ **FIGURE 93-4** TEE reveals type A dissection on gray-scale (**A**) and color Doppler (**B**) images. The *arrowheads* indicate a tear in the intimal flap, through which flow can be identified on color Doppler examination. The dissection does not extend to the aortic valve (*small arrows* indicate valve leaflets), but the dissection has caused dilation of the aortic root and therefore acute aortic regurgitation. Color Doppler image also reveals a regurgitant jet extending into the left ventricular outflow tract (*large arrow*). *(From Kapustin AJ, Litt HI. Diagnostic imaging for aortic dissection. Semin Thorac Cardiovasc Surg 2005; 17:214-223.)*

broader and more accurate aortic visualization than does TTE for improved evaluation for aortic dissection; however, TEE cannot image the distal ascending aorta and proximal aortic arch completely as the airway may be positioned between the esophagus and the aorta.[18] Catheter-based IVUS can provide imaging of the entire aorta with high sensitivity and specificity. However, it is limited in detecting the site of intimal tear, particularly in the ascending aorta.[19] IVUS is rarely used in the initial screening or follow-up of patients with aortic dissection.

Diagnosis of aortic dissection by ultrasound examination requires demonstration of the true and false lumens separated by an intimal flap. To determine the therapeutic implications, one must evaluate the involvement of the ascending aorta, the coexistence of aortic insufficiency, the site of the original tear, the characteristics of blood flow and clot formation in the false lumen, the relative position of the coronary arteries, and the involvement of the aortic arch vessels, notably the carotid arteries. Ventricular function and the presence of pericardial effusion are also important for therapeutic strategy.[3]

The advantage of ultrasonography over MRI or CT is its portability, which makes it useful at the bedside or in the operating room. However, objective and reproducible thoracic aortic evaluation with ultrasonography remains problematic given operator dependence and restricted thoracic acoustic windows. Ultrasonography, moreover, is prone to artifacts and the detection of "pseudolesions," such as reverberation artifacts, which can be misdiagnosed as aortic dissection and cause false-positive study results.[15]

Computed Tomography

CT is the most commonly used diagnostic tool in patients with suspected aortic dissection. A study from the International Registry of Acute Aortic Dissection reported that CT was used in 61% of cases as the primary diagnostic procedure for detection of aortic dissection. Ultrasonography was used in 33% of cases, followed by catheter angiography in 4.4% and MRI in 1.8%.[6] The advantages of CT scans are faster scanning, high spatial resolution, and the ability with moving table bolus chase imaging to provide extended anatomic coverage for illustration of the entire thoracoabdominal aorta. The development of multidetector technology has allowed acquisition of submillimeter-thick axial images, which can provide isotropic imaging volumes for improved postprocessed viewing of complex arterial geometries and relationships. Compared with ultrasonography, MDCT benefits from being less operator dependent, having a relative ease of use, and providing a larger field of view for improved detection of both vascular and extravascular findings. The key disadvantages of MDCT include its use of ionizing radiation and iodine-based intravenous contrast agents, which are contraindicated in certain patients.[15]

CT is highly accurate, with a sensitivity and a specificity of more than 95% reported for the diagnosis of aortic dissection.[3] Compared with ultrasonography and MRI, CT also provides an improved ability to evaluate for confounding differential diagnoses in the thorax and abdomen (Fig. 93-5).

Although major diagnostic clues are provided by contrast-enhanced CT scans, the importance of non–contrast-enhanced scans should not be overlooked. Non–contrast-enhanced CT scans can depict intimal calcifications and high-density lesions from leaking or thrombosed blood in the aortic wall, in periaortic regions, or in pleural and pericardial spaces.[20]

The main CT findings in aortic dissection include variable appearances of the true and false lumens, involvement of the ascending aorta, extension into arterial branches, and associated lesions.[15,21,22] The intimal flap divides the aortic lumen into two channels, and the true lumen is typically more opacified than the false lumen because of the higher blood pressure and faster mixing of blood with contrast material in the true lumen on early arterial phase images (Fig. 93-6). True and false lumens can be differentiated on the basis of other characteristics. The true lumen is generally posterior and left posterolateral in the ascending aorta, caudal in the aortic arch, and anterior and right anterolateral in the descending aorta. The true lumen tends to be smaller than the false lumen because of inward displacement of the intimal flap. Thrombus is commonly found in the false lumen because of its slow flow. Multiphase contrast-enhanced CT scans may show that the false lumen enhances later and washes out in a delayed fashion.[21]

Demonstration of the intimal flap on CT images is accurate and precise in the descending aorta. In contrast, the dissecting flap in the ascending aorta can be difficult to properly identify as it may be confused with aortic valve cusps on axial images or mistaken for motion artifacts of the aortic root due to cardiac or respiratory movement (Fig. 93-7). However, these artifacts can be minimized by use of a rapid scan technique and cardiac synchronization (i.e., either prospective ECG triggering or retrospective ECG gating).[23]

Magnetic Resonance

Like CT, MRI has been reported to have a sensitivity and specificity of more than 95%[3]; thus, it is a suitable alternative to catheter angiography for the diagnosis and evaluation of aortic dissection. T1- and T2-weighted black blood spin-echo MR images provide high tissue contrast between the blood pool, the vascular wall, and the adjacent soft tissues. Cine bright blood imaging provides supplemental images for improved detection of the intimal flap and extent of the true and false lumens as well as functional information about blood flow associated with the aortic dissection. Moreover, cine MR enables evaluation of the aortic valve and its function.[16]

On black blood spin-echo images, the true and false lumens are depicted as regions of signal void, and the intimal flap is seen as a linear structure of isointense signal intensity that is outlined by the flow void in the dual lumens (Fig. 93-8). The false lumen can be differentiated from the true because the flow is slower and thrombus is more likely to form. If the false lumen contains thrombus, the intimal flap may not be seen because it is not outlined by moving blood on both sides. Although MRI is superior to CT in depicting the presence of blood flow, non–contrast-enhanced MRI is sometimes unable to differenti-

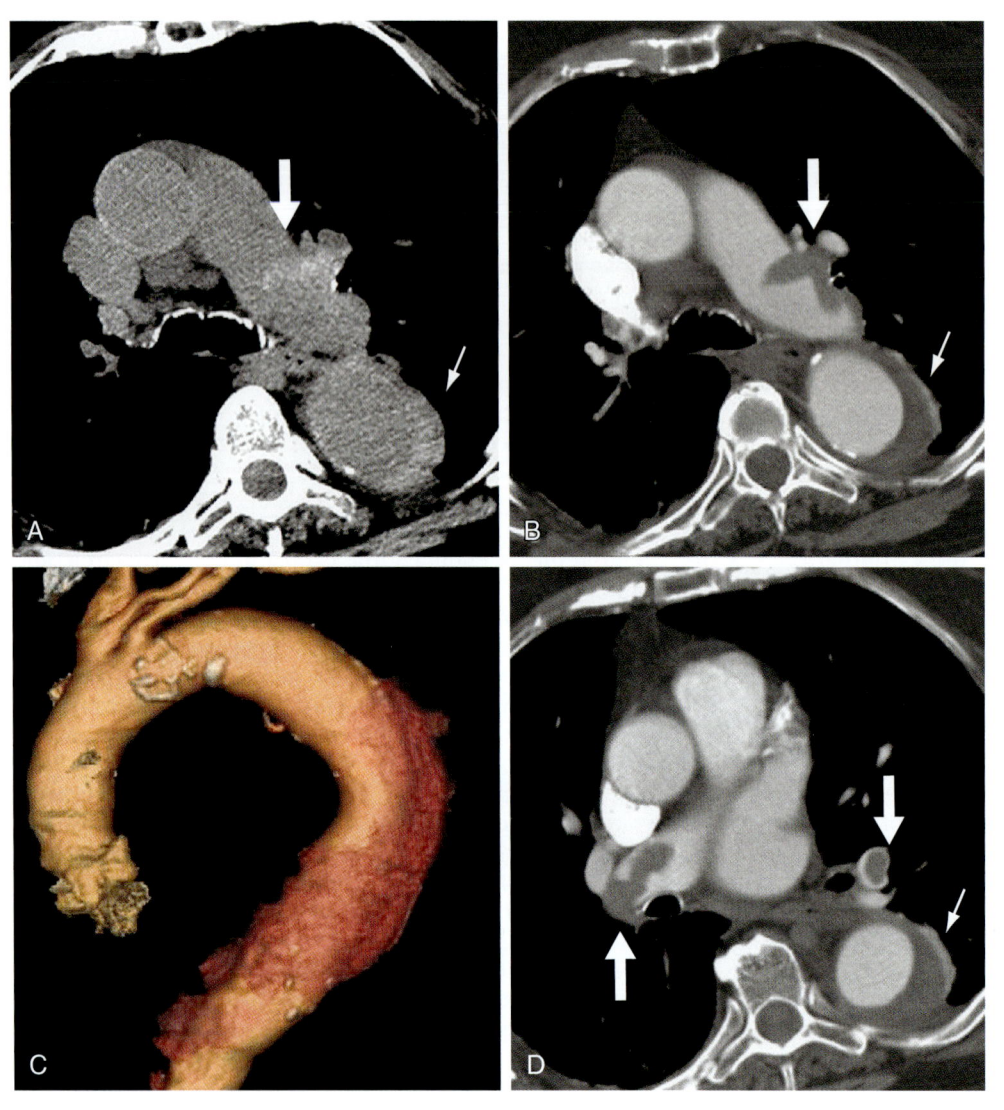

FIGURE 93-5 A patient with two reasons for chest pain. The *small arrows* indicate a crescent-shaped area of abnormal attenuation along the posterolateral wall of the descending aorta on unenhanced (**A**) and enhanced (**B** and **D**) CT, representing intramural hematoma. The hematoma is also shown in red on a volume rendered image of the same study (**C**). Images **A, B,** and **D** also reveal pulmonary emboli (*large arrows*) in both main pulmonary arteries. Rarely (as in this case), emboli can be identified on unenhanced CT (**A**), indicating that the clot was recently formed. *(From Kapustin AJ, Litt HI. Diagnostic imaging for aortic dissection. Semin Thorac Cardiovasc Surg 2005; 17:214-223.)*

ate slowly moving blood from thrombus in the false lumen.[17]

Aortic MR angiography (MRA) can be performed with time-of-flight and phase contrast techniques.[24,25] These flow-based techniques may be helpful in differentiating the signal intensities between slow blood flow and intravascular thrombus. However, the disadvantage of these techniques is relatively long scan time, which restricts their use in hemodynamically unstable patients.

Aortic MRA is more routinely performed with use of gadolinium-enhanced three-dimensional MRA.[26] Gadolinium-enhanced MRA has dramatically shortened total examination time in the diagnosis of aortic dissection and has replaced non–contrast-enhanced MRA techniques. Like contrast-enhanced CT angiography (CTA), gadolinium-enhanced MR provides arterial "luminograms" that can be postprocessed by an array of three-dimensional processing tools on an independent workstation. The advantages of gadolinium-enhanced MRA over contrast-enhanced CTA include its use of generally safer gadolinium-chelate contrast agents, lack of ionizing radiation, and production of high contrast images with fewer image sections. Furthermore, postprocessing is much faster with gadolinium-enhanced MRA than with CTA.[27] Like contrast-enhanced CTA, gadolinium-enhanced MRA can differentiate the true and false lumens according to their signal intensity differences (Fig. 93-9). The intimal flap is visualized as a line of low signal intensity with a linear or curved shape. The true lumen often has higher signal intensity than the false because of a higher concentration of contrast material during the arterial phase. The acquisition of delayed images improves depiction of thrombosis of the false lumen, which can be easily depicted as lower signal intensity.

Despite these advantages of MR techniques, MRI is rarely used as the initial imaging modality for the evaluation of aortic dissection. Data from the International Registry of Acute Aortic Dissection revealed that only 1.8% of patients with aortic dissection underwent MRI as an initial imaging test, which was less often than catheter aortography (4.4%).[6] This may be due to limited emergent availability of MRI, incompatibility with implanted metal

CHAPTER 93 ● Acute Aortic Syndrome 1293

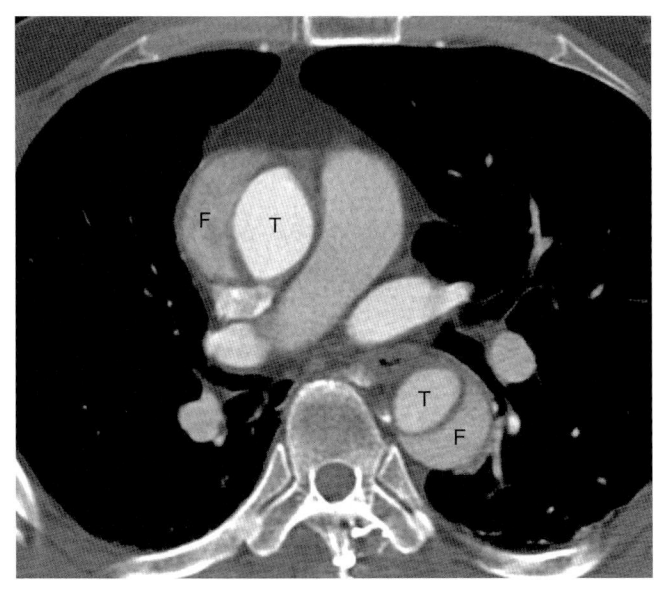

■ **FIGURE 93-6** Type A aortic dissection. The true lumen (T) is more intensely opacified than the false lumen. The false lumen (F) is anterior and right anterolateral in the ascending aorta and posterior and left posterolateral in the descending aorta. The true lumen is smaller than the false lumen, which wraps around the true lumen.

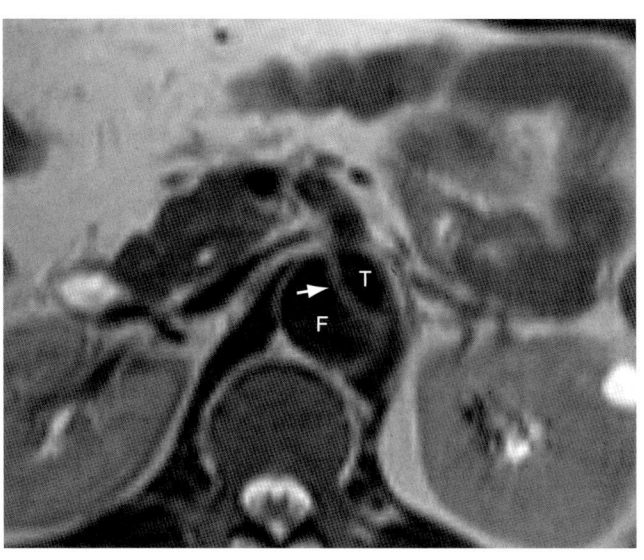

■ **FIGURE 93-8** Axial T2-weighted MR image demonstrating type B aortic dissection at the level of the superior mesenteric artery. The true (T) and false (F) lumens are depicted as the regions of signal void. The intimal flap (arrow) is seen as a linear structure of isointense signal intensity (to aortic wall) that is outlined by the flow void in double lumens.

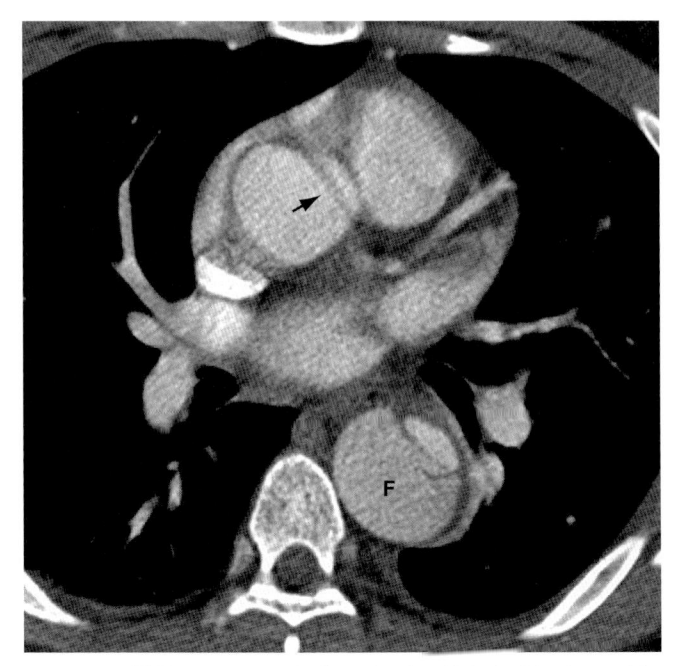

■ **FIGURE 93-7** Type B aortic dissection in which the false lumen (F) is noted on non–ECG gated, contrast-enhanced CT to be larger than the true lumen in the descending thoracic aorta. An artifactual dark linear band (arrow) mimics an intimal tear in the ascending aorta. This artifact is secondary to through-plane motion of the geometrically complex and obliquely positioned aortic root and can be minimized by ECG-gated CT acquisition. Note that genuine intimal tears are more typically oriented in the right anterolateral aspect of the ascending aorta (see Fig. 93-6).

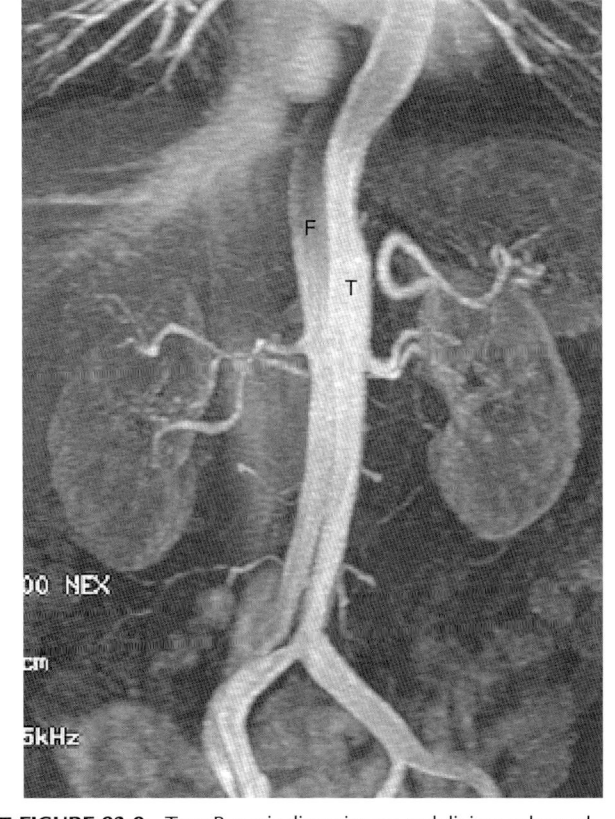

■ **FIGURE 93-9** Type B aortic dissection on gadolinium-enhanced three-dimensional MRA. On a coronal maximum intensity projection from a gadolinium-enhanced three-dimensional MRA, the intimal flap is visualized from the descending thoracic aorta to the abdominal aorta. The true lumen (T) is more intensely opacified than the false lumen (F) because of its brisker blood flow and faster filling with gadolinium-chelate contrast agent. The left renal artery and celiac trunk are supplied by the true lumen, and the right renal artery is supplied by the false lumen.

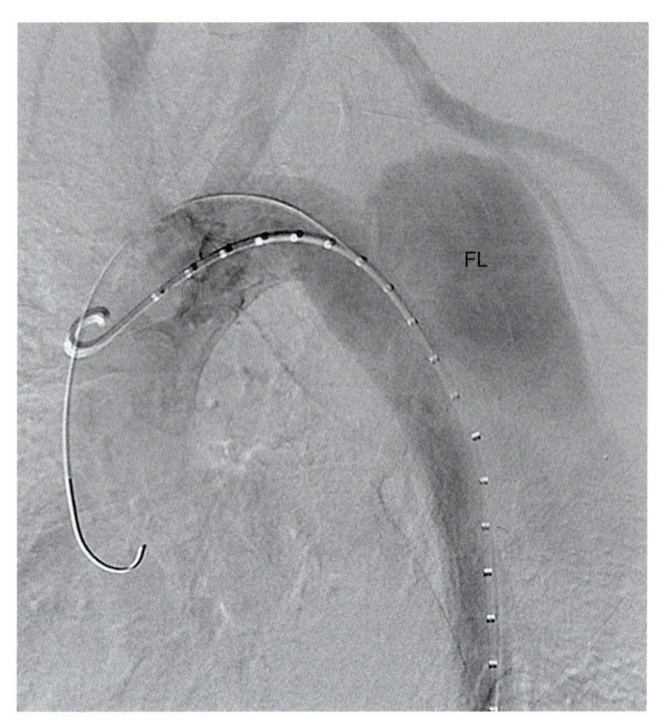

FIGURE 93-10 Catheter x-ray angiography with type B aortic dissection. Contrast enhancement is present in the true lumen. The false lumen (FL) begins at the aortic isthmus and is partially enhanced near the proximal site of the intimal tear.

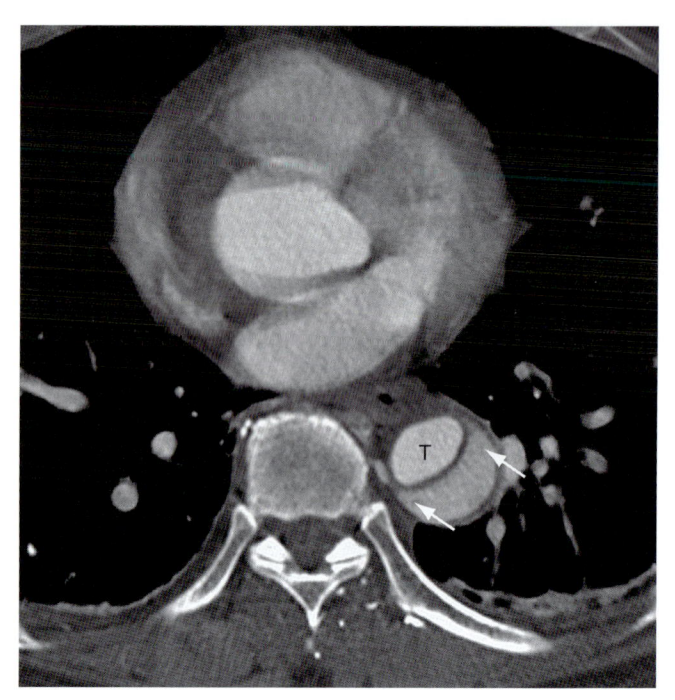

FIGURE 93-11 Type B aortic dissection. On contrast-enhanced CT, the true lumen (T) is more intensely enhanced than the false lumen because of the faster flow and mixing with contrast agent in the true lumen. The beak (*arrows*) represents the corner of the false lumen, and the beak sign is depicted in the false lumen as it wraps around the true lumen.

devices such as pacemakers and aneurysm clips, or monitoring difficulties during examination. Furthermore, MRI is not suitable in patients with hemodynamic instability. The use of MRI may also be restricted in patients with claustrophobia[15] or with renal insufficiency, in whom there is an increased risk for development of nephrogenic systemic fibrosis after the intravenous administration of gadolinium-chelate contrast agents.

Angiography

Angiographic signs of aortic dissection can be categorized as direct or indirect. Direct findings include visualization of the intimal flap or dual lumens (Fig. 93-10). Indirect findings include compression of the true lumen, thickening of the aortic wall, abnormalities of branch vessels, and aortic insufficiency.[17] The major advantage of catheter angiography is its ability to evaluate the aortic valve and extent of involvement of major aortic branches. Sensitivity and specificity of catheter angiography for diagnosis of dissection are 88% and 94%.[28]

Although catheter angiography is sensitive for the diagnosis of aortic dissection, it has recently been replaced by noninvasive modalities such as CT, ultrasonography, and MRI.[29] Proper diagnosis of aortic dissection may be difficult in situations in which the false lumen is not opacified or in which both lumens are equally opacified. The false lumen may not be opacified when it is thrombosed, when there is no intimal tear, or when the catheter tip is distal to the site of the intimal tear.[17] In addition, because catheter angiography cannot directly depict the aortic wall, it cannot accurately evaluate the size of the aorta, intramural features of the aortic wall, or periaortic complications. The higher false-negative rate, therefore, results from its inability to identify extraluminal abnormalities such as an intramural hematoma, thrombosed false lumens, and periaortic fluid collections. Because of its invasiveness and time-consuming nature, the use of catheter angiography in the diagnosis of aortic disease has been dramatically reduced.[15]

Classic Signs

On cross-sectional imaging, the "beak sign" can be seen at the corner of the false lumen, forming an acute angle with the intimomedial flap and the outer wall of the aorta (Fig. 93-11).[30] The "cobweb sign" of the medial layer sometimes persists between the intima and media, forming thin strands of medial tissue that can be seen crossing the false lumen (Fig. 93-12).[31]

Differential Diagnosis

From Clinical Presentation

Differential diagnosis includes myocardial infarction, acute pericarditis, and pulmonary embolism.[20]

From Imaging Findings

On occasion, a thrombosed false lumen can be confused with thrombus within an aneurysm sac. Similarly, slow flow in a false lumen can mimic thrombus within an aneurysm sac during arterial phase imaging.

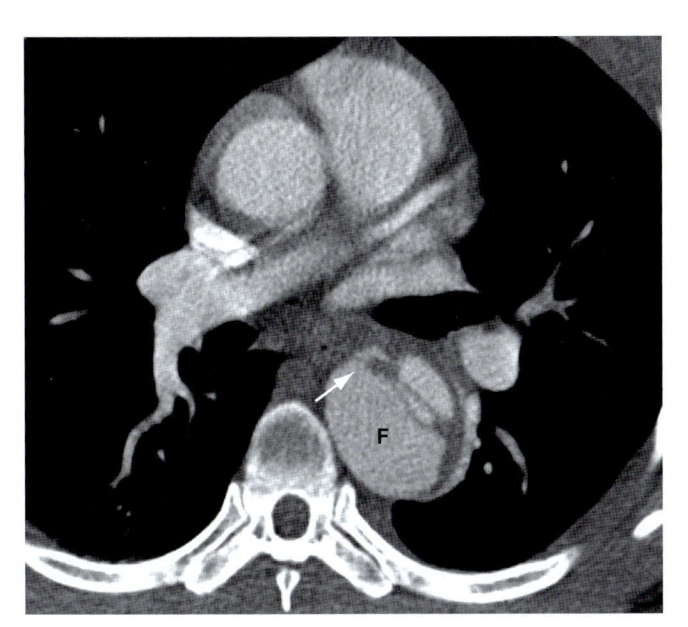

FIGURE 93-12 Type B aortic dissection. On contrast-enhanced CT, the false lumen (F) is larger than the true lumen and slightly darker than the true lumen. The cobweb sign represents thin strands of medial tissue (*arrow*) that persists between the intima and the media and crosses the false lumen.

Synopsis of Treatment Options

Medical

Aortic dissection requires immediate treatment with medical therapy or surgery, depending on the involved sites. The initial therapy is typically targeted at relieving chest pain and normalizing the systolic blood pressure to between 100 and 120 mm Hg, which may prevent further extension of the dissection or rupture of the false lumen.[32] In most patients, these results are usually achieved with morphine sulfate and intravenous β blockers, respectively. Patients who have contraindications to β blockers can receive calcium channel blockers such as verapamil or intravenous diltiazem. Most patients with type B dissections can be treated with medications alone. In patients with type A dissections, these medications may be used to prepare a patient for surgery.

Patients who are hemodynamically unstable often require intubation, mechanical ventilation, and urgent ultrasound or CT scans for confirmative diagnosis of aortic dissection. In addition, hypotensive or normotensive patients with a history of prior hypertension need to be evaluated for blood loss, pericardial effusion, or heart failure. A large pericardial effusion may induce cardiac tamponade, which requires emergent pericardiocentesis. During medical treatment, early restoration of blood flow to vital organs helps stabilize patients and improves prognosis.

Surgical/Interventional

Type A (Ascending) Aortic Dissection

Medical treatment alone is ineffective in patients with acute aortic dissections involving the ascending thoracic aorta (Stanford type A or DeBakey type I or type II). Type A dissections require urgent surgical treatment, particularly when the patient presents within the first 48 hours and if there is cerebral or visceral ischemia.[12] The mortality rate is up to 1% to 2% per hour during the first 24 to 48 hours after presentation. Patients with type A dissections may be at high risk of life-threatening complications, such as rupture of the false lumen, stroke, visceral ischemia, cardiac tamponade, and heart failure. In addition, when the dissection extends to the aortic annulus, obstruction of coronary blood flow and aortic regurgitation can occur abruptly. Therefore, the major surgical objective in type A dissection is to prevent rupture of the false lumen or development of pericardial effusion, which can lead to cardiac tamponade or death.[32]

Surgical technique varies according to involvement of the lesion in the aorta. David's and Yacoub's[33] techniques represent repair of the aortic root and preservation of the aortic valve. However, in conditions with serious anatomic injury in the aortic root, surgeons prefer to carry out complete replacement with a valved conduit and coronary artery reimplantation. This technique may prevent a second intervention or operation, and it is generally applied in cases associated with Marfan syndrome or ectasia of the aortic root.[34] When the dissection extends to the aortic arch or the descending thoracic aorta, the patient may require partial or total arch replacement because the intimal flap cannot be completely resected. A two-stage operation may be a useful technique when there is also aneurysmal dilation of the proximal descending thoracic aorta.[34] A prosthetic tube graft is first placed in the proximal descending thoracic aorta and then connected distally in the second procedure.

Medical treatment after surgery focuses on blood pressure control, with a systolic blood pressure target not to exceed 100 to 110 mm Hg. Imaging follow-up is also important to screen for development of a new dissection or formation of aneurysms at other sites of the aorta. The recurrence rate is approximately 25%, and recurrence is frequently associated with complications such as aortic rupture and death from exsanguination.[12]

Type B (Descending) Aortic Dissection

Medical treatment is acceptable in type B dissection when the lesion is stable. The objective of immediate treatment in type B dissection is control of pain and lowering of systolic blood pressure to 110 to 120 mm Hg. However, some patients with type B aortic dissection may require surgery when the patients have hemodynamic instability, intractable pain, rapid expansion of aortic diameter, and mediastinal or periaortic hematoma as signs of imminent rupture of the aorta.[12]

With the development of percutaneous approaches for the treatment of vascular disease, catheter angiography is again playing an important role in the management of aortic dissection. Endovascular treatment has recently been introduced in the minimally invasive treatment of type B dissection.[35-37] These catheter-based approaches have been used to stent across intimal tears, to treat branch vessel occlusion, and to fenestrate intimal flaps (Fig. 93-13). Exclusion of the false lumen can avoid later

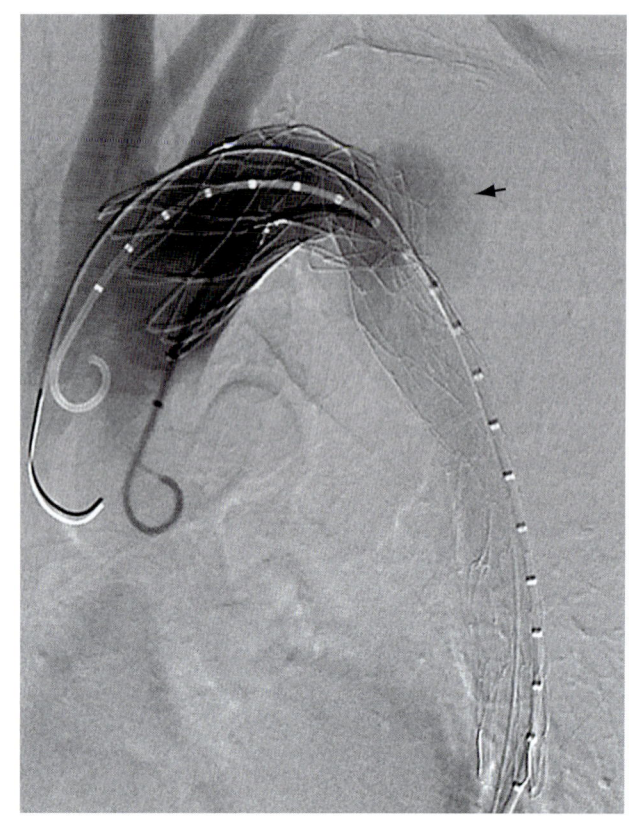

FIGURE 93-13 Stent graft treatment of type B aortic dissection. Catheter angiography shows leak of contrast material into the false lumen (*arrow*) just after deployment of the stent graft from the aortic arch to the descending thoracic aorta.

development of aneurysmal dilation and rupture. Fenestration of the intimal flap is helpful to restore perfusion to ischemic organs. This procedure is relatively safe and can yield better results than surgery in the treatment of dissection of the descending aorta.

Reporting: Information for the Referring Physician

Reporting of imaging studies performed for evaluation of aortic dissection should include the following elements:

- Stanford type A versus type B, with site of origin of intimal flap
- Extension of intimal flap to the aortic valve and into the coronary ostia, if possible on modality used
- Extension of flap into aortic branch vessels, evidence of organ or bowel ischemia
- Any direct or indirect signs of leaking or rupture
- Any regions of aneurysmal dilation of the aorta

INTRAMURAL HEMATOMA

Definition

Intramural hematoma refers to the presence of bleeding in the wall of the aorta, with visualization of acute or subacute blood clot. It is considered a forme fruste and variant form of aortic dissection. Intramural hematoma is frequently diagnosed on cross-sectional imaging during the evaluation of acute aortic syndrome.

Prevalence and Epidemiology

Intramural hematoma is reported to represent 10% to 30% of acute aortic syndromes.[9,38] Intramural hematoma of the aorta generally occurs in older patients with a history of hypertension, and it is located in the descending aorta in about 60% of cases.[39] Intramural hematoma can extend retrograde to involve the ascending aorta or anterograde to involve the descending aorta.

Etiology and Pathophysiology

The pathology of many cases of intramural hematoma is spontaneous rupture of the vasa vasorum, which results in bleeding into the aortic media. In some patients, intramural hematoma can be secondary to a penetrating atherosclerotic ulcer.[1,2] Blunt chest trauma associated with aortic wall injury sometimes causes intramural hematoma, and other causes include connective tissue disorders, Marfan syndrome, Turner syndrome, coarctation of the aorta, aortic aneurysm, pregnancy, and cocaine abuse.[40]

The morphology of the involved aortic wall may change rapidly. Bleeding into the media may be self-limited but may lead to classic aortic dissection. The rate of aortic rupture is much higher (up to 35%) in intramural hematoma than in aortic dissection because intramural hematoma usually occurs closer to the adventitia.[8] Intramural hematoma is frequently associated with mediastinal, pericardial, and pleural hemorrhage, which are related to increased permeability of the aortic wall.

Manifestations of Disease

Clinical Presentation

Symptoms in patients with intramural hematoma are similar to those of aortic dissection.

Imaging Indications and Algorithm

Recent advances in diagnostic modalities have increased recognition of aortic intramural hematoma. Diagnostic sensitivity does not differ much among TEE, CT, and MRI. In general, selection of an imaging modality depends on the physician's preference, institutional situation, and available experts. However, MDCT has been increasingly used for the diagnosis of intramural hematoma because of its benefits of improved spatial resolution and shortened scan time. However, MRI with its ability to characterize hemoglobin products may be superior for differentiation between acute and chronic bleeding.

Imaging Techniques and Findings

Radiography

Chest radiography is routinely performed in patients with intramural hematoma but is often unrevealing. In patients

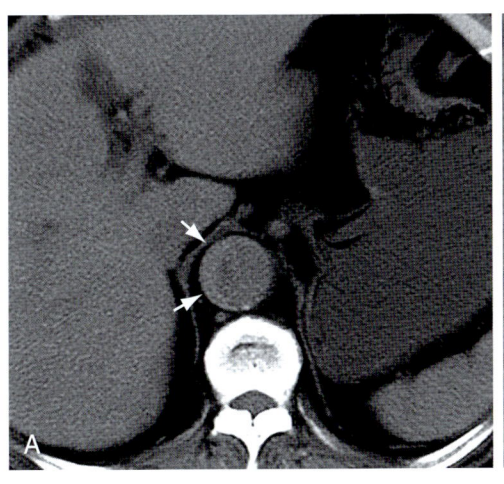

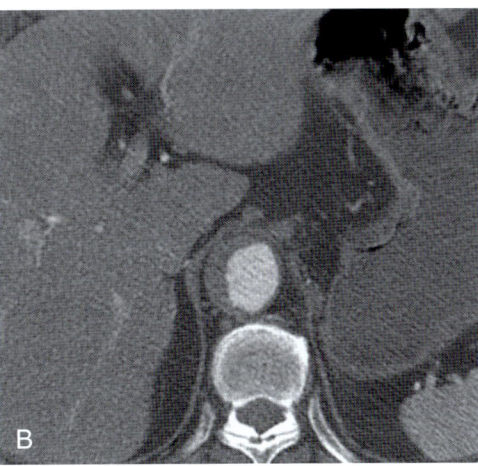

FIGURE 93-14 Intramural hematoma of the aorta. **A,** CT image before the administration of contrast material shows crescentic area of higher attenuation (*arrows*) representing intramural hematoma. **B,** This region does not enhance after injection of contrast material. On contrast-enhanced CT, the hematoma cannot be differentiated from luminal thrombus or atherosclerotic plaque, both of which also have low attenuation.

with complicated intramural hematoma, radiographs can show mediastinal widening or pleural effusion. A comparison to prior chest radiographs may be important in identifying the aortic lesion.

Ultrasonography

TEE allows direct observation of the aortic intima. Diagnostic criteria for intramural hematoma include absence of an intimal flap, no communication between false and true lumens on Doppler examination, and regional crescentic thickening of the aortic wall above 0.7 cm.[41] Recent improvements in diagnostic sensitivity of TEE enable evaluation of aortic wall thicknesses of more than 5 mm, which is sufficient for the diagnosis of intramural hematoma in patients with typical symptoms of acute aortic syndrome.

In intramural hematoma, a hypoechoic zone can sometimes be detected within the thickened aortic wall. This echolucent space represents the accumulation of blood from the vasa vasorum within the media (i.e., the intramural hematoma). However, an echolucent space is not a poor prognostic sign and is not associated with development of aortic dissection.[42]

Serial follow-up studies in patients with intramural hematoma are important for early detection of disease progression to dissection or development of complications such as mediastinal hemorrhage, pericardial effusion, and pleural effusion. Among these complications, cardiac tamponade is a clinical challenge because mortality is relatively high. Progressive accumulation of pleural effusion can occur in intramural hematoma, but this alone is not an indication for surgical intervention.[43]

Computed Tomography

CT is the most commonly used imaging technique for intramural hematoma because of its availability, accuracy, and speed. CT is beneficial for visualization of the entire aorta, diagnosis of periaortic bleeding, and evaluation of arterial branches. Intramural hematoma is visualized as crescentic or circumferential aortic wall thickening, which is manifested as high attenuation on non–contrast-enhanced CT images (Fig. 93-14A). Non–contrast-enhanced CT scans can also depict the critical complication of bleeding into the pericardium, mediastinum, or pleural spaces. Because high-attenuation areas (i.e., the intramural hematoma) are usually masked on the contrast-enhanced CT images (see Fig. 93-14B), the performance of CT before the administration of contrast material is recommended in patients with suspected acute aortic syndrome before contrast-enhanced CT.[44] High-attenuation areas along the aortic wall tend to change over time, and this noncommunicating aortic hematoma can progress to a typical dissection, aortic rupture, or hemorrhage to the mediastinal, pleural, or pericardial spaces.

Magnetic Resonance

Although crescentic wall thickening of the aorta is easily detected by MRI, the use of MRI remains controversial in patients with suspected acute aortic syndrome; the patients are often hemodynamically unstable, and the typically longer examination times of MRI may unnecessarily delay proper diagnosis and impede immediate treatment. However, its use is justified in asymptomatic and stable patients when the diagnosis of intramural hematoma has not been established by other techniques. Bleeding of the vasa vasorum can be progressive in intramural hematoma. The signal intensity of the thickened aortic wall may be variable according to the amount of methemoglobin formation. Intramural hemorrhage in the hyperacute phase can show isointense signal on the T1-weighted images and high signal intensity on T2-weighted images. For the following 1 to 2 days, intramural hematoma is visualized as areas of high signal intensity on T1- and T2-weighted images (Fig. 93-15).[45] As with CT, MR images obtained before the administration of contrast material (T1-weighted especially) are critical for proper detection of intramural hematoma.

Angiography

Catheter angiography may fail to identify intramural hematoma and is rarely the first choice for diagnosis of intramural hematoma because no intimal disruption is usually

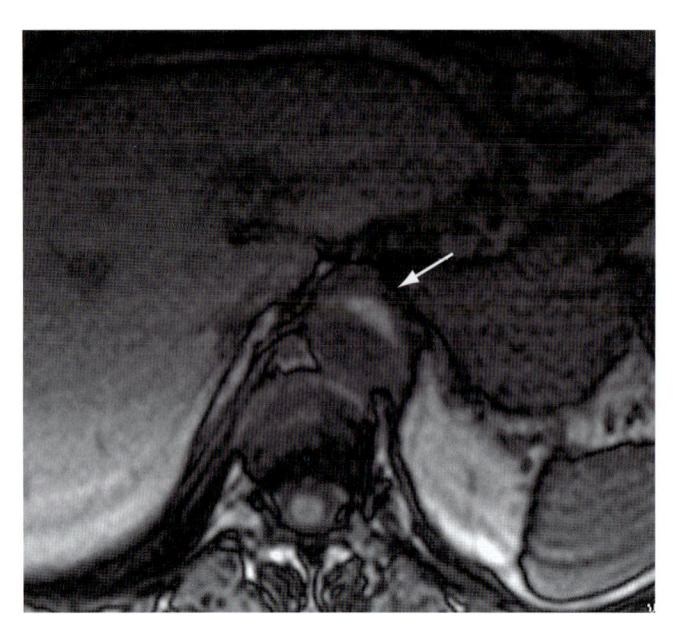

■ **FIGURE 93-15** Intramural hematoma of the aorta. Unenhanced T1-weighted MRI reveals small intramural hematoma (*arrow*) along the anterior wall of the aorta at the level of the diaphragmatic hiatus. As on unenhanced CT, acute blood products are bright on T1-weighted images. *(From Kapustin AJ, Litt HI. Diagnostic imaging for aortic dissection. Semin Thorac Cardiovasc Surg 2005; 17:214-223.)*

present. However, when the intramural hematoma is large and extensive, a thickened aortic wall may be demonstrated on catheter angiography as an indirect sign of an intramural hematoma.[46]

Classic Signs

The "crescent sign" is a crescentic area of increased attenuation on non–contrast-enhanced CT images or increased signal intensity on non–contrast-enhanced T1-weighted MR images, reflecting acute to subacute blood products within the aortic wall.

Differential Diagnosis

From Clinical Presentation

Differential diagnosis includes other acute aortic syndromes, especially aortic dissection. Other causes of chest pain, including myocardial infarction, acute pericarditis, and pulmonary embolism, should be considered.

From Imaging Findings

As with aortic dissection, thrombus within the lumen of an aortic aneurysm could be confused with intramural hematoma, although the crescent shape of intramural hematoma should point to the correct diagnosis. A slowly filling or chronically thrombosed false lumen could have an appearance similar to intramural hematoma on post–contrast-enhanced images; therefore, it is very important to obtain images before the administration of contrast material when acute aortic syndrome is suspected.

Synopsis of Treatment Options

Medical

The therapeutic strategy for intramural hematoma is similar to that for aortic dissection. Recent advances in diagnostic modalities and appropriate treatment of intramural hematoma have led to improved prognosis and survival of patients. Nevertheless, the overall mortality still remains high at 20.7%.[39]

Acute intramural hematoma involving the descending aorta only has an in-hospital mortality risk of less than 1% to 5%, similar to that seen with descending or type B dissection, and thus medical treatment is the standard of choice.[47] Evolution to localized dissection is not necessarily an indication for surgical or endovascular treatment. Acute intramural hematoma confined to the aortic arch remains a controversial subject. Evangelista and colleagues[39] stated that aggressive medical treatment alone, with a target heart rate below 60 beats/min and blood pressure below 120/80 mm Hg and at least one additional initial imaging study to exclude frank aortic dissection or early aneurysmal expansion, appears to be a reasonable strategy for management of such patients.

Intramural hematoma is often well managed with medical therapy to lower blood pressure. Prognosis in older patients with intramural hematoma is acceptable with medical therapy, perhaps because severe atherosclerosis can limit the expansion of hemorrhage with adequate blood pressure control.[48] Patients whose conditions can be stabilized with antihypertensive therapy may have a good long-term prognosis.

Surgical/Interventional

As in classic aortic dissection, the mortality rate is much higher for an intramural hematoma involving the ascending aorta than for an intramural hematoma involving the descending aorta. Regression may occur but is less common in intramural hematoma involving the ascending aorta, and surgical treatment has been favored. If there are no complications, such as persistent chest pain or periaortic bleeding, surgical intervention should take place within 24 to 72 hours.[45]

Rapid aortic dilation with signs of imminent aortic rupture and periaortic bleeding in a patient with persistent pain is an indication for endovascular treatment. Such treatment can be undertaken with good results when the ends of the stent are implanted in the healthy aortic wall and not on the hematoma.[45]

Wall configuration in acute intramural hematoma has been reported to change rapidly. Bleeding into the aortic media may be self-limited, but it is a dynamic process that may lead to classic communicating dissection, aortic rupture, rapid aneurysmal dilation of the aorta, or circumferential and longitudinal extension of the bleeding.[49] Intramural hematoma may progress to classic aortic dissection in 28% to 47% of patients and it carries a risk of aortic rupture in 20% to 45% of cases.[50] Fluid extravasation, such as pericardial and pleural effusions and mediastinal hemorrhage, is a frequent finding in patients with acute intramural hematoma. This may indicate impending aortic rupture and is considered to be an indication for emergent surgery.[51]

The size of the ascending aorta at the first examination may be important in predicting the progress of an intramural hematoma. In one study, patients with an aortic diameter of less than 5 cm experienced regression of the hematoma during medical therapy; whereas those with a larger diameter (>5 cm) had a tendency for progression to dissection or rupture.[48] A maximum thickness of a hematoma greater than 11 mm on the initial CT scan may also be a significant factor for predicting development of aortic dissection and aortic aneurysm.[42] Therefore, treatment strategies may be individualized according to the condition of the patient. Emergency surgery should be recommended in symptomatic patients, those with rapid progression during follow-up, and those with a large ascending aorta.

Reporting: Information for the Referring Physician

Reporting of imaging studies performed for evaluation of intramural hematoma should include the following elements:

- Involvement of the ascending aorta, aortic arch, or descending thoracic and abdominal aorta
- Extent of the intramural hematoma
- An opinion concerning the etiology of the intramural hematoma, if possible (i.e., trauma, penetrating atherosclerotic ulcer)
- Any direct or indirect signs of leaking or rupture
- Any regions of aneurysmal dilation of the aorta

PENETRATING ATHEROSCLEROTIC ULCER

Definition

A penetrating atherosclerotic ulcer is a condition in which an aortic atherosclerotic plaque ruptures, followed by ulcer formation and penetration through the internal elastic lamina into the aortic media.[1]

Prevalence and Epidemiology

This lesion usually affects patients who have hypertension and diffuse atherosclerosis. Penetrating atherosclerotic ulcer is more often observed in the descending aorta, which is generally more involved by atherosclerosis.[52] Involvement of the ascending aorta is rare.[20]

Etiology and Pathophysiology

The atherosclerotic ulcer is initially confined to the intima and is usually asymptomatic.[53] The progression of the intimal erosion can develop into a deep atheromatous ulcer, which penetrates through the elastic lamina into the medial layer. If an atherosclerotic ulcer penetrates into the aortic media that is very rich with the vasa vasorum, the medial layer may be exposed to pulsatile arterial flow, which can initiate hemorrhage into the media without an intimal flap. However, this lesion is mostly localized because its longitudinal propagation is limited by atherosclerotic fibrosis and calcification of the aortic wall. Further extension of penetrating atherosclerotic ulcer to the aortic adventitia can cause progressive dilation of the aorta, which leads to a pseudoaneurysm or even aortic rupture.[7]

Manifestations of Disease

Clinical Presentation

Clinical symptoms in patients with atheromatous aortic ulcers are mostly absent or nonspecific unless the lesions are associated with other pathologic changes. However, patients with penetrating atherosclerotic ulcers may present with sudden onset of retrosternal or interscapular pain that is usually similar to that of classic aortic dissection or intramural hematoma.

Imaging Indications and Algorithm

Imaging findings of penetrating atherosclerotic ulcers differ from those of acute aortic dissection. An intimal flap is absent, and a contrast-filled space is not visualized in the medial layer, although intramural hematomas are frequently associated with penetrating atherosclerotic ulcer. A penetrating atherosclerotic ulcer may be distinguished from a simple atherosclerotic plaque by the presence of a discrete ulcer crater or a focal contrast-filled outpouching (Fig. 93-16). However, ulcerated atherosclerotic

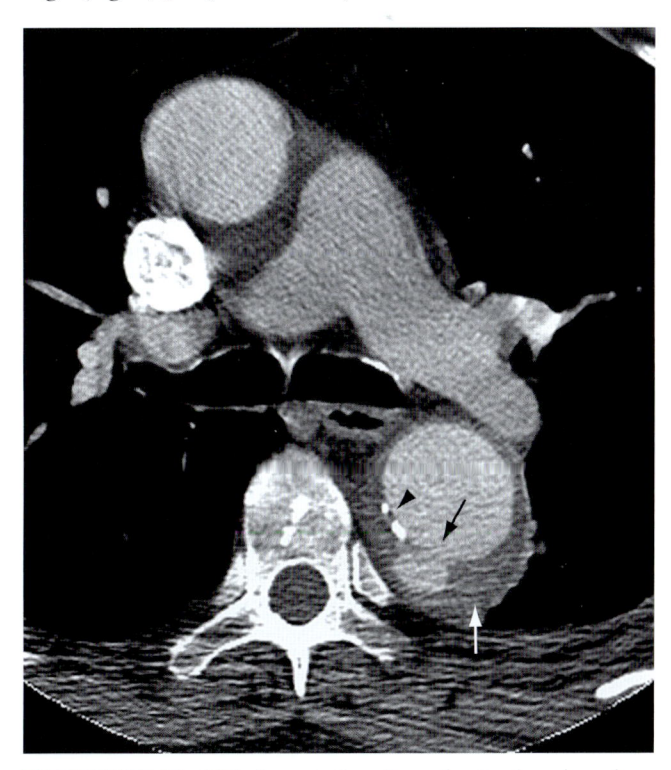

■ **FIGURE 93-16** CTA of penetrating atherosclerotic ulcer along the posterior wall of the descending aorta (*black arrow*). The *white arrow* shows an associated intramural hematoma. The *arrowhead* indicates intimal calcification. Compare with ulcerated plaque in Figure 93-17. *(From from Kapustin AJ, Litt HI. Diagnostic imaging for aortic dissection. Semin Thorac Cardiovasc Surg 2005; 17:214-223.)*

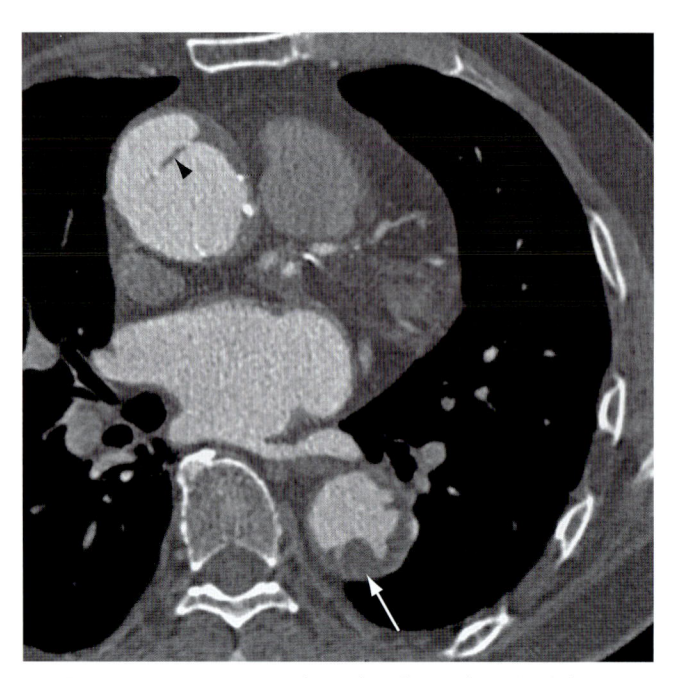

■ **FIGURE 93-17** Contrast-enhanced CT image shows irregular ulcerated atherosclerotic plaque in the descending thoracic aorta, without penetration beyond the intima (*arrow*). The ascending aorta shows aortic dissection, which has an intimal flap with spotty calcification along the luminal side of the aortic wall (*arrowhead*). Compare with penetrating atherosclerotic ulcer of the aorta in Figure 93-16.

plaque shows irregular margins of the intima without evidence of contrast material extending beyond the intimal layer (Fig. 93-17).

Imaging Techniques and Findings

Radiography

Chest radiography is relatively insensitive in patients with penetrating atherosclerotic ulcers. Chest radiographs usually have a normal appearance unless the penetrating atherosclerotic ulcer progresses to aortic dissection or aneurysm. Complications such as aortic aneurysm or fluid extravasation can change the aortic contour or show mediastinal widening or pleural effusion on plain chest radiographs. Severe calcification of the aortic wall may indicate atherosclerosis involving the aortic wall. Displaced calcification indicates that the penetrating atherosclerotic ulcer might be associated with intramural hematoma or dissection of the aorta. Comparison with prior chest radiographs may be important for identification of the aortic lesion including penetrating atherosclerotic ulcer.

Ultrasonography

TEE is relatively insensitive for diagnosis of aortic ulcers. A penetrating atherosclerotic ulcer is more difficult to identify with TEE than with CT or MR imaging.[54] However, TEE has the ability to classify the different types of aortic ulcers related to their pathogenesis. TEE can directly visualize the aortic lumen and wall and differentiates between ulcerated atherosclerotic plaques confined to the intima and penetrating atherosclerotic ulcers extending into the medial layer.[12] Ulcerated atherosclerotic plaques may demonstrate a thickened intima with irregular margins, whereas a penetrating atherosclerotic ulcer shows a discrete ulcer crater with extension beyond the intima. If the penetrating atherosclerotic ulcer is associated with intramural hematoma, the aortic wall is thickened, and intimal calcifications, if present, are displaced inward. In some patients, TEE may fail to identify the aortic ulcer and may reveal only intramural hematoma from a tiny aortic ulcer mouth.[55]

Computed Tomography

CT findings of a penetrating atherosclerotic ulcer may include a focal ulcer, intramural hematoma, displacement of calcified intima, thickened and enhancing aortic wall, pleural effusion, mediastinal fluid, or even pseudoaneurysm.[56]

CT scans performed before the administration of contrast material readily demonstrate aortic atherosclerotic plaques with ulcer craters, which are manifested as low-attenuation material along the vessel wall, with intimal calcifications frequently scattered along the luminal side of the aorta. The intramural hematoma, if it is also present, may be visualized as an area of high attenuation on the CT images obtained before contrast enhancement. Intimal calcifications can be displaced inward by surrounding intramural hematoma.[56]

Contrast-enhanced CT depicts a penetrating atherosclerotic ulcer as a focal contrast collection projecting beyond the intimal border of the aortic wall without an intimal dissection flap or false lumen (Fig. 93-18). The contrast collection may extend longitudinally up to several centimeters. Penetrating ulcers are sometimes associated with aortic wall thickening and possible mural enhancement. Massive hemomediastinum may be associated with a complicated penetrating atherosclerotic ulcer, which requires immediate surgical treatment.[20]

Magnetic Resonance

Although CT is commonly used in the initial screening of penetrating atherosclerotic ulcers, MRI can also depict a penetrating atherosclerotic ulcer as a focal contrast-filled outpouching without an intimal flap or false lumen in the aortic wall (Fig. 93-19). As in intramural hematoma, the hemorrhage associated with penetrating atherosclerotic ulcers can be demonstrated as a variable signal intensity lesion on MRI. An intramural hematoma combined with penetrating atherosclerotic ulcer is usually visualized as localized areas of high signal intensity on the T1- and T2-weighted images.

Angiography

Catheter angiography is often not the initial examination for diagnosis of penetrating atherosclerotic ulcers. If the ulcer projects tangentially from the aortic lumen, catheter angiography can show a penetrating atherosclerotic ulcer as a localized contrast-filled outpouching of the aortic

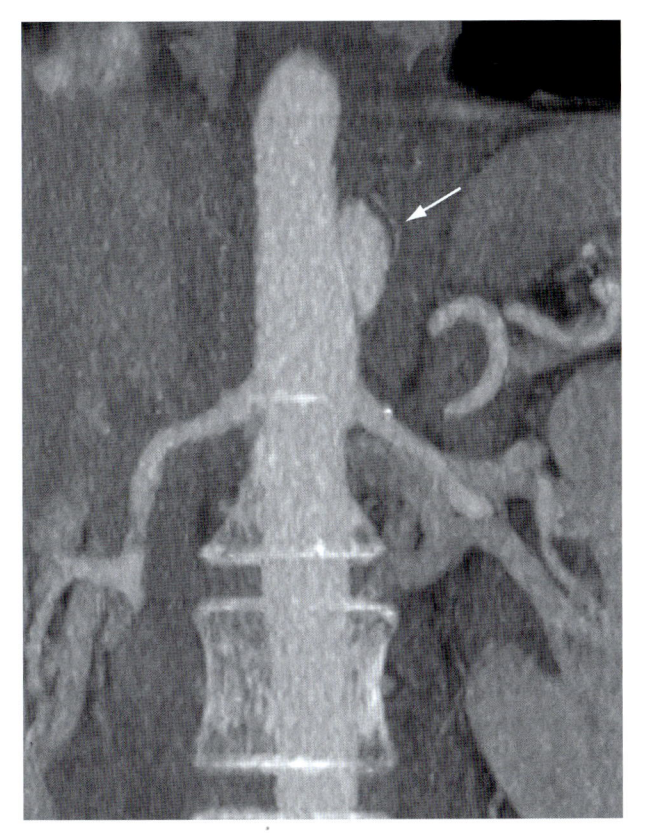

FIGURE 93-18 Multiplanar reformatted CTA reveals a penetrating atherosclerotic ulcer (*arrow*) of the proximal abdominal aorta. *(From Kapustin AJ, Litt HI. Diagnostic imaging for aortic dissection. Semin Thorac Cardiovasc Surg 2005; 17:214-223.)*

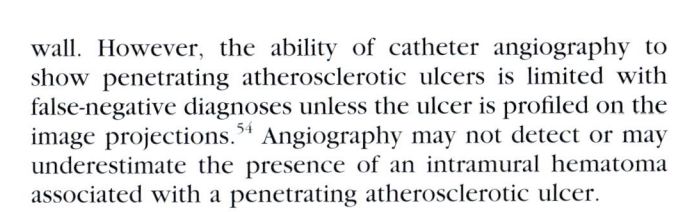

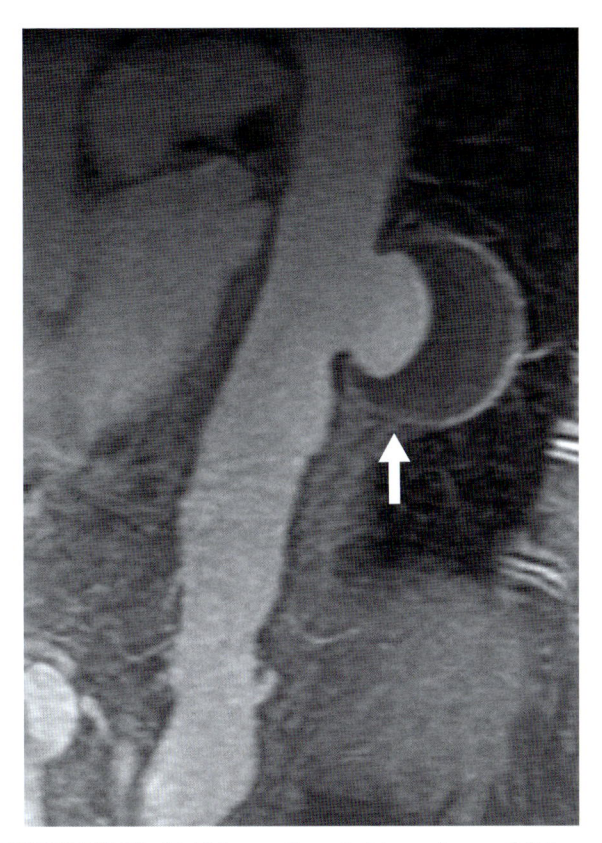

FIGURE 93-19 Multiplanar reformatted image from gadolinium-enhanced three-dimensional MRA demonstrates a partially thrombosed saccular aneurysm of the distal thoracic aorta, which probably began as a penetrating atherosclerotic ulcer. *(From Kapustin AJ, Litt HI. Diagnostic imaging for aortic dissection. Semin Thorac Cardiovasc Surg 2005; 17:214-223.)*

wall. However, the ability of catheter angiography to show penetrating atherosclerotic ulcers is limited with false-negative diagnoses unless the ulcer is profiled on the image projections.[54] Angiography may not detect or may underestimate the presence of an intramural hematoma associated with a penetrating atherosclerotic ulcer.

Differential Diagnosis

From Clinical Presentation

Differential diagnosis also includes other acute aortic syndromes, especially aortic dissection. Other causes of chest pain, including myocardial infarction, acute pericarditis, and pulmonary embolism, should be considered.

From Imaging Findings

As penetrating atherosclerotic ulcer can lead to an intramural hematoma, it is important to look for penetrating atherosclerotic ulcer whenever an intramural hematoma is identified; this etiology may alter treatment decisions. Saccular pseudoaneurysms caused by penetrating atherosclerotic ulcer may appear similar to other causes, such as mycotic aneurysms or pseudoaneurysms related to surgical anastomoses.

Synopsis of Treatment Options

Medical

Symptomatic treatment of acute penetrating atherosclerotic ulcers should be similar to that of other acute aortic syndromes. Treatment of penetrating atherosclerotic ulcers generally depends on their evolutional patterns, such as persistent symptoms, progressive dilation of the aorta, or rebleeding of the aortic wall.[12] Patients with penetrating atherosclerotic ulcers complicated by localized intramural hematoma generally undergo aggressive medical treatment in an intensive care unit.[56] Medical treatment focuses on the control of hypertension.

Surgical/Interventional

Patients with hemodynamic instability or uncontrollable pain should be recommended for surgical treatment. Patients who have developed pseudoaneurysms or aortic rupture are treated with emergency surgery.[54]

Endovascular treatment has been favored in elderly patients with atherosclerosis because of surgical risk. Indications for surgical treatment include persistent or recurrent pain, expanding intramural hematoma or pseudoaneurysm, distal embolization, and hemodynamic instability.[56] Surgical treatment of a penetrating atherosclerotic ulcer requires placement of an interposition graft at the site of the ulcer. The interposition graft is relatively extensive because it should cover the aortic wall involved by intramural hematoma, which may lead to higher morbidity such as paraplegia.[54]

Reporting: Information for the Referring Physician

Reporting of imaging studies in which penetrating atherosclerotic ulcer is diagnosed should include the following elements:

- Location of the penetrating atherosclerotic ulcer, especially if multiple ulcers are present
- Presence and extent of any associated intramural hematoma
- Description of any saccular aneurysm or pseudoaneurysm, including size and length
- Any direct or indirect signs of leaking or rupture
- Guidance for potential endovascular therapy, including
  - relationship of the penetrating atherosclerotic ulcer or pseudoaneurysm to the left subclavian, celiac, or renal arteries (i.e., proximal and distal neck length)
  - proximal and distal neck diameter
  - severe aortic or iliac artery tortuosity or calcification
  - iliac artery access diameters

RUPTURED AORTIC ANEURYSM

Definition

A ruptured aortic aneurysm is a life-threatening event requiring emergency treatment. Patients with ruptured aortic aneurysm must be diagnosed immediately. Mortality rates reach nearly 100% if treatment is delayed.

Etiology and Pathophysiology

Aortic aneurysm rupture usually occurs when the mechanical stress on the aortic wall exceeds the strength of the wall tissue.[57] The risk of rupture is closely related to the size of the aneurysm. A previous study reported that the median diameter of the aorta at the diagnosis of rupture was 6.0 cm in the ascending aorta and 7.2 cm in the descending thoracic aorta.[58] The expansion rate of aortic aneurysms may affect the risk of rupture in relation to the size of the aneurysms. The median expansion rate was much faster in patients with aneurysms of more than 4 cm in diameter (0.3 to 0.8 cm/yr) than in patients with aneurysms of less than 4 cm in diameter (0.2 cm/yr).[59] The risk of rupture may also depend on the cause of the aneurysm; rate of rupture is relatively high in mycotic aneurysms and pseudoaneurysms. In practice, ruptured aortic aneurysm is more frequently observed in the aortic arch and descending aorta, where it is more common but less life-threatening than in the ascending aorta.[20]

Manifestations of Disease

Clinical Presentation

Clinical symptoms in patients with unstable aortic aneurysm are similar to those of other acute aortic syndromes. Although patients with unstable aortic aneurysm often complain of chest or back pain, they are usually accompanied by hypotension when the aneurysm has ruptured, and, therefore, ruptured aortic aneurysm may not be routinely included as a part of acute aortic syndrome.[21]

Imaging Indications and Algorithm

Imaging in cases of suspected aneurysm rupture should proceed as expeditiously as possible to make the diagnosis and to allow appropriate emergency treatment. In cases in which clinical suspicion is high, for example, in a patient with known large aneurysm who presents with sudden onset of severe pain and hypotension, imaging may not be necessary and may delay potentially lifesaving treatment.

Imaging Techniques and Findings

Radiography

The chest film is not specific for diagnosis of ruptured aortic aneurysm. However, because ruptures of thoracic aneurysms usually extend into the mediastinum or pleural space, they are helpful in detecting mediastinal widening or pleural effusion.

Computed Tomography

CT is frequently used in the emergency department to evaluate suspected aortic disease and can accurately demonstrate the size and extent of the aneurysm or pseudoaneurysm, associated dissection of the aorta, presence and extent of mural thrombus, and other critical information about the aortic wall.[60] CT also shows mediastinal hematoma and its relationship to the aorta, pleural effusion or associated lung collapse, and rarely pericardial effusion. In an emergent situation, CT can be performed without the intravenous administration of contrast material.

The findings of aortic rupture on CT images obtained before contrast enhancement include high-attenuation thickening of the aortic wall, adjacent mediastinal hematoma, hemothorax, and hemopericardium (Fig. 93-20). Even without signs of frank rupture, demonstration of crescentic high attenuation in the thickened wall of the aorta or within the mural thrombus on CT images obtained before contrast enhancement is indicative of early aortic rupture or impending aortic rupture.[61,62] This sign represents acute hemorrhage into the preexisting mural thrombus or the aneurysm wall, which can be a potential site for rupture. Contrast-enhanced CT may demonstrate deformities of the lumen and irregular thickening of the aortic wall with or without active extravasation of contrast material into the periaortic spaces. The pattern of mural calcification can also be important, with a focal discontinuity in otherwise circumferential calcification

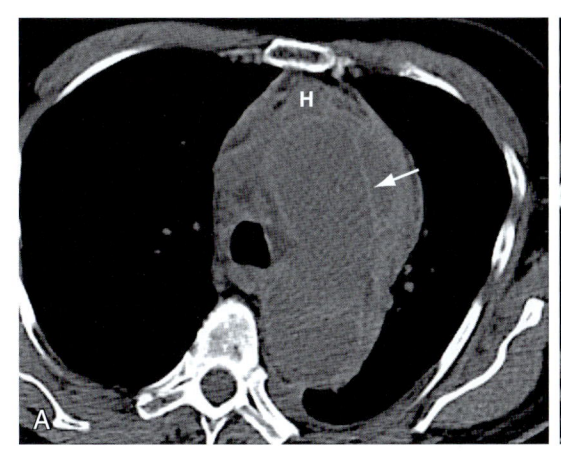

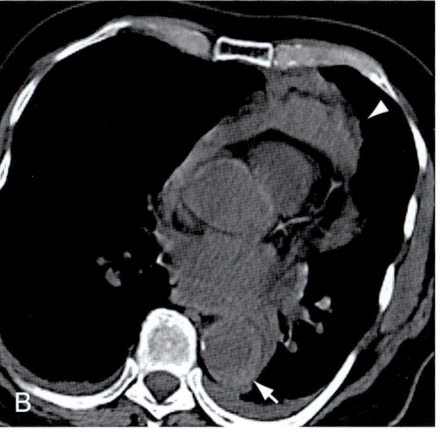

FIGURE 93-20 Ruptured aneurysmal type A dissection. CT images obtained before the administration of contrast material show (**A,** cranial) intimal flap in the ascending aorta (*arrow*) with mediastinal hematoma (H) and (**B,** caudal) hemopericardium (*arrowhead*) and an intramural hematoma in the posterolateral descending aorta (*arrow*).

depicted in patients with ruptured aortic aneurysm.[62] Draping of the posterior aspect of the aorta over the adjacent vertebral body is another sign of aortic wall insufficiency in abdominal aortic aneurysms, even in the absence of retroperitoneal hemorrhage.[63]

Magnetic Resonance

The efficacy of MRI in the diagnosis of ruptured aortic aneurysm is controversial because of examination length and monitoring difficulties in potentially unstable patients. Irregular wall thickening of the aorta can be depicted by MRI, which may show variable signal intensity according to the stages of hemorrhage. Hemorrhage within the mural thrombus or thickened aortic wall is seen as focal areas of high signal intensity on T1- and T2-weighted spin-echo MR images.[64] However, it is not clear that all areas of hemorrhage visualized on the MR images are related to the ruptured aneurysms or hyperattenuating crescent signs on CT images.

Angiography

Catheter angiography is rarely used in the diagnosis of a ruptured aortic aneurysm.

Synopsis of Treatment Options

Surgical/Interventional

Ruptured aortic aneurysm should be treated aggressively with immediate surgical repair. Although techniques have improved, surgery for ruptured aortic aneurysm is still associated with a high morbidity and mortality rate. However, a study reported that patients with ruptured aortic aneurysm had an early mortality rate of 21%.[65] This lower mortality rate suggests that most surgical patients are hemodynamically stable and are, to a certain degree, self-selected. Patients who are hemodynamically unstable do not usually survive long enough to be transported to the operating room.

Postoperative complications include paraplegia, renal failure, and other cardiopulmonary events. The development of paraplegia is the most serious complication after repair of aneurysm rupture. Paraplegia is usually due to interruption of the intercostal blood supply to the spinal cord.[7] The rate of paraplegia is much higher, with an incidence rate of 54%, in patients with aneurysm rupture than in patients without aneurysm rupture (10%). Renal failure depends on the preoperative condition of the patient; the incidence of renal impairment is reported to be between 3% and 27%.[65,66] Visceral and renal perfusion protection should be important goals in the treatment of ruptured aortic aneurysms.

KEY POINTS

- Acute aortic syndromes include aortic dissection, intramural hematoma, penetrating atherosclerotic ulcer, and ruptured aortic aneurysm.
- Whereas all may manifest with similar symptoms, imaging can differentiate among them and is important for determination of appropriate treatment and prognosis.
- CT is the preferred modality for imaging of suspected acute aortic syndrome in most cases. TEE and MRI can be used for problem solving and evaluating complications. Catheter angiography is useful for treatment.

SUGGESTED READINGS

Kapustin AJ, Litt HI. Diagnostic imaging for aortic dissection. Semin Thorac Cardiovasc Surg 2005; 17:214-223.

Macura KJ, Corl FM, Fishman EK, Bluemke DA. Pathogenesis in acute aortic syndromes: aortic dissection, intramural hematoma, and penetrating atherosclerotic aortic ulcer. AJR Am J Roentgenol 2003; 181:309-316.

Macura KJ, Corl FM, Fishman EK, Bluemke DA. Pathogenesis in acute aortic syndromes: aortic aneurysm leak and rupture and traumatic aortic transection. AJR Am J Roentgenol 2003; 181:303-307.

Nienaber CA, Eagle KA. Aortic dissection: new frontiers in diagnosis and management: Part II: therapeutic management and follow-up. Circulation 2003; 108:772-778.

Roberts DA. Magnetic resonance imaging of thoracic aortic aneurysm and dissection. Semin Roentgenol 2001; 36:295-308.

REFERENCES

1. Vilacosta I, Roman JA. Acute aortic syndrome. Heart 2001; 85:365-368.
2. Macura KJ, Corl FM, Fishman EK, Bluemke DA. Pathogenesis in acute aortic syndromes: aortic dissection, intramural hematoma, and penetrating atherosclerotic aortic ulcer. AJR Am J Roentgenol 2003; 181:309-316.
3. Zamorano JL, Perez de Isla L, Gonzalez R, et al. [Imaging diagnosis in acute aortic syndromes]. Rev Esp Cardiol 2003; 56:498-508.
4. Meszaros I, Morocz J, Szlavi J, et al. Epidemiology and clinicopathology of aortic dissection. Chest 2000; 117:1271-1278.
5. Clouse WD, Hallett JW, Jr., Schaff HV, et al. Acute aortic dissection: population-based incidence compared with degenerative aortic aneurysm rupture. Mayo Clin Proc 2004; 79:176-180.
6. Hagan PG, Nienaber CA, Isselbacher EM, et al. The International Registry of Acute Aortic Dissection (IRAD): new insights into an old disease. JAMA 2000; 283:897-903.
7. Ahmad F, Cheshire N, Hamady M. Acute aortic syndrome: pathology and therapeutic strategies. Postgrad Med J 2006; 82:305-312.
8. Coady MA, Rizzo JA, Elefteriades JA. Pathologic variants of thoracic aortic dissections. Penetrating atherosclerotic ulcers and intramural hematomas. Cardiol Clin 1999; 17:637-657.
9. Kouchoukos NT, Dougenis D. Surgery of the thoracic aorta. N Engl J Med 1997; 336:1876-1888.
10. Muna WF, Spray TL, Morrow AG, Roberts WC. Aortic dissection after aortic valve replacement in patients with valvular aortic stenosis. J Thorac Cardiovasc Surg 1977; 74:65-69.
11. Wooley CF, Sparks EH, Boudoulas H. Aortic pain. Prog Cardiovasc Dis 1998; 40:563-589.
12. Evangelista Masip A. [Natural history and therapeutic management of acute aortic syndrome]. Rev Esp Cardiol 2004; 57:667-679.
13. DeBakey ME, McCollum CH, Crawford ES, et al. Dissection and dissecting aneurysms of the aorta: twenty-year follow-up of five hundred twenty-seven patients treated surgically. Surgery 1982; 92:1118-1134.
14. Daily PO, Trueblood HW, Stinson EB, et al. Management of acute aortic dissections. Ann Thorac Surg 1970; 10:237-247.
15. Kapustin AJ, Litt HI. Diagnostic imaging for aortic dissection. Semin Thorac Cardiovasc Surg 2005; 17:214-223.
16. Shiga T, Wajima Z, Apfel CC, et al. Diagnostic accuracy of transesophageal echocardiography, helical computed tomography, and magnetic resonance imaging for suspected thoracic aortic dissection: systematic review and meta-analysis. Arch Intern Med 2006; 166:1350-1356.
17. Petasnick JP. Radiologic evaluation of aortic dissection. Radiology 1991; 180:297-305.
18. Blanchard DG, Kimura BJ, Dittrich HC, DeMaria AN. Transesophageal echocardiography of the aorta. JAMA 1994; 272:546-551.
19. Yamada E, Matsumura M, Kyo S, Omoto R. Usefulness of a prototype intravascular ultrasound imaging in evaluation of aortic dissection and comparison with angiographic study, transesophageal echocardiography, computed tomography, and magnetic resonance imaging. Am J Cardiol 1995; 75:161-165.
20. Romano L, Pinto A, Gagliardi N. Multidetector-row CT evaluation of nontraumatic acute thoracic aortic syndromes. Radiol Med (Torino) 2007; 112:1-20.
21. Bhalla S, West OC. CT of nontraumatic thoracic aortic emergencies. Semin Ultrasound CT MR 2005; 26:281-304.
22. Manghat NE, Morgan-Hughes GJ, Roobottom CA. Multi-detector row computed tomography: imaging in acute aortic syndrome. Clin Radiol 2005; 60:1256-1267.
23. Roos JE, Willmann JK, Weishaupt D, et al. Thoracic aorta: motion artifact reduction with retrospective and prospective electrocardiography-assisted multi-detector row CT. Radiology 2002; 222:271-277.
24. Urban BA, Bluemke DA, Johnson KM, Fishman EK. Imaging of thoracic aortic disease. Cardiol Clin 1999; 17:659-682, viii.
25. Roberts DA. Magnetic resonance imaging of thoracic aortic aneurysm and dissection. Semin Roentgenol 2001; 36:295-308.
26. Krinsky GA, Rofsky NM, DeCorato DR, et al. Thoracic aorta: comparison of gadolinium-enhanced three-dimensional MR angiography with conventional MR imaging. Radiology 1997; 202:183-193.
27. Liu Q, Lu JP, Wang F, et al. Three-dimensional contrast-enhanced MR angiography of aortic dissection: a pictorial essay. Radiographics 2007; 27:1311-1321.
28. Erbel R, Engberding R, Daniel W, et al. Echocardiography in diagnosis of aortic dissection. Lancet 1989; 1:457-461.
29. Cigarroa JE, Isselbacher EM, DeSanctis RW, Eagle KA. Diagnostic imaging in the evaluation of suspected aortic dissection. Old standards and new directions. N Engl J Med 1993; 328:35-43.
30. LePage MA, Quint LE, Sonnad SS, et al. Aortic dissection: CT features that distinguish true lumen from false lumen. AJR Am J Roentgenol 2001; 177:207-211.
31. Williams DM, Joshi A, Dake MD, et al. Aortic cobwebs: an anatomic marker identifying the false lumen in aortic dissection—imaging and pathologic correlation. Radiology 1994; 190:167-174.
32. Ince H, Nienaber CA. [Management of acute aortic syndromes]. Rev Esp Cardiol 2007; 60:526-541.
33. David TE, Feindel CM. An aortic valve–sparing operation for patients with aortic incompetence and aneurysm of the ascending aorta. J Thorac Cardiovasc Surg 1992; 103:617-621; discussion 622.
34. Nienaber CA, Eagle KA. Aortic dissection: new frontiers in diagnosis and management: Part II: therapeutic management and follow-up. Circulation 2003; 108:772-778.
35. Dake MD, Kato N, Mitchell RS, et al. Endovascular stent-graft placement for the treatment of acute aortic dissection. N Engl J Med 1999; 340:1546-1552.
36. Nienaber CA, Fattori R, Lund G, et al. Nonsurgical reconstruction of thoracic aortic dissection by stent-graft placement. N Engl J Med 1999; 340:1539-1545.
37. Bortone AS, Schena S, D'Agostino D, et al. Immediate versus delayed endovascular treatment of post-traumatic aortic pseudoaneurysms and type B dissections: retrospective analysis and premises to the upcoming European trial. Circulation 2002; 106:I234-I240.
38. Evangelista A, Dominguez R, Sebastia C, et al. Prognostic value of clinical and morphologic findings in short-term evolution of aortic intramural haematoma. Therapeutic implications. Eur Heart J 2004; 25:81-87.
39. Evangelista A, Mukherjee D, Mehta RH, et al. Acute intramural hematoma of the aorta: a mystery in evolution. Circulation 2005; 111:1063-1070.
40. Schlatmann TJ, Becker AE. Pathogenesis of dissecting aneurysm of aorta. Comparative histopathologic study of significance of medial changes. Am J Cardiol 1977; 39:21-26.
41. Carerj S, Cerrito M, Oreto G. Aortic intramural haematoma leading to aortic dissection. Heart 2004; 90:254.
42. Song JM, Kang DH, Song JK, et al. Clinical significance of echo-free space detected by transesophageal echocardiography in patients with type B aortic intramural hematoma. Am J Cardiol 2002; 89:548-551.
43. Song JK. Diagnosis of aortic intramural haematoma. Heart 2004; 90:368-371.
44. Mohr-Kahaly S. Aortic intramural hematoma: from observation to therapeutic strategies. J Am Coll Cardiol 2001; 37:1611-1613.
45. Evangelista Masip A. [Progress in the acute aortic syndrome]. Rev Esp Cardiol 2007; 60:428-439.
46. Bansal RC, Chandrasekaran K, Ayala K, Smith DC. Frequency and explanation of false negative diagnosis of aortic dissection by aortography and transesophageal echocardiography. J Am Coll Cardiol 1995; 25:1393-1401.
47. O'Gara PT, DeSanctis RW. Acute aortic dissection and its variants. Toward a common diagnostic and therapeutic approach. Circulation 1995; 92:1376-1378.
48. Kang DH, Song JK, Song MG, et al. Clinical and echocardiographic outcomes of aortic intramural hemorrhage compared with acute aortic dissection. Am J Cardiol 1998; 81:202-206.
49. Ohmi M, Tabayashi K, Moizumi Y, et al. Extremely rapid regression of aortic intramural hematoma. J Thorac Cardiovasc Surg 1999; 118:968-969.
50. von Kodolitsch Y, Csosz SK, Koschyk DH, et al. Intramural hematoma of the aorta: predictors of progression to dissection and rupture. Circulation 2003; 107:1158-1163.
51. Isselbacher EM, Cigarroa JE, Eagle KA. Cardiac tamponade complicating proximal aortic dissection. Is pericardiocentesis harmful? Circulation 1994; 90:2375-2378.
52. Lissin LW, Vagelos R. Acute aortic syndrome: a case presentation and review of the literature. Vasc Med 2002; 7:281-287.

53. Pauls S, Orend KH, Sunder-Plassmann L, et al. Endovascular repair of symptomatic penetrating atherosclerotic ulcer of the thoracic aorta. Eur J Vasc Endovasc Surg 2007; 34:66-73.
54. Levy JR, Heiken JP, Gutierrez FR. Imaging of penetrating atherosclerotic ulcers of the aorta. AJR Am J Roentgenol 1999; 173:151-154.
55. Movsowitz HD, David M, Movsowitz C, et al. Penetrating atherosclerotic aortic ulcers: the role of transesophageal echocardiography in diagnosis and clinical management. Am Heart J 1993; 126:745-747.
56. Kazerooni EA, Bree RL, Williams DM. Penetrating atherosclerotic ulcers of the descending thoracic aorta: evaluation with CT and distinction from aortic dissection. Radiology 1992; 183:759-765.
57. Macura KJ, Corl FM, Fishman EK, Bluemke DA. Pathogenesis in acute aortic syndromes: aortic aneurysm leak and rupture and traumatic aortic transection. AJR Am J Roentgenol 2003; 181:303-307.
58. Coady MA, Rizzo JA, Hammond GL, et al. What is the appropriate size criterion for resection of thoracic aortic aneurysms? J Thorac Cardiovasc Surg 1997; 113:476-491; discussion 489-491.
59. Guirguis EM, Barber GG. The natural history of abdominal aortic aneurysms. Am J Surg 1991; 162:481-483.
60. Ledbetter S, Stuk JL, Kaufman JA. Helical (spiral) CT in the evaluation of emergent thoracic aortic syndromes. Traumatic aortic rupture, aortic aneurysm, aortic dissection, intramural hematoma, and penetrating atherosclerotic ulcer. Radiol Clin North Am 1999; 37:575-589.
61. Mehard WB, Heiken JP, Sicard GA. High-attenuating crescent in abdominal aortic aneurysm wall at CT: a sign of acute or impending rupture. Radiology 1994; 192:359-362.
62. Siegel CL, Cohan RH, Korobkin M, et al. Abdominal aortic aneurysm morphology: CT features in patients with ruptured and nonruptured aneurysms. AJR Am J Roentgenol 1994; 163:1123-1129.
63. Schwartz SA, Taljanovic MS, Smyth S, et al. CT findings of rupture, impending rupture, and contained rupture of abdominal aortic aneurysms. AJR Am J Roentgenol 2007; 188:W57-W62.
64. Castrucci M, Mellone R, Vanzulli A, et al. Mural thrombi in abdominal aortic aneurysms: MR imaging characterization—useful before endovascular treatment? Radiology 1995; 197:135-139.
65. Lemaire SA, Rice DC, Schmittling ZC, Coselli JS. Emergency surgery for thoracoabdominal aortic aneurysms with acute presentation. J Vasc Surg 2002; 35:1171-1178.
66. Cambria RP, Davison JK, Zannetti S, et al. Thoracoabdominal aneurysm repair: perspectives over a decade with the clamp-and-sew technique. Ann Surg 1997; 226:294-303; discussion 303-295.

CHAPTER 94

Thoracic Aortic Trauma

Jonathan Balcombe and Harold Litt

Traumatic injury of the thoracic aorta is a serious and potentially fatal condition. Accurate diagnosis by imaging is essential for expeditious and potentially lifesaving management. CT angiography is the standard imaging technique because of easy availability and a high degree of accuracy. The injury involves a tear of one or more layers of the aortic wall and is usually located at the distal aortic arch or proximal descending thoracic aorta. Key imaging findings include intimal flap, pseudoaneurysm, aortic contour abnormality, and mediastinal hematoma. Intervention is almost always required and consists of either endovascular stent graft or open surgical repair.

THORACIC AORTIC TRAUMA
Etiology and Pathophysiology

Blunt aortic trauma is caused by a severe deceleration injury. The aortic arch is relatively fixed to the thoracic inlet by the brachiocephalic vessels, whereas the ascending and descending aorta are relatively mobile. During deceleration, horizontal shear forces act unequally on the relatively fixed arch and mobile ascending and descending aorta, causing extreme stress on the points of attachment of the aorta, namely, the aortic root and aortic isthmus, rendering these sites susceptible to transection (Fig. 94-1).[1] In addition, rapid deceleration may cause the vertebral column, sternum, first rib, and clavicle to compress the aorta in the region of the isthmus, contributing to the mechanism of injury.[2]

In clinical practice, the aortic isthmus is by far the most common site of aortic injury; the aortic root and ascending aorta represent 5% or less of cases (Fig. 94-2). However, in autopsy series, the ascending aorta is involved in 25% of cases.[3] This discrepancy is explained by the fact that many patients with ascending aortic injury do not survive to reach the hospital or are not stable enough for imaging because of grave complications of ascending aortic trauma, such as hemopericardium with tamponade, disruption of the aortic valve, and coronary artery dissection.

The degree of traumatic aortic injury depends on the nature of disruption of the aortic wall. Potential aortic injuries range from intimal hemorrhage, through intimal laceration and medial laceration, to complete laceration of the aorta.[1] Disruption of the intima and media results in a pseudoaneurysm. Complete laceration, with disruption of the adventitia, usually results in immediate death.

Manifestations of Disease
Clinical Presentation

A history of high-speed deceleration or blunt chest trauma should suggest thoracic aortic injury. Chest or upper back pain, dyspnea, dysphagia, absence of femoral pulses, ecchymoses of the chest wall, seat belt injuries, and fractured sternum act to increase suspicion but are frequently absent.

Imaging Indications and Algorithm

Indications for imaging are based on the mechanism of trauma and clinical signs detailed earlier. As part of a trauma series, most patients will undergo initial chest radiography but will progress immediately to CT regardless of the radiographic results, provided the patient is stable enough.

Imaging Techniques and Findings

Radiography

Plain film findings associated with aortic trauma include a widened mediastinal contour, obscuration of the aortic arch or descending aortic margin, displacement of the trachea or of a nasogastric tube (if present) to the right, and left apical cap (Fig. 94-3). Fracture of the first or second ribs may be seen as a result of the causative trauma.[4] However, each of these findings has been shown to have poor sensitivity or poor specificity. For example,

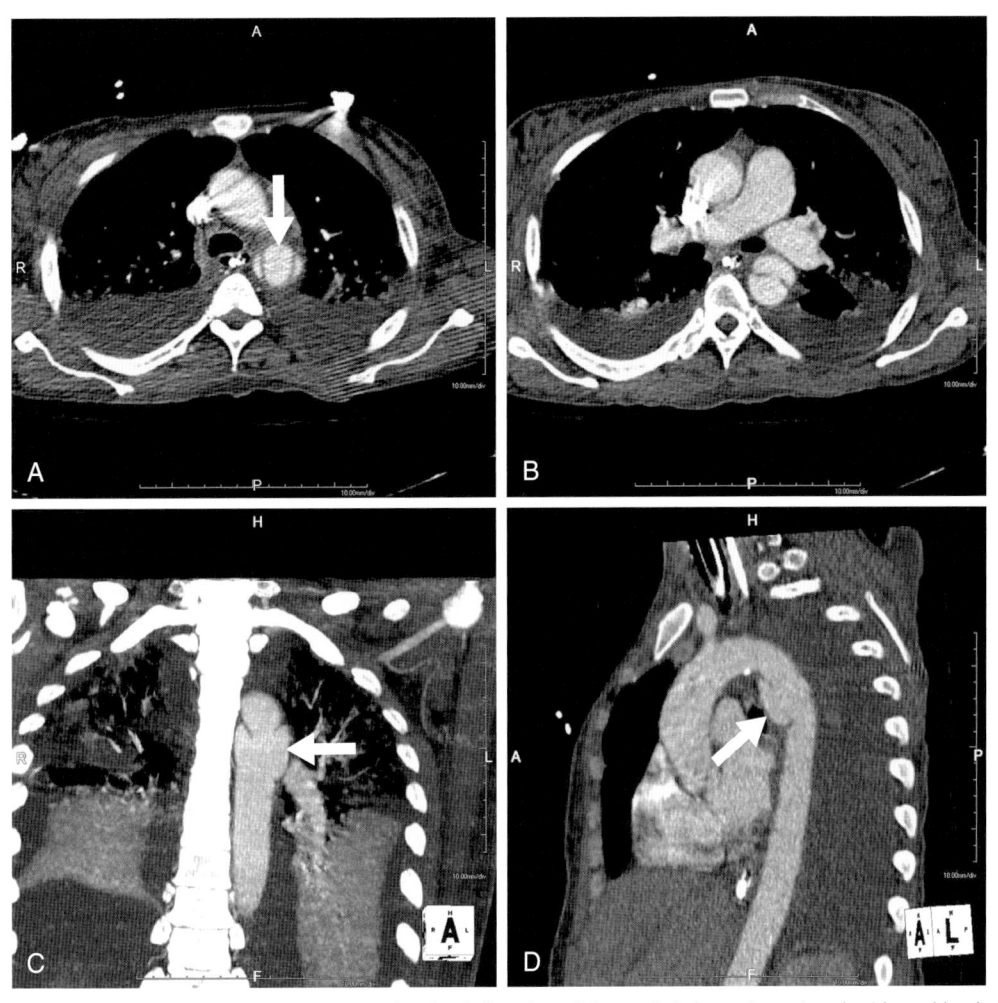

■ **FIGURE 94-1** CT demonstrates traumatic aortic injury at the classic location of the aortic isthmus (*arrow*) and evidenced by the curvilinear intimal flap (cranial to caudal, **A** and **B**). On reformatted images (oblique coronal, **C**; oblique sagittal, **D**), the resultant pseudoaneurysm (*arrow*) is much more easily appreciated.

in the trauma setting, a widened mediastinum is more commonly explained by anteroposterior positioning, lung contusion, hemothorax, and venous mediastinal bleeding, decreasing the specificity of these findings. Furthermore, in the majority of aortic injuries, the adventitia remains intact, resulting in only mild radiographic mediastinal findings, decreasing the sensitivity of plain radiography. In one study of aortic trauma, 44% of patients with subsequently proven aortic injury had a normal chest radiograph.[5] Therefore, plain radiography is not sufficiently sensitive or specific for the evaluation of aortic injury, and in the correct clinical setting, the patient should proceed directly to other modes of imaging.

Ultrasonography

Transthoracic ultrasonography has little role in the diagnosis of acute aortic trauma because it would delay CT evaluation, the preferred imaging technique. Transesophageal echocardiography (TEE), on the other hand, has the benefit of portability, which is an advantage for bedside evaluation of very unstable patients. However, in patients with suspected cervical spine injury and facial trauma, TEE is contraindicated. In addition, TEE is highly operator dependent and there is difficulty visualizing the distal ascending aorta and the aortic branch vessels. Therefore, TEE is rarely used clinically for evaluation of aortic trauma, although it may be used in some unusual cases when imaging options are limited or further confirmation is desired.

Computed Tomography

Multidetector computed tomography (MDCT) is the definitive modality for diagnosis of aortic trauma because of its speed, accuracy, postprocessing advantages, and ability to simultaneously evaluate the whole body for traumatic injury. CT angiography has been shown to have 100% sensitivity and 100% negative predictive value for traumatic aortic injury, at lower cost and with fewer complications than by catheter angiography.[6]

MDCT Technique

In most trauma centers, chest CT is performed as part of a trauma protocol that consists of an unenhanced head CT

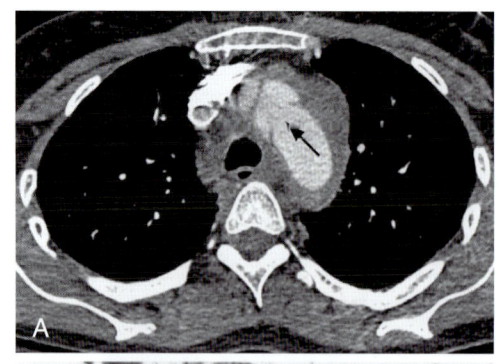

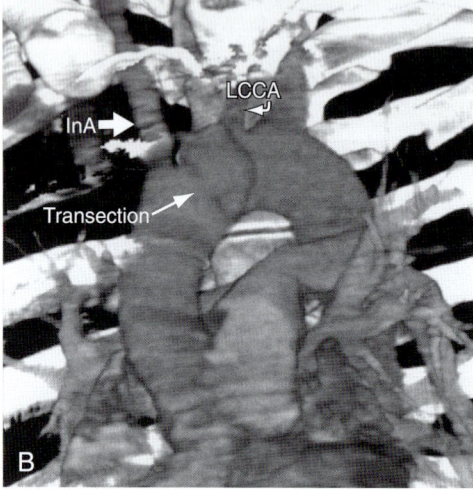

■ **FIGURE 94-2** **A,** Axial image from multidetector helical CT of the chest in a 40-year-old woman after a high-speed motor vehicle accident demonstrates aortic transection (*arrow*) with pseudoaneurysm and large periaortic hematoma containing the free aortic rupture. **B,** Volume rendered reconstruction demonstrates the location of the transection between the takeoff of the innominate artery (InA) and left common carotid arteries (LCCA). (*From Leshnower BG, Litt HI, Gleason TG. Anterior approach to traumatic mid aortic arch transection. Ann Thorac Surg 2006; 81:343-345.*)

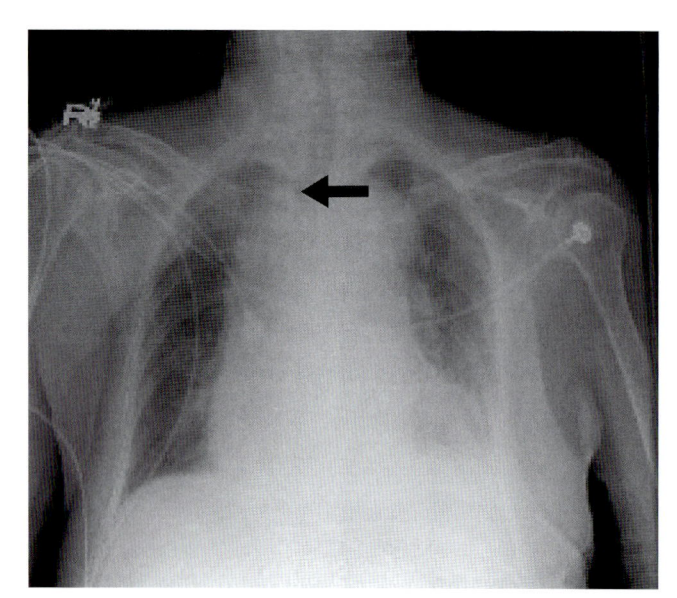

■ **FIGURE 94-3** Chest radiograph of a patient with acute traumatic aortic injury demonstrates a widened mediastinum, with deviation of the trachea to the right (*arrow*).

scan followed by an enhanced study of the chest, abdomen, and pelvis, with use of intravenous contrast material only. Evaluation of the neck can be included if cervical trauma is suspected. The chest CT scan is usually performed in the arterial phase, triggered by bolus timing from the mid-descending aorta. Images are obtained with 1-mm or thinner collimations; 3- to 5-mm axial sections are used for initial review. However, the data should be viewed in multiple planes, which can be achieved either by three-plane reconstructions generated by the CT technologist or by use of an independent workstation by the interpreting physician.

Aortic Pseudoaneurysm

Most patients with aortic trauma who survive to imaging will have a partial tear of the aortic wall. If the intima and media are torn but the adventitia remains intact, blood is forced between the layers, causing formation of a pseudoaneurysm. The imaging appearance is of a rounded bulge projecting from the aorta (Fig. 94-4). The margins are typically irregular, and there is often an intimal flap that forms a "collar" at the neck of the pseudoaneurysm. Note that the injury to the intima may extend several centimeters proximal or distal to the visualized pseudoaneurysm. The extent of the injury, especially the proximal extent, is crucial in the planning of repair because branch vessel involvement has a major influence on repair technique.

Intimal Flap

An intimal flap arises from blood dissecting through an intimal tear as described earlier. It is commonly but not always seen in association with a pseudoaneurysm. To best visualize a flap and to avoid a false-negative diagnosis, thin-section images and an appropriate window must be employed. An intimal flap can be obscured by thick-slab maximum intensity projection images or rendered undetectable by suboptimal windowing during subsequent viewing. Care must be taken to evaluate source or single-voxel multiplanar reconstruction images to ensure that an intimal flap is not present.

A potential complication of an intimal flap is the formation of thrombus, which may subsequently embolize and cause distal organ infarction.

Contour Abnormality

Whereas a pseudoaneurysm presents an obvious contour abnormality, more subtle contour changes without obvious irregularity are sometimes seen. The aortic lumen is of relatively constant diameter from the distal arch through the aortic hiatus in most patients, with the occasional exception of congenital narrowing at the isthmus, which is typically mild and smooth. A change in contour of the aorta in the setting of suspected aortic injury may represent dissection of blood into the aortic wall without a visible intimal flap. The contour of the arch and descending thoracic aorta is usually better assessed on multiplanar reconstruction or maximum intensity projection images than on axial images.

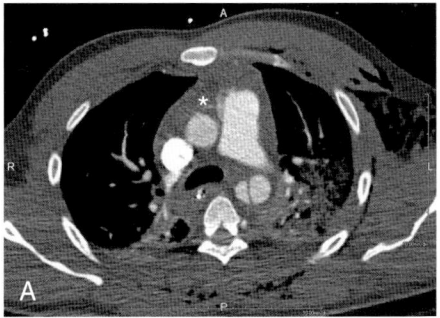

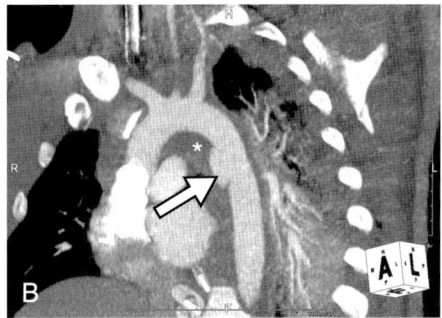

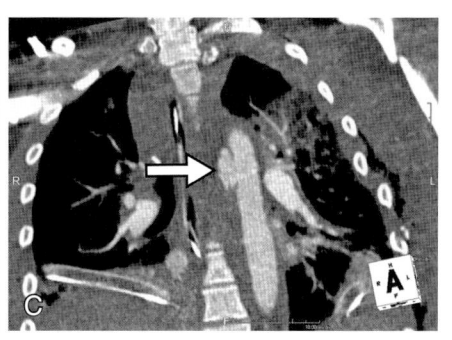

■ **FIGURE 94-4** Axial CT image in a trauma patient demonstrates an intimal flap in the proximal descending thoracic aorta (**A**). Oblique sagittal maximum intensity projection (**B**) and oblique coronal (**C**) reformatted images depict a pseudoaneurysm (*arrow*). Note extensive mediastinal hematoma (*asterisk*) diffusely engulfing the aorta, great vessels, and remainder of the mediastinal structures.

Periaortic Mediastinal Hemorrhage

Mediastinal hemorrhage is an indirect sign of thoracic aortic trauma, being attributable to aortic injury in only 12.5% of cases.[7] Arterial disruption of one of the great thoracic vessels with active contrast extravasation from the vessel into the hematoma represents a potentially catastrophic injury in which the patient would be highly unstable. Traumatic mediastinal hemorrhage, however, is most commonly caused by rupture of small mediastinal veins.

The location of mediastinal hematoma is a guide to its cause. Hematoma abutting the sternum or vertebral body should suggest fracture. Likewise, hematoma surrounding the aorta should provoke a thorough evaluation of the aorta for direct signs of injury (Fig. 94-5). Nevertheless, an isolated finding of mediastinal hemorrhage, even if it is periaortic, is unlikely to be accompanied by aortic injury if no direct sign of aortic injury is seen.[8] In addition, mediastinal hematoma can track inferiorly. The presence of retrocrural hematoma on an abdominal CT image should prompt careful evaluation of the thorax for vascular injury.

Contrast Agent Extravasation

On CT, the extravasation of contrast agent from an aortic injury is diagnosed by the presence of high-density streaks or puddles within a mediastinal hematoma, but it is a very rare finding. Such patients are extremely unstable. In one series of four patients with contrast agent extravasation from thoracic aortic trauma, none survived.[9]

Magnetic Resonance

MR can be used to depict the findings of aortic trauma (Fig. 94-6). However, the typically longer duration of the examination (relative to CT), difficulty of monitoring the patient, and relative lack of 24-hour emergent availability combine to exclude MR in most cases from evaluation for acute traumatic aortic injury. In equivocal or unusual cases, MR can be an effective problem-solving tool. The diagnosis of very small pseudoaneurysms and intimal flaps, moreover, can be challenging on MR because of the generally inferior spatial resolution compared with MDCT (Fig. 94-7).

In rare patients, severe associated traumatic injuries preclude acute treatment of an aortic injury, and a chronic pseudoaneurysm develops that may be managed conservatively. MR is an appropriate modality for close imaging follow-up of these patients (Fig. 94-8). Key sequences include ECG-gated cine steady-state free precession, three-dimensional steady-state free precession MR angiography, and gadolinium-enhanced three-dimensional MR angiogra-

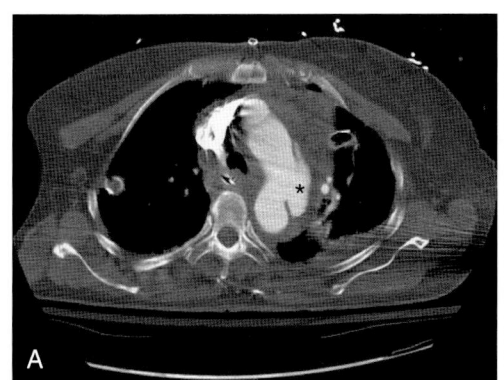

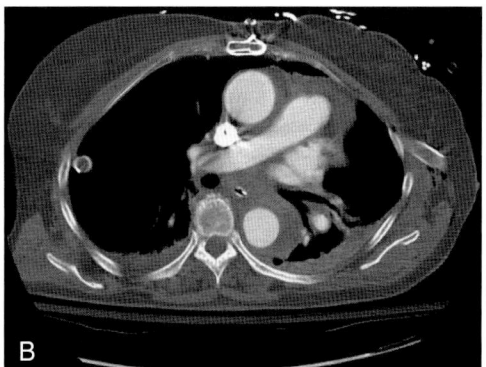

■ **FIGURE 94-5** Extensive mediastinal hematoma surrounds a traumatic aortic injury (**A**; intimal tear with pseudoaneurysm, *asterisk*). The hematoma tracks inferiorly in the mediastinum, surrounding the descending aorta (**B**). If hematoma is seen in a retrocrural location on the superior aspect of an abdominal CT image, aortic injury must be suspected.

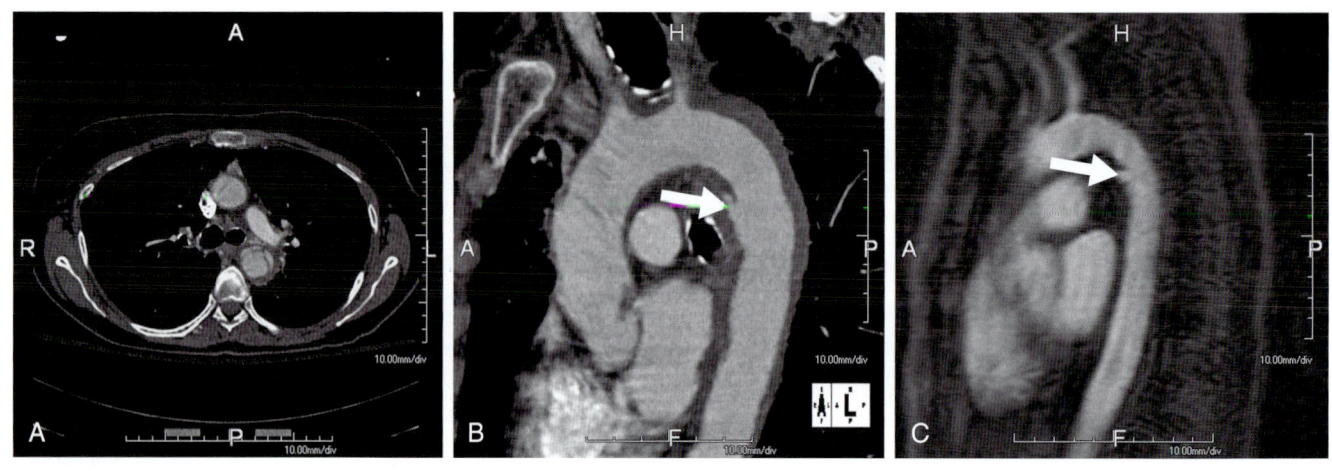

■ **FIGURE 94-6** Traumatic aortic injury with intimal flap and pseudoaneurysm as depicted on axial CT (**A**) and oblique sagittal CT (**B**, *arrow*) images. Oblique sagittal postcontrast T1-weighted MR image (**C**) obtained 1 day after CT demonstrates the same findings (*arrow*).

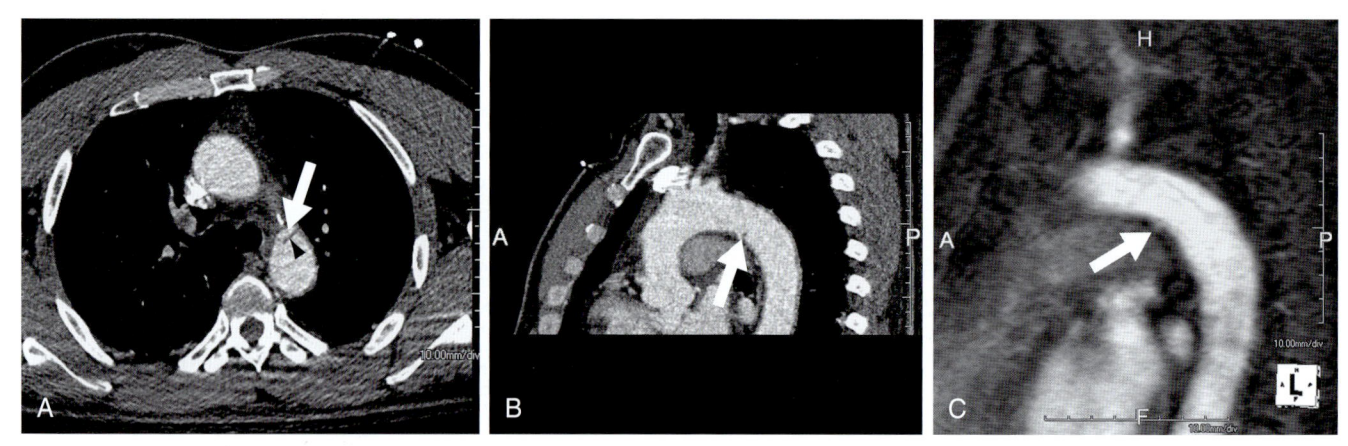

■ **FIGURE 94-7** Axial CT image (**A**) and oblique sagittal reconstruction (**B**) demonstrate a faint intimal flap (*arrowhead*) with a very small pseudoaneurysm (*arrow*). Oblique sagittal postcontrast T1-weighted MR image (**C**) acquired 1 day after CT demonstrates less clearly than on CT the small pseudoaneurysm (*arrow*) but highlights the limits of spatial resolution of MR imaging in this clinical setting.

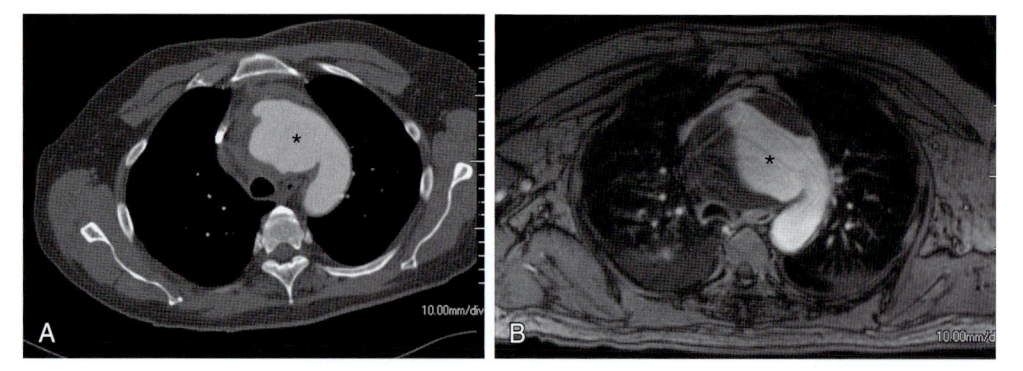

■ **FIGURE 94-8** Axial CT image (**A**) demonstrates a large acute pseudoaneurysm (*asterisk*) with surrounding mediastinal hematoma. Axial postcontrast T1-weighted MR image (**B**) acquired 3 years later shows no interval increase in size of the pseudoaneurysm (*asterisk*).

phy of the chest. ECG gating is particularly helpful for evaluation of the aortic root.

Nuclear Medicine/Positron Emission Tomography

Nuclear medicine/positron emission tomography has no role in evaluation of aortic trauma.

Angiography

Before the wide availability of CT, conventional angiography was the definitive modality for work-up of suspected aortic injury. Angiographic technique requires evaluation of the entire aorta. At least two projections are used, most commonly a 45-degree left anterior oblique view followed by a steep left anterior oblique or lateral view. Imaging findings of intimal flaps and change in aortic contour are similar to the CT findings, although care must be taken to ensure that subtle findings are not missed because of obscuration by the contrast column.

Classic Signs

Mediastinal Widening

The finding of a widened mediastinum on plain film in a patient with a history of a significant traumatic event must trigger suspicion for traumatic aortic injury. Although neither sensitive nor specific, a widened mediastinum cannot be ignored, and more definitive imaging should be pursued. Specificity may be added by deviation of the trachea to the right or indistinctness of the contour of the aortic knob.

Unfortunately, in a trauma setting or intensive care unit, plain films are often anteroposterior plain films (i.e., the x-ray tube is located anterior to the patient, and the film or film screen is placed behind the patient). On anteroposterior plain films, there is inherent artifactual widening of the mediastinal contour compared with a standard posteroanterior radiograph, making the use of this sign less effective in these settings.

Pseudoaneurysm

A traumatic pseudoaneurysm is typically seen as a rounded bulge projecting anteriorly from the juxtaductal region (junction of distal aortic arch and proximal descending aorta) of the thoracic aorta. It represents bulging of the adventitia caused by dissection of blood through an intimal and medial tear. The residual torn intima is often seen as a flap at the margin of the pseudoaneurysm. The finding of a juxtaductal pseudoaneurysm almost invariably indicates aortic trauma. The main differential diagnosis involves a ductus bump or ductus diverticulum, which is a remnant of the ligamentum arteriosum. However, the ductus diverticulum displays a smooth contour, with obtuse angles with the aortic wall, as opposed to the irregular and acutely angled pseudoaneurysm. The presence of an intimal flap confirms the presence of a pseudoaneurysm. Pseudoaneurysms outside the juxtaductal region should suggest other causes, notably infectious etiologies (mycotic aneurysm) and atherosclerosis.

Intimal Flap

An intimal flap within the lumen of the aorta, in the setting of trauma, is highly suggestive of an acute traumatic aortic injury. Alternatively, the intimal tear may represent a concomitant nontraumatic aortic pathologic process, such as aortic dissection. Findings that increase specificity for a traumatic etiology include location in the juxtaductal region of the thoracic aorta and presence of a pseudoaneurysm or mediastinal hemorrhage.

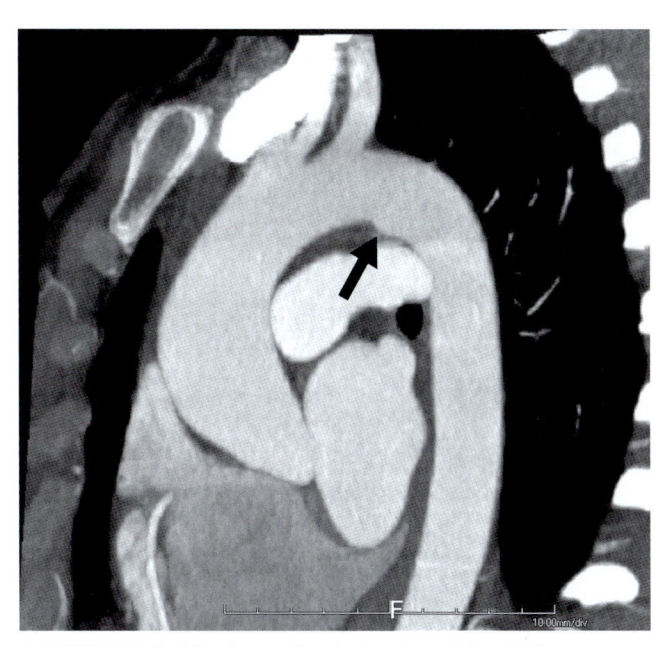

■ **FIGURE 94-9** The ductus diverticulum (*arrow*) is a shallow depression with smooth contours and obtuse margins with the aorta. This is distinct from the appearance of a traumatic aortic pseudoaneurysm (compare with Figs. 94-1 and 94-10), which has acute margins with the aorta.

Differential Diagnosis

Ductus Diverticulum

The ligamentum arteriosum, the remnant of the ductus arteriosus, inserts along the anterior undersurface of the aortic isthmus. At this location, a common variant is a small anterior bulge of the aortic lumen, known as a ductus bump or ductus diverticulum. A ductus diverticulum (Fig. 94-9) demonstrates a smooth contour and obtuse angles with the aortic wall and is distinct from the appearance of an aortic intimal tear with pseudoaneurysm (Fig. 94-10), in which there are acute angles and often an irregular contour.

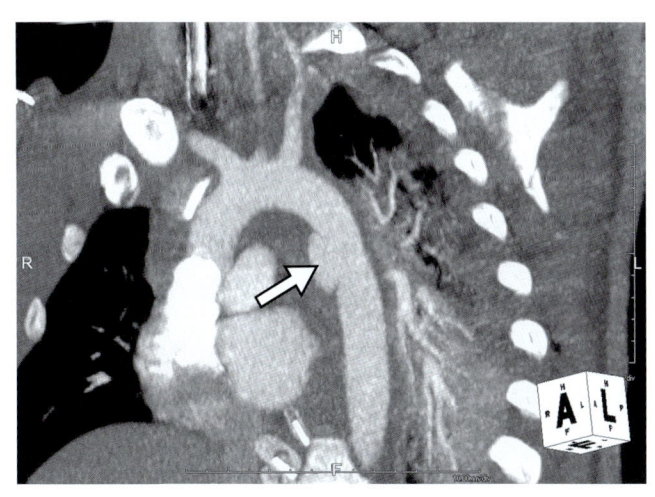

■ **FIGURE 94-10** Traumatic aortic pseudoaneuryms (*arrow*) with acute margins of a traumatic pseudoaneurysm (similar to that shown in Fig. 94-1).

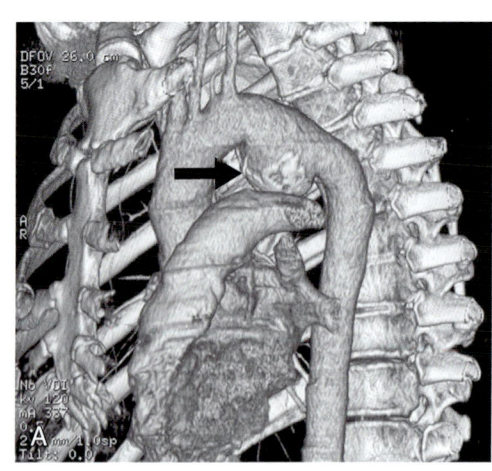

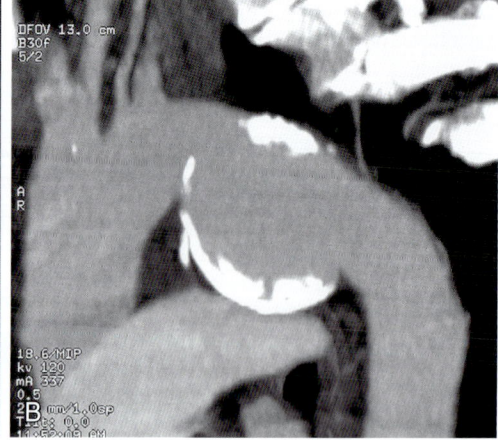

FIGURE 94-11 Volume rendered (A) and maximum intensity projection (B) images demonstrate a chronic calcified pseudoaneurysm (A, *arrow*) from a remote traumatic event.

Synopsis of Treatment Options

Medical

Identification of aortic injury is critical; 40% of patients who survive to reach the emergency department but are not diagnosed will die within 24 hours.[6] There is no role for medical management of traumatic aortic injury. However, a patient will occasionally present with an enlarging aortic pseudoaneurysm years after a traumatic event (Fig. 94-11). This is due to either a rare case of survival of a missed minor traumatic aortic injury or a known injury that was not treated surgically because of severe concomitant injury. Over time, there is gradual progression from intimal tear to pseudoaneurysm. Intervention will usually be required. In other cases, the presenting feature of a missed aortic injury may be due to thrombus formation on the damaged intima, which introduces the potential complication of distal embolization.

Surgical/Interventional

The standard therapy for traumatic aortic injury is surgical repair. The surgical approach is commonly through a left lateral thoracotomy, although unusual sites of aortic injury may require an alternative approach. For example, a mid-arch dissection may be more easily approached through a median sternotomy.[10] An open repair is associated with high morbidity and mortality, not least due to the usually extensive accompanying injuries. Emergent surgical repair carries a 15% to 50% mortality rate.[11-13] The recent introduction of endovascular techniques to treat these patients has led to a reduced mortality rate and has also enabled the treatment of patients who are not candidates for open thoracic surgery. Recent data demonstrate that use of endovascular techniques in place of open repair in aortic trauma has increased from 0% to 64% of cases from 1997 to 2007, with concomitant reduction by more than 50% in mortality and paraplegia rates.[14,15]

Endovascular stent graft placement requires a proximal aortic neck of at least 15 mm for safe graft attachment (Fig. 94-12). In the case of aortic isthmus injury, the lesion is frequently too close to the left subclavian artery to provide a suitable attachment site ("landing zone") for the stent graft. In this case, the left subclavian artery may be intentionally covered, provided patency of both vertebral arteries can be demonstrated before graft placement as

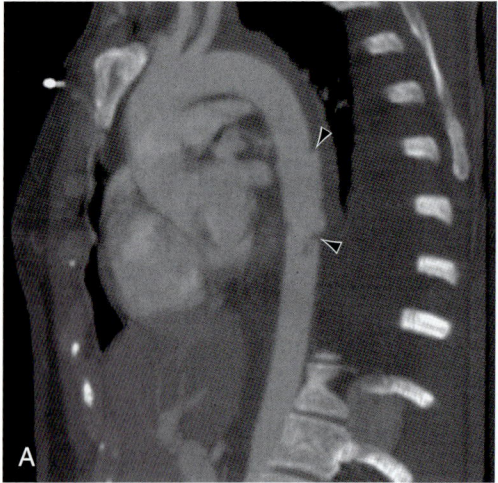

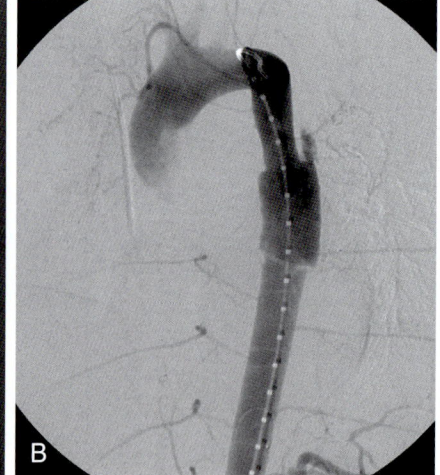

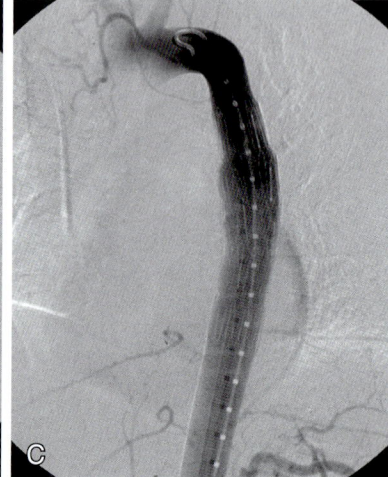

FIGURE 94-12 Traumatic aortic injury (*arrowheads*) in the mid descending thoracic aorta, distant from the arch vessels on oblique sagittal CT reconstruction (A). The injury was successfully treated with endovascular stent graft placement (before stenting, B; after stenting, C). *(Courtesy of Dr. K. Kolbeck.)*

the vertebral arteries enable collateral filling of the subclavian artery (i.e., left subclavian "steal" filling through left vertebral artery). In most patients, this will suffice. If vertebrobasilar or arm ischemia develops, a carotid-subclavian transposition or shunt can be performed.[16]

Reporting: Information for the Referring Physician

The referring physician should be informed of the imaging findings of thoracic aortic trauma in an urgent manner so that the patient may be treated without delay. Key information includes the proximal and distal extent of the lesion, as referenced to adjacent structures or branch vessels. The distance to the left subclavian artery is particularly important in determining the mode of repair; a proximal landing zone for a stent graft that does not occlude the vessel is preferred. A pseudoaneurysm should be characterized by its location, neck size, width, and depth. Presence or absence of mediastinal hematoma, and its precise location, should be noted. Rarely, active extravasation of contrast material may be seen and should be communicated to the trauma physicians immediately, before dictation of a report. The interpreting physician should also note concomitant injuries, which are not uncommon—for example, fractures, pulmonary contusion or laceration, and hemothorax. There may be associated cranial, cervical spine, or abdominal injuries.

If the imaging study is negative for aortic trauma, the report should confirm whether the study is technically adequate and correctly performed for the exclusion of such injury.

KEY POINTS

- Thoracic aortic trauma is a potentially fatal injury.
- MDCT is the definitive diagnostic tool, having replaced catheter angiography.
- Imaging findings include pseudoaneurysm, intimal flap, contour abnormality, and mediastinal hematoma.
- Therapy is most commonly by endovascular stent graft, although open surgery is a common alternative.

SUGGESTED READINGS

Alkadhi H, Wildermuth S, Desbiolles L, et al. Vascular emergencies of the thorax after blunt and iatrogenic trauma: multi-detector row CT and three-dimensional imaging. Radiographics 2004; 24:1239-1255.

Brinkman WT, Szeto WY, Bavaria JE. Overview of great vessel trauma. Thorac Surg Clin 2007; 17:95-108.

Fattori R, Buttazzi K, Russo V, et al. Evolving concepts in the treatment of traumatic aortic injury. A review article. J Cardiovasc Surg (Torino) 2007; 48:625-631.

Fisher RG, Sanchez-Torres M, Whigham CJ, et al. "Lumps" and "bumps" that mimic acute aortic and brachiocephalic vessel injury. Radiographics 1997; 17:825-834.

Hoffer E, Forauer A, Silas A, Gemery JM. Endovascular stent-graft or open surgical repair for blunt thoracic aortic trauma: systematic review. J Vasc Interv Radiol 2008; 19:1153-1164. Epub 2008 Jun 27.

Mirvis SE, Shanmuganathan K. Diagnosis of blunt traumatic aortic injury 2007: still a nemesis. Eur J Radiol 2007; 64:27-40.

Nzewi O, Slight RD, Zamvar V. Management of blunt thoracic aortic injury. Eur J Vasc Endovasc Surg 2006; 31:18-27.

Walsh SR, Tang TY, Sadat U, et al. Endovascular stenting versus open surgery for thoracic aortic disease: systematic review and meta-analysis of perioperative results. J Vasc Surg 2008; 47:1094-1098.

REFERENCES

1. Parmley LF, Mattingly TW, Manion WC, et al. Non-penetrating traumatic injury of the aorta. Circulation 1958; 17:1086-1101.
2. Crass JR, Cohen AM, Motta AO, et al. A proposed new mechanism of traumatic aortic rupture: the osseous pinch. Radiology 1990; 176:645-649.
3. Groskin SA. Selected topics in chest trauma. Radiology 1992; 183:605-617.
4. Creasy JD, Chiles C, Routh WD, et al. Overview of traumatic injury of the thoracic aorta. Radiographics 1997; 17:27-45.
5. Demetriades D, Gomez H, Velmahos GC, et al. Routine helical computed tomographic evaluation of the mediastinum in high-risk blunt trauma patients. Arch Surg 1998; 133:1084-1088.
6. Dyer DS, Moore EE, Mestek MF, et al. Can chest CT be used to exclude aortic injury? Radiology 1999; 213:195-202.
7. Sandor F. Incidence and significance of traumatic mediastinal hematoma. Thorax 1967; 22:43-62.
8. Sammer M, Wang E, Blackmore CC, et al. Indeterminate CT angiography in blunt thoracic trauma: is CT angiography enough? AJR Am J Roentgenol 2007; 189:603-608.
9. Mirvis SE, Shanmuganathan K. Diagnosis of blunt traumatic aortic injury 2007: still a nemesis. Eur J Radiol 2007; 64:27-40.
10. Leshnower BG, Litt HI, Gleason TG. Anterior approach to traumatic mid aortic arch transection. Ann Thorac Surg 2006; 81:343-345.
11. Lamme B, de Jonge IC, Reekers JA, et al. Endovascular treatment of thoracic aortic pathology: feasibility and mid-term results. Eur J Vasc Endovasc Surg 2003; 25:532-539.
12. Kato N, Dake MD, Miller DC, et al. Traumatic thoracic aortic aneurysm: treatment with endovascular stent grafts. Radiology 1997; 205:657-662.
13. Kasirajan K, Heffernan D, Langsfeld M. Acute thoracic aortic trauma: a comparison of endoluminal stent grafts with open repair and nonoperative management. Ann Vasc Surg 2003; 17:589-595.
14. Hoffer E, Forauer A, Silas A, Gemery JM. Endovascular stent-graft or open surgical repair for blunt thoracic aortic trauma: systematic review. J Vasc Interv Radiol 2008; 19:1153-1164. Epub 2008 Jun 27.
15. Demetriades D, Velmahos GC, Scalea TM, et al. Diagnosis and treatment of blunt thoracic aortic injuries: changing perspectives. J Trauma 2008; 64:1415-1418.
16. Gonzalo G, Fernández-Velilla M, Martí M, et al. Endovascular stent-graft treatment of thoracic aortic disease. Radiographics 2005;25:S229-S244.

CHAPTER 95

Thoracic Aortitis

Neil R.A. Isaac and Harold Litt

Aortitis is often characterized by inflammation of the media and adventitia.[1] Aortitis has many causes and may be related to autoimmune diseases or noninfectious causes as well as infection by microorganisms. Aortitis belongs to the group of diseases collectively known as the large-vessel vasculitides, as defined by the Chapel Hill Consensus Conference on the classification of systemic vasculitides.[2] Regardless of the source, inflammation of the aorta often results in dilation of the aortic root and aortic insufficiency. As a consequence, aortic valve replacement with aortic root reconstruction is often needed. It can be divided into an acute inflammatory phase and a chronic fibrotic phase.

Classification can be based on whether the aortitis is inflammatory. Other classification systems are based on whether the cause is associated with antineutrophil cytoplasmic antibodies. The exact cause is often difficult to define with certainty (Table 95-1).

Nonspecific aortic inflammation can also be seen in atherosclerosis. Because assessment of the vessel wall is critical in these patients, magnetic resonance angiography (MRA) or computed tomographic angiography (CTA) is preferred to conventional angiography. In general, inflammatory aortitis tends to affect the thoracic aorta rather than the abdominal aorta, whereas atherosclerosis affects the abdominal aorta.[3]

The more common diseases are discussed in this chapter.

TAKAYASU ARTERITIS
Definition

Takayasu arteritis was first described in 1908 by a Japanese ophthalmologist. This is a chronic vasculitis of unknown etiology affecting the aorta and its primary branches that can progress to ischemia or occlusion. The inflammation causes thickening of the walls of the affected arteries. The proximal aorta may become dilated secondary to inflammatory injury. Narrowings and occlusions are more common, but dilation of involved portions of the arteries can also result in myriad symptoms. Aneurysmal disease occurs in as many as 20% of patients,[4] but mostly in the descending thoracic aorta (Table 95-2).

Prevalence and Epidemiology

The majority of reported cases are in Asian patients, but there is a worldwide distribution. Women are affected in 80% to 90% of cases, with an age at onset between 10 and 40 years. In Japan, up to 150 cases occur per year,[5] whereas there are about 1 to 3 new cases per year per million in the United States and Europe.[6]

Etiology and Pathophysiology
Laboratory Findings

Laboratory findings are typically not specific. As in any inflammatory process, there can be elevation of blood acute-phase reactants, such as erythrocyte sedimentation rate and C-reactive protein. There is also usually a normocytic, normochromic anemia suggestive of a chronic disease.

Manifestations of Disease
Clinical Presentation

Usual presenting symptoms are systemic or constitutional—fatigue, weakness, arthralgias, weight loss, and low-grade fever—probably secondary to released cytokines. Vascular symptoms are rare at presentation; when they do develop, it is secondary to dilation or stenosis of the affected vessels. Classically, the disease is characterized by stenosis, but the incidence of aneurysmal lesions is increasing (30% to 50%).[7] Patients may present in heart failure secondary to aortic dilation and regurgitation. Late-phase symptoms include diminished or absent pulses, bruits, hypertension, and heart failure (Fig. 95-1). Dissection is possible, but giant cell arteritis has a higher incidence.

CHAPTER 95 • Thoracic Aortitis

TABLE 95-1 Classification of Aortitis

Infectious	Noninfectious
Syphilis	Takayasu
	Giant cell
	Nonspecific, granulomatous
	Other

TABLE 95-2 Classification of Takayasu Arteritis by the American College of Rheumatology Classification Criteria*

Age at disease onset <40 years
Claudication of the extremities
Decreased brachial artery pressure
Difference of at least 10 mm Hg in systolic blood pressure between the arms
Bruit over both subclavian arteries or the abdominal aorta
Arteriographic narrowing or occlusion of the entire aorta, its primary branches, or large arteries in proximal upper or lower extremities, not due to atherosclerosis, fibromuscular dysplasia, or other causes

*If three of six criteria are met, patients are said to have Takayasu arteritis.

Subclavian artery involvement is very common and often results in a blood pressure difference between the arms of more than 10 mm Hg. Lesions proximal to the vertebral artery may result in amaurosis fugax and subclavian steal. Up to 50% of patients have involvement of the pulmonary arteries.[8] Pulmonary artery involvement can give rise to chest pain, dyspnea, hemoptysis, and pulmonary hypertension,[9] but pulmonary function is generally not compromised despite extensive involvement, although unilateral pulmonary artery occlusion has been reported.[10] Most frequently affected arteries apart from the aorta are subclavian (90%), carotid (45%), vertebral (25%), and renal (20%).[11] Angina secondary to coronary ostial narrowing or coronary involvement is also possible. Affected arteries need to have vasa vasorum and are thus muscular, a feature lacking in peripheral arteries, which explains their lack of involvement in this condition. Patients may also present with abdominal pain, diarrhea, and skin lesions such as erythema nodosum and pyoderma gangrenosum.

Imaging Indications and Algorithm

CT is the preferred initial modality for diagnosis, although MRI is equally sensitive. MRI is useful for follow-up. Ultra-

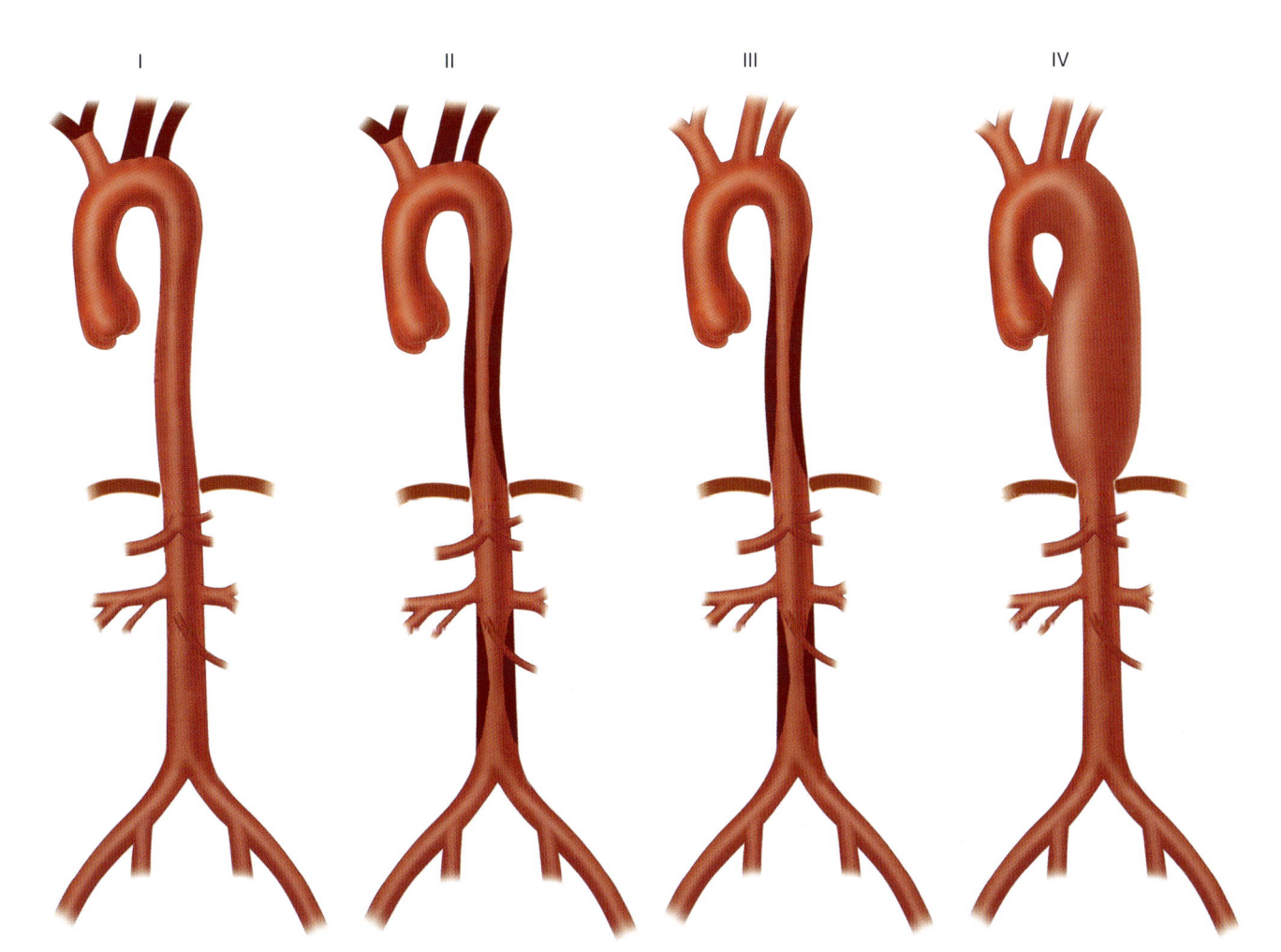

■ **FIGURE 95-1** Late-stage characteristics of Takayasu arteritis.

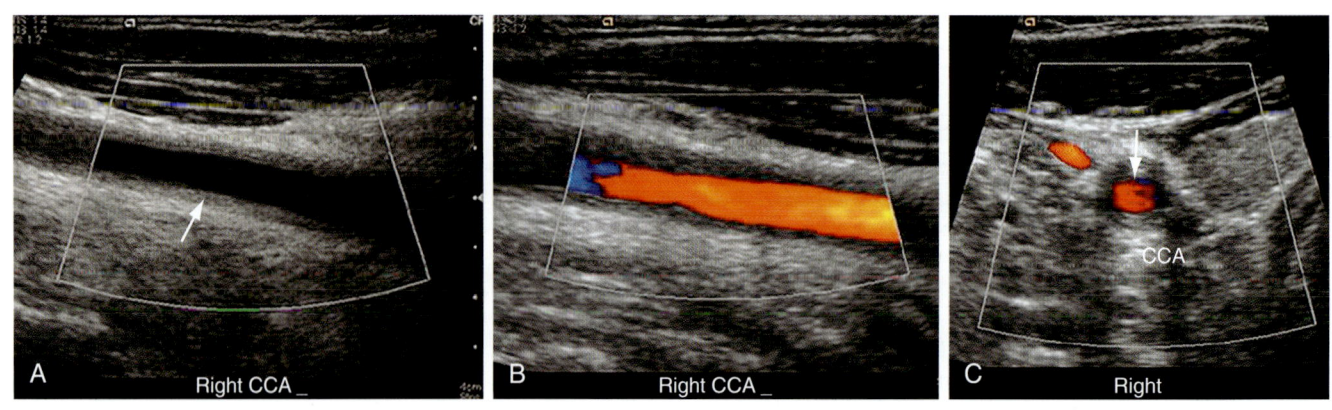

FIGURE 95-2 Takayasu arteritis. Carotid ultrasound images (**A**, gray scale; **B** and **C**, color) of a patient known to have Takayasu arteritis showing the wall thickening (*arrows*).

sonography is useful for assessment of neck vessels as well as for assessment of hemodynamics.

Imaging Techniques and Findings

Radiography

A dilated aorta or mediastinal widening may be seen from aneurysmal dilation of aortic branch vessels. The descending thoracic aorta may also have a wavy, scalloped appearance. In the late phase, calcification in the arch and descending aorta can be seen, sparing the ascending aorta.

Ultrasonography

Ultrasonography can detect perivasculitis, a rim of soft tissue around a great vessel, hypoechoic on ultrasound examination. One problem is that wall thickening may be indistinguishable from atherosclerotic plaque (Fig. 95-2). Intravascular ultrasound may detect subtle wall changes not seen on other techniques.

Echocardiography is useful to assess the ascending aorta for aneurysm formation, mural thickening, and aortic regurgitation; it can also assess pulmonary artery thickening. Transesophageal echocardiography may be useful for initial assessment of the descending thoracic aorta.

Computed Tomography

CT is usually the preferred initial examination; one can see mural calcification, and early disease detection portends a better prognosis. CT is good for detection and surveillance of arterial mural thickening, which decreases after steroid treatment. Typically, a double-ring pattern (poorly enhancing ring centrally, with a well-enhancing outside ring) can be seen. Perivasculitis, a rim of soft tissue around a great vessel that is hypodense on CT (vessel wall edema; Fig. 95-3), can also be detected. CT can also assess aortic or aortic branch vessel stenoses. The downside is ionizing radiation, especially in follow-up scans, as well as the need for iodinated contrast material, but it is a fast technique.

Magnetic Resonance

MR can detect mural thickening. It can also detect perivasculitis, a rim of soft tissue around a great vessel, along with aortic valvular thickening and pericardial effusion. Wall enhancement can be seen as an indicator of disease activity, secondary to edema and inflammation. Mural edema is seen as elevated T2 signal. Studies have shown reduced wall enhancement on follow-up, presumably secondary to reduced inflammation.[12] Three-dimensional

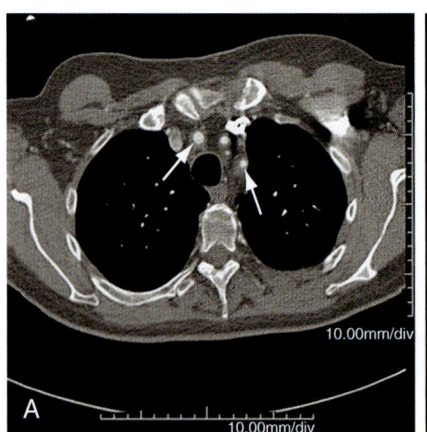

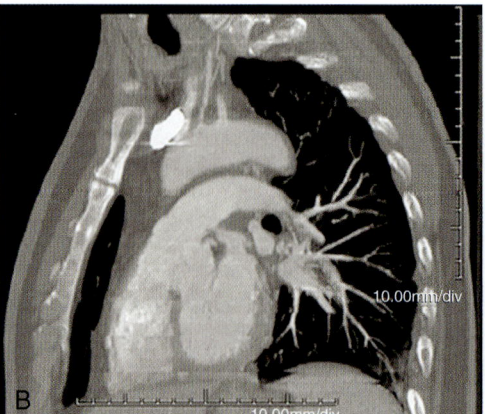

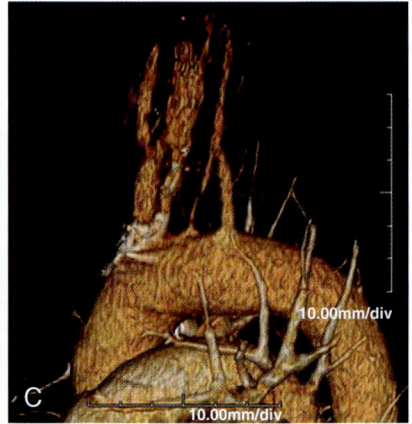

FIGURE 95-3 Takayasu arteritis. Axial (**A**), coronal (**B**), and volume rendered (**C**) CT images show diffuse involvement of the soft tissues surrounding the great vessels (*arrows*), with regions of stenosis (left common carotid) and mild dilation.

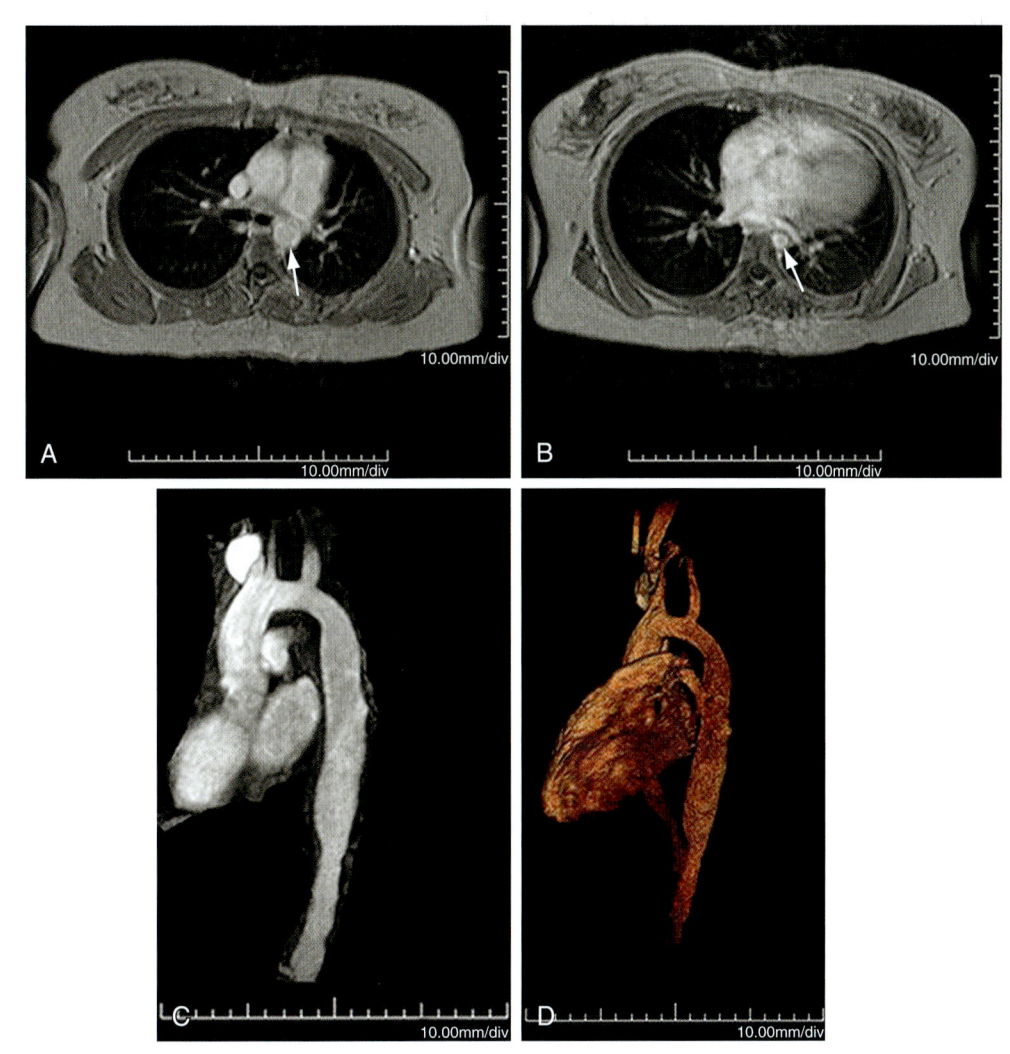

■ **FIGURE 95-4** Takayasu arteritis. **A,** Postcontrast T1-weighted gradient-echo MR image suggests subtle mural enhancement of the posterior wall of the descending thoracic aorta. **B,** Postcontrast T1-weighted gradient-echo MR image slightly lower than **A** shows a narrowing in the caliber of the descending thoracic aorta (*arrows*) from **A**. **C** and **D,** Maximum intensity projection (**C**) and volume rendered (**D**) images show the stenosis of the descending thoracic aorta as well as the mural irregularity.

MRA does have decreased sensitivity for small vessels in comparison with conventional angiography (Figs. 95-4 and 95-5). One can do cine sequences to detect aortic regurgitation. Maximum intensity projection images should be used with caution because they can exaggerate the degree of vascular stenoses. Whereas MR is a longer examination, it benefits from its lack of ionizing radiation exposure, a feature preferable for long-term surveillance of Takayasu arteritis, which typically affects younger women.

Nuclear Medicine/Positron Emission Tomography

Increased uptake of fluorodeoxyglucose (FDG) in regions of the aorta corresponds to abnormal regions on MRI.[13] Positron emission tomography (PET) should be able to distinguish mural thickening secondary to active inflammation from scar formation and can be used to assess response to treatment (Fig. 95-6).

Labeled white cells may reveal unsuspected large-vessel involvement. Gallium may also reveal large-vessel inflammation, but its sensitivity is reported as low. Perfusion defects on technetium Tc 99m albumin aggregated lung scans may also be seen if there is pulmonary artery stenosis.

Angiography

Angiography is the gold standard for evaluation of Takayasu arteritis. The examination must evaluate the thoracic and abdominal aorta; findings are most commonly seen in the aorta and its primary branches. Early changes, such as arterial wall thickening, cannot be well assessed. In the late phase, one primarily sees smooth-walled, tapered, or focally narrowed areas, usually involving the descending thoracic and abdominal aorta and the subclavian, common carotid, and renal arteries (Fig. 95-7). Late-phase dilation can be seen in the ascending aorta and right-sided brachiocephalic artery, but the walls are generally smooth, differentiating this from atherosclerotic aneurysm. Collaterals may be present as stenotic disease can be chronic. Whereas angiography can lead to angioplasty or stenting, it rarely leads to biopsy because central arteries are being imaged.

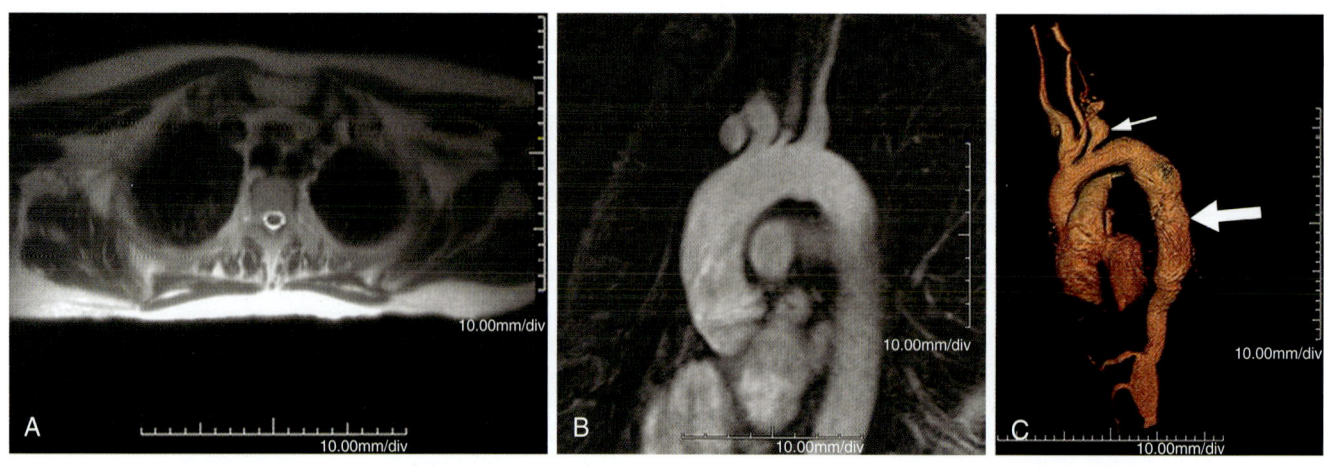

FIGURE 95-5 Takayasu arteritis. **A,** Axial T2-weighted fast spin-echo MR image reveals edema of the left subclavian artery. **B,** Sagittal oblique maximum intensity projection image from sagittal oblique contrast-enhanced three-dimensional MRA shows the mixed stenosis and dilation of the great vessels. **C,** Volume rendered image demonstrates the full extent of the disease, with regions of dilation of the descending aorta (*large arrow*) but also some stenosis and aneurysm of the left subclavian artery (*small arrow*).

Pulmonary artery evaluation is recommended only in those with pulmonary hypertension.

Synopsis of Treatment Options

Medical

Most patients are treated with intravenous or oral corticosteroids, either without or in combination with cyclophosphamide.

Surgical/Interventional

Angioplasty can be performed for stenotic (>70% or gradient >50 mm Hg) or obstructive lesions. Restenosis rates are lower when intervention is done in the relatively quiescent period or with postinterventional immunosuppressive treatment. Restenosis is reduced with stent placement.

Bypass grafts may also be used in patients with severe stenosis or occlusion of the aorta (Fig. 95-8).

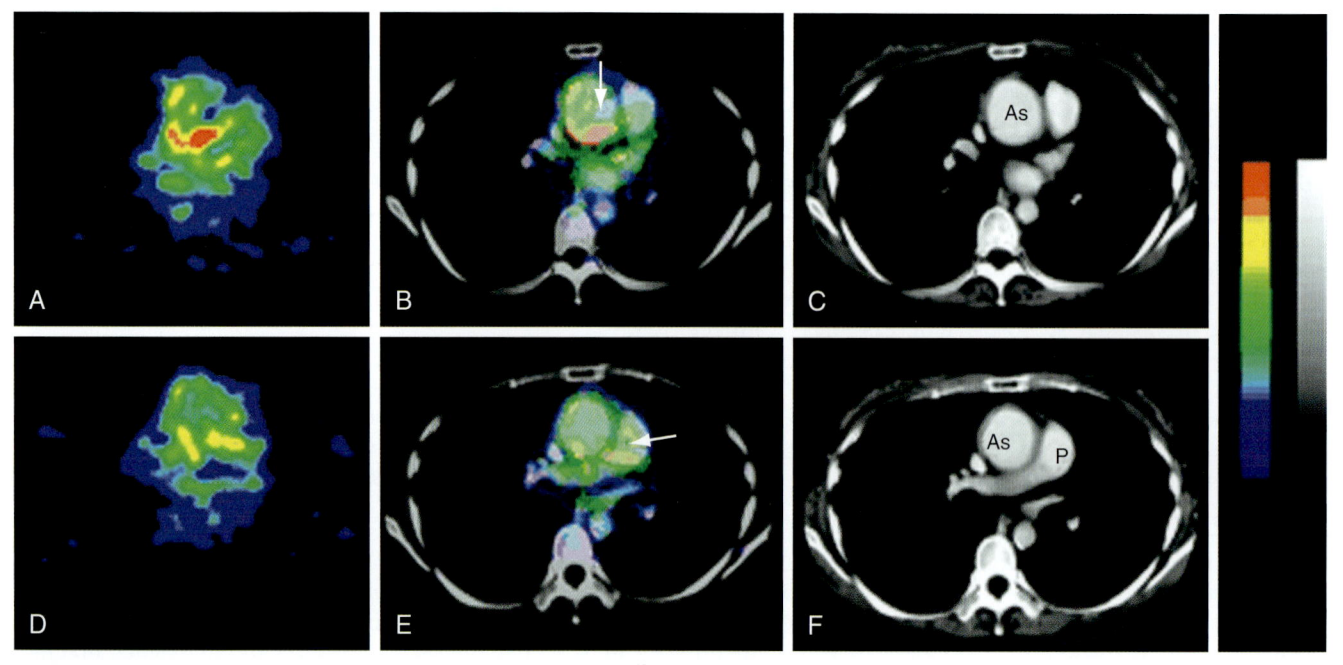

FIGURE 95-6 A 37-year-old woman with active Takayasu arteritis. ^{18}F-FDG-PET coregistered with enhanced CT revealed that ^{18}FDG accumulations were localized in the vascular wall of the ascending aorta and pulmonary artery. **A** and **D,** Axial images of ^{18}FDG-PET. ^{18}FDG accumulated in mediastinum. **B** and **E,** Coregistered PET with enhanced CT images; *arrows* indicate ^{18}FDG accumulation in ascending aorta (**B**) and pulmonary arteries (**E**). **C** and **F,** Enhanced reconstituted CT images at the same level of **A** and **D**. The ascending aorta was enlarged, causing aortic regurgitation. As, ascending aorta; P, pulmonary artery. *(From Kobayashi Y, Ishii K, Oda K, et al. Aortic wall inflammation due to Takayasu arteritis imaged with 18F-FDG PET coregistered with enhanced CT. J Nucl Med 2000; 46:917-922.)*

CHAPTER 95 • Thoracic Aortitis 1319

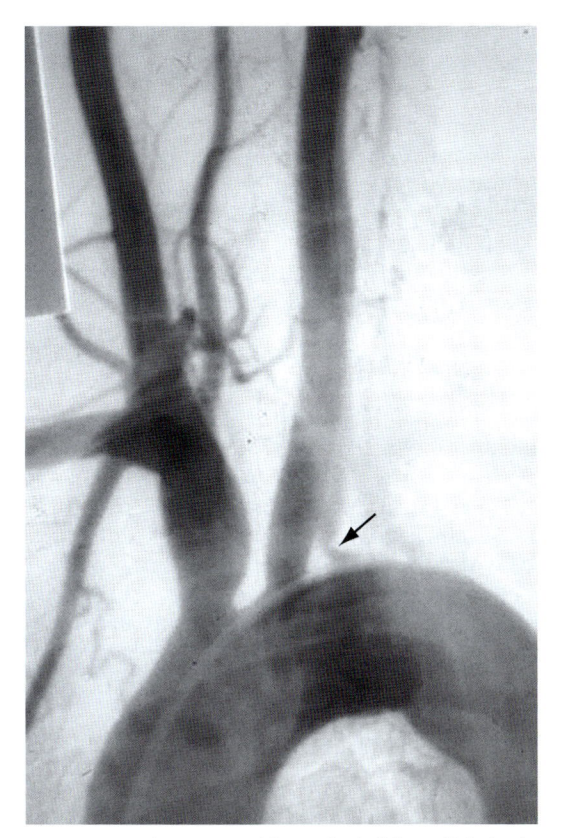

■ **FIGURE 95-7** Takayasu arteritis. Sagittal oblique digital subtraction angiography image shows the stenosis of the proximal right innominate artery and left common carotid artery. The left subclavian artery (*arrow*) is markedly stenotic or occluded proximally.

TABLE 95-3 Differential Characteristics of Takayasu Arteritis Versus Giant Cell Arteritis

Finding	Takayasu Arteritis	Giant Cell Arteritis
Female-to-male ratio	7:1	3:2
Age at onset	<40 years	>50 years
Ethnicity	Asian	European
Histopathology	Granulomatous inflammation	Granulomatous inflammation
Primary vessels involved	Aorta and branches	External carotid artery branches
Course	Chronic	Self-limited
Response to steroids	Excellent	Excellent
Surgical intervention	Common	Rare

Modified from Hunder GG. Clinical features and diagnosis of Takayasu arteritis. UpToDate 2007.

KEY POINTS

- Takayasu arteritis involves the large vessels; it affects the aorta and its primary branches.
- Inflammation causes wall thickening, which can lead to stenosis or dilation.
- There is a higher prevalence in Asian populations, and it is more common in women.
- It usually occurs in patients younger than 50 years.
- The main differential is giant cell aortitis, which can be ruled out by biopsy and the features in Table 95-3.

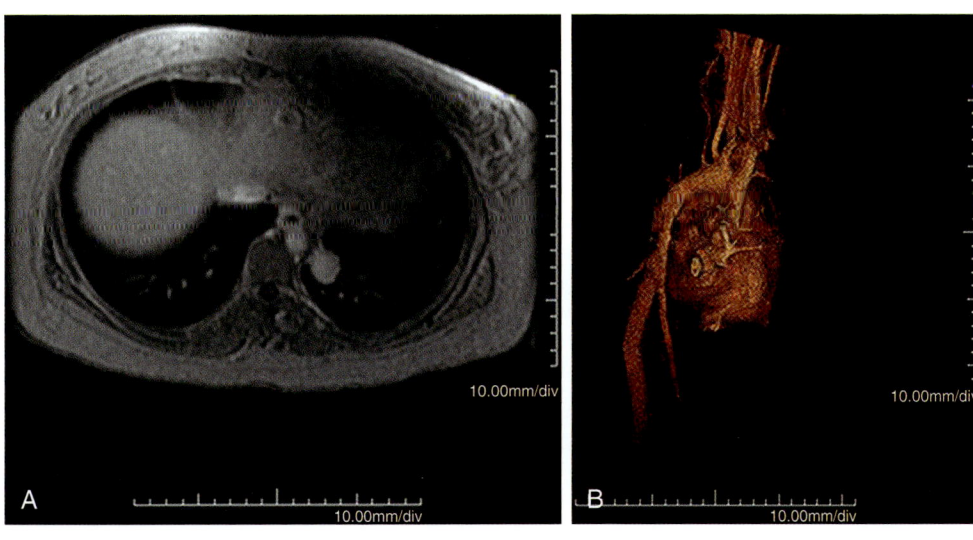

■ **FIGURE 95-8** Takayasu arteritis. **A,** Axial postcontrast T1-weighted gradient-echo image shows the aortic bypass graft centrally and the native, stenotic aorta laterally. **B,** Volume rendered image of the descending thoracic aorta shows the bypass graft, with the stenotic native vessel laterally.

TABLE 95-4 The American College of Rheumatology Criteria (1990) for the Diagnosis of Giant Cell Arteritis

Age at onset of 50 years
New headache
Abnormalities of the temporal arteries
Erythrocyte sedimentation rate of 50 mm/hr
Positive results of a temporal artery biopsy (vasculitis characterized by a predominance of mononuclear infiltrates or granulomas, usually with multinucleated giant cells)

GIANT CELL ARTERITIS

Definition

Giant cell arteritis, also known as temporal arteritis, is a chronic systemic panarteritis predominantly seen in elderly patents and affecting mainly cranial arteries. It affects large and medium-sized arteries, usually the cranial branches of arteries originating from the aortic arch and especially the temporal artery. Patients are at high risk for blindness; ischemic optic retinopathy develops in 20% to 50% of patients. Vision loss is often irreversible (Table 95-4). The etiology is unknown, but it may be autoimmune or secondary to infection; 10% to 15% of those with temporal artery involvement have aortic disease and often polymyalgia rheumatica.[14] The median time to development of aortic aneurysm after diagnosis of giant cell arteritis is 5.8 years.[15]

Prevalence and Epidemiology

Incidence in the United States is 15 to 30 cases per year per 100,000 in those older than 50 years.[16] In northern European countries, the annual incidence is more than 50 cases per 100,000.[17] Sex predilection is in women, especially of northern European descent, with a 2:1 ratio of women to men. The mean age at presentation is 72 years, and it is essentially never seen in the age group younger than 50 years.[18] A higher incidence is seen in Scandinavian countries.

Etiology and Pathophysiology

The exact etiology is unknown. The chronic inflammatory process involves the large arteries (aortic media), and the intima may wrinkle, giving a "tree bark" appearance. There is concentric intimal hyperplasia, and biopsy reveals necrotizing arteritis or a granulomatous process with multinucleated giant cells, although involvement can be patchy. Patients will have elevated inflammatory markers, such as erythrocyte sedimentation rate and C-reactive protein. There may also be a normocytic, normochromic anemia of chronic disease. Various cytokines may be released as a result of the inflammation. Some of the signs are indistinguishable from those of Takayasu arteritis.

Manifestations of Disease

Clinical Presentation

Systemic symptoms are a common presentation. Localized temporal headache of new onset is seen in at least two thirds of patients. Tenderness and decreased pulse of the temporal artery are other common signs. Presentation is usually a fever of unknown origin; 50% of patients suffer from jaw claudication.[19] A variety of visual symptoms can also occur, usually heralded by amaurosis fugax. Symptoms suggestive of aortic involvement are claudication of the upper or lower extremities, paresthesias, Raynaud phenomenon, abdominal angina, coronary ischemia, transient ischemic attacks, seizures, and aortic arch and great vessel steal phenomena. Aortic aneurysms with aortic regurgitation or dissection are possible. Dissection is more frequent with giant cell arteritis than with Takayasu arteritis. Polymyalgia rheumatica also occurs in 40% to 50% of patients.[19] Jaw claudication in patients older than 50 years is highly specific but only 40% to 50% sensitive for giant cell arteritis.[20] Giant cell arteritis is much less common in African Americans, and it affects women twice as commonly as men. Most patients present after the sixth decade, with a peak incidence between 60 and 80 years of age. Eighty-eight percent of large-vessel involvement occurs in women,[21] and large-vessel involvement sometimes occurs years after diagnosis and treatment of giant cell arteritis. Patients can also present with abdominal aortic involvement, resulting in abdominal aortic aneurysm and intestinal infarction.

Imaging Indications and Algorithm

Even if temporal artery biopsy findings are normal, one must consider great vessel giant cell arteritis as a possibility. MRA is the study of choice, especially if there are symptoms of arm claudication, although multidetector CTA could also be performed.

Imaging Techniques and Findings

Radiography

A dilated aorta may be visible on plain film.

Ultrasonography

The performance of ultrasound examination is highly operator dependent, although Doppler measurement may be useful for evaluation of extracranial vessels and can determine vessel wall thickness. Sonographic findings include a hypoechoic halo surrounding the artery, representing edema, and arterial stenoses or occlusions. Ultrasonography is also useful for assessment of aortic regurgitation or ascending aortic aneurysm, and it can be used for screening or follow-up of abdominal aortic aneurysms.

Computed Tomography

Aortic aneurysms or dissection may be detected, although these are seen in only 15% of patients. CT can discern vessel wall thickness and lumen configuration, with the ability to assess wall enhancement as a measure of inflammation and edema. Long, smooth, tapering stenoses with areas of dilation may also be seen in subclavian, axillary, and brachial arteries. CT may be useful in patients with

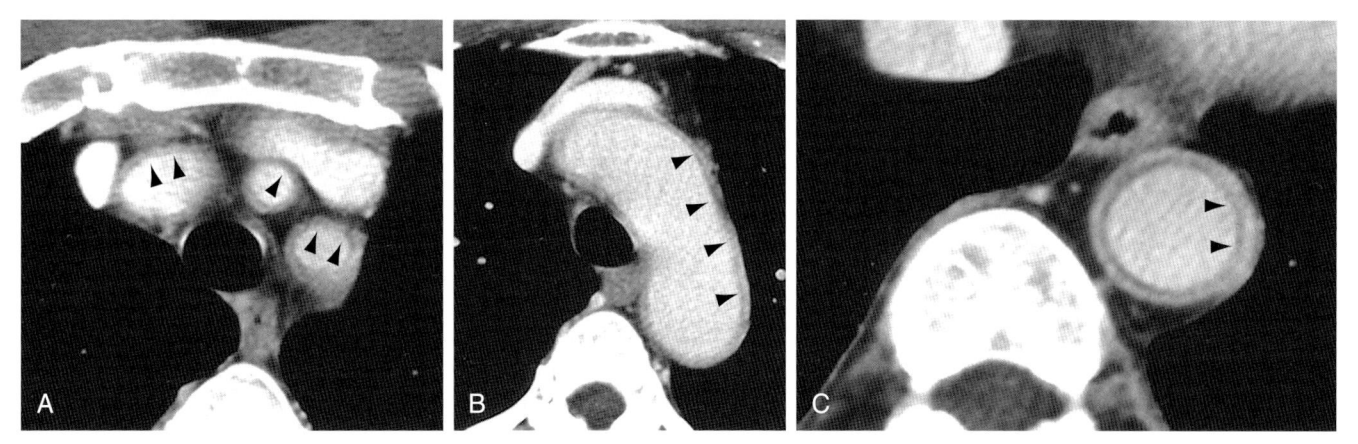

■ **FIGURE 95-9** Giant cell arteritis. **A,** Axial contrast-enhanced chest CT image shows diffuse thickening (*arrowheads*) of walls of great vessels (*left to right*, right brachiocephalic artery, left common carotid artery, left subclavian artery). **B,** Axial contrast-enhanced chest CT image shows diffuse aortic arch wall thickening (*arrowheads*). **C,** Axial contrast-enhanced chest CT image shows extension of vasculitic process to descending aorta (*arrowheads*). *(From Bau JL, Ly JQ, Borstad GC, et al. Giant cell arteritis. AJR Am J Roentgenol 2003; 181:742.)*

multiple cranial infarcts for evaluation of the arteries (Fig. 95-9).

Magnetic Resonance

MR is the study of choice, especially for diagnosis of large-vessel giant cell arteritis. MR can also identify regional temporal artery involvement with edema or enhancement, thereby guiding biopsy. Disease activity and response to treatment can also be observed, probably secondary to vessel wall edema, a sign of early inflammatory change (Fig. 95-10). Aortic aneurysms or dissection may be seen, although these are detected in only 15% of patients. MR can discern vessel wall thickness and lumen configuration, with the ability to assess wall enhancement as a measure of inflammation and edema (Fig. 95-11). Long, smooth, tapering stenoses with areas of dilation may also be seen in subclavian, axillary, and brachial arteries.

Nuclear Medicine/Positron Emission Tomography

PET is highly specific but insensitive. Whole-body techniques are not effective for evaluation of temporal artery involvement secondary to brain uptake and background in the skin, but they may be more useful in evaluation of the great vessels and for follow-up after treatment.

Angiography

Angiography is seldom used for diagnosis. Aortic root dilation, aortic regurgitation, and dissection as well as stenosis may be seen. Long, smooth, tapering stenoses with areas of dilation may also be seen in subclavian, axillary, and brachial arteries as well as in cerebral arteries (Fig. 95-12). It is sensitive but not specific. It can be used to measure intravascular blood pressures distal to stenoses, especially if there is four-limb involvement with the disease.

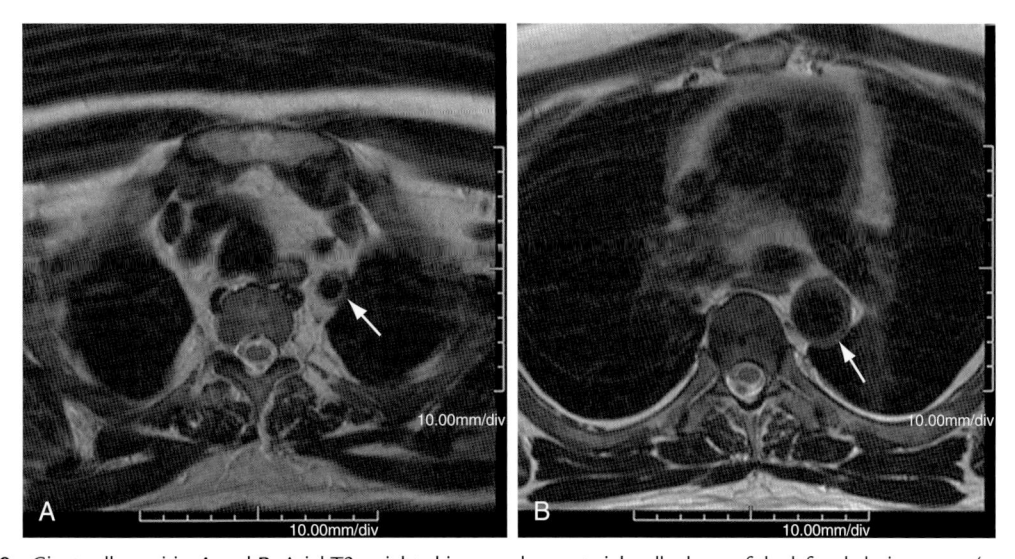

■ **FIGURE 95-10** Giant cell arteritis. **A** and **B,** Axial T2-weighted images show arterial wall edema of the left subclavian artery (*arrow*) (**A**) and descending aorta (*arrow*) (**B**), which are involved with giant cell arteritis.

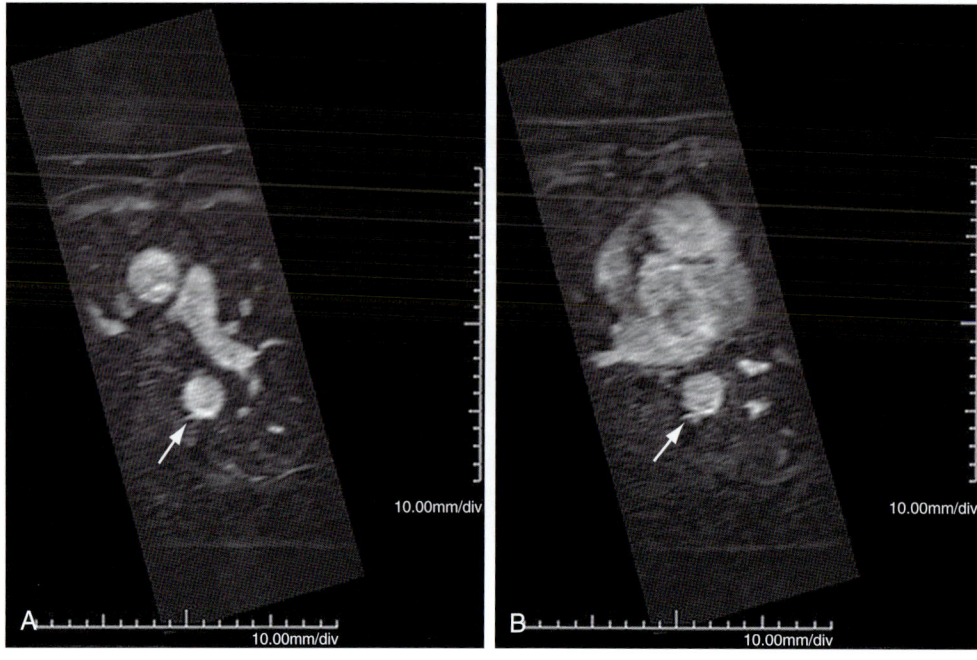

■ **FIGURE 95-11** Giant cell arteritis. Multiplanar reconstruction images (**A** and **B**) from gadolinium-enhanced three-dimensional MRA show enhancement and thickening of the posterior descending aortic wall (*arrow*) in a patient with giant cell arteritis.

Synopsis of Treatment Options

Medical

Glucocorticoids are the mainstay of treatment. Once there is clinical remission, steroids can be tapered and then discontinued. Relapses do require increased dosage and longer treatment periods.

Surgical/Interventional

Temporal artery biopsy is suggested in all cases of suspected giant cell arteritis, but the negative predictive value is at best 90%.[22]

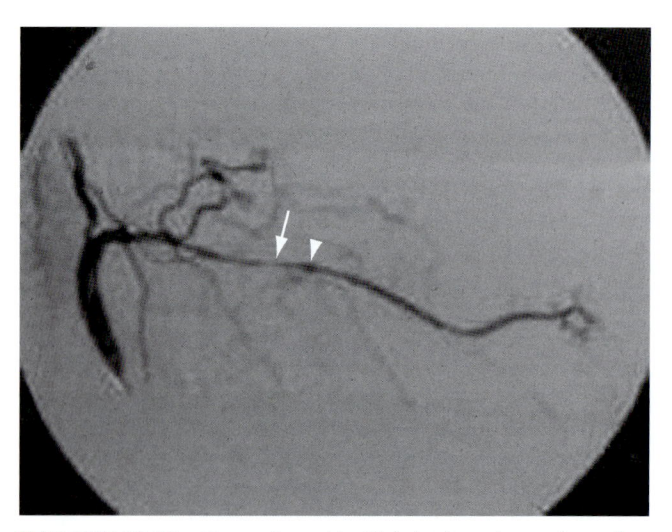

■ **FIGURE 95-12** Giant cell arteritis. Digital subtraction angiography image of the left arm shows regions of stenosis (*arrow*) and dilation (*arrowhead*) in the left subclavian artery.

KEY POINTS

- Giant cell arteritis is rare in those younger than 50 years.
- It often occurs in women of northern European descent.
- Aortic and aortic root involvement is seen in only 15%.
- Temporal artery biopsy (on the symptomatic side) is suggested in all suspected cases, and optimally, bilateral biopsy is performed.
- MRA is useful for large-vessel involvement and is the study of choice.

SYPHILITIC AORTITIS

Definition

Syphilitic aortitis is now exceedingly rare in developed countries, but it once accounted for 5% to 10% of all cardiovascular deaths. However, with the increase in sexually transmitted diseases worldwide, the incidence may increase in the future. Among untreated patients, aortitis occurs in up to 70% to 80%.[23] Cardiac complications usually occur in 10% of untreated cases. The latent period is 5 to 40 years, with disease usually occurring between 10 and 25 years (Table 95-5).

TABLE 95-5 Syphilitic Manifestations in Cardiovascular Disease

Syphilitic aortitis
Syphilitic aortic aneurysm
Syphilitic aortic valvulitis
Syphilitic coronary ostial stenosis

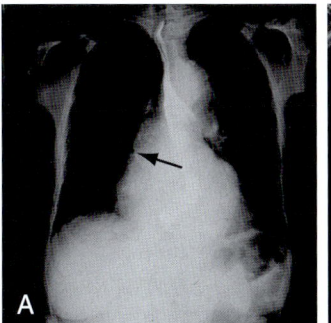

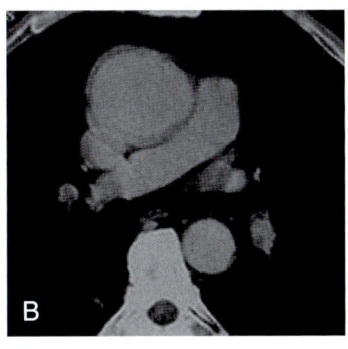

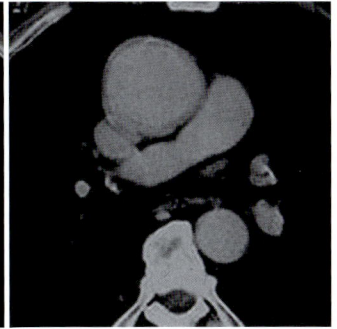

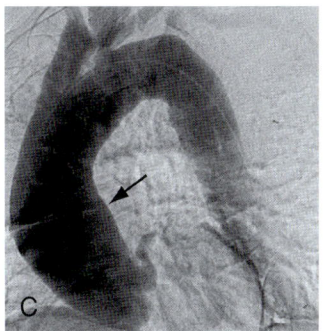

FIGURE 95-13 Syphilitic aortitis. **A,** Chest film obtained after barium ingestion in patient with syphilitic aortitis demonstrates rim calcification of the dilated ascending aorta (*arrow*). **B,** Axial CT scan after the administration of contrast material in a different patient with syphilitic aortitis shows circumferential wall thickening of the ascending aorta. **C,** Digital subtraction angiography in the same patient as in **B** shows dilated ascending aorta with wall irregularity (*arrow*).

Etiology and Pathophysiology

The initial lesion is a multifocal lymphoplasmacytic infiltrate around the vasa vasorum, extending into the media (endarteritis obliterans). Destruction of the media results in aortic dilation, which is also seen in Takayasu aortitis.

Manifestations of Disease

Clinical Presentation

Patients usually present with a combination of the aforementioned syphilitic complications, and syphilitic aortitis without aneurysm is uncommon. The aneurysms occur in the ascending aorta (47%), transverse arch (24%), abdominal aorta (7%), descending arch (5%), descending thoracic aorta (5%), multiple sites (4%), and sinus of Valsalva (<1%).[24] Commonly, syphilitic aortitis involves the sinotubular junction and also the sinuses of Valsalva, a feature different from Takayasu arteritis. Coronary ostial lesions are seen in 20% to 25% of patients with syphilitic aortitis but in only 0.1% of patients with coronary artery disease.[25] Dissection and intramural hematoma are rare. The aortitis usually involves the proximal aorta, only occasionally extending below the renal arteries.[1]

The syndrome of Döhle-Heller is tertiary syphilis: aortitis, sometimes complicated by aortic valve insufficiency; coronary stenosis; and aortic aneurysm. Men are affected more than women are.

Imaging Techniques and Findings

Radiography

The classic tree bark appearance is shared with other forms of aortitis, notably Takayasu arteritis.[26] On plain film, one may see a dense shadow, widening, and calcification of the aortic arch or possibly eggshell calcification outlining the aortic aneurysm. Calcification usually involves the ascending aorta (Fig. 95-13A).

Computed Tomography and Magnetic Resonance

Early, the wall is thickened (see Fig. 95-13B), with subsequent aneurysmal dilation and thinning. Calcification can also occur, as can aortic rupture, but dissection is rare. Aneurysms can be saccular or fusiform.

Angiography

Patients with bilateral coronary ostial lesions and no distal disease and patients with ascending thoracic aneurysms should be screened for syphilis (see Fig. 95-13C).

Synopsis of Treatment Options

Medical

Penicillin is the drug of choice, although duration and route of therapy are debatable. This is generally pursued if the infection is thought to be active.

Surgical/Interventional

Surgery may be needed for aortic valve or ascending aorta repair.

Differential Diagnosis for Thoracic Aortitis

From Clinical Presentation

- Fever of unknown origin
- Infective endocarditis
- Rheumatoid arthritis
- Multiple myeloma
- Non-Hodgkin lymphoma
- Dermatomyositis
- Systemic lupus erythematosus
- Tuberculosis
- Transient ischemic attacks
- Nonarteritic anterior ischemic optic neuropathy

From Imaging Findings (Mural Thickening and Luminal Stenosis or Aneurysm)

- Takayasu arteritis: young female patient with mural thickening, stenosis, or aneurysmal disease of the aorta and great vessels.
- Giant cell (temporal) arteritis: difficult distinction, but it can be made by history (older age of patient) and

distribution of lesions. Both involve large arteries, respond to steroids, and show granulomatous vasculitis at pathologic examination (see Table 95-3).
- Aortic dissection or intramural hematoma: intimal flap or hemorrhage in wall may be seen; predilection for aortic root or juxtaductal aortic arch.
- Tuberculosis: usually causes erosion of the vessel, resulting in true or false aneurysms.
- Atherosclerosis: older patient with mural plaque and typical risk factors (e.g., history of smoking, diabetes mellitus, obesity, hyperlipidemia).
- Ehlers-Danlos syndrome: can be associated with multiple aneurysms, which can rupture, but systemic signs of inflammation are absent.
- Ergotamine: can cause spasm of large vessels and mimic clinical findings (Fig. 95-14).
- Fibromuscular dysplasia: similar to Takayasu aortitis and more focal generally, but with no systemic symptoms.

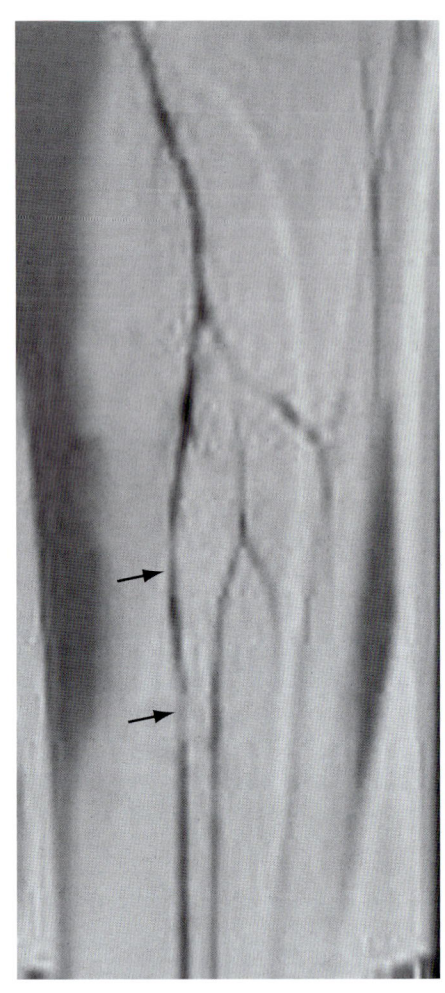

FIGURE 95-14 Ergotamine injection in left forearm on this digital subtraction angiography image shows marked stenosis of the radial artery (*arrows*), although the ulnar and brachial arteries are also involved.

SUGGESTED READINGS

Arend WP, Michel BA, Bloch DA, et al. The American College of Rheumatology 1990 criteria for the classification of Takayasu arteritis. Arthritis Rheum 1990; 33:1129-1134.
Gravanis MB. Giant cell arteritis and Takayasu aortitis: Morphologic, pathogenetic and etiologic factors. Int J Cardiol 2000; 1:S21-S33.
Jennette JC, Falk RJ, Andrassy K, et al. Nomenclature of systemic vasculitides. Proposal of an international consensus conference. Arthritis Rheum 1994; 37:187-192.
Paget SA, Leibowitz E. Giant cell arteritis. Available at: http://www.emedicine.com/med/topic2241.htm. Accessed May 21, 2008.
Tavora F, Burke A. Review of isolated ascending aortitis: differential diagnosis, including syphilitic, Takayasu's and giant cell aortitis. Pathology 2006; 38:302-308.

REFERENCES

1. Tavora F, Burke A. Review of isolated ascending aortitis: differential diagnosis, including syphilitic, Takayasu's and giant cell aortitis. Pathology 2006; 38:302-308.
2. Jennette JC, Falk RJ, Andrassy K, et al. Nomenclature of systemic vasculitides. Proposal of an international consensus conference. Arthritis Rheum 1994; 37:187-192.
3. Rojo-Leyva E, Ratliff NB, Cosgrove DM, Hoffman GS. Study of 52 patients with idiopathic aortitis from a cohort of 1204 surgical cases. Arthritis Rheum 2000; 43:901-907.
4. Weidner N. Giant cell vasculitides. Semin Diagn Pathol 2001; 18:24-33.
5. Koide K. Takayasu arteritis in Japan. Heart Vessels 1992; 7:48.
6. Arend WP, Michel BA, Bloch DA, et al. The American College of Rheumatology 1990 criteria for the classification of Takayasu arteritis. Arthritis Rheum 1990; 33:1129-1134.
7. Hotchi M. Pathological studies on Takayasu arteritis. Heart Vessels Suppl 1992; 7:11-17.

8. Nakabayashi K, Kurata N, Nangi N, et al. Pulmonary artery involvement as first manifestation in three cases of Takayasu arteritis. Int J Cardiol 1996; 54:S177.
9. Kerr GS, Hallahan CW, Giordano J, et al. Takayasu arteritis. Ann Intern Med 1994; 120:919.
10. Suzuki Y, Konishi K, Hisada K. Radioisotope lung scanning in Takayasu's arteritis. Radiology 1973; 109:133-136.
11. Shelhamer JH, Volkman DJ, Parillo JE, et al. Takayasu's arteritis and its therapy. Ann Intern Med 1985; 103:121-126.
12. Johnston SL, Lock RJ, Gompels MM. Takayasu arteritis: a review. J Clin Pathol 2002; 55:481-486.
13. Meller J, Strutz F, Siefker U, et al. Early diagnosis and follow up of aortitis with ^{18}F FDG PET and MRI. Eur J Nucl Med Mol Imaging 2003; 30:730-736.
14. Levine SM, Hellman DB. Giant cell arteritis. Curr Opin Rhematol 2002; 14:3-10.
15. Evans JM, O'Fallon WM, Hunder GG. Increased incidence of aortic aneurysm and dissection in giant cell (temporal) arteritis: a population based study. Ann Intern Med 1995; 122:502-507.
16. Huston KA, Hunder GG, Lie JT, et al. Temporal arteritis: a 25-year epidemiologic, clinical and pathologic study. Ann Intern Med 1978; 88:162-167.
17. Roque MR, Roque BL, Miserocchi E, Foster CS. Giant cell arteritis. Available at: http://www.emedicine.com/OPH/topic254.htm. Accessed May 21, 2008.
18. Smetana GW, Shmerling RH. Does this patient have temporal arteritis? JAMA 2002; 287:92.
19. Hunder GG. Clinical manifestations of giant cell (temporal) arteritis. UpToDate 2007. Available at: http://www.uptodate.com/online/content/topic.do?topicKey=vasculit/2816&selectedTitle=1~150&source=search_result. Accessed May 21, 2008.
20. Goodwin JS. Progress in gerontology: polymyalgia rheumatica and temporal arteritis. J Am Geriatr Soc 1992; 40:515-525.
21. Paget SA, Leibowitz E. Giant cell arteritis. Available at: http://www.emedicine.com/med/topic2241.htm. Accessed May 21, 2008.
22. Hall S, Persellin S, Lie JT, et al. The therapeutic impact of temporal artery biopsy. Lancet 1983; 2:1217.
23. Jackman JD, Radolf JD. Cardiovascular syphilis. Am J Med 1989; 87:425-433.
24. Heggtveit HA. Syphilitic aortitis. A clinicopathologic autopsy study of 100 cases 1950-1960. Circulation 1964; 29:346-355.
25. Yamanaka O, Hobbs RE. Solitary ostial coronary artery stenosis. Jpn Circ J 1993; 57:404-410.
26. Gravanis MB. Giant cell arteritis and Takayasu aortitis: Morphologic, pathogenetic and etiologic factors. Int J Cardiol 2000; 1:S21-S33.

CHAPTER 96

Subclavian Steal Syndrome

Dharshan Vummidi and Gautham P. Reddy

The aortic arch extends from approximately the level of the upper border of the second sternocostal articulation on the right, runs superiorly, posteriorly, and to the left in front of the trachea, where it then turns posteriorly left of the trachea and finally inferiorly on the left side of the body. The branches that conventionally arise from the arch are the right brachiocephalic artery, the left common carotid artery, and the left subclavian artery (see Chapter 71).

When stenosis or occlusion involves the subclavian artery, the vertebral artery can reverse direction to serve as a collateral pathway to reconstitute the subclavian artery, a phenomenon known as subclavian steal phenomenon, which can lead to brainstem ischemia and neurologic symptoms. This chapter will discuss the clinical manifestations, imaging evaluation, and treatment of subclavian steal.

DEFINITION

Subclavian steal syndrome is defined as stenosis or occlusion of the subclavian artery proximal to the origin of the vertebral artery, with consequent reversal of blood flow in the vertebral artery to supply the distal subclavian artery, resulting in neurologic symptoms. This reversal of flow is said to "steal" blood from the intracranial circulation, which can cause ischemia or stroke.[1] In the absence of neurologic symptoms, the constellation of findings can be called subclavian steal phenomenon.

PREVALENCE AND EPIDEMIOLOGY

Most patients with the syndrome are older than 50 years because of its association with atherosclerosis. If subclavian steal is found in young adults or children, Takayasu arteritis should be suspected.

ETIOLOGY AND PATHOPHYSIOLOGY

Atherosclerosis is the most common cause of subclavian steal syndrome. Although Takayasu arteritis is an infrequent cause of the syndrome, it occurs more commonly in people of Asian descent.[2]

Subclavian artery stenosis or occlusion proximal to the vertebral artery origin results in the alteration of vertebral artery hemodynamics. The low pressure in the subclavian system eventually results in reversal of flow in the ipsilateral vertebral artery, which serves as a source of collateral flow to the distal subclavian artery.

Vollmar and colleagues[3] have described four categories of subclavian steal phenomenon based on the vascular territories that provide and receive flow—vertebrovertebral, carotid-basilar, external carotid-vertebral, and carotid-subclavian. Another classification scheme[4] is based on the degree of hemodynamic disturbances of the vertebral artery: stage I (occult steal, decreased blood flow), stage II (partial steal, transient or partial reversal of flow), and stage III (complete steal, permanent reversal of flow).

When the collateral flow directs a large amount of flow into the subclavian artery and away from the brain, neurologic symptoms can occur. Such symptoms have been reported to occur in approximately 36% of patients.[5] Often, the circle of Willis can provide enough collateral circulation to the brainstem to avert neurologic symptoms. If the posterior communicating artery is stenotic, occluded, or absent, or if there is concomitant carotid disease, then neurologic symptoms are more likely to occur.

MANIFESTATIONS OF DISEASE

Clinical Presentation

Most patients with reversal of flow in the vertebral artery have neurologic symptoms.[5] In the absence of neurologic symptoms, patients are said to have subclavian steal phenomenon.

Neurologic symptoms of subclavian steal syndrome include lightheadedness, dizziness, vertigo, upper extremity numbness, visual alterations, transient ischemic attacks and, rarely, seizures or stroke.[6-8] Ipsilateral upper extremity exercise increases the blood flow demand in the subclavian artery and can cause transient neurologic symptoms caused by an increase in diversion of intracranial blood flow.[9]

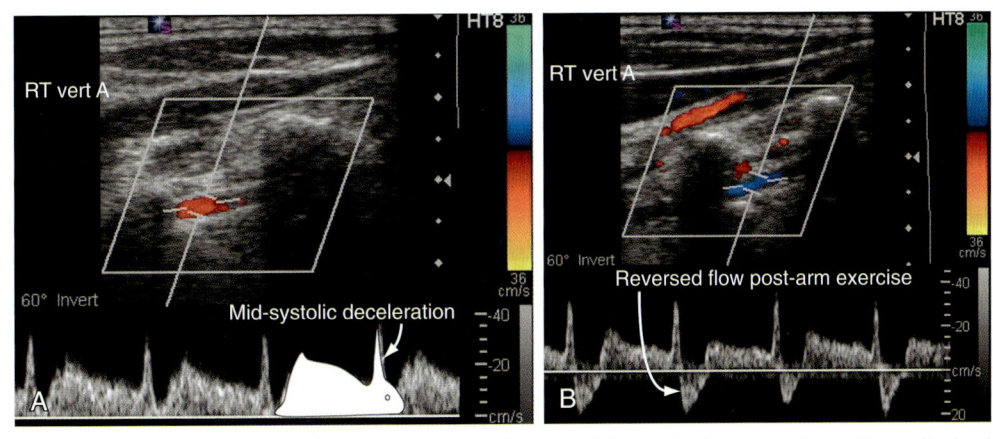

FIGURE 96-1 **A,** Occult steal. Pulsed wave Doppler spectral ultrasound image of the vertebral artery depicts mid-systolic deceleration with antegrade late systolic velocities (*white outline,* bunny rabbit sign). **B,** Partial steal. Pulsed wave Doppler spectral image (obtained after arm exercise) demonstrates mid-systolic deceleration with retrograde late systolic velocities. *(From Gosselin C, Walker PM. Subclavian steal syndrome: existence, clinical features, diagnosis and management. Semin Vasc Surg 1996; 9:93-97.)*

On physical examination, subclavian steal may manifest with a subclavian artery bruit or reduced blood pressure in the ipsilateral upper extremity, along with weakness of the radial pulse.[10]

Imaging Indications and Algorithm

Doppler sonography is the imaging modality of choice for the diagnosis of subclavian steal phenomenon. When sonography is limited, such as for the evaluation of subclavian disease, CT or MRI can be used to evaluate the anatomy. Unlike CT, MRI has the ability unequivocally to determine direction of blood flow in the vertebral artery, and it does not require ionizing radiation or iodinated contrast agent. Because of its invasiveness, angiography has a limited role in current practice, and is used primarily when percutaneous intervention is contemplated.

Imaging Techniques and Findings

Ultrasound

Sonography is the initial imaging examination when subclavian steal syndrome is suspected. Ultrasound with pulsed Doppler spectral analysis can demonstrate patency and flow direction in the vertebral artery and can establish the presence of subclavian steal.[11,12]

Subclavian steal phenomenon is associated with specific vertebral artery waveforms. There are four types of waveforms that indicate the degree of abnormal hemodynamics[11]:

- Type 1: Flow velocity at the nadir of the mid-systolic notch greater than that of end-diastole
- Type 2: Velocity in mid-systolic notch equal to end-diastole
- Type 3: Velocity in mid-systolic notch at baseline
- Type 4: Velocity in mid-systolic notch below baseline

In occult steal (Branchereau stage I),[4] the pulsed wave Doppler spectrum typically demonstrates antegrade vertebral flow with midsystolic deceleration.[11,12] The waveform may show a reversed late systolic flow as a response to reactive hyperemia in the upper extremity after arm exercise (see Fig. 96-1B). In partial subclavian steal (stage II), pulsed wave Doppler depicts partial flow reversal. The Doppler waveform in occult and partial subclavian steal has been described as the bunny rabbit sign because of its resemblance to the outline of a rabbit (Fig. 96-1A).[11,12]

In complete (stage III) subclavian steal, the pulsed wave Doppler spectrum shows complete reversal of flow in the vertebral artery (Fig. 96-2).[12]

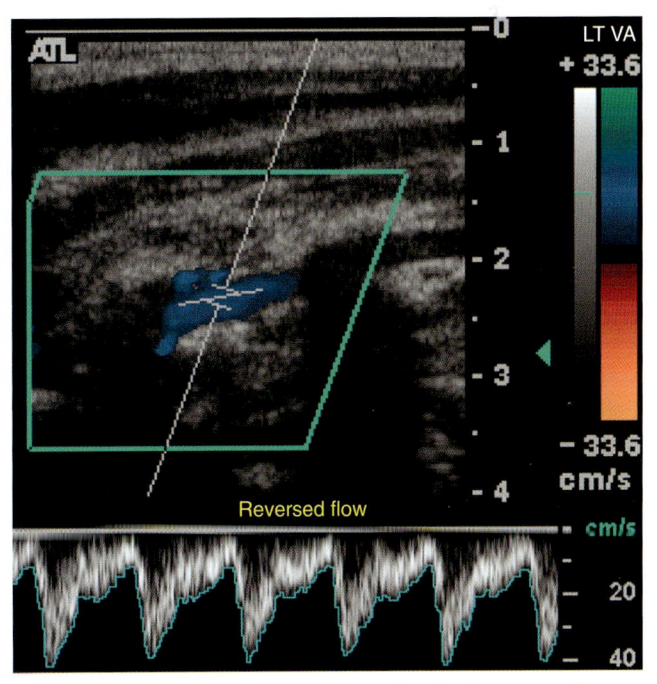

FIGURE 96-2 Complete subclavian steal. Pulsed wave Doppler spectral ultrasound of the left vertebral artery shows complete flow reversal. *(From Gosselin C, Walker PM. Subclavian steal syndrome: existence, clinical features, diagnosis and management. Semin Vasc Surg 1996; 9:93-97.)*

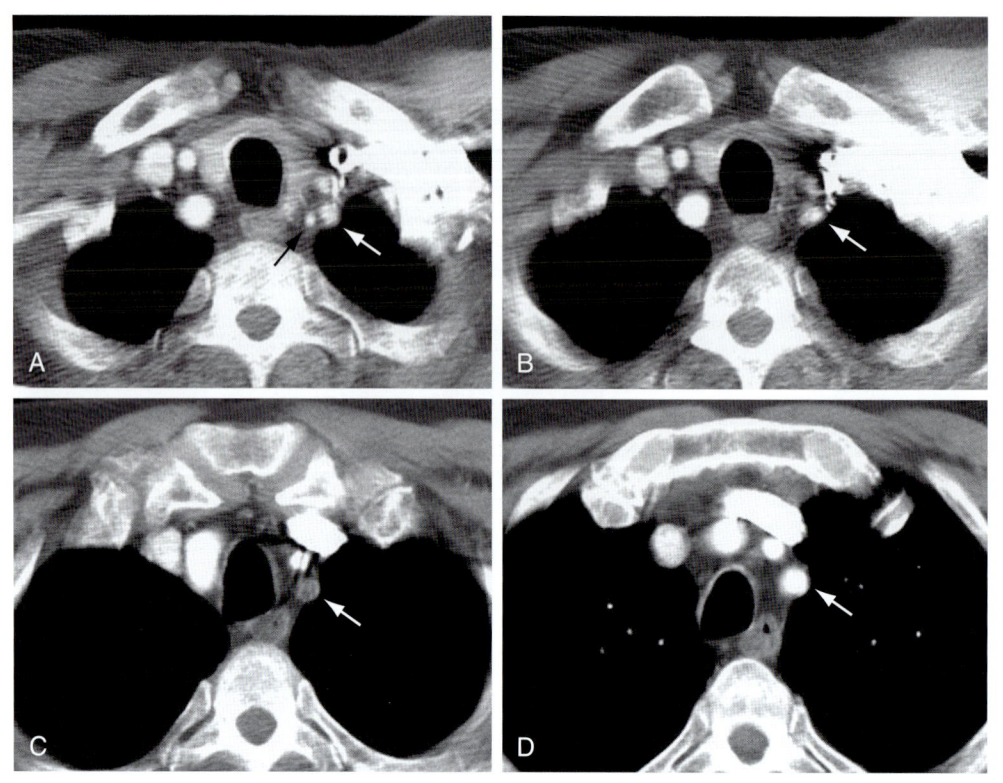

FIGURE 96-3 Subclavian steal phenomenon. Contrast-enhanced CT scan shows that the left subclavian artery (**D**, *white arrow*) is occluded beyond its origin (**C**) and reconstitutes (**B**) via the vertebral artery (**A**, *black arrow*).

Recently, transcranial Doppler ultrasound has been studied for evaluation of flow reversal in the basilar artery in the presence of retrograde vertebral artery flow.[13] Transcranial Doppler ultrasonography can be used to determine if there is reversal of basilar artery flow, which occurs in fewer than 25% of patients with retrograde vertebral flow. This is especially useful before intervention in patients with neurologic symptoms.

Computed Tomography

Contrast-enhanced computed tomography (CT) can demonstrate subclavian artery stenosis or occlusion with patency of the ipsilateral vertebral artery (Fig. 96-3).[14] The obstructive lesion is often associated with calcification. Coronal reformations are often useful to depict the site of narrowing. CT can also be used to identify indirect signs of subclavian steal phenomenon, such as poor internal mammary opacification or decreased unilateral brain perfusion.[15,16]

Magnetic Resonance Imaging

Magnetic resonance imaging (MRI) can accurately and noninvasively depict the features of subclavian steal phenomenon.[17] Contrast-enhanced magnetic resonance angiography (MRA) or noncontrast MRA can reveal the site of stenosis or occlusion (Figs. 96-4 and 96-5).[18] Time-resolved three-dimensional MRA has been described as a means of identifying reversal of vertebral artery flow.[19,20] Time-of-flight MRA has also been used to evaluate vertebral flow

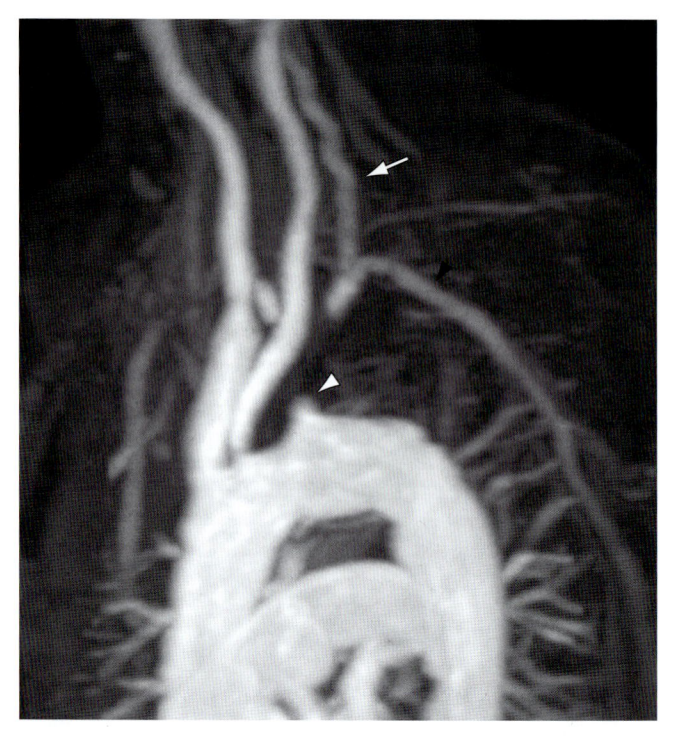

FIGURE 96-4 Subclavian steal. Contrast-enhanced MRA scan shows an atherosclerotic occlusion (*white arrowhead*) of the left subclavian artery with distal reconstitution (*black arrowhead*) via the vertebral artery (*white arrow*).

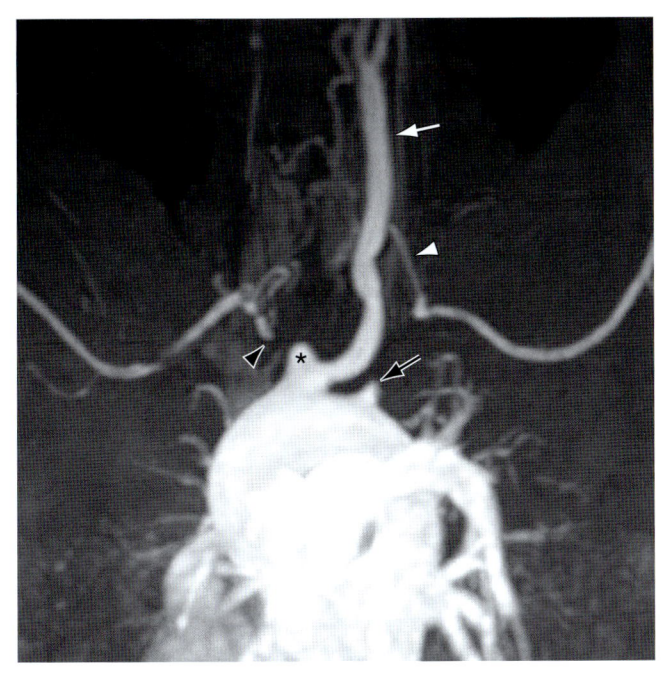

FIGURE 96-5 Subclavian steal syndrome—contrast-enhanced MRA scan in a patient with Takayasu arteritis and lightheadedness induced by upper extremity exercise. The left subclavian artery is occluded approximately 1 cm beyond its origin (*black arrow*) and reconstitutes (*black arrow*) via the vertebral artery (*white arrowhead*). Note the bovine arch, in which the left common carotid artery (*white arrow*) arises from the brachiocephalic artery (*asterisk*). The brachiocephalic artery is also occluded and the subclavian artery reconstitutes (*black arrowhead*), presumably via the vertebral artery. The right common carotid artery does not reconstitute. The left common carotid artery serves as the sole source of blood flow to the intracranial circulation, leading to neurologic symptoms.

direction, but this technique may be less reliable (Fig. 96-6).[18] Phase contrast MRI can confirm the reversal of blood flow in the vertebral artery, and velocity-encoded cine phase contrast MRI can be used to quantify velocity and flow in the vertebral and subclavian arteries (Fig. 96-7).[21] The carotid and vertebral arteries, and even the circle of Willis, can be evaluated in the same examination.

Angiography

Angiography can show stenotic or occlusive lesions in the subclavian, carotid, and vertebral arteries, as well as reversal of flow in the vertebral artery (Fig. 96-8). The use of angiography is limited by the widespread availability of ultrasound, CT, and MRI, but angiography does play an important role in the guidance of endovascular therapy.

DIFFERENTIAL DIAGNOSIS
From Clinical Presentation

- Stroke
- Intracranial tumor
- Dissection

From Imaging Findings

- Subclavian stenosis without steal
- Subclavian steal phenomenon
- Subclavian steal syndrome

SYNOPSIS OF TREATMENT OPTIONS
Medical Therapy

In the absence of symptoms, management is usually conservative.[3]

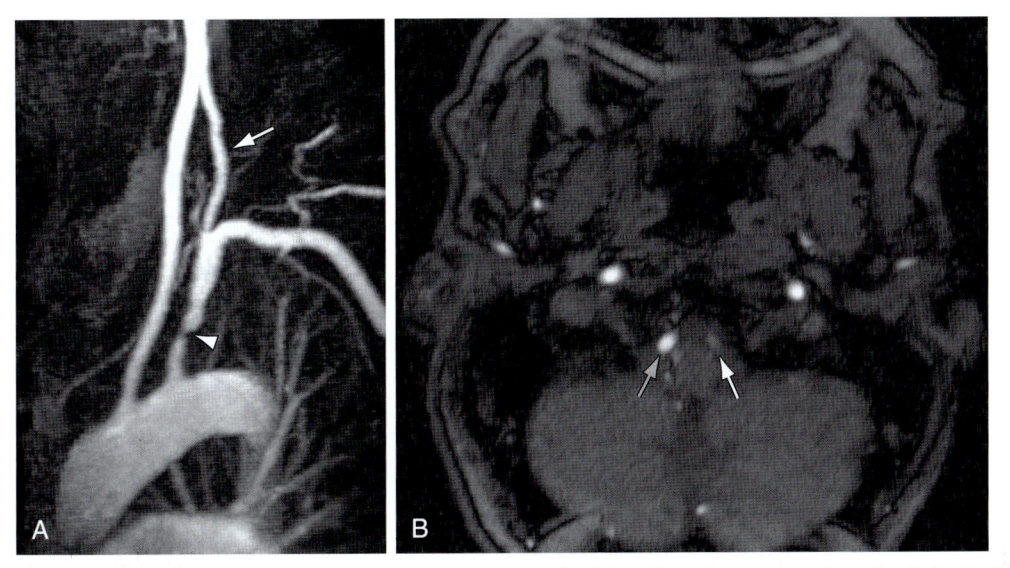

FIGURE 96-6 **A,** Contrast-enhanced MRA scan demonstrates a severe stenosis of the left subclavian artery (*arrowhead*). **B,** The left vertebral artery (*white arrow*) shows signal drop compared with the right side (*gray arrow*) on the time-of-flight MRA scan. The signal drop suggests reversal of flow on the left side.

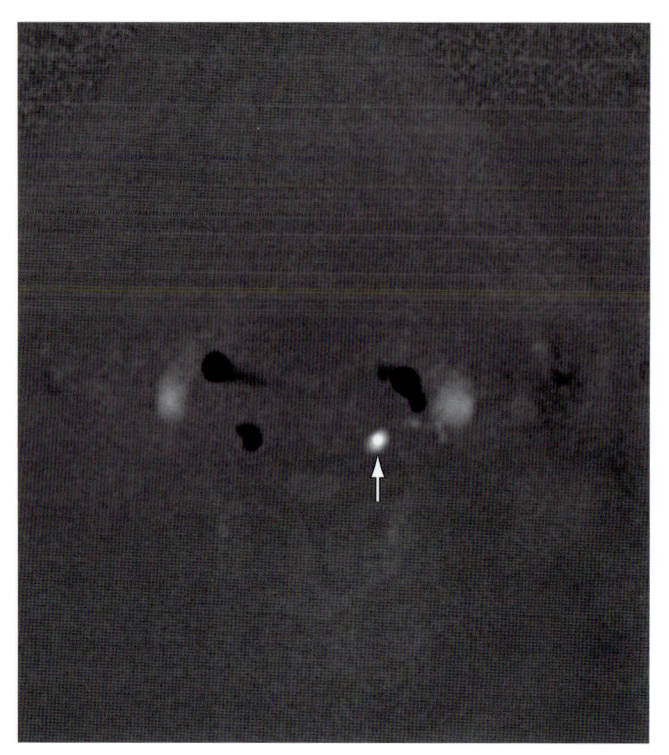

■ **FIGURE 96-7** Phase contrast MRI depicts flow reversal (*white arrow*) in the left vertebral artery in a patient with subclavian steal syndrome. The *dark circles* represent the carotid right vertebral arteries, all of which have an antegrade (cephalad) direction of flow. (*From Bitar R, Gladstone D, Sahlas D, Moody A. MR Angiography of subclavian steal syndrome: pitfalls and solutions. AJR Am J Roentgenol 2004; 183:1840-1841.*)

Surgical and Interventional Therapy

Percutaneous intervention is indicated when reversal of vertebral blood flow is detected in a symptomatic patient. Angioplasty and stenting of the subclavian artery are performed with the goal of improving blood flow to the upper extremity, thereby reverting to antegrade vertebral flow and improving intracranial blood flow.[22]

If the lesion is not amenable to endovascular intervention, surgery can be performed. Surgical options include carotid-subclavian bypass, axilloaxillary bypass, and carotid-subclavian transposition.[23,24] It is important to perform revascularization of a coexisting hemodynamically significant carotid artery.

KEY POINTS

- Subclavian steal phenomenon is characterized by subclavian artery stenosis, flow reversal in the vertebral artery.
- Neurologic symptoms are uncommon but when they are present, the complex is known as subclavian steal syndrome.
- The most common cause is atherosclerosis. In young adults and children, Takayasu arteritis is an important cause.
- Ultrasound is the mainstay of diagnosis, and MRI can depict stenoses and assess flow direction.
- Endovascular or surgical treatment is performed when the patient has neurologic symptoms.

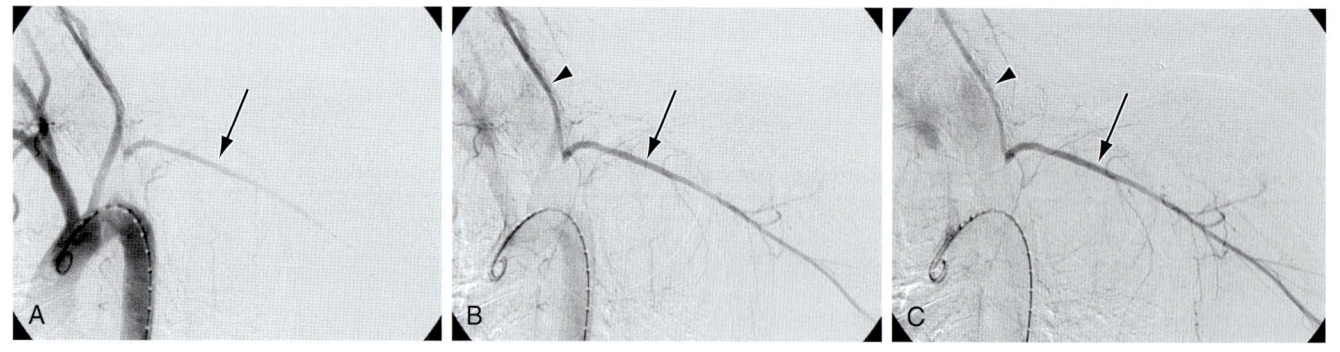

■ **FIGURE 96-8** Angiogram in a patient with subclavian steal syndrome. **A,** The left subclavian artery is occluded proximally and reconstitutes distally (*arrow*). **B,** It is evident that the vertebral artery (*arrowhead*) reconstitutes the subclavian artery (*arrow*) because the delayed image (**C**) shows less flow in the vertebral than in the subclavian artery.

SUGGESTED READINGS

Gosselin C, Walker PM. Subclavian steal syndrome: existence, clinical features, diagnosis and management. Semin Vasc Surg 1996; 9:93-97.

Bitar R, Gladstone D, Sahlas D, Moody A. MR Angiography of subclavian steal syndrome: pitfalls and solutions. AJR Am J Roentgenol 2004; 183:1840-1841.

REFERENCES

1. Reivich M, Holling HE, Roberts B, Toole JF. Reversal of blood flow through the vertebral artery and its effect on cerebral circulation. N Engl J Med 1961; 265:878-885.
2. Roldan-Valadez E, Hernandez-Martinez P, Osorio-Peralta S, et al. Imaging diagnosis of subclavian steal syndrome secondary to Takeyasu arteritis affecting a left-side subclavian artery. Arch Med Res 2003; 34:433-438.
3. Vollmar J, Elbayar M, Kolmar D, et al. Cerebral circulatory insufficiency in occlusive processes of the subclavian artery ("subclavian steal effect"). Dtsch Med Wochenschr 1965; 90:8-14.
4. Branchereau A, Magnan PE, Espinoza H, Bartoli JM. Subclavian artery stenosis: hemodynamic aspects and surgical outcome. J Cardiovasc Surg 1991; 32:604-612.
5. Hennerici M, Klemm C, Rautenberg W. The subclavian steal phenomenon: a common vascular disorder with rare neurologic deficits. Neurology 1988; 38:669-673.
6. Fields WS, Lemak NA. Joint study of extracranial arterial occlusion. VII. Subclavian steal—a review of 168 cases. JAMA 1972; 222: 1139-1143.
7. Bornstein NM, Norris JW. Subclavian steal: a harmless haemodynamic phenomenon? Lancet 1986; 2:303-305.
8. Ioannides MA, Eftychiou C, Georgiou GM, Nicolaides E. Takayasu arteritis presenting as epileptic seizures: a case report and brief review of the literature. Rheumatol Int 2009; 29:703-705.
9. Kaneko K, Fujimoto S, Okada Y, et al. SPECT evaluation of cerebral blood flow during arm exercise in patients with subclavian steal. Ann Nucl Med 2007; 21:463-470.
10. Gosselin C, Walker PM. Subclavian steal syndrome: existence, clinical features, diagnosis and management. Semin Vasc Surg 1996; 9:93-97.
11. Kliewer MA, Hertzberg BS, Kim DH, et al. Vertebral artery Doppler waveform changes indicating subclavian steal physiology. AJR Am J Roentgenol 2000; 174:815-819.
12. Tahmasebpour HR, Buckley AR, Cooperberg PL, Fix CH. Sonographic examination of the carotid arteries. Radiographics 2005; 25:1561-1575.
13. Harper C, Cardullo PA, Weyman AK, Patterson RB. Transcranial Doppler ultrasonography of the basilar artery in patients with retrograde vertebral artery flow. J Vasc Surg 2008; 48:859-864.
14. Park JH, Chung JW, Lee KW, et al. CT angiography of Takayasu arteritis: comparison with conventional angiography. J Vasc Interv Radiol 1997; 8:393-400.
15. Alegret RE, Blandon RJ, Kirsch J. Poor left internal mammary artery opacification on coronary CT angiography: an indirect sign of subclavian steal. J Vasc Interv Radiol 2008; 19:1791-1792.
16. Huang BY, Castillo M. Radiological reasoning: extracranial causes of unilateral decreased brain perfusion. AJR Am J Roentgenol 2007; 189(6 Suppl):S49-S54.
17. Van Grimberge F, Dymarkowski S, Budts W, Bogaert J. Role of magnetic resonance in the diagnosis of subclavian steal syndrome. J Magn Reson Imaging 2000; 12:339-342.
18. Bitar R, Gladstone D, Sahlas D, Moody A. MR Angiography of subclavian steal syndrome: pitfalls and solutions. AJR Am J Roentgenol 2004; 183:1840-1841.
19. Schubert R. Time-resolved, contrast-enhanced 3D MR angiography in the subclavian steal effect. Vasa 2010; 39:85-93.
20. Virmani R, Carroll R, Hung J, et al. Diagnosis of subclavian steal syndrome using dynamic time-resolved magnetic resonance angiography: a technical note. Magn Reson Imaging 2008; 26:287-292.
21. Bauer AM, Amin-Hanjani S, Alaraj A, Charbel FT. Quantitative magnetic resonance angiography in the evaluation of the subclavian steal syndrome: report of 5 patients. J Neuroimaging 2009; 19:250-252.
22. Rodriguez-Lopez JA, Werner A, Martinez R, et al. Stenting for atherosclerotic occlusive disease of the subclavian artery. Ann Vasc Surg 1999; 13:254-260.
23. Stipa S, Cavallaro A, Sciacca V, et al. Cross-over axillary by-pass. Treatment of subclavian or innominate artery obstructive lesions. Int Angiol 1987; 6:421-427.
24. Deriu GP, Milite D, Verlato F, et al. Surgical treatment of atherosclerotic lesions of subclavian artery: carotid-subclavian bypass versus subclavian-carotid transposition. J Cardiovasc Surg 1998; 39: 729-734.

CHAPTER 97

Acute Pulmonary Thromboembolic Disease

Nidhi Sharma and Tan-Lucien Mohammed

Pulmonary embolism (PE) was clinically described in the early 1800s, and von Virchow first described the connection between venous thrombosis and PE.[1,2] In 1922, Wharton and Pierson reported the first radiographic description of PE,[3] a commonly encountered entity whose diagnosis is clinically challenging because of its nonspecific symptoms.

Definition

Pulmonary thromboembolism is defined as the obstruction of the pulmonary artery or one of its branches leading to the lungs by a blood clot, usually from the leg, or foreign material causing sudden closure of the vessel. (Embolus is from the Greek *embolos*, meaning plug.) Emboli can also be composed of fat, air, or tumor tissue.

Prevalence and Epidemiology

PE is a potentially fatal condition with substantial morbidity and mortality in untreated patients. The annual incidence of pulmonary embolism is estimated to be between more than 300,000 cases, resulting in approximately 50,000 to 100,000 deaths in the United States every year.[4] Nearly 90% of PEs arise from lower extremity deep venous thrombosis (DVT). Diagnosis of pulmonary embolism remains a clinical challenge because of its nonspecific presentation. Mortality ranges from 3.5% to 15% and can be as high as 31% to 58% in the presence of shock.[5,6] Hence, prompt and accurate diagnosis is imperative because 65% of patients die within 1 hour of presentation and approximately 93% in the first 2.5 hours.[7] Since its original description, imaging has played an important role in the diagnosis of PE. For many years, ventilation-perfusion (V/Q) scintigraphy has been the main imaging modality for the evaluation of patients with suspected PE. However, with the advent of and the widespread availability of faster computed tomography (CT) scanners, CT scanning has emerged as another important diagnostic test for the evaluation of not only PE but also DVT in select patients. Thus, familiarization with various aspects of imaging evaluation is of extreme importance for the interpreting physician.

Various imaging modalities are currently available to evaluate suspected PE in routine clinical practice. We will discuss current imaging options in the remainder of this chapter.

Etiology and Pathophysiology

Three primary influences predispose a patient to thrombus formation, which form the so-called Virchow triad: (1) endothelial injury; (2) stasis or turbulence of blood flow; and (3) blood hypercoagulability.[1,2,8]

More than 90% of all PEs arise from thrombi within the large deep veins of the legs, typically the popliteal vein and the larger veins central to it.[1,2,4] The pathophysiologic consequences of thromboembolism in the lung largely depend on the cardiopulmonary status of the patient and on the size of the embolus, which in turn dictates the size of the occluded pulmonary artery.

PE has two important consequences: (1) an increase in pulmonary artery pressure produced by obstruction of flow, and possibly vasospasm caused by neurogenic mechanisms and/or release of mediators (such as thromboxane A2 and serotonin); and (2) ischemia of the downstream pulmonary parenchyma. Thus, occlusion of major vessels of more than 60% of the arterial bed suddenly increases pulmonary artery pressure, diminishes cardiac output, and causes right-sided heart failure (acute cor pulmonale) or even death. Usually, hypoxemia develops as a result of multiple mechanisms. If smaller vessels are occluded, the result is less catastrophic or the event may even be clinically silent.

MANIFESTATIONS

Clinical Presentation and Pretest Probability

Many patients with suspected PE present with nonspecific findings such as acute chest pain, and some are even asymptomatic. Some observers have suggested that because of the decline in tolerance for diagnostic uncertainty, diagnostic studies for the evaluation of PE may be overused in current practice. Pretest probability is an important concept, because the sensitivity, specificity, and predictive values of diagnostic imaging modalities are based on the pretest probability of PE, which is usually determined by clinical findings and laboratory test results.[9-11] The Wells criteria (Table 97-1)[12] and Geneva score,[13] which were devised and validated for clinical pretest probability, have been reported to have similar accuracy levels. Chagnon and colleagues[14] have shown that these methods can be used to divide patients into low-, intermediate-, and high-probability groups for PE, although neither was accurate enough to diagnose PE in individual cases.

Serum D-dimer levels can be used to gauge the presence of PE. D-dimer is a fibrin degradation product that increases with clot lysis, suggesting the presence of thrombosis. It has been shown that this test with levels above a threshold value of 0.5 mg/L has an excellent sensitivity of 95%, but the specificity is lower (38% to 83%)[15] because of elevated levels in some conditions, such as active inflammation, infection, pregnancy, malignancy, and liver failure. Of all the methods available for measurement of D-dimer levels (Table 97-2),[10] the VIDAS D-dimer assay (bioMérieux, Marcy l'Etoile, France), a rapid, quantitative, enzyme-linked immunosorbent assay (ELISA) procedure, has been reported to have a 96.4% sensitivity,[16] thus ruling out PE in the absence of a calculation of clinical pretest probability.[16,17] However, this is not routine clinical practice. Several studies[10,11,18] have demonstrated that a negative result of rapid quantitative ELISA D-dimer can be combined with the clinical probability score to exclude PE in up to 40% of patients, thereby eliminating further workup.

TABLE 97-1 Wells Clinical Decision Rule for Pulmonary Embolism

Variable	Points
Clinical signs and symptoms of deep vein thrombosis	3.0
Alternative diagnosis less likely than pulmonary embolism	3.0
Heart rate > 100/min	1.5
Immobilization (> 3 days) or surgery in the previous 4 weeks	1.5
Previous pulmonary embolism or deep vein thrombosis	1.5
Hemoptysis	1.0
Malignancy (receiving treatment; treated in the last 6 months or palliative)	1.0

Clinical probability of pulmonary embolism unlikely—4 points or less.
Clinical probability of pulmonary embolism likely—more than 4 points.
Adapted from Wells PS, Anderson DR, Rodger M, et al. Derivation of a simple clinical model to categorize patients probability of pulmonary embolism: increasing the models utility with the SimpliRED D-dimer. Thromb Haemost 2000; 83:416-420.

TABLE 97-2 Sensitivity and Specificity (%) of D-Dimer Based on Laboratory Technique

Laboratory Technique	Mean (Range)	
	Sensitivity	Specificity
ELISA	95 (85-100)	44 (34-54)
Rapid quantitative ELISA	95 (83-100)	39 (28-51)
Rapid semiquantitative ELISA	93 (79-100)	36 (23-50)
Rapid qualitative ELISA	93 (74-100)	68 (50-87)
Quantitative latex agglutination	89 (81-98)	45 (36-53)
Semi quantitative latex agglutination	92 (79-100)	45 (31-59)
Whole blood agglutination	78 (64-92)	74 (60-88)

ELISA, enzyme-linked immunosorbent assay.
Adapted from Ginsberg JS, Wells PS, Kearon C, et al. Sensitivity and specificity of a rapid whole-blood assay for D-dimer in the diagnosis of pulmonary embolism. Ann Intern Med 1998; 129: 1006-1011.

Imaging Techniques and Findings

Chest Radiography

Initially, the chest radiography findings commonly are normal. However, in later stages, the radiograph may show findings that include a Westermark sign (dilation of pulmonary vessels and a sharp cutoff), atelectasis, a small pleural effusion, and an elevated diaphragm. Although chest radiographic findings may indicate an alternate diagnosis, this study alone is not sufficient to confirm the diagnosis of PE.

Chest radiographic findings of PE can be subtle, nonspecific, and infrequently present. Among the patients in a PIOPED study without any evidence of prior cardiopulmonary disease, 84% of patients with proven PE and 66% of those without PE had abnormal chest radiographs. In an actual clinical setting, certain findings may suggest a diagnosis of PE and direct further imaging.

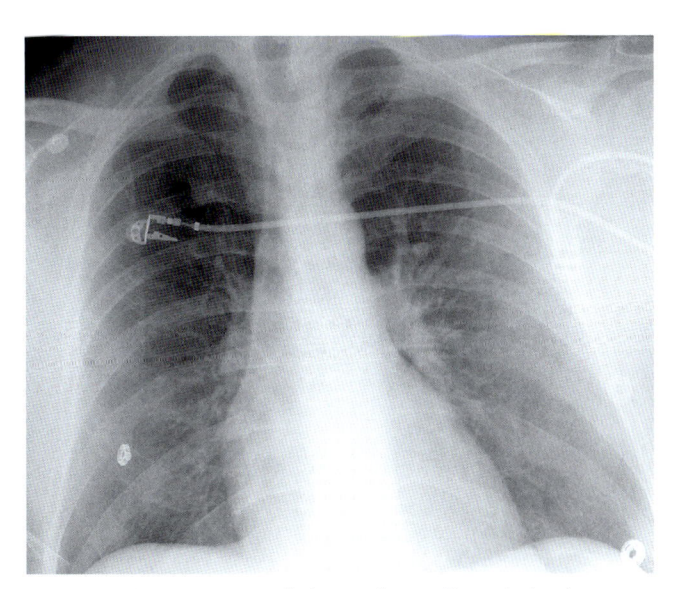

■ **FIGURE 97-1** Westermark sign on chest radiograph showing oligemia of the right lung fields in comparison to the left lung. It denotes focal peripheral lucency beyond an occluded vessel accompanied by mild dilation of central pulmonary vessels.

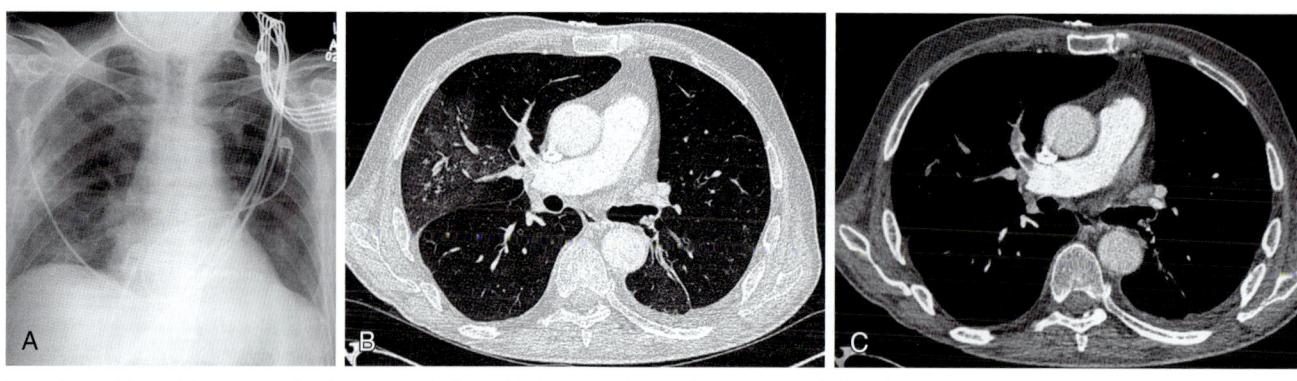

■ **FIGURE 97-2** Classic case of pulmonary embolism with Hampton hump sign showing subpleural infarct opacities on radiograph (A) and corresponding axial CT scans (B, C). *(Courtesy of Dr. Jeffrey P. Kanne, Cleveland Clinic, Cleveland, Ohio.)*

The Westermark sign (Fig. 97-1)[19] is a focal peripheral lucency beyond an occluded vessel accompanied by mild dilation of central pulmonary vessels, seen in 7% to 14% of cases of documented PE in the PIOPED study. It is a subtle finding caused by embolic obstruction or hypoxic vasoconstriction of pulmonary artery.

Another finding is enlarged central pulmonary vasculature, which can be easily missed. It may be caused by vessel distention by thrombus or by an acute rise in pulmonary arterial pressure secondary to distal emboli. A sausage-like configuration of focal enlargement of the right descending interlobar pulmonary artery caused by the physical presence of a clot has also been noted in many patients with acute PE and referred to as the knuckle sign. Hampton hump[20] is classically referred to as a conical peripheral opacity pointing toward the hilum. These are multiple, subpleural lower lobe infarcts seen as ill-defined opacities without air bronchography (Figs. 97-2 and 97-3).

Focal parenchymal abnormalities are the most commonly encountered lesions on chest radiographs in PIOPED series patients. These particularly include subsegmental atelectasis (Fleischner lines),[21] seen as linear opacities in lung bases; these are transient in nature and thought to be caused by mucus plugging, hypoventilation, or distant airway closure. Focal air space consolidation represents true pulmonary infarction, with ischemic necrosis or pulmonary hemorrhage without infarction occurring in 10% to 60% of patients. Small, unilateral, pleural effusions and diaphragmatic elevation are seen in a large number of PE patients.

In summary, the chest radiograph is often normal in patients with suspected PE. The sensitivity (33%) and specificity (59%) are low. The major role is in exclusion of conditions such as pulmonary edema, pneumonia, or pneumothorax, whose symptoms may overlap with those of PE. In addition, chest radiographs are used for correlation of the interpretation of V/Q scintigraphy results.

Lower and Upper Extremity Ultrasonography

As noted, 90% of PEs originate from thrombosis within the deep venous system of the lower extremities and are mostly clinically silent; other sources are the pelvic, renal, and upper extremity veins.[22] Significant morbidity and mortality are associated with undiagnosed DVT; thus, methods such as contrast venography (CV), magnetic resonance venography (MRV), and lower extremity ultrasonography are commonly used for its detection. Real-

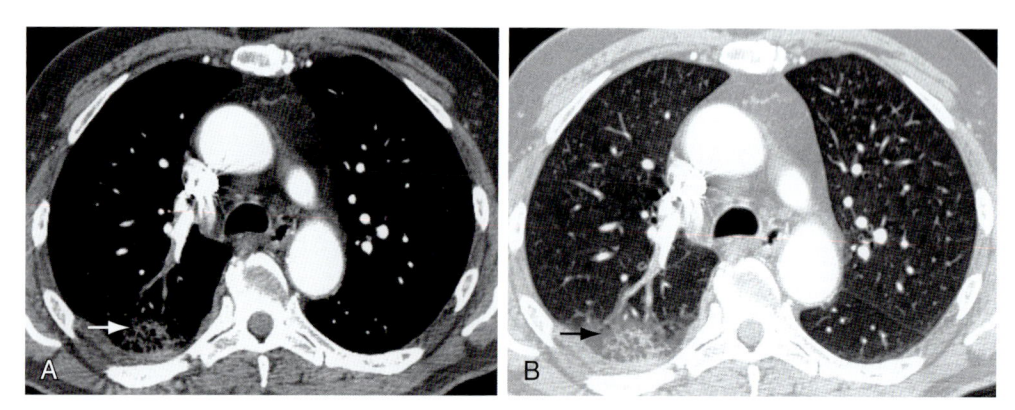

■ **FIGURE 97-3** A, B, Axial CT scans of 66-year-old patient with acute right upper lobe pulmonary embolism. B, The *arrow* points toward a developing infarct in the posterior segment of right upper lobe.

time gray scale, continuous wave and pulsed Doppler, and color Doppler imaging, along with ancillary techniques such as the Valsalva maneuver and manual blood flow augmentation, are used to image the lower extremity veins.

Acute thrombus is often anechoic with variable echogenicity, making compression ultrasonography an important tool for assessment. The diagnosis is established by lack of venous compression caused by intraluminal thrombus. Lack of appropriate response to a Valsalva maneuver also indicates thrombosis of the central veins outside the field of view. The reliability of a negative compression ultrasonography examination is high.

Spectral Doppler analysis is particularly useful for vessels that cannot be visualized directly, such as the inferior vena cava (IVC), superior vena cava (SVC), and brachiocephalic veins. Normal patent vessels show respiratory phasicity, whereas a monophasic waveform suggests venous obstruction.

Color Doppler imaging is useful to identify deeper veins such as the iliac veins and superficial femoral veins, for which direct venous compression is not possible, or for obese or swollen extremity patients. Thrombosis is identified as the absence of color flow within a vessel lumen at baseline and with augmentation; the sensitivity and specificity are 95% and 98%, respectively, for femoropopliteal DVT.[22]

Upper extremity thrombosis is screened using spectral and color Doppler techniques for veins inaccessible to direct compression. The incidence of PE with upper extremity DVT may be as high as 12% to 15%, making these diagnostic tests highly significant.

In summary, color flow Doppler imaging and compression ultrasonography have a high sensitivity (89% to 100%) and specificity (89% to 100%) for the detection of proximal DVT in symptomatic patients. However, compression ultrasonography has a low sensitivity (38%) and a low positive predictive value (26%) in patients without symptoms of DVT. Patients with positive findings for DVT can be anticoagulated irrespective of their V/Q scan results; other patients must have more invasive investigations performed to rule out PE definitively.

Ventilation-Perfusion Scintigraphy

V/Q scanning of the lungs is an important diagnostic modality for establishing the diagnosis of PE. The PIOPED classification scheme allows for a more meaningful interpretation of the V/Q scan to treat patients with anticoagulation. The scans should be interpreted primarily as a diagnostic or nondiagnostic pattern, indicating whether the patient has or does not have a high likelihood of having PE.

A normal perfusion scan excludes a diagnosis of PE, with its negative predictive value close to 100%.[23-25] It is a safe, relatively inexpensive, and widely available test that allows the acquisition of single-breath, equilibrium, and washout images. A high-probability V/Q scan (Figs. 97-4 and 97-5), in combination with high-probability clinical findings, corresponded to PE in 96% of patients, whereas a low-probability clinical assessment showed PE in only 4% of patients in a major study.[9]

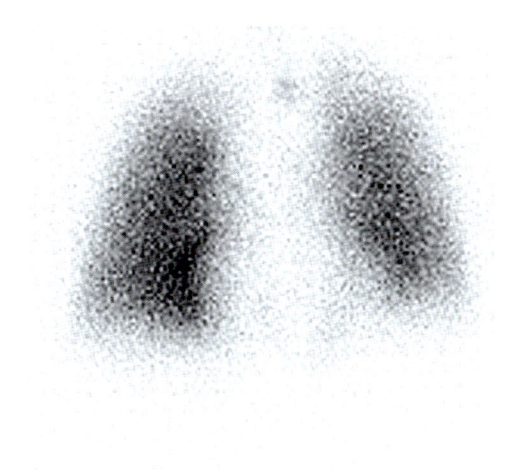

■ **FIGURE 97-4** Anterior projection of a Tc 99m diethylenetriamine pentaacetic acid (DTPA) aerosol image demonstrates relatively homogeneous ventilation. *(Courtesy of Dr. Donald Neumann, Cleveland Clinic, Cleveland, Ohio.)*

In PIOPED-1, a V/Q scan in patients with a normal chest radiograph was diagnostic in 52% of patients with suspected PE,[26] and one study has shown it to be diagnostic in 91% of patients.[27] This PIOPED group retrospectively analyzed perfusion scans alone and found the results to be equivalent to those of the V/Q technique.[28] In the PISA-PED trial,[29] only perfusion scans were obtained. These were classified according to the shape of defects, yielding sensitivity and specificity of 86% and 93%, respectively, for abnormal perfusion scans compatible with PE, with the result being dichotomous. These studies indicate that the ventilation scan can be eliminated, thus reducing cost and radiation dose. It can also be used as a preferred alternative for patients unable to undergo CT angiography.

It can be used particularly for reproductive female patients whose chest radiograph is likely to be normal and in whom the breast irradiation dose from CT angiography can be minimized using the perfusion scan only.[9,30] Another significant use is follow-up of proven PE patients undergoing anticoagulation.

Ventilation-Perfusion Single Photon Emission Computed Tomography

V/Q single photon emission computed tomography (SPECT) is a newer modality that may improve both sensitivity and specificity of the V/Q scan (Fig. 97-6). Reinartz and associates[31] analyzed 83 patients who underwent four-slice spiral CT, V/Q planar, and V/Q SPECT studies, giving sensitivity, specificity, negative predictive value (NPV), and positive predictive value (PPV) of 97%, 91%, 98%, and 90%, respectively, for SPECT techniques. This study used aerosolized technetium 99m (Tc 99m) for the ventilation portion of the V/Q scan instead of the radioisotope xenon 133. Tc 99m is five times smaller in diameter and has a 20% efficiency of pulmonary deposition in comparison to 2% for xenon 133, thus helping improve the results.[32,33] Unlike PIOPED, this study considered all the mismatched results as PE, regardless of the size. This technique has the potential to improve the interpre-

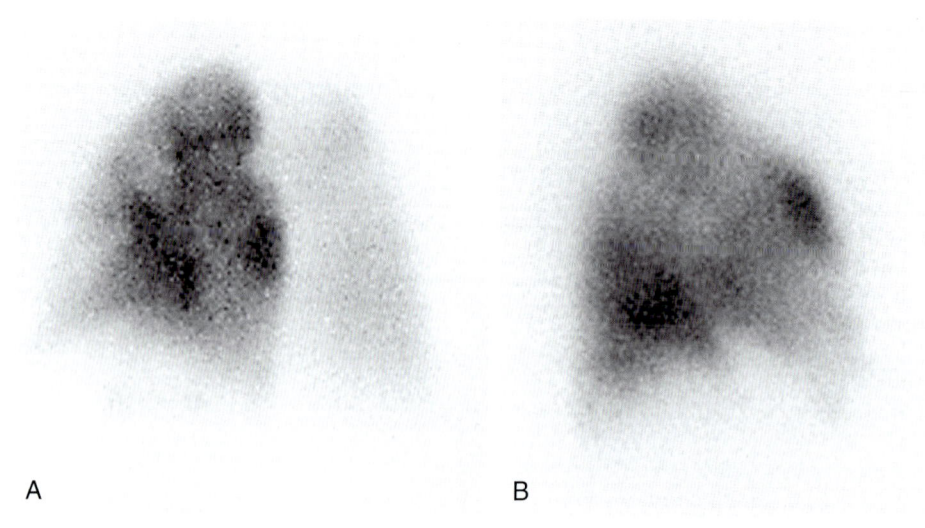

■ FIGURE 97-5 Left posterior oblique (A) and right lateral planar (B) views of Tc 99m macroaggregated albumin pulmonary perfusion scans show multiple large perfusion defects compatible with a high-probability scan in a patient with pulmonary embolism. *(Courtesy of Dr. Donald Neumann, Cleveland Clinic, Cleveland, Ohio.)*

tation of V/Q scanning by incorporating computerized interpretations.

Thus, a normal V/Q SPECT scan is a sensitive and safe test for PE evaluation and may be especially useful for renal failure patients. Initial studies using SPECT technique with Tc 99m are promising and suggest improved accuracy of V/Q scanning, but further prospective studies are needed to incorporate its use in daily practice.

Pulmonary Angiography

This method had served as a standard of reference for PE detection for decades before the advent and widespread use of CT. It was usually performed in cases of discrepancy between the clinical suspicion and results of the V/Q scan, or if there were coexisting conditions (e.g., pneumonia, lung cancer) that could result in a false-positive result. Angiography was also often performed prior to interventions such as mechanical clot fragmentation. The relative contraindications to this procedure are listed in Box 97-1.[22]

Pulmonary angiography has high specificity rates, approaching almost 100% for a filling defect or abrupt pulmonary arterial obstruction. Other findings for acute PE include delayed venous return, decreased pulmonary flow, and tortuous vessels. In the past, a negative pulmonary angiogram was thought to exclude the diagnosis of clinically significant PE, but there is currently some controversy regarding this conclusion.

Major complications (1% to 3%) associated with the procedure include respiratory distress requiring resuscitation, cardiac perforation, contrast reactions, major dysrhythmias, renal failure, and hematomas. Minor complications (5%) are contrast-induced renal dysfunction, respiratory distress, angina, minor contrast reaction, and transient dysrhythmias.

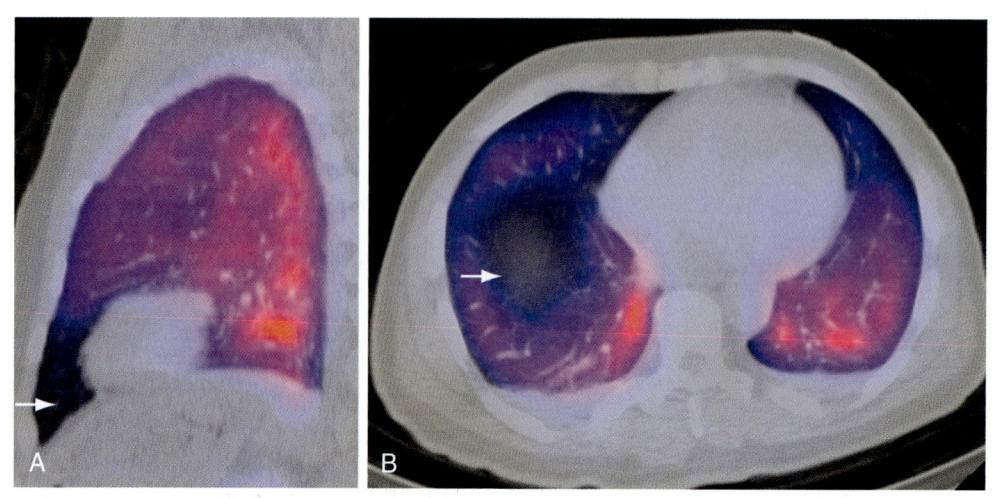

■ FIGURE 97-6 Fused sagittal (A) and transverse (B) Tc 99m macroaggregated albumin SPECT/CT tomograms of a 67-year-old male patient show lack of perfusion associated with the inferior lingular segment. Subsequently, this patient was diagnosed to have acute pulmonary embolism. *(Courtesy of Dr. Donald Neumann, Cleveland Clinic, Cleveland, Ohio.)*

> **Box 97-1 Relative Contraindications to Pulmonary Angiography**
>
> - Documented allergy to contrast materials
> - Elevated right ventricular end-diastolic pressure (greater than 20 mm Hg) and/or increased pulmonary artery pressure over 70 mm Hg
> - Left bundle branch block
> - Renal insufficiency or failure
> - Bleeding diatheses
>
> Adapted from Gotway MB, Reddy GP, Dawn SK: Pulmonary thromboembolic disease. In Webb WR, Higgins CB (eds). Thoracic Imaging. Philadelphia, Lippincott Williams & Wilkins, 2005, pp 609-629.

Computed Tomography of the Chest

CT Pulmonary Angiography

The role of a multidetector CT (MDCT) scan for the diagnosis of PE has evolved over the last decade. MDCT can visualize main, lobar, and segmental pulmonary emboli with a reported sensitivity of greater than 90%. Multidetector CT scanning can detect emboli as small as 2 mm that affect up to the seventh-order arterial division. Small subsegmental emboli may not be detected, although the advent of faster scanners has allowed even these small and likely clinically insignificant emboli to be readily seen with increasing frequency. CT has another benefit—an alternate diagnosis may be suggested in up to 57% of patients.

Single-detector helical CT pulmonary angiography (SCTA) is an older technique that is still in clinical use. It has a reported high accuracy, with sensitivity reported to range from 60% to 100% and specificity from 81% to 100%.[34,35] This technique involves the use of a single detector and x-ray source that rotate around the patient, taking multiple cross-sectional images and allowing the entire study to be completed in 25 to 30 seconds. When it was first developed it represented an important advance, because it allows over 90% of patients to hold their breaths throughout the study, thus reducing motion artifact from breathing.[36] Also, 3-mm slices can be obtained with the spiral technique which aid in higher quality imaging of the vasculature. By 2001, at many institutions, SCTA had surpassed the V/Q scan as the initial test for evaluation of PE.

There have been a few published reports challenging the accuracy of SCTA, reporting a high specificity and low sensitivity in the evaluation of PE. Most of these studies concluded that SCTA was inadequate as a single first-line test for PE evaluation, especially for acute thrombi in subsegmental pulmonary arteries and right middle lobe and lingular arteries.[34,35] Several follow-up studies were performed to determine whether the sensitivity of SCTA could be improved. Perrier and coworkers[37] found in 299 patients that SCTA combined with lower extremity ultrasonography yielded only a 70% sensitivity, despite the fact that ultrasonography yielded better false-negative rates. In another similar study, approximately 16% of the negative SCTA had positive lower extremity ultrasonography needing treatment.[38] Thus, it was suggested that a negative SCTA along with lower extremity ultrasonography was important for ruling out a diagnosis of PE.

Technical Considerations

A specific imaging protocol is designed to optimize the diagnostic information, giving particular attention to various scan parameters to obtain high-quality images. Ideally, for a helical CT scan, it must include the entire pulmonary arterial system, without the other areas of thorax, to reduce radiation exposure and keep the timing of the study optimal. A caudocranial scanning direction is beneficial because most PEs are detected in the lung bases, where the blood flow is maximal. Therefore, even if the patient loses his or her breath-hold, the degradation of scan quality from motion would most likely occur in the upper lung region, where PE occurrence is less likely. An inspiratory breath-hold is desirable because it can increase the pulmonary vascular resistance, leading to better contrast enhancement. Various concentrations of contrast agent and protocols for injection rate have been used, each with its own advantages and disadvantages. High-contrast agent concentration (300 to 360 mg/mL) with a high rate of infusion (3 mL/second or higher) is the most popular, convenient, and effective because it maximizes pulmonary artery opacification and allows the use of preloaded syringes. Typically, 2- to 3-mm collimation imaging is done with or without narrow overlapping reconstruction. This technique provides excellent image quality, but also leads to a larger data storage requirement. Additionally, it is preferable to use larger pitch values with narrower collimation. Pitch values of 1.7 to 2 are commonly used. Also, proper timing of the contrast bolus is extremely important to obtain a high-quality image. Generally, a presumptive scan delay of 20 seconds for upper extremity injections works well to obtain adequate enhancement. Rapid viewing of contiguous scans in sequence is useful in clinical practice. Multiplanar reformatted images can be useful to identify small artery abnormalities, which usually follow an oblique course, and three-dimensional reconstructions with volume rendering aid in displaying complex anatomy.[22]

Classic Findings

A diagnosis of acute PE is established when a partial intraluminal filling defect is visualized with a sharp interface surrounded by varying degree of contrast (Fig. 97-7). Eccentric or peripheral intraluminal filling defects form acute angles with the vessel wall. Acute PE thrombus attenuation measures 33 ± 14 HU, whereas that of chronic PE thrombus measures 90 ± 30 HU. There are two very reliable signs for acute PE diagnosis—a thrombus usually appears to be central in the pulmonary artery when seen in cross section (the doughnut sign). Occasionally, it may be outlined by contrast agent when imaged along its axis (railroad track sign).[22] Other findings include mosaic perfusion, right ventricular strain (Fig. 97-8), peripheral consolidation (representing pulmonary hemorrhage or infarction), and pleural effusions. Saddle embolus bridges can form across the right and left main pulmonary arteries and are a cause of sudden death (Fig. 97-9). Mosaic perfu-

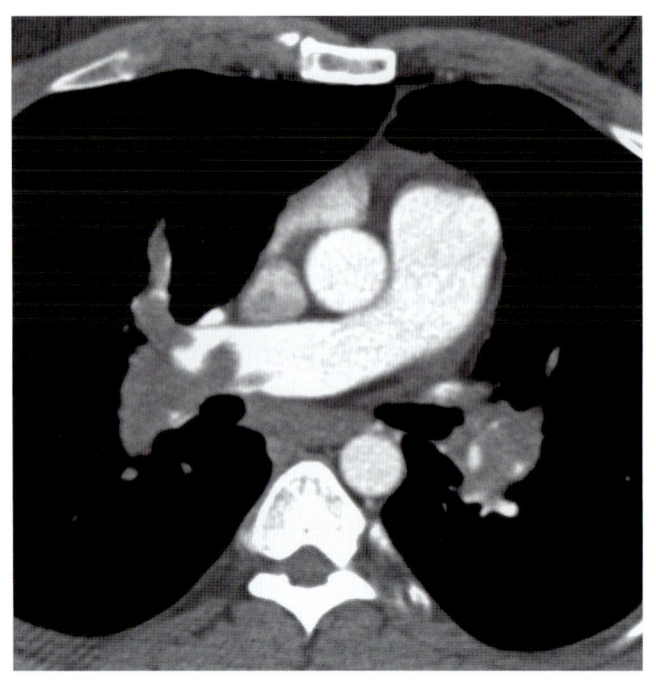

■ **FIGURE 97-7** Axial view CT scan of a 49-year-old patient depicting a massive central embolism.

sions are inhomogeneous lung opacities caused by alteration in pulmonary blood flow. The Miller method[39] is commonly used to measure the clot burden and indicates the severity of PE, but is a poor predictor of mortality. In this method, 1 point is given for a clot in each proximal artery, which is equivalent to each segment arising distally, thus resulting in a maximum score of 9 for right lung, 7 for left lung, and 16 total.

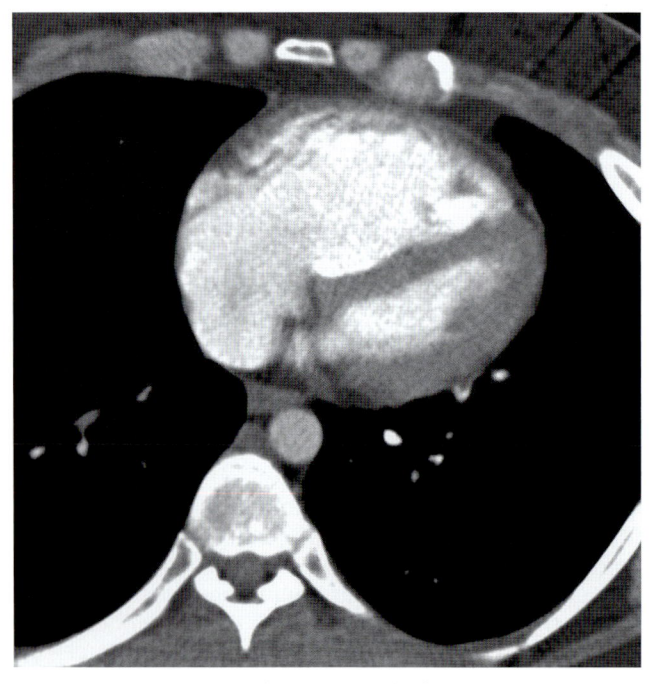

■ **FIGURE 97-8** CT scan showing marked enlargement of right ventricle, with associated compression of the left ventricle denoting right ventricular strain.

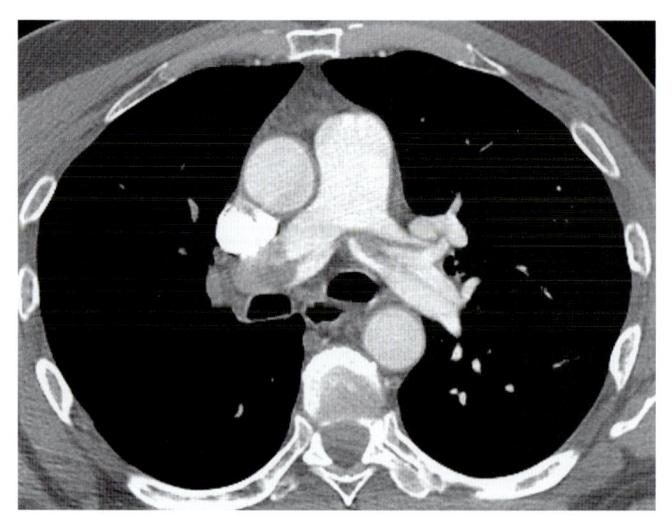

■ **FIGURE 97-9** CT scan, axial view, of a 56-year-old patient with a saddle embolus bridging across the right and left main pulmonary arteries.

Benefits and Accuracy

SCTA has high specificity rates, making a positive result highly likely to be PE. Moreover, CT directly depicts a thrombus, thereby eliminating false-positive results caused by factors such as radiation effects and extraluminal compression. CT allows imaging of the lung parenchyma, chest wall, and mediastinum, reducing the need for additional studies to make a diagnosis if PE is absent. This is important, because neither V/Q scan nor pulmonary angiography can detect other conditions reliably.

The accuracy of diagnosis depends on the size of the artery affected and the size of the emboli (clot burden). CT has a diagnostic accuracy of almost 100% for acute emboli in large pulmonary arteries. It has also been shown to have higher sensitivity and specificity in comparison to V/Q scintigraphy. A confident diagnosis can be made in 90% of patients because, even in those in whom a scan is interpreted as negative, an alternative diagnosis can be established. Furthermore, transthoracic and transesophageal echocardiography have proved to be of limited accuracy in the diagnosis of PE in an acute setting. Controversies regarding the accuracy for diagnosis have been reflected in various studies in different populations (see further discussion in the next section).

Limitations

Pooled data from numerous studies have suggested a sensitivity of 90% and specificity over 90% in cases of suspected acute PE involving main, lobar, and segmental arteries, although a wider range has been observed in many studies. Contributing to the lower sensitivity is its resolution. The sensitivity and specificity rates are particularly diminished (61% to 79% at its best) for small subsegmental emboli, which are usually uncommon in an acute setting.[34,40] Between 6% and 30% of patients with PE have isolated subsegmental emboli.[41] Thus, studies that demonstrated the lowest sensitivity rates mainly consisted of patients with small thrombi.

CT scanning leads to significant radiation exposure; for all indications, it accounts for approximately 40% to 75% of medical radiation exposure.[42,43] This increases the risk of malignancy in patients involved in serial studies. The radiation dose to the breast is of special concern. This radiation exposure is also an issue of concern for pregnant women.

Another limitation to be taken into account is reaction to the contrast medium used. Nearly 15% of patients experience mild reactions such as nausea, vomiting, and flushing.[44] Severe reactions are less frequent; these include laryngeal edema, bronchospasm, convulsions, and cardiovascular collapse (0.04% to 0.22%). The incidence of these reactions is reduced substantially by using low-osmolality contrast media. Contrast-induced nephropathy (CIN) is another important life-threatening complication. Furthermore, patients with preexisting primary conditions such as pregnancy and renal failure are contraindicated from the use of this test.

Anatomic pitfalls include normal hilar lymph nodes, which simulate acute PE, pulmonary vein artifacts being confused with arterial filling defects, partial volume averaging of anterior segmental artery creating an effect of intraluminal filling defect and, rarely, a calcified bronchus with mucoid impaction suggests a defect surrounded by contrast.

TABLE 97-3 Diagnostic Reference Standard for Prospective Investigation of Pulmonary Embolism Disorders (PIOPED) II

PE Diagnosed	PE Excluded
High-probability V/Q scan in patient without prior history of PE	Normal findings on digital subtraction pulmonary angiography
Abnormal findings on pulmonary digital subtraction angiography	Normal findings on V/Q scan
Abnormal findings on venous ultrasonography in patient with no prior history of DVT at that site and nondiagnostic V/Q scan (not normal and not high probability)	Low or very low probability V/Q scan in subject with clinical Wells score <2 and negative lower extremity ultrasonography

DVT, deep venous thrombosis; PE, pulmonary embolism; V/Q, ventilation-perfusion.
Adapted from Stein PD, Fowler SE, Goodman LR, et al. Multidetector computed tomography for acute pulmonary embolism. N Engl J Med 2006; 354: 2317-2327.

Multidetector Computed Tomography

MDCT became available for clinical use in the late 1990s and is now widely accepted as the standard of care. In this technique, multiple detectors are rotated as the patient slides through the CT scanner gantry. In its earliest form, MDCT used four scanners. However, that number gradually increased to 64-detector technology, which is widely used currently, and scanners with 256 detectors or more are or will be available in the near future. The increase in the number of detectors has led to a reduction in study time by 10 seconds and slice thickness as low as 0.5 mm, greatly contributing to higher resolution and imaging, up to sixth-order pulmonary arteries.[40] This has consequently led to improved detection of subsegmental PEs, higher sensitivity rate, and reduction in false-negative results. The coronal, sagittal, and axial reconstructions using thin axial collimation have different sensitivities and may aid in the reduction of artifacts and false-positive rates by three-dimensional visualization. Thin collimation also allows retrospective reconstruction of CT images using electrocardiographic reconstruction based on the R-R interval, which eliminates cardiac artifact and helps obtain better visualization of the coronary arteries and thoracic aorta.

Several studies have validated the use of MDCT for the evaluation of PE. The first evaluated patients with high clinical probability or an abnormal D-dimer test by the Geneva score.[45] In the second study, inpatients and outpatients were evaluated with abnormal D-dimer or PE-like clinical probability by a modified Wells score.[11]

In the PIOPED II multicenter trial, 1090 patients were enrolled; 824 underwent CT pulmonary angiography (CTPA), CT venography (CTV), and a confirmatory test. Of these, 192 patients (24%) had PE and 51 patients (6%) had an inadequate CTPA result.[46] The primary aim of PIOPED II was to determine the accuracy of MDCT for the diagnosis and exclusion of PE in suspected patients. The observed sensitivity was 83% specificity was 96%, and 87 patients (11%) had an inadequate CTV result. The combined sensitivity and specificity of CTA-CTV were 90% and 95%, respectively. This led to the conclusion that MDCT CTA-CTV is more accurate than CTPA alone for the diagnosis of PE. It also established that in the case of the clinical picture being dissonant with CTPA, further imaging should be undertaken. Because V/Q scanning was the reference test in this study, any discordance with CTPA led to the incorporation of another test, such as a positive lower extremity ultrasonography, low-probability V/Q, and low clinical probability using Wells criteria or a positive digital subtraction angiography (DSA) result. Additionally, the PIOPED investigators created a composite standard, which, if satisfied, could diagnose or exclude PE, in case MDCT was positive, with a negative angiography result. This is a powerful set of tests that can be reliably used for the exclusion of PE without pulmonary angiography or CT scanning (Table 97-3). The main limitation was the use of clinical probability as the decision point.

Limitations

Important limitations include unsatisfactory images caused by respiratory and cardiac motion. MDCT detects PEs at a subsegmental level, especially involving fifth- and sixth-order branch vessels, which have lower significance but immediate importance. They may not be of acute danger to the patient but predict a future, more severe embolism. Thus, the incidence of PE should be higher in MDCT studies than in those performed with other methods. It was 33% for the original PIOPED study,[9] whereas only 20.4% to 26% for the newer PIOPED II, Perrier, and Christopher studies.[11,45]

MDCT also exposes patients to significantly greater radiation exposure and a further increased risk of CIN; 25% of patients will have a contraindication such as pregnancy or renal insufficiency. Also, patients allergic to contrast media are contraindicated. Finally, although MDCT scanners are an excellent modality for detection of PE, the number of scans should be limited because of side effects.

Computed Tomography Venography

CTV provides the additional ability to image DVT in the pelvic veins as well as the lower extremity venous system immediately following CT angiography of the pulmonary arterial system, without administration of additional contrast. The thrombi are visible as filling defects within the veins. Such a technique not only expedites patient evaluation, but also provides a diagnostic benefit over ultrasound assessment. A large cohort study conducted by Cham and colleagues[47] has shown a 20% increase in the detection of thromboembolism when CTV was performed with contiguous, helically acquired 10-mm sections in comparison to CTA alone. As noted, a PIOPED II trial clearly reported that the sensitivity of CTA for the diagnosis of PE increased from 83% to 90% with the addition of CTV.[46] Thus, the addition of CTV is beneficial for better diagnosis and further treatment planning for patients with suspected PE undergoing CTA studies.

Magnetic Resonance Imaging

Recent advances in the field of MRI technology has made this challenging field useful for the imaging of pulmonary vascular structures. The reduction in breath-hold time to 20 seconds (as a result of the acquisition of all the images in a shorter time) had led to its increased popularity.[48] Although many challenges exist, such as a relative lack of signals in lieu of paucity of protons in chest, air, and soft tissue interface artifacts, and respiratory and cardiac motion problems, it is still attractive for two primary reasons. First, and most important, MRI overcomes the use of ionizing radiation to generate images, making it completely harmless to the patient. Hence, it is being considered safe in pregnancy as well. Secondly, intravenous contrast agents are considered less nephrotoxic.

Techniques

The three most commonly used techniques include gadolinium-enhanced magnetic resonance angiography (Gd-MRA), real-time MRI (RT-MRI), and MR perfusion.

Gd-MRA is the most commonly used method, and its protocol varies in different institutions. The signal-to-noise ratio is optimized using phased-array coils. A gradient recalled echo (GRE) localizing sequence is obtained in the transverse plane. Coronal three-dimensional spoiled gradient-recalled-echo (SPGR) MR angiography acquisition is then prescribed for transverse images. The SPGR sequence is completed during a breath-hold of 20 to 25 seconds, and the entire study is completed in 30 to 45 seconds.[22] Oudkerk and associates[49] have performed the largest study of Gd-MRA, in which 118 patients underwent Gd-MRA followed by pulmonary angiography. The reported sensitivity and specificity were 77% and 98%, respectively. The high specificity allows patients with positive results to be treated with confidence.

RT-MRI is a technique timed to take images gated to the patient's respiratory cycle and uses a principle similar to the one used in electrocardiographic-gated CT scanners. Hence, it eliminates breath-hold and also produces T-2 weighted images, allowing thrombus imaging without the use of any contrast.[50] Also, it has a higher sensitivity in comparison to Gd-MRA.

MR perfusion frequently uses gadolinium as the contrast agent, which causes a local magnetic field disturbance measured by an MR scanner. Instead of directly imaging the vascular structures, this technique generates a signal based on the volume of blood in that region. Decreased or absent blood flow suggests obstruction. Also, there is no need for breath-holding with this method.

Advantages and Limitations

In general, MR techniques are harmless and considered safe for the pregnant population as well. Also, they do not cause any end-organ toxicity effects. The major limitation is its low sensitivity rate but its combination with lower extremity imaging may improve the diagnosis. The most important contraindication for MRI is an electronic implanted device. There have been reports of fatal arrhythmias caused by cardiac pacemaker failure; hence, they are strongly contraindicated. Nerve stimulators, cardiac defibrillators, cochlear implants, insulin pumps, continuous medicine pumps, prosthetic devices, and metallic fragments such as bullets and shrapnel are among other pertinent contraindications because they may move during the course of MRI.[52] Rarely, burns have been reported in patients with tattoos.[51] Gadolinium-based contrast agents are considered to be less toxic, with an incidence of adverse events of 1.47%,[52] but they have been implicated by the U.S. Food and Drug Administration (FDA) in patients with renal failure as the cause of nephrogenic systemic fibrosis (NSF), which tends to be a progressive fatal condition.

DIFFERENTIAL DIAGNOSIS

When considering acute pulmonary thromboembolism, a reasonable differential diagnosis should include the following entities:

1. Hilar lymphadenopathy. With thicker image acquisition, adenopathy can often be confused with intraluminal filling defects. However, with the advent of faster MDCT and other advancing technologies, such as better reformatted images, their extraluminal location can be better delineated.
2. In situ thrombosis. In a recent postoperative setting, such as can be seen in pneumonectomy patients, an arterial stump or cutoff can be misconstrued as representing an acute embolus.
3. Transient contrast interruption. This frequent diagnostic dilemma is encountered when there is a lack of opacification in multiple pulmonary vessels. There will be an admixture of nonopacified blood from the IVC with deep inspiration, but the presence of nonopacified blood can also be observed on the preceding images to aid in diagnosis.
4. Pulmonary artery (PA) sarcoma. PA sarcomas are very rare malignancies of the wall of the pulmonary artery

or some other great vessel. They are often confused with an acute pulmonary embolus. It presents as a lobulated enhancing mass and should be considered when there is an emboli that is unresponsive to standard treatment
5. Tumor emboli. Emboli from primary cancers such as renal cell carcinoma, hepatoma, melanoma, and angiosarcoma can invade the IVC and/or hepatic veins. This tumor phenomenon can metastasize to the pulmonary vasculature and mimic an acute thrombus.

SYNOPSIS OF TREATMENT OPTIONS

- Anticoagulation and fibrinolysis can be used, as noted earlier (hemorrhage occurs as a complication in nearly 10% of patients).
- An IVC filter is placed if there are contraindications to drug therapy or recurrent emboli.
- Surgical endarterectomy is usually reserved for chronic organizing pulmonary emboli and not during acute presentation.

CONCLUSION

Further evaluation of proposed clinical pathways by using decision analyses, evidence-based criteria, and cost-effectiveness assessment is needed. This would help focus future clinical research, in particular regarding strategies for further imaging when CT is inconclusive or contraindicated. In addition, tests and pathways in specific patient groups have not been evaluated in detail. For example, there are many studies on the use of D-dimer testing in emergency department patients but few on its use in inpatients or intensive care unit patients. Patients with specific comorbid conditions have not been studied extensively, and preliminary data suggest specific characteristics in oncology patients, patients with chronic obstructive pulmonary disease, and others. It will be of particular importance to resolve disparate assertions regarding radiation exposure from the use of different imaging techniques.

The advances over the past several decades have significantly improved our diagnostic abilities and refined the treatment of patients with PE. However, several areas need further research and properly conducted therapeutic trials. The role of imaging and the optimal duration of anticoagulant therapy in different subgroups of patients with venous thromboembolism require further study.

What the Referring Physician Needs to Know

- The interpreting physician should diagnose and inform the referring physician about the findings of acute pulmonary embolism so that prompt medical treatment can be initiated. He or she should also specify about any right ventricular strain, if any, because this helps establish the severity of the disease.

KEY POINTS

- No telltale signs, symptoms, or laboratory studies that strongly suggest acute PE; some patients are actually asymptomatic.
- Positive D-dimer, normal range (1.5 to 2.5)—is of minimal clinical value in altering probability of disease.
- Because of declining tolerance for diagnostic uncertainty, PE studies are now overused, especially in emergency setting.
- Embolization of thrombi to pulmonary arteries usually occurs from deep veins in lower extremities or pelvis.
- Chest radiograph—10% normal (detection of disease other than PE in 70% of CT patients).
- When using MDCT, look for thrombus in pulmonary arteries; location on MDCT—acute thrombus often straddles bifurcation points.
- Look for additional signs
  - Westermark sign—focal origin because of vascular obstruction
  - Hampton hump—pleural-based, cone-shaped opacity pointing toward the hilum

SUGGESTED READINGS

Anderson DR, Kahn SR, Rodger MA, et al. Computed tomographic pulmonary angiography vs. ventilation-perfusion lung scanning in patients with suspected pulmonary embolism: a randomized controlled trial. JAMA 2007; 298:2743-2753.
Bhalla S, Lopez-Costa I. MDCT of acute thrombotic and nonthrombotic pulmonary emboli. Eur J Radiol 2007; 64:54-64.
Clemens S, Leeper KV Jr. Newer modalities for detection of pulmonary emboli. Am J Med 2007; 120(Suppl 2):S2-S12.
Gotway MB, Reddy GP, Dawn SK. Pulmonary thromboembolic disease. In Webb WR, Higgins CB (eds). Thoracic Imaging. In Pulmonary and Cardiovascular Radiology. Philadelphia, Lippincott Williams & Wilkins, 2005, 609-629.
Martine RJ, Massimo P, Lawrence RG. Management of suspected acute pulmonary embolism in the era of CT angiography: a statement from the Fleischner Society. Radiology 2007; 245:315-329.
Mir MA. Excluding pulmonary embolism with computed topographic pulmonary angiography or ventilation-perfusion lung scanning. JAMA 2007; 298:2743-2753.

Sostman HD, Stein PD, Gottschalk A, et al. Acute pulmonary embolism: sensitivity and specificity of ventilation-perfusion scintigraphy in PIOPED II study: Radiology 2008; 246:941-946.
Stein PD, Fowler SE, Goodman LR, et al. Multidetector computed tomography for acute pulmonary embolism. N Engl J Med 2006; 354:2317-2327.
Stillman AE, Oudkerk M, Ackerman M, et al. Use of multidetector computed tomography for the assessment of acute chest pain: a consensus statement of the North American Society of Cardiac Imaging and the European Society of Cardiac Radiology. Int J Cardiovasc Imaging 2007; 23:415-427.
Winer-Muram HT. Pulmonary emboli. In Gurney JW, Winer-Muram HT, Stern EJ (eds). Diagnostic Imaging: Chest. 1st ed. Salt Lake City, Amirsys; 2006:II-4-50–II-4-53.

REFERENCES

1. Boyden EA: Segmental Anatomy of the Lungs: Study of the Patterns of the Segmental Bronchi and Related Pulmonary Vessels. New York, McGraw-Hill, 1955, pp 23-32.
2. Mitchell RN, Kumar V. Hemodynamic disorders, thrombosis, and shock. In Kumar V, Cotran RS, Robbins SL (eds). Basic Pathology, 6th ed. Philadelphia, WB Saunders, 1997, pp 60-80.
3. Wharton LR, Pierson JW. Minor forms of pulmonary embolism after abdominal operations. JAMA 1922; 79:1904-1910.
4. Haines ST. Venous thromboembolism: pathophysiology and clinical presentation. Am J Health Syst Pharm 2003; 60(Suppl 7): S3-S5.
5. Wood KE. The presence of shock defines the threshold to initiate thrombolytic therapy in patients with pulmonary embolism. Intens Care Med 2002; 28:1537-1546.
6. Konstantinides S, Geibel A, Olschewski M, et al. Association between thrombolytic treatment and the prognosis of hemodynamically stable patients with major pulmonary embolism: results of a multicenter registry. Circulation 1997; 96:882-888.
7. Stein PD, Henry JW: Prevalence of acute pulmonary embolism among patients in a general hospital and at autopsy. Chest 1995; 108:978-981.
8. Virchow RLK. Thrombosis and Emboli, 1846-1856. Translated by Matzdorff AC, Bell WR. Sagamore Beach, Mass, Science History Publications, 1998.
9. The PIOPED Investigators. Value of the ventilation/perfusion scan in acute pulmonary embolism. Results of the prospective investigation of pulmonary embolism diagnosis (PIOPED). JAMA 1990; 263:2753-2759.
10. Ginsberg JS, Wells PS, Kearon C, et al. Sensitivity and specificity of a rapid whole-blood assay for D-dimer in the diagnosis of pulmonary embolism. Ann Intern Med 1998; 129:1006-1011.
11. Van Belle A, Buller HR, Huisman MV, et al. Effectiveness of managing suspected pulmonary embolism using an algorithm combining clinical probability, D-dimer testing, and computed tomography. JAMA 2006; 295:172-179.
12. Wells PS, Anderson DR, Rodger M, et al. Derivation of a simple clinical model to categorize patients probability of pulmonary embolism: increasing the models utility with the SimpliRED D-dimer. Thromb Haemost 2000; 83:416-420.
13. Wicki J, Perneger TV, Junod AF, et al. Assessing clinical probability of pulmonary embolism in the emergency ward: a simple score. Arch Intern Med 2001; 161:92-97.
14. Chagnon I, Bounameaux H, Aujesky D, et al. Comparison of two clinical prediction rules and implicit assessment among patients with suspected pulmonary embolism. Am J Med 2002; 113:269-275.
15. Stein PD, Hull RD, Patel KC, et al. D-dimer for the exclusion of acute venous thrombosis and pulmonary embolism: a systematic review. Ann Intern Med 2004; 140: 589-602.
16. Dunn KL, Wolf JP, Dorfman DM, et al. Normal D-dimer levels in emergency department patients suspected of acute pulmonary embolism. J Am Coll Cardiol 2002; 40: 1475-1478.
17. de Moerloose P., Desmarais S., Bounameaux H., et al. Contribution of a new, rapid, individual and quantitative automated D-dimer ELISA to exclude pulmonary embolism. Thromb Haemost 1996; 75:11-13.
18. Wells PS, Anderson DR, Rodger M, et al. Excluding pulmonary embolism at the bedside without diagnostic imaging: management of patients with suspected pulmonary embolism presenting to the emergency department by using a simple clinical model and D-dimer. Ann Intern Med 2001; 135:98-107.
19. Westmark N. On the roentgen diagnosis of lung embolism. Acta Radiol 19: 357-372, 1938.
20. Hampton AO, Castleman B. Correlation of postmortem chest teleroentgenograms with autopsy findings: with special reference to pulmonary embolism and infarction. AJR 1940; 43:305-326.
21. Fleischner FG. Pulmonary embolism. Clin Radiol 1962; 13:169-182.
22. Gotway MB, Reddy GP, Dawn SK. Pulmonary thromboembolic disease. In Webb WR, Higgins CB (eds). Thoracic Imaging. Philadelphia, Lippincott Williams & Wilkins, 2005, pp 609-629.
23. Kipper MS, Moser KM, Kortman KE, Ashburn WL. Long-term follow-up in patients with suspected pulmonary embolism and a normal lung scan. Chest 1982; 82:411-415.
24. Hull RD, Raskob GE, Coates G, Panju AA. Clinical validity of a normal perfusion lung scan in patients with suspected pulmonary embolism. Chest 1990; 97:23-26.
25. Van Beek EJ, Kuyer PM, Schenk BE, et al. A normal perfusion scan in patients with clinically suspected pulmonary embolism: frequency and clinical validity. Chest 1995; 108:170-173.
26. Stein PD, Alavi A, Gottschalk A, et al. Usefulness of non-invasive diagnostic tools for diagnosis of acute pulmonary embolism in patients with a normal chest radiograph. Am J Cardiol 1991; 67:1117-1120.
27. Forbes KP, Reid JH, Murchison JT. Do preliminary chest x-ray findings define the optimum role of pulmonary scintigraphy in suspected pulmonary embolism? Clin Radiol 2001; 56:397-400.
28. Stein PD, Terrin ML, Gottschalk A, et al. Value of ventilation/perfusion scans compared to perfusion scans alone in acute pulmonary embolism. Am J Cardiol 1992; 69:1239-1241.
29. Miniati M, Pistolesi M, Marini C, et al. Value of perfusion lung scan in the diagnosis of pulmonary embolism: results of the Prospective Investigative Study of Acute Pulmonary Embolism Diagnosis (PISA-PED). Am J Respir Crit Care Med 1996; 154:1387-1393.
30. Parker MS, Hui FK, Camacho MA. Female breast radiation exposure during CT pulmonary angiography. Am J Roentgenol 2005; 185:1228-1233.
31. Reinartz P, Wildberger JE, Schaefer W, et al. Tomographic imaging in the diagnosis of pulmonary embolism: a comparison between V/Q lung scintigraphy in SPECT technique and multislice spiral CT. J Nucl Med 2004;45:1501-1508.
32. Senden TJ, Moock KH, Gerald JF, et al. The physical and chemical nature of technegas. J Nucl Med 1997; 38:1327-1333.
33. Hartmann IJ, Hagen PJ, Stokkel MP, et al. Technegas versus 81mKr ventilation-perfusion scintigraphy: a comparative study in patients with suspected acute pulmonary embolism. J Nucl Med 2001; 42:393-400.
34. Goodman LR, Curtin JJ, Mewissen MW, et al. Detection of pulmonary embolism in patients with unresolved clinical and scintigraphic diagnosis: helical CT versus angiography. Am J Roentgenol 1995; 164:1369-1374.
35. Garg K, Welsh CH, Feyerabend AJ, et al. Pulmonary embolism: diagnosis with spiral CT and ventilation-perfusion scanning-correlation with pulmonary angiographic results or clinical outcome. Radiology 1998; 208:201-208.
36. Herold CJ: Spiral computed tomography of pulmonary embolism. Eur Respir J 2002; 35(Suppl):13S-21S.
37. Perrier A, Howarth N, Didier D, et al. Performance of helical computed tomography in unselected outpatients with suspected pulmonary embolism. Ann Intern Med 2001; 135:88-97.
38. Musset D, Parent F, Meyer G, et al. Diagnostic strategy for patients with suspected pulmonary embolism: a prospective multicenter outcome study. Lancet 2002; 360:1914-1920.
39. Miller GA, Sutton GC, Kerr IH, et al. Comparison of streptokinase and heparin in treatment of isolated acute massive pulmonary embolism. Br Med J 1971; 2:681-684.
40. Schoepf UJ: Diagnosing pulmonary embolism: time to rewrite the textbooks. Int J Cardiovasc Imaging 2005; 21:155-163.
41. Oser RF, Zuckerman DA, Gutierrez FR, Brink JA. Anatomic distribution of pulmonary emboli at pulmonary angiography: implications for cross-sectional imaging. Radiology 1996; 199:31-35.
42. Shrimpton PC, Edyvean S. CT scanner dosimetry. Br J Radiol 1998; 71:1-3.
43. Wiest PW, Locken JA, Heintz PH, Mettler FA Jr. CT scanning: a major source of radiation exposure. Semin Ultrasound CT MR 2002; 23:402-410.
44. Thomsen HS, Marcos SK. Management of acute adverse reactions to contrast media. Eur Radiol 2004; 14:476-481.
45. Perrier A, Roy PM, Sanchez O, et al. Multidetector-row computed tomography in suspected pulmonary embolism. N Engl J Med 2005; 352:1760-1768.
46. Stein PD, Fowler SE, Goodman LR, et al. Multidetector computed tomography for acute pulmonary embolism. N Engl J Med 2006; 354:2317-2327.
47. Cham MD, Yank Levitz DF, Henchmen CI. Thromboembolic disease detection at indirect CT venography versus CT pulmonary angiography. Radiology 2005; 234:591-594.

48. Pedersen MR, Fisher MT, van Beek EJ. MR imaging of the pulmonary vasculature—an update. Eur Radiol 2006; 16:1374-1386.
49. Oudkerk M, van Beek EJ, Wielopolski P, et al. Comparison of contrast-enhanced magnetic resonance angiography and conventional pulmonary angiography for the diagnosis of pulmonary embolism: a prospective study. Lancet 2002; 359:1643-1647.
50. Kluge A, Muller C, Hansel J, et al. Real-time MR with TrueFISP for the detection of acute pulmonary embolism: initial clinical experience. Eur Radiol 2004;14:709-718.
51. Kanal E, Borgstede JP, Barkovich AJ, et al; American College of Radiology Blue Ribbon Panel on MR Safety. ACR white paper of magnetic resonance (MR) safety: combined papers of 2002 and 2004. ACR Practice Guidelines and Clinical Standards. Available at: http://www.acr.org/SecondaryMainMenuCategories/quality_safety/guidelines/WhitePaperonMRSafetyCombinedPapersof2002and2004Doc11.aspx. Accessed September 14, 2009.
52. Niendorf HP, Haustein J, Cornelius I, Alhassan A, Clauss W: Safety of gadolinium-DTPA: extended clinical experience. Magn Reson Med 1991; 22:222-232.

CHAPTER 98

Chronic Pulmonary Embolism

Sanjeev Bhalla

Pulmonary hypertension is defined as a mean arterial pressure of greater than 25 mm Hg at rest and 30 mm Hg with exercise.[1] Symptoms are often nonspecific and include dyspnea on exertion and easy fatigability. When it is severe, pulmonary hypertension can be severely debilitating and even fatal. During the past decade, advances in diagnosis and therapeutics have markedly affected the mortality of pulmonary hypertension.[2] What was once a lethal condition without transplantation has become a condition that may be managed with various medications.

In 2003, an international multidisciplinary conference held in Venice, Italy, revisited the classification of pulmonary hypertension with a goal of classifying pulmonary hypertension into categories based on treatment algorithms that may be beneficial.[3] The result was five main categories: pulmonary arterial hypertension, pulmonary hypertension due to left-sided heart disease, pulmonary hypertension from chronic hypoxia, pulmonary hypertension due to chronic embolic disease, and pulmonary hypertension from miscellaneous causes. Of these categories, pulmonary hypertension due to chronic embolic disease is the only one that may benefit from pulmonary thromboendarterectomy and one of the only forms of pulmonary hypertension that may be cured.[4] The goal of this chapter is to highlight the imaging findings of chronic pulmonary embolism and to help delineate those patients who may benefit from surgical intervention.

CHRONIC PULMONARY EMBOLISM

Definition

Chronic pulmonary embolism is more accurately referred to as chronic thromboembolic pulmonary hypertension (CTPH) to distinguish it from chronic emboli from foreign materials, such as talc, or parasitic ova, such as schistosomiasis.[3] CTPH represents cytokine-mediated scarring of the pulmonary circulation from even one episode of acute pulmonary embolism.[5,6] The net effect of the scarring is decreased luminal volume for the pulmonary circulation. This decrease in arterial volume results in increased pulmonary pressures.

Prevalence and Epidemiology

In the age of cross-sectional imaging, CTPH may be more common than previously thought. Prior reports suggested that less than 0.1% of patients with an episode of acute pulmonary embolism will go on to develop CTPH and pulmonary hypertension.[7] More recent studies suggest that this number is an underestimation of the true incidence and prevalence. In one prospective follow-up study of 78 patients with acute pulmonary embolism, 4 patients (5%) went on to develop definite CTPH, and in another of 223 patients with acute pulmonary embolism, 3.8% went on to develop symptomatic CTPH at 2 years.[8,9] Estimations of true incidence are hindered by the large number of patients with CTPH who may not have had any history or memory of symptomatic pulmonary embolism in the past. As many as two of three patients with CTPH may not have had a documented history of acute pulmonary embolism.[6]

Etiology and Pathophysiology

CTPH is a cytokine-mediated condition that may follow even one episode of acute pulmonary embolism. This is important to consider so that it is not confused with recurrent acute pulmonary embolism, which represents either failure of anticoagulation or a manifestation of a hypercoagulable state.[6] CTPH also does not represent failure of an acute pulmonary embolism from resolution. Instead, CTPH represents the end of a cycle of in situ thrombus, scarring, and vascular remodeling that occurs after a vascular insult, usually acute pulmonary embolism.[5]

Manifestations of Disease

Clinical Presentation

Like other causes of pulmonary hypertension, CTPH usually is manifested with vague symptoms and nonspecific findings.[10,11] Patients tend to notice decrease in exercise tolerance, easy fatigability, and dyspnea on exertion. As the condition progresses, they may find that they develop dyspnea at rest. The mean time from onset of symptoms to diagnosis is about 3 years, highlighting the insidious, nonspecific nature of this process.[6,10]

Imaging Indications and Algorithm

Imaging of a patient with suspected pulmonary hypertension from CTPH is aimed at answering four main questions: (1) What is the degree of pulmonary hypertension? (2) What is the etiology of the pulmonary hypertension— is chronic pulmonary embolism the cause or is another entity more likely? (3) Are changes of chronic pulmonary embolism surgically accessible? (4) Are any new pulmonary emboli present? Imaging usually begins with a chest radiograph, which might suggest pulmonary hypertension, and quickly moves to an echocardiogram, which is used to estimate pulmonary pressures and to assess cardiac function.[12] Traditionally, ventilation-perfusion scintigraphy (V/Q scan) has been used to assess for CTPH in combination with CT to exclude interstitial lung disease.[6,12,13] At many institutions, however, the pulmonary embolism protocol CT has replaced both studies.[14] This single study, especially when it is performed on a multidetector row CT (MDCT) scanner, allows the simultaneous assessment for CTPH and interstitial lung disease.

MR may allow a noninvasive assessment of pulmonary pressures, but its routine use for exclusion of CTPH remains somewhat experimental.[15] If pulmonary hypertension is confirmed on any of the modalities, patients tend to be referred for right-sided heart catheterization so that accurate measurements of pulmonary pressures and right-sided heart hemodynamics may be performed. If CTPH is uncovered, patients may go on to pulmonary angiography to assess whether pulmonary thromboendarterectomy may be beneficial. Multiplanar postprocessing of MDCT data and thin maximum intensity projections (usually 4 to 7 mm) may provide equivalent information and avoid angiography altogether.

Imaging Techniques and Findings

Radiography

Conventional radiography may show enlargement of the right side of the heart, with increased convexity of the right border of the heart on the frontal projection and filling in of the retrosternal clear space on the lateral projection (Figs. 98-1 and 98-2). The pulmonary arteries may be enlarged. Features unique to CTPH are rarely observed.

Ultrasonography

Echocardiography will show increase in the size of the right atrium and the right ventricle as well as the main pulmonary artery. Echocardiography may be used to estimate pulmonary pressures.[16] This estimate is based on calculating the peak velocity of the tricuspid regurgitation jet and calculating a pressure based on a modified Bernoulli equation [pressure = $4 \times$ velocity^2 (velocity in meters/sec)]. This value is added to an estimate of right atrial pressure, which is based on the size of the inferior vena cava and its variation during respiration.

On occasion, echocardiography may be performed with a contrast agent or agitated saline. The left atrium and ventricle are observed to confirm the absence of any echogenic material. If any is seen, this suggests that an intracardiac right-to-left shunt is present and the intravenously injected material is shunting to the left side of the heart. The shunt could be an alternative explanation for pulmonary hypertension. Care must be taken to confirm that the shunt is not a patent foramen ovale, which can be secondary to CTPH and elevated pulmonary pressures.

Computed Tomography

CT findings can be divided into three main categories: cardiac findings, pulmonary arterial findings, and parenchymal or other findings.[17-19]

Cardiac findings, as with echocardiography, center on the effect of increased pulmonary pressures on the right ventricle and right atrium. Both chambers tend to be enlarged, and the right ventricle tends to be hypertrophied (see Figs. 98-1 and 98-2). The observation of muscle hypertrophy is important because right ventricular enlargement alone may be seen in the setting of acute pulmonary embolism. In this situation, right ventricular enlargement may be a finding of right-sided heart strain and may require more aggressive intervention or closer observation. With right-sided heart enlargement and right ventricle hypertrophy, the interventricular septum tends to straighten at first and then to bow toward the left. The interatrial septum also may eventually straighten and then bow toward the left. Rarely, intravenous contrast material may be seen entering the left atrium through a septal defect, or two thin membranes may be seen in the region of the atrial septum. These CT features of a patent foramen ovale can be subtle and, as with echocardiography, may be secondary to pulmonary hypertension from CTPH. One should not expect to see a defect on a single transaxial image in a patent foramen ovale. If one is observed, a true atrial septal defect may be present.

Pulmonary artery findings on CT are similar to the vascular findings on angiography.[18,19] These include thrombus along the vessel wall, abrupt vessel caliber change, abrupt vessel cutoff or thrombosed vessel, webs within the arteries, beaded vessels, and enlarged central vessels. The eccentric nature of the thrombus is key in distinguishing CTPH from acute pulmonary embolism (see Figs. 98-1 and 98-2). CTPH tends to be present along the wall of the vessel, with a flat or concave interface with the lumen.[17] Conversely, acute pulmonary embolism tends to be central with vessel expansion. When it is eccentric, along the vessel wall, acute pulmonary embolism is convex toward the lumen. CTPH rarely calcifies. In fact, if calcification is seen, one must strongly consider in situ thrombus formation as can be seen in pulmonary artery

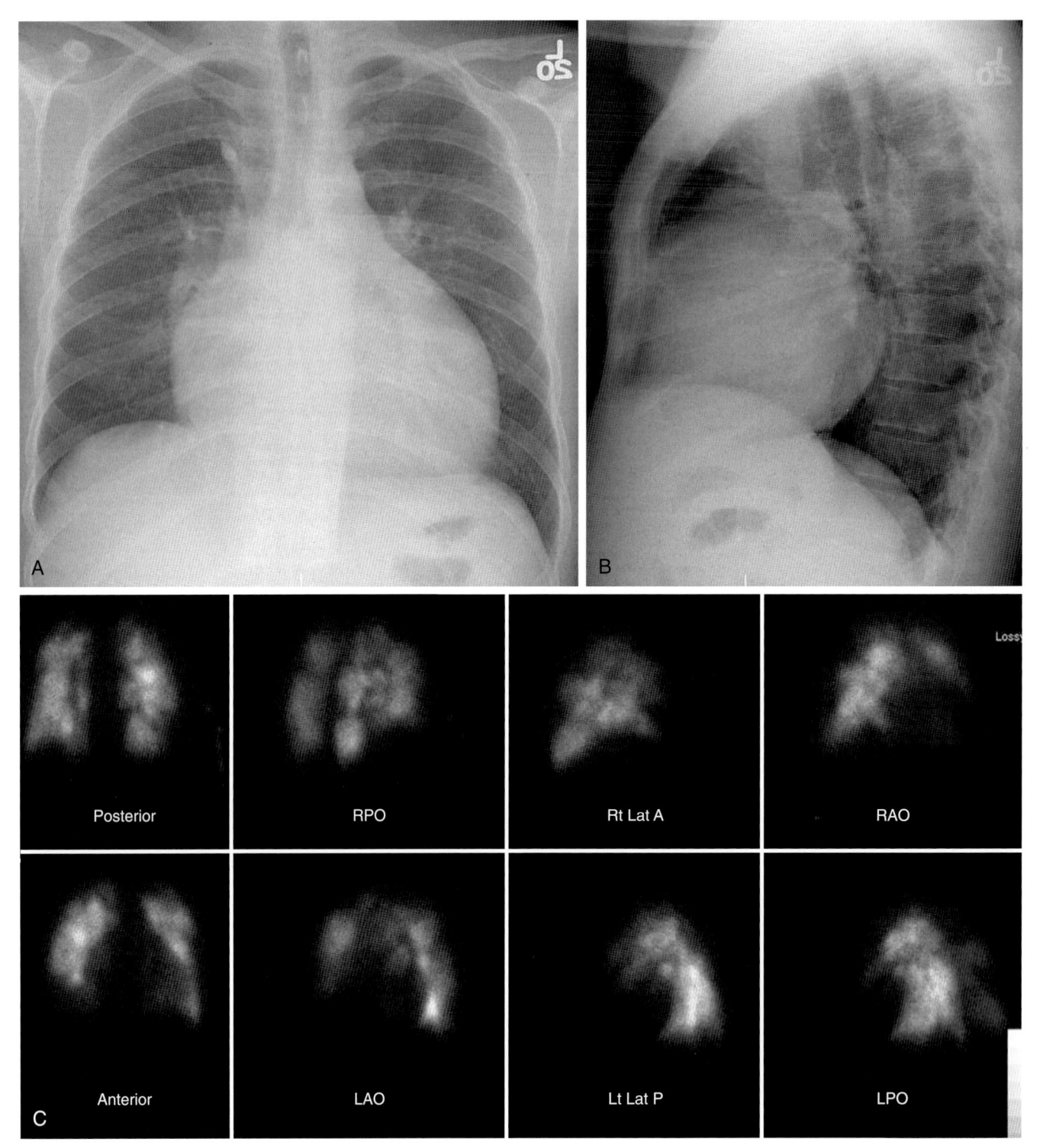

■ **FIGURE 98-1** A 38-year-old man with progressive shortness of breath after a kayaking episode 2 years ago showing the classic features of chronic pulmonary embolism. **A** and **B**, Frontal and lateral chest radiographs show large pulmonary arteries and enlarged right cardiac chambers. The radiograph suggests pulmonary hypertension but does not allow a more specific diagnosis. **C** and **D**, Perfusion (C) and ventilation (D) images from a V/Q scan show multiple wedge-shaped perfusion abnormalities with normal ventilation.

CHAPTER 98 • Chronic Pulmonary Embolism 1347

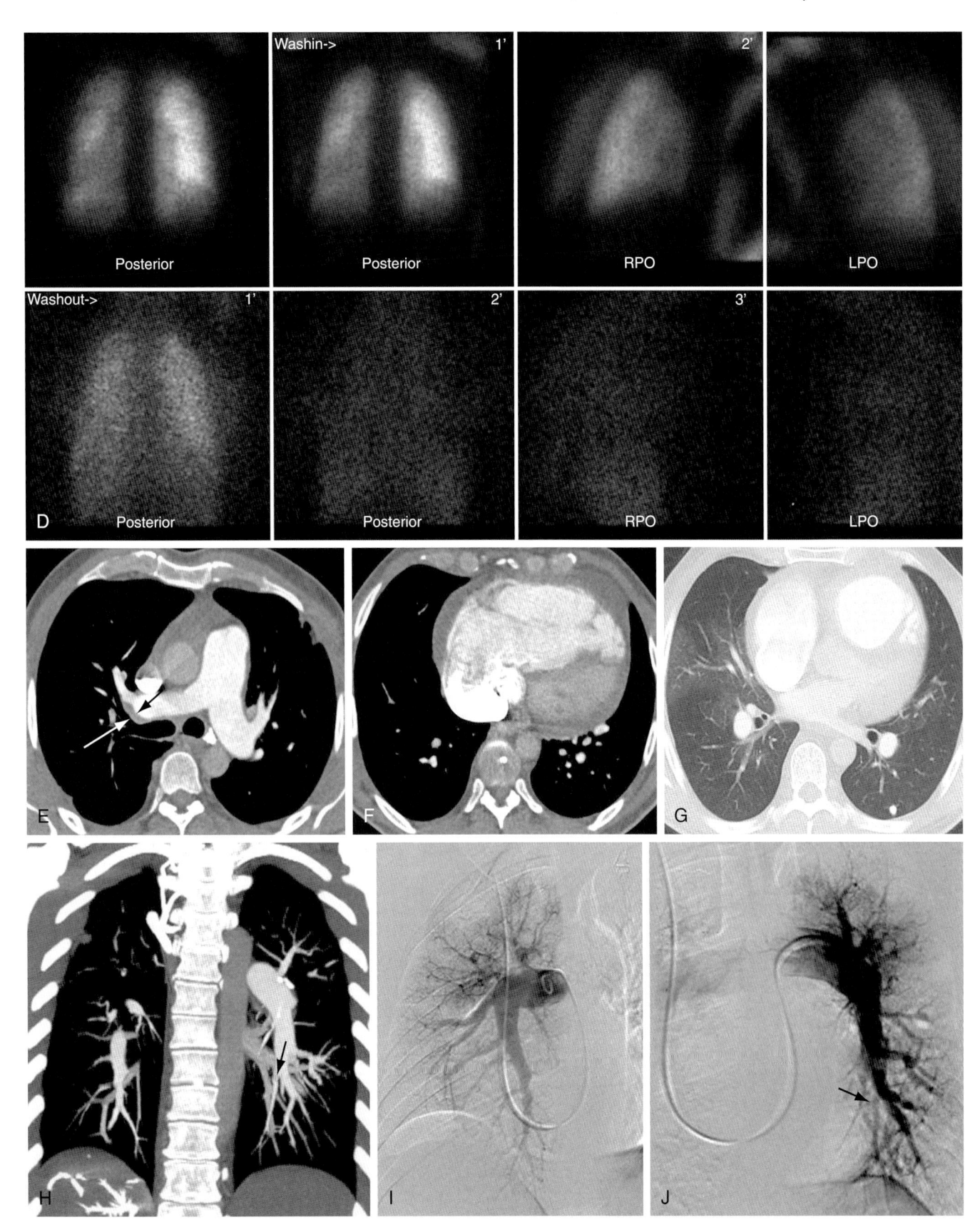

■ **FIGURE 98-1, cont'd** This study was interpreted as a "high probability" study for pulmonary embolism and, in this setting, favored chronic pulmonary embolism. No information is provided on surgical accessibility of the disease. **E** and **F**, Soft tissue windows from contrast-enhanced CT show the enlarged main pulmonary artery and an eccentric filling defect in the right pulmonary artery (*arrows* in **E**) in keeping with chronic pulmonary embolism. The enlarged right side of the heart with hypertrophy results from the severe pulmonary hypertension. **G**, Lung windows from CT show the mosaic perfusion pattern; the darker areas represent abnormal lung. **H**, Coronal thin maximum intensity projection CT image (6 mm) shows the beaded appearance of the lower lobe pulmonary arteries with a clear-cut web in the left lower lobe (*arrow*). **I** and **J**, Pulmonary angiography performed as part of preoperative planning confirms the beaded appearance of the pulmonary arteries and the web (*arrow* in **J**).

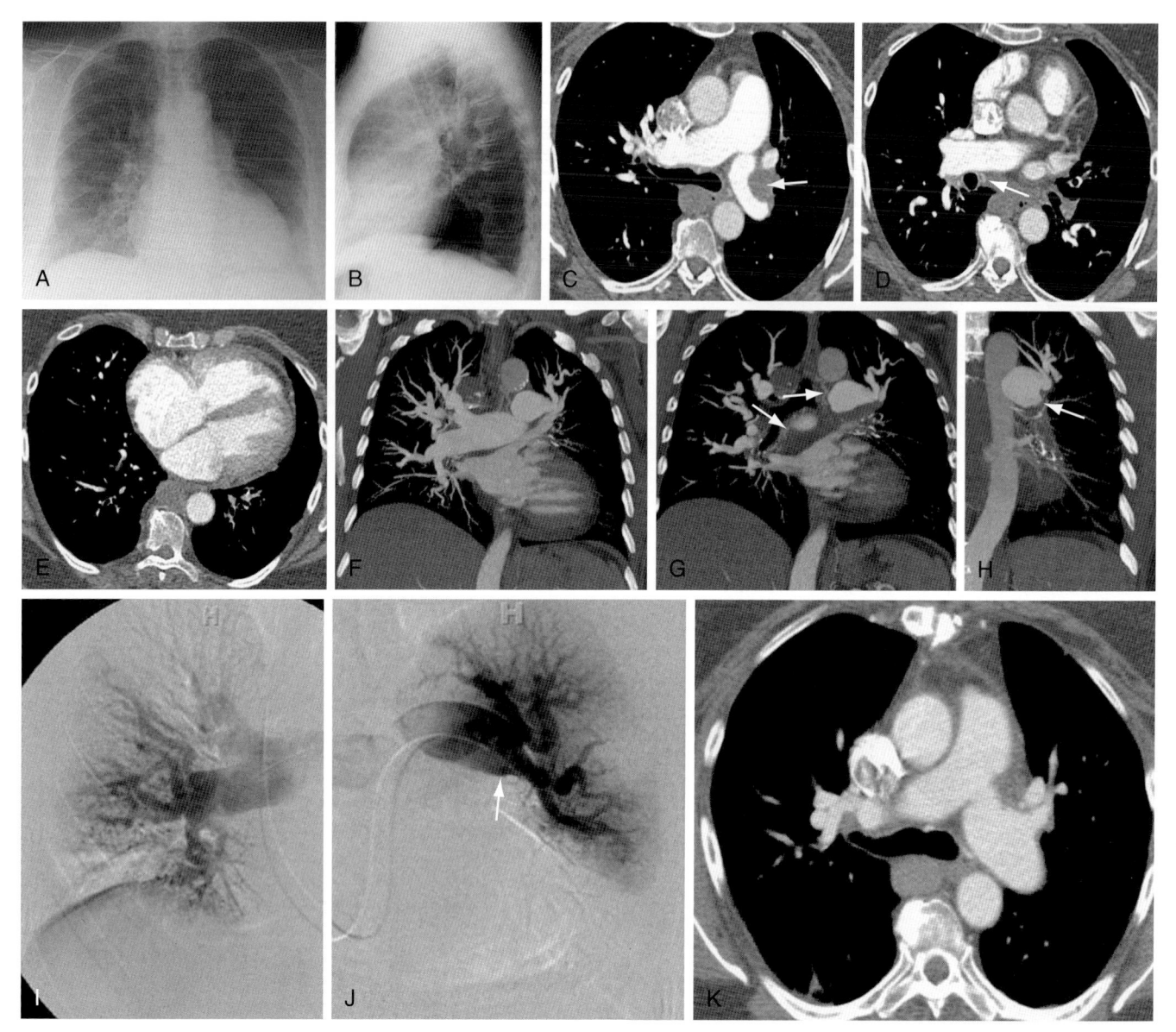

FIGURE 98-2 A 64-year-old woman with progressive dyspnea. **A** and **B,** Frontal and lateral chest radiographs show enlarged pulmonary arteries in keeping with pulmonary hypertension. **C to E,** Contrast-enhanced CT shows an eccentric thrombus (*arrow* in **C**) and enlarged bronchial arteries (*arrow* in **D**). The enlarged right side of the heart in **C** confirmed the diagnosis of pulmonary hypertension from chronic pulmonary embolism. **F to H,** Coronal thin maximum intensity projection images (6 mm) show the CT findings of chronic pulmonary embolism including beaded vessels, enlarged bronchial arteries (*arrows* in **G**), and vessel cutoff (*arrow* in **H**). In many ways, the CT findings are easier to appreciate on the coronal images. **I** and **J,** Pulmonary angiography confirms the extensive disease and exhibits the finding of "pouching" with a convex contrast column pointing away from the hilum (*arrow* in **J**). **K,** The patient was thought to be a candidate for thromboendarterectomy, and postoperative CT shows the decreased clot burden. Unfortunately, the patient had only minimal decrease in pulmonary pressures from her surgery.

aneurysms, familial pulmonary arterial hypertension, intracardiac shunts, or even mitral disease (Fig. 98-3). Many of these features are better appreciated on coronal reconstructions.

For optimal evaluation, CT angiography according to a pulmonary embolism protocol should be performed. Review of images must be done with a window setting that allows visualization of any intraluminal webs, which tend to be less than 1 mm in size. Lung windows should also be used to look for any absent vessels. Nothing is more difficult than to look for a missing vessel on soft tissue windows. The lung windows can be helpful as they show the bronchus with a thready or absent accompanying artery.

Parenchymal or other findings are useful in confirming that the patient has CTPH as an explanation for pulmonary hypertension. These include enlarged bronchial arteries, mosaic perfusion, and bronchiectasis.[20-22] The enlarged bronchial arteries tend to be variable, with only some of the arteries being enlarged. In general, these may be seen at the level of the carina as serpentine, enhancing structures near the descending aorta. They are much better delineated on coronal reconstructions. Mosaic perfusion in CTPH is a reflection of the small-vessel disease, with

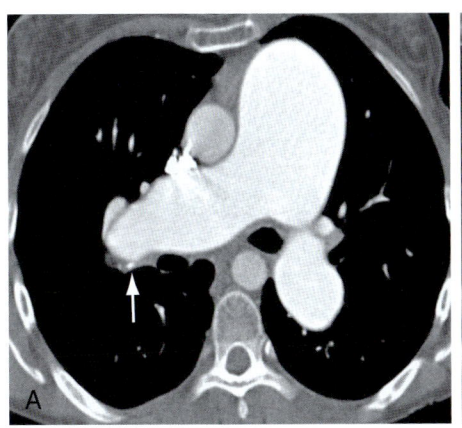

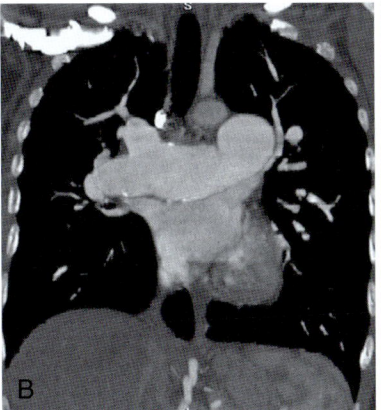

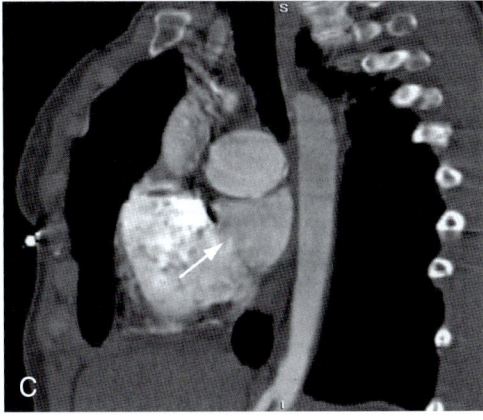

■ **FIGURE 98-3** A 45-year-old woman with severe pulmonary hypertension. **A,** Contrast-enhanced CT shows the markedly enlarged pulmonary arteries with some eccentric calcification (*arrow*). **B,** The calcifications are better seen on the coronal maximum intensity projection image. These calcifications are very unusual for chronic pulmonary embolism and should prompt one to consider an intracardiac shunt or other cause of pulmonary hypertension. **C,** Sagittal oblique reconstruction shows the very large ostium secundum atrial septal defect (*arrow*) that was responsible for these CT findings.

the darker areas representing abnormal lung with decreased vascularity. The darker lung should not demonstrate air trapping. Bronchiectasis in CTPH is a poorly understood phenomenon that has been clearly observed in the setting of CTPH. In general, the bronchiectasis is cylindrical.

Magnetic Resonance

The role of MR in the evaluation of CTPH is very much under current investigation.[15] Ideally, MR would provide a one-test answer to the severity of hypertension and the location of the emboli, if present. As with echocardiography, estimation of pulmonary pressures depends on visualization of a tricuspid regurgitation jet. The excursion of the tricuspid annulus (up to 4 cm) during the cardiac cycle can make imaging of a clear dephasing jet difficult. Using a velocity-encoded phase contrast sequence, one can then obtain images orthogonal to the jet to calculate a peak velocity, which can then be used to calculate a pressure gradient. This number can be added to an estimation of right atrial pressure based on the size of the inferior vena cava and its respiratory variation.[15,16]

MR can also be used to observe cardiac function noninvasively. By using flow quantification of the pulmonary artery just above the pulmonary valve, one can calculate a right-sided heart stroke volume. Short-axis imaging through the heart can be used to calculate right ventricle volumes and ejection fraction. These values can then be used to observe a patient's response to treatment in a noninvasive fashion. In theory, this potential for MR makes this modality eclipse the others. Unfortunately, a comprehensive MR study is longer than a CT examination, taking up to 1 hour, and typically requires repetitive breath-holding, which is often not practical in patients who may be dyspneic. Postprocessing may also be tedious and time-consuming, making this type of study impractical in a diverse, busy practice.

A third feature of MR is the analysis for a potential cause of the pulmonary hypertension. MR can allow the assessment of an intracardiac shunt and with gadolinium provides excellent depiction of the pulmonary circulation. MR findings are identical to those of CT. Mosaic intensity may also be better appreciated on postcontrast images. On occasion, MR will not show CTPH as the cause of the pulmonary hypertension but may show that the hypertension is related to an interstitial lung disease. Care must be taken to assess the lungs on all sequences.

At our institution, MR is used primarily as a method to evaluate for intracardiac shunts. We are currently using the techniques to determine whether our patients can be observed noninvasively. We do not routinely use the modality to exclude CTPH.

Nuclear Medicine/Positron Emission Tomography

Nuclear medicine for CTPH primarily relies on ventilation and perfusion (V/Q) scans. There is no role for positron emission tomography in the evaluation of CTPH. As with acute pulmonary embolism, the V/Q scan in CTPH tends to show multiple perfusion defects without ventilation abnormalities.[13,23] These "mismatches" can be used to diagnose CTPH in the presence of pulmonary hypertension. A potential pitfall is that subsegmental defects may be seen in veno-occlusive disease, fibrosis, and idiopathic pulmonary hypertension (Fig. 98-4).[24] On occasion, these defects can be difficult to separate from those of CTPH. Another shortcoming of V/Q scintigraphy is its inability to delineate location of the scars of CTPH.[23] No information about the surgical resectability of the lesions is provided by this examination. Despite these potential pitfalls, V/Q scintigraphy offers a safe, lower radiation alternative to MDCT and is still frequently used in the evaluation of pulmonary hypertension that may be secondary to CTPH.[25]

Angiography

Like MDCT and contrast-enhanced MR, angiography relies on the vascular findings of CTPH: intravascular webs, eccentric thrombus, beaded vessels, vessel cutoff, and enlarged main pulmonary artery.[26] Because imaging is performed at various points in time, another well-described

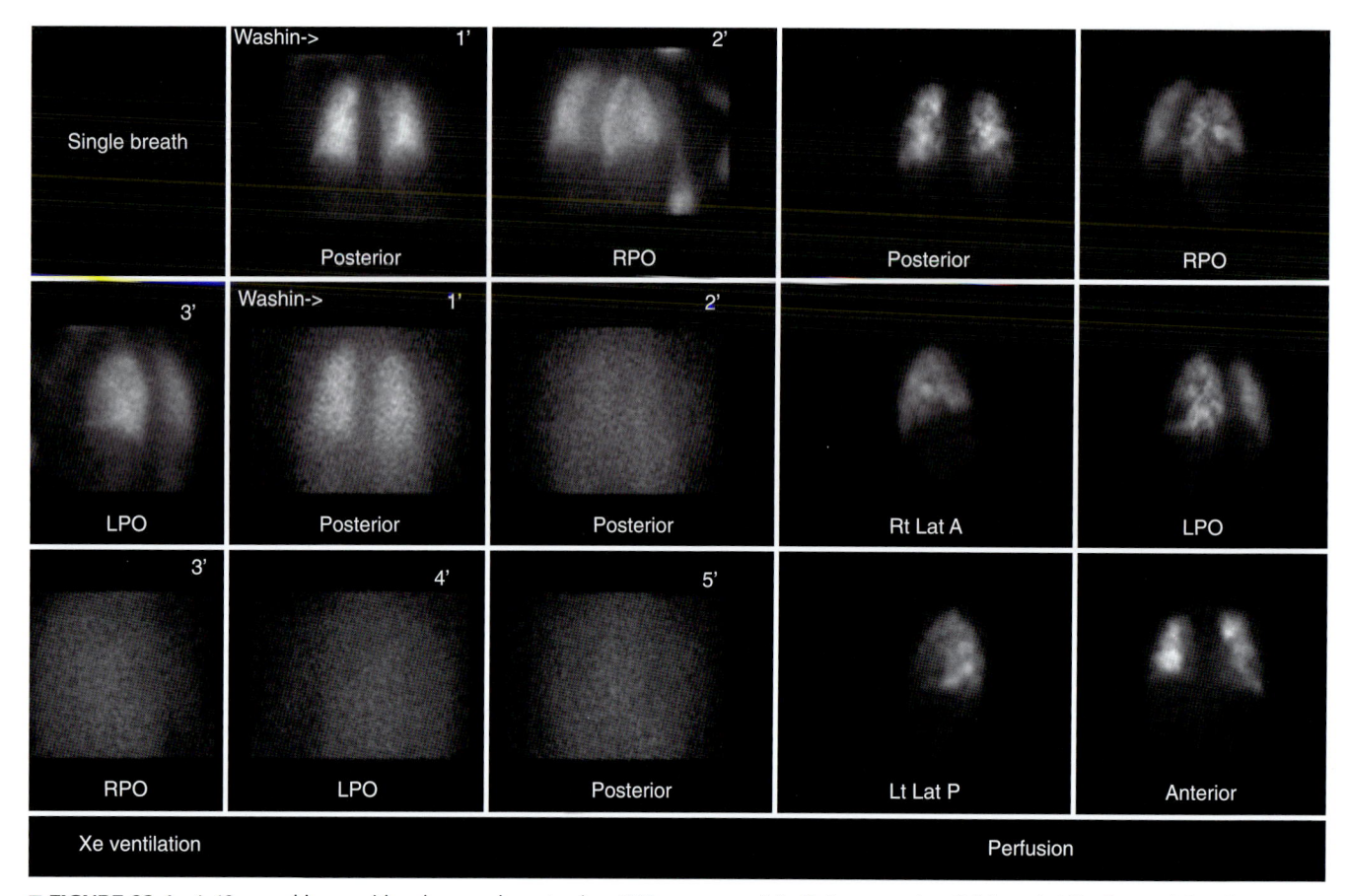

FIGURE 98-4 A 48-year-old man with pulmonary hypertension. V/Q scan was originally interpreted as "high probability," an opinion that changed when the nature of the disease was discovered—vasculitis. Vasculitis can occasionally be confused with chronic pulmonary embolism on V/Q scans.

sign, known as pouching, may be seen. In pouching, a convex, enlarged vessel is seen without initial filling of peripheral vessels. Over time, the thready peripheral vessels opacify.

An advantage of angiography is that it allows simultaneous measurements of right-sided heart and pulmonary pressures. These are still considered the gold standard measurements and are used for determination of prognosis and for follow-up of the patients.[6]

During the parenchymal phase, mosaic perfusion may be observed.

Classic Signs

Classic signs of CTPH consist mostly of enlarged pulmonary arteries centrally, with increased size of the right side of the heart, mosaic perfusion, and eccentric arterial filling defects with intravascular webs. Segmental arteries tend to be thready and may be cut off or absent.

Differential Diagnosis

From Clinical Presentation

Any cause of pulmonary hypertension may mimic CTPH clinically.[6,23] These include idiopathic pulmonary hypertension, Eisenmenger syndrome, pulmonary vasculitis, left-sided heart failure, chronic hypoxia, sarcoidosis, interstitial lung disease, fibrosing mediastinitis, and central bronchogenic cancer.

From Imaging Findings

Other conditions can mimic the angiographic findings. These include fibrosing mediastinitis and pulmonary vasculitis, such as Takayasu arteritis.[23] Both of these conditions may cause thready vessels with beading and vascular cutoffs. The key in excluding these other conditions is to look for soft tissue attenuation or lymphadenopathy on CT or MR (Fig. 98-5). Enhancement of the vessel wall may also be helpful. This finding is not present with CTPH.

Calcification of the vessel wall should also not be used as the sole diagnostic feature of CTPH. Although this finding may rarely be seen with CTPH, calcification is much more commonly seen with pulmonary hypertension from long-standing cardiac shunts, familial pulmonary hypertension, pulmonary aneurysms, or even mitral disease.

Synopsis of Treatment Options

Medical

Treatment of CTPH very much depends on the location of the scars and webs. If it is central enough, patients may

CHAPTER 98 • Chronic Pulmonary Embolism

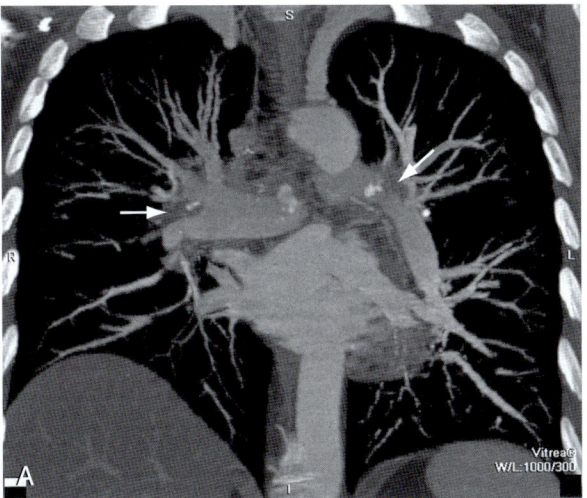

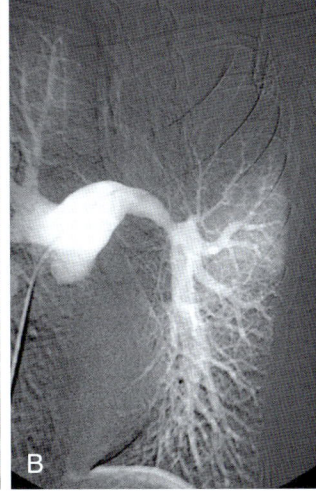

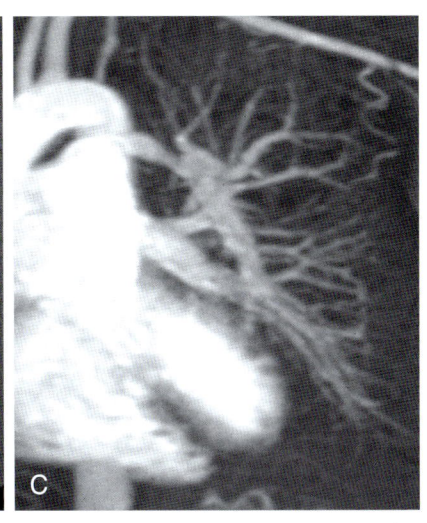

FIGURE 98-5 A 28-year-old woman with pulmonary hypertension. **A,** CT angiography shows beaded vessels with calcified soft tissue (*arrows*) that were in keeping with lymphadenopathy. These beaded vessels could be confused with chronic pulmonary embolism. **B,** Conventional angiography depicts the beaded vessels but not the extrinsic nature of the disease. **C,** MR angiography, similar to the angiography in B, also fails to show that the compression and beading are from lymphadenopathy. This patient was found to have fibrosing mediastinitis.

be referred for surgery, which can be curative.[2,4,18] If it is peripheral, CTPH will be treated similarly to pulmonary arterial hypertension. Vasodilator therapy may be all that can be offered to the patient. Because isolated peripheral disease will be treated like other causes of pulmonary arterial hypertension, one should not fear that tiny webs in small arterioles that may be missed on CT will alter treatment.

Surgical/Interventional

Surgical treatment consists of removal of the scar tissue so that the pulmonary vascular volume can be returned.[2,4,18] The surgical procedure is a pulmonary thromboendarterectomy. The boundary between what is accessible and what is not depends on the experience of the surgeon. Usually, subsegmental artery thromboendarterectomy marks the limit to where a patient may be cured. This procedure is quite different from an embolectomy, which may be used in the setting of a large acute or subacute saddle pulmonary embolism. This procedure does not require stripping of the pulmonary artery intima and is quicker.

Reporting: Information for the Referring Physician

The imager must make sure to comment on the presence of findings of CTPH and the location of these findings. Precise localization is important to guide therapy. It is not adequate to simply document the absence or presence of webs.

> ### KEY POINTS
> - CTPH represents a potentially curable cause of pulmonary hypertension.
> - CT, MR, and angiography can show the vascular findings of CTPH, including vessel cutoff, webs, beaded vessels, and eccentric thrombus.
> - CT, echocardiography, and MR also allow morphologic cardiac assessment.
> - CT also allows corroborative evidence of CTPH, including mosaic perfusion, bronchiectasis, and enlarged bronchial arteries.
> - Echocardiography and MR may allow noninvasive pressure estimation and assessment of right-sided heart function.
> - V/Q scans can be a useful screen but do not allow lesion localization to determine surgical resectability.

SUGGESTED READINGS

Frazier AA, Galvin JR, Franks TJ, Rosado-de-Christenson ML. From the archives of the AFIP: pulmonary vasculature—hypertension and infarction. Radiographics 2000; 20:491-524.

Han D, Lee KS, Franquet T, et al. Thrombotic and nonthrombotic pulmonary arterial embolism: spectrum of imaging findings. Radiographics 2003; 23:1521-1539.

Hoeper MH, Mayer E, Simonneau G, Rubin LJ. Chronic thromboembolic pulmonary hypertension. Circulation 2006; 113:2011-2020.

Simonneau G, Galiè N, Rubin LJ, et al. Clinical classification of pulmonary hypertension. J Am Coll Cardiol 2004; 43(Suppl S):5S-12S.

Wittram C, Kalra MK, Maher MM, et al. Acute and chronic pulmonary emboli: angiography-CT correlation. AJR Am J Roentgenol 2006; 186(Suppl 2):S421-S429.

REFERENCES

1. Frazier AA, Galvin JR, Franks TJ, Rosado-de-Christenson ML. From the archives of the AFIP: pulmonary vasculature—hypertension and infarction. Radiographics 2000; 20:491-524.
2. Sahara M, Takahashi T, Imai Y, et al. New insights in the treatment strategy for pulmonary arterial hypertension. Cardiovasc Drugs Ther 2006; 20.377-386.
3. Simonneau G, Galiè N, Rubin LJ, et al. Clinical classification of pulmonary hypertension. J Am Coll Cardiol 2004; 43(Suppl S):5S-12S.
4. Wray CJ, Auger WR. Evaluation of patients for pulmonary endarterectomy. Semin Thorac Cardiovasc Surg 2006; 18:223-229.
5. Moser KM, Braunwald NS. Successful surgical intervention in severe chronic thromboembolic pulmonary hypertension. Chest 1973; 64:29-35.
6. Hoeper MH, Mayer E, Simonneau G, Rubin LJ. Chronic thromboembolic pulmonary hypertension. Circulation 2006; 113:2011-2020.
7. Fedullo PF, Auger WR, Kerr KM, Rubin LJ. Chronic thromboembolic pulmonary hypertension. N Engl J Med 2001; 345:1465-1472.
8. Ribeiro A, Lindmarker P, Johnsson H, et al. Pulmonary embolism: one-year follow-up with echocardiography Doppler and five-year analysis. Circulation 1999; 99:1325-1330.
9. Pengo V, Lensing AW, Prins MH, et al. Thromboembolic Pulmonary Hypertension Study Group. Incidence of chronic thromboembolic pulmonary hypertension after pulmonary embolism. N Engl J Med 2004; 350:2257-2264.
10. Rubin LJ, Badesch DB. Evaluation and management of the patient with pulmonary arterial hypertension. Ann Intern Med 2005; 143:282-292.
11. Nauser TD, Stites SW. Diagnosis and treatment of pulmonary hypertension. Am Fam Physician 2001; 63:1789-1798.
12. Galiè N, Manes A, Branzi A. Evaluation of pulmonary arterial hypertension. Curr Opin Cardiol 2004; 19:575-581.
13. Worsley DF, Palevsky HI, Alavi A. Ventilation-perfusion lung scanning in the evaluation of pulmonary hypertension. J Nucl Med 1994; 35:793-796.
14. Coulden R. State-of-the-art imaging techniques in chronic thromboembolic pulmonary hypertension. Proc Am Thorac Soc 2006; 3:577-583.
15. Kreitner KF, Kunz RP, Ley S, et al. Chronic thromboembolic pulmonary hypertension—assessment by magnetic resonance imaging. Eur Radiol 2007; 17:11-21. Epub 2006.
16. Sallach SM, Peshock RM, Reimold S. Noninvasive cardiac imaging in pulmonary hypertension. Cardiol Rev 2007; 15:97-101.
17. Wittram C, Kalra MK, Maher MM, et al. Acute and chronic pulmonary emboli: angiography-CT correlation. AJR Am J Roentgenol 2006; 186(Suppl 2):S421-S429.
18. Heinrich M, Uder M, Tscholl D, et al. CT scan findings in chronic thromboembolic pulmonary hypertension: predictors of hemodynamic improvement after pulmonary thromboendarterectomy. Chest 2005; 127:1606-1613.
19. Han D, Lee KS, Franquet T, et al. Thrombotic and nonthrombotic pulmonary arterial embolism: spectrum of imaging findings. Radiographics 2003; 23:1521-1539.
20. Hasegawa I, Boiselle PM, Hatabu H. Bronchial artery dilatation on MDCT scans of patients with acute pulmonary embolism: comparison with chronic or recurrent pulmonary embolism. AJR Am J Roentgenol 2004; 182:67-72.
21. King MA, Bergin CJ, Yeung DW, et al. Chronic pulmonary thromboembolism: detection of regional hypoperfusion with CT. Radiology 1994; 191:359-363.
22. Remy-Jardin M, Remy J, Louvegny S, et al. Airway changes in chronic pulmonary embolism: CT findings in 33 patients. Radiology 1997; 203:355-360.
23. Dartevelle P, Fadel E, Mussot S, et al. Chronic thromboembolic pulmonary hypertension. Eur Respir J 2004; 23:637-648.
24. Thadani U, Burrow C, Whitaker W, Heath D. Pulmonary veno-occlusive disease. Q J Med 1975; 44:133-159.
25. Tunariu N, Gibbs SJ, Win Z, et al. Ventilation-perfusion scintigraphy is more sensitive than multidetector CTPA in detecting chronic thromboembolic pulmonary disease as a treatable cause of pulmonary hypertension. J Nucl Med 2007; 48:680-684.
26. Auger WR, Fedullo PF, Moser KM, et al. Chronic major-vessel thromboembolic pulmonary artery obstruction: appearance at angiography. Radiology 1992; 182:393-398.

CHAPTER 99

Pulmonary Hypertension

Michael B. Gotway

An understanding of the causes and imaging manifestations of pulmonary hypertension must begin with a firm grasp of pulmonary vascular anatomy. A brief review of the relevant anatomy and physiology of the pulmonary vascular system, particularly as it relates to an understanding of pulmonary hypertension, will be presented. Subsequently, the classification of pulmonary hypertension and individual lesions producing pulmonary hypertension will be discussed.

PULMONARY HYPERTENSION

Definition

Pulmonary hypertension (PH) is defined as a resting mean pulmonary arterial pressure more than 25 mm Hg at rest or more than 30 mm Hg with exercise. Among the various subclassifications of PH, the subgroup referred to as pulmonary arterial hypertension adds the criterion that the pulmonary capillary wedge pressure should be 15 mm Hg or less.[2]

Etiology and Pathophysiology

Anatomy and Physiology of the Pulmonary Circulation

The pulmonary circulation consists of two parallel networks, the pulmonary arterial circulation and bronchial arterial circulation.[1] The pulmonary arterial circulation consists of a series of branching arteries, arterioles, capillaries, venules, and veins. Pulmonary arteries travel adjacent to the lobar, segmental, and subsegmental airways to the level of the terminal bronchioles. The small pulmonary arteries from the subsegmental level to the terminal bronchioles possess a thick muscular media. At the level of the respiratory bronchioles and alveolar ducts, the small pulmonary arteries have lost much of the muscle within the arteriolar media as well as their external elastic membranes, and are now termed *pulmonary arterioles*, ranging in size from 10 to 150 μm. These vessels ramify further within the alveolar walls and form a rich capillary network. Capillary blood collects in venules, which progressively coalesce to form pulmonary veins. Pulmonary veins course within interlobular septa, eventually emptying into the left atrium.

The major site of resistance to pulmonary arterial blood flow occurs at the small muscular pulmonary artery and arteriole level. Caliber changes in the vessels at this level regulate pulmonary arterial pressure and are critical for optimizing ventilation and perfusion matching.

The mean arterial pressure of the pulmonary circulation is approximately one sixth that of the systemic circulation. This low pressure is maintained even with large increases in pulmonary blood flow, as occurs with exercise. This is possible because at rest, numerous pulmonary capillaries are normally not perfused and become recruited when increased pulmonary blood flow must be accommodated.

Pathogenesis

Several mechanisms may produce a decrease in the total number of small pulmonary arteries and arterioles, thereby increasing pulmonary vascular resistance and producing elevated pulmonary arterial pressure. Such mechanisms include intraluminal arterial occlusion, muscular contraction of small pulmonary arteries, vascular remodeling with wall thickening, or conditions that produce pulmonary venous hypertension. Several of these mechanisms may be operative simultaneously in patients with PH.

The pulmonary vascular endothelium actively responds to changes in oxygen tension, transmural pressure, and pulmonary blood flow, and actively participates in the regulation of pulmonary arterial pressure through the elaboration of a number of vasoactive substances, including prostacyclin, nitrous oxide, and endothelin.[3] These agents have direct effects on pulmonary vascular smooth muscle tone, promoting relaxation or vasodilation, and also may directly affect platelet function.

Various pathologic derangements may be seen in patients with PH, varying somewhat depending on the cause of PH. In general, regardless of the cause of PH, the pulmonary arteries become dilated,[1] occasionally to the point of being considered aneurysmal. Pulmonary arterial atherosclerosis, typically absent in the pulmonary arteries of normal adults, may be extensive and frequently involves smaller vessels in patients with PH. PH-related pulmonary arterial atherosclerosis histopathologically appears similar to atherosclerosis occurring in systemic arteries, although complicating features, such as necrosis, ulceration, and calcification, are relatively uncommon.

Plexogenic pulmonary arteriopathy is the term applied to a constellation of vascular changes often encountered in patients with primary PH, but may also be seen in patients with PH of other causes, including hepatic disease, connective tissue disorders, congenital cardiovascular disease, and some anorexigenic medications.[2]

Classification

There have been a number of proposed classification schemes to categorize the causes of PH. In 1998, during the Second World Symposium on Pulmonary Hypertension held in Evian, France, a clinical classification for PH was proposed (Box 99-1).[3-5] The aim of the Evian classification was to provide categories for causes of PH that shared similar pathophysiologic mechanisms, clinical presentations, and therapeutic considerations. Similar to oncologic staging considerations, such a classification was designed to allow standardization of diagnosis and treatment for patients with PH, conduction of trials with similar patient cohorts, and investigation of pathobiologic abnormalities in patient populations that are highly characterized. In 2003, the Third World Symposium on Pulmonary Arterial Hypertension, held in Venice, evaluated the usefulness of the Evian classification system and recommended some minor modifications. The Venice classification was adopted by the World Health Organization (WHO) and has been referred to as the Revised World Health Organization Classification of Pulmonary Hypertension (Box 99-2). More recently, the revised WHO-Venice classification underwent revision at the Fourth World Symposium on Pulmonary Hypertension held in Dana Point, California. The new classification system is referred to as the 2008 Dana Point Pulmonary Hypertension classification system.[6] Traditionally, pulmonary hypertension has been classified into primary versus secondary causes or precapillary and postcapillary causes; this classification scheme is still in common use, particularly among interpreting physicians, and is included here as well. The pre- and postcapillary PH classification scheme is commonly reviewed in radiology texts (Box 99-3),[1] but the 2008 Dana Point classification system is in more widespread use among clinicians and investigators dealing with PH. The 2008 Dana Point classification system will be used for this chapter.

In the 2008 Dana Point classification schemes, the category of pulmonary arterial hypertension (PAH) includes a subgroup of patients with PH without any identifiable cause, or idiopathic PAH,[6] previously referred to as primary pulmonary hypertension (PPH). Other subgroups in the category of PAH include disorders that share localization of the lesions to small, muscular pulmonary arterioles, including heritable causes of PH (e.g., patients with mutations in bone morphogenetic protein receptor 2 and activin receptor-like kinase 1), drug and toxin exposures, and associations with certain conditions, such as collagen vascular diseases, HIV-related PH, portopulmonary hyper-

---

BOX 99-1   Classification of Pulmonary Hypertension: Evian Classification

I. **PULMONARY ARTERIAL HYPERTENSION**
   a. Primary pulmonary hypertension
      i. Familial
      ii. Sporadic
   b. Pulmonary arterial hypertension related to risk factors or associated conditions
      i. Collagen vascular disease
      ii. Congenital cardiovascular shunts
      iii. Portal hypertension
      iv. HIV infection
      v. Drugs, toxins (e.g., anorexigens)
      vi. Persistent pulmonary hypertension of the newborn
      vii. Other

II. **PULMONARY VENOUS HYPERTENSION**
   a. Left-sided atrial, ventricular disease
   b. Left-sided valvular heart disease
   c. Extrinsic compression (e.g., mediastinal fibrosis, tumor, lymphadenopathy)
   d. Pulmonary veno-occlusive disease
   e. Other

III. **PULMONARY HYPERTENSION SECONDARY TO RESPIRATORY DISEASE, HYPOXIA**
   a. COPD
   b. Interstitial lung disease
   c. Sleep-disordered breathing
   d. Alveolar hypoventilation disorders
   e. Chronic exposure to high altitude
   f. Neonatal lung disease
   g. Alveolar-capillary dysplasia
   h. Other

IV. **PULMONARY HYPERTENSION SECONDARY TO CHRONIC THROMBOTIC OR EMBOLIC DISEASE**
   a. Thromboembolic arterial obstruction of proximal arteries
   b. Distal pulmonary arterial obstruction
      i. Pulmonary emboli, tumor, ova or parasites, foreign material
      ii. In situ thrombosis
      iii. Sickle cell disease

V. **PULMONARY HYPERTENSION SECONDARY TO DIRECT PULMONARY VASCULAR INSULTS**
   a. Inflammatory—schistosomiasis, sarcoidosis, other
   b. Pulmonary capillary hemangiomatosis

> **BOX 99-2 Classification of Pulmonary Hypertension: Venice-Revised WHO Classification**
>
> I. **PULMONARY ARTERIAL HYPERTENSION**
>   a. Idiopathic
>   b. Familial
>   c. Pulmonary arterial hypertension related to risk factors or associated conditions
>   i. Collagen vascular disease
>   ii. Congenital cardiovascular shunts
>   iii. Portal hypertension
>   iv. HIV infection
>   v. Drugs, toxins (e.g., anorexigens)
>   vi. Other (e.g., thyroid disorders, glycogen storage disease, Gaucher disease, hemoglobinopathies, myeloproliferative disorders, hereditary hemorrhagic telangiectasia, splenectomy)
>   d. Persistent pulmonary hypertension of the newborn
>   e. Associated with significant venous or capillary involvement
>   i. Pulmonary veno-occlusive disease
>   ii. Pulmonary capillary hemangiomatosis
>
> II. **PULMONARY HYPERTENSION WITH LEFT HEART DISEASE**
>   a. Left-sided atrial, ventricular disease
>   b. Left-sided valvular heart disease
>   c. Other
>
> III. **PULMONARY HYPERTENSION SECONDARY TO RESPIRATORY DISEASE / HYPOXIA**
>   a. COPD
>   b. Interstitial lung disease
>   c. Sleep-disordered breathing
>   d. Alveolar hypoventilation disorders
>   e. Chronic exposure to high altitude
>   f. Developmental abnormalities
>
> IV. **PULMONARY HYPERTENSION SECONDARY TO CHRONIC THROMBOTIC AND/OR EMBOLIC DISEASE**
>   a. Thromboembolic arterial obstruction of proximal arteries
>   b. Thromboembolic arterial obstruction of distal arteries
>   c. Nonthrombotic pulmonary embolism (e.g., emboli, tumor, ova or parasites, foreign material)
>   d. Other
>
> V. **MISCELLANEOUS**
>   a. Sarcoidosis, lymphangiomatosis, extrinsic vascular compression (e.g., mediastinal fibrosis, tumor, lymphadenopathy)

> **BOX 99-3 Classification of Pulmonary Hypertension: Precapillary Versus Postcapillary Etiologies**
>
> **PRECAPILLARY PULMONARY HYPERTENSION**
> - Pulmonary arterial hypertension
> - Congenital cardiovascular left to right shunts
> - Pulmonary thromboembolism
> - Nonthrombotic embolization (including tumor, particulate, and parasitic thromboemboli)
> - Chronic alveolar hypoxia.
>
> **POSTCAPILLARY PULMONARY HYPERTENSION**
> - Left-sided cardiac obstruction—left ventricular failure, systemic hypertension, mitral valvular disease, atrial myxoma, cor triatriatum, other congenital cardiac anomalies
> - Pulmonary venous obstruction—fibrosing mediastinitis
> - Pulmonary veno-occlusive disease

tension, congenital systemic to pulmonary artery shunts, schistosomiasis, and chronic hemolytic anemias. The morphologic and clinical characteristics of these disorders are similar, and they also share a clinical response to treatment with continuous infusion of epoprostenol.[5] Most patients previously diagnosed with primary pulmonary hypertension would now be classified as patients with idiopathic pulmonary arterial hypertension (IPAH) or, less commonly, heritable PH or anorexigen-induced PH (Box 99-4).[7] Persistent PH of the newborn was also recognized as a cause of PAH in the 2008 Dana Point PH classification system. The Venice-revised WHO classification system also includes another subcategory in the pulmonary arterial hypertension group, referred to as "pulmonary arterial hypertension associated with significant venous or capillary involvement." This subcategory includes pulmonary veno-occlusive disease and pulmonary capillary hemangiomatosis. In the 2008 Dana Point system, this subcategory remains a group 1 (PAH) condition, but is now referred to as "pulmonary veno-occlusive disease and/or pulmonary capillary hemangiomatosis" in recognition of the similarities between these two disorders (see Box 99-4). Both entities were classified differently in the Evian system.

The category referred to as pulmonary venous hypertension in the Evian system and as PH with left heart disease in the Venice-revised WHO system is now called pulmonary hypertension secondary to left heart disease (see Box 99-4). It includes systolic and diastolic dysfunction as well as left-sided valvular and myocardial conditions that require therapies directed at improving cardiac function or repairing or reducing valvular mechanical dysfunction, as opposed to treatment with vasodilator therapy.[5,6] In fact, epoprostenol infusion in these patients can be harmful. Pulmonary veno-occlusive disease and lesions producing extrinsic compression on pulmonary veins are included in this category in the Evian system, but were reclassified in the Venice-revised WHO system in 2003 and again in the 2008 Dana Point system.

PH secondary to hypoxia and/or lung disease (see Box 99-4) results from inadequate arterial blood oxygenation caused by chronic obstructive pulmonary disease, interstitial lung diseases, sleep-disordered breathing, alveolar hypoventilation, and residence at high altitude. Usually, the elevated pulmonary arterial pressures in these patients are fairly modest (<35 mm Hg).

Group 4 in the 2008 Dana Point PH classification system is chronic thromboembolic pulmonary hypertension (see

> **BOX 99-4** **Classification of Pulmonary Hypertension: 2008 Dana Point Classification**
>
> 1. Pulmonary arterial hypertension (PAH)
>   1.1 Idiopathic PAH
>   1.2 Heritable
>   1.2.1 Bone morphogenetic protein receptor type 2 germline mutations
>   1.2.2 Activin receptor-like kinase type 1 (endoglin) mutations, with or without hereditary hemorrhagic telangiectasia
>   1.2.3 Unknown
>   1.3 Drug- and toxin-induced
>   1.4 Associated with:
>   1.4.1 Connective tissue disease
>   1.4.2 HIV infection
>   1.4.3 Portal hypertension
>   1.4.4 Congenital heart disease
>   1.4.5 Schistosomiasis
>   1.4.6 Chronic hemolytic anemia
>   1.5 Persistent pulmonary hypertension of the newborn
> 1'. Pulmonary veno-occlusive disease and/or pulmonary capillary hemangiomatosis
> 2. Pulmonary hypertension secondary to left heart disease
>   2.1 Systolic dysfunction
>   2.2 Diastolic dysfunction
>   2.3 Valvular disease
> 3. Pulmonary hypertension secondary to hypoxia and/or lung disease
>   3.1 Chronic obstructive pulmonary disorders
>   3.2 Interstitial lung disease
>   3.3 Other pulmonary diseases with a mixed restrictive and obstructive pattern
>   3.4 Sleep-disordered breathing
>   3.5 Alveolar hypoventilation syndromes
>   3.6 Chronic exposure to high altitude
>   3.7 Developmental abnormalities
> 4. Chronic thromboembolic pulmonary hypertension
> 5. Pulmonary hypertension with unclear multifactorial mechanisms
>   5.1 Hematologic disorders: myeloproliferative disorders, splenectomy
>   5.2 Systemic disorders: sarcoidosis, Langerhans cell histiocytosis, lymphangioleiomyomatosis, vasculitis, neurofibromatosis
>   5.3 Metabolic disorders: glycogen storage disease, Gaucher disease, thyroid disorders
>   5.4 Others: obstruction by neoplasm, fibrosing mediastinitis, chronic renal failure on dialysis

PH caused by disorders of the pulmonary vasculature in the Evian system was simply referred to as the miscellaneous category in the Venice-revised WHO system, and is now called pulmonary hypertension with unclear multifactorial mechanisms in the 2008 Dana Point classification. Included in this group are a variety of disorders such as myeloproliferative diseases, splenectomy, cystic lung diseases, sarcoidosis, and metabolic disorders. External vascular compression, particularly fibrosing mediastinitis, previously considered a subcategory of pulmonary arterial hypertension in the Evian system, was moved to the miscellaneous category in the Venice-revised WHO system and is now classified as a group 5 lesion in the 2008 Dana Point system.[6]

Manifestations

Imaging Techniques and Findings

The characteristic finding of pulmonary arterial hypertension on chest radiography, CT, or MRI is dilation of the central pulmonary arteries, with rapid tapering of the pulmonary vessels as they course peripherally.[1] This pattern is present regardless of the cause of the PH.

Radiography

Chest radiography may show enlargement of the main pulmonary artery segment and dilation of the right and left interlobar pulmonary arteries in patients with PH, regardless of cause (Fig. 99-1).

Ultrasound

Echocardiography is the most commonly performed examination for the noninvasive assessment of possible PH. Echocardiography, using continuous wave or pulsed Doppler, provides noninvasive measurement of pulmonary arterial pressures and also allows detailed morphologic evaluation of the right ventricle. Furthermore, stress echocardiography assesses the hemodynamic response of the pulmonary arterial circulation in response to a variety of challenges, such as exercise or pharmacologic agents in patients with PH.

Computed Tomography

The main pulmonary arterial segment cannot be directly measured on chest radiography, but is easily measured on CT or MRI. When the main pulmonary artery segment exceeds 3 cm (Fig. 99-2), PH is often present. However, PH may be present in patients with a normal-sized main pulmonary arterial segment. The main pulmonary artery–to–ascending aortic ratio is also a useful internal indicator that can suggest enlargement of the main pulmonary artery. When the ratio of the main pulmonary artery to the aorta exceeds 1, elevated pulmonary pressures are usually present.[1]

When PH is prolonged and severe, calcification of the pulmonary arteries, usually affecting the main, right, and/or left pulmonary arteries and, less commonly, the lobar pulmonary arteries, may be present (see Fig. 99-2). This

Box 99-4).[6] In many patients with chronic thromboembolic PH, the central pulmonary arteries show emboli and/or thrombi, and such patients may benefit from pulmonary endarterectomy.[1] In other patients, emboli or thrombi are relatively distally located and are not amenable to surgical treatment. These patients may respond to chronic pulmonary vasodilator therapy, similar to patients with IPAH. Both subgroups of patients are treated with lifelong anticoagulation.

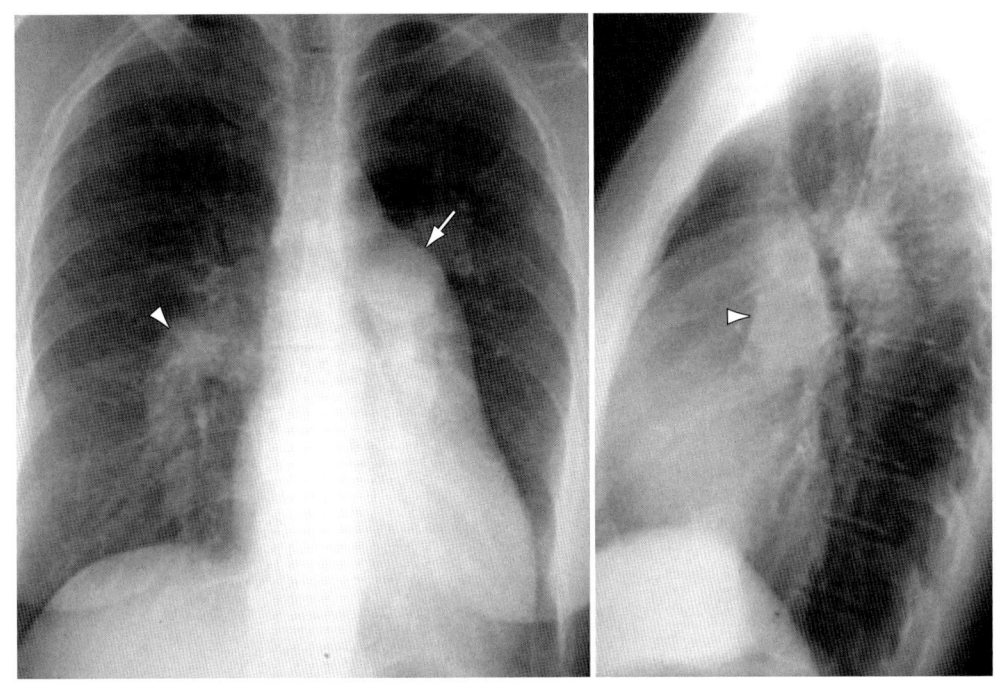

FIGURE 99-1 Frontal and lateral chest radiographs show imaging findings typical of pulmonary hypertension—enlarged main pulmonary artery (*arrow*) and enlarged right (*arrowheads*) and left pulmonary arteries that rapidly taper in the lung periphery.

finding is usually, but not invariably, associated with irreversible pulmonary vascular disease.

Patients with elevated pulmonary arterial pressures may also show right ventricular enlargement and right ventricular hypertrophy (Fig. 99-3) on cross-sectional imaging studies.[1] The right atrium and inferior vena cava may also be enlarged, and contrast reflux into the infradiaphragmatic inferior vena cava is also commonly seen.

Magnetic Resonance Imaging

MRI will show all the vascular abnormalities that thoracic CT detects in patients with PH, such as main pulmonary artery enlargement and right ventricular enlargement and hypertrophy.[1] Additionally, MRI can provide functional information equivalent to echocardiography, such as direction and velocity of blood flow, in addition to specific anatomic information. MRI techniques are well suited to

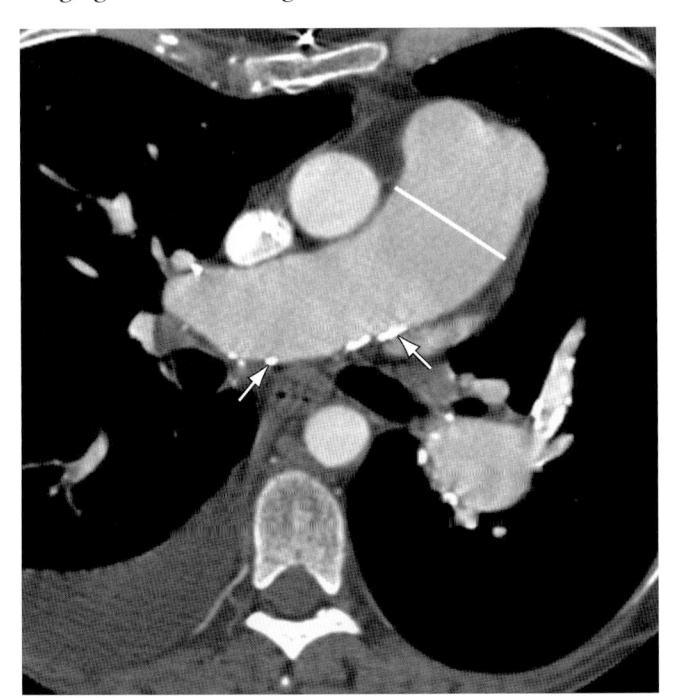

FIGURE 99-2 Axial CT scan shows transverse measurement of main pulmonary artery (*white line*). When this measurement exceeds approximately 3 cm, PH is likely. Note that the transverse dimension of the main pulmonary artery exceeds the transverse dimension of the ascending aorta at the same level. Pulmonary arterial atherosclerosis (*arrows*) is present.

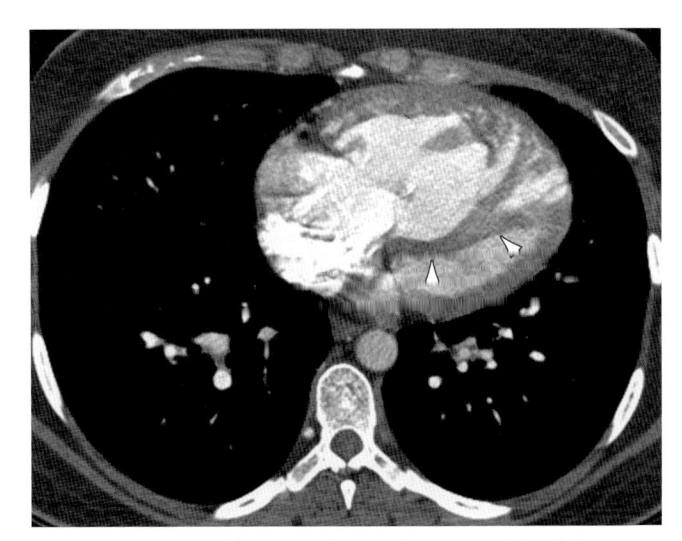

FIGURE 99-3 Axial CT scan shows enlargement of the right ventricle, with leftward bowing of the interventricular septum (*arrowheads*). Either finding may indicate elevated pulmonary arterial pressures. Note right ventricular muscular hypertrophy, indicating long-standing pulmonary arterial pressure elevation.

the evaluation of patients with PH because they allow a detailed anatomic and extensive functional examination of the entire cardiovascular system.

IDIOPATHIC PULMONARY ARTERIAL HYPERTENSION

Definition

The term *primary pulmonary hypertension* was first used in 1951 to describe hypertensive vasculopathy in the pulmonary arteries without an identifiable cause.[5] More recently, it has been recognized that patients with heritable forms of PAH and those with various conditions associated with PH, including connective tissue diseases, the use of appetite suppressant medications, portopulmonary hypertension, and HIV infection, among others, may share pathologic and clinical features similar to PPH, and were previously collectively referred to as secondary PH. The disorders encompassed by the term *secondary PH* are a fairly heterogeneous group of conditions that also include conditions affecting the pulmonary venous circulation or pulmonary parenchyma as well. The use of secondary PH has been largely abandoned because it does not provide a useful framework for the diagnosis or treatment of patients with PH. Therefore, the Venice group recommended changing the term *primary PH* to *idiopathic pulmonary arterial hypertension*; this nomenclature was adopted in the Venice-revised WHO classification system and is maintained in the 2008 Dana Point classification system.

Etiology and Pathophysiology

The cause of IPAH is unknown. The prevalence of PAH is estimated at about 15/million.[7] The disease affects females more commonly than males. The Venice-revised WHO classification system previously recognized two forms of IPAH, familial and idiopathic (sporadic). The 2008 Dana Point classification system now refers to familial PAH as heritable PAH, and considers IPAH as a separate subcategory of PAH (see Box 99-4).[6] Heritable forms of PAH account for approximately 10% of PAH cases, show autosomal dominant inheritance with incomplete penetrance, and have been localized to chromosome 2 at the locus of the bone morphogenic protein receptor type II gene.[5] Heritable PAH associated with mutations in activin receptor-like kinase type 1 may be associated with hereditary hemorrhagic telangiectasia.

The cause of IPAH remains unknown, but is generally attributable to an imbalance between vasodilating agents and vasoconstricting agents, with a relative paucity of prostacyclin and nitric oxide synthase expression and an increase in expression of endothelin-1.

Manifestations of Disease

Clinical Presentation

Patients with IPAH usually present with dyspnea on exertion. The mean age of diagnosis is approximately 37 years.[7] Other presenting symptoms include fatigue, chest pain, syncope, and occasionally cough.

Imaging Techniques and Findings

Radiography

Chest radiography in patients with IPAH typically shows enlargement of the main, right, and left pulmonary arteries (see Fig. 99-1), often with enlargement of the right ventricle (see Fig. 99-3) and right atrium.[1] CT and black blood MRI techniques will show these same findings to advantage. Occasionally, black blood MRI will show increased signal within the pulmonary arteries resulting from slow flow.

Computed Tomography

High-resolution CT (HRCT) in patients with IPAH may show inhomogeneous lung opacity resulting from differential pulmonary parenchymal perfusion (Fig. 99-4).[1] The regions of decreased pulmonary parenchymal attenuation represent areas of mosaic perfusion, and the vessels in these regions of lung may be visibly smaller than their counterparts in the regions of relatively increased lung attenuation. Although airway diseases may result in a similar pattern of mosaic perfusion, vascular and airway causes of mosaic perfusion may be distinguished using postexpiratory imaging. When caused by an obstructive airway process, regional differences in lung attenuation become accentuated with postexpiratory imaging, whereas a proportional increase in attenuation in areas of both increased and decreased attenuation will be seen in patients with pulmonary vascular disease.

Occasionally, HRCT will show centrilobular ground-glass opacities in patients with IPAH (Fig. 99-5), representing foci of hemorrhage, plexiform lesions, or cholesterol granulomas.[8]

Nuclear Medicine and Positron Emission Tomography

Ventilation-perfusion (V/Q) scintigraphy is commonly abnormal in patients with IPAH, but the findings are usually nonspecific and are often interpreted as represent-

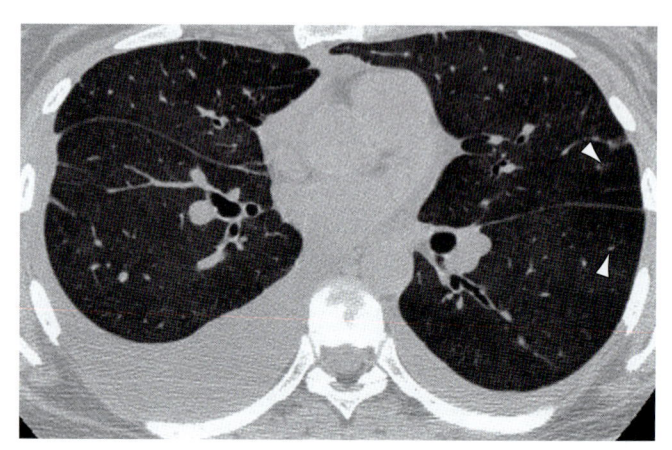

■ **FIGURE 99-4** Axial CT scan shows bilateral inhomogeneous lung opacity, consisting of areas of abnormally decreased opacity *(arrowheads),* representing mosaic perfusion, and areas of normal or increased attenuation. Note that pulmonary vessels are abnormally small in areas of decreased lung opacity.

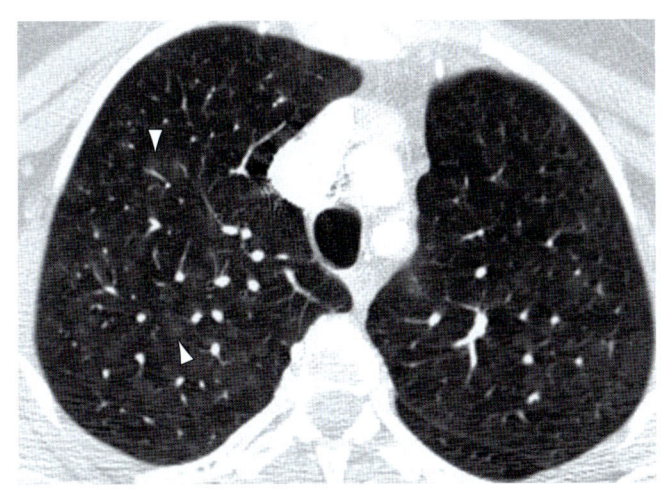

FIGURE 99-5 Axial CT scan shows areas of vaguely nodular ground-glass opacity (*arrowheads*). In some areas, these are centrilobular in distribution. Such findings may represent areas of hemorrhage, plexiform lesions, or cholesterol granulomas.

BOX 99-5 Pulmonary Arterial Hypertension: Risk Factors and Associated Conditions

Definite: appetite suppressants (e.g., fenfluramine), toxic rapeseed oil
Likely: amphetamines, L-tryptophan, methamphetamine
Possible: cocaine, chemotherapeutic agents, St. John's Wort, phenylpropanolamine
Unlikely: oral contraceptives, estrogens, cigarette smoking

---

ing a low probability for pulmonary thromboembolic disease.[1]

Angiography

Catheter pulmonary angiography in patients with IPAH shows tapering peripheral vessels with a "corkscrew" appearance, occasionally with visualization of subpleural collateral vessels.[1]

PULMONARY ARTERIAL HYPERTENSION RELATED TO RISK FACTORS OR ASSOCIATED WITH CONDITIONS

Definition

Pulmonary arterial hypertension related to associated conditions (APAH) includes PH in patients with connective tissue diseases, HIV infection, portal hypertension, congenital cardiovascular systemic to pulmonary shunts, schistosomiasis, and chronic hemolytic anemias.[6] The term *risk factors* in the category of PAH indicates any condition suspected to play a role in predisposing or facilitating the development of PAH, whereas the term *associated conditions* is used when it is impossible to determine whether a predisposing factor was present prior to the development of PAH.[5] The Evian conference in 1998 explored a number of potential risk factors and classified them according to the strength of association with PAH and the likelihood of a causal role in the development of PAH as definite, very likely, possible, or unlikely, according to the strength of available evidence in the literature (Box 99-5).

Etiology and Pathophysiology

PAH associated with connective tissue disease usually occurs in patients with systemic sclerosis, particularly those with limited forms of this disorder, such as CREST syndrome (*c*alcinosis, *R*aynaud phenomenon, *e*sophageal dysmotility, *s*clerodactyly, *t*elangiectasia).[7,9] Although most patients with systemic sclerosis do not develop clinical evidence of PAH, histopathologic changes of PAH are common in patients with systemic sclerosis. Echocardiographic studies have suggested that mild or moderate PAH is not uncommon in patients with systemic sclerosis.

HIV has not been shown to infect pulmonary circulation endothelial cells directly, so the mechanism of action of HIV-associated PAH remains unknown. The proposed mechanism in portopulmonary arterial hypertension is thought to be the incomplete hepatic degradation of humoral factors that exert vasoconstricting and inflammatory effects on the pulmonary circulation.

Intracardiac and extracardiac systemic to pulmonary (left to right) vascular shunts, including ventricular-septal defects, atrial-septal defects, partial anomalous pulmonary venous return, transposition of the great vessels, and patent ductus arteriosus, produce increased flow through the pulmonary arterial bed. The clinical severity is not related to the mechanism of shunting but rather correlates with the degree of pulmonary artery pressure elevation.

The increased pulmonary arterial flow that results from long-standing systemic to pulmonary vascular shunting produces persistently increased vasomotor tone within the pulmonary arteries, eventually leading to the development of pulmonary plexogenic arteriopathy and irreversible pulmonary vasculopathy. Eventually, the systemic to pulmonary vascular shunting may reverse, producing a pulmonary to systemic shunt, referred to as Eisenmenger syndrome.

Most patients with congenital systemic to pulmonary vascular shunts are corrected during infancy or early childhood, before the onset of severe PAH. For the infrequent patient who escapes surgical repair of the causative lesion during childhood, lung biopsy may be performed to assess the potential success for reversing the vasculopathy following surgical intervention.[1] This histopathologic grading system is called the Heath-Edwards grading system, and was originally described using a six-point scale. More recently, a three-point system has been proposed. The Heath-Edwards grading system allows prediction of disease reversibility. Grades I and II (medial hypertrophy, intimal proliferation, and neomuscularization) represent mild reversible disease. Grade III is considered borderline and is characterized by intimal fibrosis and luminal obliteration. Higher grades, corresponding with plexiform lesions, aneurysm, and necrotizing arteritis, are considered irreversible changes, and surgical correction of the abnormality is not warranted.

In prior PH classification systems, PH with schistosomiasis was previously thought to be the result of embolic obstruction of the pulmonary arteries by the organism's eggs. However, recent data suggest that PH related to schistosomiasis shares a clinical presentation and histopathologic findings similar to those of IPAH.[6]

PAH is increasingly recognized as a complication of chronic hemolytic anemias, particularly sickle cell disease; estimates of the prevalence of PAH in patients with sickle cell disease range from 10% to 30%.[7] The pathophysiology of the development of PAH in patients with sickle cell disease is likely multifactorial, including a number of disparate mechanisms, such as asplenia, chronic thromboembolic disease, pulmonary parenchymal disease from repeated episodes of inflammation and scarring, vasculopathy associated with sickle cell disease, and a relative paucity of vasodilating substances, such as nitrous oxide with an abundance of vasoconstricting agents, such as endothelin-1.

Pulmonary arterial hypertension with associated conditions shows histopathologic lesions identical to those of IPAH—arterial medial hypertrophy, intimal proliferation and fibrosis, necrotizing arteritis, and plexiform lesions. Superimposed organized thrombi may be seen, making the distinction between chronic thromboembolic pulmonary hypertension and other causes of IPAH occasionally difficult. It is the clinical scenario that defines these syndromes as distinct from IPAH and one another.

Manifestations of Disease

Clinical Presentation

Patients with PAH associated with certain conditions usually present with dyspnea on exertion. Other presenting symptoms include fatigue, chest pain, syncope, and occasionally cough. The Raynaud phenomenon may be present in certain patients, particularly those with PAH associated with connective tissue diseases such as systemic lupus erythematosus and progressive systemic sclerosis.

The incidence of PAH in patients with HIV infection is less than 1%. Patients with HIV-related pulmonary arterial hypertension have a similar presentation to patients with IPAH, except that they present at a slightly earlier age. Patients usually present while still relatively immunocompetent; the CD4 count is typically more than 200 cells/μL at presentation in most patients.

PAH associated with liver disease is typically encountered in the setting of cirrhosis and very rarely in patients with noncirrhotic portal hypertension caused by portal fibrosis or multifocal nodular hyperplasia. Most patients with cirrhosis do not develop pulmonary arterial hypertension; the frequency of this association based on hemodynamic studies is 2% to 6% of cirrhotic patients.[7] However, the frequency may be higher when considering a subset of patients with severe cirrhosis, such as those awaiting liver transplantation. Hepatic disease-related pulmonary arterial hypertension slowly improves following liver transplantation.

Many patients with congenital cardiovascular disease and systemic to pulmonary vascular shunts are asymptomatic. When symptoms are present, palpitations, shortness of breath, fatigue, cyanosis, and dyspnea on exertion are common. Heart failure may occur in some patients. Physical examinations may reveal suggestive cardiac murmurs.[10]

Imaging Techniques and Findings

Radiography

The various conditions associated with PAH show similar features on chest radiography- enlarged main and central pulmonary arteries, with rapid tapering of more peripheral vessels.[1] Right atrial and ventricular enlargement may be present. Patients with connective tissue disease–associated PAH may show evidence of fibrotic and/or inflammatory lung disease, although the latter is not invariably present.

Computed Tomography

Cross-sectional imaging studies show findings similar to those of patients with IPAH, including pulmonary arterial enlargement, right atrial and ventricular enlargement, and inhomogeneous lung opacity.[1] However, in patients with collagen vascular disease–associated PAH, fibrotic lung disease may be more readily visible on CT than chest radiography. Similarly, whereas chest radiography provides few clues to the hepatic cause in patients with portopulmonary PAH, cross-sectional imaging studies readily show features of cirrhosis in these patients. Imaging findings of PAH related to HIV are almost identical to those of IPAH and other causes of PAH.

Unlike many of the other conditions seen in patients with PAH, imaging studies in patients with PAH related to congenital systemic to pulmonary vascular shunts may show features that allow a specific diagnosis to be made. Furthermore, cross-sectional imaging studies may also provide methods that allow quantification of the degree of vascular shunting and thereby provide direction for treatment. The chronic increase in pulmonary flow causes the characteristic radiographic changes associated with pulmonary hypertension—increased size of the pulmonary trunk and central pulmonary arteries, diminished peripheral vessel caliber, and right ventricular chamber dilation. Often, the pulmonary arterial enlargement is striking, greater than that seen in other causes of PH (Fig. 99-6). It is important to note, however, that normal chamber size may represent increasing pulmonary pressures with progression toward Eisenmenger syndrome.

Thoracic CT may show calcification[1] and thrombus in the main pulmonary arteries resulting from high pressures and turbulent flow in the affected vessels. CT, particularly multislice CT pulmonary angiography, may also show abnormal vascular connections directly, such as atrial septal defects and patent ductus arteriosus. In the case of a patent ductus arteriosus, CT or MR imaging (Fig. 99-7) may reveal dilation of the patent ductus, possibly with aneurysm formation or mural calcification.

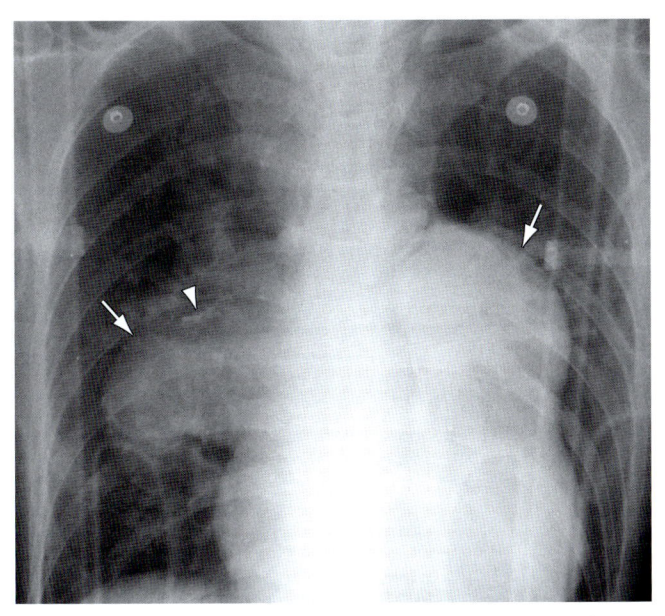

FIGURE 99-6 Frontal chest radiograph in a patient with a left to right intracardiac shunt shows massive enlargement of the central pulmonary arteries (*arrows*). Note the presence of pulmonary arterial calcification (*arrowhead*).

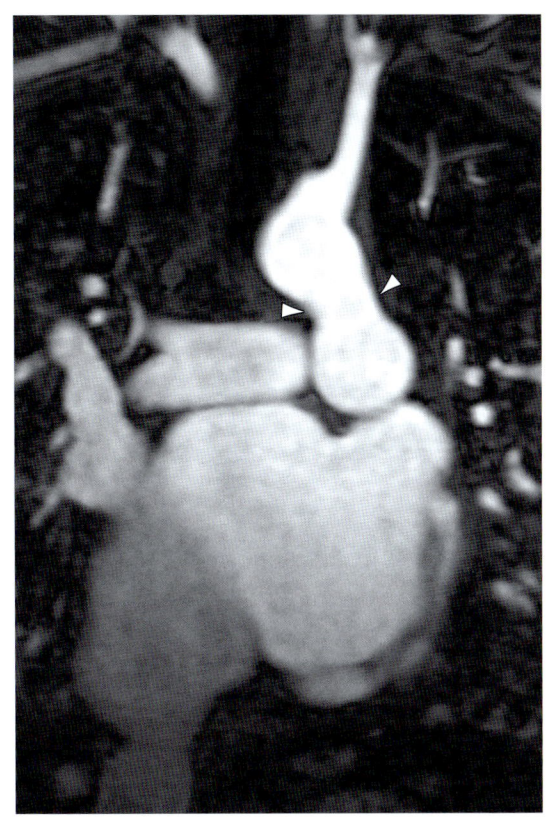

FIGURE 99-7 PH caused by congenital systemic to pulmonary shunt. This coronal three-dimensional MR angiography image shows patent ductus arteriosus (*arrowheads*).

Magnetic Resonance Imaging

MRI, in addition to revealing dilated pulmonary arteries and enlargement of the right ventricle, may also directly show abnormal atrial or ventricular connections, and abnormal intravascular or cardiac chamber signals, such as flow jets between vascular chambers of different pressure. Recently, time-resolved MRI techniques, in which a bolus of intravenous contrast is sequentially tracked through the vascular system, have been used to document successfully the anatomic derangements present in patients with systemic to pulmonary vascular shunts.

PULMONARY VENO-OCCLUSIVE DISEASE AND/OR PULMONARY CAPILLARY HEMANGIOMATOSIS

Definition

Pulmonary veno-occlusive disease (PVOD) and pulmonary capillary hemangiomatosis (PCH) were placed in separate groups in the Evian system (see Box 99-1), distinct from PAH. In the Venice-revised WHO system (see Box 99-2), PVOD and PCH were classified together as a subcategory of PAH in recognition of similarities in the clinical presentation, histopathologic features, and risk factors for disease of these two disorders. Such risk factors include use of anorexic medications, HIV infection, and scleroderma.[6] PVOD and PCH also share similarities with PAH, including reports of a familial association, but there are important differences between PAH and PVOD-PCH, especially in regard to imaging findings and treatment. Therefore, PVOD and PCH are included as group 1 lesions in the Dana Point classification of PH, but in a subcategory separate from other causes of PAH (1′; see Box 99-4).

Etiology and Pathophysiology

Pulmonary veno-occlusive disease is an idiopathic condition but has been associated with factors such as pregnancy, medications (e.g., chemotherapeutic agents [bleomycin and carmustine] and oral contraceptives), toxic ingestion, systemic lupus erythematosus, some collagen vascular diseases, and bone marrow transplantation.[11] Mutations in the bone morphogenic protein receptor-2 have also been detected in patients with PVOD. Immunologic mechanisms and viral infections have also been implicated as potential causes.

The characteristic hemodynamic feature of PVOD is normal to low pulmonary capillary wedge pressures, with normal left atrial and ventricular function and pressures.[11] PVOD affects the venous bed in a patchy distribution, accounting for the variability in the wedge pressure.

Histopathologic specimens in patients with PVOD show fibrous obliteration of small pulmonary veins and venules.[11,12] Plexiform lesions are absent, but capillary proliferation may be seen, which suggests the presence of angiogenesis. Prior episodes of infarction and hemosiderosis may be encountered. Acute or recanalized thrombi may be present.

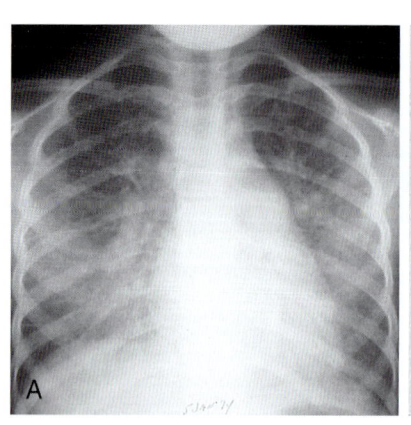

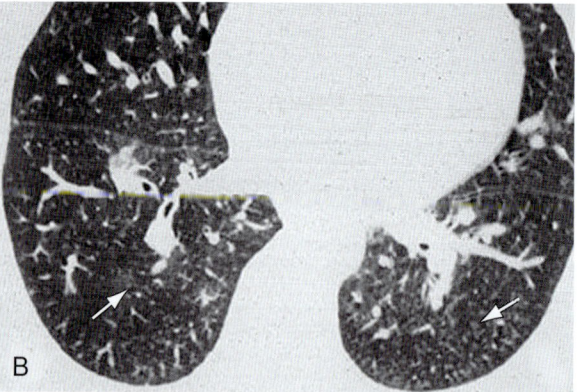

■ **FIGURE 99-8** Pulmonary arterial hypertension with significant venous or capillary involvement—pulmonary veno-occlusive disease. **A,** Frontal chest radiograph shows bilateral interstitial opacity and interlobular septal thickening suggestive of hydrostatic pulmonary edema. Note enlargement of the main pulmonary artery, suggesting elevated pulmonary pressures. **B,** Axial CT scan shows poorly defined areas of ground-glass opacity, some of which are vaguely centrilobular (*arrows*) in morphology. A few thickened interlobular septa were seen on other images. Unless interlobular septal thickening is pronounced, differentiation from other causes of pulmonary hypertension, especially pulmonary capillary hemangiomatosis (see Fig. 99-9), is difficult.

Manifestations of Disease

Clinical Presentation

PVOD is a very uncommon disease, with an estimated annual incidence of 0.1 to 0.2 patients/million persons. The age of patients affected by PVOD is wide, ranging from newborns to 70 years, but it is most commonly encountered in children and young adults.[11,13] In children and adolescents, no known gender predilection exists, but men are more commonly affected than women when PVOD manifests in young adults. Patients with PVOD present with chronic, progressive dyspnea, fatigue, and malaise, usually superimposed on other findings suggestive of PH, such as right heart failure. It has been suggested that PVOD is misdiagnosed as IPAH or chronic thromboembolic disease in a significant number of patients, which may lead to incorrect treatment.

It is important to distinguish patients with PVOD from those with interstitial lung disease because therapy for interstitial lung disease–induced pulmonary hypertension is vasodilation, which could precipitate pulmonary edema in patients with PVOD.[11] The prognosis for PVOD is poor, with most patients succumbing within 2 to 3 years of diagnosis. Treatment typically rests on heart-lung transplantation.

Imaging Techniques and Findings

Radiography

Chest radiography in patients with PVOD shows typical features of PH, but evidence of pulmonary edema is also often present (Fig. 99-8A), which is a distinguishing feature for PVOD compared with many other causes of PH.[11] Left atrial enlargement and redistribution of blood flow into the upper lobes are typically absent, allowing distinction from various causes of left-sided cardiac disease, particularly mitral stenosis.

Computed Tomography

Thoracic CT and HRCT will show normal or small central pulmonary veins, patchy dependent ground-glass opacity, smoothly thickened interlobular septa (see Fig. 99-8B), and pleural effusions.[11,13] Ground-glass opacity centrilobular nodules may be seen.[14] Mild lymphadenopathy may be present. Right-sided cardiac chambers are often enlarged, but the left atrium should not be enlarged. Multifocal air space opacities caused by pulmonary hemorrhage, air space edema, or venous infarction are uncommon. Inhomogeneous lung opacity consistent with mosaic perfusion may be present.

Nuclear Medicine and Angiography

V/Q scintigraphy in patients with PVOD will show patchy perfusion, most likely secondary to superimposed pulmonary arterial hypertension. Pulmonary angiography shows features of PH, including enlarged pulmonary arteries with peripheral pruning, but with delayed filling of the central pulmonary veins and a prolonged parenchymal enhancement phase.[11] These latter findings are secondary to the patchy obstruction of the venous system.

PULMONARY CAPILLARY HEMANGIOMATOSIS

Definition

Pulmonary capillary hemangiomatosis (PCH) is an idiopathic disorder first recognized in 1978 and characterized by capillary proliferation within the alveolar walls. The widespread vascular obstruction, centered on the pulmonary alveolar capillaries, results in PH.

Etiology and Pathophysiology

Various causes have been suggested for PCH, including congenital factors, vascular neoplasia, and autoimmune disease, and as a response to PVOD. Similar to PVOD, PCH has been noted to occur in association with various other conditions, including systemic lupus erythematosus, Takayasu arteritis, scleroderma, Kartagener syndrome, and hypertrophic cardiomyopathy. Lung biopsies in patients with PCH typically show proliferation of circumscribed capillary channels within the walls of alveoli. Intervening lung tissue is often normal.[11] The capillary proliferation results in the appearance of densely cellular alveolar walls. The proliferating capillaries compress the walls of pulmonary veins and venules, producing intimal fibrosis and secondary venous occlusion. Progressive scarring with in situ thrombosis develops, with pulmonary infarcts occurring as a result of vascular obliteration. Compensatory muscular hypertrophy of pulmonary arteries results from the foregoing processes. Like PVOD, histopathologic specimens in patients with PCH show hemosiderosis, interstitial edema, dilation of the lymphatic system, and vascular intimal fibrosis, with arterial medial hypertrophy.

Manifestations of Disease

Clinical Presentation

PCH is a rare disorder, occurring in approximately 4/million individuals.[15] The age range of patients affected by PCH is broad, 2 to 71 years, with a mean of 29 years. Males and females are affected equally. Patients typically present with fatigue and progressive shortness of breath. Cough may occasionally be present and chest pain, syncope, and digital clubbing have been reported. The clinical presentation of PCH is similar to that of PVOD, although hemoptysis may occur in patients with PCH but usually does not occur in patients with PVOD.[11] Similarly, hemorrhagic pleural effusions have been noted in patients with PCH, but typically do not occur in patients with PVOD. Other findings typically associated with PH may be present as well. As with PVOD, patients with PCH have elevated pulmonary arterial pressures but normal or near-normal pulmonary capillary wedge pressures. The prognosis of patients with PCH is rather poor, with a median survival of 3 years after diagnosis.

Imaging Techniques and Findings

Radiography

Chest radiographs in patients with PCH shows the usual findings of PH associated with bilateral, basilar reticular, and nodular opacities.[11] Unlike PVOD, interlobular septal thickening and pleural effusions are unusual and, when present, are usually less pronounced in patients with PCH compared with patients with PVOD. Enlargement of mediastinal lymph nodes has been reported in patients with PCH.

Computed Tomography

Thoracic CT shows enlargement of the main and central pulmonary arteries and right ventricle. Poorly defined centrilobular or lobular ground-glass opacities are also often present in patients with PCH (Fig. 99-9).[11] The presence of centrilobular ground-glass opacities tends to favor PCH, whereas smooth interlobular septal thickening and pleural effusions tend to favor the diagnosis of PVOD. Reports of interlobular septal thickening, pleural effusions, and lymphadenopathy in patients with PCH are noted, however, and ground-glass opacity centrilobular nodules may occur in patients with PVOD.[14] Areas of mosaic perfusion reflecting oligemia may be present. Overall differentiation of PCH from PVOD by imaging is difficult.

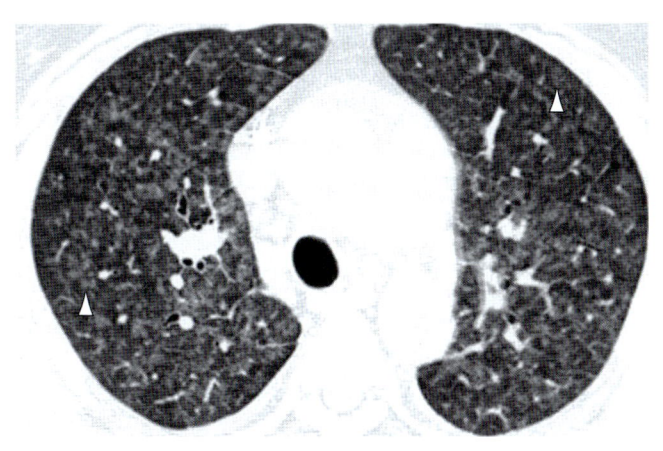

FIGURE 99-9 Pulmonary arterial hypertension with significant venous or capillary involvement—pulmonary capillary hemangiomatosis. This axial CT scan shows numerous poorly defined centrilobular nodules (*arrowheads*). A few thickened interlobular septa are present, which makes differentiation from pulmonary veno-occlusive disease challenging.

Nuclear Medicine and Angiography

V/Q typically does not show findings that specifically suggest the diagnosis of PCH. V/Q scans are often abnormal in patients with PCH,[11] but may even be interpreted as normal. Pulmonary angiography in patients with PCH is often normal or only nonspecifically abnormal.

PULMONARY HYPERTENSION WITH LEFT HEART DISEASE (PULMONARY VENOUS HYPERTENSION)

Definition

The most frequently encountered causes of PH with left heart disease, previously referred to as pulmonary venous hypertension in the Evian system and now referred to as pulmonary hypertension caused by left heart disease in the 2008 Dana Point classification of PH, include left ventricular systolic and diastolic dysfunction and valvular heart disease, such as aortic stenosis, aortic regurgitation, and mitral stenosis. An obstructing intra-atrial tumor or thrombus is an uncommon cause of elevated pulmonary arterial pressure.[1] In the case of patients with left-sided tumor or thrombus, the size of the obstructing lesion correlates with the degree of PH. Overall, left-sided cardiac disease, sometimes also referred to as nonpulmonary arterial pulmonary hypertension,[7] is probably the most common cause of pulmonary hypertension.

Etiology and Pathophysiology

Secondary PH arises when increased venous pressure requires elevated arterial pressure to allow forward flow of blood. The histopathologic changes in the arterial system are therefore secondarily caused by the increased venous pressure. Histopathologic specimens from the venous system of patients with PH related to left heart disease show vascular medial hypertrophy, interstitial thickening and edema, hemosiderosis and, occasionally, venous infarction.[1] Typically, no significant gradient is seen between the elevated pulmonary arterial pressure and pulmonary capillary wedge pressure, and pulmonary vascular resistance is normal or near normal. Occasionally, in some patients, pulmonary arterial pressure rises disproportionately to left atrial pressure in patients with pulmonary hypertension caused by left heart disease, probably as a result of vascular remodeling and/or increased pulmonary vasomotor tone.

Manifestations of Disease

Clinical Presentation

The clinical presentation of PH related to left heart disease is variable and depends on the specific disorder under consideration. Chronic left-sided cardiac diseases often present with progressive shortness of breath and exercise intolerance. Chest pain, cough, syncope, and lower extremity edema may occur. Atrial myxomas may manifest with these symptoms and may also produce symptoms of systemic embolization or constitutional symptoms, such as fever and weight loss.

Imaging Techniques and Findings

Radiography

Chest radiographs and CT scans show the characteristic findings of pulmonary venous hypertension, including interlobular septal thickening (Kerley A and B lines), pleural effusion, and air space opacity representing alveolar edema (Fig. 99-10).

Ultrasound

Echocardiography is the most common imaging method used for the evaluation of left-sided cardiac disease or suspected cardiac tumors. Echocardiography provides useful functional cardiac information, such as estimates of chamber volume and pressure and stroke volume. Echocardiography also has the ability to determine the degree of functional impairment caused by the size of a cardiac mass lesion, the degree of valvular dysfunction caused by the lesion, and the lesion's mobility.

Computed Tomography

If pulmonary arterial hypertension has developed, the central pulmonary arteries will also be enlarged. In addition to the foregoing findings, mitral stenosis may result in ossified nodules within the pulmonary parenchyma.

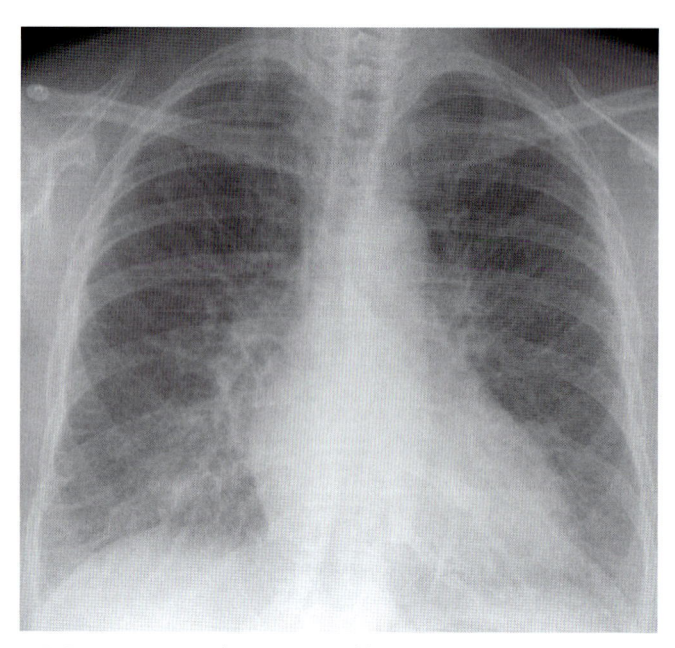

■ **FIGURE 99-10** Pulmonary arterial hypertension with left heart disease—pulmonary edema. This frontal chest radiograph shows interstitial thickening and interlobular septal thickening.

Atrial myxomas, if calcified, may be occasionally seen within the left atrium on chest radiographs. On contrast-enhanced thoracic CT (Fig. 99-11) or MRI scans, myxomas appear as filling defects within a cardiac chamber, most commonly the left atrium and often attached to the interatrial septum or anterior leaflet of the mitral valve.

Magnetic Resonance Imaging

MRI also shows the location and morphology of cardiac masses, such as atrial myxomas, to advantage. MRI also provides valuable functional data analogous to that obtained with echocardiography. MRI is not limited by acoustic windows, unlike echocardiography, and provides a comprehensive anatomic and physiologic assessment of the heart and central cardiovascular system. Delayed enhancement techniques provide additional insight into the cause and prognosis of a number of left-sided lesions that could produce PH, in particular valvular disease, cardiomyopathy, and cor triatriatum.

Synopsis of Treatment Options

Medical Treatment

Typically, treatment of PH caused by left heart disease is directed at the cause of left heart failure; the best example of success with this strategy is balloon valvotomy for mitral stenosis.[9] When right heart failure develops in patients with PH caused by left heart disease, the prognosis is poor. In these patients, prognosis is most closely associated with the degree of pulmonary artery pressure elevation and right ventricular, rather than left ventricular, ejection fraction.

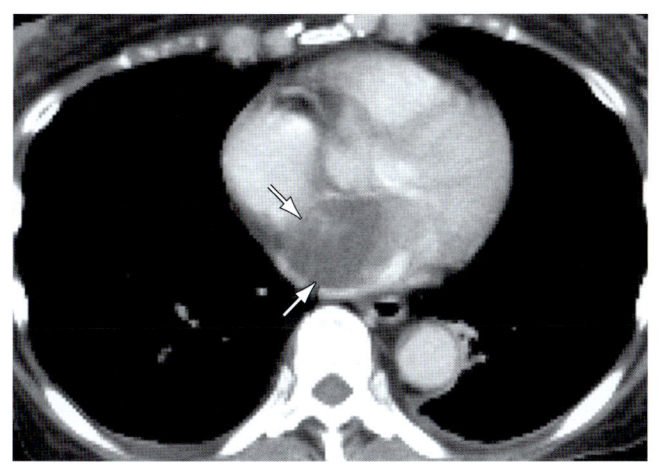

FIGURE 99-11 Pulmonary arterial hypertension with left heart disease—left atrial myxoma. This axial CT scan shows a low attenuation filling defect (*arrows*) within the left atrium. The lesion attaches to the interatrial septum and prolapses through the mitral valve.

PULMONARY HYPERTENSION CAUSED BY LUNG DISEASES AND/OR HYPOXIA

Disorders producing lung disease and/or hypoxia that result in PH have in common the final common pathway of chronic alveolar hypoxia. Such disorders include chronic obstructive pulmonary disease (COPD, including emphysema and bronchiectasis), various interstitial lung diseases, alveolar hypoventilation syndromes, sleep-disordered breathing (sleep apnea), and developmental abnormalities. These disorders produce hypoxia, with or without associated acidosis, through various combinations of ventilation-perfusion mismatching, shunt, or alveolar hypoventilation. Other mechanisms that may play a role in the development of PH caused by lung diseases or hypoxia include polycythemia, alveolar-capillary membrane destruction, systemic arterial shunting of blood through bronchial artery–pulmonary artery anastomoses, and pulmonary thromboemboli.

Definition

COPD includes several conditions—emphysema, chronic bronchitis, asthma, and bronchiectasis—that share the basic characteristic of poorly reversible air flow obstruction on forced expiration. Among causes of COPD, smoking-related conditions are most common. Ventilation-perfusion mismatching is the primary mechanism of hypoxemia in COPD, and regional alveolar hypoxia produces hypoxic vasoconstriction and increased resistance in the pulmonary arterial vasculature.

Interstitial lung diseases are a heterogeneous group of pulmonary disorders characterized by inflammatory and fibrotic destruction of the pulmonary parenchyma.

Prevalence and Epidemiology

The prevalence of pulmonary hypertension in patients with COPD is uncertain, but is related to disease severity.[7] In most patients with COPD, pulmonary hypertension is mild (mean pulmonary arterial pressure [mPAP] < 35 mm Hg) and treatment is directed at the COPD itself rather than pulmonary hypertension. The onset of PH in the COPD patient is associated with a poor prognosis, with a 5-year survival of only 10% in patients with pulmonary artery pressures higher than 45 mm Hg.

PH is fairly common among patients with interstitial lung diseases, including those with idiopathic pulmonary fibrosis. The exact prevalence of PH in patients with idiopathic pulmonary fibrosis is uncertain, but has been estimated to be as high as 40% using echocardiographic assessment.[7]

Etiology and Pathophysiology

The PH that results from the aforementioned mechanisms that produce hypoxia is exacerbated by the alveolar capillary destruction that is also present in patients with COPD. Various biologic mechanisms influence the development of pulmonary hypertension in patients with COPD, and some researchers think that severe pulmonary hypertension may be a disorder that occasionally manifests in patients with COPD as much as it is a condition resulting from COPD.[7]

PH associated with interstitial lung diseases in part results from chronic hypoxemia. Fibrotic restriction of pulmonary vessels, limiting their distensibility, and reduction of the vascular surface area may also potentially play a role. In the case of connective tissue diseases, the development of PH may be related to immunologic mechanisms. Hypoxia-mediated pulmonary arteriolar vasoconstriction is present and is often associated with vascular inflammation. Eventually, pulmonary vascular remodeling occurs, and thrombotic angiopathy and perivascular fibrosis may be present in patients with PH and interstitial lung disease. In patients with idiopathic pulmonary fibrosis undergoing lung transplantation, explanted lungs often show thickening of the walls of pulmonary arteries and veins, with areas of vascular narrowing resulting from dense fibrosis. However, obliteration of small veins and venules may also be seen outside areas of dense fibrosis.

As with COPD, the degree of PH in patients with idiopathic pulmonary fibrosis is typically modest although, again like COPD, a small subset of patients with idiopathic pulmonary fibrosis may have more marked pulmonary arterial pressure elevations.[7] The correlation between measurements of lung variables and severity of pulmonary hypertension is poor in patients with idiopathic pulmonary fibrosis, suggesting that there may be more to the development of PH than the mere degree of pulmonary fibrotic disease would predict.

The ability of thoracic CT to predict PH (mPAP > 25 mm Hg) in patients with idiopathic pulmonary fibrosis has been questioned. Considering a main pulmonary artery measurement of 29 mm or higher as abnormal, the sensitivity of this measurement for the detection of elevated pulmonary arterial pressure on right heart catheterization may exceed 85%,[16] but at the expense of insufficient specificity and negative predictive value.[17,18]

Sleep-disordered breathing is a term that includes a number of sleep-related breathing disorders, such as central sleep apnea, obstructive sleep apnea, and nocturnal desaturation (>10% of total time spent sleeping with arterial oxygenation <90%). The prevalence of sleep-disordered breathing may be as high as 4% in middle-aged men. Sleep-disordered breathing and other alveolar hypoventilation syndromes result in chronically depressed P_{O_2} and elevated P_{CO_2}. The chronic hypoxemia produces pulmonary arterial vasoconstriction, vascular remodeling,[3] and increased pulmonary arterial resistance, resulting in PH.

Manifestations of Disease

Clinical Presentation

For both COPD and interstitial lung diseases, the clinical presentation is dominated by the presence of the lung disease, and pulmonary hypertension may not be recognized until cor pulmonale develops. Sleep-disordered breathing is often suggested by the presence of loud snoring, daytime sleepiness, and poor-quality or restless sleep.

Imaging Techniques and Findings

Radiography

The chest radiographic appearance of PH caused by COPD and chronic alveolar hypoxia is similar to other causes of PH—enlarged central pulmonary arteries with rapid peripheral tapering. Right-sided cardiac chamber enlargement may also be present.

Computed Tomography

The presence of abnormally large lung volumes and other signs of COPD are key to diagnosing obstructive lung disease as the cause of PH. Such findings are relatively easy to recognize on cross-sectional imaging, particularly thoracic CT. Basilar reticulation, linear opacities, honeycombing, and diminished lung volumes suggest the presence of interstitial lung disease in the setting of PH. No specific imaging features suggest the diagnosis of sleep-disordered breathing, although such patients are often obese. The diagnosis of sleep-disordered breathing is typically established using clinical and laboratory criteria.

CHRONIC THROMBOEMBOLIC PULMONARY HYPERTENSION

Definition

In the 2003 Venice PH classification (see Box 99-2), chronic thromboembolic pulmonary hypertension (CTEPH) included a heterogeneous group of disorders producing pulmonary arterial obstruction, such as chronic thromboemboli, foreign bodies, and tumors.[6] However, it is now recognized that there are significant differences in the clinical presentation, imaging findings, and management of patients with chronic thromboembolic disease compared with patients with nonthrombotic pulmonary arterial embolic disease. Additionally, the Venice classification system (see Box 99-2) recognized two subgroups of CTEPH: (1) proximal disease, accessible to pulmonary thromboendarterectomy; and (2) distal disease, which is not accessible to surgical therapy. However, the distinction between proximal and distal chronic thromboembolic disease is not always clear and general agreement regarding what constitutes proximal and distal disease is lacking. Therefore, in the 2008 Dana Point PH classification, CTEPH is regarded as resulting from thromboemboli and has been maintained as a group 4 lesion, but nonthrombotic emboli are now considered group 5 lesions (PH with Unclear Multifactorial Etiologies; see Box 99-4). Additionally, the distinction of proximal and distal disease in the Venice PH classification (see Box 99-2) has been abandoned. From a radiologist's viewpoint, however, it nevertheless remains useful to consider nonthrombotic emboli at the same sitting as CTEPH, because often nonthrombotic emboli will be encountered as pulmonary arterial filling defects during pulmonary CTA studies. Therefore, recognizing that nonthrombotic emboli are classified as group 5 lesions in the Dana Point PH classification system, particulate, tumor, and parasitic emboli will be discussed here.

Etiology and Pathophysiology

Thromboemboli have numerous sources, including the deep veins of the pelvis and thigh, the right atrium, indwelling catheters, or septic thromboemboli in patients with endocarditis involving the tricuspid or pulmonic valves.[1] Acute thromboembolic disease can produce transient pulmonary arterial pressure elevations, but sustained elevations are more likely a consequence of chronic thromboembolic disease, which may occur in up to 4% of patients with acute emboli.[6,7]

Thromboemboli induce pulmonary arterial hypertension by occluding the pulmonary vascular bed. This process may occur through numerous repeated small thromboembolic episodes, a few large embolic episodes that fail to resolve completely, or the development of in situ thrombosis in small vessels and proximal migration of pulmonary arterial thrombosis, with secondary endothelial changes and cellular hyperplasia, vascular webs, and incomplete remodeling of thromboemboli.[19] There are data to suggest that the latter mechanism plays some role in the development of CTEPH. The common event leading to the development of elevated pulmonary arterial pressures is cytokine-mediated pulmonary arterial scarring resulting from lysis of pulmonary thromboemboli.

Histopathologically, chronic emboli may organize, resulting in vascular channels interspersed with connective tissue. Fibrous bands and webs, representing organizing thrombi, are present,[1] often in association with fresh thromboemboli. The elevated pulmonary pressures also produce the characteristic histopathologic changes of medial hypertrophy and intimal proliferation and luminal obliteration, often in association with atherosclerosis. Plexogenic lesions are occasionally present in patients with chronic thromboembolic PH.[7]

Manifestations of Disease

Clinical Presentation

Patients at high risk for the development of CTEPH include oncologic patients, patients with chronic cardiac or pulmonary disease, and patients with clotting disorders. Patients with CTEPH typically present with dyspnea on exertion, cough, chest pain, and syncope.[1] Anticardiolipin antibody may be found in 10% of patients with CTEPH,[7] but the only other consistent abnormality of the coagulation and fibrinolytic systems identified in patients with CTEPH is an elevated level of factor VIII. The onset of PH in patients with chronic thromboembolic disease generally portends a poor prognosis.

Imaging Techniques and Findings

Radiography

Chest radiographs may be normal early in the course of the development of CTEPH. Later in the disease course, the characteristic findings of pulmonary arterial hypertension, including enlargement of the main, right, and left pulmonary arteries, are seen. Subpleural opacities, representing recent or remote pulmonary infarction, may be encountered.

Computed Tomography

Helical CT pulmonary angiography is the study of choice for the evaluation of central CTEPH. The main pulmonary artery is often enlarged. Eccentric filling defects adjacent to the vessel wall, representing organizing thrombi, are characteristic of chronic thromboembolic disease. Such thrombi may calcify. The eccentric nature of organizing thrombi may be shown to advantage with multiplanar reformatted imaging. Organizing thrombi may undergo recanalization, in which case CT will show small foci of contrast within an occluded vessel. Linear intraluminal filling defects, representing intravascular webs, may be also seen. Abrupt narrowing of pulmonary arteries with reduction in arterial diameter is common in patients with chronic thromboembolic PH, and pulmonary CT angiography (CTA) may also show markedly hypertrophied bronchial arteries in these patients.[1] Enlargement of the right ventricular and right atrium is common.

HRCT may show bilateral, geographically distributed inhomogeneous lung opacity in patients with CTEPH, representing mosaic perfusion.[1] The vessels in the regions of decreased pulmonary parenchymal attenuation are often visibly smaller than their counterparts in the areas of normal or increased parenchymal attenuation. Small foci of subpleural consolidation, representing areas of prior pulmonary infarction, may also be evident.

Magnetic Resonance Imaging

Findings of central CTEPH on MRI and MRA are similar to those encountered on CT. Chronic, organized thrombi appear as very low signal foci adjacent to the vascular wall on T1-weighted or black blood images[1] as well as flow-sensitive sequences, such as gradient echo or balanced fast-field echo (FFE) images. Vascular webs and stenoses and hypertrophied bronchial arteries may be visible. MRI provides the additional benefit of accurate assessment of right ventricular performance, and improvements in right ventricular ejection fraction and peak systolic pulmonary arterial flow velocity may be seen in surgically treated patients with CTEPH. Velocity-encoded cine phase contrast MRI has been used to assess the degree of bronchopulmonary shunt volume through hypertrophied bronchial arteries before and after surgical pulmonary endarterectomy, and it has been reported that reduction of bronchopulmonary shunt volume represents a favorable response to surgical therapy in patients with CTEPH.[20]

Nuclear Medicine and Positron Emission Tomography

V/Q scanning is often interpreted as high probability in patients with chronic thromboembolic PH, although scintigraphy may underestimate the degree of hemodynamic derangement associated with CTEPH. Furthermore, in the original PIOPED series,[21] the positive predictive value of a high-probability V/Q scan interpretation decreased from 91% to 74% for patients with a history of thromboembolic disease, representing a loss of specificity in the high-probability scan interpretation. Other studies have shown high sensitivity and specificity for V/Q scintigraphy for the detection of chronic thromboembolic disease, but the limitations of this technique often favor helical CT pulmonary angiography as the test of choice in the diagnostic evaluation of these patients. Nevertheless, expert consensus recommendations have usually indicated that V/Q scintigraphy may be used to screen patients for suspected CTEPH as a result of reports indicating that V/Q scintigraphy is more sensitive for the detection of CTEPH amenable to surgical therapy.[22] A normal or very low-probability scan result excludes CTEPH, whereas a high-probably scan result usually prompts catheter pulmonary angiography.[7] Investigators at the University of California, San Diego, who have the most experience in the evaluation and treatment of patients with CTEPH, use a combination of transthoracic echocardiography, V/Q scintigraphy, right heart catheterization, and catheter pulmonary angiography in the preoperative assessment of patients suspected of CTEPH.[19]

Angiography

Pulmonary angiography typically shows vascular tortuosity, webs, bands, stenoses, pouching defects, and abrupt vascular truncation or occlusions in patients with CTEPH.[1]

Synopsis of Treatment Options

Medical Treatment

The treatment of CTEPH depends on the extent of the thrombus burden in the pulmonary circulation. If thromboemboli are shown within the lobar arteries or more proximally, the patient is considered an appropriate candidate for surgical thromboembolectomy.[1] Thromboemboli distal to the proximal segmental vessels are usually not amenable to surgical resection, and medical management is the preferred treatment. Medical therapies typically used for patients with CTEPH who are not suitable candidates for surgery include oral anticoagulation, digitalis, calcium channel blockers, and PAH-specific medical therapy (e.g., prostacyclin analogues, endothelin receptor antagonists). In some cases, balloon angioplasty of affected pulmonary arteries or lung transplantation may be performed for inoperable patients with CTEPH.[23]

Surgical or Interventional Therapy

Surgical pulmonary thromboendarterectomy is an effective treatment for properly selected patients with CTEPH, and often provides significant immediate improvement in symptoms and pulmonary hemodynamics. However, surgical pulmonary thromboendarterectomy can be associated with significant morbidity and mortality, and another 10% to 15% of patients who undergo the procedure may fail to have substantial reductions in pulmonary vascular resistance.[23] In the hands of experienced surgeons, the mortality related to surgical pulmonary thromboendarterectomy is approximately 4% to 7%.[24] The best outcomes following surgical pulmonary thromboendarterectomy are seen with patients treated at centers with recognized experience in the surgical management of CTEPH, concordance between preoperative pulmonary vascular resistance and anatomic extent of disease, preoperative pulmonary vascular resistance less than 1000 to 1200, absence of a number of comorbid conditions (e.g., splenectomy) and a significant decrease in pulmonary vascular resistance following surgery. It has been suggested that a postoperative residual pulmonary vascular resistance of more than 500 dyn $\cdot$ s $\cdot$ cm^{-5} is associated with a mortality of just over 30% in patients undergoing surgical pulmonary thromboendarterectomy, whereas the mortality for these patients is less than 1% when the postoperative pulmonary vascular resistance falls below 500 dyn $\cdot$ s $\cdot$ cm^{-5} following surgery. Preoperative imaging assessment is essential for segregating those patients who stand a might benefit from surgical pulmonary thromboendarterectomy from those who will not. When visible central thromboemboli are present on multislice computed tomography pulmonary angiography (msCTPA) or catheter pulmonary angiography, it is more likely that patients will have improvements in pulmonary vascular resistance after pulmonary thromboendarterectomy. However, the amount of central thromboembolic material does not necessarily correlate with mPAP; some patients with central disease will not respond well to surgical pulmonary thromboendarterectomy, whereas others without central disease may have favorable results with surgery. The cause of this discrepancy is uncertain but suggests that factors other then mere vascular obstruction are involved in the development of chronic thromboembolic pulmonary hypertension.

NONTHROMBOTIC EMBOLIZATION
Etiology and Pathophysiology

Nonthrombotic emboli may result from tumor emboli, parasitic embolization, or embolization of foreign material (e.g., mercury, talc) into the pulmonary arterial circulation, producing pulmonary hypertension.

Tumor Embolization

As many as 25% of patients with solid malignancies may have microemboli that ultimately lodge in the pulmonary circulation.[1] The most frequent cause of tumor microembolization is gastric carcinoma, but breast, ovarian, lung, renal, hepatocellular, and prostate malignancies may also produce tumor emboli. Most emboli preferentially occlude small arteries and arterioles, with the exception of atrial myxomas and renal carcinomas, which may form larger, more centrally located thromboemboli.

Parasitic Embolization

In the Venice PH classification system (see Box 99-2), PH resulting from schistosomiasis was classified as a group V lesion, PH caused by chronic thrombotic or embolic disease.[6] However, in the 2008 Dana Point PH classification scheme (see Box 99-4), PH caused by schistosomiasis has been reclassified as a group 1 lesion. Nevertheless, pulmonary schistosomiasis will be discussed here because it is convenient to consider the various causes of nonthrombotic pulmonary emboli together.[25]

Pulmonary schistosomiasis is most commonly the result of infection with *Schistosoma mansoni*, which is endemic in the Middle East, Africa, and South America.[1] A latency period of 5 years or more after the onset of infection typically occurs before cardiopulmonary disease is seen. Secreted ova migrate into the lungs via portal-systemic collaterals and lodge in medium-sized muscular pulmonary arteries and arterioles. In the pulmonary circulation, the ova elicit an inflammatory reaction that results in medial hypertrophy, granuloma formation, intimal hyperplasia, collagen deposition and fibrosis, and eventually obliterative arteritis. An associated eosinophilic alveolitis may be present.

Particulate Embolization

Pulmonary arterial embolization with talc most commonly occurs in intravenous drug users. When intravenous drug users abuse medications containing talc, they inject a suspension containing crushed tablets, which are intended for oral use, and the injected talc embolizes small pulmonary arterioles.[1] The talc may then migrate from the pulmonary vasculature into the surrounding interstitium, where its presence elicits a foreign body granulomatous response. Vascular thrombosis with recanalization, intimal hyperplasia, medial arterial hypertrophy, fibrosis, and refractile talc particles are present in histopathologic specimens.

Intravascular mercury embolization may also produce PH. Following injection, mercury embolizes small vessels and eventually migrates from the vessel into the surrounding pulmonary interstitium, where the metal elicits an inflammatory granulomatous response producing vascular obstruction and eventually PH.

Manifestations of Disease

Clinical Presentation

Tumor Embolization

Because tumor emboli are quite small, symptoms directly related to tumor embolization are uncommon. If the embolic load is high enough, patients may present with dyspnea on exertion, chest pain, hypoxemia, cough, syncope, and even cor pulmonale.[1]

Parasitic Embolization

Presenting symptoms of parasitic embolization include hepatosplenomegaly, right heart symptoms, dyspnea, and cough. Patients with cardiopulmonary schistosomiasis always have cirrhosis and portal hypertension.[1]

Particulate Embolization

Pulmonary talcosis may produce few symptoms, but patients may present with chronic, progressive shortness of breath, cough, and dyspnea on exertion.[1] Symptoms may progress even after cessation of drug abuse.

Mercury may be injected into the vascular system accidentally or intentionally.[1] Intentional mercury injection most often occurs as the consequence of a suicide attempt.

Imaging Techniques and Findings

Radiography

Tumor Embolization

Chest radiographs in patients with intravascular tumor embolization are often normal. When abnormal, findings resembling those of pulmonary lymphangitic carcinomatosis are commonly seen.[1]

Parasitic Embolization

Chest radiography in patients with parasitic embolization shows findings consistent with pulmonary arterial hypertension.[1] Small nodules, representing parasitic granulomas, may be seen. Pulmonary infarction is rarely seen as a result of parasitic embolization. Contrast-enhanced thoracic CT may show embolized organisms directly in the pulmonary arteries or right-sided cardiac chambers (Fig. 99-12). Thoracic CT or MRI can also show the presence, location, and morphology of cardiac or pericardial parasitic infection directly, as may occur with echinococcosis.

Particulate Embolization

The chest radiographic findings of mercury embolization include fine, branching, symmetric nodules that result from intra-arterial mercury deposits. Metal deposits may also collect within the heart, particularly at the apex of the right ventricle.[1]

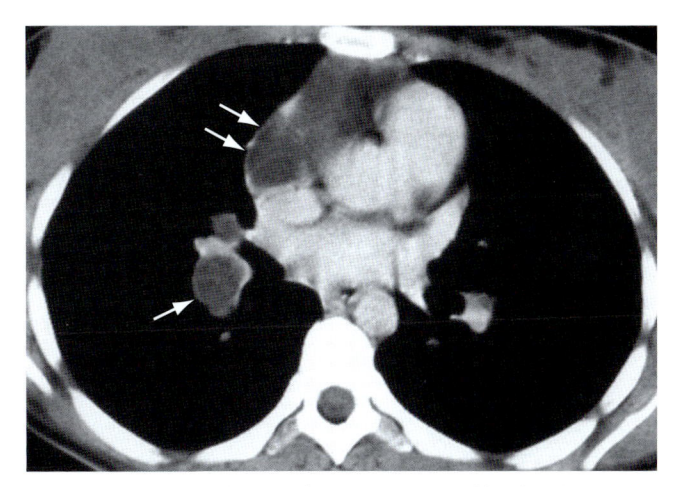

FIGURE 99-12 Pulmonary hypertension caused by chronic thromboembolic or embolic disease—parasitic emboli. This axial CT scan in a patient with echinococcosis shows low attenuation masses expanding the right lower lobe pulmonary artery (*single arrow*) and right atrium (*double arrows*).

Chest radiographs in patients with talc embolization show diffuse bilateral small nodular (2 to 3 mm) opacities throughout the lung parenchyma.[1] Perihilar conglomerate masses associated with fibrosis, producing retraction of lung parenchyma and relative hyperlucency in the lower lung, may be seen in some patients; these findings may resemble progressive massive fibrosis.

Computed Tomography

Tumor Embolization

In addition to the characteristic cross-sectional imaging findings of PH and thromboembolism noted, thoracic CT scans in patients with tumor emboli may reveal lymphadenopathy, findings consistent with lymphangitic carcinomatosis, and peripheral wedge-shaped opacities representing pulmonary infarction.[1] When emboli affect larger vessels, such as subsegmental pulmonary arteries, thoracic CT may reveal a beaded appearance of these vessels (Fig. 99-13). When smaller vessels are affected, such as at the centrilobular level, beading and nodularity may be observed, and the affected vessels may assume a branching configuration, resembling "tree in bud" opacity.

Parasitic Embolization

HRCT in patients with parasitic embolization may show nodules, interstitial prominence and thickening, and ground-glass opacity in combination with the classic findings of PH.[1]

Particulate Embolization

Thoracic CT scans in patients with pulmonary talcosis often show numerous micronodules, with or without patchy ground-glass opacity. Upper lobe fibrotic opacities, resembling progressive massive fibrosis, may be present.[1] These fibrotic opacities may show high attenuation caused by the presence of talc.

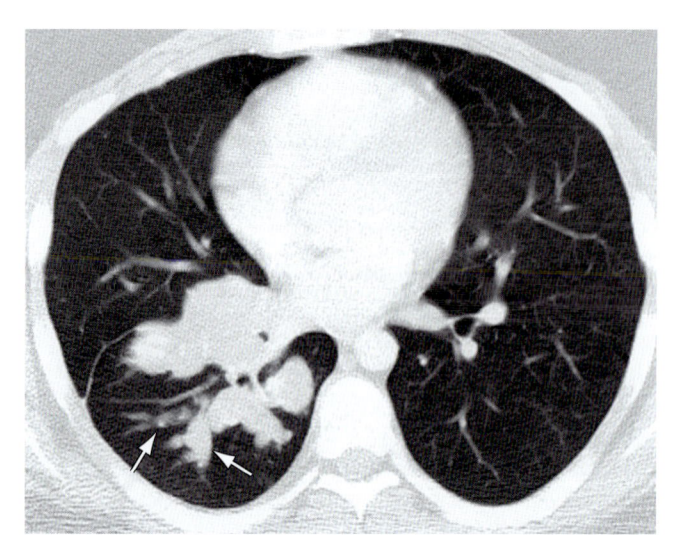

FIGURE 99-13 Pulmonary hypertension caused by chronic thromboembolic or embolic disease—tumor emboli. This axial CT scan in a patient with osteosarcoma shows expanded, bead-like right lower lobe pulmonary arteries (*arrows*), consistent with pulmonary arterial tumor embolization.

Nuclear Medicine and Angiography

Tumor Embolization

V/Q scintigraphy may reveal subsegmental unmatched perfusion defects, indistinguishable from thromboembolic disease.[1] Pulmonary angiography may show a delayed arterial phase, intravascular filling defects, and peripheral pruning.

PULMONARY HYPERTENSION WITH UNCLEAR MULTIFACTORIAL MECHANISMS

Definition

In the 2003 Venice-revised WHO classification of PH (see Box 99-2), a number of inflammatory and idiopathic causes that may be associated with PH were classified under the category "miscellaneous." Included in this category are various conditions such as sarcoidosis, lymphangiomatosis, and extrinsic pulmonary venous compression. The latter may be caused by malignancy, such as mediastinal and hilar lymphadenopathy or tumor, but inflammatory causes, in particular fibrosing mediastinitis, may also elevate pulmonary pressures through pulmonary arterial and/or venous compression or obliteration. These conditions have been categorized as group 5 lesions in the 2008 Dana Point PH classification system (see Box 99-4). Other conditions that may be associated with PH, including hematologic abnormalities and metabolic abnormalities previously classified as group I lesions in the 2003 Venice system, as well as a number of systemic disorders, have been included in this group as well.[6]

The first subcategory of the group 5 2008 Dana Point classification of PH (see Box 99-4) includes hematologic conditions, such as myeloproliferative diseases, essential thrombocytosis, polycythemia vera, chronic myeloid leukemia, and splenectomy.[6] Various mechanisms may result in PH in patients with these conditions, including congestive heart failure, high cardiac output, asplenia, or mechanical pulmonary arterial obstruction caused by circulating megakaryocytes. Several other systemic conditions in group 5 include sarcoidosis, Langerhans cell histiocytosis, lymphangioleiomyomatosis, pulmonary vasculitis, and neurofibromatosis. The mechanisms postulated to produce PH in patients with sarcoidosis include capillary bed destruction resulting from fibrosis, pulmonary artery and venous compression secondary to lymphadenopathy, and granulomatous inflammation directly involving the pulmonary vessels, especially the veins. PH in patients with end-stage Langerhans cell histiocytosis is common and may be related to a combination of pulmonary parenchymal destruction, hypoxemia, and vasculopathy. PH is relatively uncommon in patients with lymphangioleiomyomatosis but, when present, may be the result of hypoxemia caused by capillary destruction produced by the cystic lesions characteristic of this condition.

Also in group 5 of the 2008 Dana Point classification of PH (see Box 99-4) are a number of metabolic disorders, such as Gaucher disease, glycogen storage disease, and thyroid conditions such as hyper- and hypothyroidism.[6] Various mechanisms for the development of PH in these conditions include hypoxemia, pulmonary parenchymal disease, portocaval shunts (in the case of type Ia glycogen storage disease), and capillary blockade by Gaucher cells. Precisely how thyroid disorders produce PH are unclear, but an association between autoimmune thyroid disease and PAH raises the possibility of a linked genetic pathogenesis.

The last subcategory of group 5 in the 2008 Dana Point classification (see Box 99-4) includes a number of disorders that produce mechanical obstruction of the pulmonary arteries and/or veins, including central obstructing tumors, metastatic microvascular obstruction, and fibrosing mediastinitis.[6] Also included in this category is PH associated with end-stage renal disease in those on long-term hemodialysis. Tumor microvascular obstruction has been reviewed previously, and centrally obstructing tumors are usually readily apparent as a cause of symptoms suggesting PH. Fibrosing mediastinitis may present with suggestive thoracic imaging findings and will be discussed in detail in the next sections.

Fibrosing Mediastinitis

Etiology and Pathophysiology

Fibrosing mediastinitis (FM) represents a progressive proliferation of collagenous and fibrous tissue within the mediastinum, producing encasement and compression of mediastinal structures. Granulomatous infections, particularly *Histoplasma capsulatum* and *Mycobacterium tuberculosis*, are among the most common causes of FM.[1]

The deposition of fibrous tissue in FM commonly affects relatively soft and deformable structures, such as the systemic veins within the mediastinum, trachea and central airways, esophagus, pulmonary arteries, and pulmonary veins. PH may result when fibrous encasement of the pulmonary arteries or draining pulmonary veins occurs, with the former often mistaken for chronic thromboembolic disease. Pulmonary venous obstruction occurs in a patchy distribution, producing wide variations in pulmonary capillary wedge pressure measurements,[1] although usually the wedge pressure is elevated. Cardiac catheterization studies typically show normal left heart size and pressures.

Manifestations of Disease

Clinical Presentation

Common symptoms in patients with FM depend on the structures most severely involved. Patients often present with nonspecific symptoms of pulmonary venous hypertension, including dyspnea and hemoptysis.[1] The treatment for FM is limited. If localized pulmonary venous involvement predominates, surgical treatment may be effective. Steroids have shown minor efficacy.

Imaging Techniques and Findings

Radiography

Chest radiography often shows widening of the mediastinum, with hilar prominence and calcified lymph nodes. Findings of pulmonary venous hypertension, including interlobular septal thickening and air space consolidation representing alveolar edema, may be present. FM may result in airway stenoses that present with lobar volume loss.[1]

Computed Tomography

Thoracic CT will reveal extensive infiltration of the mediastinum with abnormal soft tissue. FM caused by *Histoplasmosis capsulatum* usually produces extensive lymph node calcification, readily identifiable by CT. Often, the abnormal mediastinal and hilar soft tissue resembles lymph nodes, and the diagnosis of FM may be mistaken for lymphadenopathy. Similarly, FM and chronic thromboembolic disease may superficially resemble one another. Contrast-enhanced CT in patients with FM may show extensive collateral vein formation resulting from fibrotic involvement of systemic thoracic veins, such as the superior vena cava or azygos vein. Pulmonary artery compression may also be directly visualized. Pulmonary venous infarcts, appearing as subpleural wedge-shaped consolidations may be seen in patients with pulmonary venous involvement.[1]

Magnetic Resonance Imaging

On MRI scans, FM often manifests as homogeneous soft tissue with intermediate signal intensity on T1-weighted imaging, with variable signal on T2-weighted imaging. Both increased and decreased signal may be encountered simultaneously on T2-weighted imaging, with the decreased T2 signal probably related to calcification or fibrotic tissue, whereas the increased T1 signal is thought to be related to areas of active inflammation. Enhancement of the infiltrating mediastinal soft tissue, often rather heterogeneous, following gadolinium administration is typical.

Nuclear Medicine and Positron Emission Tomography

V/Q scintigraphy may show focal unmatched perfusion defects. Unilateral lack of perfusion of one lung has been reported in patients with FM.

Angiography

Catheter pulmonary angiography findings depend on the location of obstruction. If the arterial circulation is primarily affected, asymmetric narrowing of the pulmonary arteries will be present. When pulmonary veins are primarily affected, venous phase angiography will show stenoses, dilation, or obstruction in combination, often near the junction of the affected vein and the left atrium.[1]

KEY POINTS

- Pulmonary hypertension is classified according to the 2008 Dana Point classification system, which recognizes five major categories—pulmonary arterial hypertension, pulmonary hypertension secondary to left heart disease, pulmonary hypertension secondary to hypoxia and/or lung disease, chronic thromboembolic pulmonary hypertension, and pulmonary hypertension with unclear multifactorial mechanisms.
- Pulmonary hypertension, regardless of cause, typically manifests on imaging as enlarged central pulmonary arteries with rapid tapering.
- Imaging features specific to a particular diagnosis may be evident in selected cases.

SUGGESTED READINGS

Diller GP, Gatzoulis MA. Pulmonary vascular disease in adults with congenital heart disease. Circulation 2007; 115:1039-1050.

Frazier AA, Galvin JR, Franks TJ, et al. From the archives of the AFIP: pulmonary vasculature: hypertension and infarction. Radiographics 2000; 20:491-524.

Keogh AM, Mayer E, Benza RL, et al. Interventional and surgical modalities of treatment in pulmonary hypertension. J Am Coll Cardiol 2009; 54:S67-S77.

McLaughlin VV, Archer SL, Badesch DB, et al. ACCF/AHA 2009 expert consensus document on pulmonary hypertension. A report of the American College of Cardiology Foundation Task Force on Expert Consensus Documents and the American Heart Association developed in collaboration with the American College of Chest Physicians; American Thoracic Society, Inc; and the Pulmonary Hypertension Association. J Am Coll Cardiol 2009; 53:1573-1619.

Reddy GP, Gotway MB, Araoz PA. Imaging of chronic thromboembolic pulmonary hypertension. Semin Roentgenol 2005; 40:41-47.

Rossi SE, Goodman PC, Franquet T. Nonthrombotic pulmonary emboli. AJR Am J Roentgenol 2000; 174:1499-1508.

Simonneau G, Robbins IM, Beghetti M, et al. Updated clinical classification of pulmonary hypertension. J Am Coll Cardiol 2009; 54:S43-S54.

REFERENCES

1. Frazier AA, Galvin JR, Franks TJ, et al. From the archives of the AFIP: pulmonary vasculature: hypertension and infarction. Radiographics 2000; 20:491-524.
2. Badesch DB, Abman SH, Simonneau G, et al. Medical therapy for pulmonary arterial hypertension: updated ACCP evidence-based clinical practice guidelines. Chest 2007; 131:1917-1928.
3. Farber HW, Loscalzo J. Pulmonary arterial hypertension. N Engl J Med 2004; 351:1655-1665.
4. Galie N, Torbicki A, Barst R, et al. Guidelines on diagnosis and treatment of pulmonary arterial hypertension. The Task Force on Diagnosis and Treatment of Pulmonary Arterial Hypertension of the European Society of Cardiology. Eur Heart J 2004; 25:2243-2278.
5. Simonneau G, Galie N, Rubin LJ, et al. Clinical classification of pulmonary hypertension. J Am Coll Cardiol 2004; 43:5S-12S.
6. Simonneau G, Robbins IM, Beghetti M, et al. Updated clinical classification of pulmonary hypertension. J Am Coll Cardiol 2009; 54:S43-54.
7. McLaughlin VV, Archer SL, Badesch DB, et al; American College of Cardiology Foundation Task Force on Expert Consensus Documents; American Heart Association; American College of Chest Physicians; American Thoracic Society, Inc; Pulmonary Hypertension Association. ACCF/AHA 2009 expert consensus document on pulmonary hypertension. A report of the American College of Cardiology Foundation Task Force on Expert Consensus Documents and the American Heart Association developed in collaboration with the American College of Chest Physicians; American Thoracic Society, Inc; and the Pulmonary Hypertension Association. J Am Coll Cardiol 2009; 53:1573-1619.
8. Nolan RL, McAdams HP, Sporn TA, et al. Pulmonary cholesterol granulomas in patients with pulmonary artery hypertension: chest radiographic and CT findings. AJR Am J Roentgenol 1999; 172:1317-1319.
9. Chin KM, Rubin LJ. Pulmonary arterial hypertension. J Am Coll Cardiol 2008; 51:1527-1538.
10. Diller GP, Gatzoulis MA. Pulmonary vascular disease in adults with congenital heart disease. Circulation 2007; 115:1039-1050.
11. Frazier AA, Franks TJ, Mohammed TL, et al. From the archives of the AFIP: pulmonary veno-occlusive disease and pulmonary capillary hemangiomatosis. Radiographics 2007; 27:867-882.
12. Resten A, Maitre S, Humbert M, et al. Pulmonary hypertension: CT of the chest in pulmonary venoocclusive disease. AJR Am J Roentgenol 2004; 183:65-70.
13. Swensen SJ, Tashjian JH, Myers JL, et al. Pulmonary venoocclusive disease: CT findings in eight patients. AJR Am J Roentgenol 1996; 167:937-940.
14. Resten A, Maitre S, Humbert M, et al. Pulmonary arterial hypertension: thin-section CT predictors of epoprostenol therapy failure. Radiology 2002; 222:782-788.
15. El-Gabaly M, Farver CF, Budev MA, Mohammed TL. Pulmonary capillary hemangiomatosis imaging findings and literature update. J Comput Assist Tomogr 2007; 31:608-610.
16. Tan RT, Kuzo R, Goodman LR, et al. Utility of CT scan evaluation for predicting pulmonary hypertension in patients with parenchymal lung disease. Medical College of Wisconsin Lung Transplant Group. Chest 1998; 113:1250-1256.
17. Zisman DA, Karlamangla AS, Ross DJ, et al. High-resolution chest CT findings do not predict the presence of pulmonary hypertension in advanced idiopathic pulmonary fibrosis. Chest 2007; 132:773-779.
18. Chen H, De Marco T, Golden JA, Gould MK: Utility of CT for predicting pulmonary hypertension in patients with parenchymal lung disease: Similar results, different conclusion? Chest 2008; 133:1053-1054.
19. Thistlethwaite PA, Kaneko K, Madani MM, Jamieson SW. Technique and outcomes of pulmonary endarterectomy surgery. Ann Thorac Cardiovasc Surg 2008; 14:274-282.
20. Reddy GP, Gotway MB, Araoz PA. Imaging of chronic thromboembolic pulmonary hypertension. Semin Roentgenol. 2005; 40:41-47.
21. The PIOPED Investigators. Value of the ventilation/perfusion scan in acute pulmonary embolism. Results of the prospective investigation of pulmonary embolism diagnosis (PIOPED). JAMA 1990; 263:2753-2759.
22. Tunariu N, Gibbs SJ, Win Z, et al. Ventilation-perfusion scintigraphy is more sensitive than multidetector CTPA in detecting chronic thromboembolic pulmonary disease as a treatable cause of pulmonary hypertension. J Nucl Med 2007; 48:680-684.
23. Rubin LJ, Hoeper MM, Klepetko W, et al. Current and future management of chronic thromboembolic pulmonary hypertension: from diagnosis to treatment responses. Proc Am Thorac Soc 2006; 3:601-607.
24. Keogh AM, Mayer E, Benza RL, et al. Interventional and surgical modalities of treatment in pulmonary hypertension. J Am Coll Cardiol 2009; 54:S67-S77.
25. Rossi SE, Goodman PC, Franquet T. Nonthrombotic pulmonary emboli. AJR Am J Roentgenol 2000; 174:1499-1508.

CHAPTER 100

Pulmonary Edema

Michael B. Gotway

Pulmonary edema is frequently classified as hydrostatic edema (e.g., cardiogenic pulmonary edema) or edema caused by increased capillary permeability (e.g., noncardiogenic pulmonary edema or capillary leak). Often, chest radiographs of patients with pulmonary edema are not as easily classified in such a dichotomous fashion. The following pulmonary edema classification has been proposed to better accommodate the histopathologic, physiologic, and radiographic findings of these patients[1]:

1. Hydrostatic pulmonary edema
2. Permeability edema associated with diffuse alveolar damage (DAD)
3. Permeability edema without associated DAD
4. Mixed pulmonary edema patterns

HYDROSTATIC PULMONARY EDEMA

The main physiologic derangement in patients with hydrostatic pulmonary edema is an imbalance between intra-and extravascular hydrostatic and capillary oncotic pressures, often the result of pulmonary venous hypertension.

Etiology and Pathophysiology

Among the various potential causes of pulmonary venous hypertension, left heart failure is overwhelmingly the most common. Other potential causes include left atrial, mitral valvular, or pulmonary venous obstruction and volume overload in patients with renal failure or iatrogenic hypervolemia. Less commonly, low intravascular oncotic pressure resulting from hypoalbuminemia, typically in patients with liver failure or nephrotic syndrome, may produce interstitial fluid accumulation. Often, multiple mechanisms are operative in a given patient.

Manifestations of Disease

Clinical Presentation

Course and Clearing of Hydrostatic Pulmonary Edema

The chest radiograph usually becomes abnormal with the appearance of clinical symptoms in patients with hydrostatic pulmonary edema. However, it may show abnormalities before clinical symptoms appear and, conversely, clinical symptoms may appear prior to the development of radiographic abnormalities. This phenomenon is often referred to as lag (clinical lag or radiographic lag, respectively), and may occur with the development or during resolution of hydrostatic pulmonary edema. The radiographic lag phase of alveolar edema resolution in particular may be pronounced.

Interstitial edema may change or clear within hours of treatment, whereas alveolar edema may require a longer time to clear. Whereas most patients who develop hydrostatic pulmonary edema will develop interstitial edema first, followed by alveolar edema, some patients will present first with alveolar edema. In contrast, however, as alveolar edema resolves, it does not clear by forming interstitial edema. In fact, it is not uncommon to see a paradoxical increase in pleural effusions as interstitial or alveolar edema clears.

Imaging Techniques and Findings

Radiography

The chest radiographic findings of hydrostatic pulmonary edema are detailed in Box 100-1. These findings are all more reliably distinguishable on posteroanterior (PA) and lateral chest radiographs than on portable radiographs,

> **BOX 100-1 Thoracic Imaging Findings in Hydrostatic Pulmonary Edema**
>
> **CHEST RADIOGRAPHY**
> Cardiomegaly
> Pulmonary venous enlargement
> Widened vascular pedicle
> Azygos vein distention
> Interstitial edema
>
> - Vascular indistinctness
> - Interlobular septal thickening
> - Peribronchial cuffing
> - Subpleural edema
>
> Pleural effusion
>
> **THORACIC CT**
> Cardiomegaly
> Pulmonary venous enlargement
> Vascular engorgement
> Bronchial wall thickening
> Ground-glass opacity
> Centrilobular nodules, often with ground-glass attenuation
> Smooth interlobular septal thickening
> Pleural effusions, fissure thickening pericardial effusion

but commonly patients with the greatest likelihood of hydrostatic pulmonary edema will be imaged using an anteroposterior technique (AP). AP techniques can make the diagnosis of hydrostatic pulmonary edema difficult because heart magnification, resulting from the considerably shorter focus-film distance as well as projectional magnification, can render determination of cardiac size unreliable, particularly in patients with low lung volumes. Additionally, pulmonary vascular congestion is difficult to determine accurately in nonerect patients because upper lobe vessels frequently normally appear larger than lower lobe vessels for patients imaged in a supine or semierect position. Furthermore, azygos vein dilation, often considered an indicator of elevated right atrial pressure, is a common and potentially normal finding on supine radiographs. Finally, pleural effusions often appear only as hazy attenuation projecting over lungs in patients imaged in a supine or semierect position. However, this appearance is not specific for pleural effusion and can be seen with extensive posterior atelectasis because anterior aerated lung superimposes on the increased opacity of the posteriorly located atelectatic lung. This pattern is often seen in severely ill patients and patients in the intensive care unit, which is the same patient population at risk for hydrostatic pulmonary edema.

The first chest radiographic signs of pulmonary venous hypertension include pulmonary vascular redistribution, appearing as equalization of the size of the upper and lower lobe vessels, which progresses to the upper lobe vessels becoming larger than those in the lower lobes (a reversal of the normal situation). In the acute setting, this phenomenon is seen with left atrial (wedge) pressures in the range of 12 to 19 mm Hg.[2] In chronically compensated patients, such as those with mitral stenosis, upper and lower lobe vascular equalization and reversal will occur with left atrial pressures between 15 to 25 mm Hg.[2] As the physiologic derangements worsen, pulmonary venous hypertension progresses to frank interstitial pulmonary edema, with the development of interlobular septal thickening, often referred to as Kerley A and B lines (Fig. 100-1A), perihilar indistinctness and vascular haze (see Fig. 100-1B), peribronchial cuffing (see Fig. 100-1C), and subpleural edema (see later).[2] Findings of interstitial edema usually are apparent on the chest radiograph, with left atrial pressures of 20 to 25 mm Hg in the acutely ill patient and 25 to 30 mm Hg in chronically compensated patients.[2] At higher left atrial pressures, frank alveolar edema occurs, with spillage of fluid into the air spaces. In these patients, the chest radiograph will show an air space consolidation pattern (see Fig. 100-1D) and acinar nodules,[2] often superimposed on findings of interstitial edema. The relationship between left atrial (pulmonary capillary wedge) pressure and radiographic findings is not precise, and the radiographic findings often lag behind the physiological changes. Furthermore, stepwise progression through these phases is not always seen, and some imaging findings of hydrostatic edema may be present in the absence of others.

CT

On thoracic CT, findings of hydrostatic pulmonary edema include those seen on chest radiographs, such as cardiomegaly, vascular engorgement, and pleural effusions. Findings of interstitial edema (see later), are also apparent and are more readily appreciable with thoracic CT, particularly high-resolution CT (HRCT), than with chest radiography. Bronchial wall thickening, smooth interlobular septal thickening (Fig. 100-2), and ground-glass opacity (often with hazy, poorly defined centrilobular nodules) are highly suggestive of hydrostatic pulmonary edema.

Classic Signs

Interstitial Edema

The findings of interstitial edema on chest radiography (see Box 100-1) are usually readily visible with CT scanning and, in addition to the findings noted, ground-glass opacity and centrilobular nodules are frequently present in patients with hydrostatic pulmonary edema.

Interlobular Septal Thickening (Kerley A and B lines)

Both Kerley A and B lines represent thickened interlobular septae. Kerley B lines are horizontal linear opacities, 1 to 2 cm in length, in contact with the pleural surface. Kerley B lines are most readily visible in the inferior and lateral aspects of the thorax, near the lateral costophrenic sulcus (see Fig. 100-1A). The regular appearance of Kerley B lines in the lung bases is the result of the regular organization of pulmonary lobules at the lung bases.

Kerley A lines also represent interlobular septal thickening but are relatively uncommon compared with Kerley B lines. Kerley A lines are obliquely oriented linear opaci-

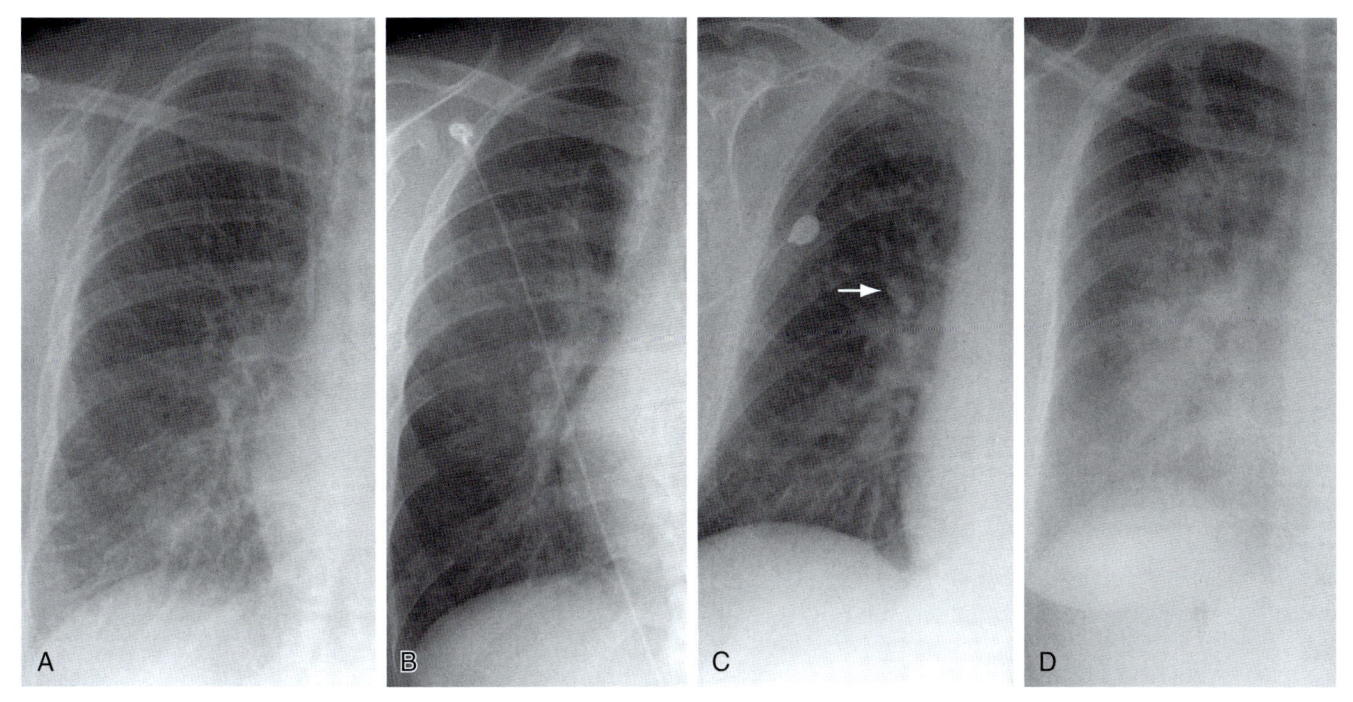

FIGURE 100-1 Chest radiographic findings of interstitial (A-C) and alveolar (D) edema. **A,** Interlobular septal thickening. **B,** Perihilar "haze." **C,** Peribronchial cuffing (*arrow*). **D,** Consolidation (alveolar edema).

ties several centimeters long, radiating outward from the central or perihilar lung. Kerley A lines have a somewhat different appearance from Kerley B lines because of the different organization of secondary lobules within the central lung.

The interlobular septal thickening resulting from hydrostatic pulmonary edema is readily visualized on thoracic CT, especially HRCT. Interlobular septal thickening in patients with hydrostatic pulmonary edema is smooth and often most readily visualized in the lung bases and in the pulmonary apices (Fig. 100-2). Poorly defined, ground-glass attenuation centrilobular nodules or lobular ground-glass opacity often coexists.

Vascular Indistinctness and Perihilar Haze

In patients with pulmonary venous hypertension and interstitial edema, fluid transudating from the vessels surrounds the vessels and blurs their margin on chest radiographs, rendering the vascular margins indistinct.

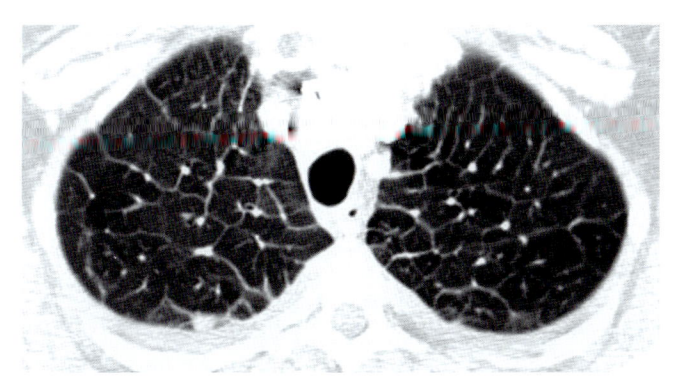

FIGURE 100-2 Interstitial pulmonary edema—interlobular septal thickening. This axial CT scan shows a pronounced linear pattern in the apices.

Pulmonary vascular indistinctness is frequently most visible in the lower lobes and may be present before Kerley lines are apparent.

Perihilar haze is a term occasionally used to refer to poor definition of and slightly increased opacity surrounding the perihilar vessels; it manifests as perihilar vascular indistinctness with a hazy or ground-glass appearance (see Fig. 100-1B). Although not always easily recognizable, perihilar haze can be a useful finding that suggests hydrostatic pulmonary edema in patients with lower lobe atelectasis.

Peribronchial Cuffing

Peribronchial cuffing represents bronchial wall thickening, possibly accompanied by a variable amount of peribronchial interstitial fluid. Peribronchial cuffing is most readily recognizable in the central and perihilar regions of lung, when bronchi are seen in cross section (see Fig. 100-1C). Peribronchial cuffing may also be seen as a tram-track appearance when bronchi are visualized in longitudinal section. Peribronchial cuffing may also appear as nonspecific thickening of the interstitium radiating outward from the hilum. On thoracic CT, peribronchial thickening or cuffing usually appears as bronchial wall thickening. Peribronchial cuffing may represent a finding of interstitial edema in the proper clinical setting, but is not specific for that diagnosis; peribronchial inflammation or tumor may also produce this finding.

Subpleural Edema

The subpleural interstitium is contiguous with the peribronchovascular interstitium through the peripheral centrilobular interstitium and interlobular septa. When fluid accumulates within interlobular septa, this fluid may track into the subpleural interstitium, creating thickening of this compartment as well. On chest radiography and thoracic CT, subpleural edema appears as fissural thickening.

Ground-Glass Opacity

An abnormal increase in lung water may produce an overall increase in haziness in the pulmonary parenchyma, often with decreased lung volumes because of diminished pulmonary compliance. This haziness may create the appearance of ground-glass opacity (increased attenuation without obscuration of the underlying vascular bundles) on chest radiographs, although this finding is usually difficult to appreciate. However, ground-glass opacity caused by interstitial edema is readily recognizable on HRCT, and may occasionally appear as centrilobular nodules.

Air Space (Alveolar) Edema

As factors producing interstitial edema progress, eventually interstitial fluid will begin to accumulate within the air spaces, producing air space edema. Because the edema fluid replaces air within the alveoli, air space edema represents a form of air space consolidation and appears as a confluent opacity (see Fig. 100-1D), which may be accompanied by air space or acinar nodules.

Distribution of Hydrostatic Edema

Hydrostatic edema may assume a number of different distributions, although a symmetric perihilar and basilar predominant distribution is most common. A distinct perihilar distribution of hydrostatic edema is often referred to as a bat wing or butterfly distribution, and is often seen when edema fluid accumulates rapidly. Uncommonly, hydrostatic edema will accumulate in a reverse bat wing distribution reminiscent of other causes of peripheral lung opacity. Other variations in the distribution of hydrostatic edema are frequently recognized (Box 100-2).[2]

BOX 100-2   Atypical Distributions of Pulmonary Edema

Unilateral or asymmetric pulmonary edema
- Ipsilateral abnormalities
  - Gravitational decubitus positioning
  - Re-expansion edema
  - Pulmonary vein atresia, stenosis, obstruction, or occlusion
  - Congenital or acquired systemic to pulmonary artery shunt (e.g., Blalock-Taussig shunt)
- Contralateral abnormalities
  - Pulmonary artery occlusion pulmonary embolism, tumor, mediastinal fibrosis
  - Pulmonary arterial stenosis or interruption
  - Pulmonary arterial hypoplasia (Swyer-James syndrome)

Right upper lobe edema with papillary muscle rupture or dysfunction
Upper lobe edema

PERMEABILITY EDEMA WITH DIFFUSE ALVEOLAR DAMAGE

Etiology and Pathophysiology

Permeability edema results from injury to the capillary endothelium from a wide variety of insults, and causes the alveolar-capillary membrane unit to become leaky. Such leaks allow protein and fluid to move from the vascular spaces into the alveoli. Unlike interstitial and alveolar hydrostatic pulmonary edema, which is low in protein content, permeability edema in the air spaces is high in protein, which prolongs retention of fluid transudated into the air spaces and is therefore comparatively slow to clear. Histopathologically, depending on the enticing insult, diffuse alveolar damage may coexist.

Manifestations of Disease

Clinical Presentation

Adult Respiratory Distress Syndrome

The adult respiratory distress syndrome (ARDS) is a form of diffuse pulmonary parenchymal lung injury associated with noncardiogenic pulmonary edema that results in hypoxemic respiratory failure.[3] Histopathologically, ARDS is characterized by DAD. ARDS represents a constellation of clinical and physiologic findings that are thought to represent a single common process. The diagnostic criteria based on the American-European Consensus Conference for ARDS[4] is as follows:

1. Multilobar, bilateral pulmonary opacities on chest radiography
2. Acute onset
3. Pulmonary capillary wedge pressure <18 mm Hg (or no clinical evidence for left atrial hypertension)
4. Arterial partial pressure of oxygen/fraction of inspired oxygen (PaO_2/FIO_2) <200

When the PaO_2/FIO_2 ratio is <300, the term *acute lung injury* is often used. Acute lung injury is considered a milder version of diffuse lung injury, which may or may not progress to full ARDS.

Histopathologically, ARDS is characterized by DAD. The exact mechanism of injury that brings about DAD is not known, but undoubtedly free radicals and cellular infiltration with expression of proteolytic enzymes and cytokines play a prominent role in the resulting tissue damage. A wide variety of insults may result in ARDS (Box 100-3).

Histopathologic Abnormalities and Stages in Patients with Adult Respiratory Distress Syndrome

The histopathologic findings in patients with ARDS have been described in three overlapping stages (Box 100-4):

1. Acute exudative stage
2. Subacute proliferative stage
3. Chronic fibrotic stage

BOX 100-3 Potential Causes of Adult Respiratory Distress Syndrome

DIRECT PULMONARY INJURY
- Toxic gas or fume inhalation
- Drug exposures
- Aspiration
- Pneumonia
- Pulmonary contusion
- Reperfusion injury (following lung transplantation)
- Fat embolism
- Near-drowning

INDIRECT PULMONARY INJURY
- Sepsis
- Multiple trauma
- Pancreatitis
- Drug overdose
- Multiple blood transfusions
- Shock
- Cardiopulmonary bypass

The histopathologic findings in these stages are similar regardless of the cause of ARDS. In the exudative stage, the predominant histopathologic pattern is DAD, with hyaline membrane formation associated with high protein content. Neutrophilic infiltration, hemorrhage, epithelial cell injury, and macrophage accumulation are also seen.

BOX 100-4 Stages of Adult Respiratory Distress Syndrome (ARDS)

ARDS: Diffuse pulmonary parenchymal lung injury associated with noncardiogenic pulmonary edema producing hypoxemic respiratory failure histopathologically characterized by diffuse alveolar damage (DAD)

Diagnostic criteria from the American-European Consensus Conference for ARDS

- Multilobar, bilateral pulmonary opacities on chest radiography
- Acute onset
- Pulmonary capillary wedge pressure <18 mm Hg (or no clinical evidence for left atrial hypertension)
- Arterial partial pressure of oxygen/fraction of inspired oxygen (PaO_2/FIO_2) <200

Stages and imaging findings

- Acute exudative stage (days 1-8)
  - Patchy ground-glass opacity, air space consolidation, evolves rapidly; dependent atelectasis; minimal or no effusion
- Subacute proliferative stage (starts as early as day 7, possibly even day 1 to day 30)
  - Air space consolidation regresses; linear and reticular opacities develop; ground-glass opacity may persist; traction bronchiectasis, architectural distortion
- Chronic fibrotic stage (day 8 on)—most pulmonary opacities clear; anterior lung fibrosis may remain

---

This phase lasts for approximately 5 to 7 days. The exudative stage is sometimes subdivided into an early phase, which occurs hours after the insult, and in which endothelial cell edema, capillary congestion, interstitial edema, and hemorrhage occur. In the late exudative phase, which occurs several days following the inciting insult, DAD with hyaline membrane formation is seen, associated with type I pneumocyte necrosis and protein-rich alveolar edema fluid.[3]

Imaging Techniques and Findings

Radiography

Imaging Findings During Exudative Phase of Adult Respiratory Distress Syndrome

Thoracic imaging studies early in the exudative phase may be normal, again reflecting a radiographic latent period, or lag phase. Later in the exudative phase, multifocal bilateral patchy opacities, usually ground-glass opacity and air space consolidation, will be seen. These opacities may be accompanied by air bronchogram formation (generally uncommon in patients with hydrostatic pulmonary edema). These opacities progress over the following days, and become increasingly confluent until the involved portions of all lobes bilaterally. Dependent atelectasis is commonly present. Radiographic opacities in patients with ARDS during the exudative phase may show a somewhat more peripheral predominance than in patients with hydrostatic pulmonary edema. Pleural effusions are uncommon and, when present, are smaller than in patients with hydrostatic pulmonary edema. Interlobular septal thickening is uncommon, and may be a useful feature for distinguishing patients with ARDS from those with hydrostatic edema. Similarly, patients with ARDS often have a normal heart size, whereas those with hydrostatic pulmonary edema will show cardiomegaly.

Because of severe hypoxemia, almost all patients with ARDS undergo mechanical ventilation. The positive pressure used during mechanical ventilation will increase lung volumes and create the appearance of improvement in the radiographic opacities, but usually this finding does not reflect true clearing of fluid from the alveoli. Because the alveoli are filled with protein-rich fluid, numerous inflammatory cells, and hyaline membranes, true radiographic clearing will be prolonged. Mechanical ventilation in patients with ARDS may result in complications, particularly because the lungs are very poorly compliant. Pneumomediastinum and pneumothorax are not uncommon.

The HRCT findings of the various stages of ARDS have been described. In the exudative phase, patchy areas of ground-glass opacity (Fig. 100-3) and air space consolidation are common. These opacities initially tend to predominate in the dependent lung regions. Patchy multifocal opacities may rapidly evolve to diffuse opacities later in the exudative phase and as the proliferative phase progresses. Pleural effusions, if present, are small. Mild interlobular septal thickening may occur, but is less pronounced than in patients with hydrostatic pulmonary edema.

Although the various causes of ARDS are generally radiographically indistinguishable, the temporal sequence

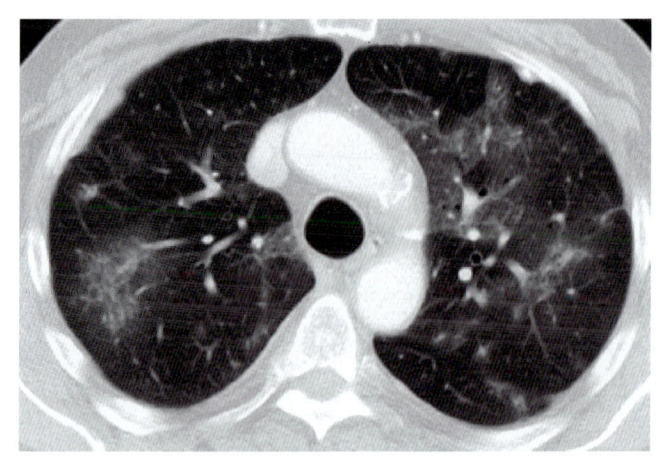

FIGURE 100-3 Adult respiratory distress syndrome (ARDS), exudative stage. This axial thoracic CT scan shows patchy areas of ground-glass opacity and mild reticulation in a patient with developing ARDS. Hours later, the patient deteriorated and was intubated.

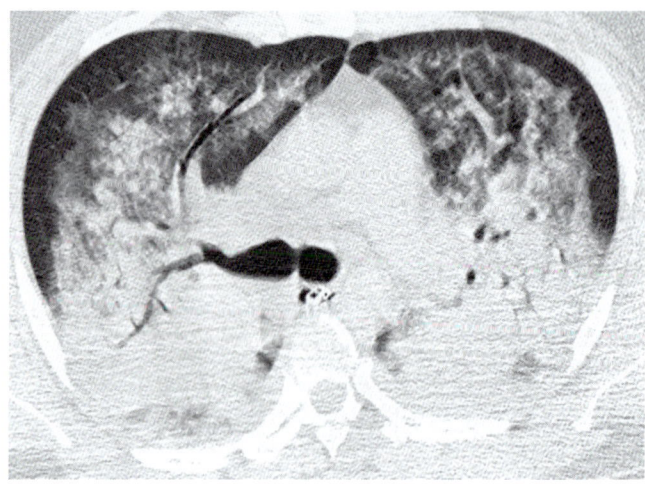

FIGURE 100-4 Adult respiratory distress syndrome, proliferative stage. This axial CT scan shows bilateral ground-glass opacity and consolidation, somewhat posteriorly dependent, with a background of mild reticulation.

of films and presence of certain patterns can provide clues to the insults leading to ARDS. A sequence of films initially showing focal air space consolidation, perhaps suggesting community-acquired pneumonia, which subsequently shows development of multifocal bilateral opacities consistent with ARDS, suggests a primary lung insult causing ARDS. Furthermore, in patients with ARDS resulting from pulmonary disease, consolidation and ground-glass opacity are equally prevalent and pulmonary abnormalities are commonly asymmetric, reflecting the presence of the underlying causative pulmonary insult. In contrast, for patients with an extrapulmonary cause of ARDS, ground-glass opacity predominates and symmetric lung involvement is the rule.

The proliferative phase of ARDS occurs from 7 to 30 days following the onset of ARDS. During this phase, hyaline membranes become organized, pulmonary capillaries are obliterated, and collagen deposition begins. The amount of pulmonary edema fluid and inflammatory cell infiltration decreases. Recent studies have actually indicated that fibroproliferation may begin almost simultaneously with the onset of ARDS, rather than occurring sequentially in stages.

Imaging Findings During the Proliferative Phase of ARDS

After 1 week, air space consolidation begins to regress and linear and reticular opacities become more prominent (Fig. 100-4). Ground-glass opacity may persist. The imaging findings are not specific, but indicate development of a coarser, more organized appearance, which tends to reflect the underlying histopathologic changes. Traction bronchiectasis and bronchiolectasis and architectural distortion may appear. Patients with ARDS in the exudative or early proliferative phases who have more widespread findings of fibrosis, such as traction bronchiectasis, generally require prolonged ventilatory support, are at higher risk for ventilator-associated lung injury, and have higher mortality.

The chronic fibrotic phase of ARDS may begin as early as 8 days following the initial insult, but is more commonly encountered in patients who survive 1 month or longer. In patients who survive ARDS more than 30 days, many of these histopathologic abnormalities resolve, and areas of fibrosis, architectural distortion (Fig. 100-5), and even honeycombing are seen on imaging studies. Ground-glass opacity may persist, but is often associated with coarse reticulation architectural distortion, and reflects the presence of fibrosis rather than edema, hyaline membrane formation, and inflammatory cell infiltration, as in the exudate and proliferative phases. The HRCT findings may show a striking anterior lung involvement (see Fig. 100-5), perhaps because of sparing of the posterior atelectatic lung from the adverse effects of mechanical ventilation, such as high ventilatory pressures and high oxygen tension. If this hypothesis is correct, the prevalence of anterior lung fibrosis in survivors of ARDS may be altered in the future with the use of prone ventilation for the treatment of ARDS patients.

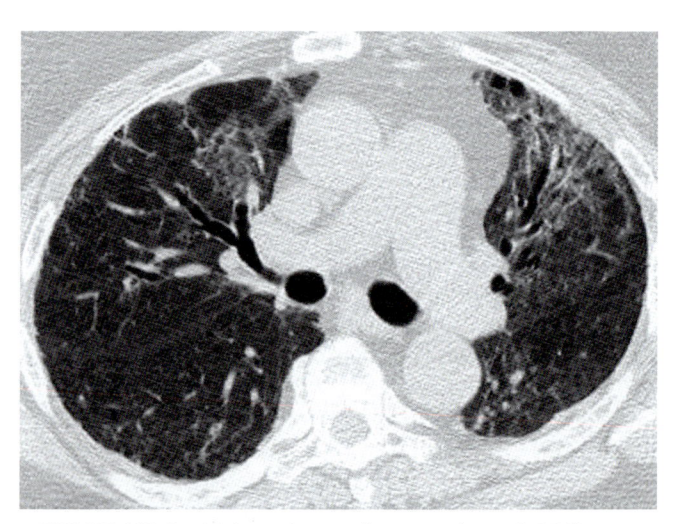

FIGURE 100-5 Adult respiratory distress syndrome (ARDS), chronic stage. This axial CT scan in an ARDS survivor shows patchy ground-glass opacity and coarse reticulation with traction bronchiectasis, consistent with anterior lung fibrosis.

PERMEABILITY PULMONARY EDEMA WITHOUT DIFFUSE ALVEOLAR DAMAGE

Permeability pulmonary edema without DAD may be encountered in patients with reactions to various drugs (such as interleukin-2 treatment), transfusion reactions, infectious causes (e.g., hantavirus pulmonary syndrome), heroin overdose,[1] or other insults that may result in ARDS, such as air emboli or toxic shock syndrome.

Imaging Techniques and Findings
Radiography

Patients with pulmonary edema unaccompanied by DAD may present with chest radiographic and thoracic CT abnormalities resembling those of hydrostatic edema. Interlobular septal thickening is often a prominent feature, whereas air space consolidation is less conspicuous or absent altogether. Unlike ARDS, permeability edema without DAD may clear rapidly on chest radiographs.

MIXED EDEMA

A combination of hydrostatic pulmonary edema and permeability edema, termed *mixed edema*, may be seen in the presence of conditions producing increased intravascular pressure and capillary endothelial injury. This pattern of edema may be seen in patients with re-expansion pulmonary edema, high-altitude pulmonary edema, and neurogenic pulmonary edema, among other less commonly encountered situations (Box 100-5).

Imaging Techniques and Findings
Radiography

Chest radiography in patients with conditions producing mixed edema shows features typically associated with hydrostatic pulmonary edema as well as the multifocal or diffuse lung opacities typically encountered in permeability edema. It is therefore both nonspecific and difficult to interpret accurately.

NEUROGENIC PULMONARY EDEMA

Etiology and Pathophysiology

Neurogenic pulmonary edema occurs in patients with head trauma, intracranial hemorrhage, increased intracranial pressure, seizures, or other acute neurologic conditions producing intracranial hypertension.[1] Drug overdoses, particularly opiates, barbiturates, and alcohol, may also produce neurogenic pulmonary edema. The mechanism of neurogenic pulmonary edema formation includes sympathetic discharge caused by CNS injury, resulting in systemic vasoconstriction, elevated systemic blood pressure and, subsequently, elevated left ventricular pressure and dysfunction. Because the alveolar edema fluid is protein-rich and pulmonary capillary wedge pressures are often normal, some element of capillary leak is also present. Therefore, neurogenic pulmonary edema shows a histopathologic pattern of both hydrostatic and permeability pulmonary edema, representing a mixed edema pattern.

Manifestations of Disease
Clinical Presentation

The edema fluid may appear very quickly, within minutes to hours of the responsible episode.

Imaging Techniques and Findings
Radiography

Chest radiographs show multifocal, bilateral air space consolidation (Fig. 100-6), often predominating in the upper lobes,[1] with normal heart size or no pleural effusion. Radiographic opacities show clearing within 1 to 2 days.

RE-EXPANSION PULMONARY EDEMA

Rapid re-expansion of lung after collapse for at least several days, usually caused by a large pleural effusion or

---

BOX 100-5 Causes of Mixed Pulmonary Edema

Neurogenic pulmonary edema
Re-expansion edema
High-altitude pulmonary edema
Reperfusion edema following lung transplantation
Edema associated with tocolytic therapy
Postpneumonectomy or postvolume reduction edema
Air embolism
Volume overload, renal failure, or congestive heart failure in patients with ARDS

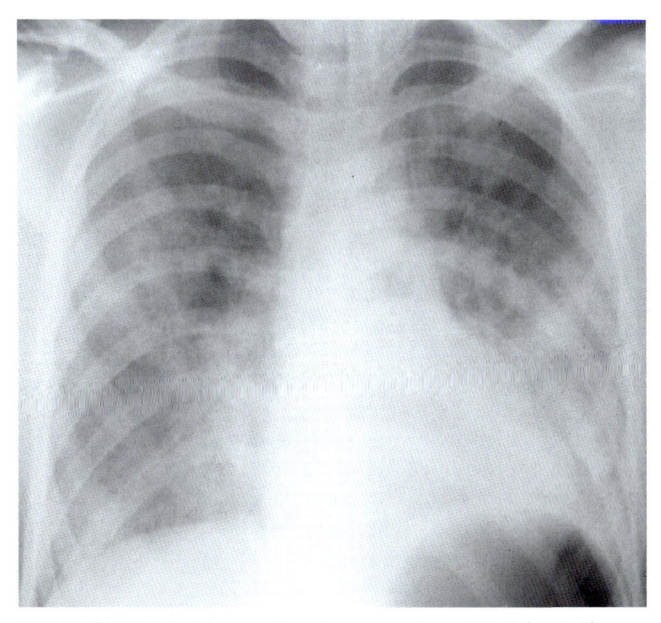

■ **FIGURE 100-6** Neurogenic pulmonary edema. This frontal chest radiograph in a patient with subarachnoid hemorrhage shows bilateral pulmonary opacity without widening of the vascular pedicle or features suggesting hydrostatic edema.

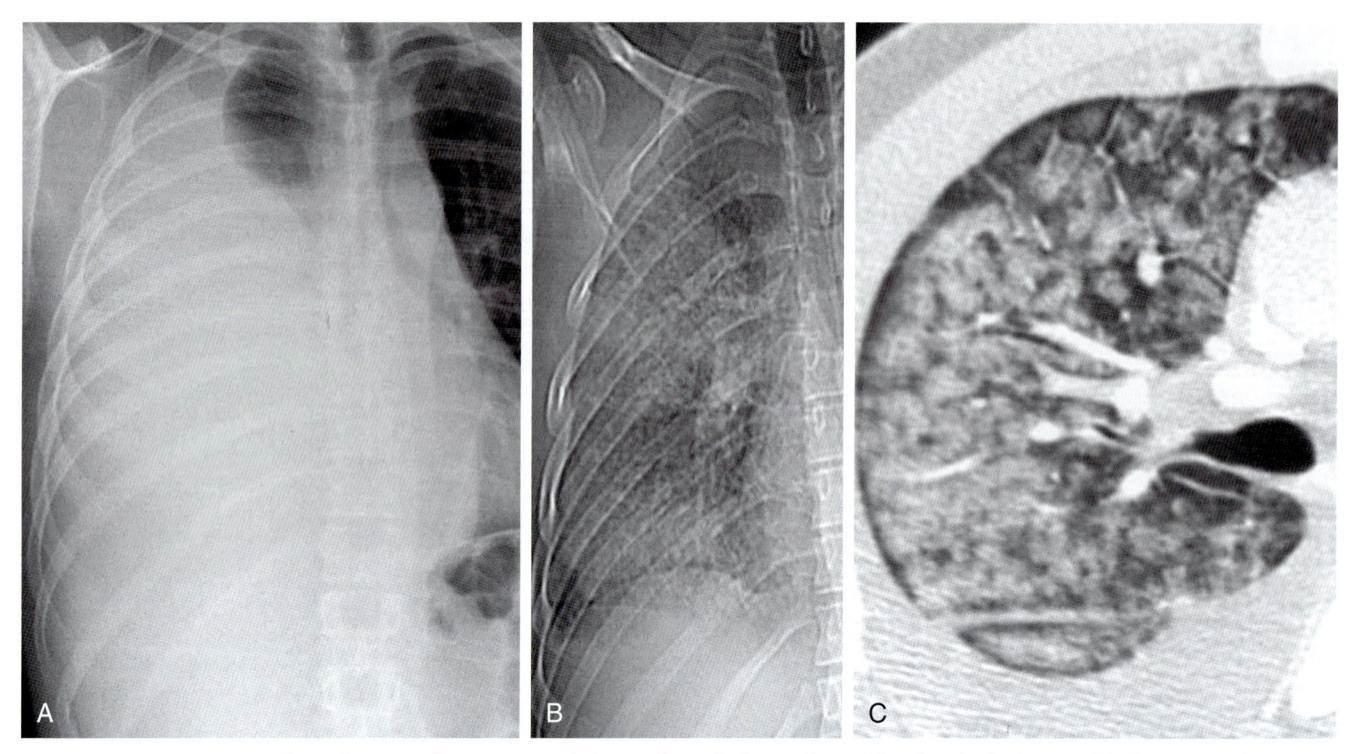

■ FIGURE 100-7 Re-expansion pulmonary edema. **A,** Frontal chest radiograph shows a large right pleural effusion. **B,** Digital scout view from thoracic CT scan after thoracentesis, when patient developed shortness of breath, shows development of consolidation, ground-glass opacity, and linear opacities. **C,** Thoracic CT scan shows ground-glass opacity centrilobular nodules and smooth interlobular septal thickening.

pneumothorax, may produce edema in the re-expanded lung. This process is referred to as re-expansion pulmonary edema.

Etiology and Pathophysiology

The mechanism of re-expansion pulmonary edema includes a combination of several factors. First, diminished perfusion in the collapsed lung results in decreased surfactant production and decreased pulmonary compliance, requiring a more negative intrapleural pressure to achieve inflation of the collapsed lung. Additionally, pulmonary collapse increases vascular resistance. These factors favor the production of hydrostatic pulmonary edema when the pulmonary collapse is relieved. Additionally, the hypoxemia that accompanies the prolonged pulmonary collapse and hypoperfusion results in the release of free radicals that produce capillary endothelial injury, causing permeability edema that worsens from the increased perfusion that occurs with reperfusion. The production of free radicals that gain access to the blood stream may also explain the occasional occurrence of re-expansion pulmonary edema that develops in regions of lung that were not severely collapsed, and even pulmonary parenchyma on the contralateral side. Temporarily decreased pulmonary lymphatic or venous return may also play a role in re-expansion pulmonary edema.

Risk factors for the development of re-expansion pulmonary edema include prolonged pulmonary collapse (usually at least 72 hours), a large-volume pleural space-occupying process (>1500 mL fluid), and coexistent cardiovascular disease.

Manifestations of Disease

Clinical Presentation

Re-expansion pulmonary edema usually occurs within 2 to 4 hours of lung re-expansion, often after rapid removal of the space-occupying process within the pleural space, but may progress for 1 to 2 days.

Imaging Techniques and Findings

Radiography and CT

Thoracic imaging studies will show the abnormality producing the pulmonary collapse, usually a large pleural effusion (Fig. 100-7) or pneumothorax, that subsequently undergoes drainage. The history will usually suggest that a large volume of fluid or air was removed, and that the pleural process has usually been present for a number of days. Within hours of the drainage procedure, increased opacity, usually ground-glass opacity or air space consolidation, develops within the expanded lung (see Fig. 100-7B). HRCT will also show ground-glass opacity (see Fig. 100-7C) and air space consolidation within the affected lung. The pathologic and radiographic findings associated with re-expansion pulmonary edema usually resolve within a few days to a week.

Synopsis of Treatment Options

Re-expansion edema is usually self-limited but, in some patients, symptoms such as fever, nausea, vomiting, worsening dyspnea, chest pain, and cough with frothy sputum can be severe and even fatal. Treatment of re-expansion pulmonary edema is usually supportive, with supplementary oxygen and ventilatory support as required. Prevention of re-expansion pulmonary edema revolves around slow removal of the pleural effusion or pneumothorax over a period of days, as well as optimization of cardiovascular disease treatment before thoracentesis. As a general rule, for long-standing pleural effusions, one should avoid removing more than 1500 mL during the first thoracentesis procedure.

HIGH-ALTITUDE PULMONARY EDEMA

Etiology and Pathophysiology

Pulmonary edema may develop in some individuals after rapid ascent to high altitude, usually at altitudes higher than 10,000 feet. Pulmonary edema usually develops between 12 hours and 3 days after ascent,[1] usually in the first day. Less commonly, high-altitude pulmonary edema develops in people with prolonged residence at a high altitude.

Manifestations of Disease

Clinical Presentation

Reduction in the partial pressure of oxygen in inspired air is responsible for the development of high-altitude pulmonary edema. The drop in partial pressure of oxygen that occurs at high altitude produces severe hypoxic vasoconstriction in the pulmonary arterial bed but, in susceptible individuals, this vasoconstriction is nonuniform. This inhomogeneous vasoconstriction response results in high-volume shunting of blood into pulmonary vessels unprotected by hypoxic vasoconstriction, producing severe elevations in pulmonary arterial pressure and resulting in pulmonary edema.[1] Both hydrostatic and permeability pulmonary edema mechanisms are present in patients with high-altitude pulmonary edema.

Imaging Techniques and Findings

Radiography

Chest radiographs show patchy air space consolidation, which may be unilateral (often the right side) or bilateral, usually without pleural effusion or cardiomegaly. Histopathologically, hyaline membrane formation with protein-rich edema fluid is present and capillary thrombi and hemorrhage may be seen, but high-altitude pulmonary edema does not result from the same inflammation-driven process that produces ARDS.

Synopsis of Treatment Options

Supplemental oxygen administration or return to sea level results in resolution within 1 to 2 days,[1] and radiographic findings clear rapidly with appropriate treatment.

BOX 100-6 Radiographic Differentiation of the Types of Pulmonary Edema

Hydrostatic pulmonary edema

- Cardiomegaly
- Interlobular septal thickening
- Symmetric pleural effusions
- Rapid appearance, change, and clearing
- Air bronchograms *not* common or prominent

Permeability edema with diffuse alveolar damage (DAD)

- Radiographic appearance of opacities delayed for hours after clinical presentation; resolution prolonged
- Multifocal or diffuse opacities; air bronchograms common
- Interlobular septal thickening *not* common
- Pleural effusions uncommon

Permeability edema without DAD

- Rapid onset and resolution
- Interlobular septal thickening
- Minimal air space consolidation

Mixed edema

- Suggestive clinical context
    - Neurogenic pulmonary edema (intracranial pathology)
    - Re-expansion edema (rapid drainage of pneumothorax or pleural effusion)
    - High-altitude pulmonary edema
    - Reperfusion edema following lung transplantation
    - Edema associated with tocolytic therapy (preterm labor treatment)
    - Postpneumonectomy or postvolume reduction edema, air embolism (e.g., CNS surgery, trauma, lung biopsy, catheter malfunction or dislodgment)

Differential Diagnosis

From Clinical Presentation

The clinical presentation may provide strong evidence favoring one pattern over the other, but distinguishing between permeability edema without DAD and mixed edema is often not possible. Fortunately, however, permeability edema without DAD and mixed edema tend to occur in suggestive clinical scenarios, which may indicate the correct diagnosis.

From Imaging Findings

Differentiating among the various histopathologic patterns of edema on imaging studies can be challenging. Imaging features favoring one pattern over another are detailed in Box 100-6. Often, presumptive treatment for hydrostatic pulmonary edema with radiographic reassessment is useful—hydrostatic pulmonary edema will improve rapidly, whereas the time course to resolution for permeability edema with diffuse alveolar damage is prolonged.

KEY POINTS

- Pulmonary edema may be classified into four distinct categories: hydrostatic pulmonary edema, permeability edema associated with diffuse alveolar damage, permeability edema without associated diffuse alveolar damage, and mixed pulmonary edema patterns.
- Hydrostatic pulmonary edema is typically characterized on thoracic imaging studies by findings suggesting pulmonary venous hypertension and interstitial edema: peribronchial cuffing, perihilar indistinctness and vascular haze, subpleural edema and, in particular, interlobular septal thickening. Cardiomegaly and pleural effusions are often present.
- Imaging features of interstitial edema are less prominent in nonhydrostatic causes of pulmonary edema.

SUGGESTED READINGS

Gluecker T, Capasso P, Schnyder P, et al. Clinical and radiologic features of pulmonary edema. Radiographics 1999; 19:1507-1531.

Higgins CB. Essentials of Cardiac Radiology and Imaging. Philadelphia, JB Lippincott, 1992.

REFERENCES

1. Gluecker T, Capasso P, Schnyder P, et al. Clinical and radiologic features of pulmonary edema. Radiographics 1999; 19:1507-1531.
2. Higgins CB. Essentials of Cardiac Radiology and Imaging. Philadelphia, JB Lippincott, 1992.
3. Donati SY, Papazian L. Role of open-lung biopsy in acute respiratory distress syndrome. Curr Opin Crit Care 2008; 14:75-79.
4. Bernard GR, Artigas A, Brigham KL, et al. The American-European Consensus Conference on ARDS. Definitions, mechanisms, relevant outcomes, and clinical trial coordination. Am J Respir Crit Care Med 1994; 149:818-824.

CHAPTER 101

Pulmonary Hemorrhage and Vasculitis

Michael B. Gotway

A large number of conditions may result in pulmonary hemorrhage (Table 101-1). Broadly speaking, pulmonary hemorrhage may originate in the airways or lung parenchyma. Airway-related pulmonary hemorrhage is commonly the result of bronchitis, bronchiectasis, or malignancy, whereas parenchymal hemorrhage may result from pulmonary infarction, necrotizing pneumonias, toxic inhalational injury, malignancy, or causes of diffuse alveolar hemorrhage, with or without pulmonary vasculitis.

DIFFUSE ALVEOLAR HEMORRHAGE

Etiology and Pathophysiology

Diffuse alveolar hemorrhage (DAH) is present when the cause of the hemorrhage primarily affects the alveolar capillary surface. Causes of DAH may be divided into conditions associated with inflammation of the pulmonary capillaries, referred to as capillaritis, and those without capillaritis, so-called bland DAH (see Table 101-1). Pulmonary capillaritis refers to alveolar interstitial inflammation consisting of neutrophil accumulation associated with fibrinoid necrosis, producing injury to the basement membrane and resulting in leaky capillaries. Repeated bouts of inflammation and hemorrhage result in the deposition of hemosiderin-laden macrophages. In patients with bland DAH, red blood cells fill the alveoli in the absence of capillary inflammation. Note that there is occasionally some overlap in this classification system; Goodpasture syndrome, collagen vascular disease, and systemic lupus erythematosus may be associated with pulmonary hemorrhage with or without pulmonary capillaritis. For DAH with capillaritis, autoantibodies directed against the alveolar basement membrane produces direct damage or basement membrane injury results from immune complex deposition.

Manifestations of Disease

Clinical Presentation

The clinical manifestations of DAH with or without capillaritis are relatively similar, and consist of cough, dyspnea, and hemoptysis, usually over a few days' or weeks' duration. Note that the absence of hemoptysis does not exclude DAH because hemoptysis may occur later in the course of a patient's presentation, or occasionally will not be seen at all, even with extensive alveolar bleeding. However, at least with extensive bleeding, the patient's hematocrit usually falls; when combined with extensive thoracic imaging findings and the proper clinical context, this should suggest the correct diagnosis. As a result of repeated hemorrhage, iron deficiency anemia may be present. In patients with DAH associated with connective tissue or rheumatologic syndromes, inflammation in other organ systems, such as sinusitis, arthritis, and glomerulonephritis, may be present. Increasingly bloody sequential bronchoalveolar lavage, often with hemosiderin-laden macrophages, confirms the diagnosis of DAH, but is not specific for the underlying insult producing the hemorrhage. In particular, when pulmonary-renal syndromes are responsible for DAH, red cell casts and proteinuria are often found in the urine. The erythrocyte sedimentation rate is frequently elevated in patients with DAH, but is a nonspecific finding.

Diagnosis

The diagnosis of DAH is usually suspected on the basis of the rapid interval appearance of bilateral pulmonary opacities in an anemic patient with cough, shortness of breath, and hemoptysis, often in the context of a condition known to be associated with alveolar hemorrhage. Diffusing capacity of carbon monoxide is characteristically elevated

TABLE 101-1 Differential Diagnosis of Pulmonary Hemorrhage

Cause	Features
Airway	Bronchitis
	Bronchiectasis
	Endobronchial lesions (benign or malignant)
	Malignancy
Parenchyma	
Diffuse alveolar hemorrhage with capillaritis	Wegener's granulomatosis
	Microscopic polyangiitis
	Goodpasture syndrome
	Connective tissue diseases
	Systemic lupus erythematosus
	Antiphospholipid antibody syndrome
	Behçet syndrome
	Henoch-Schönlein purpura
	Pauci-immune glomerulonephritis
	Drug-induced
	Mixed cryoglobulinemia
Diffuse alveolar hemorrhage without capillaritis	Idiopathic pulmonary hemosiderosis
	Systemic lupus erythematosus
	Coagulation disorders
	Pulmonary veno-occlusive disease
	Pulmonary capillary hemangiomatosis
	Diffuse alveolar damage
	Mitral stenosis
	Drug-induced (penicillamine)
	Lymphangioleiomyomatosis
	Tuberous sclerosis
	Hematopoietic stem cell transplantation
	Leukemia
Other	Pulmonary arteriovenous malformation

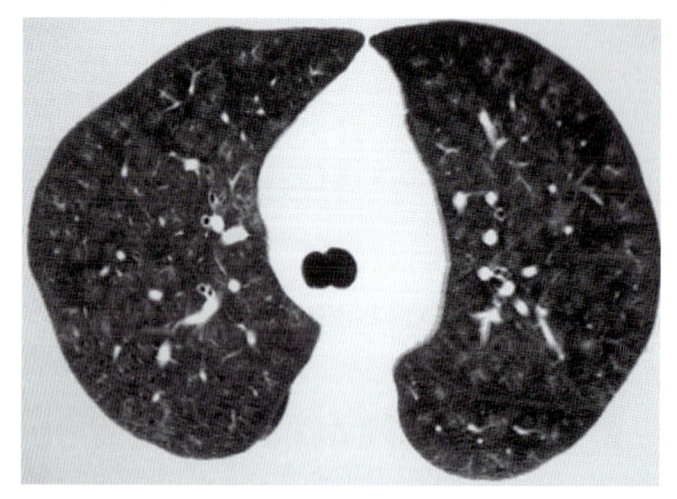

■ **FIGURE 101-1** Diffuse alveolar hemorrhage: centrilobular nodules. This axial CT scan shows diffuse ground-glass opacity centrilobular nodules found to represent pulmonary hemorrhage on biopsy.

and may specifically suggest the diagnosis of DAH, but the diagnosis usually requires confirmation with progressively bloody fluid on bronchoalveolar lavage. Occasionally DAH may be the manifestation of an underlying condition, and further diagnostic testing will then be directed at identifying the cause of DAH. A number of specific diseases associated with DAH will be discussed in the remainder of this chapter.

Imaging Techniques and Findings

Radiography

Chest radiography in patients with DAH of any cause will show focal, multifocal, or diffuse ground-glass opacity and/or consolidation, usually in the presence of a normal heart size and without pleural effusion. Findings often predominate in the dependent regions of lung and, in most patients, appear relatively quickly. A reverse bat wing appearance may occasionally be seen. Shortly after the appearance of lung opacities, a linear and reticular network may be evident superimposed on the regions of ground-glass opacity, representing interlobular septal thickening. The pulmonary opacities clear slowly over a period of 7 to 14 days if there are no superimposed processes or repeated episodes of alveolar hemorrhage. Recurrent bouts of alveolar hemorrhage may produce areas of fibrosis and scarring, manifesting on chest radiography as areas of coarse linear and reticular opacity with architectural distortion.

CT

CT and high-resolution CT (HRCT) typically show multifocal or diffuse bilateral ground-glass opacity and consolidation. Ground-glass attenuation poorly defined nodules (Fig. 101-1) may occur. Often, a network pattern of smooth interlobular septal thickening is superimposed in the regions of ground-glass opacity.

VASCULITIS

The histopathologic hallmark of vasculitis is the presence of angiocentric inflammation, usually extending through all layers of blood vessel walls. Fibrinoid necrosis and perivascular fibrosis are also commonly present, and may ultimately lead to vascular obliteration and occlusion. Both leukocytoclastic (neutrophil-predominant) and granulomatous (lymphocyte-predominant) vasculitic patterns may occur. Most pulmonary vasculitides share the common pathogenesis of immune complex deposition in the vessel wall, with activation of complement and cellular chemotaxis, leading to an enzymatic and inflammatory cascade that ultimately produces vascular damage. The whole process may be antigen-driven, which may explain the association of a number of vasculitides with viral infections and collagen vascular disorders. However, some granulomatous vasculitides may be the result of cell-mediated immunity rather than immune complex deposition. A number of vasculitides may affect the thorax, the lung in particular. The main histopathologic derangement of vasculitides affecting the lung is capillaritis, perhaps associated with inflammation of slightly larger vessels (Table 101-2).

WEGENER'S GRANULOMATOSIS

First described in 1936, Wegener granulomatosis (WG) is a clinical syndrome characterized by a necrotizing granulomatous vasculitis involving the upper and lower respiratory tract and kidneys. WG is the most common vasculitis to affect the lungs.

CHAPTER 101 • Pulmonary Hemorrhage and Vasculitis 1385

TABLE 101-2 Common Causes of Pulmonary Vasculitis

Location	Cause
Large vessels (aorta and major branch vessels)	Takayasu arteritis Giant cell (temporal) arteritis Behçet syndrome*
Medium-sized vessels (visceral arteries)*†	Polyarteritis nodosa Kawasaki disease Behçet syndrome*
Small vessels (arterioles, capillaries, venules, distal intraparenchymal small arteries leading to arterioles)	Wegener's granulomatosis Microscopic polyangiitis Isolated pulmonary capillaritis Churg-Strauss syndrome Henoch-Schönlein purpura Mixed cryoglobulinemia

*Some overlap in level of involvement may occur, particularly with either large or small vessel vasculitides involving medium-sized vessels.
†Visceral arteries = coronary, hepatic, mesenteric, and renal arteries

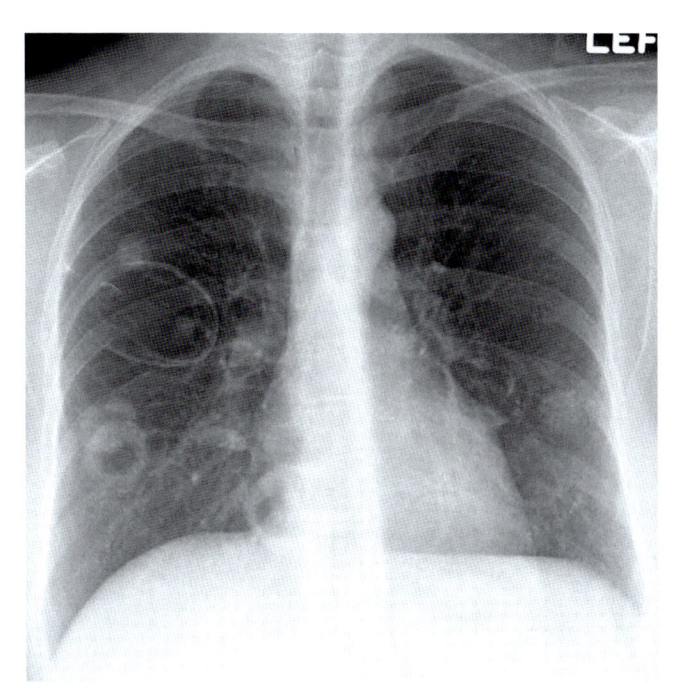

FIGURE 101-2 Wegener's granulomatosis, lung cavities. This frontal chest radiograph shows multiple cavities of variable wall thickness. Solid nodules are also present bilaterally.

Prevalence and Epidemiology

WG is a rare condition that occurs more commonly in whites but with an almost equal gender incidence, perhaps slightly more common in men. WG may occur at any age, even adolescence, but is most commonly encountered in patients between 35 and 55 years of age.

Manifestations of Disease

Clinical Presentation

Patients with WG typically present with fever and upper respiratory symptoms, such as nasal discharge and sinus symptoms. Constitutional symptoms, such as fatigue, weight loss, and malaise, are common. Cough, hemoptysis, shortness of breath and chest pain are common in patients with pulmonary involvement. Skin lesions, hearing loss, and ulcers in the oral and nasal cavities may occur. C-ANCA antibodies (antineutrophil cytoplasmic autoantibodies) with PR-3 specificity are elevated in more than 90% of patients with WG. C-ANCA antibodies are relatively specific for WG, but may be seen in microscopic polyangiitis, although protoplasmic-staining antineutrophil cytoplasmic antibodies (p-ANCA) is more suggestive of the latter. P-ANCA antibodies are seen in about 25% of patients with WG.

Imaging Techniques and Findings

Radiography

Chest radiographs are abnormal in up to 85% of patients with WG at some point during the course of the illness. The most characteristic imaging manifestation of WG is multiple, usually bilateral, nodules or masses typically measuring 2 to 4 cm, often associated with cavitation (Fig. 101-2). Pulmonary opacities and cavities in patients with WG may occasionally be much larger. WG-related pulmonary cavities often have a rather thick, irregular internal wall, and air-fluid levels are occasionally seen. Ground-glass opacity surrounding the cavities is a frequent finding and is usually caused by adjacent alveolitis or pulmonary hemorrhage.

CT

Thoracic CT scanning in patients with WG also typically shows multiple bilateral nodules and/or masses,[1] and is far more sensitive for the detection of cavitation than chest radiography. In fact, most nodules measuring more than 2 cm in patients with WG will show cavitation on CT (Fig. 101-3). Nodules and cavities in patients with WG have no particular zonal predilection, and are somewhat randomly distributed throughout the lungs.

Patchy multifocal or diffuse ground-glass opacities, often with areas of consolidation,[1] is the second most common thoracic imaging manifestation of WG, and may occur in the absence of pulmonary nodules. These opacities are usually the result of pulmonary hemorrhage. Occasionally, areas of consolidation may be subpleural or peribronchiolar in distribution, simulating organizing pneumonia; the so-called atoll or reverse halo sign may also be seen (Fig. 101-4).

Tracheobronchial wall thickening and narrowing may be present in patients with WG,[1] and may even lead to atelectasis. Typically, airway involvement in patients with WG predominates in the subglottic region and extends a variable distance caudally (Fig. 101-5). The airway wall thickening is circumferential and often nodular and irregular, occasionally resulting in tracheobronchial stenosis. The tracheobronchial thickening may occasionally calcify.

Pleural effusions and lymphadenopathy may occur in patients with WG, but are nonspecific findings and are relatively uncommon overall.

Pulmonary parenchymal opacities in patients with WG may resolve during treatment. Cavities may occasionally

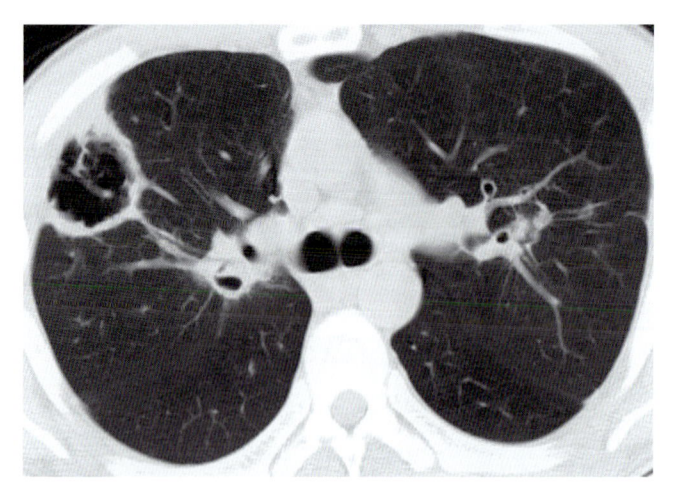

FIGURE 101-3 Wegener's granulomatosis, lung cavity. This axial CT scan shows an irregular-appearing subpleural right lung cavity of indeterminate wall thickness.

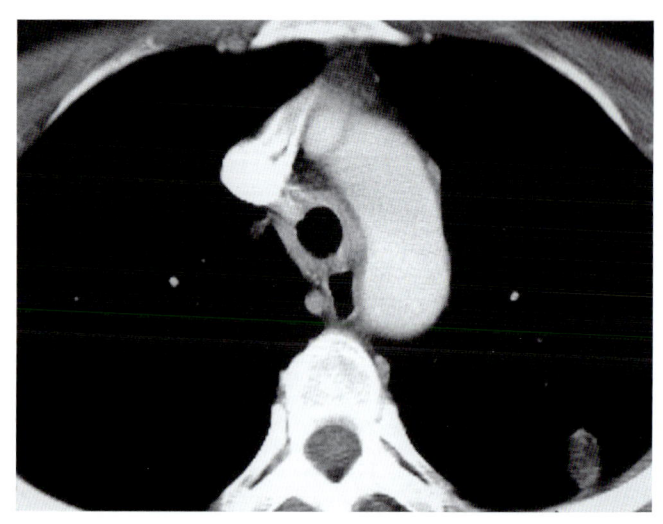

FIGURE 101-5 Wegener's granulomatosis, diffuse tracheobronchial thickening. This axial CT scan shows circumferential, noncalcified tracheal thickening.

even enlarge during treatment, although wall thickness usually becomes progressively thinner and the internal wall character becomes smoother.

Differential Diagnosis

From Clinical Presentation

A number of serologic abnormalities may be seen in patients with WG, including anemia, elevated rheumatoid factor, and elevated erythrocyte sedimentation rate, and other uncommon serologic test results. Most of these laboratory findings are fairly nonspecific. Recurrent alveolar hemorrhage is common in patients with WG, is often subclinical and may lead to the detection of hemosiderin-laden macrophages on bronchoscopy with lavage. The most useful test for the evaluation of patients with WG is the c-ANCA antibody, which is elevated in more than 90% of patients with WG. C-ANCA antibody titers may also be used to follow disease course. Although c-ANCA antibody titers may be elevated in other diseases, in the proper clinical context and with suggestive radiologic features, the diagnosis of WG can be confidently established when c-ANCA antibodies are present.

The term *limited Wegener's granulomatosis* refers to a clinical syndrome essentially identical to the full-blown WG syndrome but without systemic (especially renal) involvement clinically; upper respiratory tract manifestations are usually present. Histopathologically, WG manifestations are often present in the viscera of patients with limited WG, and therefore it is probably appropriate to consider limited WG as one end of the spectrum of WG rather than as a separate condition.

MICROSCOPIC POLYANGIITIS

Microscopic polyangiitis is a small-vessel vasculitis[2] that closely resembles polyarteritis nodosa, except that the latter usually involves medium-sized vessels, often involves abdomen viscera, and rarely produces DAH.

Manifestations of Disease

Clinical Presentation

The average age of onset is about 50 years, and men are more commonly affected than women.[2] Fever and constitutional symptoms, such as weight loss and malaise, are common in patients with microscopic polyangiitis. Patients also often complain of myalgias and arthralgias, and individually affected organ systems may also produce particular symptoms. For example, involvement of the gastrointestinal tract may produce diarrhea and bleeding, whereas involvement of the skin may produce dermatologic manifestations, such as purpura and splinter hemorrhages. Peripheral neuropathy may occur. Shortness of breath, cough, and hemoptysis are the more common symptoms of thoracic involvement, and hemoptysis may be life-threatening.

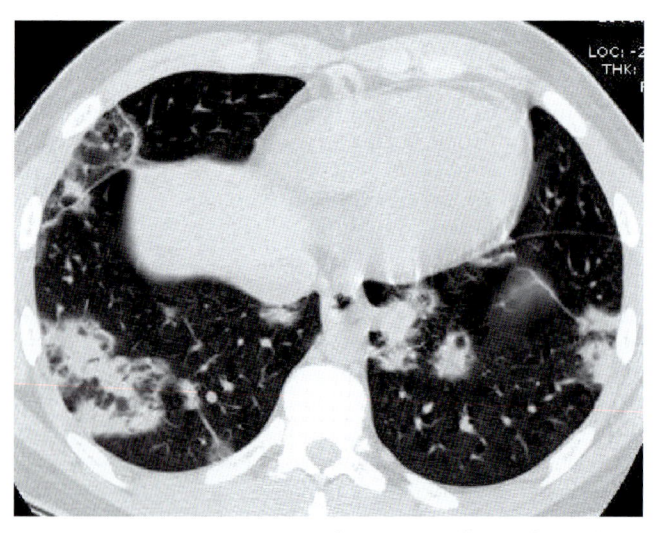

FIGURE 101-4 Wegener's granulomatosis, atoll sign. This axial CT scan shows bilateral subpleural opacities with central ground-glass attenuation and peripheral consolidation, consistent with the atoll or reverse ground-glass halo sign. The appearance is suggestive of organizing pneumonia.

Imaging Techniques and Findings
Radiography

Chest radiographs typically show multifocal bilateral areas of ground-glass opacity and/or consolidation related to alveolar hemorrhage.

CT

HRCT will show multifocal areas of ground-glass opacity, possibly with consolidation; smooth interlobular septal thickening may be associated with the areas of ground-glass opacity. Poorly defined ground-glass opacity centrilobular nodules, reflecting prior pulmonary hemorrhage and the presence of hemosiderin-laden macrophages, may be seen. Pleural effusion may occur, but is uncommon.

Differential Diagnosis
From Clinical Presentation

Patients with microscopic polyangiitis typically have elevated erythrocyte sedimentation rates, and other rheumatologic markers, such as rheumatoid factor and antinuclear antibody, may be elevated. These findings are ultimately nonspecific. An elevated p-ANCA antibody directed against myeloperoxidase is associated with microscopic polyangiitis and may be diagnostic in the context of the proper clinical and imaging findings. However, p-ANCA antibodies may be elevated in other vasculitides, such as Churg-Strauss syndrome and pauci-immune capillaritis. Therefore, a tissue diagnosis, usually obtained from the lung via surgical lung biopsy, is often required.

BEHÇET SYNDROME

Behçet syndrome is a rare condition characterized by the combination of mucosal aphthous stomatitis, uveitis, genital ulcers, and skin lesions,[3] particularly erythema nodosum, and is a systemic multisystem disorder that may also be associated with arthritis, meningoencephalitis, thrombophlebitis, and cutaneous vasculitis.

Etiology and Pathophysiology

The cause of Behçet syndrome is unknown. Some have speculated that a virus may be responsible, whereas others have implicated an immunologic mechanism as the cause. Histopathologically, a small-vessel vasculitis is present caused by extensive inflammation of vessel walls with plasma cells and lymphocytes.[3] Larger vessel involvement may also occur, resulting in aneurysm formation. Venous thrombosis may also be present.

Manifestations of Disease
Clinical Presentation

Males are much more commonly affected than females in patients with Behçet syndrome. The typical age of diagnosis is 20 to 30 years, and Behçet syndrome is most commonly encountered in the Middle East, Mediterranean countries, and Japan.[3] Patients usually present with chronic remitting oral and genital ulcers and skin lesions, especially erythema nodosum, as well as uveitis. A number of systemic manifestations are common in Behçet syndrome, including arthritis, neuropathy, thrombophlebitis, and aneurysm formation. Thoracic involvement usually occurs in the setting of established disease, with patients complaining of chest pain, shortness of breath, cough, and hemoptysis. Hemoptysis may be massive and life-threatening and is the cause of death in up to 39% of patients.

Imaging Techniques and Findings
Radiography

Chest radiographs in patients with Behçet syndrome may show multifocal or diffuse bilateral air space opacities in patients with thoracic symptoms and hemoptysis; these findings are nonspecific and resemble those of other causes of DAH.[3] Much more characteristic of Behçet syndrome is the presence of pulmonary artery aneurysms. On chest radiographs, pulmonary artery aneurysms appear as central hilar prominence or perihilar rounded opacity of variable size (Fig. 101-6A).[3] Aneurysms may grow rapidly, and therefore a rapid change in the appearance of the hilum may be suggestive of aneurysm development in the proper context. The margins of the aneurysms may be poorly defined because of surrounding pulmonary hemorrhage.

CT

CT is clearly much more sensitive for the detection and characterization of pulmonary artery aneurysms (see Fig. 101-6B), and may even detect thrombosed pulmonary artery aneurysms that would be difficult to detect by catheter pulmonary angiography. Behçet syndrome may closely resemble another condition associated with the development of pulmonary artery aneurysms and venous thrombosis, Hughes-Stovin syndrome.

Thrombotic complications are also common in patients with Behçet syndrome and may involve the great veins of the thorax and the proximal pulmonary arteries.[3] Pulmonary arterial thrombosis or emboli, as well as vasculitis, may produce pulmonary infarction, which usually manifests on chest radiographs or CT scans as a subpleural wedge-shaped consolidation.

Pleural effusions may occur in patients with Behçet syndrome, possibly caused by venous thrombosis or pulmonary infarction. Occasionally, the effusion may be chylous in nature.

TAKAYASU ARTERITIS

Takayasu arteritis is an uncommon large-vessel vasculitis that primarily affects the aorta and its branch vessels, including the coronary arteries, and occasionally the pulmonary arteries. Several classification schemes for Takayasu arteritis have been advanced (see later), and criteria for diagnosis have also been established (Table 101-3).

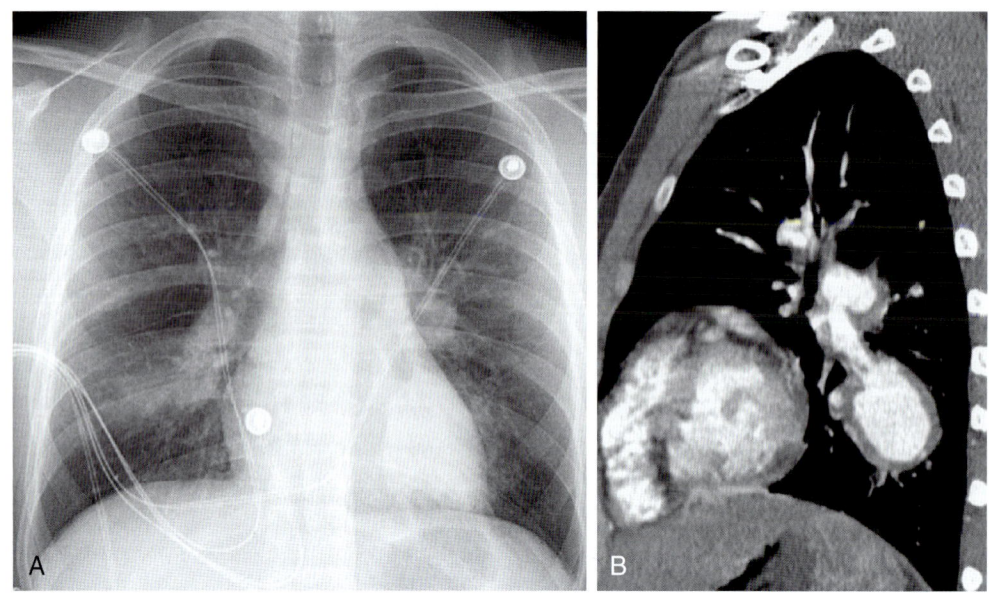

FIGURE 101-6 Behçet syndrome, pulmonary artery aneurysm. **A,** Frontal chest radiograph shows rounded, poorly defined opacity in the left retrocardiac region representing a pulmonary artery aneurysm. The poorly defined nature of the lesion suggests surrounding hemorrhage. A smaller lesion is present on the right. **B,** Sagittal thoracic CT scan shows pulmonary artery aneurysm in left lower lobe.

Prevalence and Epidemiology

Takayasu arteritis usually occurs in patients younger than 40 years and shows a strong predilection for women, who account for 80% to 90% of cases. The highest disease prevalence has been reported in Asia, especially Japan, although it may be underreported in Europe and North America.[4]

Etiology and Pathophysiology

An immunologic mechanism is thought to be responsible for Takayasu arteritis. The possibility of a heritable cause or hormonal influences has also been considered.[4]

TABLE 101-3 Diagnostic Criteria for Takayasu Arteritis

Criterion	Definition
Age of disease onset ≤40 yr	Development of signs or symptoms attributable to Takayasu arteritis at age 40 or younger
Extremity claudication	Muscular fatigue, pain, discomfort involving one or more of the extremities with exercise, particularly upper extremities
Decreased brachial artery pulse	Diminished brachial artery pulse
Differential blood pressure	Blood pressure differential between two arms of 10 mm Hg or more
Vascular bruits	Bruit detectable on auscultation over subclavian arteries or abdominal aorta
Arteriographic abnormalities	Narrowing or occlusion of the aorta, major branch vessels of the aorta, or large vessels of the extremities unrelated to atherosclerosis, fibromuscular dysplasia, or similar process

Manifestations of Disease

Clinical Presentation

Classically, Takayasu arteritis has been divided into early (prepulseless) and late (pulseless) phases. Late-phase Takayasu arteritis may be further subclassified as classic pulseless disease (type I), a mixed type (type II), an atypical coarctation type (type III), and a dilated type (type IV). Most patients present with a form of late-phase disease.

During the early, inflammatory stage, fever, pain in the region of the inflamed vessels, myalgias, fatigue, and malaise are common. On physical examination, bruits or diminished pulse over the involved vessels may be detected. Ischemic symptoms may result when vascular stenoses or occlusions are present. When the brachiocephalic vessels are involved, neurologic symptoms may dominate the clinical picture.[4]

In the late occlusive phase, ischemic symptoms are the primary manifesting features, including angina, claudication, syncope, and visual impairment.[4]

Imaging Techniques and Findings

CT

CT is useful for the early diagnosis of Takayasu arteritis because it allows evaluation of arterial wall thickness rather than just the luminal diameter. This is especially important because early diagnosis and treatment are associated with improved prognosis in patients with Takayasu arteritis. The findings of Takayasu arteritis on CT and CT angiography (CTA) include stenoses, occlusions, aneurysms (Fig. 101-7), and concentric arterial wall thickening affecting the aorta and its branches, as well as the the pulmonary arteries. Occasionally, coronary artery aneu-

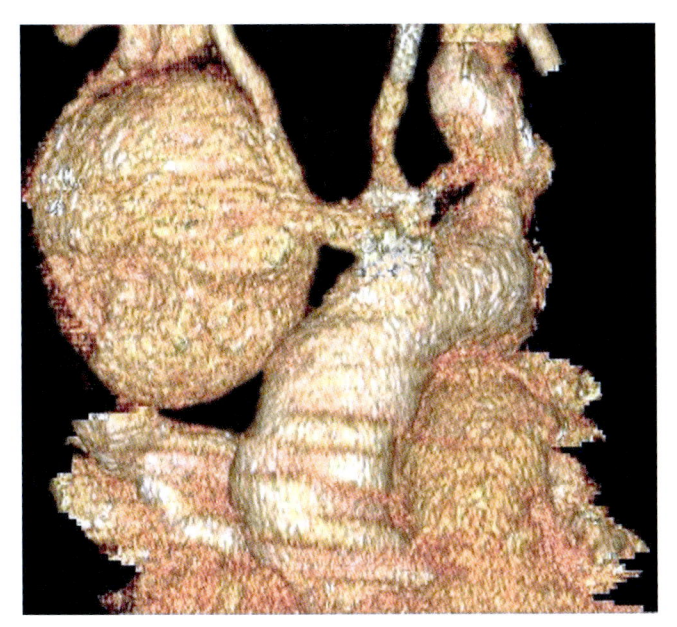

CHAPTER 101 ● *Pulmonary Hemorrhage and Vasculitis* **1389**

■ **FIGURE 101-7** Takayasu arteritis, arterial aneurysm. This volume rendered thoracic CT image shows a large right subclavian artery aneurysm.

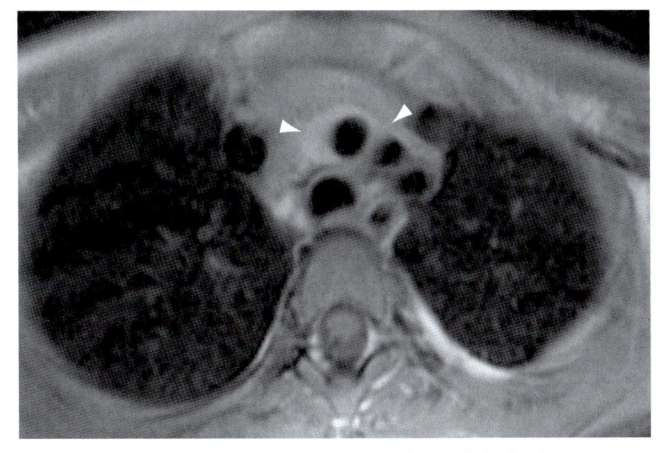

■ **FIGURE 101-8** Takayasu arteritis, vascular wall thickening and enhancement. This postcontrast T1-weighted image shows circumferential intense enhancement of the thickened brachiocephalic artery wall (*arrowheads*).

rysms may be seen. In late-stage Takayasu arteritis, extensive vascular calcification may occur.[4] Limitations of CT include the need for iodinated contrast material and ionizing radiation, which may be particularly important given the typically young age of patients with Takayasu arteritis.

MRI

Advantages of MRI include the lack of need for ionizing radiation and iodinated contrast material, making MRI ideal for the serial evaluation of patients with Takayasu arteritis who are undergoing treatment. Furthermore, techniques such as cine MRI may show significant cardiovascular functional and hemodynamic abnormalities in patients with Takayasu arteritis, particularly aortic regurgitation. As with CT, MRI is useful for early diagnosis because of its ability to evaluate arterial wall thickness rather than just luminal narrowing.

Findings of Takayasu arteritis on MRI include mural thrombi, signal alterations within and surrounding inflamed vessels (Fig. 101-8), fusiform vascular dilation or frank aneurysm formation, thickened aortic valvular cusps, multifocal stenoses, and concentric thickening of the aortic wall. MRI may also show pericardial effusions and signal abnormalities within the pericardium, representing fluid and granulation tissue.[4] The main disadvantages of MRI in patients with Takayasu arteritis include difficulty in visualizing small branch vessels and poor visualization of vascular calcification. MRI is also expensive, and is frequently less available in regions in which Takayasu arteritis is most prevalent.

MR angiography provides detailed vascular information, including the location, degree, and extent of stenoses, as well as the presence of aneurysms. The patency of surgical bypass grafts may also be readily assessed.[4]

Angiography

Angiography has traditionally been the primary procedure for the diagnostic evaluation of Takayasu arteritis. Angiography often demonstrates long, smooth, tapered stenoses that range from mild to severe (Fig. 101-9). Arterial occlusions may be present, and collateral vessels or the subclavian steal phenomenon may be seen. Angiography is useful for guiding and evaluating interventional procedures, such as angioplasty or stent placement. However,

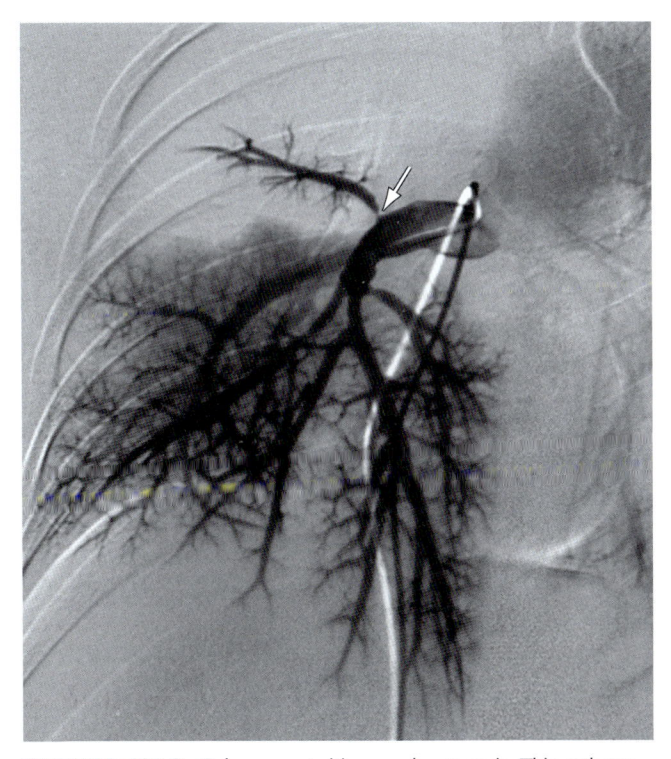

■ **FIGURE 101-9** Takayasu arteritis, vascular stenosis. This catheter pulmonary angiogram shows several stenoses, one high grade (*arrow*), in the right pulmonary arterial system.

angiography is invasive, may require a large amount of iodinated contrast material, delivers a substantial radiation dose, and can be difficult to perform in patients with long-segment stenoses or heavy arterial calcification. Additionally, angiography does not depict changes in wall architecture as well as cross-sectional techniques, and cannot differentiate between vascular narrowing caused by acute mural inflammation from that caused by chronic transmural fibrosis. Importantly, ischemic complications resulting from angiography in patients with Takayasu arteritis may be substantial, possibly because blood coagulation activity is increased in these patients.

Differential Diagnosis

From Clinical Presentation

Because histopathologic specimens are seldom available because of the large vessels commonly affected and because the histopathologic appearance of Takayasu arteritis can mimic that of other vasculitides, including temporal arteritis, the diagnosis of Takayasu arteritis is largely based on the combination of clinical information, laboratory evaluation, and diagnostic imaging.

CHURG-STRAUSS SYNDROME

Churg-Strauss is a rare vasculitis of unknown cause, with an incidence of 2.4/million. As with many other vasculitides, an immunologic mechanism is suspected.

Prevalence and Epidemiology

Churg-Strauss syndrome most commonly affects men with asthma, usually in their late 30s through 50 years of age.[5] Multiorgan involvement is common, with the skin, lungs, peripheral nerves, heart, and abdominal viscera potentially affected. Pansinusitis and allergic rhinitis are common as well.

Manifestations of Disease

Clinical Presentation

The following three stages of Churg-Strauss syndrome have been described:

1. Adult-onset asthma and sinusitis
2. Eosinophilic infiltration of the lungs and abdominal viscera
3. Vasculitis, presenting as cardiomyopathy or pericarditis, glomerulosclerosis, neuritis, and/or palpable purpura

Anemia is frequent as well. Cardiomyopathy is a common cause of death in patients with Churg-Strauss syndrome. A limited form of Churg-Strauss syndrome, with involvement of one organ system only, similar to limited Wegener's granulomatosis, has been described. In such patients, the lung is rarely involved, and usually the gastrointestinal tract is affected.

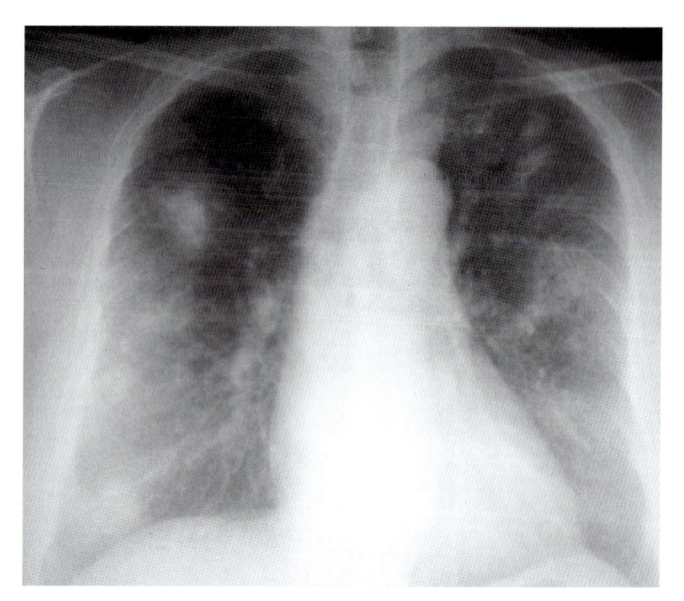

■ **FIGURE 101-10** Churg-Strauss syndrome. This frontal chest radiograph shows multifocal bilateral pulmonary opacities, some nodular in appearance. Biopsy and clinical presentation indicated a diagnosis of Churg-Strauss syndrome.

Imaging Techniques and Findings

Radiography

Chest radiographs are commonly abnormal in patients with Churg-Strauss syndrome, usually showing transient, nonsegmental, occasionally subpleural, consolidation.[5] No particular zonal predilection has been noted. Occasionally, pulmonary opacities may be nodular in configuration (Fig. 101-10), somewhat resembling Wegener's granulomatosis but, unlike Wegener's granulomatosis, cavitation does not usually occur.

CT

Thoracic CT findings in patients with Churg-Strauss syndrome include bilateral, subpleural ground-glass opacity or consolidation often accompanied by small centrilobular nodules.[5]

Differential Diagnosis

From Clinical Presentation

As with other vasculitides and numerous inflammatory processes, the erythrocyte sedimentation rate is usually elevated. Blood hypereosinophilia is usually present, typically more than 10% of the peripheral white blood cell count. The American College of Rheumatology diagnostic criteria for Churg-Strauss syndrome are presented in Box 101-1. Note that the presence of vasculitis is not among these criteria, because the presence of extravascular tissue eosinophilia is a more sensitive indicator of disease.

GIANT CELL ARTERITIS

Giant cell arteritis is a large-vessel granulomatous arteritis that affects the aorta and large arteries of the head and neck. Giant cell arteritis has a predilection for affecting

BOX 101-1   Diagnostic Criteria for Churg-Strauss Syndrome

Asthma
Eosinophilia >10%
History of allergy
Neuropathy (mono-or poly-)
Migratory or transient pulmonary opacities
Paranasal sinus abnormalities

branches of the external carotid artery—hence the other term frequently used for giant cell arteritis, *temporal arteritis*. The ophthalmic artery and vertebral arteries are also commonly involved. Intracranial vessels are not involved because they lack an internal elastic lamina. Genetic, immunologic, and infectious causes have all been postulated.

Manifestations of Disease

Clinical Presentation

Patients with giant cell arteritis often present with headache, malaise, joint aches, jaw claudication, fatigue, and polymyalgia rheumatica. Characteristically, pain on palpation over the temporal artery may be present. Patients are usually 50 years of age or older.

Imaging Techniques and Findings

Ultrasound

Ultrasound may show a hypoechoic halo involving the temporal artery, representing vascular wall edema.

CT

Giant cell arteritis may produce visible thickening and enhancement of the walls of the affected large arteries, usually in a patchy fashion. These findings are best appreciated on unenhanced and enhanced (Fig. 101-11) CT studies. Stenoses and occlusions may occur. Bilateral pleural effusions may be seen, and a reticular and nodular pulmonary parenchymal pattern has been described. A larger nodular pattern has also been reported in patients with giant cell arteritis, but because there is some overlap between the pattern and areas of involvement in giant cell arteritis and other systemic vasculitides, such as Wegener's granulomatosis and Churg-Strauss syndrome, it is not clear whether pulmonary nodules truly represent a manifestation of giant cell arteritis.

CONNECTIVE TISSUE DISEASES AND SYSTEMIC LUPUS ERYTHEMATOSUS

Etiology and Pathophysiology

DAH with or without capillaritis may occur in patients with systemic lupus erythematosus (SLE) and various connective tissue disorders. Immune complex deposition

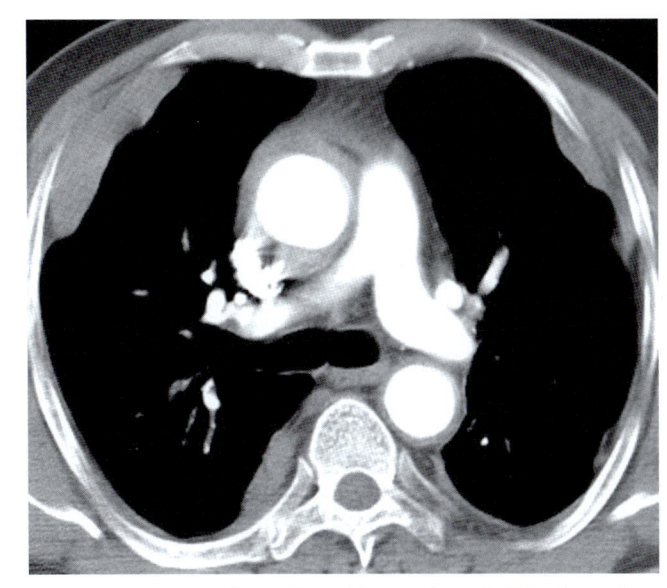

FIGURE 101-11   Giant cell arteritis, vascular wall thickening and enhancement. This postcontrast thoracic CT scan shows thickening and enhancement of the wall of the aorta.

within the alveolar interstitium and intra-alveolar vessels may be found in such patients. Most affected SLE patients have lupus renal involvement at the time of diagnosis.

Manifestations of Disease

Clinical Presentation

DAH with pulmonary capillaritis has occasionally been seen in patients with rheumatoid arthritis, polymyositis, scleroderma, and mixed connective tissue syndromes. DAH may be the initial manifestation of disease in some patients with connective tissue diseases, whereas in others it may be a late manifestation of disease. The clinical presentation of DAH in the setting of connective tissue disorders resembles other causes of alveolar hemorrhage.

Imaging Techniques and Findings

CT

The imaging manifestations of DAH in the setting of connective tissue disease are similar to those of DAH in other clinical settings—multifocal or diffuse, usually bilateral, air space opacities, often a combination of ground-glass opacities and consolidation and often acute in onset. HRCT shows multifocal bilateral ground-glass opacity, often with smooth interlobular septal thickening; chronic or recurrent episodes may show poorly defined ground-glass attenuation centrilobular nodules. In patients with SLE, DAH should be distinguished from acute lupus pneumonitis. The latter is more common than DAH in SLE and usually manifests with multifocal or diffuse air space opacities, but usually with evidence of serosal membrane inflammation, such as pleural and pericardial effusions.

NECROTIZING SARCOID GRANULOMATOSIS

Necrotizing sarcoid granulomatosis is a rare disorder characterized by the following[6]:

1. Sarcoid-like granulomas on histopathologic specimens, usually associated with granulomatous vasculitis of small- and medium-sized arteries and veins and necrosis
2. Diffuse pulmonary nodules or opacities, but no mediastinal or hilar lymphadenopathy
3. A benign clinical course, with spontaneous remission or remission following therapy with corticosteroids

Imaging Techniques and Findings
Radiography

On chest radiographs, necrotizing sarcoid granulomatosis has been reported to show multiple, bilateral small (10-mm) circumscribed nodules. The presentation may resemble a miliary pattern, although large nodules have also been reported as a manifestation of necrotizing sarcoid granulomatosis. Other reported appearances of necrotizing sarcoid granulomatosis include bilateral areas of air space consolidation, a solitary pulmonary nodule, and pleural effusion.

CT

HRCT will typically show that the nodules are distributed in a perilymphatic pattern, similar to classic sarcoidosis. Nodules may coalesce and cavitation may occur.

Differential Diagnosis
From Clinical Presentation

It is unclear whether necrotizing sarcoid granulomatosis represents a separate disease entity or is an unusual reaction in patients with sarcoidosis. Because necrotizing granulomas often have an infectious cause, it is very important that such causes be excluded before the diagnosis of necrotizing sarcoid granulomatosis is considered.

IDIOPATHIC PULMONARY HEMOSIDEROSIS

Etiology and Pathophysiology

The cause of idiopathic pulmonary hemosiderosis (IPH), sometimes referred to as idiopathic pulmonary hemorrhage, is unknown. Some have postulated an immune-mediated mechanism, given the fact that IPH has occasionally been found in the setting of other autoimmune diseases, such as celiac disease. Others have suggested a genetic cause because some patients with IPH have been found to have familial associations. Allergy to cow's milk protein (Heiner disease) has also been considered, but no common underlying mechanism for the development of IPH has been elucidated.

Manifestations of Disease
Clinical Presentation

IPH usually affects children and, much less commonly, young adults; children younger than 10 years are most commonly affected. Males are more commonly affected than females, at least with adult-onset disease. Patients with IPH characteristically present with hemoptysis. Other nonspecific symptoms, such as fever, cough, chest pain, shortness of breath, and iron deficiency anemia, may be present.[7] Hemoptysis is not invariably seen. In some cases, the onset of disease is insidious, whereas in others, disease onset is acute. Some patients develop lymphadenopathy and hepatosplenomegaly.[7] Later in the course of disease, with repeated episodes of hemorrhage, pulmonary fibrosis may develop, associated with other signs and symptoms, such as digital clubbing and progressive dyspnea or decreased exercise tolerance.

Imaging Techniques and Findings
Radiography

Patients with IPH usually present with patchy, bilateral air space opacities with air bronchograms as a result of pulmonary hemorrhage. Findings may predominate in the mid and lower lungs and perihilar regions. Often, the pattern superficially resembles that of cardiogenic pulmonary edema, except that the vascular pedicle is usually not widened and cardiomegaly should be absent. Pleural effusions are also less common in patients with IPH than in patients with cardiogenic pulmonary edema. Asymmetric pulmonary opacities may occur in patients with IPH and, although rare, unilateral disease has been reported. The apices and costophrenic angles tend to be spared.

Over time, serial chest radiography characteristically shows pulmonary abnormalities evolving from ground-glass opacity and consolidation to areas of linear and reticular abnormalities. These abnormalities may resolve over a 1- to 2-week period. However, with repeated episodes of pulmonary hemorrhage, the areas of reticulation and linear abnormality may persist, often associated with architectural distortion, and represent developing pulmonary fibrosis.

CT

CT and HRCT in patients with IPH show findings typical of pulmonary hemorrhage—multifocal, bilateral, patchy or diffuse ground-glass opacities, with or without areas of air space consolidation associated with smooth interlobular septal thickening (Fig. 101-12). Findings tend to favor the dependent regions of the lung. Poorly defined ground-glass centrilobular nodules may be seen.

Differential Diagnosis
From Clinical Presentation

The diagnosis of IPH is one of exclusion. To consider the diagnosis of IPH, other causes of pulmonary hemorrhage

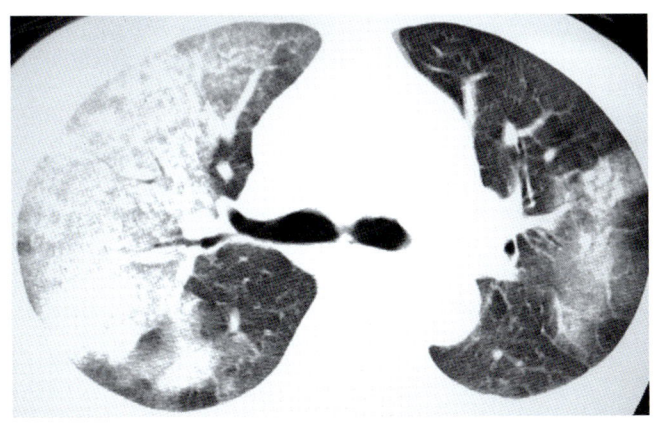

FIGURE 101-12 Idiopathic pulmonary hemosiderosis (IPH). This axial CT scan shows multifocal bilateral ground-glass opacity associated with mild interlobular septal thickening.

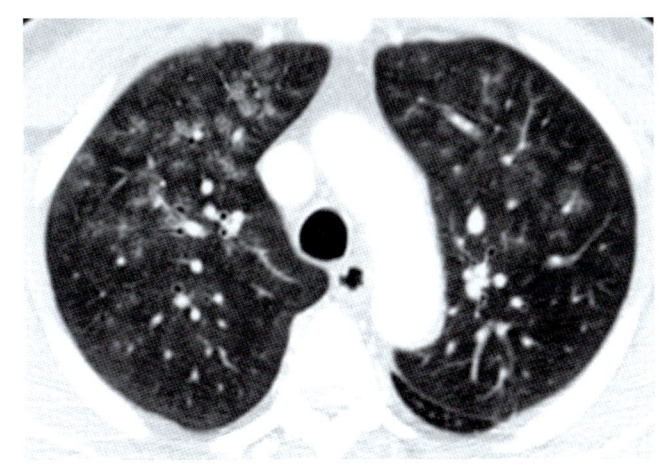

FIGURE 101-13 Goodpasture syndrome. This axial CT scan shows multifocal ground-glass opacity centrilobular nodules consistent with hemorrhage.

must be addressed and excluded through a combination of imaging studies, careful clinical history and physical examination demonstrating repeated episodes of pulmonary hemorrhage associated with recurrent chest radiographic opacities consistent with pulmonary hemorrhage, and a series of laboratory examinations to rule out the possibility of other causes of pulmonary hemorrhage. Often, renal biopsy is required to obtain tissue for immunofluorescence and electron microscopy to exclude pulmonary-renal syndromes.

GOODPASTURE SYNDROME

Etiology and Pathophysiology

Goodpasture syndrome is caused by anti–basement membrane autoantibodies directed against type IV collagen located in the basement membrane of the alveoli and glomeruli. Alveolar hemorrhage with hemosiderin-laden macrophages is present within pulmonary tissue. With recurrent hemorrhage, pulmonary fibrosis eventually develops. Interstitial inflammation may also be present. Immunofluorescence usually shows linear staining of the alveolar wall, usually caused by IgG antibody. The same pattern may be seen on renal biopsy and is often better appreciated with renal tissue specimens than with pulmonary specimens. The typical renal lesion seen in patients with Goodpasture syndrome is focal segmental necrotizing glomerulonephritis with crescent formation.

Manifestations of Disease

Clinical Presentation

Patients with Goodpasture syndrome are usually young adults, more often men. The main presenting complaint is hemoptysis, although this symptom is not invariably present. Typically, the hemoptysis in patients with Goodpasture syndrome develops before the onset of renal disease. Other common symptoms include fever, chest pain, shortness of breath, and fatigue. Hematuria and hypertension may occur in some patients, but these findings are unusual. At some point, an active urine sediment will occur, including proteinuria, and cellular or granular cell casts in the urine. This particular finding, in the setting of pulmonary hemorrhage or diffuse pulmonary opacities, is very suggestive of a pulmonary-renal syndrome, such as Goodpasture syndrome. In most patients, pulmonary and renal disease are present, but in a small percentage of patients, pulmonary disease without renal involvement may occur, as may the reverse.

The overall survival rate of Goodpasture syndrome is about 50%, with most deaths caused by DAH, often precipitated by pulmonary infection.

Imaging Techniques and Findings

Radiography

Patients with Goodpasture syndrome usually present with patchy, bilateral air space opacities with air bronchograms related to pulmonary hemorrhage, very similar to IPH or other causes of DAH, with or without pulmonary capillaritis. Findings are often somewhat gravitationally dependent, predominating in the mid and lower lungs. As with IPH, the vascular pedicle is usually not widened and cardiomegaly should be absent; pleural effusions are also uncommon. The apices and costophrenic angles tend to be spared.

As with IPH or any cause of DAH, over time, serial chest radiographs characteristically show pulmonary abnormalities resolving, with areas of linear and reticular abnormalities developing, typically over a 1- to 2-week period, in the regions previously affected with ground-glass opacity and consolidation. With repeated episodes of pulmonary hemorrhage, the areas of reticulation and linear abnormality may persist, often associated with architectural distortion, representing developing pulmonary fibrosis.

CT

CT and HRCT in patients with Goodpasture syndrome show findings typical of pulmonary hemorrhage—multifocal, bilateral, patchy or diffuse ground-glass opacities (Fig. 101-13), with or without areas of air space consolidation associated with smooth interlobular septal thickening. Findings tend to favor the dependent regions of lung. Poorly defined ground-glass centrilobular nodules are common.

Differential Diagnosis

From Clinical Presentation

The diagnosis of Goodpasture syndrome is usually suspected when a young patient presents with hemoptysis and bilateral opacities on chest radiographs associated with urinalysis showing cellular or granular cell casts. Immunofluorescence or enzyme-linked immunosorbent assay confirmation of circulating or tissue anti–basement membrane antibodies is typically performed to establish the diagnosis. The diagnosis is usually confirmed with tissue from the kidney because the absence of proven pulmonary involvement does not exclude the diagnosis and, frequently, the linear pattern of immunofluorescence is more readily recognizable on renal, rather than pulmonary, biopsies.

KEY POINTS

- Pulmonary vasculitis may involve small, medium, or large vessels.
- Pulmonary vasculitis of any cause may present with pulmonary hemorrhage resulting from the presence of capillaritis.
- Other suggestive imaging features are occasionally evident in specific causes of pulmonary vasculitis.

SUGGESTED READINGS

Chae EJ, Do KH, Seo JB, et al. Radiologic and clinical findings of Behçet disease: comprehensive review of multisystemic involvement. Radiographics 2008; 28:e31.

Gotway MB, Araoz PA, Macedo TA, et al. Imaging findings in Takayasu's arteritis. AJR Am J Roentgenol 2005; 184:1945-1950.

Hiller N, Lieberman S, Chajek-Shaul T, et al. Thoracic manifestations of Behçet disease at CT. Radiographics 2004; 24:801-808.

Schwarz MI, Brown KK. Small vessel vasculitis of the lung. Thorax 2000; 55:502-510.

Semple D, Keogh J, Forni L, Venn R. Clinical review: vasculitis on the intensive care unit—part 1: diagnosis. Crit Care 2005; 9:92-97.

REFERENCES

1. Lee KS, Kim TS, Fujimoto K, et al. Thoracic manifestation of Wegener's granulomatosis: CT findings in 30 patients. Eur Radiol 2003; 13:43-51.
2. Collins CE, Quismorio FP Jr. Pulmonary involvement in microscopic polyangiitis. Curr Opin Pulm Med 2005; 11:447-451.
3. Hiller N, Lieberman S, Chajek-Shaul T, et al. Thoracic manifestations of Behçet disease at CT. Radiographics 2004; 24:801-808.
4. Gotway MB, Araoz PA, Macedo TA, et al. Imaging findings in Takayasu's arteritis. AJR Am J Roentgenol 2005; 184:1945-1950.
5. Kim YK, Lee KS, Chung MP, et al. Pulmonary involvement in Churg-Strauss syndrome: an analysis of CT, clinical, and pathologic findings. Eur Radiol 2007; 17:3157-3165.
6. Lazzarini LC, de Fatima do Amparo Teixeira M, Souza Rodrigues R, Marcos Nunes Valiante P. Necrotizing sarcoid granulomatosis in a family of patients with sarcoidosis reinforces the association between both entities. Respiration 2008; 76:356-360
7. Susarla SC, Fan LL. Diffuse alveolar hemorrhage syndromes in children. Curr Opin Pediatr 2007; 19:314-320.

PART SEVENTEEN

The Abdominal Vessels

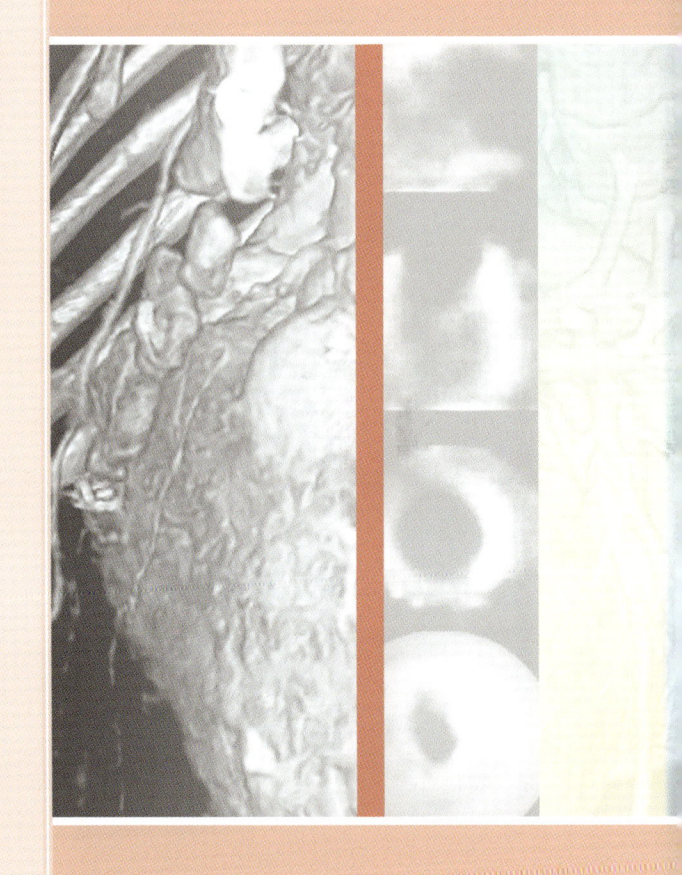

CHAPTER 102

The Abdominal Aorta

Martin L. Gunn, Jonathan H. Chung, Michelle M. Bittle, and Jeffrey H. Maki

INTRODUCTION

Modern advances in noninvasive imaging of the aorta, including multidetector row computed tomography (MDCT), magnetic resonance angiography (MRA), and CT-positron emission tomography (CT-PET) have almost completely replaced diagnostic catheter angiography. Coupled with these advances has been the development of minimally invasive treatments of aortic disease, especially endovascular aortic aneurysm repair.

TECHNIQUES

The choice of imaging technique used to evaluate the aorta is determined by patient and disease-specific indications. Plain radiography has a limited role except following endovascular stent graft placement. Ultrasound has been shown to be an effective screening tool and has the advantages of portability, price, absence of ionizing radiation, or potentially nephrotoxic contrast. MDCT has much greater spatial resolution than any other cross-sectional modality and offers the added advantage of clear demonstration of visceral organs and extremely rapid image acquisition. Magnetic resonance imaging (MRI) techniques can provide additional physiologic information such as flow quantification. There is increasing evidence that PET-CT may be useful in the evaluation of the inflammatory and the noninflammatory aortic aneurysm.

CT Techniques

With recent advances in MDCT technology, routine acquisition of a high resolution isotropic volumetric dataset at the peak of contrast enhancement is easily achieved. There are several advantages to MDCT, but perhaps the greatest is the ability to analyze and display the aorta and branch vessels in any plane and to perform three-dimensional volume rendering for improved visualization and vascular diagnosis.

Using MDCT, a helical volume is acquired with a detector collimation of between 0.5 and 1.5 mm, and reconstructed with a similar thickness using a matrix size of 512 × 512 or greater. The use of tube current modulation techniques (e.g., automated exposure control) reduces radiation exposure compared to fixed-tube current techniques. For MDCT angiography, increased vascular enhancement can be achieved by reducing the kVp to 100 keV (or 80 keV in smaller patients) because this increases photon attenuation by iodinated contrast and moves the mean energy closer to the k-edge of iodine (33.2).[1]

Prior to acquisition of the arterial phase images, a noncontrast CT image set can be obtained. This is particularly useful where significant vascular calcification is expected, or in instances in which intramural hematoma is a differential consideration. Proper timing of the CTA volume acquisition with peak arterial contrast enhancement is critical for optimal arterial illustrations. For detection of associated parenchymal abnormalities, scar tissue, and endoleaks, the addition of delayed phase images can also be helpful. If multiple phases are used routinely, acquisition of those additional phases using lower radiation dose techniques should be considered to minimize patient radiation exposure doses.

After the patient is scanned, the dataset can be sent to a postprocessing workstation for both two-dimensional and three dimensional image reconstruction, and for evaluation of the aorta and branch vessels in a double-oblique true axial plane.

MRI Techniques

Coils and Patient Position

Patients are imaged supine, ideally in a 1.5T or 3.0T MR scanner. Arms should be placed above the patient's head, or folded across the chest to prevent wrap artifact (also known as *image aliasing artifact*).

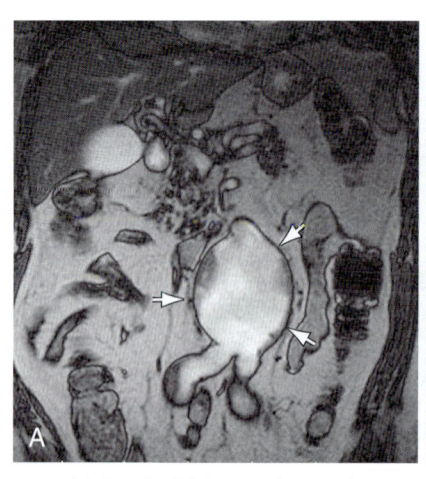

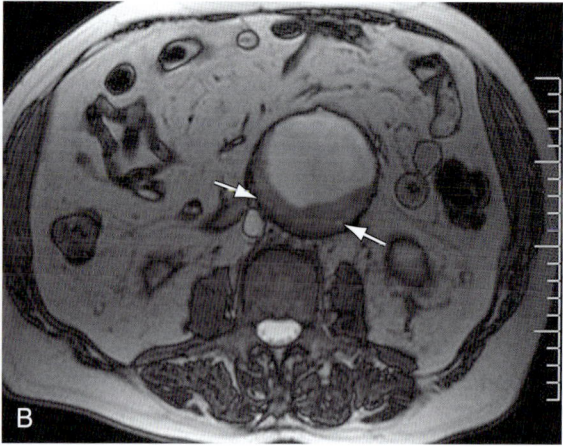

■ **Figure 102-1** Coronal (**A**) and axial (**B**) steady-state free precession sequence. A rapid breath-hold sequence without intravenous gadolinium, providing an overview of the aneurysm (*arrows*) location, relationship to major branch vessels, size, and internal contents.

Coil Choice

Signal-to-noise ratio (SNR) can be maximized with a surface phased array torso coil, positioned to cover the region from the suprarenal abdominal aorta to the iliac vessels. More than one coil may be used in series to maximize range in the *z*-axis.

The extra SNR, greater signal uniformity, and number of coil elements provided by phased array torso coils enable the use of parallel imaging techniques, higher spatial resolution, more rapid signal processing (if there are enough receiver channels), and lower doses of intravenous contrast. In obese or especially tall patients, a body coil can be employed, although this will result in lower SNR.

MR Pulse Sequences

Precontrast Techniques

Localizers: During a breath-hold, localizers are initially obtained in the sagittal, coronal, and axial planes. Performing localizers during breath-hold ensures that the intra-abdominal organs will be located in a similar place to the post-gadolinium sequences which are typically acquired using breath-holding. Localizers can be performed using a variety of sequences, but nongated two-dimensional steady-state free precession sequences (SSFP) provide good tissue contrast and bright-blood images of vessels. Alternatively, HASTE (half-Fourier acquisition single shot turbo spin echo) or SSFSE (single shot fast spin echo) sequences can be performed, which provide a single breath-hold overview of the abdominal organs, with rapidly flowing blood appearing black.

Precontrast Sequences

Axial T1 Weighted Sequences: To survey the intra-abdominal structures, axial T1 weighted images are useful. These can be performed as breath-hold in and out of phase sequences, or using a double inversion fast spin echo technique to eliminate signal from slowly flowing blood. Precontrast T1-weighted images are particularly important for evaluation of the aortic wall for possible pathologies, such as intramural hematoma, which may have high T1 signal related to the presence of hemorrhage. Axial T2 fast spin echo sequences (usually with fat suppression) can also be performed from the diaphragm to the iliac crests to evaluate mass lesions and fluid collections around grafts.

Steady-State Free Precession: Steady-state free precession sequences (also termed *balanced-FFE, true-FISP,* and *FIESTA*) are rapid, have high intrinsic contrast resolution, and have been shown to be accurate in evaluating renal artery stenosis,[2] aneurysm sac contents (Figure 102-1),[3] thoracic aortic dissection, and aneurysm.[4] These sequences can be performed with breath-hold techniques or free breathing with navigator gating, and they provide an overview of the aneurysm sac and surrounding contents.

Velocity Encoded Cine MR Techniques: Unlike the thoracic aorta, velocity encoded cine MR techniques (also known as *cine phase contrast MR*) are not widely used in the abdominal aorta. However, in cases of abdominal aortic coarctation or stenosis, these techniques may assist in quantifying the hemodynamic severity of the obstruction.

Postcontrast MRA: Following contrast injection, the abdominal aorta is scanned using a 3D spoiled gradient echo pulse sequence. The sequence should be optimized to acquire a near isotropic voxel size of 1 to 1.5 mm, in approximately 10 to 15 seconds.

CONTRAST MEDIA

A bolus of intravenous gadolinium-chelate contrast agent for MRA, or of iodinated contrast agent for CTA, is typically injected through a peripheral vein followed by a saline flush. The aim of MRA or CTA of the abdominal aorta, as with MRA and CTA elsewhere in the body, is to achieve peak arterial enhancement during the critical imaging periods, which for CTA is during the whole helical acquisition, and for MRA, is during the acquisition of the central lines of k-space. Proper synchronization of imaging for the arterial transit of the bolus through the target vascular bed will ensure optimal arterial illustration.

The time that it takes for a contrast bolus to pass from the site of intravenous injection until it reaches the abdominal aorta varies widely between individuals, from as little as 10 seconds to as long as 60 seconds. Consequently, varying techniques are available to synchronize MR and CT acquisition with peak arterial enhancement.

Contrast Media Dose

For abdominal aortic CTA, doses of up to 150 mL of nonionic contrast delivered at 3 to 6 mL per second have been routinely used in the past. However, with rapid acquisition techniques, doses as low as 50 mLs have been used, especially in smaller patients.[5] For MRA, a typical gadolinium-chelate contrast agent dose is 0.2 mmol/kg injected at 2 mL/sec.

Empiric Bolus Timing Techniques

These "best guess" techniques estimate the patients circulation time based on general population rates, and can be modified by patient age and size. This technique works in about 85% of cases. To achieve more consistent results, a higher dose of contrast agent or a slower injection rate is typically used.

Timing Bolus Techniques

A small "test-bolus" (0.5 to 4 mL of gadolinium-chelate contrast agent or 10 to 20 mL of iodinated contrast agent) is administered followed by a saline flush at the same injection rate as the main bolus. From the beginning of contrast injection, images through the proximal abdominal aorta are obtained every 1 to 2 seconds for approximately 30 to 40 seconds. A time-intensity (MR) or time-attenuation (CT) curve can be generated using a region of interest (ROI) over the aorta, and the time to peak enhancement can be calculated. The circulation time and the time to inject the contrast are used to calculate the scan delay, which should correlate with the acquisition of the central k-space data (MR) or the helical CT data acquisition. For MRA, the formula used to determine scan delay depends on the relative timing for central k-space data acquisition and depends on whether a sequential, centric, reverse centric, or other means of k-space ordering is used.

Bolus Detection/Triggering Methods

Bolus detection methods monitor the arrival of the full contrast bolus using a series of 2D images or low-dose CT sections, which are acquired every few seconds over the vessel of interest. When adequate vascular enhancement is achieved, the CT or MRI acquisition is initiated. Triggering can be manual (the technologist or radiologist starts the acquisition when contrast can be seen to arrive in the aorta) or automatic by software detection. With automatic triggering, an ROI is placed on the aorta, and the software commences the acquisition (in MRI, usually using centric ordered k-space acquisition) when aortic enhancement reaches a predetermined threshold.

MRA: K-Space

For MR angiography, there are a variety of k-space acquisition schemes. Common ways of filling k-space for an MRA include sequential and centric phase ordering. In sequential k-space filling, the central lines of k-space are filled during the middle part of the acquisition period. To maximize contrast resolution, and therefore enhancement, it is best that the scan delay should lead to the maximum of enhancement in the middle of the acquisition window. In centric k-space filling, the central lines of k-space are filled in the first part of the acquisition period. Hence, the scan delay should be equal to the circulation time to ensure match of key image data with peak arterial contrast enhancement, If a bolus detection method is used for MRA, a centric ordered k-space scheme is typically used to ensure improved synchronization of the central k-space data acquisition with bolus arrival into the target vascular bed.

By using time-resolved magnetic resonance imaging (TR-MRA) techniques, the dynamics of blood flow in the abdominal vessels can be demonstrated in a way similar to conventional angiography. In TR-MRA, there is oversampling of central k-space, which is acquired every 2 to 8 seconds for 1 to 3 minutes after gadolinium injection, without the need of a timing bolus. Time-resolved MRA has been shown to be an effective means of classifying endoleaks following endovascular repair.[6]

ABDOMINAL AORTIC ANEURYSM

Abdominal aortic aneurysm (AAA) is enlargement of the abdominal aorta above a diameter of 3 cm.[7]

Prevalence and Epidemiology

Abdominal aortic aneurysms are nearly five times more common in men than in women and almost twice as common in people of European descent than African Americans. The prevalence of aneurysm is also increased in those with a family history of AAA, and is strongly related to a history of smoking.[8] Other risk factors include age, coronary artery disease or another manifestation of atherosclerosis, high cholesterol, and hypertension. In a large ultrasound screening study,[9] an abdominal aortic aneurysm was detected in approximately 5% of males older than 65 years. Ruptured AAA occurs in 1% to 3% of men per year aged 65 years or more, and mortality is 70% to 95%. Left untreated, AAA leads to death in about one third of patients.[8]

Etiology and Pathophysiology

Although the exact etiology of AAA remains unclear, it appears that degradation of elastin, collagen, and other structural proteins in the aortic wall is a major factor.[10] Atherosclerosis is considered to play an important role in the etiology, likely via chronic inflammation in the aortic wall. An imbalance of T-helper and T-suppressor lymphocytes leads to a proliferation of B-lymphocytes. Elastin-derived peptides (EDPs), which are breakdown products of medial elastin, are thought to be the initiating and propagating antigen in this process. Chronic inflammation leads to excess matrix metalloproteinases and degradation of medial elastin and collagen.[11] However, the etiology is unquestionably multifactorial. Current research suggests that genetic, environmental, hemodynamic, and immunologic factors all contribute to the development of aneurysms.

Clinical Manifestations of Disease

Most AAAs are asymptomatic and are discovered incidentally on routine physical examination or during other imaging studies. Patients with ruptured AAAs often present with an abrupt onset of back pain as well as abdominal pain and tenderness. Patients may present critically ill. Most will have a pulsatile abdominal mass. Rupture has a high mortality rate, with 25% mortality prior to arriving at the hospital and an overall 30-day survival rate of approximately 10%.[12]

The rate of aneurysm growth increases with increasing diameter in concordance with Laplace law. Aneurysms smaller than 4 cm grow at 2 to 4 mm/year, those measuring 4 to 5 cm grow at 2 to 5 mm per year, and aneurysms >5 cm grow at 3 to 7 mm per year.[13] The risk of rupture increases with aneurysm size and rate of aneurysm expansion. In the U.K. Small Aneurysm Trial,[14] aneurysms with a cross-sectional diameter of 5 to 5.9 cm in size had an annual risk of rupture of 6.5%. Elective AAA repair carries a 4% to 6% mortality. Recommendations[10] suggest elective repair of aneurysms greater than 5.5 cm in males, and greater than 4.5 to 5 cm in women. Aneurysm length is not thought to be associated with rupture risk.[15]

Imaging Indications and Algorithm

The U.S. Preventive Services Task Force (USPSTF)[16] recommends screening for AAA in men aged 65 to 75 years of age who have ever smoked. It can also be considered in patients with a strong family history of AAA. Ultrasound is the modality of choice for screening in most patients. Its advantages include the absence of intravenous contrast, absence of ionizing radiation, and relatively low cost.

For asymptomatic and smaller aneurysms, ultrasound surveillance is recommended (Table 102-1). For aneurysms >4.5 cm, CT or MRI offer the advantages of greater measurement accuracy, better depiction of the suprarenal aorta and branch vessels, and superior reproducibility versus ultrasonography.

Imaging Techniques and Findings

Radiography

The presence of calcification in the abdominal aortic wall, although commonly present, is not invariable. Moreover, a tortuous and calcified aorta may mimic an AAA. A lateral radiograph (Fig. 102-2) may depict aortic calcification more clearly. However, radiographs are unreliable for diameter measurements of the aortic wall and are not recommended for diagnosis or surveillance.[17]

TABLE 102-1 Rescreening Intervals for Asymptomatic AAAs

Diameter up to	Re-image aorta in
<3.5 cm	5 years
<4.0 cm	2 years
<4.5 cm	1 year
<5 cm	6 months
5-5.5 cm	3-6 months*

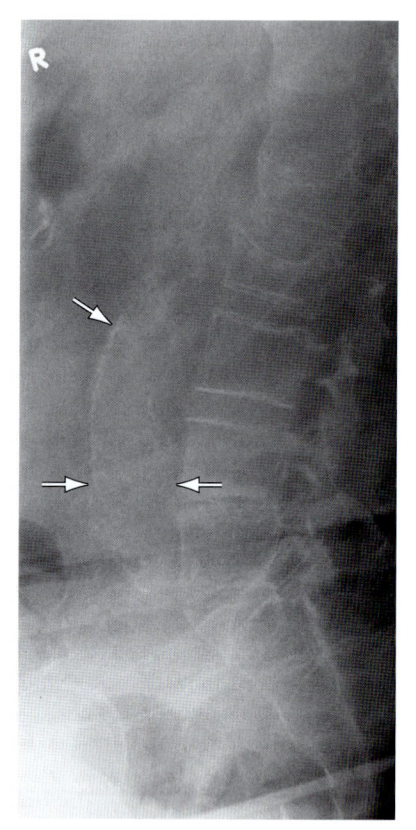

*Also consider referral to a vascular surgeon.
Derived from Isselbacher EM. Thoracic and abdominal aortic aneurysms. Circulation 2005; 111(6):816-828.

■ **Figure 102-2** Lateral radiograph of an abdominal aortic aneurysm. Fusiform dilation of the infrarenal aorta with calcification of the intima (*arrows*). The superior and inferior extent of the aneurysm sac are not visible.

Ultrasonography

Examination of the abdominal aorta is an essential component of a complete abdominal ultrasound study, and should be examined in all patients presenting with acute abdominal pain. Abdominal aortic aneurysms should be detectable by sonography in up to 100% of patients.[18]

The aorta appears on ultrasound as a hypoechoic tubular structure with echogenic walls (Fig. 102-3A). The anterior and posterior walls of the aneurysm are usually better seen than are the lateral walls. Mural thrombus (see Fig. 102-3B) has low to medium echogenicity and is attached to the margins of the aortic wall. At times, mural thrombus will have a lamellated appearance. Thrombus

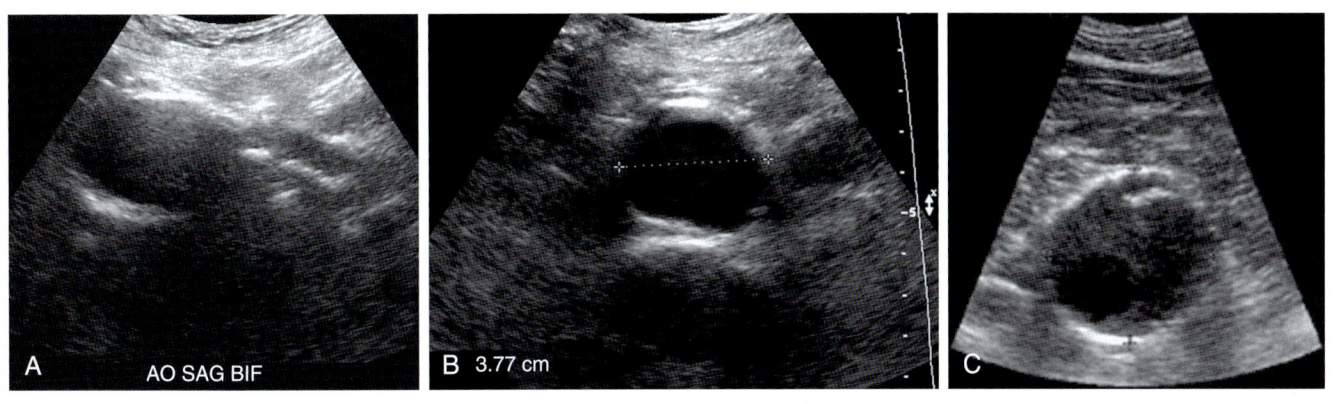

Figure 102-3 **A** and **B,** Abdominal aortic aneurysm on ultrasound. Transverse and sagittal ultrasound images of the aorta demonstrate a small aortic aneurysm, not appropriate for surgical repair. **C,** Abdominal aortic aneurysm containing mural thrombus. Measurements of the aneurysm are from outer wall to outer wall, not the caliber of the patent lumen.

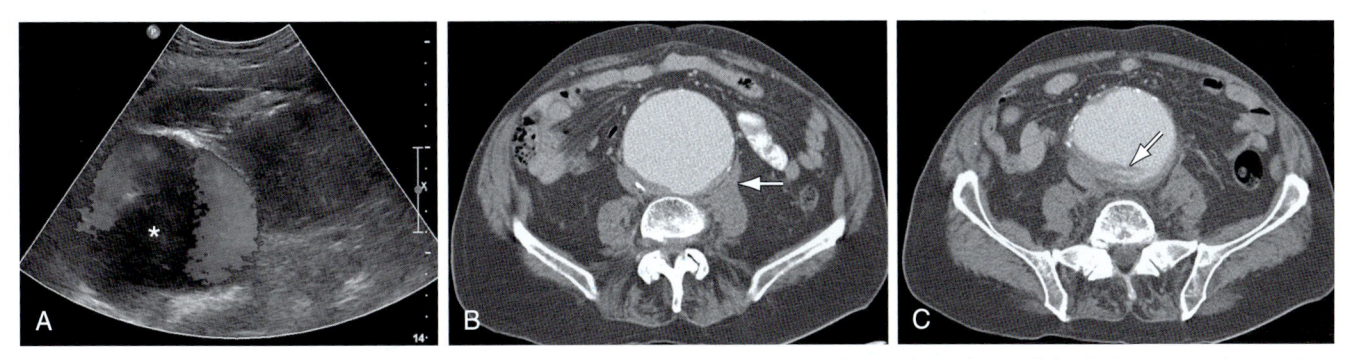

Figure 102-4 Bedside ultrasound (**A**) and subsequent CT (**B** and **C**) on a hypotensive patient with a pulsative abdominal mass. On ultrasound, a 9 cm aneurysm (*asterisk*) was diagnosed, but retroperitoneal blood was not suspected. On subsequent CT (**B**), a small periaortic hematoma was identified (*arrow*), in addition to a "draped aorta sign" of a deficient posterior wall. More inferiorly (**C**), a small fissure has formed within the posterior aspect of intramural thrombus (*arrow*). Ultrasound is not accurate in excluding small retroperitoneal ruptures.

that appears to "flutter" during the cardiac cycle may be at risk of embolization.

Ultrasound measurements of abdominal aortic aneurysms are accurate and repeatable. The measurements are taken from the outer-to-outer wall of the aorta in a plane perpendicular to the long axis of the aorta.

In suspected aneurysm rupture, a bedside ultrasonogram may be helpful for those patients who are too unstable for CT, or if CT is not readily available. Ultrasound scanning may assist in determining the aneurysm size and the presence of retroperitoneal or intraperitoneal fluid (Fig. 102-4), although the role of ultrasonography in identifying impending rupture is limited.[19]

CT and MRI

Compared to ultrasonography, CT and MRI (Fig. 102-5) provide superior depiction of the extent and shape of the aneurysm, involvement of the renal, mesenteric, and iliac arteries, and the suprarenal abdominal and thoracic aorta. On average, ultrasound underestimates aneurysm size by 3 to 9 mm compared to CT angiography.[20] Due to their excellent contrast resolution and multiplanar capabilities, CT and MR angiography are now the mainstay of aneurysm characterization prior to endovascular or surgical repair. CT is the modality of choice for the evaluation of suspected rupture of the abdominal aorta[19]; usually it can be performed within minutes, and has clear benefits in showing alternative causes of acute abdominal pain. Contrast-enhanced CT provides information about the lumen size, location, extent, relationship to branch vessels, presence of active contrast extravasation, and complications secondary to aneurysm rupture.

Signs of Rupture, Impending Rupture, and Contained Rupture

Noncontrast CT is useful in demonstrating the presence of an abdominal aortic aneurysm, maximum aneurysm size, and the presence of retroperitoneal hemorrhage. A high attenuating crescent within the wall of aneurysm (Figs. 102-6 and 102-7) is a sign of impending or frank aneurysm rupture.[21] A high attenuation crescent is denser than the psoas muscles (on enhanced CT) and the lumen (on nonenhanced CT scans).

The most common finding in aneurysm rupture is a retroperitoneal hematoma adjacent to the abdominal aortic aneurysm (see Figs. 102-4, 102-7, and 102-8). This blood usually tracks into the pararenal and perirenal spaces (Fig. 102-9). Active extravasation (Figs. 102-9 and 102-10) is frequently visualized on contrast-enhanced CT images. The "draped aorta sign," where the abdominal aorta is closely applied to the spine with lateral "draping" of the aneurysm around the vertebral body (see Fig.

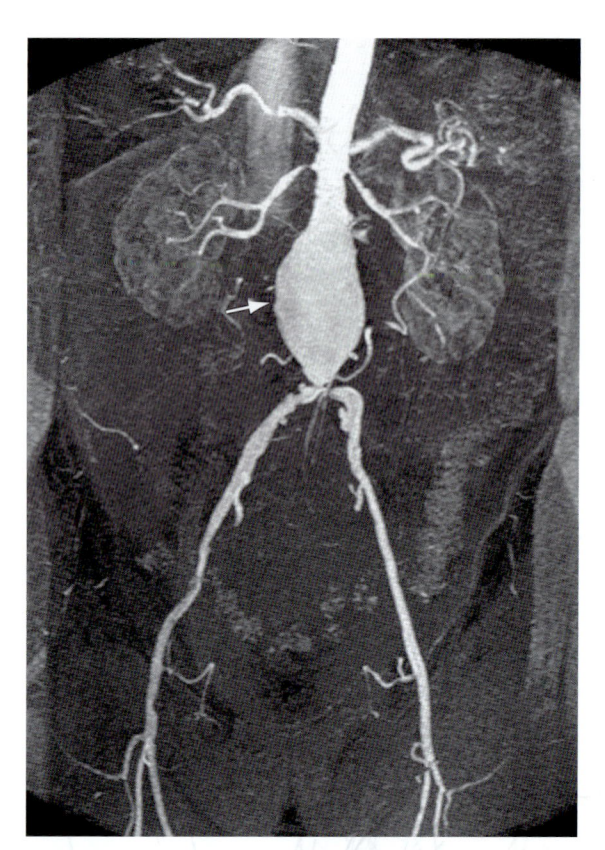

■ **Figure 102-5** Infrarenal abdominal aortic aneurysm (*arrow*) demonstrated on maximum intensity projection (MIP) reconstruction of a gadolinium-enhanced MRA. The neck of the aneurysm and relationship to the renal arteries is clearly shown, as are the associated stenoses of the renal arteries and common iliac arteries.

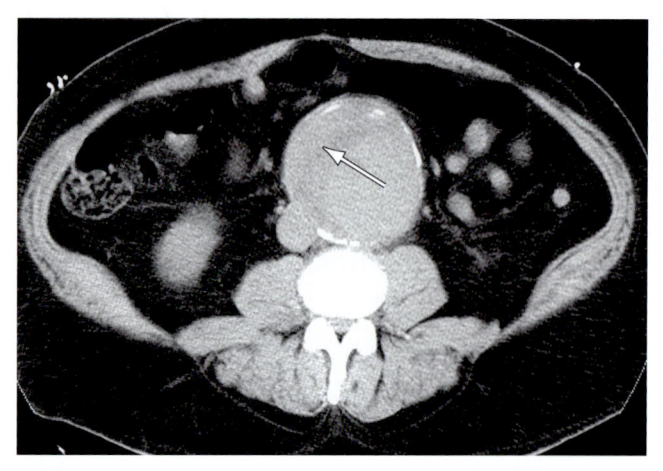

■ **Figure 102-6** Noncontrast CT of the abdomen demonstrates a high-density crescent in the periphery of the aneurysmal wall suggesting impending rupture (*arrow*).

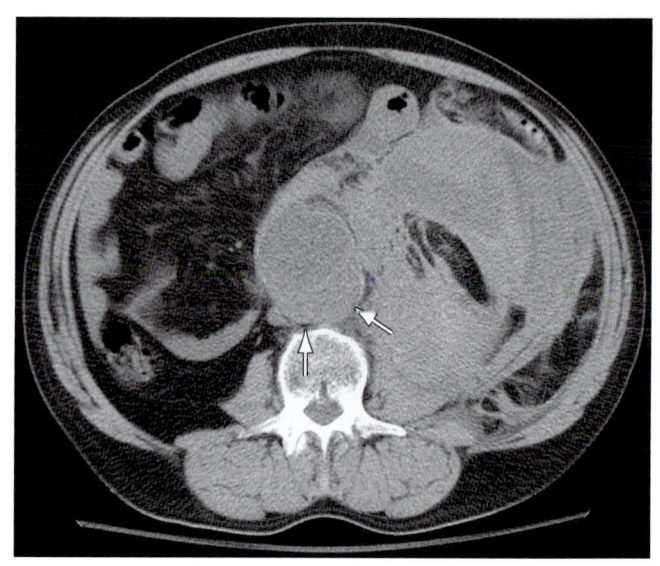

■ **Figure 102-7** In patients unable to receive intravenous contrast, noncontrast CT is useful in evaluating the presence of an aneurysm and retroperitoneal hematoma. A large left heterogeneous retroperitoneal hematoma is present on noncontrast abdominal CT. Crescentic hyperattenuating thrombus is also present within the posterior wall (*arrows*).

102-4), has been described as a finding of a deficient posterior wall of the aorta and a contained leak.[22] Other sites of rupture include the bowel (most commonly the duodenum), and inferior vena cava (Fig. 102-11).[23] Signs of AAA rupture, impending rupture, and contained rupture are (1) periaortic and retroperitoneal hemorrhage; (2) contrast extravasation; (3) high attenuating crescent sign; and (4) draped aorta sign.

FDG-PET

Recent evidence suggests that increased aortic wall metabolism, as measured by FDG-PET, may suggest increased rupture risk. Increased metabolism may represent increased activation of inflammatory cells in the aortic wall, which leads to increased degradation of elastin and collagen in the aneurysm wall.[24] Pilot studies examining the role of FDG-PET-CT in asymptomatic and symptomatic AAAs,[25] have demonstrated increased activity in those with symptomatic AAAs, and increased activity in focal areas of increased inflammation and collagen degradation.

Differential Diagnosis

Nonruptured AAAs are often asymptomatic. Pain associated with a ruptured aneurysm is nonspecific. Other diagnoses which could manifest similarly include biliary disease, renal colic, diverticulitis, pancreatitis, cardiac ischemia, and mesenteric ischemia.

The imaging findings of AAA are pathognomonic in the correct clinical situation. The differential diagnosis of atherosclerotic AAA includes mycotic aneurysms and traumatic pseudoaneurysms.

Treatment Options

Medical

Medical therapy is usually instituted in patients with smaller aneurysms not treated surgically or endovascularly. Smoking cessation is paramount because smoking plays a major role in aneurysm growth.[26,27] Although the effect of hypertension and dyslipidemia on aneurysm growth and rupture are unknown, treating these

CHAPTER 102 • The Abdominal Aorta 1403

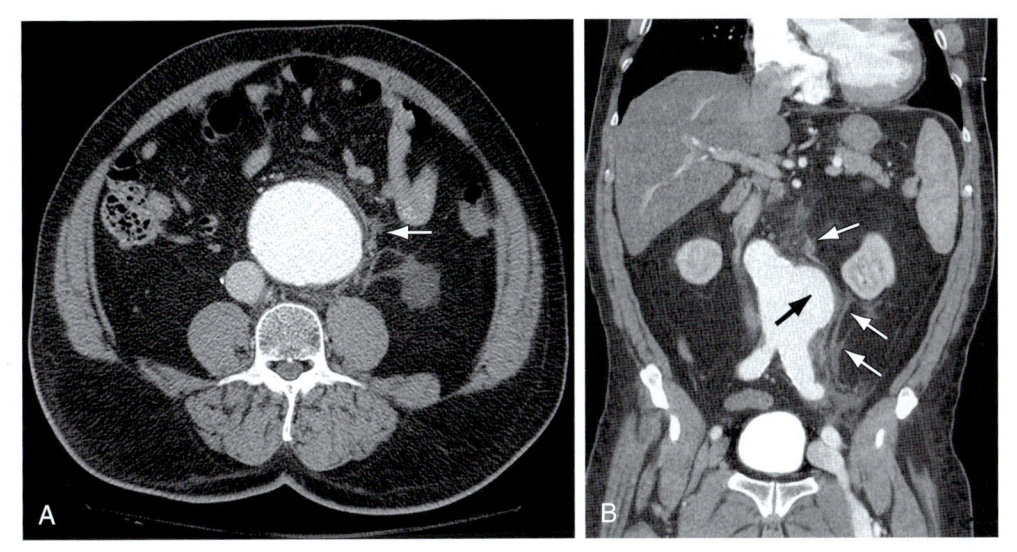

■ **Figure 102-8** **A**, Early rupture of an abdominal aortic aneurysm. Contrast-enhanced axial CT of the abdomen shows a large abdominal aortic aneurysm with adjacent fat stranding (*arrow*) suggesting aortic leak or impending rupture. **B**, Contrast-enhanced coronal CT of the abdomen demonstrates a saccular aneurysm of the infrarenal aorta (*black arrow*) with adjacent fat stranding (*white arrows*) suggesting aortic leak or impending rupture.

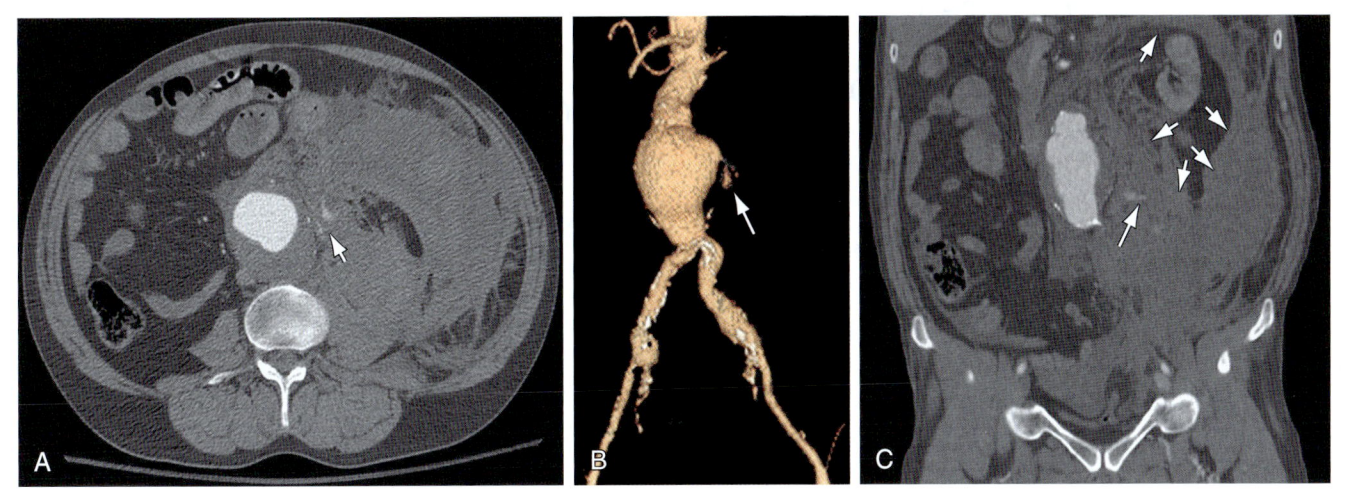

■ **Figure 102-9** **A** and **B**, Ruptured abdominal aortic aneurysm. Contrast-enhanced axial CT and VR images of the abdomen demonstrate a saccular infrarenal abdominal aortic aneurysm with frank rupture into the left retroperitoneum. Active contrast extravasation is also present (*arrows*). **C**, Contrast-enhanced coronal CT of the abdomen demonstrates a saccular infrarenal abdominal aortic aneurysm with a massive left retroperitoneal hemorrhage (*thin arrows*). Active contrast extravasation is again present (*thick arrow*). Sparing of the perinephric space excluded the kidney as the bleeding source.

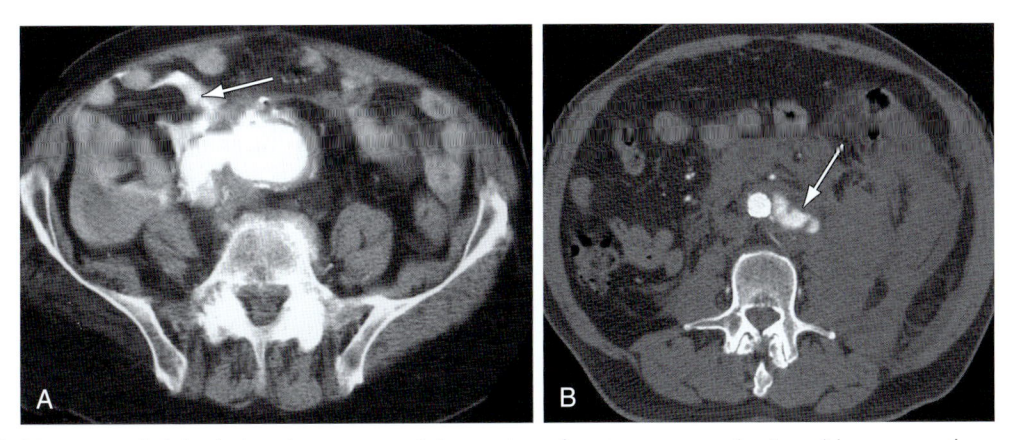

■ **Figure 102-10** Two ruptured abdominal aortic aneurysms. **A**, Intraperitoneal contrast extravasation (*arrow*) is uncommonly encountered. **B**, More commonly retroperitoneal extravasation is seen (*arrow*).

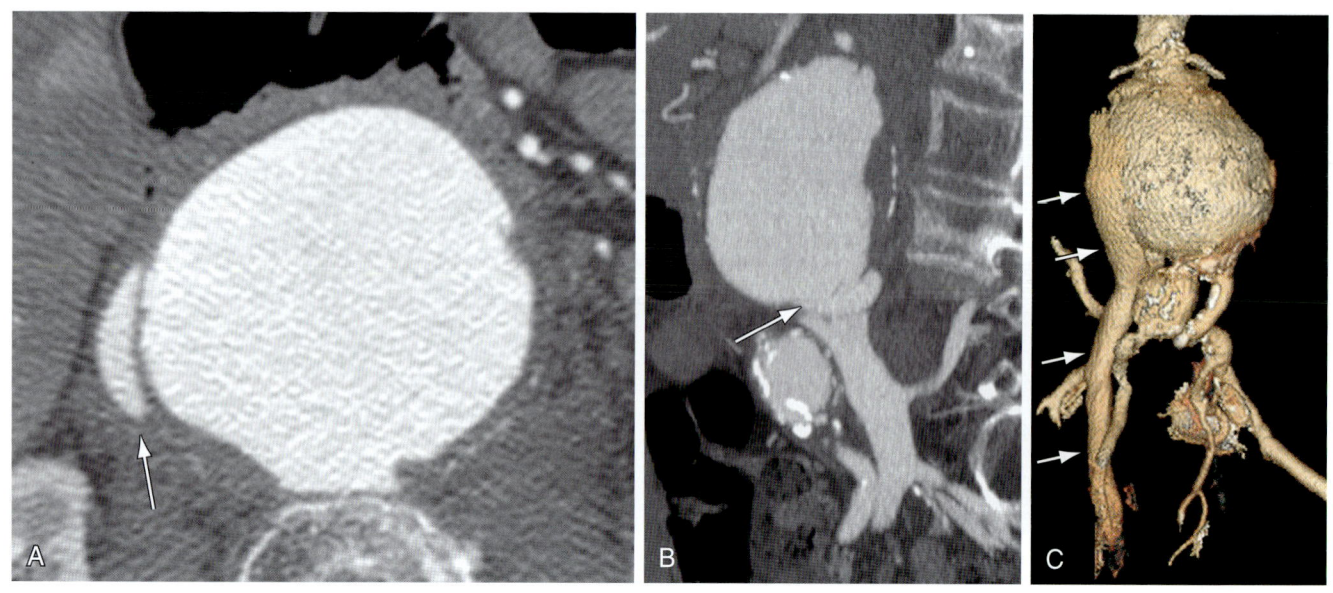

Figure 102-11 **A,** Abdominal aortic aneurysm with a fistula between the aorta and inferior vena cava. Axial images from arterial phase of a contrast-enhanced CTA demonstrates a large infrarenal abdominal aortic aneurysm; a crescentic structure just lateral to the aorta demonstrates enhancement during this arterial phase study *(arrow)*. **B,** Sagittal reconstruction demonstrates a fistula connection between the abdominal aortic aneurysm and the inferior vena cava *(arrow)*. **C,** Volume rendered AP image of the aorta demonstrates contrast filling the right iliac vein and the lower IVC *(arrows)*.

conditions may prolong survival. Statin therapy has been shown to reduce mortality and slow aneurysm growth.[26] β-blockers may slow the expansion rate of aneurysms.[28]

Surgical/Interventional

In patients requiring surgery, options for open repair include the traditional transabdominal route or the recently popularized retroperitoneal approach. Surgical complications include acute renal failure, distal embolization, infection, aortoenteric fistula, colonic ischemia, and vascular injury. The complication rate has decreased with better surgical techniques. In patients with concomitant cardiorespiratory conditions, perioperative pneumonia, atelectasis, myocardial ischemia, and arrhythmia are not uncommon. Endovascular stent repair may also be performed because it is less invasive and more appropriate in poor surgical candidates. However, the long-term outcome of patients after endovascular repair is not yet known.

INFLAMMATORY AORTIC ANEURYSM

A variant of aortic aneurysm, inflammatory abdominal aortic aneurysms (IAAAs) are characterized by peri-aneurysmal fibrosis and adhesions and are a surgical challenge. Surgical repair is associated with a higher morbidity and mortality than surgery for degenerative AAAs.

Definition

Inflammatory abdominal aortic aneurysms are defined by the presence of a thickened aneurysm wall, marked peri-aneurysmal and retroperitoneal fibrosis, and dense adhesions of adjacent abdominal organs.[11]

Prevalence and Epidemiology

IAAAs constitute approximately 3% to 10% of abdominal aortic aneurysms. Male sex and smoking are both strong risk factors, with a male-to-female ratio ranging from 6:1 to 30:1. From 77% to 100% of patients smoke.[11] Other risk factors include northern European descent and autoimmune disease.

Etiology and Pathophysiology

Like AAA, the etiology of IAAAs is multifactorial. Current understanding suggests a common immune-mediated inflammatory pathogenesis shared with degenerative AAA, but in IAAA, the inflammation is more pronounced. White blood cells in the aortic wall cause degradation of the extracellular matrix by releasing proteolytic enzymes and cytokines. Based on this knowledge, steroid and other anti-inflammatory agents have been found by some to inhibit aneurysm growth. Some have postulated a role of infection in the aortic wall. Suggested agents include herpes simplex virus, cytomegalovirus, and *Chlamydia* organisms.

CLINICAL MANIFESTATIONS OF DISEASE

Unlike degenerative AAAs, in which back or flank pain is present in a minority of patients, a great majority of patients with IAAAs have back pain. In patients with a known aneurysm, the classic triad of back pain, weight loss, and elevated erythrocyte sedimentation rate (ESR) is highly suggestive of an inflammatory aneurysm.

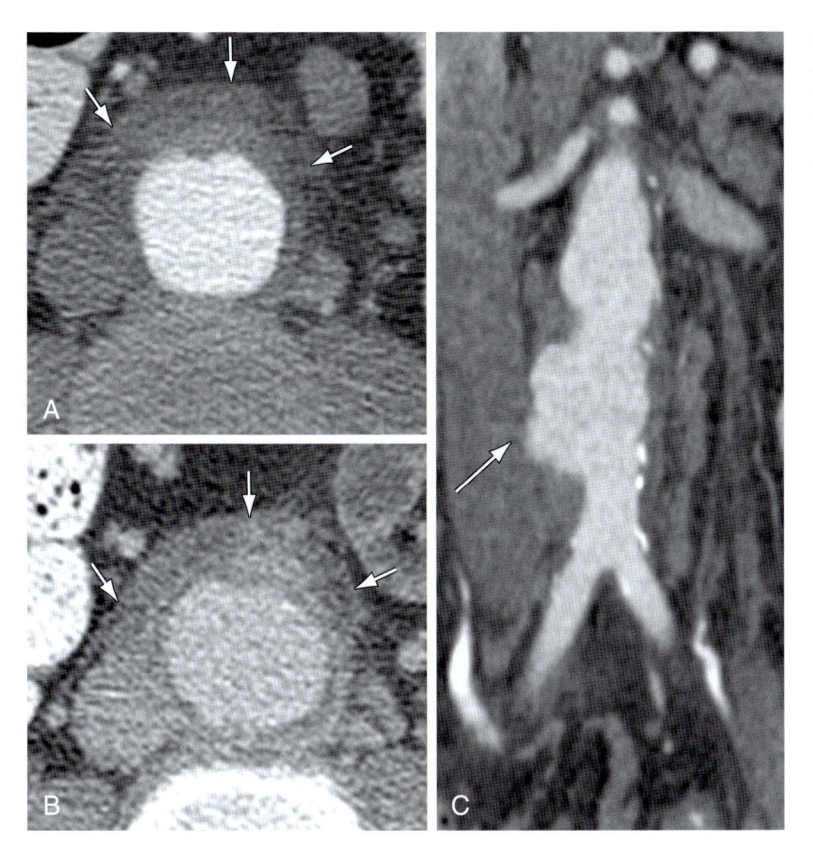

■ **Figure 102-12** **A** and **B,** Inflammatory abdominal aortic aneurysm. Axial images from arterial phase of contrast-enhanced CTA demonstrates a small saccular, infrarenal abdominal aortic aneurysm with an irregular soft tissue rim (*arrows*) which undergoes enhancement. There is relative sparing of its posterior margin consistent with an inflammatory abdominal aortic aneurysm. **C,** Coronal reformat demonstrates the saccular aneurysm (*arrow*) to better detail.

Imaging Techniques and Findings

Ultrasound

Sonographic signs include aortic dilation, thickened and echogenic aortic wall, and a hypoechoic periaortic cuff measuring 1 to 1.5 cm.[29]

CT and MRI

MDCT and MRI are the mainstays in the investigation of suspected inflammatory abdominal aortic aneurysms. CT accurately distinguishes IAAA from AAA in 93.7% of cases.[30] Signs include a thickened, calcified aortic wall surrounded by a low density soft tissue mass (Figs. 102-12 and 102-13). There is relative sparing of the posterior wall of the aorta. The inflammatory soft tissue surrounding the aorta undergoes contrast enhancement in both CT and MRI (Fig. 102-14). On CT, periaortic inflammatory soft tissue generally has lower density than acute blood, helping differentiation from acute AAA rupture. CT and MRI are useful to assess associated effects on adjacent structures, such as ureteric encasement, hydronephrosis, inferior vena cava narrowing, and bowel involvement. Ureteric involvement is present in approximately 25% of cases (see Fig. 102-13) at presentation.[11]

Differential Diagnosis

From the Clinical Presentation

If back or abdominal pain is the presenting feature, the clinical differential is very broad. On clinical examination, if a pulsatile abdominal mass is noted, traditional AAA should be considered.

From the Imaging Findings

The imaging findings of inflammatory AAA must be differentiated from Takayasu arteritis and giant cell arteritis. Cogan syndrome may also cause an aortitis but is very rare (associated with visual and vestibulo-auditory symptoms).[31]

Treatment Options

Medical

When there is extensive periaortic inflammation with involvement of surrounding organs, surgical repair is much more challenging, and a nonoperative approach may be prudent. Steroid therapy may reduce the inflammatory process, but steroid use is not universally accepted. The rupture rate of IAAA with nonoperative management may be lower than in noninflammatory AAAs.

Surgical

An operative or endovascular approach is taken whenever possible. Although associated with a higher perioperative mortality than noninflammatory AAAs, 30-day surgical mortality rates have fallen and are now in the upper end of the 3% to 10% range. A transperitoneal approach is most popular.

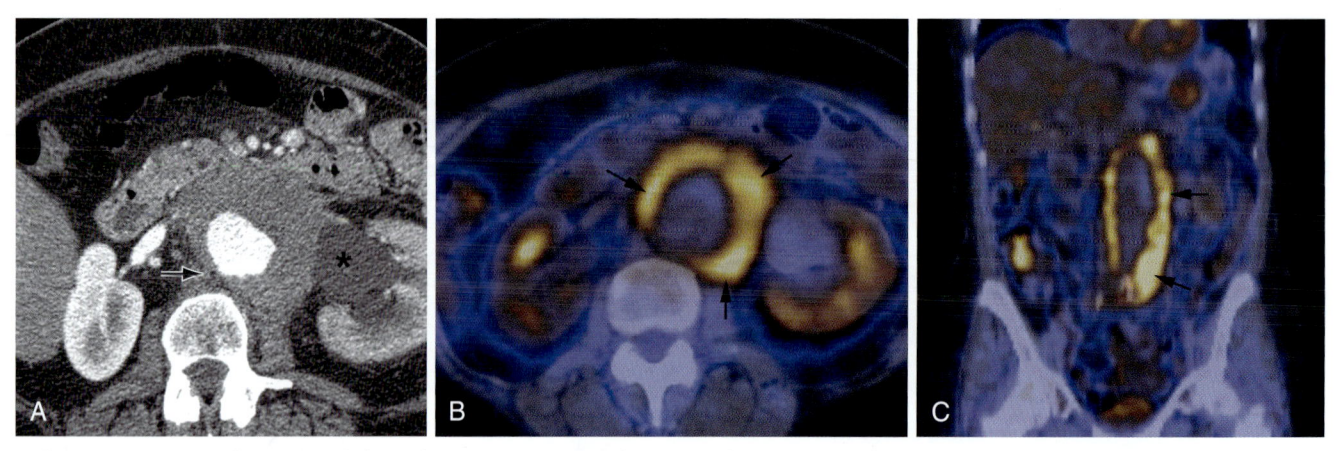

Figure 102-13 **A,** Inflammatory abdominal aortic aneurysm. Axial contrast-enhanced CT (**A**) demonstrates thick periaortic soft tissue thickening with relative sparing of the posterior aorta (*arrow*). There is obstruction of the left ureter, with left hydronephrosis (*asterisk*) and left renal hypoperfusion. Axial and coronal images from fused FDG-PET CT (**B,C**) demonstrate avid uptake within the periaortic soft-tissue thickening (*arrows*) consistent with inflammation.

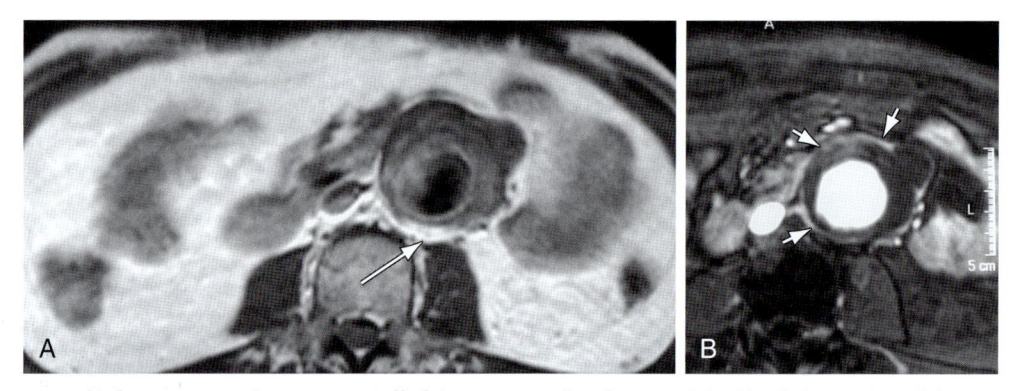

Figure 102-14 MRI of inflammatory aortic aneurysm. Cuff of tissue surrounding the aorta (**A**) with relative sparing of the posterior wall (*arrow*). Following intravenous gadolinium (**B**), there is enhancement of the cuff and the surrounding soft tissues (*arrows*).

Depending on the degree of ureteric obstruction, nephrostomy tubes, ureteric stenting, and even ureterolysis may be considered to manage renal failure. Even after surgical resection, complete regression of retroperitoneal fibrosis occurs in the minority of cases, and long-term therapy with ureteric stenting and immunosuppressive therapy may be necessary.

Endovascular

Endovascular repair of AAAs has shown promising early and mid-term results and is appealing in high-risk patients, especially when technical difficulties are anticipated due to periaortic inflammation and fibrosis. Only small case series have been reported. In a meta-analysis of 46 patients treated with endovascular repair,[32] there was no periprocedural mortality. The primary technical success rate of 95.6%, was associated with medium term regression in aneurysmal sac size, reduced periaortic fibrosis, and improvement in renal impairment.[32]

MYCOTIC AORTIC ANEURYSM

Mycotic aortic aneurysms (also known as *infected aortic aneurysms*) represent a minority of AAAs. Their diagnosis may be difficult. They have a higher incidence of rupture and are challenging to treat. Perioperative morbidity and mortality is also higher than in noninfected AAAs.

Prevalence and Epidemiology

Mycotic AAAs are rare, representing 0.7% to 2.6% of all aortic aneurysms.[33] They are associated with immunosuppression and chronic comorbid conditions, such as diabetes or renal failure.[34]

Etiology and Pathophysiology

Staphyloccccus aureus and *Salmonella* are the most common organisms. Previously common organisms such as *Streptococcus pyogenes*, pneumococcus, and *Enterococcus* are less common with widespread antibiotic use. The organism may infect the vessel wall either via the vaso vasorum or by implantation in diseased vessel wall (e.g., intimal injury, ulcerated plaque, or mural thrombus).

Clinical Manifestations of Disease

Most patients have nonspecific symptoms including fever and pain. Diagnosis is challenging until late in the disease. Even with recent advances, a high rate of aneurysm rupture has been reported (50% to 85%).[34]

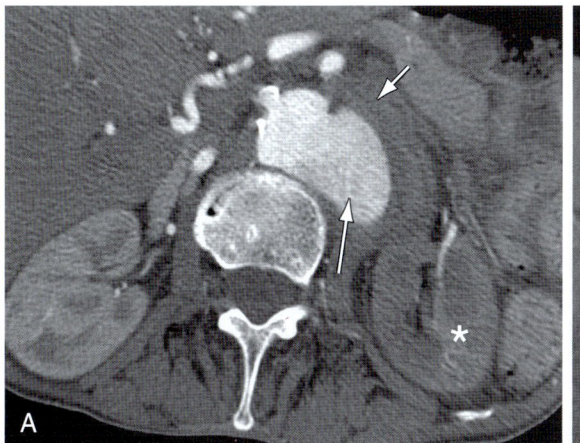

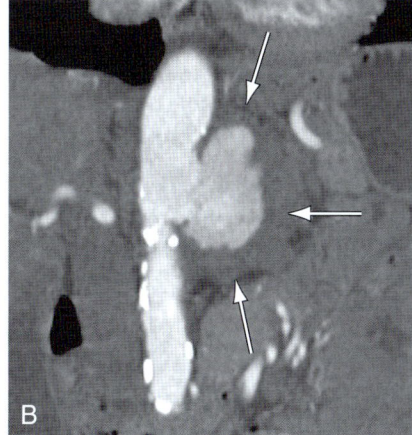

■ **Figure 102-15** **A,** Large saccular aneurysm in a patient presenting with abdominal, back pain, and fever. Axial images from contrast-enhanced CT demonstrates a large saccular aneurysm (*white arrows*) projecting from the left aspect of the superior abdominal aorta. Mural wall thickening is also present. The left kidney is underperfused, implying involvement of the left renal artery (*asterisk*). **B,** Coronal images demonstrates the saccular aneurysm (*arrows*) in better detail.

Imaging Findings

The imaging findings of mycotic aneurysms are similar across all modalities including ultrasound, CT scan, MRI, and angiography.

CT and MRI

Approximately two thirds of infected aortic aneurysms involve the abdominal aorta, although most also involve the suprarenal or thoraco-abdominal aorta. Aneurysms are mostly saccular (95%) (Fig. 102-15) and may have an irregular contour. In the largest published series,[33] about 50% of patients had a periaortic soft tissue mass, soft tissue stranding, and/or fluid surrounding the aneurysm. One of the characteristic features of infected aortic aneurysm is rapid progression. Periaortic gas, adjacent vertebral body destruction, and psoas muscle abscesses are also signs of infection and additional clues of a mycotic AAA.

Angiography

The same findings identified on cross-sectional imaging may be identified on angiography. However, given the wide availability of CT, catheter arteriography is being used less often in the setting of suspected mycotic aneurysm.

Nuclear Medicine

Increased uptake can be seen on leukocyte, gallium, or PET scan in the infected portions of the aorta. In one series, increased scintigraphic uptake was seen in 86% of mycotic aortic aneurysms.[33]

Treatment Options

Medical

Parenteral antimicrobial therapy is mandatory in all mycotic aneurysms. Patients are treated for at least 6 weeks and until inflammatory markers normalize.[35] Some suggest treating patients with antibiotics for life.[36] Initial treatment is empiric. After microorganism susceptibility testing has been performed, more specific agents can be started.

Surgical/Interventional

In cases of suprarenal mycotic aortic aneurysms, in situ repair or reconstruction is the preferred surgery.[37] In-situ bypass reconstruction is the procedure of choice in infected infrarenal aortic aneurysms. Critically ill patients who cannot tolerate surgery can be treated with endovascular repair until definitive intervention can be performed.[38,39]

COMPLICATIONS OF ENDOVASCULAR AORTIC ANEURYSM REPAIR

Major complications from endovascular aortic aneurysm repair occur in approximately 5% of cases. Endoleak, or contrast enhancement of the aneurysm sac following endovascular aortic aneurysm repair (EVAR) is much more common and occurs in 30% to 40% of patients acutely and in 20% to 40% during routine follow-up. Endoleaks are defined as blood flow within the aortic sac, but outside the stent graft lumen. A "primary endoleak" occurs within 30 days of implantation, and a "secondary endoleak" occurs after 30 days.

Prevalence and Epidemiology

Early endoleaks, according to the EUROSTAR registry, occur in 18% of patients. These are usually graft related, and seal spontaneously. A meta-analysis of endoleaks following EVAR revealed a total of 24% of patients experiencing endoleaks, with the majority (66%) present immediately after stent graft placement. These most commonly arose from the distal stent attachment site, and were persistent.[40]

Etiology and Pathophysiology

Endoleaks are classified according to the site and cause of the leak (Table 102-2). Deficient sealing at the proximal or distal end of the stent graft causes type I endoleaks. Primary type I endoleaks are usually caused by difficult anatomy (e.g., angulated aneurysm neck), a noncircular landing zone, malpositioning, or underdilation of the stent graft. Secondary type I leaks may be caused by aneurysm remodeling, stent graft migration, or progressive dilation of the neck.[41] Systemic blood pressure occurs within the aortic sac in type 1 endoleaks, and there is persistent tension on the aortic wall.

Type II endoleaks are due to retrograde filling of the aneurysm sac from branch arteries, usually the lumbar arteries or inferior mesenteric artery (Fig. 102-16). About 40% of type II endoleaks will seal spontaneously, and the risk of aneurysm expansion and rupture with type II endoleaks is lower than with types I or III.

Type III endoleaks are caused by a failure in the structure of the graft: junctional separation of the modular components of the graft, holes in the fabric, and tears due to strut failure. As in type I endoleaks, the aneurysm sac is exposed to full systemic pressure in type III endoleaks, and hence, intervention is usually necessary.

Type IV endoleaks are due to graft fabric porosity. These may be seen temporarily at the time of endograft placement.

Type V endoleak, also known as endotension, is continuing expansion of the aneurysm in the absence of a confirmed endoleak. Endotension may be due to an undiagnosed endoleak or due to the accumulation of serous fluid in the sac due to ultra-filtration through the graft pores.

Imaging Indications and Algorithm

Due to the absence of long-term clinical data on stent-graft performance, it is generally accepted that life-long imaging surveillance is necessary.[42] However, the ideal surveillance strategy has been widely debated. The Society of Interventional Radiology Device Forum,[43] recommends four views of the abdomen (AP, lateral, and oblique) performed after placement of the graft, and every 6 months for at least 2 years. In addition, imaging with CTA, MRI, or ultrasound should be considered at baseline. If no complications are present, surveillance should be repeated every 6 months for 2 years, and then yearly.[43] Some investigators[42,44] have used AP and lateral radiographs and CTA at less frequent intervals.

Imaging Techniques and Findings

Radiography

Radiography plays a useful role in the evaluation for stent graft expansion; migration, kinking, dislocation, and hook or tent fracture can be identified.[45] Although multiplanar reformations on CT allow characterization of many of

TABLE 102-2 Classification of Endoleaks

I	Attachment site leak (proximal, distal, or iliac occluder)
	A. Proximal
	B. Distal
	C. Iliac occluder
II	Collateral vessel leak(s)
	A. Single vessel
	B. Two or more vessels
III	Graft failure, junctional leak, or disconnection fabric disruption
	A. Junctional separation (modular devices)
	B. Endograft defect
IV	Graft-wall porosity
V	Endotension

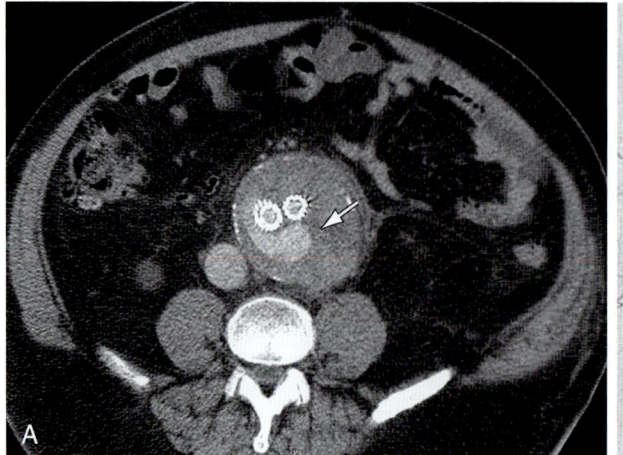

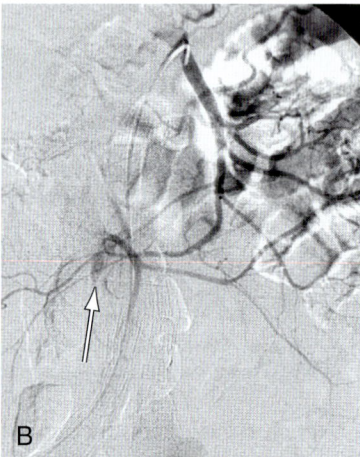

Adapted from Golzarian J, Valenti D. Endoleakage after endovascular treatment of abdominal aortic aneurysms: Diagnosis, significance and treatment. Eur Radiol 2006; 16(12):2849-2857.

■ **Figure 102-16** Type II endoleak after endovascular repair. Late phase contrast-enhanced axial CT (**A**) of the abdomen demonstrates contrast (*arrow*) in the excluded portion of an abdominal aortic aneurysm. **B**, Selective catheter inferior mesenteric arteriography demonstrates extravasation of contrast overlying the aortic endograft (*arrow*), consistent with a type II endovascular leak.

these complications, plain radiographs have the advantage because they are less susceptible to artifact from metallic prostheses.

Stent migration usually involves caudal migration of the proximal end, whereas the distal end of the stent is more likely to move cranially. Care should be taken to avoid parallax error when assessing for migration.[45] Kinking or deformity of the stent often accompanies migration.

Ultrasound

Techniques used for endoleak surveillance include color duplex ultrasound (CDU) and contrast enhanced ultrasound (CEUS) using a micro-bubble agent. Overall, studies have shown a greater sensitivity for endoleak detection when contrast-enhanced ultrasound is used. Reported sensitivities vary widely, ranging from 12% to 100%, likely because sonography for endoleaks is operator and experience dependent.[44]

Computed Tomography

MDCT remains the widely accepted gold standard for endoleak detection. Advantages of CT include multiplanar reconstructions, reproducibility, and fast speed of acquisition. A multiphasic technique is recommended, comprising precontrast imaging, an arterial phase, and a "delayed phase" acquired 60 to 120 seconds following the beginning of contrast injection. Delayed phase imaging has been shown to detect endoleaks not seen on the arterial phase, especially smaller endoleaks and type II endoleaks. It has been suggested that noncontrast CT can be omitted from examinations after the baseline examination to reduce radiation dose.

MRI

MRI is particularly suitable for the surveillance of nitinol stents, which have fewer artifacts on MRI. Stainless steel stents and elgiloy stents can cause extensive artifacts on MRI such that they may preclude proper visualization of the abdominal aortic lumen.[42] Studies have shown MRI to be at least as sensitive for endoleak detection as CT. MRI is typically performed using dynamic gadolinium-enhanced MRA (Fig. 102-17) using timing similar to CTA.

Treatment Options

Type I endoleaks: Proximal type I endoleaks should be repaired if fully supported grafts are used. Unsupported grafts with a proximal type I endoleak can be observed for up to 6 months if no sac expansion is noted. All distal type I endoleaks should be repaired when detected.

Type II endoleaks: Type II endoleaks noted on initial postoperative CT scan can be safely observed for 6 months in the absence of sac expansion. Most of these leaks are benign. However, if a new type II leak is detected or if there is sac expansion, coil embolization of the feeding vessel(s) should be considered.

Type III endoleaks: Coil embolization at the time of detection should be considered for all type III endoleaks.

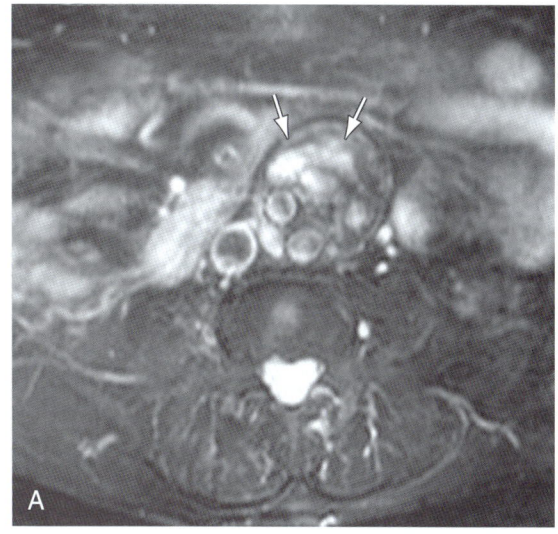

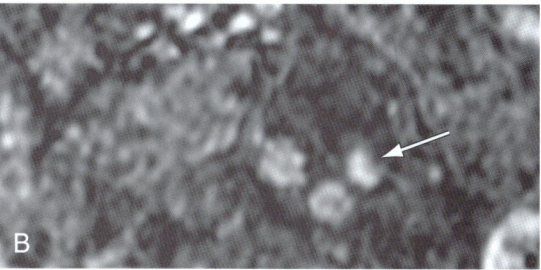

■ **Figure 102-17** Type II endoleak demonstrated with MRA. Axial T2 weighted sequence (**A**) demonstrates the heterogeneous signal of blood products and flow artifacts within the native sac (*arrows*). Following gadolinium (**B**), the endoleak is visible adjacent to one of the iliac limbs (*arrow*).

Type V endoleaks (endotension): Treatment of endotension is controversial. After careful exclusion of overt type I through III endoleaks, surgical revision should at least be considered.[46,47] Secondary endografting is more appropriate in critically sick patients who are poor surgical candidates.

TRAUMATIC ABDOMINAL AORTIC INJURY

Prevalence and Epidemiology

Abdominal aortic injuries are rare, and represent only 4% to 6% of aortic injuries. These injuries are commonly associated with high-speed motor vehicle accidents and have been linked to steering wheel injury to the lower abdomen and the use of lap-belt restraints.[48]

Etiology and Pathogenesis

The mechanism of injury is thought to be due to direct compression of the aorta against the spine, although other theories implicate stretching of the aortic wall from increased intraluminal pressure and aortic distraction from hyperflexion.

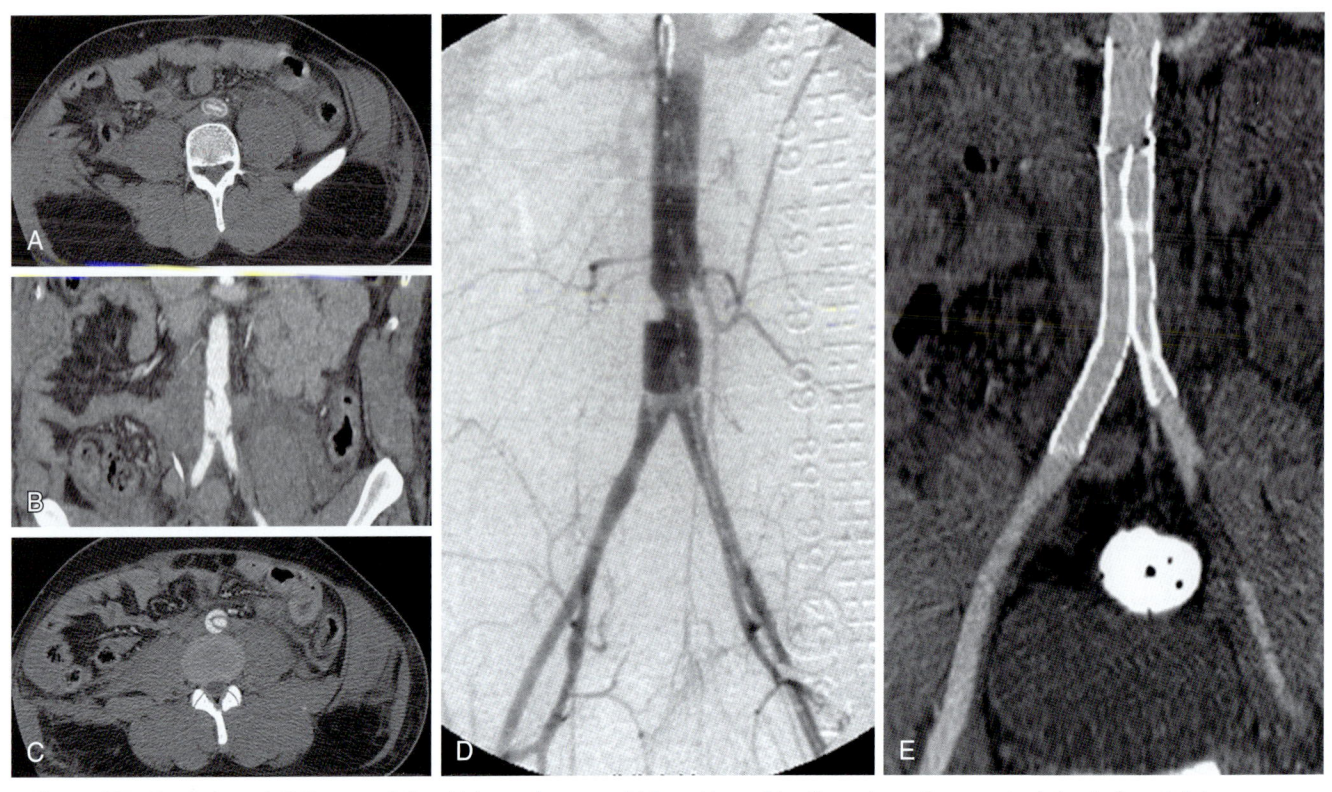

■ **Figure 102-18** A through E, Young male in a high-speed motor vehicle accident with a "stretch type" traumatic abdominal aortic injury. Intimomedial flaps at the level of the IMA and aortic bifurcation on axial and coronal CT are well demonstrated on catheter angiography (**D**). Owing to the presence of an associated bowel injury, endovascular repair (**E**) was performed.

Clinical Manifestations of Disease

Acute manifestations include symptoms of acute arterial insufficiency, an acute abdomen, or neurologic deficits. The lesion may be asymptomatic when there are no associated injuries to produce an acute abdomen or when there is a nonocclusive intimal flap.

Imaging Techniques and Findings

Radiography

As opposed to the thoracic aorta which can be screened readily with chest radiography, there is no good plain film screening modality for abdominal aortic injuries.

CT and MRI

On CT, the direct signs of abdominal aortic injuries include intimal flaps, irregular aortic morphology, focal enlargement of the aorta, and contrast extravasation.[49] Periaortic retroperitoneal hematoma may also be present. Abdominal aortic injuries are typically limited in length. The most commonly injured sites are at the level of the inferior mesenteric artery, renal arteries, and between the IMA and bifurcation (Fig. 102-18).[50] Given long acquisition times, MRI is not appropriate for imaging of aortic trauma in the acute setting.

Angiography

Catheter arteriogram of the aorta is the gold standard to confirm abdominal aortic injury.

Treatment Options

Treatment is necessary, except for those with minimal intimal disruptions. Surgical treatment is associated with an overall mortality of 27%. Because of the high incidence of associated bowel injury, surgical placement of a prosthetic graft at the time of initial laparotomy risks graft infection. Endoluminal treatment of aortic injuries using uncovered stents provides excellent results with inframesenteric aortic dissections.[50] For those cases of contained transection, both covered and uncovered stents have been employed successfully.

ACUTE AORTIC OCCLUSION

Acute occlusion of the abdominal aorta is a vascular emergency, usually resulting from a saddle embolus or thrombosis. It has a high mortality rate (75%) with conservative treatment.[51]

Etiology and Pathophysiology

Acute aortic occlusion may result from an aortic saddle embolus, thrombosis of preexisting atheromatous plaque, thrombosis of a small abdominal aortic aneurysm, or

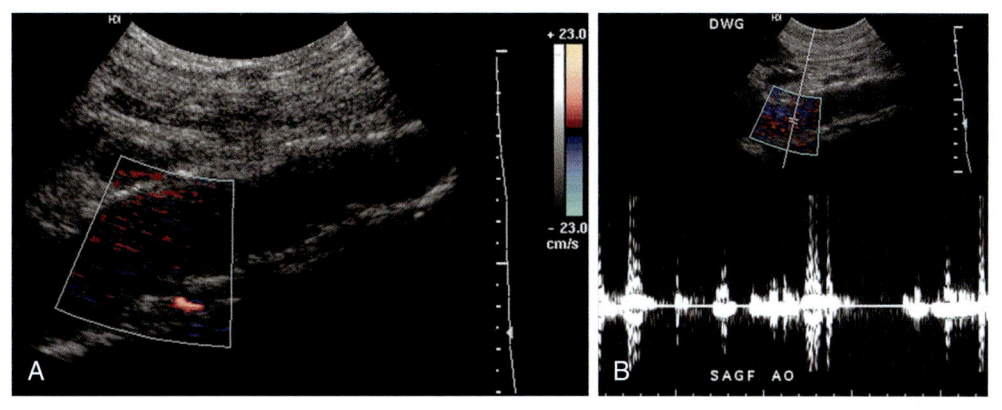

Figure 102-19 Color (**A**) and spectral Doppler of acute aortic occlusion. With high color gain settings, just noise is visible on color Doppler. No flow was present on spectral Doppler (**B**).

thrombosis related to aortic dissection. The high mortality likely results from the absence of collateral pathways at the time of presentation and common comorbid conditions such as cardiac disease (61%).[51]

Clinical Manifestations of Disease

The absence of both femoral pulses in a patient without significant atherosclerosis risk factors is highly suggestive of the diagnosis.[49] Patients may present with paralysis mimicking acute spinal cord compression, and a subsequent delay in diagnosis may increase mortality. Coexistent cardiac arrhythmias suggest a saddle embolus.

Imaging Indications and Algorithm

When acute aortic occlusion is suspected, CT is the most appropriate imaging modality given its wide availability and quick acquisition. If iodinated contrast is contraindicated (contrast allergy), MRI and ultrasound (Fig. 102-19) can also be used.

CT and MRI

On CT, acute aortic occlusion is manifested by the absence of contrast enhancement of the aorta distal to the occlusive site (Figs. 102-20 and 102-21). Collateral vessels will be largely absent. Secondary ischemia in bowel or solid organs may also be present due to global decreased perfusion or to small cardiac emboli. Cardiac sources of emboli are sometimes seen (Fig. 102-20). When present, abdominal aortic aneurysms are well evaluated by CT.

Findings in MRI are similar to those seen on CT. Noncontrast bright blood or black blood sequences may be useful when contrast cannot be administered. When present, abdominal aortic aneurysms are well evaluated by MRI. Given its long acquisition time, MRI is often not appropriate in acute presentations.

Angiography

An abrupt interruption of flow in the aorta at the level of the occlusion with a relative absence of arterial collaterals suggests the diagnosis. Abdominal aortic aneurysms may be occult on angiography if there is significant mural thrombus.

Treatment Options

Acute aortic occlusion is a surgical emergency. Heparin should be started to prevent further propagation of clot. Surgical procedures include transfemoral embolectomy (most useful in cases of saddle embolus) and bypass procedures.

TAKAYASU ARTERITIS

Takayasu arteritis (TA), also known as nonspecific aortitis, is a chronic inflammatory disorder that affects the aorta, branch vessels, and the pulmonary arteries. Progressive vascular occlusion with systemic ischemic symptoms usually ensue.

Etiology and Pathogenesis

The exact etiology of TA remains unclear, although infections, autoimmune and genetic factors may play a role. T cells and natural killer cells, which infiltrate the vessel wall, play a role in vascular injury; antiendothelial antibodies have also been reported.[52] Moreover, certain human leukocyte antigen (HLA) alleles, such as HLA-B52, HLA-B39, and HLA-DRB1*1301 have been associated with the disease in certain ethnic groups and in certain clinical situations.[53]

Histologically, TA is associated with a panarteritis in the acute phase. Mononuclear cell infiltrates occur in the adventitia with cuffing of the vasa vasorum, and the media is infiltrated by lymphocytes and the occasional giant cells. During the chronic phase of the disease, there is thickening of the vessel wall with fibrosis of the adventitia, destruction of the media, and intimal proliferation with secondary luminal narrowing. Medial destruction, without significant intimal fibrosis, can lead to aneurysm formation. Involvement is usually patchy, with intervening "skipped areas."

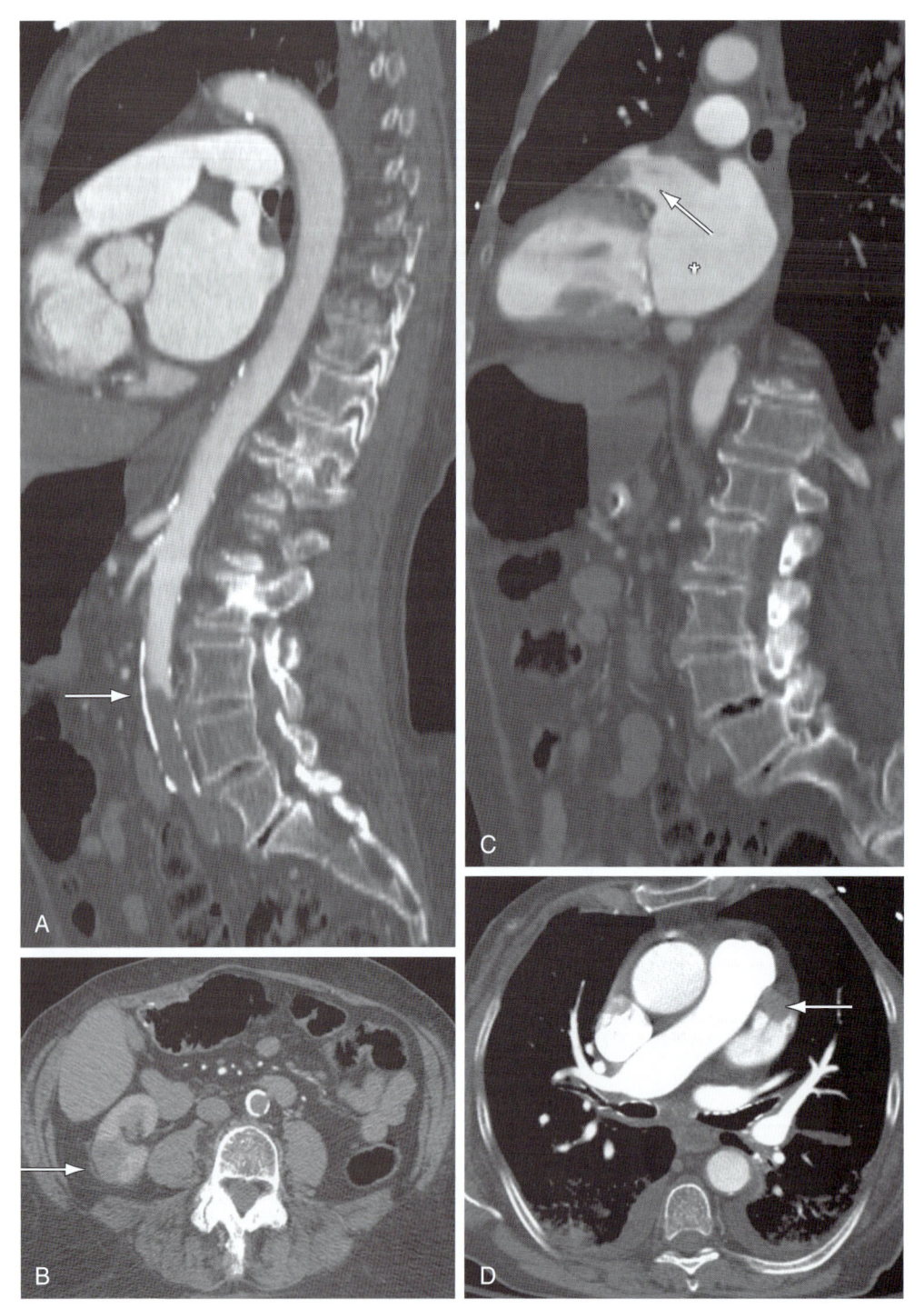

Figure 102-20 **A,** Contrast-enhanced CTA in a 91-year-old woman with long-standing atrial fibrillation who presented with white, pale, and pulseless legs. Abrupt cutoff of contrast within the infrarenal abdominal aorta (*white arrow*) is accompanied by infarction of the right kidney (**B,** *thin arrow*). This suggests a more proximal embolic source. **C** and **D,** CT of the chest in the same patient demonstrates left atrial enlargement (*asterisk*) and thrombus in the left atrial appendage (*white arrow*).

Prevalence and Epidemiology

Takayasu disease predominantly affects young women, with a mean age of diagnosis of 35 years, although nearly 20% of cases present after the age of 40.[53] It has been most commonly reported in people of Asian descent.

Clinical Manifestations

Three clinical phases are described in TA: an early "pre-pulseless" systemic phase, a later occlusive phase, and a final "burned out" phase. The phases usually overlap. Most patients present during the occlusive phase of disease.

During the "prepulseless" phase, diagnosis is difficult because patients have nonspecific signs including fever, weight loss, and arthralgias. In the occlusive phase, ischemic complications dominate: claudication, angina, visual impairment, and syncope. The American College of Rheumatology has developed classification criteria for Takayasu disease.[54]

Differential Diagnosis

The differential diagnosis depends on patient symptoms and signs. Other vasculitides should be the main consideration if there is multisystemic inflammation.

Imaging Indications and Algorithm

Ultrasound

Characteristic long segments of smooth, homogeneous, mildly echogenic circumferential wall thickening are present. This has been called the "macaroni phenomenon."[55] Unlike atherosclerosis, the wall is not irregular, and there are few, if any, calcifications.

Especially in the extracranial carotid arteries, ultrasonography has been shown to be accurate in the assessment of arterial wall thickness measurements and surveillance of wall thickness following steroid treatment. Intravascular sonography provides high spatial resolution imaging to assess for early or subtle wall changes.

CT and MRI

Both the vessel wall and lumen are well evaluated on CT and MRI. Therefore, these techniques have advantages for the detection of early disease. Concentric arterial wall thickening is seen early on. With continued inflammation, vascular stenoses, occlusions, and aneurysms develop (Fig. 102-22).

Not only does MRI enable assessment of vessel wall involvement, it is ideal for serial follow-up in young patients. Patients can be comprehensively evaluated with MRI without the risks of ionizing radiation. The pulmonary arteries and extracranial arteries, as well as the aorta, can be evaluated. Findings described with MRI and MRA include increased T2 signal around inflamed vessels, aortic wall thickening, vascular dilation, multifocal stenoses, and collateral vessels.[56]

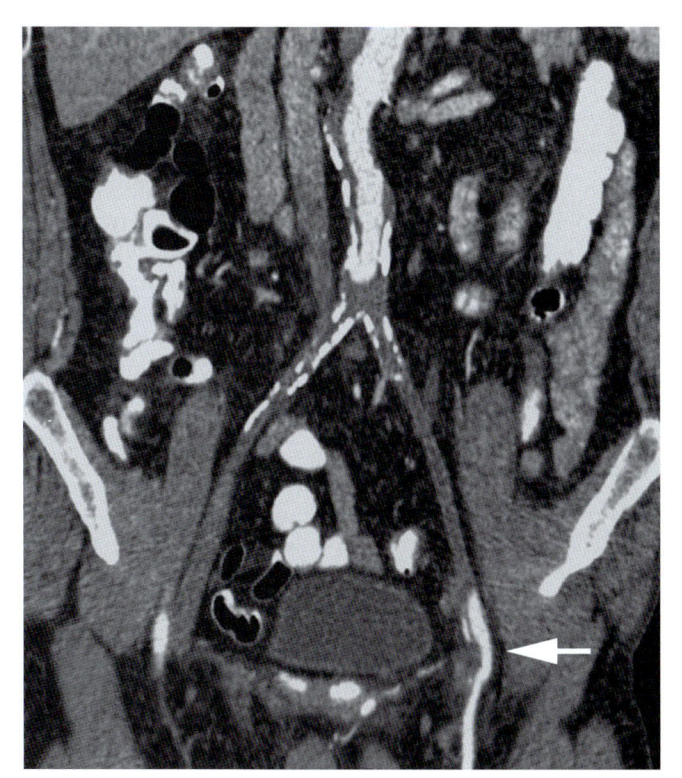

■ **Figure 102-21** Curved planar reformat of chronic aortic occlusion in an 81-year-old male. The rounded contour of the aortic occlusion and collateral filling of the left external iliac artery (*arrow*) is consistent with chronic occlusion.

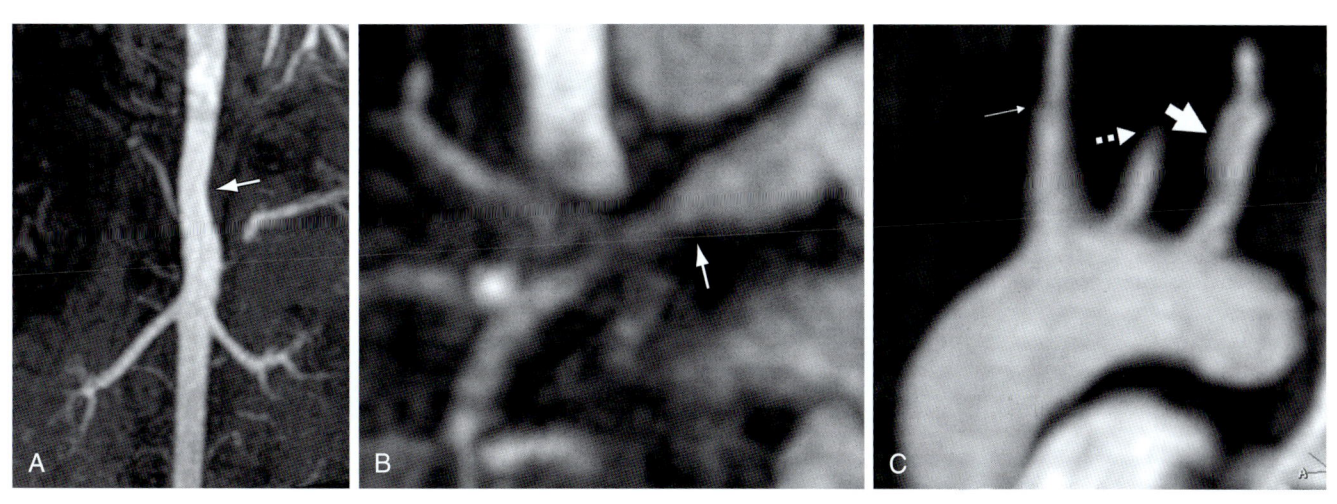

■ **Figure 102-22** Takayasu arteritis. Irregular narrowing of the suprarenal abdominal aorta (**A**) is accompanied by right pulmonary artery stenosis (**B**). In addition, there is occlusion in C (*dotted arrow*), stenosis (*small arrow*), and focal aneurysm formation (*large arrow*) of the branches of the aortic arch.

Arteriography

Arteriography is the traditional gold-standard technique for TA. Like CTA, and MRA, angiography demonstrates smooth-walled, focal, narrowed areas and collateral pathways. However, arteriography is superior in that it better depicts very small vessels and can directly measure pressure differences. Intravascular ultrasound can be used to assess for early changes.

PET

^{18}F-fluorodeoxyglucose positron emission tomography (^{18}FDG-PET) and ^{18}FDG-PET co-registered with contrast enhanced CT have recently been suggested as a means of evaluating the early changes of TA, and showing the distribution of inflammatory activity in the aorta and its branches,[57] with high diagnostic accuracy.[58] The uptake pattern in the early stages of disease is linear and continuous.[58] Uptake becomes more patchy in later disease.

Treatment Options

Medical

Glucocorticoids are the primary treatment for TA, usually arresting disease progression and systemic inflammation. Arterial stenosis may reverse unless there has been associated fibrosis of the aortic wall.[59] In cases refractory to steroids, trials of methotrexate, azathioprine, or other immunomodulators can be initiated.

Surgical

Percutaneous angioplasty or surgical bypass grafts may be considered in cases where significant ischemic symptoms and irreversible arterial stenosis are present. Given its less invasive nature, percutaneous angioplasty is currently the first-line invasive measure. However, surgical intervention is often required in cases of long stenosis or heavy fibrosis.

GIANT CELL ARTERITIS (TEMPORAL ARTERITIS)

Giant cell arteritis is the most common idiopathic vasculitis of the large- and medium-sized arteries. It classically affects the temporal artery and other cranial vessels, although the aorta may be affected.

Prevalence and Epidemiology

The prevalence of giant cell arteritis in the United States is approximately 160,000 cases (approximately 0.06%), which is likely an underestimate given that many patients have subclinical disease.[60] Affected patients tend to be older than 50 years of age.

Etiology and Pathophysiology

Alhough both the humoral and cellular immune system are involved in the pathogenesis of giant cell arteritis, cell-mediated processes are paramount.[61] The initial activating factor is unknown; autoantigens, infectious agents, and toxins have been implicated. Transmural inflammation of the arteries results in eventual luminal occlusion through intimal hyperplasia of branch vessels of the aorta. However, in the aorta, inflammation results in aneurysm formation, dissection, and rupture.

Differential Diagnosis

Other vasculitides should be the main consideration if there is multisystemic inflammation.

Clinical Manifestations of Disease

Almost all patients with giant cell arteritis demonstrate signs of systemic inflammation: anorexia, weight loss, fever, malaise, and night sweats. Abrupt visual disturbances and jaw claudication occur commonly. Approximately one third of patients will have polymyalgia rheumatica. Inflammatory markers are typically elevated. Diagnosis is typically achieved through temporal artery biopsy.

Imaging Indications and Algorithm

Abdominal aortic aneurysms and dissection associated with giant cell arteritis may be detected on CT, MRI, and angiography. Abnormal FDG-PET uptake may also be helpful in the setting of giant cell arteritis.

Imaging Techniques and Findings

CT and MRI

Abdominal aortic aneurysms, dissections, and rupture can be detected with CT or MRI. On CT, associated mural aortic thickening (Fig. 102-23) (possibly representing inflammatory tissue proliferation) may also be present.[62] On MRI, high mural signal on fluid-sensitive sequences and mural wall enhancement within the aorta may represent active inflammation.[63]

Angiography

Catheter angiography remains the gold standard in the evaluation of arterial vasculitis. Aortic aneurysm, dissection, and rupture can be readily diagnosed with this modality. However, given the availability of noninvasive imaging modalities with less radiation exposure, catheter arteriography is being used less frequently in the diagnosis of giant cell arteritis.

PET

FDG-PET is a sensitive marker for large vessel vasculitis and may be a contributory tool in the diagnosis and follow up of giant cell arteritis. Increased uptake may be present in the walls of the aorta and branch vessels, most often in a linear continuous pattern.[58] The degree of FDG-PET uptake in the aortic wall may correlate with the degree of aortic inflammation.[58] In addition, increased FDG uptake may correlate with aortic enlargement.[64]

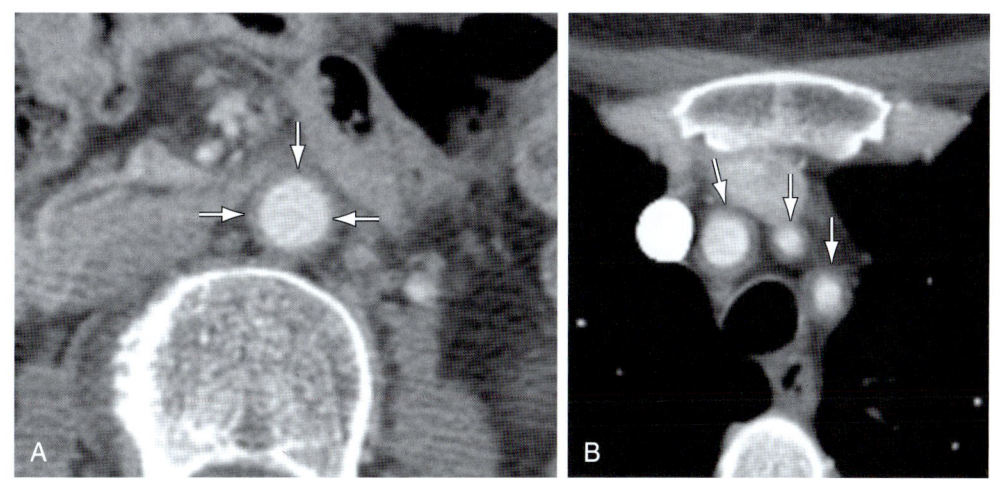

Figure 102-23 Vessel wall thickening in a 71-year-old woman with giant cell arteritis and a chronically elevated erythrocyte sedimentation rate. Axial contrast-enhanced CT demonstrates circumferential soft tissue thickening of the abdominal aortic wall (**A**, *arrows*) and branch vessel of the aortic arch (**B**, *arrows*).

Treatment Options

Medical

Treatment with glucocorticoids can be started promptly if giant cell arteritis is suspected. Temporal artery biopsy should be considered. Even with a negative arterial biopsy result, if there is high clinical suspicion for giant cell arteritis, glucocorticoid treatment should be continued.

Surgical and Interventional

The natural history of giant cell arteritis is not known. Currently, treatment recommendations are based on criteria for aortic repair in atherosclerotic abdominal aortic aneurysms. Abdominal aortic aneurysms larger than 5.5 cm that are growing rapidly or demonstrating dissection, are repaired. Open repair has been the intervention of choice. Endovascular repair may be a viable option in the treatment of abdominal aortic aneurysms related to giant cell arteritis.[65]

AORTOENTERIC FISTULAS

Abdominal aortoenteric fistulas (AEF) are direct communications between the abdominal aorta and the gastrointestinal tract.

Prevalence and Epidemiology

Approximately 80% of aortoenteric fistulas arise in the duodenum, and about 60% of these arise in the third part.[66] Outside the duodenum, the jejunum, sigmoid colon, stomach, and ileum can be involved. Aorta-duodenal fistulas following surgical repair of a prior aortic aneurysm (secondary) are more common than de novo aorta-duodenal fistulas from an abdominal aortic aneurysm (primary). Aorta-duodenal fistulas occur approximately 0.4% to 2.4% of the time following aortic aneurysm surgery. They can manifest soon after surgery or years later.

Etiology and Pathogenesis

The propensity for fistula to the duodenum likely relates to the location of the third part of the duodenum, which is fixed in the retroperitoneum just anterior to the aorta. Aortic expansion and inflammation likely lead to duodenal inflammation, and eventual fistulization. Failure of separation of the bowel from the graft, accompanied by mechanical pulsations of the prosthetic graft, can lead to pressure necrosis of the bowel. Infection may also play a role. Primary aortoenteric fistulas arise from atherosclerotic aneurysms, mycotic aneurysms, and traumatic pseudoaneurysms, as well as many other inflammatory and neoplastic diseases of the aorta and gastrointestinal tract.

Clinical Manifestations of Disease

The classic clinical triad consists of gastrointestinal hemorrhage, abdominal pain, and a pulsatile abdominal mass, but this is found in a minority of patients. Patients may present with an initial small "herald" bleed (hematemesis or hematochezia), and later develop uncontrollable bleeding leading to exsanguination. Alternatively, there may be recurrent intermittent gastrointestinal bleeding. Associated constitutional symptoms occur—likely related to concomitant periaortic infection.

Imaging Indications and Algorithms

Because patients with aortoenteric fistulas can quickly exsanguinate, CT is used most commonly. Endoscopy is also performed. Ultrasound, nuclear medicine studies, and MRI do not reliably detect aortoenteric fistulas.

CT

There may be significant overlap in the CT appearance of periaortic infection and aortoenteric fistulas. In both cases, ectopic gas (Fig. 102-24), periaortic fluid, periaortic soft tissue thickening, bowel wall thickening, periaortic

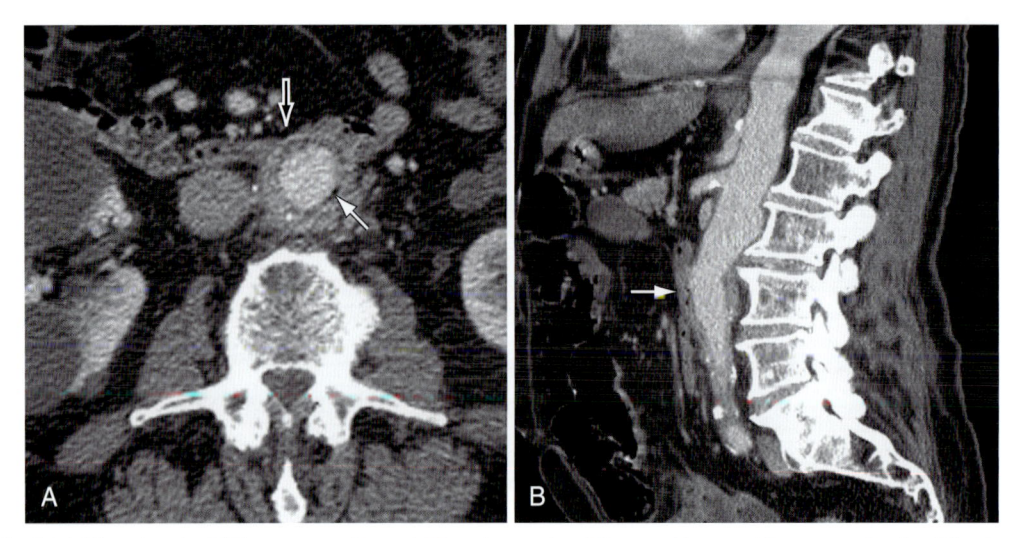

■ **Figure 102-24** Axial (**A**) and sagittal (**B**) contrast-enhanced CT angiogram in a 78-year-old man with an aortoduodenal fistula who presented with hematemesis. He had an open aneurysm repair ten years earlier. Gas is present within the aortic sac (*white arrow*). The proximal end of the aortic graft is surrounded by soft tissue and is inseparable from the third part of the duodenum (*open arrow*). On duodenoscopy, aortic graft material was seen eroding through the posterior wall of the duodenum.

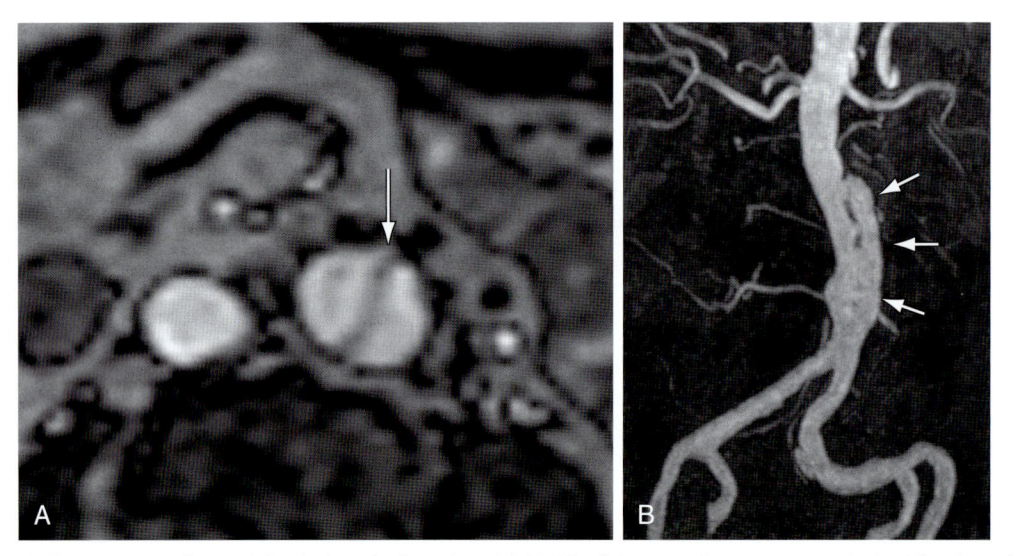

■ **Figure 102-25** **A**, Spontaneous primary abdominal aortic dissection. Axial MPR of the aorta demonstrates an intimal flap (*arrow*). The right lumen is the true lumen. **B**, Coronal MIP of the aorta demonstrates the left false lumen (*arrows*) of the aortic dissection.

fat plane obliteration, and pseudoaneurysms may be present.[67] To definitively diagnose aortoenteric fistula, blood or contrast leaking into bowel must be visualized. The presence of a secondary aortoenteric fistula can also be inferred if the aortic graft is seen within bowel lumen.[68]

Treatment Options

Surgical treatment and antibiotic treatment are paramount. In cases of secondary fistulas, the infected graft is removed and extra-anatomic bypass is placed. Infected graft removal and in situ graft replacement has also been proposed as an alternative. Primary fistulas can be treated similarly. Endovascular repair may be a temporizing step in patients too ill for immediate surgery.[69]

ABDOMINAL AORTIC DISSECTION

Abdominal aortic dissection consists of an entry tear in the inner layers of the wall of the abdominal aorta, allowing blood to flow between the mural layers. Spontaneous abdominal aortic dissections not associated with thoracic aortic dissection are extremely rare, representing approximately 2% of all aortic dissections.

In a review of the literature by Farber and colleagues,[70] about 40% of spontaneous abdominal aortic dissections were associated with AAA. Abdominal aortic dissection may be the result of atheromatous disease; conversely, the dissection may cause aneurysm formation due to a weakened wall. Abdominal aortic dissections generally originate at or below the level of the renal arteries (Fig. 102-25).

They may be iatrogenic (e.g., as a complication of vascular catheterization), traumatic, or spontaneous. Like thoracic dissection, isolated aortic dissection is associated with hypertension.[71] Marfan syndrome has not been associated with abdominal aortic dissection. Patients usually present with back pain, peripheral ischemia, and signs of distal embolization but may be asymptomatic. A pulsatile abdominal mass is usually present.

Because of its low incidence, the natural history is unknown, although rupture has been reported in up to 25% of patients in one study.[70] In uncomplicated cases, medical management typically consists of blood pressure control and vasodilators. Treatment may include open or endovascular repair in patients with major aortic branch occlusion, aortic expansion, extension of the dissection, and aortic rupture.

KEY POINTS

- **Abdominal aortic aneurysm**
  - Strongly related to smoking
  - Elective repair of aneurysms 5.5 cm in "average" males and 4.5 to 5 cm in women
  - Signs of impending/contained rupture: high attenuation crescent sign, draped aorta sign
  - Signs of rupture: contrast extravasation, periaortic hematoma or fat stranding
- **Inflammatory abdominal aortic aneurysm**
  - Cuff of inflammatory soft tissue, similar in density to the psoas muscles and undergoing contrast enhancement
  - Sparing of the posterior wall of the aorta
  - Encasement or obstruction of the ureters, bowel, or inferior vena cava (IVC)
- **Infected/mycotic aortic aneurysm**
  - Saccular contour and rapid growth
  - Periaortic soft tissue mass, stranding, or fluid
- **Complications of endovascular aortic aneurysm**
  - Type II endoleaks are most common.
  - Type I, III leaks should be treated. Type II leaks should be treated if they are new or if there is associated sac expansion.
- **Traumatic abdominal aortic injury**
  - CT is the most appropriate imaging modality.
  - Direct findings include intimal flaps, irregular aortic morphology, focal enlargement of the aorta, and contrast extravasation.
  - Usually requires surgical/endovascular treatment unless limited to the intima.
- **Acute aortic occlusion**
  - Acute loss of both femoral pulses without known significant atherosclerosis risk factors
  - Abrupt interruption of flow at the level of the aortic occlusion with a relative absence of arterial collaterals
  - Imaging may reveal a cardiac source
- **Takayasu arteritis**
  - Chronic inflammatory disorder of the aorta, branch vessels, and pulmonary arteries.
  - Concentric arterial wall thickening followed later by vascular stenoses, occlusions, and aneurysms.
  - Treatment primarily involved glucocorticoids; angioplasty or surgical intervention.
  - Giant cell arteritis (temporal arteritis).
  - Idiopathic vasculitis affecting the large- and medium-sized arteries.
  - Diagnoses usually requires a temporal artery biopsy.
  - Abdominal aortic aneurysms, dissections, and rupture may be present.
  - Aortic wall thickening, mural edema, and enhancement.
- **Aortoenteric fistulas**
  - Most often secondary to surgical aortic repair.
  - Third portion of the duodenum the most common area affected.
  - Periaortic infection almost always coexists.
  - Contrast extravasation into bowel or an aortic graft within the bowel.
  - Ectopic gas, periaortic fluid, periaortic soft-tissue thickening, bowel wall thickening, periaortic fat plane obliteration, and pseudoaneurysms common.

SUGGESTED READINGS

Gotway MB, et al. Imaging findings in Takayasu's arteritis. AJR Am J Roentgenol 2005; 184(6):1945-1950.

Hellmann DB, Grand DJ, Freischlag JA. Inflammatory abdominal aortic aneurysm. JAMA 2007; 297(4):395-400.

Isselbacher EM. Thoracic and abdominal aortic aneurysms. Circulation 2005; 111(6):816-828.

Rakita D, et al. Spectrum of CT findings in rupture and impending rupture of abdominal aortic aneurysms. Radiographics 2007; 27(2):497-507.

Sakalihasan N, Hustinx R, Limet R. Contribution of PET scanning to the evaluation of abdominal aortic aneurysm. Semin Vasc Surg 2004; 17(2):144-153.

Screening for abdominal aortic aneurysm: recommendation statement. Ann Intern Med 2005; 142(3):198-202.

Stavropoulos SW, Charagundla SR. Imaging techniques for detection and management of endoleaks after endovascular aortic aneurysm repair. Radiology 2007; 243(3):641-655.

REFERENCES

1. Kalva SP, et al. Using the K-edge to improve contrast conspicuity and to lower radiation dose with a 16-MDCT: a phantom and human study. J Comput Assist Tomogr 2006; 30(3):391-397.
2. Maki JH, et al. Steady-state free precession MRA of the renal arteries: breath-hold and navigator-gated techniques vs. CE-MRA. J Magn Reson Imaging 2007; 26(4)966-973.
3. Schwope RB, et al. MR angiography for patient surveillance after endovascular repair of abdominal aortic aneurysms. AJR Am J Roentgenol 2007; 188(4):W334-W340.
4. Pereles FS, et al. Thoracic aortic dissection and aneurysm: evaluation with nonenhanced true FISP MR angiography in less than 4 minutes. Radiology 2002; 223(1):270-274.

5. Cohen EI, et al. Time-resolved MR angiography for the classification of endoleaks after endovascular aneurysm repair. J Magn Reson Imaging 2008; 27(3)500-503.
6. Kubo S, et al. Thoracoabdominal-aortoiliac MDCT angiography using reduced dose of contrast material. AJR Am J Roentgenol 2006; 187(2):548-554.
7. Johnston KW, et al. Suggested standards for reporting on arterial aneurysms. Subcommittee on Reporting Standards for Arterial Aneurysms, Ad Hoc Committee on Reporting Standards, Society for Vascular Surgery and North American Chapter, International Society for Cardiovascular Surgery. J Vasc Surg 1991; 13(3):452-458.
8. Lederle FA, et al. Prevalence and associations of abdominal aortic aneurysm detected through screening. Aneurysm Detection and Management (ADAM) Veterans Affairs Cooperative Study Group. Ann Intern Med 1997; 126(6)441-449.
9. Multicentre aneurysm screening study (MASS): cost effectiveness analysis of screening for abdominal aortic aneurysms based on four year results from randomised controlled trial. BMJ 2002; 325(7373):1135.
10. Isselbacher EM. Thoracic and abdominal aortic aneurysms. Circulation 2005; 111(6)816-828.
11. Tang T, et al. Inflammatory abdominal aortic aneurysms. Eur J Vasc Endovasc Surg 2005; 29(4)353-362.
12. Brown PM, et al. Selective management of abdominal aortic aneurysms in a prospective measurement program. J Vasc Surg 1996; 23(2):213-220; discussion 221-222.
13. Hallin A, Bergqvist D, Holmberg L. Literature review of surgical management of abdominal aortic aneurysm. Eur J Vasc Endovasc Surg 2001; 22(3):197-204.
14. Mortality results for randomised controlled trial of early elective surgery or ultrasonographic surveillance for small abdominal aortic aneurysms. The UK Small Aneurysm Trial Participants. Lancet 1998; 352(9141):1649-1655.
15. Siegel CL, et al. Abdominal aortic aneurysm morphology: CT features in patients with ruptured and nonruptured aneurysms. AJR Am J Roentgenol 1994; 163(5)1123-1129.
16. U.S. Preventive Services Task Force. Screening for abdominal aortic aneurysm: recommendation statement. Ann Intern Med, 2005; 142(3):198-202.
17. Julius Grollman, M.A.B., Thomas Casciani, Antoinette S. Expert Panel on Vascular Imaging: Gomes, Stephen R. Holtzman, Joseph F. Polak, David Sacks, William Stanford, Michael Jaff, Gregory L. Moneta. American College of Radiology ACR Appropriateness Criteria: Pulsatile Abdominal Mass. 2005 2005 [cited 2008 December 2, 2008]; Available from: http://www.acr.org/SecondaryMainMenuCategories/quality_safety/app_criteria/pdf/Vascular/PulsatileAbdominalMassDoc13.aspx.
18. Rumack CM, Wilson SR, Charboneau JW. Diagnostic Ultrasound. 3rd ed. St. Louis, 2005. Elsevier Mosby. 2 v. (xxiv, 2080, xxxiv).
19. Rakita D, et al. Spectrum of CT findings in rupture and impending rupture of abdominal aortic aneurysms. Radiographics 2007; 27(2):497-507.
20. Sprouse LR, 2nd, et al. Comparison of abdominal aortic aneurysm diameter measurements obtained with ultrasound and computed tomography: Is there a difference? J Vasc Surg 2003; 38(3):466-471; discussion 471-472.
21. Mehard WB, Heiken JP, Sicard GA. High-attenuating crescent in abdominal aortic aneurysm wall at CT: a sign of acute or impending rupture. Radiology 1994; 192(2):359-362.
22. Halliday KE, al-Kutoubi A. Draped aorta: CT sign of contained leak of aortic aneurysms. Radiology 1996; 199(1):41-43.
23. Schwartz SA, et al. CT findings of rupture, impending rupture, and contained rupture of abdominal aortic aneurysms. AJR Am J Roentgenol, 2007; 188(1):W57-W62.
24. Sakalihasan N, Hustinx R, Limet R. Contribution of PET scanning to the evaluation of abdominal aortic aneurysm. Semin Vasc Surg 2004;17(2):144-153.
25. Reeps C, et al. Increased 18F-fluorodeoxyglucose uptake in abdominal aortic aneurysms in positron emission/computed tomography is associated with inflammation, aortic wall instability, and acute symptoms. J Vasc Surg 2008;48(2):417-423; discussion 424.
26. Powell JT, Greenhalgh RM. Clinical practice. Small abdominal aortic aneurysms. N Engl J Med 2003; 348(19):1895-1901.
27. Wilmink TB, Quick CR, Day NE. The association between cigarette smoking and abdominal aortic aneurysms. J Vasc Surg 1999; 30(6):1099-1105.
28. Gadowski GR, Pilcher DB, Ricci MA. Abdominal aortic aneurysm expansion rate: effect of size and beta-adrenergic blockade. J Vasc Surg 1994; 19(4):727-731.
29. Cullenward MJ, et al. Inflammatory aortic aneurysm (periaortic fibrosis): radiologic imaging. Radiology 1986; 159(1)75-82.
30. Iino M, et al. Sensitivity and specificity of CT in the diagnosis of inflammatory abdominal aortic aneurysms. J Comput Assist Tomogr 2002; 26(6):1006-1012.
31. Hellmann DB, Grand DJ, Fielschlag JA. Inflammatory abdominal aortic aneurysm. JAMA 2007; 297(4):395-400.
32. Puchner S, et al. Endovascular therapy of inflammatory aortic aneurysms: a meta-analysis. J Endovasc Ther 2005; 12(5):560-567.
33. Macedo TA, et al. Infected aortic aneurysms: imaging findings. Radiology 2004; 231(1):250-257.
34. Oderich GS, et al. Infected aortic aneurysms: aggressive presentation, complicated early outcome, but durable results. J Vasc Surg 2001; 34(5):900-908.
35. Cina CS, et al. Ruptured mycotic thoracoabdominal aortic aneurysms: a report of three cases and a systematic review. J Vasc Surg 2001; 33(4):861-867.
36. Katz SG, Andros G, Kohl RD. Salmonella infections of the abdominal aorta. Surg Gynecol Obstet 1992;175(2):102-106.
37. Chan FY, et al. In situ prosthetic graft replacement for mycotic aneurysm of the aorta. Ann Thorac Surg 1989; 47(2):193-203.
38. Corso JE, Kasirajan K, Milner R. Endovascular management of ruptured, mycotic abdominal aortic aneurysm. Am Surg 2005; 71(6):515-517.
39. Koeppel TA, et al. Mycotic aneurysm of the abdominal aorta with retroperitoneal abscess: successful endovascular repair. J Vasc Surg 2004; 40(1):164-166.
40. Schurink GW, Aarts NJ, van Bockel JH. Endoleak after stent-graft treatment of abdominal aortic aneurysm: a meta-analysis of clinical studies. Br J Surg 1999; 86(5):581-587.
41. Golzarian J, Valenti D. Endoleakage after endovascular treatment of abdominal aortic aneurysms: diagnosis, significance and treatment. Eur Radiol 2006; 16(12):2849-2857.
42. Stavropoulos SW, Charagundla SR. Imaging techniques for detection and management of endoleaks after endovascular aortic aneurysm repair. Radiology 2007; 243(3):641-655.
43. Geller SC, Imaging guidelines for abdominal aortic aneurysm repair with endovascular stent grafts. J Vasc Interv Radiol 2003; 14(9 Pt 2): S263-S264.
44. Manning BJ, O'Neill SM, Haider SN, et al. Duplex ultrasound in aneurysm surveillance following endovascular aneurysm repair: a comparison with computed tomography aortography. J Vasc Surg 2008; 49(1):60-65.
45. Fearn S, et al. Follow-up after endovascular aortic aneurysm repair: the plain radiograph has an essential role in surveillance. J Endovasc Ther 2003; 10(5):894-901.
46. Kougias P, et al. Successful treatment of endotension and aneurysm sac enlargement with endovascular stent graft reinforcement. J Vasc Surg 2007; 46(1):124-127.
47. Veith FJ, et al. Nature and significance of endoleaks and endotension: summary of opinions expressed at an international conference. J Vasc Surg 2002; 35(5):1029-1035.
48. Roth SM, et al. Blunt injury of the abdominal aorta: a review. J Trauma 1997; 42(4):748-755.
49. Bhalla S, Menias CO, Heiken JP. CT of acute abdominal aortic disorders. Radiol Clin North Am 2003; 41(6):1153-1169.
50. Gunn M, Campbell M, Hoffer EK. Traumatic abdominal aortic injury treated by endovascular stent placement. Emerg Radiol 2007; 13(6):329-331.
51. Surowiec SM, et al. Acute occlusion of the abdominal aorta. Am J Surg 1998; 176(2):193-197.
52. Maffei S, et al. Takayasu's arteritis: a review of the literature. Intern Emerg Med 2006; 1(2):105-112.
53. Maksimowicz-McKinnon K, Hoffman GS. Takayasu arteritis: what is the long-term prognosis? Rheum Dis Clin North Am 2007; 33(4):777-786, vi.
54. Arend WP, et al. The American College of Rheumatology 1990 criteria for the classification of Takayasu arteritis. Arthritis Rheum 1990; 33(8):1129-1134.

55. Schmidt WA, Gromnica-Ihle E. What is the best approach to diagnosing large-vessel vasculitis? Best Pract Res Clin Rheumatol 2005; 19(2): 223-242.
56. Gotway MB, et al. Imaging findings in Takayasu's arteritis. AJR Am J Roentgenol 2005; 184(6):1945-1950.
57. Kobayashi Y, et al. Aortic wall inflammation due to Takayasu arteritis imaged with 18F-FDG PET coregistered with enhanced CT. J Nucl Med 2005; 46(6):917-922.
58. Walter MA. [(18)F]fluorodeoxyglucose PET in large vessel vasculitis. Radiol Clin North Am 2007; 45(4):735-744, viii.
59. Kerr GS. Takayasu's arteritis. Rheum Dis Clin North Am 1995; 21(4):1041-1058.
60. Anchishkin AI, Khodyreva V, Kurilov EN. [An organizational model for the activities of microbiology laboratories]. Zh Mikrobiol Epidemiol Immunobiol 1991; (5):79.
61. Weyand CM, Goronzy JJ. Medium- and large-vessel vasculitis. N Engl J Med 2003; 349(2):160-169.
62. Agard C, et al. Aortic involvement in recent-onset giant cell (temporal) arteritis: a case-control prospective study using helical aortic computed tomodensitometric scan. Arthritis Rheum 2008; 59(5) 670-676.
63. Narvaez J, et al. Giant cell arteritis and polymyalgia rheumatica: usefulness of vascular magnetic resonance imaging studies in the diagnosis of aortitis. Rheumatology (Oxford), 2005; 44(4):479-483.
64. Blockmans D, et al. Relationship between fluorodeoxyglucose uptake in the large vessels and late aortic diameter in giant cell arteritis. Rheumatology (Oxford) 2008; 47(8):1179-1184.
65. Baril DT, et al. Endovascular treatment of complicated aortic aneurysms in patients with underlying arteriopathies. Ann Vasc Surg 2006; 20(4):464-471.
66. Lemos DW, et al. Primary aortoduodenal fistula: a case report and review of the literature. J Vasc Surg 2003; 37(3):686-689.
67. Low RN, et al. Aortoenteric fistula and perigraft infection: evaluation with CT. Radiology 1990; 175(1):157-162.
68. Hagspiel KD, et al. Diagnosis of aortoenteric fistulas with CT angiography. J Vasc Interv Radiol 2007; 18(4):497-504.
69. Saers SJ, Scheltinga MR. Primary aortoenteric fistula. Br J Surg 2005; 92(2):143-152.
70. Farber A, et al. Spontaneous infrarenal abdominal aortic dissection presenting as claudication: case report and review of the literature. Ann Vasc Surg 2004; 18(1):4-10.
71. Trimarchi S, et al. Acute abdominal aortic dissection: insight from the International Registry of Acute Aortic Dissection (IRAD). J Vasc Surg 2007; 46(5):913-919.

CHAPTER 103

Postendograft Imaging of the Abdominal Aorta and Iliac Arteries

Thomas G. Vrachliotis, Kostaki G. Bis, and Lisa M. Dias

The primary complication of abdominal aortic aneurysm (AAA) is acute rupture, a frequently lethal event.[1] As a rule, even large abdominal aortic aneurysms are asymptomatic until rupture occurs.[2,3] In the United States, a ruptured abdominal aortic aneurysm is the 10th leading cause of death in patients older than 55 years. Risk of rupture is directly related to aneurysmal size, with a 5% to 10% annual risk of rupture for AAAs measuring between 5 and 6 cm. There is controversy regarding the exact size at which an aneurysm should be repaired. Surgical repair has been advocated for AAAs reaching 5.0 to 5.5 cm in size by several authors; however, open surgical repair is a major operation, with an overall operative mortality ranging between 4% and 8.4%.[3,4] Endovascular repair of abdominal aortic aneurysms with the use of stent grafts has emerged as a new imaging-guided procedure (Fig. 103-1). The use of stent grafts for repair of AAA in humans was first described in 1991 by Parodi and colleagues,[5] who constructed devices from Palmaz stents and a standard woven polyethylene terephthalate surgical graft material.

Similarly, the natural course of an iliac artery aneurysm (IAA) consists of progressive expansion with eventual rupture. Involvement of iliac arteries is seen in 10% to 20% of patients with AAAs.[6] IAA is defined as enlargement of the iliac artery to a diameter of more than 1.5 cm. The natural course of an IAA consists of progressive expansion with eventual rupture, and the risk of rupture increases with aneurysm size.[7] Surgical repair should be recommended for isolated IAAs larger than 3.0 to 3.5 cm in diameter.[8,9] A variety of minimally invasive therapeutic options have now become available (e.g., coil embolization, stent graft placement; Fig. 103-2), and choosing an appropriate option is essential for achieving optimal long-term results and reducing potential complications.[10]

The ultimate goal of endovascular repair of AAA and IAA with a stent graft is the same as for surgical repair—that is, depressurization and exclusion of the aneurysm sac from the circulation to prevent rupture. The dominant limiting factor in patient selection is the stent graft itself.[11,12] Each device has specific and relatively restrictive requirements with regard to the diameter, length, and angulation of the proximal and distal attachment sites, and to the ability of the iliofemoral arteries to accommodate the stent graft delivery systems. A certain length of non-aneurysmal infrarenal aortic length, depending on the device used, must be present for proper placement of the proximal attachment of the stent graft. Aortic neck angles more than 45 degrees may pose problems with implantation and may stress the device. Trapezoidal, conical, or thrombus-filled aortic necks may cause device instability. Additionally, the iliofemoral vessels must have a certain (device-dependent) caliber and straightness. Patients who do not fit the device cannot be treated.[13]

POSTOPERATIVE ASSESSMENT

Depending on the outcome and general condition of the patient immediately postendograft placement, short-term hospitalization in the intensive care unit may be desirable. Vital signs as well as urine output are continuously monitored for 24 hours. Patients are usually ambulatory within 24 hours after the procedure and are discharged on the third or fourth day after the procedure.

Endograft placement is relatively new, and studies regarding its long term efficacy are still being performed to define its clinical role better. In the Endovascular Aneurysm Repair (EVAR) trial 1,[14] the 30-day mortality rate for endovascular repair was 1.7% and the corresponding rate for open repair was 4.7% ($P < .001$). At 4 years, the

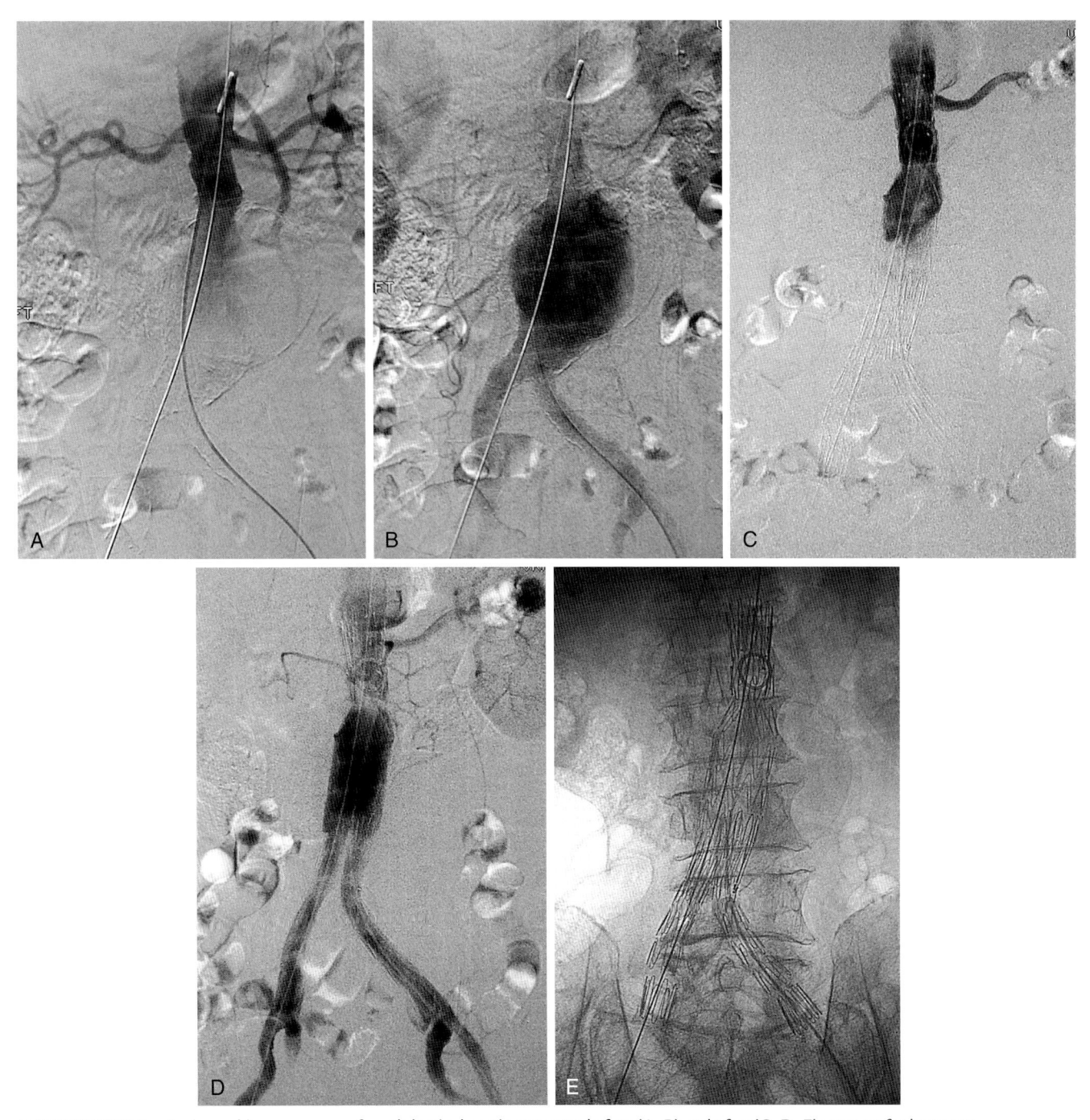

FIGURE 103-1 Angiographic appearance of an abdominal aortic aneurysm before (A, B) and after (C, D, E) stent graft placement.

aneurysm-related mortality rate in the group of patients who underwent endovascular repair was half that of the group of patients who underwent open repair ($P = .04$), but there was no significant difference in mortality from any cause (26% for endovascular repair and 29% for open repair). However, a higher percentage of patients (20%) who underwent endovascular repair required reinterventions (compared with 6% in the open-repair group). Therefore, although perioperative mortality was higher in patients who underwent open repair, a higher percentage of patients in the endovascular repair group required reinterventions, and there was no significant difference in 4-year mortality rates between the two groups.

In the Dutch Randomized Endovascular Aneurysm Management (DREAM) trial,[13] the 30-day mortality rate was significantly lower in patients who had undergone endovascular repair compared with those who had undergone open repair. However, the overall survival rate was not significantly different between the two groups at 2 years. Although aneurysm-related death was more frequent in patients who had undergone open repair, reinterventions were required more often in patients who had undergone endovascular repair. These results corroborate those of the EVAR trial 1. In the EVAR trial 2,[16] 338 patients with AAA who were not candidates for open repair were randomly assigned to undergo endovascular repair or no

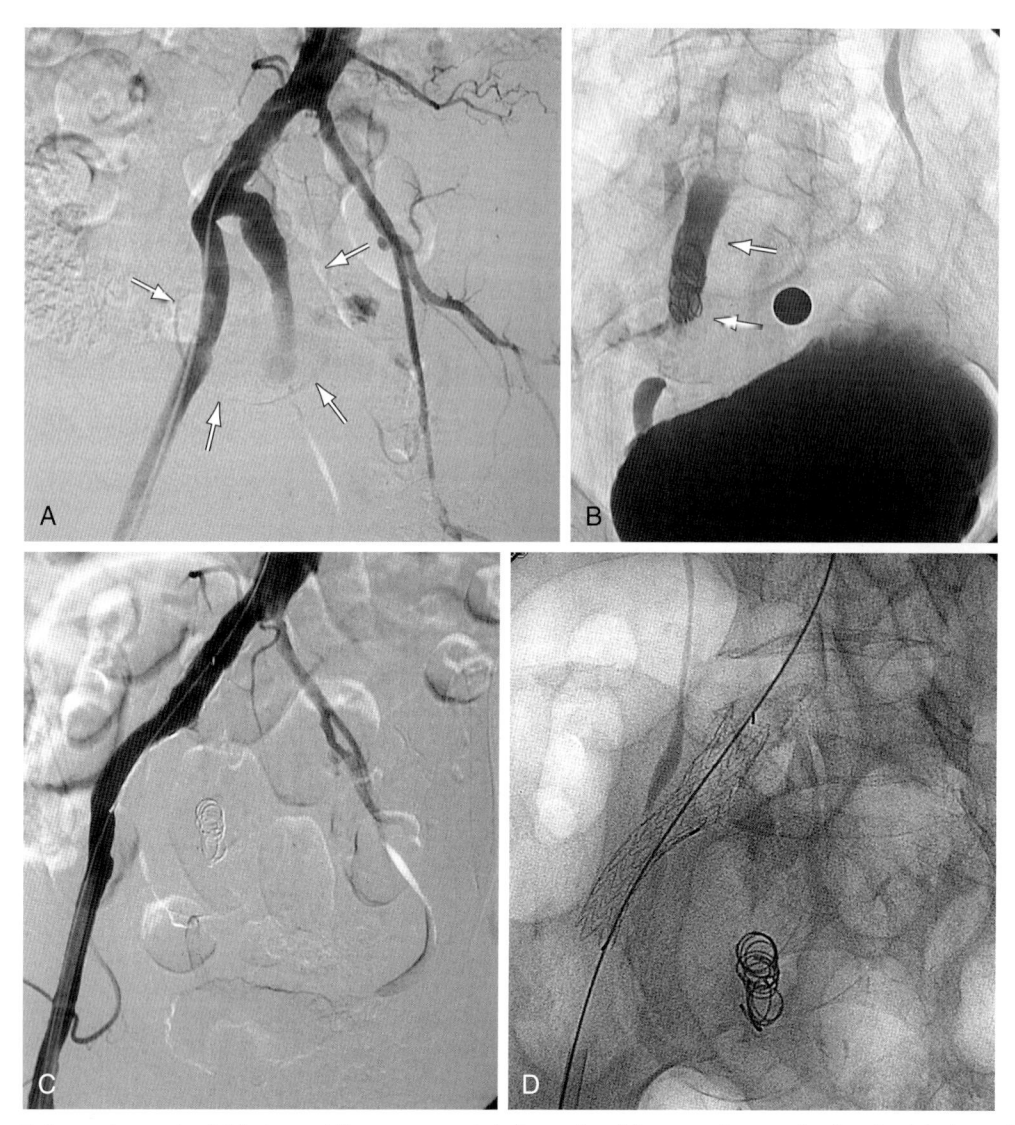

FIGURE 103-2 Endovascular repair of right internal iliac aneurysm. **A,** Left anterior oblique arteriogram showing the right internal liac artery aneurysm (*arrows*). **B,** After successful placement of coils, there is stagnant flow within the aneurysmal lumen of the right internal iliac artery. **C,** Subsequent placement of a stent graft across the right internal iliac artery origin excludes inflow to the aneurysm. The combination of proximal sealing of the aneurysm with the stent graft and distal occlusion of the artery, thus preventing retrograde flow from the contralateral iliac artery, results in total exclusion of the aneurysm from the circulation. **D,** Plain completion radiograph showing the coils and supporting wire mesh of the stent graft.

intervention. No benefit of endovascular repair was apparent during follow-up. Complications and subsequent interventions were more frequent in the group of patients who underwent endovascular repair. Therefore, the benefit of endovascular repair in patients who are not surgical candidates appears unclear.

Successful endovascular repair of AAA and IAA remains technically challenging despite continued improvement in device design. As noted, additional interventions may be required before or during stent graft placement.[13] Primary technical success is defined on an intent to treat basis and requires the following: (1) successful insertion and deployment of the graft without the need for surgical conversion; (2) no perioperative mortality; (3) absence of type I or III endoleak; and (4) freedom from limb obstruction or occlusion, up to 24 hours postoperatively. Clinical success of stent grafting is defined as technical success in conjunction with freedom from aneurysm-related death, type I or III endoleak, graft infection or thrombosis, aneurysm rupture, conversion to open repair, or graft migration during the life of the patient.[17]

Occlusion of branch vessels arising from the proximal neck, aneurysm sac, or iliac arteries is the most common preprocedural intervention.[13,18] This is done to provide appropriate attachment sites or prevent retrograde perfusion of the aneurysm sac after placement of the stent graft. Contralateral common iliac artery occlusion is required when inserting an aortounilateral iliac artery stent graft. In a patient with a common or internal IAA, embolization of the internal iliac artery is required before stent graft is deployed across its origin into the ipsilateral external iliac artery (Fig. 103-3). Interventions such as angioplasty or stent placement may also be required during insertion of a stent graft to accommodate large delivery systems better.[13] Angioplasty to dilate conduit artery stenoses should be performed at the time of the stent graft proce-

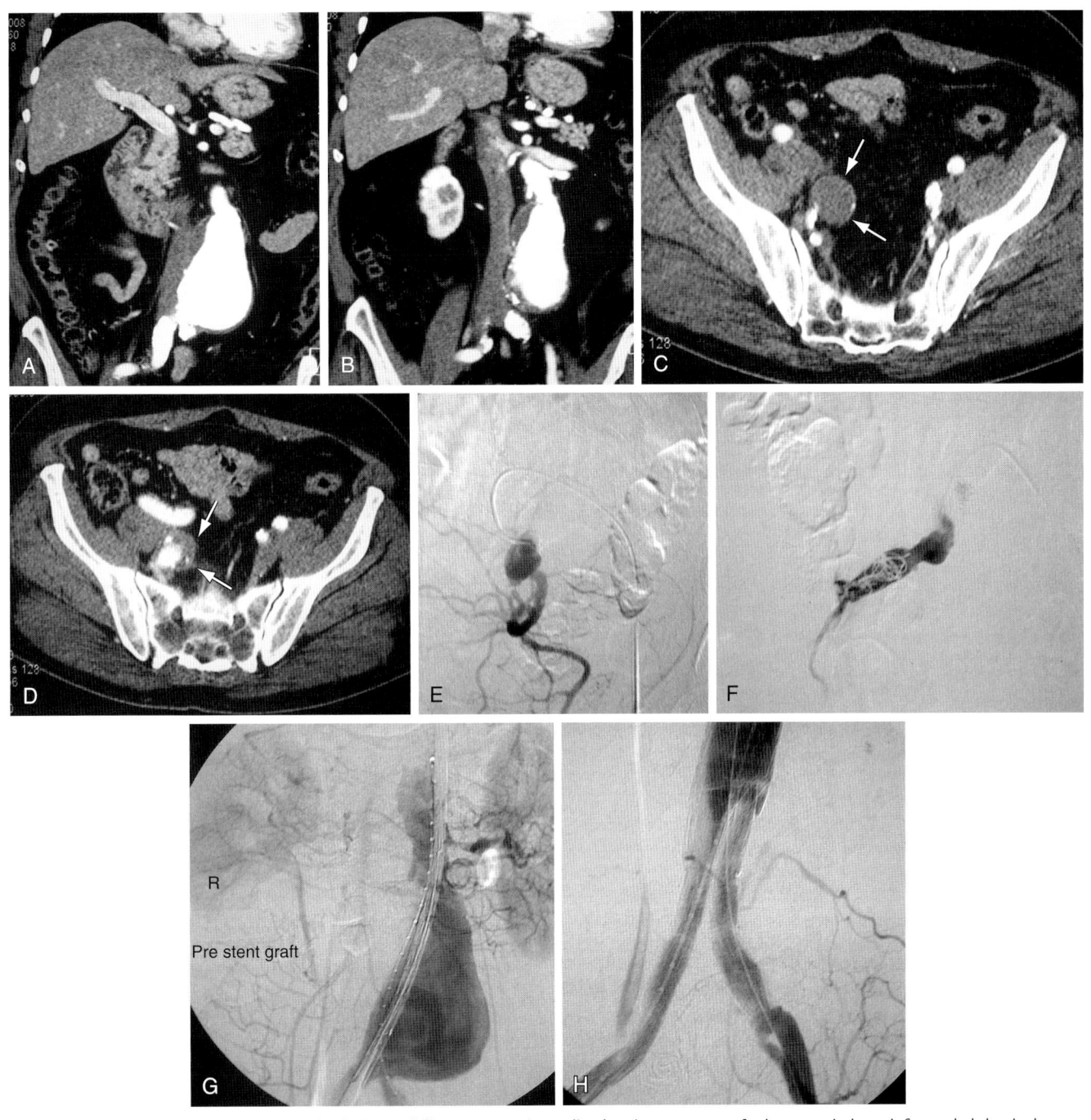

FIGURE 103-3 Endovascular repair of right internal iliac aneurysm immediately prior to stent graft placement in large infrarenal abdominal aortic aneurysm. This coronal multiplanar reformation (MPR) image was obtained with CT angiography. **A, B,** Infrarenal abdominal aortic aneurysm. **C, D,** Axial contrast-enhanced CT images showing the right internal iliac artery aneurysm. **E, F,** After successful coil placement, stent graft placement to treat the aortic aneurysm was performed (**G, H**).

dure, not before. At times, the main body of the graft may have to be inserted through the contralateral side from the one initially planned if difficulties are encountered during its insertion because of a stenosis (Fig. 103-4). The threshold for stent placement to repair a traumatic dissection (Figs. 103-5 to 103-7) caused by a large delivery system or to buttress the iliac limb of an unsupported stent graft should be low. Aortounilateral iliac artery stent grafts require a surgical femoral to femoral bypass graft to perfuse the pelvis and limb contralateral to the stent graft. A vascular plug to occlude flow through the contralateral common iliac artery should be placed immediately prior to the surgical femoral to femoral bypass.

Successful insertion of an aortic stent graft is achieved in more than 95% of procedures in carefully selected patients and appropriately chosen devices. The most common cause of a failed procedure is the inability to insert a device through diseased or tortuous iliac arteries, especially with devices with large profiles. Misplacement of the stent graft, failure to deploy, or acute and irrevers-

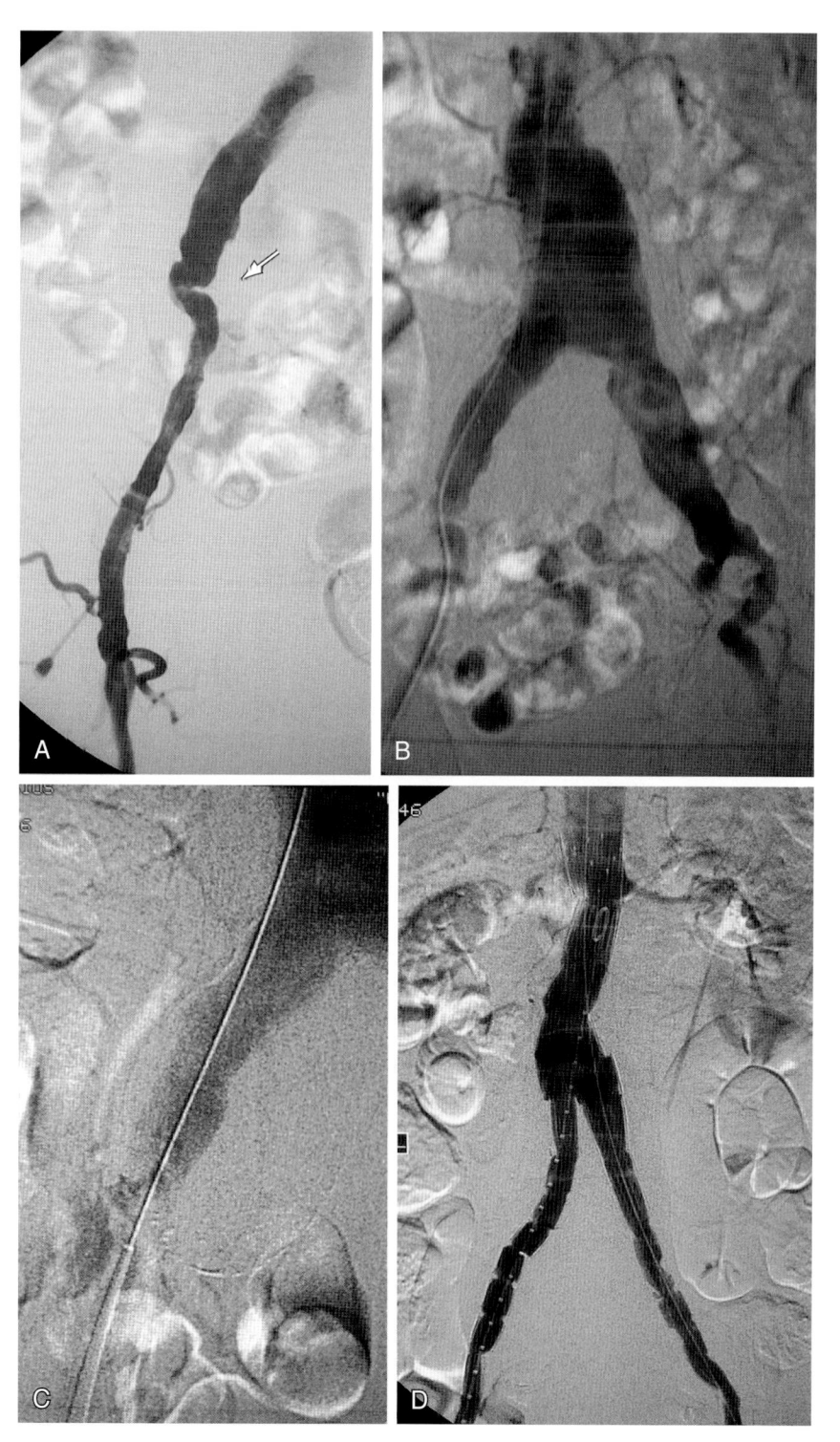

FIGURE 103-4 Tight right external iliac artery stenosis preventing advancement of delivery system of the body of the stent graft. **A,** Right iliac system preprocedural angiogram showing a stenotic area (*arrow*) in the external iliac artery. The ipsilateral right internal iliac artery was occluded. **B,** During the procedure, the delivery system of the main body of a Zenith-Cook stent graft could not be advanced, despite several attempts of experienced operators. It was decided to insert the main body from the contralateral side. **C,** The final angiogram showed a good result.

ible occlusion (Fig. 103-8) are unusual events but may require urgent open surgical repair. This is termed a *surgical conversion* and is associated with a higher morbidity than conventional open surgical repair.

When compared with open surgery, there are definite early advantages to stent graft repair of an AAA. The procedure poses less hemodynamic stress than traditional open surgical repair, which is an important consideration in older patients. Blood loss is lower with stent graft repair compared with open surgery (average, 400 vs. 1200 mL), and the use of the intensive care unit becomes the exception rather than the rule. Patients are able to ambulate the next day, and hospital stays are reduced from 7 to 10 days (open surgery) to 2 to 3 days (stent graft repair). The 30-day mortality rate in large stent graft series ranges from 0.7% in low-risk populations to 15.7% in high-risk

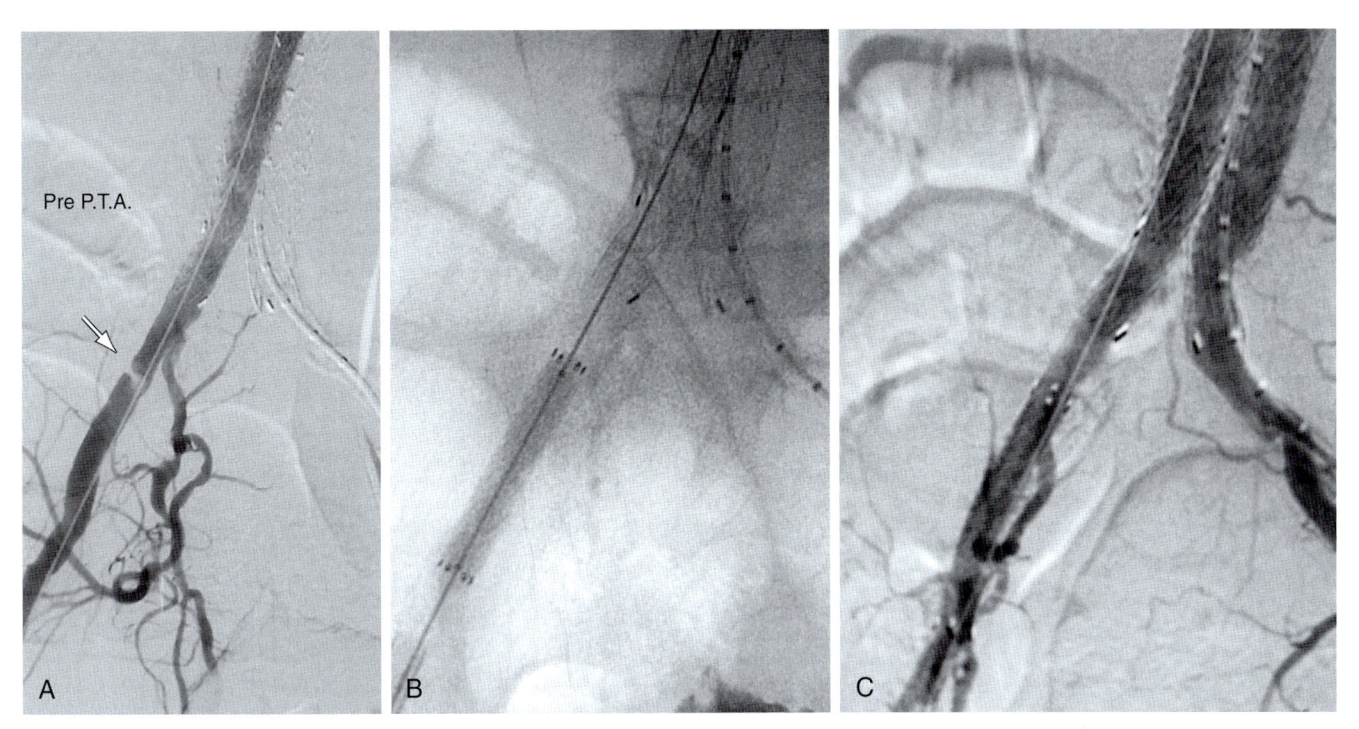

CHAPTER 103 • Postendograft Imaging of the Abdominal Aorta and Iliac Arteries   1425

FIGURE 103-5 Non–flow-limiting dissection in right external iliac artery treated with stent placement. **A,** After successful placement of a stent graft for abdominal aortic treatment, completion arteriogram demonstrates a non–flow-limiting dissection in the right external iliac artery. **B, C,** A self-expandable stent was successfully placed with a good result. P.T.A., percutaneous transluminal angioplasty.

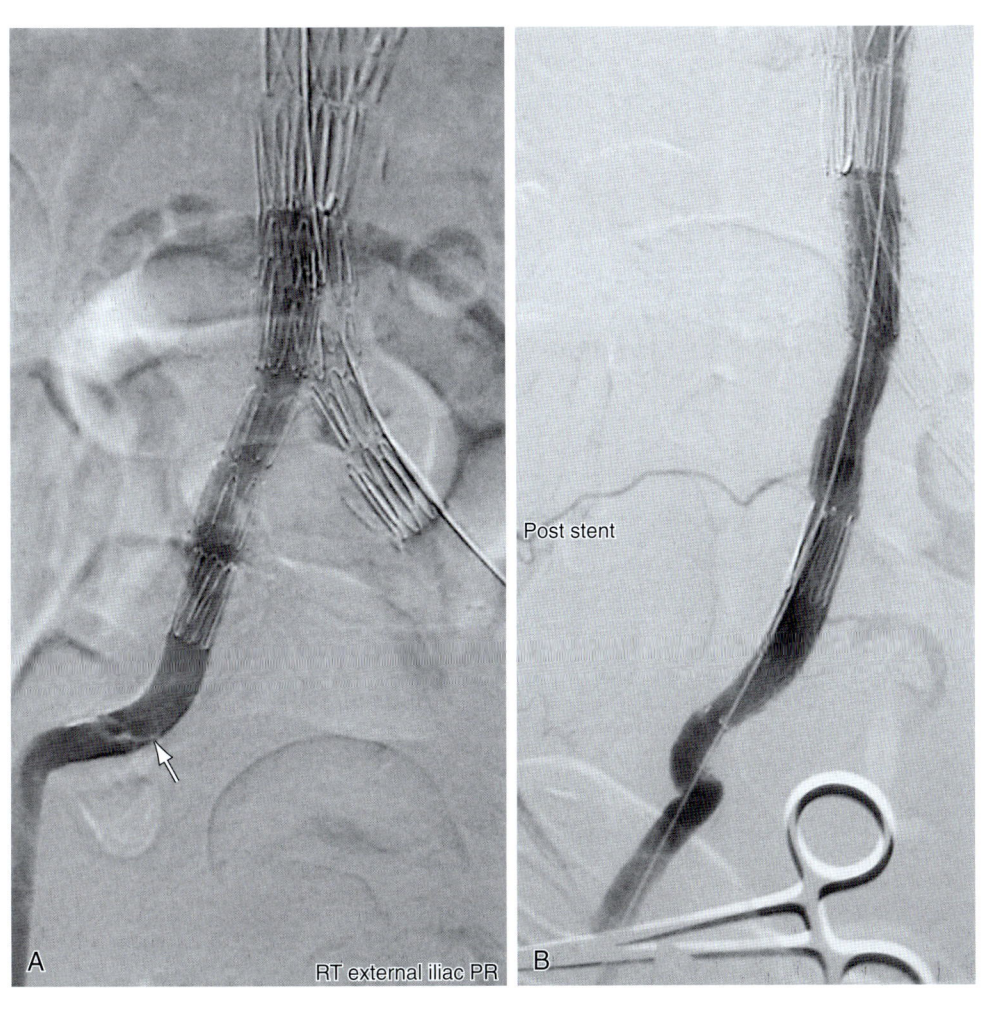

FIGURE 103-6 Non–flow-limiting dissection in right external iliac artery treated with stent placement. **A,** After successful placement of a stent graft for abdominal aortic treatment a non–flow-limiting dissection in the mid–right external iliac artery (*arrow*) was noted. **B,** A self-expandable stent was successfully placed with good result.

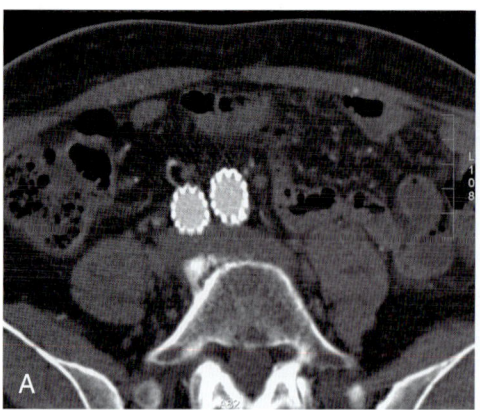

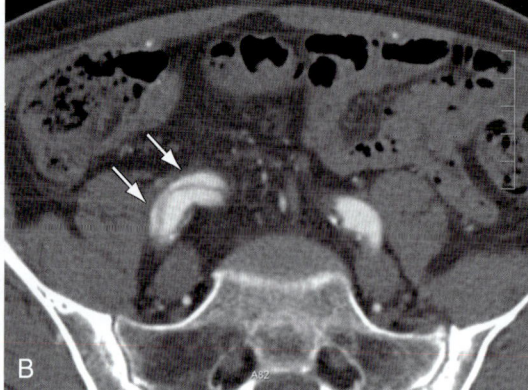

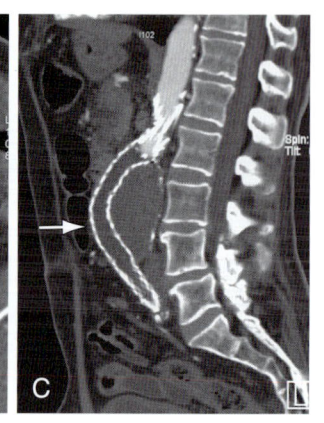

FIGURE 103-7 Postprocedural iliac dissection with subsequent iliac limb thrombosis. **A,** Follow-up CT scan obtained 1 month after aortic bi-iliac stent graft implantation reveals patency at the level of both iliac limbs. **B,** More distally, just below the landing zone on the right, an intimal flap is identified within the distal right common iliac artery (*arrows*). This was not immediately addressed and led to the development of complete occlusion of the stented right iliac artery, requiring subsequent femoral to femoral bypass graft placement. **C,** The completely occluded graft is identified on the sagittal multiplanar reformation (MPR) image (*arrow*).

patients. These statistics compare favorably with those associated with surgical repair of abdominal aortic aneurysm.

Death during a stent graft procedure is very rare. Acute intraprocedural rupture of an AAA during stent graft placement with successful outcome has been reported but is also rare. Complications such as multiorgan system failure, myocardial infarction, bowel infarction, stroke, pulmonary embolism, and peripheral arterial embolism have all been described after stent graft procedures, but most early complications are minor and mainly consist of injuries to access arteries or issues related to groin incisions.[13]

As noted, complete exclusion of the aneurysm sac is the goal of stent graft placement and the definition of early clinical success.[19] Figure 103-9 demonstrates the expected anatomic appearance after successful deployment of a stent graft on CT angiography.

Endoleak

Persistent opacification of the aneurysm sac after insertion of a stent graft is termed an *endoleak* and is classified by cause and time of occurrence.[20] This classification of endoleaks is described in Table 103-1. Most early endoleaks are currently types II and IV. Type I leaks can be minimized by careful patient selection and preprocedural measurements. Tube stent grafts may have a higher rate of type I leak, particularly at the distal attachment site, than bifurcated stent grafts and today are used for selected patients only. Large attachment leaks that result in continued pressurization of the aneurysm sac indicate a failed procedure and may leave the patient at risk for subsequent AAA rupture. Because more than 50% of small endoleaks will resolve spontaneously, their management is usually expectant.[13] Although many early endoleaks disappear within 6 months, reappearance of leaks and delayed appearance of new leaks can occur at any time. Stabilization of aneurysm size or even shrinkage and avoidance of secondary endovascular procedures or open surgery are considered measures of long-term success.

The presence of an endoleak is correlated with less reduction in the diameter of the sac and occasionally even with slight enlargement. After endovascular repair, an increase in the aneurysm sac diameter of less than 0.5 cm is considered acceptable. A greater degree of enlargement should prompt treatment of the endoleak using endovascular means or surgical conversion. The currently reported rate of long-term surgical conversion caused by persistent endoleak and aneurysm expansion is low.[13] Conversion caused by aneurysm expansion with no visible leak is even less frequent, but both indications may become more common as long-term follow-up experience is accumulated. Additional complications such as thromboses, stent migration, and visceral organ infarctions can also be demonstrated. Finally, because atherosclerotic disease can progress over time, it is imperative to evaluate the aortic visceral tributaries for disease progression.

Clinical Presentation

Following successful placement of an abdominal aortic stent graft, the patient will require evaluation of the aneurysm sac size and perfusion to detect changes in the diameter of the vessels at the sites of attachment, changes in stent graft morphology, endoleaks, and detection of new aneurysms. These are usually asymptomatic and will be discovered during routine follow-up examinations. Certainly, however, more severe complications such as stent graft limb occlusion, peripheral embolization, or wound infection will present with early and sound symptomatology and will require immediate attention.

Imaging Indications and Algorithm

Three questions must be answered for every patient who has had endovascular treatment with a stent graft:

1. What is the status of the size of the aneurysm?
2. Has the stent graft migrated?
3. Is there an endoleak?

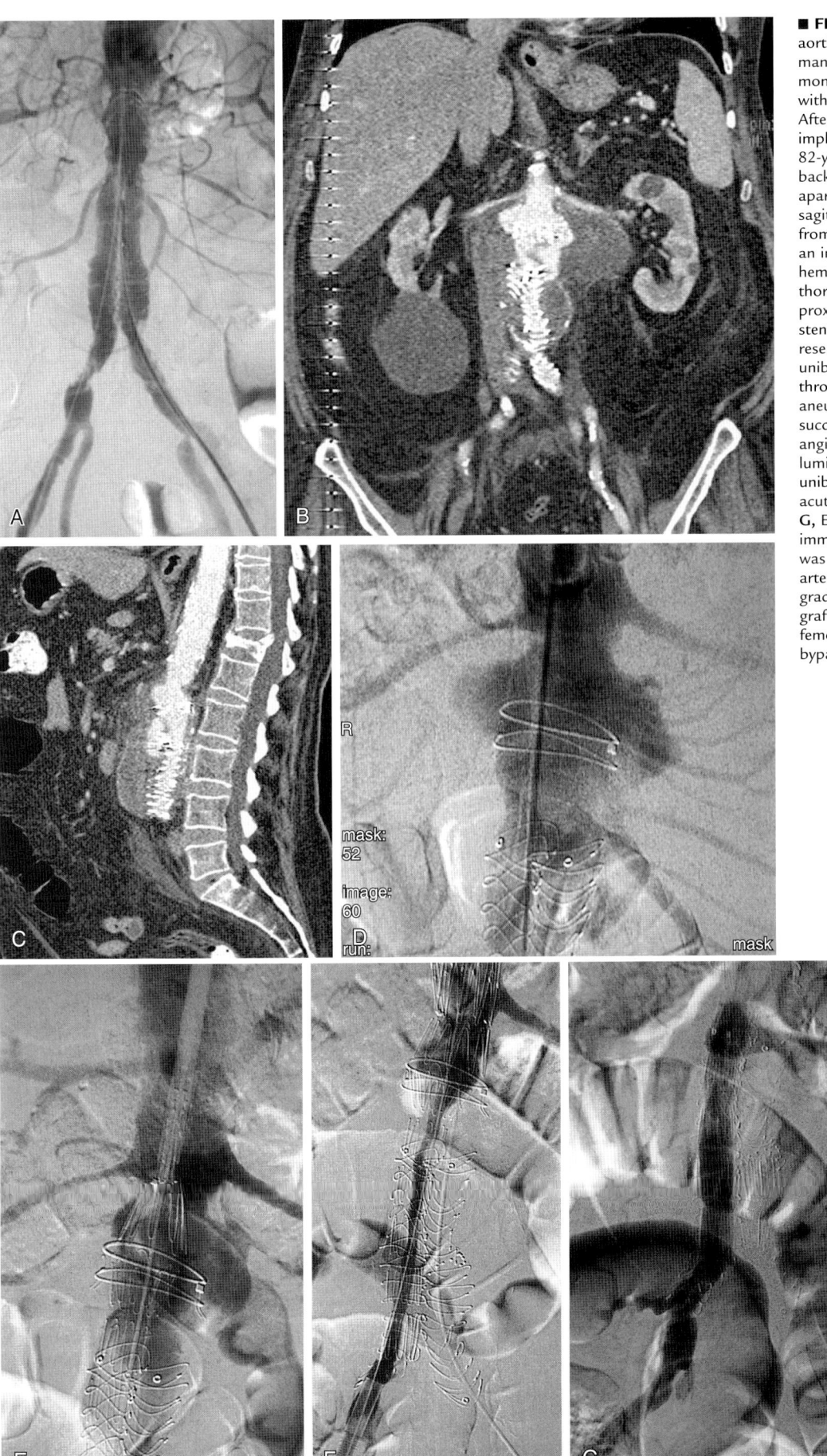

FIGURE 103-8 Abdominal aortic aneurysm in an 82-year-old man after endovascular repair 8 months previously, now presenting with back pain after trauma. **A**, After uneventful stent graft implantation, 8 months ago, this 82-year-old man presented with back pain after falling in his apartment. Coronal (**B**) and sagittal (**C**) reconstructed images from contrast-enhanced CT show an infrarenal retroperitoneal hematoma, as well as a lower thoracic vertebrae fracture. **D**, The proximal attachment site of the stent graft was now aneurysmal, resembling a type I endoleak. **E**, A unibody stent graft was advanced through the right limb to seal the aneurysm neck proximally and was successfully deployed. **F**, Control angiogram showed, however, luminal narrowing within the unibody stent graft consistent with acute thrombus formation. **G**, Embolectomies were immediately performed and flow was restored. During repair of the arteriotomy, however, flow gradually diminished, indicating graft occlusion. A right axillary-femoral and right to left femoral bypass was performed.

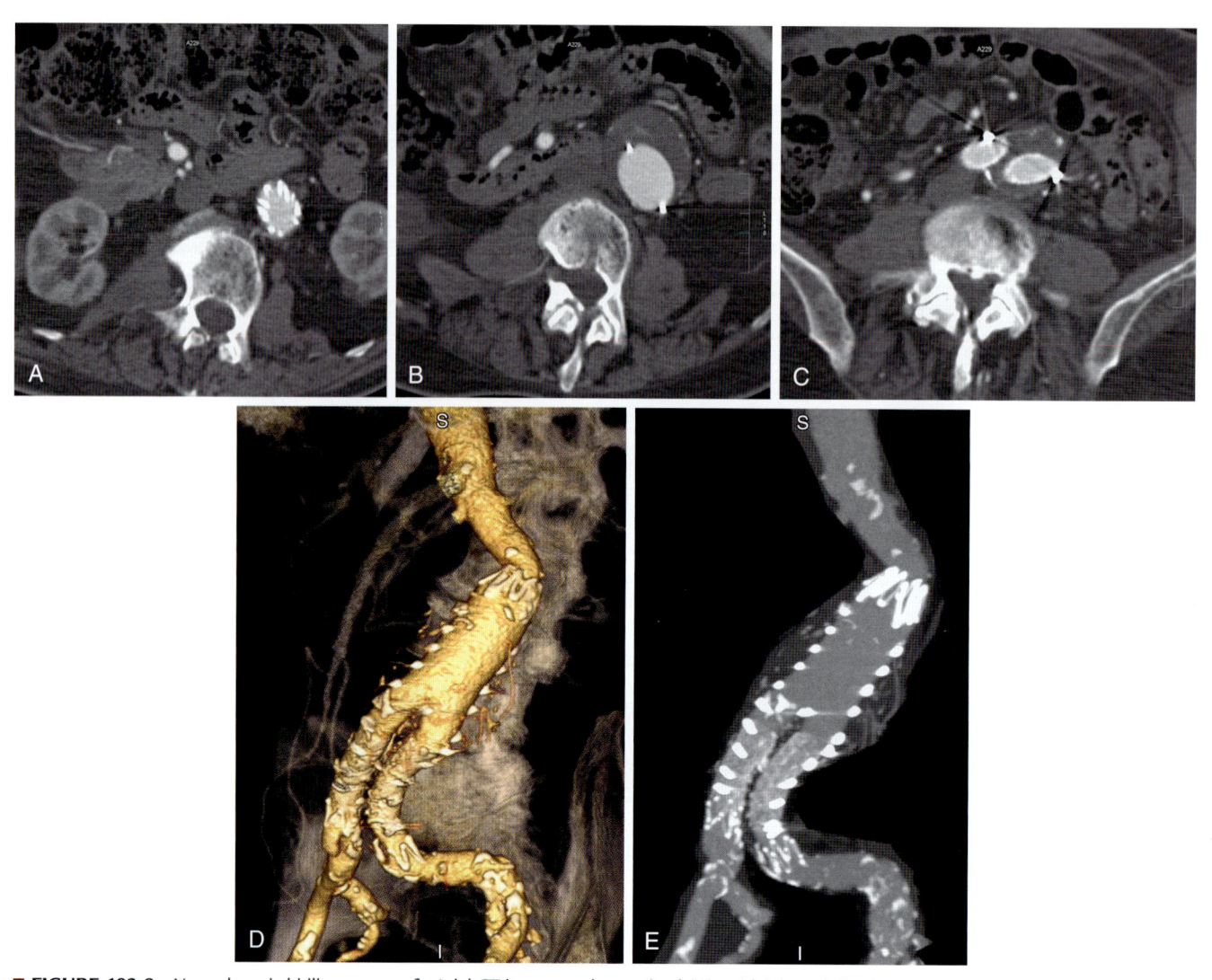

FIGURE 103-9 Normal aortic bi-iliac stent graft. Axial CT images at the proximal (**A**), mid (**B**), and distal (**C**) aspects of the stent graft reveal the different components of this stent graft. At the proximal and distal landing zones, the typical corrugated wire mesh is identified and best displayed on the coronal volume rendered image (**D**) as well as a coronal maximum intensity projection (**E**).

TABLE 103-1 Endoleak Classification

Type of Endoleak	Features
I	Lack of complete seal between stent graft and vessel wall at attachment sites
II	Back-filling of aneurysm sac via branch vessels such as lumbar or inferior mesenteric arteries
III	Leaks at connections of modular components, device disruption, fabric tears
IV	Extravasation of contrast material through interstices in the graft material
V	Endotension
Primary endoleak	Immediate or less than 30 days postimplantation
Secondary endoleak	More than 30 days postimplantation

Modified from Kaufman JA, Geller SC, Brewster DC, et al. Endovascular repair of abdominal aortic aneurysms: Current status and future directions. AJR Am J Roentgenol 2000; 175:289-302.

The purpose of endovascular aneurysm repair is to prevent aneurysm rupture, which is why it is imperative to monitor the status of the aneurysm sac after repair. This is most often done with CT angiography (CTA). Recently, volumetric analysis comparing preoperative and postoperative CT imaging has proven useful in following these patients. Because aneurysms in the postendograft period change configuration in their longitudinal as well as axial dimensions, volumetric analysis may provide a more sensitive method for determining whether an aneurysm is enlarging, shrinking, or remaining stable. It is important to determine whether the stent graft is in the same position as it was placed in the operating room. Migration and device failure can occur without the presence of an endoleak or any other signs or symptoms. For example, a fracture of a hook or barb at a proximal attachment site could eventually lead to proximal migration. Failures at attachment sites and the graft itself can manifest as endoleaks, and these failures require immediate attention and repair. Collateral endoleaks can have a benign self-limiting

■ **FIGURE 103-10** Aneurysm sac decrease after stent deployment for abdominal aortic aneurysm. **A,** An axial CT image obtained 1 month after stent graft deployment reveals the aneurysm sac surrounding the iliac components of the stent graft. **B,** Follow-up CT study 1 year after stent graft deployment at the same anatomic level reveals significant decrease in size of the aneurysm sac.

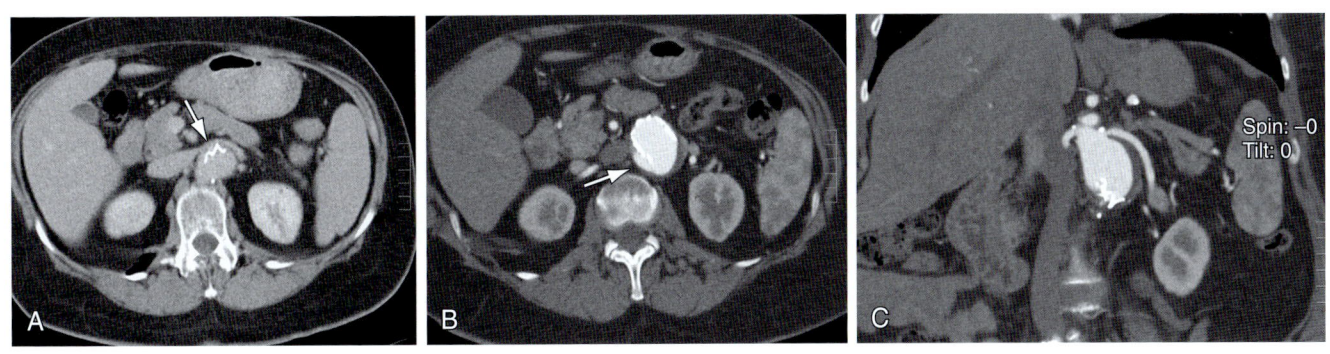

■ **FIGURE 103-11** Aneurysm development at and above proximal landing zone. **A,** An axial CT image obtained after an aortic stent graft deployment for abdominal aortic aneurysm reveals the cephalad margin of the aortic stent component (*arrow*), with no evidence of aneurysm. **B,** An axial CT image obtained several years after stent deployment at approximately the same level reveals aneurysm development at the cephalad margin of the stent, with associated endoleak posterolaterally on the right (*arrow*). **C,** A coronal multiplanary formation reveals an infrarenal aneurysm between the renal arteries and cephalad margin of the stent graft.

course or can lead to aneurysm enlargement and rupture. Identifying these problems early may prevent catastrophic failures.

Imaging Techniques and Findings

Imaging plays a pivotal role in preprocedural patient evaluation, during the procedure of stent graft implantation, and for patient follow-up. The follow-up of patients with stent grafts requires evaluation of AAA sac size (Fig. 103-10) and perfusion, stent graft patency, changes in diameter of the vessels at the sites of endograft attachment (Fig. 103-11), changes in stent graft morphology, changes in stent graft position (Fig. 103-12), and detection of new aneurysms. The imaging requirements are different from those after surgical repair of an AAA, in which imaging is limited in scope and frequency.

Techniques

The single most useful imaging test that allows rapid assessment of patients with stent grafts is contrast-enhanced multidetector CT (MDCT).[13] A sample CTA protocol used is shown in Table 103-2. The crucial issue after stent graft placement is correlation of sac opacification from any cause with pressure within the aneurysm sac, because continued pressurization results in continued risk of AAA rupture.[21] There is no easy way to obtain sac pressures in a noninvasive manner and, furthermore, it has been suggested that lack of visualization of contrast material within the aneurysm sac does not guarantee lack of pressurization.[13] Contrast-enhanced CT scans are sensitive for the detection of endoleaks, although use of color flow Doppler sonography has been advocated. Essentially, all patients with stent grafts should be followed up for life with contrast-enhanced CT. In addition, although abdominal radiographs are invaluable tools for assessment of the integrity of the metallic components of the stent graft, the integrity of the metallic components can be assessed on CT studies through volume-rendered and maximum intensity projection images.

As noted earlier, the critical issue after stent graft implantation is correlation of sac opacification from any cause with pressure within the aneurysm sac because

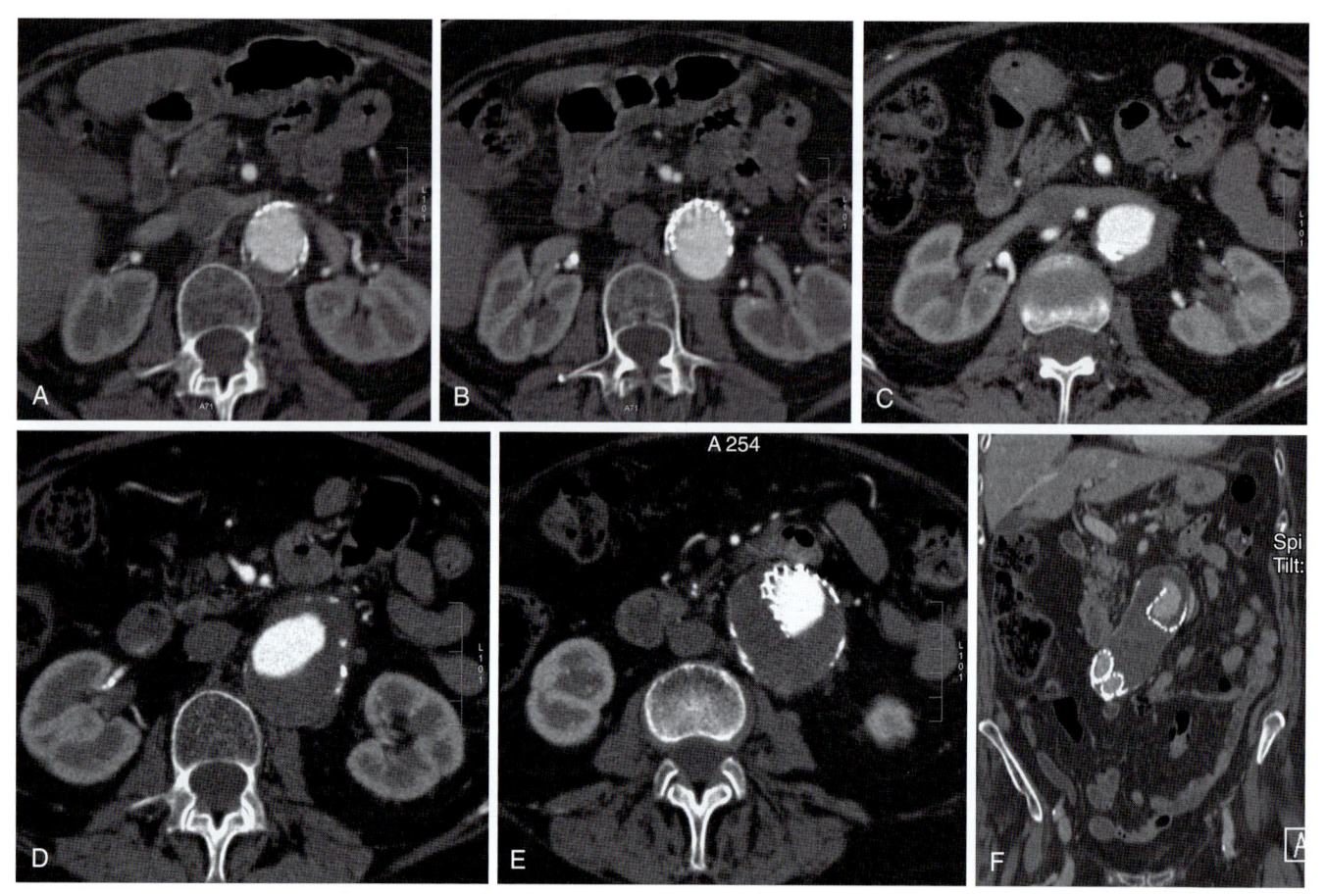

FIGURE 103-12 Stent migration with aneurysm enlargement. **A, B,** Axial CT images at and immediately below the left renal vein reveal the cephalad margin of the aortic stent graft component. **C, D,** On follow-up, axial CT images at and immediately below the left renal vein did not reveal evidence of the cephalad aspect of the aortic stent component. The aorta has significantly enlarged in the interval. **E,** Rather, the cephalad margin of the aortic stent component is seen at a much more inferior level on an axial CT image obtained at the level of the lower poles of the kidneys. **F,** This is best visualized on a coronal multiplanar reformation.

TABLE 103-2 CT Angiography: Prestent and Poststent Protocol

Parameter	Protocol
Anatomic region	1. T12 to symphysis pubis; coned field of view (FOV), 200 mm 2. Full FOV
Oral contrast	None
IV contrast, volume, and type	80-100 mL (iodinated contrast with 370 mg I/mL) or 120 mL (iodinated contrast with 350 mg I/mL)
Respiratory phase	Inspiration
Injection rate	4 mL/sec
Scan delay	1. Arterial phase with bolus trigger in upper abdominal aorta 2. 2-min delay
kVp and effective mAs	100 kVp (body mass index [BMI] ≤ 29), 120 kVp (BMI = 30-44), 140 kVp (BMI ≥ 45); variable mAs based on body proportions
Detector configuration (detector collimation in mm)	64 (0.6) 16 (0.75) 10 (0.75)
Pitch	0.9 (64 slice) 0.9 (16 slice) 0.55 (10 slice)
Slice thickness/reconstruction interval	1. 1.0 mm/0.5 mm 2. 2.0 mm/2.0 mm
Kernel	B30
Three-dimensional reconstruction	Send 1- × 0.5-mm data for three-dimensional reconstructions.
Special instructions	All poststent studies require precontrast imaging abdomen/pelvis 5 × 0.5

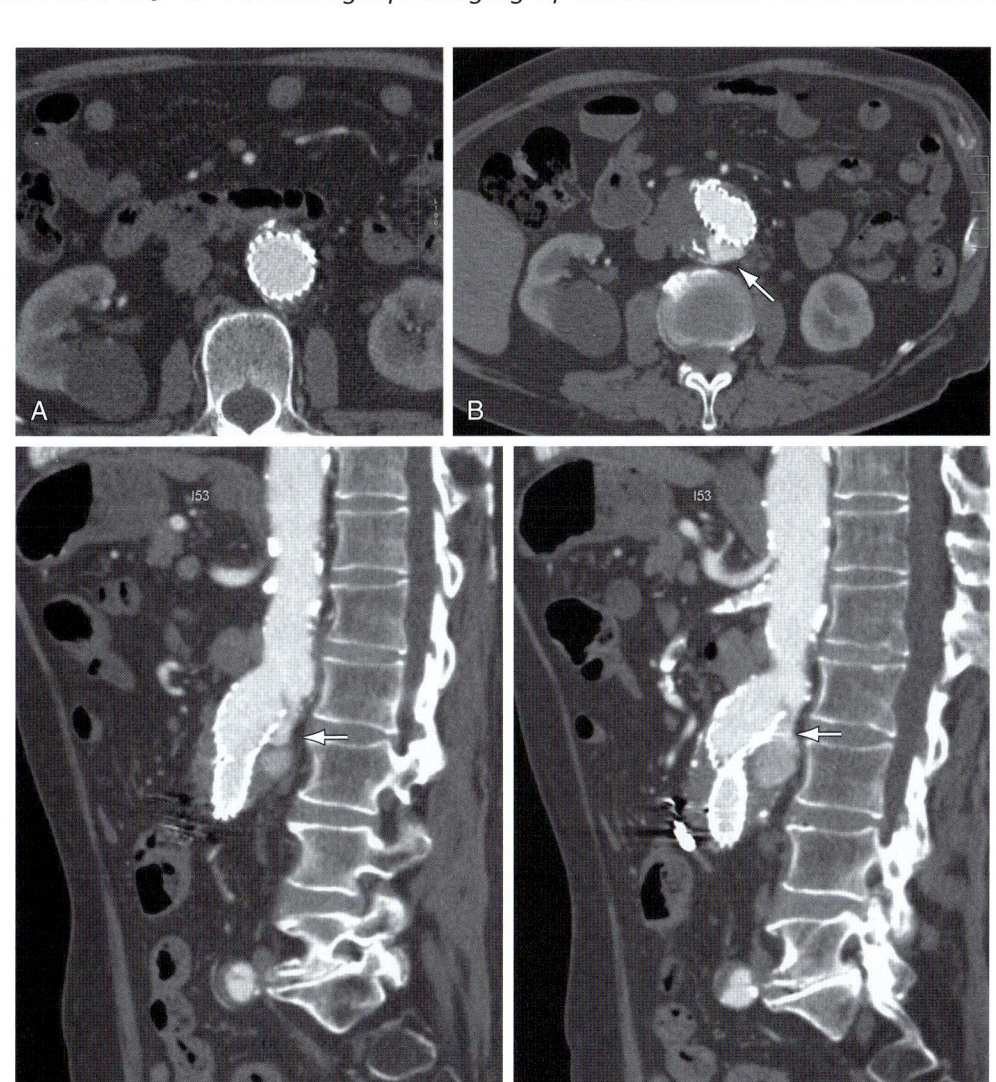

FIGURE 103-13 Type I endoleak at the proximal landing zone caused by aneurysm development. **A,** Axial CT images soon after aortic bi-iliac stent graft deployment reveal an aorta measuring 3 cm, with no endoleak. **B,** On follow-up examination, axial CT images revealed progression in dilation of the upper abdominal aorta, with evidence of endoleak (*arrow*) seen posteriorly. **C, D,** Sagittal MPR images show origin of the endoleak (*arrow*) posterior to the proximal landing zone.

continued pressurization results in continued risk of aneurysm rupture. Therefore, the scope of postendograft imaging of abdominal aortic aneurysms is directed toward early detection of any factor that will compromise the configuration of vascular anatomy. These include endoleaks, graft thrombosis, graft kinking, graft infection, graft occlusion, shower embolism, colon necrosis, dissection, and hematomas.

Complications and Their Detection

Endoleaks

Complete exclusion of the aneurysm sac is the goal of stent graft placement and the definition of early clinical success. The most common complication after stent graft implantation is leakage of blood into the aneurysm sac. Endoleak is defined as blood flow outside the lumen of the stent graft and contained within the aneurysm sac as demonstrated on contrast-enhanced CT, contrast-enhanced MR, duplex ultrasonography, or conventional x-ray catheter arteriography, and are classified by type (see Table 103-1). Rates of endoleak after endovascular repair of aortic aneurysms range between 2.4% to 45.5%.[13,22]

Type I endoleaks include those caused by inadequate proximal or distal graft fixation, resulting in lack of complete seal between the stent graft and vessel wall (Figs. 103-13 and 103-14). Type II endoleaks are defined by retrograde flow originating from aneurysm sac side branches, such as lumbar or inferior mesenteric arteries, back into the aneurysm sac (Figs. 103-15 to 103-18). Type III endoleaks include grafts that developed prosthetic graft holes after implantation or that sustained a separation of one or more of the modular components that formed the completed graft (Fig. 103-19). Type IV endoleaks include extravasation of contrast material through interstices in

1432 PART SEVENTEEN • *The Abdominal Vessels*

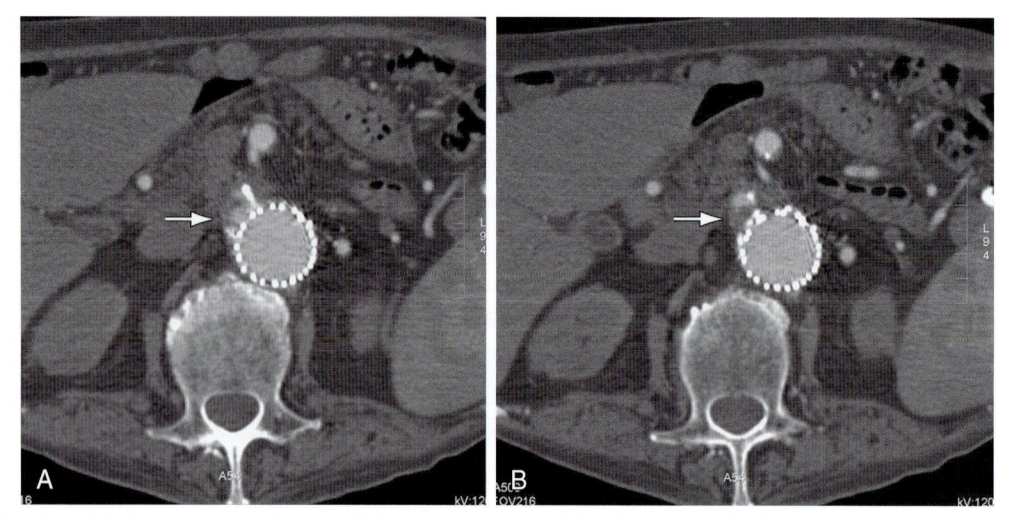

■ **FIGURE 103-14** Pseudoleak caused by renal artery origin aneurysm. **A, B,** Axial CT images reveal enhancement outside the aortic stent. This does not represent an endoleak but indicates enhancement of a renal artery origin aneurysm. **B,** The axial CT reveals continuation of the proximal right renal artery (*arrow*).

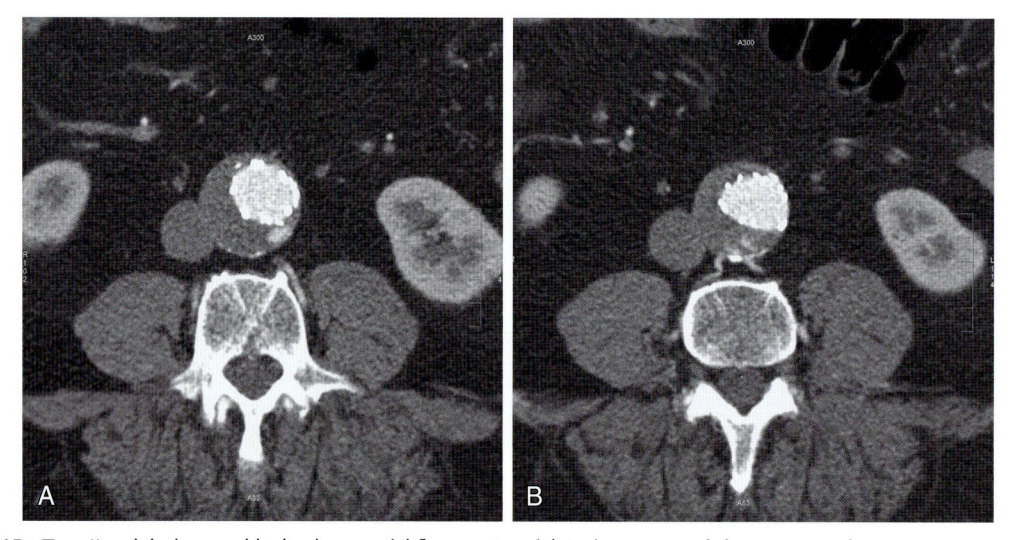

■ **FIGURE 103-15** Type II endoleak caused by lumbar arterial flow. **A, B,** Axial CT images reveal the presence of contrast consistent with endoleak posterior to the stent graft caused by inflow from the lumbar arteries.

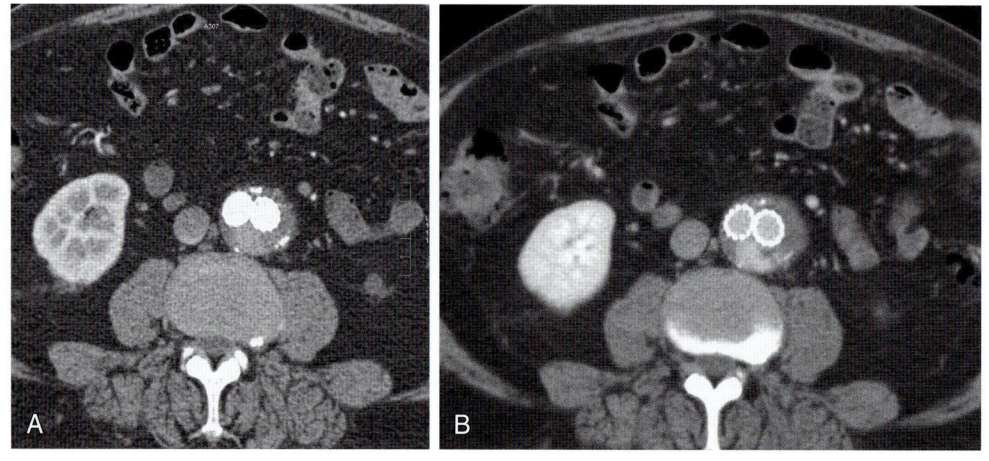

■ **FIGURE 103-16** Type II endoleak best seen on delayed acquisition postcontrast. Early **(A)** and delayed **(B)** acquisition postcontrast reveal the posterior endoleak. This was not appreciated on the early arterial phase data acquisition.

CHAPTER 103 ● *Postendograft Imaging of the Abdominal Aorta and Iliac Arteries* 1433

■ **FIGURE 103-17** Type II endoleak best seen on delayed acquisition postcontrast. Early (A) and delayed (B) acquisition postcontrast reveal the anterior endoleak. This was not appreciated on the early arterial phase data acquisition.

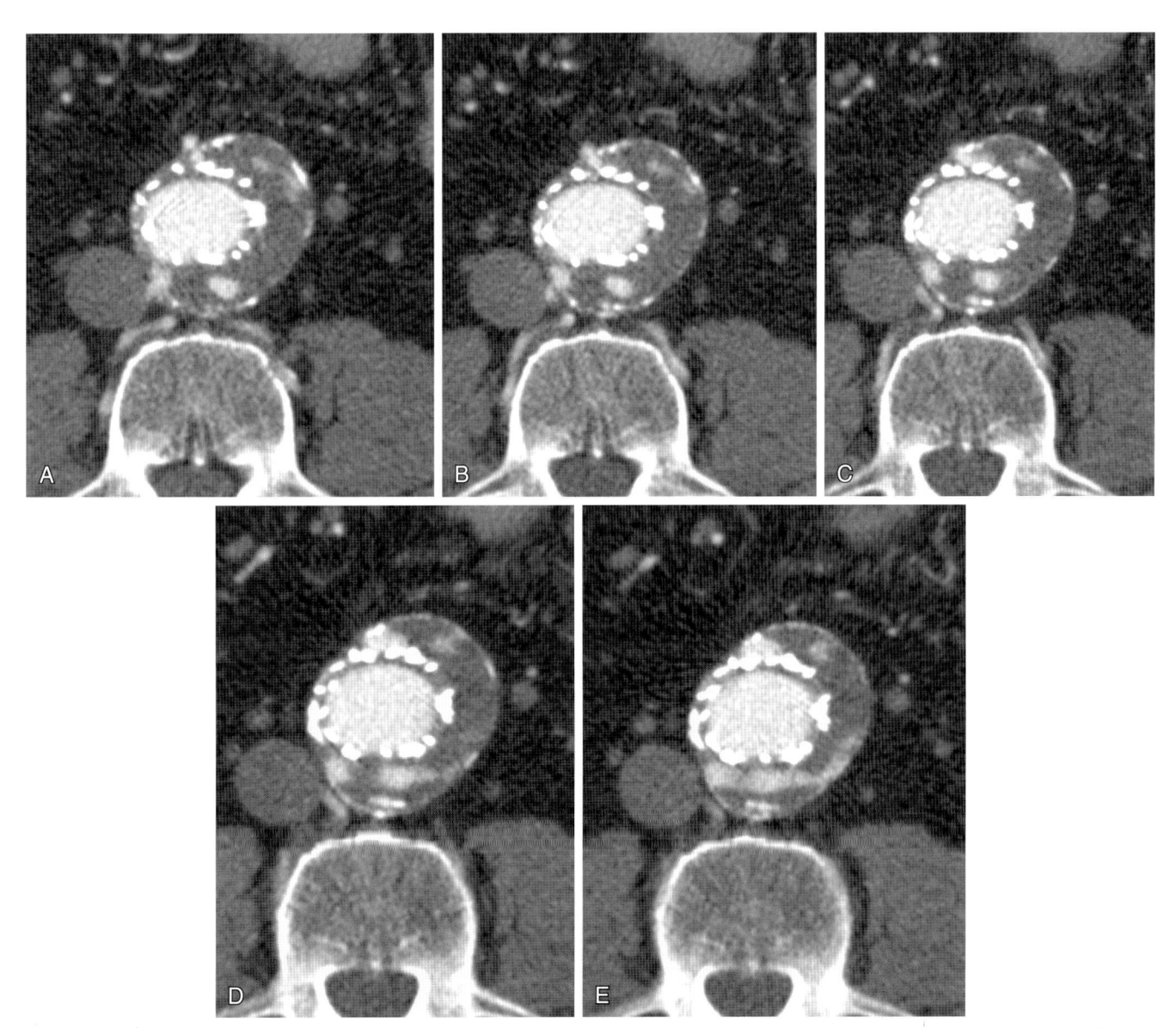

■ **FIGURE 103-18** Type II endoleak from the inferior mesenteric and lumbar arteries. A-D, Serial CT images reveal evidence of endoleak involving the aneurysm sac anteriorly and posteriorly. Serial image examination reveals enhancement anteriorly caused by flow from the inferior mesenteric artery and posteriorly from the lumbar arteries.

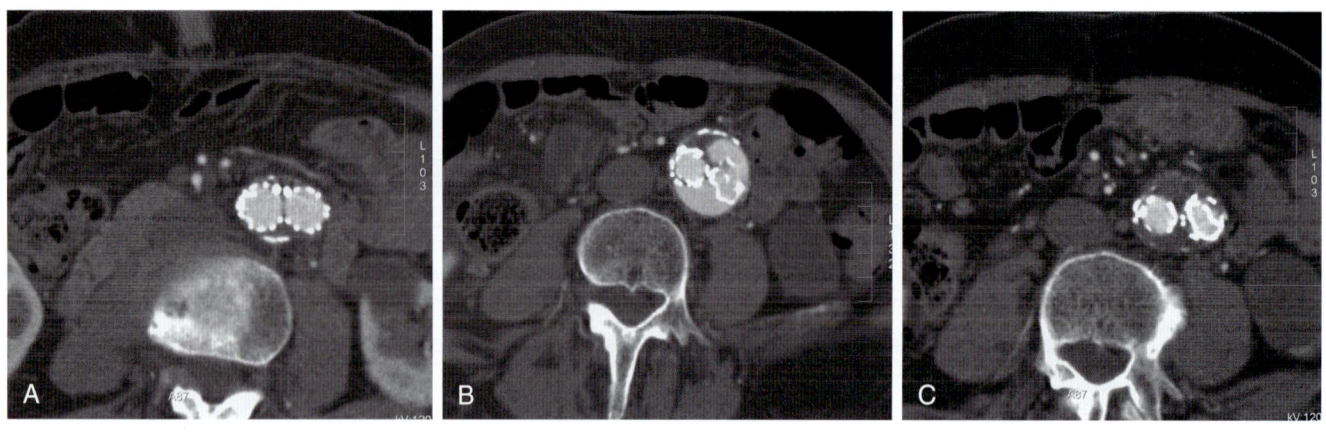

FIGURE 103-19 Type III endoleak. **A-C,** Axial CT images reveal focal endoleak anterolaterally at the junction between the aortic and iliac stent components.

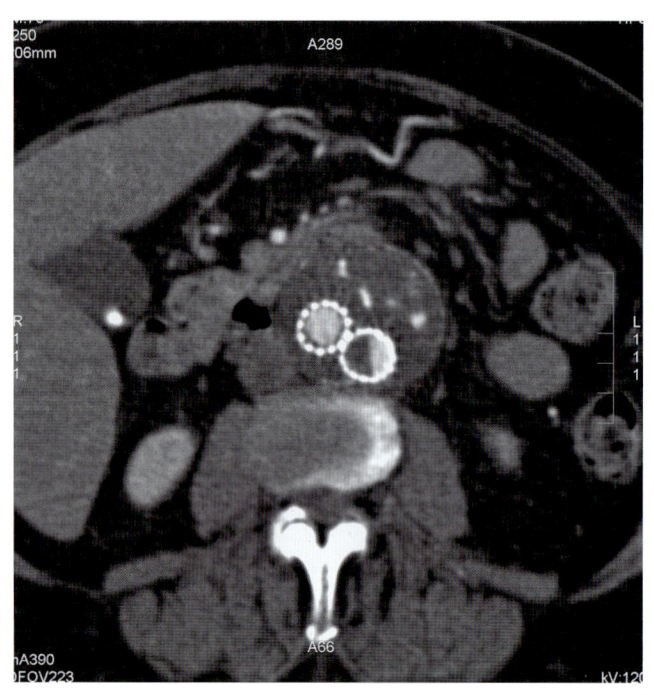

FIGURE 103-20 Partial thrombosis of stented iliac limb. This axial CT image reveals partial thrombosis of the left iliac limb of the stent graft.

the graft material. Endotension, or a type V endoleak, is evident when the aneurysmal sac increases in size without a definite demonstration of an endoleak on imaging studies.

Graft Thrombosis

On contrast-enhanced CT scans, graft thrombosis is recognized as a nonenhancing intraluminal, parietal, circular, or semicircular area within the stent graft (Figs. 103-20 to 103-23; see Fig. 103-8). Parietal thrombi within the stent graft are reported to occur at rates of 3% to 19%. The prognosis for these parietal thrombi varies from spontaneous shrinkage to development of complete thrombosis, thus necessitating follow-up studies at short intervals.[23]

Graft Kinking

When large aneurysms decrease in diameter after endovascular repair, they also decrease in length. Therefore, the three-dimensional space in which the stent graft is contained decreases its volume, which may lead to the development of a kink in the stent graft. Axial CT images cannot adequately depict the shape of the stent graft, but maximum intensity projection or multiplanar reconstruction images can better demonstrate the graft kinking. Kinking is more prone to occur in unsupported portions of the stent graft or can be associated with distal migration of the proximal portion of the stent graft.

Graft Infection

Graft infection, a rare event after endovascular stent graft implantation, is associated with considerable mortality and morbidity rates. Although fever, leukocytosis, elevation of C-reactive protein, and perigraft air are frequently observed immediately after implantation, these findings do not represent evidence of systemic or graft infections. Periprosthetic thickening with soft tissue attenuation at follow-up CT does not always indicate graft infection, and the diagnosis of graft infection may be difficult to establish. Graft infection is occasionally observed some time after the procedure and is suspected on the basis of clinical symptoms and CT findings. A combination of administration of systemic antibiotics and surgery is typically necessary to obtain successful therapeutic results. The outcome of no treatment of aortic stent graft infection or treatment with exclusive antibiotics is invariably fatal. The principle in such surgical treatment is total excision of the infected graft.[23]

Graft Occlusion

Graft occlusion is a relatively rare event after stent graft implantation. Decreased blood flow into the stent graft, caused by the inability of the stent graft to bend along a tortuous infrarenal aorta, may lead to graft occlusion. Occlusion of the iliac graft limb caused by emboli from the left atrium has been reported. Occlusion of the aortic portion of a bifurcated stent graft 4 months after

■ **FIGURE 103-21** Aortic bi-iliac stent graft with circumferential thrombus development within aortic lumen. Axial (**A**) as well as coronal MPR (**B**) images reveal moderate circumferential thrombus within the aortic component of this stent graft. There is no endoleak.

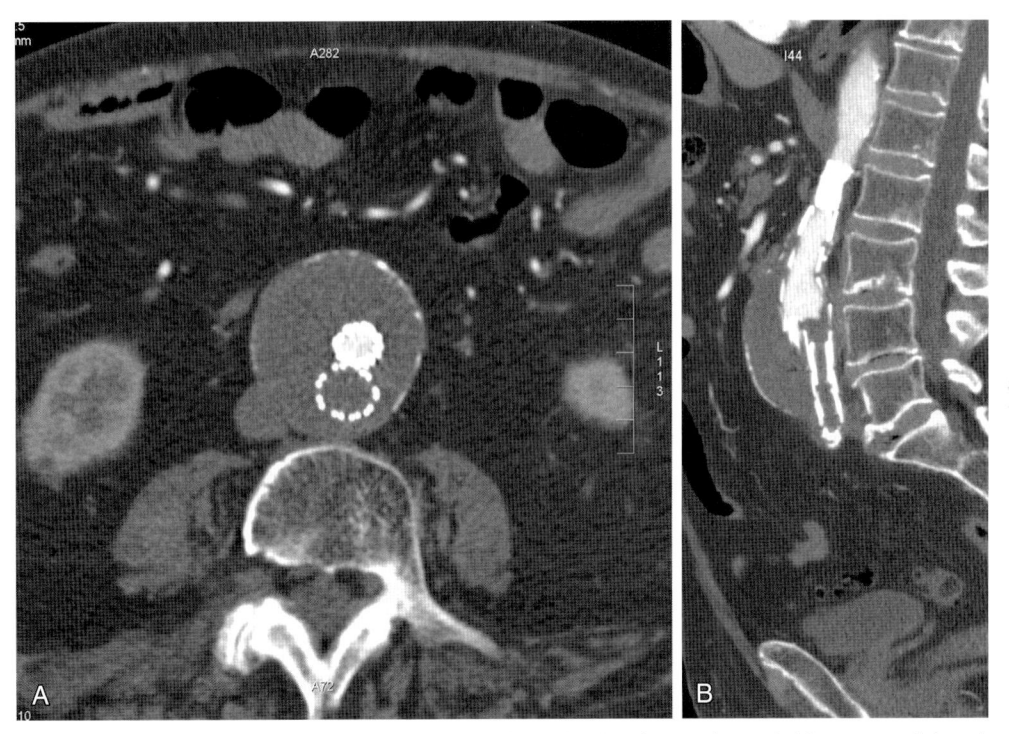

■ **FIGURE 103-22** Thrombotic occlusion of the left limb of the stent graft. Axial (**A**) and coronal MPR (**B**) images reveal thrombotic occlusion of the left iliac limb of the stent graft.

implantation has been described, associated with distal kinking of the left iliac limb.[23]

Shower Embolism

Shower embolism is one of the most serious, possibly fatal complications after conventional repair of infrarenal abdominal aortic aneurysm and is relatively rare. Shower embolism occurs more frequently after endovascular aneurysm repair than after conventional open surgery. Shower embolism after endovascular procedures is reported at rates of 4% to 17% and was fatal in all reported cases.[24]

Colon Necrosis

Colon ischemia, or necrosis, is a feared complication of endovascular stent graft implantation to treat infrarenal abdominal aortic aneurysm. This will occur if both internal iliac arteries and the inferior mesenteric artery are

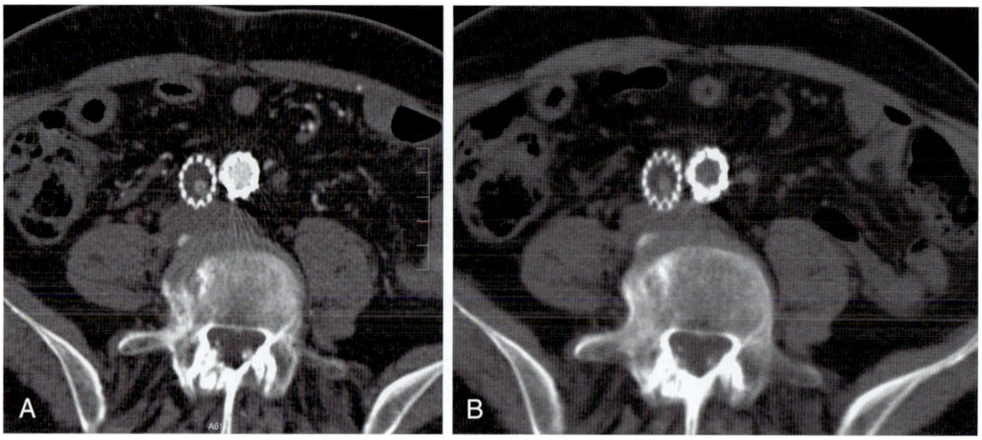

FIGURE 103-23 Calcified occluded stent graft mimicking focal patency. **A,** An axial CT image postcontrast reveals thrombosis of the iliac stent component on the right, with an apparent focal region of increased attenuation suggesting residual patency. **B,** The noncontrast CT scan, however, reveals the similar density indicating focal thrombus calcification. The iliac limb on the right was completely occluded, requiring femoral to femoral bypass graft placement.

occluded by the stent graft, in which case colon ischemia necessitating sigmoid colon resection may be needed.[25] Intraprocedural hypoperfusion of both internal iliac arteries and occlusion of a widely patent inferior mesenteric artery by the stent graft may result in sigmoid colon necrosis, with subsequent hemicolectomy.[23] It has been reported that a widely patent inferior mesenteric artery may be an exclusion criterion for endovascular treatment.[26] There is not, however, sufficient evidence to support this.[23]

Dissection

Aortic or iliac artery dissection caused by a retrograde injury from delivery system introduction has been described. However, no treatment is necessary in cases in which the patient is asymptomatic and hemodynamically stable. Alternatively, placement of a stent can be considered, if applicable (see Figs. 103-5 to 103-7).

Hematoma at the Arteriotomy Site

Hematoma at the arteriotomy site can develop on grounds of hypocoagulability and may require surgical repair. Small hematomas at the arteriotomy sites, however, are not unusual postsurgical findings and will resolve over time with no need for intervention.[27]

POSTOPERATIVE MANAGEMENT

As noted, surveillance of stent graft patients is critical to determine long-term performance of the devices. This is usually accomplished with contrast-enhanced CT at 30 days, 6 months, and then annually for the life of the patient. The goals of these scans are to determine the response of the aneurysm sac to the placement of the endograft and to identify the presence or absence of endoleaks. An endoleak is defined as blood flow outside the lumen of the stent graft and contained within the aneurysm sac as demonstrated on contrast-enhanced CT, contrast-enhanced MR, duplex ultrasonography, or conventional x-ray catheter arteriography. Endoleaks after endovascular repair of aortic aneurysm range from 2.4% to 45.5%.[13] Persistent endoleak is considered a therapeutic failure. Its detection, therefore, is of primary importance because it is associated with increased pressure within the aneurysmal sac, thus increasing the risk of aneurysmal rupture. Endoleaks can appear during the first 30 days after implantation, in which case they are termed *primary*. *Secondary endoleaks* are the ones that occur during subsequent follow-up. The reappearance of an endoleak after its spontaneous resolution or after it was treated is termed a *recurrent endoleak*.[13,28] Type I endoleaks, also called *attachment site endoleaks*, are repaired immediately after diagnosis because this represents a direct communication between the aneurysm sac and arterial blood under systemic pressure. These leaks are usually corrected by further securing the attachment sites with angioplasty balloons, stents, or stent graft extensions. They can be minimized by careful patient selection and accurate preprocedural measurements.

Type II endoleaks are the most commonly identified endoleaks and there is controversy regarding optimal management. A type II endoleak is retrograde flow into the aneurysmal sac from patent side branches, usually the lumbar arteries and/or a patent inferior mesenteric artery. A risk factor that predisposes to type II endoleak formation is the number of patent side branch vessels, including lumbar arteries and the inferior mesenteric artery. The greater the number of patent side branches, the greater the likelihood of leak formation. Preprocedural embolization of patent lumbar or inferior mesenteric arteries is not performed routinely. Treatment of all type II endoleaks has been advocated because the increasing pressure within the aneurysm sac may promote sac rupture. Others, however, have recommended that unless the aneurysm sac is expanding, clinical observation is sufficient because many small type II endoleaks will seal spontaneously; this practice is most widely accepted.[29] The treatment of type II endoleaks can be performed using percutaneous embolization, such as with a microcatheter that is advanced through collateral vessels and into the vessel that communicates with the aneurysm sac, usually the inferior mesenteric artery or a lumbar artery, if possible. Metallic coils are then used to embolize the vessel near its communication with the aneurysm. However, recurrences using this technique are very common. A percutaneous translumbar approach has also been described; this involves direct puncture of the aneurysm sac at the level of the endoleak using a 19-gauge, 20-cm needle. Embolic agents are then administered through the access needle. The most commonly used embolic agents are stainless steel or platinum coils. Liquid embolic agents such as n-butyl cyanoacrylate have also been successfully used.[30]

Type III endoleaks are caused when there is a structural failure with the stent graft and modular attachment points—for example, when an iliac limb becomes separated from the main body of the stent graft. When such an endoleak occurs, there is direct communication between systemic arterial blood and the aneurysm sac, which must be repaired immediately on diagnosis. Such endoleaks can usually be corrected by bridging the defect with a stent graft extension. These leaks are believed to be the most dangerous because of rapid repressurization of the aneurysm sac.

Type IV endoleaks are uncommon with grafts used currently but are usually seen during the immediate post-deployment angiogram (as an aneurysm sac blush) while patients are fully anticoagulated. These leaks are self-limited and no treatment is needed; they resolve after the patient's coagulation status is normalized after endovascular repair of an AAA.

At present, the management and treatment of endoleaks remain a work in progress, despite advances in stent graft technology. There is general agreement on the need to treat patients with type I and III endoleaks. However, there is no consensus regarding management of type II endoleaks and reports on their natural course, with or without treatment, will continue to accumulate. More and continued investigations are needed to determine when and how patients with endoleaks are managed after endovascular aneurysm repair.

In summary, a successful stent graft procedure should result in successful implantation of the device, thereby preventing aneurysm rupture by permanently excluding the aneurysm from the arterial circulation while retaining long-term device patency. Early results are promising, but the future role of this treatment modality is not certain. Imaging will continue to have a pivotal role in the preprocedural evaluation of patients with abdominal aortic aneurysms and surveillance of their repairs.

KEY POINTS

- Endovascular treatment of abdominal aortic aneurysms has been accepted as an alternative to conventional open surgery in carefully selected patients.
- Patients with stent grafts should have lifelong follow-up, both clinically and radiologically.
- Contrast-enhanced CT (typically CTA) is the preferred imaging modality for follow-up of these patients.
- Various complications may occur after endovascular implantation of a stent graft, and many of these can be treated by interventionalists.
- Some complications are potentially fatal and interpreting physicians need to be familiar with their appearance.
- Awareness and understanding of potential complications should help ensure a safe and successful procedure.

SUGGESTED READINGS

Bashir MR, Ferral H, Jacobs C, et al. Endoleaks after endovascular abdominal aortic aneurysm repair: management strategies according to CT findings. AJR Am J Roentgenol 2009; 192:W178-W186.

Chaikof EL, Blankensteijn JD, Harris PL, et al; Ad Hoc Committee for Standardized Reporting Practices in Vascular Surgery of The Society for Vascular Surgery/American Association for Vascular Surgery. Reporting standards for endovascular aortic aneurysm repair. J Vasc Surg 2002; 35:1048-1060.

Davis M, Taylor PR. Endovascular infrarenal abdominal aortic aneurysm repair. Heart 2008; 94:222-228.

Eliason JL, Clouse WD. Current management of infrarenal abdominal aortic aneurysms. Surg Clin North Am 2007; 87:1017-1033.

Eliason JL, Upchurch GR Jr. Endovascular abdominal aortic aneurysm repair. Circulation 2008; 117:1738-1744.

Kaufman JA, Geller SC, Brewster DC, et al. Endovascular repair of abdominal aortic aneurysms: current status and future directions. AJR Am J Roentgenol 2000; 175:289-302.

Lovegrove RE, Javid M, Magee TR, Galland RB. A meta-analysis of 21,178 patients undergoing open or endovascular repair of abdominal aortic aneurysm. Br J Surg 2008; 95:677-684.

REFERENCES

1. Dardik A, Burleyson G, Bowman H, et al. Surgical repair of ruptured abdominal aortic aneurysms in the state of Maryland: factors influencing outcome among 527 recent cases. J Vasc Surg 1998; 28:413-421.
2. Hallett JJ, Bower T, Cherry K, et al. Selection and preparation of high-risk patients for repair of abdominal aortic aneurysms. Mayo Clin Proc 1994; 69:763-768.
3. Ernst C. Abdominal aortic aneurysm. N Engl J Med 1993; 328:1167-1172.
4. Hodges TC, Cronenwett J. Abdominal aortic and iliac artery aneurysms: clinical presentation, natural history, and indications for intervention. In Perler BA, Becker GJ (eds). Vascular Intervention: A Clinical Approach. New York, Thieme, 1998, pp 339-350.
5. Parodi J, Palmaz J, Barone H. Transfemoral intraluminal graft implantation for abdominal aortic aneurysms. Ann Vasc Surg 1991; 5:491-499.
6. Krupski WC, Selzman CH, Floridia R, et al. Contemporary management of isolated iliac aneurysms. J Vasc Surg 1998; 28:1-11.
7. Sekkal S, Cornu E, Christides C, et al. Iliac artery aneurysms: sixty-seven cases in forty-eight patients. J Mal Vasc 1993; 18:13-17.
8. Brunkwall J, Hauksson N, Bengtsson H, et al. Solitary aneurysm of the iliac artery system: an estimate of their frequency of occurrence. J Vasc Surg 1989; 10:381-384.
9. Richardson JW, Greenfield LJ. Natural history and management of iliac aneurysms. J Vasc Surg 1988; 8:165-171.

10. Sakamoto I, Sueyoshi E, Hazama S, et al. Endovascular treatment of iliac artery aneurysms. Radiographics 2005; 25:S213-S227.
11. Armon M, Yusuf S, Latief K, et al. Anatomical suitability of abdominal aortic aneurysms for endovascular repair. Br J Surg 1997; 84:178-180.
12. Treiman G, Lawrence P, Edwards WJ, et al. An assessment of the current applicability of the EVT endovascular graft for treatment of patients with an infrarenal abdominal aortic aneurysm. J Vasc Surg 1999; 30:68-75.
13. Kaufman JA, Geller SC, Brewster DC, et al. Endovascular repair of abdominal aortic aneurysms: current status and future directions. AJR Am J Roentgenol 2000; 175:289-302.
14. EVAR Trial Participants. Endovascular aneurysm repair versus open repair in patients with abdominal aortic aneurysm (EVAR trial 1): randomised controlled trial. Lancet 2005; 365:2179-2186.
15. Blankensteijn JD, de Jong SECA, Prinssen M, et al. Two-year outcomes after conventional or endovascular repair of abdominal aortic aneurysms. N Engl J Med 2005; 352:2398-2405.
16. EVAR Trial Participants. Endovascular aneurysm repair and outcome in patients unfit for open repair of abdominal aortic aneurysm (EVAR trial 2): randomised controlled trial. Lancet 2005; 365:2187-2192.
17. Lee C, Kaufman J, Fan C-M, et al. Clinical outcome of internal iliac artery occlusions during endovascular treatment of aorto-iliac aneurysmal diseases J Vasc Interv Radiol 2000; 11:567-571.
18. Ahn S, Rutherford R, Johnston K, et al. Reporting standards for infrarenal endovascular abdominal aortic aneurysm repair. J Vasc Surg 1997; 25:405-410.
19. White G, May J, Waugh R, et al. Type III and type IV endoleak: toward a complete definition of blood flow in the sac after endoluminal abdominal aortic aneurysm repair. J Endovasc Surg 1998; 5:305-309.
20. Marin ML, Hollier LH, Ellozy SH, et al. Endovascular stent graft repair of abdominal and thoracic aortic aneurysms: a ten-year experience with 817 patients. Ann Surg 2003; 238:586-595.
21. Rozenblit A, Marin M, Veith F, et al. Endovascular repair of abdominal aortic aneurysm: value of postoperative follow-up with helical CT. AJR Am J Roentgenol 1995; 165:1473-1479.
22. Görich J, Rilinger N, Soldner J, et al. Endovascular repair of aortic aneurysm: treatment of complications. J Endovasc Surg 1999; 6:136-146.
23. Mita T, Arita T, Matsunaga N, et al. complications of endovascular repair for thoracic and abdominal aortic aneurysm: an imaging spectrum. Radiographics 2000; 20:1263-1278.
24. Thompson MM, Smith J, Naylor AR, et al. Microembolization during endovascular and conventional aneurysm repair. J Vasc Surg 1997; 25:179-186.
25. Yusuf SW, Whitaker SC, Chuter TAM, et al. Early results of endovascular aortic aneurysm surgery with aortouniiliac graft, contralateral iliac occlusion, and femorofemoral bypass. J Vasc Surg 1997; 25:165-172.
26. Blum U, Langer M, Spillner G, et al. Abdominal aortic aneurysms: preliminary technical and clinical results with transfemoral placement of endovascular self-expanding stent grafts. Radiology 1996; 198:25-31.
27. Mialhe C, Amicabile C, Becquemin JP. Endovascular treatment of infrarenal abdominal aneurysms by the Stentor system: preliminary results of 79 cases. J Vasc Surg 1997; 26:199-209.
28. Chaikof EL, Blankensteijn JD, Harris PL, et al; Ad Hoc Committee for Standardized Reporting Practices in Vascular Surgery of The Society for Vascular Surgery/American Association for Vascular Surgery. Reporting standards for endovascular aortic aneurysm repair. J Vasc Surg 2002; 35:1048-1060.
29. Zarins CK, White RA, Hodgson KJ, et al. Endoleak as a predictor of outcome after endovascular aneurysm repair: AneuRx multicenter clinical trial. J Vasc Surg 2000; 32:90-107.
30. Baum RA, Stavropoulos SW, Fairman RM, Carpenter JP. Endoleaks after endovascular repair of abdominal aortic aneurysms. J Vasc Interv Radiol 2003; 14:1111-1117.

CHAPTER 104

Open Repair of Abdominal Aortic Aneurysms and Postoperative Assessment

Lisa M. Dias, Kostaki G. Bis, and Thomas Vrachliotis

Most surgeons agree that repair should be considered for abdominal aortic aneurysms (AAAs) larger than 50 to 55 mm in diameter. Open surgical repair was the mainstay of treatment for AAA until the 1990s. This procedure is associated with a low mortality rate in select patients. However, it is also a major operation, with the potential for significant blood loss, stress on the cardiopulmonary system, and a prolonged hospital stay. In particular, patients who have significant comorbidities have a significantly increased mortality risk associated with the procedure. In such patients, endovascular repair may be considered.

A limitation of endovascular repair, however, is that patients with certain types of vascular anatomy are not candidates for the procedure. For example, some length of nonaneurysmal infrarenal aorta (depending on the device used) must be present for placement of the proximal attachment of the endovascular graft. Most operators prefer that the neck have a minimum caliber of 1.5 cm. Aortic neck angles more than 45 degrees are often problematic for proper endograft implantation and may result in excessive stress on the device. Trapezoidal, conical, or thrombus-filled aortic necks may cause device instability. Additionally, the iliofemoral vessels must have a certain (device-dependent) caliber and straightness. In a healthy patient with any of these limitations of anatomy, open surgical repair may be the preferred option.

Open repair of an AAA involves attaching a tube or bifurcated graft within the aneurysm sac. Occasionally, however, the native AAA is excluded from the graft and remains intact posterior to the aortic graft. The transperitoneal or the retroperitoneal approach may be used. In one study, there was no significant difference in mortality rates between the two procedures, and although retroperitoneal repair was associated with less frequent respiratory failure, it was also associated with more frequent wound complications.[1]

There are no strict anatomic contraindications to open repair of an AAA. However, there are many anatomic variations that must be taken into account. Coexisting aneurysms of the common iliac artery, especially if larger than 3 cm, should undergo exclusion during AAA repair. Attention should also be given to possible aneurysms of the hypogastric and external iliac arteries. The common and external iliac arteries may be severely affected by atherosclerotic disease, and may require arterial bypass grafting.[2] Many pararenal aortic aneurysms are now repaired via the open surgical technique because of the frequent lack of a proximal implantation site sufficient for endovascular repair. These aneurysms require greater exposure than infrarenal aneurysms, and are technically more demanding. Repair of juxtarenal, pararenal, or suprarenal aneurysms require suprarenal clamping, which are associated with increased risk for renal damage because of ischemia.

Subsequent sections in this chapter will delineate the postoperative assessment of patients who have undergone open repair of AAAs, postoperative complications that they may encounter, indications and algorithms for imaging these patients, characteristic imaging findings, and, finally, postoperative management.

POSTOPERATIVE ASSESSMENT

Early Postoperative Complications

On the first postoperative day after open repair of an AAA, hypotension and cardiac and respiratory dysfunction are the most likely complications to occur. Between days 1 and 3, the most common complications are congestive heart failure, pulmonary embolism, and respiratory failure. Pneumonia occurs most commonly between 4 and 7 days following surgery. The incidence of renal failure peaks within the initial 3 days following surgery and between 1 and 4 weeks postoperatively.[2] A midline transabdominal incision is associated with higher postoperative rates of pulmonary complications, persistent ileus, and incisional hernias.

Overall, perioperative complications occur in up to 30% of patients. The organs most commonly affected are the heart, lungs, and kidneys. Cardiac-related complications, including arrhythmia, infarction, and congestive heart failure, occur in about 10% to 15% of patients after elective aneurysm repair. Perioperative renal dysfunction predicts a poorer prognosis and correlates with poor preoperative renal function. Insufficient management of pulmonary disease is also associated with a poorer prognosis.[2]

Early postoperative complications also include groin infections (in 2% to 3%), thromboembolism to the kidneys and lower extremities, and hemorrhage. Peripheral ischemia develops in less than 1% of patients postoperatively, but may occur because of damage to diseased arteries during cross clamping, iliac dissection, or peripheral embolization from aortic plaque. Spinal cord ischemia, which may result in paralysis, can occur secondary to a variety of differing factors. The artery of Adamkiewicz may arise below L3 in a minority of patients and ligation of a lumbar artery in the aneurysm sac in such a patient may lead to spinal cord ischemia. An additional cause is suprarenal or supraceliac cross clamping that compromises the spinal cord circulation. Small bowel infarction and colonic ischemia occur in 0.15% and 1% of patients undergoing elective AAA repair, respectively. Colonic ischemia most commonly develops because of ligation of the inferior mesenteric artery.[2]

Because of the course of the ureter over the iliac vessels, the ureter may be injured during open repair of AAAs. The ureter may have a variant course in patients with renal anomalies such as horseshoe kidney, further raising the likelihood for its injury. Ureteral fistulas with resulting urinomas may occur. Options for repair of ureteral injury include placement of a stent and reimplantation of the injured ureter into the bladder.[2]

Late Postoperative Complications

A common late postoperative complication is sexual dysfunction, including impotence and retrograde ejaculation. Erectile dysfunction may occur because of poor flow through the internal pudendal artery as a result of narrowing or occlusion, ligation of the internal iliac artery, an embolus or emboli in the distal pudendal arteries, or injury to the sympathetic nerves in the fascia surrounding the aorta. Other late complications include pseudoaneurysm formation, graft thrombosis, infection, aortoenteric fistula, aneurysm rupture, colonic ischemia, and peripheral embolism. These complications may affect up to 10% of patients.[2]

Aortic neck dilation is a concern after endovascular and open surgical repair. After open repair, aortic neck dilation may lead to para-anastomotic aneurysm formation or rupture. The suprarenal aorta is of particular concern in fenestrated and branched stent grafts.

Postoperative Mortality and Survival

The postoperative mortality rate for elective open repair is approximately 5%; it is lower in younger healthier patients and higher in older at-risk patients. Risk factors that increase a patient's risk of mortality following open aneurysm repair include advanced age, female gender, and any associated comorbidities. Additional factors include the experience of the operating surgeon, need for urgent (rather than elective) repair, and hospital volume (hospitals with higher surgical volumes generally have a lower mortality rate than those with lower volumes).[2]

Five-year survival of patients after successful elective open AAA repair is 60% to 70% and the 10-year survival rate is approximately 40%. These survival rates are lower than those of matched patients without AAAs, and the increased mortality is mostly to the result of manifestations of atherosclerosis, especially coronary artery disease.[3]

The few published reports of pararenal aortic aneurysm repair describe mortality rates that vary from 0% to 15.4%. Renal morbidity rates are high in such patients.[4] In one study, there was a higher risk of overall perioperative mortality for patients who underwent open repair of juxtarenal and pararenal aortic aneurysms compared with those who underwent open repair of infrarenal aortic aneurysms (12% and 3.5%, respectively; $P < .02$).[5]

The mortality for ruptured AAA ranges from 15% to 50%, often caused by hemorrhagic shock, acute renal failure, myocardial infarction, respiratory insufficiency, or multiorgan failure.[6] Mortality following open repair of a ruptured AAA is 30% to 40%.

Surgical Conversion from Endovascular Repair

Conversion from endovascular to open repair may be required for a number of reasons (Table 104-1).[7] Older age, presence of chronic obstructive pulmonary disease (COPD), wider infrarenal necks, and larger aneurysms have been associated with a higher rate of conversion. In one study, the mortality rate of patients who underwent emergency conversion operations was 40%.[8]

Clinical Presentation

The vast majority of AAAs are clinically silent. Often, AAAs are detected incidentally during abdominal ultrasonography. AAA rupture should be suspected particularly in patients with known AAAs who present with pain in the low back, flank, abdomen, or groin. On physical examination, a palpable, pulsatile abdominal mass may be detected. Abdominal bruits may reflect renal or visceral arterial stenosis.

Bleeding from a ruptured AAA often leads to hypovolemic shock, the signs of which include hypotension, tachycardia, cyanosis, and altered mental status. Flank ecchymosis (the Grey-Turner sign) may be apparent, and reflects retroperitoneal hemorrhage.

TABLE 104-1 Reported Reasons for Conversion from Endoluminal Graft (ELG) to Open Repair

Primary Conversion	Secondary Conversion
Inability to gain access	Persistent endoleak
Aortic rupture	Aortic rupture
Failed deployment	Sealed endoleak with continued AAA expansion
Irreversible twisting of a nonmodular ELG	Apparently successful repair with continued expansion
Migration of ELG causing obstructed flow	Infection in the ELG
Endograft thrombosis	Renal arteries covered by the endograft

From Myers K, Devine T, Barras C, Self G. Endoluminal versus open repair for abdominal aortic aneurysms 2009. Available at: http://www.fac.org.ar/scvc/llave/interven/myers/myersi.htm. Accessed October 6, 2009.

Aortoenteric Fistula

Although the classic array of symptoms in patients with an aortoenteric fistula following aortic graft repair of AAA consists of GI bleeding, pain, and sepsis, most patients do not present in this way. Some patients present with a herald bleed followed by temporary stoppage and then severe hemorrhage. An aortoduodenal fistula develops when an AAA ruptures into the fourth portion of the duodenum. These patients may present with a herald upper gastrointestinal bleed followed by severe hemorrhage.

Aortic Graft Infection

In cases of aortic graft infection occurring within 4 months of surgery, the patient may present with fever and a high white blood cell (WBC) count. Associated septicemia, wound infection, and graft dysfunction from thrombosis or hemorrhage from the anastomotic site may occur. Infections that occur more than 4 months postoperatively may present with more subtle signs and symptoms, and a fever may be absent. Such patients have a higher likelihood of presenting with signs of complications from their aortic graft infection, such as pseudoaneurysm, aortoenteric fistula, hydronephrosis, or osteomyelitis.[9]

Aortoiliac Occlusive Disease

Stenosis at the distal anastomosis is a common reason for failure of bypass repair for aortoiliac occlusive disease. Symptoms include recurrent lower extremity claudication.

Aortocaval Fistula

An aortocaval fistula develops when an AAA ruptures into the vena cava, producing an arteriovenous fistula. Patients with an aortocaval fistula most commonly present with abdominal pain, back pain, and dyspnea. They often have hematuria and acute renal insufficiency. On physical examination, a machinery-type abdominal bruit may be auscultated, and an abdominal thrill may be palpated. Additional signs include tachycardia and peripheral edema.

Anastomotic Pseudoaneurysms

An anastomotic pseudoaneurysm is a potential late complication after repair of an AAA. It does not contain all the layers normally present in an arterial wall and are at risk for rupture. Anastomotic pseudoaneurysms most commonly result from arterial degeneration or infection.[10] They may be aortic, iliac, or femoral. Degenerative anastomotic pseudoaneurysms may present in 0.2% to 15% of patients after AAA repair.[11-13] One study[10] found the most common manifestations of such pseudoaneurysms to be bleeding caused by rupture (30%) and sequelae of chronic limb ischemia (25%). Pseudoaneurysms may also manifest with symptoms caused by compression of adjacent structures or acute limb ischemia, or as an asymptomatic pulsatile mass.

Imaging Indications and Algorithm

Abdominal Ultrasound

Abdominal ultrasound is often used for screening but also for preoperative and postoperative evaluation of AAAs. On ultrasound, the size of an AAA can be measured; this serves as a good method to follow patients with smaller AAAs that do not meet the size criteria for surgery. If performed by trained personnel, ultrasound has a high sensitivity (approaching 100%) and specificity (approximately 96%) for the detection of infrarenal AAAs.[14]

Advantages of ultrasound compared with other modalities include its lack of exposure to intravenous contrast and ionizing radiation and its low cost. However, ultrasound is limited in its ability to demonstrate the relationship of the proximal AAA to the renal arteries, and it is also limited in its ability to demonstrate the presence or absence of associated internal iliac artery aneurysms. Ultrasound is an operator-dependent modality and is often suboptimal in patients who are obese or of large body habitus and in patients with excessive overlying bowel gas may obscure proper visualization of the abdominal aorta.

Computed Tomography and Computed Tomographic Angiography

In cases of planned open repair of an AAA, a preoperative contrast-enhanced CT scan is usually adequate. Contrast-enhanced CT and, in particular, CT angiography (CTA), are the primary imaging modalities for illustration and evaluation of AAAs and for the postoperative assessment of AAAs. CT and CTA are noninvasive methods that can be used to detect thrombus within the aneurysm, thus making them more accurate in sizing the full extent of AAAs (i.e., wall to wall dimension) than conventional x-ray catheter angiography. Conventional x-ray angiography may yield a falsely low estimate of aneurysm size by demonstrating only the inner luminal diameter of the aneurysm when there is thrombus adherent to the wall of the AAA. CT can demonstrate coexisting aneurysms of the iliac vessels, determine the relationship of an AAA to the renal vessels, reveal venous and renal anomalies (e.g., a retroaortic left renal vein and horseshoe kidney), and demonstrate incidental but perhaps significant intra-abdominal pathology not related to the AAA.

The clinical limitations of CT include its risks related to the use of iodinated contrast (e.g., anaphylactoid contrast reactions, contrast-induced nephropathy) and the need to subject the patient to ionizing radiation exposure. CT of patients with certain metallic implanted devices may also be problematic secondary to metallic artifacts, which may obscure proper visualization of pertinent vascular regions.

Conventional X-Ray Catheter Angiography

Select patients with AAAs, such as those with suspected mesenteric ischemia, peripheral vascular occlusive disease or peripheral vascular aneurysms, renovascular hypertension, renal anomalies such as horseshoe kidney, or thoracoabdominal aneurysms, should undergo conventional angiography. Angiography may also be performed prior to planned endovascular repair to evaluate tortuous proximal aneurysm necks and tortuous iliac arteries.[15]

Risks of catheter angiography include catheter-related complications and exposure to iodinated contrast media and ionizing radiation. As noted, catheter angiography may yield a falsely low estimate of aneurysm size.

Magnetic Resonance Imaging and Magnetic Resonance Angiography

MRI (and MR angiography, MRA) can also be useful for the evaluation of AAAs prior to open repair, especially in patients with known iodinated contrast allergy or renal insufficiency, because MRI does not require the administration of iodinated contrast media. MRI with MRA can provide the necessary information for proper surveillance of postoperative complications such as pseudoaneurysm formation, thrombosis, graft infection, and fistulas.

The limitations of MRI include its high cost, the fact that MRI is contraindicated in patients with certain implanted devices (such as indwelling pacemakers), and the long acquisition times associated with MRI, which make it an inappropriate study for the evaluation of medically unstable patients. The use of gadolinium chelate contrast agents for MRI or MRA can be an issue in patients with known allergy to gadolinium or with severe renal insufficiency, in whom there may be an increased albeit small risk for nephrogenic systemic fibrosis (NSF).

Imaging Techniques and Findings

Abdominal Ultrasound

Abdominal ultrasound can detect an aneurysm and investigate its size and location. As noted, ultrasound is limited in its ability to demonstrate the relationship of the proximal AAA to the renal arteries, and it is also limited in its ability to demonstrate the presence or absence of associated internal iliac artery aneurysms.[16]

Ultrasonographic imaging of the abdominal aorta should include imaging in the transverse and longitudinal planes. The maximum diameter of the AAA, proximal and distal extent, length and diameter of the proximal neck, diameter of the common iliac arteries, and diameter of the hypogastric arteries can be determined. Often, a B-mode ultrasound study is sufficient. Occasionally, color and Duplex scanning are useful, such as in the identification of an aortocaval fistula.[15]

Computed Tomography and Computed Tomographic Angiography

CT, especially CTA, can detect extension of an aneurysm into the iliac vessels, delineate the relationship of an aneurysm to the renal vasculature, and demonstrate the presence of renal anomalies and intra-abdominal pathology, such as masses.[15] CT is particularly well suited for imaging the postoperative aorta following aortic graft repair.

Typically, a non–contrast-enhanced CT is performed initially to cover the abdomen and pelvis. No oral contrast is given so as not to interfere with subsequent postprocessing of the contrast-enhanced CTA. Oral water-soluble contrast, however, is helpful for the evaluation of a suspected aortoenteric fistula in a patient who is not actively bleeding. In patients with normal renal function, contrast-enhanced CT using a CTA protocol (120 kVp, variable mAs, depending on body size, pitch 1, 0.6 to 0.75 collimation, 1-mm reconstructions every 0.5 mm for postprocessing, automated bolus detection for arterial phase acquisition) is typically performed. A delayed-phase acquisition (90 to 120 seconds postcontrast, 2- to 3 mm-reconstructions) is also carried out to evaluate the abdomen and pelvis.

Conventional X-Ray Catheter Angiography

Digital subtraction angiography (DSA) provides high-resolution images of the aorta, demonstrates the presence of significant stenoses in visceral and iliofemoral arteries, and can demonstrate tortuosity of the proximal neck of an AAA and of the iliac arteries.

Magnetic Resonance Imaging and Magnetic Resonance Angiography

Like CT, MRI with MRA can demonstrate intraluminal thrombus and detect intra-abdominal pathology. Also, MRI can differentiate perigraft fibrosis or thrombus from fluid (e.g., that caused by infection) through the use of T2- and T1-weighted postcontrast sequences. However, the sensitivity of MRI for the detection of aortic graft infection remains unclear.

The protocol for postoperative assessment should include MRI (axial T1-weighted precontrast and postcontrast and T2-weighted [with fat suppression] sequences) and contrast-enhanced three-dimensional MRA. The ability of MRI and MRA to evaluate the proximal aspect of AAAs accurately, detect stenoses larger than 50% at the origin of the renal arteries, and assess patency of the superior mesenteric artery has been well established.[16]

Normal Postoperative Appearance Following Open Surgical Repair

In a patient who has undergone an open surgical repair of an AAA, the graft may be seen as a round, well-

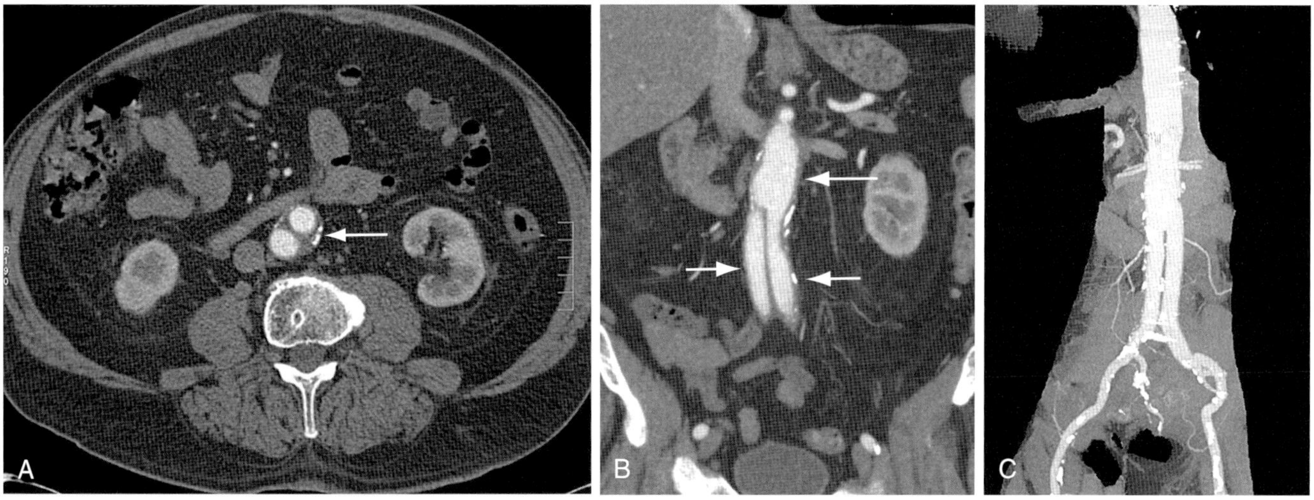

FIGURE 104-1 Normal aortic bi-iliac bypass graft wrapped with native calcified aortic wall. **A,** Axial CTA image demonstrates the two iliac limbs surrounded by the native calcified aortic wall (*arrow*). Intervening low-attenuation thrombus is also present. **B,** The coronal multiplanar reformation (MPR) image shows the aortic graft component (*long arrows*) attached to the native aorta via end-to-end anastomosis. The opposed iliac graft components (*short arrows*) are also seen. **C,** The maximum intensity projection (MIP) image shows the end-to-end infrarenal anastomosis of the aortic graft.

demarcated structure within the aneurysmal sac. After intravenous contrast administration on CT, the graft is seen as an enhancing tubular structure surrounded by the native aorta in cases of proximal end-to-end anastomosis (Fig. 104-1). In cases of end-to-side proximal anastomosis, the enhancing graft may be seen running ventral and parallel to the nonenhancing diseased or aneurysmal aorta, which is now collapsed (Figs. 104-2 and 104-3). The graft bifurcation is at a higher level compared with the now occluded native bifurcation in cases of aortic-bi-iliac or aortobifemoral grafts. In cases of more complicated grafts such as combined unilateral aortoiliac with or without femoral to femoral bypass, knowledge of surgical history helps the interpreting physician to follow the graft as an enhancing tubular structure from the site of the proximal to distal anastomosis. MRA (Fig. 104-4) is also well suited for imaging the aortic and iliac graft components after surgery.

Aortocaval Fistula

An aortocaval fistula is discovered in 2% to 4% of ruptured AAAs and requires immediate surgical repair. Most (90%) of these occur between the aortic bifurcation and iliac veins or distal vena cava. Duplex ultrasound demonstrates high-velocity flow in the inferior vena cava or the left renal vein. CT may demonstrate early filling of the subjacent venous system during the arterial phase of CTA acquisition.

Aortic Graft Infection

Aortic graft infection occurs in 1% to 5% of reconstructions.[17] This complication has mortality rates of 25% to 75%.[18] Aortic graft infection may lead to graft occlusion and anastomotic hemorrhage, which may lead to aortoenteric fistula.

Graft infection may occur from a few days to many years after surgery. CT is considered the imaging modality of choice for the diagnosis of graft infection (Figs. 104-5 to 104-8). One study has shown that CT has a sensitivity of 94% and specificity of 85% for the detection of perigraft infection, with or without associated aortoenteric fistula, when the criteria of perigraft fluid, perigraft soft tissue density, ectopic gas, pseudoaneurysm, or focal bowel wall thickening were used.[19] CT-CTA can demonstrate persistent perigraft soft tissue density, fluid, and gas, characteristics associated with graft infection. However, abnormal perigraft soft tissue density may also represent hematoma, fibrosis, and/or postoperative changes. In this regard, MRI may be helpful because it has improved soft tissue contrast resolution and the improved ability to differentiate between subacute and chronic hematomas, thrombus, and fibrosis from perigraft fluid resulting from graft infection (Fig. 104-9).

Although the normal graft has surrounding fat attenuation in the early postoperative period, there should be less than 5 mm of soft tissue attenuation between the aneurysm wall and underlying graft. Persistent fluid or soft tissue attenuation around the graft may persist for up to 3 months after surgery. Similarly, pockets of gas around the graft may be present for up to 10 days after surgery, but persistence after about 4 weeks postsurgery suggests infection.[20]

Duplex ultrasound or CTA can confirm the occlusion and also reveal perigraft fluid, consistent with infection. MRI, however, has higher specificity for differentiating thrombus and fibrosis from fluid related to infection and can be used in difficult cases.

A recent study has shown that positron emission tomography (PET)-CT has a sensitivity of 93%, specificity of 91%, positive predictive value of 88% and negative predictive value of 96% for the diagnosis of vascular graft infection.[21] PET alone, although highly sensitive, has low specificity and limited anatomic localization.

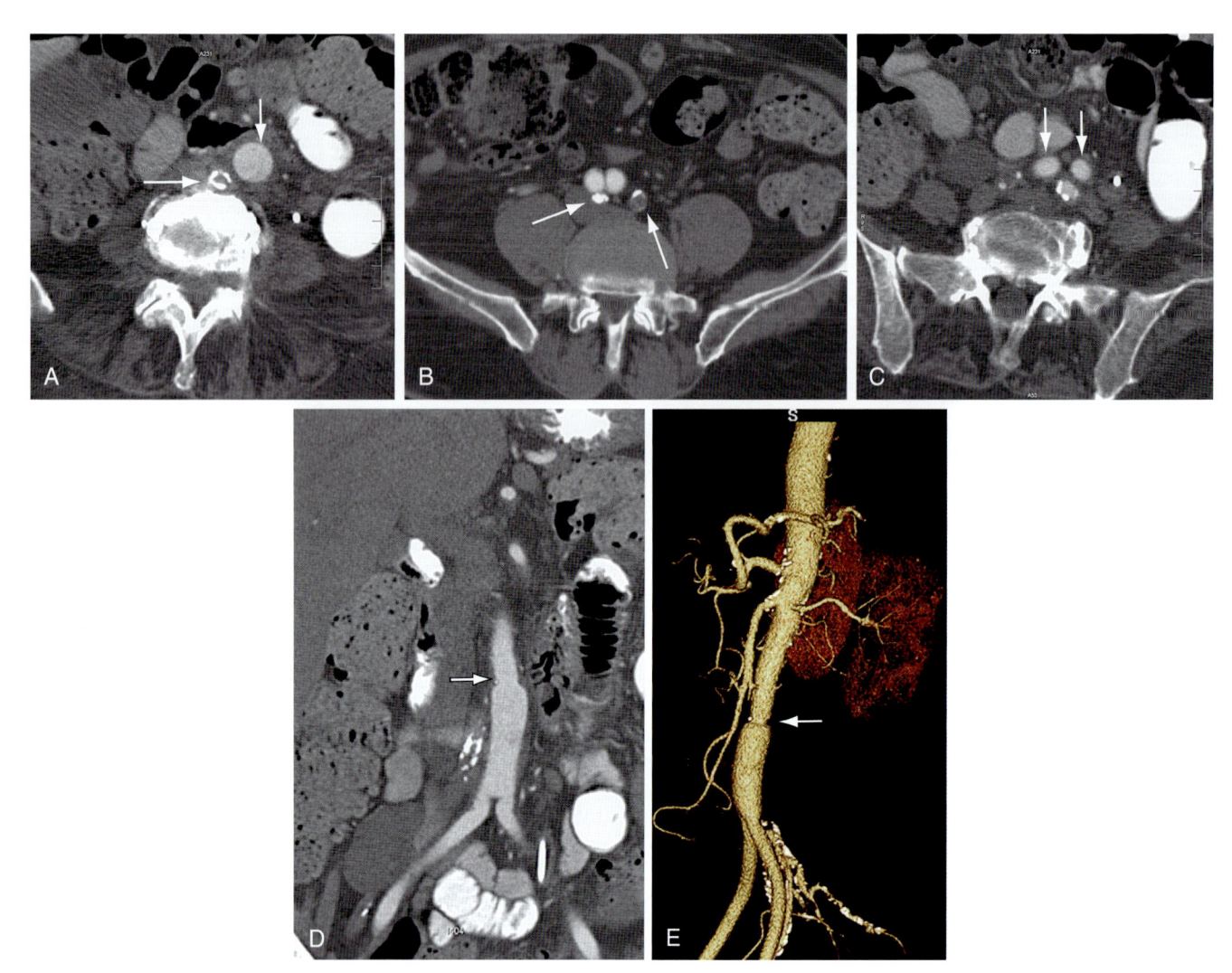

FIGURE 104-2 Normal aortic bifemoral bypass-graft (occluded native aorta excluded posteriorly). **A,** Axial CTA image at the level of the aortic graft demonstrates enhancement of the graft (*short arrow*) with no surrounding fluid. The occluded native aorta is demonstrated posteriorly (*long arrow*). **B,** Axial CTA image demonstrates the enhancing proximal femoral limbs with the native occluded iliac arteries noted posteriorly (*arrows*). **C,** Axial CTA image more inferiorly demonstrates the patent limbs anteriorly (*arrows*) with retrograde flow into native iliac artery on the left. A coronal MPR image (**D**) and volume rendered image (**E**) demonstrate the end-to-end anastomosis at the level of the aorta (*arrow*).

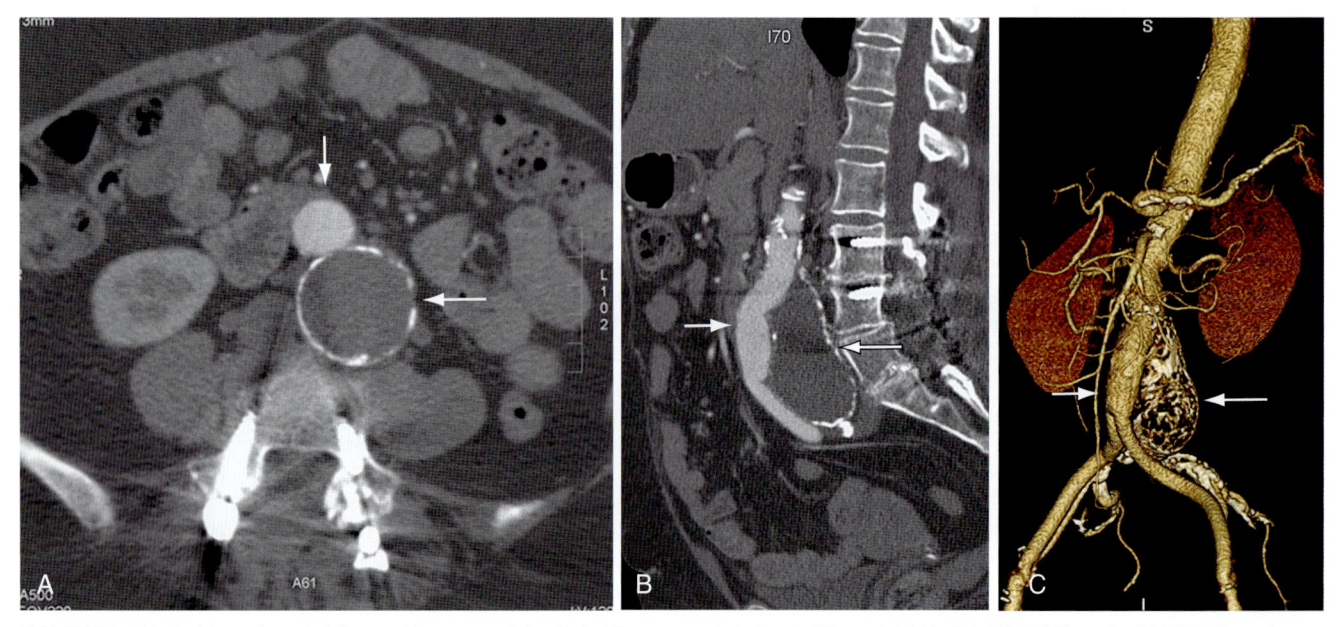

FIGURE 104-3 Normal aortic bifemoral bypass graft (excluded from posteriorly located ligated AAA). Axial CTA (**A**), sagittal MPR (**B**), and oblique volume rendered images (**C**) show the enhancing aortic graft component (*short arrows*) lying anterior to the thrombosed ligated AAA (*long arrows*).

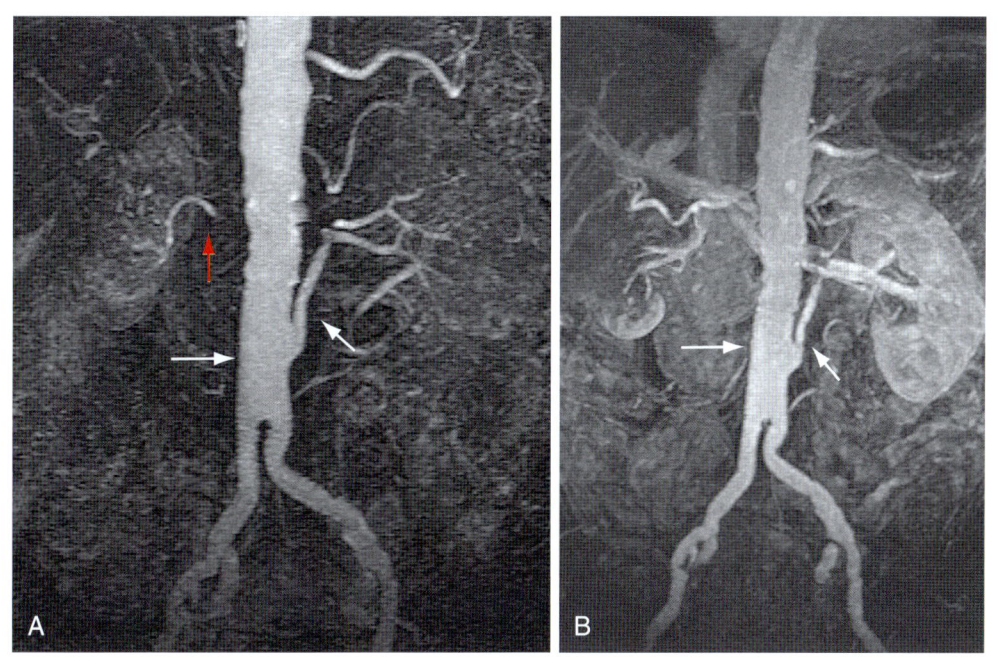

■ **FIGURE 104-4** Aortic bi-iliac bypass graft with left renal artery reimplantation and right-sided renal artery occlusion with renal infarction. Coronal early arterial phase **(A)** and venous phase **(B)** MRA images demonstrate the graft (*long arrows*) and reimplanted left renal artery (*short arrow*). There is proximal occlusion of the right renal artery (*red arrow*). **B,** Delayed-phase acquisition demonstrates a left renal nephrogram and infarction of the right kidney with lack of enhancement sparing the lower pole.

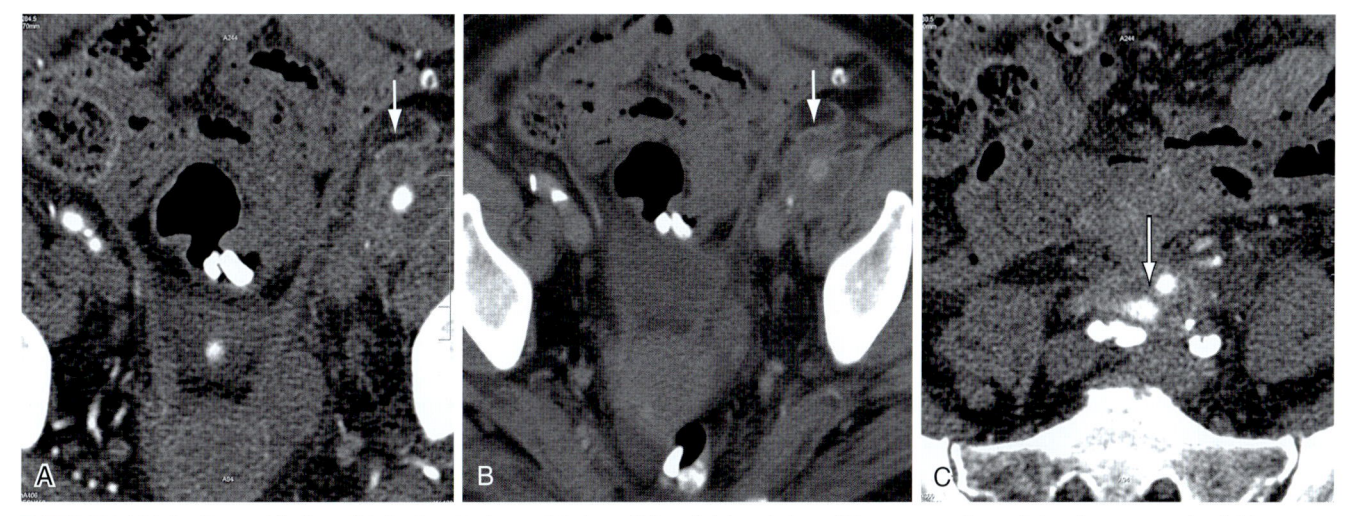

■ **FIGURE 104-5** Femoral limb graft infection. Early arterial phase **(A)** and delayed-phase **(B)** contrast-enhanced CTA images reveal a fluid collection around the left femoral limb within the iliac fossa (*arrows*). Findings represent an abscess. Surrounding abscess wall enhancement is also identified. **C,** Fluid (*arrow*) extended proximally surrounds both proximal femoral graft limbs.

Aortoenteric Fistula

Secondary aortoenteric fistula is a rare but severe complication after abdominal aortic surgery, with mortality rates approaching 100%. This type of fistula accounts for most aortoenteric fistulas. They often result from infection near the proximal anastomosis between the aorta and prosthesis. It is estimated that 80% of secondary aortoenteric fistulas involve the duodenum; typically, its third and fourth parts are affected. These fistulae may occur at any time between 2 weeks and many years after surgery. The annual incidence ranges from 0.6% to 2%.[18]

Although contrast-enhanced CT using a CTA protocol (Figs. 104-10 and 104-11) is the favored diagnostic modality,[18] its sensitivity and specificity vary (from 40% to 90% and 33% to 100%, respectively). CT conducted with oral water-soluble contrast before and after contrast-enhanced CTA is preferred for patients who are not actively bleeding to delineate the fistula from the overlying duodenum (see Fig. 104-10). Prior to intervention, other modalities (e.g., endoscopy, radionuclide studies, angiography) may be needed to arrive at the diagnosis. Conventional x-ray catheter angiography may be combined with embolization and/or stent placement for therapy.

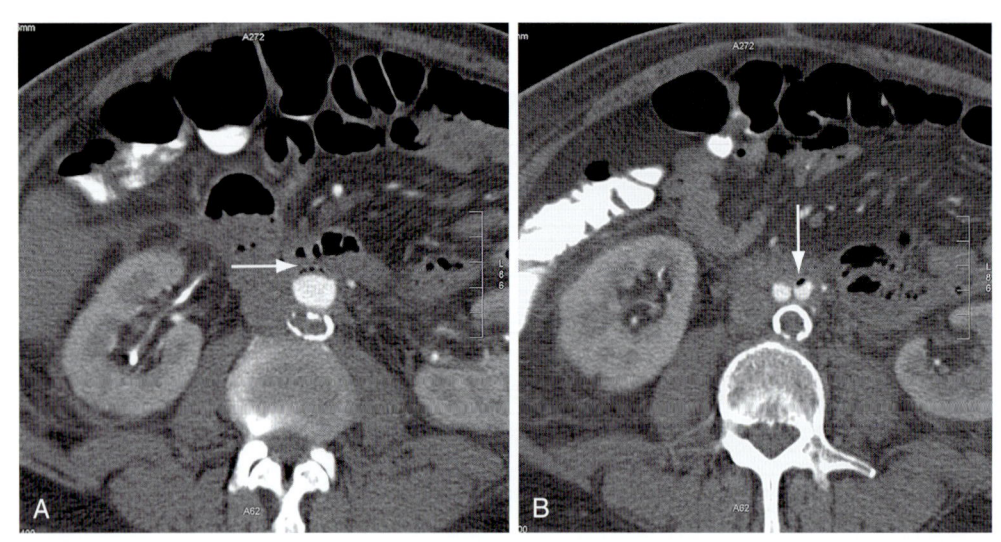

■ **FIGURE 104-6** Aortic bifemoral bypass graft infection. Axial contrast-enhanced CTA images reveal gas within the wall of the graft at the level of the aorta (**A**), as well as at the level of the proximal femoral limb on the left (**B**) (*arrows*). Surrounding ill-defined infiltration indicates inflammatory response. The occluded aorta is excluded posterior to the aortic graft.

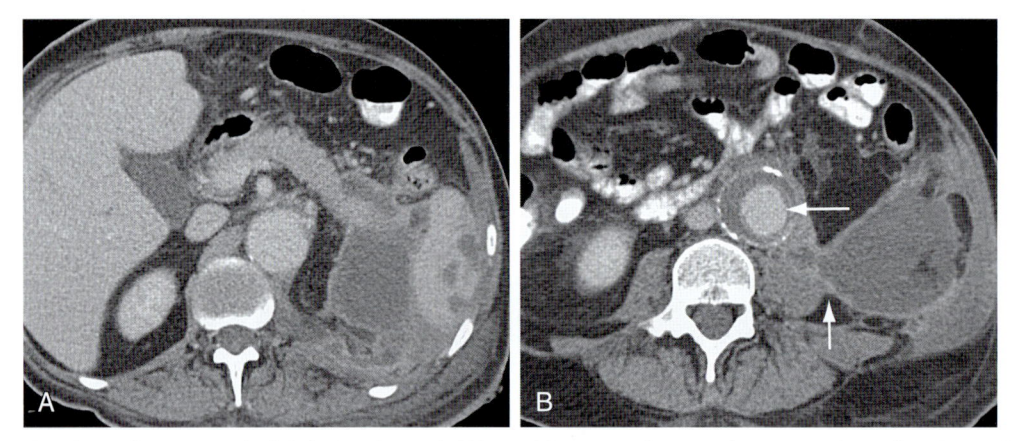

■ **FIGURE 104-7** Infected pseudocyst secondarily infecting the aortic bifemoral bypass graft. **A,** Axial contrast-enhanced CT image demonstrates a pseudocyst surrounding the pancreatic tail and portions of the spleen; the latter demonstrates segmental regions of infarctions. **B,** This fluid collection extended inferiorly into the iliac fossa as well as medially and was incorporated with the ventral margin of the psoas major muscle (*short arrow*) and with the wall of the left lateral aortic aneurysm wall (*long arrow*). The aortic graft is wrapped by the native aortic wall and moderate intervening abnormal fluid is present, indicating graft infection.

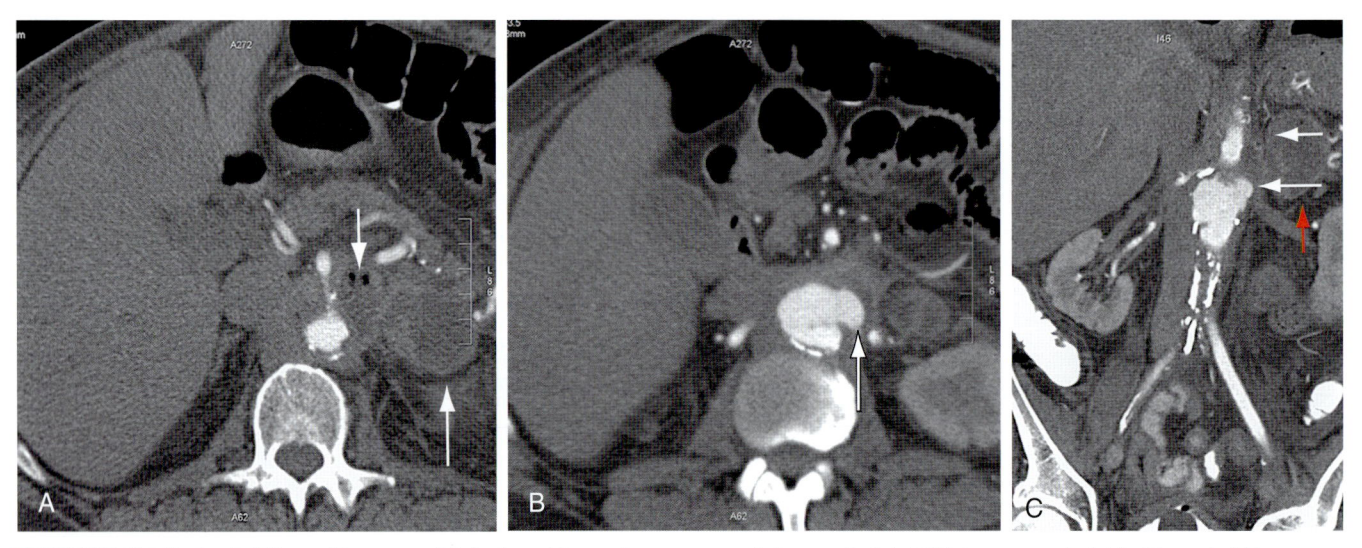

■ **FIGURE 104-8** Aortic bifemoral bypass graft infection with pseudoaneurysm and abscess. **A,** Axial CTA image reveals fluid with gas bubbles (*short arrow*) around the aorta, partially encasing the superior mesenteric artery. An abscess extending into the left periaortic area is also seen (*long arrow*). **B,** Axial CTA image near the anastomosis reveals a focal hypodense crescent of fluid surrounding a pseudoaneurysm (*arrow*). **C,** This is better appreciated on a coronal MPR image. The pseudoaneurysm (*long arrow*) is seen on the left. Fluid with a surrounding enhancing wall is also identified (*short arrow*). The periaortic abscess is also partially identified on the left (*red arrow*).

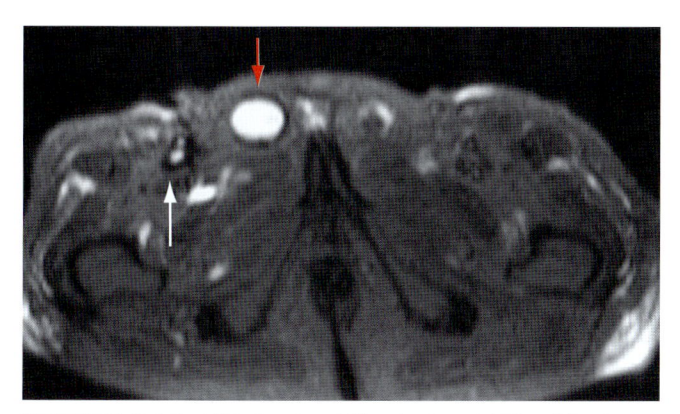

FIGURE 104-9 MRI of perigraft fibrosis. An axial T2-weighted image in a patient with graft anastomosis to the femoral artery shows low signal intensity (*arrow*) around the vessels, consistent with postoperative fibrosis. Fluid, on the other hand, demonstrates high signal intensity on T2-weighted sequences, as noted within the right inguinal canal (*red arrow*).

Many other entities, such as retroperitoneal fibrosis, infected aortic aneurysm, aortitis and, most commonly, perigraft infection, may mimic aortoenteric fistula. Features that suggest aortoenteric fistula include periaortic or intra-aortic gas, breach of the aortic wall, loss of fat planes, extravasation of aortic contrast agent into the bowel lumen or para-aortic space, retroperitoneal hematoma, and hematoma in the bowel wall or lumen. Perigraft air is more often seen in association with aortoenteric fistula than with aortic graft infection alone. The most specific feature of aortoenteric fistula is extravasation of intravenously administered contrast agent from the aorta into the bowel lumen.[19] Similarly, extravasation of oral water-soluble contrast from the bowel into or around the aortic graft is a specific feature of aortoenteric fistula. Ectopic gas should not persist after 3 to 4 weeks postsurgery, which suggests infection and/or fistula formation to bowel.[19]

Aortoiliac Occlusive Disease

One study has investigated the sensitivity and specificity of color flow and Duplex ultrasound compared with digital subtraction angiography for determining the presence of stenosis at the distal anastomosis of aortoiliac and aortofemoral bypasses in long-term follow-up of 103 patients.[23] Color flow imaging had a sensitivity of 89% in identifying the presence and location of distal anastomotic stenosis and a specificity of 95% of ruling out significant lesions. CTA and MRA (Fig. 104-12) can also be used for the investigation of graft thromboses and stenoses.

After aortoiliac surgery with Y grafts, dynamic CT has been shown to detect neointima formation, occlusion of the limbs of the bifurcation graft, and dilation and patency of the prosthesis, and correlates well with clinical findings in assessing for graft occlusion.[24] MRA can be used as an alternative.

Renal Infarction

Renal infarction as it pertains to this discussion may have various causes, such as surgical trauma, embolism caused by catheter manipulation, or arterial thrombosis from an AAA. On CT, renal infarctions often appear as cortically based, wedge-shaped areas of hypodensity. A capsular rim sign refers to a kidney that is diffusely hypodense except for its rim, which enhances normally because of the latter's blood supply from capsular arteries. Ultrasound may demonstrate a focal area of increased echogenicity associated with an absent or tardus parvus Doppler waveform. Renal scintigraphy may show a focal photopenic area corresponding to the area of infarction. Finally, focal arterial filling defects may be seen on catheter angiography, or there may be delayed filling of the renal arteries on a catheter abdominal aortogram.

A remote renal infarct may appear as a focal area of decreased attenuation with cortical atrophy caused by scarring on CT (Fig. 104-13) or MRA (see Fig. 104-4) images.

Anastomotic Pseudoaneurysms

CT is the imaging modality of choice for the evaluation of anastomotic aortic pseudoaneurysms. A pseudoaneurysm appears as a collection of flowing blood in continuity with major arteries; it may also contain thrombus (Fig. 104-14). Hematomas or adjacent fluid collections may be apparent. Angiography may be used to evaluate the anatomy of a pseudoaneurysm further.

Ultrasound is often the first modality used to evaluate a pulsatile abdominal mass that may represent a pseudoaneurysm. On gray-scale sonography, pseudoaneurysms appear as anechoic structures associated with an artery. On pulsed Doppler, pseudoaneurysms often show turbulent flow in a "to-and-fro" pattern throughout the cardiac cycle, representing flow into the pseudoaneurysm during systole and flow out of the pseudoaneurysm during diastole.[25]

POSTOPERATIVE MANAGEMENT

Most patients are followed postoperatively in the surgical intensive care unit. The patient's hemodynamic profile is monitored continuously. Coagulation studies, complete blood count (CBC) and serum chemistries, and electrocardiograms are typically assessed. Patients with high or intermediate risk factors have troponin I levels drawn at 24 hours postprocedure and again at 96 hours postprocedure, or prior to discharge. Deep venous thrombosis and gastric ulcer prophylaxis are also typically initiated following surgical repair.[2]

Aortoenteric Fistula

Antibiotics and urgent surgery are indicated in cases of aortoenteric fistula. The goals of surgery are to achieve cessation of bleeding, remove the aortic graft, and establish circulation to peripheral vessels via extra-aortic bypass. The intestinal communication can be repaired if it is smaller than 3 cm or resected if it is larger than 3 cm. An omental or peritoneal flap is created as a precaution against recurrent fistulas.

1448 PART SEVENTEEN • *The Abdominal Vessels*

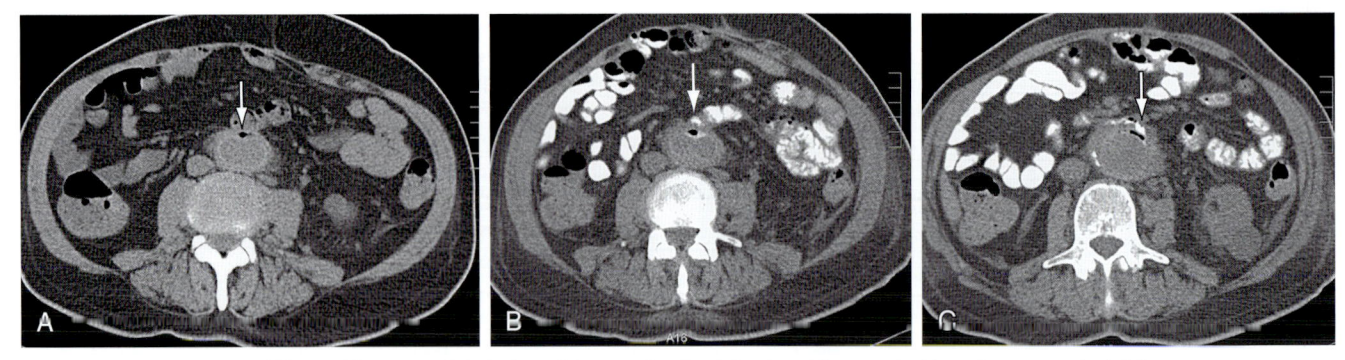

■ **FIGURE 104-10** Aorta bifemoral bypass graft infection with aorta duodenal fistula, without and with oral contrast. **A,** Axial non–contrast-enhanced CT image (because of renal insufficiency) demonstrates a gas bubble surrounding the aortic graft (*arrow*). A loop of bowel is noted overlying this. Hazy infiltration of the periaortic fat is seen. Non–IV contrast-enhanced CT was repeated following oral water-soluble contrast. **B,** At the same level, the gas bubble with surrounding extravasated contrast is identified (*arrow*). **C,** At a higher level, a CT image demonstrates the fistulous communication with the transverse portion of the duodenum (*arrow*). Gas is also noted around the aortic graft. This highlights the importance of the use of water-soluble oral contrast to delineate these fistulas.

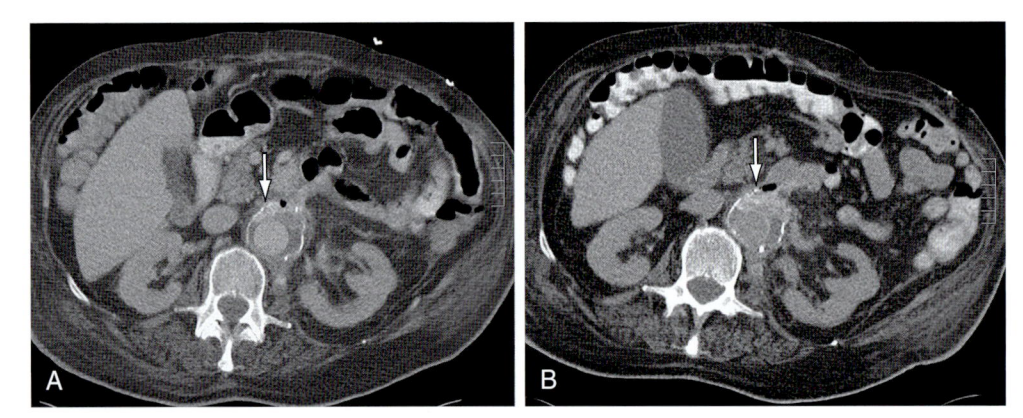

■ **FIGURE 104-11** Aortic bifemoral surgical graft with infection and aortoduodenal fistula. Axial CT images without IV contrast (because of renal insufficiency) but with oral water-soluble contrast demonstrate an air-fluid collection (**A, B**) anteriorly within the native aortic aneurysm wall surrounding the underlying graft. Ill-defined higher attenuation represents extravasated diluted contrast (*arrows*) entering via the aortoduodenal fistula.

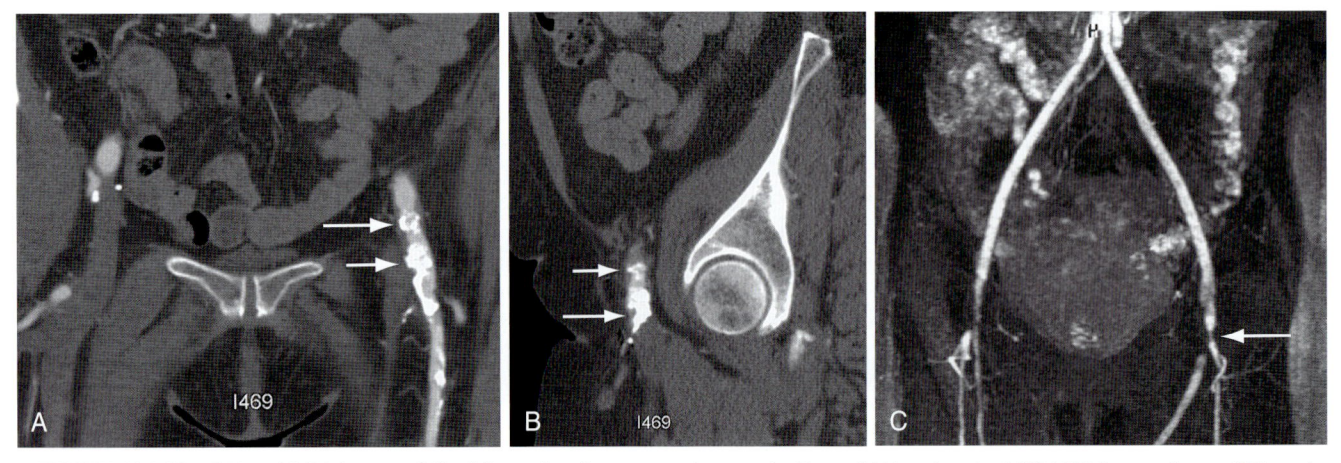

■ **FIGURE 104-12** CTA and MRA images of distal femoral graft anastomosis stenosis. Coronal (**A**) and sagittal (**B**) MPR images from a CTA study demonstrate significant calcified atheromatous plaque (*arrows*) causing severe stenosis on follow-up examination. Heavily calcified plaque, however, can result in acoustic shadowing on ultrasound examination and blooming artifact on CT studies. These artifacts from calcified plaque may result in interpretation errors, but are not present with MRA. **C,** The underlying lumen with stenosis (*arrow*) is better appreciated in this case with MRA.

Aortic Graft Infection

The most common organism responsible for aortic graft infection is *Staphyloccus aureus*; such infections often present in the early postoperative period. Most specimens that demonstrate white blood cells but are culture-negative contain *Staphylococcus epidermidis*. Antibiotic therapy is not usually curative. Previously, such infections were treated with excision of the graft with extra-anatomic reconstruction. However, aortic replacement with femoropopliteal veins has been proposed and has demonstrated reduced mortality and reinfection rates.[26]

Anastomotic Pseudoaneurysms

Surgical repair of anastomotic aortic pseudoaneurysms involves resection followed by placement of an interposition graft or vascular bypass. Endovascular repair is a good alternative,[27] particularly for patients with multiple comorbidities. Some patients are not candidates for stent graft placement because of unusual anatomy or technical limitations of the stent graft.

> **KEY POINTS**
>
> - Although perioperative mortality is higher in patients undergoing open repair of an AAA, reinterventions are more common in matched patients undergoing endovascular repair, and long-term mortality does not significantly differ between the groups.
> - Anatomic considerations and comorbidities must be taken into account when deciding between endovascular and open repair for a patient with an AAA that meets the criteria for treatment.
> - The postoperative mortality rate for elective open repair is approximately 5%.
> - Most AAAs are asymptomatic; when they rupture, a patient may present with acute abdominal, flank, or back pain.
> - Most AAAs are detected incidentally by abdominal ultrasonography.
> - A CT scan is the preoperative imaging study of choice prior to open repair.
> - MRI/MRA and/or conventional x-ray catheter angiography may be helpful for preoperative imaging in select patients.
> - Postoperative management of patients after open repair of an AAA includes careful monitoring of hemodynamic and respiratory status and electrolytes, and the implementation of preventive measures, such as prophylaxis for deep venous thrombosis and gastric ulcer.
> - Various postoperative complications may occur after open repair, including but not limited to, the following: aortoenteric fistula, aortic graft infection, aortocaval fistula, aortoiliac occlusive disease, ischemic colitis, and renal infarction. CT-CTA is the postoperative imaging study of choice for imaging after open surgical repair of an AAA.

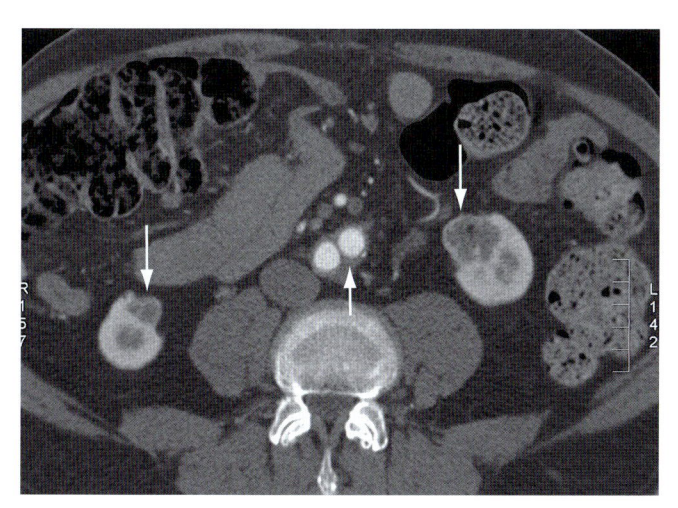

■ **FIGURE 104-13** Aortic bifemoral bypass graft with bilateral lower pole renal infarctions. An axial contrast-enhanced CT demonstrates the two limbs of an aortic bifemoral bypass graft (*short arrow*). Bilateral lower pole renal infarctions are demonstrated with focal atrophy and diminished enhancement (*long arrows*).

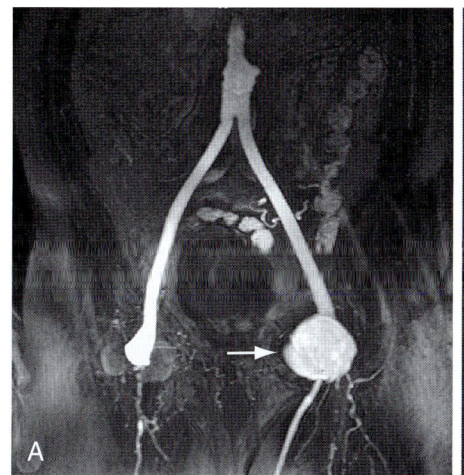

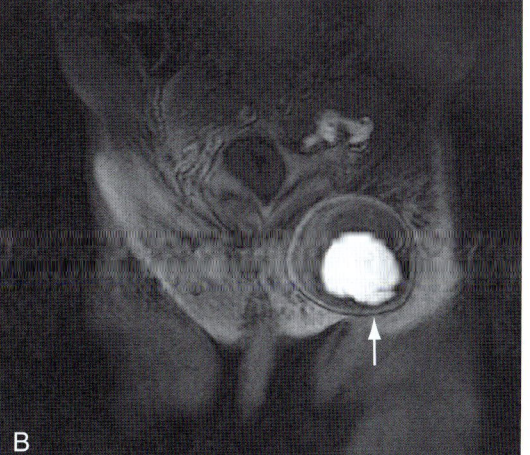

■ **FIGURE 104-14** Femoral graft anastomosis pseudoaneurysm. A coronal MIP image (**A**) and the coronal source image (**B**) from an MRA study demonstrate an aortic bifemoral bypass graft with a large pseudoaneurysm (*arrow*) arising from the femoral anastomosis site. Thrombus lining the pseudoaneurysm wall (*arrow*) is best displayed on the source image.

SUGGESTED READINGS

Almahameed A, Latif AA, Graham LM. Managing abdominal aortic aneurysms: treat the aneurysm and the risk factors. Cleve Clin J Med 2005; 72:877-888.

Blankensteijn JD, de Jong SECA, Prinssen M, et al. Two-year outcomes after conventional or endovascular repair of abdominal aortic aneurysms. N Engl J Med 2005; 352:2398-2405.

EVAR Trial Participants. Endovascular aneurysm repair and outcome in patients unfit for open repair of abdominal aortic aneurysm (EVAR trial 2): randomised controlled trial. Lancet 2005; 365:2187-2192.

EVAR Trial Participants. Endovascular aneurysm repair versus open repair in patients with abdominal aortic aneurysm (EVAR trial 1): randomised controlled trial. Lancet 2005; 365:2179-2186.

Hellmann DB, Grand DJ, Freischlag JA. Inflammatory abdominal aortic aneurysm. JAMA 2007; 297:395-400.

Kent KC, Zwolak RM, Jaff MR, et al. Screening for abdominal aortic aneurysm. J Vasc Surg 2004;39:267-269.

Low RN, Wall SD, Jeffrey RB, et al. Aortoenteric fistula and perigraft infection: evaluation with CT. Radiology 1990; 175:157-162.

Orton DF, Leveen RF, Saigh JA, et al. Aortic prosthetic graft infections: radiologic manifestations and implications for management. Radiographics 2000; 20:977-993.

Upchurch GR Jr, Schaub TA. Abdominal aortic aneurysm. Am Fam Physician 2006;73:1198-1204.

REFERENCES

1. Quinones-Baldrich WJ, Garner C, Caswell D, et al. Endovascular, transperitoneal, and retroperitoneal abdominal aortic aneurysm repair: results and costs. J Vasc Surg 1999; 30:59-67.
2. Zelenock GB, Huber TS, Messina LM, et al (eds). Mastery of Vascular and Endovascular Surgery. Philadelphia, Lippincott, Williams & Wilkins, 2006.
3. Zarins CK, Gewertz BL. Atlas of Vascular Surgery, 2nd ed. Philadelphia, Churchill Livingstone, 2005.
4. Jean-Claude JM, Reilly LM, Stoney RJ, et al. Pararenal aortic aneurysms: the future of open aortic aneurysm repair. J Vasc Surg. 1999; 29:902-912.
5. Faggioli G, Stella A, Freyrie A, et al. Early and long-term results in the surgical treatment of juxtarenal and pararenal aortic aneurysms. Eur J Vasc Endovasc Surg 1998; 15:205-211.
6. Miani S, Giorgetti PL, Giordanengo F, Tealdi D. Ruptured abdominal aortic aneurysms: factors affecting the early postoperative outcome. Panminerva Med 1998; 40:309-313.
7. Cuypers PW, Laheij RJ, Buth J. Which factors increase the risk of conversion to open surgery following endovascular abdominal aortic aneurysm repair? The EUROSTAR collaborators. Eur J Vasc Endovasc Surg 2000; 20:183-189.
8. Böckler D, Probst T, Weber H, Raithel D. Surgical conversion after endovascular grafting for abdominal aortic aneurysms. J Endovasc Ther 2002; 9:111-118.
9. Valentine RJ. Diagnosis and management of aortic graft infection. Semin Vasc Surg 2001; 14: 292-301.
10. Marković DM, Davidović LB, Kostić DM, et al. Anastomotic pseudoaneurysms. Srp Arh Celok Lek 2006; 134:114-121.
11. Hallett JW Jr, Marshall DM, Petterson TM, et al. Graft-related complications after abdominal aortic aneurysm repair: Reassurance from a 36-year population-based experience. J Vasc Surg 1997; 25:277-284.
12. Edwards JM, Teefey SA, Zierler RE, Kohler TR. Intra-abdominal paraanastomotic aneurysms after aortic bypass grafting. J Vasc Surg 1992; 15: 344-353.
13. Nevelsteen A, Suy R. Anastomotic false aneurysms of the abdominal aorta and the iliac arteries. J Vasc Surg 1989; 10: 595.
14. Kent KC, Zwolak RM, Jaff MR, et al. Screening for abdominal aortic aneurysm. J Vasc Surg 2004; 39:267-269.
15. Mansour MA, Labropoulos N (eds). Vascular Diagnosis. Philadelphia, Elsevier, 2005.
16. Tennant WG, Hartnell GG, Baird RN, et al. Radiological investigation of abdominal aortic aneurysm disease: comparison of 3 modalities in staging and the detection of inflammatory change. J Vasc Surg 1993; 17:703-709.
17. Seeger JM. Management of patients with prosthetic vascular graft infection. Am Surg 2000; 66:166-167.
18. Reilly LM, Altman H, Lusby RJ, et al. Late results following surgical management of vascular graft infection. J Vasc Surg 1984; 1:36-44.
19. Low RN, Wall SD, Jeffrey RB, et al. Aortoenteric fistula and perigraft infection: evaluation with CT. Radiology 1990; 175:157-162.
20. Orton DF, Leveen RF, Saigh JA, et al. Aortic prosthetic graft infections: radiologic manifestations and implications for management. Radiographics 2000; 20:977-993.
21. Keidar Z, Engel A, Hoffman A, et al. Prosthetic vascular graft infection: the role of ^{18}F-FDG PET/CT. J Nucl Med 2007; 48:1230-1236.
22. Mark AS, Moss AA, McCarthy S, McCowin M. CT of aortoenteric fistulas. Invest Radiol 1985; 20:272-275.
23. de Gier P, Sommeling C, van Dulken E, et al. Stenosis development at the distal anastomosis of prosthetic bypasses for aortoiliac occlusive disease. Incidence and accuracy of colour flow duplex in the diagnosis. Eur J Vasc Surg 1993; 7:237-244.
24. Tuchmann A, Hruby W. CT in aortobifemoral Y grafts. Cardiovasc Intervent Radiol 1985; 8:187-190.
25. Brown PM, Kim VB, Lalikos JF, et al. Autologous superficial femoral vein for aortic reconstruction in infected fields. Ann Vasc Surg 1999; 13:32-36.
26. Bhargava S. Textbook of Color Doppler Imaging. New Delhi, India, Jaypee Brothers, 2004.
27. Laganà D, Carrafiello G, Mangini M, et al. Endovascular treatment of anastomotic pseudoaneurysms after aorto-iliac surgical reconstruction. Cardiovasc Intervent Radiol 2007; 30:1185-1191.

CHAPTER 105

Magnetic Resonance Imaging of Vascular Disorders of the Abdomen

Marcel Santos, Bobby Kalb, and Diego Martin

INTRODUCTION

Methodology

Optimized imaging of the abdominal vasculature should provide diagnostic evaluation of the vessels and the soft tissues in the same examination. This allows for a more comprehensive diagnostic assessment of the etiology and the end-organ soft tissue effects of an underlying vascular disorder. MRI should be considered the imaging modality of choice for most applications owing to optimal inherent contrast resolution and the ability to obtain high spatial resolution vascular imaging with greater overall safety when compared to CT or digital subtraction angiography (DSA), taking radiation and contrast risks into account. MR angiographic imaging may be accomplished using three-dimensional contrast-enhanced MR angiography (3D CE MRA). Morphologic images are also acquired to serve as a supplement to contrast-enhanced vascular imaging in addition to providing relevant soft tissue detail. MRI can also provide robust vascular and soft tissue imaging even in uncooperative patients.

Arterial Imaging

MR evaluation of the abdominal vasculature includes accurate assessment of the arteries and veins, and the optimal imaging method differs for each. For the arterial system, 3D CE MRA is the imaging method of choice. This technology involves the acquisition of a coronal 3D data set that produces images with high spatial resolution and a high signal-to-noise ratio (SNR). A precontrast mask is acquired before the administration of gadolinium (Gd)-chelate contrast agent, and the examination is repeated at specified time points after the administration of Gd to capture vessel enhancement in the early arterial and a more delayed venous phase. The precontrast mask can then be subtracted from the postcontrast acquisitions to produce images of only the vasculature. Although this subtraction technique produces an additive effect with respect to image noise, subtraction of the background soft tissues provides potential benefits in image contrast, in addition to eliminating any image wrap artifact in the phase-encoded direction. However, evaluation of the unsubtracted source data has other advantages, facilitating evaluation of the soft tissues and the vasculature within the same set of images, including superior evaluation of disorders within the vessel walls. For example, the outer wall of a partially thrombosed aneurysm can be identified on the source MRA images, providing a more accurate assessment of size and morphology than a subtracted data set that shows only the patent lumen. This example highlights an inherent disadvantage to conventional angiography, in which only the injected, contrast-filled, patent portion of the vessel lumen can be visualized. 3D CE MRA has the flexibility to provide angiographic-type images with high spatial resolution in addition to evaluation of the vessel wall for improved evaluation of disorders such as partially thrombosed dissections and aneurysms. 3D CE MRA images may also be postprocessed using maximum intensity projection (MIP), rendered into different projections with multiplanar reformations (MPR), useful in the evaluation of the origin and bifurcation of the abdominal vessels. Other postprocessing techniques include shaded surface display and volume rendering, but we have found these to have less value in the evaluation of the abdominal vasculature.

One relative disadvantage to 3D CE MRA is a sensitivity to motion, which results from acquisition times that typically extend into the range of 12 to 15 seconds. This feature of 3D CE MRA generally necessitates acquiring the images during a breath-hold. Timing the breath-hold commands for the patient requires consideration of bolus timing, as proper contrast bolus timing is essential for arterial phase acquisitions. Different techniques of contrast bolus timing have been developed to ensure that image acquisition is initiated at the time of maximal contrast concentration in the vessels of interest, coinciding with the time that the central portion of k-space (which controls image contrast) is acquired. These methods include test bolus injection, real-time bolus tracking, and automated triggering methods. Additional advances involve the use of centric and elliptical k-space ordering, to acquire the central k-space data toward the beginning of the acquisition. These developments have greatly simplified timing of the arterial phase images. For example, real time bolus triggering can be performed when the contrast bolus is tracked using near real time reconstruction at a rate of 0.5 to 1 second per image. The operator starts the contrast injection and then uses bolus tracking images to monitor arrival of the contrast. When the operator sees the contrast bolus approaching the vessels of interest, the patient can be given breath-hold commands and the 3D MRA sequence is initiated. This approach depends on the image contrast being captured at the beginning of the acquisition. For abdominal arterial phase imaging, an optimal approach is for the operator to begin patient breath-hold instructions when the bolus track images show the contrast filling the left ventricle and entering the ascending aorta. The 3D MRA arterial phase images may then be initiated after 3 seconds, providing adequate time for the patient to suspend respiration. Partial Fourier imaging (exploiting the fact that one half of k-space closely mirrors the other half) and parallel processing (using separate inputs from each coil element of the surface coils to provide spatial information, allowing further k-space undersampling) have allowed marked reduction in image acquisition time and reduction of image motion artifacts. Improved gradient performance of newer MR systems has led to shortened repetition (TR) and echo (TE) times with resultant further decreases in acquisition time and image artifacts. This methodology allows for reproducible, high-quality images even in patients with depressed cardiac function and altered flow dynamics.

Venous and Soft Tissue Imaging

Whereas CE 3D MRA is the imaging method of choice for evaluation of the arterial system, venous imaging has different challenges requiring alternative approaches. Standard 3D MRA GRE uses higher flip angles and results in excellent contrast only when the Gd concentration is sufficiently high. In the venous system, standard 3D MRA GRE may result in poor signal and poor image contrast owing to hemodilution of the Gd contrast agent in the venous system. MIP and MPR images of the venous system are also less useful due to persistent arterial enhancement, rendering cluttered views of veins obscured by adjacent and overlying arteries. However, another family of 3D GRE sequences is ideal for imaging of the venous system. Sequences in this 3D GRE family include volumetric interpolated breath-hold examination (VIBE, Siemens Medical Solutions), T1-weighted high resolution isotropic volume examination (THRIVE, Philips Medical Systems) and liver acquisition with volume acceleration (LAVA-xv, General Electric); these yield volumetric acquisitions that may be acquired or reconstructed in any plane and provide excellent soft tissue detail in addition to robust imaging of the vasculature. By using a low flip angle, these 3D GRE sequences yield higher signal and contrast from lower concentrations of Gd, as found in the veins. Even several minutes after Gd administration, excellent signal intensity can be achieved from the venous structures. Thus, acquisition of venous phase images is made straightforward by being relatively insensitive to variations in timing delay. The images show arteries and veins and are complementary to traditional MRA, also providing detailed evaluation of the vessel walls and the soft tissues of the abdomen. This is in contrast to CT, in which suboptimal timing of image acquisition, combined with inherent CT limitations of image contrast on more delayed venous phase-delayed images, often results in poor contrast enhancement within the venous structures. 3D GRE images may be acquired or interpolated to less than 3 mm in- and out-of-plane resolution, providing visibility of smaller vessels. Concurrent soft tissue evaluation allows diagnosis of not only the patient's vascular pathology, but also of related soft tissue disorders, such as from ischemia, tumor infiltration, metastases, and evaluation of vessel wall and mural thrombus. Precontrast imaging is also useful to differentiate Gd enhancement from intrinsic T1 high signal owing to blood products or proteinaceous fluid.

3D CE MRA and 3D GRE imaging are the major components involved in vascular imaging of the abdomen. However, as described, associated soft tissue detail is critical, especially in imaging of the abdominal vasculature where the consequences of vessel pathology are often quite serious. Comprehensive evaluation of the abdominal vessels should then include an additional small number of selected sequences for morphologic evaluation. The two most useful sequences are single shot T2W (HASTE) sequences with and without fat saturation, and also sequences that use steady-state magnetization, such as True FISP (TFISP). These are rapid, 2D sequences that allow robust imaging even with marked patient motion and do not add a significant time penalty to the overall imaging examination time. In addition to providing alternative views of soft tissue contrast, they offer a back-up evaluation of the vasculature that does not require the administration of Gd chelate. T2W images employ a "black blood" method to evaluate the vessels, as magnetized spins exit the imaged slice between RF excitation and readout in vessels with flowing blood. Thrombosed vessels will not demonstrate this signal void that is seen with flowing blood. More consistent black blood T2W images may be obtained with double inversion recovery T2W images that are often employed in cardiac imaging. In contrast, TFISP sequences employ a "bright blood" method of vascular contrast, but without the administration of Gd. The presence of unspoiled, steady-state magnetization in this sequence brings out high signal in blood, even in the setting of slow flow. Intraluminal thrombus is depicted as relatively lower signal within the vessel lumen, providing an alternate method for vascular analysis. Both of these sequences are also helpful for evaluation of aneurysm size and morphology, and hold up well, even in a free-breathing patient. The combination of 3D CE MRA, 3D GRE, T2W, and TFISP sequences provides a comprehensive evaluation of vascular and soft tissue pathology that is not available in other imaging modalities.

Gadolinium Agent Use and Safety

Concerns regarding the use of Gd-chelate contrast agents in the setting of renal disease have arisen since the initial description of a new disease, nephrogenic systemic fibrosis (NSF),[1] and the subsequent correlation between prior Gd-chelate contrast agent exposure and development of NSF in patients with severe renal dysfunction.[2] The current understanding of NSF is that nearly all cases have been attributed to exposure to gadodiamide (Omniscan) in more than 90% of peer-reviewed published cases, with the remainder of NSF cases associated with gadoversetamide (Optimark) or gadopentetate dimeglumine (Magnevist) exposure. Gadodiamide has relatively lower conditional stability, and it is believed that prolonged exposure to this agent, as occurs in the setting of reduced renal clearance, leads to greater chelate ligand dissociation and deposition of free gadolinium in tissues, including skin, leading to activation of the fibrotic process associated with NSF. NSF is primarily a disease affecting patients with severely impaired renal function (less than 15 mL/min) and mostly affecting patients on dialysis.[1] Furthermore, NSF risk and severity appears to correlate with higher single and cumulative total gadodiamide dose.[3] However, the risk of NSF using low dose, high relaxivity linear agents or high conditional stability cyclic agents appears immeasurably small; there remain no documented cases of NSF in the peer-reviewed literature with any of these other agents. Given concerns regarding NSF, we currently use a dose of 0.05 to 0.1 mmol/kg of a more stable high relaxivity linear or macrocyclic Gd-chelate contrast agent, mixed with an equal volume of normal saline. The contrast is then injected at a rate of 2 mL/s, followed by at least 20 mL of saline flush using a dual-chamber injector, which allows for a continuous influx of gadolinium during imaging. Our current understanding of NSF, and of contrast-induced nephropathy (CIN) associated with iodinated CT contrast, supports preferential use of contrast enhanced MRI over CT in patients with impaired renal function.[4] Not yet published data documenting immeasurably low risk of higher cumulative dose administrations of high conditional stability cyclic agents may help to further define these dosage recommendations.

Cirrhosis and Portal Hypertension

Definition

Chronic liver disease and cirrhosis induce extensive intra-abdominal vascular changes that are easily detected with MRI. The strength of MRI in this clinical setting is the concurrent parenchymal and soft tissue imaging that is unmatched by other imaging modalities. This soft tissue detail, together with vascular evaluation, provides a comprehensive analysis of the etiology and subsequent effects of various pathologic processes affecting the abdominal vasculature.

Etiology and Pathophysiology

Portal hypertension is an end-stage pathophysiologic state that arises from a variety of causes, all with a common thread of inducing increased resistance to portal venous flow into the hepatic sinusoids. Causes of portal hypertension include prehepatic (portal and mesenteric thrombosis), hepatic (intrinsic liver disease) and posthepatic (outflow obstruction of the draining hepatic veins). By far, the most common of these etiologies is intrinsic liver dysfunction, usually caused by viral hepatitis or alcohol. Regardless of the etiology, repeated liver injury induces changes of hepatic fibrosis which cause mechanical obstruction to portal flow in the hepatic sinusoids. There is also an alteration in the vasoactive substances present in the liver, which causes vasoconstriction of the portal vasculature. This common pathway of hepatic injury leading to portal inflow resistance causes predictable morphologic changes in the portal and mesenteric vasculature that are diagnostic of portal hypertension.

The parenchymal and vascular changes seen with MRI parallel the pathophysiologic changes occurring within the portal venous system, and are reflective of the underlying resistance to portal flow in the hepatic sinusoids. Chronic liver disease induces vasoconstriction within the hepatic microcirculation, owing to a relative lack of nitrous oxide (NO) and the action of potent vasoconstrictors.[5] The larger portal venous branches dilate in a compensatory effort to increase portal flow. The reduction in NO within the hepatic microcirculation is reversed in the splanchnic vasculature,[5] which also dilates in an attempt to increase portal flow and overcome developing resistance. An enlarged portal vein, superior mesenteric vein (SMV), and splenic vein are clear indicators of portal hypertension (Fig. 105-1). Flow in the portal vein, normally directed into the liver (hepatopetal) eventually reverses direction away from the liver (hepatofugal). These altered flow dynamics are most commonly assessed with ultrasound, although MRI has the capability to provide additional functional measures of portal flow that better correlate with the severity of cirrhosis and portal hypertension when compared with ultrasound.[6] Continued increased resistance to portal flow in the hepatic sinusoids results in shunting of portal blood to the systemic venous system at predictable locations. Shunted blood pools at these sites of portosystemic anastomosis, causing the formation of varices.

Manifestations of Disease

Clinical Presentation

Patients often have a history of predisposing factors, such as alcohol abuse or viral (hepatitis B and/or C) infection. Clinical symptoms usually manifest with the development of portal hypertension, and include edema, ascites, and bleeding from varices and decreased production of clotting factors by the liver. The Child-Turcotte-Pugh score is a clinical scoring system that is used to grade severity of disease, and takes into account the presence or absence of encephalopathy, ascites, and the bilirubin, albumin, and INR levels.

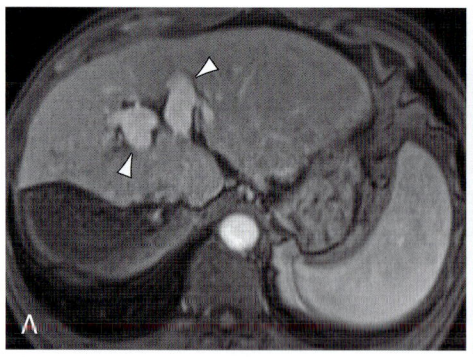

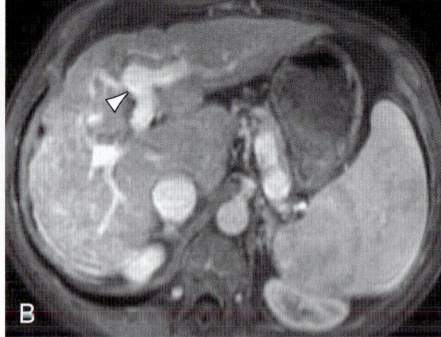

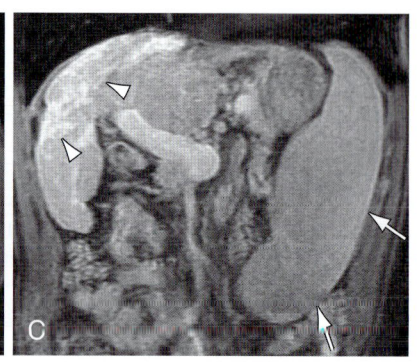

FIGURE 105-1 Enlarged portal vasculature in the setting of portal hypertension. Arterial (**A**) and 70-second (**B**) postcontrast 3D GRE images show enlargement of the portal venous branches (*arrowheads*). Coronal delayed postcontrast 3D GRE image (**C**) again demonstrates dilation of the main portal vein with hepatic fibrosis (*arrowheads*) and a massively enlarged spleen (*arrows*), all morphologic changes occurring secondary to underlying portal hypertension.

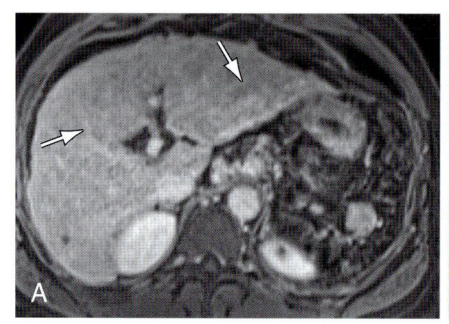

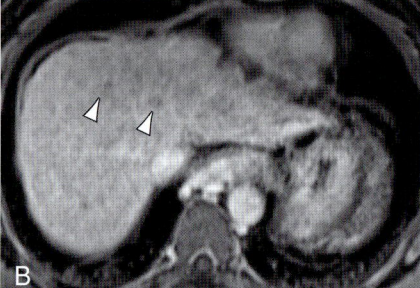

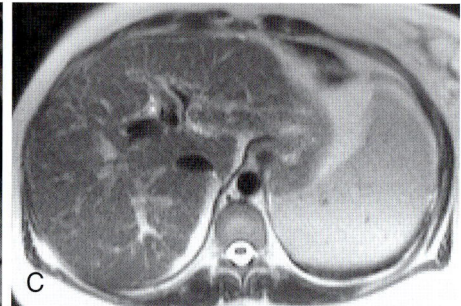

FIGURE 105-2 Chronic liver disease with fibrosis. Delayed, postcontrast 3D GRE images (**A, B**) demonstrate a coarse, reticular pattern of enhancement (*arrows*) representing fibrotic bands that surround small, regenerating nodules (*arrowheads*) in the setting of chronic liver disease. These fibrotic bands demonstrate increased signal on T2W images (**C**).

Imaging Indications and Algorithm

MRI has the unique ability to characterize underlying hepatic parenchymal changes prior to the development of frank portal hypertension. The hepatic fibrosis caused by repeated liver injury is seen on delayed phase, 3D GRE images, showing a fine or coarse reticular pattern of enhancement in the underlying hepatic parenchyma (Fig. 105-2). This reticular parenchymal enhancement can identify fibrotic liver disease before morphologic changes of cirrhosis and portal hypertension develop. This is a powerful tool in that it allows for an earlier, more aggressive treatment plan in patients at high risk for chronic liver disease. Conventional catheter angiography assesses strictly vascular morphology, which only typically becomes abnormal with more advanced disease and cannot evaluate parenchymal changes of fibrosis. CTA can also provide a noninvasive method of evaluating both vessels and soft tissues; however, it lacks the underlying contrast resolution to adequately assess fibrotic changes in the hepatic parenchyma. In addition, CTA and catheter angiography employ the use of ionizing radiation, a concern especially in the setting of chronic liver disease, which often requires repeated, multiphase imaging. MR is the only modality with the contrast and spatial resolution to fully assess the vasculature and hepatic parenchyma, with the added benefit of not employing ionizing radiation. Currently, early detection of fibrotic liver disease is primarily diagnosed through biopsy, but the use of MR to grade liver fibrosis may reduce the need for liver biopsy, which carries risks of hepatic injury, bleeding, and infection.

Imaging Techniques and Findings

MR

The most dangerous consequence of portosystemic shunting is bleeding from esophageal varices (Fig. 105-3). Varices may be identified within the esophageal wall (termed *esophageal varices*) or surrounding the esophagus (termed *paraesophageal varices*), although both drain the portal system via the left gastric (cardinal) vein. Additional common sites of variceal formation within the abdomen due to portosystemic shunting include gastric and retroperitoneal varices, spontaneous splenorenal shunts, and recanalized paraumbilical veins. Recanalized paraumbilical veins drain into the epigastric veins along the undersurface of the abdominal wall, often forming a mesh of dilated varices surrounding the umbilicus termed *caput medusa* (Fig. 105-4). Identification of paraumbilical varices are important in that the draining meshwork of superficial veins along the anterior abdominal wall must be avoided during diagnostic and therapeutic paracenteses that are often performed in patients with chronic liver disease. Although less common, intrahepatic portosystemic (venovenous shunts) may also occur in the setting of chronic liver disease as a result of increased portal

CHAPTER 105 • Magnetic Resonance Imaging of Vascular Disorders of the Abdomen

FIGURE 105-3 Esophageal and paraesophageal varices. Axial 3D GRE images (A, B) demonstrate enlarged venous structures contained within (*arrowhead*) and also surrounding (*arrow*) the esophageal wall. Coronal 3D GRE image (C) again demonstrates extensive paraesophageal varices at the gastroesophageal junction, a cause of major morbidity and mortality in the setting of portal hypertension.

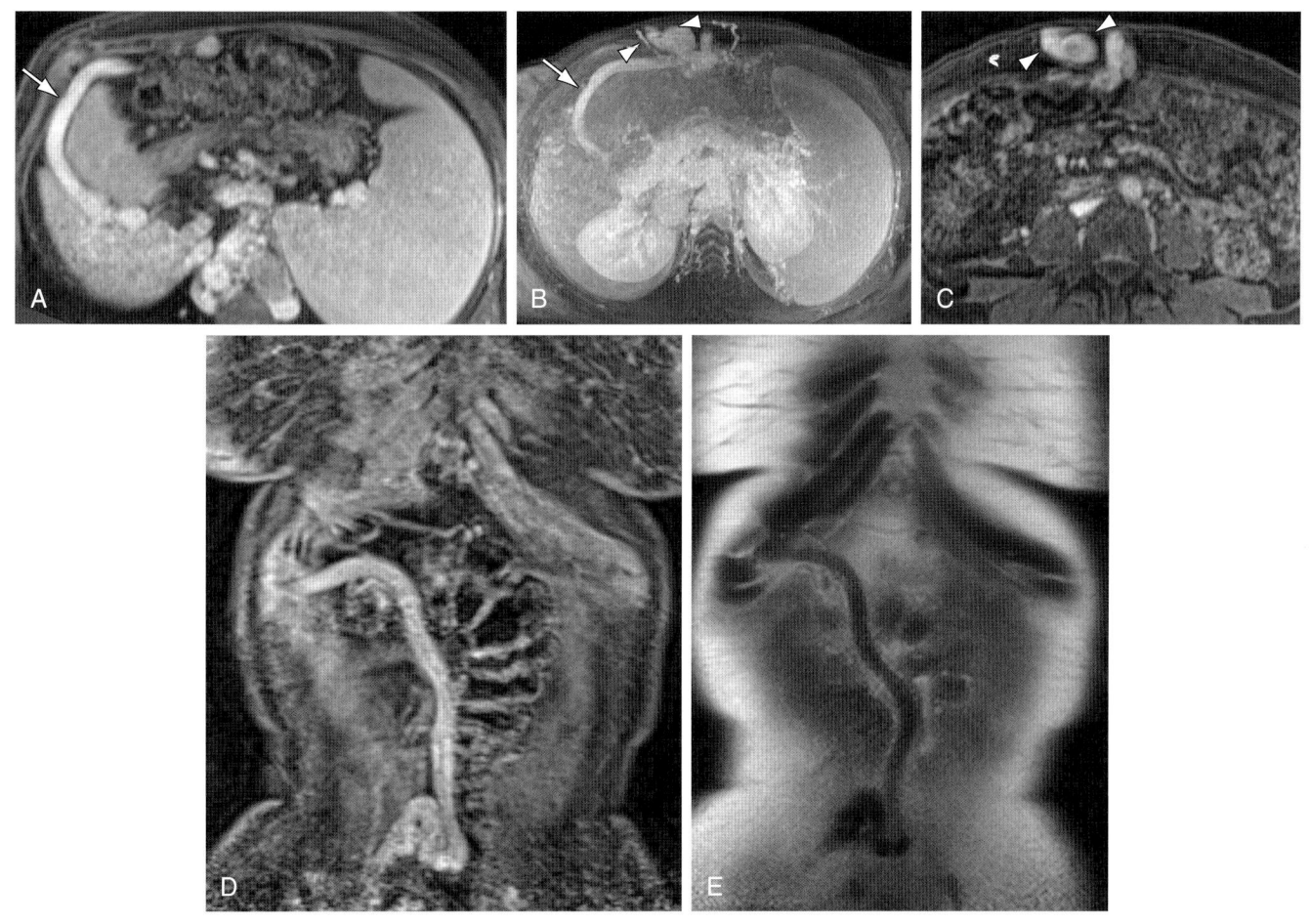

FIGURE 105-4 Recanalized paraumbilical vein and caput medusa. Axial 3D GRE (A) and MIP images (B) demonstrate an enlarged, recanalized paraumbilical vein (*arrow*), which drains to a large meshwork of superficial veins (*arrowheads*) surrounding the umbilicus (C). Coronal 3D GRE image (D) again demonstrates this site of portosystemic shunting, whereas coronal T2W image (E) provides an alternate "black-blood" method for vascular analysis.

resistance. These shunts have been described at the microscopic level[7] and can also be identified with MR (Fig. 105-5). Other etiologies of intrahepatic portosystemic shunting include congenital malformations and rupture of a portal vein aneurysm into a hepatic vein, whereas post-traumatic shunts are most often associated with surgical interventions such as transhepatic catheter placement.

In addition to portosystemic shunting, chronic liver injury and fibrosis also causes arterioportal shunting, either secondary to underlying tumor (hepatocellular carcinoma) or cased by the parenchymal changes of fibrosis itself. These arterioportal shunts manifest on MR as small, linear- or wedge-shaped blushes of enhancement on arterial phase imaging, most often located along a capsular

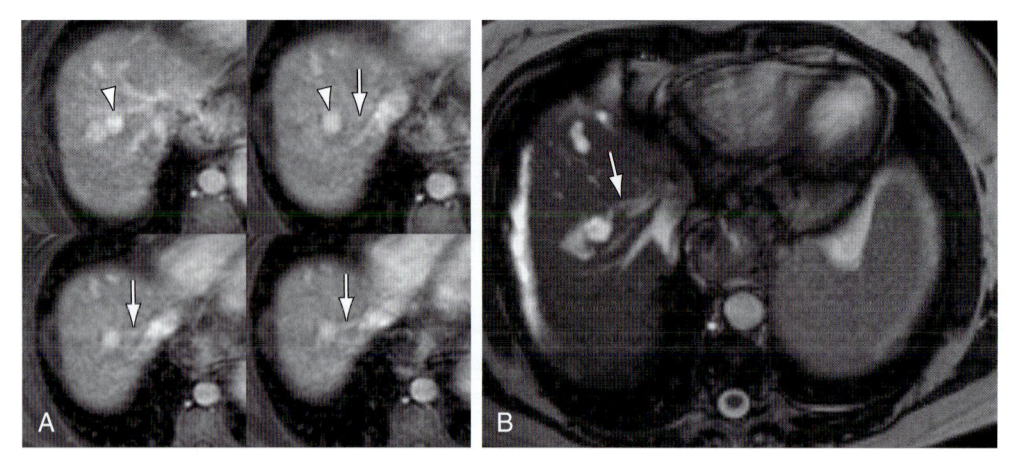

■ **FIGURE 105-5** Veno-venous (intrahepatic) shunt. Anomalous connection (*arrows*) between the enlarged portal vein (*arrowheads*) and the IVC is well demonstrated on delayed postcontrast 3D GRE images (**A**), and a noncontrast TFISP image (**B**) also clearly demonstrates the shunt (*arrow*).

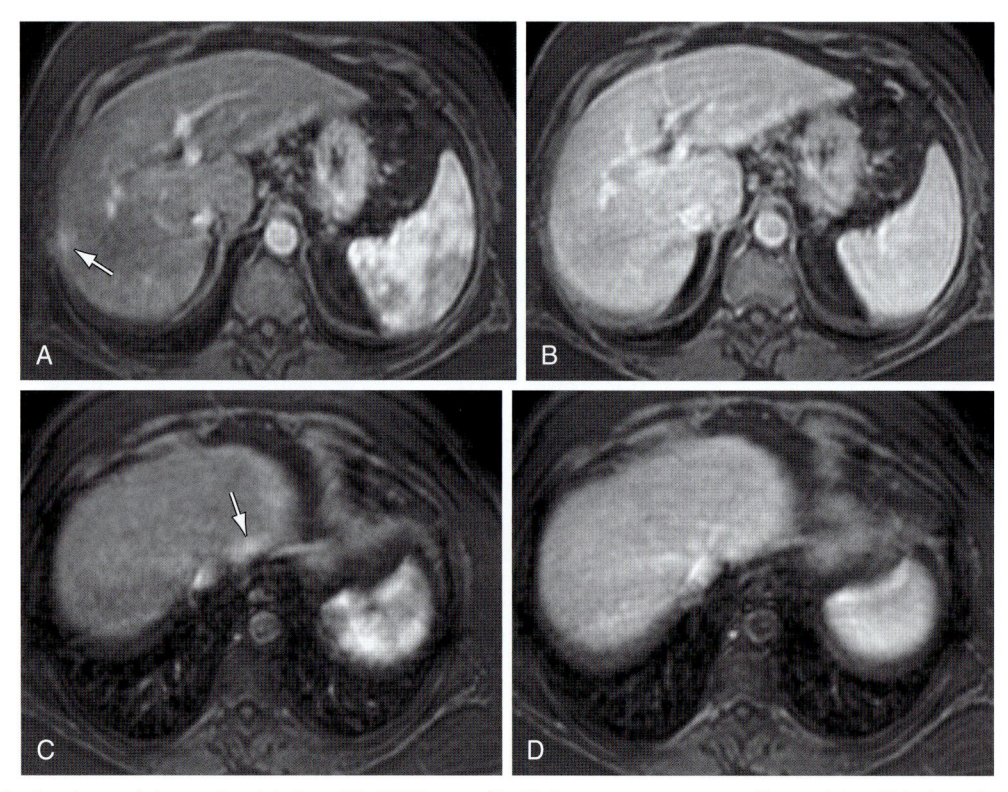

■ **FIGURE 105-6** Arterioportal shunts. Arterial phase 3D GRE images (**A, C**) demonstrate non–mass-like, peripheral blushes of arterial enhancement (*arrows*). These areas become isointense on delayed 3D GRE images (**B, D**), without washout or rim enhancement that would be expected with hepatocellular carcinoma. These findings are in keeping with small vascular perfusion anomalies.

surface (Fig. 105-6). These foci of enhancement may be mistaken for a small tumor on CT owing to a relative lack of contrast resolution. However, MRI can more easily differentiate these small arterioportal shunts (APS) from hepatocellular carcinoma (HCC) in the majority of cases because the APS will show a more linear- or wedge-shaped morphology and will not demonstrate the washout and rim enhancement typical of HCC. Arterioportal shunts may also occur in settings other than chronic liver disease, such as trauma, iatrogenic (postbiopsy or surgery), congenital anomalies, or aneurysm rupture.[8] APS are associated with both benign (hemangiomas) and malignant (HCC) hepatic tumors.[9] APS also contribute to the flow changes seen in portal hypertension. Studies examining flow characteristics in the portal vein with intermittent occlusion of the hepatic artery have demonstrated that APS are a factor in hepatofugal flow of the portal vein in the setting of chronic liver disease.[10]

Differential Diagnosis from Imaging Findings

The imaging findings for cirrhosis and portal hypertension are pathognomonic and one of the goals of imaging is to establish an etiology, determining if the liver disease is

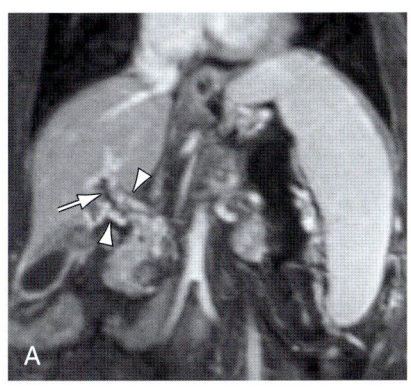

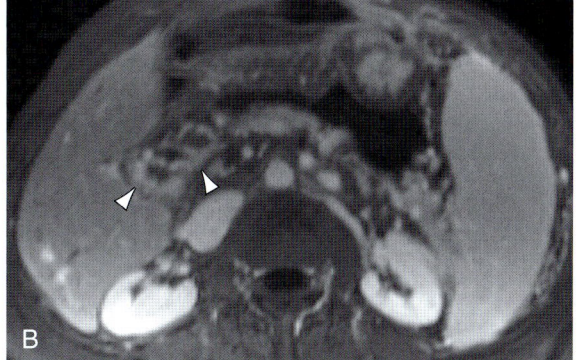

FIGURE 105-7 Cavernous transformation of the portal vein. Coronal (**A**) and axial (**B**) 3D GRE images demonstrate low-signal intensity thrombus (*arrow*) in the portal vein, with the development of multiple, serpiginous venous collaterals (*arrowheads*) extending into the liver hilum.

caused by prehepatic, intrinsic hepatic, or posthepatic causes. Imaging also serves to grade disease and provide a pathway for tumor surveillance.

Synopsis of Treatment Options

Medical

Medical treatment consists of managing the patient's fluid and nutritional status, in addition to treating underlying causes such as hemochromatosis and Wilson's disease.

Surgical/Interventional

Transjugular intrahepatic portosystemic shunts are often placed to decompress the portal circulation, with less morbidity and mortality than surgically created shunts. The treatment of choice for decompensated cirrhosis is liver transplantation.

KEY POINTS

- Causes of portal hypertension include prehepatic, intrinsic, and posthepatic causes.
- Vascular changes include dilation of the portal and mesenteric vasculature with development of portosystemic collateral vessels.
- MRI can evaluate the underlying hepatic parenchymal abnormalities in addition to vascular changes of portal hypertension.

Portal and Mesenteric Thrombosis

Definition

Thrombosis of the portal circulation can be a life-threatening condition that manifests with nonspecific clinical symptoms, and the diagnosis is usually dependent on imaging. Thrombosis of the SMV causes venous outflow obstruction and bowel ischemia, which may progress to pneumatosis and frank infarction.

Etiology and Pathophysiology

Thrombosis of the portal vein may be idiopathic, iatrogenic, or secondary to adjacent infection and/or inflammation, and is a cause of prehepatic portal hypertension. Portal thrombosis is also common in the setting of portal hypertension due to intrinsic liver disease, likely caused by altered flow dynamics in the setting of sinusoidal obstruction. Predisposing factors include prior surgery, infection, or hypercoagulable states.

Manifestations of Disease

Clinical Presentation

Clinical presentation may be acute or chronic and involves nonspecific symptoms such as abdominal pain, nausea, vomiting, and anorexia. As such, imaging plays a key role in the diagnosis.

Imaging Techniques and Findings

MR

Intraluminal thrombus within the SMV is well demonstrated on MRI with 3D GRE images, providing a noninvasive method for diagnosis (Fig. 105-7). In addition, evaluation of the end-organ effects of mesenteric occlusion is important because the clinical picture varies between acute and chronic presentations, and not all patients require surgery. Bowel pathology can be evaluated concurrently with the vasculature using MRI, with ischemia demonstrating increased signal on fat saturated T2W images secondary to inflammation and edema caused by venous congestion. The presence of bowel ischemia as identified by MR may prompt more aggressive therapy, with both percutaneous and intraoperative catheter-directed therapy demonstrating good results.[11] Thrombosis of the splenic vein is a cause of isolated gastric varices and has been treated with splenectomy in the past, although percutaneous therapy has also been successful.

Differential Diagnosis

From Clinical Presentation

Due to nonspecific symptomatology, the differential diagnosis is often quite broad on a clinical basis.

From Imaging Findings

Evaluation with postcontrast 3D GRE sequences allows direct identification of intraluminal thrombus within the SMV and portal vein, allowing for a specific diagnosis.

Synopsis of Treatment Options

Medical

Medical therapy includes supportive care and identification and treatment of the underlying cause. In addition, patients receive systemic anticoagulation with follow-up imaging. Systemic thrombolytic therapy is not widely employed.

Surgical/Interventional

Surgical clot decompression is performed in cases with an acute, life-threatening presentation, with signs of bowel infarction or peritonitis. This also allows the resection of infarcted segments of bowel. However, percutaneous therapy with catheter-directed thrombolysis has also been performed with good results in patients without symptoms of bowel perforation, either alone or with surgical assistance.

KEY POINTS

- Due to nonspecific clinical symptoms, imaging is critical for the diagnosis of portal and mesenteric thrombus.
- MRI (including postcontrast 3D GRE images) is well-suited for identification of the intraluminal thrombus and the end-organ effects of mesenteric occlusion.
- Portal thrombosis often occurs in the setting of chronic liver disease owing to altered flow dynamics.

Malignant Hepatic Neoplasms

Definition

Thrombus developing in the portal vein may be bland (due to the causes described earlier) or be secondary to tumor thrombus. In the vast majority of cases, tumor thrombus within the portal vein and its intrahepatic branches is due to one of two primary hepatic malignancies: hepatocellular carcinoma and cholangiocarcinoma.

Prevalence and Epidemiology

The incidence of primary liver cancer has been steadily increasing over the past 20 years, primarily due to an increase in the number of hepatocellular carcinomas.

Etiology and Pathophysiology

Risk factors for HCC include cirrhosis, viral infection, and alcohol abuse. Patients with chronic bile duct obstruction, infection, primary sclerosing cholangitis, or congenital bile duct malformations are at an increased risk for cholangiocarcinoma.

Manifestations of Disease

Clinical Presentation

Vascular invasion by tumor again produces nonspecific symptoms that are often identical to bland thrombus, again emphasizing the importance of imaging in the diagnosis. Patients will often present with predisposing factors such as cirrhosis, viral infection, or chronic biliary obstruction.

Imaging Techniques and Findings

MR

MRI has been shown to be highly sensitive and specific for HCC,[12] a tumor that is strongly associated with chronic liver disease. In the well-defined, focal type of HCC, defined MR features include an arterial enhancing lesion that demonstrates washout with rim enhancement on delayed images. The tumor washes out to become hypointense to adjacent liver parenchyma, a direct result of the differential vascular supply between tumor (fed primarily by hepatic artery) and adjacent liver parenchyma (fed primarily by portal vein). T2 signal, if elevated, supports the diagnosis, although this is not a necessary feature. These imaging features are distinct from intrahepatic cholangiocarcinoma (IHC), the second primary hepatic malignancy that tends to invade hepatic vasculature. MRI is also the imaging modality of choice for the evaluation of IHC. After the administration of gadolinium chelate, the tumor does not avidly enhance on arterial phase images, but demonstrates gradual accumulation of contrast on delayed imaging, likely due to leakage of gadolinium into the interstices of the tumor over time. IHC is usually associated with ill-defined T2 signal, and at least some degree of biliary ductal dilation is usually present. Both of these neoplasms invade intrahepatic portal and hepatic venous branches, a finding especially common in the infiltrative type of HCC. The distinction between tumor thrombus and bland thrombus in the setting of these neoplasms is important, especially in the setting of HCC when liver transplantation is considered. The diagnosis of tumor thrombus can be made with the use of 3D GRE sequences. Bland thrombus has no associated vascularity and will not have any signal on postgadolinium imaging, producing images of a black clot. Tumor thrombus, alternatively, will take up gadolinium on delayed imaging, which can be easily demonstrated with comparison to precontrast images. Any enhancement within a thrombus associated with these tumors is indicative of vascular tumor invasion (Fig. 105-8).

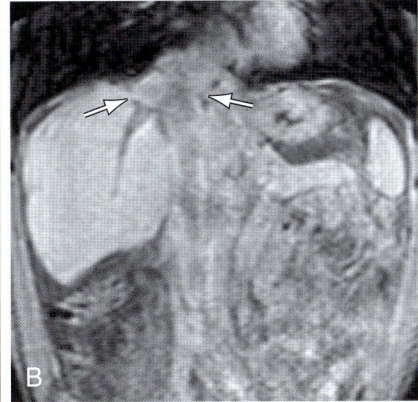

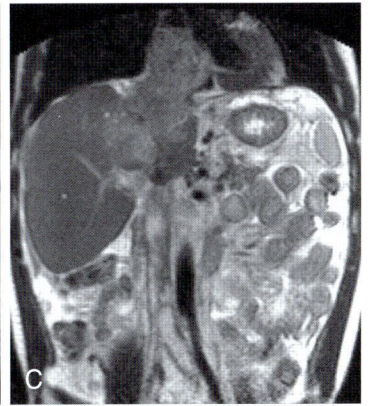

CHAPTER 105 ● Magnetic Resonance Imaging of Vascular Disorders of the Abdomen

FIGURE 105-8 Hepatocellular carcinoma with vascular invasion. An ill-defined hepatic tumor is demonstrated on axial postcontrast 3D GRE (**A**), with coronal 3D GRE images showing thrombus (*arrows*) extending into the hepatic veins and IVC (**B**). This clot shows enhancement after Gd administration in keeping with tumor thrombus. Vascular involvement is also well demonstrated on coronal T2W image (**C**), with loss of normal signal void secondary to tumor thrombus extending into the right atrium.

Differential Diagnosis from Imaging Findings

Vascular tumor invasion is from a primary neoplasm, either HCC or cholangiocarcinoma in the vast majority of cases. Because the imaging appearances of these neoplasms are markedly different with MRI, diagnostic specificity is not usually a problem.

Synopsis of Treatment Options

Medical

For unresectable disease, chemotherapy is the mainstay of medical treatment, in addition to supportive care.

Surgical/Interventional

HCC meeting the Milan criteria is treated with liver transplantation, whereas unresectable disease is often managed in a palliative manner by percutaneous chemo-embolization. The treatment of choice for cholangiocarcinoma is resection, although extensive portal and mesenteric tumor invasion will likely exclude surgery.

KEY POINTS

- Tumor thrombus demonstrates enhancement on postcontrast 3D GRE images, as opposed to bland thrombus which appears black.
- Hepatocellular carcinoma (HCC) and intrahepatic cholangiocarcinoma (IHC) are the two primary liver neoplasms associated with portal vein invasion.
- HCC and IHC have very different imaging and perfusion characteristics on MRI, allowing clear differentiation between the tumor types in the majority of cases.

Liver Transplantation

Prevalence and Epidemiology

There were nearly 6,000 deceased and living donor liver transplants performed in 2007, although there are more than 16,000 people on the waiting list at the time of this writing. Careful postoperative care and imaging of the post-transplant population is important to ensure graft survival.

Manifestations of Disease

Clinical Presentation

Liver transplantation is the treatment of choice for patients with end-stage liver disease, and is also intended as a curative procedure for patients with HCC meeting specific imaging criteria.[13] Patency of the portal and mesenteric vasculature is critical in the pretransplant cirrhotic patient because portal thrombosis will hasten liver failure. In addition, extension of thrombus into the SMV directly affects the technical feasibility of liver transplantation. If the patent portion of the SMV is large enough, the surgeon may attempt an interposition graft from the SMV to the transplanted liver. If, however, the patent SMV tributaries are small or replaced by varices, liver transplantation is not technically feasible. MRI is an excellent technique to evaluate mesenteric thrombosis and the technical feasibility of transplantation, providing accurate evaluation of vessel size and varices.

Imaging Indications and Algorithm

Detailed preoperative knowledge of a patient's hepatic vascular anatomy is of paramount importance, especially in the setting of living-donor liver transplantation (LDLT), a more common occurrence especially in the pediatric setting. In this clinical scenario, accurate depiction of the donor vasculature is just as important as recipient

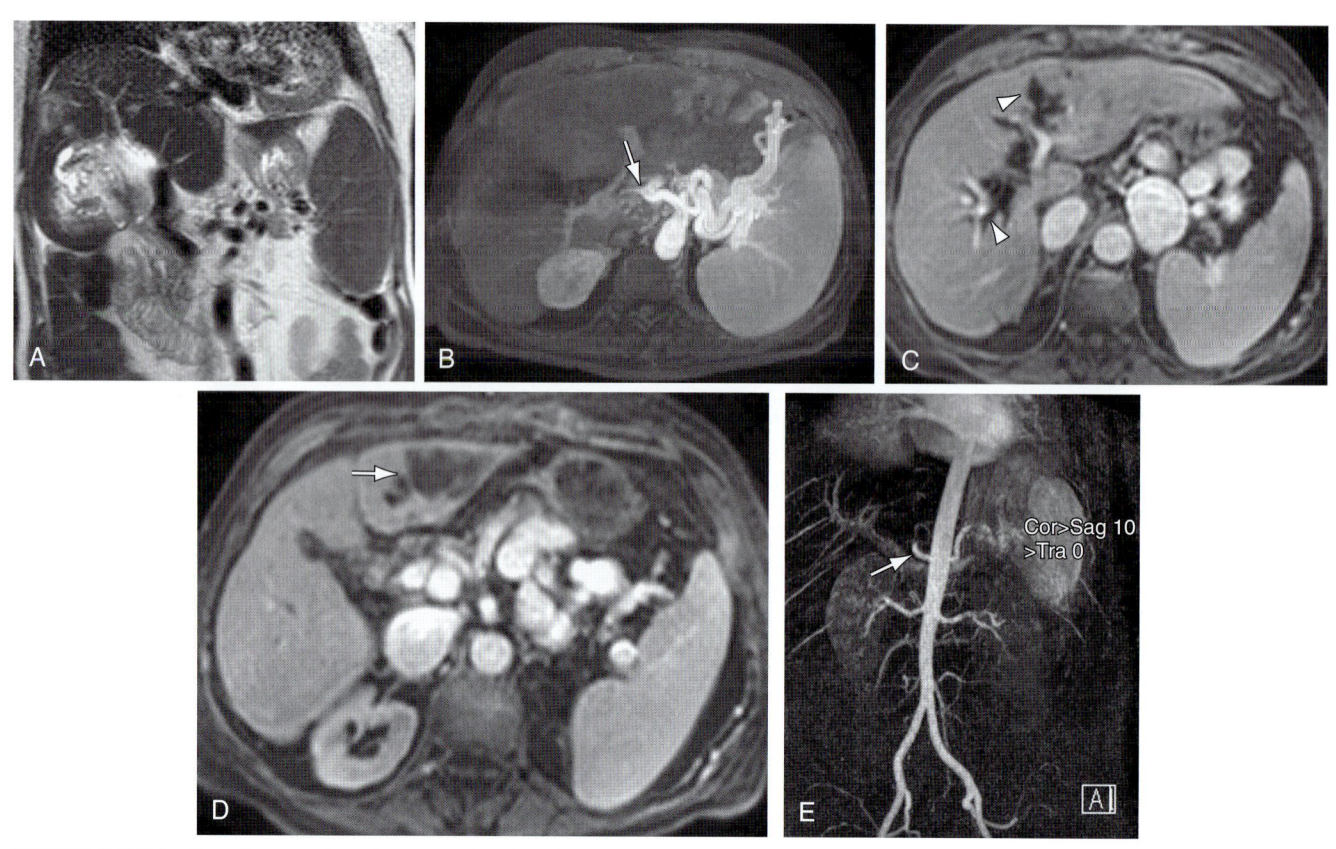

FIGURE 105-9 Hepatic artery thrombosis (HAT) and resultant parenchymal abscess postorthotopic liver transplantation. Coronal (**A**) fat suppressed T2W HASTE images show a large, complex intrahepatic fluid collection. The etiology of this abscess is demonstrated on postgadolinium 3D GRE arterial phase MIP images (**B**), showing occlusion of the hepatic artery (*arrow*). A second case of HAT with resultant intrahepatic biliary ductal dilation (**C,** *arrowheads*) and biloma formation (**D,** arrow) is clearly demonstrated on axial 3D GRE image. Hepatic artery thrombosis (*arrow*) is confirmed on CE 3D GRE MIP image (**E**).

evaluation, especially to reduce postsurgical morbidity and mortality in a previously healthy population.

Imaging Techniques and Findings

MR

MR has been shown to be equivalent to CTA in the preoperative evaluation of hepatic vascular anatomy,[14] but with the added benefits of improved parenchymal soft tissue evaluation compared to CT and also the lack of ionizing radiation, an especially important issue in the pediatric population. Of note, liver transplantation is usually performed with intent to cure and not as a palliative procedure. In this setting, cumulative radiation dose is a consideration, especially in patients with chronic liver disease who undergo surveillance imaging. MRI provides a superior imaging modality for evaluation of parenchymal and vascular changes associated with liver disease without contributing to cumulative radiation doses in a patient set to undergo curative surgery.

MRI performs quite well in the vascular assessment of the postoperative transplanted liver. In the immediate postoperative setting, complex and hemorrhagic blood products are often identified in and around the surgical bed. The most serious immediate postoperative complication is hepatic artery thrombosis, which occurs at variable rates from 3% to 9% and is more common with LDLT in centers with less experience.[15] MRI not only directly detects hepatic artery thrombosis (HAT), but also the resultant changes in the hepatic parenchyma related to arterial devascularization. The consequences of acute hepatic artery thrombosis are severe and often require retransplantation to avoid graft loss. More commonly, HAT results in defined biliary complications because the sole vascular supply of the biliary system is via the hepatic artery in graft livers. These biliary complications include ductal dilation, biloma formation, and sepsis secondary to a resultant cholangitis (Fig. 105-9). MRI can also demonstrate the acute hepatic inflammation that is associated with bile stasis and infection[16] better than any other imaging modality. Thromboses of the IVC, hepatic and portal veins are less common complications, but also are well assessed with 3D GRE imaging. Another rare vascular complication is the splenohepatic arterial steal syndrome. This is characterized by arterial malperfusion and ischemic damage of the hepatic graft caused by diversion of blood flow to a markedly enlarged spleen. Splenohepatic arterial steal syndrome may ultimately result in graft loss if it is recognized too late. A post-transplantation splenectomy represents a successful therapeutic approach for this condition. Even in the absence of pathology, a transplanted liver may be identified with MR by reproducible mild narrowing at the IVC and portal vein anastomosis with mild susceptibility artifact at the IVC anastomosis (Fig. 105-10).

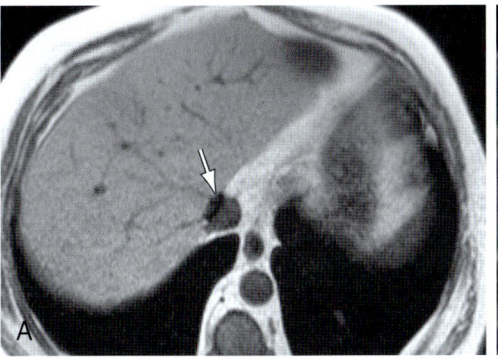

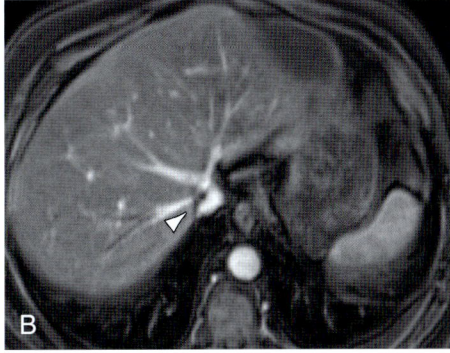

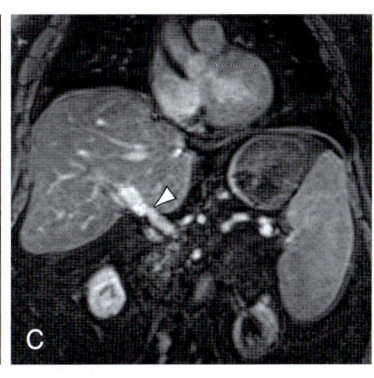

■ **FIGURE 105-10** Normal post liver transplant MR. Susceptibility artifact is seen at the IVC anastomosis on 2D T1 FLASH (**A**, *arrow*) image due to prior transplant, resulting in mild, expected narrowing of the IVC at this site on postcontrast 3D GRE (**B**, *arrowhead*) image. Coronal 3D GRE (**C**) of a normal post-transplant liver also shows mild narrowing at the portal vein anastomosis (*arrowhead*), and the transplant hepatic parenchyma demonstrates normal perfusion. Residual changes of portal hypertension, including an enlarged spleen, persist.

KEY POINTS

- Liver transplantation is the treatment of choice for patients with end-stage liver disease and HCC meeting specific criteria.
- Thrombosis of the portal vein and SMV will directly affect the feasibility of transplantation, and preoperative imaging is critical.
- Hepatic artery thrombosis is an important post-transplant complication that results in biliary necrosis.

Budd-Chiari Syndrome

Definition

Budd Chiari syndrome is a posthepatic cause of portal hypertension in which hepatic venous outflow obstruction (anywhere from the level of the hepatic venules to the right atrium) causes hepatic sinusoidal congestion.

Prevalence and Epidemiology

Budd-Chiari occurs equally in men and women, usually presenting in the 3rd and 4th decade.

Etiology and Pathophysiology

Sinusoidal congestion induces inflammation and fibrosis, leading to the common endpoint of hepatic fibrosis and portal hypertension from resistance to portal inflow. The etiology of this syndrome is variable, and includes vascular webs, venous tumor invasion (especially by HCC), inflammation (especially Behçet syndrome) and iatrogenic causes, although an underlying hypercoagulable disorder is present in most cases.[17]

Manifestations of Disease

Clinical Presentation

Budd-Chiari may manifest acutely with fulminant hepatic failure, encephalopathy, and ascites, with biopsy demonstrating rapid hepatocellular necrosis. However, in the majority of cases, the presentation is subacute or chronic in nature because some hepatic venous outflow may be preserved by draining through a variety of accessory hepatic veins. These patients present with more advanced changes of cirrhosis and chronic liver disease, with a more gradual onset of symptomatology from portal hypertension.

Imaging Techniques and Findings

MR

The diagnosis of Budd Chiari depends on evaluation of the hepatic venous outflow system in addition to the associated parenchymal changes, and MR is the modality best suited for evaluation of both areas. Evaluation of the venous system is performed with postcontrast 3D GRE sequences in axial and coronal planes. Venous patency can also be assessed on additional imaging sequences, such as evaluating vascular signal on TFISP imaging and "black blood" flow void on T2W images. The ability to assess vessel patency on additional imaging sequences provides an inherent level of redundancy within the image acquisition that contributes to the high sensitivity and specificity of MR compared to CT. Parenchymal changes in Budd-Chiari are also well evaluated with MR. The most consistent feature is marked hypertrophy of the caudate lobe (sometimes quite massive) due to its separate drainage into the IVC, thus sparing the caudate from the effects of venous outflow obstruction (Fig. 105-11). In the acute setting, the liver is usually enlarged secondary to edema, whereas in the chronic setting there is atrophy of the peripheral aspects of the liver and sparing of the caudate. Postcontrast 3D GRE images demonstrate decreased perfusion of the peripheral aspects of the liver secondary to altered flow dynamics induced by liver injury. An additional parenchymal finding is the presence of focal nodules in the liver parenchyma. These nodules are termed "large regenerative nodules" or "multiacinar regenerative nodules"[18] and correlate to nontumorous liver parenchyma surrounded by variable amounts of fibrous stroma.[18] These nodules characteristically show no distinctive enhancement features compared with adjacent liver parenchyma or arterial phase images.

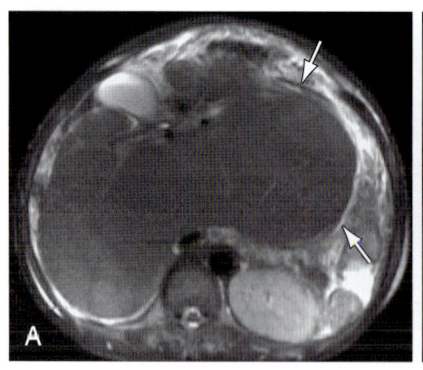

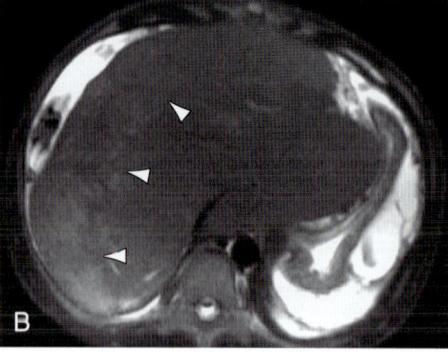

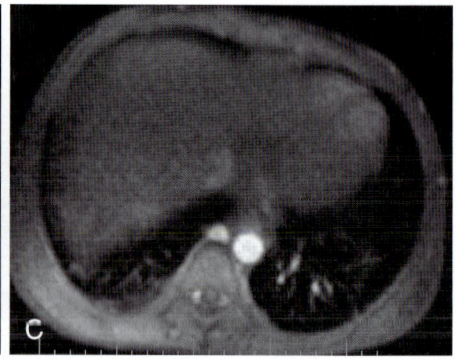

■ **FIGURE 105-11** Hepatic changes of Budd Chiari. Axial fat-saturated T2 HASTE images (**A, B**) demonstrate massive enlargement of the caudate lobe (**A**, *arrows*). Patchy increased T2 signal is present along the periphery of the liver (**B**, *arrowheads*) due to hepatic congestion and edema, with relative sparing of the more central portions of the liver. Saturation-recovery postcontrast Turbo FLASH (**C**) demonstrates no enhancement of the occluded hepatic veins and intrahepatic IVC.

Differential Diagnosis

From Clinical Presentation

Other etiologies for acute, fulminant hepatic failure and chronic liver disease are clinical considerations, but can often be excluded with imaging.

From Imaging Findings

The diagnosis of Budd-Chiari should be differentiated from a distinct entity termed *hepatic veno-occlusive disease*. Seen most often in the post–stem-cell transplant setting, this is an inflammatory process that results in the destruction of the vascular endothelium of the hepatic venules.

Synopsis of Treatment Options

Medical

Supportive care and aggressive treatment of any underlying causes are the mainstay of medical management. Anticoagulation with heparin followed by warfarin is also employed

Surgical/Interventional

Because a large majority of these patients present with advanced-stage liver disease and portal hypertension, liver transplantation is usually the only effective treatment, although placement of a TIPS may allow for a bridge to transplantation. Some centers have performed TIPS and catheter-directed thrombolysis in specific clinical scenarios.

KEY POINTS

- Hepatic venous outflow obstruction results in sinusoidal congestions and liver injury.
- Vascular patency and underlying parenchymal changes are best evaluated with MRI, including changes of portal hypertension.
- Liver transplantation is the treatment of choice.

Splanchnic Artery Aneurysm

Definition

Splanchnic artery aneurysms can be divided into true aneurysms and pseudoaneurysms.

Prevalence and Epidemiology

True aneurysms represent a rare disorder, with an incidence between 0.1% to 2%. The visceral arteries most prone to true aneurysm formation are the splenic (Fig. 105-12) and hepatic arteries, having approximately 60% and 20% relative incidence, respectively. Splenic artery aneurysms are encountered in two distinct patient populations—women with multiple pregnancies and patients with portal hypertension. Other causes of splenic artery aneurysms include mycotic infection, fibromuscular dysplasia, and congenital causes. True aneurysms are most commonly located in the distal third of the splenic artery (75%), followed by the middle third (20)%. Hepatic artery aneurysms, in contrast, are seen most often in patients with hypertension, fibromuscular dysplasia, or polyarteritis nodosa. Seventy-seven percent of hepatic aneurysms are isolated to the segment proximal to the liver, whereas 20% have combined intra- and extraparenchymal involvement; 3% are localized exclusively within liver.[20]

Pseudoaneurysms are secondary to a disruption of the vessel wall, with blood contained only by the thin, outer adventitia. They are usually the result of trauma, iatrogenic injury, or pancreatitis. Splenic artery pseudoaneurysms are especially associated with severe, acute pancreatitis secondary to its intimate anatomic relationship with the pancreas. The rupture rate of pseudoaneurysms is significantly higher than that of true aneurysms, owing to the lack of all three vessel wall layers, and therapeutic intervention is the rule.

Etiology and Pathophysiology

Pseudoaneurysms are usually due to trauma, iatrogenic injury, or adjacent inflammation. True aneurysms are usually congenital, due to an inherent weakness in the vessel wall.

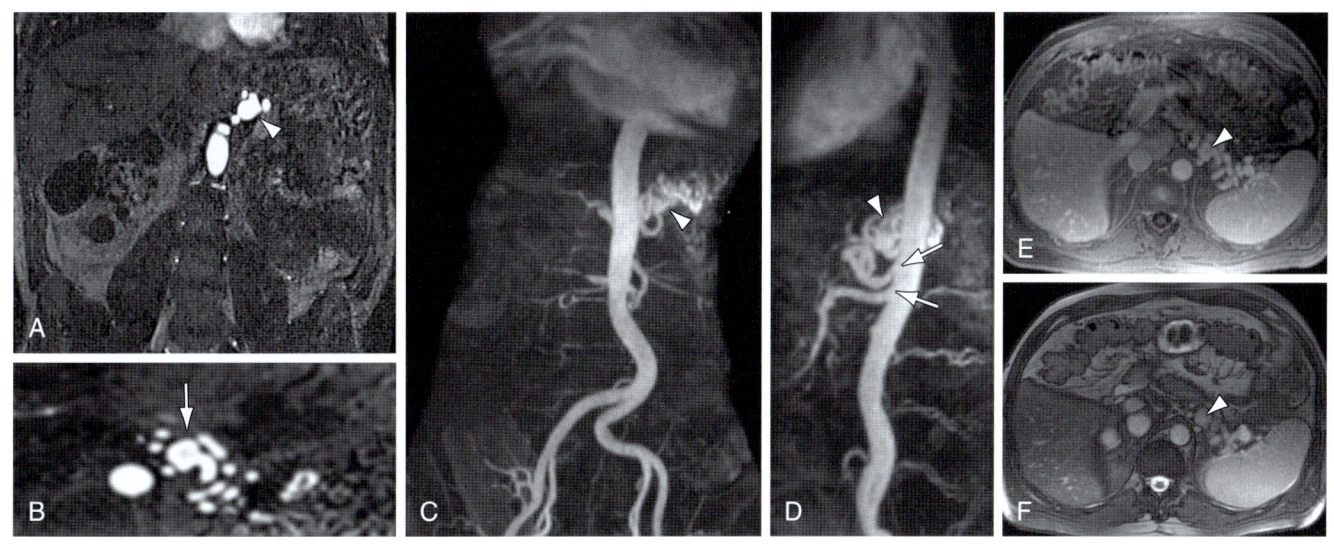

■ **FIGURE 105-12** Splenic artery aneurysm incidentally found with prerenal transplant MRI. Coronal (**A**) and axial reformatted (**B**) 3D CE MRA demonstrate a 2 cm splenic artery aneurysm. MIP images obtained from the source data (**C, D**) show the splenic artery is markedly tortuous (*arrowheads*), making it difficult to identify the aneurysm. The remainder of the vasculature is also well demonstrated, with a normal aorta and patent origins of the celiac trunk and superior mesenteric artery (**D,** *arrows*). Axial 3D postcontrast GRE (**E**) and True-FISP (**F**) images also show the aneurysm well (*arrowheads*), serving as back-up images for the arterial system, in addition to excluding perianeurysmal complications, such as inflammation and rupture.

Manifestations of Disease

Clinical Presentation

Patients may present with vague clinical symptomatology, but acute rupture leads to hemodynamic instability and substantial perioperative morbidity and mortality, underscoring the importance of therapy at the time of diagnosis, even if the patient is asymptomatic.[19]

Imaging Techniques and Findings

MR

MRI is highly sensitive for the detection of splanchnic artery aneurysms, which may be detected on CE 3D MRA or 3D GRE imaging. 3D GRE images better depict the aneurysm wall and associated thrombus, and are more helpful for distinguishing true from false aneurysms. Important preoperative information that is depicted with MR includes the type and location of the aneurysm, diameter and extent along the vessel, involvement of branch vessels, presence of mural thrombus, and whether the aneurysm has already ruptured.[21] Morphologic imaging, including T2W images and TFISP, are also important for aneurysm assessment. Hepatic and gastroduodenal aneurysms may manifest with obstructive jaundice secondary to compression of the biliary tree, which is demonstrated well with T2W images (Fig. 105-13). Mycotic aneurysms show perianeurysmal inflammation, which is depicted as surrounding high signal on fat-suppressed T2W images.

Differential Diagnosis from Clinical Presentation

Other etiologies of gastrointestinal bleeding, such as angiodysplasia, diverticulitis, or carcinoma may be considered clinically.

Synopsis of Treatment Options

Medical

Medical therapy includes supportive management and blood transfusions in the case of active hemorrhage.

Surgical/Interventional

Because the natural course of splanchnic artery aneurysms (especially pseudoaneurysms) may lead to rupture, MRI is critical in providing the correct diagnosis to prompt therapy and treatment planning. Although therapy is clearly mandated in patients with asymptomatic aneurysms or contained rupture (pseudoaneurysms), the following asymptomatic lesions also warrant intervention: (1) splenic artery aneurysms in patients with the potential to become pregnant or requiring liver transplantation; (2) common or proper hepatic artery aneurysms in patients with polyarteritis nodosa or fibromuscular dysplasia; and (3) splenic or hepatic artery aneurysms greater than 2.0 cm in diameter.[22] Percutaneous treatment with aneurysm coiling has demonstrated excellent results compared to surgery and should be the first line of therapy.

KEY POINTS

- Splanchnic artery aneurysms are divided into true (congenital) or pseudoaneurysms (secondary to vessel wall disruption).
- MRA best evaluates the patent aneurysm lumen, whereas postcontrast 3D GRE images provide information about the vessel wall and mural thrombus.
- Prompt therapy (either percutaneous or surgical) is necessary for pseudoaneurysms and certain true aneurysms.

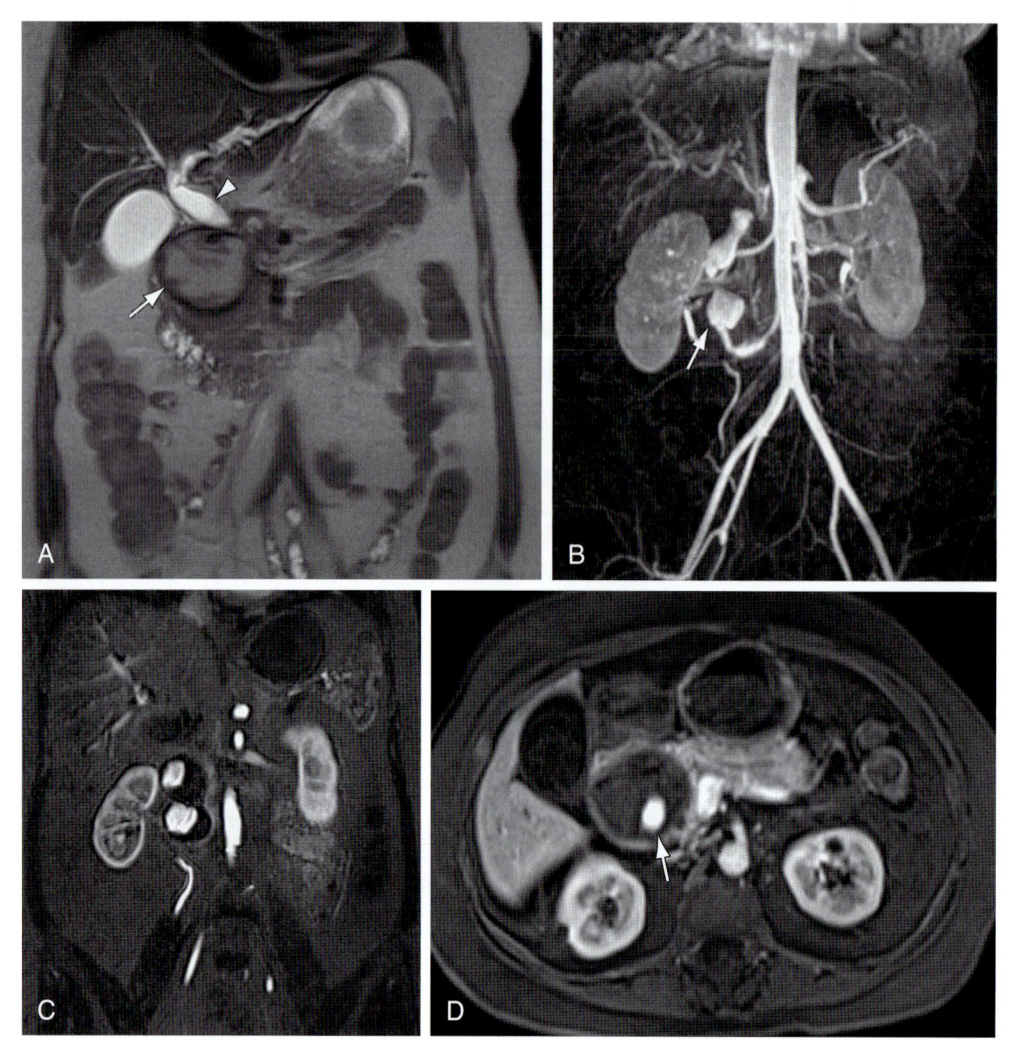

■ **FIGURE 105-13** Gastroduodenal pseudoaneurysm. Coronal single-shot T2 HASTE (**A**) demonstrates a complex rounded mass (*arrow*) with hypointense signal at the periphery due to blood products. T2W images also show compression of the common bile duct by the mass (*arrowhead*), causing intra and extrahepatic biliary ductal dilation. Coronal CE 3D MRA MIP image (**B**) shows the irregular, bilobed pseudoaneurysm arising from the gastroduodenal artery, with shunting of blood from a branch of the superior mesenteric artery (*arrow*). The MRA source image (**C**) better demonstrates the peripheral, thrombosed portions of the aneurysm. 3D GRE images (**D**) not only demonstrate the patent lumen (*arrow*), but also best demonstrate the wall and extensive mural thrombus.

Pancreatic Pathology: Vascular Involvement

Definition

Pancreatic adenocarcinoma is an infiltrative tumor that often presents at a later stage of diagnosis as a poorly vascularized mass.

Etiology and Pathophysiology

Because of the intimate relationship between the pancreatic body and the splenic vein, inflammatory and neoplastic processes in this region often result in narrowing and/or occlusion of the splenic vein. The most common etiologies for acute pancreatitis include biliary stone disease and alcohol abuse, although there are a large number of additional causes, including medications and idiopathic etiologies.

Manifestations of Disease

Clinical Presentation

Patients with pancreatic adenocarcinoma present with vague clinical symptoms that are often silent early in its course, leading to an advanced stage at final diagnosis. Symptoms arise due to mass effect from the tumor on the biliary system, causing obstructive jaundice (often painless). Acute pancreatitis, on the other hand, manifests with abdominal pain and anorexia, and there is often a history of alcohol abuse or gallstones.

Imaging Indications and Algorithm

MRI of the pancreas continues to evolve with improvement in rapid-acquisition breath-hold or breathing-independent imaging techniques. MR should be considered

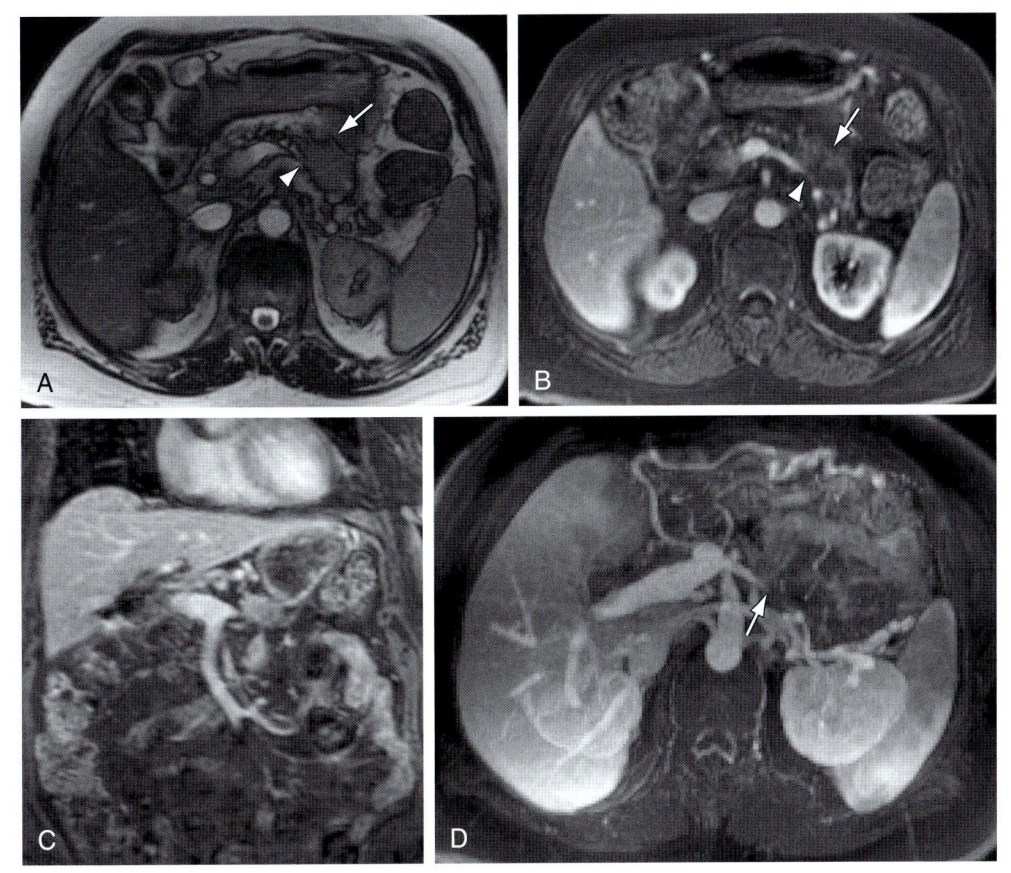

■ **FIGURE 105-14** Pancreatic adenocarcinoma. Axial TFISP (**A**) demonstrates a focal mass (*arrow*) in the pancreatic tail, whereas arterial phase 3D GRE (**B**) images show the tumor (*arrow*) has poor vascular perfusion, a finding consistent with poorly differentiated adenocarcinoma. Tumor obliterates the adjacent splenic vein (*arrowheads*). Splenic vein invasion is also well depicted on coronal 3D GRE (**C**) and axial 3D GRE MIP image (**D**, *arrow*).

essential in the imaging evaluation of pancreatic disease, and particularly for optimal presurgical identification, characterization, and staging of pancreatic masses. High resolution CE 3D MRA can easily define arterial vascular anatomy for presurgical planning, and MR assessment of vascular infiltration by tumor reaches a sensitivity and specificity of 83% and 96%, respectively, comparable to CT and endoscopic sonography evaluation.[23] MR also offers concurrent, superior, soft tissue imaging that defines tumor size, invasion into adjacent soft tissue structures, pancreatic and biliary ductal obstruction, and also venous invasion by tumor.

Imaging Techniques and Findings

MR

The most common presentation is that of biliary ductal obstruction from tumor in the pancreatic head, at which point assessment of the adjacent portal vein, SMV and SMA are critical if surgical resection is attempted. Evaluation depends on a combination of the coronal MRA source data and 3D GRE images. Vascular tumor infiltration is assumed on the basis of either vessel caliber reduction, vessel encasement (90% circumferential involvement) or vessel occlusion.[24] Extensive vascular collaterals may also be demonstrated. Pancreatic adenocarcinoma may also arise within the tail, typically presenting as a larger mass with local infiltration (Fig. 105-14) that commonly encases or occludes the splenic vein, and may invade the splenic hilum, leading to extensive infarction of the spleen.

Although pancreatic adenocarcinoma is an infiltrative tumor that invades adjacent vasculature, there are several additional pancreatic neoplasms that may compress the splanchnic vasculature owing to overall size and morphology. These include cystic neoplasms of the pancreas, either serous cystadenomas, or mucinous cystadenomas/cystadenocarcinomas. If occurring in the pancreatic head, they more commonly cause compression of the biliary tree, but occasionally these lesions can also compress local vessels, especially the portal confluence. Differentiation of tumor type, in addition to assessment of vascular involvement, is best performed with MR.

Inflammatory processes of the pancreas also commonly involve the adjacent vasculature. This is seen in the setting of acute pancreatitis, which is a well-known cause of splenic vein thrombosis (Fig. 105-15), and has also been reported in at least 20% of patients with chronic pancreatitis. Occlusion of the splenic vein is often seen in association with collateralized venous flow into extensive peripancreatic and perisplenic varices. Splenic vein thrombosis is also a well-known cause of isolated gastric varices, and less commonly a cause of esophageal or colonic varices. Postcontrast 3D GRE imaging is the best sequence

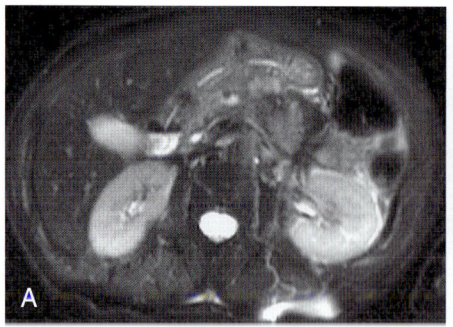

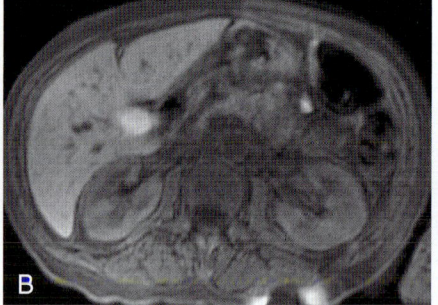

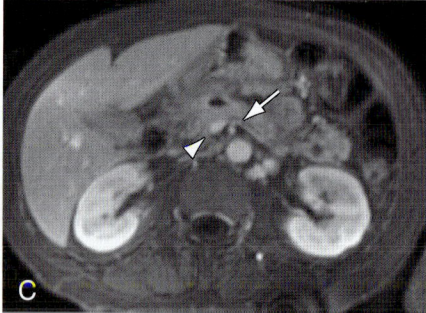

FIGURE 105-15 Acute pancreatitis. Peripancreatic edema is present on axial fat-suppressed T2W HASTE (**A**), whereas precontrast 3D GRE (**B**) image shows loss of the normal increased pancreatic T1 signal. Postgadolinium 3D GRE (**C**) shows a narrowed portal vein confluence (*arrowhead*) and thrombosis of the splenic vein (*arrow*).

for depiction of splenic vein thrombosis and associated collateral flow from varices. The splenic artery may also be secondarily involved in cases of severe pancreatitis, with the formation of aneurysms and pseudoaneurysms secondary to vascular endothelial breakdown from the adjacent inflammatory process. Pseudocysts may erode into the adjacent splenic artery or vein, causing life-threatening episodes of hemorrhage.

In addition to the identification of vascular involvement, MR is also able to delineate parenchymal changes of acute and chronic pancreatitis. Acute pancreatitis demonstrates edema and inflammation in and around the pancreas and retroperitoneum, manifested as increased signal on fat-saturated T2W images. Chronic pancreatitis, in contrast, shows loss of normal T1 signal within the pancreatic parenchyma, and persistent enhancement on delayed imaging secondary to fibrosis. Additional morphologic images are helpful for diagnosing the etiology of the pancreatitis, such as from stone disease or tumor. Evaluation of the parenchymal and vascular changes of acute and chronic pancreatitis in the same imaging examination provides a comprehensive evaluation that is important for diagnosis and clinical management.

Differential Diagnosis

From Clinical Presentation

Clinical symptoms are usually nonspecific, although painless jaundice is concerning for pancreatic adenocarcinoma.

From Imaging Findings

Focal pancreatitis at times may mimic an aggressive neoplasm, but evaluation of dynamic, contrast-enhanced MRI, in combination with fat-saturated T2W images, can make the correct diagnosis in the vast majority of cases.

Synopsis of Treatment Options

Medical

Pancreatitis is treated with supportive care, especially fluid replacement. Chronic pancreatitis may require enzyme replacement.

Surgical/Interventional

The treatment of choice for pancreatic adenocarcinoma is a Whipple procedure, and preoperative MRI is important to establish resectability. Repetitive, chronic pancreatitis may require surgical drainage such as a Frey procedure to provide symptom relief.

KEY POINTS

- The close relationship of the pancreas to the SMA, SMV, splenic and portal vein causes vascular compromise in a variety of pancreatic pathologies.
- Vascular involvement is best demonstrated with a combination of MRA and 3D GRE images.
- MRI also provides excellent soft tissue imaging which allows evaluation of the underlying neoplastic or inflammatory etiology.

Splenic Infarction

Prevalence and Epidemiology

Splenic infarcts are often seen in the setting of chronic liver disease, likely due to relative ischemia produced by a massively enlarged spleen. Other clinical settings with a predisposition to splenic infarction include arterial emboli (most commonly of cardiac origin), sickle cell anemia, infiltrative disorders such as Gaucher disease, hematological malignancies, collagen vascular diseases, and rarely, splenic torsion.[25]

Etiology and Pathophysiology

Branches of the splenic artery are noncommunicating end arteries, and the spleen does not have the dual blood supply of the liver. Because of this, occlusion of splenic artery branches often leads to focal splenic infarction.

Manifestations of Disease

Clinical Presentation

Splenic infarction is a relatively common occurrence, and at times, the acute event causes symptoms referable to the

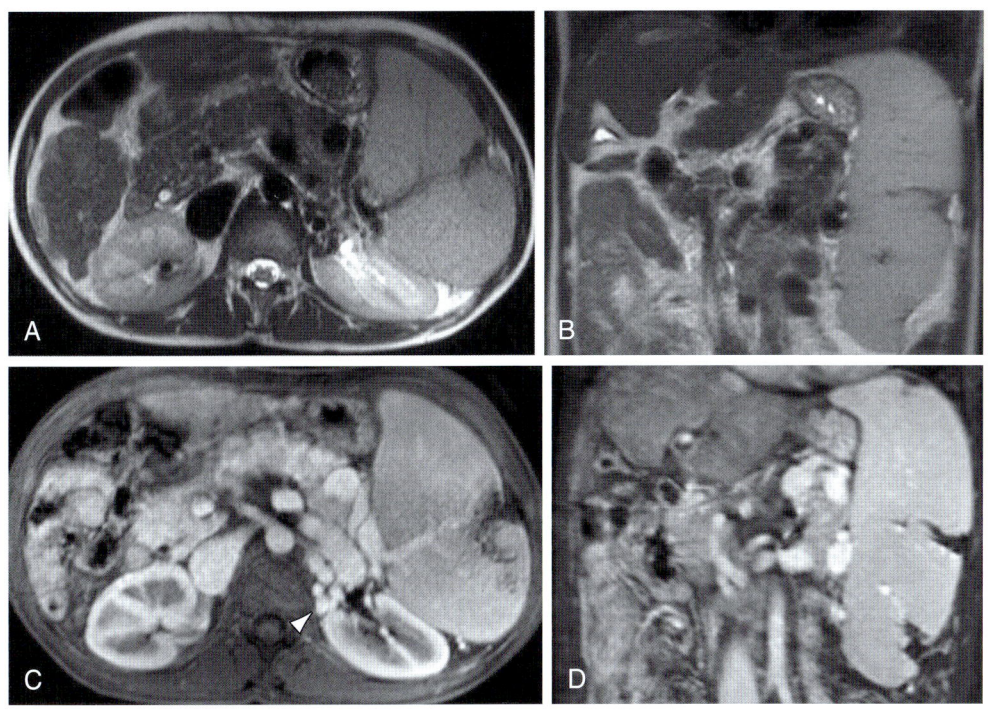

FIGURE 105-16 Splenic infarcts. Axial (**A**) and coronal (**B**) T2 HASTE images show a massively enlarged spleen with multiple peripheral, wedge-shaped areas of hypointense signal. These areas show no perfusion on axial (**C**) and coronal (**D**) postcontrast 3D GRE images. Also note the splenorenal shunt (**C,** *arrowhead*), another indication of portal hypertension in this cirrhotic patient.

left upper quadrant. However, it is more frequently asymptomatic, with residual features seen only on future imaging studies.

Imaging Techniques and Findings

MR

On MRI, splenic infarcts are seen as peripheral wedge-shaped or linear defects that exhibit decreased signal intensity on both T1W and T2W images. These areas show no internal perfusion after the administration of Gd, most clearly defined on delayed postcontrast images (Fig. 105-16). Complications of splenic infarctions include abscess, splenic pseudocyst formation, splenic rupture and hemorrhage—all features that are easily depicted with MRI. Rarely, the entire spleen may be infarcted, demonstrating diffuse low-signal intensity on T1W images, inhomogeneous high-signal intensity on T2W, and an enhancing capsule on postgadolinium images.

Differential Diagnosis from Imaging Findings

Wedge-shaped perfusion defects within the spleen are highly specific for splenic infarction.

Synopsis of Treatment Options

Medical

Often supportive care is all that is necessary.

Surgical/Interventional

Surgical therapy may be considered in the case of a complete splenic infarction that has been secondarily infected, requiring resection or drainage.

KEY POINTS

- Splenic artery branches are noncommunicating end arteries, with occlusion leading to segmental infarction.
- Infarctions occur most often in the setting of splenomegaly and sickle cell disease.
- MRI demonstrates a wedge-shaped perfusion defect that is highly specific for infarction. Complications of splenic infarction are also well evaluated with MRI.

Polyarteritis Nodosum

Definition

Polyarteritis nodosum (PAN) is a vasculitis of small- to medium-sized arteries presenting as a systemic and multi-organ disease.

Manifestations of Disease

Clinical Presentation

The skin, joints, gastrointestinal tract, kidneys, and nervous system are often simultaneously affected. PAN does not characteristically affect single vessels, although there have been reports of single intra-abdominal vessel involvement involving the hepatic and splenic arteries.

Imaging Techniques and Findings

MR

The most characteristic finding on MRA is multiple small, peripheral aneurysms, tending to occur at branch points of the affected arteries due to necrosis of the internal elastic lamina of the small- and medium-sized arteries. Other less specific findings include arterial stenosis, thrombosis, and occlusion.

Differential Diagnosis from Imaging Findings

The differential diagnosis includes a vasculitis from drug abuse, mycotic aneurysms, Takayasu arteritis, and vasculitis associated with connective tissue disorders.[26]

Hereditary Hemorrhagic Telangiectasia

Definition

Hereditary hemorrhagic telangiectasia (HHT), or Osler-Weber-Rendu disease, is an autosomal dominant disorder characterized by telangiectases and arteriovenous malformations (AVM) of the skin and mucosa, but may potentially involve every organ.

Imaging Techniques and Findings

MR

Hepatic involvement occurs in 8% to 31% of cases, and MR images can identify hepatic AVMs and associated features, such as a prominent feeding hepatic artery, dilated portal and/or hepatic veins, and collateral supply involving the gastric, pancreaticoduodenal, splenic, mesenteric and renal vasculature. MR imaging is also used in the staging and follow-up of these abnormalities in patients with HHT.[27]

AVMs can also uncommonly occur in the spleen. Reports of splenic AVMs have described patients presenting with massive diarrhea, ascites, abdominal pain, and signs of portal hypertension. MRI can demonstrate these lesions as multiple, serpiginous flow voids on T2W images and extensive, serpentine enhancement on 3D GRE images. Dilated feeding vessels in association with AVMs are also common, and are easily depicted on MR.[20]

Trauma

Prevalence and Epidemiology

Besides blunt and penetrating traumatic injury, iatrogenic injury is a common cause of vascular pathology, resulting in stenosis, thrombosis, and pseudoaneurysm formation.

Manifestations of Disease

Imaging Indications and Algorithm

The role of MRI in patients with acute traumatic injury to the abdomen is less well defined, and CT remains the primary imaging modality in this scenario, primarily due to speed and ease of accessibility. However, MR may be useful in selected cases of traumatic injury. Settings that may benefit from an increased use of MR imaging include the pediatric population, in which trauma patients are often subject to pan-body CT in addition to multiple follow-up examinations. There is an increased lifetime radiation risk in children relative to adults, and the use of CT in the trauma setting may be overused, especially in the pediatric population.[28] Other clinical settings include that of underlying allergy to iodinated contrast, or in the setting of chronic renal disease. The risk of contrast-induced nephropathy (CIN) is an important consideration in patients with chronic renal disease. CIN occurs at a rate of approximately 3% in the general population, but increases to 12% to 33% with underlying diabetes and chronic renal disease. In addition, CIN nephropathy has been shown to correlate with increased morbidity and mortality, even if renal dysfunction is transient.[29] Consideration of MRI in selected cases such as these would limit patient morbidity induced by imaging and is also useful as a problem-solving modality.

Imaging Techniques and Findings

MR

The spleen is the most commonly ruptured organ in blunt trauma, accounting for approximately 40% of abdominal organ injuries. The spleen is particularly susceptible to injury due to its complex ligamentous attachments and spongy parenchymal consistency. MR signal characteristics of splenic subcapsular or intraparenchymal hematomas include intrinsically increased T1 signal with decreased T2 signal secondary to the degradation products of hemoglobin. Splenic contusion and infarction are depicted as focal areas of hypoperfusion, with a lack of enhancement on postgadolinium GRE images.

MRI combined with MRA can also readily identify vascular complications of the abdominal vessels as a complication of different surgeries and procedures (Fig. 105-17). Bile duct injury in the setting of laparoscopic cholecystectomy is a well-known complication. Because biliary injuries sustained during laparoscopic cholecystectomy are known to occur more proximally compared to open cholecystectomy, a higher incidence of concomitant hepatic arterial injury has been described.[30] This complication is potentially lethal and often requires partial hepatectomy or liver transplantation. MRA and magnetic resonance cholangiography (MRCP) can be performed emergently in patients with a suspicion of biliary and vascular injury, allowing the simultaneous evaluation of both the biliary tree and the hepatic vascular supply in these patients.

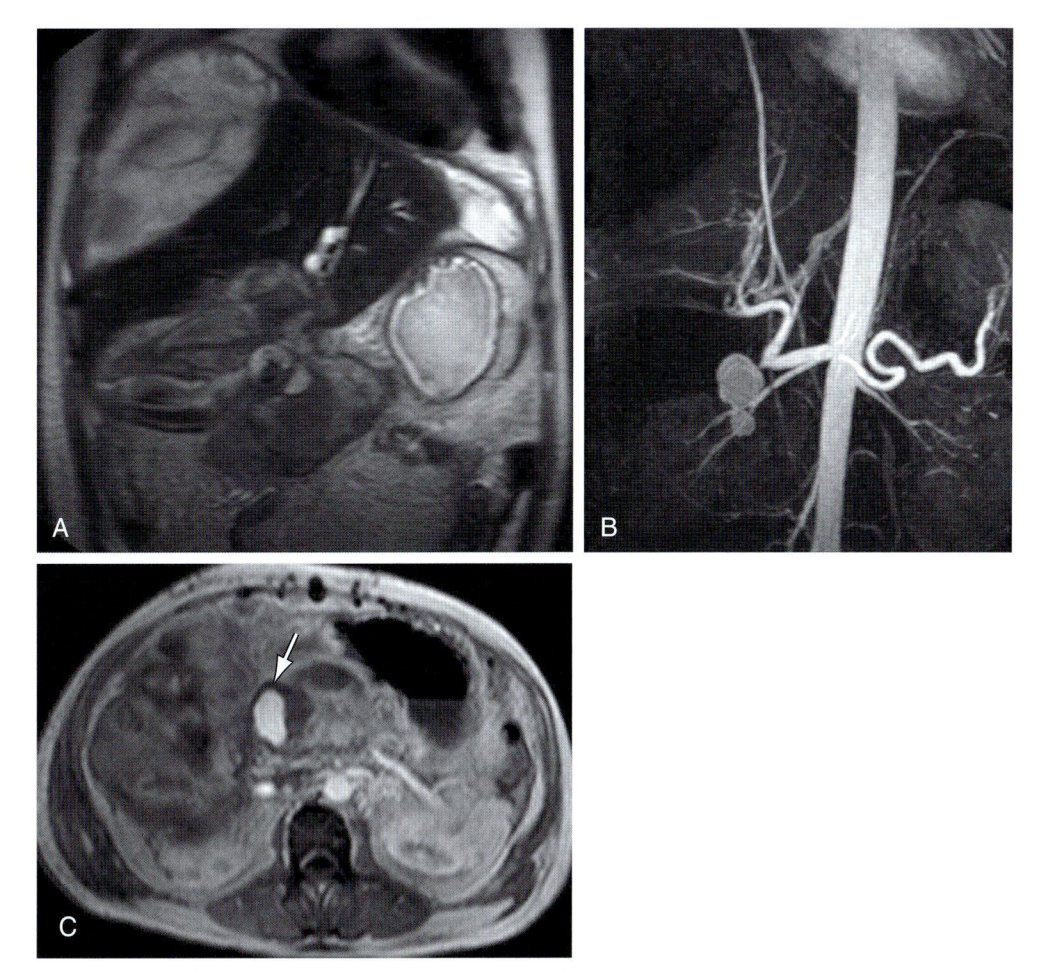

FIGURE 105-17 Gastroduodenal (GDA) pseudoaneurysm, postresection of a pancreatic tail neuroendocrine tumor. Coronal T2W HASTE (**A**) shows a massive subcapsular liver hematoma with heterogeneous signal intensity. Postcontrast 3D CE MRA coronal (**B**) image demonstrates the patent lumen of a lobulated GDA pseudoaneurysm. The extent of the pseudoaneurysm is well depicted on postcontrast 3D GRE (**C,** *arrow*) image, with the surrounding hematoma that communicates with subcapsular hepatic space.

Differential Diagnosis from Clinical Presentation

Traumatic injury often presents with a relevant antecedent history, but must be kept in the differential considerations in all patients presenting with pain or altered mental status.

Synopsis of Treatment Options

Medical

Supportive therapy with fluid resuscitation is important. Often, visceral organ injury may be managed with purely supportive care if the patient is hemodynamically stable.

Surgical/Interventional

Hemodynamic compromise will often prompt surgery, with the aim to control active bleeding and repair injuries from penetrating trauma. However, percutaneous therapy, including vessel coiling and embolization, has emerged as the first-line treatment of choice in trauma patients with active bleeding from blunt trauma.

> **KEY POINTS**
> - CT remains the first-line modality of choice in trauma patients, although MRI should be considered in select patient populations (such as children), chronic renal disease, and pregnancy.
> - The spleen is the most commonly injured intra-abdominal organ in blunt trauma, with blood products demonstrating characteristic signal intensities on MRI.
> - Iatrogenic vascular injury, along with associated parenchymal sequelae, are best imaged with MRI.

SUGGESTED READINGS

Hogspiel KD, Leung DA, Angle JF, et al. MR angiography of the mesenteric vasculature. Radiol Clin North Am 2002; 40:867-886.

Martin DR, Brown MA, Semella RC. Primer on MR imaging of the abdomen and pelvis. John Wiley & Sons, Inc., Hoboken, NJ, 2005.

Nael K, Laub G, Finn JP. Three-dimensional contrast-enhanced MR angiography of the thoraco-abdominal vessels. Magn Reson Imaging Clin North Am 2005; 13:359-380.

REFERENCES

1. Cowper SE, Su LD, Bhawan J, et al. Nephrogenic fibrosing dermopathy. Am J Dermatopathol 2001; 23:383-393.
2. Marckmann P, Skov L, Rossen K, et al. Nephrogenic systemic fibrosis: suspected causative role of gadodiamide used for contrast-enhanced magnetic resonance imaging. J Am Soc Nephrol 2006; 17:2359-2362.
3. Lauenstein TC, Salman K, Morreira R, et al. Nephrogenic systemic fibrosis: center case review. J Magn Reson Imaging 2007; 26:1198-1203.
4. Martin DR. Nephrogenic systemic fibrosis: A radiologist's practical perspective. Eur J Radiol 2008; 66(2):220-224.
5. Garcia-Tsao G. Portal hypertension. Current opinion in gastroenterology 2006; 22:254-262.
6. Annet L, Materne R, Danse E, et al. Hepatic flow parameters measured with MR imaging and Doppler US: correlations with degree of cirrhosis and portal hypertension. Radiology 2003; 229:409-414.
7. Villeneuve JP, Dagenais M, Huet PM, et al. The hepatic microcirculation in the isolated perfused human liver. Hepatology (Baltimore, Md) 1996; 23:24-31.
8. Gabriel S, Maroney TP, Ringe BH. Hepatic artery-portal vein fistula formation after percutaneous liver biopsy in a living liver donor. Transplantation Proc 2007; 39:1707-1709.
9. Byun JH, Kim TK, Lee CW, et al. Arterioportal shunt: prevalence in small hemangiomas versus that in hepatocellular carcinomas 3 cm or smaller at two-phase helical CT. Radiology 2004; 232:354-360.
10. Wachsberg RH, Bahramipour P, Sofocleous CT, Barone A. Hepatofugal flow in the portal venous system: pathophysiology, imaging findings, and diagnostic pitfalls. Radiographics 2002; 22:123-140.
11. Kaplan JL, Weintraub SL, Hunt JP, et al. Treatment of superior mesenteric and portal vein thrombosis with direct thrombolytic infusion via an operatively placed mesenteric catheter. Am Surg 2004; 70:600-604.
12. Lauenstein TC, Salman K, Morreira R, et al. Gadolinium-enhanced MRI for tumor surveillance before liver transplantation: center-based experience. AJR Am J Roentgenol 2007; 189:663-670.
13. Mazzaferro V, Regalia E, Doci R, et al. Liver transplantation for the treatment of small hepatocellular carcinomas in patients with cirrhosis. N Engl J Med 1996; 334:693-699.
14. Lee MW, Lee JM, Lee JY, et al. Preoperative evaluation of the hepatic vascular anatomy in living liver donors: comparison of CT angiography and MR angiography. J Magn Reson Imaging 2006; 24:1081-1087.
15. Salvalaggio PR, Modanlou KA, Edwards EB, et al. Hepatic artery thrombosis after adult living donor liver transplantation: the effect of center volume. Transplantation 2007; 84:926-928.
16. Martin DR, Seibert D, Yang M, et al. Reversible heterogeneous arterial phase liver perfusion associated with transient acute hepatitis: findings on gadolinium-enhanced MRI. J Magn Reson Imaging 2004; 20:838-842.
17. Zimmerman MA, Cameron AM, Ghobrial RM. Budd-Chiari syndrome. Clin Liver Dis 2006; 10:259-273, viii.
18. Brancatelli G, Federle MP, Grazioli L, et al. Large regenerative nodules in Budd-Chiari syndrome and other vascular disorders of the liver: CT and MR imaging findings with clinicopathologic correlation. AJR Am J Roentgenol 2002; 178:877-883.
19. Grego FG, Lepidi S, Ragazzi R, et al. Visceral artery aneurysms: a single center experience. Cardiovasc Surg (London) 2003; 11:19-25.
20. Pilleul F, Forest J, Beuf O. Magnetic resonance angiography of splanchnic artery aneurysms and pseudoaneurysms [in French]. Journal de radiologie 2006; 87:127-131.
21. Pilleul F, Beuf O. Diagnosis of splanchnic artery aneurysms and pseudoaneurysms, with special reference to contrast-enhanced 3D magnetic resonance angiography: a review. Acta Radiol 2004; 45:702-708.
22. Berceli SA. Hepatic and splenic artery aneurysms. Semin Vasc Surg 2005; 18:196-201.
23. Catalano C, Pavone P, Laghi A, et al. Pancreatic adenocarcinoma: combination of MR imaging, MR angiography and MR cholangiopancreatography for the diagnosis and assessment of resectability. Eur Radiol 1998; 8:428-434.
24. Pavone P, Laghi A, Catalano C, et al. MR imaging of pancreatic neoplasms. Tumori 1999; 85:S6-10.
25. Paterson A, Frush DP, Donnelly LF, et al. A pattern-oriented approach to splenic imaging in infants and children. Radiographics 1999; 19:1465-1485.
26. Adajar MA, Painter T, Woloson S, Memark V. Isolated celiac artery aneurysm with splenic artery stenosis as a rare presentation of polyarteritis nodosum: a case report and review of the literature. J Vasc Surg 2006; 44:647-650.
27. Willinek WA, Hadizadeh D, von Falkenhausen M, et al. Magnetic resonance (MR) imaging and MR angiography for evaluation and follow-up of hepatic artery banding in patients with hepatic involvement of hereditary hemorrhagic telangiectasia. Abdom Imaging 2006; 31:694-700.
28. Fenton SJ, Hansen KW, Meyers RL, et al. CT scan and the pediatric trauma patient—are we overdoing it? J Pediatr Surg 2004; 39:1877-1881.
29. Dangas G, Iakovou I, Nikolsky E, et al. Contrast-induced nephropathy after percutaneous coronary interventions in relation to chronic kidney disease and hemodynamic variables. Am J Cardiol 2005; 95:13-19.
30. Ragozzino A, Lassandro F, De Ritis R, Imbriaco M. Value of MRI in three patients with major vascular injuries after laparoscopic cholecystectomy. Emerg Radiol 2007; 14:443-447.

CHAPTER 106

Renal Artery Hypertension

Tim Leiner

The classic studies by Goldblatt in the 1930s have shown that renal artery stenosis (RAS) is the underlying cause of renovascular hypertension (RVH).[1] Although only 5% of cases of hypertension can be attributed to RAS, it is a potentially curable cause of hypertension. In most cases, RVH is caused by atherosclerotic RAS or fibromuscular dysplasia (FMD).[2] Atherosclerosis accounts for 70% to 90% of cases of RAS and usually involves the ostium and proximal third of the main renal artery.[2,3] Fibromuscular dysplasia (FMD) frequently involves the distal two thirds of the renal artery and its branches. It is most often characterized by aneurysmal dilations interspersed with localized narrowings presenting as a so-called string of beads or string-of-pearls appearance on angiography.[4]

Together, atherosclerosis and FMD constitute primary renal artery disease. Conversely, there are many diseases with secondary involvement of the renal arteries causing small vessel and intrarenal vascular disease. The latter category of diseases, also called secondary renal artery disease is, however, beyond the scope of this chapter.

Intra-arterial digital subtraction angiography (IA-DSA) is traditionally regarded as the definitive test to diagnose the presence of RAS. However, both the invasive nature of IA-DSA and the difficulty in assessing the pathophysiologic significance of stenotic lesions have encouraged the search for widely available noninvasive or minimally invasive diagnostic tests. In addition, IA-DSA is not a perfect test for the detection of RAS because it is subject to substantial interobserver variation.[5]

With the introduction of contrast-enhanced magnetic resonance angiography (CE-MRA), multidetector computed tomography angiography (MDCTA), and color Doppler ultrasonography, alternatives for IA-DSA have emerged. In this chapter, an overview of these techniques is provided, as well as a discussion of their relative merits and shortcomings.

RENAL ARTERY STENOSIS
Atherosclerotic Renal Artery Disease

Atherosclerosis accounts for the vast majority of cases of RAS and usually involves the ostium or proximal renal artery. This form of RAS is more prevalent in patients with advanced atherosclerosis, such as older patients and patients with diabetes mellitus, coronary artery disease, and/or peripheral arterial occlusive disease.

Fibromuscular Dysplasia

FMD is a relatively uncommon cause of RAS in comparison to atherosclerosis. Principal forms of FMD include intimal fibroplasia (5% of cases), medial hyperplasia (uncommon), medial fibrodysplasia (85% of cases), and perimedial dysplasia (10% of cases). The cause of FMD remains unknown at present. It is thought that about 10% to 30% of cases of RAS are caused by FMD. It had been thought that FMD is more often encountered in young women between 15 and 50 years of age, but because it is not a lethal disease, older women may also have the disease.

PREVALENCE AND EPIDEMIOLOGY
Atherosclerotic Renal Artery Disease

The prevalence of RAS in the general population is low. Among patients diagnosed with hypertension, RAS is present in 1% to 6%.[6] On the other hand, atherosclerotic RAS is a common and progressive disease in patients with preexisting manifestations of atherosclerosis or clinical clues suggestive of RAS (see later, "Imaging Indications and Algorithm"). In selected cohorts of patients, such as those undergoing coronary or peripheral angiography, the prevalence of atherosclerotic RAS may increase to more than 20%. Among patients with atherosclerotic RAS, progressive stenosis has been reported in 51% of renal arteries 5 years after diagnosis (including 18% of initially normal vessels). Only 3% to 16% of renal arteries became totally occluded and renal atrophy of more than 60% developed in 21% of patients with RAS.[2]

Fibromuscular Dysplasia

FMD is responsible for 10% to 30% of cases of RAS.[2-4] In one of the largest studies on imaging of RAS, the Dutch Renal Artery Diagnostic Study in Systolic Hypertension (RADISH),[7] the prevalence of FMD, as shown by IA-DSA, was 27 of 356 patients (7.6%), all of whom were referred for imaging of the renal arteries because of therapy-resistant hypertension and/or clinical clues suggestive of RAS, including a baseline blood pressure higher than 95 mm Hg. In this study, FMD comprised 38% of all cases of RAS.

ETIOLOGY AND PATHOPHYSIOLOGY

The relationships between renal artery stenosis, hypertension, and renal excretory disfunction are not straightforward but are complex. Renal artery stenosis may occur as an isolated finding or in combination with hypertension, renal insufficiency, or both. The underlying pathophysiologic mechanisms are incompletely elucidated. Current understanding[2,8] is that a decrease in renal perfusion pressure activates the renin-angiotensin system, which leads to the release of renin and the production of angiotensin II. This, in turn, has a direct effect on sodium excretion, sympathetic nerve activity, intrarenal prostaglandin concentrations, and nitric oxide production. When all these factors are present, the end result is renovascular hypertension. When hypertension is sustained, plasma renin levels may decrease, partially explaining the limitations of renin measurements for identifying patients with renovascular hypertension; this phenomenon is referred to as reverse tachyphylaxis.

MANIFESTATIONS OF DISEASE

Clinical Presentation

RAS is one of the most common secondary causes of hypertension in the adult population, especially among those with other risk factors for the development of atherosclerosis. Laboratory studies are neither sensitive nor specific for the diagnosis of RAS. However, laboratory measurement of renal function should be performed to exclude other potential secondary causes of hypertension.

In addition to hypertension, patients may present with ischemic nephropathy. Ischemic nephropathy is defined as an obstruction of renal blood flow that leads to ischemia and excretory dysfunction.[9] The pathophysiology of ischemic nephropathy is not fully understood but it is present when the serum creatinine level is elevated because of loss of renal mass as a consequence of long-standing hypertension. In general, loss of more than 50% of renal mass is usually associated with elevated creatinine levels. It is estimated that ischemic nephropathy is present in up to 24% of patients with unexplained chronic or progressive renal failure.

A more acute presentation of the renal artery stenosis is acute, or flash, pulmonary edema. RAS should be suspected in such patients, especially when there are signs of uncontrolled hypertension or ischemic nephropathy or other clinical clues suggestive of RAS.

Imaging Indications and Algorithm

The rational use of noninvasive imaging techniques to detect RAS is important to maximize the diagnostic performance of the test. It is well known in epidemiology that positive and negative predictive values depend on the prevalence of disease. A general rule of thumb is that diagnostic tests perform better when the prevalence of disease is higher. Therefore, clinical clues are used to increase the a priori chances of a patient having RAS (Fig. 106-1). Clinical clues suggestive of RAS include the following: are the presence of diastolic blood pressure of 95 mm Hg or higher; an epigastric, subcostal, or flank bruit; sudden, accelerated, or malignant hypertension; unilateral small kidney; hypertension in children or young adults (prior to age 35) or adults older than 55 years; hypertension and unexplained impairment of renal function; sudden worsening of renal function in a patient with known hypertension; hypertension refractory to three or more appropriate antihypertensive drugs; impairment of renal function in response to angiotensin-converting enzyme inhibitor; and the presence of extensive occlusive disease in the coronary, cerebral, and/or peripheral circulation.[3] Using these clinical clues, the prior probability of RAS can be increased to approximately 20% or higher.[7,10]

There are many noninvasive methods used to assess the presence of RAS. Currently used modalities are duplex and Doppler ultrasonography (DUS), magnetic resonance angiography (MRA), and CT angiography (CTA), as well as nuclear medicine tests such as captopril renography. At present, however, there is no consensus on the best noninvasive method for screening for renal artery hypertension. Captopril renal scintigraphy was historically a very popular study that has been replaced at many sites by Doppler ultrasound because of its lack of ionizing radiation exposure and broad availability. In the late 1990s and early 2000s, there was much excitement about MRA and CTA, but the first large-scale truly blinded trials yielded disappointing sensitivities and specificities for the detection of RAS. In retrospect, this was likely the result of a suboptimal choice of imaging parameters—mainly, spatial resolution that was too low. Today, this is no longer an issue because over the past 7 or 8 years spatial resolution has improved dramatically for CTA and MRA techniques, and there is nearly universal consensus that these methods can reliably detect and rule out the presence of RAS. Therefore, invasive catheter angiography remains the gold standard for renal artery imaging but is relegated primarily for therapeutic intervention or diagnosis in cases in which noninvasive studies are not definitive. In clinical practice, individual sites have developed their own imaging algorithms based on clinical access to scanning equipment, available expertise, and/or a specific population.

Apart from determining which technique is best for the detection of RAS, there is an ongoing and controversial discussion about the value of imaging techniques. It has recently been shown in several large trials that invasive treatment of RAS by endovascular or surgical means, rather than medical therapy, does not improve renal function in many patients (see later). The future challenge of imaging in RAS is therefore not only to detect RAS reliably, but also to identify patients for whom invasive intervention might still be of added value over medical therapy alone.

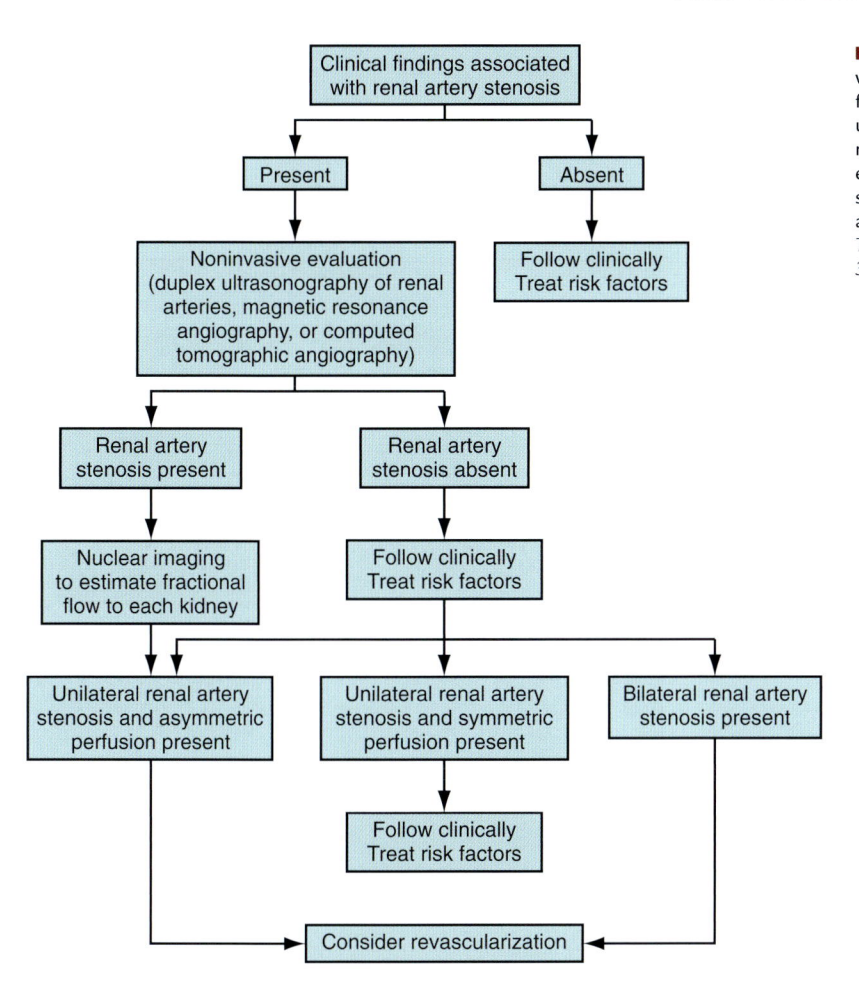

■ **FIGURE 106-1** Algorithm for evaluating patients in whom renal artery stenosis is suspected. Clinical follow-up includes periodic reassessment with duplex ultrasonography, magnetic resonance angiography, and nuclear imaging to estimate fractional blood flow to each kidney. The treatment of risk factors includes smoking cessation and the use of aspirin, lipid-lowering agents, and antihypertensive therapy. *(From Safian RD, Textor SC. Renal-artery stenosis. N Engl J Med 2001; 344:431-442.)*

Imaging Techniques and Findings

Once a patient has been identified as being at high risk for RAS the choice of the best diagnostic test remains controversial.

Radiography

Apart from incidental discovery of calcified atherosclerotic plaque formation in the perirenal aorta or renal arteries, there is no role for radiography in the work-up of suspected RAS.

Ultrasound

Ultrasonography has traditionally been used for imaging renal parenchyma, detection of nephrolithiasis, and hydronephrosis. In the past decade, with the advent of color Doppler techniques, ultrasonography has been applied with increasing success to diagnose RAS.

Ultrasonographic examination of the renal arteries is entirely noninvasive because it does not require injection of contrast medium. In contrast to CE-MRA and MDCTA, however, it does require fasting for 8 hours prior to the examination.[11]

RAS can be detected by color DUS using peak systolic velocity in a stenosis or by poststenotic flow phenomena. Most researchers have used 180 to 200 cm/sec at the point of maximum stenosis as the cutoff point to establish 50% or higher RAS[12] (Fig. 106-2). However, because of obesity, excessive bowel gas, or inability of the patient to sustain a breath-hold, about 10% to 20% of the examinations are unsuccessful. In addition, a study by Nchimi and colleagues[13] has demonstrated that the accuracy of DUS for the detection of accessory renal arteries is still low. An indirect approach to assessing the severity of RAS is by measuring acceleration in intrarenal arteries distal to a stenosis and the presence of a tardus-parvus waveform. The tardus-parvus phenomenon is used to describe a change in the Doppler blood flow velocity waveform that may be found downstream from significant arterial stenoses. Tardus refers to delayed or prolonged early systolic acceleration (more than 0.07 second[14]), and parvus refers to diminished amplitude and rounding of the systolic peak.[15] By combining direct and indirect measurements, the diagnostic yield may be increased.

The most widely used ultrasonographic parameter to assess the functional significance of RAS is the resistance index (RI). The RI can be calculated from a Doppler spectrum, and is defined by the equation

$$RI = 1 - (\text{minimum diastolic velocity}/\text{maximum systolic velocity})$$

Velocities are measured by obtaining Doppler signals from segmental arteries, typically in the upper, middle, and lower portions of each kidney (Fig. 106-3). When measuring the RI, it is important to keep in mind that

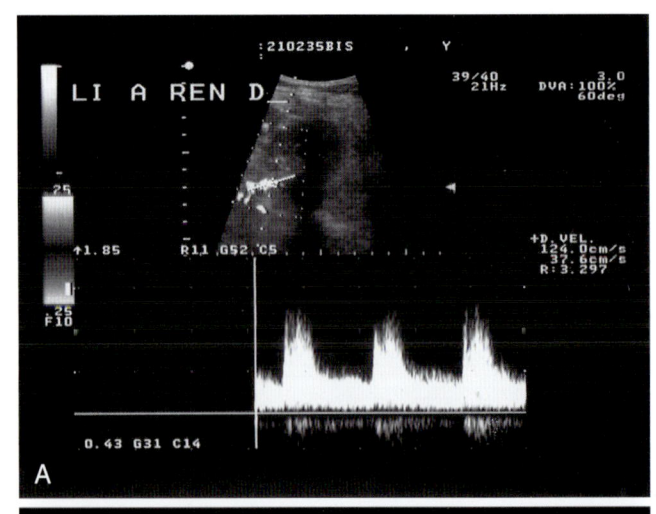

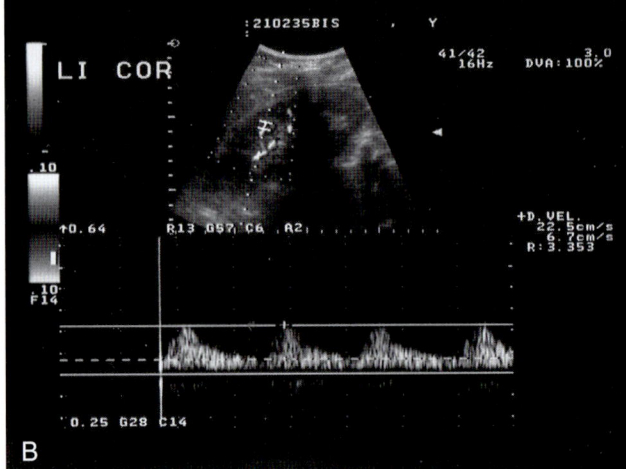

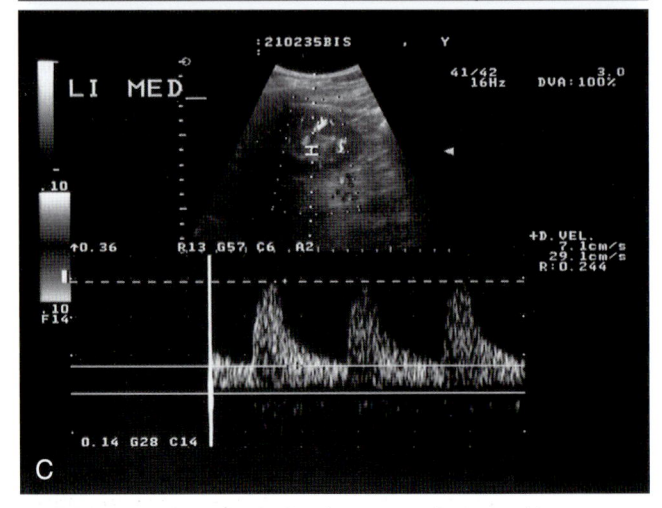

■ **FIGURE 106-2** Color duplex ultrasonography (printed in gray scale) in a 69-year-old female patient with unexplained hypertension and suspected left renal artery stenosis. The peak systolic velocity in the left renal artery was 124.0 cm/sec (**A**), indicating a normal renal artery. Velocities measured in the left renal cortex (**B**) and medulla (**C**) also indicate normal renal perfusion.

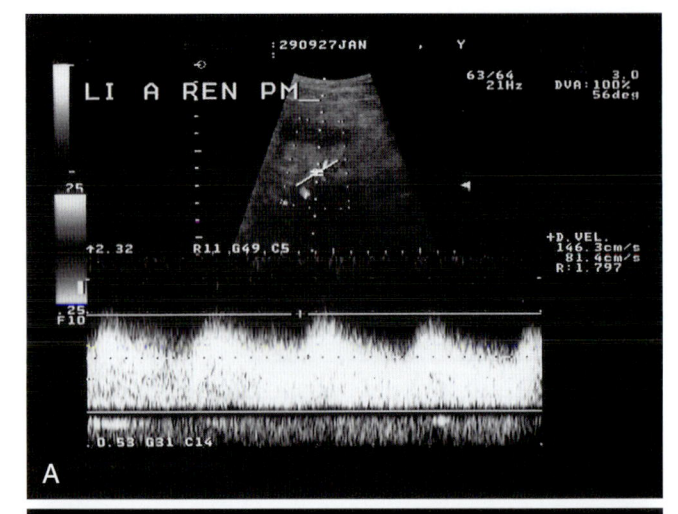

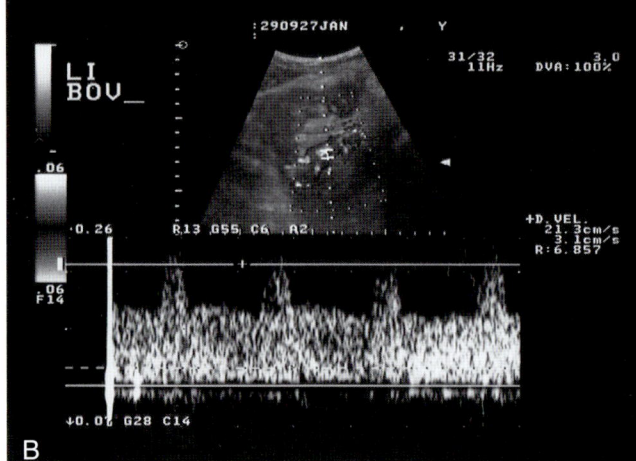

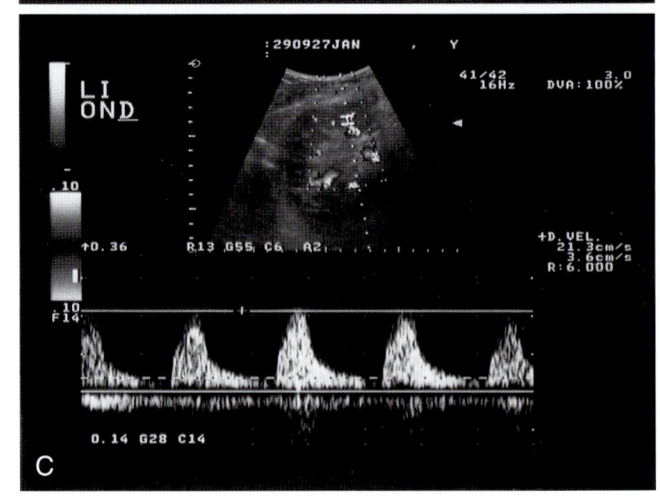

■ **FIGURE 106-3** Color duplex ultrasonography (printed in gray scale) in a 70-year-old male patient with moderate left renal artery stenosis (<50% luminal narrowing). **A**, The peak systolic velocity measured at the point of maximum stenosis in the left renal artery was 146.3 cm/sec. The resistance index (RI) is increased in both the upper (**B**) and lower pole (**C**) arteries (RI upper = 1 − [3.1/21.3] = 0.85; RI lower = 1 − [3.6/21.3] = 0.83).

pulse rates below 50 or above 70 beats/min, or measuring during inspiration or a Valsalva maneuver, may lead to less accurate measurements. Radermacher and associates[16] have shown that in patients with 50% or greater stenosis in at least one renal artery, RI values above 0.80 are highly sensitive and specific to identify patients in whom angioplasty or surgery will not improve renal function, blood pressure, or kidney survival. However, a potential source of bias in this study was that only in patients in which ultrasound detected 50% or greater RAS was therapy considered. In addition, it is not known whether elevated RI values alone are predictive of therapeutic failure. The same group showed that an RI value above 0.80 measured at least 3 months after transplantation is associated with poor subsequent allograft performance and death.[17]

The diagnostic accuracy of color DUS is moderate to high, depending primarily on the expertise of the vascular laboratory. Reported sensitivities and specificities are generally in the 80% to 90% range. In a meta-analysis comparing different noninvasive diagnostic tests for RAS, the accuracy of ultrasonography for the detection of RAS was shown to be significantly lower than that of CE-MRA and MDCTA.[18] A well-known drawback of ultrasonography is the large interobserver variation, although in expert laboratories with dedicated ultrasonographers, this may not be a prohibitive problem.[19] Intravenous microbubble contrast agents may improve diagnostic accuracy and success rates.[20] DUS may become an interesting alternative to CTA and MRA because of concerns about the effects of administration of iodinated and MR contrast media.

Computed Tomography

Over the past decade, multidetector CT (MDCT) of the vascular system has become firmly integrated into clinical routine. With the recent introduction of MDCT scanners, with which up to 320 slices can be acquired in parallel, CTA has evolved even further. MDCT systems are equipped with two or more parallel detector arrays and always use a synchronously rotating tube and detector array.[21,22] To provide sufficient vessel to background contrast, up to 150 mL of 300 mg I/mL or up to 85 mL of 400 mg I/mL nonionic contrast medium is needed. Injection speeds range from 2 to 6 mL/sec. Faster acquisitions require less total contrast medium.[23]

The need to acquire data during breath-hold and careful, individualized synchronization of contrast injection with acquisition are technical aspects of CTA that are similar to those of CE-MRA (see later, "Magnetic Resonance Imaging"). With the fastest CT scanners, timing of data acquisition becomes even more critical because the imaging time becomes substantially shorter, and the contrast bolus may be missed if mistimed.[23] Currently, the spatial resolution of CTA is superior to that of CE-MRA. The typical resolution used for renal artery imaging when using multidetector row systems is $0.6 \times 0.6 \times 1.0$ mm^3 (left-right direction × anteroposterior direction × craniocaudal/slice direction). With increasing numbers of detector rows, resolution in the slice direction can be decreased even further.

Because CT uses ionizing radiation, there are concerns about radiation exposure, especially in younger patients, who have a relatively higher prevalence of FMD. In addition, CTA requires the injection of nephrotoxic and potentially allergenic contrast media. Cochran and coworkers[24] analyzed adverse events in 90,473 administrations of iodinated contrast media and found that of 10 severe reactions (0.02%) and one death in 5 years of using nonionic contrast media, seven reactions occurred in patients after helical CT angiography. Petersein and colleagues[25] have reported similar rates of adverse events in a cohort of 60,213 patients given a modern nonionic contrast agent.

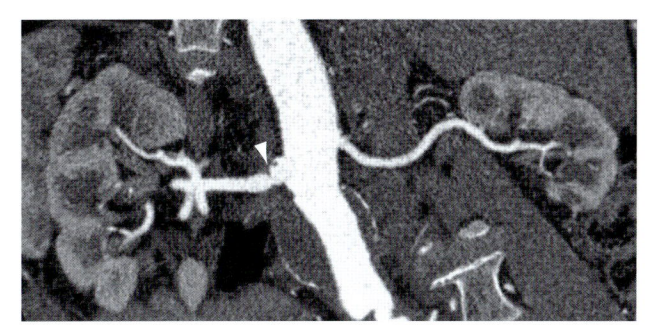

■ **FIGURE 106-4** MDCTA scan of a 50-year-old male patient referred for therapy-resistant hypertension. The curved multiplanar reformations of both renal arteries show moderate luminal narrowing in the proximal right renal artery. Images were acquired using a 64-channel system (2- × 32- × 0.6-mm detector configuration; Somatom Sensation Cardiac 64, Siemens Medical Solutions USA, Malvern, Pa) using 1-mm section thickness.

CTA has been successfully used for the assessment of atherosclerotic RAS (Fig. 106-4). The diagnostic accuracy of CTA is high and similar to that of CE-MRA, as was confirmed by results of meta-analysis noted earlier.[18] Beregi and associates[26] have investigated the diagnostic accuracy of helical CTA in 20 patients with angiographically proven FMD and were able to detect the FMD in all patients accurately. A similar study in 21 patients has recently been published by Sabharwal and coworkers.[27] The results of these studies must be interpreted with caution because they involved only patients who already had FMD. As is the case with CE-MRA, little additional data are available about the prospective accuracy of CTA for the detection of FMD in patients with therapy-resistant hypertension. An example of a 64-detector row CT scan of FMD is shown in Figure 106-5.

The results of these CTA studies are, however, in contrast with the results of a large multicenter study from the Netherlands in which the validity of CE-MRA and CTA were prospectively investigated in 356 patients suspected of having RVH, using IA-DSA as the standard of reference.[7] Two panels of three observers each judged CE-MRA and CTA examination results; they were blinded for each others' results and the results of all other imaging modalities. Overall, sensitivity ranged from 61% to 69% for CTA and from 57% to 67% for CE-MRA. Specificity ranged from 89% to 97% for CTA and from 77% to 90% for CE-MRA. Additional analyses revealed that selecting a subgroup of patients with a high prevalence of RAS could increase the diagnostic performance of both tests, but not to levels that were commonly reported in the literature. Possible explanations for these discrepant findings are suboptimal technique, low overall disease prevalence, a high proportion of patients with FMD, and imperfect standard of reference.

Magnetic Resonance Imaging

Because of the relative ease of use and high reliability, CE-MRA is the preferred MR technique for the detection of RAS.[28] In addition, phase contrast MRA or MR flow measurements might provide supplemental functional data on renal artery blood flow.

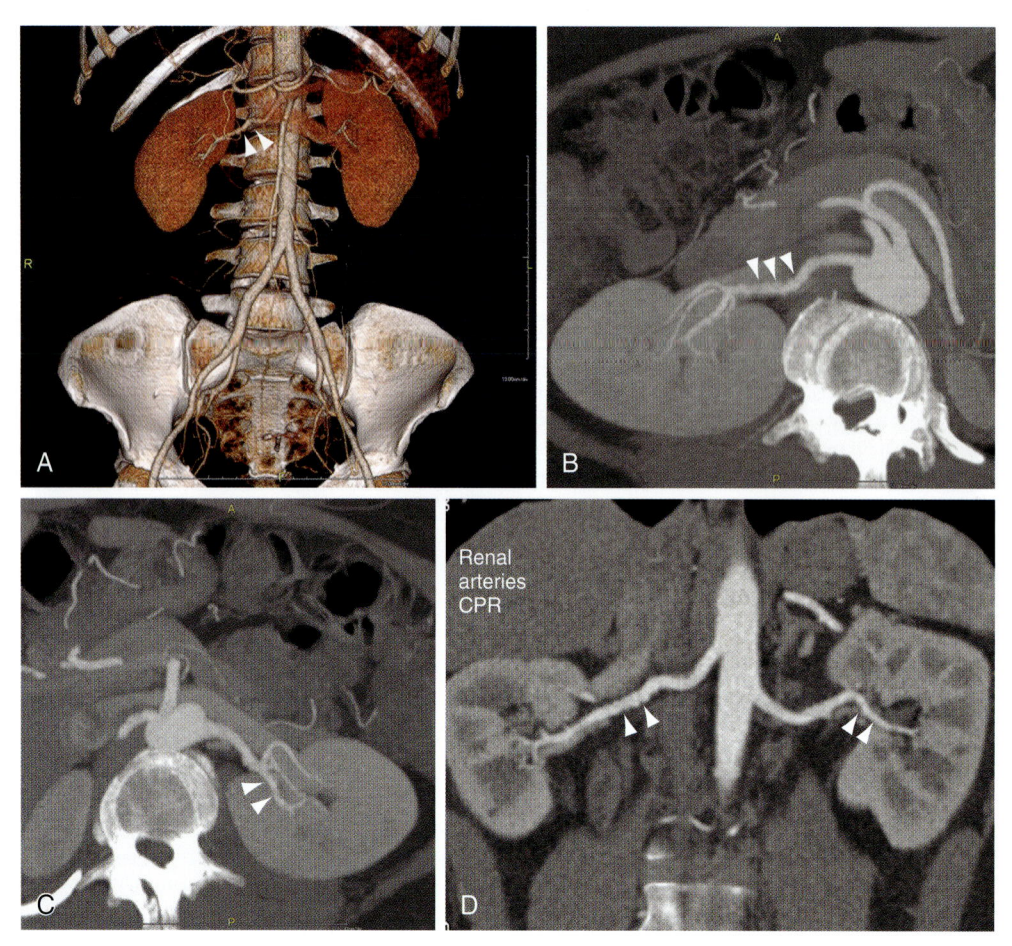

FIGURE 106-5 MDCTA scan of a 44-year-old female patient referred for pretransplantation workup as a living renal donor. Both the volume rendering (**A**) and the source images (**B-D**) support the incidental finding of bilateral renal artery FMD (*arrowheads*). Images were acquired using a 64-channel system (2- × 32- × 0.6-mm detector configuration; Somatom Sensation Cardiac 64, Siemens Medical Solutions USA, Malvern, Pa) using 1-mm section thickness and 0.7-mm reconstruction interval. 60 mL of iopamidol, 370 mg I /mL, were injected at 5 mL/sec. (*Courtesy of Dr. Dominik Fleischmann, Department of Radiology, Stanford University Medical Center, Stanford, Calif.*)

In CE-MRA, the renal arteries are imaged in the coronal plane during initial arterial passage of a 0.1- to 0.2-mmol/kg dose of a traditional (0.5 M) extracellular gadolinium chelate contrast medium. Because of the increase in T1 of tissue at 3.0 T, the contrast media dose can be reduced relative to that used for CE-MRA at 1.5 T.[29] For best results, patients are required to hold their breath during the acquisition, which typically lasts about 10 to 20 seconds, depending on the resolution and other technical factors related to system performance. Contrast medium is injected at speeds up to 3.0 mL/sec, followed by 25 mL saline flush, and typical spatial resolution in current reports is approximately 1.0 × 1.0 × 1.0-2.0 mm^3 (craniocaudal frequency direction × left-right phase-encoding direction × anteroposterior slice direction) or better. Using this approach, the abdominal aorta and renal arteries, including accessory arteries, can be visualized with high accuracy (Fig. 106-6). Arteries can usually be evaluated down to the proximal part of the segmental arteries. Distal segmental and interlobar branches cannot be evaluated reliably at this time.[28,30]

To obtain a study with maximum arterial and minimum venous enhancement, it is very important to ensure careful synchronization of peak arterial contrast concentration, with sampling of central k-space profiles.[31] This is typically done by performing a timing sequence with 1 to 2 mL of contrast medium prior to the contrast-enhanced acquisition, or by the use of real-time bolus monitoring software. With the latter technique, the entire contrast bolus is injected and simultaneously monitored by the operator or the MR scanner and, when sufficient enhancement is present in the descending aorta, the MR fluoroscopy sequence is aborted, the patient is given a breath-hold command, and the three-dimensional CE-MRA acquisition is started. A third option, available on the most advanced systems, is the use of a time-resolved technique to obtain a series of high spatial resolution three-dimensional volumes by using view-sharing techniques.[32]

Because of the risk of motion artifacts, it is important to limit breath-hold length. Motion artifacts may occur when patients are unable to sustain the breath-hold because the acquisition is too long, and even while performing a breath-hold, the kidneys are subject to linear caudocranial motion.[30] Application of parallel imaging technology can lead to higher spatial resolution CE-MRA and/or shorter acquisition durations.[33]

Both nonenhanced (two-dimensional time-of-flight [TOF] and phase-contrast [PC]), as well as CE-MRA tech-

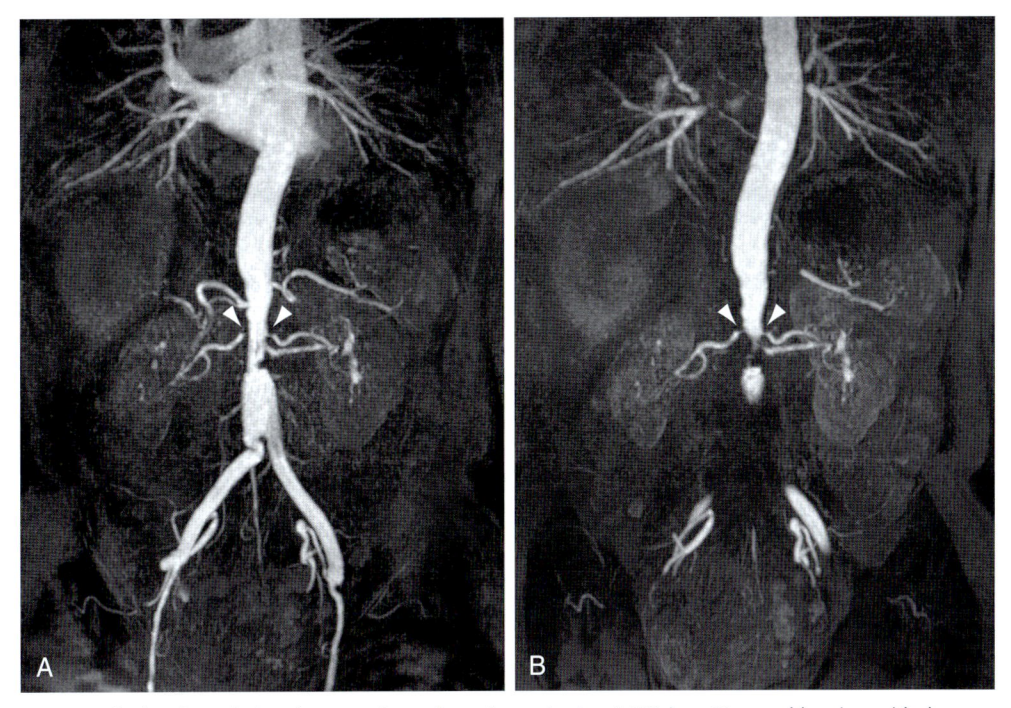

FIGURE 106-6 **A,** MRA displayed as whole-volume maximum intensity projection (MIP) in a 65-year-old patient with therapy-resistant hypertension on the basis of bilateral high-grade renal artery stenosis (*arrowheads*). The patient had undergone prior aortobifemoral bypass grafting for aortic occlusion. **B,** Thin-slab subvolume MIP better shows the bilateral stenoses. Also note that the stenosis of the right renal artery is overestimated on the whole-volume MIP in **A.**

niques, have been investigated for the detection of RAS. The results of these studies were summarized in a meta-analysis by Vasbinder and colleagues.[18] Of the 306 studies published up to mid-2000, in which the utility of renal MRA was investigated, 18 studies were performed because of clinical suspicion of RVH; they used explicitly defined criteria for the presence of RAS and IA-DSA as the standard of reference test. Reported sensitivities and specificities for the detection of atherosclerotic RAS in these CE-MRA studies were uniformly high.

The reported sensitivity of CE-MRA for the visualization of accessory renal arteries is more than 90%.[34,35] At present, one study has been published that specifically investigated the utility of CE-MRA for the detection of FMD. Willoteaux and associates[36] retrospectively analyzed the accuracy of CE-MRA in comparison to IA-DSA in 25 subjects with angiographically proven FMD. They evaluated the sensitivity, specificity, and accuracy of CE-MRA for the detection of FMD-associated stenosis, string-of-pearls sign, and aneurysm formation. Although the sensitivity for FMD-associated stenosis in their study was only 68%, the sensitivity for the detection of the string-of-pearls sign and aneurysm formation was 95% and 100%, respectively. The overall sensitivity and specificity for the diagnosis FMD were 97% and 93%. However, although overt cases of FMD can be diagnosed with CE-MRA (Fig. 106-7), it is generally believed that CE-MRA currently cannot detect FMD with high accuracy in the presence of only subtle anatomic changes.

The favorable results of these CE-MRA studies are, however, in contrast with the results of the previously noted large multicenter RADISH study from the Netherlands, in which the sensitivity ranged from 57% to 67% and specificity ranged from 77% to 90% for CE-MRA.[7] Strikingly similar results were obtained in a more recent multicenter trial by Soulez and coworkers,[37] who investigated the diagnostic performance of CE-MRA for the detection of RAS using IA-DSA as the reference standard in 268 patients with hypertension and/or suspected renal artery stenosis. Sensitivity, specificity, and accuracy for the detection of 51% or more RAS on a patient level in this study ranged from 65.2% to 79.9%, 81.3% to 91.4% and 73.6% to 83.8%, respectively.

Recently, there has been much interest in non–contrast-enhanced balanced steady-state free precession (SSFP)–based techniques as alternatives for CE-MRA. Although these techniques are promising,[38] there are limited data with regard to their diagnostic accuracy and clinical utility. Preliminary data have indicated that the value of these techniques lies in their high negative predictive value.[39]

Nuclear Medicine and Positron Emission Tomography

The diagnosis of RAS on nuclear scintigraphy relies primarily on its ability to detect abnormalities in renal function rather than the anatomic depiction of arterial narrowing, as with CTA and MRA. Although both CT and MRA have shown potential for assessment of renal perfusion and/or function, these methods remain investigational and have yet to be widely applied in clinical practice. Thus, although nuclear medicine techniques are not ideal for the anatomic detection of renal artery stenosis, they are well suited to quantify renal function to determine the functional severity of a stenosis.[18]

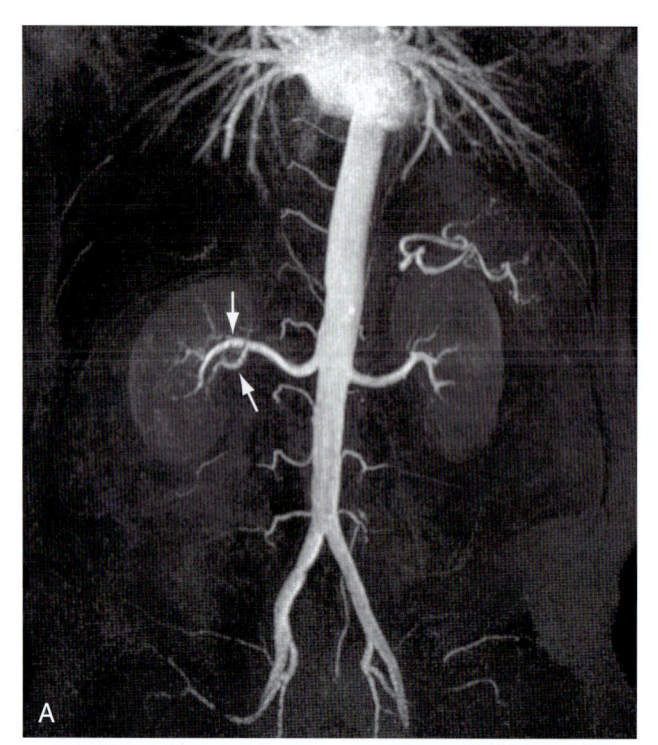

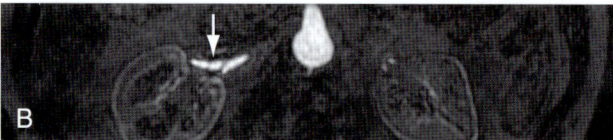

FIGURE 106-7 Therapy-resistant hypertension in a 50-year-old man. **A,** Coronal whole-volume maximum intensity projection (MIP) shows multiple consecutive luminal irregularities in the branches of the right renal artery (*arrows*), compatible with fibromuscular dysplasia. **B,** Transverse reformation confirms finding and better shows septae in the vessel. The patient was subsequently referred for DSA, where the finding was confirmed and the renal artery was dilated (not shown).

There are numerous radionuclide techniques for studying kidney function. Nuclear techniques are the most reliable way to determine the true glomerular filtration rate (GFR); there are tracers that are exclusively cleared by glomerular filtration (e.g., ^{51}Cr-EDTA, ^{99m}Tc-DTPA, ^{99m}Tc-MAG3). These types of agents can be used not only to determine GFR, but also to determine individual kidney function, also known as split renal function). Parameters that can be determined are differential blood flow, divided and regional renal function, and mean intrarenal transit time. A specific test that is sometimes still used to assess the significance of a suspected renal artery stenosis is the captopril scan, or captopril renography. In this test, the patient is imaged prior to and after having been given a 25- to 50-mg dose of captopril. In cases of hemodynamically significant RAS, uptake of the radionuclide tracer will fall after captopril administration because renal perfusion drops in response to inhibition of the renin-angiotensin system. However, in a meta-analysis comparing the diagnostic accuracy of different tests for the detection of RAS, nuclear medicine techniques performed poorly compared with CTA and CE-MRA, using IA-DSA as the standard of reference.[18]

Except for one study of 18 patients, there is a paucity of data in the literature on positron emission tomography (PET) techniques for the assessment of RAS.[40] On the other hand, a recent experimental study has demonstrated proof of concept of imaging the angiotensin II subtype 1 receptor in the context of RAS.[41]

In clinical practice, most nuclear techniques are relatively time-intensive from the patients' perspective and therefore are mostly used if Doppler ultrasonography, CTA, and CE-MRA are inconclusive or contraindicated (Fig. 106-8). An exception is assessment of renal transplant function, for which nuclear medicine techniques are still widely used. It is expected that in the near future, direct receptor imaging using PET techniques will enter the clinical arena.

Angiography

At present, IA-DSA is still widely regarded as the definitive test to diagnose the presence of RAS (Figs. 106-9 and 106-10). However, both the invasive nature of IA-DSA and the difficulty in assessing the pathophysiologic significance of stenotic lesions have encouraged the search for widely available noninvasive or minimally invasive diagnostic tests (see earlier). At present, these alternative tests are widely accepted in the medical community. In clinical practice, IA-DSA is mainly used in cases of equivocal findings with one of the noninvasive modalities. Our experience is that the number of diagnostic IA-DSA examinations specifically aimed at establishing the presence of RAS has dropped dramatically over the past decade. Currently, this test is rarely used for the diagnosis of RAS. IA-DSA for therapeutic intervention still remains the standard of care for patients with RAS in whom the decision has been made to perform percutaneous revascularization.

Classic Signs

The classic sign of renal artery stenosis is a focal narrowing or occlusion in the ostium or proximal third of the renal artery if the lesion is of atherosclerotic origin. The classic presentation of FMD-associated RAS is the string-of-beads or string-of-pearls sign.

DIFFERENTIAL DIAGNOSIS
From Clinical Presentation

The main differential diagnosis in patients with therapy-resistant hypertension caused by RAS is essential hypertension. Other diagnostic considerations that should be taken into account are acute renal failure, azotemia, glomerulonephritis, nephrosclerosis, and hypersensitivity nephropathy. These conditions can usually be distinguished by laboratory findings.

From Imaging Findings

There are several diseases that may present with RAS, apart from atherosclerosis and FMD. RAS has been described in association with Takayasu disease[42] and developmental hypoplasia of the infrarenal aorta.[43] This latter condition is rare and usually presents in childhood. Other diseases that may lead to RAS are neurofibromatosis, tuberous

CHAPTER 106 • Renal Artery Hypertension 1479

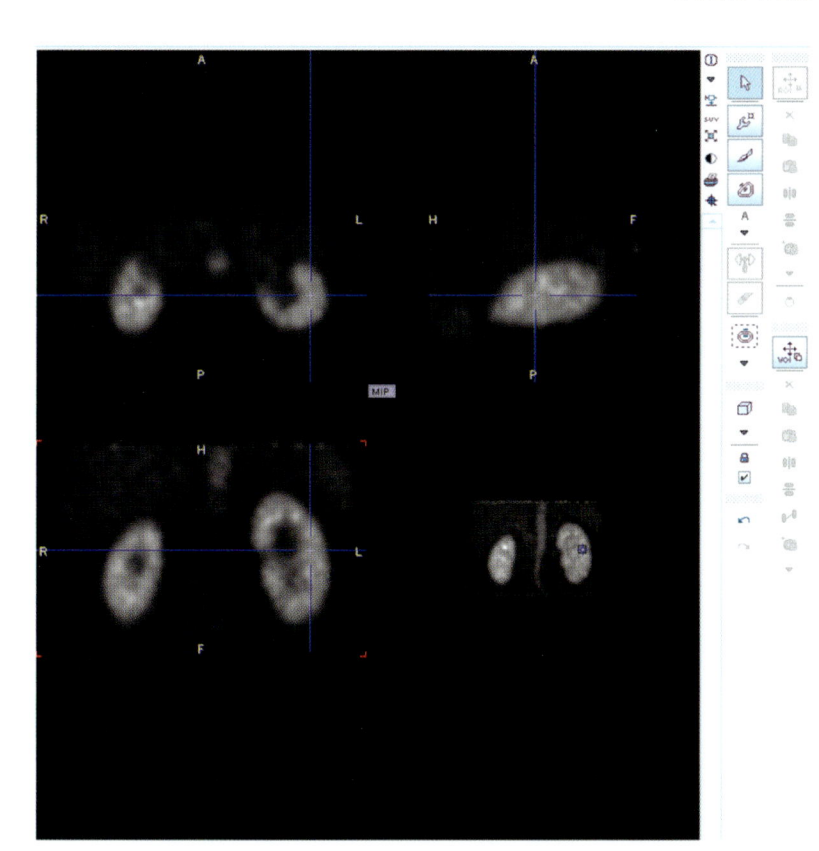

■ **FIGURE 106-8** Maximum intensity projections of ^{68}Ga-EDTA excretion in the kidneys (≈100-MBq dose) in a 58-year-old man with therapy-resistant hypertension and suspected renal artery stenosis on the basis of differences in kidney size. These represent a sum of images obtained at different time points after injection of the label (11 10-second images followed by five 20-second images). Inulin clearance was 110 mL/min/1.73 m². No renal artery stenosis was found by DSA. *(Courtesy of Dr. Audrey Habets and Dr. Jaap Teule, Maastricht University Medical Center, Department of Nuclear Medicine, Maastricht, the Netherlands.)*

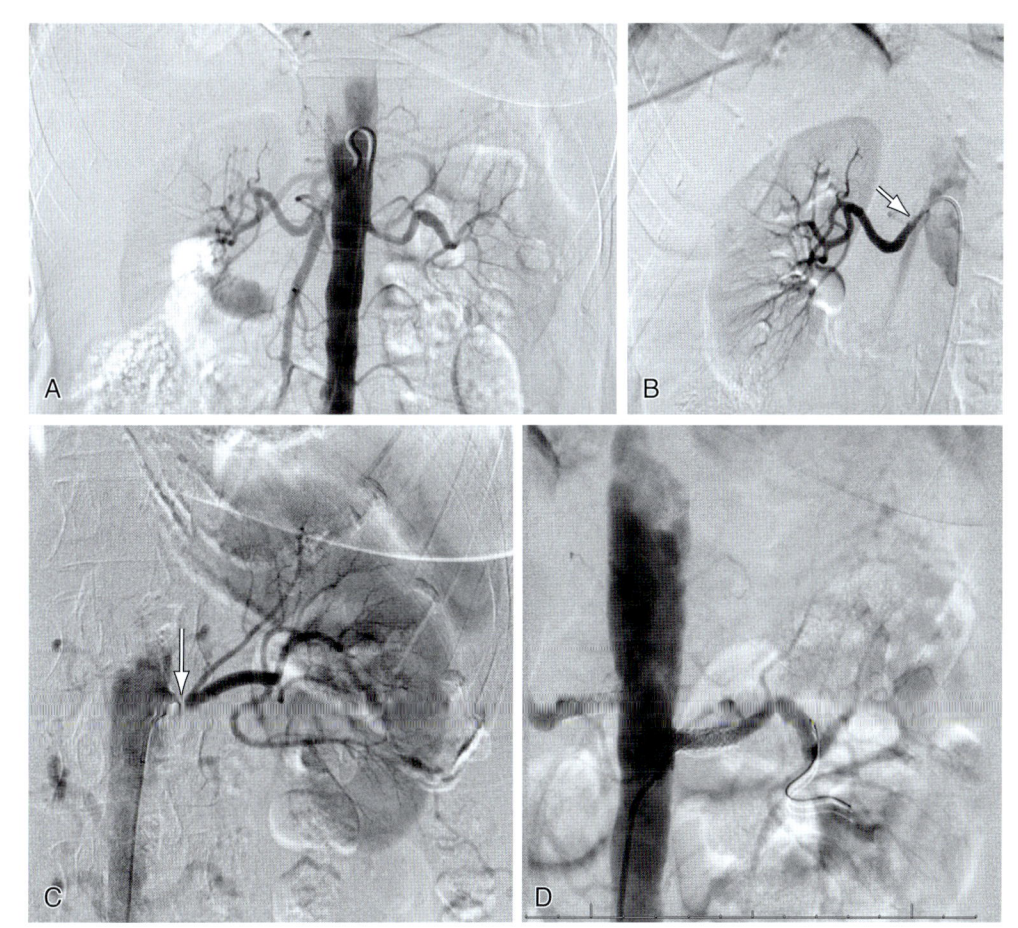

■ **FIGURE 106-9** DSA scan in a 55-year-old female patient with bilateral moderate renal artery stenoses. **A,** Nonselective DSA may obscure adequate depiction of renal artery origin, as is the case on the right side in this patient. Selective catheterization and depiction of the right (**B**) and left (**C**) renal arteries confirms presence of stenoses (*arrows*). **D,** Poststenting, both renal arteries are widely patent.

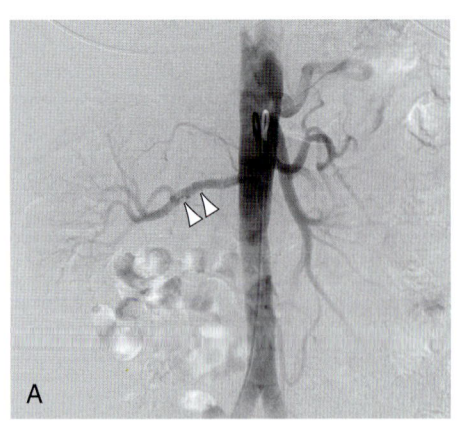

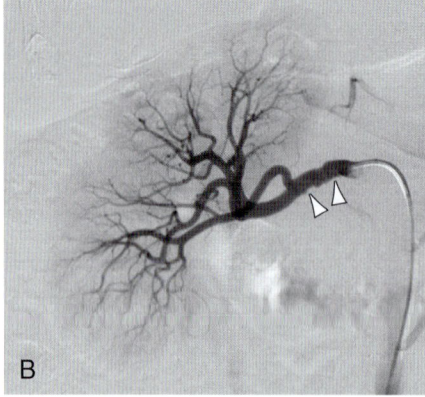

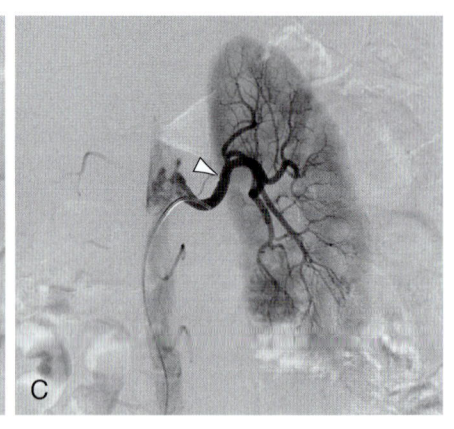

FIGURE 106-10 Bilateral fibromuscular dysplasia in a 59-year-old woman. **A**, On first inspection, the nonselective DSA scan shows only luminal irregularities of the right renal artery (*arrowheads*). However, selective DSA of both the right (**B**) and left (**C**) renal arteries demonstrates the characteristic but subtle luminal irregularities associated with FMD in both renal arteries (*arrowheads*), underscoring that selective DSA of individual renal arteries should always be performed. These subtle findings might also easily be missed at MRA and CTA when suboptimal spatial resolution protocols are used. This patient underwent balloon dilation of both renal arteries.

sclerosis, and various space-occupying lesions. Finally, an acutely angulated renal artery may impede renal artery flow.

SYNOPSIS OF TREATMENT OPTIONS

Medical Treatment

The standard medical treatment of patients with RAS is usually a combination of different antihypertensive medications consisting of β blockers and angiotensin-converting enzyme inhibitors and/or angiotensin receptor blockers. The most appropriate regimen is the subject of continuous discussions and is beyond the scope of this chapter. For an excellent overview, see the review article by Textor.[8]

Surgical or Interventional Management

One of the most hotly debated issues in contemporary medicine is whether there is a long-term beneficial effect of renal artery dilation in patients with RAS compared with optimal medical treatment alone. The rapid increase in the number of percutaneous renal revascularizations, in patients with therapy-resistant hypertension and in those in whom RAS is accidentally discovered, is in sharp contrast with the limited evidence of its efficacy. It was once assumed that the mere presence and subsequent endovascular treatment of RAS of more than 50% luminal narrowing would improve renal function, but several randomized trials have shown that this is not necessarily the case, and only certain patients will benefit from intervention.[44-49]

Several clinical trials aimed at elucidating the optimal treatment strategy in patients with RAS are currently underway or in the final phase of follow-up. The conventional wisdom—that is, to dilate and/or stent in the presence of 50% or greater RAS—was greatly challenged in 2000 with the appearance of the results of the DRASTIC study by van Jaarsveld and colleagues,[48] who found no difference at 12-month follow-up in 106 patients with RAS and hypertension randomized between medical antihypertensive therapy and angioplasty. The Dutch study of stent placement and blood pressure and lipid lowering to prevent the progression of renal dysfunction caused by atherosclerotic ostial stenosis of the renal artery has just completed enrollment and results of a 2-year follow-up are expected shortly.[50] The large-scale ASTRAL trial will compare renal function in 750 patients with RAS randomized to medical management or revascularization[51] and is specifically powered to detect a reduction in the decline of renal function of more than 20%, as assessed by reciprocal serum creatinine determinations over time. The final ongoing trial is the 1000-patient CORAL study,[52] which aims to address a similar question as in the ASTRAL trial.

Common to all these studies is the selection of patients based on only the presence of RAS, not taking into account the functional consequences of the stenosis nor the degree of renal impairment. Future trials combining MRA and functional MR techniques into a single examination will have to be carried out to investigate whether such a protocol leads to the optimal selection of patients for whom revascularization therapy is indeed beneficial. Apart from these considerations, the detection and differentiation of renal parenchymal disease independently from the presence of RAS may be another suitable indication for functional MRI techniques. Larger single-center studies on this topic are currently being undertaken.

Current thinking is that patients with RAS alone may benefit from revascularization to prevent the loss of renal mass and excretory function. In patients with RAS and hypertension, hypertension is seldom cured by revascularization, except in those with FMD. In patients with RAS and chronic renal failure, renal revascularization may improve or stabilize renal function.

REPORTING: INFORMATION FOR THE REFERRING PHYSICIAN

When reporting a study of the kidneys and renal arteries, there are several points that should be mentioned. The referring clinician should receive information on kidney size and whether or not the renal cortex has a normal thickness and appearance. Any lesions in the kidney, including cysts, should be mentioned. When evaluating the renal arteries, the interpreting physician should note the number of renal arteries and from which vessel(s) they originate, including the presence of accessory arteries and the location and severity of any lumen-encroaching lesions. Measurements should preferably be made perpendicular to the center lumen line and the report should state whether stenosis was measured in plane (usually in the coronal acquisition plane), or as surface area. The latter is preferred, because it correlates significantly better with the degree of stenosis as seen with IA-DSA and intravascular ultrasonography.[53]

KEY POINTS

- In more than 90% of patients with unexplained hypertension, there is no evidence of renal artery stenosis.
- Clinical clues are essential for the best selection of patients suspected of having renal artery stenosis for whom the additional information obtained with imaging exceeds the negative effects of such tests.
- Renal artery stenosis is almost always the result of atherosclerosis or, less commonly, fibromuscular dysplasia.
- There is conflicting and very limited evidence with regard to the clinical efficacy of renal artery dilation when a stenosis is present. Most likely this is because of the current inability to discriminate a priori patients who may benefit from percutaneous intervention from those who do not.
- Renal artery stenosis measurements should preferably be made perpendicular to the renal artery center lumen line; the report should state whether stenosis was measured in plane (usually in the coronal acquisition plane) or as surface area.

SUGGESTED READINGS

Leiner T. Magnetic resonance angiography of abdominal and lower extremity vasculature. Top Magn Reson Imaging 2005; 16:21-66.

Michaely HJ, Sourbron S, Dietrich O, et al. Functional renal MR imaging: an overview. Abdom Imaging 2007; 32:758-771.

Miyazaki M, Lee VS. Nonenhanced MR angiography. Radiology 2008; 248:20-43.

Robbin ML, Lockhart ME, Barr RG. Renal imaging with ultrasound contrast: current status. Radiol Clin North Am 2003; 41:963-978.

Safian RD, Textor SC. Renal-artery stenosis. N Engl J Med 2001; 344:431-442.

Schoenberg SO, Prince MR, Knopp MV, Allenberg JR. Renal MR angiography. Magn Reson Imaging Clin North Am 1998; 6:351-370.

Slovut DP, Olin JW. Fibromuscular dysplasia. N Engl J Med 2004; 350:1862-1871.

Textor SC. Renovascular hypertension update. Curr Hypertens Rep 2006; 8:521-527.

REFERENCES

1. Laragh J. Harry Goldblatt 1891-1977. Trans Assoc Am Physicians 1978; 91:24-27.
2. Safian RD, Textor SC. Renal-artery stenosis. N Engl J Med 2001; 344:431-442.
3. Working Group on Renovascular Hypertension. Detection, evaluation, and treatment of renovascular hypertension. Final report. Arch Intern Med 1987; 147:820-829.
4. Slovut DP, Olin JW. Fibromuscular dysplasia. N Engl J Med 2004; 350:1862-1871.
5. Schreij G, de Haan MW, Oei TK, et al. Interpretation of renal angiography by interpreting physicians. J Hypertens 1999; 17:1737-1741.
6. Simon N, Franklin SS, Bleifer KH, Maxwell MH. Clinical characteristics of renovascular hypertension. JAMA 1972; 220:1209-1218.
7. Vasbinder GB, Nelemans PJ, Kessels AG, et al. Computed tomographic angiography and magnetic resonance angiography for the diagnosis of renal artery stenosis: a comparative study with digital subtraction angiography. Results of the renal artery diagnostic imaging study in hypertension (RADISH). Ann Intern Med 2004; 141:674-682.
8. Textor SC. Renovascular hypertension update. Curr Hypertens Rep 2006; 8:521-527.
9. Dean RH, Tribble RW, Hansen KJ, et al. Evolution of renal insufficiency in ischemic nephropathy. Ann Surg 1991; 213:446-455.
10. Krijnen P, van Jaarsveld BC, Steyerberg EW, et al. A clinical prediction rule for renal artery stenosis. Ann Intern Med 1998; 129:705-711.
11. Rabbia C, Valpreda S. Duplex scan sonography of renal artery stenosis. Int Angiol 2003; 22:101-115.
12. Radermacher J, Chavan A, Schaffer J, et al. Detection of significant renal artery stenosis with color Doppler sonography: combining extrarenal and intrarenal approaches to minimize technical failure. Clin Nephrol 2000; 53:333-343.
13. Nchimi A, Biquet JF, Brisbois D, et al. Duplex ultrasound as first-line screening test for patients suspected of renal artery stenosis: prospective evaluation in high-risk group. Eur Radiol 2003; 13:1413-1419.
14. De Cobelli F, Venturini M, Vanzulli A, et al. Renal arterial stenosis: prospective comparison of color Doppler US and breath-hold, three-dimensional, dynamic, gadolinium-enhanced MR angiography. Radiology 2000; 214:373-380.
15. Kliewer MA, Tupler RH, Carroll BA, et al. Renal artery stenosis: analysis of Doppler waveform parameters and tardus-parvus pattern. Radiology 1993; 189:779-787.
16. Radermacher J, Chavan A, Bleck J, et al. Use of Doppler ultrasonography to predict the outcome of therapy for renal-artery stenosis. N Engl J Med 2001; 344:410-417.
17. Radermacher J, Mengel M, Ellis S, et al. The renal arterial resistance index and renal allograft survival. N Engl J Med 2003; 349:115-124.
18. Vasbinder GB, Nelemans PJ, Kessels AG, et al. Diagnostic tests for renal artery stenosis in patients suspected of having renovascular hypertension: a meta-analysis. Ann Intern Med 2001; 135:401-411.

19. Baumgartner I, Behrendt P, Rohner P, Baumgartner RW. A validation study on the intraobserver and interobserver reproducibility of renal artery duplex ultrasound. Ultrasound Med Biol 1999; 25:225-231.
20. Robbin ML, Lockhart ME, Barr RG. Renal imaging with ultrasound contrast: current status. Radiol Clin North Am 2003; 41:963-978.
21. Prokop M. Protocols and future directions in imaging of renal artery stenosis: CT angiography. J Comput Assist Tomogr 1999; 23(Suppl 1):S101-S110.
22. Prokop M. General principles of MDCT. Eur J Radiol 2003; 45(Suppl 1):S4-S10.
23. Fleischmann D. MDCT of renal and mesenteric vessels. Eur Radiol 2003; 13(Suppl 5):M94-M101.
24. Cochran ST, Bomyea K, Sayre JW. Trends in adverse events after IV administration of contrast media. AJR Am J Roentgenol 2001; 176:1385-1388.
25. Petersein J, Peters CR, Wolf M, Hamm B. Results of the safety and efficacy of iobitridol in more than 61,000 patients. Eur Radiol 2003; 13:2006-2011.
26. Beregi JP, Louvegny S, Gautier C, et al. Fibromuscular dysplasia of the renal arteries: comparison of helical CT angiography and arteriography. AJR Am J Roentgenol 1999; 172:27-34.
27. Sabharwal R, Vladica P, Coleman P. Multidetector spiral CT renal angiography in the diagnosis of renal artery fibromuscular dysplasia. Eur J Radiol 2007; 61:520-527.
28. Schoenberg SO, Prince MR, Knopp MV, Allenberg JR. Renal MR angiography. Magn Reson Imaging Clin North Am 1998; 6:351-370.
29. Michaely HJ, Kramer H, Oesingmann N, et al. Intraindividual comparison of MR-renal perfusion imaging at 1.5 T and 3.0 T. Invest Radiol 2007; 42:406-411.
30. Vasbinder GB, Maki JH, Nijenhuis RJ, et al. Motion of the distal renal artery during three-dimensional contrast-enhanced breath-hold MRA. J Magn Reson Imaging 2002; 16:685-696.
31. Maki JH, Chenevert TL, Prince MR. Three-dimensional contrast-enhanced MR angiography. Top Magn Reson Imaging 1996; 8:322-344.
32. Michaely HJ, Sourbron S, Dietrich O, et al. Functional renal MR imaging: an overview. Abdom Imaging 2007; 32:758-771.
33. Weiger M, Pruessmann KP, Kassner A, et al. Contrast-enhanced 3D MRA using SENSE. J Magn Reson Imaging 2000; 12:671-677.
34. Bakker J, Beek FJ, Beutler JJ, et al. Renal artery stenosis and accessory renal arteries: accuracy of detection and visualization with gadolinium-enhanced breath-hold MR angiography. Radiology 1998; 207:497-504.
35. Shetty AN, Bis KG, Kirsch M, et al. Contrast-enhanced breath-hold three-dimensional magnetic resonance angiography in the evaluation of renal arteries: optimization of technique and pitfalls. J Magn Reson Imaging 2000; 12:912-923.
36. Willoteaux S, Faivre-Pierret M, Moranne O, et al. Fibromuscular dysplasia of the main renal arteries: comparison of contrast-enhanced MR angiography with digital subtraction angiography. Radiology 2006; 241:922-929.
37. Soulez G, Pasowicz M, Benea G, et al. Renal artery stenosis evaluation: diagnostic performance of gadobenate dimeglumine-enhanced MR angiography—comparison with DSA. Radiology 2008; 247:273-285.
38. Miyazaki M, Lee VS. Nonenhanced MR angiography. Radiology 2008; 248:20-43.
39. Maki JH, Wilson GJ, Eubank WB, et al. Navigator-gated MR angiography of the renal arteries: a potential screening tool for renal artery stenosis. AJR Am J Roentgenol 2007; 188:W540-W546.
40. Shreve P, Chiao PC, Humes HD, et al. Carbon-11-acetate PET imaging in renal disease. J Nucl Med 1995; 36:1595-1601.
41. Xia J, Seckin E, Xiang Y, et al. Positron-emission tomography imaging of the angiotensin II subtype 1 receptor in swine renal artery stenosis. Hypertension 2008; 51:466-473.
42. Leiner T. Magnetic resonance angiography of abdominal and lower extremity vasculature. Top Magn Reson Imaging 2005; 16:21-66.
43. Prakken FJ, Kitslaar PJ, van de Kar N, et al. Diagnosis of abdominal aortic hypoplasia by state-of-the-art MR angiography. Pediatr Radiol 2006; 36:57-60.
44. Cheung CM, Hegarty J, Kalra PA. Dilemmas in the management of renal artery stenosis. Br Med Bull 2005; 73-74:35-55.
45. Ives NJ, Wheatley K, Stowe RL, et al. Continuing uncertainty about the value of percutaneous revascularization in atherosclerotic renovascular disease: a meta-analysis of randomized trials. Nephrol Dial Transplant 2003; 18:298-304.
46. Plouin PF, Chatellier G, Darne B, Raynaud A. Blood pressure outcome of angioplasty in atherosclerotic renal artery stenosis: a randomized trial. Essai Multicentrique Medicaments vs Angioplastie (EMMA) Study Group. Hypertension 1998; 31:823-829.
47. van de Ven PJ, Kaatee R, Beutler JJ, et al. Arterial stenting and balloon angioplasty in ostial atherosclerotic renovascular disease: a randomised trial. Lancet 1999; 353:282-286.
48. van Jaarsveld BC, Krijnen P, Pieterman H, et al. The effect of balloon angioplasty on hypertension in atherosclerotic renal-artery stenosis. Dutch Renal Artery Stenosis Intervention Cooperative Study Group. N Engl J Med 2000; 342:1007-1014.
49. Webster J, Marshall F, Abdalla M, et al. Randomised comparison of percutaneous angioplasty vs continued medical therapy for hypertensive patients with atheromatous renal artery stenosis. Scottish and Newcastle Renal Artery Stenosis Collaborative Group. J Hum Hypertens 1998; 12:329-335.
50. Bax L, Mali WP, Buskens E, et al. The benefit of STent placement and blood pressure and lipid-lowering for the prevention of progression of renal dysfunction caused by Atherosclerotic ostial stenosis of the Renal artery. The STAR-study: rationale and study design. J Nephrol 2003; 16:807-812.
51. Mistry S, Ives N, Harding J, et al. Angioplasty and STent for Renal Artery Lesions (ASTRAL trial): rationale, methods and results so far. J Hum Hypertens 2007; 21:511-515.
52. Murphy TP, Cooper CJ, Dworkin LD, et al. The Cardiovascular Outcomes with Renal Atherosclerotic Lesions (CORAL) study: rationale and methods. J Vasc Interv Radiol 2005; 16:1295-1300.
53. Schoenberg SO, Rieger J, Weber CH, et al. High-spatial-resolution MR angiography of renal arteries with integrated parallel acquisitions: comparison with digital subtraction angiography and US. Radiology 2005; 235:687-698.

CHAPTER 107

Renal Arteries: Computed Tomographic and Magnetic Resonance Angiography

Danny Kim, Sooah Kim, and Vivian Lee

INTRODUCTION

Renal computed tomographic angiography (CTA) and magnetic resonance angiography (MRA) have become clinically important diagnostic tools. Technological advancements are primarily responsible for their rapid development. The implementation of multidetector row array and slip-ring gantry design have propelled CT technology.[1] In the past few years, there has been tremendous progress in the development of MR hardware and sequence design, high-performance gradients, parallel imaging techniques, and advanced torso phased-array coils enabling faster scanning and improved image quality. In contrast to CT, MR scanning does not utilize ionizing radiation, avoids exposure to nephrotoxic iodinated contrast material, and demonstrates the capability to provide functional information.[2] Alternatively, CT scanning is more widely available and less expensive. Ultimately, although digital subtraction angiography (DSA) remains the gold standard for diagnosing renovascular disease, the diagnostic accuracy of renal CTA and MRA and their ability to offer a reliable, less invasive alternative to diagnostic DSA have fueled their widespread adoption. In this chapter, the technical considerations for performing a renal CTA and MRA will be reviewed.

DESCRIPTION OF TECHNICAL REQUIREMENTS

Renal CTA

Renal CTA is best performed with a multidetector row CT (MDCT) scanner, especially one with at least 64 detector rows. A dual-chamber power injector and a dedicated 3D workstation are also recommended. On-going CT hardware and software development have focused on optimizing image quality while minimizing radiation exposure and improving coordination of the scan with contrast material administration.[1]

Renal MRA

Renal MRA can be successfully performed on nearly all currently available high-performance MR scanners. It is recommended that renal MRA be performed on a high field MR scanner with at least 1.5 Tesla (T) field strength and equipped with high performance gradient subsystems (e.g., 40 mT/sec slew rates), using a dedicated torso phased-array coil, an MR compatible power injector with the availability of supplemental oxygen for patients who may have breath-holding difficulty.

TECHNIQUES

Indications

The most common indications for renal artery CTA and MRA include evaluation for renal artery stenosis and evaluation of potential living kidney donors.[1-3] Other common indications include presurgical planning for ureteropelvic junction (UPJ) obstruction, renal tumor evaluation, assessment of congenital anomalies, and trauma.[1,8]

Renal Artery Stenosis

Renal artery stenosis most commonly occurs secondary to atherosclerosis.[4,5] Atherosclerotic disease generally occurs in older patients. Often, there is generalized or diffuse atherosclerotic plaque formation with concomitant involvement of the aorta and the ostium or proximal segment of the main renal artery (Fig. 107-1).[4,5] The second most common etiology is fibromuscular dysplasia (FMD)

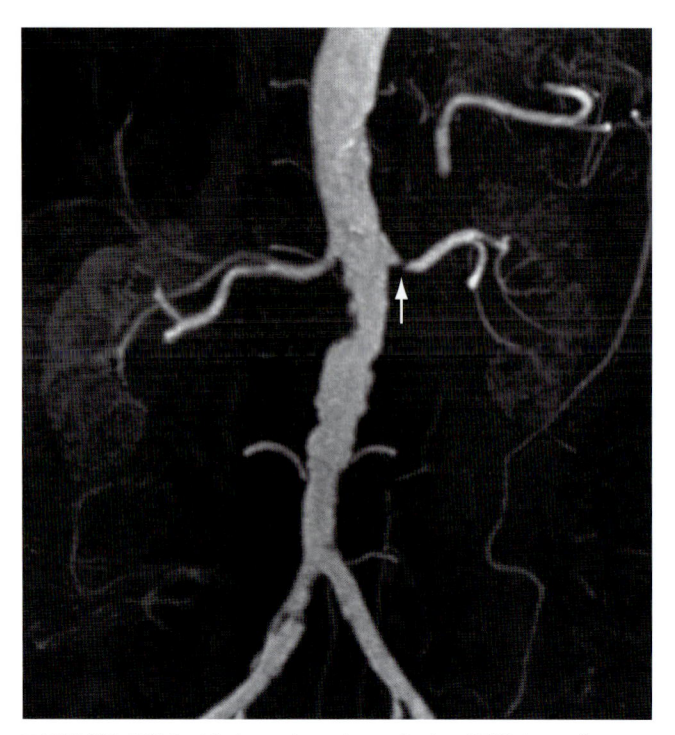

FIGURE 107-1 Maximum intensity projection (MIP) image from a renal MRA demonstrating atherosclerotic disease of the abdominal aorta and severe stenosis of the left renal artery (*arrow*).

which is found in younger patients, typically females.[2,4,5] As opposed to atherosclerotic disease, the middle and distal segments of the main renal artery tend to be more affected in FMD (Fig. 107-2).[2,4,5]

The clinical presentation of patients with renal artery stenosis may include abrupt onset or intractable hypertension, acute or chronic azotemia, angiotensin converting enzyme inhibitor induced azotemia, asymmetric renal size, and congestive heart failure in patients with normal ventricular function.[2] CTA demonstrates a sensitivity up to 90% and a specificity up to 97% in the detection of hemodynamically significant renal artery stenosis.[6] MRA demonstrates a sensitivity of 88% to 100% and a specificity of 70% to 100% in the diagnosis of renal artery stenosis, especially for severe stenosis greater than 70%.[2] Following therapeutic angioplasty and/or stenting for renal artery stenosis, CTA and MRA may also be helpful for the surveillance of renal artery restenosis.

Renal Donor Evaluation

Many renal transplantations are performed with living renal donors because of the insufficient availability of cadaveric kidneys.[7] Accurate evaluation of the renal vasculature, parenchyma, and collecting system is critical for determining suitability of the donor kidney for transplantation and for preoperative planning.[7-10] In many medical centers, donor nephrectomy is now performed laparoscopically to diminish morbidity for the donor.[7-10] Consequently, accurate preoperative evaluation has become even more important to minimize the likelihood for unexpected intraoperative vascular complications from unexpected anatomic variants. More than one third of patients may possess anatomic variants (Fig. 107-3).[5,7-10] This statis-

FIGURE 107-2 Maximum intensity projection (MIP) image from a renal MRA demonstrating fibromuscular dysplasia of the right renal artery (*arrow*).

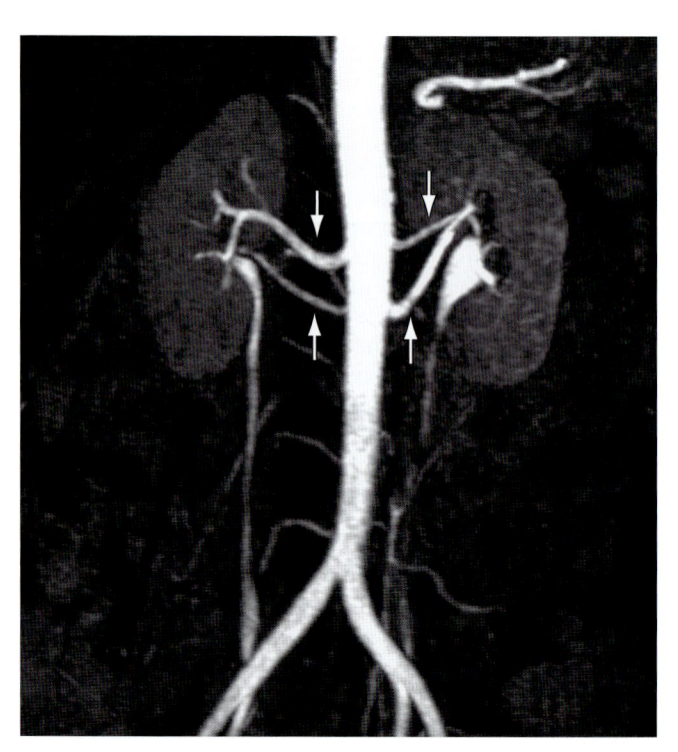

FIGURE 107-3 Maximum intensity projection (MIP) image from a renal MRA demonstrating two bilateral renal arteries (*arrows*).

tic highlights the importance of accurate preoperative assessment.

Preoperative Planning

In preoperative planning for congenital UPJ obstruction surgery, the CTA or MRA is one component of the diagnostic imaging evaluation. The renal and vascular anatomy, etiology of obstruction, functional significance of obstruction and concomitant conditions will determine the treatment approach.[11] The CTA or MRA can typically identify a crossing vessel that is responsible for extrinsic compression of the UPJ resulting in obstruction.[11] CTA demonstrates a sensitivity of 91% to 100% and a specificity of 96% to 100% in the detection of crossing vessels.[11] MRA demonstrates an accuracy of 86% in the detection of a crossing vessel.[11] The presence of a crossing vessel may necessitate a more invasive surgical approach to treat the UPJ obstruction.[11]

Renal Tumor Evaluation

Renal tumor evaluation is another indication for renal artery CTA and MRA. The vascular features of the tumor may assist staging of the tumor and presurgical planning.[11] For instance, renal cell carcinoma may invade the renal vein and extend into the inferior vena cava, which necessitates a substantially longer and more extended surgical approach. Renal cell carcinoma extension into the venous system is typically well assessed by CTA and MRA. Also, the detection of accessory renal arteries or possibly extracapsular feeding arteries of a renal malignancy are important preoperative determinations because knowledge of their presence will minimize intraoperative bleeding complications, especially for laparoscopic nephrectomies, which are becoming increasingly popular surgeries.[11]

Contraindications

Renal CTA

The contraindications for renal CTA include impaired renal function, known allergy to iodinated contrast material and pregnancy. Also, caution is advised in diabetic patients taking metformin hydrochloride. The development of acute renal impairment secondary to contrast-induced nephropathy may prohibit proper clearance of metformin, which is eliminated through the kidneys, and result in lactic acidosis.[12] These patients should discontinue use of metformin for at least 48 hours following administration of iodinated contrast material.[12] Metformin may be resumed after 48 hours if the patient's renal function is normal.[12]

Renal MRA

The concerns and contraindications for renal MRA are those typical to MRI and include a functioning cardiac pacemaker (note that MRI has been safely performed in some patients with cardiac pacemakers but proper physician supervision is necessary), the presence of metallic elements in the body (cerebral aneurysm clips, shrapnel in critical locations of the body, etc.), inability to lie flat for the duration of the examination, claustrophobia, advanced renal failure, first trimester pregnancy. If MR contrast agents are used for renal CE MRA, then proper screening of the patient for known allergy to gadolinium-based contrast material or severe renal impairment should also be performed.

Recently, a rare and potentially life-threatening condition called nephrogenic systemic fibrosis (NSF) has been reported in patients with advanced renal failure receiving gadolinium-based contrast material.[13,14] This disease is characterized by fibrosis of the skin and connective tissues throughout the body. Patients may develop skin thickening to such an extent that it results in decreased joint mobility. Fibrosis may also occur in other parts of the body including the diaphragm, musculature of the lower abdomen and extremities, and the pulmonary vasculature. The clinical course of NSF is progressive and may be fatal. At the present time, no treatment has been identified. Consequently, extreme caution is advised in administering gadolinium-based contrast material in those patients with advanced renal failure. At our institution, we do not recommend the use of gadolinium-chelate contrast agents in patients with glomerular filtration rate (GFR) < 30 mL/min/1.73 m².

Technique Description

Renal CTA

The New York University renal CTA protocol is outlined in Table 107-1. Two important factors in performing a renal CTA examination are the selection of scan parameters for optimization of sufficient volume of anatomic coverage for the highest spatial resolution possible within a reasonable scan period, and the administration of iodinated contrast medium for sufficient opacification of the aorta and renal arteries during imaging. Multidetector row array technology and slip-ring gantry design allow volumetric coverage from the upper abdominal aorta through the common iliac arteries within one breath-hold. The data set may be reconstructed at different slice thicknesses to review the images. For a renal CTA, the data set are reconstructed with overlapping thin slices to enable improved data postprocessing on a 3D workstation.

TABLE 107-1 New York University Renal CTA Protocol

Scan Parameters for a 64-slice MDCT Scanner	
Range	Top of kidneys through iliac crests
Collimation	64 × 0.6
Slice thickness	1 mm
Increment	0.5 mm
Pitch	0.9
Rotation time	0.5 sec
kVp	120 (Caredose)
mAs	280
CTDI vol	20.2 mGy
IV contrast dose	1.5 mL/kg (minimum 100 mL)
IV contrast infusion	3-4 mL/sec
Scan delay	Bolus tracking at the level of T12 (threshold of 150 HU)

CTDI vol, CT dose index of scanned volume.

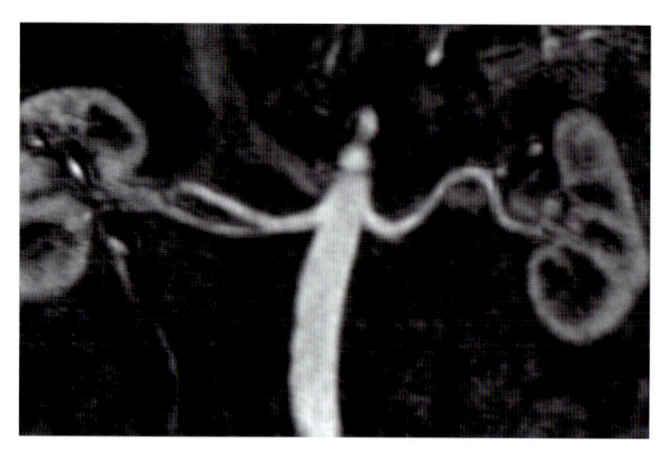

FIGURE 107-4 Multiplanar reformation (MPR) image from a renal MRA demonstrating bilateral renal arteries.

The most critical element of performing a renal CTA examination is coordination of the scan delay with the arterial arrival of the intravenous contrast bolus.[1] Ideally, the scan is obtained during peak contrast opacification of the aorta and renal arteries (Fig. 107-4). The contrast infusion duration should approximate the scan acquisition time.[1] Faster scans require less contrast material. However, the drawback of using less contrast material is the shortened duration of the contrast bolus, which increases the challenge for proper coordination of imaging with opacification of the arteries. That is to say, if scanning is too fast, imaging may occur prior to complete opacification of the target vasculature, resulting in suboptimal arterial contrast enhancement and poor arterial visualization. Alternatively, if scanning is slow or performed too late, images would illustrate the venous phase of the bolus with suboptimal arterial enhancement. Consequently, it is important to accurately determine circulation time to achieve an optimal scan.

There are three methods to determine the patient's circulation time for proper scan delay determination.[1] The first method is selecting an empiric scan delay. This method is the least reliable because various factors influence circulation time such as IV catheter location, injection rate, cardiac output, patient body habitus, and patient positioning. The second method is performing a timing bolus scan. In this technique, a small test dose of contrast material, 10 to 15 mL, is infused at a rate of 3 to 4 mL/sec followed by repetitive scans obtained at the level of the upper abdominal aorta at 2-second intervals. The plot of abdominal aortic attenuation versus time will reveal the time of peak enhancement and, consequently, the correct scan delay time for synchronization of CTA acquisition with peak abdominal aortic (and, by inference, renal arterial) enhancement. The main drawbacks with this technique include the higher volume of contrast administered and the additional ionizing radiation dose associated with the timing bolus. The third method is bolus tracking at the level of the upper abdominal aorta. This is the technique used at our institution. In this technique, a region of interest is selected in the upper abdominal aorta at approximately the level of the celiac artery. Following contrast administration, repetitive scans are obtained at this level until a target threshold attenuation of 150 HU is achieved. When the threshold is achieved, the CTA scan is initiated. Although this technique results in a lesser amount of contrast administered than the timing bolus technique, the additional nondiagnostic ionizing radiation dose is comparable to that required for a timing test bolus scan. The drawback with this technique is the time lag between contrast opacification exceeding the threshold and actual initiation of the scan. Generally, this time lag is approximately 6 to 8 seconds. In order to counteract this unavoidable delay, a lower threshold value may be used to trigger the CTA scan. However, this determination is somewhat arbitrary and susceptible to error. For instance, selecting too low a threshold may initiate the scan before peak opacification is achieved. Alternatively, selecting too high a threshold may miss the peak enhancement phase or not trigger the scan at all. Consequently, optimizing the timing for CTA scanning with arrival of the contrast bolus in the target vascular territory requires careful attention to the specific hardware and software configurations at the host site and to the individual patient that is to undergo the CTA.

Renal MRA

The New York University renal MRA protocol is outlined in Table 107-2. Each of these sequences will be briefly reviewed. The patient is placed in the supine position and intravenous access is obtained in the upper extremity. A phased-array coil is positioned over the abdomen and centered over the kidneys. The phased-array coil permits implementation of parallel imaging techniques, which can shorten acquisition times and increase image resolution. The arms are propped up anterior to the level of the coil to avoid wrap-around artifact. Breath-holding instructions are reviewed with the patient to improve compliance.

The T1-weighted in- and opposed-phase gradient-recalled echo (GRE) pulse sequence provides T1-weighted images for evaluation of renal and adrenal lesions. At our

TABLE 107-2 New York University Renal MRA Protocol

Sequence	Plane
T1-weighted in- and opposed-phase GRE (include adrenals and kidneys)	Axial
HASTE	Axial
VIBE (include entire kidneys)	Axial
3D FLASH	Coronal
	Scan parameters at 1.5 T
	TR: 3.1 msec
	TE: 1.16 msec
	Flip angle: 25 degrees
	Slice thickness: 1.2 mm
	Matrix size: 256 × 512
Timing Run	Axial
	Performed at level of renal arteries
3D FLASH	Coronal
	Two measures 7 seconds apart
	Standard timing formula
VIBE	Axial

GRE: gradient-recalled echo; HASTE: half-Fourier acquisition single-shot turbo spin echo; VIBE: volumetric interpolated breath-hold examination; FLASH: fast low angle shot.

institution, T1-weighted spin-echo (SE) or fast spin-echo (FSE) sequences are not used for renal imaging secondary to the longer acquisition time requirements compared to that for GRE pulse sequences. Short repetition time (TR) and short echo time (TE) are used to achieve T1-weighting. In- and opposed-phase GRE pulse sequences, also known as chemical shift imaging, enable the detection of significant fat within voxels secondary to the signal cancellation that occurs on opposed-phase GRE images. This, in turn, enables the detection of fat within renal and/or adrenal lesions. For instance, this techniques enables the detection of microscopic or intravoxel fat within adrenal adenomas.[15]

The half-Fourier acquisition single-shot turbo spin echo sequence (HASTE, Siemens Medical Solutions, Malvern, PA) is a long echo train imaging technique that enables acquisition of T2-weighted images in less time than conventional SE sequences.[16] This pulse sequence is a single-shot technique that fills just over 50% of k-space in one echo train.[16] The remainder of k-space is mathematically filled based on the symmetric properties of k-space. The acquisition times are generally less than 1 second permitting essentially motion-free T2-weighted images. This technique is useful in uncooperative patients or patients who cannot adequately breath-hold. The main drawback, however, is the low signal-to-noise ratio. In this protocol, the HASTE images are mainly used for delineation of the anatomy and assessment of the renal collecting systems.

At our institution, we also perform the volumetric interpolated breath-hold examination technique (VIBE, Siemens Medical Solutions), which is a 3D T1-weighted fat-suppressed GRE pulse sequence that provides high spatial and temporal resolution imaging.[17] This volumetric acquisition is performed before and after intravenous contrast administration to allow accurate detection and characterization of adrenal and renal lesions. The complete volume of the adrenal glands and kidneys may be imaged within a single breath-hold to minimize respiratory and other motion artifacts and allow advanced 3D image postprocessing.

Contrast-Enhanced 3D MRA

Renal MRA is best achieved using contrast-enhanced 3D MRA using a 3D fast spoiled GRE pulse sequence (e.g., Fast Low Angle Shot or FLASH, Siemens Medical Solutions).[16] This volumetric acquisition is performed during the arterial phase of the contrast bolus and can reliably provide high spatial resolution vascular illustration of the abdominal aorta and renal arteries. The extremely short TR value of this pulse sequence produces high T1 contrast.[16,17]

In order to accurately image the renal arteries during the arterial phase, the circulation time must be determined for the individual patient because the circulation time can vary significantly from patient to patient. Different methods can be used to accomplish this task. At our institution, we use a preliminary timing bolus scan to estimate scan delay times necessary for the MRA examination.[18] In this protocol, a 1 mL test dose of gadolinium-chelate contrast agent is infused followed by a 20 mL saline flush; both infused at a rate of 2 mL/sec with an MR-compatible power injector. At the same time, axial images are acquired at the level of the upper abdominal aorta, at the celiac artery, at 2-second intervals. From these images, the time for peak enhancement of the aorta may be determined. The actual scan delay depends on the k-space scheme of the 3D MRA pulse sequence and the period that the central k-space data is being acquired. For a sequential 3D MRA acquisition, the center of k-space is filled during the middle of the acquisition time, the following formula may be used to calculate the scan delay: T (scan delay) = T (circulation time) + $\frac{1}{2}$ T (contrast infusion) − $\frac{1}{2}$ T (acquisition time). The circulation time is the time for peak enhancement of the aorta. Contrast infusion time is the duration of the contrast infusion (10 sec for 20 mL of contrast infused at 2 mL/sec). Acquisition time is approximately 20 seconds. If a centric phase ordering is used, the central lines of k-space are acquired at the beginning of data acquisition and scan delay is typically timed by simply adding 2 seconds to the circulatory time. The addition of 2 seconds minimizes the risk for ringing artifacts that can occur if central k-space views are sampled during the rapid rise in gadolinium concentration.[19] It is preferred that the central k-space views, therefore, be acquired during the plateau phase (i.e., more stable period) of the contrast enhancement curve.

If the contrast-enhanced 3D MRA is suboptimal, there are several additional imaging options that can be performed to ensure a diagnostic result. One is to perform a renal 3D phase contrast (PC) MRA.[20] This can be performed during free breathing and using an axial prescription. Vascular signal intensity on 3D PC MRA is actually quite good after Gd-chelate contrast agent administration.[21] Yet another option is to perform a postcontrast 3D SSFP MRA. On 3D SSFP, arterial signal intensity is also very high after Gd-chelate contrast administration; however, venous structures also will have high signal intensity.[22]

New Developments in MRA

Noncontrast enhanced MRA techniques, such as ECG-gated balanced steady-state free precession (true-FISP, Siemens Medical Solutions; FIESTA, General Electric Healthcare, Waukesha, WI; balanced FFE, Philips Medical Systems, Andover, MA) with or without arterial spin labeling (ASL), have mainly been applied for research purposes. However, interest in noncontrast MRA techniques has been increasing because of the risks of nephrogenic systemic fibrosis (NSF) in patients with advanced renal failure who receive gadolinium contrast material.

A noncontrast enhanced 3D SSFP MRA with fat suppression was originally developed for whole heart coronary artery imaging but is a valuable technique for body MRA. 3D SSFP can be cardiac gated and respiratory gated, typically using navigator echo gating. Of course, 3D SSFP can also be obtained without cardiac or respiratory gating during a breath-hold. Image contrast in 3D SSFP is determined by the T2/T1 ratio which produces bright blood imaging with minimal reliance on inflow effects for signal generation. Consequently, both arteries and veins have high signal intensity. For renal MRA examinations, saturation bands over the kidneys and inferior vena cava can reduce venous signal.[23] Application of a slab-selective inversion prepulse can also suppress the signal from the renal parenchyma and the renal veins.[24]

ASL is frequently used for perfusion measurements in the brain, and also has been applied for renal perfusion measurement and renal artery imaging.[25,26] ASL can be combined with fast MRA imaging methods. The ASL technique relies on spin-tagging the blood upstream of the area of interest to provide vessel contrast. With alternate acquisition of the tagged and nontagged images and subtracting these two data sets, a bright blood image, without background signal, can be obtained. ASL imaging can also be produced by using a combination of a spatially nonselective inversion recovery pulse and a spatially selective tagged pulse. The combination of ASL with SSFP technique provides bright blood angiographic images, without venous signal and with high signal-to-noise ratio, suitable for renal artery imaging. The combination of cardiac-triggered, navigator-gated, 3D SSFP technique with a cylindrical (pencil beam) 2D selective spin-labeling inversion pulse, tagging the blood in the suprarenal aorta, demonstrated comparable quality to contrast-enhanced MRA images.[26] The main limitation of this technique is the requirement of high velocity flow. ASL works best where there is fast flow such as within the carotid, renal, or pulmonary arteries. It is less effective in regions of slow flow, such as within the peripheral arteries, where blood in the imaging volume is not being adequately replaced by tagged blood.

Pitfalls and Solutions

CTA Pitfalls and Solutions

For CTA, lack of coordination between contrast infusion and scan acquisition may yield a poor quality examination. Solutions to minimize this pitfall include checking the patient's intravenous injection site and the MR compatible power injector to ensure proper functioning, relaxing the position of the arms to prevent venous kinking and prolonged bolus transit times, and using a saline chaser following the contrast infusion to prevent pooling of contrast material within the catheter tubing and peripheral veins.[1]

MRA Pitfalls and Solutions

For MRA, parallel imaging with multichannel systems offers the potential to decrease imaging times without sacrificing spatial resolution in those patients who have difficulty breath-holding.[16] More than one receiver coil is required, with each coil having its own receiver channel. This technique uses the difference in signal detected by receiver coils positioned over different parts of the body. By incorporating the differences in sensitivity of multiple coils to detect signal from the same source, information regarding spatial localization may be obtained and may reduce the number of phase-encoding steps required to produce an image. Consequently, imaging times will be decreased. Two main techniques of parallel imaging are known as SMASH, simultaneous acquisition of spatial harmonics, and SENSE, sensitivity encoding.[16] There are several issues that should be considered when incorporating these techniques. First, special coils must be designed with independent coil elements having their own receiver channels. Second, accuracy of coil sensitivity measurements may be difficult to determine. Third, extensive computational time is required to integrate the independent data from multiple channels. Finally, the signal-to-noise ratio will be decreased inversely with the acceleration factor because of the under-sampling of k-space.

Image Interpretation

Postprocessing

Examination of the 3D CTA or MRA data set requires specialized 3D postprocessing software. For CTA, the reconstruction parameters must be selected to create the source data. For MRA data, no specific reconstruction parameters need to be chosen because the raw data is the source data. When the source data is loaded, an unlimited number of projections, different slice thicknesses, and orientations may be displayed using most commercially available CTA and/or MRA postprocessing software.

The most commonly used postprocessing techniques include multiplanar reformation (MPR), maximum intensity projection (MIP), and 3D volume rendering (VR).[1,2,6,27,28] Each of these visualization techniques possesses different strengths and limitations and a more detailed description can be found in Chapter 83. In any case, the source data should be routinely evaluated to corroborate specific findings.

MPR presents the source data in any desired plane to maximize visualization of the vascular anatomy (Fig. 107-5). The limitation of this technique is that the renal

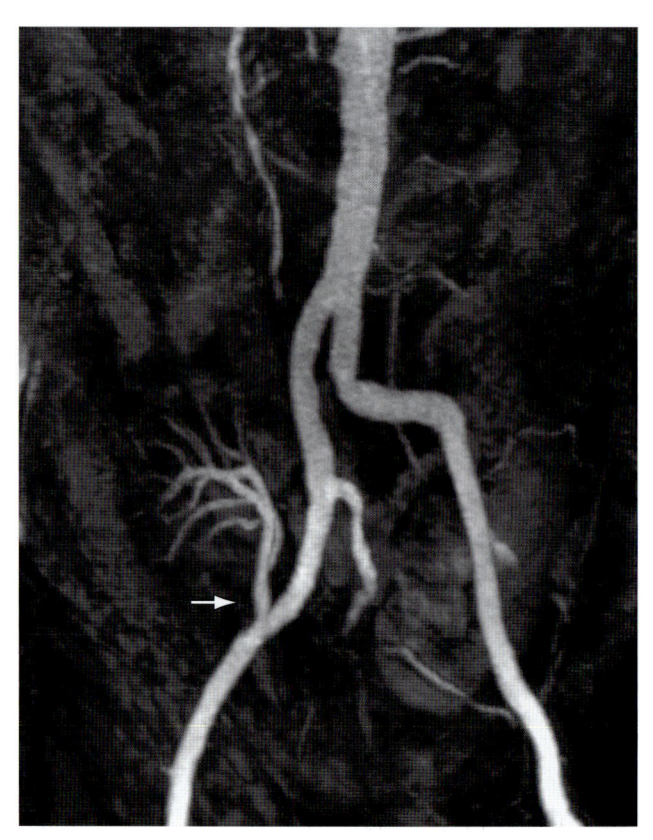

■ **FIGURE 107-5** Maximum intensity projection (MIP) image from a renal MRA demonstrating a right lower quadrant transplant renal artery arising from the right external iliac artery (*arrow*).

artery must lie in the same plane. Because the renal artery may be tortuous in course, segments of the artery may course in and out of the visualization plane resulting in the appearance of pseudostenoses.[6] Proper visualization of arterial branch points may also present a similar challenge at tortuous segments. Curved planar reformation (CPR), a modification of the MPR technique, may be used to overcome this limitation. CPR presents the source data in a single voxel tomogram that follows a curved path.[6] The curved path may be manually or automatically designated along the course of the renal artery. This modified technique allows complete visualization of the renal artery in one plane of section. The major limitation of this technique is dependence on accurate designation of the course of the renal artery. If the curve does not accurately follow the renal artery, false stenoses (i.e., pseudostenoses) may be erroneously created. In addition, because the images are only a single voxel in thickness, small or thin structures may not be included in the tomogram image.[6] To avoid this potential pitfall, an orthogonal plane may be helpful to visualize a more complete representation of the vessel anatomy.

MIP presents the source data in a selected plane by using a simple algorithm.[27] First, the operator selects a desired visualization plane. Then, the value of each voxel is determined by the maximum value along an array directed perpendicular to the imaging plane and through the volumetric data set. This value represents the maximum density for CTA images and maximum signal intensity for MRA images. The 3D data set is converted to a representative 2D projection image (Fig. 107-6). The limitation of this technique is the loss of depth information because voxels with lower values are overlooked and only maximum values are displayed.[27] Overlapping structures often may confound interpretation. One solution to ease interpretation is the creation of MIP images in multiple projections at different angles around the data set to create a 3D effect. For CTA images, any structure with a density greater than intravenous contrast, such as bone, calcification and metal, has the potential to obscure visualization of the vascular anatomy. One solution to avoid this pitfall is to use a smaller selected volume of the original data set, or a sub-volume MIP. For a subvolume MIP, the 2D projection is generated using a subset of the total 3D data (i.e., a thin slab of the volumetric data set) corresponding to the expected plane of the renal arteries. On CTA, this technique can be useful for removing bony structures from the image data set. However, similar to the limitations of MPR, the vascular anatomy must lie within the slab to avoid the generation of pseudostenoses. On CTA, even with these techniques, however, the ostial calcification from atherosclerosis may make it very challenging to separate calcification from the luminal contrast, precluding accurate grading of an ostial renal artery stenosis. MRA offers a few advantages over CTA in this regard. One advantage is that calcification causes a signal void (i.e., no MR signal) and thus will not obscure luminal anatomy. The second advantage of MRA is its ability to acquire precontrast and postcontrast images and perform a subtraction of the volumetric data set. By subtracting the precontrast data set from the postcontrast data set, the resulting postprocessed data set will contain only information regarding the distribution of contrast material. As a result, the MIP images will allow easier visualization of the arterial anatomy without the interference of adjacent structures.

3D VR presents the source data in a 3D format by incorporating the values of each voxel to construct the image data set.[1,2,6,27,28] Unlike MIP images, depth information is preserved. Various filters may be applied to the source data to create different colors or degrees of opacity corresponding to each voxel value. In this manner, certain voxel values may be emphasized or minimized to evaluate specific structures. For instance, CTA images may be created that render the bony structures relatively transparent to facilitate visualization of the vascular anatomy (Fig. 107-7). In addition to preserving depth information, 3D VR provides an excellent overview of the anatomic relationships within the data set. Accessory renal arteries and unexpected anatomic variants may be easier to appreciate with these images. The limitation of this technique is the potential to create or overlook pathology because many of the attributes of the image are arbitrarily determined. For instance, the colors and degrees of transparency are user-defined variables and may be vulnerable to error.

Fishman and colleagues found MIP images to be useful for many CTA applications, but rely on 3D VR images for interpretation secondary to its superior ability to differentiate soft tissues and accurately depict 3D anatomic relationships.[27] Mallouhi and colleagues found that 3D VR for renal MRA offered three advantages over MIP: a higher positive predictive value for detecting clinically significant

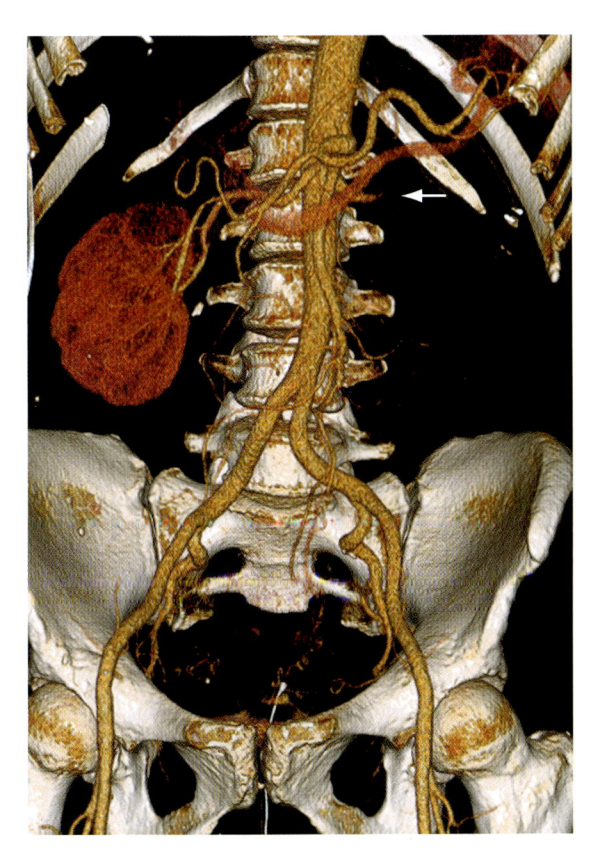

■ **FIGURE 107-6** 3D volume rendered image from a renal CTA demonstrating occlusion of the left renal artery (*arrow*).

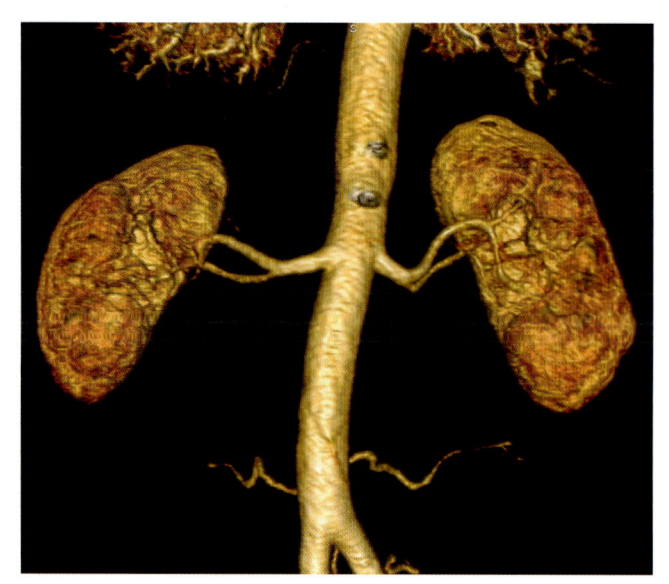

FIGURE 107-7 3D volume rendered image from a renal CTA demonstrating bilateral branching renal arteries with incorporation of a bone removal algorithm.

renal artery stenosis, better correlation with DSA, and improved delineation of the renal artery.[28]

Reporting

The radiologic interpretation for both renal CTA and MRA should include a description of the imaging protocol. The aorta should be described in regard to its course, caliber, and presence of pathology (atherosclerotic disease, aortic aneurysm, aortic dissection, etc.). The renal arteries should be described in terms of their number, course, caliber, and presence of pathology. For renal artery stenosis, the segment of vessel involved, length of stenosis, and grading of degree of stenosis should be reported. Finally, other nonvascular findings such as renal size, renal parenchymal assessment, and other incidental findings should be included.

KEY POINTS

- Renal CTA and MRA offer a viable, less invasive alternative to conventional catheter digital subtraction angiography.
- Renal MRA does not use ionizing radiation, avoids exposure to nephrotoxic iodinated contrast material, and has the ability to provide functional information.
- Renal CTA is more widely available and is less expensive.
- Renal CTA and MRA demonstrate high diagnostic accuracy in the detection of renal artery stenosis and an important role in the evaluation of living renal donors and preoperative planning for renal surgery.
- The most critical element of performing a renal CTA examination is coordination of the scan delay with intravenous contrast administration.
- New developments in renal MRA may permit improved noncontrast MRA options.
- Advanced postprocessing techniques, such as multiplanar reformation (MPR), maximum intensity projection (MIP) and 3D volume rendering (VR), possess different strengths and limitations.
- Evaluation of the source data for renal CTA and MRA is recommended to corroborate findings on postprocessed images.

SUGGESTED READINGS

Fishman EK, Ney DR, Heath DG, et al. Volume rendering versus maximum intensity projection in CT angiography: What works best, when and why. RadioGraphics 2006; 26:905-922.

Hussain SM, Kock MCJ, Ijzermans JNM, et al. MR imaging: A "one-stop shop" modality for preoperative evaluation of potential living kidney donors. RadioGraphics 2003; 23:505-520.

Kawamoto S, Montgomery RA, Lawler LP, et al. Multi-detector row CT evaluation of living renal donors prior to laparoscopic nephrectomy. RadioGraphics 2004; 24:453-466.

Zhang H, Prince MR. Renal MR angiography. Magn Reson Imaging Clin N Am 2004; 12:487-503.

REFERENCES

1. Chow LC, Rubin GD. CT angiography of the arterial system. Radiol Clin N Am 2002; 40:729-749.
2. Zhang H, Prince MR. Renal MR angiography. Magn Reson Imaging Clin N Am 2004; 12:487-503.
3. Kang PS, Spain JW. Multidetector CT angiography of the abdomen. Radiol Clin N Am 2005; 43:963-976.
4. Kawashima A, Sandler CM, Ernst RD, et al. CT evaluation of renovascular disease. RadioGraphics 2000; 20:1321-1340.
5. Urban BA, Ratner LE, Fishman EK. Three-dimensional volume-rendered CT angiography of the renal arteries and veins: Normal anatomy, variants, and clinical applications. RadioGraphics 2001; 21:373-386.
6. Kocakoc E, Bhatt S, Dogra V. Renal multidetector row CT. Radiol Clin N Am 2005; 43:1021-1047.
7. Israel GM, Lee VS, Edye M, Krinsky GA, et al. Comprehensive MR imaging in the preoperative evaluation of living donor candidates for laparoscopic nephrectomy: Initial experience. Radiology 2002; 225:427-432.
8. Hussain SM, Kock MCJ, Ijzermans JNM, et al. MR imaging: A "one-stop shop" modality for preoperative evaluation of potential living kidney donors. RadioGraphics 2003; 23:505-520.
9. Kawamoto S, Montgomery RA, Lawler LP, et al. Multi-detector row CT evaluation of living renal donors prior to laparoscopic nephrectomy. RadioGraphics 2004; 24:453-466.
10. Sahani DV, Rastogi N, Greenfield AC, et al. Multi-detector row CT in evaluation of 94 living renal donors by readers with varied experience. Radiology 2005; 235:905-910.
11. Shah O, Taneja SS. Renal imaging: What the urologist wants to know. Magn Reson Imaging Clin N Am 2004; 12:387-402.
12. Rasuli P, French GJ, Hammond DI. Metformin hydrochloride all right before, but not after, contrast medium administration. Radiology 1998; 209:586.

13. Sadowski EA, Bennett LK, Chan MR, et al. Nephrogenic systemic fibrosis: risk factors and incidence estimation. Radiology 2007; 243:148-157.
14. Marckmann P, Skov L, Rossen K, et al. Nephrogenic systemic fibrosis: suspected causative role of gadodiamide used for contrast-enhanced magnetic resonance imaging. J Am Soc Nephrol 2006; 17:2359-2362.
15. Merkle EM, Nelson RC. Dual gradient-echo in-phase and opposed-phase hepatic MR imaging: a useful tool for evaluating more than fatty infiltration or fatty sparing. RadioGraphics 2006; 26:1409-1418.
16. Lee VS, Cardiovascular MRI. Physical Principles to Practical Protocols. Philadelphia, Lippincott Williams & Wilkins, 2005.
17. Rofsky NM, Lee VS, Laub G, et al. Abdominal MR imaging with a volumetric interpolated breath-hold examination. Radiology 1999; 212:876-884.
18. Earls J, Rofsky N, DeCorato D, et al. Hepatic arterial-phase dynamic gadolinium-enhanced MR imaging: optimization with a test examination and a power injector. Radiology 1997; 202:268-273.
19. Maki JH, Prince MR, Londy FJ, Chenevert TL. The effects of time varying intravascular signal intensity and k-space acquisition order on three-dimensional mr angiography image quality. J Magn Reson Imaging 1996; 6(4):642-651.
20. Hood MN, HO VB, Corse WR. Three-dimensional phase-contrast magnetic resonance angiography: a useful clinical adjunct to gadolinium-enhanced three-dimensional renal magnetic resonance angiography. Mil Med 2002; 167(4):343-349.
21. Bass JC, Prince MR, Londy FJ, Chenevert TL. Effect of Gadolinium on phase-contrast MR angiography of the renal arteries. AJR Am J Roentgenol 1997; 168(1):261-266.
22. Foo TK, Ho VB, Marcos HB, et al. MR Angiography using steady-state free precession. Magn Reson Med 2002; 48(4):699-706.
23. Coenegrachts KL, Hoogeveen RM, Vaninbroukx JA, et al. High-spatial-resolution 3D balanced turbo field-echo technique for MR angiography of the renal arteries: initial experience. Radiology 2004; 231:237-242.
24. Wyttenbach R, Braghetti A, Wyss M, et al. Renal artery assessment with nonenhanced steady-state free precession versus contrast-enhanced MR angiography. Radiology 2007;245:186-195.
25. Fenchel M, Martirosian P, Langanke J, et al. Perfusion MR imaging with FAIR true FISP spin labeling in patients with and without renal artery stenosis: Initial experience. Radiology 2006; 238:1013-1021.
26. Spuentrup E, Manning WJ, Börnert P, et al. Renal Arteries: Navigator-gated balanced fast field-echo projection MR angiography with aortic spin labeling: Initial experience. Radiology 2002; 225:589-596.
27. Fishman EK, Ney DR, Heath DG, et al. Volume rendering versus maximum intensity projection in CT angiography: What works best, when and why. RadioGraphics 2006; 26:905-922.
28. Mallouhi A, Schocke M, Judmaier W, et al. 3D MR angiography of renal arteries: comparison of volume rendering and maximum intensity projection algorithms. Radiology 2002; 223:509-516.

CHAPTER 108

Renal Artery Scintigraphy

Lina Mehta, James K. O'Donnell, and Peter Faulhaber

Renovascular hypertension (RVH) secondary to renal artery stenosis (RAS) can be a challenging diagnosis to make. The presence of RAS does not necessarily imply RVH. There are many radiologic methods of investigating RAS, including Doppler ultrasound, computed tomography, magnetic resonance imaging, nuclear renography, and angiography. Most imaging modalities assess renal artery stenosis, but the functional information provided by nuclear renography augmented with an angiotensin-converting enzyme inhibitor (ACEI) allows for the detection of renovascular hypertension.

In patients with a hemodynamically significant reduction in renal artery caliber, there is a reduction in renal perfusion pressure distal to the stenosis. This results in the activation of the renin-angiotensin-aldosterone system, whereby renin is released from the juxtaglomerular apparatus, and a cascade of events occurs that ultimately leads to peripheral vasoconstriction, blood volume increase, and an elevation in blood pressure. Notably, renin converts angiotensinogen to angiotensin I and angiotensin I is then converted to angiotensin II through a process that requires ACE. In the kidney, angiotensin II results in the preferential constriction of efferent arterioles, which raises the pressure gradient across the glomerular capillary membrane and maintains the glomerular filtration rate (GFR). In patients with RVH, the administration of an ACEI blocks the conversion of angiotensin I to angiotensin II, thereby lowering the degree of vasoconstriction in the efferent arterioles, dropping the transcapillary pressures, and resulting in decreased GFR. There is also an increase in the creatinine level, which is the most common reason for pursuing a diagnosis of renal vascular disease. Decreased GFR can be assessed using nuclear scintigraphy and is the underlying mechanism for the diagnosis of RVH by ACEI scintigraphy.[1]

TECHNICAL REQUIREMENTS

ACEI scintigraphy is performed with one head of a gamma camera. The field of view should include at least the kidneys and bladder. A large field of view camera is preferred so that the heart and blood pool clearance can be assessed. Ideally, continuous blood pressure monitoring should be performed and personnel trained in basic cardiopulmonary resuscitation should be immediately available in case of hypotension. An intravenous line can be placed for hydration, and should be used for those patients who are at high risk of cardiac disease and those receiving intravenous enalaprilat.

TECHNIQUES

Indications

ACEI renography can be used to assess for the presence of renovascular hypertension caused by renal artery stenosis. It is most cost-effective when used in a patient population with a high prevalence of RVH.[2] Many imaging modalities exist for the evaluation of renal artery stenosis, but renography may be particularly useful for those with known contrast allergy and in whom assessment of functional significance of a stenotic vessel is desired. The success of this technique is based on the inhibition of the conversion of angiotensin I to angiotensin II following the administration of an ACEI, with subsequent reduction in the GFR, and consequently a change in the radiopharmaceutical pattern of uptake and clearance in comparison to a baseline study.

Contraindications

Patients receiving an ACEI can experience significant hypotension; administration of an ACEI warrants proper clinical monitoring. Blood pressure should be carefully measured, with a baseline blood pressure established prior to the administration of the ACEI; subsequent blood pressure measurements should be performed at 5- to 15-minute intervals following drug administration and prior to discharge. Patients should not be discharged home unless their blood pressure is at least 70% of their baseline blood pressure. Chronic ACEI use can reduce the sensitivity of the study and a short-acting ACEI should be held for 3 days before the study and a longer acting ACEI should be held for 5 to 7 days. Chronic diuretic use may be associated with dehydration, leading to an increased risk of hypotension when the ACEI is administered; it should therefore be stopped a few days before the study. Calcium channel blockers have been reported to cause false-positive results and cessation prior to the study should also be considered.[3] Many patients referred for this study will be at high risk for cardiovascular disease, however, and if hypertension is severe, antihypertensive use can be maintained with the understanding that there may be a mild reduction in the overall sensitivity of the study.

DESCRIPTION OF THE PROCEDURE

The initial patient screening should include a thorough patient history that includes listing of all medications and a review of any relevant imaging studies. Whenever possible, patients who have a history of chronic use of ACEI and diuretics should have these medications held prior to the study.

Oral captopril or intravenous enalaprilat may be used, although captopril is used more commonly. The oral captopril dose is 25 to 50 mg in adults, and 1 mg/kg in children, with a maximum dose of 50 mg. The captopril tablet is generally crushed and dissolved in water to ensure better gastric absorption. Peak systemic concentrations of captopril occur around 60 minutes after administration and then begin to decrease; therefore, the radiopharmaceutical is injected 60 minutes following captopril administration. Patients receiving oral captopril should avoid solid foods for at least 4 hours prior to administration to aid gastric absorption, although normal hydration should be continued.

Enalaprilat is administered intravenously over 3 to 5 minutes, with a dose of 40 μg/kg and a maximum dose of 2.5 mg. The radiopharmaceutical may be given 15 minutes following enalaprilat administration and the intravenous line should be maintained, because enalaprilat administration may be associated with more significant hypotension. The use of enalaprilat avoids the problem of uneven or incomplete gastric absorption, which could be an issue with captopril. In addition, the shorter waiting period prior to injection may also lead to a shorter study duration than when using oral captopril. Although enalaprilat and captopril are both thought to be suitable for the evaluation of RVH, enalaprilat is associated with a greater risk of hypotension. Captopril is generally more widely used and therefore will be discussed in this chapter.

Patients should be appropriately hydrated, because dehydration can affect renal perfusion curves.[4] Patients with renin-dependent RVH may experience a drop in systolic blood pressure when the ACEI is administered, a drop that may be more severe if the patient is dehydrated. Hydration will also help decrease radiation dose to the bladder wall[5] and to the surrounding reproductive organs by diluting the radioactivity in the bladder. Patients can receive oral or intravenous hydration, although intravenous hydration is generally preferred with enalaprilat. Oral hydration is generally 7 mg/kg of water and IV hydration, 10 mg/kg, with a maximum administered volume of 500 mL of normal saline over 30 minutes; both are initiated following ACEI administration.

A baseline blood pressure reading should be taken and recorded prior to administration of the medication. Four sequential blood pressure measurements are taken and recorded in the patient's record at 15-minute intervals during the hour following captopril administration, prior to radiopharmaceutical administration. At the culmination of the study, a final blood pressure reading should be taken prior to discharge home. Patients receiving enalaprilat should have blood pressure measured every 5 minutes during the examination. The patient should void when the waiting period comes to an end, prior to imaging, because a full bladder may affect emptying of the upper tract[6] and could also lead to premature termination of the study if the patient needs to void during imaging.

The patient is then brought into the scan room and positioned supine on the imaging table with the camera located posteriorly to ensure that the kidneys are lying at the same depth, which could be affected with the patient semirecumbent or sitting.[7] Once the patient is positioned appropriately, imaging begins with the intravenous injection of the radiopharmaceutical. The study should be dynamic, with the first series generally consisting of 1 sec/frame for 1 minute to assess early perfusion, the second series consisting of 5 sec/frame for 24 frames, and the final functional sequence, 30 sec/frame for 60 frames, for a total imaging time of approximately 30 minutes. The patient should void at the end of the study to reduce radiation dose to the kidneys, bladder, and pelvic organs. A postvoid bladder residual can also be calculated with a postvoid image consisting of a single 60-sec/frame image.

Dose infiltration can affect the results of the study. Correction for infiltration can be done by imaging the injection site and qualitatively or quantitatively assessing the injection dose. A quantitative evaluation is performed by determining the ratio of infiltrated counts to the original counts in the injected dose; with this method, syringe counts should be calculated prior to injection. A qualitative assessment is done visually. Assessment of a region of interest over the abdominal aorta during the immediate postinjection perfusion phase can also provide information about the quality of the injection bolus.

The study can be performed as either a 1- or 2-day protocol. The 1-day protocol requires the patient to visit the imaging department only once, but the length of time spent may be longer than with the 2-day protocol.

The 1-day protocol begins with a baseline study using a 1-mCi dose of radiopharmaceutical (37 MBq). This is followed by the ACEI-augmented study with a higher radionuclide dose of 5 to 10 mCi (185 to 370 MBq) to supersede any residual activity from the baseline study. It is helpful to obtain a single static postvoid image of the kidneys and bladder prior to the second injection of the radiopharmaceutical to assess how much, if any, residual activity remains, because residual activity could interfere with interpretation of the second imaging sequence.

Many departments begin the 2-day protocol with the ACEI-augmented study because a normal study will indicate a low likelihood of renovascular hypertension, obviating the need for the patient to return for a baseline determination. An abnormal augmented study will require the patient to return on a subsequent day for a baseline scan, at least 24 hours following the ACEI scan, to ensure that the baseline dose of technetium has decayed. Given this decay, both parts of the examination can be performed with 3 to 5 mCi (111 to 185 MBq) of the radiotracer, leading to better count statistics and better image resolution.

Following radiotracer injection, the loop diuretic furosemide may also be administered intravenously to clear radiotracer activity from the collecting system, reducing retention which could otherwise confound quantitative assessment.

Either technetium 99m mercaptoacetyltriglycine (^{99m}Tc-MAG3), a tubularly secreted agent, or technetium 99m diethylenetriaminepentaacetic acid (^{99m}Tc-DTPA), a glomerular agent, can be used for ACEI imaging. ^{99m}Tc-MAG3 has a higher renal extraction rate and is therefore preferred by many institutions, particularly for patients with elevated creatinine levels. Iodohippurate sodium I 123 (^{123}I-OIH), also a tubularly secreted agent, can be used in a similar fashion, but is not commercially available in the United States or Canada.

PITFALLS AND SOLUTIONS

ACEI renography is best used in patients with normal or almost normal serum creatinine levels to ensure adequate renal concentration of the radiopharmaceutical. A poorly functioning kidney could lead to difficulty in interpretation because a kidney must be able to extract enough radiopharmaceutical to show a change in function when the ACEI is administered. ^{99m}Tc-MAG3 has a higher renal extraction than ^{99m}Tc-DTPA and is therefore preferred for patients with impaired renal function. Bilateral renal insufficiency can lead to a similar problem. Chronic administration of certain antihypertensives can reduce specificity of the examination and these medications may need to be held prior to the study.

IMAGE INTERPRETATION

Postprocessing

Whole renogram curves should be obtained over each kidney and cortical regions of interest (ROIs) can also be assessed to exclude any pelvocaliceal tracer retention, which could interfere with study interpretation by introducing artificial counts into the calculations. Background subtraction should also be performed using a background ROI. Renal curves are generated from the renal ROIs and the time to maximum counts (T_{max}), as shown on the curves, is an important parameter in the diagnosis of RAS. Computer quantification can aid in interpretation and has been found to be useful in reducing false-positive results in patients with mildly abnormal perfusion at baseline.[8]

Reporting

The scintigraphic diagnosis of RAS is made when a change is seen on the ACEI-augmented scan from baseline. Diagnostic criteria will vary based on the radiotracer used. Decreases in GFR as a result of ACEI administration generally do not affect tubular uptake and secretion; therefore, initial tracer uptake is not affected with ^{99m}Tc-MAG3 but will be affected with glomerularly secreted agents, such as ^{99m}Tc-DTPA. With agents such as ^{99m}Tc-DTPA, the main diagnostic finding with ACEI-augmented scans and RVH is an overall drop in function, although other findings such as delayed time to peak uptake, more than a 10% drop in differential function, and less than a 10% drop in GFR can also be seen. The most useful criterion for the diagnosis of RVH is unilateral cortical retention in the affected kidney, which can be seen with both agents, although more commonly with ^{99m}Tc-MAG3.

Results from ACEI scintigraphy are reported as low, intermediate, or high probability for RAS (Fig. 108-1). A normal ACEI renogram indicates a low probability (less than 10%) of renal artery stenosis and these patients generally do not need further work-up for RVH or a baseline scan. A scan is read as having an intermediate probability for RVH when the baseline scan is abnormal but does not demonstrate change following the ACEI challenge. These patients generally are found to have ischemic nephropathy, often with a small shrunken kidney. ACEI-augmented scans are also read as intermediate probability in the face of bilateral cortical retention, as commonly seen with renal insufficiency, and in patients with only very small changes in function in relation to the baseline study. With both ^{99m}Tc-DTPA and ^{99m}Tc-MAG3, a change in differential function of greater than 10% is considered high probability for RAS, whereas a change from 5% to 9% is considered intermediate probability. Depending on the radiotracer, high-probability scans—those that demonstrate reductions in function, changes in differential function, delayed time to peak, and/or increased cortical retention—indicate a greater than 90% likelihood of RAS. These patients are likely to benefit from vascular intervention.

Bilateral cortical retention is more often caused by dehydration or a hypotension artifact rather than bilateral renal artery stenosis. Unilateral retention can be quantitatively assessed in several ways:

1. An increase in the 20/peak (ratio of cortical activity at 20 minutes to the amount of peak activity) or 20/3 ratio (count activity at 20 minutes divided by the activity at 3 minutes).
2. An increase of at least one grade in the renogram curve (Fig. 108-2). Renogram curves are scored from 0 to 4, with 0 reflecting a normal scan and thus a low probability of RVH, and 4 reflecting complete renal failure, with no extraction of the radiotracer, and thus a high probability of RVH. Grades 1 through 3 reflect progressive worsening from baseline, with increasing grade indicating more corresponding profound changes.
3. An increase in time to maximum parenchymal uptake (T_{max}) of at least 2 to 3 minutes.

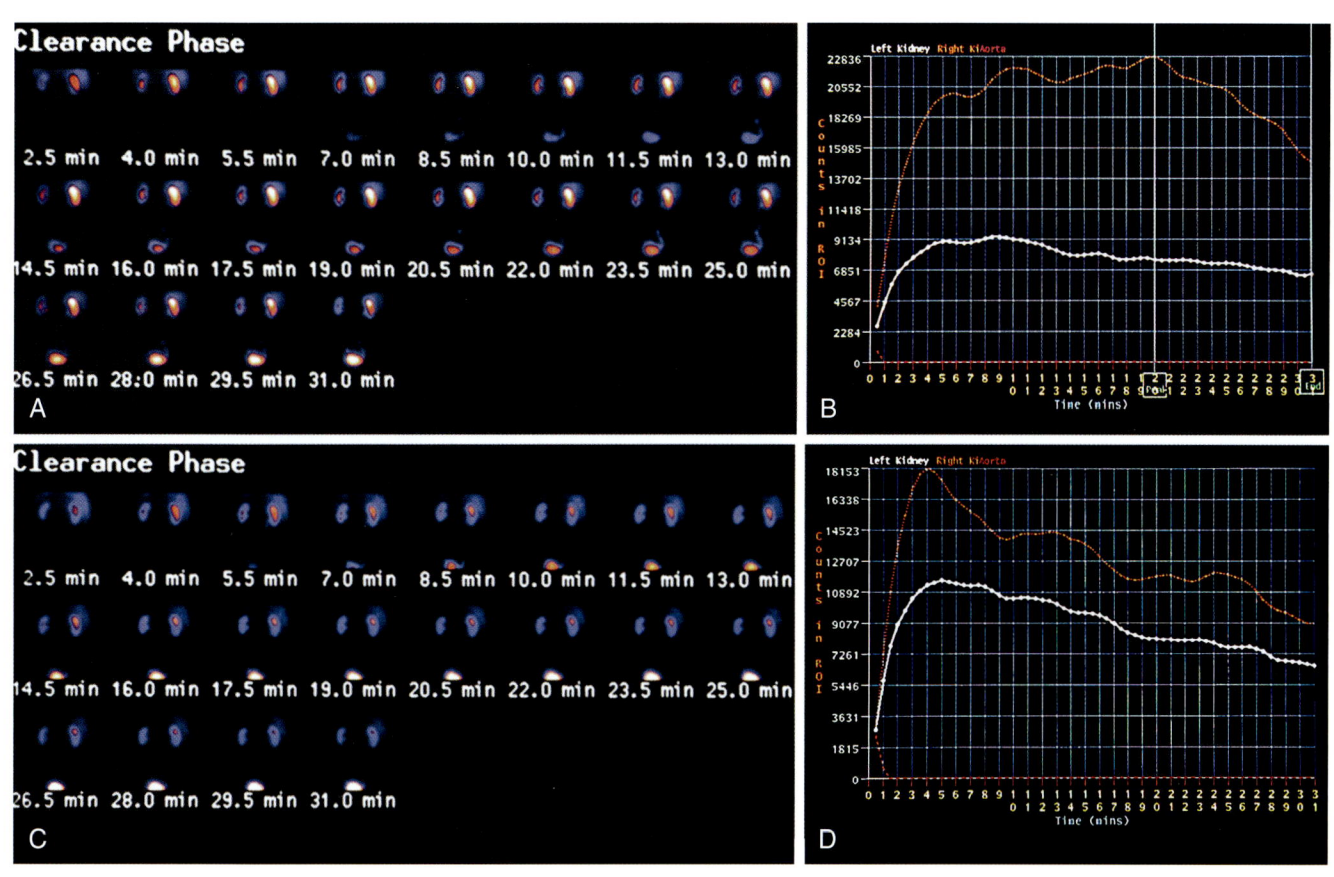

FIGURE 108-1 Positive captopril-augmented ^{99m}Tc-MAG3 renal scintigraphy. **A,** The captopril study was performed first and revealed asymmetric renal function and bilateral cortical retention. **B,** A baseline scan shows continued renal asymmetry but with normalization of right renal function and a small change in the left. The left kidney was interpreted as indeterminate for RAS, and further work-up revealed it to be small in size. The right kidney was interpreted as having a high probability for RAS.

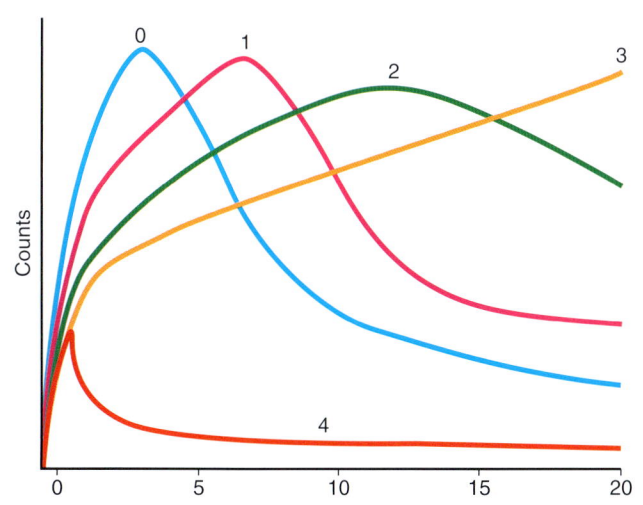

FIGURE 108-2 In the presence of RVH, renogram patterns will change following the administration of ACE inhibitors. Patterns are scored from 0 to 4, with 0 reflecting a normal curve and a low probability of RVH, and 4 indicating complete renal failure, with no washout and a high probability for RVH. The curves can be summarized as follows: grade 0, normal curve; grade 1, peak mildly delayed (longer than 5 minutes) and with delayed excretion; grade 2, very delayed uptake but some washout; grade 3, extremely delayed uptake with no washout; grade 4, complete renal failure, in which the blood pool moves through the kidney in the vascular phase, with no extraction phase. *(From Ziessman HA, O'Malley JP, Thrall JH. Nuclear Medicine: The Requisites, 3rd ed. Philadelphia, Mosby, 2006, p 237.)*

4. A change of 10% or more in differential function, the amount each kidney contributes to overall function. This finding is less common with ^{99m}Tc-MAG3 than with ^{99m}Tc-DTPA. It is a significant finding and, when present, is considered high probability for RVH. A change of 5% to 9% is considered intermediate.
5. With ^{99m}Tc-DTPA, a reduction in the glomerular filtration rate by 10% or more is also considered to be high probability for RVH.

KEY POINTS

- ACEI-augmented nuclear scintigraphy can be used to diagnose renovascular hypertension noninvasively.
- ACEI-augmented scintigraphy can be performed as a 1- or 2-day protocol.
- ACEI-augmented studies are assigned a likelihood of RAS, depending on changes in comparison to baseline studies.

SUGGESTED READINGS

Taylor AT, Blaufox MD, Dubovsky EV, et al. Society of Nuclear Medicine Procedure Guideline for Diagnosis of Renovascular Hypertension, version 3.0, June 20, 2003. Available at: http://www.health.gov.il/download/forms/pg_ch16.pdf. Accessed December 1, 2009.

Taylor A, Nally J, Aurell M, et al. Consensus report on ACE inhibitor renography for detecting renovascular hypertension. J Nucl Med 1996; 37:1876-1882.

REFERENCES

1. Taylor A, Nally J, Aurell M, et al. Consensus report on ACE inhibitor renography for detecting renovascular hypertension. J Nucl Med 1996; 37:1876-1882.
2. Blaufox MD, Middleton ML, Bongiovanni J, et al. Cost efficacy of the diagnosis and therapy of renovascular hypertension. J Nucl Med 1996; 37:171-177.
3. Ludwig V, Martin WH, Delbeke D. Calcium channel blockers: a potential cause of false-positive captopril renography. Clin Nucl Med 2003; 28:108-112.
4. Jung HS, Chung YA, Kim EN, et al. Influence of hydration status in normal subjects: fractional analysis of parameters of Tc-99m DTPA and Tc-99m MAG3 renography. Ann Nucl Med 2005; 19:1-7.
5. Dimitrou PA, Tsinikas DT, Depaskouale AK, et al. The effect of hydration on the dose to the urinary bladder wall during technetium-99m diethylene triamine penta-acetic acid renography. Eur J Nucl Med 1992; 19:765-769.
6. O'Reilly P, Aurell M, Brittonn K, et al. Consensus on diuretic renography for investigating the dilated upper renal tract. J Nucl Med 1996; 37:1872-1876.
7. Taylor A, Lewis C, Giacometti A, et al. Improved formulas for the estimation of renal depth in adults. J Nucl Med 1993; 34:1766-1769.
8. Gruenewald SM, Collins LT. Renovascular hypertension: quantitative renography as a screening test. Radiology 1983; 149:287-291.

CHAPTER 109

Sonography of the Renal Vessels

Rajesh Sharma and Vikram S. Dogra

Sonography of renal vessels in modern practice combines the use of gray-scale, color Doppler, power Doppler, and contrast-enhanced ultrasound imaging. Duplex sonography of renal vessels is a common screening modality for the evaluation of hypertensive patients worldwide because it is the most inexpensive and noninvasive imaging method. Duplex sonography has proven to be a good modality for the assessment of flow in renal and intrarenal vessels and enables measurement of flow parameters that are significant in many kidney diseases. Renal artery stenosis is the most common curable cause of hypertension and of end-stage renal disease as well. Sonography plays a vital role in the detection of renal artery stenosis and occlusion, and in the follow-up of renal stents and renal allografts. In addition, sonography of renal vessels is used to evaluate numerous other conditions, such as renal vein thrombosis and renal tumors. Renal Doppler ultrasound also provides valuable information regarding urinary tract obstruction and various other renal parenchymal diseases.

TECHNICAL REQUIREMENTS

Successful sonography of renal vessels requires the use of gray-scale sonography, tissue harmonics, color flow imaging, power Doppler, and spectral Doppler wave analysis. Additionally, ultrasound contrast agents can aid in the sonographic evaluation of renal vessels. In adult patients, a transducer frequency range between 3.5 and 5 MHz is required, whereas in pediatric patients a higher transducer frequency range can be used.[1,2] Transducers with higher frequencies, of 6 to 8 MHz or more, are used to evaluate renal allografts because of their superficial location as compared with native kidneys. The highest transducer frequency that will provide the best resolution should be selected, depending on the depth of penetration required.[3]

Patients should fast or be on a clear liquid diet starting at midnight the day before the examination.[2] Patients should also be encouraged to drink at least two 8-oz glasses of water the previous night and the morning of the examination.[4] An oral dose of simethicone, an antigas medication, may be helpful in reducing bowel gas.

TECHNIQUES

Renal vascular ultrasound is indicated for a broad range of renal arterial and venous indications (Box 109-1). Clinically, renal arterial indications are more common, notably for the evaluation of possible renal artery stenosis. Select indications are detailed later. There are no known contraindications for the sonography of renal vessels.

Renal Artery Stenosis

The detection of renal artery stenosis in hypertensive patients (i.e., evaluation for renal vascular hypertension) represents the overwhelming indication in most practices. Renal artery stenosis (RAS) is estimated to be responsible for less than 5% of cases of hypertension. However, because it is one of the few treatable causes of hypertension, second only to the secondary hypertension caused by the use of oral contraceptives in women,[5] it remains a common indication for renal artery imaging. About one quarter to one third of all patients with RAS eventually develop ischemic nephropathy. Renovascular hypertension is also responsible for the development of end-stage renal disease in 20% of patients. RAS is also seen in approximately 7% of all patients who have cardiovascular diseases (e.g., atherosclerosis, myocardial infarction, congestive heart failure). Its association with stroke has also been reported. Atherosclerosis is the most common cause of RAS, with fibromuscular dysplasia representing a distant second, but other entities such as Takayasu arteritis can also result in renal artery stenosis.

Atherosclerotic Renal Artery Stenosis

Atherosclerotic RAS usually involves the ostium and proximal segment (proximally within 2 cm) of renal arteries. Bilateral atherosclerotic RAS can be seen in a significant number with some case series reporting it in 50% of

1497

> **BOX 109-1 Indications for Renal Vascular Ultrasound**
>
> - Recent onset of hypertension in patients younger than 25 years
> - Sudden, abrupt onset of hypertension in patients older than 45 or 50 years
> - Malignant or accelerated hypertension or grade 3 or 4 hypertensive retinopathy; diastolic BP > 110 mm Hg
> - Hypertension resistant to usual three-drug (or more) therapy
> - Sudden exacerbation of previously well-controlled hypertension
> - Onset of hypertension within the last 2 years
> - Deteriorating renal function in hypertensive patients
> - Patients with aortic aneurysm or vasculitis or arteritis
> - Unexplained azotemia
> - Azotemia in response to administration of angiotensin-converting enzyme (ACE) inhibitors
> - Unexplained hypokalemia
> - Small atrophic kidney (unilateral) with reduced renal function
> - Flash pulmonary edema or recurrent flash pulmonary edema without cardiac explanation
> - Unexplained congestive heart failure
> - Preoperative assessment for suitability of renal transplant
> - Postoperative assessment of renal allograft for vascular complications
> - Follow-up for adequacy of the renal artery flow after percutaneous angioplasty or surgical bypass
> - Follow-up of the renal artery for stent patency in all cases
> - Detection of restenosis after endovascular therapy
> - Monitoring of the renal functional response to reperfusion and prediction of clinical outcome after renal artery revascularization
> - Assessment of the renal vein in all cases of renal mass
> - Seeing the extent of renal vein thrombosis in renal cell cancer (RCC) and adrenal masses
> - Renal trauma
> - Patients in whom MRA is problematic or contraindicated
> - Patients with renal disease in whom MDCT angiography is problematic or contraindicated (e.g., poor renal function or first trimester of pregnancy)
>
> **RELATIVE INDICATIONS**
>
> - Assess cases of obstructive uropathy in which gray-scale sonography is equivocal and noncontrast abdominal CT is contraindicated, as for pregnant patients.
> - Assess tumor vascularity and grade of vascularity in small renal masses.
> - Assess kidneys in diabetic nephropathy.
> - Assess kidneys in lupus nephropathy.
> - Differentiate transient renal arterial ischemia from arterial infarction.
> - Predict oligohydramnios in post–term pregnancy.

patients. Atherosclerotic RAS is invariably associated with atherosclerotic changes in the aorta.

Atherosclerotic RAS is mostly progressive, because 20% to 50% of patients with 50% stenosis of renal arteries show progression of the disease within a few years, and 12% to 20% of those having greater than 75% RAS end up with complete occlusion within a year (Figs. 109-1 to 109-9). If RAS patients are left untreated, then in addition to worsening renovascular hypertension, 5% to 16% of these patients will progress to complete occlusion of the renal artery. Even in cases of unilateral RAS, damage to the other kidney in the form of nephrosclerosis caused by increased systemic blood pressure will occur if RAS is left untreated.

Fibromuscular Dysplasia

Fibromuscular dysplasia (FMD) results in RAS involving mainly the mid or distal part, and sometimes the intrarenal branches, of the renal artery (Fig. 109-10). FMD is almost eight times more commonly seen in females than males and usually occurs in younger individuals. FMD represents a collection of vascular diseases that affect the intima, media, and adventitia. It generally accounts for less than 10% of cases of RAS. FMD can be classified according to the layer of the arterial wall involved. Clinically, FMD involves the renal artery in three forms, with most (up to 90% of patients) having medial fibroplasia, which typically affects patients younger than 35 years. About one third of patients with medial fibroplasia show progression of the disease, but complications such as dissection and thrombosis are rarely seen.

The classic appearance of FMD, which is seen in 85% of patients, is known as the string of beads appearance, as seen angiographically. An endovascular ultrasound study of FMD by Gowda and colleagues[6] has challenged the status of renal angiography as the gold standard for RAS in FMD patients. Other findings of FMD, such as a fibrous diaphragm, may not be seen sonographically; however, focal narrowing of the main artery caused by medial or adventitial hyperplasia might be seen.

Takayasu Arteritis

Takayasu arteritis, or nonspecific arteritis, is associated with stenosis (and occlusion) of the aorta and renal arteries (Figs. 109-11 to 109-15). This disease is more prevalent in Far Eastern and Southeast Asian countries.[7] The disease is classified into four types, with each type assigned to the vessels involved: aortic arch, thoracoabdominal aorta and its branches, both aortic arch and thoracoabdominal aorta, and pulmonary arteries.[8] The thoracoabdominal type is more common in the Indian subcontinent and Southeast Asia, as is middle aortic syndrome. The disease predominantly involves the media of the vessel and then progresses to cause fibrosis of intima and the adventitia. Most of the patients present during adulthood, very frequently during the third decade of life.

Renal Artery Thrombosis

A renal artery can be occluded by atherosclerotic embolism, thromboembolism, thrombus in situ, aortic dissection, or vasculitis. Renal artery embolism is a common cause of renal insufficiency in older patients, especially those with atherosclerosis. Renal artery thromboembolism can occur in association with a variety of conditions, such

Text continued on p. 1505

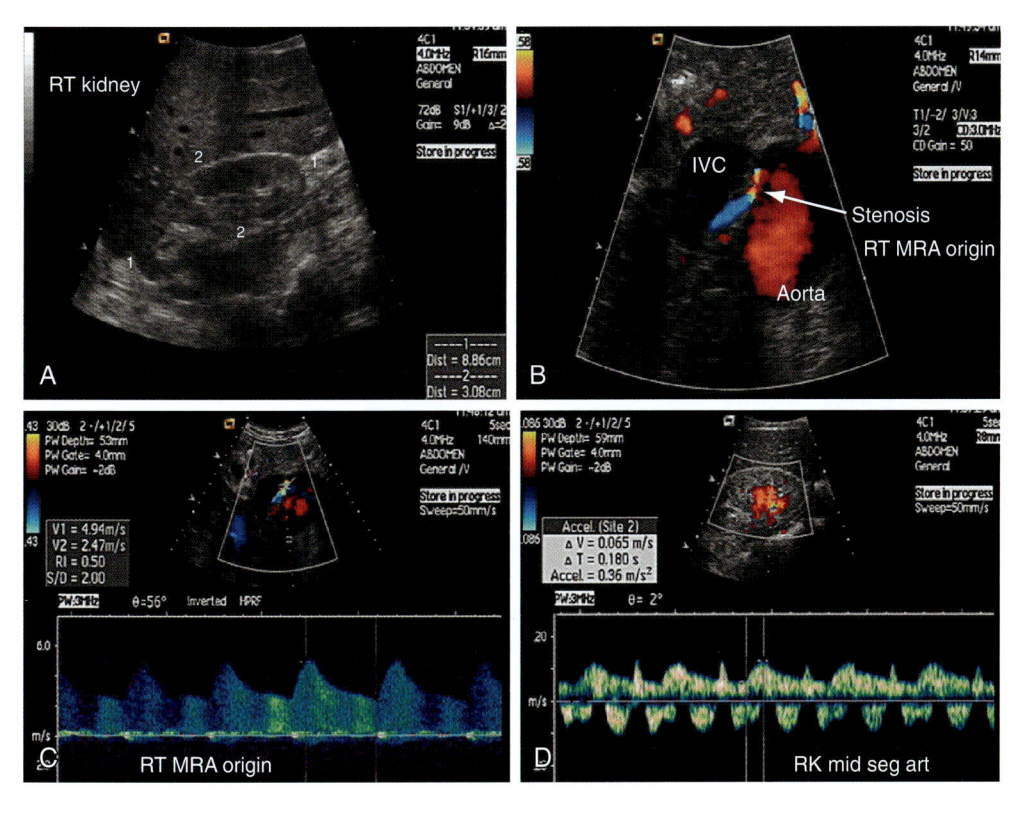

CHAPTER 109 • *Sonography of the Renal Vessels* 1499

■ **FIGURE 109-1** Atherosclerotic renal artery stenosis at the level of origin of right renal artery. **A,** Longitudinal gray-scale image in right lateral decubitus position reveals the longitudinal dimension of the right kidney to be 8.86 cm. The left kidney measured 10.6 cm in the longitudinal plane (not shown). **B,** Color Doppler image reveals an area of color aliasing (*arrow*) at the origin of the right renal artery, suggestive of stenosis of the origin of the right main renal artery (RTMRA). **C,** Pulse wave Doppler imaging at the origin of the right renal artery reveals a peak systolic velocity of 4.94 m/sec. **D,** Pulse wave Doppler of the middle segmental artery reveals an acceleration time of 0.18 seconds, acceleration index of 0.36 m/sec^2, and pulsus tardus parvus waveform.

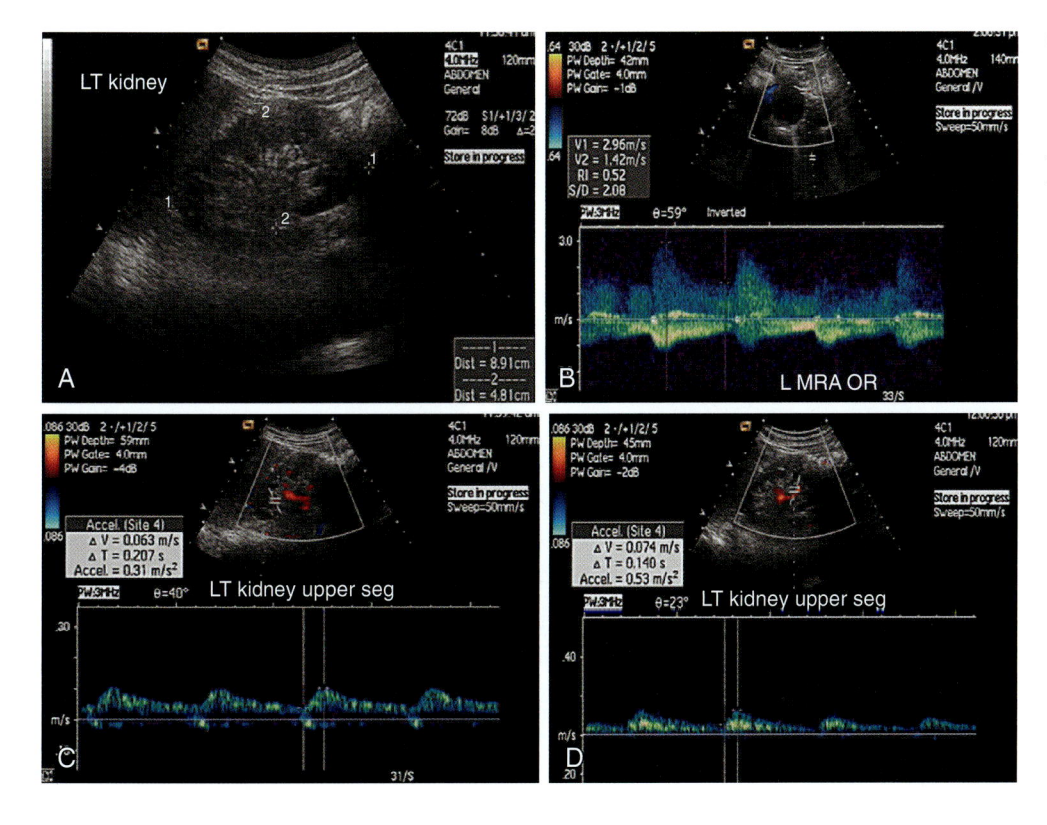

■ **FIGURE 109-2** Atherosclerotic renal artery stenosis at the origin of left renal artery (**A**) has resulted in small (8.91-cm) left kidney (**B**) and increased peak systolic velocity. The pulsus tardus parvus waveform of upper segmental artery is seen (**C, D**).

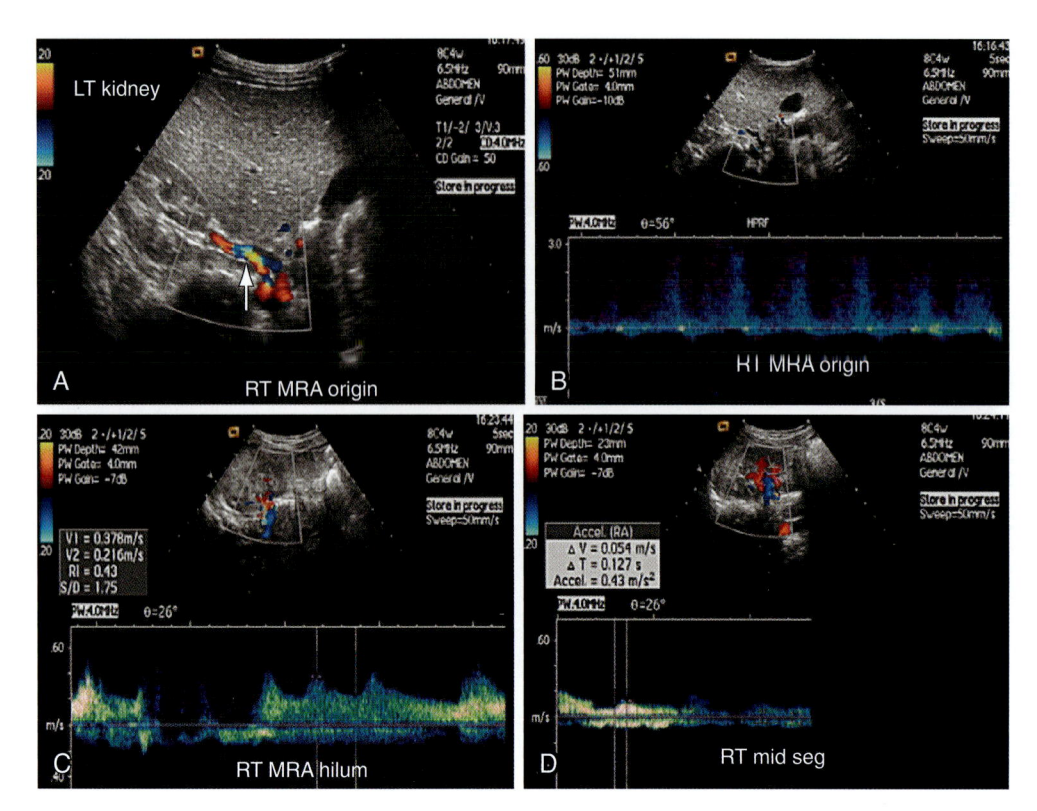

FIGURE 109-3 **A,** Stenosis (*arrow*) at the origin of the right renal artery, with increased peak systolic velocity in the renal artery at the origin **(B)** of the renal artery and hilum **(C)**. **D,** Tardus parvus waveform in middle segmental artery.

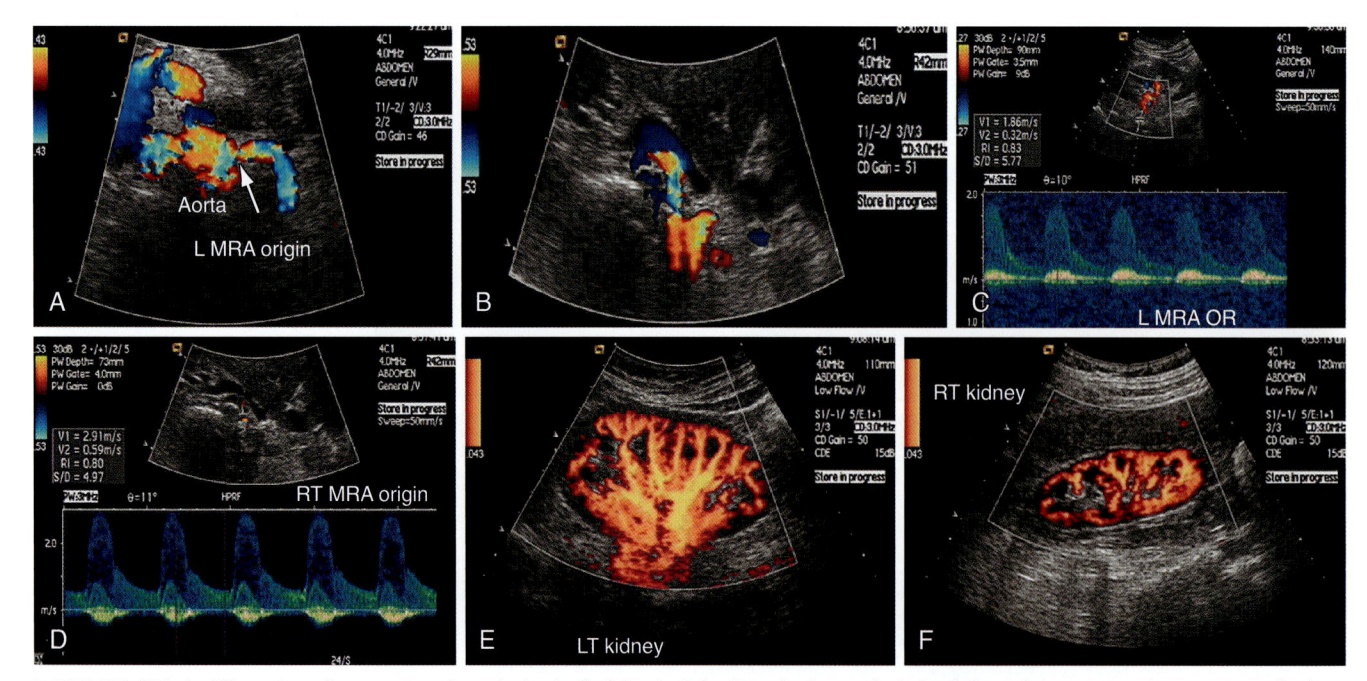

FIGURE 109-4 Bilateral renal artery stenosis at the level of origin. **A,** Color Doppler image depicting left renal artery stenosis as an area of color aliasing (*arrow*). **B,** Color Doppler image of right renal artery stenosis. Spectral waveform analysis shows peak systolic velocities of 1.86 m/sec (left renal artery) **(C)** and 2.91 m/sec (right renal artery) **(D)**. Also shown are the perfusion images of the left **(E)** and right **(F)** kidneys.

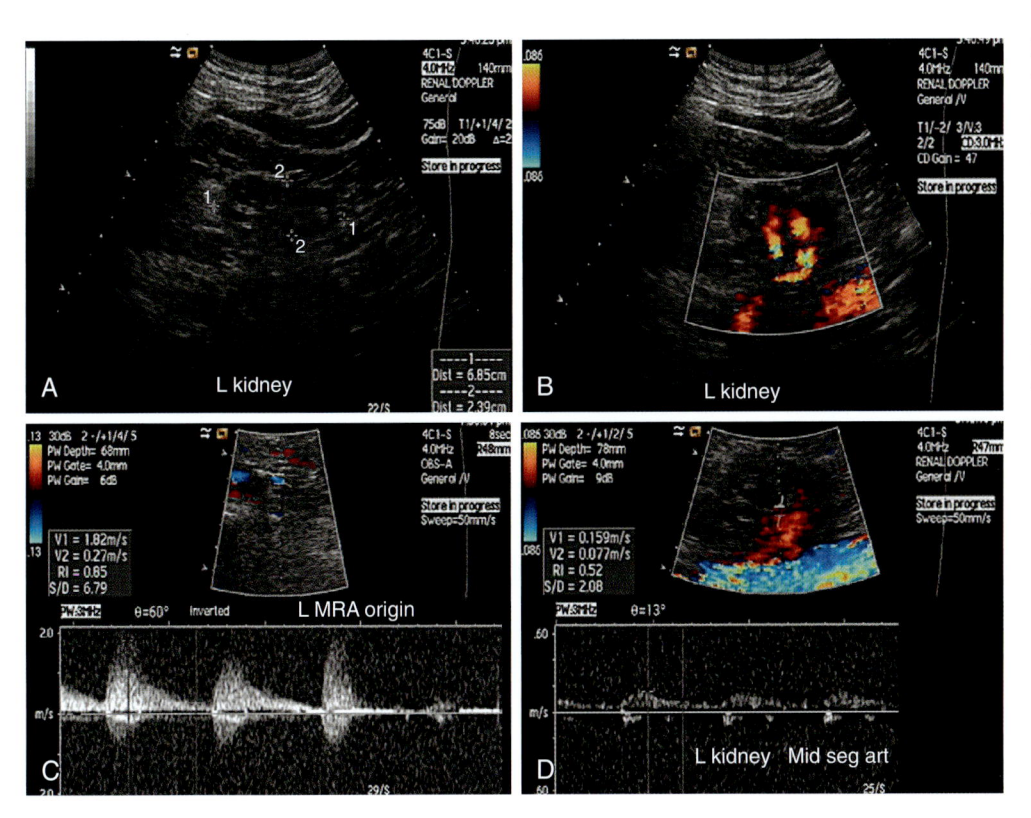

CHAPTER 109 • *Sonography of the Renal Vessels* 1501

■ **FIGURE 109-5** Critical renal artery stenosis. **A,** Gray-scale longitudinal image shows longitudinal dimension of left kidney (6.85 cm). **B,** Color Doppler image acquired in lateral decubitus position. **C,** Spectral waveform at the level of origin of renal artery shows a PSV of 1.82 m/sec. **D,** Spectral waveform of middle segmental artery reveals a tardus parvus waveform supporting the diagnosis of a hemodynamically significant renal artery stenosis.

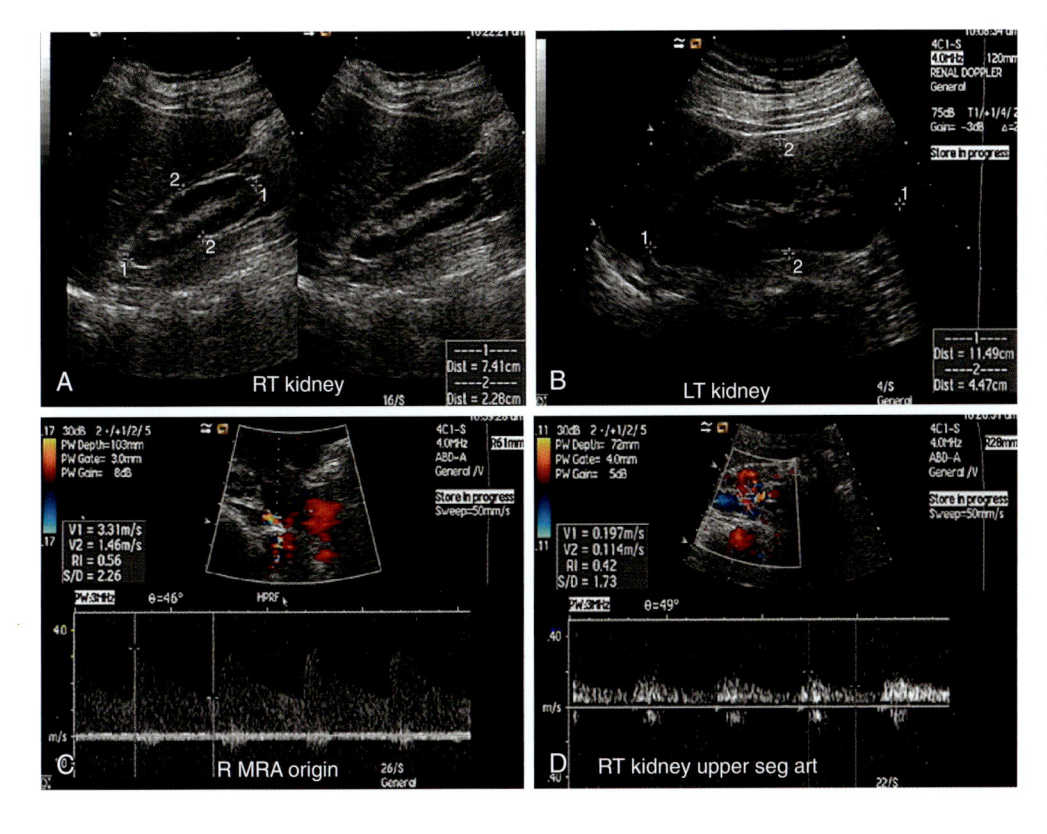

■ **FIGURE 109-6** Right renal artery stenosis at the origin of right renal artery. Gray-scale longitudinal images of right **(A)** and left **(B)** kidneys reveal considerable differences in the longitudinal dimensions of both kidneys. **C,** Spectral Doppler image reveals a PSV of 3.31 m/sec at the origin of the right renal artery. **D,** Spectral waveform of right upper segmental artery reveals pulsus tardus parvus waveform.

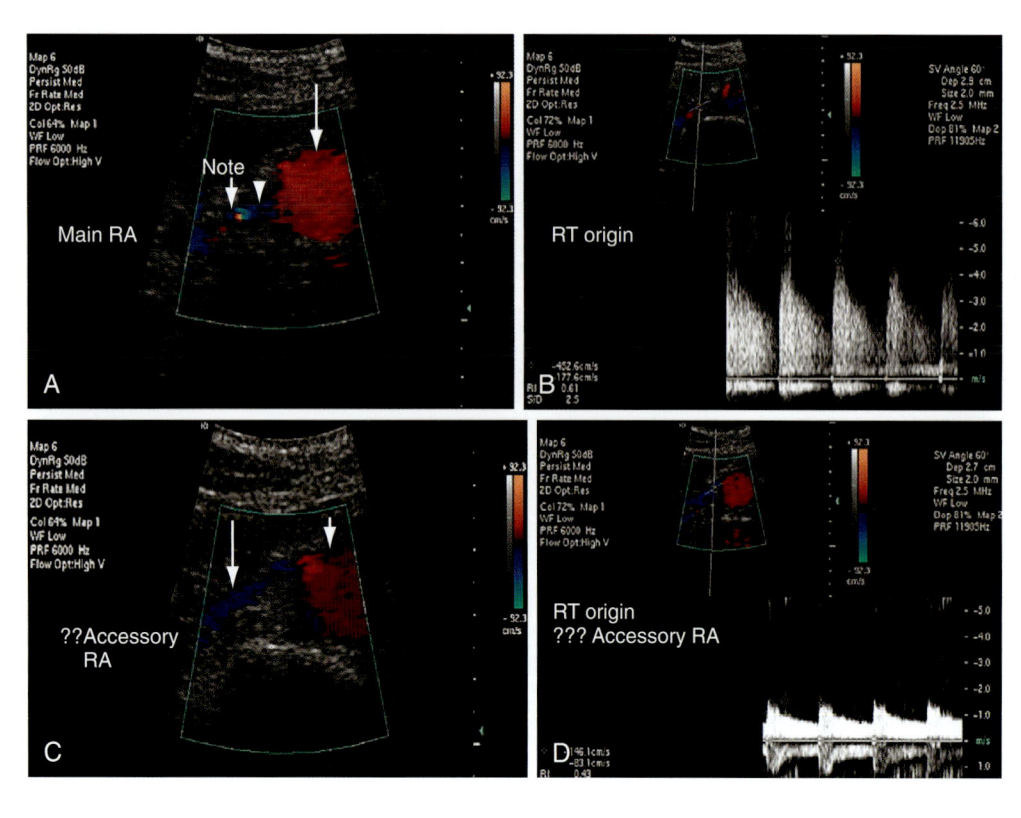

■ **FIGURE 109-7** Stenosis of main renal artery with normal accessory artery. **A,** Color aliasing (*short arrow*) is seen in the proximal segment (*arrowhead*) of the right renal artery. **B,** Pulse wave Doppler image of the proximal segment of main renal artery reveals a peak systolic velocity of 452 cm/sec. **C,** Accessory renal artery (*long arrow*) is seen arising from the aorta (*short arrow*). **D,** Pulse wave Doppler ultrasound image of the accessory renal artery reveals a normal peak systolic velocity of 145.1 cm/sec.

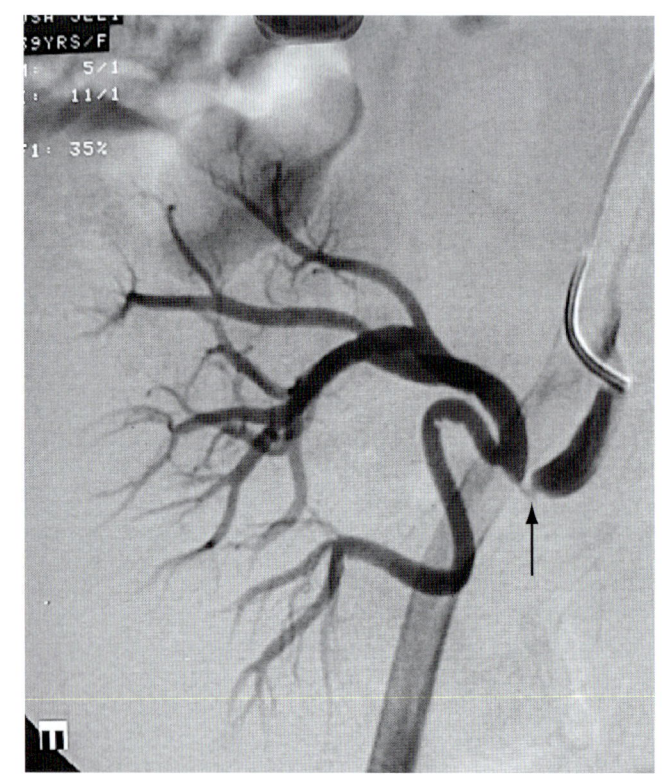

■ **FIGURE 109-8** A 36-year-old female patient presented with deteriorating renal function after renal transplantation. Renal angiography reveals stenosis of the middle segment of the renal artery supplying the allograft (*arrow*).

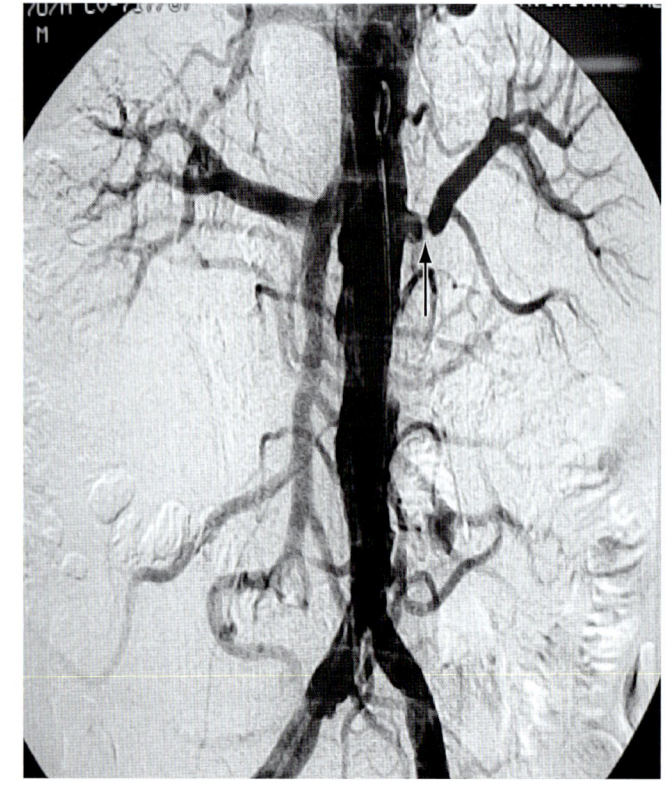

■ **FIGURE 109-9** Renal angiogram shows stenosis (*arrow*) in the proximal segment of left renal artery. (*Courtesy of Dr. Gurpreet Singh Gulati, New Delhi, India.*)

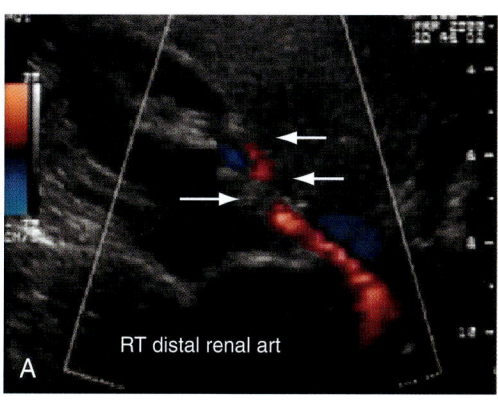

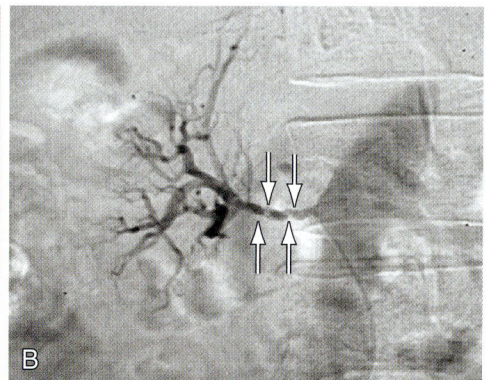

■ **FIGURE 109-10**
Fibromuscular dysplasia (FMD). **A,** Color Doppler image of an FMD patient shows stenosis (*arrows*) of the distal segment of right renal artery. **B,** Renal angiogram of another FMD patient shows the classic string of beads appearance (*arrows*). (**A,** courtesy of Dr. Mukund Joshi, Mumbai, India; **B,** courtesy of Dr. Gurpreet Singh Gulati, New Delhi, India.)

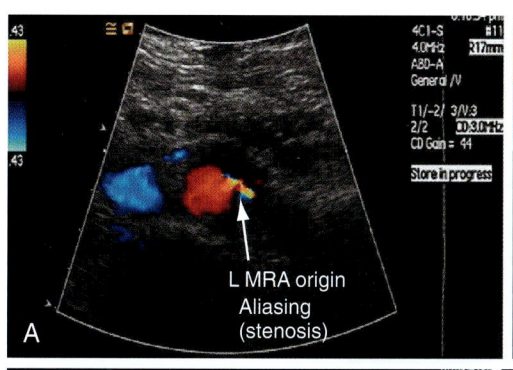

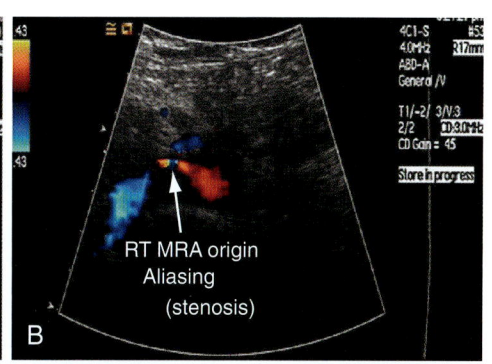

■ **FIGURE 109-11** Takayasu arteritis in a young female patient presenting with bilateral renal artery stenosis along with aortic stenosis (not shown here). Color aliasing (*arrow*) is seen at the site of stenosis of the left (**A**) and right (**B**) renal arteries. Spectral analysis shows PSV of 3.09 m/sec, left renal artery (**C**) and 3.22 m/sec, right renal artery (**D**).

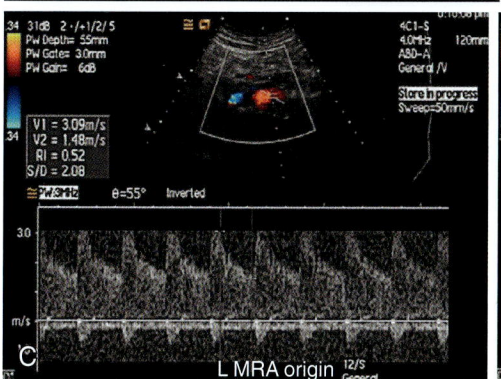

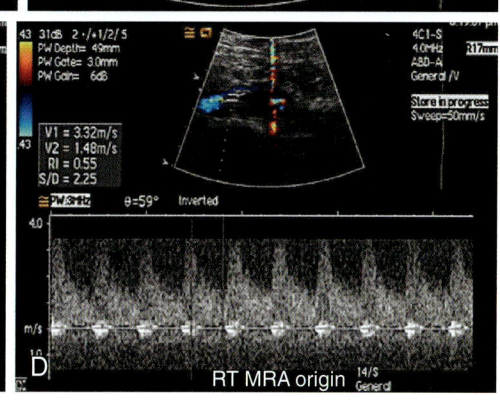

■ **FIGURE 109-12** Aortitis in a 17-year-old male involving the aorta and both renal arteries. **A, B,** Color Doppler images of the right renal artery (RA) and left renal artery (LRA). Spectral waveforms of the left renal artery at the hilum (**C**) and right intrarenal artery (**D**) reveal elevated PSVs.

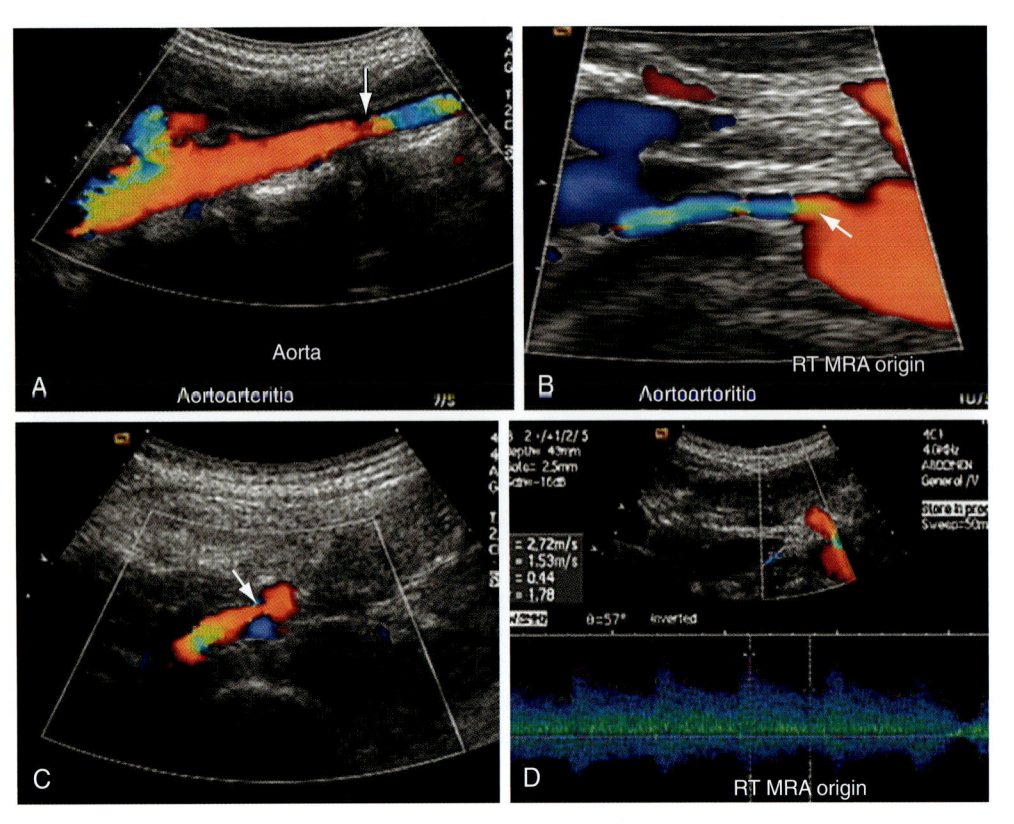

■ **FIGURE 109-13** Aortitis in a female patient. **A,** Color Doppler image shows aortic stenosis (*arrow*). **B,** Color Doppler image shows stenosis at the origin of right renal artery (*arrow*). **C,** Color Doppler image shows stenosis (*arrow*) of the left renal artery. **D,** Spectral analysis of right renal artery shows an elevated PSV of 2.72 m/sec.

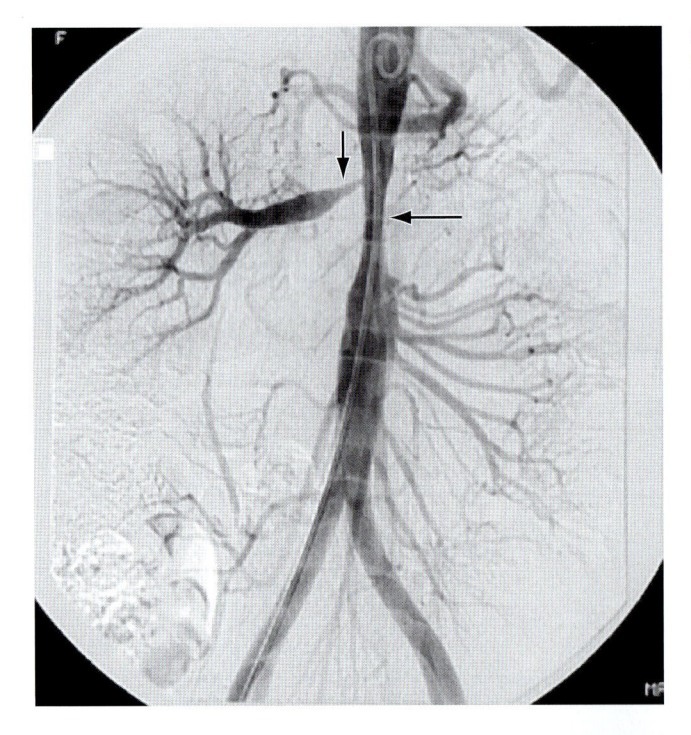

■ **FIGURE 109-14** Renal catheter angiogram in a patient with aortitis shows smooth, long-segment stenoses of the abdominal aorta (*long arrow*) and right renal artery (*short arrow*).

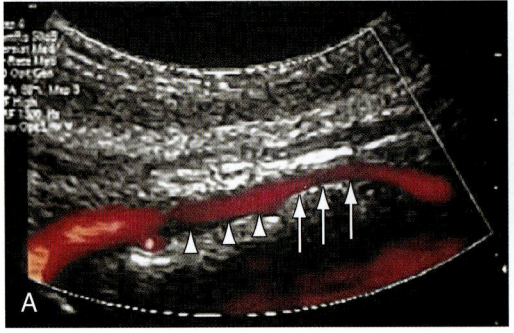

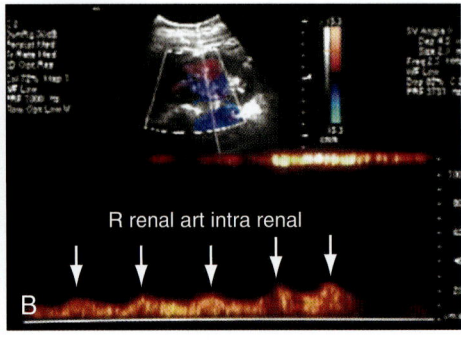

■ **FIGURE 109-15** Aortitis. **A,** Color Doppler image of aorta in longitudinal plane shows smooth long segment of narrowing of the aorta, with areas of moderate (*arrowheads*) to severe stenosis (*arrows*). **B,** Spectral waveform of right middle segmental artery shows tardus parvus waveform pattern (*arrows*). (*Courtesy of Dr. Mukund Joshi, Mumbai, India.*)

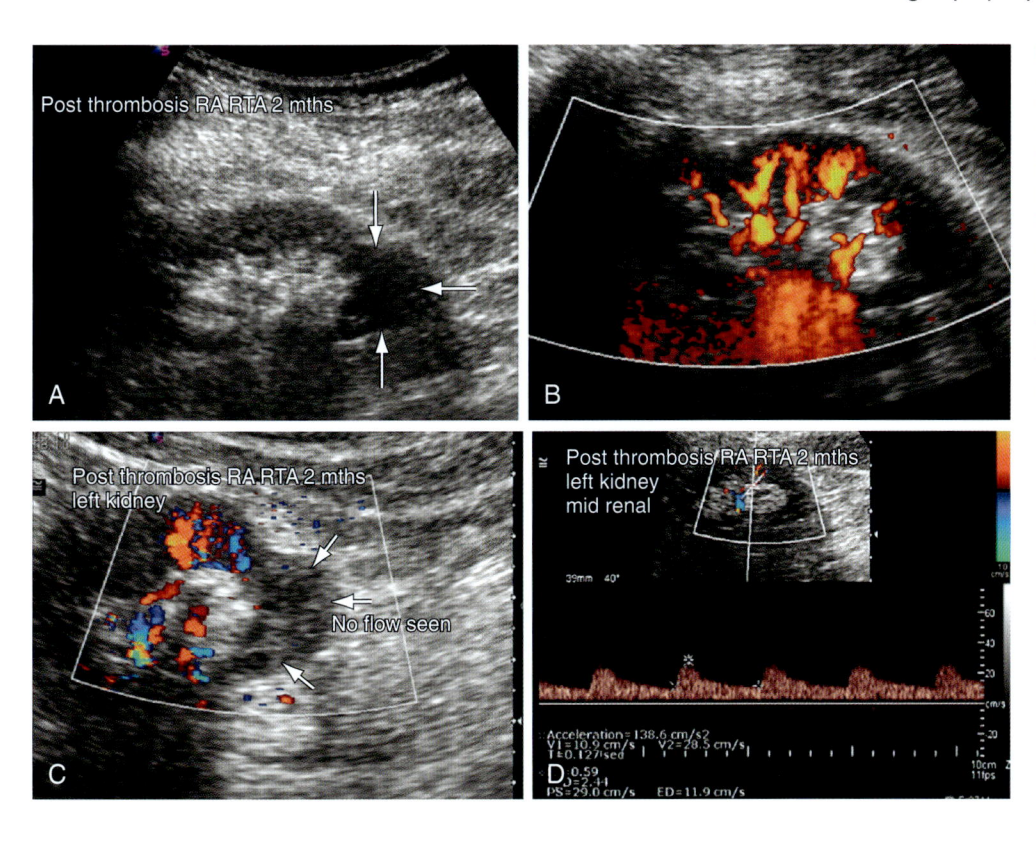

■ FIGURE 109-16 Follow-up (after 2 months) case of renal artery thrombosis subsequent to a traffic accident. **A**, Longitudinal gray-scale image shows a slightly hypoechoic area (*arrows*) in the lower pole of the kidney. **B**, Perfusion image shows no perfusion in the lower pole. **C**, Color Doppler image shows no flow in the lower pole (*arrows*). **D**, Spectral waveform of middle segmental artery. *(Courtesy of Dr. T.H.S. Bedi, DCA Imaging Centre, New Delhi, India.)*

as aortic aneurysm, myocardial infarction, bacterial endocarditic, aseptic vegetations, and even paradoxical emboli originating in the right heart caused by congenital heart diseases such as atrial septal defect (ASD; Fig. 109-16).

Renal Vein Thrombosis

Renal vein occlusion can occur because of thrombus formation, intraluminal tumor, or external compression of the renal vein. The predisposing factors for renal vein thrombosis (RVT) are nephrotic syndrome, membranous glomerulonephritis, hypercoagulable states, abdominal surgery, dehydration, trauma, renal cell carcinoma and, rarely, hypereosinophilic syndrome (Figs. 109-17 and 109-18).[9-13] Renal vein thrombosis is commonly seen in patients with nephrotic syndrome and can present as acute or chronic RVT. RVT occurs in up to 40% of patients of nephrotic syndrome caused by membranous glomerulopathy, membranoproliferative glomerulonephritis, and amyloidosis. RVT is frequently bilateral in cases of nephrotic syndrome.

Intraluminal extension of tumor into the renal vein can occur with renal malignancy, notably renal cell carcinoma, but also may be seen with renal lymphoma, transitional cell carcinoma, and adrenal tumors such as Wilms' tumor.[14,15] Extension of the thrombus from ovarian veins into the renal vein can also occur.[16]

Renal Transplant Assessment

Renal transplantation is becoming routine practice and evaluation presents a particular challenge. Ultrasound is an ideally suited modality for renal transplant assessment because of its relatively lower cost and excellent ability to assess the transplant noninvasively without the need for ionizing radiation or the use of iodinated contrast agents, with their inherent nephrotoxicity concerns. Further discussion of renal transplant imaging can be found in Chapter 112.

TECHNIQUE DESCRIPTION

Sonography of the renal vessels includes evaluation of the main renal arteries, intrarenal arteries, main renal veins, abdominal aorta, and renovascular function, including overall renal perfusion.

Anatomic Considerations

Renal Arteries

Both renal arteries arise from the abdominal aorta approximately 1 to 1.5 cm below the origin of the superior mesenteric artery and at the level of the superior border of the L2 vertebra, with the origin of the left renal artery (LRA) slightly inferior to the right renal artery (RRA; Fig. 109-19). The RRA arises from the anterolateral aspect of the aorta at approximately the 10 o'clock position and the left main renal artery arises from the posterior or lateral aspect of the aorta at about the 4 o'clock position. The RRA courses anterolaterally in its proximal few centimeters, and then courses posterior to the inferior vena cava (IVC) and eventually follows a posterolateral course towards the right kidney (Figs. 109-20 and 109-21). Sonographically, it is identified as the largest vessel seen posterior to the inferior vena cava. The LRA runs a shorter

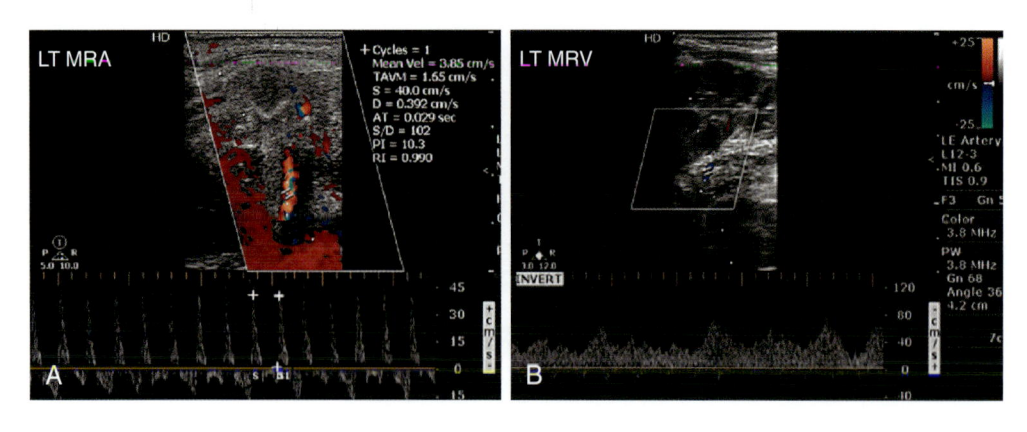

■ **FIGURE 109-17** Renal vein thrombosis in a 2-day-old neonate. **A,** Pulse wave Doppler image shows increased mean velocity (3.85 m/sec) in the renal artery and increased RI (0.99). **B,** Follow-up pulse wave Doppler image 2 weeks after systemic thrombolysis. The spectral waveform in the left renal vein is suggestive of its patency. *(Courtesy of Dr. Gurpreet Singh Gulati, New Delhi, India.)*

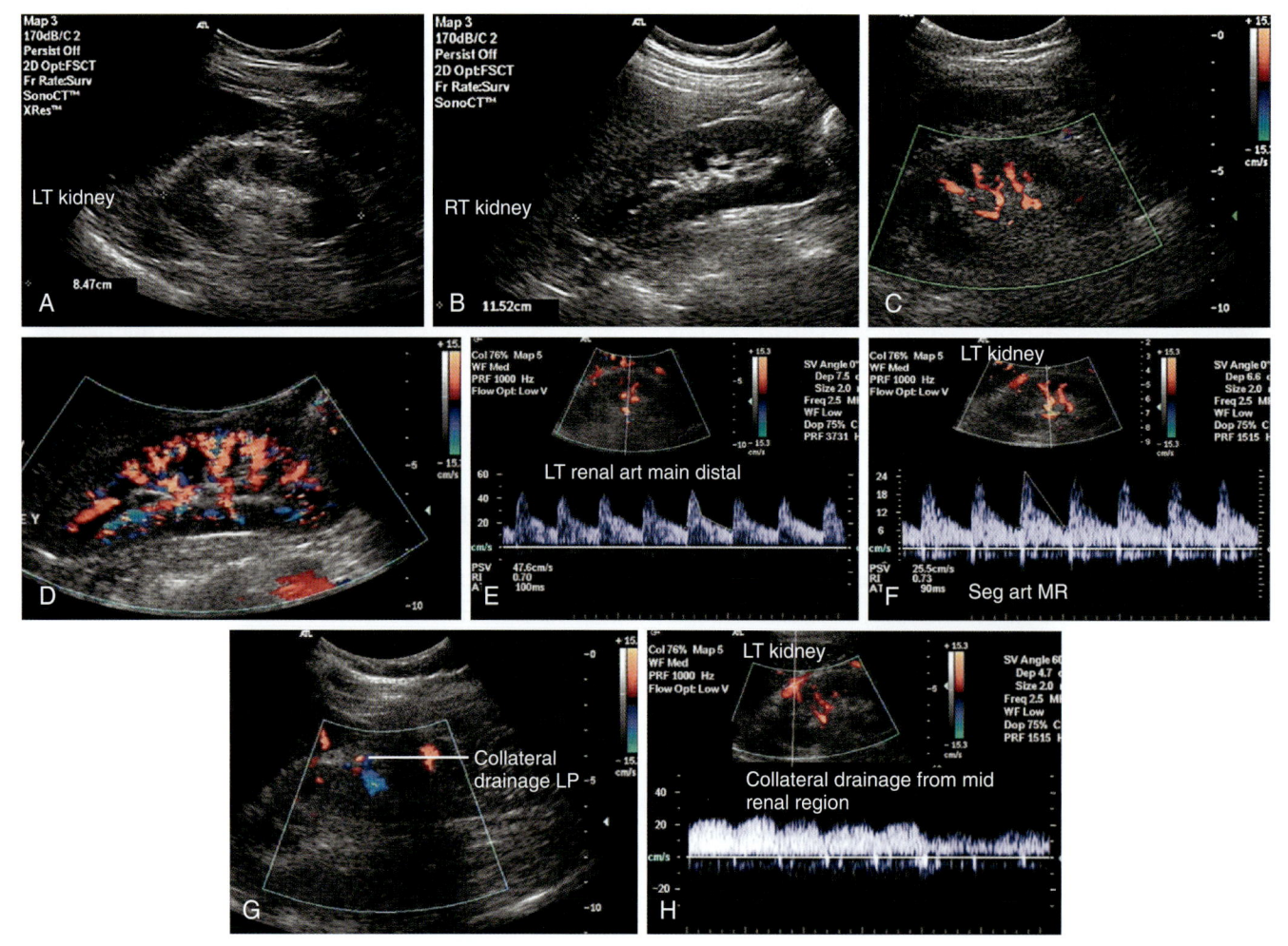

■ **FIGURE 109-18** Follow-up evaluation at 6 months in a patient with a history of left renal vein thrombosis demonstrates collateral venous drainage. Gray-scale longitudinal images of the left **(A)** and right kidney **(B)** show significant differences between the longitudinal dimensions of both kidneys. Color Doppler images of the left kidney **(C)** and right kidney **(D)** reveal only residual flow in the midpole of the left kidney but normal flow in the right kidney. **E, F,** Color Doppler and spectral waveform images of left main renal artery **(E)** and left middle segmental artery **(F)**. **G,** Collateral venous drainage is seen in the midpole of the left kidney. **H,** Spectral waveform of collateral venous drainage of the left kidney. *(Courtesy of Dr. T.H.S. Bedi, DCA Imaging Centre, New Delhi, India.)*

FIGURE 109-19 Color Doppler image acquired by the midline transverse approach shows origin of both renal arteries from aorta.

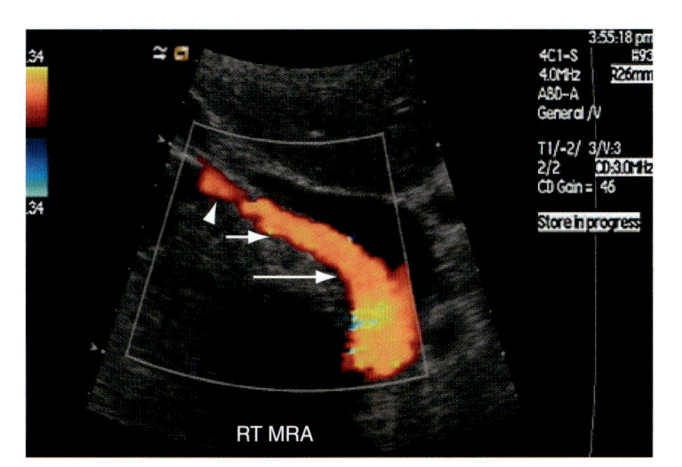

FIGURE 109-20 Color Doppler image shows proximal (*long arrow*), middle (*short arrow*) and distal (*arrowhead*) segments of the right renal artery.

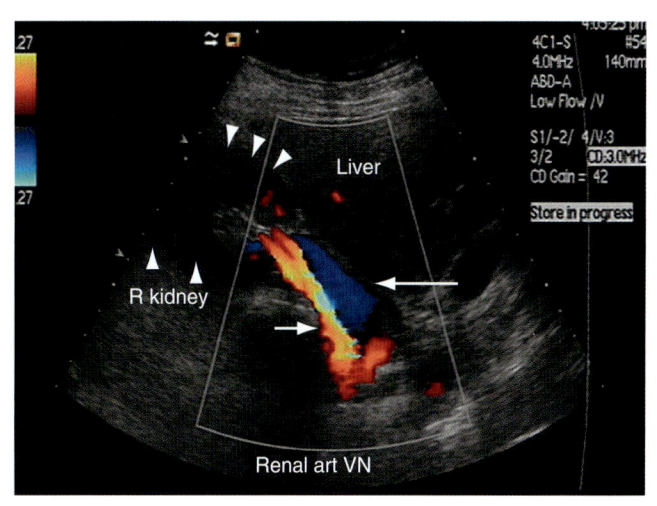

FIGURE 109-21 Color Doppler image acquired in the left lateral decubitus position by the intercostal approach by using the liver and right kidney (*arrowheads*) as acoustic windows. The right renal vein (*long arrow*) lies anterior to the right renal artery (*short arrow*).

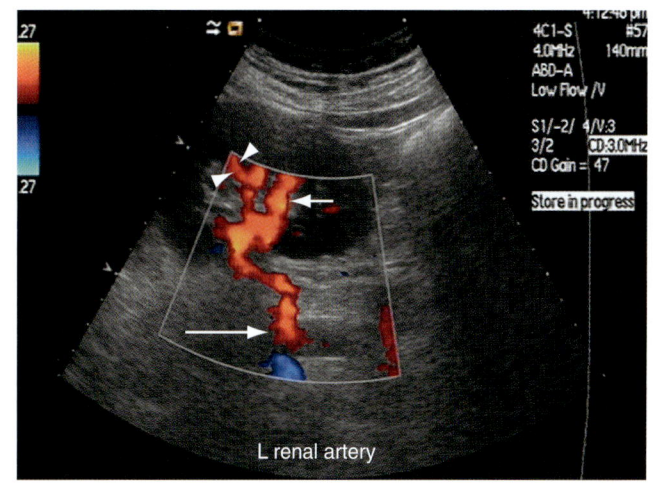

FIGURE 109-22 Color Doppler image in the left lateral decubitus position using the left kidney as acoustic window. The left renal artery (*long arrow*) enters the renal hilum and divides into segmental arteries (*short arrow*), and the segmental artery gives rise to interlobar arteries (*arrowheads*).

course and passes between the superior mesenteric artery and the left adrenal vein (Fig. 109-22). Bannister and associates[17] have reported accessory renal arteries in approximately 25% to 30% of individuals; however, most imaging studies have reported these in from 12% to 22% of patients (Fig. 109-23). The accessory renal arteries can arise from the aorta or iliac arteries. The rate of successful imaging of the accessory renal artery varies between 0% and 24%. In the presence of a normal main renal artery, a concerted attempt should be made to search for these vessels because stenosis of an accessory renal artery can similarly result in renovascular hypertension.[18-20] The small caliber of the main renal artery is an indirect clue to the presence of the accessory renal artery.[21]

Intrarenal Arteries: Segmental, Interlobar, and Arcuate Arteries

After entering the hilum, the main renal arteries split into anterior and posterior divisions. The arteries in these divisions give rise to segmental arteries, usually four, that supply each of the four vascular regions of the kidney—apical, anterior, posterior, and inferior. The segmental arteries give rise to lobar and interlobar arteries that travel between the medullary pyramids (Fig. 109-24). After traversing the corticomedullary junction, interlobar arteries give rise to arcuate arteries. Arcuate arteries give rise to the cortical and medullary branches, which supply the cortex and medulla, respectively. Most of the blood flow (90%) to the kidney goes to the cortex, with only 10% flowing into the medulla.

Renal Veins

The right renal vein lies anterior to the right main renal artery and runs in a posterior to anterior direction to end in the IVC. On sonography, the left renal vein appears larger than the right in a supine position. The left adrenal vein, left gonadal vein, and lumbar veins are tributaries of the left renal vein (Fig. 109-25). The left renal vein runs a horizontal course and is placed anterior to the aorta and posterior to the superior mesenteric artery. The left renal vein ends at the IVC at the level of the L1 vertebra. The

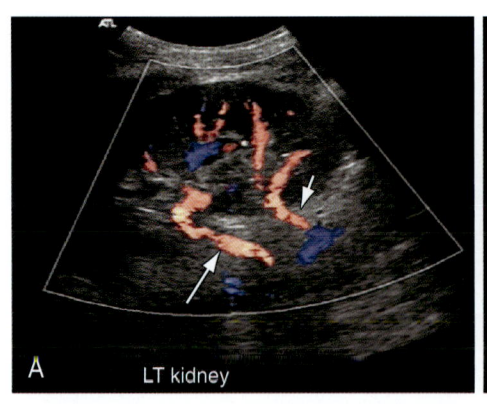

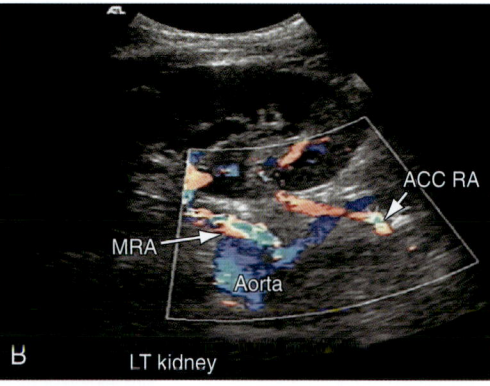

■ FIGURE 109-23 A, Accessory renal artery (*short arrow*) and left main renal artery (*long arrow*) are seen supplying the left kidney. B, Left main renal artery (*long arrow*) and accessory renal artery (*short arrow*) are seen arising from aorta.

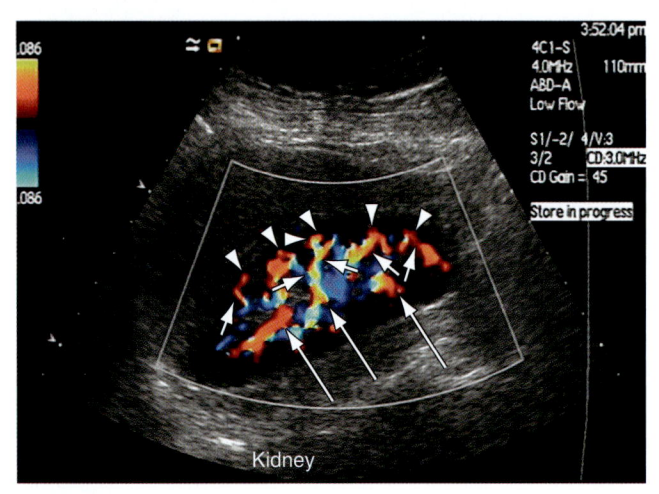

■ FIGURE 109-24 Normal intrarenal vessels. Segmental arteries (*long arrows*) give rise to the interlobar arteries (*short arrows*), which further give rise to the arcuate arteries (*arrowheads*).

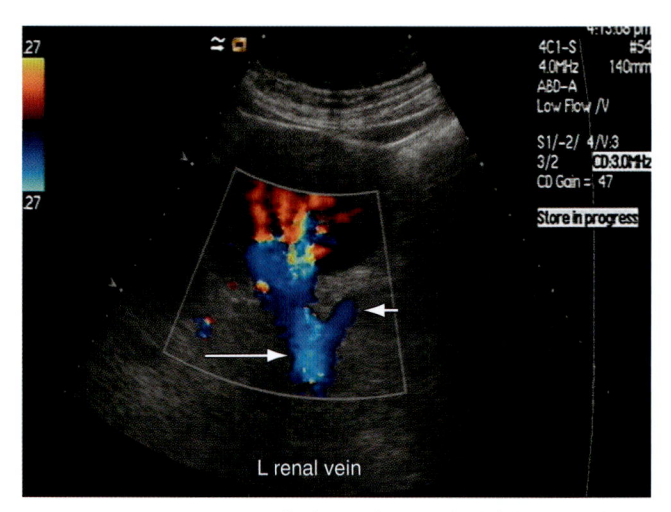

■ FIGURE 109-25 Longitudinal scan through the left kidney in the right lateral decubitus position. The left renal vein arises from the hilum of the left kidney (*long arrow*). The left adrenal vein (*short arrow*) drains into the left renal vein. Blood flow in the renal and adrenals veins is blue because the direction of blood flow is away from the transducer.

left renal vein can be retroaortic in 0.5% to 3.7% of patients, but has been reported to be as high as 25%.[2,22]

Abdominal Aorta

Sonography of renal vessels is always preceded by sonography of the aorta.[2,4,14] The presence of atherosclerotic plaque in the aorta increases the possibility of atherosclerotic ostial stenosis of the renal arteries. To see the presence of atherosclerotic plaque in the abdominal aorta, the aorta should be scanned in its entirety—that is, from the origin of the celiac artery to the bifurcation of the aorta into the common iliac arteries. The ostium of the superior mesenteric artery and the celiac artery should also be assessed. In addition to atherosclerotic plaque, the aorta is also evaluated for any aneurysm, stenosis, coarctation, or features of aortic arteritis (Figs. 109-26 and 109-27).[7] Examination of the aorta should include evaluation in the sagittal, transverse, and coronal planes. If bowel gas interferes with the visualization of the aorta, the transducer can be placed in paramedian longitudinal planes, and medial sweeps of the transducer can then be made to facilitate visualization of the aorta.

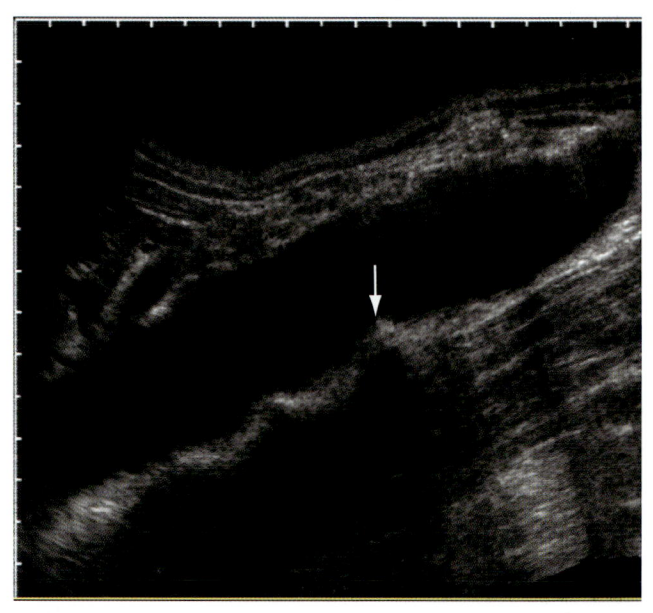

■ FIGURE 109-26 Gray-scale longitudinal scan of the aorta in supine position reveals an aortic aneurysm along with atherosclerotic changes (*arrow*).

Functional Ultrasound Assessment

After this initial overview, the second part of the examination should include color flow and spectral imaging of the aorta and renal vessels. For proper color flow assessment, the parameters of the machine have to be calibrated for every patient. To do this, an area of laminar flow in the aorta is identified and this window is used to adjust color gain, pulse repetition frequency, and wall filter (Fig. 109-28). The peak systolic velocity and end-diastolic velocity of the aorta are recorded just below the level of origin of the superior mesenteric artery by keeping a Doppler angle of insonation of less than 60° C.[23] The peak systolic velocity of the aorta is used to calculate the renal artery aortic ratio (RAR; Fig. 109-29). After taking these measurements, the ostium of the renal arteries is identified just inferior and caudal to the origin of the superior mesenteric artery.

Technical Considerations

The gray-scale sonography of the renal arteries is initially done from the midline transverse plane with a slight rotation of the transducer laterally on either side to visualize the entire length of the renal arteries. The transducer is placed at the midpoint between the xiphoid process and umbilicus. If overlying bowel gas interferes with the examination, the transducer is swept in a cranial or caudal direction to look for the vessel. If this fails, then the liver can be used as an acoustic window to scan the proximal and middle segments of both renal arteries. The distal segment of both renal arteries is scanned, along with the intrarenal vessels, by the respective lateral and flank approaches by using the ipsilateral kidneys as acoustic windows. In children, sometimes the longitudinal span from a lateral and flank approach can help visualize both renal arteries.

Main Renal Arteries

Both renal arteries are assessed by gray-scale sonography for any area of narrowing of the lumen, calcification, or atherosclerotic plaque. The diameter of the main renal artery is also assessed in its proximal segment (proximal 2 cm). Color flow Doppler is then used to visualize any areas of turbulence and color aliasing. Both renal veins are also assessed for patency, along with the examination of renal arteries.

As far as color Doppler and spectral wave imaging of the renal arteries is concerned, the ideal transducer position is one in which the direction of blood flow in the vessel is parallel to the ultrasound beam and the Doppler angle of insonation is almost 0 degrees. Practically, this is only possible in very thin and cooperative patients who can hold their breath reliably. A normal spectral waveform in the renal artery is that of low resistance with continuous forward diastolic flow (Fig. 109-30).

Color Doppler and spectral waveform assessment of the proximal segment of the RRA is done by placing the transducer in a transverse plane, slightly to the right of midline and rotating it toward the left kidney (see Fig. 109-19). This results in a Doppler angle of nearly 0 degrees and blood flow is seen as red because its direction is toward the transducer. If the anterior transverse approach is not successful, the patient is rotated 45 degrees to the right anterior oblique position. A right subcostal approach is adapted by using the liver as an acoustic window to analyze the proximal part of the RRA. By following this

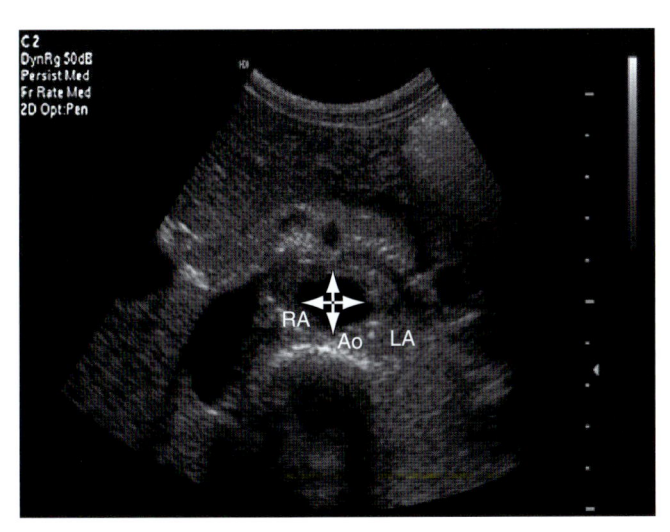

■ **FIGURE 109-27** Gray-scale image of the aorta acquired in the midline transverse plane in a patient with aortitis. There is irregular narrowing (*arrows*) of the lumen of the aorta (Ao).

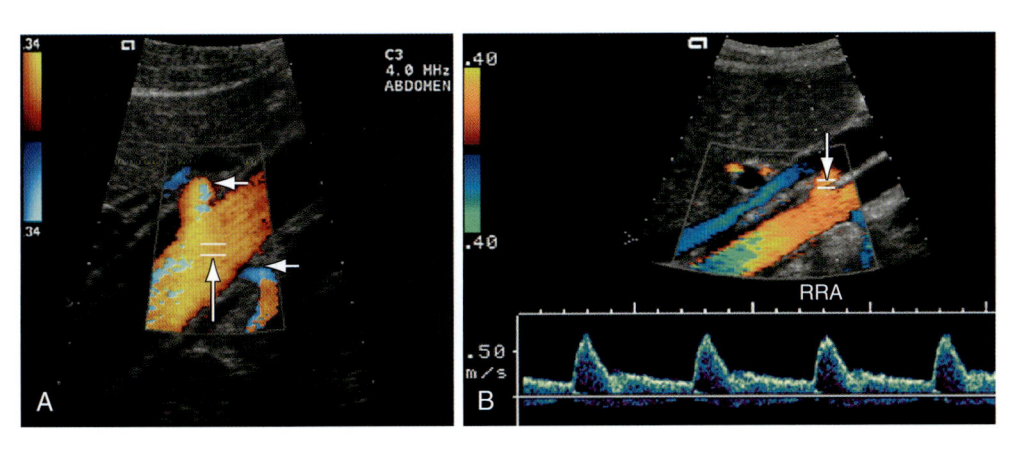

■ **FIGURE 109-28** The RAR is the ratio of the PSV of the aorta and renal artery. **A,** Color Doppler image of the aorta shows the sampling gate (*long arrow*) placed at an area of laminar flow in the aorta, which is usually at the level of origin of the renal arteries (*short arrows*). **B,** Color and pulse wave Doppler image shows the sampling gate (*arrow*) in the proximal segment of renal artery (also see Fig. 109-36).

approach, the color flow in the proximal segment of the RRA will again appear as red, but the Doppler angle of insonation will be increased (the aim should be to keep the angle as low as possible and never allow it to exceed 60 degrees).

Color Doppler imaging and spectral measurements of the middle segment of the RRA are done by using an anterior transverse approach. The transducer is placed slightly to the left of midline and rotated toward the right so that blood flow of the middle segment of the right renal artery is parallel to the ultrasound beam. The flow of blood in the middle segment of the RRA is seen as blue because the blood flow is away from the transducer.

The proximal and middle segments of the LRA are studied by using an anterior approach, with the transducer located slightly to the right side of midline. The transducer is placed in a transverse plane and rotated (4 or 5 o'clock) toward the left side so that the blood flow in the proximal and middle segments of the LRA is parallel to the beam of transducer. The flow of blood in the proximal and middle segments of the LRA will be seen as blue because it is moving away from the transducer (Fig. 109-31). Moreover, the angle of insonation will also be low. If this anterior approach is unsuccessful, a lateral approach through the liver is used. In this approach, the transducer is placed in a transverse plane and directed toward the left side to visualize the proximal two thirds of the LRA. If the proximal and middle segments of the LRA are not optimally visualized by these positions, these are studied by placing the patient in a right lateral decubitus position and approached laterally by using the left kidney as an acoustic window. Sometimes, pediatric patients are placed in the right lateral decubitus position; a longitudinal scan through the left kidney provides a good view for adequate visualization of both renal arteries. The distal segment of the RRA is studied by placing the patient in the left lateral decubitus position and using a lateral longitudinal and flank scanning approach. Similarly, the distal segment of the LRA is studied by placing the patient in the right lateral decubitus position and using a lateral longitudinal and flank scanning approach to perform Doppler imaging. In situations in which other approaches to assess the proximal and middle segments of renal arteries fail because of bowel gas, morbid obesity, or inability to hold the breath, the lateral approaches in decubitus positions are used to assess the proximal two thirds of both renal arteries.

An additional approach that yields a banana or banana peel view is also popular with renal sonographers (Fig. 109-32). The patient is placed in a left lateral decubitus

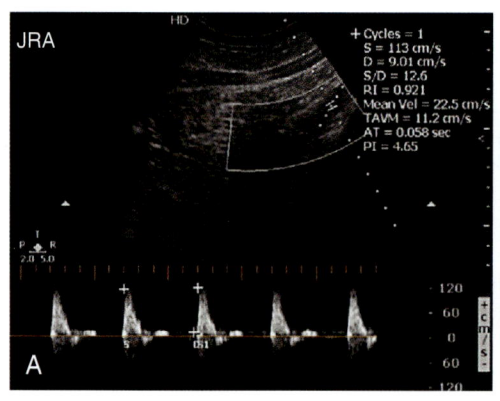

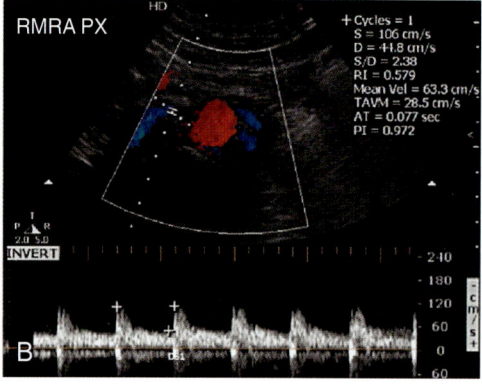

■ **FIGURE 109-29** Normal peak systolic velocity measurement. **A,** Peak systolic velocity of the aorta is 113 cm/sec. **B,** PSV at the origin of right renal artery is 106 cm/sec in another patient. Compare with the RAS patient shown in Figure 109-36.

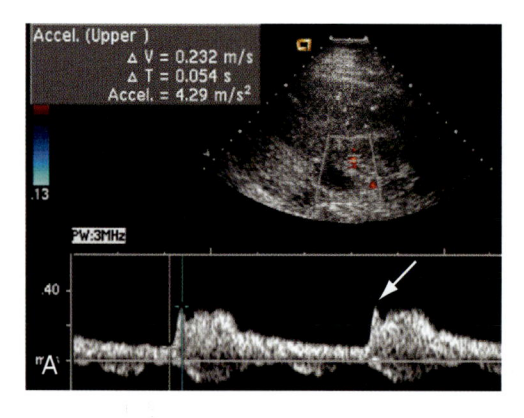

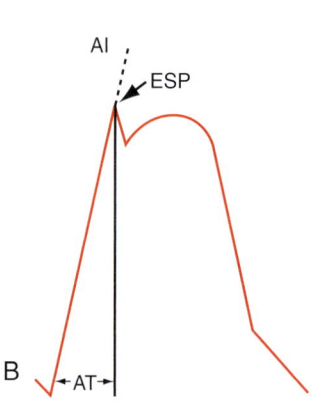

■ **FIGURE 109-30** Normal spectral waveform. **A,** Spectral waveform pattern in main renal artery is of low impedance with continuous forward diastolic flow and a characteristic early systolic peak (*arrow*) at the end of the systolic rise. **B,** Sketch of normal spectral waveform of main renal artery. AI, acceleration index; AT, acceleration time; ESP, early systolic peak.

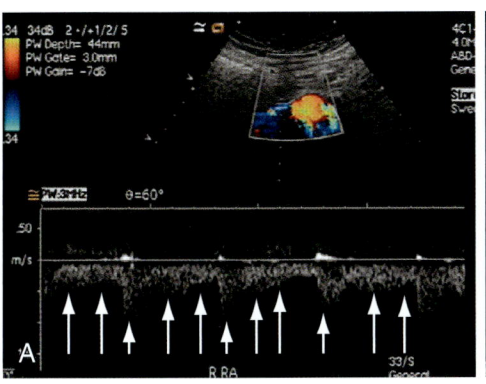

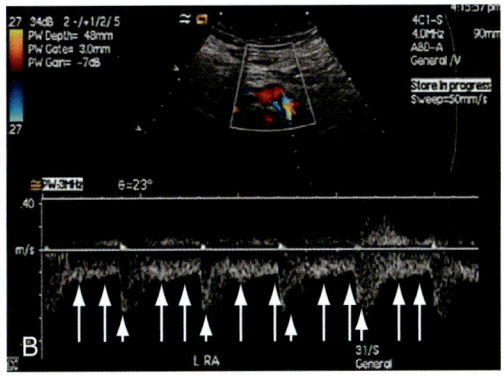

FIGURE 109-31 Midline transverse sampling. The spectral waveforms of the proximal segments of the right (**A**) and left (**B**) renal arteries show a low-resistance waveform, with an early sytolic peak and flow throughout the diastole.

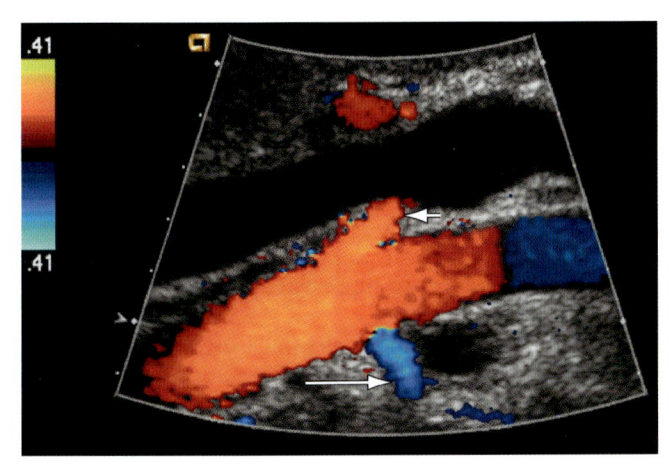

FIGURE 109-32 Banana peel view of the aorta and origin of both renal arteries. The transducer is placed on the right side. The blood flow in the right renal artery (*short arrow*) is toward it and hence is shown in red, whereas flow in the left renal artery (*long arrow*) is away from the transducer and is shown in blue.

position and the transducer is placed anterior to the anterior paraspinal muscles, with a longitudinal orientation of the scanning plane to identify the aorta. The transducer is adjusted slightly in an anterior or posterior direction so that both renal arteries are seen arising from the aorta and coming toward the transducer. The banana peel view is especially useful in older patients, in whom stenosis caused by atherosclerosis is expected in the ostium of the renal arteries. In case of failure of all approaches for optimum visualization of the renal arteries, the patient can be asked to lie prone and the examination can be attempted by using the kidneys as acoustic windows on both sides.

Peak systolic and end-diastolic velocities (see Table 109-1) are obtained at the origin, proximal segment, and middle segment of both renal arteries with a Doppler angle of insonation of 60 degrees or less. These are usually done by anterior approaches. After taking these samples, the distal part of the renal arteries is sampled for peak systolic and end-diastolic velocities in a lateral decubitus position with the use of a 0-degree angle of insonation. The RAR is calculated by comparing the peak systolic aortic flow velocity with the peak systolic velocity of the renal artery.

Intrarenal Arteries

Imaging of the intrarenal vessels is done by the flank approach by placing the patient in a lateral decubitus position (left lateral decubitus for RRA and right lateral decubitus for LRA). Before sampling intrarenal vessels, a perfusion scan of the kidney should be obtained.

Sampling of the intrarenal arteries is done in the upper, middle, and lower poles of the kidney by color Doppler guidance. By taking a Doppler angle of insonation of 0 degree, using the lowest velocity scale and lowest wall filter setting, and adjusting the smallest Doppler gate width, a good spectral waveform is typically obtained (Fig. 109-33). Peak systolic and end-diastolic velocities are recorded for the intrarenal arteries. Spectral traces of the intrarenal arteries are used for calculation of acceleration time (AT) and acceleration index (AI; see Table 109-1). The software installed in almost all modern ultrasound machines automatically performs these calculations. Acceleration time is the time from the beginning of the systole upstroke to the systolic peak and AI is the gradient of this upstroke (see Fig. 109-30B).[24-26]

Renal Morphology

No evaluation of renal vessels is complete without assessment of kidney size, shape, and echo texture. Longitudinal measurement of the kidney in the cephalocaudal plane should always be performed. In case of a normal-sized kidney, and a very small diameter main renal artery (less than 5 mm), there is every likelihood that an accessory, supernumerary, or polar renal artery supplies the kidney.[21] This criterion for the presence of an accessory renal artery in a smaller sized main renal artery of a normal sized kidney is useful in some patients with renovascular hypertension, but does not eliminate the necessity of performing magnetic resonance angiography (MRA) or catheter angiography before renal transplantation and surgical correction of the abdominal aorta. Therefore, to see any accessory renal arteries, longitudinal and transverse sweeps of the transducer are done in the decubitus position. Several helpful suggestions from Li and coworkers[27] are that the sample line should be parallel to the direction of the jet stream of the vessel, the sample gate should be

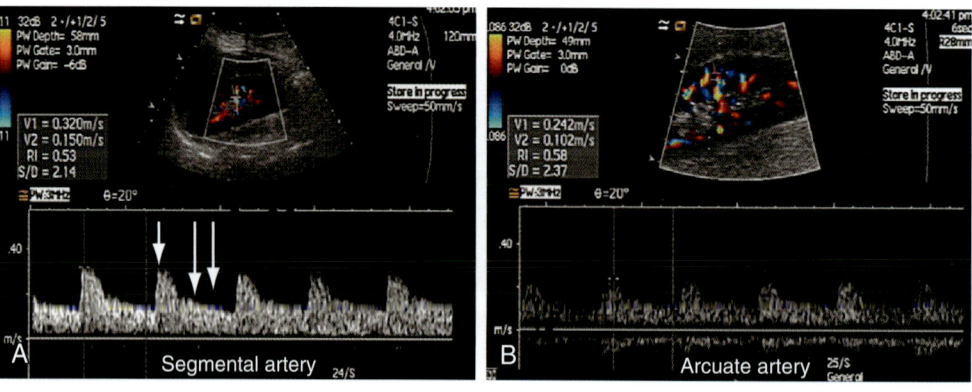

FIGURE 109-33 Lateral decubitus renal imaging. **A,** Waveform of a segmental artery recorded in the lateral decubitus position after placing the sampling gate (=) at the segmental artery. The normal waveform shows a sharp systolic upstroke (*short arrow*) and forward flow throughout the cardiac cycle (*long arrows*). **B,** Normal spectral waveform of arcuate artery acquired by the lateral decubitus approach. The peak systolic velocity decreases as vessels are traced proximally to distally (i.e., peripherally from the main renal artery to the arcuate arteries). In healthy subjects, the renal artery PSV > segmental artery PSV > interlobar artery PSV > arcuate artery PSV.

placed at the most stenotic site, and repeated samples around the turbulent signals should be taken.

PITFALLS AND SOLUTIONS

Complete evaluation of main renal arteries may not be possible because of obesity, interference of bowel gas, respiratory motion or the inability to suspend respiration, transmitted aortic pulsation, and difficulty in measuring the Doppler angle. In addition, other pitfalls include the inherent difficulties of imaging small vessels, the posterior location of mid and distal arteries, and failure to make a good acoustic window. There is a 10% to 20% failure rate for complete examination of both renal arteries from their ostium to the hilum of the kidneys.[28] Other pitfalls of sonography include shadowing from plaque, interobserver variation, and the presence of accessory arteries. Technical factors that may limit renal evaluation include pulse repetition frequency and wall filter frequency, actual flow velocity and Doppler angle of insonation, and choice of transducers used. Tortuosity and kinking of the renal artery and a Doppler angle of more than 60 degrees can result in a false-positive RAS.

The following can help overcome above-mentioned pitfalls:

1. Ultrasound contrast agents can improve visualization of the renal arteries.[29]
2. If complete sampling of the main renal artery is not possible, then sampling of the intrarenal arteries (without RAR and renal artery peak systolic velocity) is used for evaluation.
3. In addition to gray-scale and color Doppler sonography, power Doppler imaging can be done because it is independent of the angle of insonation. It allows visualization of low poststenotic velocities and improves visibility of tortuous or kinked vessels or of vessels lying perpendicular to the ultrasound beam.[30]

The renal resistive index (RI) is not specific and depends on many variables, such as the site of measurement and intra-abdominal pressure, pulse rate, age of the patient, the sonographer's skill, presence of other renal diseases such as diabetes, hypertensive nephrosclerosis, acute renal failure, and urinary obstruction with hydronephrosis.[31] An increased pulse rate (more than 70 beats/min) lowers the RI, whereas a pulse rate less than 50 beats/min increases the RI.

The compliance index, which measures pulsating renal blood flow distribution using power Doppler, is technically simple and independent of many variables for RI. The compliance index considers multiple interlobular arteries, rather than a single large artery.[32]

A difference of mean RIs between both kidneys of more than 5% can be used as a criterion for diagnosing RAS of more than 50%.[33] A difference of mean RIs of both kidneys has been used by a few researchers in cases of unilateral RAS, but this cannot be used in cases of bilateral stenosis, renal artery disease, single kidney, or renal allograft.

The lack of an early systolic peak has a low sensitivity for moderate stenosis. The waveform is dependent on the maintenance of vessel compliance, which limits its effectiveness in older patients with atherosclerosis.

The RAR is often inaccurate in patients with concomitant abdominal aortic pathology. It can be elevated in cases of aortic aneurysm and decreased cardiac contractility, or depressed in cases of significant atherosclerotic changes in the aorta.

There is considerable interobserver variation in the measurement of AT. Some observers measure it as time from the beginning of the systole to the first peak, others measure it up to the first inflection point, and some measure it to the second or maximum peak.[26]

There have been a large number of false-negative and false-positive cases of RAS on sonography. The false-negative cases can result from a variety of causes, such as multifocal or diffuse but severe RAS, segmental RAS, small atrophic kidneys, accessory renal artery stenosis, or distal renal artery stenosis. False-positive RAS cases also occur in patients with aortic stenosis or with conditions leading to increased cardiac output, such as hyperthyroidism.[27]

Renal artery angiography still remains the gold standard for the evaluation of renal arteries. MRA of the renal arteries offers a good alternative for patients, in addition to multidetector computed tomography (MDCT) angiography of renal vessels. MRA is a useful noninvasive method for assessing renal arteries that has the advantage of three-dimensional views. The limitations of MRA are its relatively higher cost and suboptimal ability to evaluate most patients who have undergone renal stenting, typically using stents made of Nitinol or platinum.[23] Contrast-enhanced MR imaging (MRI), however, is useful for the diagnosis of infarctions, ranging from small ones caused by vasculitis to segmental or global infarctions caused by renal artery occlusion. Sometimes, in cases of arteriovenous (AV) fistulas or pseudoaneurysms, the perifistular vibration may limit the assessment on ultrasound; MRI may be helpful in these cases.

Sonography may not be able to diagnose renal vein thrombosis in some native kidneys that develop rich collaterals that lead to a normal venous flow within the kidney. A wrong diagnosis of RVT can be made if there is a very sluggish flow for any reason. MRA can be used as an alternative. MRI for significant RAS has a sensitivity of 88% to 100% and specificity of 71% to 99%.[34]

Pitfalls of Sonography of Allograft Renal Vein Thrombosis

Sonography may not be able to diagnose RVT in some cases. Transplant nephrectomy may become essential in these cases because of the development of infarction and secondary infection. MRI could diagnose renal vein thrombosis in these cases and prompt thrombectomy might salvage the allograft.

Vascular compliance of recipient arteries affects the Doppler RI of the interlobular and segmental arteries of renal allograft. RI is not a very good parameter for assessing the allograft kidney because this depends on the vascular stiffness of the transplant recipient's arterial bed. Atherosclerotic changes in the recipient's renal artery can lead to an increased RI. Color Doppler indices such as the RI of the allograft mostly represent the compliance of central vessels of the host rather than the indices of the allograft, so these cannot always be correlated with allograft function. Contrast-enhanced sonography offers a potential solution for allograft evaluation by providing rapid and complete visualization of renal arteries.

IMAGE INTERPRETATION

Diagnosis of Renal Artery Stenosis

Renal artery stenosis is considered significant when the internal diameter of the renal artery is reduced more than 60%, although some use the more conservative threshold of 50%.[34] The location of RAS is often ostial, but it may occur in any segment of the main renal artery (proximal, middle, or distal), in an accessory renal artery, or in segmental arteries. The diagnosis of RAS can be made on sonography by two criteria (Box 109-2), direct and indirect.

BOX 109-2 Criteria for Hemodynamically Significant Renal Artery Stenosis in Native Vessels (>60% Stenosis)

DIRECT CRITERIA

Peak systolic velocity (PSV) > 180 m/sec in main renal artery
Renal artery aortic ratio (RAR) > 3.0 to 3.5
Resistive index (RI) > 0.7

INDIRECT CRITERIA

Renal artery interlobar artery ratio (RIR) > 5
Acceleration time (AT) > 0.07 second
Acceleration index (AI) > 3 m/sec^2
Parvus tardus waveform pattern in intrarenal vessels

Direct Criteria

Direct criteria for the diagnosis of RAS include an intrastenotic increased velocity of blood flow, poststenotic turbulence, color aliasing phenomenon, increased peak systolic velocity (PSV), increased ratio of PSV of the renal artery to the PSV of the aorta (renal-aortic ratio, or RAR), increased ratio of the PSV in the renal artery to the PSV in the interlobar arteries (renal artery interlobar artery ratio or RIR) in addition to the gray-scale findings (Figs. 109-34 to 109-36). A PSV more than 180 to 200 cm/sec and RAR more than 3.5 are diagnostic of RAS. An RI more than 0.7 predicts a poor outcome after revascularization.

Indirect Criteria

Indirect criteria for the diagnosis of RAS are acceleration index (AI) less than 300 cm/sec, AT more than 0.07 second, resistive index (RI), pulsatility index (PI), demonstration of a pulsus parvus tardus waveform in intrarenal vessels, and spectral broadening (Figs. 109-37 and 109-38).

Diagnostic Accuracy of Sonographic Criteria

A meta-analysis by Williams and colleagues[35] has evaluated the test performance of Duplex sonographic parameters for screening for hemodynamically significant RAS. In their comprehensive review of the literature, they identified 88 studies involving a total of slightly more than 8,000 patients who had renal sonographic evaluation to determine PSV, AT, AI and renal-aortic radio (RAR) for the diagnosis of RAS. PSV was found to be the single measurement with the highest performance characteristics and with sensitivity of 85%, specificity of 92%, and diagnostic odds ratio of 60.9%. The RAR was noted to provide a sensitivity of 78%, specificity of 89%, and odds ratio of 29.3% for RAS diagnosis. The AT was found to have a sensitivity of 78%, specificity of 89%, and diagnostic odds ratio of 29.3%; the AI was found to have a sensitivity of 78%, specificity of 89%, and diagnostic odds ratio of 29.3%. Interestingly, the combination of PSV with other measurements did not increase accuracy.

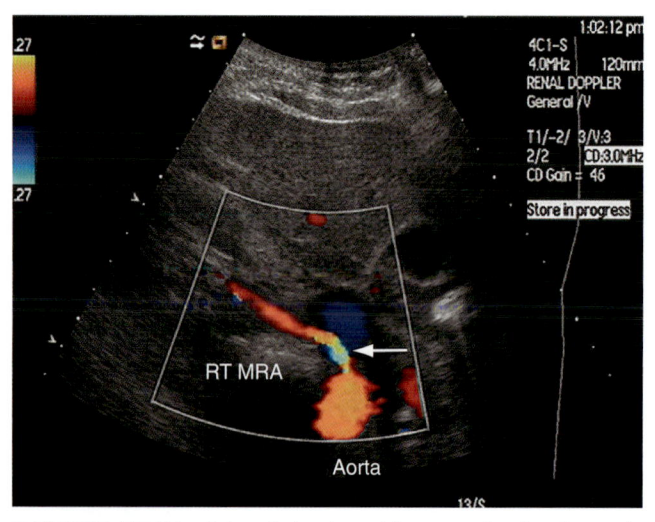

FIGURE 109-34 Color aliasing (*arrow*) is seen at the site of stenosis and at the poststenotic region of the proximal segment of the right main renal artery (RTMRA).

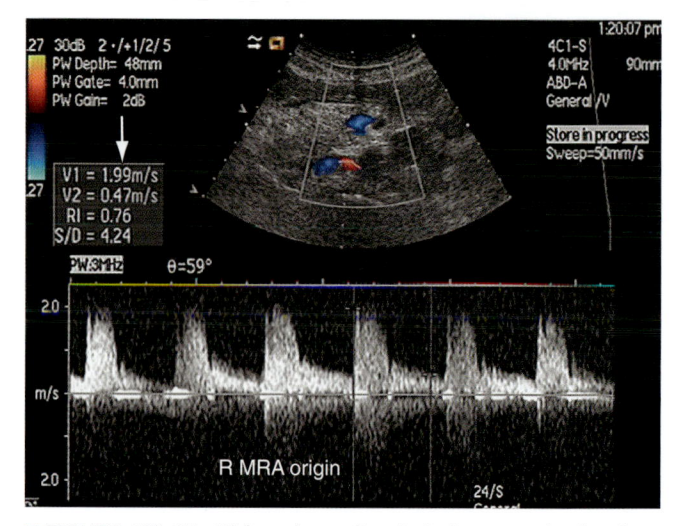

FIGURE 109-35 High peak systolic velocity is seen at the site of stenosis of the proximal segment of the right renal artery (*arrow*). The PSV is 1.99 m/sec.

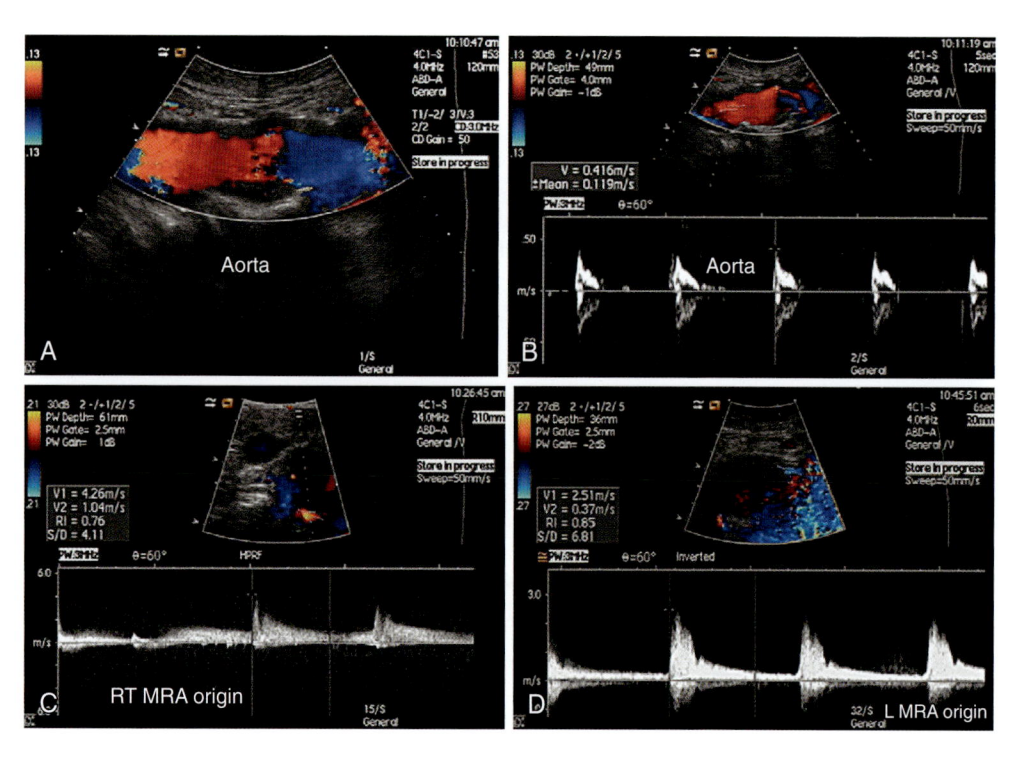

FIGURE 109-36 Color (**A**) and spectral (**B**) Doppler images of the aorta reveal a PSV of 0.416 m/sec. Color and spectral Doppler images of the right (**C**) and left (**D**) renal arteries reveal elevated PSVs of 4.26 m/sec and 2.5 m/sec, respectively, consistent with bilateral RAS. The RAR was more than 3.5 on both sides (right, 4.260/0.416; left, 2.510/0.416).

Other Diagnostic Findings

On gray-scale sonography, atherosclerotic plaque in the renal artery can be hyperechoic or hypoechoic, and sometimes calcified. These changes could present as circumferential hyperechoic wall thickening of variable size or can be irregular shapes. There could be focal narrowing of the lumen of the renal artery. In cases of hemodynamically insignificant stenosis, there may be only a small reduction in the luminal diameter. The string of beads sign could be demonstrated in the middle or distal segment of the renal artery, suggestive of FMD, and there could be poststenotic dilation or even a focal aneurismal dilation. At times, there is a significant difference (more than 1.5 cm) in the longitudinal dimensions of both kidneys in addition to the asymmetry of cortical thickness in cases of RAS.

Postangioplasty Renal Artery Assessment

Patients who undergo renal angioplasty consequent to a diagnosis of RAS still have a 15% restenosis rate (Figs. 109-39 to 109-44). The follow-up for evaluation of patency of renal artery is therefore important. Intimal hyperplasia

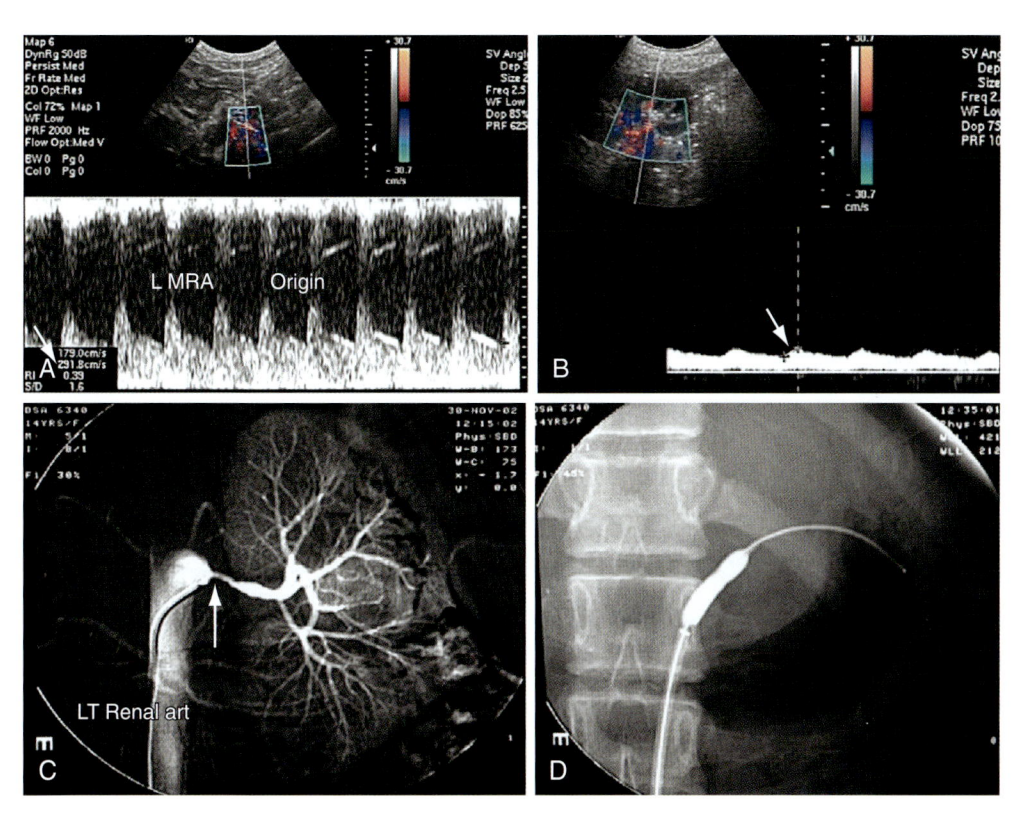

FIGURE 109-37 Patient with severe hypertension. **A,** Doppler images reveal increased PSV of 291 cm/sec (*arrow*) at the origin of left renal artery. **B,** Spectral waveform analysis reveals tardus parvus waveform (*arrow*) and increased AT in a segmental artery. **C,** Renal angiogram reveals stenosis (*arrow*) of the proximal segment of the left renal artery. **D,** Balloon angioplasty was performed with success in this patient.

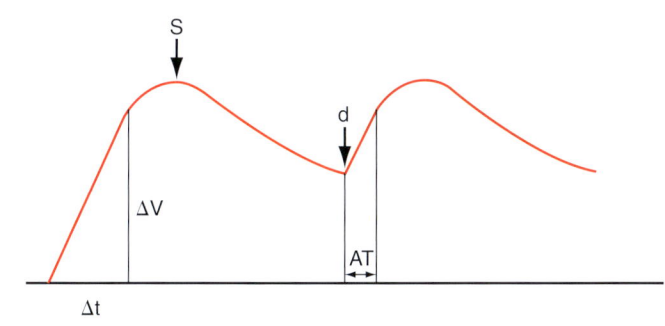

FIGURE 109-38 Tardus parvus waveform of intrarenal vessel (segmental artery) in a patient with renal artery stenosis. Increased AT is seen with loss of ESP (S).

is a common cause for in-stent restenosis and can be detected by enhanced PSV within a stent. Whenever there is enhanced PSV and deteriorating renal function, repeat renal angiography should be performed to assess for restenosis.

Diagnosis of Renal Artery Aneurysm

A renal artery aneurysm can involve the main renal artery or a branch of the renal artery. On gray-scale sonography, a hypoechoic mass is seen, showing a color flow signal on Doppler imaging. In cases of calcified aneurysms, the calcification is easily identified by gray-scale sonography. Calcified aneurysms can be thrombosed or patent, and therefore a Doppler sonography appearance would be seen accordingly.[14]

Diagnosis of Renal Artery Thrombosis

Thrombosis of the renal artery or its branches can lead to infarction in kidneys. Renal infarctions are mostly peripherally located in native kidneys. Acute renal failure and acute pancreatitis are two conditions that lead to multiple bilateral peripheral infarctions. Gray-scale sonography of the infarction shows these as hypoechoic areas. Doppler sonography shows a complete loss of Doppler signal within these hypoechoic areas.

In atherosclerosis, renal artery thrombosis (RAT) is characterized by a mute renal artery with a signal in the proximal renal artery and a tardus parvus pattern in intrarenal arteries. In cases of renal trauma, a mute renal artery can be seen in addition to the presence of an arterial stump. Other conditions leading to RAT can have different combinations of the features of RAT.

Diagnosis of Renal Vein Thrombosis

Renal vein occlusion caused by any pathology mostly leads to an initial increase in the size of the kidney. Gray-scale sonographic appearance of the kidney in renal vein occlusion is variable and nonspecific. The usual appearance is a hypoechoic cortex, with loss of corticomedullary differentiation.[14] On gray-scale sonography, the renal vein thrombus in the native kidney is typically echogenic—a thrombus full of solid echogenicity or with strip echogenicity. A partial or complete filling defect within the lumen of the main renal vein may be seen. Color Doppler imaging typically shows a mute renal vein, with absent or few intrarenal venous flow signals, with the renal vein associated with increased renal arterial resistance.

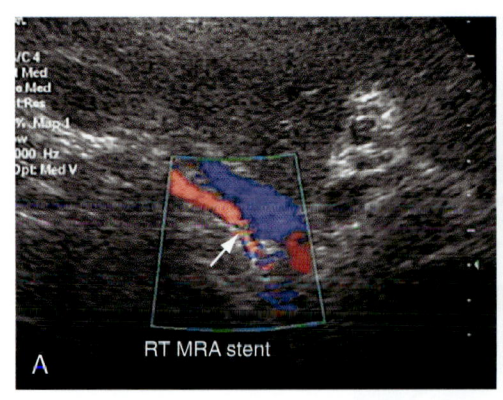

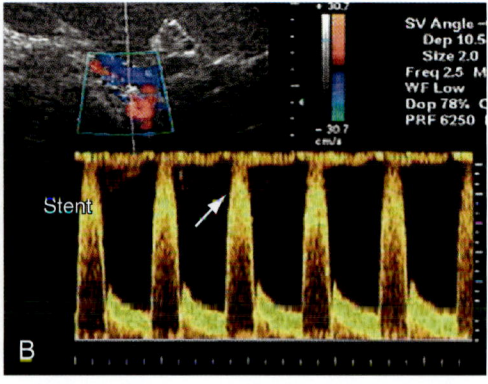

FIGURE 109-39 In-stent renal artery stenosis. **A,** Color aliasing (*arrow*) is seen at the level of the stent in the right renal artery. **B,** Pulse wave Doppler image reveals increased PSV (*arrow*) consistent with in-stent stenosis.

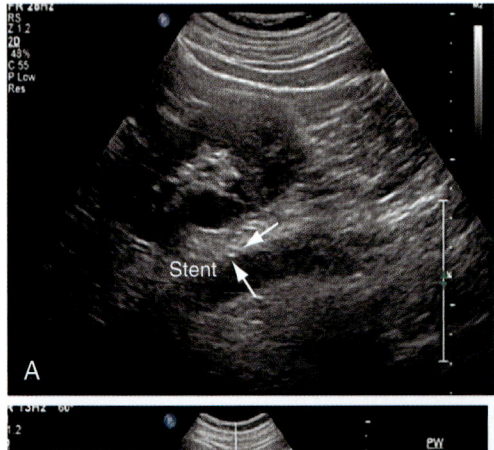

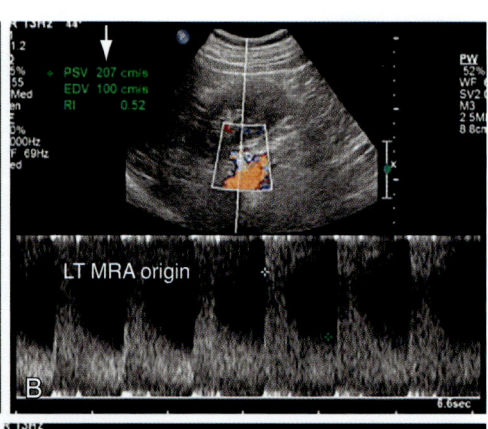

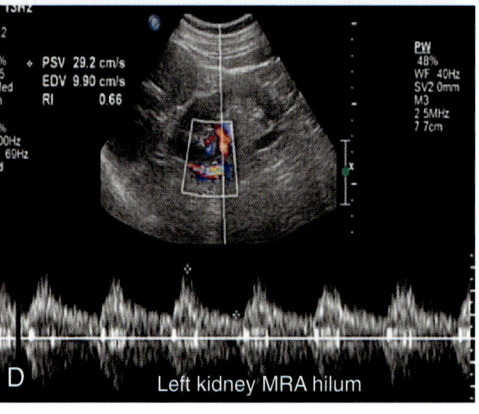

FIGURE 109-40 In-stent renal artery stenosis. **A,** Gray-scale image of the stent (*arrows*) in the left renal artery. **B,** Color Doppler image PSV of 207 cm/sec (*arrow*) at the origin of the left renal artery. **C, D,** Spectral waveforms of the left renal artery at the hilum (**C**) and middle segmental artery (**D**).

Sometimes, a small trickle of flow around the clot may be seen. Reverse diastolic flow in the intrarenal arteries is seen in RVT patients, but this feature has a low sensitivity for the diagnosis. In acute RVT, the clot may appear as hypoechoic or anechoic and hence is sometimes missed on gray-scale imaging; however, color Doppler imaging will usually help visualize the RVT.

RVT in native kidneys can manifest in diverse clinical presentations (acute, subacute, chronic). Acute renal vein thrombosis is a common vascular complication in neonates as a result of dehydration, sepsis, fetal distress, polycythemia, maternal diabetes, or umbilical vein catheterization. In neonates, thrombosis mostly starts from the arcuate or interlobular veins, commences into the interlobar veins, and eventually into the main renal vein. The initial stage of involvement of interlobar and interlobular veins persists for a few days and is characterized by the appearance of echogenic streaks on gray-scale ultrasonography. The kidney appears swollen and echogenic, with an echo-poor medulla. After the initial week, the kidney becomes increasingly swollen and heterogeneous in appearance, along with a loss of corticomedullary differentiation. The appearance of reduced echogenicity at the apex of the renal papilla and an echo-poor halo around the involved pyramid can also be seen in the initial acute phase. Some of these neonates may recover from this initial stage of thrombosis with only small focal areas of residual scarring but those who do not recover end up with an atrophic small kidney. The extension of the thrombus into the main renal vein and IVC is easily seen

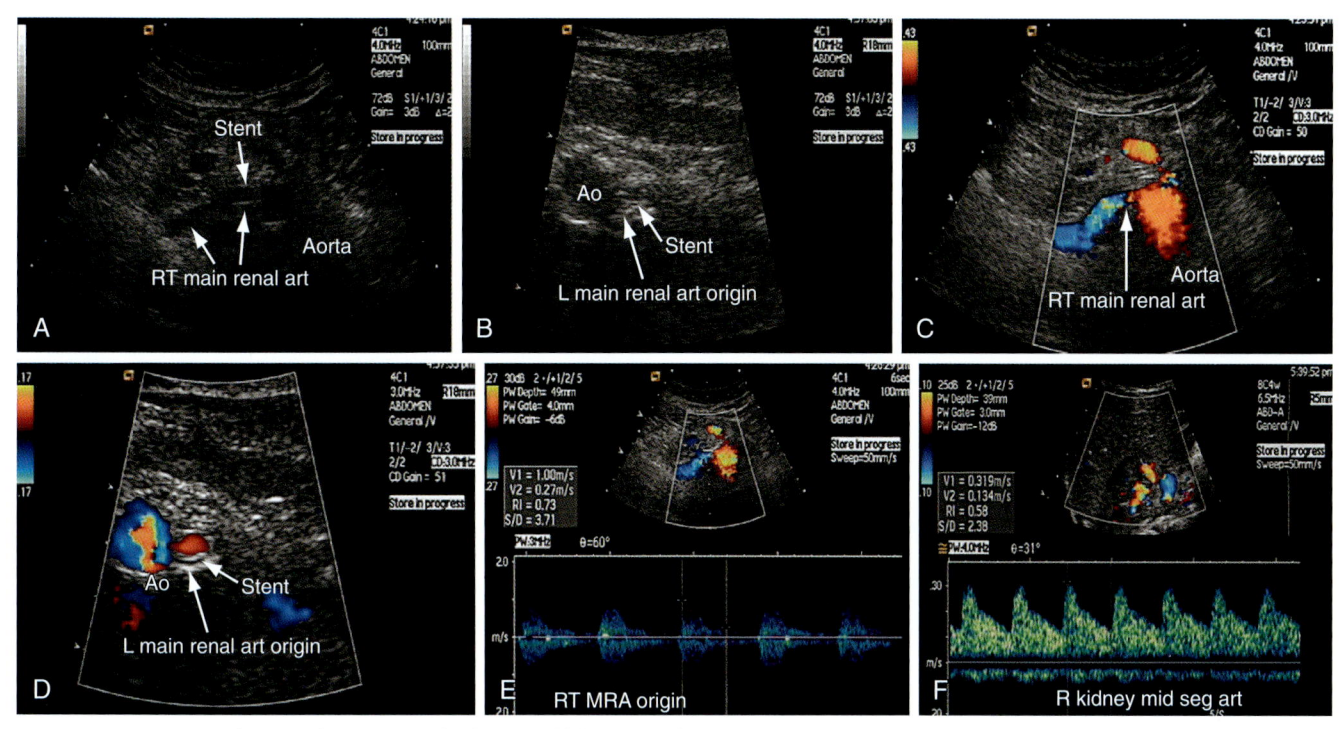

CHAPTER 109 • *Sonography of the Renal Vessels* 1517

■ **FIGURE 109-41** Evaluation of a patient with a history of bilateral renal artery stenosis after angioplasty and stenting. **A, B,** Gray-scale images show stent (short *arrows*) in the right renal artery (*long arrow*) and left renal artery (*long arrow*). Color Doppler images show flow and patency of the renal artery stents (C, right renal artery; D, left renal artery). The spectral waveforms of the right renal artery (**E**) and right middle segmental artery (**F**) are normal, confirming a patent right stent.

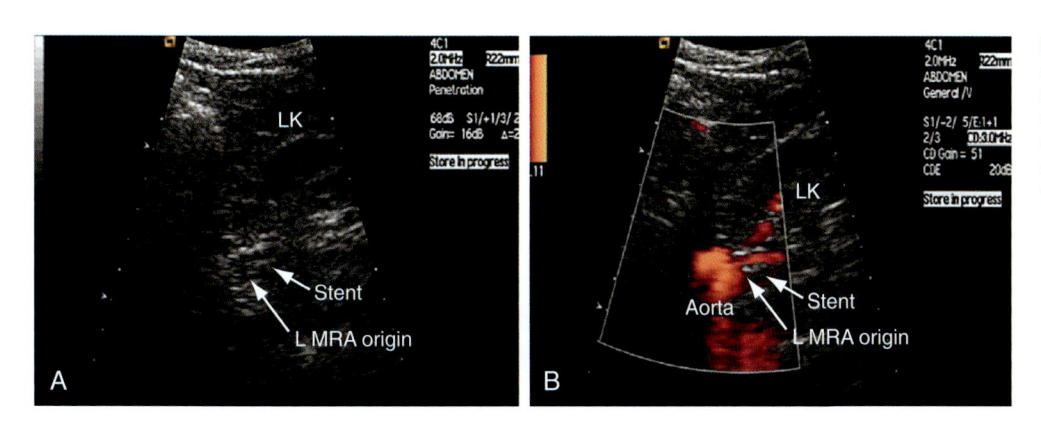

■ **FIGURE 109-42** Evaluation of stent patency. **A,** Gray-scale image shows a stent (*arrows*) at the origin of the left main renal artery (LMRA). **B,** Power Doppler image depicts the patency of the stent (*arrows*).

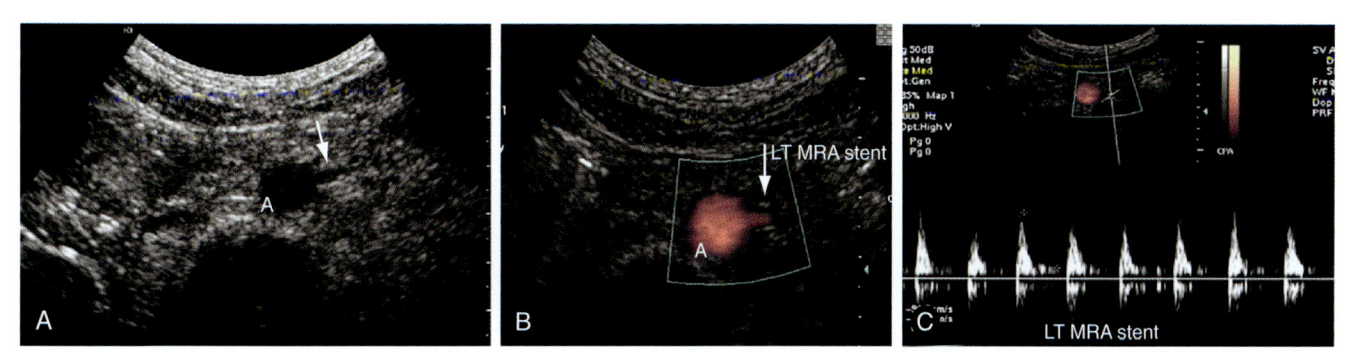

■ **FIGURE 109-43** Evaluation of stent patency in a second patient. The stent is in the proximal segment of the left renal artery. **A,** Gray-scale image acquired by midline tranverse approach shows a stent (*arrow*) in the proximal segment of the left renal artery, **B,** Power Doppler image shows the patency of the stent. **C,** Pulse wave Doppler image shows the normal spectral waveform of the renal artery. The peak systolic velocity is 90.7 cm/sec.

on gray-scale sonography, with the thrombus appearance ranging from echo-poor to highly echogenic or calcified (retracted thrombus). Because the left adrenal vein is a tributary of the left renal vein, there are patients who have RVT along with adrenal hemorrhage because of the direct passage of the thrombus from the renal to the adrenal vein. Bilateral adrenal hemorrhages along with RVT can also present in some patients.

Color Doppler imaging and spectral imaging help in the diagnosis of RVT. The initial stage of RVT shows a lack of flow and pulsatility in the intrarenal and main renal veins, with an increased RI and renal arterial diastolic flow. Retraction of the thrombus and formation of collaterals around the hilum and capsule may occur in the first few days, leading to the detection of some flow on color Doppler imaging of the renal vein. These events also lead to poor sensitivity and poor specificity of RI in these patients. The detected flow should therefore be analyzed for any pulsatility, because reduced or absent pulsatility points to obstruction of flow.[16]

Acute RVT can also be seen in children, often resulting in hemorrhagic renal infarction. In addition to the other predisposing conditions (see earlier), renal vein occlusion has also been reported to be associated with gangrenous appendicitis in children. Gray-scale imaging of RVT in acute cases typically exhibits increased renal size in addition to demonstrating a thrombus in the renal vein.

Chronic renal vein thrombosis leads to decreased renal size and increased parenchymal echogenicity caused by fibrosis. Gradual or chronic RVT occurs in older patients.

Renal vein thrombosis is frequently associated with a few malignancies, such as renal cell carcinoma (Fig. 109-45). In patients with renal cell carcinoma, tumor extension into the renal veins (21% to 35%) and into the IVC (4% to 10%) is a common feature.[15] In particular, tumor extending into the right renal vein is three times more likely to extend into the IVC as compared with the left renal vein. The operative treatment approach of renal cell carcinoma with or without venous extension does not change if it extends only up to the right renal vein or lateral segment of left renal vein. However, if a tumor

FIGURE 109-44 Postprocedure catheter angiogram following stenting in a patient with RAS.

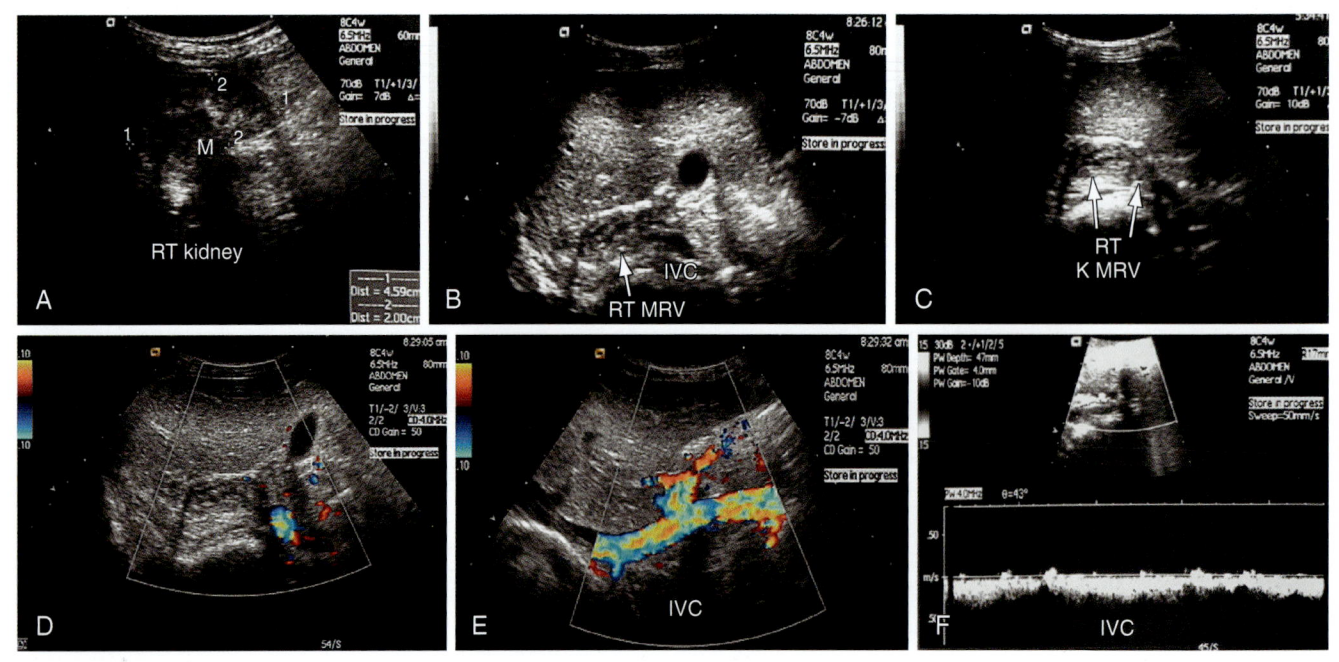

FIGURE 109-45 Chronic renal vein thrombosis in a 6-year-old boy with pheochromocytoma. Gray-scale images show a small right kidney (**A**) with renal vein thrombosis (*arrows*) (**B, C**). **D,** Color Doppler image shows no flow in the right renal vein. **E,** Color flow images demonstrate normal flow in the inferior vena cava (IVC). **F,** Similarly, the spectral waveform in the IVC is normal.

BOX 109-3 Normal Values of Parameters in Allograft Renal Transplant Vessels

PSV of main renal artery (normal) < 200 cm/sec
PSV of main renal artery (indeterminate) = 200-250 cm/sec
Renal vein flow velocity = 40-60 cm/sec
RI (normal) < 0.7
RI (indeterminate) = 0.7-0.8
RAR > 3.5 (indicates 60% stenosis)[24]
PSV > 150 cm/sec (indicates 50% RAS)[24]
PSV > 180 cm/sec (indicates 60% RAS)[24]
Sensitivity, 89%-98%; specificity, 90%-98%[24]
50% RAS: PSV > 200 cm/sec, RAR > 2.5 (best Duplex)
PSV < 200 cm/sec and RAR < 0.5 exclude severe (70%) RAS (best Duplex)

BOX 109-4 Criteria for Renal Artery Stenosis in Allograft Vessels

1. Presence of color aliasing at the site of stenotic segment
2. Focal frequency shift of more than 7.5 kHz (with 3.5-MHz transducer)
3. PSV > 200 to 250 cm/sec
4. Velocity gradient between stenotic and poststenotic segments = 2:1
5. RI > 0.8
6. Tardus parvus waveform in renal parenchyma

extends into the IVC or involves the medial segment of the left renal vein, the operative procedure is more extensive, requiring modification; thus, the exact extent of the venous extension of a tumor on imaging is essential for preoperative planning. On gray-scale sonography the tumor venous extension is seen as an intraluminal lesion, with homogeneous low or medium echogenicity within the distended renal vein. On occasion, renal vein thrombosis can be differentiated from the extension of tumor into the renal vein by the demonstration of color flow in small blood vessels within the tumor, which would be absent in bland thrombus.

In addition to the intraluminal causes of blockage of renal veins, external compression of renal veins by various retroperitoneal and abdominal pathologies is also seen in clinical settings. The important causes of external compression of renal veins are acute pancreatitis, lymph node enlargement, and retroperitoneal fibrosis. The external compression of the vascular pedicle predisposes patients to RVT.

Vascular Evaluation of Renal Transplants

Allograft renal vessels can be easily visualized sonographically because of their superficial location as compared with native renal vessels. Gray-scale sonographic assessment of an allograft kidney is important before the sonography of renal vessels is carried out. Renal size is assessed in the orthogonal planes and renal volume is calculated. Renal volume serves as a reference tool for all future sonographic examination of allograft and allograft vessels. Doppler and spectral imaging of the allograft renal vessels and ipsilateral external iliac artery are done to view the patency of renal vessels and the anastomotic site and to view any focal area of color aliasing. Doppler and spectral sonography of the main renal vein and intrarenal vessels (interlobar arteries) are also carried out. The parameters to be measured are PSV, AT, RI, pulsatility index, and ratio of PSV of the iliac artery and main renal artery (Boxes 109-3 and 109-4). The normal flow in an allograft renal artery is low-resistance flow. The RI is increased in allograft rejection because of edema, and serial measurements are required to monitor the allograft. Sometimes, there can be a normal RI in allograft rejection. Other features of

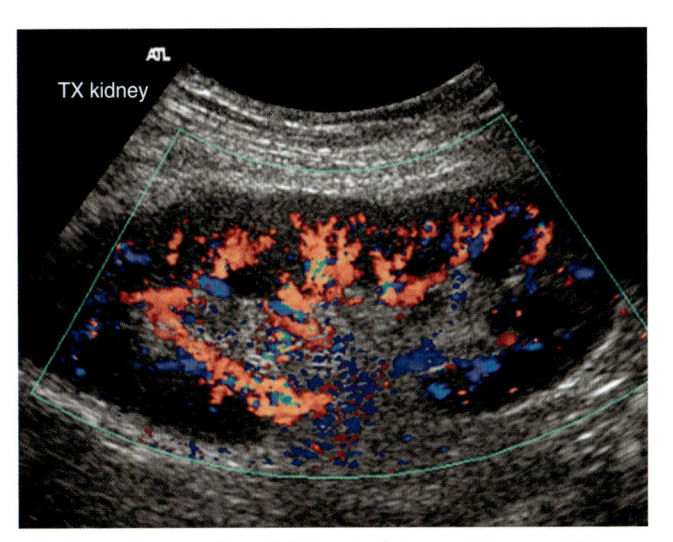

FIGURE 109-46 Allograft kidney in a 40-year-old woman. This longitudinal color Doppler image shows decreased flow in the cortical regions of the upper and lower poles of the allograft. *(Courtesy of Dr. T.H.S. Bedi, DCA Imaging Centre, New Delhi, India.)*

graft rejection include a high-resistance waveform, with minimal or absent diastolic flow, narrow systolic peak, with the second peak higher than the first, and flow reversal in early diastole. The pulsatility index (PI) and RI above 1.8 and 0.7, respectively, are abnormal.[14]

Power Doppler imaging shows alterations of small vessels in the cortex in the early stages of rejection and therefore is more sensitive. The flow can be patchy or completely absent in the cortex (Figs. 109-46 and 109-47). The absence of these signs on power Doppler imaging does not rule out acute graft rejection. Chronic rejections take months to occur and result in a smaller kidney, with reduced visualization of intrarenal vessels.

RAS is the most common vascular complication of allografts and accounts for 75% of all of these (Fig. 109-48). It affects 1% to 10% of all allografts. Stenosis of an allograft renal artery usually occurs during the first year of renal transplantation, although cases can present for the first time even 3 years after transplantation. Stenosis is usually seen at the site of anastomosis, although stenosis proximal or distal to anastomosis can also occur. Proximal stenosis is exclusively caused by atherosclerotic disease of the donor vessel, whereas stenosis of the anastomosis site is caused by a perfusion injury or suture-related issues, such as a reaction to suture material or a faulty suture technique. Stenosis distal to the anastomosis is primarily caused by rejection, although mechanical factors such as compression, renal artery kink, or turbulent flow can also cause stenosis. Kinks of the renal transplant artery with normal intra-arterial pressures do not progress to threaten graft function, even up to 5 years after transplantation. End to end anastomoses have three times more risk of stenosis than end to side anastomoses.

Gray-scale sonography of an allograft RAS reveals focal narrowing of the lumen and mural thickening. Mural calcification can also be seen. Focal color aliasing is seen at the site of stenosis on color Doppler imaging. Spectral examination reveals spectral broadening and a tardus parvus waveform in addition to the increased peak systolic velocity. A PSV more than 250 cm/sec is very suggestive of RAS. Ultrasound is considered a screening modality, so a stenosis diagnosed by ultrasound has to be further confirmed by MRI, CTA, or angiography.

Renal artery thrombosis in renal allografts is associated with hyperacute transplant rejection, anastomotic occlusion, arterial kinking, and arterial intimal tear. If extensive, renal artery occlusion can occur, resulting in segmental or global infarction of the kidney (Fig. 109-49). On gray-scale sonography, segmental infarction appears as a focal or diffuse hypoechoic area with either well-defined echogenicity or with margins. Color Doppler imaging reveals wedge-shaped areas with no flow signals. Global infarction of the entire kidney results in an enlarged, swollen, hypoechoic kidney, with no arterial or venous blood flow. Acute pyelonephritis and rupture of the allograft can also mimic these findings on ultrasound imaging.

Other vascular complications of renal transplants, such as AV fistulas and pseudoaneurysms, are seen consequent to percutaneous graft biopsies. AV fistulas have turbulent flow in the small artery coupled with color aliasing in the involved vein (Fig. 109-50). There is a high-velocity, low-resistance waveform in the involved artery, with arteriali-

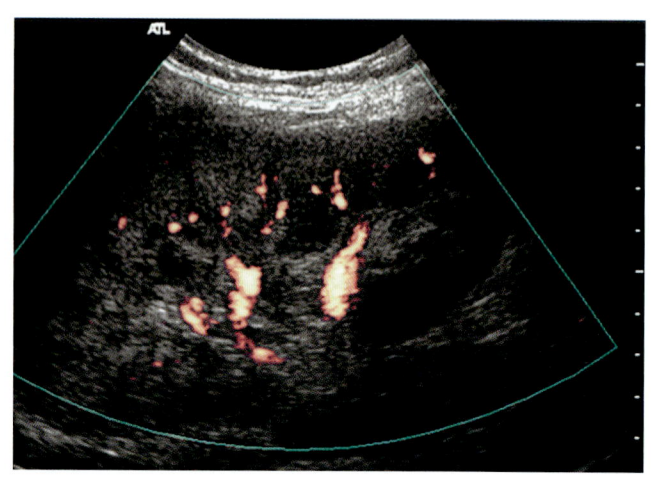

■ **FIGURE 109-47** Graft rejection in a 46-year-old man after renal transplantation. This color flow image shows very little flow in the allograft kidney. *(Courtesy of Dr. T.H.S. Bedi, DCA Imaging Centre, New Delhi, India.)*

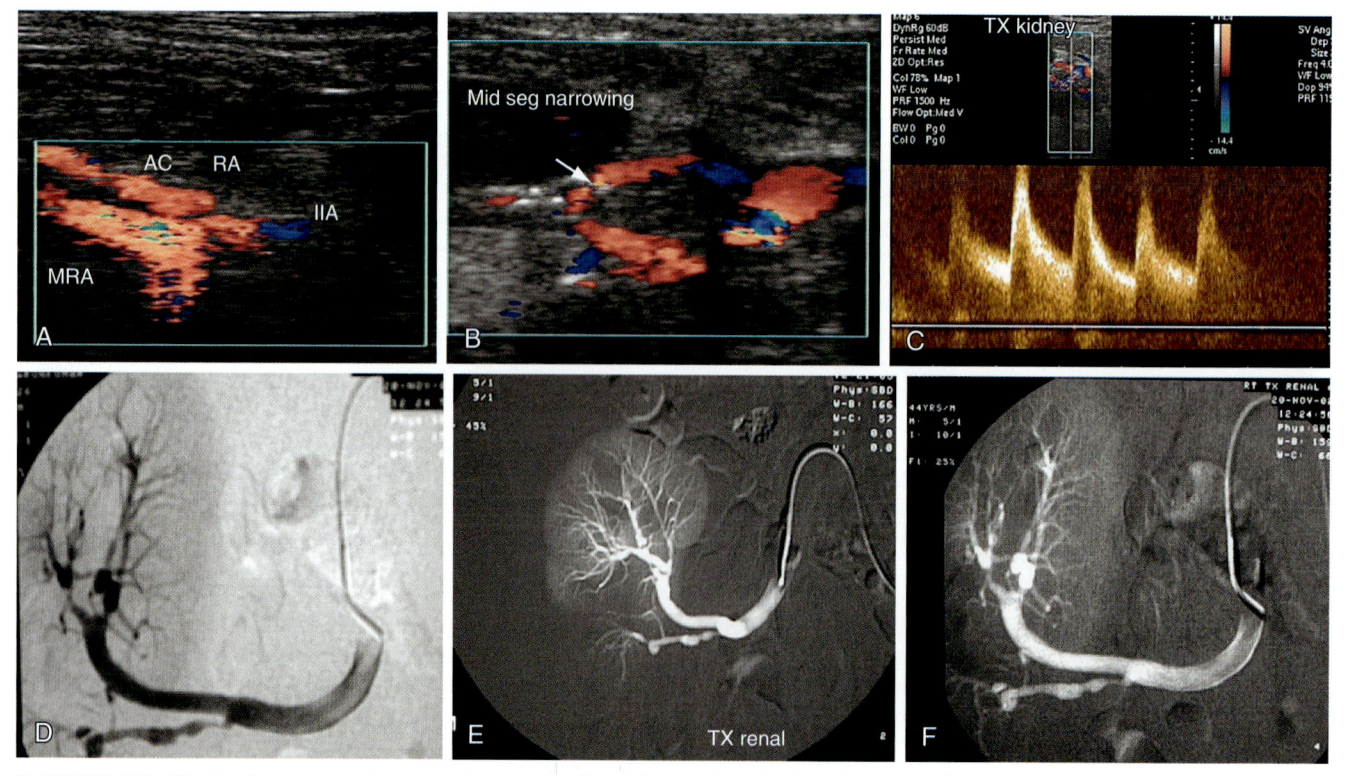

■ **FIGURE 109-48** Renal artery stenosis in a renal transplantation patient. **A, B,** Color Doppler images show a stenosis of the middle segment of the main renal artery *(arrow)*. **C,** Spectral waveform of the main renal artery reveals increased PSV. **D** through **F,** Renal angiography confirmed the diagnosis. AC RA, accessory renal artery; IIA, internal iliac artery; MRA, main renal artery.

zation of the draining vein. Areas of disorganized color outside the walls of the vessels are seen in AV fistulas because of the phenomenon of perifistular vibration. Pseudoaneurysms appear as cystic structures on gray-scale imaging and exhibit high flow within their confines on color Doppler imaging.

RVT can occur in the first week after transplantation, although it is seen in fewer than 5% of cases. RVT can have multiple causes, such as hypovolemia, clot progression from the iliac vein, faulty surgical technique, or external compression by collections (Fig. 109-51). The increased prevalence of RVT on the left side is because of compression of the left common iliac vein between the sacrum and left common iliac artery. This phenomenon is called silent iliac artery compression. On gray-scale imaging, an echogenic thrombus is seen inside a dilated renal vein in cases of complete RVT. Allograft vessels are not able to develop collateral venous drainage, so Doppler sonography shows reversed diastolic flow in the renal artery along with no flow in the renal vein. This type of reversed flow in the renal artery is also seen in acute pyelonephritis, but venous flow is normal. In cases of partial RVT, there is reduced venous flow along with a nonspecific increase in arterial resistance.

Renal transplant torsion is one of the rare complications, characterized by rotation of an allograft around its own vascular pedicle. This may eventually lead to loss of the graft if prompt surgical correction is not done.

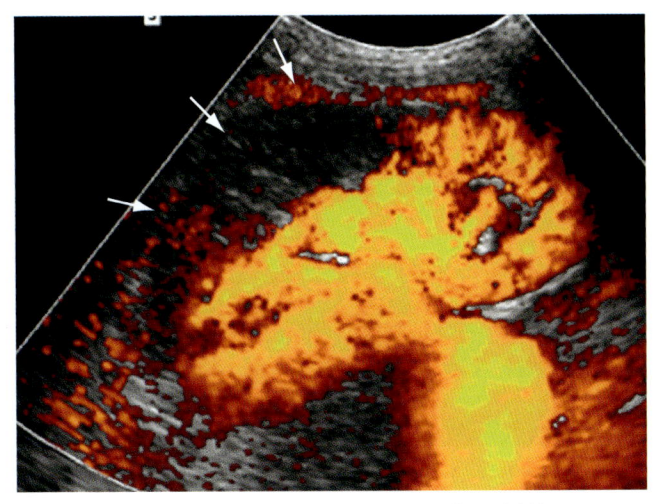

■ **FIGURE 109-49** Segmental infarction in an allograft kidney. Perfusion scan of the allograft kidney shows segmental infarction (*arrows*) in the midpole of the allograft. *(Courtesy of Dr. T.H.S. Bedi, DCA Imaging Centre, New Delhi, India.)*

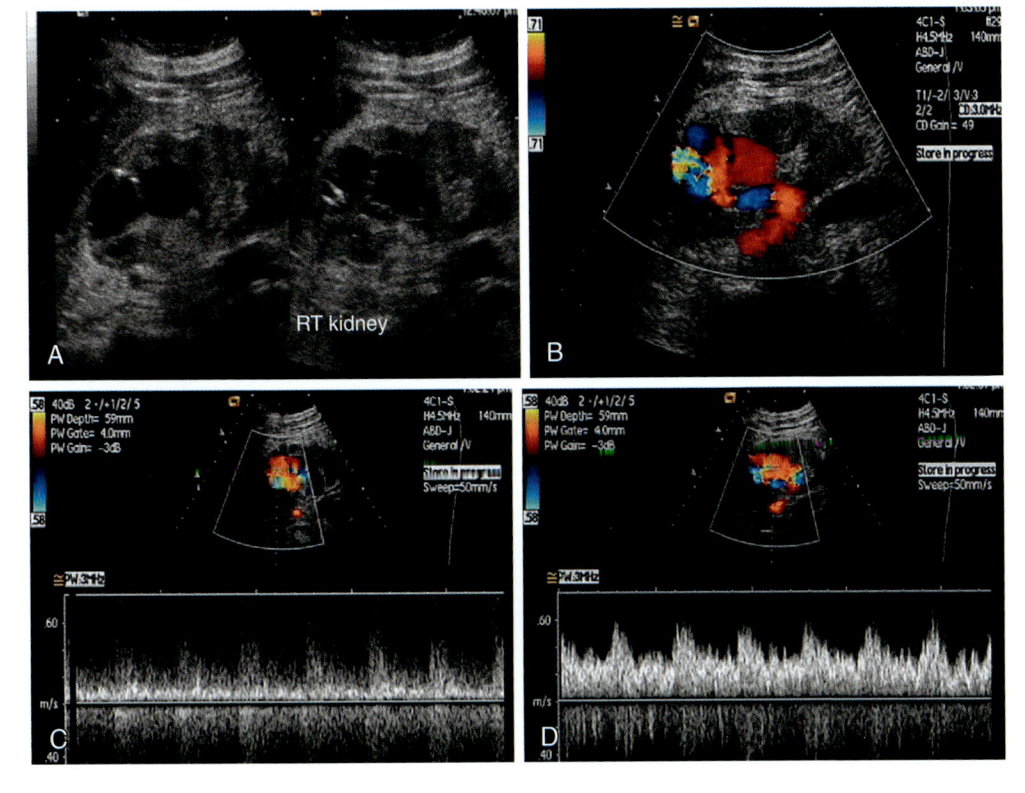

■ **FIGURE 109-50** Arteriovenous fistula in a male patient consequent to renal biopsy. **A,** Gray-scale longitudinal scan of kidney reveals cystic areas in the right kidney. **B,** Color flow Doppler image reveals turbulent flow within this area of mixed arteriovenous flow pattern. Color flow (**C**) and spectral waveform images (**D**) show increased PSV (6 m/sec).

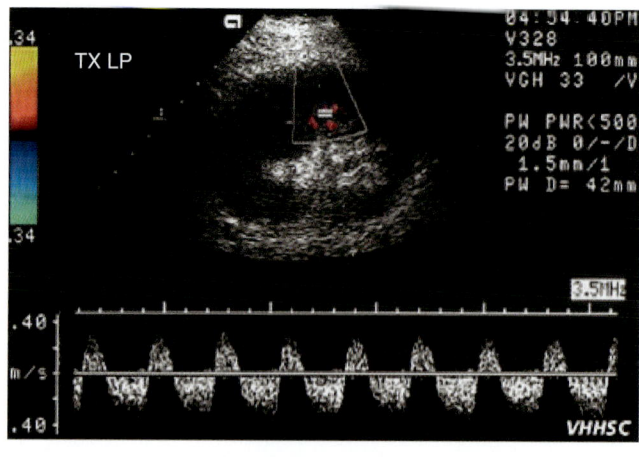

FIGURE 109-51 Color Doppler and spectral waveform images of a patient with renal vein occlusion of the allograft kidney.

KEY POINTS

- In skilled hands, renal ultrasound can accurately diagnose renal artery stenosis.
- Renal artery stenosis is one of the few treatable causes for hypertension and is typically secondary to atherosclerosis, or much less commonly, to fibromuscular dysplasia.
- Ultrasound provides not only morphologic vascular evaluation but the ability to provide blood flow velocity information, such as PSV, RI, RAR, IR, AT, AI, and a waveform that can be used to diagnose significant renal artery stenosis.
- Peak systolic velocity is the single duplex measurement that yields the highest diagnostic performance.

SUGGESTED READINGS

Akbar SA, Jafri ZH, Amendola MA, et al. Complications of renal transplantation. Radiographics 2005; 25:1335-1356.

Bradley DL, James EM, Charboneau JW, et al. Current applications of color Doppler imaging in the abdomen and extremities. Radiographics 1989; 9:599-631.

Helenom O, Rody FE, Correas JM, et al. Color Doppler US of renovascular disease in native kidneys. Radiographics 1995; 15:833-854.

Helenon O, Correas JM, Chabriais, et al. Renal vascular Doppler imaging: clinical benefits of power mode. Radiographics 1998; 18:1441-1454.

Langer JE, Jones LP: Sonographic evaluation of the renal transplant. Ultrasound Clin 2007; 2:73-88.

Lee HY, Grant ED: Sonography in renovascular hypertension. J Ultrasound Med 2002; 21:431-441.

Moukaddam H, Pollak J, Scoutt LM. Imaging of renal artery. Ultrasound Clin 2007; 2:455-475.

Singh AK, Sahani DV. Imaging of the renal donor and transplant recipient. Radiol Clin North Am 2008; 46:79-93.

Soulez G, Oliva EL, Turpin S, et al. Imaging of renovascular hypertension: respective values of renal scintigraphy, renal Doppler US, and MR angiography. Radiographics 2000; 20:1355-1368.

Staub D, Canevascini R, Huegli RW, et al. Best Duplex-sonographic criteria for the assessment of renal artery stenosis—correlation with intra-arterial pressure gradient. Ultraschall Med 2007; 85:45-51.

Zubarav AV. Evaluation of renal vessels. Eur Radiol 2001; 11:1902-1915.

REFERENCES

1. de Hann MW, Kroon AA, Flobbe K, et al. Renovascular disease in patients with hypertension: detection with duplex ultrasound. J Hum Hypertension 2002; 16:501-507.
2. Herman MG, Gardin JM, Jaff M, et al. Guidelines for the noninvasive vascular laboratory testing: a report from the American Society of Echocardiography and the Society for Vascular Medicine and Biology. Vasc Med 2006; 11:183-200.
3. Tublin ME, Bude RO, Platt JE. The resistive index in renal Doppler sonography. AJR Am J Roentgenol 2003; 180:885-892.
4. Soares GM, Murphy TP, Singha MS, et al. Renal artery duplex ultrasonography as a screening and surveillance tool to detect renal artery stenosis. J Ultrasound Med 2006; 25:293-298.
5. Cardosa CM, Xavier SS, Lopez GE, Brunini TMC. Direct Duplex scanning parameters in the diagnosis of renal artery stenosis: a study to validate and optimize cut-off points. Arq Brasiel Cardiol 2005; 87:286-293.
6. Gowda M, Loeb AL, Crouse LJ, Kramer PH. Complementary roles of color flow Duplex imaging and intravascular ultrasound in the diagnosis of renal artery fibromuscular dysplasia: should renal arteriography serve as the "gold standard"? J Am Coll Cardiol 2003; 41:1305-1311.
7. Rao SA, Mandalan KR, Rao VR. Takayasu's arteritis: initial and long-term follow-up in 16 patients after percutaneous transluminal angioplasty of the descending thoracic and abdominal aorta. Radiology 1993; 189:173-179.
8. Lupi-Herrera E, Sanchez TG, Marcushamer J, et al. Takayasu's arteritis: clinical study of 107 patients. Am Heart J 1977; 93:94-103.
9. Kliewer MA, Tupler RH, Hertzberg BS, et al. Doppler evaluation of renal artery stenosis: interobserver agreement in the interpretation of waveform morphology. AJR Am J Roentgenol 1994; 162:1371-1376.
10. Zucchelli PC. Hypertension and atherosclerotic renal artery stenosis: diagnostic approach. J Am Soc Nephrol 2002; 13:S184-S186.
11. Garcia-Criado A, Gilabert R, Nicolau C. Value of Doppler sonography for predicting clinical oucome after renal artery revascularization in atherosclerotic renal artery stenosis. J Ultrasound Med 2005; 24:141-1647.
12. Platt JF, Rubin JM, Ellis JH. Diabetic nephropathy: evaluation with renal duplex Doppler US. Radiology 1994; 190:343-346.
13. Platt JF, Rubin JM, Ellis JH. Lupus nephritis: predictive value of conventional and Doppler US and comparison with serologic and biopsy parameters: Radiology 1997; 203:82-86.
14. Zwiebel WJ, Pellerito J. Ultrasound assessment of native renal vessels and renal allografts. In Zwiebel WJ, Pellerito J. Introduction to Vascular Ultrasonography, 5th ed. Philadelphia, Elsevier Saunders, 2005, pp 611-636.
15. Habboub HK, Abu Yousef MM, William RD, et al. Accuracy of color Doppler sonography in assessing venous thrombus extension in renal cell carcinoma. Am J Roentgenol 1997; 168:267-271.
16. Hibbert J, Howlett DC, Greenwood KL, et al. The ultrasound appearances of neonatal renal vein thrombosis. Br J Radiol 1997; 70:1191-1194.
17. Bannister LH, Berry MM, Williams PL (eds). Gray's Anatomy, 37th ed. London, Churchill Livingstone, 1989, pp 1407-1409.
18. Berland L, Koslin B, Routh W, Keller F. Renal artery stenosis: prospective evaluation of diagnosis with color duplex US compared with angiography. Radiology 1990; 174:421-423.

19. Desberg A, Pauster D, Lammert G, et al. Renal artery stenosis: evaluation with color Doppler flow imaging. Radiology 1990; 177:749-753.
20. Haplen EJ, Nazarian LN, Wechsler RJ, et al. US, CT and MR evaluation of accessory renal arteries and proximal arterial branches. Acta Radiol 1999; 6:299-304.
21. Aytac SK, Yigit H, Sancak T, Ozcan H. Correlation between diameter of the main renal artery and the presence of an accessory renal artery. J Ultrasound Med 2003; 22:433-439.
22. Yagci B, Tavasli B, Karabulut N, Kiroglu Y. Clinical significance and renal hemodynamics of incidentally detected retroaortic left renal vein: assessment with venous Doppler sonography. Br J Radiol 2008; 81:187-191.
23. Soares GM, Murphy TM, Singha MS, et al. Renal artery duplex ultrasonography as a screnning and surveillance tool to detect renal artery stenosis. J Ultrasound Med 2006; 25:293-298.
24. House MK, Dowling RJ, King P, Gibson RN. Using Doppler sonography to reveal renal artery stenosis. AJR Am J Roentgenol 1999; 173:761-765.
25. Li JC, Yuan Y, Qin W, et al. Evaluation of the tardus-parvus pattern in patients with atherosclerotic and nonatherosclerotic renal artery stenosis. J Ultrasound Med 2007; 26:419-426.
26. Gottlieb RH, Snitzer EL, Hartley DF, et al. Interobserver and intraobserver variation in determining intrarenal parameters by Doppler sonography. AJR Am J Roentgenol 1997; 168:627-631.
27. Li JC, Wang L, Jiang YX, et al. Evaluation of renal artery stenosis with velocity parameters of Doppler sonography. J Ultrasound Med 2006; 25:735-742.
28. Turi ZG, Jaff MR. Renal artery stenosis: searching for the algorithms for the diagnosis and treatment. J Am Coll Cardiol 2003; 41:1312-1315.
29. Claudon M, Plauin PE, Baxter GM, et al. Renal arteries in patients at risk of renal arterial stenosis: multicenter evaluation of the echo-enhancer SH U508A at color and spectral Doppler US. Radiology 2000; 214:739-746.
30. Manganaro A, Ando G, Salvo A, et al. A comparision of power Doppler with conventional sonographic imaging for the evaluation of renal artery stenosis. Cardiovasc Ultrasound 2004; 2:1.
31. Radermacher J, Mengel M, Ellis S, et al. The renal arterial resistive index and renal allograft survival. N Engl J Med 2003; 349:115-124.
32. Nago M, Murase K, Saeki H, et al. Pulsating renal blood flow distribution measured using power Doppler ultrasound: correlation with hypertension. Hypertens Res 2002; 25:697-702.
33. Schwerk WB, Restrepo IK, Stellwaag M, et al. Renal artery stenosis: grading with image-directed Doppler US evaluation renal resistive index. Radiology 1994; 190:785-790.
34. Grenier N, Haugher O, Cimpean A, Perot V. Update of renal imaging. Semin Nucl Med 2006; 36:3-15.
35. Williams GJ, Macaskill P, Chan SF, et al. Comparative accuracy of renal duplex sonographic parameters in the diagnosis of renal artery stenosis: paired and unpaired analysis. AJR Am J Roentgenol 2007; 188:798-811.

CHAPTER 110

Inferior Vena Cava and Its Main Tributaries

Carlos Cuevas, Manjiri Dighe, and Mariam Moshiri

INTRODUCTION

The inferior vena cava (IVC) and major tributary veins are retroperitoneal structures with unique anatomic and developmental characteristics that offer special challenges for clinical and radiologic assessment. Even though the clinical assessment of IVC pathology presents several limitations, the revolutionary advances we have seen in computed tomography (CT) and magnetic resonance imaging (MRI) technology allow us to achieve excellent noninvasive assessments of these structures. The emergence of CT and MRI for vascular imaging has facilitated the transitioning of x-ray catheter angiography from merely a diagnostic tool to a viable less invasive percutaneous therapeutic replacement for complex open surgical interventions.

Multidetector row CT (i.e., MDCT) has become the modality of choice for IVC assessment. The fast scanning speeds that they can obtain has reduced motion artifacts to a minimum and enabled quick extended coverages of body anatomy, notably for rapid assessment of the heart, IVC, and pelvic veins. Another advantage of modern advanced MDCT scanners is their isotropic voxel resolution, allowing improved multiplanar reformation of image data (i.e., axial, coronal, sagittal, or oblique) with high spatial resolution, providing excellent anatomic assessment of complex anatomic relationships that can often be the case when evaluating vascular anatomy of abdominal organs.

MRI assessment of the IVC has also been improved with recent advances. The new phased array coils built with 12 and 16 channels can deliver better coverage of the abdomen and pelvis and provide increased signal-to-noise ratio. It is always important to keep in mind that MRI examinations do not expose the patient to ionizing radiation.

In this chapter, we will discuss the anatomy and pathology of the IVC, starting with the anatomic variants, then we will review tumoral disease affecting the IVC and finally, we will discuss some liver transplantation and interventions.

Inferior Vena Cava

Normal Anatomy and Congenital Anomalies

The IVC extends from the confluence of the common iliac veins at the level of L5 vertebral body, to the right atrium of the heart in right prevertebral location, next to the abdominal aorta and is surrounded by a rich network of lymphatic vessels (Fig. 110-1). It is partially covered anteriorly by the peritoneal membrane. The retroperitoneal space where the IVC is located can communicate with the perirenal spaces and the anterior and posterior interfascial spaces.[1]

The shape of the IVC varies from round to ovoid or even flat depending on a multitude of factors such as intrathoracic pressure, blood volume status, or the presence of congestive heart failure. The IVC receives a number of tributaries including common iliac, lumbar, renal, right adrenal, and hepatic veins. The IVC lies between the liver and the diaphragm and cephalad courses medially to enter the right atrium. At this level, a fat pad (continuous with the retroperitoneal fat) can be seen in many normal patients in an inferomedial location, sometimes bulging into the lumen of the IVC. This fat should not be considered pathologic and should not generate any further work-up studies.

Congenital anomalies of the IVC generally include abnormal position of the IVC or absence of IVC. The most common IVC anomalies are: (1) left IVC, (2) duplicated IVC, (3) azygos continuation of IVC, (4) circumaortic left renal vein, (5) retroaortic left renal vein, (6) circumcaval or retrocaval ureter, (7) duplicated right renal vein,

CHAPTER 110 • Inferior Vena Cava and Its Main Tributaries

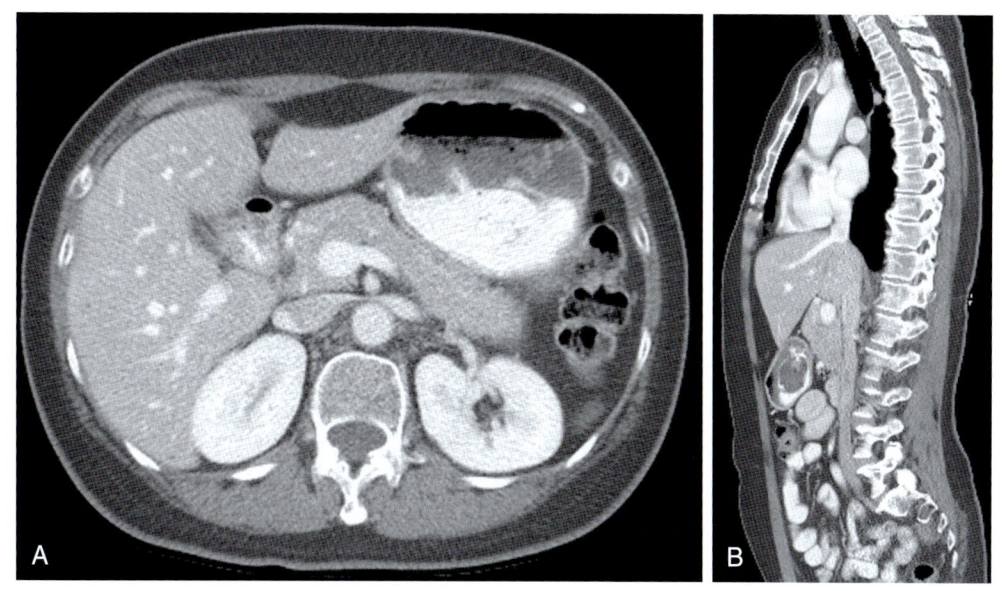

■ **FIGURE 110-1** Normal IVC. **A,** Contrast-enhanced CT of the abdomen depicts axial images at the level of the renal veins showing normal location and size of the IVC located to the right of the aorta. This image, obtained at portal-venous phase at the level of the left renal vein, shows heterogeneous luminal enhancement due to mixing of the renal vein blood with the inferior IVC blood. **B,** Sagittal reformat of the same study shows IVC segments with different luminal enhancement due to the normally observed different timing of the contrast return. Therefore we recommend imaging with longer delays (2 to 4 minutes) in order to obtain more homogeneous luminal enhancement.

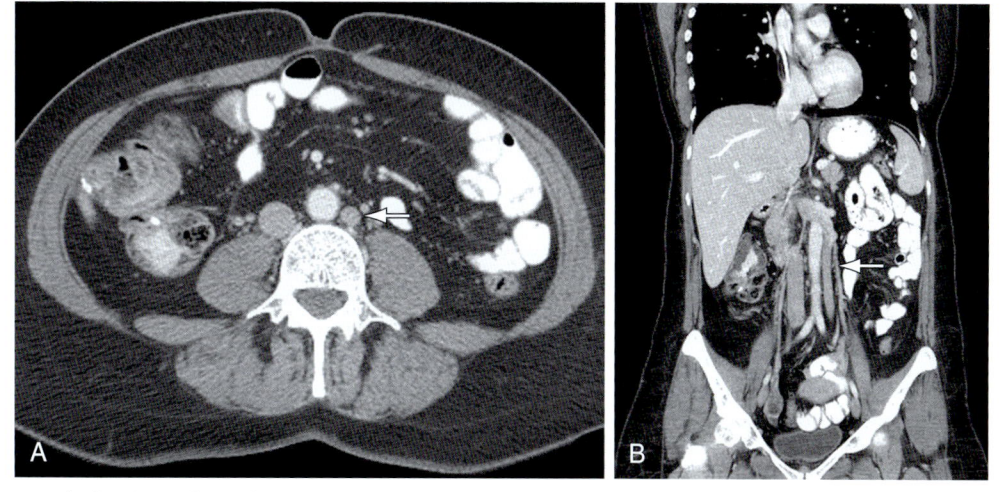

■ **FIGURE 110-2** IVC duplication (infrarenal). Contrast-enhanced CT shows two IVC—one on each side of the aorta. The left sided IVC originates in the left iliac vein and drains into the left renal vein (*arrows*) to join the right IVC (I) and form a single vein superior to the renal vessels.

(8) absence of infrarenal or entire IVC, (9) duplicated IVC with retroaortic right renal vein and hemiazygos continuation of the IVC, and (10) duplication of IVC with retroaortic left renal vein and azygos continuation of the IVC.

Left IVC: The infrarenal IVC is located to the left of the abdominal aorta, then it joins the left renal vein which then crosses anterior to the abdominal aorta and along with the right renal vein forms the normal right-sided prerenal IVC.

Duplicated IVC: There are two IVCs below the level of the renal veins—each connected to the ipsilateral common iliac vein. The left IVC joins the left renal vein, which then crosses anterior to the abdominal aorta and drains into the right IVC (Fig. 110-2). There may be variants in this anatomy and there may be significant discrepancy in the size of the two IVCs.

Azygos continuation of IVC: The infrarenal portion of IVC receives blood from the renal veins. It passes posterior to the diaphragmatic crura, enters the thorax as the azygos vein, and then joins the superior vena cava at the azygos arch. The hepatic and right adrenal veins drain directly into the right atrium. The gonadal veins drain into the ipsilateral renal veins. The right renal artery crosses abnormally anterior to the IVC (Fig. 110-3).

Circumaortic left renal vein: There are two left renal veins. The superior-anterior renal vein receives the adrenal vein and crosses the aorta anteriorly to join the IVC. The second renal vein is approximately 1 to 2 cm more inferior and posterior. It receives the left gonadal vein and crosses posterior to the aorta to join the IVC (Fig. 110-4).

Retroaortic left renal vein: The renal vein crosses posterior to the aorta to join the IVC.

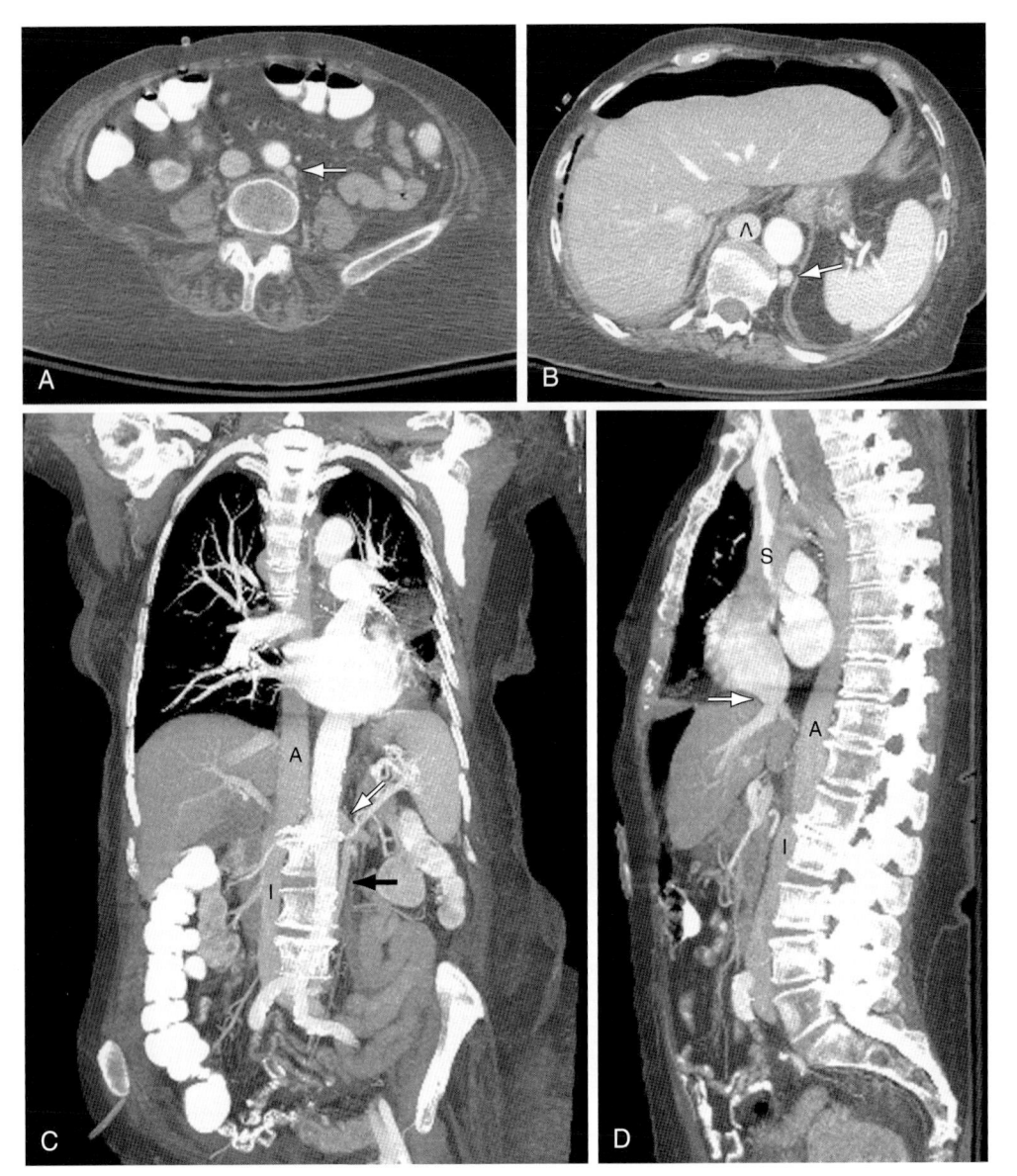

■ **FIGURE 110-3** Azygos-hemiazygos continuation of the IVC with duplication of the infrarenal IVC. **A**, Contrast-enhanced CT axial images show infrarenal IVC (I) and a smaller duplicated left IVC (*arrow*) that arises from the left iliac vein. **B**, CECT at a higher level demonstrates the absence of the intrahepatic portion of the IVC, which continues through the azygos vein (A) in retrocrural location. The image also shows a large hemiazygos vein (*arrow*) that arises from the left renal vein as continuation of the left IVC. **C**, Thick coronal MIP reformat shows the duplicated infrarenal IVC with the left (*arrow*) draining into the left renal vein and crossing behind the aorta (*black arrow*). The right IVC (I) continues through the azygos vein (A) above the level of the renal veins. **D**, Sagittal MIP reformat shows the azygos (A) continuation of the right IVC and how it connects to the SVC (S) through the azygos arch. Note the absence of the intrahepatic IVC and how the hepatic veins drain directly into the right atrium (*arrow*).

Circumcaval ureter (also known as retrocaval ureter): The anomaly always occurs on the right side. The proximal right ureter courses posterior to the IVC, emerges to the right of the aorta, and lies anterior to the right iliac vessel.

Duplicated right renal vein: There is presence of two right renal veins, one anterior and one posterior, usually at the same level.

Partial or complete absence of IVC: The variants of this anomaly include complete absence of the entire IVC which may include the iliac veins as well and partial absence of IVC with preservation of the suprarenal segment. In either case, the iliac veins join to form enlarged ascending lumbar veins. If the entire IVC is absent, the anterior paravertebral collateral vessels convey the blood return to the azygos and hemiazygos veins. If the suprarenal IVC is present, it receives blood from the renal veins. With partial or complete absence of the IVC, large gonadal and parauterine veins can be seen.

Duplication of IVC with retroaortic right renal vein and hemiazygos continuation of the IVC: There are two IVCs below the level of the renal veins. The right IVC joins the right renal vein, which crosses posterior to the aorta to drain in the left IVC. The left IVC then passes posterior to the diaphragmatic crura and continues into the thorax as the hemiazygos vein. There may be a significant size difference between the two vessels. In the thorax, the hemiazygos vein may have any of these different drainage

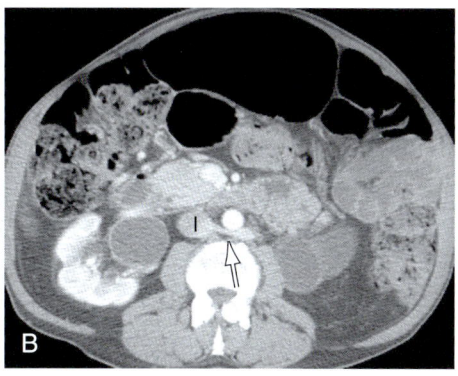

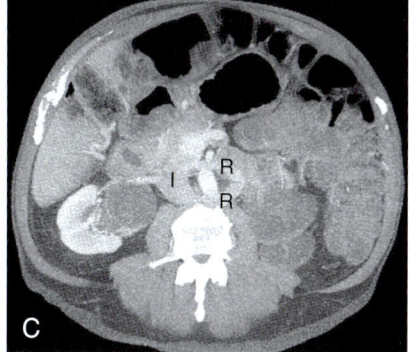

FIGURE 110-4 Circumaortic left renal vein. **A,** CECT of the abdomen shows a left renal vein crossing anterior to the aorta (*arrow*). The origin of a second, posterior left renal vein is visualized (*arrowhead*). **B,** CECT of the abdomen shows the posterior left renal vein (*arrow*) crossing behind the abdominal aorta 1 cm caudad to the anterior left renal vein. **C,** Axial oblique MIP shows both renal veins (R) surrounding the aorta.

pathways: (1) it crosses posterior to the aorta at about T8 to T9 to join the rudimentary azygos vein; (2) it joins a persistent left SVC and drains into the coronary vein; (3) an accessory hemiazygos continues to join the left brachiocephalic vein.

Duplication of IVC with retroaortic left renal vein and azygos continuation of IVC: There are two infrarenal IVCs. The left IVC joins the left renal vein which then crosses posterior to the aorta to join the right IVC. It passes posterior to the diaphragmatic crura and enters the thorax as azygos vein. It then joins the superior vena cava at its normal location in the right paratracheal space. The hepatic segment may not be truly absent. It drains directly into the right atrium.

Prevalence and Epidemiology

Deviations in the complex embryogenesis of the IVC may result in an overall 4% of anatomic variants in the general population. Duplicated IVC occurs in 0.2% to 3%, left IVC in 0.2% to 0.5%, azygos continuation of the IVC in 0.6%, circumaortic left renal vein in 8.7%, retroaortic left renal vein in 2.1%. The remaining congenital IVC anomalies are rare.

Etiology and Pathophysiology (Including any Special Anatomic Considerations)

Genetic factors may play a role in IVC anomalies because having a first-degree relative with an IVC anatomic anomaly is considered a risk factor.

Embryogenesis

Knowledge of the IVC embryogenesis is necessary for a better understanding of the IVC anatomic aberrations. The IVC is composed of four segments which form during the 6 to 8 weeks postconception.[2,3] This is due to continuous appearance and regression of three paired embryonic veins, which include the posterior cardinal veins, the subcardinal veins, and the supracardinal veins. The first step in this complex process is the formation of the posterior supracardinal and more anterior subcardinal veins. Then, the most caudal segment of the right supracardinal vein becomes the infrarenal vena cava. The hepatic segment of IVC is derived from the vitelline vein, which conveys blood from the viscera. The suprarenal segment is formed via a subcardinal-hepatic anastomosis. The renal segment forms via anastomosis of the right supra-subcardinal and post-subcardinal veins. The infrarenal segment arises from the right supracardinal vein.

Congenital anomalies of IVC are due to interruption of normal regression or lack of development of the different segments. The circumaortic venous ring and retroaortic left renal vein are related to aberrant development of the renal segment. Azygos continuation of the IVC results when there is a developmental anomaly involving the suprarenal segment.

Early in embryogenesis, there are two renal veins for each kidney: ventral and dorsal. Normally, the dorsal renal vein involutes as the anterior persists as the main renal vein in adult patients. Anatomic anomalies can occur if the involution of the dorsal veins does not occur, including retrocaval and circumaortic left renal vein and duplication of right renal vein.

Manifestations of Disease

Clinical Presentation

Patients with IVC anatomic aberrations are most commonly asymptomatic and the anomaly is discovered fortuitously during an imaging study ordered to assess other problems. Nevertheless, complications sometimes occur directly related to the presence of anatomic aberrations.

With retroaortic left renal vein, an increased incidence of testicular varicoceles has been reported, presumably due to compression of the left renal vein by the abdominal aorta. With the circumcaval ureter type, there could be partial right ureteral obstruction or recurrent urinary tract infection. With the absence of infrarenal IVC or entire IVC, patients may present with venous insufficiency of the lower extremities or idiopathic deep venous thrombosis. Approximately 5% of patients younger than 30 years with idiopathic deep venous thrombosis show IVC absence on CT. Almost 10% of these patients with a coexisting thrombophilia have congenital absence of the IVC.[4]

In female patients, enlarged gonadal and pelvis veins can simulate pelvic congestion syndrome. Anatomic variants of the IVC can be seen in association with other anomalies. Azygos continuation, in particular, can be associated with significant congenital heart disease.

Imaging Indications and Algorithm

The symptomatic patients would require evaluation of the venous system in the lower extremity and the urinary system. The best imaging consideration would be CT with multiplanar reformation. The detection of anatomic variants in the renal veins is particularly important at the time of surgical planning for kidney donation. Although the diagnosis of left renal vein variants is easy to detect, in the right kidney the findings of a double vein can be more subtle and sometimes may be overviewed.

Although the diagnosis of IVC anatomic aberrations may be suspected with abdominal ultrasonography, the assessment is usually limited due to their deep location, difficult insonation angle for Doppler studies, and/or the presence of bowel gas that may obscure key segments of the veins. The compression performed during a standard abdominal ultrasonographic examination may also cause collapse of some veins, making the anatomic assessment even more limited. The superior anatomic assessment provided by MRI or MDCT of the abdomen and pelvis makes them the modalities of choice at the time of making the final diagnosis. The advantages of these two modalities are among the following:

- Cross-section images provide the best diagnosis of the patency of the veins.
- Multiplanar images (axial, coronal, sagittal, and oblique) better demonstrate the extent of IVC anomalies and their relationship with other anatomic structures.
- Maximum intensity projection (MIP) reconstructions or 3D volume rendering may also be useful to demonstrate complex anatomic relationships.
- Intravenous contrast media may be administered to confirm venous patency, presence of a stenosis, visualization of collaterals, and/or venous tumor invasion.

There are some risks involved in the use of MDCT, including the ones related to ionizing radiation and the use of intravenous contrast media. MRI risks are related to those associated with the magnetic field but also to that of intravenous contrast agent administration if performed. X-ray catheter angiography is indicated primarily for therapeutic purposes such as installing an IVC filter, taking a biopsy of an intraluminal mass, or installing a stent to treat a venous stenosis.

Imaging Techniques and Findings

Radiography

Plain radiographs of the abdomen and pelvis have no role in the anatomic assessment of the IVC because they are unable to differentiate the veins from other retroperitoneal soft tissues. They may provide gross information though, of the relative location of foreign bodies such as filters, and catheters installed within the IVC.

Ultrasound Imaging

Ultrasound imaging with color flow Doppler imaging can be diagnostic for a variety of IVC anomalies. The key is to properly identify the abdominal venous structures (i.e., IVC), its location, its number, and its connections. With azygous continuation of the IVC, the infrahepatic IVC can be seen draining into the azygos vein with direct hepatic venous drainage into the right atrium. With left IVC, the IVC is positioned to the left of the abdominal aorta. In duplicated IVC, two vertical venous vascular structures can be seen adjacent to and paralleling the abdominal aorta. On Doppler, one IVC will drain the left renal vein.

Circumaortic left renal vein: A circumaortic left renal vein may be difficult to see on Doppler imaging because the two veins do not join the IVC at the same level.

Retroaortic left renal vein: A retroaortic left renal vein may be difficult to see on Doppler imaging. One could see a renal vein crossing behind the abdominal aorta to join the IVC. In more complex IVC anomalies, such as duplication of IVC with retroaortic right renal vein and hemiazygos continuation of the IVC or complete absence of the IVC, ultrasonography may be unable to fully delineate all venous connections and CT or MRI may be required. A circumcaval ureter is also typically not seen on ultrasound images unless there is hydroureter.

CT Scan

CT is a very useful modality to evaluate IVC anomalies because of its ability to generate volumetric data quickly for multiplanar reformation.

Technique: To study the anatomy of the IVC, the CT protocol should include imaging of the chest, abdomen, and pelvis with the use of an intravenous iodinated contrast agent. It is recommended to ensure that there is at least a 2-minute delay between intravenous contrast administration and CT scanning because this will improve the likelihood for homogeneous enhancement of the IVC. If CT is begun at the traditional portal venous phase (65 to 70 sec delay), the infrarenal IVC may have poor luminal enhancement owing to the relatively longer delay necessary for the venous return from the pelvis and inferior extremities to the IVC. The suprarenal IVC, moreover, may show heterogeneous enhancement because of mixing of the contrast bolus returning from the renal veins.

MR

Similar anatomic detail can be seen on MRI as is seen on CT. Steady-state free precession (SSFP; also termed *b-FFE*, Philips Medical Systems; FIESTA, General Electric Healthcare; True-FISP, Siemens Medical Solutions) pulse sequences are "bright blood" techniques that are particularly good for illustrating abdominal veins. SSFP, especially performed in cine mode, is useful for identification of central venous thrombosis. This technique does not require the intravenous administration of gadolinium-chelate contrast agents.

"Black blood" MRI pulse sequences, in which the vessel lumen is dark secondary to the washout phenomenon (also termed *flow void*) associated with moving spins (i.e., flowing blood that washes out of the imaging slice prior to sampling of the echo). Examples of this technique include T4-weighted spin echo and single shot T2-weighted imaging (e.g., SSFSE, HASTE), which can provide excellent anatomic assessment almost free of motion artifacts.

Gadolinium-enhanced MRI is arguably the most reliable method to assess vascular patency. We recommend postcontrast imaging using a 3D T1-weighted gradient sequence (e.g., LAVA, THRIVE, or VIBE). Because MRI does not expose the patient to ionizing radiation, it is possible to acquire multiple series of images postcontrast injection, including axial, coronal, and sagittal planes with different timing for more homogeneous luminal enhancement.

Angiography

X-ray catheter angiography studies provide limited anatomic information. In our institution, they are used mostly for therapeutic procedures. Anatomic variants should be diagnosed prior to angiographic procedures in the IVC or otherwise may cause confusion and prolong fluoroscopic time at the time of the intervention, therefore for therapy planning purposes, we recommend the use of CT or MRI.

Reporting: Information for the Referring Physician

IVC and renal vein anatomic variants have minimal increased risk for medical complications such as thrombus or embolism, but are particularly important to identify in patients planning to undergo surgical or percutaneous interventions because their identification can aid in procedure planning and reduce likelihood of complications. Recommendations for clinicians are

1. Obtain a complete anatomic assessment with CT or MRI of the relevant location (i.e., chest, abdomen, and/or pelvis).
2. Inform the patient and other physicians of the presence and kind of anatomic variant. The patient should be informed to also alert any treating physician.
3. Provide the information when requesting an imaging examination because this may aid in selecting the proper protocol for the imaging examination.

TUMORS OF THE IVC AND MAIN TRIBUTARIES

Prevalence and Epidemiology

Primary IVC tumors (leiomyosarcomas) are very rare with only one large series published in the literature.[5] It is more common to see tumors invading the IVC through its tributary veins arising from separate abdominal organs. One of the most common causes of neoplastic invasion of the IVC lumen is the renal cell carcinoma (RCC) that can be seen invading the IVC through the renal vein in 4% to 10% of the cases. Hepatocellular carcinoma (HCC) frequently invades the portal vein but also on rare occasions can invade the IVC through the hepatic veins. Primary adrenocortical carcinoma is a rare adrenal tumor that invades the IVC. Multiple other retroperitoneal tumors can compress and invade the IVC, including lymphomas, metastasis of gonadal or uterine tumors, pheochromocytomas, and other retroperitoneal sarcomas.

Etiology and Pathophysiology (Including any Special Anatomic Considerations)

Leiomyosarcomas of the IVC arise from the smooth muscle cells in the vessel wall. They can arise in any segment of the IVC and can extend intraluminally to the right atrium of the heart. Two thirds of the leiomyosarcomas appear predominantly as extraluminal growth and the other one third appear mostly as intraluminal tumors. Both types can cause obstruction of the IVC and consequently, can cause venous congestion of the abdominopelvic organs and lower extremities. The venous congestion caused by the tumor can cause acute organ failure of the liver, kidneys, and other organs depending on its location, growth rate, and the development of bland thrombus aggravating the problem. Right adrenocortical carcinomas directly invade the IVC through the adrenal veins. Because the left adrenal veins drain to the left renal vein, left adrenal tumors reach the IVC through this pathway.

Manifestations of Disease

Clinical Presentation

IVC Obstruction Syndrome

The patients typically present lower extremity edema and subcutaneous collateral veins in the abdominal wall. If the tumor obstructs the hepatic segment of the IVC, it may manifest as **Budd-Chiari syndrome** with abdominal pain, hepatomegaly, and ascites due to obstruction of the hepatic veins.

Abdominal Mass

Palpable, painful mass could be the presentation for some tumors (i.e., renal cell carcinoma or large retroperitoneal sarcomas).

Pulmonary Embolism

Occasionally IVC tumors may cause embolism to the pulmonary arteries and produce cardiorespiratory symptoms including chest pain, tachycardia, and dyspnea.

Imaging Indications and Algorithm

Best Imaging Modality

Contrasted MRI or CT of the abdomen and pelvis is the modality of choice for the assessment of these complex tumors.[6-8] The scanning protocol should include the right atrium of the heart as well as the entire pelvis and common femoral veins. Early postcontrast phases (arterial and portal-venous) may demonstrate heterogeneous luminal enhancement due to admixing artifacts at the level of the renal veins that can obscure tumor or produce a false positive diagnosis of IVC thrombus; therefore additional 2- to 4-minute delayed images are recommended, which will provide more homogeneous luminal enhancement for improved ability to detect the presence or absence of intraluminal tumor or thrombus.

Recommendations

- Obtain multiplanar images: axial, coronal and sagittal.
- Include the entire heart: accurate assessment of the proximal extension of the tumor is very important for surgical planning. Invasion of the right atrium will make the tumor unresectable.
- When indicated, obtain a CT scan of the chest to rule out pulmonary embolism and detect the presence of lung metastasis that may change management. PET-CT can be useful in staging some tumors (not hepatocellular carcinoma).
- Intraoperative ultrasonography: could be useful to determine proximal extension of the tumor at the time of surgery.

Imaging Techniques and Findings

Radiography

Although abdominal radiographs can sometimes demonstrate the presence of a large calcified retroperitoneal mass, there are no specific signs of IVC invasion on plain films and, therefore, it is very limited for retroperitoneal tumor detection and characterization.

Ultrasound Imaging

Ultrasonography can detect the presence of tumor in the IVC, but in many cases, the anatomic assessment is incomplete owing to multiple limiting factors because of characteristics of the IVC anatomy. The deep location in the abdomen requires the use of low-frequency transducers with less spatial resolution and low signal-to-noise ratio. The surrounding bowel gas and bone may obscure key segments of the IVC and its tributaries. The position of the IVC in 90-degree angle with the ultrasound beam makes the color and spectral Doppler examination equivocal and limited. In summary, although in some cases ultrasound imaging can diagnose correctly the presence of IVC tumors, most of the times conclusions are limited by the technical challenges of the anatomy and, therefore, other studies are necessary to confirm the diagnosis.

Real time gray-scale US: can demonstrate an intraluminal mass and the presence of expansion of the IVC. It can demonstrate primary liver, renal and adrenal tumor.

Intraoperative US: is useful to assess proximal extension of the tumor and possible heart involvement.

Color Doppler: Can show the absence of flow caused by the thrombus that can be partially occluding the lumen or causing complete obstruction, sometimes with presence of collateral veins. Color blooming may obscure partial thrombus.

CT

Technique: pre- and multi-phase postcontrast CT is necessary to differentiate bland nonenhancing thrombus from enhancing tumor, but both may coexist in the same patient. A chest CT should be considered to look for pulmonary metastases and/or pulmonary embolism. Abdominal and pelvic CT should be performed with 2- and 4-minute delayed phases following the intravenous administration of iodinated contrast agent to obtain homogeneous luminal enhancement. The examination should include the heart and common femoral veins. We recommend producing coronal and sagittal reconstructions to better demonstrate the extension of the tumor and its relation to other anatomic structures that can be key at the time of surgical planning.

CT Findings

Intraluminal leiomyosarcoma: presents as a tumor thrombus in the lumen of the vessel. This solid neoplasm shows contrast enhancement in postinjection images. The tumor thrombus characteristically produces expansion of the IVC and can also occlude the lumen, causing venous congestion in the proximal organs such as the liver or kidneys (Fig. 110-5). Lack of a known primary tumor suggests the diagnosis of primary leiomyosarcoma of the IVC.

Extraluminal leiomyosarcoma and other retroperitoneal neoplasms: Other retroperitoneal tumors that can occlude the IVC and its tributaries include lymphomas, metastasis (ovary, testis, uterus, and others) and primary leiomyosarcomas of predominant extraluminal growth. Often these tumors are indistinguishable from each other and only a histologic analysis can differentiate them. The presence of fat density tissue may suggest a liposarcoma. Diffuse lymphadenopathy points to lymphoma. Unfortunately, the presence of calcifications is not specific for any particular kind of retroperitoneal tumor.

Adrenocortical carcinoma: Presents as a large heterogeneous adrenal mass typically with venous invasion.[10] It usually compresses and displaces adjacent organs such as the kidney or liver and it can be confused with renal cell carcinoma or hepatocellular carcinoma. For this particular point, the use of sagittal or coronal reconstructions can be useful to determine the origin of the mass. As mentioned previously, the right adrenal veins drain directly into the IVC but the left adrenal carcinoma invades the IVC through the left renal vein, potentially being confused with venous invasion from renal cell carcinoma arising from the upper pole of the left kidney.

Renal cell carcinoma: typically presents as a solid, heterogeneous renal mass that can extend into the renal veins and IVC (Fig. 110-6).[8,9] There may be gonadal vein invasion. This tumor also can display direct retroperitoneal extension and lymph node metastasis.

Hepatocellular carcinoma: is a solid hepatic tumor that is most commonly seen in patients with cirrhosis. After contrast injection, it typically enhances in the arterial phase and washes out in the delay phase. It invades

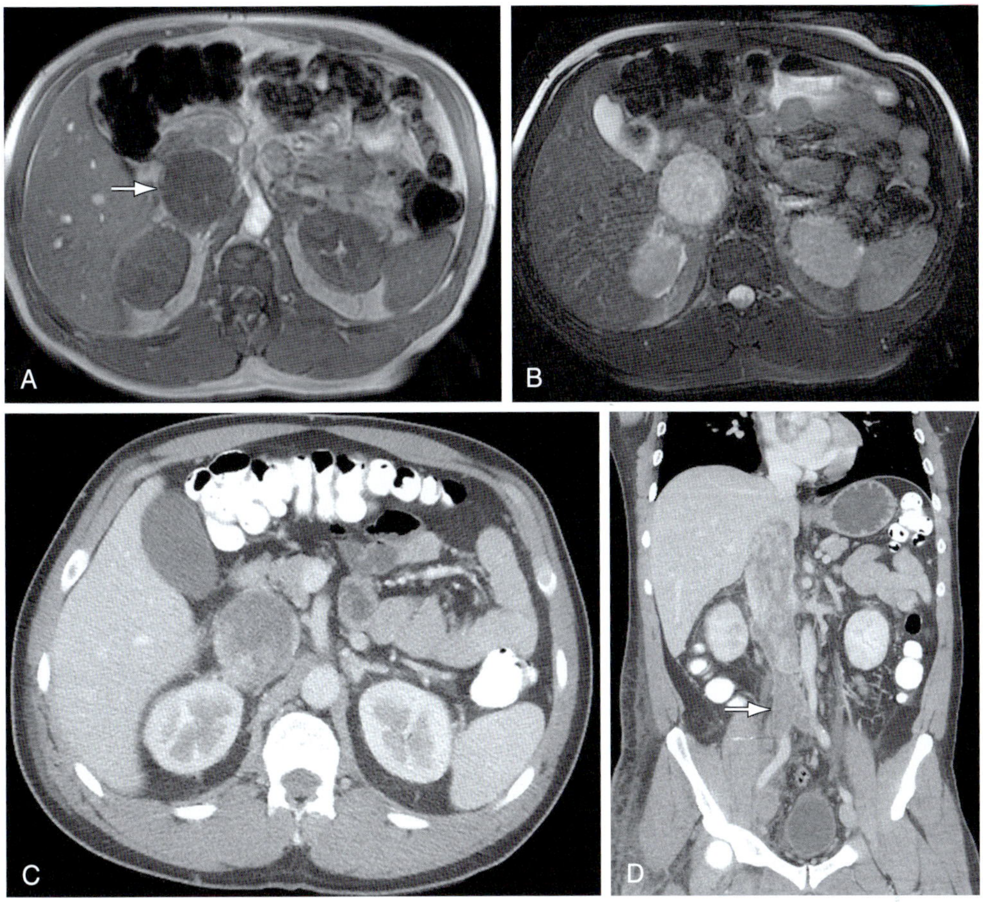

FIGURE 110-5 Primary leiomyosarcoma of the IVC. **A,** Axial T1-weighted MRI of the abdomen demonstrates a hypointense tumor expanding the IVC lumen (*arrow*). T2 fat saturated MRI shows high signal in the IVC tumor (**B**). Contrast-enhanced CT of the abdomen in axial (**C**) and coronal (**D**) images show that the thrombus in the IVC enhances heterogeneously as well as expands the vein. The more inferior component of the thrombus does not enhance or enlarge the vein and, therefore, is consistent with bland thrombus (*arrow*).

the IVC through the hepatic veins.[11] As other tumoral thrombus, it typically expands the veins (Fig. 110-7).

MR

Technique: Although nonenhanced MRI sequences can show the presence of tumor thrombus in the IVC, pre- and post-gadolinium MRI pulse sequences are ideal for the detection, characterization, and assessment of disease extent. It also is useful to characterize the primary lesion when the tumor is originated in an adjacent organ such as the liver or kidney.

SSFP and single shot T2-weighted pulse sequences can be used to demonstrate the presence of tumor without the use of gadolinium-chelate contrast agent. Using SSFP, one can detect the presence of intraluminal tumor; using single shot T2-weighted images, one can evaluate the venous mass and its relationship with the wall of the vein and the adjacent structures. The tumor thrombus has typically a heterogeneous elevated signal on T2-weighted images. We recommend acquiring sequences in axial, coronal, and sagittal planes for better assessment of the extension of the lesion.

Multiphase, pre- and post-gadolinium-enhanced three-dimensional T1-weighted imaging with fat saturation (e.g., LAVA, THRIVE, VIBE) is a very useful MRI technique. Tissue enhancement helps to differentiate a solid tumor from nonenhancing bland thrombus. Subtraction techniques can be used to demonstrate tumoral enhancement or bland thrombus nonenhancement. Postcontrast multiphase images should be obtained: Early phase (arterial and portal-venous) can show better the solid organs in the abdomen and a late phase (2 to 4 min) for infrarenal IVC assessment. Multiplanar images (axial, coronal, and sagittal) should be obtained for better anatomic assessment.

Nuclear Medicine/PET

Primary IVC sarcoma, adrenocortical carcinoma, and renal cell carcinoma are in general FDG avid tumors in PET imaging. Therefore PET can be used to detect and characterize pulmonary or systemic metastasis in these cases. PET imaging does not have a role in hepatocellular carcinoma staging because the well differentiated hepatocellular carcinomas are not FDG avid.

Angiography

Angiographic techniques are mostly used for interventions, including biopsy, IVC stent, or filter placement and

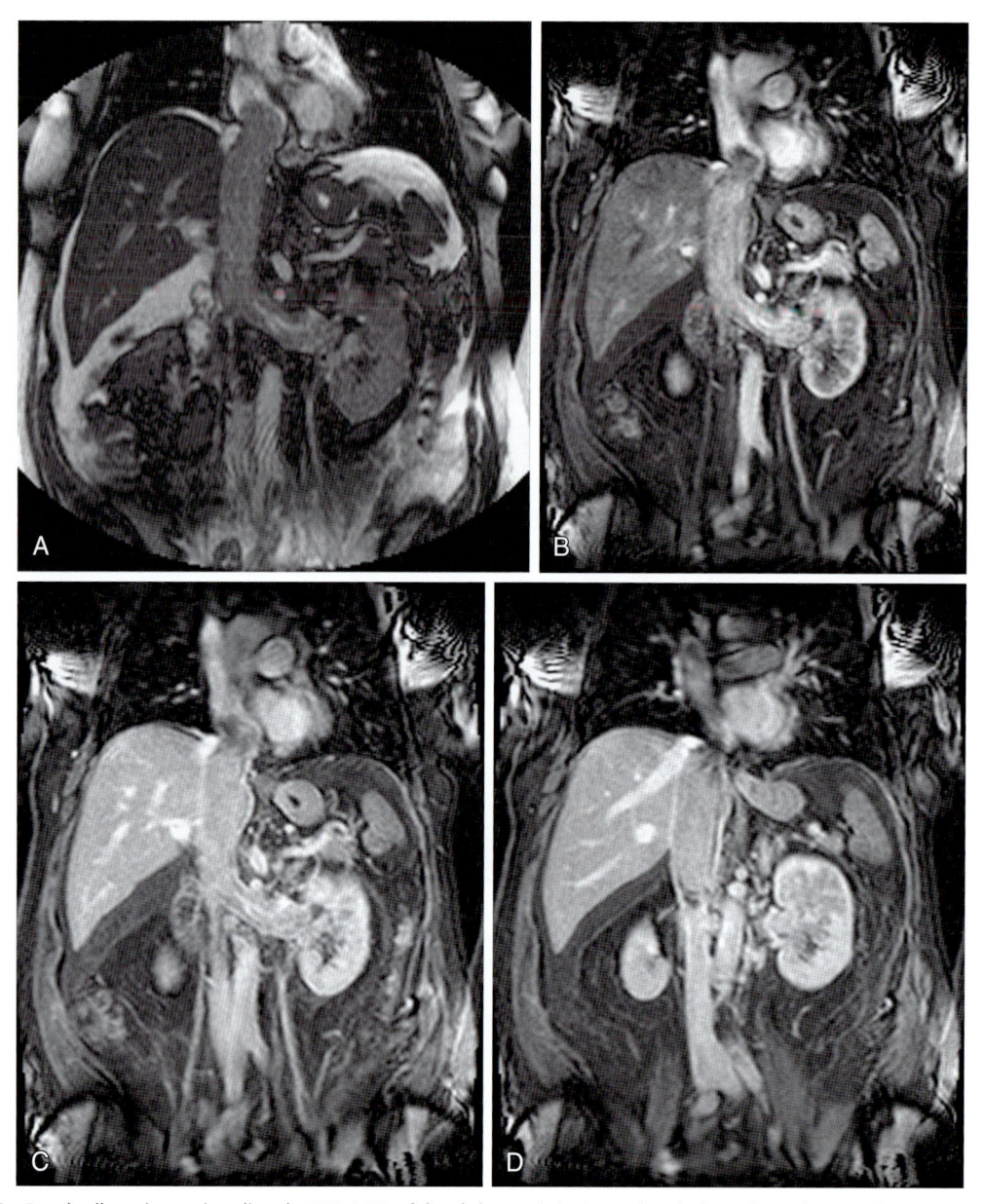

FIGURE 110-6 Renal cell carcinoma invading the IVC. MRI of the abdomen (**A**). Coronal T2 balanced steady-state free precession shows RCC thrombus extending through the left renal vein, IVC, and protruding into the right atrium of the heart. The patient has developed ascites due to partial obstruction of the hepatic veins without causing thrombosis. Arterial phase CE MRI (**B**) shows tumor thrombus enhancement. Five-minute delay CE MRI (**C, D**) images demonstrate tumor enhancement and vessel expansion—both specific signs of tumor thrombus. The primary left renal mass and the patency of the infrarenal IVC are better demonstrated in a more posterior plane (**D**).

angioplasty for IVC stenosis. The invasiveness of the angiographic studies and the limited information of only intraluminal anatomy makes them a less preferred technique for purely diagnostic imaging compared with noninvasive tomographic techniques such as CT or MRI.

DIFFERENTIAL DIAGNOSIS

From Clinical Presentation

Benign differential diagnosis for clinical symptoms includes primary Budd Chiari syndrome, benign IVC thrombosis or external compression, cirrhosis, and congestive heart disease.

From Imaging Findings

Heterogeneous enhancement of the IVC due to mixing contrast media at the level of the renal veins can cause the false appearance of IVC thrombosis. Budd-Chiari syndrome from benign causes such as thrombophilia or vascular webs can also be confused with tumor thrombus; the absence of thrombus enhancement and no vessel expansion are important signs to differentiate them from tumoral thrombus.

External compression of the IVC from benign causes are retroperitoneal fibrosis, liver edema, inflammatory pseudotumor, and retroperitoneal fat herniation into the suprahepatic IVC.

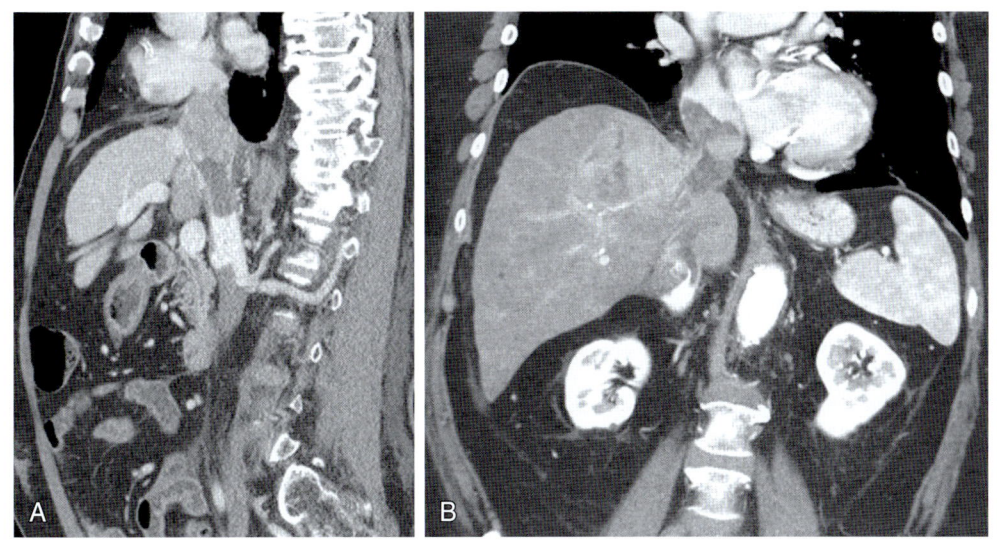

■ **FIGURE 110-7** HCC invading the IVC through the hepatic veins. **A,** CECT. Sagittal reconstruction. Note the presence of a nonenhancing, nontumoral thrombus component inferior to the enhancing tumor invading the IVC. The tumor expands the vessel and extends into the right atrium. **B,** Coronal CECT of another patient shows HCC invading large portions of the right atrium.

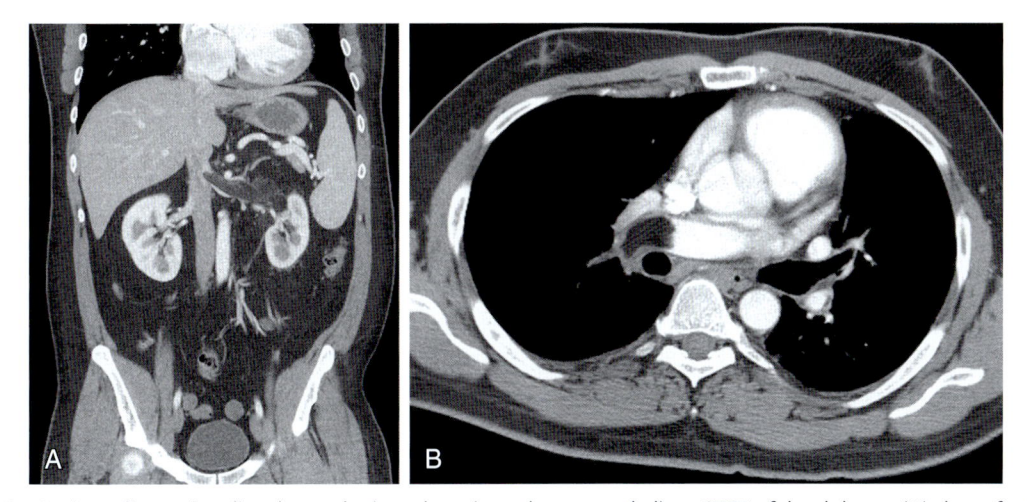

■ **FIGURE 110-8** Angiomyolipoma invading the renal vein and causing pulmonary embolism. CECT of the abdomen (**A**) shows fat-density tumor invading the renal vein consistent with a surgically proven angiomyolipoma. Although the invasion of the veins may suggest a malignant nature, this is a benign tumor. CECT of the chest of the same patient (**B**) shows a large fat density embolism in the right pulmonary artery caused by a portion of detached tumor.

Renal angiomyolipoma can be a benign cause of renal vein invasion and can be easily diagnosed demonstrating fat tissue in the tumor thrombus (Fig. 110-8).

SYNOPSIS OF TREATMENT OPTIONS
Medical
No curative medical treatment is available for sarcomas or carcinomas invading the IVC. Palliative experimental chemotherapy can be tried.

Surgical/Interventional
Surgical resection is the only option of curative treatment. Published 5-year survival of patients with tumor resection of renal cell carcinoma with IVC invasion is 32% to 64% in patients without distant metastasis. Survival of patients with primary leiomyosarcoma is short, depending on stage and grade of the tumor. Without surgery, the survival of a patient with malignant thrombus of the IVC is only a few months, usually aggravated by acute pulmonary embolism.

Reporting: Information for the Referring Physician
IVC tumors can be considered a relative emergency. Appropriate staging and detection of acute complications (i.e., pulmonary embolism, liver or renal failure) should be made and imaging plays a central role in these two tasks. It is also crucial that the chest, abdomen, and pelvis have been examined with the adequate MRI or CT protocols, otherwise the studies should be repeated.

It is very important for the surgical planning to describe accurately the proximal extension of the tumor, if there are signs of IVC wall invasion, and if there is evidence of distant metastasis. It is of main importance also to distinguish between tumor and nontumor thrombus that can coexist in the same case.

IVC COMPLICATIONS IN ORTHOTOPIC LIVER TRANSPLANTATION ANATOMY

Definition

The liver is transplanted in an orthotopic position, that is, the native liver is removed and the donor liver is transplanted in the normal anatomical site.[12] Because of the firm attachment of the retrohepatic inferior vena cava (IVC) to the caudate lobe, the most direct method of removal is to take the IVC with it. An end-to-end anastomosis is then performed between the recipient and donor IVC. In order to minimize complications arising from the clamping of the portal vein and IVC during the operation, a veno-venous bypass must be performed. Another type of IVC anastomosis performed is the "piggy-back" anastomosis. In this technique, the liver is lifted off the IVC, by dividing the short caudate veins. The suprahepatic IVC of the implanted liver is then anastomosed to the hepatic venous confluence of the recipient by an end-to-side anastomosis and the donor infrahepatic IVC is tied off. The main advantage of this technique is that it does not need the veno-venous bypass because the recipient IVC is not clamped. Although the procedure is both technically difficult and time-consuming, there is one less anastomosis to perform.

In living or pediatric transplants, a split-liver transplantation is performed, where the donor liver may be provided or the donor liver may be reduced to a right lobe (segments 5 through 8), left lobe (segments 1 through 4) or left lateral segment (segments 2 and 3). With the first two, the cava is preserved, allowing either the caval replacement or piggy-back technique to be employed. The left lateral segment reduction is performed in spilt-liver transplants only and involves removal of the IVC; thus the piggy-back method is necessary.[13]

Prevalence and Epidemiology

Liver transplantation has become the method of choice for treatment of patients with irreversible severe liver dysfunction.[13] Today, liver transplantation is a standardized treatment modality for well-defined indications.[14] According to the United Network of Organ Sharing (UNOS), to-date 97,166 liver transplants have been performed. It is increasingly successful with 1-year patient survival rate of approximately 84% and 3-year survival rate of 76%.[14] IVC complications in orthotopic liver transplantation, that is, stenosis and thrombosis, are diagnosed in fewer than 1% of transplant cases.[15]

Manifestations of Disease

Clinical Presentation

Clinical features in IVC or hepatic stenosis include hepatomegaly, ascites, and pleural effusions. Some patients are clinically asymptomatic and imaging abnormality may be the first sign of a problem. Hepatic venous outflow obstruction presents clinically with elevated liver enzymes, Budd-Chiari syndrome, or coagulation disorders.

Imaging Indications and Algorithm

Ultrasound imaging is the modality of choice for imaging post liver transplantation patients. CT and MRI may be used as well.

Imaging Techniques and Findings

Ultrasound Imaging

On ultrasound findings, the normal hepatic vein and IVC have a triphasic waveform. Ultrasound findings in IVC thrombosis are absent flow within the vein on color Doppler with no spectral Doppler flow. An intraluminal echogenic thrombus can also be seen in complete or partial thrombosis of the IVC. In IVC stenosis, there is a three- to fourfold increase in velocity as compared to the prestenotic segment. The velocity in the IVC has to be measured at the sites of anastomosis, suprahepatic and infrahepatic, in end-to-end anastomosis and at the end-to-side anastomosis in piggy-back anastomosis (Figs. 110-9 and 110-10). A significant caval stenosis may result in

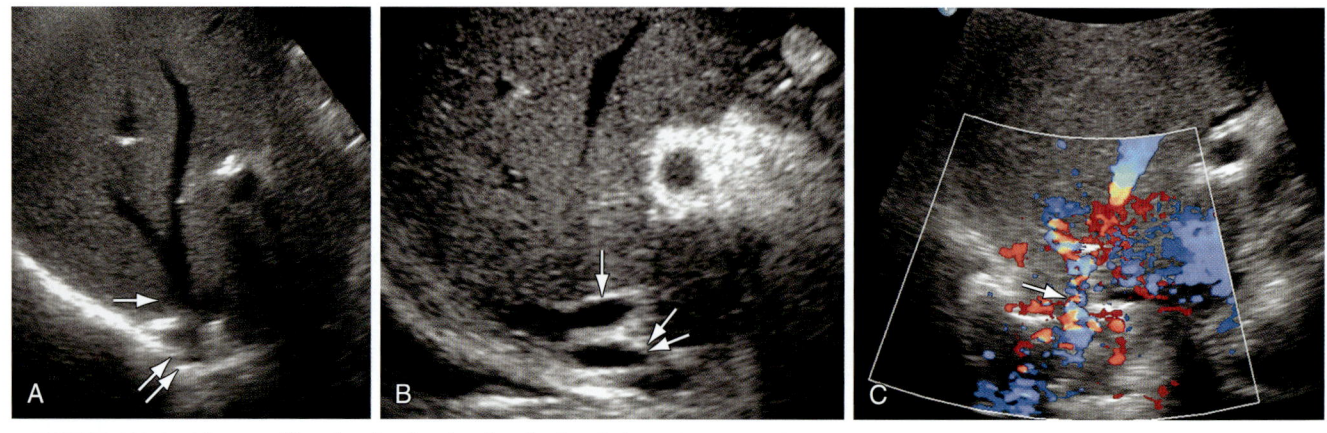

FIGURE 110-9 Ultrasound imaging showing the piggy-back technique of anastomosis in transverse (**A**) and sagittal (**B**) images. Donor IVC (*long white arrow*) and recipient IVC (*double white arrows*) are shown. **C,** Color Doppler showing the correct site of measurement of the velocity in the piggy-back anastomosis (*arrow*).

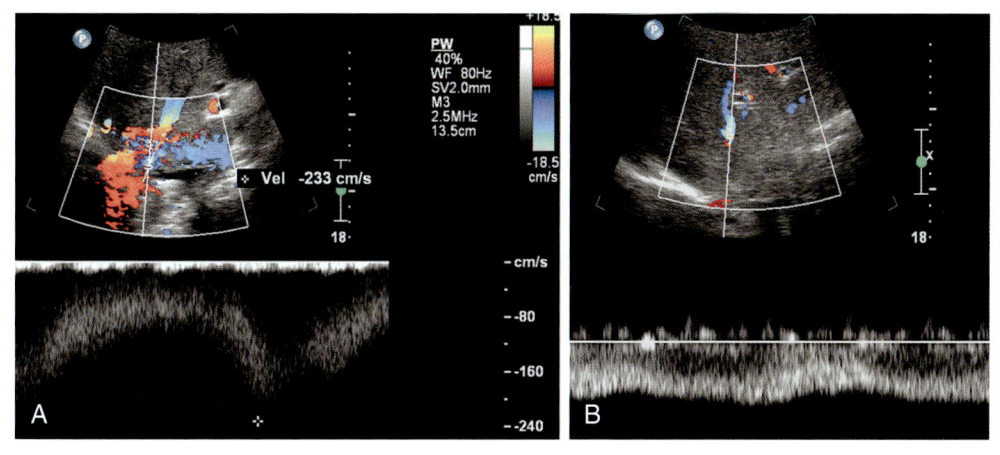

FIGURE 110-10 **A,** Spectral Doppler showing an increased velocity in the area of anastomosis and **B,** monophasic waveform in the hepatic vein consistent with stenosis.

reversed flow or absence of phasicity in the hepatic veins.[16]

CT
CT can differentiate between stenosis and occlusion or thrombosis of the hepatic veins and IVC. Contrast administration is essential.

MR
MR can also differentiate between stenosis and occlusion or thrombosis of the hepatic veins and IVC, however contrast administration is essential.

Nuclear Medicine/PET
Nuclear medicine/PET is not used for imaging vascular complications in post–liver transplantation patients.

Angiography
Angiography is definitive in diagnosing IVC stenosis and can provide treatment at the same time as well. Pressure gradients can be measured in the IVC and the atrium during angiography. Percutaneous treatment for IVC stenosis and thrombosis includes angioplasty and/or stenting (Figs. 110-11 and 110-12).

Classic Signs
- Increased velocity in the IVC at the anastomotic site
- Monophasic waveforms in the hepatic veins
- Ascites

Differential Diagnosis
From Clinical Presentation
The clinical differential diagnosis of IVC obstruction/stenosis post–liver transplantation includes portal hypertension, hepatic vein stenosis, portal vein stenosis, and liver transplant rejection.

From Imaging Findings
IVC compression from enlarged liver.

Synopsis of Treatment Options
Medical
Diuretics may be administered but treatment is primarily interventional.

Surgical/Interventional
Percutaneous intervention using angioplasty and/or stenting.

Reporting: Information for the Referring Physician
Important information for referring physicians:

- Increased velocity at the IVC anastomotic site
- Monophasic waveforms in the hepatic veins

IVC THROMBOSIS
Definition
IVC thrombosis can be caused by a variety of factors, some of which are mentioned subsequently with the most common etiology being extension of the thrombus from the lower limb deep venous thrombosis (DVT) into the IVC. Iliac vein compression syndrome (IVCS), also known as May-Thurner syndrome, is the result of compression of the left common iliac vein between the right common iliac artery and overlying vertebrae. It is not an infrequent source of venous abnormalities in the left lower extremity. The true prevalence of this disorder is unknown.

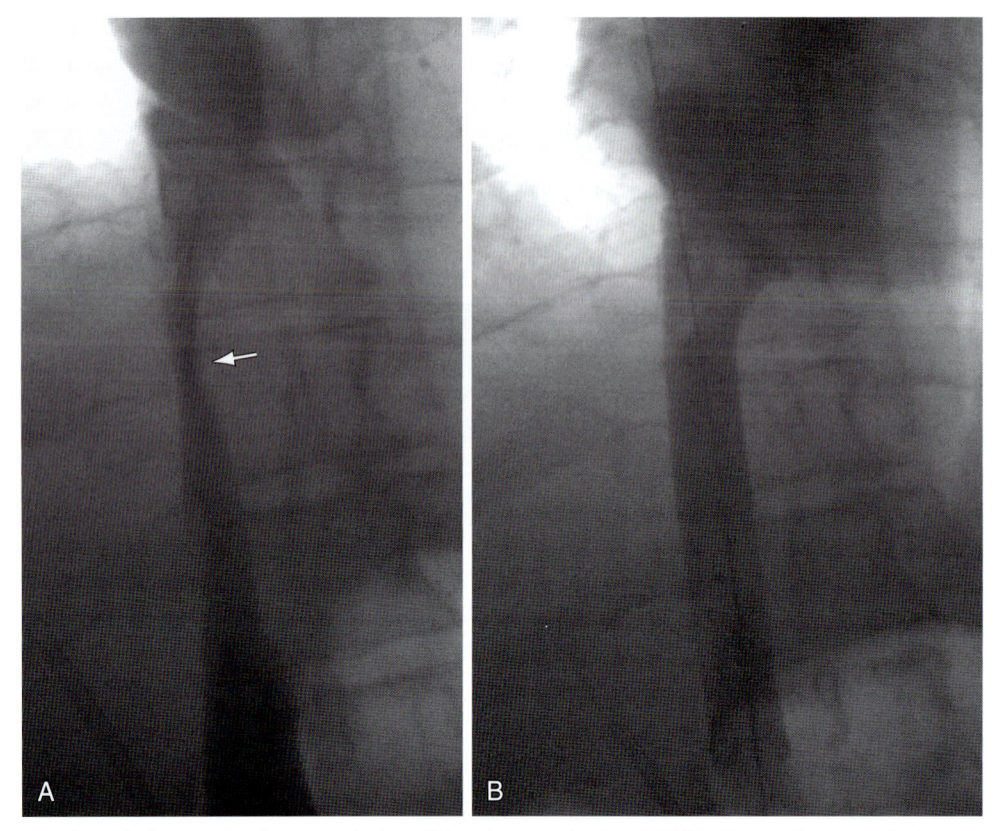

FIGURE 110-11 Angiography images showing preangioplasty (**A**) and postangioplasty IVC (**B**). Stenosis is present in the preangioplasty image (*arrow*), and the IVC appears of normal caliber in the postangioplasty image.

Prevalence and Epidemiology

The exact number of patients who have IVC thrombosis remains elusive because of the clinical variability in presentation. By compiling information from several epidemiologic studies that investigated DVT prevalence, the estimated rate of IVC thrombosis in patients with DVT is 4% to 15%; in the United States, 6,600 to 74,000 cases of IVC thrombosis occur each year.

Etiology and Pathophysiology (Including any Special Anatomic Considerations)

The variety of underlying etiologies for IVC thrombosis is extensive and listed in Table 110-1. IVC thrombosis can result from extension of a DVT, but also can be secondary to other factors such as tumor invasion/extension, external compression, hematoma/trauma, coagulation dysfunction, iatrogenic causes, and other miscellaneous etiologies.

Manifestations of Disease

Clinical Presentation

Patients with IVC thrombosis may present with a spectrum of signs and symptoms. Patients may present with symptoms that are predominantly thrombotic in origin or predominantly embolic in nature. Additionally, the thrombotic findings are dependent on the degree of occlusion of the cava and on the location between the iliac confluence and the right atrium. The classic presentation of IVC thrombosis includes bilateral lower extremity edema with dilated, visible superficial abdominal veins. The most common clinical presentation in iliocaval compression syndrome is left lower extremity deep vein thrombosis. Rarely, a patient with IVCS can present with obstruction of venous outflow without deep vein thrombosis.

Imaging Indications and Algorithm

Presence of bilateral leg edema and pulmonary embolism are common indications for imaging the IVC.

Imaging Techniques and Findings

Ultrasound Imaging

A filling defect is seen in the IVC which appears echogenic in an acute thrombus with a distended IVC. A chronic thrombus appears hypoechoic with decreased size of the IVC lumen.[17] Doppler ultrasound examinations show monophasic flow without respiratory variation distal to the compression and a significant increase in flow velocity at the point of arterial compression in the common iliac vein in patients with May-Thurner syndrome. DVT may be seen in the left lower extremity on ultrasonography in patients with May-Thurner syndrome.

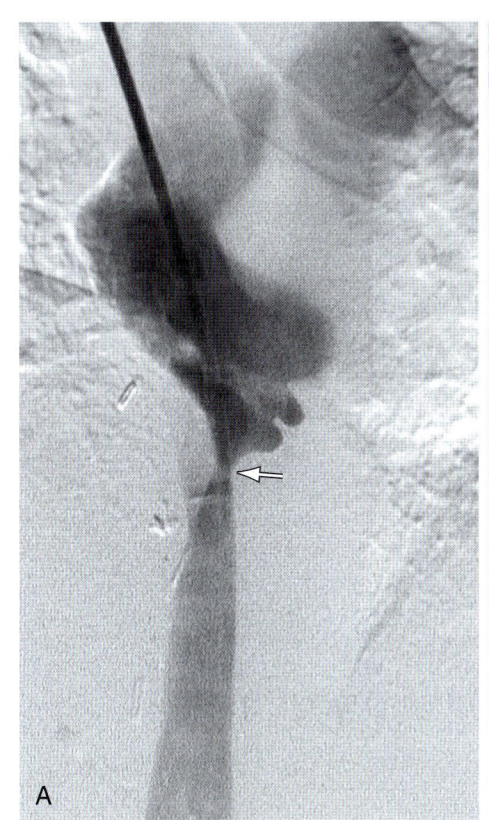

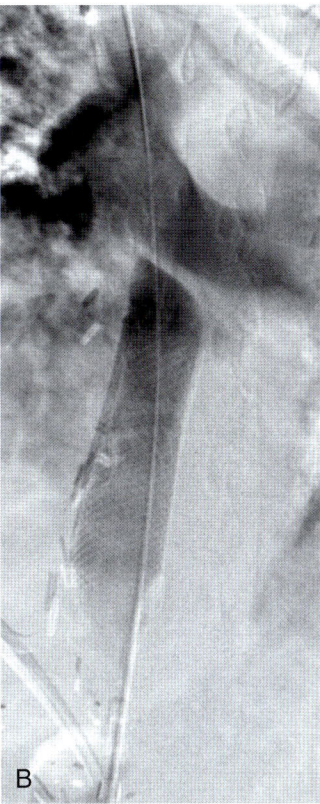

■ **FIGURE 110-12** Angiography image (**A**). Pre-stent placement showing the narrowed caliber of the IVC (*arrow*) and **B,** postangioplasty image showing a stent in the IVC with improved caliber.

CT

Definitive diagnosis of venous thrombosis by CT depends on demonstration of an intraluminal thrombus. Whereas a fresh thrombus has a density similar to or higher than that of circulating blood, an old thrombus is of lower density than the surrounding blood on noncontrast CT scans. When the occlusion is complete, the involved segment remains unenhanced on postcontrast CT scans. In case of chronic occlusion, the IVC may become atrophic and calcified. In partial IVC occlusion, the thrombus is seen as a filling defect surrounded by enhanced blood. A "pseudothrombus" artifact is seen due to nonopacified blood flow mixing with enhanced blood giving an artifactual filling defect appearance (Fig. 110-13). CT has 100% sensitivity and 96% specificity in detecting DVT when compared to conventional venography (Fig. 110-14).[18] In patients with May Thurner syndrome, pelvic CT images in the transverse plane show iliac vein compression by the overlying right common iliac artery in patients with left-sided deep vein thrombosis.[19] In case of complete caval obstruction, extensive venous collaterals may also be identified.

MR

On spin-echo (SE) images, venous thrombus appears as a region of persistent intraluminal signal which can be

TABLE 110-1 Potential Causes for IVC Thrombosis

Deep venous thrombosis
Tumors
  Renal cell carcinoma
  Seminoma
  Teratoma
  Retroperitoneal leiomyosarcoma
  Adrenal cortical carcinoma
  Renal angiomyolipoma
Compression
  Aneurysm of the abdominal aorta
  Hepatic abscess
  Pancreatic pseudocyst
  Acute pancreatitis
Hematoma/trauma
  Psoas hematomas and other hematomas of the retroperitoneum
Dysfunctional coagulation system
Iatrogenic
  Hepatic transplantation
  Dialysis access
  Femoral venous catheters
  Pacemaker wires
  Vena caval filters
Other causes
  Developmental anomalies of the IVC
  Retroperitoneal fibrosis
  Pregnancy
  Oral contraceptives

IVC, inferior vena cava.

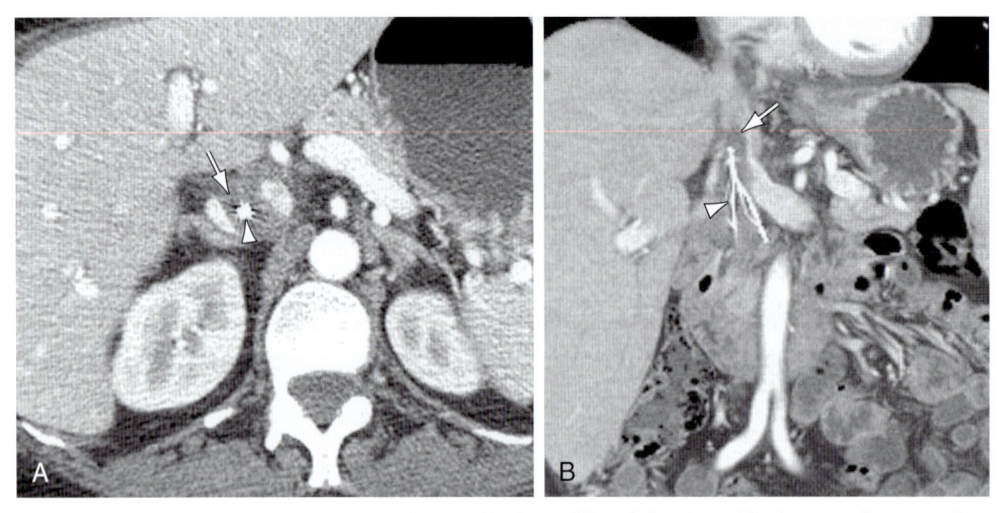

FIGURE 110-13 Axial (**A**) and coronal (**B**) postcontrast CT images showing a filling defect (*arrow*) in the IVC adjacent to the IVC filter (*arrowhead*) consistent with a thrombus.

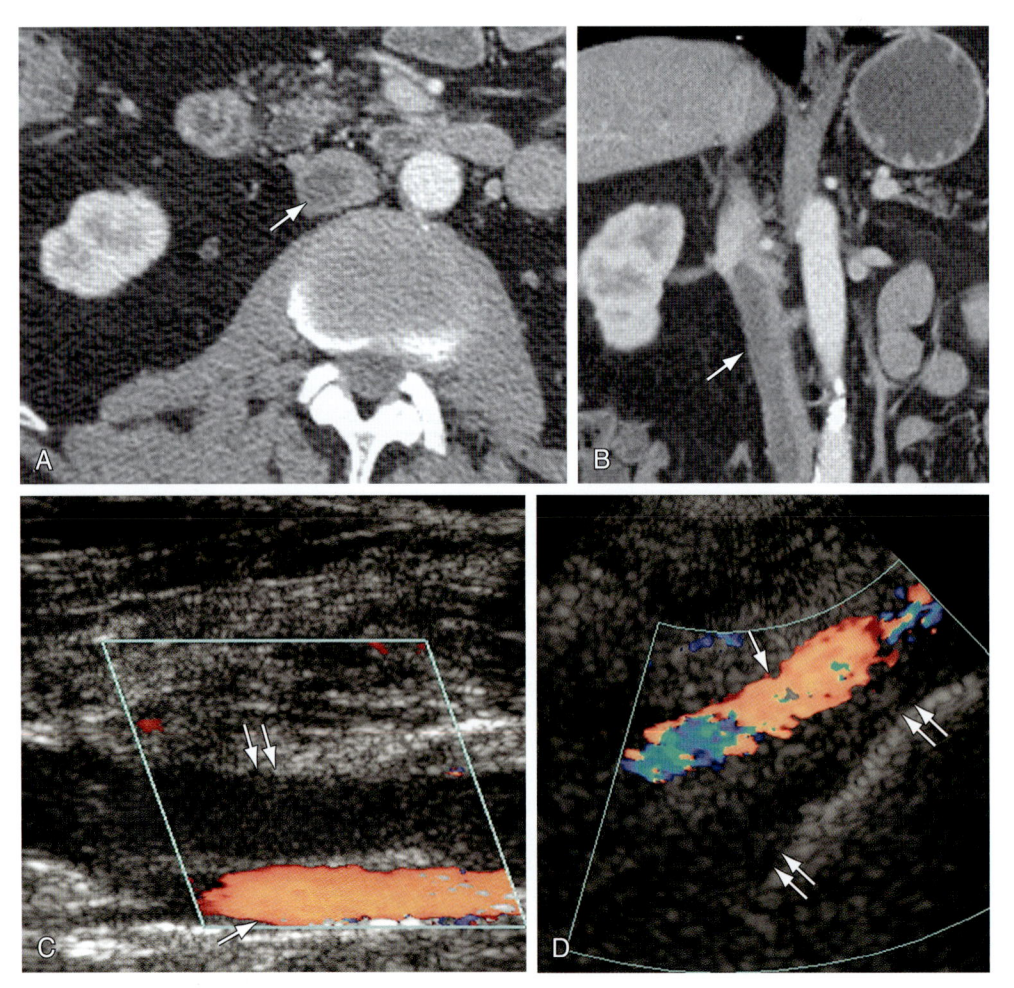

FIGURE 110-14 Axial (**A**) and coronal (**B**) postcontrast CT shows a thrombus (*arrow*) in the infrarenal IVC due to extension of deep venous thrombosis. Ultrasound images showing the thrombus (double arrows) in the same patient in the popliteal vein (**C**) and in the common iliac vein (**D**). The *top arrow* in **D** indicates the patent artery adjacent to the veins.

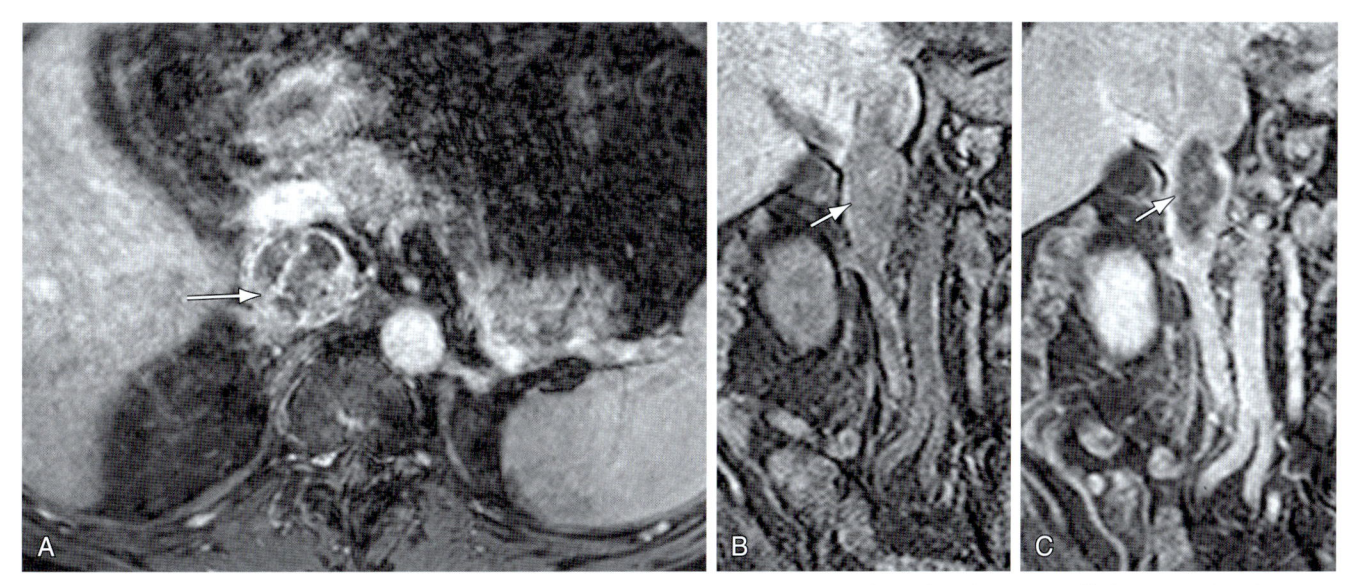

FIGURE 110-15 MR showing the tumor thrombus in the IVC. **A**, Axial postcontrast image shows the enhancement (*black arrow*) within the tumor thrombus. Coronal precontrast (**B**) and postcontrast (**C**) images show the filling defect (*white arrow*) in the IVC with enhancement in the thrombus.

confused with slow flowing blood which can also appear as high signal intensity. On SSFP or gradient recalled echo (GRE) images, venous thrombus appears as an area of lower signal intensity. SSFP and GRE pulse sequences are faster than SE imaging and hence are preferred if gadolinium-chelate contrast agents cannot be administered because of a contraindication.[20] Acquisition of SSFP (or GRE) in cine mode using ECG gating will help differentiate flow artifacts from true thrombus. On cine MR, thrombus will appear as fixed intraluminal filling defects that persist throughout the cardiac cycle. Alternatively, flow artifacts will not persist and will be seen only on a few phases of the cardiac cycle. On gadolinium-enhanced MRI, in addition to a filling defect in complete thrombosis, lack of enhancement is seen in a bland thrombus; however, enhancement is seen in a tumor thrombus (Fig. 110-15). In addition, there will be focal dilation of the vena cava in an acute thrombosis and presence of venous collateral vessels in chronic thrombosis.

Nuclear Medicine/PET

PET study may show increased uptake if the thrombosis is due to a tumor thrombus; however, PET is not used to diagnose IVC thrombosis.

Differential Diagnosis

From Clinical Presentation

The differential considerations for IVC thrombosis include renal dysfunction, liver dysfunction, external compression of the IVC from tumor masses, and fluid overload.

From Imaging Findings

The main differential consideration for IVC thrombosis is normal blood flow (i.e., admixing of nonopacified blood on contrast-enhanced CT; flow artifacts from normal blood flow on MRI).

Synopsis of Treatment Options

Medical

Medical management can include anticoagulation therapy and thrombolytic agents.

Anticoagulation

Heparin or warfarin may be used to prevent propagation of thrombus. Therapy is usually converted to oral anticoagulation with warfarin, but the time course of warfarin therapy is empiric.

Thrombolytic Agents

Most thrombolytic agents have been reported in the treatment of IVC thrombosis. The relative merits of thrombolytic therapy must be weighed against the risks of hemorrhagic complications. Urokinase, tissue-type plasminogen activator (tPA), and streptokinase have all been used. Typically, delivery is catheter-directed with or without a pulse spray. Patients require concurrent heparin therapy; however, tPA protocols do not use concurrent heparin because of the risk of bleeding complications.[21]

Surgical/Interventional

Surgical therapy encompasses caval interruption and thrombectomy. Currently, both of these modalities are being used less frequently. Several endovascular interventional modalities are available to treat IVCT. The optimal result can often be obtained by using a combination of these options as follows: (1) percutaneous balloon angioplasty, (2) Wallstents, and (3) Z stents.

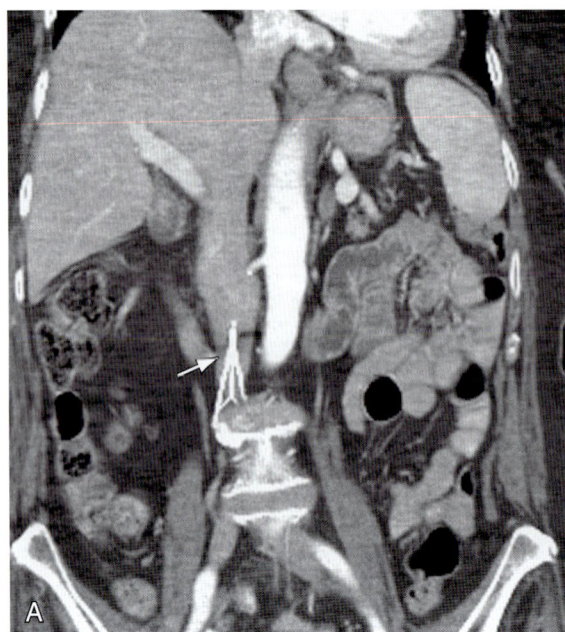

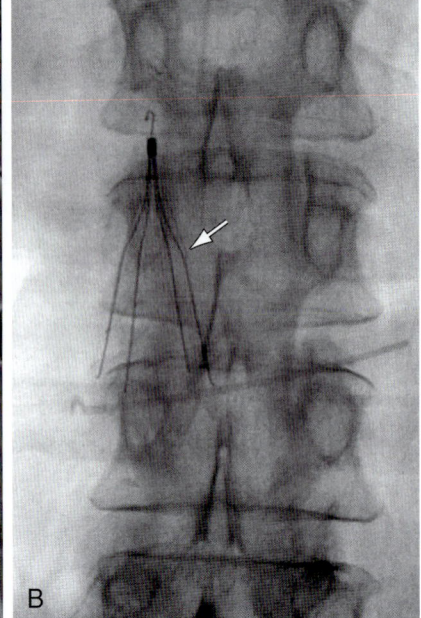

FIGURE 110-16 IVC filter (*arrow*) with correct placement as seen on coronal CT reformat (**A**) and angiography (**B**).

Reporting: Information for the Referring Physician

The report to the referring physician should include comment on the following:

1. The extent of IVC thrombosis
2. The presence of tumor thrombus
3. The presence of any external masses compressing the IVC

IVC INTERVENTIONS
Definitions

IVC intervention includes angioplasty, placement of stents and filters, biopsy, and shunt creation. *IVC angioplasty* or *stenting* is performed to bypass areas of occlusion or stenosis. *Inferior vena cava filters* are used to prevent pulmonary embolism (PE) in patients with contraindications to, complications of, or failure of anticoagulation therapy and patients with extensive free-floating thrombi or residual thrombi following massive PE. *IVC biopsies* are performed for tissue diagnosis in cases with suspected tumor thrombi or primary IVC malignancies. IVC biopsy can be performed by transcatheter aspiration,[22] brush biopsy, and scoop biopsy.[23] *IVC shunt* is the surgical anastomosis between portal and systemic veins and the surgical anastomosis between the portal vein and the vena cava.

Etiology and Pathophysiology (Including any Special Anatomic Considerations)

Inferior vena cava syndrome causes accumulated ascites and edema in the lower limbs, scrotum, and abdominal wall. Placement of a stent in the narrowed area of the vena cava with prompt dilation of the vascular lumen and correction of venous flow decreases venous pressure distal to the stenosis and results in improvement of congestive symptoms.[24]

IVC Filters

Choice of access site depends on a patient's anatomy, the site of venous thromboemboli, and the type of filters available. Generally, the right internal jugular vein or the right femoral vein is the preferred route, but left-sided venous approaches or approaches from arm veins can be used in some circumstances (Fig. 110-16). Ultrasound scanning can be used to confirm entry site and to guide puncture in difficult cases. After local anesthetic injection, the subcutaneous tissues are infiltrated and the vein is punctured under strict antiseptic conditions. A cavogram is performed to confirm anatomy and the presence or absence of intraluminal filling defects and to identify the renal veins and anatomical variants. Conscious sedation with midazolam and fentanyl can be used. Following the cavogram, the diameter of the IVC is calculated; most filters cannot be placed if the cava is larger than 28 mm, the exception being the bird's nest filter. The filter is usually placed below the renal veins but can be placed in a suprarenal position when there is renal vein thrombosis or thrombus extending proximal to the renal veins, during pregnancy, and when there is thrombus proximal to an indwelling filter. The procedure usually takes less than 60 minutes.[25]

IVC Shunts

Different types of IVC shunts include the side-to-side portocaval shunt and the mesocaval shunt.

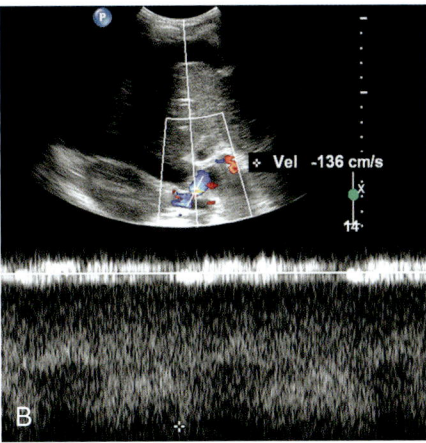

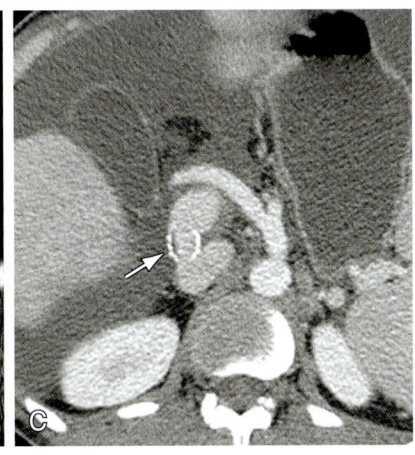

FIGURE 110-17 Ultrasound image in a patient with a portocaval shunt (**A**). Color Doppler image shows an area of aliasing (*double arrows*) in the shunt with high velocity seen on spectral Doppler (**B**), and stent (*arrow*) placed in the portocaval shunt as seen on CT (**C**).

Side-to-Side Portacaval Shunt (SSPCS). This shunt may be performed for hepatic venous obstruction due to isolated hepatic vein thrombosis (Fig. 110-17). The data on SSPCS for hepatic vein obstruction is somewhat limited—an earlier review reported only two studies with more than 10 patients each.[26] The reservation against performing SSPCS in patients with hepatic vein thrombosis is the likely technical difficulty in approximating the portal vein to the infrahepatic vena cava in the presence of a hypertrophied caudate lobe. Another argument is that because a portacaval shunt involves hepatic hilar dissection, it may increase the technical difficulties if a subsequent liver transplantation is needed because of progression of liver disease. Despite these reservations, excellent long-term graft patency and symptom-free survival of 81% to 94% has been reported in series from dedicated centers.

Mesocaval Shunt (MCS). MCS is the preferred shunt in the setting of isolated hepatic vein thrombosis in many studies.[27] Advantages of MCS are its technical simplicity and avoidance of hilar dissection. The prerequisite for this shunt is a patent IVC and it provides an effective hepatic decongestion even in those patients in whom an enlarged caudate lobe presses on the IVC.[28] The shunt can be an autologous internal jugular vein or prosthetic (Dacron or PTFE). The main disadvantage of the Dacron grafts is high incidence (up to 50% or more in some series) of postoperative thrombosis, whereas the reported long-term patency of the internal jugular vein grafts exceeds 80%.[29] Reported 5-year survival after MCSs for hepatic venous outflow obstruction ranges between 57% and 95%. Because the mesocaval shunt is a partial shunt (portal vein flow is maintained), there is a low rate of encephalopathy, rebleeding, and improved quality of life.

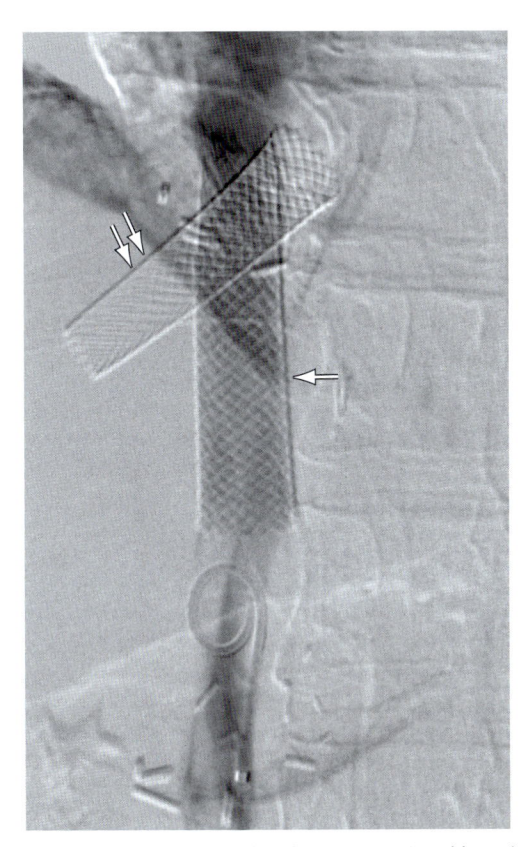

FIGURE 110-18 Stents placed in the IVC (*arrow*) and hepatic vein (*double arrows*) for stenosis in a post-liver transplantation patient.

IVC Stents

IVC stents are placed routinely to bypass areas of occlusion or stenosis (Fig. 110-18). Placement of long-standing indwelling venous catheters or creation of surgical anastomoses in patients undergoing liver transplantation increases the risk of IVC stenosis. Percutaneous stent insertion can produce rapid and sustained relief of symptoms, either as a primary treatment or in patients in whom other methods have failed or symptoms have recurred. Since this technique was first reported in 1986, it has become widely used in the palliation of IVC obstruction.

KEY POINTS

- **Inferior Vena Cava**
  - Best diagnostic clue to the congenital anomalies of IVC is malposition or absence of parts or all of IVC.
  - Circumaortic left renal vein is the most common type, followed by retroaortic left renal vein. Next most common types are duplicated IVC and left IVC; this is followed by azygos continuation of IVC.
  - Best imaging diagnostic tool is CT with multiplanar reformation.
  - Top differential diagnosis is adenopathy and retroperitoneal mass.
  - Patients are usually asymptomatic. Those with duplicated IVC can present with recurrent PE. Those with absence of IVC can present with lower extremity venous insufficiency.
  - Preoperative anatomic delineation is necessary in all cases.
- **Tumors of the IVC and main tributaries**
  - Primary versus secondary tumor invasion of the IVC
  - Tumor thrombus versus nontumoral thrombosis of the IVC
  - Multiphase, multiplanar contrasted CT or MRI is indicated. Include chest (heart and pulmonary arteries) and abdomen-pelvis.
  - Surgical resection is the only curative treatment and can be attempted in patients without distant metastasis.
- **IVC complications in orthotopic liver transplantation anatomy**
  - Monophasic waveforms in the hepatic veins
  - Increased velocity at the IVC anastomotic site
  - Exclude compression from enlarged liver or other focal lesions such as fluid collection
- **IVC thrombosis**
  - Assess extent of IVC thrombosis
  - Exclude presence of tumor thrombus
  - Watch out for artifact from nonopacified blood

SUGGESTED READINGS

Bass JE, Redwine MD, Kramer LA, et al. Spectrum of congenital anomalies of the inferior vena cava: cross-sectional imaging findings. Radiographics. May-Jun 2000; 20(3):639-652.

Chung J, Owen RJ. Using inferior vena cava filters to prevent pulmonary embolism. Can Fam Physician. Jan 2008; 54(1):49-55.

Crossin JD, Muradali D, Wilson SR. US of liver transplants: normal and abnormal. Radiographics. Sep-Oct 2003; 23(5):1093-1104.

Cuevas C, Raske M, Bush WH, et al. Imaging primary and secondary tumor thrombus of the inferior vena cava: multi-detector computed tomography and magnetic resonance imaging. Curr Probl Diagn Radiol. May-Jun 2006; 35(3):90-101.

Sheth S, Fishman EK. Imaging of the inferior vena cava with MDCT. AJR Am J Roentgenol. Nov 2007; 189(5):1243-1251.

Vaidya S, Dighe M, Kolokythas O, Dubinsky T. Liver transplantation: vascular complications. Ultrasound Q. Dec 2007; 23(4):239-253.

REFERENCES

1. Gore RM, Balfe DM, Aizenstein RI, Silverman PM. The great escape: interfascial decompression planes of the retroperitoneum. AJR Am J Roentgenol 2000; 175(2):363-370.
2. Phillips E. Embryology, normal anatomy, and anomalies. In Ferris EJ, Hipona FA, Kahn PC, et al. (eds). Venography of the Inferior Vena Cava and its Branches. Baltimore, Williams & Wilkins, 1969, pp 1-32.
3. Bass JE, Redwine MD, Kramer LA, et al. Spectrum of congenital anomalies of the inferior vena cava: cross-sectional imaging findings. Radiographics 2000; 20(3):639-652.
4. Gayer G, Luboshitz J, Hertz M, et al. Congenital anomalies of the inferior vena cava revealed on CT in patients with deep vein thrombosis. AJR Am J Roentgenol 2003; 180(3):729-732.
5. Mingoli A, Cavallaro A, Sapienza P, et al. International registry of inferior vena cava leiomyosarcoma: analysis of a world series on 218 patients. Anticancer Res 1996; 16(5B):3201-3205.
6. Cuevas C, Raske M, Bush WH, et al. Imaging primary and secondary tumor thrombus of the inferior vena cava: multi-detector computed tomography and magnetic resonance imaging. Curr Probl Diagn Radiol 2006; 35(3):90-101.
7. Sheth S, Fishman EK. Imaging of the inferior vena cava with MDCT. AJR Am J Roentgenol 2007; 189(5):1243-1251.
8. Sheth S, Scatarige JC, Horton KM, et al. Current concepts in the diagnosis and management of renal cell carcinoma: role of multidetector CT and three-dimensional CT. Radiographics 2001; 21 Spec No:S237-S254.
9. Russo P. Renal cell carcinoma: presentation, staging, and surgical treatment. Semin Oncol 2000; 27(2):160-176.
10. Ng L, Libertino JM. Adrenocortical carcinoma: diagnosis, evaluation and treatment. J Urol 2003; 169(1):5-11.
11. Okada Y, Nagino M, Kamiya J, et al. Diagnosis and treatment of inferior vena caval invasion by hepatic cancer. World J Surg 2003; 27(6):689-694.
12. Corbally MT, Rela M, Heaton ND. Standard orthotopic operation, retransplantation and piggybacking. In Williams R, Portmann B, Tan KC (eds). The Practice of Liver Transplantation. London, Churchill Livingstone, 1995, pp135-142.
13. Starzl TE. Liver transplantation. Gastroenterology 1997; 112(1):288-291.
14. Keeffe EB. Summary of guidelines on organ allocation and patient listing for liver transplantation. Liver Transpl Surg 1998; 4(5 Suppl 1):S108-S114.
15. Nghiem HV, Tran K, Winter TC, 3rd, et al. Imaging of complications in liver transplantation. Radiographics 1996; 16(4):825-840.
16. Glanemann M, Settmacher U, Langrehr JM, et al. Portal vein angioplasty using a transjugular, intrahepatic approach for treatment of extrahepatic portal vein stenosis after liver transplantation. Transpl Int 2001; 14(1):48-51.
17. Park JH, Lee JB, Han MC, et al. Sonographic evaluation of inferior vena caval obstruction: correlative study with vena cavography. AJR Am J Roentgenol 1985; 145(4):757-762.

18. Baldt MM, Zontsich T, Stumpflen A, et al. Deep venous thrombosis of the lower extremity: efficacy of spiral CT venography compared with conventional venography in diagnosis. Radiology 1996; 200(2):423-428.
19. Oguzkurt L, Tercan F, Pourbagher MA, et al. Computed tomography findings in 10 cases of iliac vein compression (May-Thurner) syndrome. Eur J Radiol 2005; 55(3):421-425.
20. Erdman WA, Weinreb JC, Cohen JM, et al. Venous thrombosis: clinical and experimental MR imaging. Radiology 1986; 161(1):233-238.
21. Girard P, Hauuy MP, Musset D, et al. Acute inferior vena cava thrombosis. Early results of heparin therapy. Chest 1989; 95(2):284-291.
22. Wendth AJ, Jr., Garlick WB, Pantoja GE, Shamoun J. Transcatheter biopsy of renal carcinoma invading the inferior vena cava. J Urol 1976; 115(3):331-332.
23. Kishi K, Sonomura T, Terada M, Sato M. Scoop biopsy of intracaval tumor thrombi: a preliminary report of a minimally invasive technique to obtain large samples. Eur J Radiol 1997; 24(3):263-268.
24. Furui S, Sawada S, Kuramoto K, et al. Gianturco stent placement in malignant caval obstruction: analysis of factors for predicting the outcome. Radiology. 1995; 195(1):147-152.
25. Chung J, Owen RJ. Using inferior vena cava filters to prevent pulmonary embolism. Can Fam Physician 2008; 54(1):49-55.
26. Pisani-Ceretti A, Intra M, Prestipino F, et al. Surgical and radiologic treatment of primary Budd-Chiari syndrome. World J Surg 1998; 22(1):48-53; discussion 53-44.
27. Slakey DP, Klein AS, Venbrux AC, Cameron JL. Budd-Chiari syndrome: current management options. Ann Surg 2001; 233(4):522-527.
28. Fisher NC, McCafferty I, Dolapci M, et al. Managing Budd-Chiari syndrome: a retrospective review of percutaneous hepatic vein angioplasty and surgical shunting. Gut 1999; 44(4):568-574.
29. Stipa S, Thau A, Schillaci A, et al. Mesentericocaval shunt with the internal jugular vein. Surg Gynecol Obstet 1978; 146(3):391-399.

CHAPTER 111

Vascular Imaging of Hepatic Transplantation

Maitraya K. Patel and Steven S. Raman

With more than 6000 surgeries performed in 2008,[1] liver transplantation is the current treatment of choice for many causes of progressive acute and chronic end-stage liver disease. In the United States, liver transplantation typically involves harvesting of an organ from a deceased donor (orthotopic liver transplantation). However, demand for liver transplantation is increasingly outstripping the supply of cadaveric livers, and transplantation of a portion of the liver from a live donor (i.e., living related donor) is increasing in popularity. Knowledge of recipient and live donor hepatic vascular anatomy is critical for proper preoperative planning for transplantation.

Major indications for liver transplantation include viral cirrhosis, alcoholic cirrhosis, acute liver failure, Budd-Chiari syndrome, trauma, biliary cirrhosis (primary or secondary), and sclerosing cholangitis. Congenital disorders include congenital hepatic fibrosis, cystic fibrosis, neonatal hepatitis, biliary atresia, and several inborn errors of metabolism.

Although malignant disease is a contraindication to transplantation in most other solid organs, liver transplantation offers the only potential cure for primary, low- and moderate-volume hepatocellular carcinoma. The overall 5-year survival in this setting is expected to be 70%, with a recurrence rate below 15%. Compared with hepatocellular carcinoma, transplantation for cholangiocarcinoma is controversial because 5-year survival rates are much lower (20% to 30%) and recurrence rates are much higher. Transplantation for metastatic liver lesions is generally not performed; rare exception is made for metastatic carcinoid and other neuroendocrine tumors.[2]

PRETRANSPLANTATION WORK-UP
Imaging of Liver Transplant Recipients

The radiologic evaluation of a potential candidate for orthotopic liver transplantation primarily focuses on an assessment of the degree of cirrhosis (liver size and morphology, presence of ascites) and patency and caliber of the portal vein and associated feeding veins (splenic vein and superior mesenteric vein) to determine whether a suitable site for venovenous anastomosis between the donor liver and recipient portal vein or feeding branches exists. Because of the greatly increased risk for development of hepatocellular carcinoma in cirrhotic livers, most centers perform routine sonographic surveillance for early detection of hepatocellular carcinoma. Whereas ultrasonography is sensitive in the evaluation of portal vein caliber, patency, and direction of flow, its operator-dependent nature limits its sensitivity for detection of hepatocellular carcinoma (20% to 40% for lesions smaller than 3 cm).[3]

Dynamic contrast-enhanced (multiphase) multidetector computed tomography (CT) and magnetic resonance imaging (MRI) enable rapid, whole-liver evaluation during arterial and portal venous phases of intravenous contrast enhancement, allowing a comprehensive assessment of the hepatic artery and the portal, splenic, and superior mesenteric veins as well as major collateral veins. In general, both contrast-enhanced CT and MRI are more sensitive than sonography for detection of hepatocellular carcinoma lesions larger than 2 cm (sensitivity, 74% to 96%). The 2-cm size is important because by the Model for End-Stage Liver Disease scoring system, cirrhotic patients with 2-cm or larger lesions are assigned priority for liver transplantation. Although both multiphase CT and MRI are less sensitive for detection of hepatocellular carcinoma lesions smaller than 2 cm, they are better than ultrasonography, which has sensitivities as low as 20% for these lesions.[4-9] MRI benefits from its ability to provide additional lesion characterization for further differentiation of the myriad types of liver nodules in cirrhotic livers based on signal intensity (e.g., T1 and T2) and contrast enhancement characteristics. Multiphase CT and MR examinations can determine vascular patency and are superior to ultrasound examination in the characterization of the recipient vascular anatomy.

Imaging of Potential Living Donors for Hepatic Transplantation

As an alternative to cadaveric liver transplantation, which is not an option in many European and Asian countries and usually entails a long wait time in many regions of the United States, living related and living donor hepatic transplantations have been advocated to expand the pool of available hepatic allografts. In adult-to-adult living donor transplantation, the right lobe (segments V, VI, VII, and VIII) is resected and transplanted. In adult-to-pediatric liver donation, the left lateral segment (segments II and III) is transplanted into the pediatric recipient. However, because of concerns of donor safety in the United States, fewer than 250 adult living donor hepatic transplantations were performed in 2007.[10]

At most centers performing this procedure, a thorough imaging evaluation of the donor liver is performed before surgery. This includes evaluation of the hepatic vasculature, bile ducts, hepatic lobar volume, and any possible diffuse (typically fat or iron deposition) or focal liver disease. A description of the size and branching pattern of these donor vessels is necessary in evaluation of the donor vasculature (hepatic arteries, hepatic veins, and portal veins) and bile ducts. Assessment of donor liver itself includes quantitative measurement of hepatic lobar volume and of some diffuse liver diseases, such as hepatic steatosis or siderosis. Detection and characterization of incidental liver lesions (typically cysts or hemangiomas) are necessary. Each component of this evaluation can be performed with either CT or MR by angiographic, parenchymal, and bile duct–specific imaging.

At a minimum, acceptable adult-to-adult donor liver volume criteria include a ratio between right lobe graft weight and recipient body weight of 0.8% or an estimated liver volume of 40% in an idealized whole liver. The healthy donor adult can function on a minimum of at least 30% residual liver volume without risking donor hepatic decompensation. These percentages are for a presumed normal liver free of diffuse liver disease. The most common unrecognized diffuse liver disease identifiable in the general population is macrovesicular hepatic steatosis, which may affect the liver diffusely or in a patchy, localized, and nodular fashion. Causes include obesity, steroid use, diabetes mellitus, and metabolic syndrome. With either CT or MR, steatosis may be detected and graded accurately in the absence of coexistent siderosis. In general, livers with less than 5% to 10% of macrovesicular steatosis are considered acceptable. Another form of common and unrecognized diffuse liver disease is diffuse siderosis. When both steatosis and siderosis are present, both CT and MR become unreliable for quantification, and a liver biopsy may be required.

In an adult-to-adult living donor transplantation, the entire donor right lobe is resected along a surgical plane surrounding the middle hepatic vein. In the United States, the middle hepatic vein is typically preserved in the donor, and the resection is usually 1 cm to the right of the middle hepatic vein from the dome of the liver to the portal bifurcation and gallbladder fossa. In the recipient, the right hepatic vein, right portal vein, and right hepatic artery will provide the vascular anastomoses in the graft. However, in some centers, especially outside the United States, the middle hepatic vein is resected along with the right lobe, and thus the resection plane is to the left of the middle hepatic vein.

Approximately 55% of patients have a conventional right and left hepatic artery arising from a common hepatic artery (Michel type I, Fig. 111-1).[11,12] However, in the remaining 45% of patients, there can be a wide range of hepatic artery variations (Fig. 111-2) that can be described by the Michel classification (Table 111-1). Proper identification of hepatic artery anatomy in the donor is critical for surgical planning and minimization of postoperative complications in both the donor and recipient. A donor may be rejected when aberrant arterial anatomy is also associated with other biliary and venous variants, which in combination result in an increased complexity of the operation.

Ideal portal venous anatomy has the right portal vein branching from the main portal vein (Fig. 111-3) and not from the left portal vein. Cases in which portal venous branches to segment IV arise from the right anterior portal vein may be a contraindication to transplantation.

Ideal hepatic venous anatomy has the single dominant right hepatic vein available for anastomosis without significant (>5 mm diameter branch veins) hepatic venous branches draining into the now-missing middle hepatic vein. However, many variants in hepatic venous drainage exist. Hepatic venous branches larger than 5 mm that drain the right posterior lobe (VII and VI) and insert into the inferior vena cava (IVC) may require separate venous anastomoses in the recipient to prevent hepatic segmental

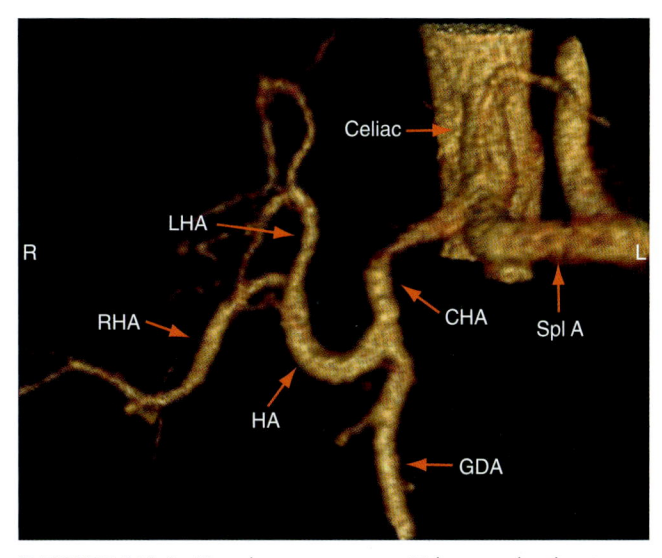

FIGURE 111-1 Hepatic artery anatomy. Volume rendered three-dimensional image from CTA of typical normal hepatic anatomy in which the right hepatic artery (RHA) and left hepatic artery (LHA) arise from the hepatic artery (HA). CHA, common hepatic artery; GDA, gastroduodenal artery; Celiac, celiac artery; Spl A, splenic artery.

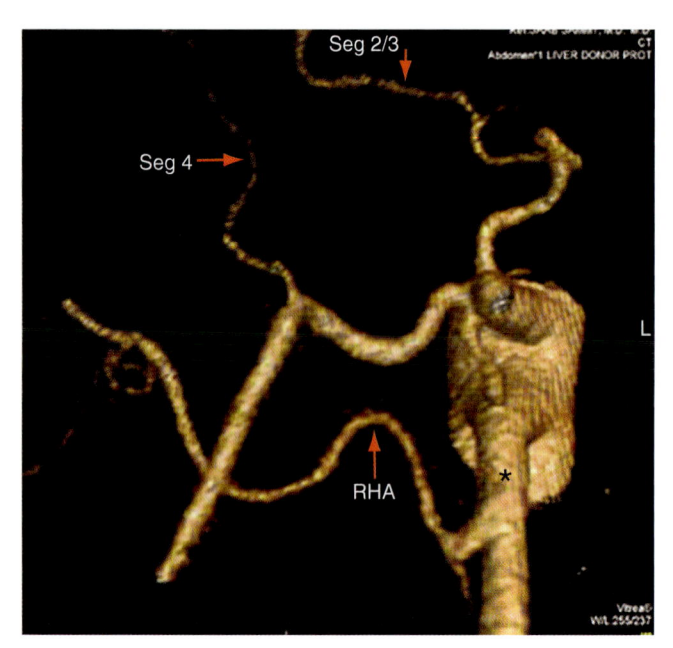

FIGURE 111-2 Replaced right hepatic artery. Volume rendered three-dimensional image from CTA in a patient with a replaced right hepatic artery (RHA) arising from the superior mesenteric artery (asterisk).

Table 111-1	Michel Classification of Arterial Variants
Type 1	Normal anatomy: proper hepatic artery dividing into sole right and left hepatic arteries
Type 2	Left hepatic artery replaced to the left gastric artery
Type 3	Right hepatic artery replaced to the superior mesenteric artery
Type 4	Both right and left hepatic arteries replaced
Type 5	Accessory left hepatic artery
Type 6	Accessory right hepatic artery
Type 7	Accessory right and left hepatic arteries
Type 8	Proper hepatic artery originating from the superior mesenteric artery combined with an accessory left hepatic artery
Type 9	Proper hepatic artery arising from the superior mesenteric artery
Type 10	Proper hepatic artery arising from the left gastric artery

From Artioli D, Tagliabue M, Aseni P, et al: Detection of biliary and vascular anatomy in living liver donors: value of gadobenate dimeglumine enhanced MR and MDCT angiography. Eur J Radiol. In press.

congestion or bleeding and subsequent liver dysfunction. Hepatic venous branches larger than 5 mm that drain the right anterior lobe branches (VIII and V) into the middle hepatic vein will invariably transect the surgical resection plane and probably require separate venous anastomoses to also prevent complications such as hepatic venous congestion in the recipient.[13,14]

SURGICAL ANATOMY (CADAVERIC LIVER TRANSPLANTATION)

The hepatic artery anastomosis is typically a branch patch anastomosis formed at the origin of the gastroduodenal artery from the common hepatic artery in the recipient and at the origin of the splenic artery from the celiac trunk in the donor (Fig. 111-4). In some instances, a donor anastomosis is made at the celiac axis with use of an aortic patch (Carrel patch).[15,16] On occasion, an aortic jump graft will be formed from the donor common and external iliac arteries joined to the recipient abdominal aorta in an end-to-side anastomosis and to the hepatic artery of the donor by a branch patch anastomosis. This technique can be used in cases of small native hepatic artery or celiac artery stenosis in which an adequate inflow cannot be ensured.

When there is variant donor hepatic artery anatomy, modification of normal technique is required. For example, in Michel type III variant (a replaced right hepatic artery from the superior mesenteric artery, the most common arterial variant; see Fig. 111-2),[17] a primary anastomosis between the donor celiac artery with an aortic patch and the recipient branch patch at the gastroduodenal artery takeoff and a secondary anastomosis between the replaced right hepatic artery and the proximal stump of the donor splenic artery can be performed.[15] In situations of variant hepatic arterial anatomy in the recipient, such as a replaced right hepatic artery, the larger of the two inflow vessels is used.[16]

The portal vein anastomosis is typically an end-to-end anastomosis between the donor and recipient portal veins.[18] A venous jump graft between the donor portal vein to the recipient superior mesenteric vein may be needed in cases of portal vein thrombosis or prior portal venous surgery.[16] Rarely, arterialization of the portal vein, in which the donor portal vein is anastomosed to the arterial vessels of the recipient, has been performed when a suitable visceral venous anastomosis is impossible because of extensive thrombus.[19]

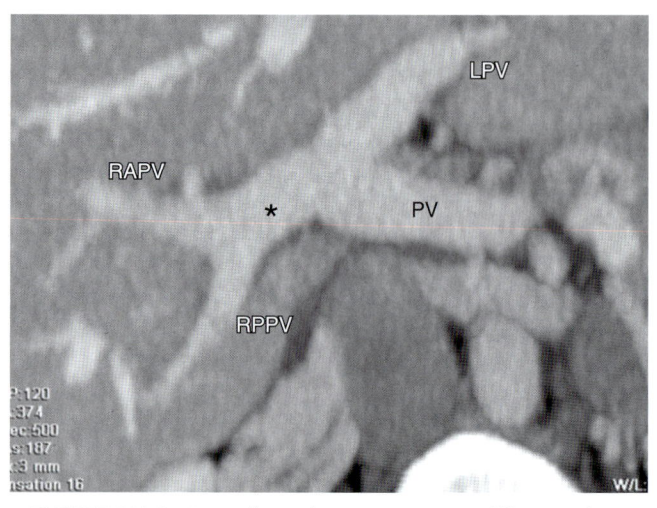

FIGURE 111-3 Normal portal venous anatomy. Oblique maximum intensity projection image from portal CTA demonstrates normal portal vein (PV) bifurcation into left portal vein (LPV) and right portal vein (asterisk). RAPV, right anterior portal vein; RPPV, right posterior portal vein.

■ **FIGURE 111-4** Hepatic artery branch patch anastomosis. CTA (**A**, coronal reformations; **B**, volume rendered three-dimensional image) illustrates a typical hepatic artery anastomosis, a branch patch anastomosis, formed at the origin of the gastroduodenal artery from the common hepatic artery in the recipient (*arrow*) and at the origin of the splenic artery from the celiac trunk in the donor.

For the caval anastomosis, the IVC is transected above and below the intrahepatic segment during cadaveric hepatectomy, and an end-to-end anastomosis is made between the upper and lower margins of the IVC in the recipient.[16] In the "piggyback" technique, a single end-to-end anastomosis is made between the donor hepatic vein–IVC stump and the recipient's common hepatic vein stump off the IVC (Fig. 111-5).[18] This technique is preferred at some institutions because IVC flow is not interrupted during most of the operation, thus reducing inherent operative risk as well as obviating the need for venovenous bypass.[20]

COMPLICATIONS AFTER LIVER TRANSPLANTATION

Orthotopic liver transplantation is a technically complex procedure with inferior vena caval, portal venous, and hepatic arterial vascular anastomoses. A variety of short- and long-term complications may arise. Of particular relevance to interpreting physicians are the vascular complications, which are among the most frequent causes of early acute graft failure.[21] The transplant team is particularly sensitive to the patency of the allograft vessels in the immediate postoperative period in patients with signs of bile leak or sepsis or more commonly a persistent elevation in serum liver enzymes. When any of these are suspected, ultrasonography with color, power, and spectral Doppler imaging is immediately performed. If sonography is inconclusive or suggests arterial stenosis or occlusion, MR angiography (MRA) or CT angiography (CTA) is typically performed to determine the extent of these potentially morbid vascular complications to enable revascularization with endovascular interventional procedures.

Both CTA and MRA are performed for definitive evaluation of vascular complications after liver transplantation, with a sensitivity reported to be 100%, specificity between 74% and 96%, and negative predictive value of 100%.[22-27]

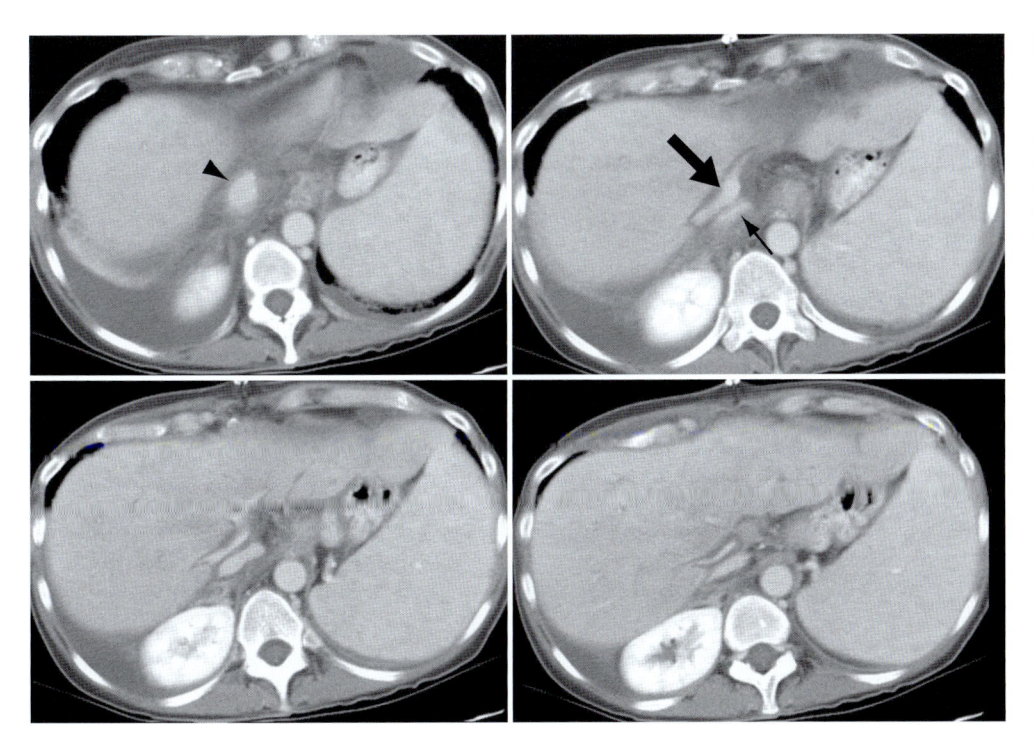

■ **FIGURE 111-5** Piggyback caval anastomosis. CTA demonstrates a piggyback caval anastomosis, which is a single end-to-end anastomosis (*arrowhead*) of the donor hepatic vein–IVC stump (*large arrow*) and the recipient's common hepatic vein stump off the recipient IVC (*small arrow*).

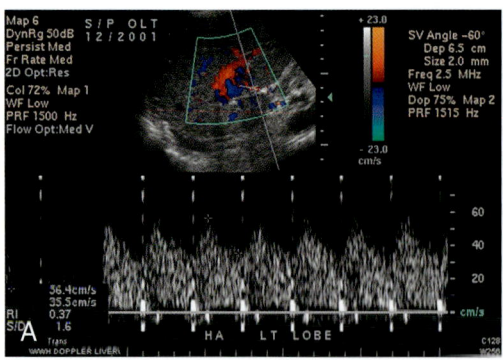

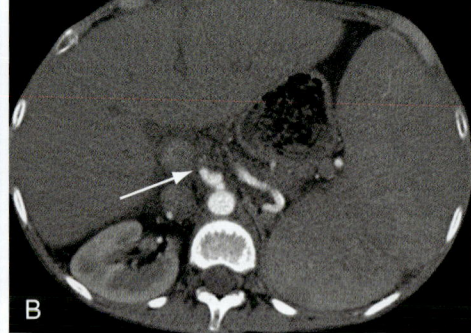

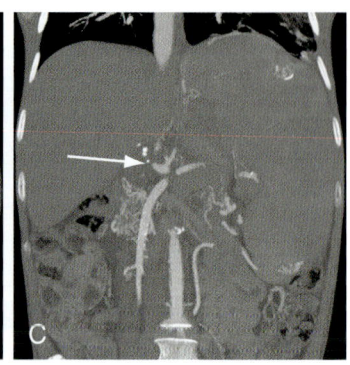

FIGURE 111-6 Hepatic artery thrombosis. **A,** Spectral Doppler ultrasound image demonstrates a tardus et parvus waveform in the left hepatic artery of a patient after an orthotopic liver transplantation. **B,** Axial CTA image demonstrates the development of a hepatic artery thrombosis (*arrow*). **C,** Coronal reformatted image from the same CTA confirming the hepatic artery thrombosis (*arrow*).

Although no studies directly comparing their performance exist in the post-transplantation setting, the latest generation of CT and MR equipment with optimized imaging protocols is generally regarded as equivalent in terms of their ability to evaluate vascular complications. CTA is usually more widely available with regard to equipment and expertise, and it can be a more reliable examination in uncooperative patients with fewer limitations on motion of the patient. Its major limitation is in those patients for whom iodinated contrast material cannot be administered for concern of nephrotoxicity or severe contrast allergy. In a minimally cooperative patient, contrast-enhanced three-dimensional MRA is a robust examination that allows assessment of hepatic vessels and hepatic parenchyma. The biliary tree is also easily assessed with the use of MR cholangiopancreatography sequences incorporated into a single examination. Its major limitations are an increased susceptibility to erratic respiratory motion, the possible overestimation of vascular stenosis due to slow flow or surgical clips–related susceptibility artifact,[28] and a small chance of inducing potentially progressive and debilitating intravenous gadolinium–associated nephrogenic systemic fibrosis in post-transplantation patients with severe acute renal failure (glomerular filtration rate <30 mL/min/1.73 m^2).[29]

Hepatic Artery

With an occurrence between 5% and 12% of adult patients and up to 42% of pediatric patients, presumably owing to small size of the transplant vessel, hepatic artery thrombosis is the most frequent and most serious vascular complication after liver transplantation.[21,27,30] Although the liver parenchyma has dual arterial and portal venous blood supply, the hepatic artery alone perfuses the biliary tree of the transplanted liver.

Hepatic artery thrombosis generally develops within the first 3 months after transplantation.[30] Risk factors for development of hepatic artery thrombosis include small native hepatic arteries, use of a Roux-en-Y biliary reconstruction, length of cold ischemia and operative times, volume of blood and plasma products used intraoperatively, and use of aortic conduits in arterial reconstruction.[15,31]

Clinical presentation of hepatic artery thrombosis can be variable, depending on the time and severity of hepatic injury related to hepatic artery thrombosis. The most devastating is fulminant hepatic necrosis, which occurs in up to 33% of patients with hepatic artery thrombosis. Patients have rapid decompensation of liver synthetic function, fever, sepsis, hypotension, and coagulopathy, which can necessitate retransplantation. Somewhat more variable in nature are the biliary tract complications resulting from hepatic arterial ischemia or infarction. These include intrahepatic biliary strictures, intrahepatic bile leaks or bilomas, and biliary necrosis in up to 60% of cases of anastomotic hepatic artery stenosis and in up to 80% of cases of hepatic artery thrombosis.[32] The clinical presentation of patients is variable. Some patients may present with intermittent episodes of sepsis without a clear source, presumably caused by focal abscesses in areas of infarcted liver or biliary necrosis. Others may remain asymptomatic or mildly symptomatic, with a diagnosis of hepatic artery thrombosis made incidentally.

For suspected postoperative hepatic artery thrombosis, ultrasonography is usually the first imaging modality performed because of its speed and portability. In addition to gray-scale two-dimensional imaging, color, power, and spectral Doppler ultrasound examinations may be performed to maximize chances of evaluating arterial flow. In experienced hands, ultrasonography has achieved up to 92% sensitivity for detection of hepatic artery thrombosis. Spectral Doppler findings include progressively decreased to absent diastolic flow, decreased slope and amplitude (tardus et parvus) of the peak systolic velocity, and finally absence of the hepatic waveform altogether. If this process is prolonged, the development of intrahepatic arterial collateral vessels can lead to a false-negative examination.[33] However, these collateral intrahepatic arterial vessels are often not completely normal, also often demonstrating a tardus-parvus waveform. CTA (Fig. 111-6) or MRA studies are usually relied on to confirm ultrasound findings and to determine the extent of the problems. False-positive diagnoses by Doppler study can be due to severe hepatic edema, hypotension, high-grade hepatic arterial stenosis, or technical limitations.

By CTA or MRA, arterial thrombosis of the hepatic artery (Fig. 111-7) or of other vessels (celiac artery, Fig.

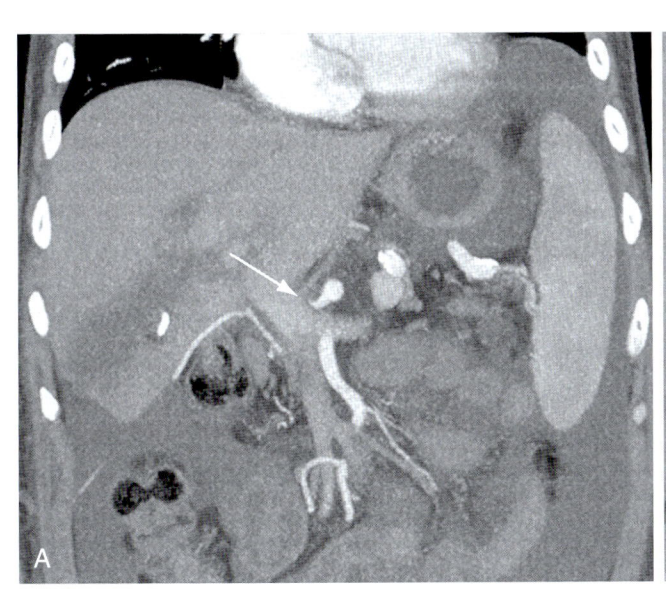

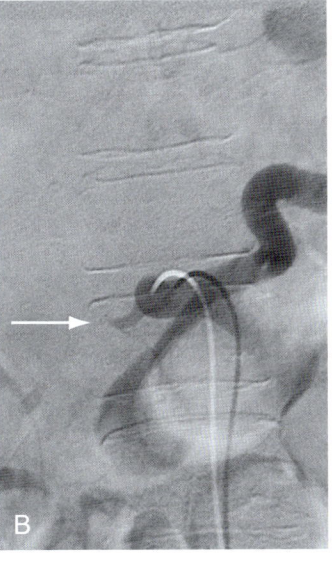

FIGURE 111-7 Hepatic artery thrombosis. **A**, Coronal reformatted image from CTA demonstrates hepatic artery thrombosis (*arrow*) in an orthotopic liver transplantation patient. **B**, Conventional x-ray hepatic angiography confirms the hepatic artery thrombosis (*arrow*).

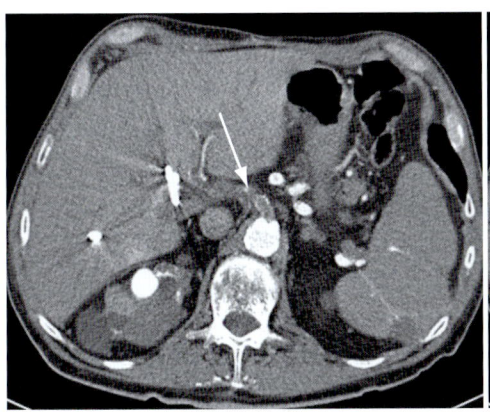

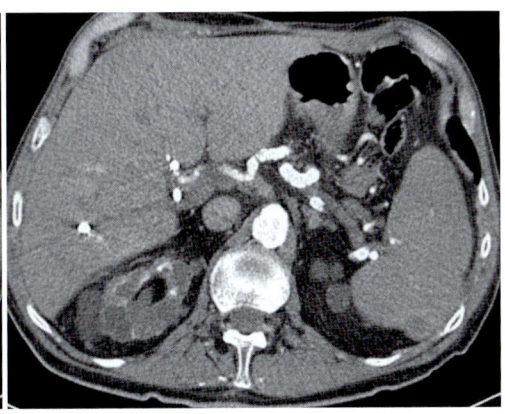

FIGURE 111-8 Celiac artery thrombosis. Axial images from CTA demonstrate thrombosis in the celiac artery (*arrow*). The hepatic artery and splenic artery remain patent.

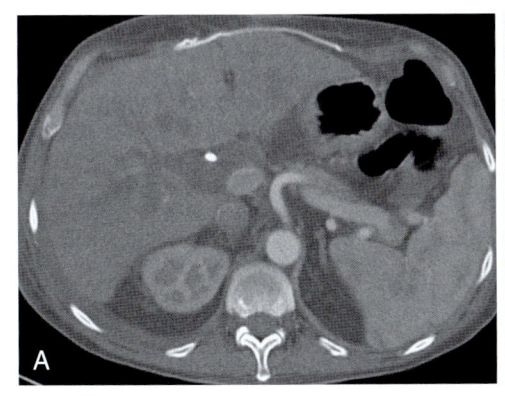

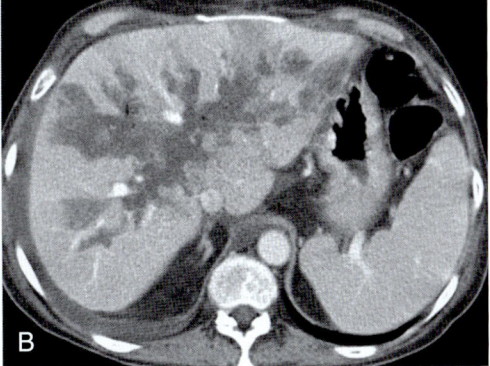

FIGURE 111-9 Hepatic artery thrombosis and biliary necrosis. **A**, Axial image from CTA of an orthotopic liver transplantation patient in hepatic arterial phase. The hepatic artery is not seen in its expected location because of thrombosis. **B**, Corresponding portal venous phase image demonstrating biliary necrosis.

111-8) is readily diagnosed. Hepatic arterial thrombosis can be diagnosed by the lack of contrast media opacification of the hepatic artery or graft. Hepatic artery thrombosis is often associated with hepatic and biliary complications (Figs. 111-9 to 111-12). Intrahepatic collateral vessels can be seen if progression toward hepatic artery thrombosis is advanced.

Because hepatic artery thrombosis may be clinically manifested with a spectrum of mild to severe clinical symptoms, its treatment varies correspondingly. In fulminant hepatic failure, the patient is resuscitated and listed for retransplantation. If thrombosis is acute and patients are symptomatic or minimally symptomatic, operative exploration with arterial reconstruction is performed. If the celiac artery inflow is adequate, thrombectomy with revision of the thrombosed segment may be performed without arterial reconstruction. If the inflow is inadequate, revascularization with an end-to-side anastomosis with the aorta or an interposition arterial graft is performed (Figs. 111-13 and 111-14). In some centers, percutaneous

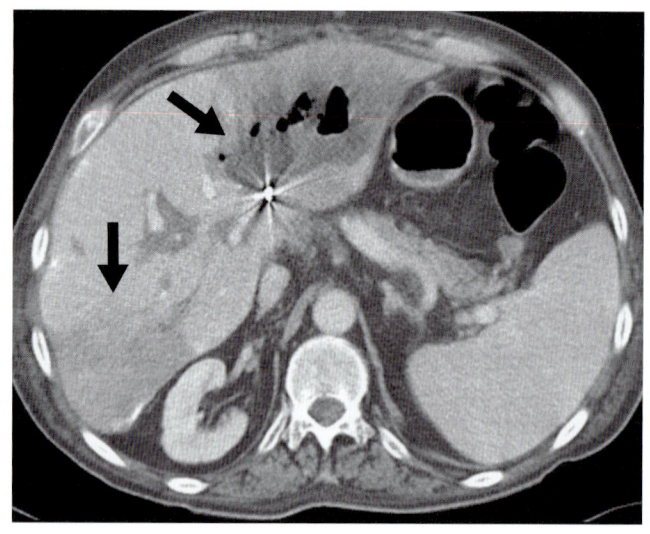

FIGURE 111-10 Hepatic artery thrombosis associated with hepatic infarction and necrosis. Venous phase from CTA demonstrates hepatic infarcts (*arrows*) and necrosis in a patient with hepatic artery thrombosis after an orthotopic liver transplantation.

catheter-mediated thrombolysis, with or without angioplasty and stenting, is performed in those patients who are asymptomatic or minimally symptomatic. This technique works best in acute or subacute thromboses. Percutaneous management of biliary complications may be sufficient, but retransplantation may be required when diffuse biliary injury and breakdown are accompanied by infection. If the thrombosis is late and the patient is asymptomatic, the patient may be expectantly observed with no intervention performed because hepatic arterial collateral vessels may be sufficient.[34-36]

Hepatic artery stenosis is a common vascular complication of orthotopic liver transplantation, with a prevalence between 5% and 11%.[25,30,37] It can be difficult to diagnose because many cases progress to hepatic artery thrombosis by the time clinical symptoms develop. Hepatic artery stenosis most often occurs at the vascular anastomosis. Early clinical findings may be manifested by biliary dysfunction or graft failure progressing to cholangitis or areas of ischemic infarcts.

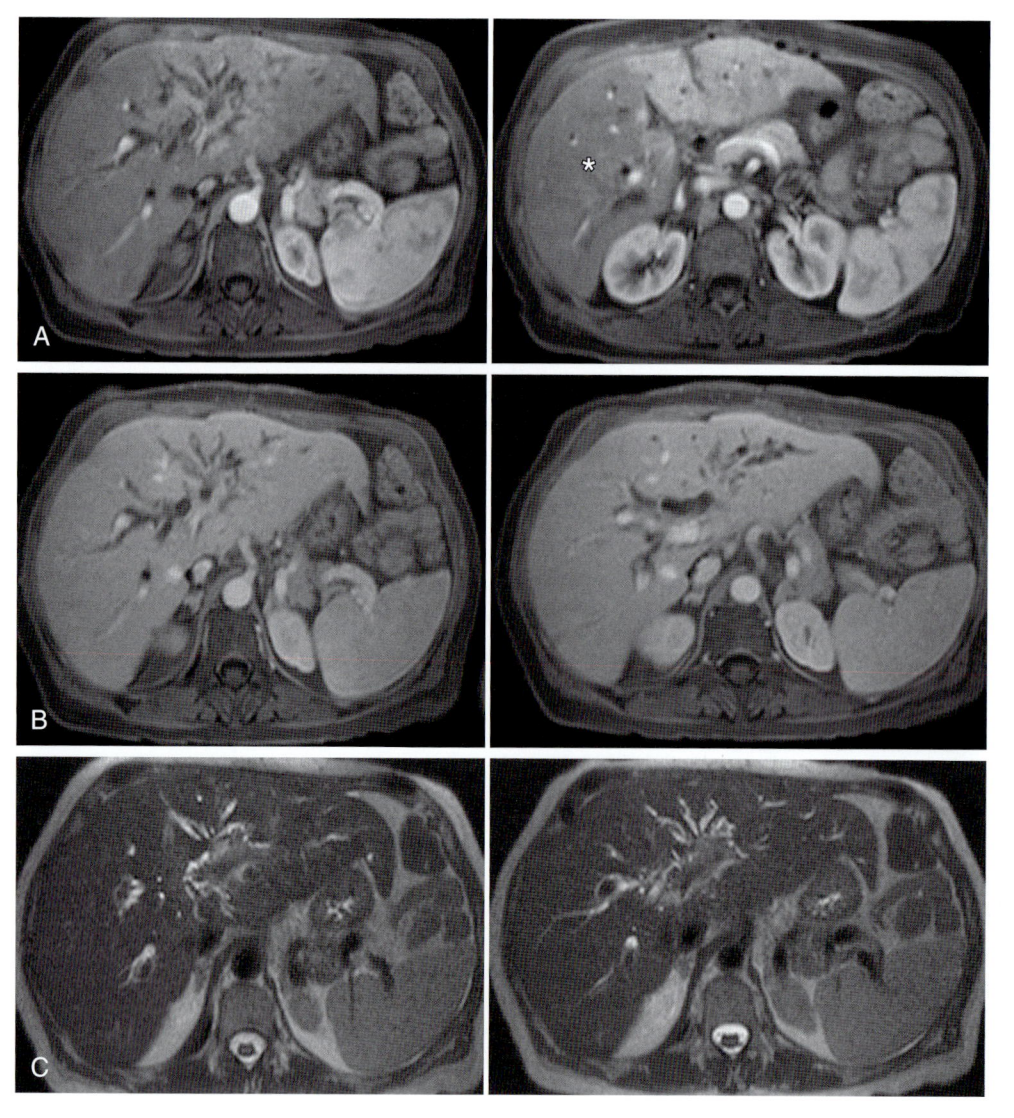

FIGURE 111-11 Hepatic artery thrombosis with associated hepatic and biliary findings. Hepatic artery thrombosis in an orthotopic liver transplantation patient is seen on MR to be associated with altered hepatic perfusion and biliary dilation. **A**, Postcontrast T1-weighted two-dimensional gradient-echo images with fat saturation in an early arterial phase reveal diminished perfusion (*asterisk*). **B**, Postcontrast T1-weighted two-dimensional gradient-echo images with fat saturation in a venous phase reveal dilated dark biliary ducts. **C**, Bright dilated biliary ducts are also noted on T2-weighted images.

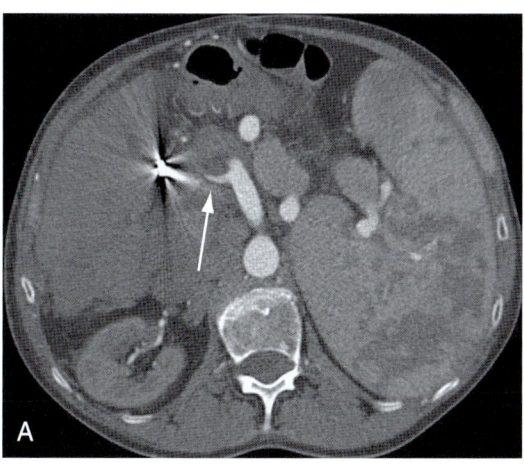

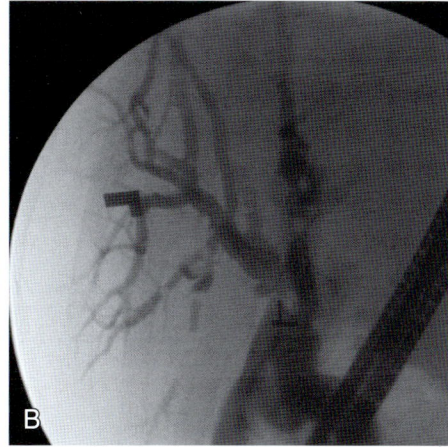

FIGURE 111-12 Hepatic artery thrombosis associated with biliary necrosis. **A,** CTA demonstrates hepatic artery thrombosis (*arrow*) in an orthotopic liver transplantation patient. **B,** Subsequent endoscopic retrograde cholangiopancreatography image demonstrates development of biliary necrosis.

Doppler ultrasound study is frequently performed in the evaluation of hepatic artery stenosis. Elevation of blood flow velocities by twofold to threefold at the hepatic artery anastomosis, increased downstream diastolic flow, and downstream tardus-parvus arterial waveforms within intrahepatic arteries are diagnostic criteria. Mild degrees of stenosis, however, may have normal Doppler findings. CTA and MRA are more direct methods for anatomic assessment of the anastomosis and are sensitive in the evaluation for stenosis. Both CTA and MRA can overestimate the degree of narrowing.[22,25,26,38] Stenosis at the celiac axis should be assessed in all cases during evaluation of the hepatic arterial inflow (Figs. 111-15 to 111-17).

In patients who are symptomatic or who have a long-segment stenosis, operative revision may be performed. Otherwise, hepatic artery stenosis can be successfully treated with angioplasty, which can improve graft survival by preventing progression to arterial thrombosis.[39-41]

Hepatic artery pseudoaneurysm (Fig. 111-18) is a rare complication of liver transplantation. Often at the vascular anastomosis, and frequently mycotic in nature, it is at increased risk for rupture. A pseudoaneurysm can be intrahepatic or peripheral after biopsy, instrumentation, or infection.[16,30] It can be treated surgically or by transarterial embolization.

Portal Vein

Portal vein thrombosis (Figs. 111-19 and 111-20) is an uncommon complication after orthotopic liver transplantation. Seen in 1% to 3% of cases, it can develop as late as 5 years after transplantation.[18,21-23,25,30] Causes include surgical technique, misalignment or excessive vessel length, hypercoagulable states, previous portal vein surgery, and thrombus formation from portal venous bypass cannula used at transplantation. By ultrasound examination, echogenic thrombus within the portal vein is demonstrated. In some acute settings, the thrombus can be anechoic. In all instances, color Doppler and spectral analysis should be performed. On CT and MR, portal vein thrombosis is evident with lack of contrast media enhancement, either complete or partial, within the portal vein. MR has the added ability to detect thrombus without the need for contrast media by bright blood pulse sequences such as steady-state free precession. Postoperative venous aneurysms can also be seen (Fig. 111-21).

Portal vein thrombus in the early post-transplantation setting can be manifested by graft failure, ascites, intestinal congestion, and gastrointestinal bleeding. Mortality is high in this setting; it can be treated by thrombectomy and in some instances may require retransplantation. Late portal vein thrombus can be treated with anticoagulation therapy if graft function is preserved. In some instances, a portacaval shunt may be required.

Portal vein stenosis (Fig. 111-22) can be an incidental finding or can be manifested by symptoms of portal hypertension.[30] In interpreting studies, however, it is important to note that size discrepancy between the donor and recipient portal vein can cause an apparent anastomotic

FIGURE 111-13 Patent hepatic arterial conduit. Volume rendered image from CTA in a patient after an orthotopic liver transplantation reveals a patent hepatic arterial graft conduit (*arrow*).

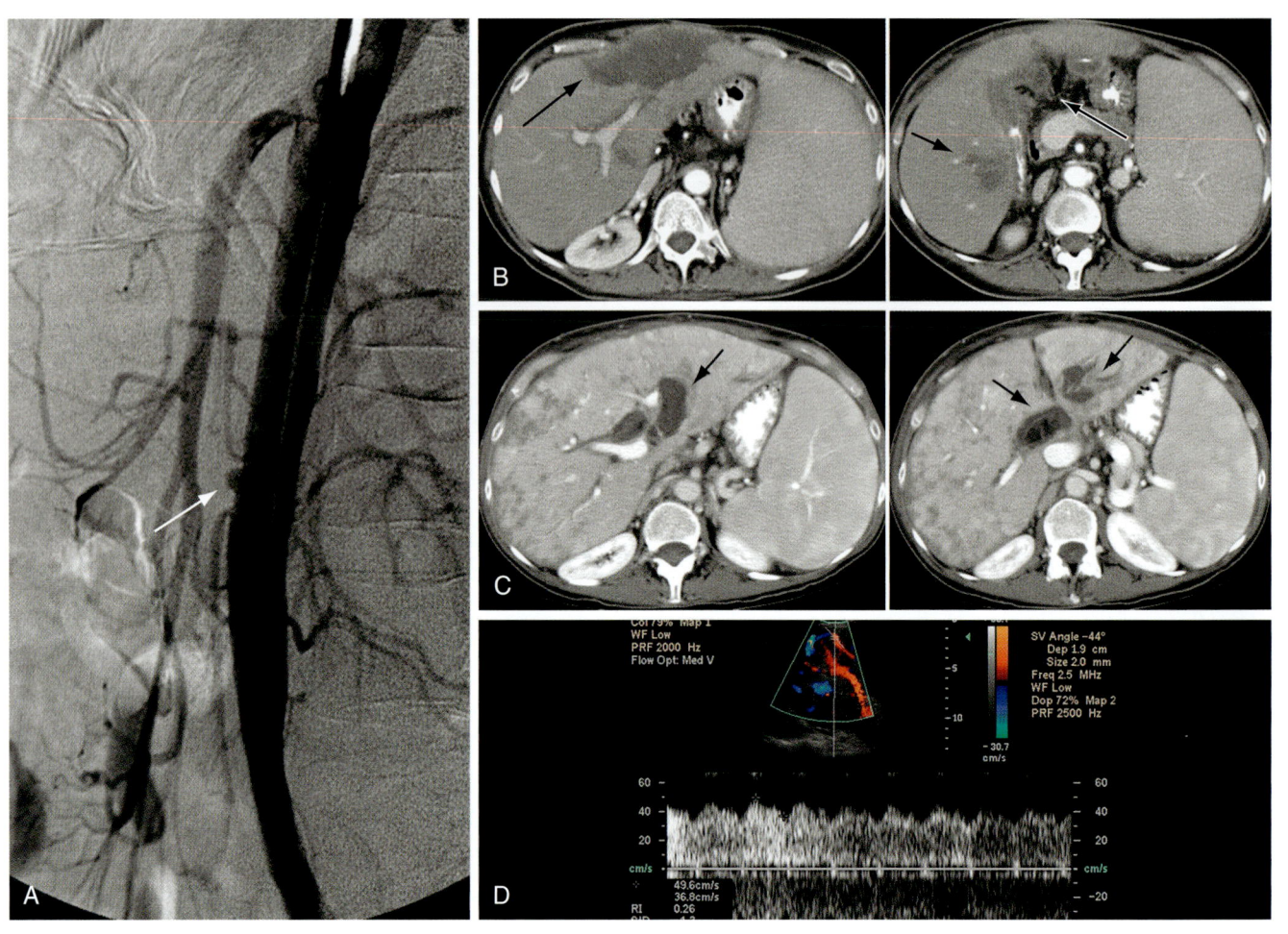

FIGURE 111-14 Thrombosed hepatic artery conduit. **A,** Fluoroscopic abdominal aortogram demonstrates an abrupt cutoff of a hepatic artery conduit (*arrow*), indicating thrombosis, in a patient after an orthotopic liver transplantation. **B,** CTA in the same patient shows multiple hepatic infarcts (*arrows*). **C,** Follow-up CTA reveals the development of biliary dilation and bilomas (*arrows*). **D,** Corresponding spectral Doppler ultrasound image with tardus et parvus waveform in the right hepatic artery.

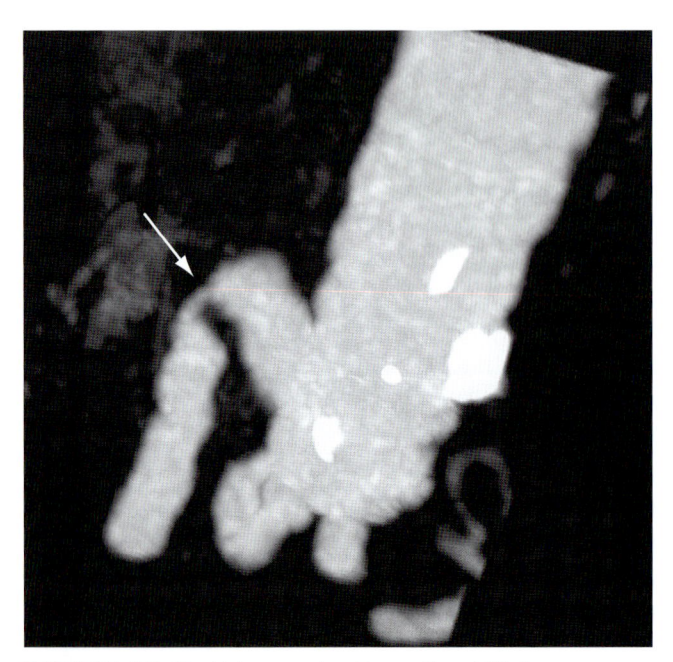

FIGURE 111-15 Volume rendered image from CTA demonstrates stenosis of the hepatic artery (*arrow*) in an orthotopic liver transplantation patient.

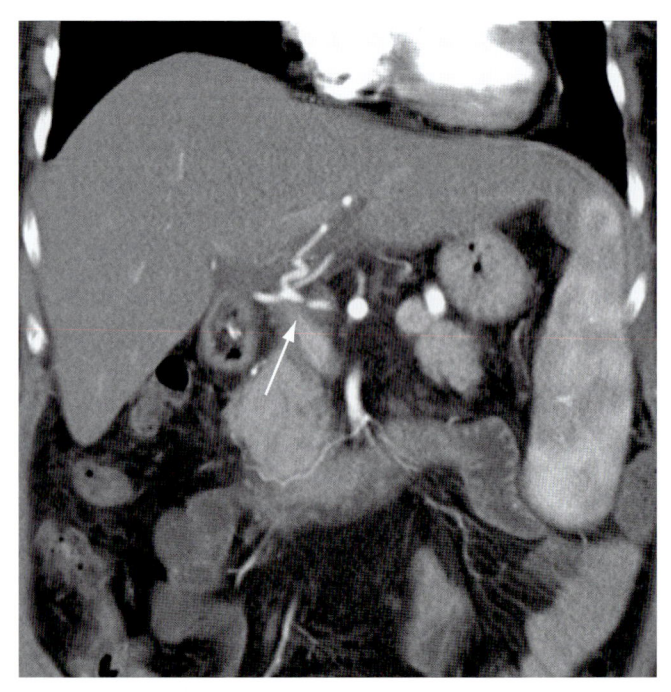

FIGURE 111-16 CTA demonstrates a high-grade hepatic artery stenosis (*arrow*) in a patient who had undergone an orthotopic liver transplantation.

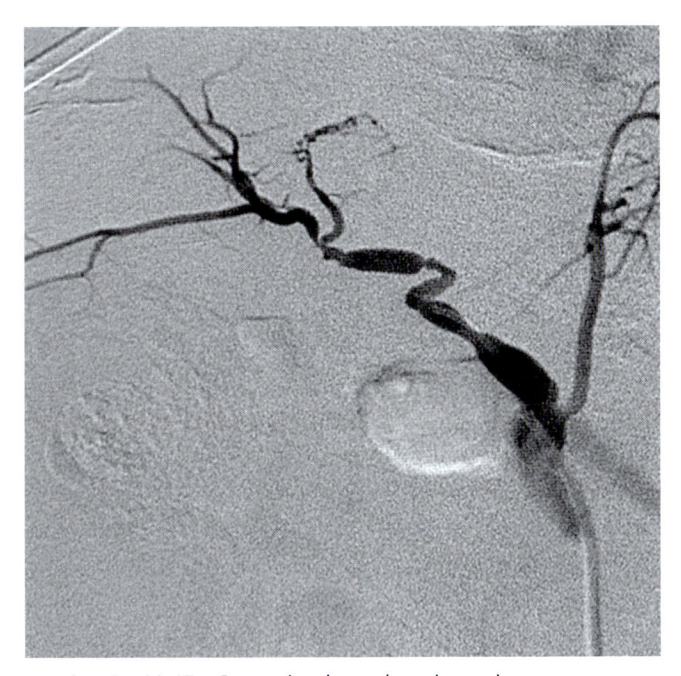

FIGURE 111-17 Conventional x-ray hepatic arteriogram demonstrates hepatic artery stenosis in an orthotopic liver transplantation patient.

stenosis. By Doppler ultrasound examination, an elevation in the velocity at the anastomosis by three or four times suggests a hemodynamically significant stenosis. Both CTA and MRA can demonstrate anastomotic narrowing. If it is not associated with other stigmata of portal hypertension, it is nonspecific in terms of hemodynamic significance. In evaluating the functional significance of an anastomotic narrowing, portal venography should be performed. A pressure gradient of 5 mm Hg or higher is compatible with a significant stenosis. Symptomatic stenosis can be treated by segmental portal vein resection or percutaneously by angioplasty with or without stent placement (Figs. 111-23 and 111-24).[39,42]

Hepatic Veins and Inferior Vena Cava

IVC stenosis is rare, occurring in less than 1% of transplants.[23,30] It is caused by technical problems related to surgery or compression by fluid collections.[42] The clinical findings in significant IVC stenosis include hepatomegaly, pleural effusions, ascites, and extremity edema.[16] A hemodynamically significant stenosis at the anastomosis may be manifested as a threefold to fourfold increase in velocity by spectral ultrasound examination. There may be dampened or reversed flow within the hepatic veins in a significant supracaval stenosis. With CTA or MRA, lack of or

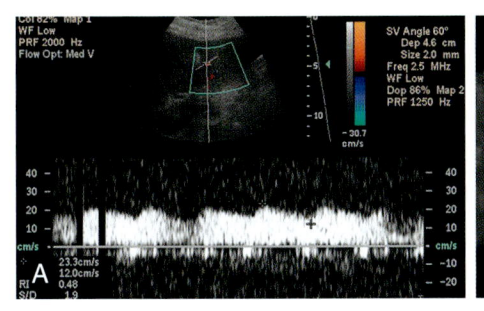

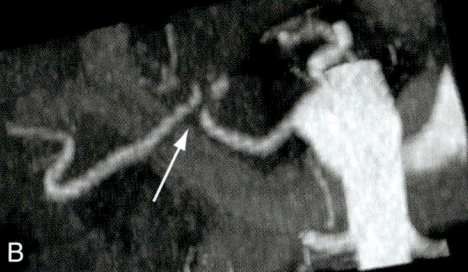

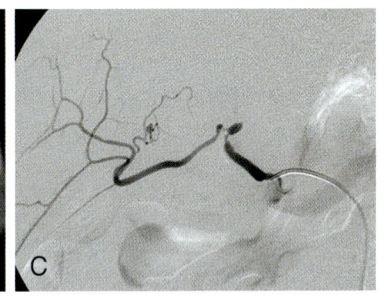

FIGURE 111-18 Hepatic artery stenosis after an orthotopic liver transplantation. A, Spectral Doppler ultrasound interrogation of the left hepatic artery in an orthotopic liver transplantation patient demonstrates a tardus et parvus waveform. B, Volume rendered image from CTA demonstrates severe hepatic artery stenosis with small pseudoaneurysm (*arrow*). C, Conventional x-ray hepatic angiography confirms the hepatic artery stenosis and pseudoaneurysm seen on CTA.

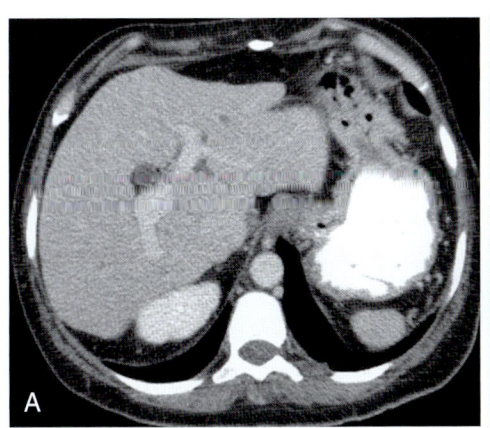

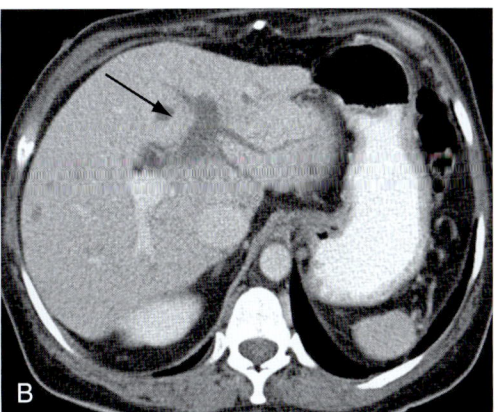

FIGURE 111-19 Portal vein thrombosis. A, Initial CTA examination after transplantation demonstrated a patent left portal vein. B, Follow-up CTA examination reveals new thrombus (*arrow*) in the left portal vein.

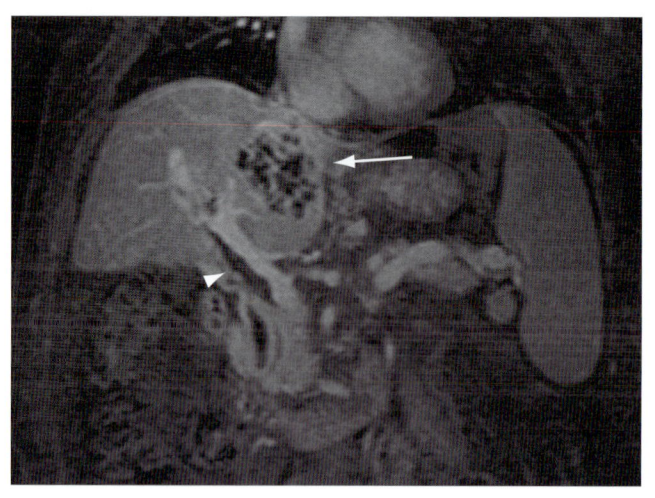

■ **FIGURE 111-20** Coronal gadolinium-enhanced three-dimensional MRA with nonocclusive thrombus in the main portal vein (*arrowhead*) as well as right hepatic lobe abscess (*arrow*) in a patient after an orthotopic liver transplantation.

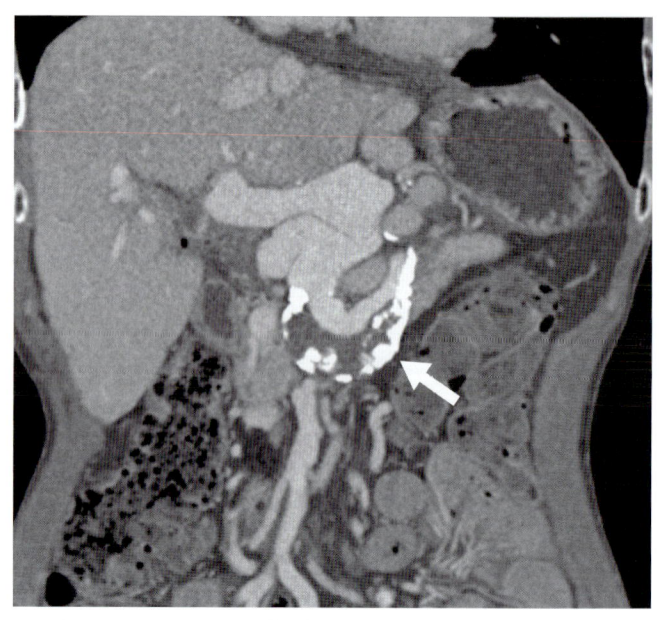

■ **FIGURE 111-21** Coronal reformatted image from CTA reveals an extrahepatic portal vein and splenic vein aneurysm containing calcified thrombus (*arrow*) in an orthotopic liver transplantation patient.

partial opacification of portions of the IVC due to thrombus or narrowing of the caval anastomosis can be seen (Figs. 111-25 to 111-28). As in portal vein stenosis, care must be taken not to mistake size discrepancy at the anastomosis between donor and recipient vessels for a hemodynamically significant stenosis (see Fig. 111-26). If a hemodynamically significant stenosis is suspected, venography should be performed to determine the presence of a significant pressure gradient. If one is found, angioplasty and stent placement can be successful.[39]

In cases of a piggyback caval anastomosis, there is an increased risk for venous outflow obstruction. Presumptive causes include direct compression of the vein by a graft that is too large, twisting of the venous anastomosis by a graft that is too small, surgical factors such as tight sutures, and, in late cases, intimal hyperplasia and fibrosis. Endovascular treatment with balloon-expandable stents can be an effective treatment in these cases.[43]

CONCLUSION

Orthotopic liver transplantation is the standard treatment of many causes of acute and chronic liver diseases. Because of the complex vascular reconstruction required for successful transplantation, vascular complications, predominantly hepatic artery thrombosis and stenosis, are among the most common causes of acute and delayed graft failure. CTA and MRA are sensitive techniques in the evaluation and diagnosis of abnormalities involving the transplant vasculature.

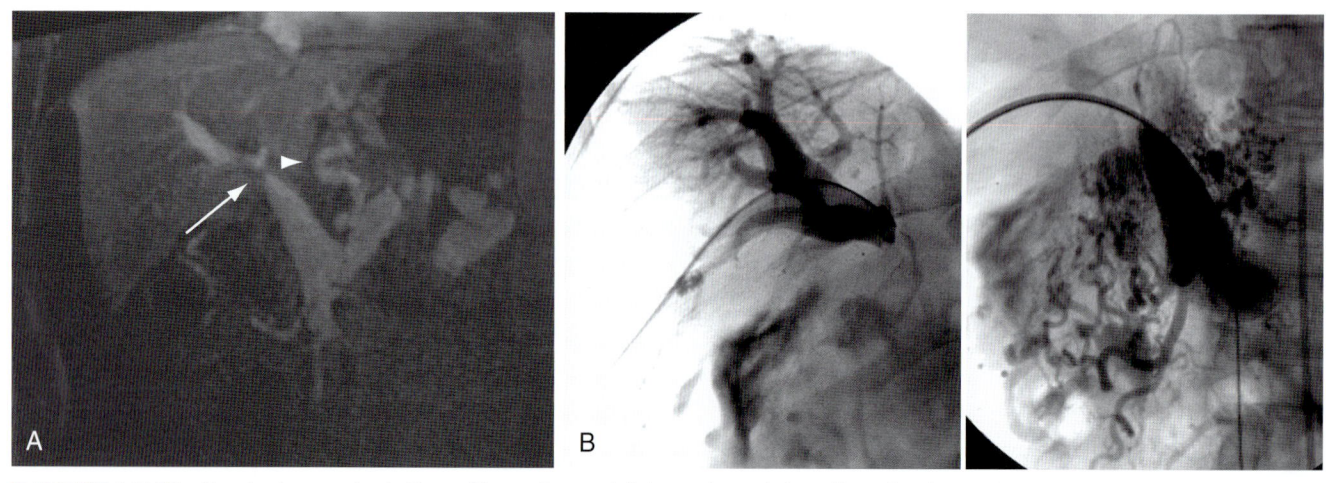

■ **FIGURE 111-22** Portal vein stenosis. **A,** Coronal image from gadolinium-enhanced three-dimensional MRA demonstrates an extrahepatic portal vein stenosis (*arrow*) in an orthotopic liver transplantation patient. Note collateral vessel (*arrowhead*). **B,** Conventional x-ray portal venogram confirms the findings on MRA. Note abundant collateral vessels. Venoplasty was performed.

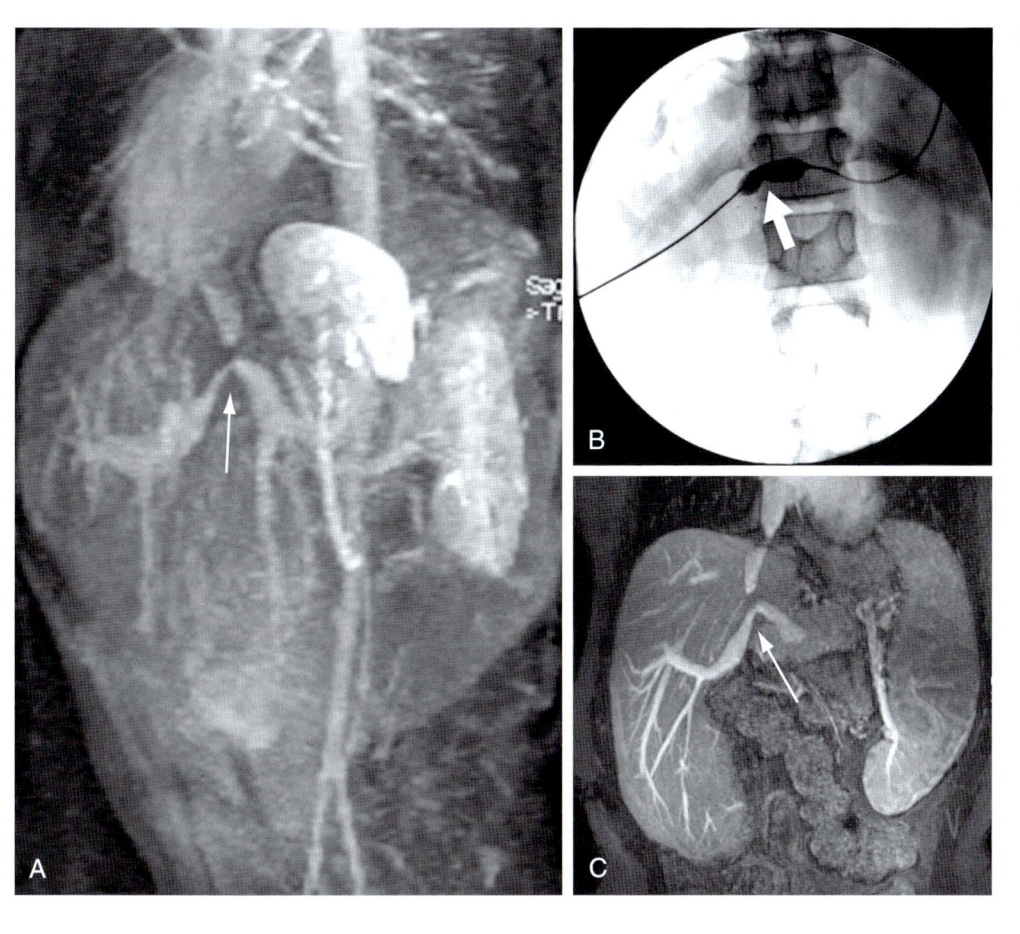

■ **FIGURE 111-23** Portal vein stenosis. **A,** Gadolinium-enhanced three-dimensional MRA demonstrating extrahepatic portal vein stenosis (*arrow*) in an orthotopic liver transplantation patient. **B,** On corresponding x-ray fluoroscopic image during venoplasty, a stenotic waist (*arrow*) in the portal vein is seen. The stenosis was associated with a portal venous pressure gradient from 12 mm Hg to 1 mm Hg. **C,** Follow-up three-dimensional gradient-echo MRA demonstrates reduction of the portal vein stenosis (*arrow*).

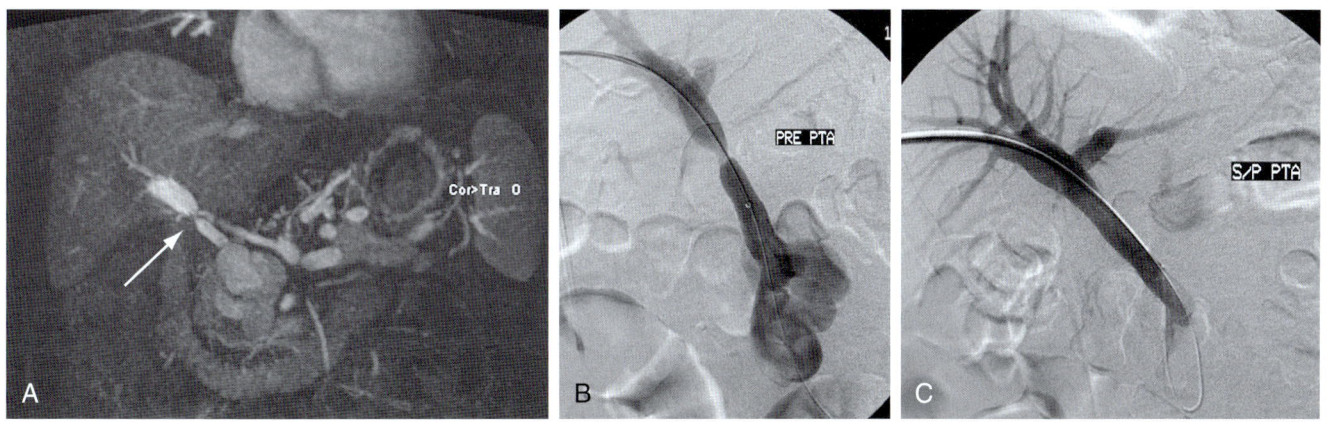

■ **FIGURE 111-24** Portal vein stenosis. **A,** Coronal gadolinium-enhanced three-dimensional MRA demonstrates stenosis of the extrahepatic portal vein in a patient after an orthotopic liver transplantation. **B,** Conventional x-ray portal venogram confirmed the stenosis, and venoplasty was undertaken. **C,** Postvenoplasty x-ray portal venogram revealed reduction of the portal vein stenosis.

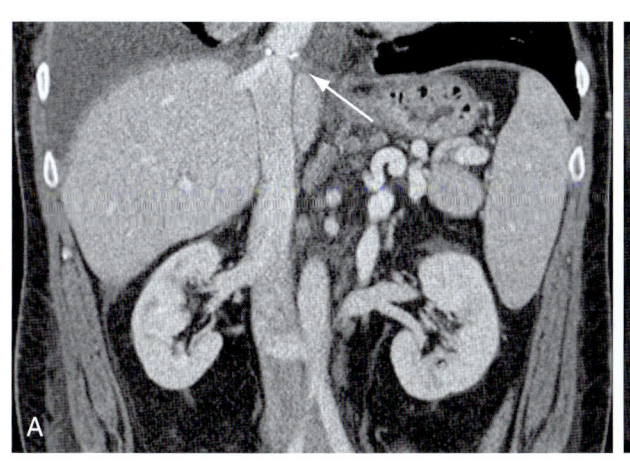

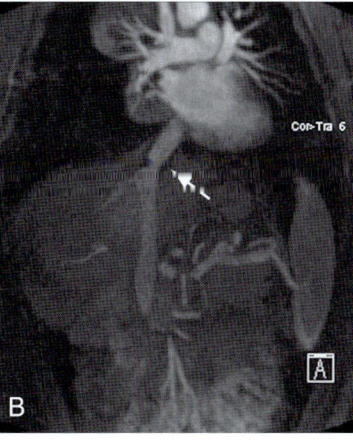

■ **FIGURE 111-25** IVC stenosis. **A,** Coronal reformatted image from CTA demonstrates a suprahepatic IVC anastomotic stenosis (*arrow*) in a patient after orthotopic liver transplantation. Note that a right pleural effusion is also present. **B,** The IVC anastomotic stenosis (*arrow*) is seen also on a corresponding gadolinium-enhanced three-dimensional MRA image.

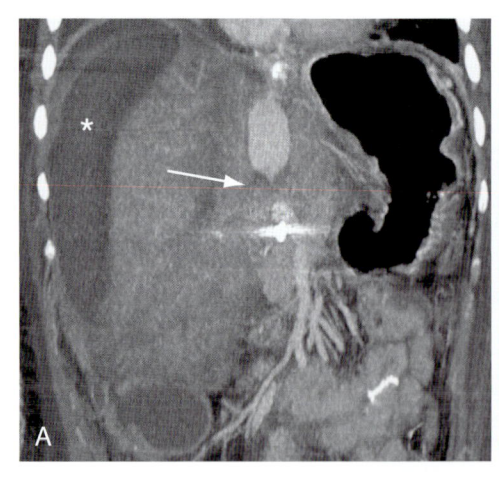

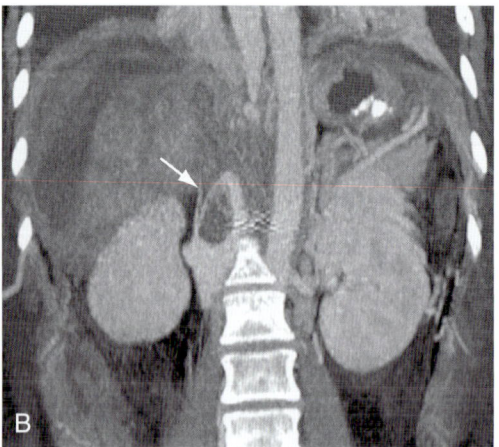

■ **FIGURE 111-26** IVC stenosis and thrombosis. Coronal reformatted images from CTA in a patient after an orthotopic liver transplantation reveal an infrahepatic IVC stenosis (**A**, *arrow*) and caval thrombosis (**B**, *arrow*). Note that ascites (**A**, *asterisk*) is also present.

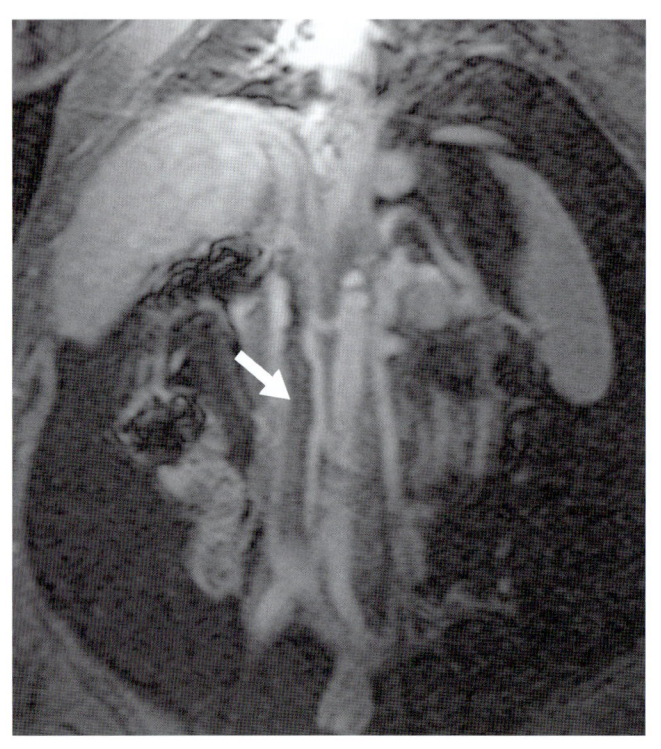

■ **FIGURE 111-27** Coronal gadolinium-enhanced T1-weighted two-dimensional gradient-echo image with fat saturation demonstrates extensive IVC thrombosis (*arrow*) as a result of a supracaval anastomotic stricture.

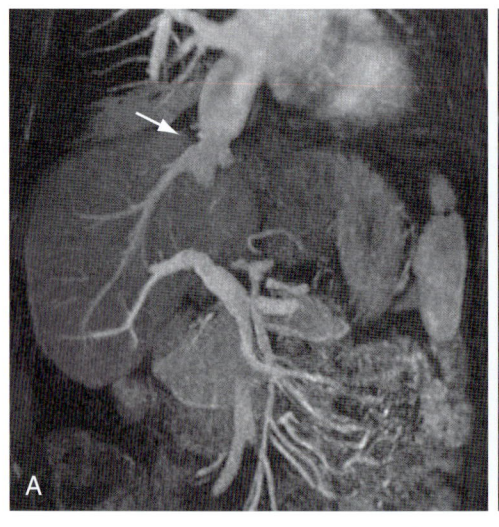

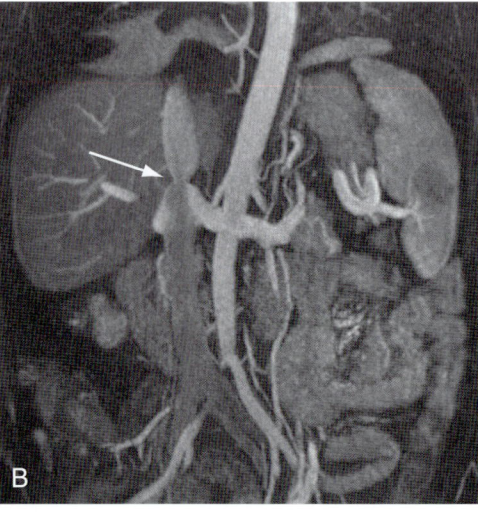

■ **FIGURE 111-28** Coronal gadolinium-enhanced three-dimensional MRA reveals mild and clinically insignificant narrowings of the suprahepatic IVC anastomosis (**A**, *arrow*) and infrahepatic IVC anastomosis (**B**, *arrow*).

KEY POINTS

- Liver transplantation is the primary treatment of many fulminant acute and chronic liver diseases as well as of certain hepatic malignant neoplasms.
- In the pretransplantation setting, multidetector CT or CTA and dynamic contrast-enhanced MR or MRA are used primarily for surgical anatomic assessment, evaluation of vascular patency, and detection of focal or diffuse liver lesions.
- In the limited instances of living related liver donor transplantation, radiologic evaluation of the donor liver vascular anatomy by CT or MR angiography is mandatory.
- Spectral and color Doppler ultrasound studies are often performed as an initial screening examination in the evaluation for complications in the post-transplantation setting, predominantly because these are rapid, portable examinations that can provide useful although limited information.
- Multidetector CT or CTA and dynamic contrast-enhanced MR or MRA are more reliable whole-liver examinations. They provide a complete assessment of each surgical vascular anastomosis in the evaluation for post-transplantation vascular complications.
- The most common and serious vascular complications are hepatic artery thrombosis and stenosis. Portal vein, hepatic vein, and inferior vena caval thrombosis and stenosis occur less frequently.
- Conventional angiography may be indicated for further evaluation or treatment.

SUGGESTED READINGS

Alonso-Torres A, Fernandez-Cuadrado J, Pinilla I, et al. Multidetector CT in the evaluation of potential living donors for liver transplantation. Radiographics 2005; 25:1017-1030.

Limanoud P, Raman SS, Ghobial RM, et al. Preoperative imaging of adult-to-adult living related liver transplant donors. J Comput Assit Tomogr 2004; 28:149-157.

Onofrio AC, Singh AH, Uppot RN, et al. Vascular and biliary variants in the liver: implications for liver surgery. Radiographics 2008; 28:359-378.

Pannu HK, Maley WR, Fishman EK. Liver transplantation: preoperative CT evaluation. Radiographics 2001; 21:S133-S146.

Saad WE, Orloff MC, Davies MG, et al. Postliver transplantation: vascular and biliary surgical anatomy. Tech Vasc Interv Radiol 2007; 10:172-190.

Sahani D, Mehta A, Blake M, et al. Preoperative hepatic vascular evaluation with CT and MR angiography: implications for surgery. Radiographics 2004; 24:1367-1380.

Schroeder T, Malago M, Debatin JF, et al. "All-in-one" imaging protocols for the evaluation of potential living liver donors: comparison of magnetic resonance imaging and multidetector computed tomography. Liver Transpl 2005; 11:776-787.

REFERENCES

1. Organ Procurement and Transplantation Network. Available at: http://optn.transplant.hrsa.gov/.
2. Lehnert T. Liver transplantation for metastatic neuroendocrine carcinoma: an analysis of 103 patients. Tranplantation 1998; 66:1307-1312.
3. Bennett GL, Krinsky GA, Abitbol RJ, et al. Ultrasound detection of hepatocellular carcinoma and dysplastic nodules in patients with cirrhosis: correlation of pretransplant ultrasound findings and liver explant pathology in 200 patients. AJR Am J Roentgenol 2002; 179:175-180.
4. Taouli B, Krinsky GA. Diagnostic imaging of hepatocellular carcinoma in patients with cirrhosis before liver transplantation. Liver Transpl 2006; 12:S1-S7.
5. Krinsky GA, Lee VS, Theise ND, et al. Transplantation for hepatocellular carcinoma and cirrhosis: sensitivity of magnetic resonance imaging. Liver Transpl 2002; 8:1156-1164.
6. Krinsky GA, Lee VS, Theise ND, et al. Hepatocellular carcinoma and dysplastic nodules in patients with cirrhosis: prospective diagnosis with MR imaging and explantation correlation. Radiology 2001; 219:445-454.
7. Hanna RF, Kased N, Kwan SW, et al. Double-contrast MRI for accurate staging of hepatocellular carcinoma in patients with cirrhosis. AJR Am J Roentgenol 2008; 190:47-57
8. Ronzoni A, Artioli D, Scardina R, et al. Role of MDCT in the diagnosis of hepatocellular carcinoma in patients with cirrhosis undergoing orthotopic liver transplantation. AJR Am J Roentgenol 2007; 189:792-798.
9. Brancatelli G, Baron RL, Peterson MS, Wallis M. Helical CT screening for hepatocellular carcinoma in patients with cirrhosis: frequency and causes of false-positive interpretation. AJR Am J Roentgenol 2003; 180:1007-1014.
10. Anselmo DM, Baquerizo A, Geevarghese S, et al. Liver transplantation at Dumont-UCLA Transplant Center: an experience with over 3,000 cases. Clin Transpl 2001; 179-186.
11. Sahani D, Mehta A, Blake M, et al. Preoperative hepatic vascular evaluation with CT and MR angiography: implications for surgery. Radiographics 2004; 24:1367-1380.
12. Onofrio AC, Singh AH, Uppot RN, et al. Vascular and biliary variants in the liver: implications for liver surgery. Radiographics 2008; 28:359-378.
13. Limanond P, Raman SS, Ghobrial RM, et al. Preoperative imaging in adult-to-adult living related liver transplant donors: what surgeons want to know. J Comput Assist Tomagr 2004; 28:149-157.
14. Alonso-Torres A, Fernandez-Cuadrado J, Pinilla I, et al. Multidetector CT in the evaluation of potential living donors for liver transplantation. Radiographics 2005; 25:1017-1030.
15. Ishigami K, Zhang Y, Rayhill S, et al. Does variant hepatic artery anatomy in a liver transplant recipient increase the risk of hepatic artery complications after transplantation? AJR Am J Roentgenol 2004; 183:1577-1584.
16. Nghiem HV, Tran K, Winter TC III, et al. Imaging of complications in liver transplantation. Radiographics 1996; 16:825-840.
17. Hiatt JR, Gabbay J, Busuttil RW. Surgical anatomy of the hepatic arteries in 1000 cases. Ann Surg 1994; 220:50-52.
18. Quiroga A, Sebastia C, Margarit C, et al. Complications of orthotopic liver transplantation: spectrum of findings with helical CT. Radiographics 2001; 21:1085-1102.
19. Stange BJ, Glanemann M, Nussler NC, et al., Indication, technique and outcome of portal vein arterialization in orthotopic liver transplantation. Transplant Proc 2001; 33:1414-1415.
20. Khan S, Silva MA, Tan YM, et al. Conventional versus piggyback technique of caval implantation; without extra-corporeal venovenous bypass. A comparative study. Transpl Int 2006; 19:795-801.
21. Varotti G, Grazi GL, Vetrone G, et al. Causes of early acute graft failure after liver transplantation: analysis of a 17-year single centre experience. Clin Transplant 2005; 19:492-500.

22. Brancatelli G, Katyal S, Federle MP, Fontes P. Three-dimensional multislice helical computed tomography with the volume rendering technique in the detection of vascular complications after liver transplantation. Transplantation 2002; 73:237-242.
23. Stafford-Johnson DB, Hamilton BH, Dong Q, et al. Vascular complications of liver transplantation: evaluation with gadolinium enhanced MR angiography. Radiology 1998; 207:153-160.
24. Finn JP, Edelman RR, Jenkins RL, et al. Liver transplantation: MR angiography with surgical validation. Radiology 1991; 179: 265-269.
25. Glockner JF, Forauer AR, Solomon H, et al. Three-dimensional gadolinium enhanced MR angiography of vascular complications after liver transplantation. AJR Am J Roentgenol 2000; 174:1447-1453.
26. Kim BS, Kim TK, Jung DJ, et al. Vascular complications after living related liver transplantation: evaluation with gadolinium-enhanced three-dimensional MR angiography. AJR Am J Roentgenol 2003; 181:467-474.
27. Legmann P, Costes V, Tudoret L, et al. Hepatic artery thrombosis after liver transplantation: diagnosis with spiral CT. AJR Am J Roentgenol 1995; 164:97-101.
28. Pandaripande PV, Lee VS, Morgan GR, et al. Vascular and extravascular complications of liver transplantation: comprehensive evaluation with three-dimensional contrast-enhanced volumetric MR imaging and MR cholangiopancreatography. AJR Am J Roentgenol 2001; 177:1101-1107.
29. Sadowski EA, Bennett LK, Chan MR, et al. Nephrogenic systemic fibrosis: risk factors and incidence estimation. Radiology 2007; 243:148-157.
30. Wozney P, Zajko AM, Bron KM, et al. Vascular complications after liver transplantation: a 5 year experience. AJR Am J Roentgenol 1986; 147:657-663.
31. Silva MA, Jambulingham PS, Gunson BK, et al. Hepatic artery thrombosis following orthotopic liver transplantation: a 10-year experience from a single centre in the United Kingdom. Liver Transpl 2006; 12:146-151.
32. Orons PD, Sheng R, Zajko AB. Hepatic artery stenosis in liver transplant recipients: prevalence and cholangiographic appearance of associated biliary complications. AJR Am J Roentgenol 1995; 165: 1145-1149.
33. Hall TR, McDiarmid SV, Grant EG, et al. False-negative duplex Doppler studies in children with hepatic artery thrombosis after liver transplantation. AJR Am J Roentgenol 1990; 154:573-575.
34. Sheiner PA, Varma CV, Guarrera JV, et al. Selective revascularization of hepatic artery thromboses after liver transplantation improves patient and graft survival. Transplantation 1997; 64:1295-1299.
35. Bhattacharjya S, Gunson BK, Mirza DF, et al. Delayed hepatic artery thrombosis in adult orthotopic liver transplantation—a 12-year experience. Transplantation 2001; 71:1592-1596.
36. Langnas AN, Marujo W, Stratta RJ, et al. Hepatic allograft rescue following arterial thrombosis. Role of urgent revascularization. Transplantation 1991; 51:86-90.
37. Glockner JF, Forauer AR. Vascular or ischemic complications after liver transplantation. AJR Am J Roentgenol 1999; 173:1055-1059.
38. Vignali C, Bargellini I, Cioni R, et al. Diagnosis and treatment of hepatic artery stenosis after orthotopic liver transplant. Transplant Proc 2004; 36:2771-2773.
39. Raby N, Kirani J, Thomas S, et al. Stenoses of vascular anastomosis after hepatic transplantation: treatment with balloon angioplasty. AJR Am J Roentgenol 1991; 157:167-171.
40. Abbasoglu O, Levy MF, Vodapally MS, et al. Hepatic artery stenosis after liver transplantation—incidence, presentation, treatment, and long term outcome. Transplantation 1997; 63:250-255.
41. Saad WE, Davies MG, Sahler L, et al. Hepatic artery stenosis in liver transplant recipients: primary treatment with percutaneous transluminal angioplasty. J Vasc Interv Radiol 2005; 16:795-805.
42. Ito K, Siegelman ES, Stolpen AH, Mitchell DG. MR imaging of complications after liver transplantation. AJR Am J Roentgenol 2000; 175:1145-1149.
43. Wang SL, Sze DY, Busque S, et al. Treatment of hepatic venous outflow obstruction after piggyback liver transplantation. Radiology 2005; 236:352-359.

CHAPTER 112

Vascular Imaging of Renal and Pancreatic Transplantation

Alexander B. Steever, Martin R. Prince, Priscilla A. Winchester, and Joan C. Prowda

The use of kidney transplantation to treat end-stage renal disease in the United States has steadily increased from 43/million in 1996 to 55.5/million in 2005. The most recent data (2006) show that there are now more than 103,000 Americans living with a renal transplant and more than 9,400 with a pancreas or kidney-pancreas transplant, up from 55,000 and 4,000, respectively, in 1996.[1] Imaging plays a major role in the surveillance of transplant complications. In this chapter, the vascular complications associated with renal and pancreatic transplantation are discussed.

VASCULAR EVALUATION OF RENAL TRANSPLANT RECIPIENTS

Transplant Renal Artery Stenosis

Hemodynamically significant stenosis of the transplant renal artery (transplant renal artery stenosis [TRAS]) is defined as a 50% or greater narrowing of the lumen. Some investigators divide stenoses into grades of mild, moderate, severe, and critical, usually corresponding to narrowings of less than 50%, 50% to 70%, 70% to 90%, and more than 90%.

Prevalence and Epidemiology

TRAS has been reported in 1% to 23% of cases, with most series finding 2% to 10% of renal transplants are complicated by TRAS.[2,3] It is usually a relatively late complication, occurring from 3 months to 2 years or more after transplantation.

Etiology and Pathophysiology

TRAS is most common at the anastomosis or most proximal segment of the donor artery and the risk is directly related to technique. Cadaveric transplants are typically harvested with an aortic patch from which the single or multiple renal arteries arise. The patch can then be anastomosed with its arterial origins end to side on the external iliac artery. Grafts from living donors, who cannot sacrifice an aortic patch, are typically anastomosed end to end to the internal iliac artery. When living donor grafts with multiple renal arteries must be used, the accessory arteries may be reconstructed to flow from the main renal artery, anastomosed separately, or anastomosed to the inferior epigastric artery (Fig. 112-1). End-to-end anastomoses have a threefold greater risk of stenosis.

Contributing causes of stenosis in end to end anastomoses are thought to be abnormal fluid dynamics and abrupt changes in caliber. Other more general causes or precipitants of stenosis include faulty suture technique, clamp injury, and kinking of the artery. In addition, atherosclerosis can occur or progress in the donor artery. An association with stenosis has also been shown among patients who have experienced episodes of acute rejection possibly caused by a component of endothelial injury from rejection of the graft artery. An additional association with cytomegalovirus infection has been reported.[4] Finally, a stenosis of the recipient artery, usually the external iliac or common iliac artery, proximal to the anastomosis may have hemodynamic effects on the kidney, similar to stenosis of the graft artery.

Manifestations of Disease

Clinical Presentation

Stenosis presents in the transplant kidney much like it does in native kidneys, with hypertension and decreasing renal function. However, 60% to 80% of recipients have preexisting hypertension, so the diagnosis of TRAS should be suspected when there is worsening or new hypertension that does not respond to medication or is associated

A

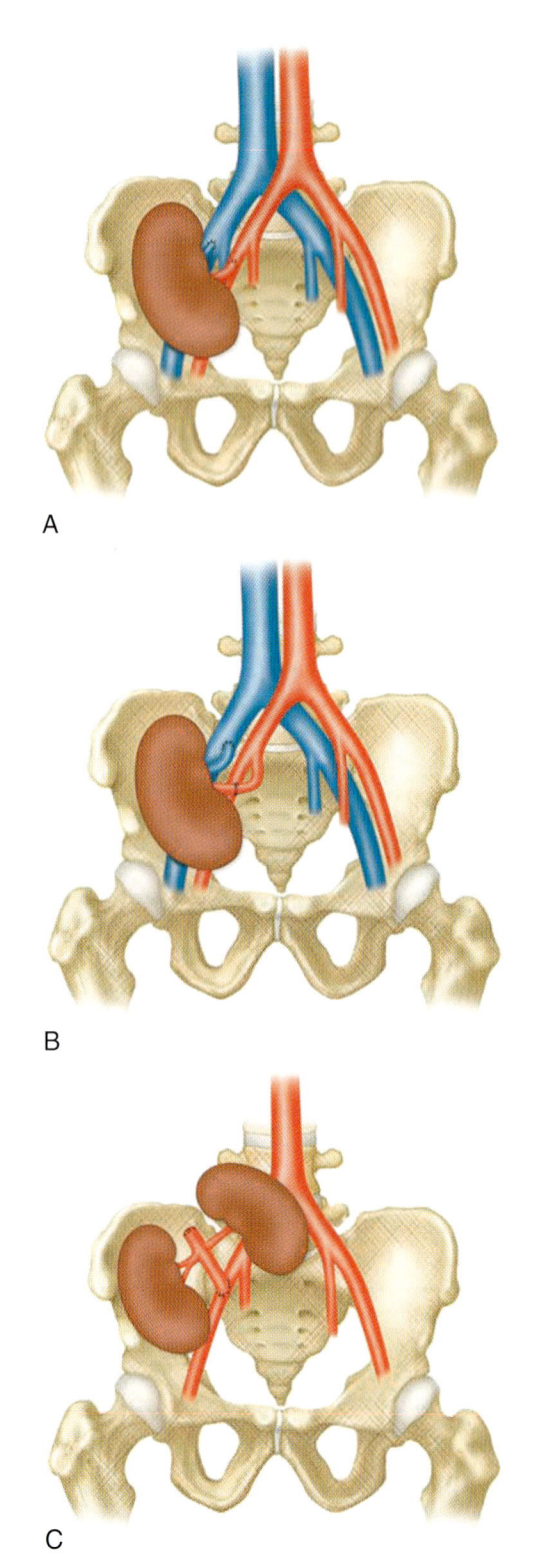

B

C

■ **FIGURE 112-1** **A,** Transplant artery anastomosed to external iliac artery (end to side). **B,** Transplant artery anastomosed to internal iliac artery end to end. **C,** Donor aorta anastomosed to external iliac artery end to side with two donor kidneys (typically from a pediatric cadaver).

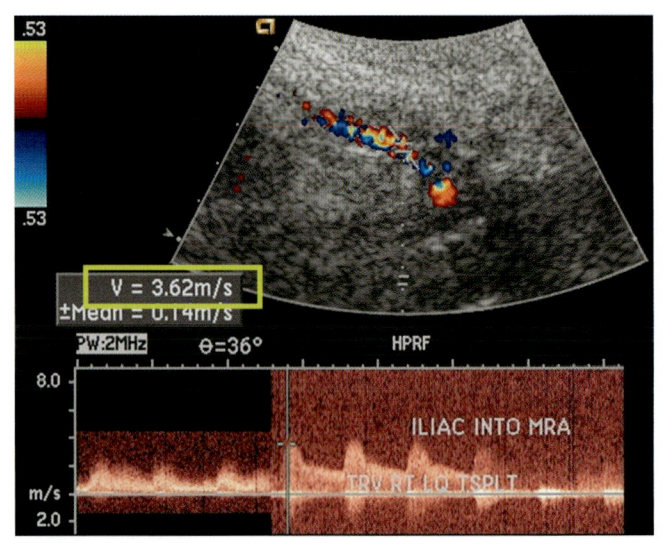

■ **FIGURE 112-2** High-velocity flow with spectral broadening indicating severe stenosis of transplant artery end-to-side anastomosis to the external iliac artery.

Imaging Indications and Algorithm

In cases of suspected TRAS, ultrasound with Doppler interrogation of the vasculature is used as the initial test. Ultrasound is typically the easiest, fastest, and least expensive to obtain. However, accurate measurements indicating a stenosis can be technically difficult to obtain secondary to poor acoustic windows and/or operator skill. Magnetic resonance angiography (MRA) is used in cases in which the ultrasound is equivocal or nondiagnostic, or when direct anatomic visualization is required (see later). MRA offers very high sensitivity and specificity in a noninvasive test. Catheter angiography with angioplasty is used for definitive diagnosis and treatment. CT angiography can demonstrate a stenosis but is generally avoided in patients with renal transplants because of the risk of nephropathy from iodinated contrast.

Imaging Techniques and Findings

Radiography

Inspection of an abdominal radiograph is valuable to note the presence and approximate location of stents, surgical clips, or other material that might interfere with subsequent imaging. This is especially true for MRA, in which local loss of signal because of clip artifact is a well-recognized pitfall.

Ultrasound

Like native renal artery stenosis, the diagnosis of TRAS is made with ultrasound by demonstrating a focal area of aliasing on color Doppler imaging from turbulence caused by the stenosis and an elevated peak systolic velocity through the stenosis more than 2.5 m/sec on spectral Doppler imaging (Fig. 112-2).[5] Because of the proximity of the allograft to the body wall in the anterior pelvis, the main artery can often be visualized in its entirety, aiding the chances of confirming the diagnosis. Power Doppler,

with a decline in renal function. Other clinical indications include worsened function after the administration of an angiotensin-converting enzyme inhibitor (ACEI) or angiotensin receptor blocker, diuretic-resistant peripheral edema, and a new bruit over the allograft.

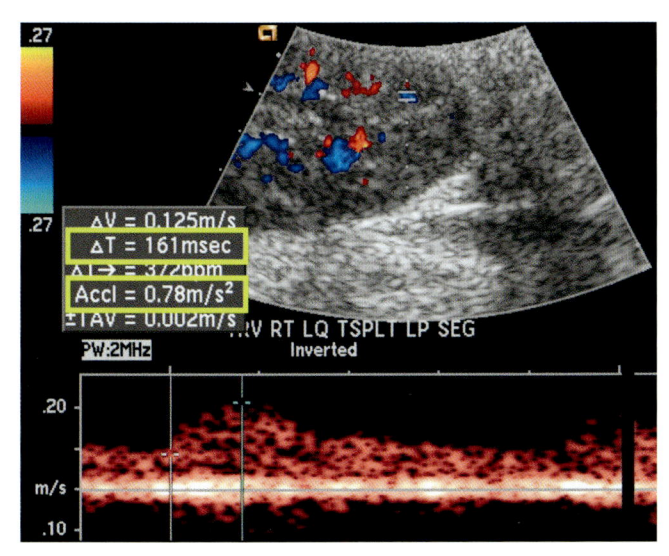

FIGURE 112-3 Low-resistance flow and tardus-parvus waveform with delayed systolic peak detected on Doppler ultrasound of intrarenal arcuate artery.

with its high sensitivity to flow in all directions, is helpful to localize and map the artery for further evaluation with color Doppler and placement of the spectral Doppler gate. However, transplant arteries are typically much more tortuous than native renal arteries. This makes the setting of accurate angle correction on spectral Doppler more difficult and sometimes almost impossible. Furthermore, a range of elevated velocities has been shown in transplant arteries, even when stenosis is not suspected or proven not to be present, particularly if there is tortuosity.[6] When there is no significant curvature, an elevated velocity may reflect elevated velocity in the external iliac artery. In these cases, a ratio of velocities in the main transplant artery and external iliac artery less than 1.8 is unlikely to be stenosis.

As in native renal stenosis, the characteristic parvus-tardus waveform of the intrarenal arteries downstream from a stenosis can support the diagnosis. This is reflected in spectral broadening of the arterial waveform, retarded acceleration less than 1.5 m/sec^2, and increased acceleration time more than 0.08 to 0.10 second (Fig. 112-3) However, these findings have been shown to be less specific than peak systolic velocity and should be used to support the diagnosis based on peak systolic velocity.[7] Resistive and pulsatility indices can also be lowered in TRAS but are only nonspecific indicators of graft dysfunction.

Computed Tomography

This is not commonly used to assess transplant renal artery stenosis due to the nephrotoxicity of iodinated contrast.

Magnetic Resonance Imaging

MRI can demonstrate TRAS with a high degree of accuracy. In multiple series, gadolinium (Gd)-enhanced three-dimensional MRA has been shown to have a sensitivity of 67% to 100% and a specificity of 75% to 100% for hemodynamically significant stenosis (Table 112-1). Although technically challenging on older scanners, the examinations have become routine with state of the art 1.5-T scanners.

Gd-enhanced MRA is performed with a three-dimensional spoiled gradient echo pulse sequence. With a fast repetition time (TR), multiple three-dimensional acquisitions (i.e., multiphase), each taken during a single breath-hold, can be obtained in approximately 2 minutes. Acquiring the first set before the administration of gadolinium allows for image mask subtraction of the precontrast image data set from postcontrast data sets, which can then be processed on a dedicated three-dimensional workstation for improved imaging using a variety of postprocessing visualization tools, such as multiplanar reformation, maximum intensity projection (MIP), and volume rendering. Careful timing of the contrast bolus to synchronize peak arterial Gd concentration with central k-space data acquisition is essential and is usually achieved by automated triggering or MR fluoroscopy sequences. Using phased-array surface coil arrays with parallel imaging helps shorten the duration of center of k-space to minimize artifacts and maximize resolution and anatomic coverage for a comfortable breath-hold time. Twofold acceleration is possible with eight coils and four- or five-fold acceleration works well with 32 coils. High resolution is necessary to resolve the renal artery adequately, with slice thickness preferably less than 3 mm zero interpolation down to less than 1.5 mm, and in-plane resolution less than 2 mm. The Gd dose should be kept at 0.1 mmol/kg or less to minimize risk of nephrogenic systemic fibrosis (NSF) in case the glomerular filtration rate (GFR) is less than 30 mL/min. Promising new noncontrast renal MRA techniques are also emerging but are not yet validated.

Review of source images, as well as review of three-dimensional postprocessed projectional views, is necessary to make the appropriate diagnosis. MIPs and multiplanar reformations using variable thicknesses allow for direct visualization through the lumen of the transplant renal artery, the anastomosis, the iliac arteries, and usually the first-order branch arteries (Fig. 112-4). It is the ability to manipulate the volumetric data of MRA that makes it so effective. This is especially true in tortuous vessels, which are typical in renal transplants. Shaded surface volume renderings can be especially helpful to visualize the anatomy in the case of tortuous vessels.

An effective complement to Gd-enhanced MRA is three-dimensional phase contrast MRA. This sequence achieves the MR signal, and therefore contrast, from protons moving across flow-encoding gradients. The signal is velocity-encoded at a certain upper threshold so that superfast flow at severe stenoses nulls the signal. Although the sequence acquisition time is long (typically 5 to 8 minutes), phase contrast MRA can be performed on a small field of view, either in the area of the transplant renal artery or any area of suspicion during imaging. Confirming suspected stenoses by demonstrating loss of signal on phase contrast helps eliminate false-positives. The combination of Gd-enhanced MRA and phase contrast MRA has been shown to increase specificity from 88% to 100%.[8]

TABLE 112-1 Accuracy of Magnetic Resonance Angiography

Study (Year)*	No. of Patients	Technique	Sensitivity (%)	Specificity (%)
Renal MRA				
Kent (1991)	23	2D TOF	100	94
Debatin (1991)	33	2D PC	80	91
	33	2D TOF	53	97
Servois (1994)	21	2D TOF	70	78
Hertz (1994)	16	2D TOF	91	94
Loubeyre (1994)	53	3D TOF	100	76
Prince (1995)	19	3D Gd	100	93
De Cobelli (1996)	50	3D PC	94	94
Silverman (1996)	37	Cine PC	100	93
de Haan (1996)	38	3D PC	93	95
Snidow (1996)	47	3D Gd	100	89
Holland (1996)	63	3D Gd	100	100
Steffens (1997)	50	3D Gd	96	95
Rieumont (1997)	30	3D Gd	100	71
De Cobelii (1997)	55	3D Gd	100	97
Bakker (1998)	50	3D Gd	97	92
Hany (1998)	103	3D Gd	93	90
Thornton (1999)	62	3D Gd	88	98
Schoenberg (1999)	26	3D Gd	94-100	96-100
Thornton (1999)	42	3D Gd	100	98
Miller (1999)	32	3D PC	93	81
Cambria (1999)	25	3D Gd + PC	97	100
Ghantous (1999)	12	3D Gd	—	100
Gilfeather (1999)	54	3D Gd		SD: MRA = 6.9%, Angio = 7.5%; MRA overestimates = 21%; MRA underestimates = 14%
Westenberg (1999)	17	3D PC-PSL		Correlation coef = 0.90
Nelson (1999)	5	3D TOF	71	95
Lee (2000)	35	Cine PC	50	78
		+ ACE	67	84
Marchand (2000)		3D Gd	88-100	71-100
Shetty (2000)	51	3D Gd	96	92
Winterer (2000)	23	3D Gd	100	98
Weishaupt (2000)	20	blood pool 3D	82	98
Bongers (2000)	43	3D Gd	100	94
		Captopril renogram	85	71
Volk (2000)	40	Time-resolved 3D Gd	93	83
Oberholzer (2000)	23	3D Gd at 1 T	96	97
Korst (2000)	38	3D Gd	100	85
De Corbelli (2000)	45	3D Gd	94	93
		Doppler US	71	93
Mittal (2001)	26	3D Gd	96	93
Voiculescu (2001)	36	3D Gd	96	86
Qanadli (2001)	41	3D Gd	97	64
		Doppler + captopril	69	82
		Captopril scintigraphy	41	82
Hood (2002)	21	3D Gd	100	74
Schoenberg (2002)	23	3D Gd + cine PC		97% agreement with DSA
Krause (2002)	71	Time-resolved MRA	75	95.7
Willmann (2003)	46	3D Gd	92-93	99-100
Vasbinder (2004)	356	3D Gd	62	84
Patel (2005)	34	3D Gd	87	69
Eklöf (2006)	58	3D Gd	93	91
Maki (2007)	20	SSFP	100	85
Rountas (2007)	58	3D Gd	90	94
Kittner (2007)	273	3D Gd	76-91	59-75
McGregor (2008)	145	3D Gd		
Stacul (2008)	26	3D Gd	77	69
Transplant Renal MRA				
Gedroyc (1992)	50	TOF	83	97
Smith (1993)	34	3D TOF	100	95
Johnson (1997)	11	3D Gd	67	88
		3D PC	60	76
		2D TOF	47	81
		3D Gd + PC	100	100
Luk (1999)	9	3D Gd	?	100
Ferreiros (1999)	24	3D Gd	100	98
Jain (2005)	29	3D Gd	100	96
Stecco (2007)	49	0.5-T 3D Gd	75	75

2D, two-dimensional; 3D, three-dimensional; ACE, angiotensin-converting enzyme; PC, phase contrast MRI imaging; SD, standard deviation; SSFP, steady-state free precession imaging; TOF, time of flight mass spectrometry.
*Full study references are available online at expertconsult.com.

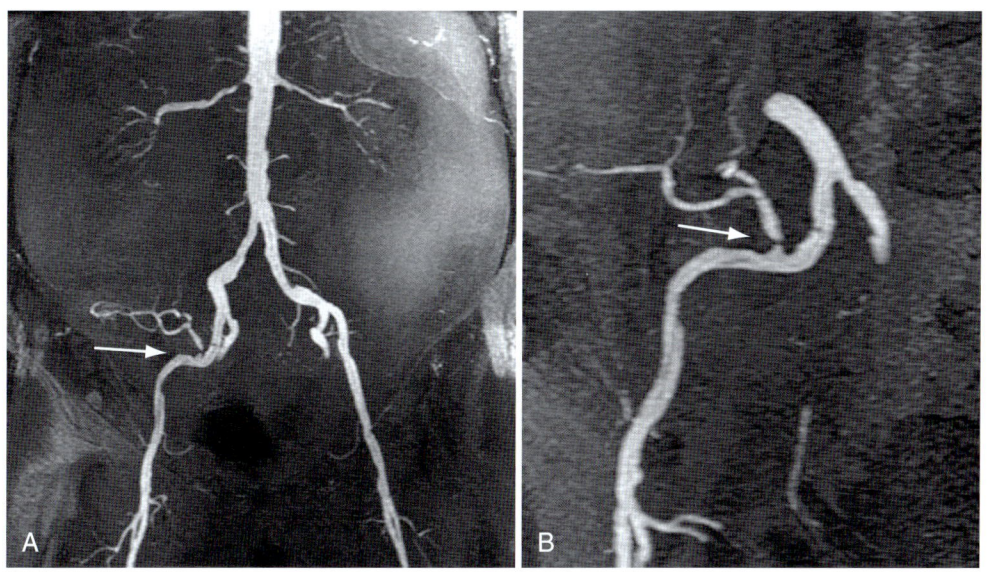

FIGURE 112-4 Severe stenosis at transplant artery end-to-side anastomosis onto external iliac artery. **A,** Anteroposterior (AP) MIP of entire imaging volume. **B,** Oblique subvolume MIP oriented for optimal display of transplant renal artery.

The limit of MRA resolution for stenosis is typically at the level of the segmental first-order branch vessels. DSA is superior in its ability to detect segmental artery stenosis. Furthermore, intrarenal arteries are typically obscured by enhancement of the renal parenchyma with MRA. However, because MRA is an anatomic image that directly displays the vessels, similar to digital subtraction angiography (DSA), it offers many advantages over the detection of secondary findings of TRAS with Doppler ultrasound (US). For example, kinked or tortuous arteries that are technically challenging or impossible with Doppler US can be evaluated with the volumetric data sets of MRA. Iliac artery stenosis proximal to the transplant artery anastomosis is an uncommon cause of TRAS (pseudo-TRAS) that is much more easily identified with MRA (Fig. 112-5). Because of the shortage of grafts, en bloc transplantation of two kidneys of limited function such as from the cadavers of older patients or two small kidneys from pediatric cadavers, has gained acceptance (see Fig. 112-1C). In these cases, not only is the anatomy more complicated, but secondary findings of velocity or ratios of velocities have not been proven to be reliable indicators of TRAS. Direct anatomic imaging also allows for the detection of other pathologies that may be the cause of patient symptoms, such as infarctions, artery or vein thrombosis, urinary collecting system complications, or a perinephric collection. It can also be helpful for preoperative planning, even when DSA is already indicated.

The major limitation of MRA in the detection of TRAS is metal artifact from surgical clips. This can often be identified as a focus of complete signal dropout with an adjacent bright focus of displaced signal. In cases of suspected recurrence in treated stenoses, the presence of an endovascular stent usually limits the ability to make the diagnosis with MRA because of artifact. MRA is effective only when the stented segment of the artery is shown to be widely patent, because loss of signal caused by artifact cannot be discriminated from a recurrent stenosis.

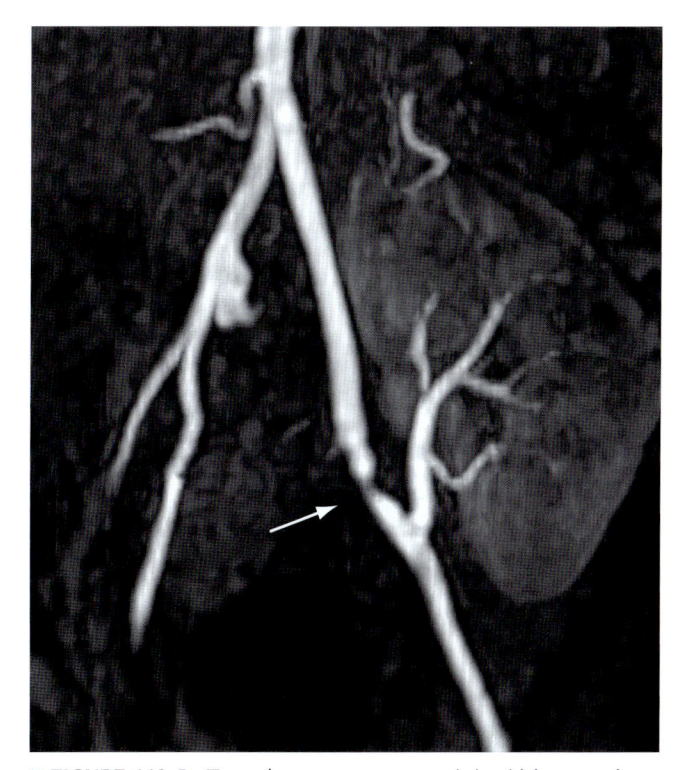

FIGURE 112-5 Transplant artery anastomosis is widely patent but there is external iliac artery anastomosis proximal to the transplant artery (*arrow*). This is a site where the artery was injured from a clamp during transplantation surgery.

A recent concern in the use of Gd-enhanced MRI is NSF. This is very rare, but is a debilitating and largely untreatable disease thought to be related to the deposition of gadolinium in the skin after dissociation from the chelated form used in MRI contrast agents. The Gd dose should be kept at 0.1 mmol/kg or less to minimize the risk of NSF in case the GFR is low (see earlier). Other risks for NSF include a concomitant inflammatory state, such as recent surgery or deep venous thrombosis, and the elevated phosphate levels of patients in renal failure. Although the large majority of cases have been reported in patients on dialysis, a GFR less than 30 mL/min is a relative contraindication for the administration of Gd chelate contrast agents. When the need to determine the diagnosis or exclusion of TRAS outweighs the risk of NSF, steps should be taken to ensure that the patient is well hydrated, that acute inflammatory states have passed before MRA is performed, that low-dose or noncontrast protocols are attempted first and, most importantly, that patients on dialysis are dialyzed immediately after receiving gadolinium (within 24 hours).

Nuclear Medicine and Positron Emission Tomography

Although a decline in renal function after the administration of an ACE inhibitor can indicate TRAS, an ACE inhibitor challenge during scintigraphy is relatively contraindicated because of reports of ACE inhibitor–induced acute renal failure, in some cases irreversible. Additionally, the specificity is less than in US, MRA, and DSA.[9]

Angiography

Catheter angiography with iodinated contrast is the gold standard for the diagnosis of transplant renal artery stenosis. It offers the highest resolution available for visualizing stenoses, including stenoses in branch renal arteries. Additionally, hemodynamic significance can be directly tested after crossing a stenosis with a catheter. A pressure gradient across a focal or a segmental stenosis more than either 10% or 10 mm Hg indicates hemodynamic significance. As an invasive test, however, catheter angiography has the highest associated risk, with mild expected morbidity and occasional severe unexpected morbidity. It is also the most expensive.

Differential Diagnosis

Failure of a renal transplant can also result from causes such as transplant rejection, toxicity from medications (especially cyclosporine), dehydration, or deteriorating cardiac function.

Treatment Options

Medical Treatment

In general, medical management of renal transplantation focuses on ensuring that there is no rejection and on managing hypertension.

Surgical and Interventional Management

The treatment of choice is percutaneous transluminal angioplasty (PTA), with stenting reserved for PTA failures. A postangioplasty pressure measurement is used to document successful repair of a stenosis. Placement of a metallic stent after angioplasty reduces the risk of restenosis.[10] In one retrospective study, 94% of PTAs were technically successful and 82% were clinically successful, with a significant reduction in mean diastolic pressure and significant improvement in renal function.[11]

Reporting: Information for the Referring Physician

MRA reports need to indicate kidney size, infarcts, perinephric collections, hydronephrosis, transplant artery anastomosis type, number and any stenosis, with grading of stenosis as mild, moderate, or severe, iliac arteries, transplant renal vein and iliac vein, magnitude transplant enhancement, excretion of gadolinium into the collecting system, status of native kidneys, and assessment for any native renal masses.

> **KEY POINTS**
> - Transplant renal artery stenosis is suspected with hypertension and/or declining renal function and is important to determine for maximizing transplant life.
> - MRA is the technique of choice for assessing renal and pancreas transplant arteries and veins.
> - Always review source images in addition to MIPs and volume renderings.

Arteriovenous Fistula and Pseudoaneurysm

Arteriovenous fistula (AVF) is an abnormal communication between an artery and vein. In the setting of renal transplantation, the vast majority of AVF are intrarenal, occurring between small, parenchymal vessels and are an acute complication of needle passage during core biopsy. Because of the crucial clinical value of biopsy results when there is a decline in renal transplant function, this is considered an acceptable risk. Pseudoaneurysms (PSAs) are saclike communications within an artery. PSA involving renal transplants are also almost exclusively caused by small vessel injury during biopsy. Although rare, AVFs and PSAs involving the main renal vessels, iliac vessels, and between transplant vessels and nearby pelvic vessels can occur and, as elsewhere in the body, are usually the result of complications of surgery, injury, or infection.

Prevalence and Epidemiology

AVFs are common, occurring in approximately 17% of biopsies in a prospective trial. Of these, 50% will spontaneously occlude within 48 hours and another 25% within 4 weeks.[12] The remaining 25% may persist for at least 1 year and often longer. Postbiopsy PSAs have an incidence of approximately 5% and are found in the vicinity of AVFs in most cases.

Etiology and Pathophysiology

Although no large trial has been undertaken, the risks for the development of AVFs and PSAs are thought to be hypertension, renal medullary disease, multiple needle passes, and deep or central biopsies.[13] Deep or central biopsies (i.e., more than 1 to 2 cm from the surface of the kidney), are probably more likely to injure larger vessels,

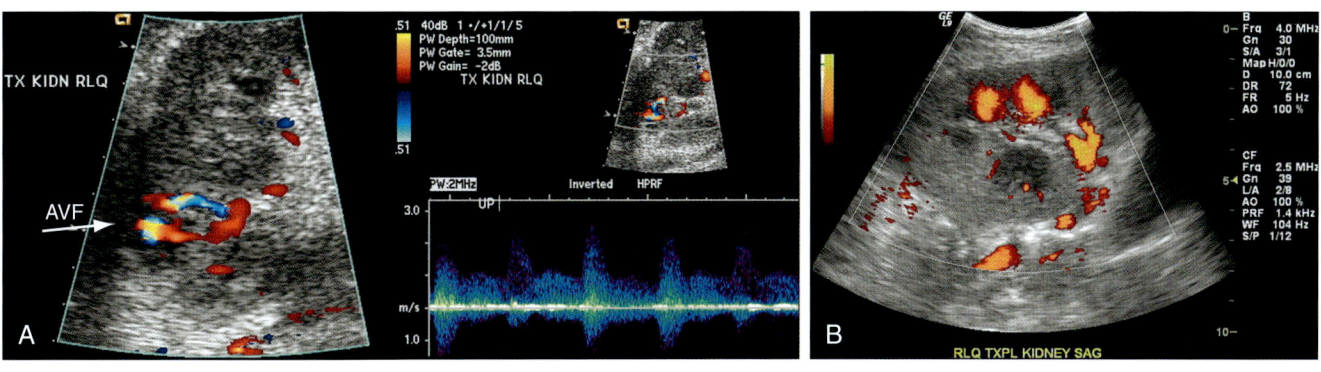

FIGURE 112-6 **A,** Ultrasound shows an AVF (*arrow*) following renal biopsy. Note the spectral broadening from the high velocity flow. **B,** Doppler ultrasound in another patient with AVF following renal biopsy.

leading to larger, higher flow AVFs, which are more likely to be clinically significant.

Manifestations of Disease

Clinical Presentation

Most AVFs and PSAs are clinically irrelevant. Clinically significant AVFs are usually those that do not spontaneously occlude and that often enlarge over time. Symptoms related to postbiopsy AFVs are most commonly hemorrhage, in the form of macroscopic hematuria, and hypertension. A decline in renal function can be seen and is thought to be caused by localized ischemia in the parenchyma surrounding the fistula from a vascular steal phenomenon, whereby renal blood is preferentially diverted or shunted from the renal parenchyma. Enlarging AVFs or PSAs are at risk for rupture. AVFs with high-flow shunting can impair cardiac function.

Imaging Indications and Algorithm

Ultrasound guidance during biopsy of renal transplants is the standard of care. At the conclusion of the needle passes, an investigation for AVF should be performed while the ultrasound probe is in position. Whereas a small amount of hematuria after biopsy is expected, persistent hematuria, flank pain, or other symptoms usually prompts ultrasound investigation for AVF. The decision to follow up to ensure resolution of the AVF is made on clinical grounds and can also be done with ultrasound. Contrast-enhanced three-dimensional MRA is useful for complicated cases for which direct anatomic imaging of an AVF or PSA is needed, such as for interventional or surgical planning. Contrast-enhanced three-dimensional MRA is also used to investigate rare nonintrarenal AVF or PSA. Catheter angiography is usually performed only in the setting of treatment procedures.

Imaging Technique and Findings

Ultrasound

Color-flow Doppler and point spectral Doppler imaging are the mainstays of diagnosing AVF and PSA with ultrasound. Although real-time ultrasound may show an anechoic focus corresponding to an enlarged vein or a PSA sac, this is usually only the case with large or extrarenal lesions. The most common finding is a focal area of increased color saturation caused by tissue vibration around the AVF.[14] Once this area has been localized, spectral Doppler investigation of the feeding artery usually shows increased velocity, with increased diastolic flow and spectral broadening (Fig. 112-6). The draining vein almost always shows increased pulsatility because of arterialization, but this finding by itself can be seen in other problems, such as right heart failure. The arterial and venous spectral findings should be compared with branch vessels in other segments of the transplant kidney to increase specificity. PSAs appear as an area of swirling, turbulent flow on color Doppler. There is biphasic to and fro flow through the neck of the cavity on spectral Doppler.

Magnetic Resonance Angiography

Contrast-enhanced three-dimensional MRA can demonstrate an AVF or PSA anatomically. The hallmark of an AVF is an early draining vein on the arterial phase of imaging. With the use and manipulation of MIPs, the actual fistulous connection can often be visualized. Similarly, a PSA can be demonstrated, including the size and dimensions of the neck and any thrombosed portions of the lesion (Fig. 112-7). Time-resolved three-dimensional MRA provides multiple sequential data sets that can provide visualization of early arterial filling of these vascular lesions.

Angiography

Catheter angiography using digital subtraction can image AVFs or PSAs anatomically and is performed during treatment as described below.

Treatment Options

Most AVFs and PSAs spontaneously resolve or are of no clinical consequence. In the subset requiring therapy, AVFs and PSAs are usually treated with microcoil embolization after superselective catheter placement to allow for maximal sparing of the renal parenchyma (Fig. 112-8). Treatment with coil embolization has been recommended if bleeding, hematuria, or continued enlargement persists after 72 hours, if an AVF has not resolved after 30 days to prevent loss of transplant function, or if there are significant cardiovascular effects.

In a retrospective study of short- and long-term outcomes, technical relief (imaging findings of PSA or AVF) and symptomatic relief were achieved in 12 of 12 patients with superselective coil embolization.[13] Estimated loss of renal parenchyma was less than 10% for nine patients and less than 20% for three patients. Chronic ischemia caused by AVF, leading to loss of most function, is treated with transplant nephrectomy.

> **KEY POINTS**
> - AVFs are relatively common but most are clinically irrelevant and spontaneously occlude.
> - Ultrasound can be used to diagnose AVFs and PSAs and follow them as necessary.
> - MRA is useful for complicated cases or when more anatomic information is required, such as treatment planning.
> - Coil embolization is used in clinically significant cases and is almost always effective.

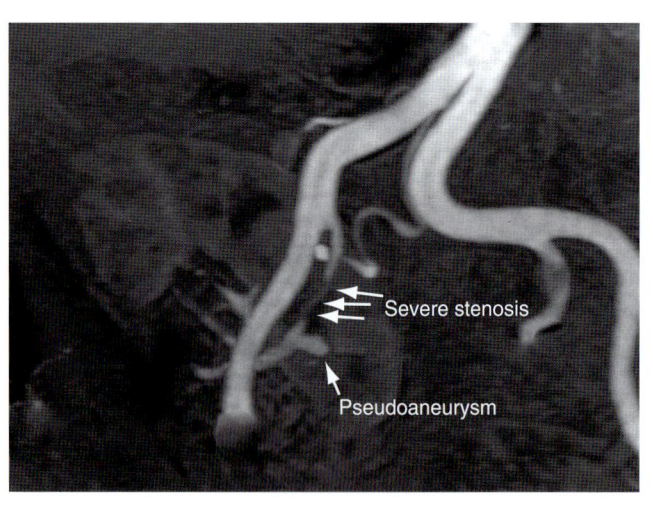

FIGURE 112-7 Three-dimensional Gd MRA shows a severe stenosis at the end-to-end renal transplant anastomosis to right internal iliac artery. Note also a small pseudoaneurysm (*bottom arrow*) just distal to the anastomotic stenosis (*top arrows*).

Transplant Renal Artery and Vein Thrombosis

Primary renal artery or venous thrombosis is a known complication of transplantation. Thrombosis usually results in graft loss, except in rare cases when it is treated with timely emergent thrombectomy.[15]

Prevalence and Epidemiology

Renal graft thrombosis is usually seen in the postoperative period, occurring within 2 days in 62% of cases and within 10 days in 90% of cases in a survey of 134 consecutive cases.[16] The overall incidence is 0.2% to 3.5% for arterial thrombosis and 0.3% to 3% for venous thrombosis.[17]

Etiology and Pathophysiology

Renal graft thrombosis is usually caused by technical problems during surgery, such as vascular kinking, torsion, or intimal dissection. Additionally, renal vein thrombosis may be caused by compression, such as by postoperative peritransplant fluid collections. Other risks for arterial or venous thrombosis include hypotension, hypovolemia, and a hypercoagulable state.

Manifestations of Disease

Clinical Presentation

Graft thrombosis usually presents with sudden anuria. Venous thrombosis is typically associated with swelling and tenderness over the graft, whereas arterial thrombosis is generally painless. Arterial thrombosis is rapidly followed by venous thrombosis and infarction of the transplanted kidney.

Imaging Indications and Algorithm

Cases of suspected graft thrombosis are usually first evaluated with ultrasound, which can be done rapidly, often in the recovery area. MRI with MRA is more sensitive and

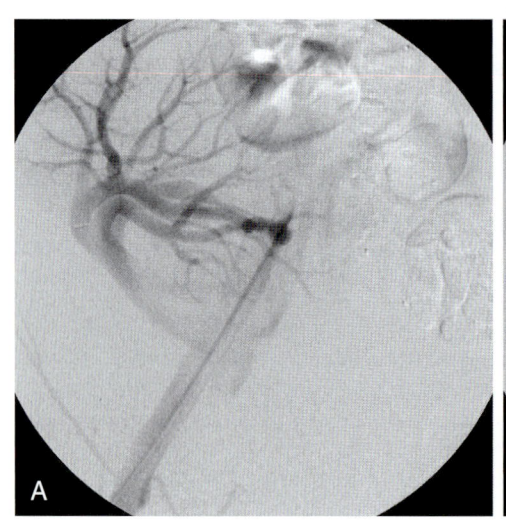

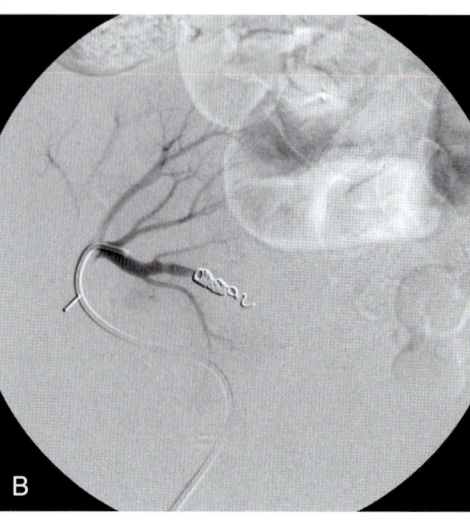

FIGURE 112-8 Coil embolization of an arteriovenous fistula following transplant biopsy. **A,** Pre-embolization DSA shows a fistula and early draining vein. **B,** Postembolization the coils are visible but the fistula is obliterated.

specific for differentiating graft thrombosis from rejection. It is essential to avoid delays in treatment. But there are cases of successfully treated thrombosis after the diagnosis was made on MRI following a nondiagnostic ultrasound.[15]

Imaging Techniques and Findings

Ultrasound

Graft artery thrombosis is diagnosed by an absence of flow in the main artery and vein. Graft vein thrombosis shows echogenic thrombus in the occluded or partially flowing vein. A swollen hypoechoic kidney is usually an associated finding in venous thrombosis. An elevated arterial resistive index is usually also seen because of the lack of collateral outflow in transplant kidneys, but this is nonspecific, because it is also seen in rejection or acute tubular necrosis. Reversal of diastolic arterial flow on spectral Doppler, once thought to be diagnostic of venous thrombosis, is also nonspecific.

Magnetic Resonance Angiography

Renal artery thrombosis manifests as nonfilling or nonvisualization of the artery in the arterial phase of contrast-enhanced (CE) MRA, followed by global nonperfusion of the graft in the parenchymal or venous phases. Segmental infarctions caused by segmental artery thrombosis can also be exquisitely demonstrated on MRA. The finding of loss of corticomedullary differentiation on T1-weighted images has also been described, but is a nonspecific finding that is also seen in rejection and cyclosporine toxicity, for which biopsy remains necessary for definitive diagnosis.

A lack of filling of the vein on delayed CE-MRA phases, sometimes with a thin rim of enhancement probably representing the wall of the vein, is diagnostic of renal vein thrombosis. This can be more difficult to demonstrate as the gadolinium bolus is diluted. Careful localizing of the vessels prior to contrast administration, using a bright blood imaging technique, notably steady-state free precession (SSFP) imaging, is helpful to ensure inclusion of vascular structures in the field of view. There may be a loss of the normal flow void on T2-weighted images. A secondary finding of renal vein thrombosis is a delayed and persistent nephrogram. Diagnosing more proximate thrombosis in the iliac vein or inferior vena cava is another advantage of CE-MRA.

Classic Signs

Reversal of diastolic flow on spectral Doppler imaging, once thought to be diagnostic of renal vein thrombosis, is now known to be nonspecific.

Treatment Options

Medical Management

Cases of segmental thrombosis or apparent partial thrombosis have been successfully treated with anticoagulation.

Surgical and Interventional Management

If performed in time, surgical thrombectomy or catheter-directed thrombectomy can salvage a kidney transplant. However, in most cases, the graft is infarcted, requiring surgical transplantectomy.

> **KEY POINTS**
> - Renal artery or vein thrombosis occurs in up to 6% of cases, usually in the first 10 days.
> - Most cases lead to graft loss because of complete infarction, but salvage with emergent thrombectomy is possible.
> - Ultrasound imaging is usually the first-line modality because it can be performed rapidly and portably. However, MRI with MRA is more sensitive and specific.

Vascular Evaluation of Living Renal Donors

The increase in living donors providing kidneys for transplantation makes careful screening of these otherwise healthy individuals important. Physicians must first ensure that the donor will be left with a fully functional kidney and that the donated kidney does not harbor occult disease. Second, surgeons would like to know the vascular anatomy prior to the harvesting procedure, especially given the high rate of renal vasculature variability. Increasing use of laparoscopic techniques for harvesting, with their more limited view, makes prior anatomic imaging even more important. When both kidneys have a single artery and vein, transplant surgeons prefer to use the left kidney because of its longer renal vein. However, the right kidney is preferred if it has an overall simpler vasculature allowing simpler anastomoses, which minimizes ischemia time.

Prevalence and Epidemiology

The overall prevalence of multiple renal vessels has been reported to be from 30% to 49% of patients, with bilaterally occurring multiple vessels in 17%.[18,19]

Manifestations of Disease

Imaging Indications and Algorithm

Previously, work-up of living renal donors included DSA for mapping of the vasculature prior to harvesting. More recently, noninvasive modalities have become accurate enough to make this assessment. Furthermore, other aspects of the work-up, such as screening for parenchymal or urothelial disease, can be accomplished with a single test. Multidetector CT angiography and CE-MRA have both been shown to be highly sensitive for the detection of main renal arteries and veins, with 100% sensitivity on CT angiography (CTA) and 97% to 100% sensitivity on MRA. CTA has been more sensitive in delineating small accessory renal vessels, such as 1- to 2-mm arteries, with a sensitivity of 100% compared with 20% to 66% for MRA on older MR scanners.[20,21] More recently, state of the art MR scanners using parallel imaging for higher resolution and fluoroscopic triggering to ensure accurate bolus timing have shown comparable accuracy to CTA.[22] CTA, however, is more sensitive to calculi and urothelial lesions. This must be weighed against the much smaller risks of Gd chelate contrast agent use for CE-MRA versus the risks associated with iodinated contrast use and ionizing radiation exposure associated with CTA.

Imaging Techniques and Findings
Computed Tomography

Multidetector CT with a rapid contrast bolus and imaging in arterial, parenchymal, and excretory phases provides excellent delineation of the renal vasculature, including accessory vessels, with almost 100% sensitivity. Thin slice reformations are used to allow for improved three-dimensional postprocessing. MIP is the most superior and time-efficient format to evaluate the vasculature, but the source data should be reviewed because it is the most accurate for small accessory vessels. Renal vein variants, such as retroaortic or circumaortic veins, and early arterial branching (within 2 cm of the origin of the artery) should be noted because they will change the surgical approach. A precontrast set of images is usually obtained to exclude occult renal calculi, a relative contraindication to donation. The parenchyma should be evaluated for masses, cysts, or scarring. Imaging during the excretory phase is usually performed throughout the entire collecting system to screen for occult urothelial lesions or variants. For example, completely duplicated ureters will usually lead to harvesting of the contralateral kidney but partially duplicated ureters may not.

Magnetic Resonance Angiography

Dynamic CE-MRA is almost as accurate as CTA for detection of the main renal vessels and their variations and is comparable for detection of accessory arteries larger than 1 to 2 mm. As with CTA, evaluation of MIPs and source images should be performed. An excretory phase of imaging should be performed (MR urography) and can detect ureteral duplications. MRI is not sensitive to small urothelial lesions, unlike CT urography; however, these lesions are rare in healthy renal donors. The sensitivity of MRI for urothelial lesions can be improved by injecting furosemide (e.g., 10 mg dose) after the Gd chelate contrast agent and performing a T1-weighted three-dimensional spoiled gradient-recalled echo (SPGR) sequence to image the distended collecting system. MRI is not sensitive to small renal calculi. The advantage of MRA is the relative safety of Gd chelate contrast and its lack of associated ionizing radiation exposure, which a similar multiphase CT urogram would require. Thus, MRA may be the modality of choice in patients with a contraindication to iodinated contrast or younger patients who have greater long-term risk of malignancy related to lifetime cumulative ionizing radiation exposure.

Angiography

DSA is more sensitive to fibromuscular dysplasia (FMD) than CTA or MRA, specifically mild disease in the proximal arterial segment and mild or moderate disease in first-order branches. For the general population, the risk of rendering the donor to a single kidney afflicted with FMD is thought to be less than the risks associated with an invasive procedure. DSA could be considered if the potential donor is at greater than average risk for FMD.

Reporting Information for the Referring Physician

Evaluation of renal donors should include the following: number of main renal arteries and veins; presence of accessory or polar vessels; presence of early branching arteries less than 2 cm from the origin; venous variants including retroaortic veins, circumaortic veins, or large draining gonadal or lumbar veins; vascular pathology such as stenosis, FMD, or aortic aneurysm; parenchymal lesions; calculi; and urothelial variants or lesions. Also, report any parenchymal abnormalities including scarring, cysts, or tumors, as well as the length of each kidney.

> **KEY POINTS**
> - CTA is the most accurate noninvasive modality for evaluating the potential renal donor vasculature.
> - Arterial and venous variations are common, will affect the surgical approach to harvesting the kidney, and should be evaluated with both three-dimensional postprocessed and source images.
> - MRA is a relatively safer alternative to CTA, but is less sensitive for certain factors that may affect donor evaluation or surgical approach, such as accessory arteries smaller than 1 to 2 mm, calculi, and small urothelial lesions.

VASCULAR EVALUATION OF PANCREAS TRANSPLANT RECIPIENTS

Pancreas transplantation is a definitive treatment for type 1 diabetes mellitus and is usually performed along with renal transplantation for end-stage renal disease. Depending on underlying causes and available donor organs, pancreas transplantation is divided into simultaneous pancreas and kidney transplantation (SPK), pancreas after kidney transplantation (PAK), and pancreas transplantation alone (PTA).

Prevalence and Epidemiology

SPK is the most common, accounting for approximately 85% of cases, and PAK and PTA account for approximately

10% and 5% of cases, respectively.[23] Improving techniques and therapies have led to increasing viability of pancreas transplants with half-lives of 143, 77, and 90 months for the pancreas portion of SPK, PAK, and PTA transplantations, respectively, performed in 1998 and 1999.

Etiology and Pathophysiology

Pancreas transplantation can be performed with systemic bladder drainage or portal-enteric drainage, with the latter preferred. Systemic bladder drainage uses donor portal vein segment drainage into the external or common iliac vein with a segment of the duodenum, including the ampulla of Vater, anastomosed to the bladder. Portal-enteric drainage uses anastomosis to the portal system, usually via the superior mesenteric vein and drainage to the small intestine, sometimes via a roux-en-Y limb. Because of the dual arterial supply of the pancreas, anastomosis of blind-ending segments of the splenic and superior mesenteric artery to the external or common iliac artery is accomplished via a donor Y graft. The Y graft is formed from the donor common iliac bifurcation into the internal and external iliac arteries.

Vascular complications are more common in pancreatic transplants than in any other solid organ and are the most common cause of early failure.[24] Venous thrombosis is the most common vascular dysfunction. Other vascular complications include arterial thrombosis, pseudoaneurysm, arteriovenous fistula, and stenosis.

Manifestations of Disease

Clinical Presentation

Most vascular complications present within a few days of transplantation with an acutely elevated serum glucose level, sometimes accompanied with an elevated serum amylase level and abdominal pain. However, these findings are nonspecific and can be caused by other complications, such as rejection or graft pancreatitis.

Imaging Indications and Algorithm

As in renal transplantation, ultrasound is the initial diagnostic modality of choice because of speed and portability. CT is useful to visualize peritransplant collections, but the iodinated contrast needed to visualize the vasculature is relatively contraindicated when there is a renal transplant present. MRI-MRA is the modality of choice for definitive diagnosis because it allows for excellent evaluation of the vasculature and can demonstrate infarction versus other possible causes of graft dysfunction, including hydronephrosis and peritransplant collections.

Imaging Techniques and Findings

Ultrasound

Color and spectral Doppler ultrasound can usually identify the iliac vessels, donor Y graft, and main graft vessels when the pancreas transplant is visualized.[25] However, because of its intraperitoneal location, the graft may be obscured by bowel. As in renal transplants, power Doppler is useful to identify vessels, but diagnosis of venous or arterial thrombosis requires demonstration of a lack of flow on spectral Doppler. A lack of venous flow in combination with reversed or severely dampened diastolic arterial flow has been shown to be highly accurate for venous thrombosis.[26] Similarly, arteriovenous fistulas and pseudoaneurysms appear on color Doppler as tissue vibration surrounding a high-flow artery and draining vein or swirling flow within a saccular outpouching from the artery, respectively, but should be confirmed with typical spectral Doppler waveforms.

Computed Tomography

CT with iodinated contrast can demonstrate vascular complications of pancreatic transplantation but should be avoided when a transplanted kidney is also present.

Magnetic Resonance Angiography

Because of the complex vascular anatomy, CE-MRA, with three-dimensional volumetric data sets, is the modality of choice to evaluate the vascular complications of pancreas transplantation. In a recent study using state of the art high-resolution three-dimensional CE-MRA, all surgically or angiographically proven vascular complications, including venous and arterial thrombosis, arteriovenous fistula, pseudoaneurysm, and stenoses, were diagnosed.[27] Occasional false-positives, especially overgrading stenoses, still occur. Direct anatomic visualization of lesions, as in renal transplants, is accomplished with manipulation of MIPs and correlation with the source images. All main vessels and 85% of first-order branches can be visualized. Additional MRI sequences, including parenchymal enhancement, can be used to rule out other causes of graft dysfunction, such as enzymatic leak or peritransplant collections and to assess for possible infarction or infection of the graft.

KEY POINTS

- Venous thrombosis is the most common vascular complication of pancreatic transplantation and usually occurs within the first week.
- Ultrasound can often visualize the graft and its vasculature quickly and portably.
- MRI-MRA is the modality of choice on which to base treatment decisions because of its high accuracy for visualizing the complex pancreas transplant anatomy and its facility for evaluating for other causes of graft dysfunction.

SUGGESTED READINGS

Bruno S, Giuseppe R, Ruggenenti P. Transplant renal artery stenosis. J Am Soc Nephrol 2004; 15:134-141.

Dobos N, Roberts DA, Insko EK, et al. Contrast-enhanced MR angiography for evaluation of vascular complications of the pancreatic transplant. Radiographics 2005; 25:687-695.

Hernandez D, Rufino M, Armas S, et al. Retrospective analysis of surgical complications following cadaveric kidney transplantation in the modern transplant era. Nephrol Dial Transplant 2006; 21:2908-2915.

Hussain SM, Kock MCJM, Ijzermans JNM, et al. MR imaging: a "one-stop shop" modality for preoperative evaluation of potential living kidney donors. Radiographics 2003; 23:505-520.

Kawamoto S, Montgomery RA, Lawler LP, et al. Multi-detector row CT evaluation of living renal donors prior to laparoscopic nephrectomy. Radiographics 2004; 24:453-466.

Nikolaidis P, Amin RS, Hwang CM, et al. Role of sonography in pancreatic transplantation. Radiographics 2003; 23:939-949.

REFERENCES

1. 2008 Annual Report of the U.S. Organ Procurement and Transplantation Network and the Scientific Registry of Transplant Recipients: Transplant Data 1998-2006. Rockville, Md, Health Resources and Services Administration, Healthcare Systems Bureau, Division of Transplantation, 2008.
2. Tarzamni MK, Argani H, Nurifar M, Nezami N. Vascular complication and Doppler ultrasonographic finding after renal transplantation. Transplant Proc 2007; 39:1096-1102.
3. Fernández-Nájera JE, Beltrán S, Aparicio M, et al. Transplant renal artery stenosis: association with acute vascular rejection. Transplant Proc 2006; 38:2404-2405.
4. Audard V, Matignon M, Hemery F, et al. Risk factors and long-term outcome of transplant renal artery stenosis in adult recipients after treatment by percutaneous transluminal angioplasty. Am J Transplant 2006; 6:95-99.
5. Baxter GM, Ireland H, Moss JG, et al. Colour Doppler ultrasound in renal transplant stenosis: which Doppler index? Clin Radiol 1995; 50:618-622.
6. Loubeyre P, Abidi H, Cahen R, Minh VAT. Transplanted renal artery: detection of stenosis with color Doppler US. Radiology 1997; 203:661-665.
7. Williams GJ, Macaskill P, Chan SF, et al. Comparative accuracy of renal duplex sonographic parameters in the diagnosis of renal artery stenosis: paired and unpaired analysis. 2007; AJR Am J Roentgenol 188:798-811.
8. Stafford Johnson DB, Lerner CA, Prince MR, et al. Gadolinium-enhanced magnetic resonance angiography of renal transplants. MRI 1997; 15:13-20.
9. Glicklich D, Tellis VA, Quinn T. Comparison of captopril scan and Doppler ultrasonography as screening tests for transplant renal artery stenosis. Transplantation 49: 217-219, 1990.
10. Da Silva RG, Lima VC, Amorim JE, et al. Angioplasty with stent is the preferred therapy for posttransplant renal artery stenosis. Transplant Proceed 34: 514-515, 2002.
11. Patel NH, Jindal RM, Wilkin T, et al. Renal arterial stenosis in renal allografts: retrospective study of predisposing factors and outcome after percutaneous transluminal angioplasty. Radiol 219: 663-667, 2001.
12. Brandenburg VM, Frank RD, Riehl J. Color-coded duplex sonography study of arteriovenous fistulae and pseudoaneurysms complicating renal allograft biopsy. Clin Nephrol 2002; 58:398-404,.
13. Loffroy R, Guiu B, Lambert A, et al. Management of post-biopsy renal allograft arteriovenous fistulas with selective arterial embolization: immediate and long-term outcomes. Clin Radiol 2008; 63:657-665.
14. Renowden SA, Blethyn J, Cochlin DL. Duplex and colour flow sonography in the diagnosis of post-biopsy arteriovenous fistulae in the transplant kidney. Clin Radiol 1992; 45:233-237,.
15. Kim HS, Fine DM, Atta MG. Catheter-directed thrombectomy and thrombolysis for acute renal vein thrombosis. J Vasc Interv Radiol 2006; 17:815-822,.
16. Penny MJ, Nankivell BJ, Disney APS, et al. Renal graft thrombosis, a survey of 134 consecutive cases. Transplant 1994; 58:565-569,.
17. Bakir N, Sluiter WJ, Ploeg RJ, et al. Primary renal graft thrombosis. Nephrol Dial Transplant 1996; 11:140-147,.
18. Geissing M, Kroencke TJ, Taupitz M, et al. Gadolinium-enhanced three-dimensional magnetic resonance angiography versus conventional digital subtraction angiography: which modality is superior in evaluating living kidney donors? Transplantation 2003; 76: 1000-1006.
19. Halpern EJ, Mitchell DG, Wechsler RJ, et al. Preoperative evaluation of living renal donors: comparison of CT angiography and MR angiography. Radiology 2000; 216:434-439,.
20. Kim T, Murakami T, Takahashi S, et al. Evaluation of renal arteries in living renal donors: comparison between MDCT angiography and gadolinium-enhanced 3D MR angiography. Radiat Med 2006; 24:617-624.
21. Bhatti AA, Chugtai A, Haslam P, et al. Prospective study comparing three-dimensional computed tomography and magnetic resonance imaging for evaluating the renal vascular anatomy in potential living renal donors. BJU Int 2005; 96:1105-1108.
22. Gluecker TM, Mayr M, Schwarz J, et al. Comparison of CT angiography with MR angiography in the preoperative assessment of living kidney donors. Transplantation 2008; 86:1249-1256.
23. Gruessner AC, Sutherland DEC. Long-term results after pancreas transplantation. Transplant Proceed 2007; 39:2323-2325.
24. Benedetti E, Sileri P, Gruessner AC, Cicalese L. Surgical complications of pancreas transplantation. In Hakim N, Stratta R, Gray D (eds). Pancreas and Islet Transplantation. New York, Oxford University Press, 2002, pp 155-165.
25. Snider JF, Hunter DW, Kuni CC, et al. Pancreatic transplantation: radiologic evaluation of vascular complications. Radiology 1991; 178:749-753.
26. Foshager MC, Hedlund LJ, Troppmann C, et al. Venous thrombosis of pancreatic transplants: diagnosis by duplex sonography. AJR Am J Roentgenol 1997; 169:1269-1273.
27. Hagspiel KD, Nandular K, Pruett TL, et al. Evaluation of vascular complications of pancreas transplantation with high-spatial-resolution contrast-enhanced MR angiography. Radiology 2007; 242:590-599.

PART
EIGHTEEN

The Lower Extremity Vessels

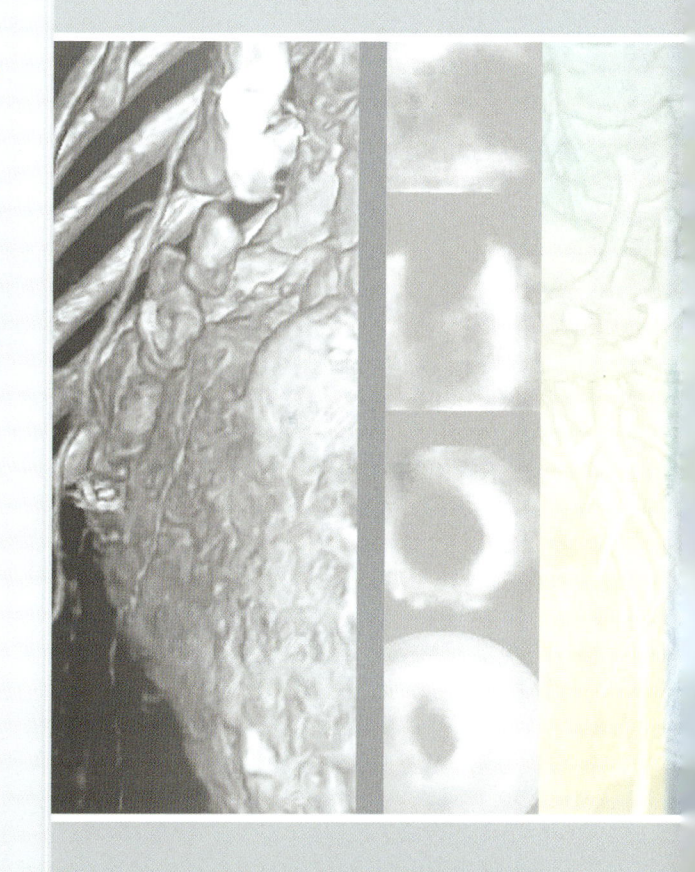

CHAPTER 113

Peripheral Artery Disease

Benjamin M. Jackson and Jeffrey P. Carpenter

Peripheral arterial disease, most often a result of atherosclerosis, occurs in approximately 10% of the adult population and affects more than 10 million people in the United States alone.[1] Most frequently, patients present with claudication. Less often, patients suffer from critical limb ischemia. Risk of illness or death from other cardiovascular causes in these patients with chronic limb ischemia is greatly increased, making peripheral arterial disease an important marker for atherosclerotic cardiovascular disease in general.[2]

Meanwhile, among the most common vascular surgical emergencies is acute lower extremity ischemia. Sudden-onset occlusion of any major artery is manifested with symptoms and signs that must be recognized and acted on to salvage the involved limb.

ACUTE LIMB ISCHEMIA

Definition

Acute limb ischemia occurs when a leg or foot suffers from inadequate blood flow to maintain vital metabolic functions. Both arterial embolism and arterial (or bypass graft) thrombosis commonly precipitate acute limb ischemia.

Prevalence and Epidemiology

The incidence of acute limb ischemia is approximately 1.7/10,000 per year.[3] Patients presenting with a pulseless extremity suffer amputation rates as high as 10% and mortality rates of 5% to 15%.[4,5] These patients are characteristically at high risk for perioperative complication and are medically fragile (Table 113-1).

Etiology and Pathophysiology

Limb ischemia can result acutely from a variety of causes (Table 113-2). Sudden-onset acute pain is indicative of an embolic event; a history of chronic pain or claudication before the acute ischemic episode is suggestive of a thrombotic etiology. Graft occlusions are slightly more common than thromboses of native arteries. Thrombotic occlusions are approximately six times more common than embolic events.

Native artery thrombosis occurs at sites of atherosclerotic lesions, where there is flow disturbance resulting in turbulence and a thrombogenic surface for platelet aggregation. Thrombosis causing complete occlusion can occur in even mildly stenotic atherosclerotic vessels. In cases of native artery occlusion without an underlying luminal lesion, consideration must be given to other causes of thrombosis, such as hypovolemia, hypercoagulable states including malignant neoplasms, and blood dyscrasias.

Bypass graft thrombosis has become the most frequent cause of acute lower extremity ischemia. Intimal hyperplasia and valvular hyperplasia are the most common causes of thrombosis in native conduit bypasses. In prosthetic grafts, acute thrombosis is most commonly due to kinking across joints or to the thrombogenicity of the graft material itself.[6]

Manifestations of Disease

Clinical Presentation

Patients commonly present within hours of the onset of pain. Lower extremity ischemia presents with six *p*'s—pain, pallor, paresthesias, paralysis, pulselessness, and poi-

TABLE 113-1 Incidence of Medical Comorbidities in Patients Presenting with Acute Limb Ischemia

Comorbidity	Incidence (%)			
	Rochester Trial (N = 114)	TOPAS-1 Trial (N = 213)	TOPAS-2 Trial (N = 544)	Total (N = 871)
Cerebrovascular disease	NR	15.4	11.5	11.6
Congestive heart failure	NR	15.5	12.5	13.3
Coronary artery disease	56.1	47.1	42.5	45.4
Diabetes mellitus	28.1	36.7	29.0	30.8
Hypercholesterolemia	31.6	29.6	23.5	26.0
Hypertension	63.2	60.9	69.6	60.3
Malignancy	NR	11.9	11.5	11.6
Tobacco history	51.8	79.3	77.5	74.6

NR, not reported; TOPAS, thrombolysis or peripheral arterial surgery.
From Ouriel K. Acute ischemia and its sequelae. In Rutherford RB (ed). Vascular Surgery, 5th ed. Philadelphia, WB Saunders, 2000.

TABLE 113-2 Causes of Acute Limb Ischemia

Embolism (often to an arterial bifurcation)
Thrombosis
    At site of preexisting atherosclerotic lesion
    Of a preexisting aneurysm
    In normal artery as a result of hypercoagulability
Bypass graft occlusion
    Anastomotic stenosis due to intimal hyperplasia

kilothermia. In general, limb ischemic symptoms and signs will be present at a level one joint below the acute occlusive phenomenon; for example, common femoral artery occlusion will result in foot and calf pain. Normal proximal and contralateral pulse examination findings are indicative of an embolic event in an otherwise normal vascular tree. In contrast, evidence of diffuse chronic atherosclerotic disease suggests a thrombotic etiology of the acute ischemia.

Muscle and nerve tissues are able to tolerate no more than 6 hours of profound ischemia. The patient will experience a variable sensory deficit. In extreme cases, the affected limb will be insensate to even penetration of a needle into the muscles of the foot or calf; use of a sterile 19-gauge needle may allow the clinician to objectively determine whether any sensation remains. Paralysis (motor deficit) is a poor prognostic sign indicating relatively profound ischemia. Deficits in dorsiflexion and plantar flexion of the foot, which are accomplished by the muscles of the leg, are indicative of more extensive ischemia and a more proximal occlusive arterial lesion than are weakness and paralysis of the intrinsic muscles of the foot.

Because of its acuity and thus the absence of adequate preformed collateral arteries, arterial embolization is the classic situation resulting in acute arterial occlusion and acute limb ischemia. The anatomic distribution of arterial embolism is depicted in Figure 113-1. The embolus most frequently lodges at an arterial bifurcation.

In the patient with bilateral lower extremity ischemia and absent femoral pulses, the most common clinical scenario is saddle embolus to the aortic bifurcation. The

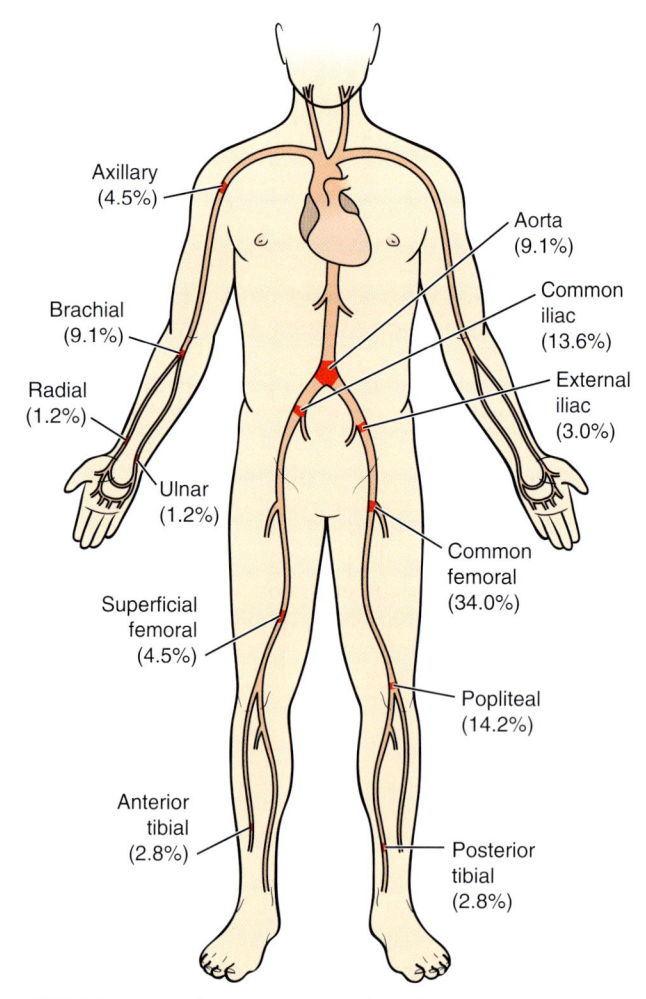

■ **FIGURE 113-1** The most common sites of arterial embolic occlusions.

patient will complain of sudden onset of bilateral buttock and lower extremity pain. Mottling of the lower extremities and lower abdomen, sometimes up to the umbilicus, will be evident on physical examination. The diagnosis in these patients is too frequently missed, probably because of the bilateral nature of the ischemic insult. Even in the

TABLE 113-3 Clinical Categorization of Acute Limb Ischemia

Category	Description and Prognosis	Findings		Doppler Signals	
		Sensory Loss	Muscle Weakness	Arterial	Venous
I Viable	Not immediately threatened	None	None	Audible	Audible
IIa Marginally threatened	Salvageable if promptly treated	Minimal (toes) or none	None	Inaudible	Audible
IIb Immediately threatened	Salvageable with immediate revascularization	More than toes, associated with rest pain	Mild, moderate	Inaudible	Audible
III Irreversible	Major tissue loss or permanent nerve damage inevitable	Profound, anesthetic	Profound, paralysis (rigor)	Inaudible	Inaudible

From Rutherford RB, Baer JD, Ernst C, et al. Recommended standards for reports dealing with lower extremity ischemia: revised version. J Vasc Surg 1997; 26:517.

setting of absent femoral pulses, patients are often evaluated for possible neurologic or neurosurgical problems, resulting in a delay of diagnosis and appropriate therapy. This disease can carry with it a poor prognosis, with a 27% mortality in one modern series.[7]

The most common site of clinically significant embolism in the lower extremity is the common femoral artery bifurcation.[8] Patients with common femoral artery embolism will experience foot and calf pain. Finally, an embolus to the popliteal artery will result in absent pedal pulses and an ischemic foot.

Approximately 90% of the time, arterial emboli arise in the heart.[9] Atrial fibrillation results in a dilated, noncontractile left atrial appendage, which predisposes to thrombus formation and—on spontaneous or therapeutic cardioversion—thromboembolism. Left ventricular thrombus may also form, for instance, adjacent to a noncontractile left ventricular segment after myocardial infarction, in a left ventricular aneurysm, or in the setting of dilated cardiomyopathy. Saddle emboli, which lodge at the aortic bifurcation and cause bilateral lower extremity ischemia, are most commonly the result of left ventricular thrombus. Thromboembolism from heart valves are less common today than in the past owing to the relative decrease in prevalence of rheumatic heart disease. Bacterial endocarditis can result in septic emboli that may cause both acute ischemia and infection of the distal vessel wall, which in turn results in mycotic aneurysm. Atheroemboli may arise from either the thoracic or the abdominal aorta. Finally, in some 5% of cases, the source of embolism is never identified.

Clinical Categorization of Acute Limb Ischemia

Since 1997, the Rutherford criteria have been used to grade the clinical severity of acute limb ischemia.[16] These grades, as summarized in Table 113-3, are indicative both of whether emergent surgical intervention is indicated and of whether the limb is salvageable. Most commonly, category I represents an acute occlusion in a chronically narrowed artery, with well-formed collaterals. Category II represents a limb that is salvageable with immediate therapy or intervention. In the case of irreversible ischemia, category III, the patient will present with profound vascular and neurologic deficits; the limb may be in a state of rigor mortis and will require amputation.

Before imaging studies, in patients with acute limb ischemia, laboratory studies are indicated. In particular, and in anticipation of imaging studies with use of nephrotoxic contrast agents, a serum creatinine concentration should be obtained. If a hypercoagulable state is suspected, a hypercoagulable profile should be sent before institution of any anticoagulation. An electrocardiogram will aid in the diagnosis of atrial fibrillation and will provide some information as to the patient's cardiac status. Assessment of the patient's cardiac risk for general anesthesia by the Goldman index or other scale may be useful.[11]

Doppler examination of the lower extremity may be useful, with attention to both arterial and venous signals. When arterial signals are present in the ankle, at either the dorsalis pedis or the posterior tibial artery, the ankle-brachial index should be measured. The absence of venous "hums" indicates more severe ischemia.

In limbs ischemic for 4 to 6 hours, significant reperfusion injury and swelling may occur. Swelling may result in increased compartment pressures, typically presenting earliest in the anterior compartment of the leg, which has both a significant mass of slow-twitch red muscle fibers and a strong encasing fascial envelope. The contents of the anterior compartment include the deep peroneal nerve, the tibialis anterior muscle, and the anterior tibial artery; compartment syndrome with accompanying tissue necrosis in this distribution classically results in footdrop.

Whereas some surgeons will elect to observe a transiently ischemic limb for signs of compartment syndrome postoperatively, in the setting of more than 6 hours of profound ischemia, many perform four-compartment fasciotomies prophylactically at the time of revascularization. If one elects to observe the patient's leg, any increased pain, especially with passive plantar flexion of the foot, or loss of sensation in the first web space of the foot (sensory distribution of the deep peroneal nerve) should prompt reevaluation. Compartment pressures may be measured by a Stryker needle (Stryker Instruments, Kalamazoo, MI) or other device. Compartment pressure of greater than 30 mm Hg can result in tissue ischemia and necrosis. Patients demonstrating hypotension or shock, those requiring pressors, those with absent flow through the popliteal artery at presentation, and younger patients with greater muscle mass and fewer arterial collaterals are

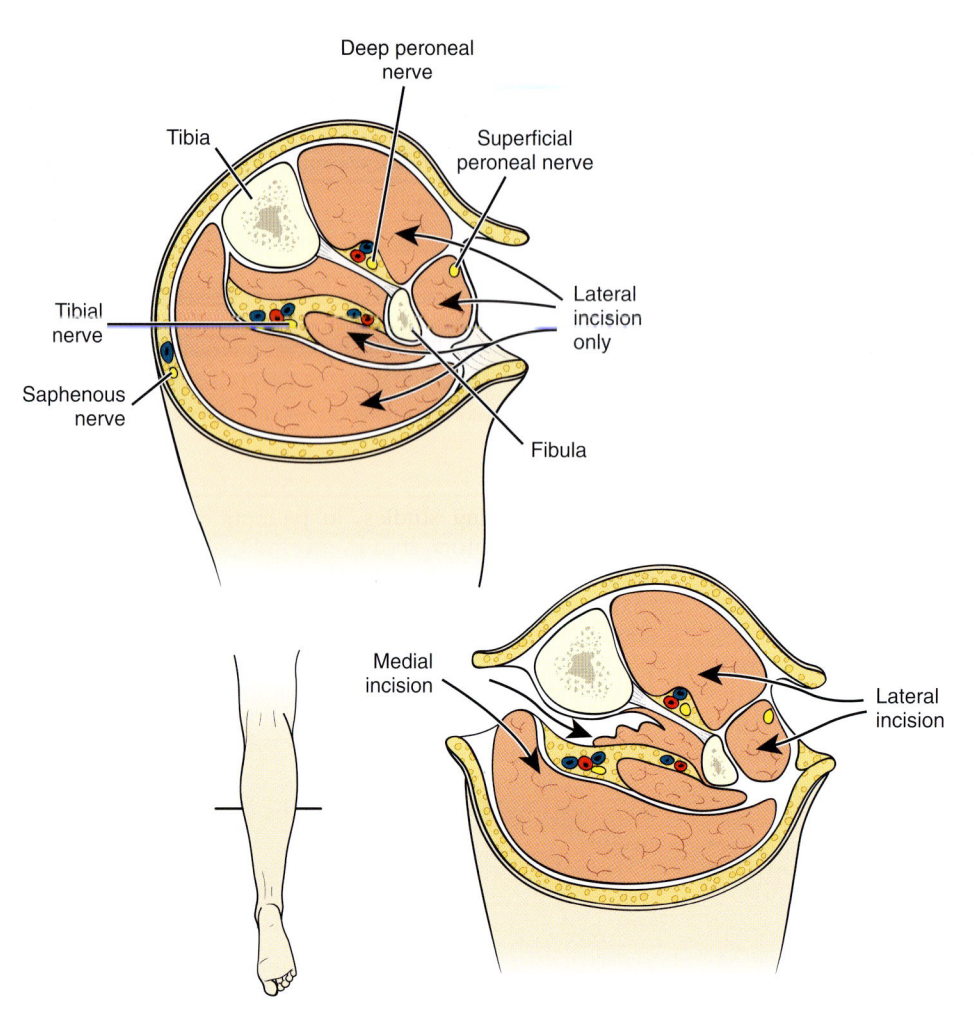

FIGURE 113-2 Four-compartment fasciotomy of the leg is usually performed through both medial and lateral incisions, but it can be performed through a lateral incision only. *(From Velmahos GC, Toutouzas KG. Vascular trauma and compartment syndromes. Surg Clin North Am 2002; 88:1.)*

at increased risk for development of compartment syndrome. Four-compartment fasciotomy is usually performed through both a medial and a lateral incision (Fig. 113-2). The incisions are left open for subsequent delayed primary closure or skin grafting.

Rhabdomyolysis can occur in patients whose limbs have suffered significant ischemia-reperfusion injury from arterial occlusion. This clinical entity should be suspected in patients with acute limb ischemia demonstrating increased muscle pain and weakness, renal failure, or hyperkalemia. Useful laboratory tests include urinalysis and serum creatine kinase concentration. The urine dip will be positive for blood, whereas the microscopic urinalysis will not demonstrate significant numbers of red blood cells; urinalysis will also demonstrate casts and myoglobin. Treatment consists of volume expansion (with goal urine output of 1 to 2 mL/kg/hr) and alkalinization of the urine with sodium bicarbonate infusion. If the patient does not succumb to the primary illness or acute renal failure, renal compromise in those patients suffering rhabdomyolysis generally resolves.

Imaging Indications and Algorithm

Arteriography is the gold standard for diagnosis and anatomic evaluation of acute limb ischemia. However, other imaging modalities at times merit consideration.

Imaging Techniques and Findings

Ultrasonography

Duplex ultrasonography can be a valuable adjunctive study in the setting of acute limb ischemia. It can localize the site of occlusion, especially in bypass grafts. If the equipment and a capable operator are available in the emergency department setting, duplex ultrasound examination can identify and localize stenoses, dissections, thrombi, emboli, and atherosclerotic plaques.

Computed Tomography

Computed tomographic angiography (CTA) is also capable of identifying occlusive disease and arterial anatomy for operative planning, but it requires the administration of intravenous contrast material.

Magnetic Resonance

Magnetic resonance angiography (MRA) is often useful and indicated in the setting of class I and IIa acute limb ischemia and excels at identifying patent tibial arteries as potential bypass targets. In addition, intravenous gadolinium is much less nephrotoxic than iodinated contrast material.

Angiography

A patient suffering from acute limb ischemia should not undergo a separate diagnostic angiogram if any delay in revascularization might result in limb loss. Access for diagnostic arteriography should be established at a site distant from the presumed occlusion to avoid any subsequent need for thrombolytic delivery in the region of the arteriotomy. Arteriography is often performed intraoperatively in the setting of a pulseless extremity.

The arteriogram should include examination of both inflow and outflow anatomy as well as study of the runoff vessels into the foot. In the case of embolic ischemia, arteriography will demonstrate minimal atherosclerotic disease, a sharp cutoff of the artery at the site of occlusion, and few collateral vessels. Meanwhile, if the acute event is thrombotic in nature, angiography will most often reveal diffuse atherosclerotic disease, irregular and tapered cutoffs, and a well-developed collateral circulation.

Differential Diagnosis

Acute arterial occlusion causing acute limb ischemia is difficult to confuse with other pathologic conditions. That said, there are some not uncommon pitfalls in patients presenting with pulseless, cool, painful extremities. In patients suffering from aortic bifurcation saddle embolus, the diagnosis is frequently missed, as discussed before. These patients are often evaluated for possible neurologic or neurosurgical problems owing to the bilateral paralysis on presentation, resulting in a delay of diagnosis and appropriate therapy. Aortic dissection can cause acute arterial insufficiency of one or both legs and must be considered in any patient presenting with a cold pulseless limb and abdominal, back, or chest pain.[12] Finally, acute venous thrombosis causing phlegmasia cerulea dolens can manifest as a painful, cold, pulseless extremity; however, massive swelling should alert the physician to the correct diagnosis.[13]

Synopsis of Treatment Options

Medical

Acute limb ischemia is a surgical disease; however, attention to the patient's medical and overall condition is essential. Maintenance intravenous fluids should be initiated and the patient kept *nil per os*. A Foley catheter should be inserted to monitor urine output. Consideration should be given to either oral acetylcysteine[14] or bicarbonate infusion[15] if the patient has chronic renal insufficiency or diabetes because diagnostic or completion angiography will likely be indicated.

Temperature extremes and fluctuations should be avoided; cold temperatures cause vasoconstriction, and heat causes increased tissue metabolic demands. Transfusion and optimization of cardiac output should be accomplished whenever these might result in improved oxygenation of the affected limb.

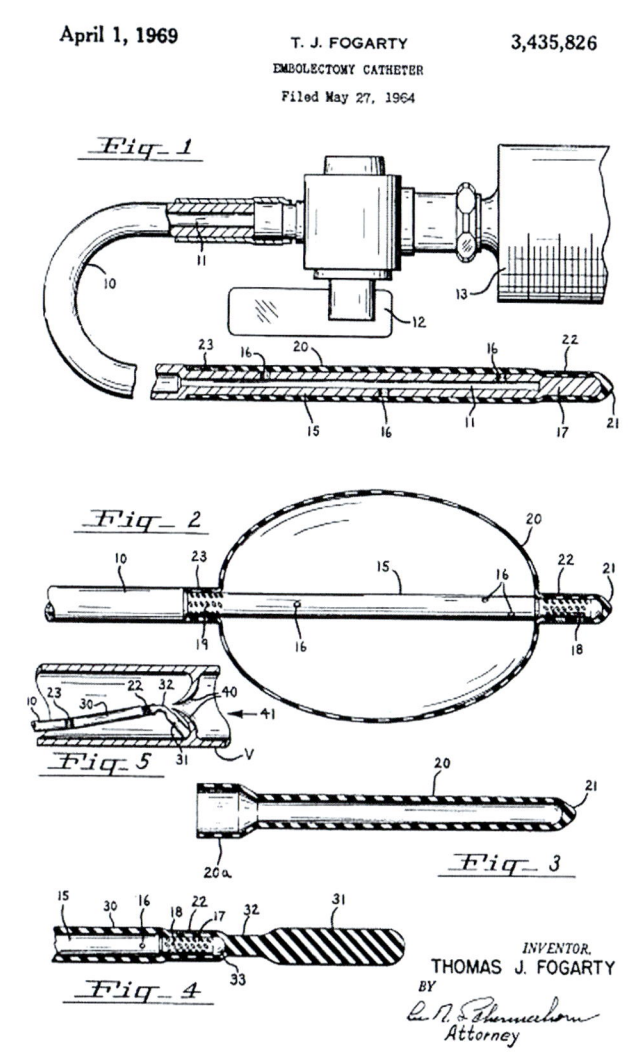

FIGURE 113-3 Original patent application for Fogarty embolectomy catheter. *(From archives of U.S. Patent and Trademark Office, with permission.)*

Surgical/Interventional

Intra-arterial or catheter-directed thrombolysis or fibrinolysis has proved effective and beneficial in a variety of clinical scenarios involving acute limb ischemia.[16-18] However, in a number of situations, thrombolytics are absolutely contraindicated; these include recent surgery or trauma, recent stroke, active bleeding diathesis, and recent history of gastrointestinal bleeding. In some cases, percutaneous aspiration or mechanical thrombectomy is used before and in conjunction with thrombolysis. It is essential that any stenoses revealed on arteriography after thrombolysis be treated with angioplasty, bypass graft revision, or revascularization. In the interim from completion of thrombolysis until intervention directed at flow-limiting lesions, heparin infusion must be continued.

Before 1963 and the introduction of Thomas J. Fogarty's balloon embolectomy catheter (Fig. 113-3), only 23% of patients suffering embolic vascular occlusion were treated surgically with embolectomy. Subsequent to the introduction of this catheter and continuing today, most of these patients undergo surgical embolectomy, which

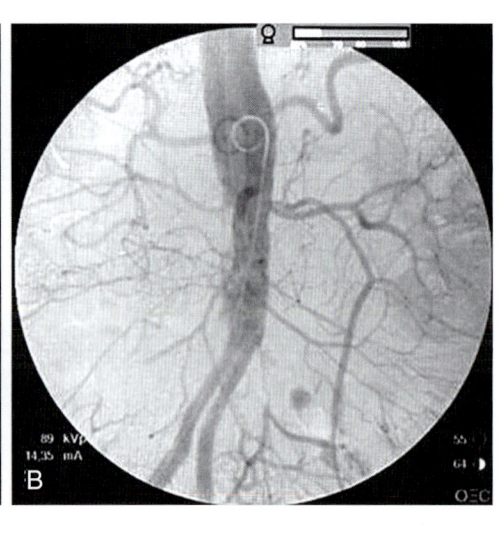

FIGURE 113-4 **A,** Occluded left limb of an abdominal aortic stent graft. Wire access to the aorta was accomplished from the patient's groin bilaterally. Stents were placed in the newly patent left iliac limb to displace residual thrombus and to treat any stenoses that might have contributed to the thrombosis. **B,** Completion angiogram.

now—along with systemic anticoagulation—is the mainstay of therapy.

Aortic occlusion may result from aortic saddle embolus, in situ thrombosis of an atherosclerotic abdominal aorta, thrombosis of an abdominal aortic aneurysm, or aortic dissection. It is important to establish the etiology of aortic occlusion because balloon catheter embolectomy through a femoral cutdown (see later) is usually successful in the setting of saddle embolus but is infrequently helpful in patients with in situ thrombosis of a chronically diseased abdominal aorta. In the latter scenario, the limbs are usually not profoundly ischemic owing to the chronic nature of the disease and resulting extensive collateralization; these patients may require aortobifemoral grafting to reestablish lower extremity perfusion.

Acute unilateral iliac occlusion can occur in patients having undergone prior aortic aneurysmorrhaphy with a bifurcated graft, prior aortobifemoral reconstruction, or prior abdominal aortic stent grafting. In these situations, the surgeon may be able to restore patency of the graft limb with balloon thrombectomy performed from a groin incision, but a technical problem in the affected limb and graft stenosis must be suspected and subsequently addressed (Fig. 113-4).[19] If limb patency cannot be reestablished, femoral-femoral or axillofemoral bypass is indicated.

Symptomatic popliteal aneurysms generally present with limb ischemia—from aneurysm thrombosis or distal thromboembolism—rather than with rupture. The diagnosis should be suspected in any patient with acute or chronic ischemia of the leg and a palpable firm pulseless (in the case of thrombosis) or pulsatile mass behind the knee. Duplex ultrasound examination can confirm the diagnosis. Angiography, MRA, and CTA are useful for operative planning. Treatment of a popliteal aneurysm presenting with acute limb ischemia consists of emergent catheter-directed thrombolysis to reestablish distal arterial patency[20] and subsequent surgical exclusion and bypass; resection of the aneurysm is not necessary. There is also an emerging experience with covered stents for treatment of popliteal aneurysms.[21] Half of patients will have bilateral popliteal aneurysms, and one third of patients with a popliteal aneurysm will have a coincident abdominal aortic aneurysm; therefore, these patients should be screened for coexisting aneurysmal disease.

In patients suffering from thrombotic arterial occlusions and in those whose thromboembolism cannot be extracted or lysed, arterial bypass grafting may be necessary to treat stenotic or occluded vascular segments. Surgical arterial bypass and other revascularization procedures are detailed in Chapter 114.

CHRONIC LIMB ISCHEMIA

Definition

Atherosclerosis resulting in peripheral arterial disease is the most common cause of chronic limb ischemia. Chronic limb ischemia presents as a spectrum of disease from asymptomatic to claudication to critical limb ischemia. This spectrum is encapsulated in two similar staging systems for peripheral arterial disease: Fontaine stages and Rutherford categories (Table 113-4).

Symptomatic patients with peripheral arterial disease generally present with either intermittent claudication or critical limb ischemia. Intermittent claudication is defined as muscle discomfort in the lower limb reproducibly produced by exercise and relieved by rest within 10 minutes. Critical limb ischemia is defined as persistent, recurring ischemic rest pain requiring opiate analgesia for at least 2 weeks with ulceration or gangrene of the foot or toes. Hence, Rutherford categories 4 through 6 comprise those patients with critical limb ischemia.[1]

Of course, there is significant overlap between critical limb ischemia and acute limb ischemia. However, the rational construct differentiating patients with immediately threatened limbs and those with chronically threatened legs is clinically useful.

Prevalence and Epidemiology

Intermittent claudication has a prevalence of approximately 3% in 40-year-olds and about 6% in 60-year-olds. Claudication often is not progressive; revascularization is required in less than one quarter of patients at 10 years, and amputation is required in approximately 2% of patients

TABLE 113-4 Fontaine Stages and Rutherford Categories of Peripheral Arterial Disease of the Limbs

Fontaine		Rutherford		
Stage	Clinical	Grade	Category	Clinical
I	Asymptomatic	0	0	Asymptomatic
IIa	Mild claudication	I	1	Mild claudication
IIb	Moderate to severe claudication	I	2	Moderate claudication
		I	3	Severe claudication
III	Ischemic rest pain	II	4	Ischemic rest pain
IV	Ulceration or	III	5	Minor tissue loss
	gangrene	III	6	Major tissue loss

From Norgren L, Hiatt WR, Dormandy JA, et al; TASC II Working Group. Inter-Society Consensus for the Management of Peripheral Arterial Disease (TASC II). J Vasc Surg 2007; 45(Suppl S):S5-S67.

at 5 years. However, continued smoking or coexistent diabetes portends worse clinical outcomes for claudicants, including more frequent eventual amputation. The outcome of intermittent claudication at 5 years is summarized in Figure 113-5.

Critical limb ischemia has an incidence in the United States of approximately 1000 new cases per 1 million population. Figure 113-6 summarizes risk factors for the development of critical limb ischemia in patients with peripheral arterial disease. More than half of patients with critical limb ischemia undergo attempts at revascularization as definitive treatment; regardless, significant numbers of patients lose their limbs or die within 1 year (Fig. 113-7).

Risk factors for peripheral arterial disease include smoking, diabetes, hypertension, chronic renal insufficiency, African-American race, male sex, hyperlipidemia, and hyperhomocysteinemia.

Again, the importance of chronic limb ischemia as a marker for atherosclerotic cardiovascular disease cannot be overstated. The 5-year mortality rate is 30% for patients with claudication and 70% for patients with critical limb ischemia.

Etiology and Pathophysiology

Peripheral arterial disease most commonly results from atherosclerosis of the distal arterial tree (i.e., aortic

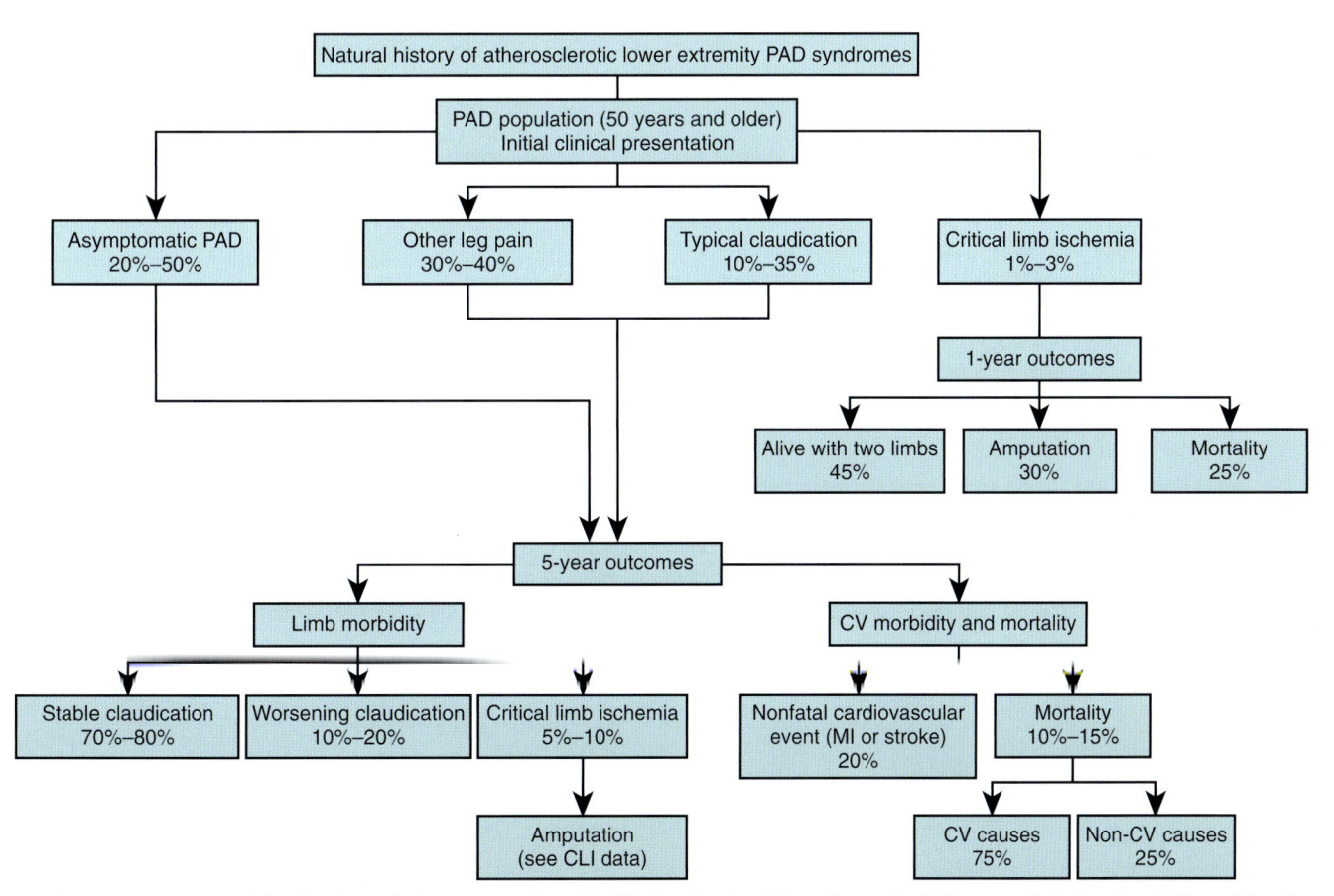

■ **FIGURE 113-5** Fate of the claudicant during 5 years. CLI, critical limb ischemia; CV, cardiovascular; MI, myocardial infarction; PAD, peripheral arterial disease. *(From Hirsch AT, Haskal ZJ, Hertzer NR, et al. ACC/AHA 2005 guidelines for the management of patients with peripheral arterial disease. J Am Coll Cardiol 2006; 47:1239-1312.)*

bifurcation and below) and is manifested typically as intermittent claudication. Patients with intermittent claudication have normal blood flow to the limb at rest; but with exercise, the occlusive arterial disease prevents proper augmentation of blood flow, resulting in insufficient oxygen delivery to the muscles and the symptoms of claudication. Critical limb ischemia represents more advanced occlusive peripheral arterial disease in which oxygen delivery to the lower limb is suboptimal even at rest.

Manifestations of Disease

Clinical Presentation

Intermittent Claudication

Patients with intermittent claudication describe fatigue, aching, or cramping in the muscles of the leg that develops after walking a consistent established distance (or other exercise) and that resolves with rest. These symptoms most often appear in the calf but can affect the thigh or buttocks. The anatomic site of pain frequently corresponds to the level of occlusive disease; symptoms typically present in muscle groups one joint level below the region of arterial occlusion. Thus, calf muscle claudication is most commonly due to superficial femoral artery occlusion; hip, thigh, or buttock claudication is most commonly due to more proximal aortoiliac disease.

A complete physical examination should focus on cardiovascular diseases. The blood pressure should be measured in both arms and the ankle-brachial index in each leg. Auscultation is performed to assess for cardiac disease. The abdomen is palpated in an attempt to detect an abdominal aortic aneurysm as a potential embolic source (although physical examination is only 50% sensitive for abdominal aortic aneurysms 4 to 5 cm in diameter).

The peripheral vascular examination comprises palpation of the radial, ulnar, brachial, carotid, femoral, popliteal, dorsalis pedis, and posterior tibial pulses. Especially prominent femoral or popliteal pulses should suggest aneurysm disease. Auscultation of the carotid, abdominal aorta, and iliac arteries and femoral artery can suggest occlusive vascular disease. In addition, the skin of the legs should be assessed for skin color, temperature, or decreased hair growth and the muscles of the leg for ischemic atrophy.

Normal leg pulses do not rule out intermittent claudication as the diagnosis of a patient's complaints; for instance, isolated internal iliac occlusive disease may cause buttock claudication (and impotence in men). In addition, in claudicants, pulses may be palpable at rest but absent with exercise; ankle-brachial indices can be performed before

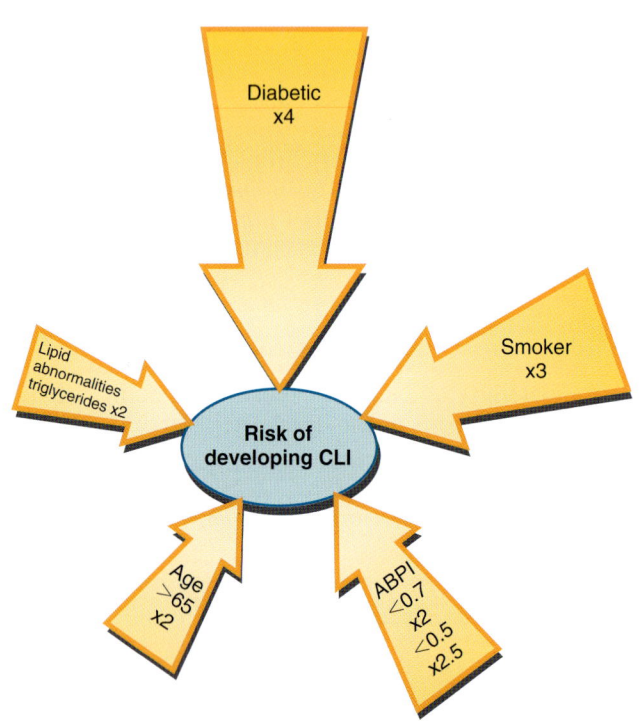

■ **FIGURE 113-6** Approximate magnitude of the effect of risk factors on the development of critical limb ischemia in patients with peripheral arterial disease. ABPI, ankle-brachial pressure index; CLI, critical limb ischemia. (From Norgren L, Hiatt WR, Dormandy JA, et al; TASC II Working Group. Inter-Society Consensus for the Management of Peripheral Arterial Disease [TASC II]. J Vasc Surg 2007; 45[Suppl S]:S5-S67.)

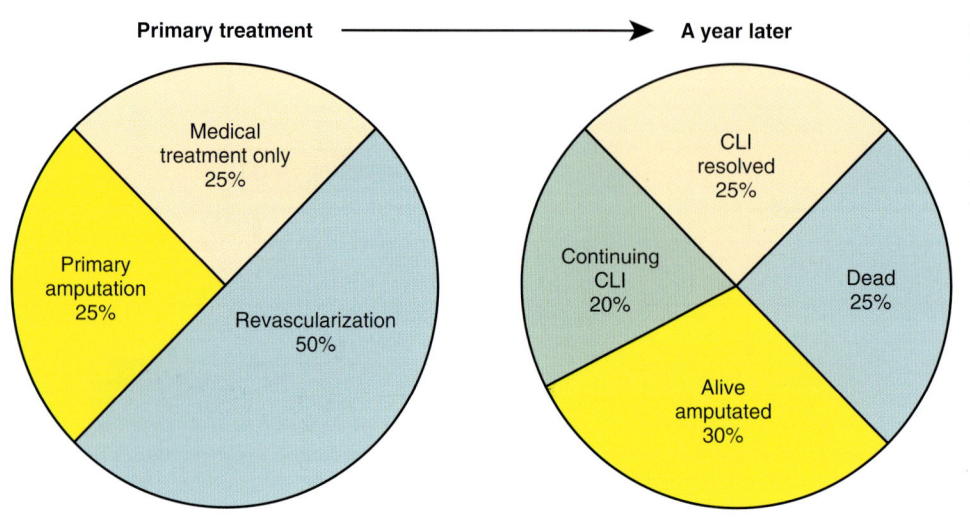

■ **FIGURE 113-7** Fate of patients presenting with critical leg ischemia (CLI). (From Norgren L, Hiatt WR, Dormandy JA, et al; TASC II Working Group. Inter-Society Consensus for the Management of Peripheral Arterial Disease [TASC II]. J Vasc Surg 2007; 45[Suppl S]:S5-S67.)

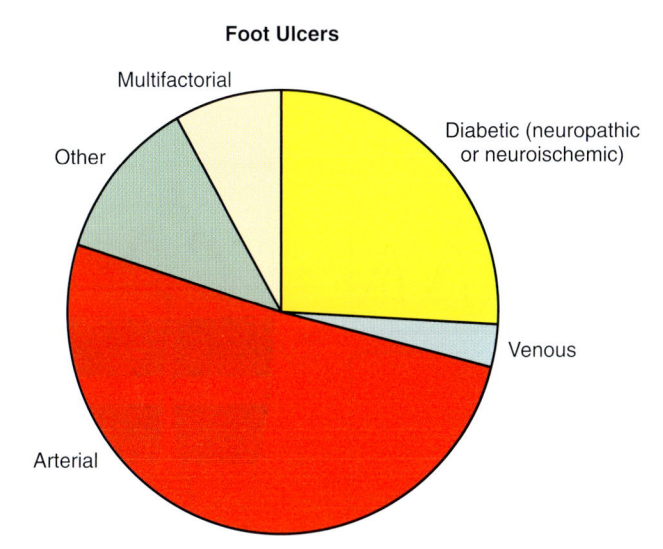

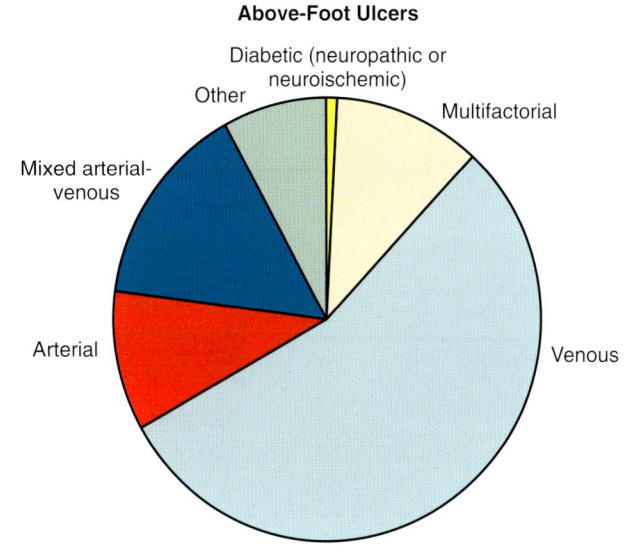

FIGURE 113-8 The causes and frequencies of lower limb ulcers. *(From Norgren L, Hiatt WR, Dormandy JA, et al; TASC II Working Group. Inter-Society Consensus for the Management of Peripheral Arterial Disease [TASC II]. J Vasc Surg 2007; 45[Suppl S]:S5-S67.)*

and immediately after exercise (usually on a treadmill) to document the claudication.

As suggested before, ankle-brachial indices constitute a first diagnostic test in patients thought to have intermittent claudication. First, the systolic blood pressure is measured in each arm, and the higher is taken as the brachial pressure. The cuff is then placed on the calf, inflated, and then slowly deflated; the highest pressure at which the Doppler signal—at either the posterior tibial or dorsalis pedis—becomes audible again marks the ankle pressure. A ratio of 1.0 is normal; an ankle-brachial index of less than 0.9 is clearly abnormal.

Critical Limb Ischemia

Patients with critical limb ischemia present with some combination of ischemic rest pain, nonhealing ulcers, and gangrene. Ischemic rest pain is severe, is intolerable, sometimes improves with lowering of the affected limb (dangling the foot over the edge of the bed), and is responsive only to narcotic analgesics. The pain is often worst at night (when the limb is elevated), sometimes wakes the patient from sleep, and is sometimes transiently relieved by rubbing the foot.

Except in cases of diabetic neuropathy and resulting anesthesia of the foot, patients with tissue loss of the lower extremity also often present with pain, localized to the wound. Ulcers and gangrene usually affect the toes, the heel and ankle, and, in severe cases, the distal foot proper. Ulcers are often initiated by minor trauma (e.g., ill-fitting shoes) or other injury (e.g., burn injury from attempts at warming a chronically painful cold foot).

In those patients with critical limb ischemia and diabetes mellitus, the peripheral neuropathy often contributes to the trauma initiating ulcer formation and to the delayed recognition of the wound by the patient. The microvascular derangement of diabetes predisposes to nonhealing of these wounds and to the subsequent development of infection (wet gangrene). Complications of diabetic foot ulcers, including gangrene, are the most common cause of nontraumatic leg, foot, and toe amputation. Up to 15% of diabetic patients will suffer from a foot ulcer during their lives, and 15% to 25% of these will require an amputation at some level.

The location and appearance of the ulcer or gangrene can provide the astute clinician a suggestion as to the etiology of the wound. For example, as indicated in Figure 113-8, calf ulcers are more often reflective of venous disease than of peripheral arterial disease.

The putative diagnosis of critical limb ischemia should be confirmed by measuring ankle-brachial indices. Symptoms of rest pain commonly occur in patients with ankle pressures below 50 mm Hg. Peripheral arterial disease often impairs healing in leg ulcers caused by trauma, venous insufficiency, or neuropathy, and augmented blood flow (above that which would cause rest pain) is required to heal wounds or infections; therefore, ankle pressures below 70 mm Hg are suggestive of critical limb ischemia in patients with ulcers or gangrene.

Subsequently, pulse volume recordings may be performed by use of a plethysmograph in a vascular laboratory. This device measures volume changes in the limb at various levels with multiple blood pressure cuffs. Pulse volume recordings can localize arterial occlusive disease with up to 85% accuracy compared with angiography. Figure 113-9 demonstrates pulse volume recordings in a patient with unilateral superficial femoral artery occlusion before and after angioplasty and stenting of the superficial femoral artery.

Imaging Indications and Algorithm

In patients with peripheral arterial disease in whom revascularization is indicated or considered, radiologic studies should be entertained. Angiography is the gold standard, but it is invasive and expensive. Duplex ultrasound exami-

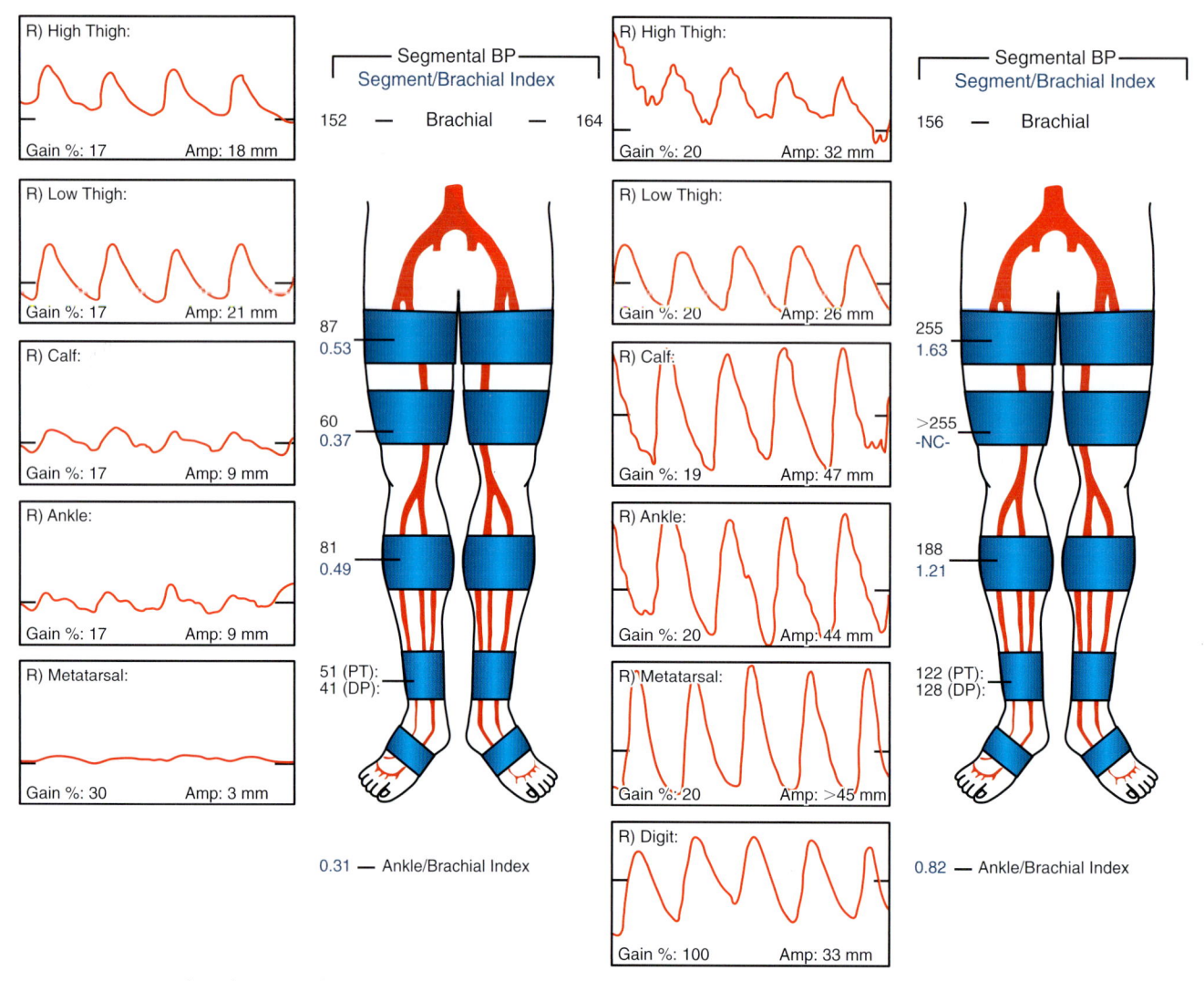

FIGURE 113-9 Pulse volume recordings in a patient with superficial femoral artery occlusion, before (*left*) and after (*right*) recanalization, angioplasty, and stenting.

nation is very useful in a defined clinical milieu. Meanwhile, both CTA and MRA are noninvasive cross-sectional imaging studies that afford imaging of the aorta, iliac, and lower extremity runoff arteries in a single study and are therefore often of great clinical utility in patients with chronic limb ischemia.

Imaging Techniques and Findings

Radiography

In patients with wet gangrene, plain radiography, by demonstrating subcutaneous or intramuscular air, can suggest but not rule out "gas gangrene" or necrotizing infection. In patients with any deep ulcer or gangrenous wound, plain films may be useful to evaluate for osteomyelitis—in which case there may be soft tissue swelling, loss of fascial planes, periosteal thickening and elevation, and osteopenia—although MRI and bone scan have higher sensitivity for detection of osteomyelitis.

Ultrasonography

Duplex ultrasonography is noninvasive and does not require the administration of contrast material or other medication. It is highly sensitive and specific for identification of stenoses in bypass grafts. It is sometimes less effective at imaging calcified vessels and tibial arteries. Ultrasound studies are somewhat dynamic and technologist dependent by their very nature, and thus objective results and images are not as portable or reproducible as in other imaging modalities. Nevertheless, Duplex ultrasonography is greater than 80% sensitive and specific for iliac, femoropopliteal, and infrapopliteal disease.[22]

Computed Tomography

CTA is often the initial anatomic imaging study of choice in patients with symptomatic peripheral arterial disease. Truly three-dimensional imaging and image reconstruction is possible. However, calcified arterial plaques cause a "blooming artifact" and can make assessment of arterial patency in regions of significant calcium difficult or impossible. Likewise, preexisting arterial stents can cause significant artifact. Intravenous iodinated contrast material must be administered in significant doses (approximately 150 mL is normally used for a study of the abdominal arteries and bilateral lower limb runoff vessels), making this study less useful in those with chronic renal insufficiency. Often, an anatomically focused catheter x-ray arteriography will require a much smaller dose of iodinated contrast agent.

Magnetic Resonance

MRA excels at identifying patent tibial arteries as potential bypass targets. In addition, peripheral MRA can be performed without iodinated contrast agents as needed for peripheral CTA and x-ray angiography. However, peripheral MRA is best performed with gadolinium-chelate contrast agents, which does have rare but serious adverse events, notably nephrogenic systemic fibrosis. Truly three-dimensional imaging and image reconstruction is possible with MRA. Unfortunately, patients with implanted metal devices or retained metal objects may not be able to undergo MR imaging. In addition, recent reports and concern relative to gadolinium-induced nephrogenic systemic fibrosis have limited its applicability in patients with severe chronic renal insufficiency who are not on dialysis.

Angiography

The expense and risks of arteriography—including contrast allergic reaction, contrast-related renal failure, arterial dissection, atheroembolization, pseudoaneurysm, arteriovenous fistula, and bleeding—are not insignificant. However, this technique is unsurpassed for providing a "road map" for revascularization, and it is often accomplished in one procedure with endovascular or open revascularization.

Differential Diagnosis

The causes of chronic leg ischemia apart from atherosclerosis include arteritis, popliteal artery entrapment, mucinous cystic degeneration, Buerger disease (thromboangiitis obliterans), Takayasu disease, aortic coarctation, popliteal aneurysm (with secondary thromboembolism), other embolic disease, fibromuscular dysplasia, pseudoxanthoma elasticum, thrombosis of persistent sciatic artery, endofibrosis of the external iliac artery (iliac artery syndrome in cyclists), and primary arterial tumors.

The differential diagnosis of intermittent claudication includes venous insufficiency, nerve root compression (sciatica or lumbar radiculopathy), symptomatic Baker cyst, chronic compartment syndrome (usually in heavily muscled athletes), spinal stenosis, hip arthritis, ankle arthritis, and foot arthritis.

In the case of critical limb ischemia with tissue loss, other causes of or factors contributing to the ulcer or gangrene must be considered. These include diabetes, venous insufficiency, neuropathies, musculoskeletal abnormalities causing disturbance in gait or mobility, infection, conventional trauma, calciphylaxis, and debility of any cause contributing to pressure or decubitus ulceration.[23]

Synopsis of Treatment Options

Medical

Modification of risk factors for atherosclerosis and hence for peripheral arterial disease is recommended to all patients with intermittent claudication or critical limb ischemia. These measures may include smoking cessation, cholesterol lowering with diet modification and prescription of statin medications, reduction of hemoglobin A_{1c}, treatment of hypertension, and institution of antiplatelet therapy.

The treatment goals for patients with intermittent claudication are to relieve symptoms and to improve exercise capacity and the ability to perform activities of daily living. The treatment strategy may incorporate exercise rehabilitation as well as one of any number of medications demonstrated to improve exercise tolerance and quality of life, including cilostazol and pentoxifylline.

The goals of therapy for patients with critical limb ischemia are to relieve pain, to heal ulcers, to prevent limb loss, to improve quality of life, and to prolong survival. To accomplish amputation-free survival, most patients will require revascularization. While work-up is under way and in those patients in whom revascularization is not an option, pain control and ulcer healing are primary therapeutic goals.

Surgical/Interventional

In the case of severe intermittent claudication that has an impact on a patient's livelihood or ability to perform activities of daily living, revascularization is sometimes indicated. Recent advances in and widespread adoption of endovascular therapy for peripheral arterial disease have lowered the threshold—in some practices—for attempted revascularization in patients with intermittent claudication. Meanwhile, revascularization is indicated and necessary in those patients with critical limb ischemia. Specific approaches and techniques for revascularization are discussed in Chapter 114.

Infection of the gangrenous toes, heel, foot, or leg in diabetic patients and in those with critical limb ischemia is often polymicrobial and present anywhere in the spectrum of local superinfection of preexisting ulcers to gas gangrene or necrotizing fasciitis of the leg. Principles of care include the initiation of broad-spectrum intravenous antibiotics until the organisms and their sensitivities are defined and the coverage can be narrowed. Débridement of infectious and gangrenous or necrotic tissue is essential. Amputation is seldom required but must be considered in certain cases. Revascularization is undertaken when the infection is under control.

Frequently, toe or forefoot amputations are undertaken to eliminate necrotic or infected tissue. When they are combined with temporally proximal revascularization, these amputations are classified as salvage procedures, allowing limb salvage in patients with ischemic gangrene of the foot. Not uncommonly in diabetic patients, toe amputation will be undertaken in the setting of unrevascularizable peripheral arterial disease or minimal peripheral arterial disease; diabetic neuropathy and vasculopathy are the causes of these gangrenous toes, and revascularization is not indicated.

Major amputation (below the knee or above the knee) is indicated when overwhelming infection threatens the patient's life, when rest pain cannot be controlled or alleviated, or in the setting of a necrotic or gangrenous "dead" foot.

> **KEY POINTS**
> - Peripheral arterial disease is the most common etiology of both chronic limb ischemia and acute limb ischemia.
> - Acute limb ischemia is a surgical emergency and is most often due to thromboembolus or acute thrombotic occlusion of a native artery or bypass graft.
> - Chronic limb ischemia can be manifested as either intermittent claudication or critical limb ischemia.
> - The mainstay of treatment for intermittent claudication is exercise therapy.
> - Revascularization is typically indicated in cases of critical limb ischemia that present with either rest pain or lower extremity ulcers or gangrene.

SUGGESTED READINGS

Kasirajan K, Ouriel K. Acute limb ischemia. In Rutherford R (ed). Vascular Surgery, 6th ed. Philadelphia, Elsevier, 2005, pp 959-971.

Norgren L, Hiatt WR, Dormandy JA, et al; TASC II Working Group. Inter-Society Consensus for the Management of Peripheral Arterial Disease (TASC II). J Vasc Surg 2007; 45(Suppl S):S5-S67.

Perera GB, Lyden SP. Current trends in lower extremity revascularization. Surg Clin North Am 2007; .87:1135-1147, x.

White C. Intermittent claudication. N Engl J Med 2007; 356:1241-1250.

REFERENCES

1. Norgren L, Hiatt WR, Dormandy JA, et al; TASC II Working Group. Inter-Society Consensus for the Management of Peripheral Arterial Disease (TASC II). J Vasc Surg 2007; 45(Suppl S):S5-S67.
2. Golomb BA, Dang TT, Criqui MH. Peripheral arterial disease: morbidity and mortality implications. Circulation 2006; 114:688-699.
3. Davies B, Braithwaite BD, Birch PA, et al. Acute leg ischaemia in Gloucestershire. Br J Surg 1997; 84:504-508.
4. Dormandy J, Heeck L, Vig S. Acute limb ischemia. Semin Vasc Surg 1999; 12:148.
5. Kasirajan K, Ouriel K. Acute limb ischemia. In Rutherford R (ed). Vascular Surgery, 6th ed. Philadelphia, Elsevier, 2005, pp 959-971.
6. Ouriel K, Shortell CK, Green RM, et al. Differential mechanisms of failure of autogenous and non-autogenous bypass conduits: an assessment following successful graft thrombolysis. Cardiovasc Surg 1995; 3:469.
7. Woratyla S, Darling RC III, Lloyd W, et al. Acute and chronic aortic occlusion: analysis of outcome. Proceedings of the Eastern Vascular Society 1998; 12:82.
8. Pfeiffer RB III, O'Mara CS. Peripheral arterial embolus. In Cameron JL (ed). Current Surgical Therapy, 8th ed. Philadelphia, Elsevier, 2004, pp 817-820.
9. Abbott W, Maloney R, McCabe C, et al. Arterial embolism: a 44 year perspective. Am J Surg 1982; 143:460.
10. Rutherford RB, Baer JD, Ernst C, et al. Recommended standards for reports dealing with lower extremity ischemia: revised version. J Vasc Surg 1997; 26:517.
11. Goldman L, Caldera DL, Nussbaum SR, et al. Multifactorial index of cardiac risk in noncardiac surgical procedures. N Engl J Med 1977; 297:845-850.
12. Ince H, Nienaber CA. Diagnosis and management of patients with aortic dissection. Heart 2007; 93:266-270.
13. Perkins JM, Magee TR, Galland RB. Phlegmasia caerulea dolens and venous gangrene. Br J Surg 1996; 83:19-23.
14. Tepel M, van der Giet M, Schwarzfeld C, et al. Prevention of radiographic-contrast-agent-induced reductions in renal function by acetylcysteine. N Engl J Med 2000; 343:180-184.
15. Merten GJ, Burgess WP, Gray LV, et al. Prevention of contrast-induced nephropathy with sodium bicarbonate: a randomized controlled trial. JAMA 2004; 291:2328-2334.
16. Ouriel K, Shortell C, DeWeese JA, et al. A comparison of thrombolytic therapy with operative revascularization in the initial treatment of acute peripheral arterial ischemia. J Vasc Surg 1994; 19:1021.
17. Weaver FA, Camerota AJ, Youngblood M, et al. Surgical revascularization versus thrombolysis for non-embolic lower extremity native artery occlusions: results of a prospective randomized trial. The STILE Investigators: Surgery versus Thrombolysis for Ischemia of the Lower Extremity. J Vasc Surg 1996; 24:513.
18. Ouriel K, Veith FJ, Sasahara AA. Thrombolysis or peripheral arterial surgery: phase I results. TOPAS Investigators. J Vasc Surg 1996; 23:64.
19. Milner R, Golden MA, Velazquez OC, et al. A new endovascular approach to treatment of acute iliac limb occlusions of bifurcated aortic stent grafts with an exoskeleton. J Vasc Surg 2003; 37:1329-1331.
20. Carpenter JP, Barker CF, Roberts B, et al. Popliteal artery aneurysms: current management and outcome. J Vasc Surg 1994; 19:65-72.
21. Mohan IV, Bray PJ, Harris JP, et al. Endovascular popliteal aneurysm repair: are the results comparable to open surgery? Eur J Vasc Endovasc Surg 2006; 32:149-154.
22. Koelemay MJ, den Hartog D, Prins MH, et al. Diagnosis of arterial disease of the lower extremities with duplex ultrasonography. Br J Surg 1996; 83:404-409.
23. Sumpio BE. Foot ulcers. N Engl J Med 2000; 343:787-793.

CHAPTER 114

Lower Extremity Operations and Interventions

T. Gregory Walker, Sanjeeva P. Kalva, and John A. Kaufman

A variety of surgical and endovascular interventions may be used in treating the different disease entities that affect the lower extremity arterial circulation. The dominant disease process is atherosclerosis; this may be manifested as stenotic, occlusive, or aneurysmal disease. Other entities affecting this vascular distribution are trauma (blunt, penetrating, and iatrogenic), neoplasm, inflammation (vasculitis and infection), and congenital abnormalities. Treatment options for many of these processes include surgery, catheter-based endovascular procedures, and a combination of both. Therapies may be further subdivided into those designed for revascularization and those for exclusion. Revascularization procedures primarily deal with stenotic or occlusive disease processes, whereas exclusion procedures focus on entities such as aneurysms, arteriovenous malformations or fistulas, vascular neoplasms, and arterial injuries. In some cases, a combination of exclusion and revascularization is required to effectively deal with the disease process.

Vascular surgical procedures have traditionally been the "gold standard" against which newer technologies and their long-term results have been measured. Whereas open vascular surgical procedures have continued to undergo refinements and expansions of clinical indications, endovascular or catheter-based interventions have had an almost explosive growth of new technology and broadened indications and have increasingly gained acceptance as the primary treatment in a variety of applications. There are now long-term data for many of these endovascular procedures that compare favorably with the traditional open surgical operations.[1-6] Some of the newer technologies continue to evolve and are likely to have expanding indications. The decision process for selection of open versus endovascular treatment, as well as which endovascular option, involves consideration of the specific disease entity, the medical condition and age of the patient, the anatomic constraints, and the durability of the procedure in question.

REVASCULARIZATION PROCEDURE: VASCULAR BYPASS SURGERY

Description and Special Anatomic Considerations

Vascular bypass surgery involves placement of a conduit to serve as an alternative vascular pathway to a diseased or obstructed arterial bed. Vascular surgical conduits are anatomically classified on the basis of the locations of the proximal and distal anastomoses. The most common infrainguinal bypass is the femoropopliteal bypass, between the common femoral and the popliteal arteries (Fig. 114-1A,B). The distal anastomosis may be to either the above-knee or the below-knee segment of the popliteal artery (Fig. 114-1C). Conduits are further defined according to the material from which they are constructed. They may be native, such as an autogenous vein or artery, or they may be prosthetic, such as expanded polytetrafluoroethylene (ePTFE) or Dacron. The native greater saphenous vein is preferred for bypass surgery in the lower extremity because it performs better than any other conduit choice. However, it may not always be an available option because donor veins may be diseased or may have been previously harvested for other vascular procedures, such as coronary artery bypass surgery. Other autogenous veins used as vascular conduits include the short saphenous vein, the femoral vein (also known as the superficial femoral vein) within the thigh, and the basilic and cephalic veins of the upper extremity.

The autogenous greater saphenous vein conduits can be further subdivided into in situ and reversed vein grafts. Use of an in situ vein graft involves mobilization of only the proximal and distal ends of the vessel while allowing most of the vein to remain within its vascular bed. The venous valves must be incised, and venous tributaries arising from the in situ graft must be ligated. Proximal and distal anastomoses to the artery are then created at the

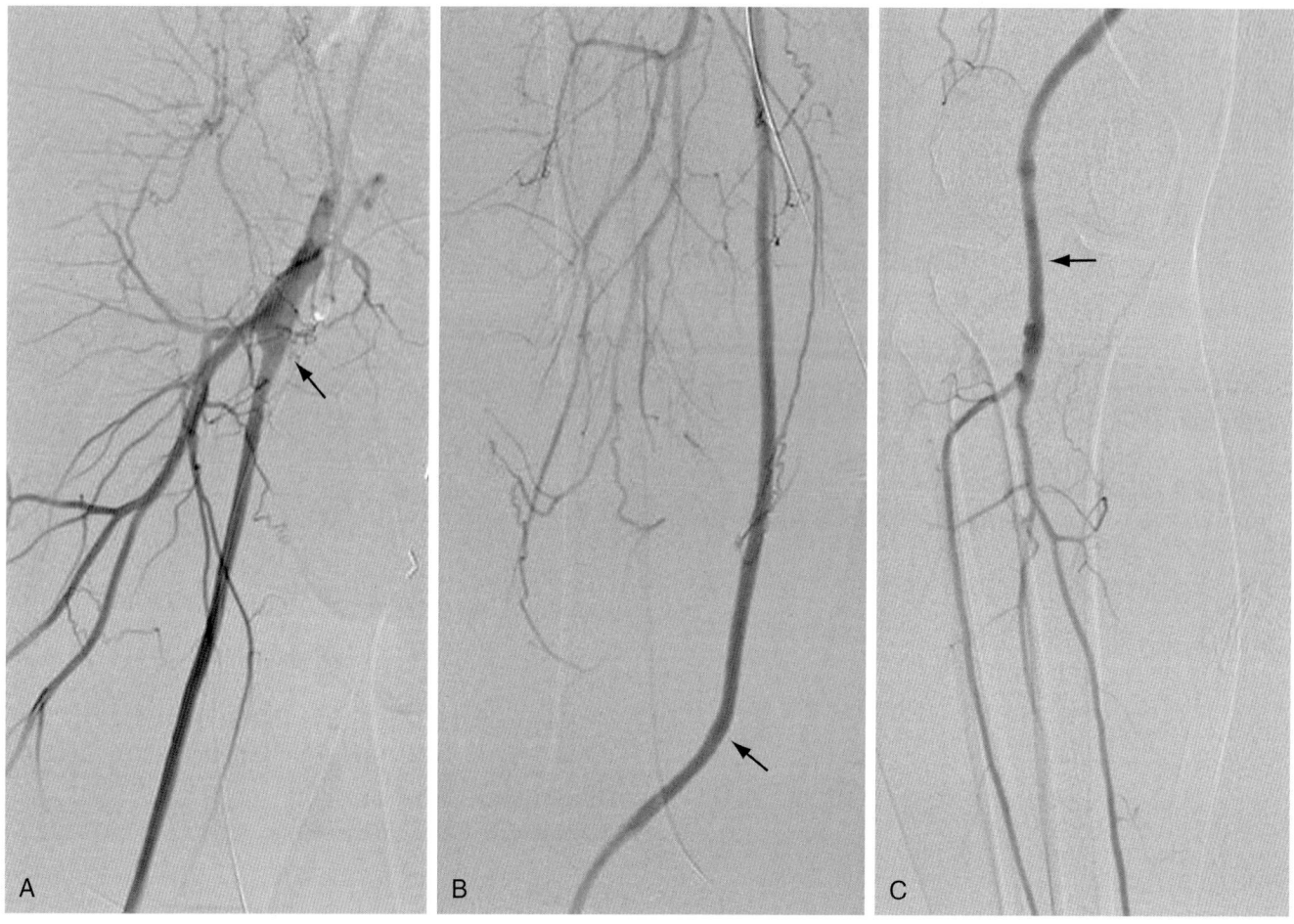

FIGURE 114-1 Femoropopliteal bypass graft. Images (**A** to **C**, cranial to caudal) from a right leg arteriogram show the proximal anastomoses (**A**, *arrow*) of a femoropopliteal bypass graft and the course of the graft (**B**, *arrow*) in the medial right thigh. The distal anastomosis of this femoropopliteal bypass graft is to the below-knee segment of the popliteal artery (**C**, *arrow*). Note the focal bulges (**C**, *arrowhead*) in the graft where venous valves were present in this in situ saphenous vein graft. These valves would have been excised with a valvulotome at the time of bypass surgery.

mobilized ends of the in situ graft. A reversed saphenous vein graft must first be carefully harvested from the thigh, with ligation of all tributary vein branches. The vein is reversed during the bypass procedure, which allows unobstructed flow through the venous valves. Because of the reversal of the vein, the smaller distal end of the harvested vein is anastomosed to the larger caliber proximal artery, a situation that has generated a variety of surgical strategies to deal with the mismatch. Some surgeons use a harvested saphenous vein in a nonreversed fashion after incising the valves.

Prosthetic grafts typically are used for aortobifemoral and extra-anatomic bypass surgery, such as axillofemoral or cross-femoral bypass graft surgery; when they are used for femoropopliteal bypass surgery, long-term patency is significantly improved when the distal anastomosis is to the above-knee rather than the below-knee segment of the popliteal artery. There are relatively poor results for distal revascularization with prosthetic grafts. If bypass to the below-knee popliteal arterial segment is necessary, an autogenous vein graft is indicated; if the greater saphenous vein is not an option as a conduit, other autogenous veins may be used. Composite grafts that use a prosthetic above the knee coupled with an autogenous graft to cross the joint and to anastomose to the below-knee segment are also used.

Prosthetic grafts have certain advantages, including ease of use, shortened surgical times, and less extensive operative dissection. The disadvantages relative to autogenous grafts include higher frequencies of intimal hyperplasia, thrombosis, and anastomotic stenoses. There are also higher rates of graft infections, material deterioration, and anastomotic pseudoaneurysms than in their native counterparts.

The lack of a completely satisfactory prosthetic substitute for the greater saphenous vein has led to the use of other biologic conduits, such as human umbilical vein, arterial or venous homografts, and xenografts. There are certain inherent problems, such as aneurysmal degeneration (Fig. 114-2), and long-term patency issues that are unique to these biografts, and results remain mixed compared with prosthetic grafts.[7]

Extra-anatomic bypass refers to grafts that are constructed in anatomic locations that are significantly different from the normal location of the diseased arteries that are being bypassed. Typical examples are the cross-femoral (femorofemoral) and axillofemoral bypass grafts (Figs. 114-3 to 114-5). These were originally designed for

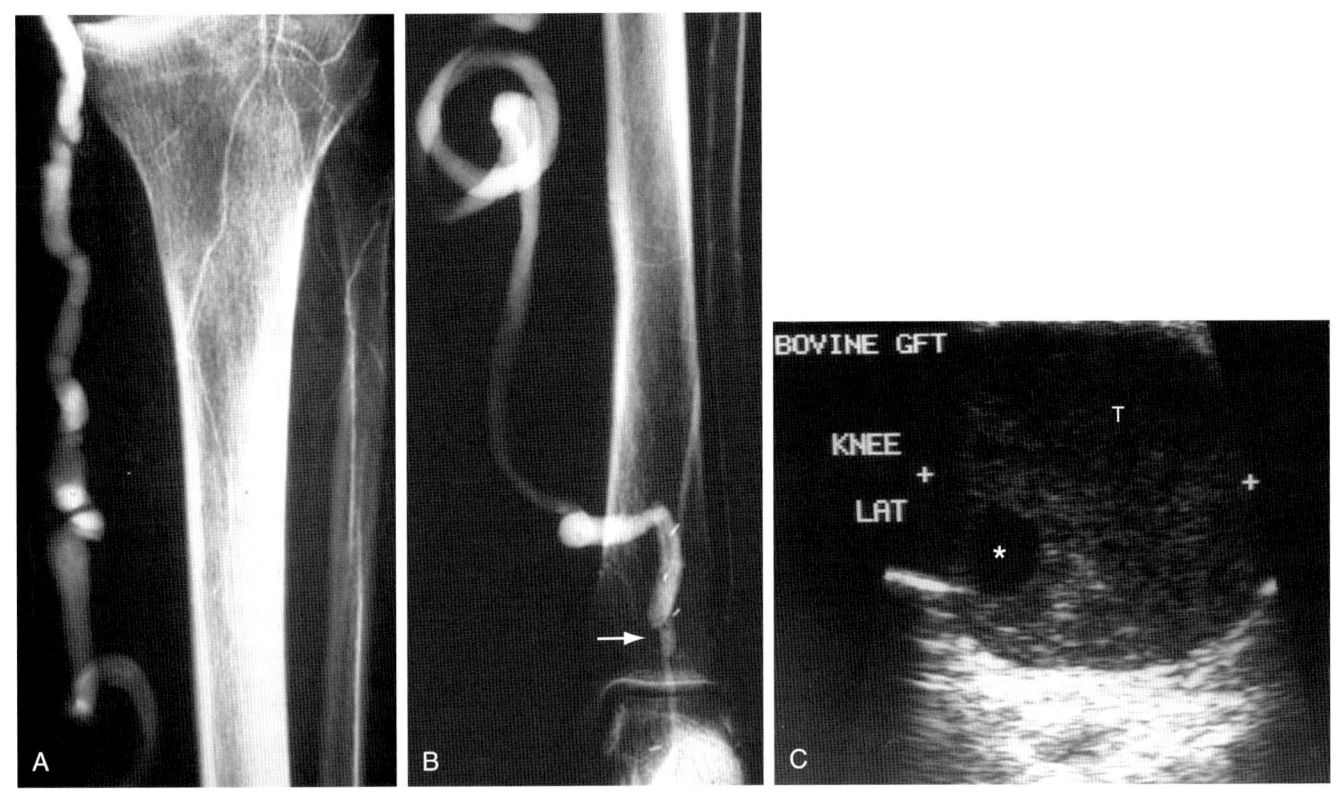

CHAPTER 114 • *Lower Extremity Operations and Interventions* 1587

■ **FIGURE 114-2** **A** and **B,** This bovine xenograft used for distal bypass to the dorsalis pedis artery (*arrow*) underwent severe degeneration, as seen in this arteriogram. There are multiple stenoses and aneurysms present in the graft as a result of the degeneration. This is an inherent problem in both xenografts and homografts. **C,** Gray-scale ultrasound image of the bovine xenograft at knee level demonstrates that there is marked aneurysmal degeneration with considerable laminar thrombus (T) and an eccentric patent lumen (*asterisk*).

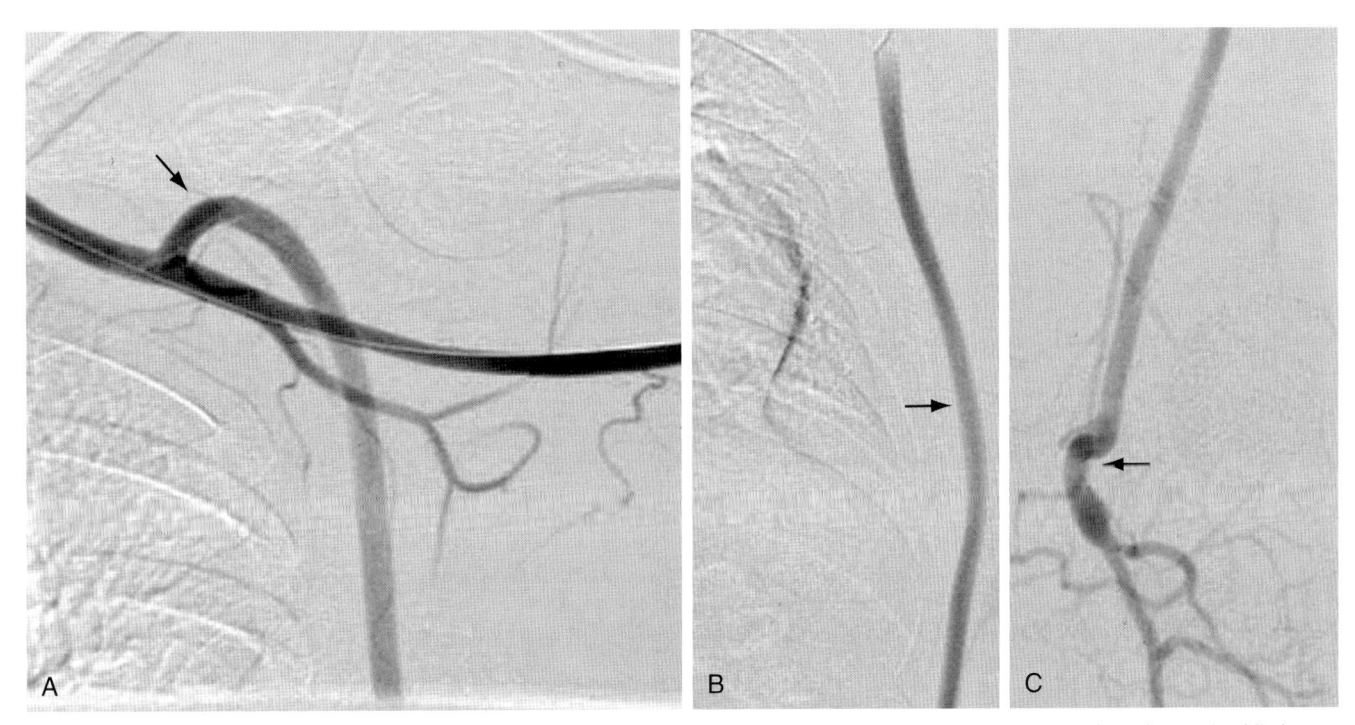

■ **FIGURE 114-3** Axillofemoral bypass graft. Digital subtraction angiography (DSA) images (**A** to **C,** cranial to caudal) show the proximal limb (**A,** *arrow*) of an axillofemoral bypass graft, the thoracic course (**B,** *arrow*) of the axillofemoral bypass graft, and the distal anastomoses to the profunda femoral artery (**C,** *arrow*). A femorofemoral bypass graft (not shown) was also constructed in this patient.

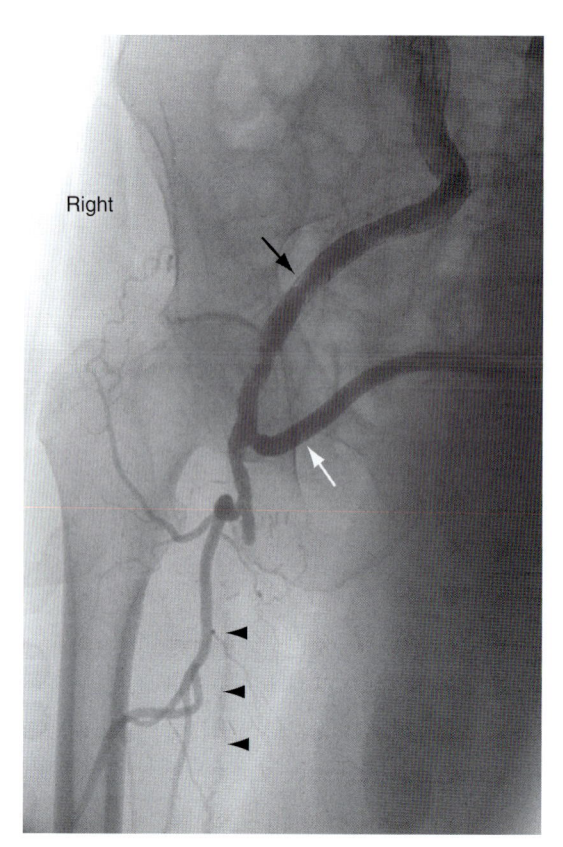

FIGURE 114-4 Conventional x-ray arteriogram shows a right-to-left femorofemoral bypass graft (*white arrow*). The study also reveals an inflow stenosis (*black arrow*) in the right external iliac artery stent graft and occlusion of the heavily calcified native superficial femoral artery (*arrowheads*) in this patient who had also previously undergone a femoropopliteal bypass graft. This patient will require correction of the inflow abnormality and either thrombolysis of the bypass graft or surgical revision.

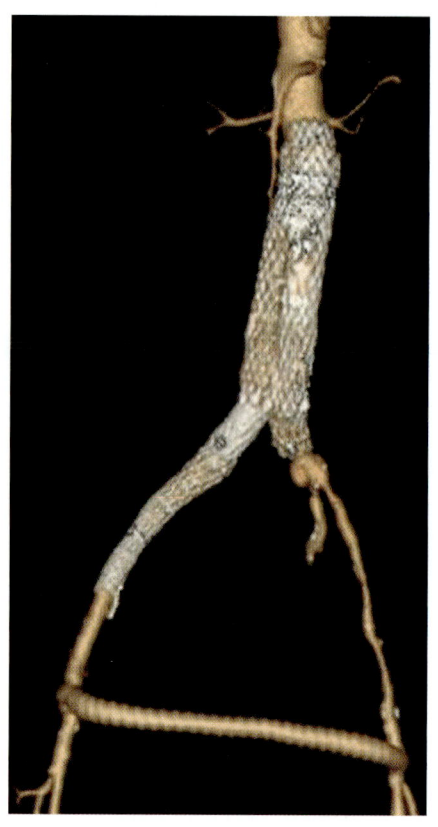

FIGURE 114-5 CTA shows a right-to-left femorofemoral bypass graft constructed in a patient who had previously undergone endovascular repair of an abdominal aortic aneurysm and subsequently had occlusion of the left limb of the graft.

patients too ill to undergo direct aortofemoral bypass or to replace grafts that were infected; these are still the primary indications. In addition, they now often serve as adjuncts to endovascular repair of abdominal aortic aneurysms (EVAR), particularly in the category of aorto-uni-iliac EVAR. These grafts are usually constructed of prosthetic material and generally have somewhat lower long-term patency than more traditional vascular bypass grafts, such as the aortobifemoral bypass graft. The obturator bypass (Fig. 114-6) was developed to replace femoropopliteal bypass surgery in patients with groin infections involving the native arteries or previously placed grafts and in patients with other complicating circumstances in the groin, such as trauma or previous radiation treatment. This bypass can be constructed with prosthetics or with autogenous vein.[8]

Indications

Patients with lower extremity peripheral arterial disease that is manifested as claudication are typically managed medically, with an emphasis on lifestyle and risk factor modification coupled with an exercise regimen. Although many patients will show symptomatic improvement, a large number will have progression of disease. In addition, compliance of patients with such a management strategy is generally poor. Disabling, lifestyle-limiting claudication or progression to critical limb ischemia, characterized by rest pain or tissue loss, may eventually occur and thus require either infrainguinal bypass surgery or endovascular revascularization.

Patients with peripheral arterial disease may be classified by both a clinical description of the symptoms and objective testing criteria by the Rutherford categories of chronic limb ischemia (Table 114-1). These aid in prognosis and treatment planning.

The anatomic location of the peripheral arterial disease affects the choice of a surgical or endovascular procedure. Arterial bypass remains the standard for revascularization and is indicated in patients with long-segment chronic total occlusion of the superficial femoral artery, chronic total occlusion of the popliteal artery and proximal trifurcation vessels, diffuse, severe multiple stenoses or occlusions that involve the entirety of the superficial femoral artery, and recurrent stenoses or occlusions after two or more prior endovascular treatments.

Contraindications

Arterial bypass surgery is contraindicated if there is insufficient inflow or outflow to maintain patency of the vascular conduit. Before bypass, therefore, some type of imaging (CT angiography [CTA], MR angiography [MRA], or catheter angiography) is generally performed for delineation of arterial anatomy and to identify an appropriate target artery for distal anastomoses. If there is no target vessel or there is uncorrected inflow disease, arterial bypass surgery will have a poor outcome.

A conduit should not be constructed in an actively infected tissue bed. An infection should be aggressively treated to resolution; if vascularity is insufficient to allow healing, extra-anatomic bypass or amputation should be considered.

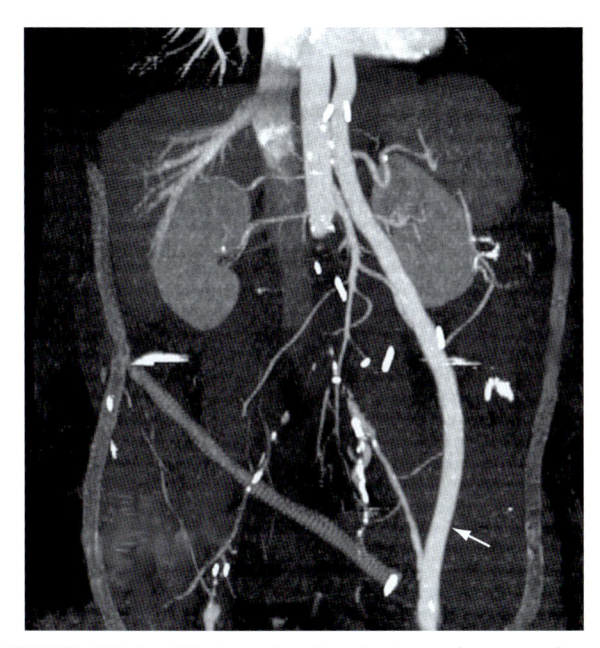

■ **FIGURE 114-6** CTA shows that there has been placement of an obturator bypass (*arrow*) in this patient who has previously had placement of an axillofemoral and right-to-left femorofemoral bypass, followed by a left axillofemoral bypass graft. Both procedures eventually failed because of chronic infection in the left inguinal region, necessitating the obturator bypass.

Outcomes and Complications

Long-term graft patency, limb salvage, and mortality are the primary reported endpoints for revascularization procedures. Relief of symptoms is subjective and thus more difficult to accurately quantify and assess.

Graft patency is described as primary, assisted primary, and secondary. Primary patency indicates that no additional procedures have been performed that involve the vascular conduit, including any graft extensions that may be required for progression of disease distally. Assisted primary patency includes any minor revisions or endovascular treatments of lesions that threaten graft patency. If the graft has thrombosed and patency is restored by thrombolysis, thrombectomy and revision, or other means, this is considered secondary patency.

Complications and lesions that threaten vascular conduit longevity include infection, development of anastomotic stenoses (Fig. 114-7) or pseudoaneurysms, progression of disease distal to the graft resulting in inadequate outflow, failure to incise all valves or to ligate all venous side branches within an in situ bypass graft, intimal hyperplasia, poor conduit quality, and degeneration of the graft. Such complications will require open surgical or endovascular correction.

Local complications, including hemorrhage, infection, and graft thrombosis, may occur at the time of the initial surgery. Hemorrhage is usually related to an anastomotic problem, such as a suture line disruption, or to a poorly ligated side branch (arterial or venous). Graft infections commonly result from hospital-acquired organisms in the early period and are increased in the presence of hematoma, lymphocele, or wound infection. Graft infections occurring more than 3 months after the bypass are usually due to microorganisms such as normal skin flora. Infections are manifested on imaging studies as perigraft fluid collections and may be confirmed with CT- or ultrasound-guided aspiration followed by culture and sensitivity testing. Special culture techniques may be required.

TABLE 114-1 Rutherford Categories of Chronic Limb Ischemia

Grade	Category	Clinical Description	Objective Criteria
0	0	Asymptomatic	Normal treadmill or reactive hyperemia test
	1	Mild claudication	Completes treadmill test; ankle pressure after exercise >50 mm Hg, but 20 mm Hg less than brachial
I	2	Moderate claudication	Between categories 1 and 3
	3	Severe claudication	Cannot complete treadmill test; ankle pressure <50 mm Hg after exercise
II	4	Ischemic rest pain	Resting ankle pressure <40 mm Hg; flat or barely pulsatile ankle or metatarsal pulse volume recording; toe pressure <30 mm Hg
III	5	Minor tissue loss; nonhealing ulcer Focal gangrene with diffuse pedal ischemia	Resting ankle pressure <60 mm Hg; flat or severely dampened ankle or metatarsal pulse volume recording; toe pressure <40 mm Hg
	6	Major tissue loss extending above transmetatarsal level; functional foot unsalvageable	Same as category 5

From Kaufman JA. Lower extremity arteries. In Kaufman JA, Lee MJ. The Requisites: Vascular and Interventional Radiology. Philadelphia, Mosby, 2004, p 421.

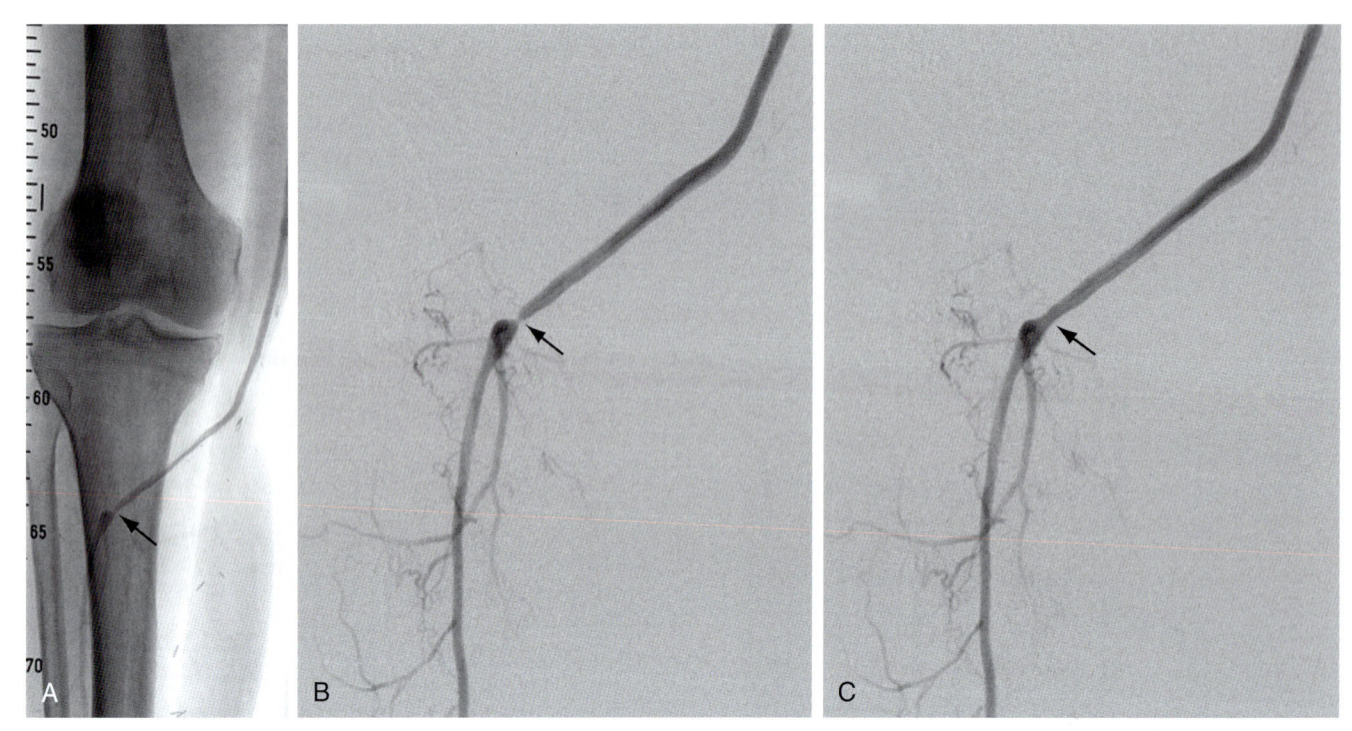

FIGURE 114-7 **A,** DSA reveals a stenosis (*arrow*) of an in situ femoropopliteal bypass graft at the distal anastomoses to the below-knee popliteal artery. **B,** Magnified DSA arteriogram delineates the high-grade distal anastomotic stenosis more clearly. **C,** The anastomotic stenosis was treated with balloon angioplasty, successfully eliminating the stenosis and maintaining graft patency. This is an example of assisted primary patency.

TABLE 114-2 Above-Knee Femoropopliteal Grafts

Primary Patency*	1 month	6 months	1 year	2 years	3 years	4 years
Reversed saphenous vein	99	91	84	82	73	69
Arm vein	99	—	82	65	60	60
Human umbilical vein	95	90	82	82	70	70
ePTFE	—	89	79	74	66	60

*All patencies expressed as percentages; all series published since 1981.
From Mills JL Sr. Infrainguinal bypass. In Rutherford RB (ed). Vascular Surgery, 6th ed. Philadelphia, WB Saunders, 2005, p 1166.

TABLE 114-3 Below-Knee Femoropopliteal Grafts

Patency*	1 month	6 months	1 year	2 years	3 years	4 years
Primary						
In situ or reversed saphenous vein	95-98	87-90	80-84	76-79	73-78	68-77
Secondary						
Arm or in situ vein	97	96	83-96	83-89	73-86	70-81
Human umbilical vein	88	82	77	70	61	60
ePTFE	96	80	68	61	44	40
Limb Salvage						
In situ or reversed saphenous vein	97-99	92-97	90-94	84-88	83-86	75

*All patencies expressed as percentages; all series published since 1981.
From Mills JL Sr. Infrainguinal bypass. In Rutherford RB (ed). Vascular Surgery, 6th ed. Philadelphia, WB Saunders, 2005, p 1166.

The outcomes of various infrainguinal bypass procedures with use of currently available vascular conduits are summarized in Tables 114-2 to 114-4. With regard to extra-anatomic bypass grafts, the long-term patency rates are typically lower than for the anatomically positioned grafts. The obturator bypass graft for infrainguinal occlusive disease has reported patency rates of 73% and 57% at 1 and 5 years, respectively, which are somewhat lower than with conventional femoropopliteal bypass.[8]

TABLE 114-4 Infrapopliteal Grafts

Patency*	1 month	6 months	1 year	2 years	3 years	4 years
Primary						
In situ or reversed saphenous vein	92-94	81-84	77-82	70-76	66-74	62-68
Secondary						
In situ or reversed saphenous vein	93-95	89-90	84-89	80-87	78-84	76-81
Arm vein	94		73	62	58	
Human umbilical vein	80	65	52	46	40	37
ePTFE	89	58	46	32		21
Limb Salvage						
In situ or reversed saphenous vein	95-96	88	85-91	83-88	82-83	82-83
ePTFE	—	76	68	60	56	48

*All patencies expressed as percentages; all series published since 1981.
From Mills JL Sr. Infrainguinal bypass. In Rutherford RB (ed). Vascular Surgery, 6th ed. Philadelphia, WB Saunders, 2005, p 1166.

Imaging Findings

Preoperative Planning

Determination of the appropriate bypass procedure depends on both the arterial inflow and the distal target vessel. Imaging of the pelvis is mandatory to exclude any iliac artery steno-occlusive disease. Any significant arterial inflow lesions should be corrected before construction of the infrainguinal vascular conduit. In addition, any disease that involves the origin and proximal portion of the profunda femoral artery should be identified and corrected. Detailed runoff information is necessary for determination of the appropriate target vessel for the distal anastomosis of the vascular conduit. Selection of the distal target should ideally allow all hemodynamically significant disease to be bypassed and provide for at least a single continuously patent runoff artery.

Postoperative Surveillance

Surveillance of bypass grafts is critical to ensure long-term patency given that a relatively high percentage of vascular conduits develop problems that threaten longevity. Early identification of any stenoses that may potentially compromise the graft may allow treatment before the graft progresses to thrombosis. The simplest and most effective surveillance tool is duplex ultrasonography coupled with ankle-brachial index measurement. The initial study is generally obtained within the first month of surgery; serial examinations are then performed every 3 months for the first year, every 6 months for the next 2 years, and then annually.

A failing graft caused by a focal lesion may have an elevated peak systolic velocity (>300 cm/sec) or a velocity ratio above 3.5 to 4.0; the velocity ratio is defined as the peak systolic velocity distal to the lesion divided by the peak systolic velocity proximal to the lesion. If low-flow velocities (peak systolic velocity <45 cm/sec) gradually develop throughout the graft or the ankle-brachial index drops by more than 0.15, other imaging, such as CTA, MRA, or catheter angiography, may be necessary.

Although a variety of problems may lead to a failing graft, the most common one in the first 2 years is intimal hyperplasia. Later culprits are inflow and outflow lesions, which cause reduced blood flow in the graft and manifest as stenoses or occlusions on imaging studies, and progression of disease in the distal runoff vessels, resulting in lack of outflow.

REVASCULARIZATION PROCEDURE: ENDOVASCULAR TREATMENT OF STENOSIS AND OCCLUSIONS

Description and Special Anatomic Considerations

Both percutaneous transluminal angioplasty and intravascular stent placement have become widely accepted as primary treatment of infrainguinal peripheral arterial disease so that endovascular treatments now have an extremely important role in its management. Application of endovascular therapies remains a dynamic process as currently available technology evolves and new treatment devices and options are introduced (e.g., atherectomy, covered stents, cryoplasty, drug-eluting stents, lasers, biodegradable stents).

The most frequently employed endovascular treatment options are angioplasty and intravascular stent placement. Angioplasty may be used as a stand-alone primary therapy (Figs. 114-8 and 114-9) or may be combined with stent placement. Stents provide an intravascular scaffold for the vessel lumen and are available in a variety of materials, configurations, and delivery systems. Stents may be constructed from stainless steel, platinum, Elgiloy, and nitinol and may be combined with ePTFE or Dacron to produce a covered stent endoprosthesis or "stent graft." Noncovered stents may be constructed with "open" or "closed cell" designs, which influence stent flexibility, conformability, radial strength, fracture resistance, and restenosis rates. In addition, there are balloon-mounted and self-expanding stents available in both the noncovered and covered groups (Figs. 114-10 and 114-11). Balloon-mounted stents are typically sized to correspond to the desired diameter of the vessel lumen, whereas self-

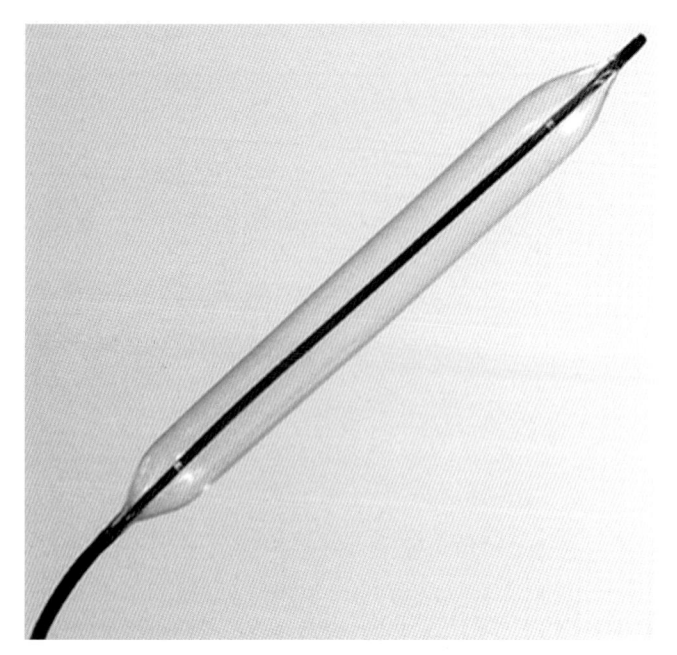

FIGURE 114-8 Angioplasty balloons are available in various lengths and diameters and have varying burst pressures, depending on the material from which they are constructed. This is a noncompliant balloon, meaning that the balloon will retain a tubular shape and will not conform to the vessel luminal characteristics by expanding beyond the manufacturer's predetermined maximum diameter.

expanding stents are usually oversized and may require secondary angioplasty to achieve a satisfactory diameter.

Given the decreased restenosis rates in the coronary arteries that have resulted from use of drug-eluting stents, there has been considerable enthusiasm for extending the application to treatment of the lower extremity arteries. Initial results have been mixed, but clinical trials remain ongoing.

Atherectomy involves a catheter-based atherosclerotic plaque excision system consisting of two components: a low-profile monorail excision catheter and a palm-sized power drive unit. A tiny rotating blade housed near the catheter tip is exposed when activated, removing and capturing thin shavings of plaque from the arterial wall into a collection chamber. Atherectomy thus permits "debulking" of atheroma from the lesion and may be used as a primary therapy or in combination with other endovascular treatment options. Catheters vary in diameter and tip length to accommodate various lesions (Figs. 114-12 and 114-13).

Cryoplasty is an angioplasty-based technology that uses liquid nitrous oxide as the balloon inflation medium, which lowers the balloon surface temperature to −10° C. Theoretically, cryoplasty causes an altered plaque response in which, as a result of freezing, microfractures form and weaken the plaque, contributing to a more uniform vessel dilation and less injury to the media. There may also be less elastic recoil and an induction of cellular apoptosis through freezing (Fig. 114-14).[9,10]

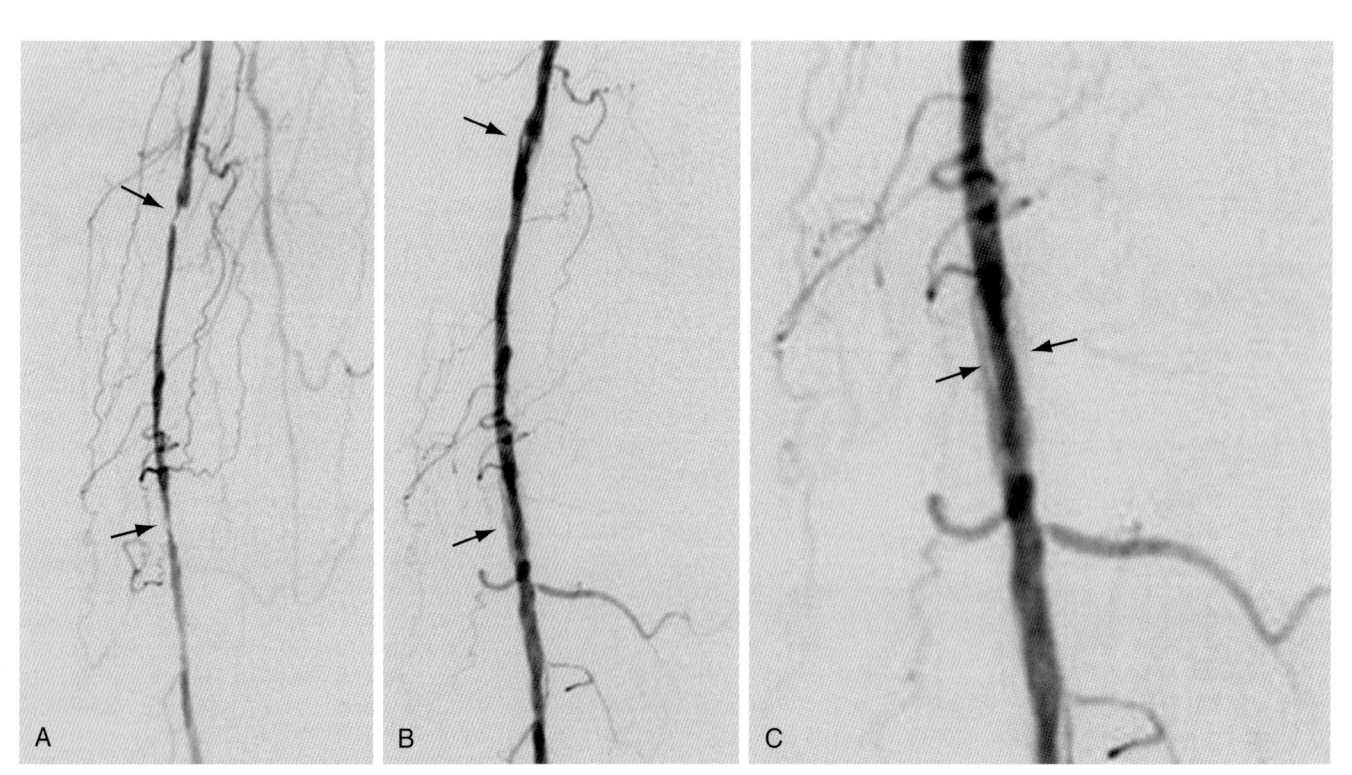

FIGURE 114-9 **A,** DSA image shows two stenoses (*arrows*) in the mid and distal superficial femoral artery. **B,** After angioplasty, there is restoration of a normal luminal caliber in the treatment areas (*arrows*). **C,** Magnification view of the distal treatment zone in **B** after angioplasty shows small linear contrast collections (*arrows*) paralleling the vessel lumen. These represent "cracks" or fissures within the plaque that have resulted from the angioplasty. The mechanism is that of a controlled fracture of the plaque, often accompanied by stretching of the muscular media. Over time, this usually remodels and assumes a more normal appearance.

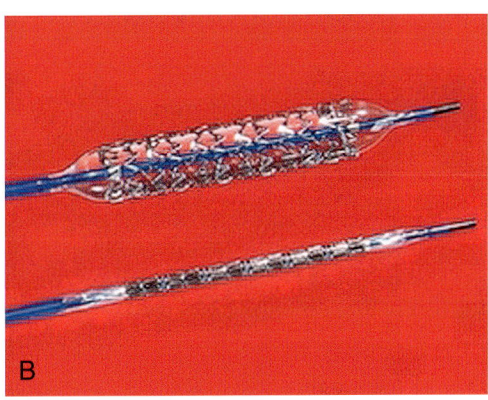

FIGURE 114-10 Noncovered stents are available as either self-expanding (**A**) or balloon mounted (**B**). The self-expanding stent is typically oversized relative to the native artery to be treated, whereas the balloon-mounted stent is more precisely sized to the native vessel diameter.

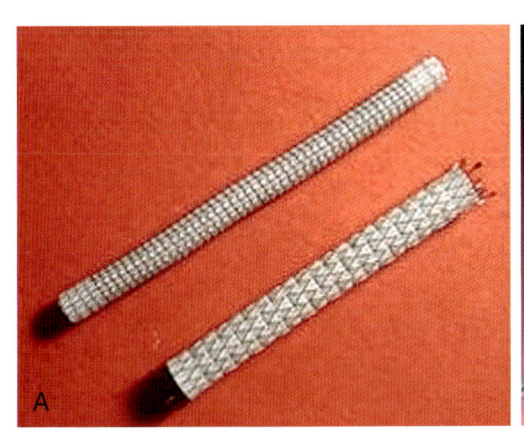

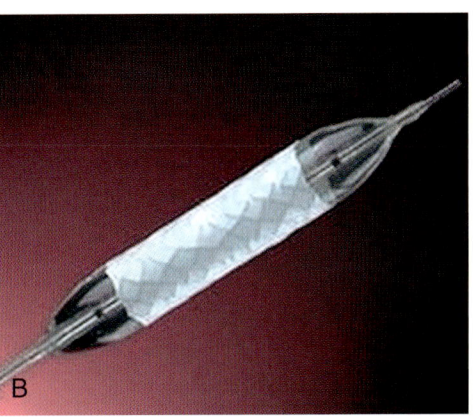

FIGURE 114-11 Covered stents (stent grafts or vascular endoprostheses) are available as either self-expanding (**A**) or balloon mounted (**B**).

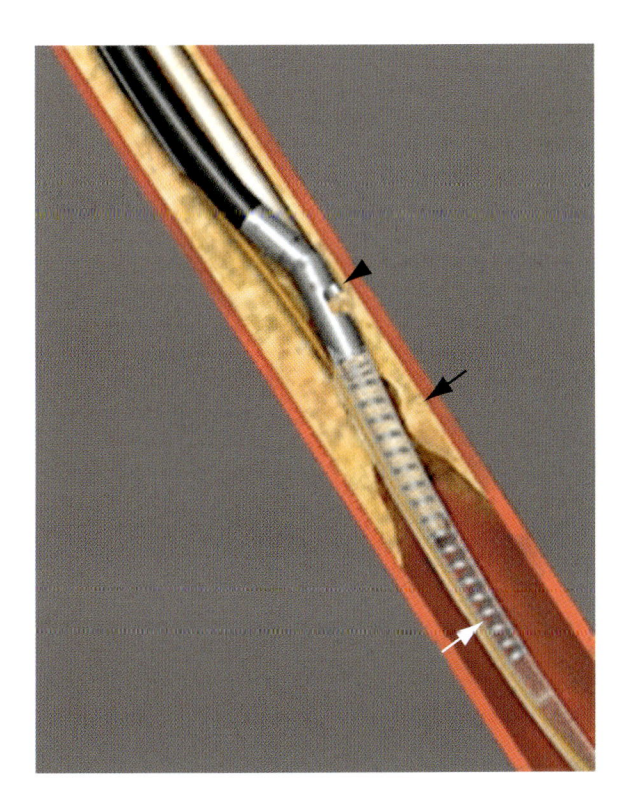

FIGURE 114-12 Graphic of the FoxHollow SilverHawk atherectomy catheter shows the cutting blade (*arrowhead*) within the cutting window engaging the atheroma (*black arrow*). As thin shavings of atheroma are excised, they are collected in the nose cone (*white arrow*) at the catheter tip.

Another angioplasty-based technology is cutting balloon angioplasty, in which multiple small atherotomes (microsurgical blades) are fixed longitudinally on the outer surface of a noncompliant balloon. These expand radially during balloon inflation, delivering longitudinal incisions into the plaque and the vessel. Theoretically, there should be advantages to cutting balloon angioplasty through reduction of vascular injury by scoring of the vessel and the plaque longitudinally rather than by causing an uncontrolled disruption of the atherosclerotic plaque. However, in a randomized trial of 1385 coronary lesions, there was no significant difference between cutting and standard angioplasty at 6-month follow-up in angiographic and clinical results. The primary endpoint of angiographic restenosis at 6 months was 31.4% in the cutting balloon angioplasty group versus 30.4% in the standard group. This trial showed that cutting balloon angioplasty is equivalent in safety and efficacy endpoints to standard angioplasty, but it did not prove superiority for the general pool of percutaneous coronary intervention patients.[11]

There are varying opinions as to the optimal endovascular treatment strategy for infrainguinal lesions with regard to angioplasty alone, angioplasty accompanied by primary stenting, and the use of noncovered versus covered stents. Treatment options depend on the route of arterial access; the type, length, and location of the lesions; the presence or absence of inflow disease; the quality of the runoff vessels distal to the lesions; the overall clinical status of the patient; and the skills and long-term success

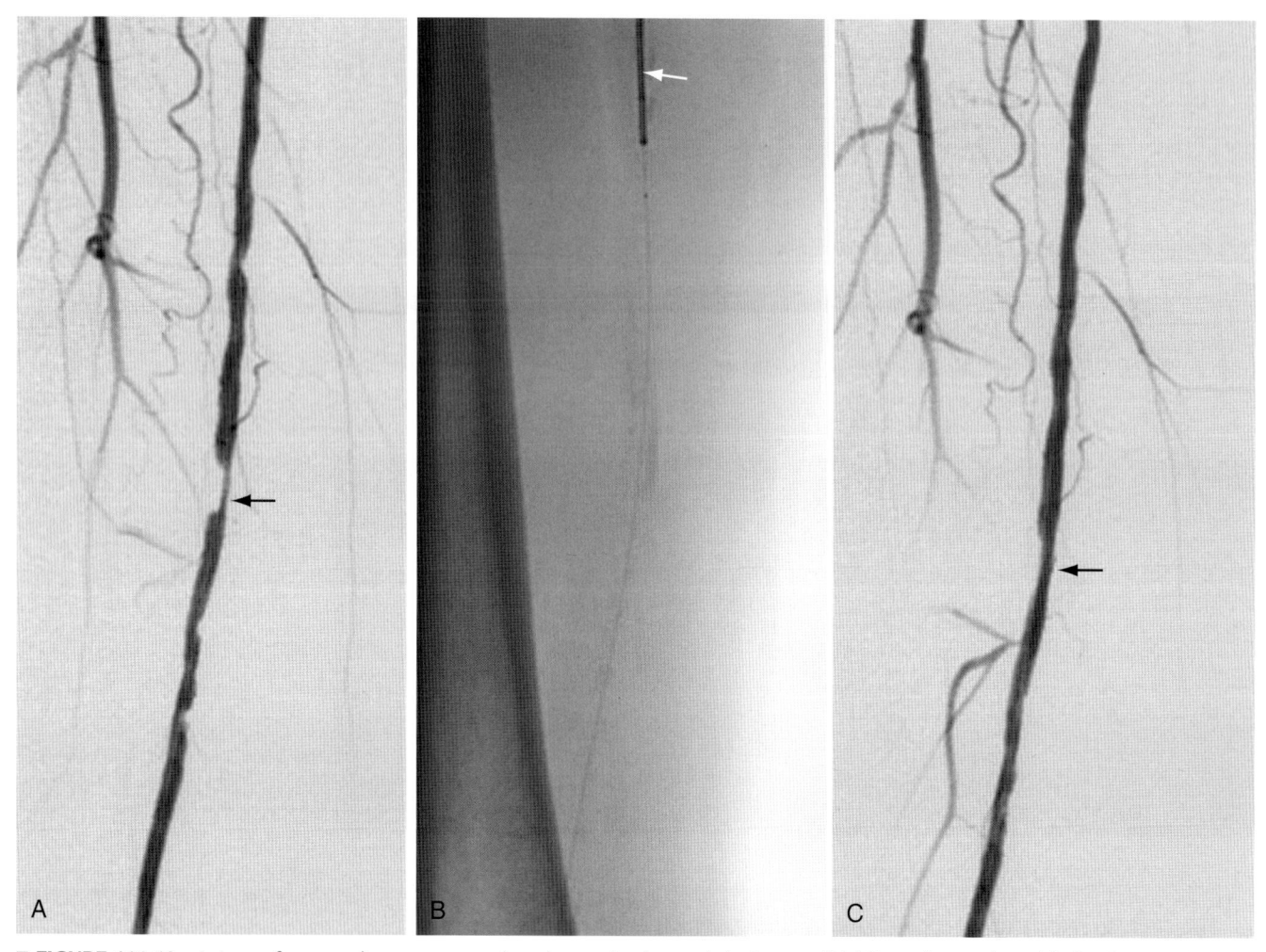

■ **FIGURE 114-13** **A,** Image from an atherectomy procedure shows a focal stenosis in the superficial femoral artery (*arrow*) before intervention. **B,** A guide wire has been advanced across the stenosis, and the atherectomy catheter (*arrow*) has been introduced. **C,** After the atherectomy, there is an almost completely normal appearance to the artery at the site of the previous stenosis (*arrow*).

rates of the operator. The cost associated with endovascular procedures is also a consideration; generally, these technologies are substantially more expensive than open surgical revascularization procedures.

Infrainguinal lesions may be treated either with an ipsilateral antegrade femoral artery puncture or from the contralateral approach, with the catheter and wire advanced across the aortic bifurcation to gain access to the arteries of the affected limb. The successful use of the latter approach depends on the distal aortic and pelvic arterial anatomy; tortuous or stenotic iliac arteries or an acutely angled aortic bifurcation may significantly complicate the negotiation of the catheter into the treatment area. This approach may be necessary for treatment of lesions that involve the common femoral or the proximal superficial or profunda femoral arteries.

Indications

Determination of which lesions are appropriate for endovascular treatment versus traditional surgical revascularization continues to be an evolving and sometimes controversial process. Addressing these concerns has resulted in multidisciplinary attempts to categorize lesions, to stratify the risks and benefits of endovascular treatment, and to propose treatment guidelines. In 1994, the American Heart Association proposed percutaneous transluminal angioplasty guidelines for endovascular versus surgical treatment. These have since been revised as longer follow-up data have become available and as intravascular stents have been incorporated into endovascular treatment regimens.

The TransAtlantic Inter-Society Consensus Working Group (TASC) developed another classification system in 2000[12] and addressed both aortoiliac and infrainguinal occlusive disease, with the latter guidelines limited to femoropopliteal disease. These guidelines were updated in 2007[13] and reflect the expanded role of endovascular therapy as a primary option in the treatment of vascular occlusive disease (Table 114-5).

Treatment choices may be influenced by the nature of the lesion to be treated. In general, short segmental stenoses respond well to angioplasty and may not require stent placement unless a significant arterial dissection or intimal flap occurs. Long-segment, diffusely diseased, or heavily calcified lesions may require stent placement to achieve and to maintain patency. Chronic total occlusions that have been successfully recanalized may also be treated

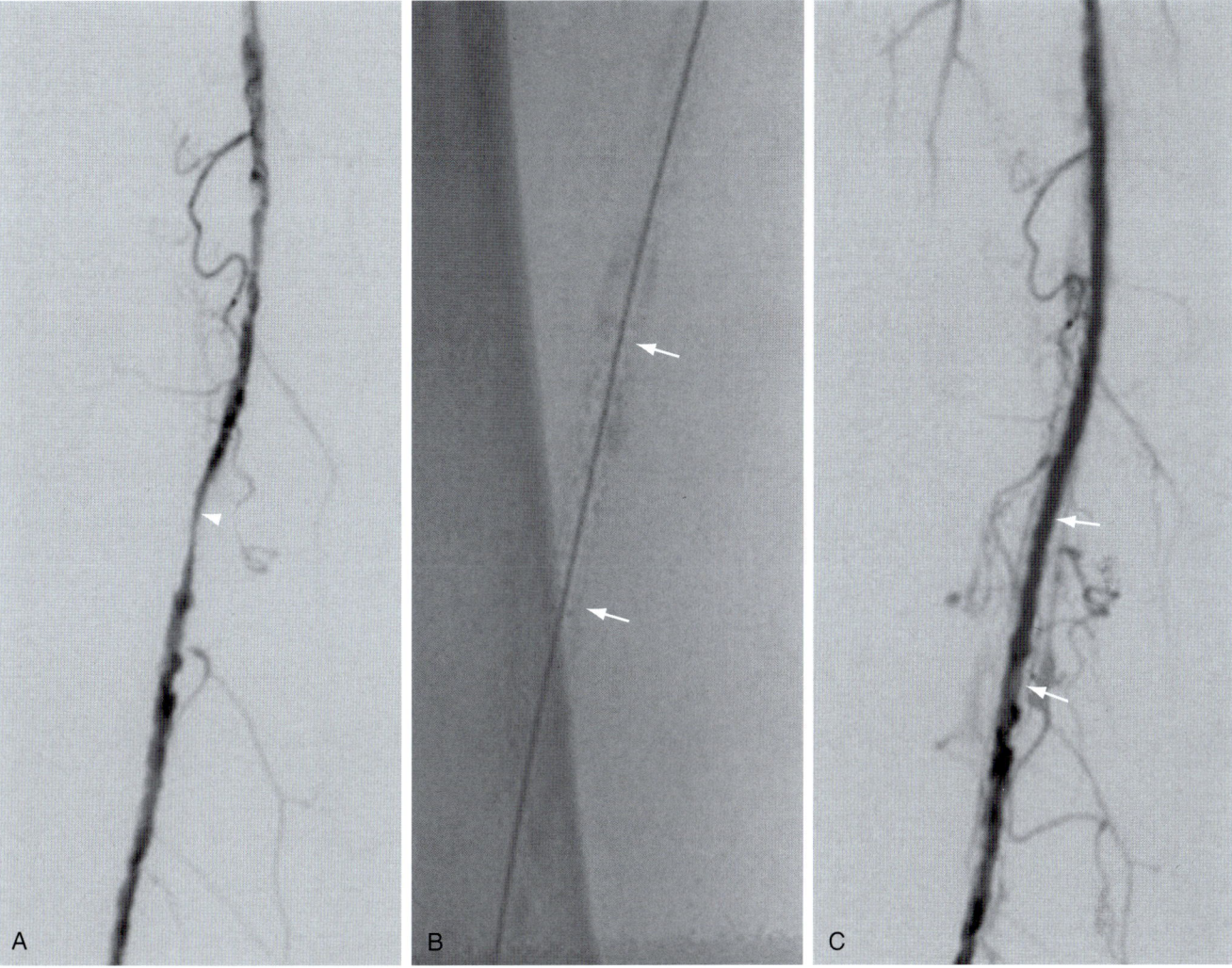

■ **FIGURE 114-14** **A**, Image from a cryoplasty procedure shows a high-grade superficial femoral artery stenosis (*arrowhead*) on the diagnostic DSA arteriogram. **B**, Fluoroscopic spot film shows that the cryoplasty balloon (*arrows*) is inflated within the stenotic area; note the atherosclerotic calcification adjacent to the cryoplasty balloon. **C**, After cryoplasty, there is a normal caliber to the arterial lumen in the treatment zone (*arrows*).

TABLE 114-5 TransAtlantic Inter-Society Consensus (TASC II) Recommendations (Femoropopliteal Arterial Disease)

Lesion Category	Lesion Characteristics	Treatment Recommendation
Type A	Single stenosis ≤10 cm in length Single occlusion ≤5 cm in length	Endovascular treatment
Type B	Multiple lesions (stenoses or occlusions), each ≤5 cm Single stenosis or occlusion ≤15 cm not involving the infrageniculate popliteal artery Single or multiple lesions in the absence of continuous tibial vessels to improve inflow for a distal bypass Heavily calcified occlusion ≤5 cm in length Single popliteal stenosis	Endovascular treatment preferred, but comorbidities, patient's preference, and operator's long-term success rates must be considered in decision
Type C	Multiple stenoses or occlusions totaling >15 cm with or without heavy calcification Recurrent stenoses or occlusions that need treatment after two endovascular interventions	Surgery preferred for good-risk patients, but comorbidities, patient's preference, and operator's long-term success rates must be considered in decision
Type D	Chronic total occlusions of common femoral artery or superficial femoral artery (>20 cm, involving the popliteal artery) Chronic total occlusion of popliteal artery and proximal trifurcation vessels	Surgery

Data from Norgren L, Hiatt WR, Dormandy JA, et al; TASC II Working Group. Inter-Society Consensus for the Management of Peripheral Arterial Disease (TASC II). J Vasc Surg 2007; 45(Suppl S):S5-S67.

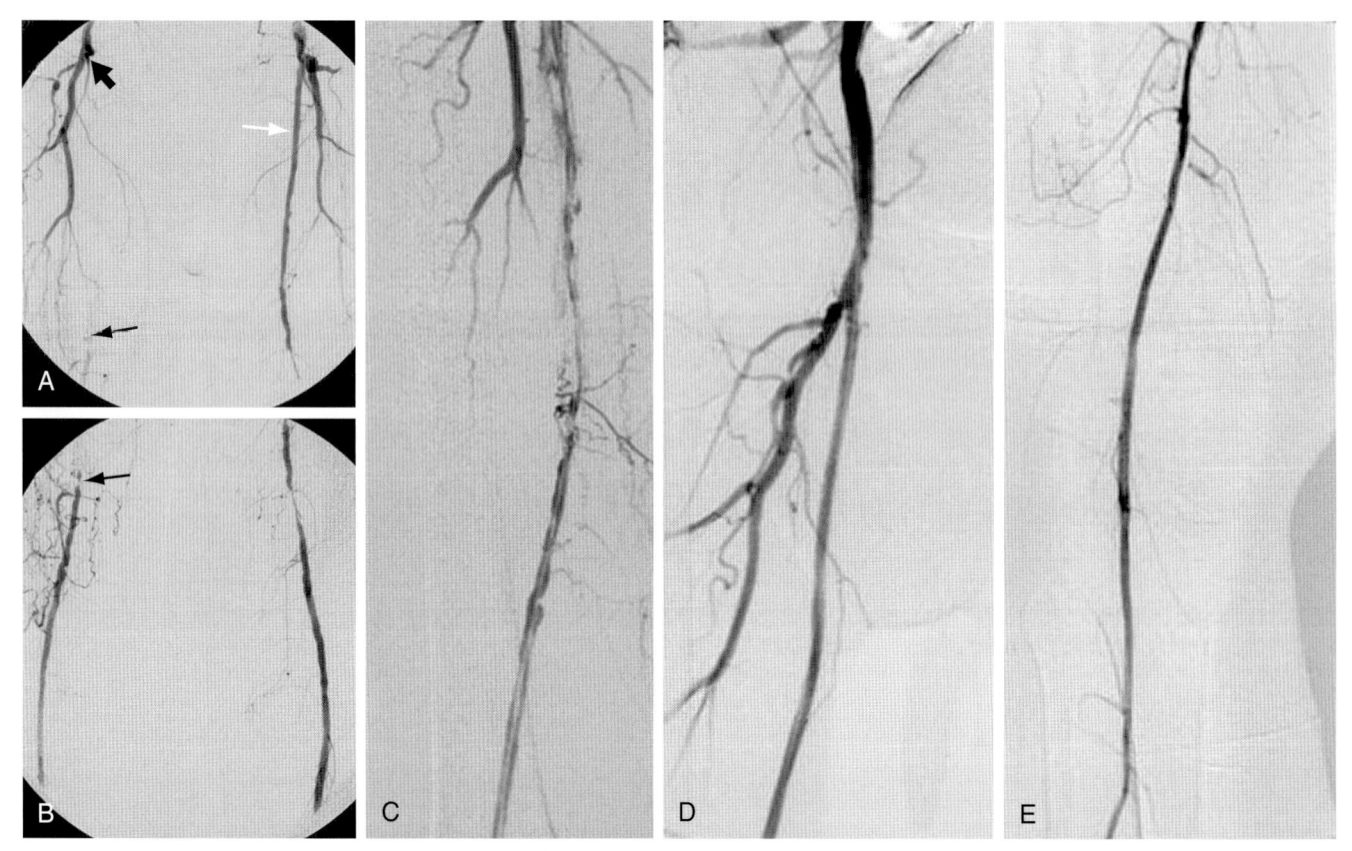

FIGURE 114-15 **A,** DSA image of the proximal thighs shows occlusion of the right superficial femoral artery (*thick black arrow*) at the femoral bifurcation, with distal reconstitution (*black arrow*) at the adductor hiatus. This is a characteristic pattern of distribution in superficial femoral artery occlusive disease. Note that the left superficial femoral artery is patent (*white arrow*). **B,** DSA image of the distal thighs shows the reconstitution of a relatively disease free above-knee popliteal artery (*arrow*). **C,** After subintimal guidewire passage and angioplasty of the superficial femoral artery occlusion, patency has been restored, but there is an irregular appearance to the vessel. This is likely to have a very poor patency rate. **D** and **E,** DSA images after placement of covered stents in the recanalized superficial femoral artery show a much more uniform appearance to the treated area both proximally (**D**) and distally (**E**). Covered rather than noncovered stents were chosen because of the lengthy subintimal guidewire passage that was necessary during the initial part of the recanalization procedure.

with either angioplasty or intravascular stent placement (Fig. 114-15). Once again, the lesion length and other characteristics may dictate the choice of treatment. Furthermore, when intravascular stents are used for treatment of recanalized chronic total occlusions, the operator must determine whether the noncovered or covered stent option is appropriate. If a lengthy subintimal guidewire passage has occurred during the recanalization process, a covered stent may be a better treatment option. The decision of whether to use a covered or noncovered stent may also be influenced by the necessity of preserving collateral vessels or by potential stent encroachment on a side branch or vessel origin. Noncovered stents allow continued perfusion of collaterals or side branches, whereas covered stents will occlude these vessels.

Contraindications

As with open vascular bypass surgery, the quality of the runoff distal to the treatment zone is a significant factor in predicting initial and long-term patency in the endovascular treatment of occlusive disease. Similarly, the characteristics of the lesion greatly affect outcomes of endovascular revascularization procedures as the aim of these procedures is essentially to repair a diseased arterial segment in situ as opposed to bypass or replacement of the diseased segment. Excessively long segments of heavily calcified, diffuse atherosclerotic disease typically are better managed with traditional surgical revascularization, unless such surgery poses an unacceptably high risk because of comorbidities. The indiscriminate application of endovascular techniques based solely on whether it is technically possible to treat a given lesion, as opposed to a patient-oriented approach, generally leads to poor outcomes. Furthermore, the endovascular specialist must consider whether the immediate or eventual failure of an endovascular procedure will preclude a later open surgical revascularization. A strategy of preserving surgical options for a patient with peripheral vascular disease should therefore be considered at the time of endovascular treatment. For example, endovascular treatment of a long segmental superficial femoral artery occlusion is acceptable if the popliteal artery is preserved as a distal target vessel should bypass surgery become necessary because of eventual endovascular failure.

Outcomes and Complications

Early experiences with stainless steel balloon-mounted stents in treating superficial femoral artery atherosclerotic disease showed no significant benefit over angioplasty alone, but more recent studies comparing angioplasty

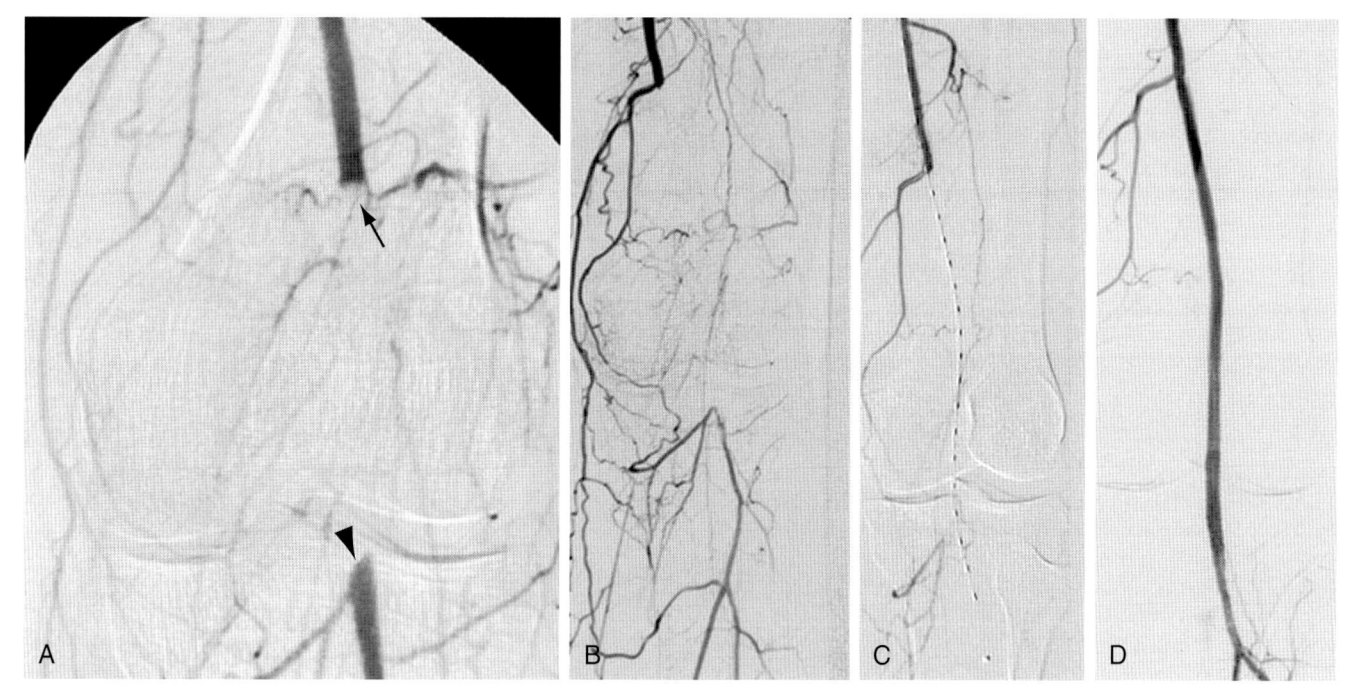

FIGURE 114-16 **A**, Acute arterial occlusion. DSA image of the left popliteal artery shows a segmental occlusion at knee joint level. There is a meniscus (*black arrow*) at the proximal margin of the occlusion and an oblique margin (*arrowhead*) distally. In addition, there are no large collateral vessels evident. This appearance is typical of an acute embolic occlusion, and the treatment is very different from that of a chronic total occlusion. Embolic occlusion is often manifested as an acutely ischemic limb and may constitute a surgical emergency. **B**, Chronic arterial occlusion. DSA image of the popliteal artery in a patient with chronic popliteal artery occlusion. The proximal end of the occlusion ends in well-developed collaterals that then reconstitute the distal runoff vessels. There is a convex end to the proximal occlusion rather than the meniscoid filling defect that is seen with an acute embolus (compare with **A**). **C** and **D**, DSA images during catheter-directed thrombolysis of the chronic occlusion demonstrate the multiple side-hole infusion catheter that was successfully passed through the occlusion, and a core wire with multiple miniature ultrasound transducers was placed through the catheter (**C**). The multiple radiopaque markers represent the transducers, which act to relax the fibrin strands of the thrombus and thus increase the surface area that is exposed to the catheter-infused thrombolytic agent. After successful thrombolysis, patency was restored, but because of intimal irregularity, a flexible covered stent was placed in the popliteal artery (**D**).

with self-expanding nitinol stents have shown decreased restenosis rates with primary stenting.[1-3] Other studies have reported superiority of ePTFE-covered stents over angioplasty alone.[4] Many centers now use endovascular revascularization procedures as a first-line therapy in appropriate patients with chronic occlusive disease and reserve open surgical bypass for endovascular failures.[5,6] A recent randomized trial that compared use of covered stents with femoropopliteal bypass surgery using a prosthetic vascular conduit for treatment of superficial femoral artery occlusive disease showed no significant difference in 1-year patency rates.[6]

There is a paucity of good clinical data regarding the use of more recently introduced technologies, such as atherectomy, cryoplasty, and drug-eluting stents. There are published data for single-center experiences as well as clinical registries for these devices, which it is hoped will aid in defining the role of these new options in treating lower extremity occlusive disease.

Thus, although there are no good long-term data for the endovascular treatment of superficial femoral artery occlusive disease, there are ongoing clinical trials that are attempting to address which endovascular therapies may have better patency rates and longevity. Given the variety of endovascular treatment options available and the lack of long-term data for every available therapy, appropriate science-based treatment algorithms are problematic and are continually evolving.

There is no doubt that endovascular treatment will continue to be integral in treating lower extremity peripheral arterial disease. It is likely to have an even more expanded role as technology continues to improve and long-term data become more available.

Imaging Findings

The distribution and characteristics of the arterial lesions to be treated with one of the numerous endovascular techniques may aid in determining which treatment modality may be most appropriate and have the highest potential for success. Factors such as lesion length, vessel diameter, amount of calcification, anatomic location, presence or absence of collaterals, quality of inflow and distal runoff, and potential routes of access must all be considered in the decision process. In addition, it is important to base the choice of whether to proceed with an endovascular treatment on the clinical situation rather than on anatomic characteristics alone. Some patients may benefit more from an exercise program or a surgical bypass than from angioplasty, stenting, or other endovascular therapies.

Understanding of the disease process that has resulted in the pathologic changes is also important in determining the optimal intervention. The appropriate treatment for embolic occlusion, for example, will differ considerably from the treatment of a chronic total occlusion (Fig. 114-16A,B). Various pathologic entities may have

TABLE 114-6 Clinical Categories of Acute Limb Ischemia

Category	Definition	Prognosis	Physical Examination		Doppler Signals	
			Sensory Loss	Muscle Weakness	Arterial	Venous
I	Viable	Not immediately threatened	None	None	+	+
II	Threatened					
IIa	Marginally	Salvageable with prompt treatment	Minimal	None	Occasional	+
IIb	Immediately	Salvageable with immediate treatment	Rest pain	Mild to moderate	Rare	+
III	Irreversible	Major permanent tissue loss	Anesthetic	Paralysis	−	−

From Kaufman JA. Lower extremity arteries. In Kaufman JA, Lee MJ. The Requisites: Vascular and Interventional Radiology. Philadelphia, Mosby, 2004, p 432.

characteristic appearances (e.g., stenotic vs. aneurysmal disease), whereas others may appear similar (e.g., various vasculitides).

A high-quality imaging study such as CTA, MRA, or catheter angiography, depicting the arterial anatomy, is necessary for determination of the appropriate intervention. During the endovascular procedure, angiographic images are obtained to evaluate the progress of the intervention, to determine the appropriate endpoint, and to assess for any untoward events (such as vessel dissection, perforation, and distal embolization). It is extremely important during any intervention to document the status of the runoff anatomy before and after treatment.

REVASCULARIZATION PROCEDURE: SURGICAL THROMBOEMBOLECTOMY

Description and Special Anatomic Considerations

Lower extremity arterial occlusions resulting from distal embolization or acute thrombosis may manifest as a profoundly ischemic limb and constitute a surgical emergency. Initially, the underlying cause of the occlusion should be determined (e.g., cardiac embolus from atrial fibrillation or myocardial infarction versus in situ thrombosis associated with atherosclerosis). The patient's clinical history and the nature of the symptoms frequently suggest the etiology of the occlusion. Embolic occlusions usually cause more severe ischemia because of the lack of collaterals, whereas thrombosis in the presence of preexisting disease may be better tolerated because there are established collaterals. The decision about appropriate imaging, such as angiography, is based on the clinical status of the limb, the presumed etiology of the occlusion, and the need to visualize distal runoff. Imaging is important in management as it localizes the level of obstruction, determines if there are multiple levels of occlusion, assesses for inflow and outflow disease, and guides the appropriate site for the arteriotomy. Surgical intervention is usually the primary consideration in treating acute limb ischemia, although endovascular treatment options are available. Surgical thrombectomy with Fogarty balloon catheters is often an effective treatment, but if it is unsuccessful, vascular bypass surgery may be necessary. Some patients may also require surgical fasciotomy if a compartment syndrome has developed. Endovascular options are appropriate when the limb is sufficiently perfused to allow pharmacologic or mechanical thrombolysis.

Treatment of an acutely thrombosed surgical bypass graft may be influenced by additional factors, such as progression of disease involving the native inflow or outflow arteries and the nature of the vascular conduit itself.

Indications

The clinical presentation of the patient and the severity of the limb ischemia usually dictate the appropriate therapy. A classification system for categorization of the acutely ischemic limb serves to direct the intervention. This classification is detailed in Table 114-6.

Contraindications

Thrombolytic therapy may have advantages over surgical thrombectomy, particularly in the treatment of thrombosed surgical vein conduits. Fogarty balloon embolectomy may damage the endothelium of a vein graft and thus increase potential thrombogenicity. Synthetic conduits, however, usually respond well to surgical thromboembolectomy. Patients who have profound limb ischemia are at a high risk for limb loss and thus require rapid revascularization. One must be vigilant for life-threatening reperfusion syndrome; profound acidosis, hyperkalemia, myoglobinuria, renal failure, and even death may occur. Primary amputation may be more appropriate in some patients with irreversible limb ischemia.

Outcomes and Complications

Surgical thromboembolectomy of an acutely ischemic limb with an inflatable balloon catheter is considered a relatively minor and technically simple operation. However, there may be high perioperative mortality that can be attributed to serious underlying cardiac disease or to the consequences of reperfusion of the ischemic limb and subsequent release of toxic metabolites. On occasion, pulmonary emboli may result from secondary venous thrombi, or there may be reactive hyperemia after successful revascularization that may increase cardiac workload of the heart and cause acute cardiac failure. There are studies that report a 30-day mortality exceeding 20% and amputation rates above 10% after arterial embolectomy. Several studies have also shown that older patients have a higher mortality rate,[14] and mortality is greater with proximal occlusions than with distal occlusions.[15-18] A short duration of symptoms before embolectomy has been reported to increase mortality, whereas other authors have found no effect on mortality. According to Levy and Butcher,[14] severe ischemia did not increase the mortality rate, whereas Balas and colleagues[19] concluded the opposite. Many studies report higher amputation rates when embolectomy was delayed[14,15,19]; other authors have found no adverse effect of delayed treatment.[20-22] High amputation rates have also been associated with age, advanced arteriosclerotic disease,[19] severe ischemic symptoms, and thrombotic compared with embolic occlusion.[23] In addition, there is a worse prognosis the more distally the occlusion is located, and the prognosis is also worse with common femoral emboli than at other sites.

Imaging Findings

Patients with clinical evidence of acute embolic or thrombotic occlusion may require emergent CTA or catheter angiography, followed by thromboembolectomy and subsequent endovascular or surgical interventions and vascular reconstruction if there is profound limb ischemia. For patients with moderate ischemia (TASC acute limb ischemia category IIa), initial diagnostic angiography should be performed, followed by primary thrombectomy and subsequent intraoperative angiography with immediate endovascular or operative treatment of remaining vascular problems. As an alternative therapeutic option, if the limb remains well perfused, catheter-directed thrombolytic infusion therapy may be appropriate in selected patients, with the intention of subsequent limb revascularization or unmasking of relevant disease that may allow endovascular or surgical vascular reconstruction.

In either situation, it is important to have preoperative or intraoperative images of the arterial inflow, the compromised vascular segments, and the outflow anatomy. In cases of embolic occlusion, there may be multiple areas of involvement, and emboli may be bilateral. In addition, if the emboli are from a cardiac source, compromise of the renal or mesenteric vasculature must be excluded. Thus, the clinical presentation of the patient will dictate the scope and proper choice of imaging.

REVASCULARIZATION PROCEDURE: CATHETER-DIRECTED OR PHARMACOMECHANICAL THROMBOLYSIS

Description and Special Anatomic Considerations

In contrast to the surgical management of thromboembolic disease, endovascular therapy employs both mechanical and pharmacologic methods for thrombolysis. With regard to the pharmacologic approach, a catheter is introduced into the occluded segment and a drug is infused that activates plasminogen and thus initiates thrombolysis. A variety of thrombolytic agents have been used, including streptokinase, urokinase, and recombinant tissue plasminogen activator (alteplase, tPA) and its derivative (reteplase, r-PA). The first two agents are now infrequently used for intra-arterial thrombolysis, mainly because of improvements in available agents. The newer plasminogen activating agents are now the agents of choice, with the activity of these agents enhanced in the presence of fibrin. All of these agents eventually fragment and dissolve thrombus and generally are most effective in the presence of acute or subacute thrombosis. When thrombosis is chronic and well organized, thrombolysis is much less successful.

For intra-arterial pharmacologic thrombolysis to be most effective, a catheter must first be advanced across the occluded segment; inability to cross the thrombosed segment generally indicates a more chronic process that will probably respond poorly to thrombolysis. A variety of infusion catheters are available; the majority are constructed with multiple side holes that allow maximal exposure of the surface area of the thrombus to the pharmacologic agent. Thrombolysis may be accelerated by the forceful pulsed injection of the fibrinolytic agent directly into the clot. Newer catheter systems combine pharmacologic with mechanical thrombolysis by use of ultrasound or rheolytic technologies to enhance drug activity (Fig. 114-16C,D).

There are also percutaneous mechanical thrombectomy devices available that are designed to achieve thrombolysis without use of pharmacologic agents. These devices use a variety of techniques that include forceful fluid jets, suction, lasers, ultrasound, rotating baskets or coils, and impellers. Whereas many of these were originally designed for declotting of dialysis grafts, they are often used intra-arterially.

Indications

Catheter-directed thrombolysis is indicated in the lower extremities when there is symptomatic acute or subacute thrombotic arterial occlusion. It is also used in the treatment of occluded surgical bypass grafts or endovascular stents, for restoration of patency; often, thrombolysis will demonstrate a high-grade stenosis that has progressed to thrombotic occlusion and may be treated with angioplasty or stenting.

Mechanical thrombectomy devices are most effective in fresh thrombus and are often used in patients with a contraindication to pharmacologic thrombolysis. They may also be used in combination with a pharmacologic agent to rapidly reduce the volume of thrombus and thus shorten the duration of treatment.

Contraindications

Thrombolysis is contraindicated in patients in whom there is irreversible limb ischemia because the reperfusion will result in severe metabolic consequences. Patients who are currently experiencing active bleeding, have recently undergone major surgery, have had recent stroke or craniotomy, or have primary or metastatic brain tumors generally are poor candidates for pharmacologic thrombolysis because of the potential for significant bleeding complications. A profoundly ischemic limb may be inappropriate for thrombolysis because the time requirements for successful treatment may be prohibitive; these patients require rapid restoration of arterial circulation to avoid limb loss. Surgical intervention with thromboembolectomy and bypass may therefore be more appropriate in such patients.

Outcomes and Complications

The success of pharmacomechanical thrombolysis is highest in short-segment occlusions that are acute or subacute (<6 months). Technical success, which is defined as recanalization of the artery and restoration of antegrade blood flow, with less than 5% residual thrombus, can be achieved in a high percentage of patients. Clinical success rates, in which there is a return to pre-thrombosis baseline status, vary, depending on whether the treatment involves the native arterial circulation, an autogenous or synthetic surgical bypass graft, or a thrombosed intravascular stent. Although graft patency can initially be restored in most patients, the 5-year primary patency rate is low, even with close surveillance. Even with surgical graft revision after successful thrombolysis, there is a 5-year primary patency rate of only around 50%, probably due to a combination of progression of disease and permanent vessel wall damage. In addition, if there is no distal runoff beyond the occluded segment, patency usually will not be maintained after thrombolysis, either alone or in combination with surgery.

The major complications of thrombolytic therapy include hemorrhage (access site and elsewhere), reperfusion syndrome, distal embolization, pericatheter thrombosis, and allergic or idiosyncratic drug reactions.

Imaging Findings

Thrombolytic therapy is performed only after a diagnostic study such as CTA, MRA, or catheter angiography has documented the extent of disease and the quality of the arterial runoff. The diagnostic study can also aid in determining the optimal approach (e.g., antegrade puncture vs. contralateral access) for introduction of the thrombolytic infusion catheter or mechanical device. Once thrombolysis is initiated, intermittent repeated imaging of the treatment zone is necessary for evaluation of the response to therapy. The duration of thrombolytic therapy may be prolonged because long infusion times are sometimes required for restoration of patency. It is also important that the cause of the thrombosis (e.g., anastomotic stenosis, distal progression of disease, graft degeneration) be demonstrated on the imaging study and corrected by the appropriate surgical or endovascular means.

One should always re-evaluate the runoff anatomy after catheter-directed or mechanical thrombolysis; distal embolization of embolic or thrombotic debris may occur during treatment.

EXCLUSION PROCEDURE: SURGICAL EXCISION AND VASCULAR BYPASS

Description and Special Anatomic Considerations

Aneurysms of the lower extremity arteries, although less common than in the thoracoabdominal aorta, are nonetheless an important disease process that may require surgical revascularization. Such aneurysms include degenerative or true aneurysms, in which all layers of the arterial wall are involved, and pseudoaneurysms, which do not include all layers. Pseudoaneurysms are often iatrogenic or post-traumatic. The choice of bypass surgery or endovascular repair depends on the aneurysm location and the clinical presentation. Iatrogenic post-catheterization pseudoaneurysms commonly involve the common femoral artery and are generally treated percutaneously, with certain exceptions as discussed later.

Vascular trauma involves the lower extremities in up to one third of patients. It may be either blunt or penetrating; treatment varies according to the type and extent of injury. Small intimal injuries or arteriovenous fistulas may spontaneously resolve, whereas major injuries may require open repair that involves vascular reconstruction or bypass. Injuries to small branch vessels may be amenable to coil embolization. Several other entities may require arterial surgical excision and vascular bypass.

Popliteal Artery Entrapment

With popliteal artery entrapment, functional or anatomic forms of the entity may be present. The functional form is caused by hypertrophy of the calf muscles and resultant compression of the neurovascular structures in the popliteal canal with exercise; it is seen in highly trained athletes, such as runners. This is a transient phenomenon, therefore, and typically does not result in injury to the popliteal artery. In the anatomic form, the popliteal artery has an abnormal anatomic relationship to the calf muscles (gastrocnemius and popliteus), causing muscle compression of the artery during exercise. This eventually results in thickening and fibrosis and may progress to aneurysm formation, arterial thrombosis, or distal embolization. This form occurs more often in men and at a later age (fifth decade) than the functional form. Four types of anatomic entrapment are described on the basis of the relationship of the artery to the calf muscles. A fifth type is used to describe venous entrapment, and the functional form of entrapment is termed the sixth type.

Arterial Adventitial Cystic Disease

Adventitial cystic disease is an unusual and rare entity in which the popliteal arterial lumen is compressed by cystic accumulations of mucinous fluid within the adventitia. Men are predominantly affected during the fourth and fifth decades. It was previously believed that operative cyst evacuation was ineffective and that this entity always required surgical excision and bypass. However, this has now become the preferred treatment in patients in whom there is no arterial occlusive process and is used with increasing frequency. Aspiration of the cysts under ultrasound or CT guidance has had disappointing results because there is usually rapid reaccumulation of fluid.

Arteriovenous Fistula and Malformation

Arteriovenous fistulas (AVFs) and vascular anomalies such as venous or arteriovenous malformations are also

FIGURE 114-17 Arteriovenous fistula. DSA image obtained during popliteal angiography shows simultaneous filling of the popliteal artery (*arrow*) and vein (*arrowhead*), indicating an arteriovenous communication. This was an iatrogenic arteriovenous fistula as a result of a retrograde popliteal artery puncture performed during an endovascular procedure.

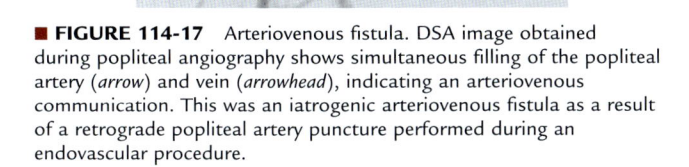

managed by exclusion procedures. AVFs may be managed surgically through ligation of the involved vessels, but endovascular treatment with embolization or covered stent placement has become the treatment of choice in many of these lesions (Fig. 114-17). Vascular anomalies are also generally treated by transcatheter delivery of embolic agents, although there are cases in which combined endovascular and surgical techniques have been effectively used.

Indications

Popliteal artery aneurysms are degenerative in more than 90% of cases and are bilateral in 60% to 70%. Thrombosis of the aneurysm or distal embolization of mural thrombus occurs far more frequently than rupture, which is the least frequent complication (Fig. 114-18). Popliteal artery aneurysms should be treated before the patient becomes symptomatic because nearly 50% of patients with asymptomatic aneurysms will develop distal ischemia within 5 years. Treatment is indicated in all symptomatic aneurysms and in asymptomatic aneurysms more than 2 cm in diameter. Surgical excision and bypass is the traditional treatment; the vascular conduit options include autogenous and prosthetic.

Pseudoaneurysms of the common femoral artery occur more frequently than true aneurysms and are frequently related to catheterization procedures or vascular anastomoses. Post-catheterization pseudoaneurysms may often be treated nonoperatively, whereas surgical revision is required if the anastomotic aneurysm is of sufficient size. Small femoral pseudoaneurysms that are a result of catheterization procedures may be treated with percutaneous thrombin injection. This has largely replaced ultrasound compression of the pseudoaneurysm as the preferred treatment. Pseudoaneurysms involving the brachial or axillary arteries are generally treated with surgical evacuation and primary arterial repair as necessary; even a small pseudoaneurysm may potentially compress adjacent nerves, with resultant sensory and motor deficits. Furthermore, thrombin injection can potentially result in upper extremity arterial thrombosis or distal embolization to the hand or digits.

True degenerative common femoral artery aneurysms larger than 2.5 cm are typically treated with surgical excision and bypass. Other true degenerative aneurysms that occur in the lower extremities are much less common; when they are identified in the superficial femoral artery, profunda femoral artery, or tibial artery, an evaluation should be initiated for an unusual etiology, such as the Ehlers-Danlos syndrome (Fig. 114-19).

Popliteal artery entrapment is manifested as exercise-induced calf and foot claudication; when these symptoms are present in a young person with no risk factors for atherosclerotic disease, this diagnosis should be considered. With the functional form, the ankle-brachial index is normal at rest, whereas it is abnormal in up to 30% of individuals with the anatomic form. As previously noted, when this entity is left untreated, there may be progression to aneurysm formation, arterial occlusion, or distal embolization. All patients with entrapment of types I to V are typically offered surgery when they are diagnosed. At exploration, if the popliteal artery is patent and undamaged, treatment is confined to resection of the entrapment mechanism. In the presence of arterial disease, the popliteal artery is resected and replaced with a saphenous vein graft after resection of the entrapment. Treatment of the functional form is much less well defined; surgical intervention is individualized.

Patients who are diagnosed with adventitial cystic disease and who fail to respond to surgical cyst evacuation or in whom there has been progression to arterial occlusion require arterial bypass. The adjacent greater or small saphenous veins are the conduits of choice.

Whereas conservative management may be appropriate for small iatrogenic AVFs, early surgical or endovascular repair is indicated in most AVFs of a traumatic nature. Several studies show that less morbidity and mortality is associated with early repair than with delayed treatment; delayed treatment may allow the development of significant venous hypertension. Treatment of vascular malformations is dictated by the patient's symptoms.

Contraindications

As previously noted, anastomotic pseudoaneurysms require surgical revision if they are sufficiently large. Currently, there are no satisfactory endovascular treatment options as pseudoaneurysms associated with vascular

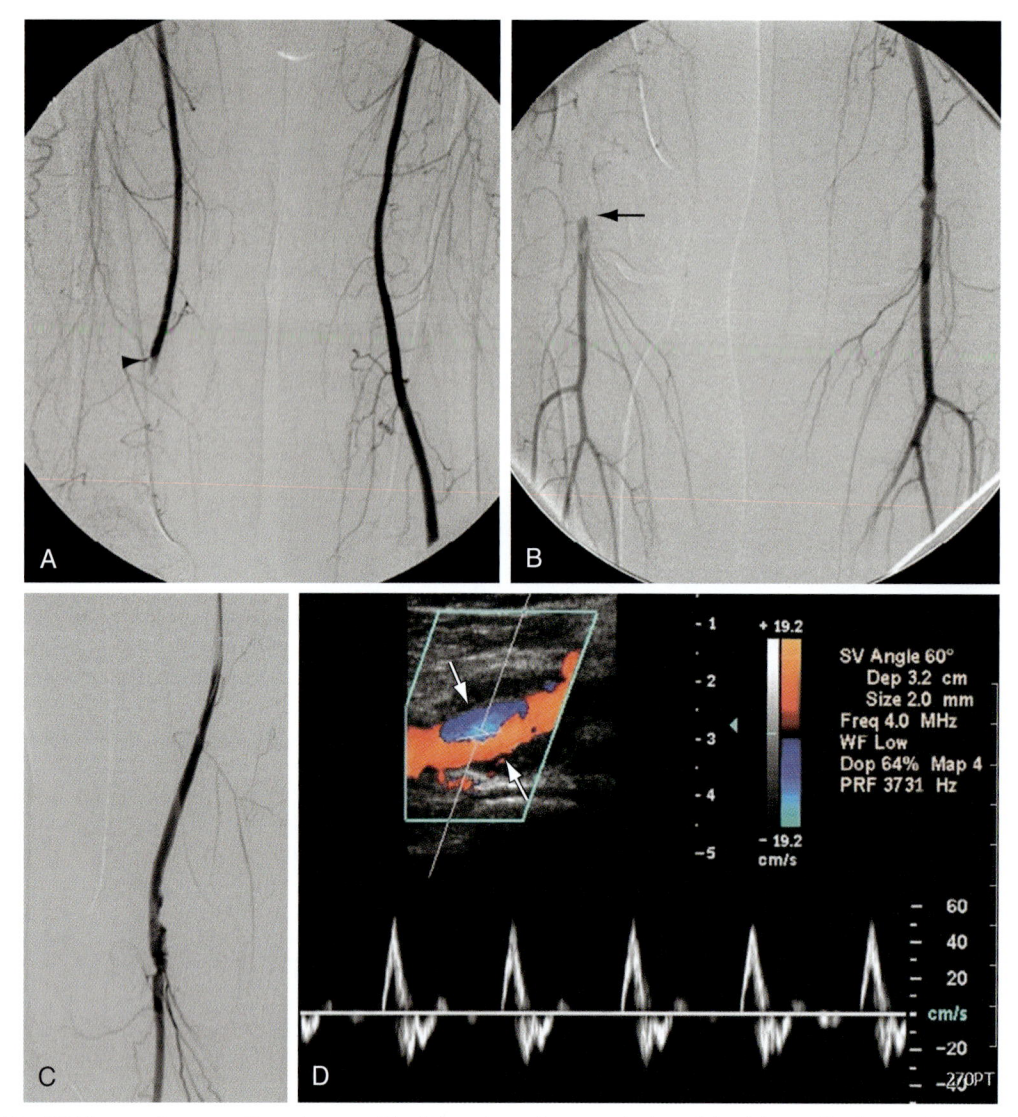

■ **FIGURE 114-18** DSA images from runoff arteriogram of both legs show abrupt occlusion of the right popliteal artery (**A**, *arrowhead*) at the adductor hiatus with distal reconstitution (**B**, *arrow*) at patellar level. The poorly developed collaterals are consistent with the history of acute right leg ischemia. There is also some slight irregularity to the contour of the left popliteal artery. After catheter-directed thrombolysis, patency is restored to the popliteal artery (**C**), but there is an irregular contour. The clinical presentation and the bilateral popliteal artery irregularity prompted further evaluation with ultrasound to assess for popliteal artery aneurysm. Duplex color flow Doppler ultrasound image (**D**) obtained after the successful thrombolysis procedure shows a patent central channel within a thrombus-containing right popliteal artery aneurysm (*white arrows*).

anastomoses result from disruption at the suture site. Pseudoaneurysms that occur spontaneously may be mycotic, and these would therefore also require surgical repair. Similarly, extremely large iatrogenic post-catheterization pseudoaneurysms that cause significant mass effect (e.g., claudication, neuropathy, limb ischemia, skin necrosis) should be treated surgically. Very small iatrogenic pseudoaneurysms (1.5 cm or less) associated with catheterization procedures may be observed for continued expansion. If they remain stable, without continued expansion, treatment may be unnecessary. Continued enlargement, however, generally mandates intervention. Larger pseudoaneurysms, with a sufficiently narrow "neck" between the true arterial lumen and the pseudoaneurysm, may be treated with thrombin injection when they involve the femoral arteries. If there is a very large or nonexistent neck to the pseudoaneurysm, this should be considered an arterial laceration and should be surgically repaired because it is unlikely that it can be effectively managed by more conservative means. Similarly, even relatively small pseudoaneurysms of the upper extremity arteries should be surgically treated, given the significant potential for adverse outcomes if they are observed or percutaneously treated.[24]

Adventitial cystic disease does not respond well to ultrasound- or CT-guided cyst aspiration. The cyst lining continues to secrete the mucinous fluid, with resultant recurrence of the arterial compression.

Outcomes and Complications

Symptomatic aneurysms of the lower extremities that present with either acute thrombosis or significant distal embolization have much worse surgical outcomes than

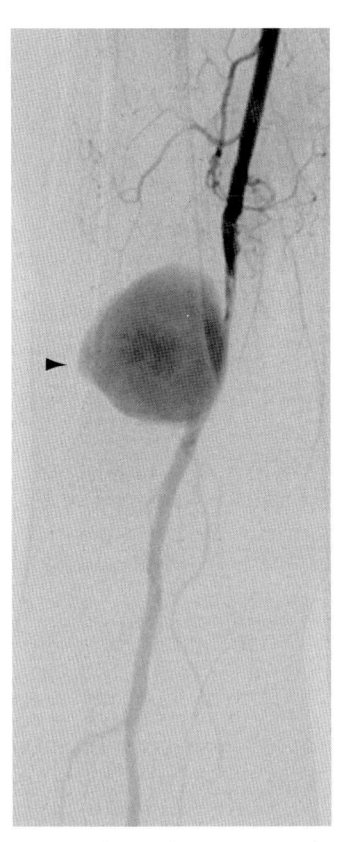

FIGURE 114-19 DSA image shows an eccentric saccular aneurysm (*arrowhead*) arising from the popliteal artery in a patient with Ehlers-Danlos syndrome.

those aneurysms that are electively treated. With regard to popliteal artery aneurysms, a recent review of consecutive patients who underwent surgical repair in two vascular surgery units between 1988 and 2006 in the United Kingdom reported 5-year primary graft patency, secondary graft patency, limb salvage, and patient survival rates of 75%, 95%, 98%, and 81%, respectively. The 10-year primary graft patency rates were significantly lower for emergency cases (59%) compared with elective cases (66%).[9] There are increased amputation rates and substantially higher morbidity and mortality associated with emergency treatment of peripheral aneurysms. In addition, adjunctive procedures, such as preoperative or intraoperative thrombolysis, may be necessary. Thrombolysis may be problematic in a severely ischemic limb, however, as there may be insufficient perfusion to allow the time required for successful thrombolysis. Also, during the thrombolysis procedure because there is fragmentation of the clot and resultant passage of small fragments distally into the smaller runoff arteries, there may be further worsening of the ischemia. This may then necessitate emergent surgical intervention. Such complications of thrombolysis are typically seen more frequently in patients undergoing thrombolysis for acute thrombosis of a peripheral arterial aneurysm than in patients in whom thrombolysis is performed for thrombotic or embolic occlusion of atherosclerotic occlusive lesions or thrombosed bypass grafts. When complications occur in association with thrombolytic therapy for acutely thrombosed aneurysms, amputation rates are high. This is particularly true if there is significant runoff disease or the thrombolysis procedure is excessively lengthy.

Treatment of patients with popliteal artery entrapment syndrome in whom significant arterial degenerative changes have occurred requires arterial bypass, as previously noted. There are reports of long-term patency exceeding 10 years in patients treated with saphenous vein bypass grafts. Because there is no definite correlation between the duration of the popliteal artery entrapment and the development of degenerative changes in the artery, surgical release of the entrapment is indicated at the time of diagnosis.

Cases of adventitial cystic disease that have progressed to arterial occlusion and have been treated with either operative cystotomy or complete cystectomy followed by arterial bypass with a vein graft are reported to have better long-term outcomes than those treated with cyst aspiration, thrombolysis, and angioplasty. The angioplasty approach has resulted in early recurrence because there is continued secretion by the cyst.

Surgical treatment of anastomotic pseudoaneurysms has patency rates similar to those of the initial primary surgery, provided there has been no disease progression in the runoff anatomy at or distal to the anastomoses. Similarly, there are excellent surgical results for primary repair of a post-catheterization pseudoaneurysm.[24]

Successful surgical or endovascular repair of a post-traumatic AVF is largely dependent on the complexity of the fistula, the anatomic location, and whether the abnormality is acute or chronic. Results are generally less satisfactory in chronic, complex, and centrally located AVFs.

Imaging Findings

Preoperative imaging of lower extremity aneurysms or pseudoaneurysms allows both diagnosis and treatment planning. The length and extent of the aneurysm, the amount of intraluminal thrombus, the inflow and runoff anatomy, and the relationship to adjacent structures should be delineated. In cases of popliteal artery aneurysms presenting with acute thrombosis or distal embolization, clear definition of the runoff circulation is essential for treatment planning. Thrombolysis or intraoperative embolectomy may be necessary if no runoff vessels can be identified. In addition, imaging confirmation of a thrombosed popliteal artery aneurysm is necessary. Because angiography will demonstrate only the arterial lumen, a thrombosed aneurysm may not be suspected if there is insufficient mural calcium. Other imaging modalities, such as ultrasonography, MR, or CT, may be necessary for confirmation. Similarly, a popliteal artery aneurysm that contains significant intraluminal thrombus may not be clearly appreciated as aneurysmal without supplemental imaging (see Fig. 114-18D).

For post-catheterization pseudoaneurysms, imaging is necessary to identify the size and depth of the pseudoaneurysm and the depth, width, and length of the track that connects to the "feeding" artery from which the pseudoaneurysm arose. Adjacent venous structures should be evaluated for any evidence of deep venous thrombosis from expansion of the hematoma that may be associated with the pseudoaneurysm. A post-catheterization pseu-

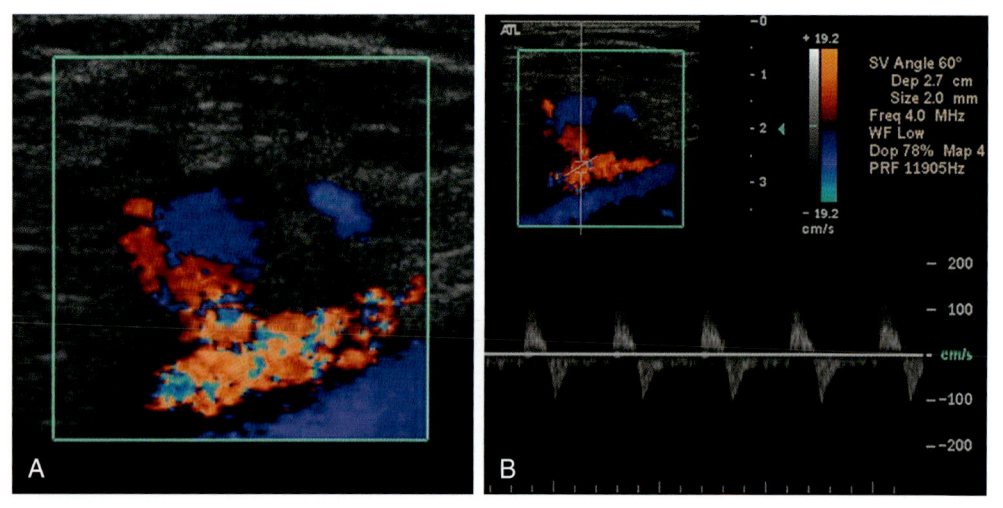

FIGURE 114-20 **A,** Color Doppler ultrasound image of an iatrogenic post-catheterization femoral artery pseudoaneurysm shows turbulent swirling flow within a sac that expands and contracts with the cardiac cycle, referred to as a yin-yang pattern. **B,** Doppler arterial waveform analysis also reveals the to-and-fro waveform that is characteristic of a pseudoaneurysm.

doaneurysm has a typical color Doppler ultrasound appearance in which there is a turbulent swirling flow pattern within a sac that expands and contracts with the cardiac cycle. Pulsed wave Doppler demonstrates a to-and-fro waveform (Fig. 114-20). If management involves thrombin injection, imaging is generally performed both during and after treatment to ensure precise needle placement within the pseudoaneurysm, complete thrombosis of the sac, and preserved patency of the feeding artery.[24]

In patients with popliteal artery entrapment syndrome, clinical examination with "stress maneuvers," such as forced plantar flexion or sometimes dorsiflexion, may produce significant reduction in the distal pulses. Imaging with continuous wave Doppler study, MRI, and angiography may be employed for diagnosis, but these also require an intraprocedural provocative stress maneuver for confirmation.

Adventitial cystic disease has a characteristic appearance on imaging studies as a result of cystic compression of the popliteal artery. Both ultrasound and MR images clearly demonstrate the cystic structures within the arterial wall and the mass effect on the adjacent artery. The angiographic appearance is that of a "spiral-shaped" stenosis and is unique to this entity (Fig. 114-21).

EXCLUSION PROCEDURE: ENDOVASCULAR METHODS OF EXCLUSION OR OCCLUSION

Description and Special Anatomic Considerations

Lower extremity aneurysms have been traditionally treated with surgical excision and bypass. However, with the continuing refinements in covered stent graft endoprostheses and the expanding role of this technology, endoluminal bypass has been offered as an alternative treatment for peripheral arterial aneurysmal disease. This is a treatment modality that is considered investigational by many operators at present because no long-term data are currently available. Present data suggest that endovascular repair of popliteal artery aneurysms offers medium-term benefits similar to those of the traditional surgical repair. There are valid concerns about short-term graft thrombosis and increased reintervention rates compared with open surgery.

In contrast, endovascular treatment of iatrogenic post-catheterization pseudoaneurysms is a well-established therapy, with excellent long-term data available.[24] With certain exceptions noted in the section on surgical treatment of these pseudoaneurysms, percutaneous thrombin injection is the preferred management.

Endovascular exclusion procedures are also well established in the treatment of post-traumatic or iatrogenic AVFs and vascular anomalies such as tumors and vascular malformations. Traumatic AVFs may result from stab or gunshot wounds or may be caused by blunt trauma. These injuries are less common in the lower extremities than in the neck, thoracic outlet, and upper extremities. Iatrogenic AVFs are generally related to catheterization procedures but may also be associated with surgical operations. AVFs may be treated by endovascular means with use of agents such as coils, covered stents, or mechanical occluders (e.g., Amplatzer plug). Vascular anomalies are categorized by both the type of vascular channel (arterial, venous, or lymphatic) and the flow dynamics (high-flow or low-flow). The high-flow anomalies include arteriovenous malformations, hemangiomas, and AVFs; low-flow anomalies include venous, capillary, and lymphatic malformations. Like AVFs, vascular anomalies are treated with embolization, sclerotherapy, or a combination of both modalities. Embolization is typically used in high-flow malformations; sclerotherapy is used primarily in low-flow anomalies and for the primary treatment of the nidus of a high-flow malformation after vascularity has been reduced by embolization.

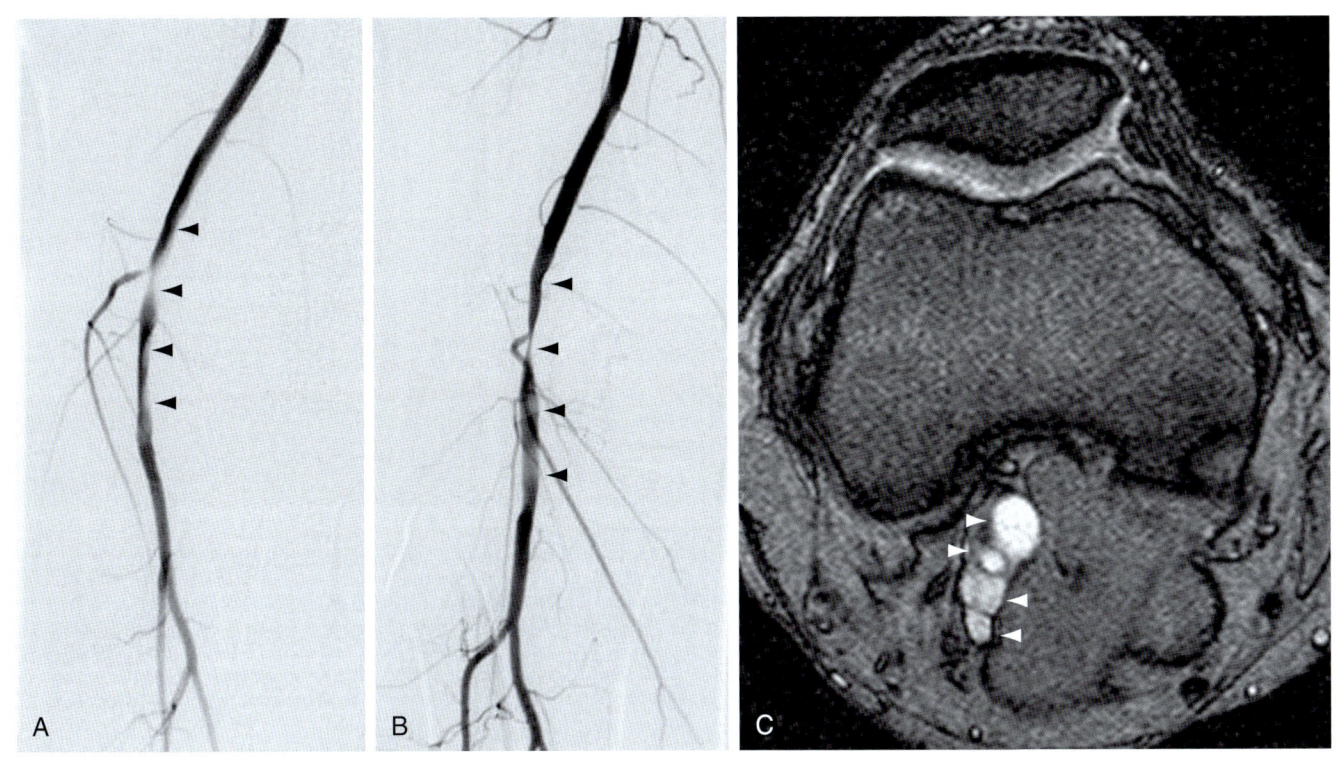

FIGURE 114-21 DSA images in oblique (**A**) and frontal (**B**) projections show a long "spiral-shaped" stenosis (*arrowheads*) of the popliteal artery, which is characteristic of cystic adventitial disease. Axial T2-weighted MRI (**C**) of the knee in the same patient shows multiple cysts (*arrowheads*) compressing the popliteal arterial lumen and thus causing the characteristic angiographic appearance.

Indications

The indications for endovascular exclusion of lower extremity arterial aneurysms are the same as those for traditional surgical excision and bypass. Many clinicians currently view the endovascular exclusion option as an inferior therapy compared with open surgery because of relatively frequent associated thrombosis. At present, it is typically reserved for older patients or those with significant medical comorbidities. Thrombolysis may be required for peripheral aneurysms that become symptomatic because of thromboembolic complications to reestablish patency and distal perfusion before any surgical or additional endovascular intervention.

Endovascular treatment of iatrogenic post-catheterization arterial pseudoaneurysms is indicated when there is continued expansion of a small (<1.5 cm) pseudoaneurysm or there are symptoms related to mass effect.

Contraindications

If there are insufficient proximal and distal disease-free arterial segments adjacent to a peripheral arterial aneurysm, there will not be adequate fixation zones for secure attachment of the endoprosthesis. This may result in either migration of the endoprosthesis or failure to exclude the aneurysm, with a resultant endoleak. Many investigators think that aneurysms occurring in areas where there is complex motion, such as the hip or knee, may have better long-term results when they are treated surgically.

Pseudoaneurysms that are extremely large or are mycotic in etiology should be surgically treated, as previously noted. This applies to both anastomotic and post-catheterization pseudoaneurysms.

Outcomes and Complications

For endovascular repair of peripheral aneurysms to be accepted as a valid alternative to open repair, it must be equivalent or superior to the accepted standard.[25-28] Mohan and coworkers[29] reported a cumulative primary patency rate of 74.5% and a cumulative secondary patency rate of 83.2% at 24 and 36 months, respectively. Tielliu and colleagues[30] reported overall 3- and 5-year patency rates of 77% and 70% for primary patency and 86% and 76% for secondary patency, respectively, in 73 popliteal artery aneurysms treated by endovascular means. This group found that the use of clopidogrel (75 mg daily) was a significant predictor of the success of a popliteal artery stent graft. In these two series, the use of versatile and flexible new stent grafts for endovascular popliteal artery aneurysm repair yielded patency results that are comparable to those of conventional open surgical repair, which has an average 5-year graft patency of 70% to 80%.[29-31]

There have been more than 45 series reporting the safety and efficacy of thrombin injection for post-catheterization pseudoaneurysms, with a 97% overall cumulative success rate. Potential complications include thrombosis of the underlying native artery, distal embolization of thrombotic material, deep venous thrombosis, allergic reaction to the thrombin, local erythema, and infected abscess. The complication rate is extremely low, however, with a reported overall incidence of 1.3% and an embolic rate of 0.5%.[24]

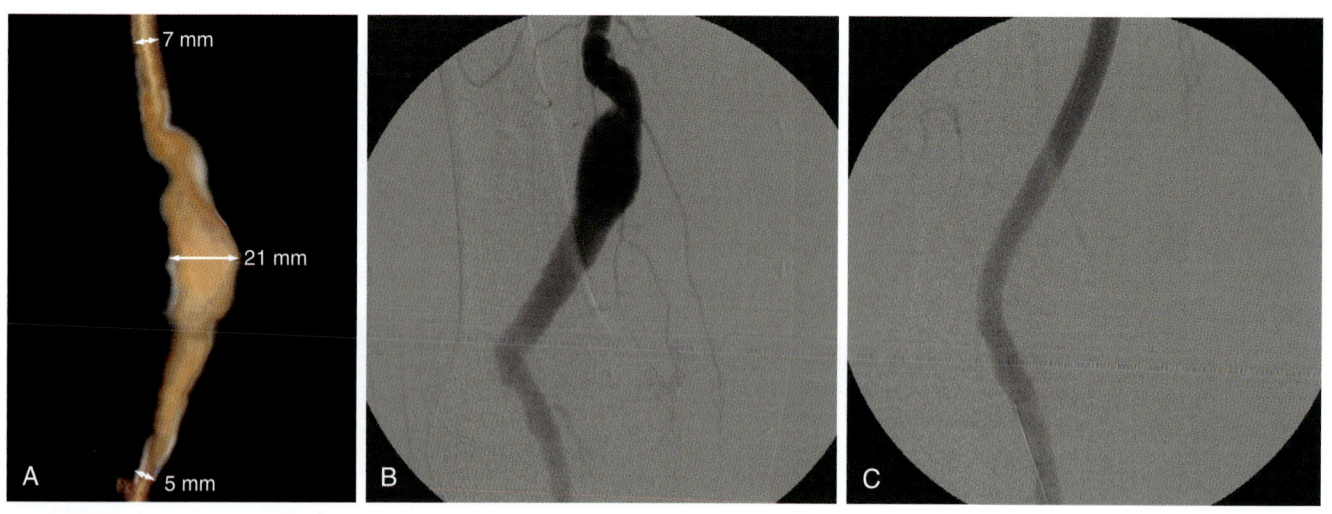

FIGURE 114-22 **A,** Three-dimensional volume rendered reformatted image of a popliteal artery aneurysm as seen on CTA is useful for depicting the morphology of the aneurysm. In this case, the aneurysm measurements and those of the segments above and below the aneurysm are less accurate than if they were measured directly on axial images; the opacity settings on this three-dimensional volume rendered image depict only the contrast-filled portion of the arterial lumen and do not account for any intraluminal thrombus. However, length measurements would be accurate because they can be obtained as centerline measurements. **B,** Intraoperative arteriogram depicts the morphology of the popliteal artery aneurysm before endovascular repair. It clearly demonstrates that there are no critical arterial branches arising from the aneurysm or from the treatment zone where the endoprosthesis will be placed. **C,** Angiographic image obtained after the deployment of the endoprosthesis reveals its correct placement that extends between the disease-free segments of the popliteal artery cephalad and caudad to the aneurysm. The stent graft was gently distended at each attachment site with an angioplasty balloon after deployment.

Endovascular treatment results for vascular anomalies are largely dependent on the type of malformation. Arteriovenous malformations have a high recurrence rate if they are treated with proximal embolization. Use of a technique in which outflow of the dominant draining vein is occluded, followed by central sclerosis of the nidus of the malformation, is the most effective treatment method. Unfortunately, some patients experience significant tissue ischemia as a result of treatment; complications such as skin or soft tissue necrosis, nerve damage, non-target embolization, pulmonary embolism, and coagulopathies may occur. Somewhat better results are generally achieved with venous and lymphatic malformations.

Imaging Findings

As with surgical exclusion procedures, successful endovascular treatment requires appropriate preoperative imaging. The morphology of the aneurysm and of the adjacent arterial segments and the distal runoff should be clearly defined. This will allow both appropriate sizing and optimal placement of the endoprosthesis. This can be accomplished with CTA, MRA, or conventional catheter angiography. If CTA is performed preoperatively, one may obtain volume rendered three-dimensional images of the aneurysm through the use of postprocessing and reformatting software (Fig. 114-22A). Images such as these allow one to view the aneurysm in multiple projections and to obtain "centerline" measurements that allow more accurate determination of the appropriate length of the endoprosthesis. Accurate intraoperative imaging is also essential for accurate endovascular aneurysm repair. Iodinated contrast medium is injected either through an intravascular sheath or through a catheter that has been positioned proximal to the aneurysm so that angiographic images are obtained. Anteroposterior and lateral angiographic views are generally obtained to delineate the aneurysm morphology intraprocedurally and to assess for any branch vessels that arise within the treatment zone. Angiography of the runoff arterial anatomy is also obtained to verify the quality and patency of the vasculature. After endovascular treatment, the proximal and distal attachments and the course of the prosthesis should be clearly demonstrated. Delayed images should be obtained to assess for an endoleak. The distal runoff anatomy should once more be evaluated; any compromise may significantly affect the long-term outcome (Fig. 114-22B,C and Fig. 114-23).

Iatrogenic or post-traumatic pseudoaneurysms must also be clearly defined, particularly the relationship of neck and the parent feeding artery. After treatment, one should document complete thrombosis of the pseudoaneurysm and patency of the adjacent native vascular structures (Fig. 114-24).

It is essential to clearly define the complex arterial and venous anatomy of an arteriovenous malformation before and after treatment. The images that are obtained before treatment should demonstrate the feeding arteries, the nidus, and the major draining veins as clearly as possible; this will allow optimal treatment planning. As with any vascular intervention, the post-treatment images should document both the results of the procedure and the status of the adjacent vascular structures.

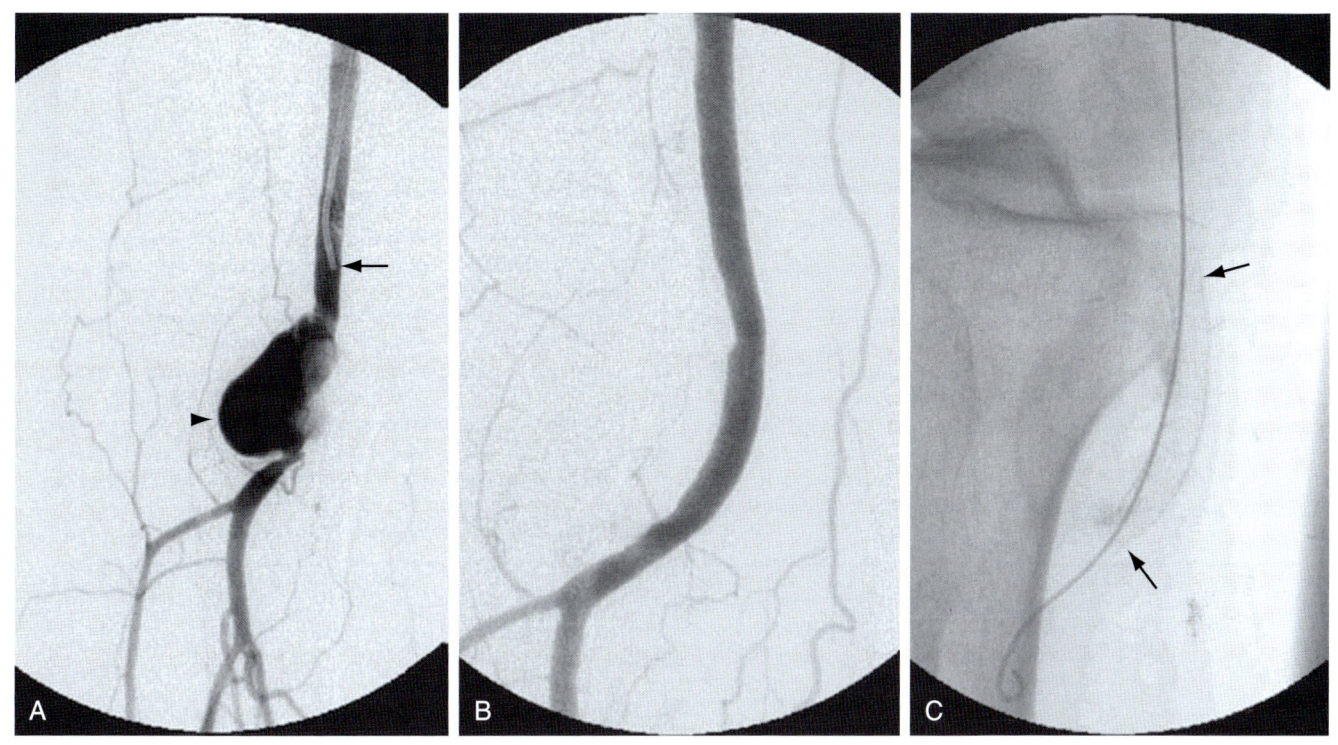

CHAPTER 114 • Lower Extremity Operations and Interventions 1607

■ **FIGURE 114-23** **A,** This angiographic image shows a catheter with the tip (*arrow*) in the distal end of a previously placed femoropopliteal artery bypass graft, above a distal anastomotic popliteal artery pseudoaneurysm (*arrowhead*). **B,** In the postdeployment angiographic image, placement of the covered stent graft is confirmed. After gentle angioplasty at the proximal and distal attachment sites, the graft is fully distended and there is no filling of the pseudoaneurysm, indicating successful exclusion, with no endoleak. The runoff arterial anatomy distal to the endoprosthesis remained intact (not shown). **C,** The deployed endoprosthesis (*arrows*) can be seen as very flexible and conforming to the course of the distal bypass graft and the popliteal artery as they cross the knee joint. Note the relatively poor radiopacity of this stent graft and the lack of radiopaque markers at either end of the graft. These factors must be considered during deployment to ensure precise placement of the endoprosthesis.

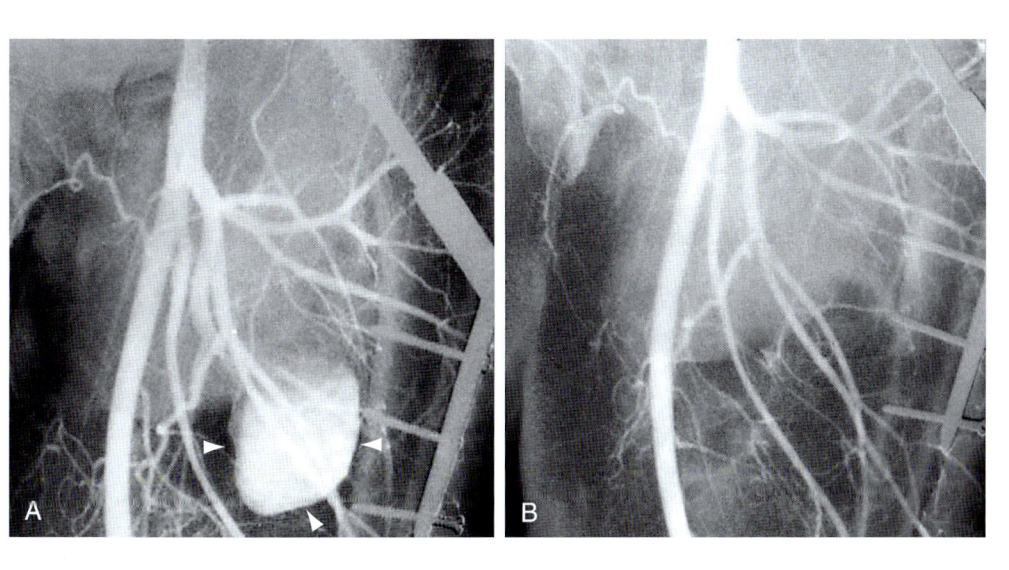

■ **FIGURE 114-24** Left femoral arteriogram (**A**) shows a large iatrogenic pseudoaneurysm (*arrowheads*) arising from the profunda femoral artery as a result of an arterial injury during an orthopedic procedure. The location of this pseudoaneurysm would make open surgical repair very difficult. Angiographic image (**B**) after transcatheter treatment with a combination of embolization coils and thrombin shows that the pseudoaneurysm has been successfully thrombosed and the surrounding vasculature preserved.

KEY POINTS

- Arterial bypass remains the standard for revascularization.
- Arterial bypass is indicated in patients with long-segment chronic total superficial femoral artery occlusion, chronic total popliteal artery or proximal trifurcation vessel occlusion, diffuse multiple stenoses or occlusions involving the entire superficial femoral artery, and recurrent stenoses or occlusions after two or more prior endovascular treatments.
- Surveillance of bypass grafts is critical to ensure long-term patency, given that a relatively high percentage of vascular conduits develop problems that threaten longevity. The simplest and most effective surveillance tool is duplex ultrasonography coupled with ankle-brachial index measurement.
- Determination of which lesions are appropriate for endovascular treatment versus traditional surgical revascularization continues to be an evolving and sometimes controversial process.
- The characteristics of the lesion greatly affect outcomes of endovascular revascularization procedures as the aim of these procedures is essentially to repair a diseased arterial segment in situ as opposed to bypass or replacement of the diseased segment.
- In general, short segmental stenoses respond well to angioplasty and may not require stent placement, whereas long-segment, diffusely diseased, or heavily calcified lesions may require stent placement to achieve and to maintain patency.
- The indiscriminate application of endovascular technique based solely on whether it is technically possible to treat a given lesion, as opposed to a patient-oriented approach, generally leads to poor outcomes.
- Symptomatic aneurysms of the lower extremities that present with either acute thrombosis or significant distal embolization have much worse surgical outcomes than do those aneurysms that are electively treated.

SUGGESTED READINGS

Bunting TA, Garcia LA. Peripheral atherectomy: a critical review. J Interv Cardiol 2007; 20:417-424.

Eskelinen E, Lepäntalo M. Role of infrainguinal angioplasty in the treatment of critical limb ischaemia. Scand J Surg 2007; 96:11-16.

Galland RB. Popliteal aneurysms: from John Hunter to the 21st century. Ann R Coll Surg Engl 2007; 89:466-471.

Lopera JE, Trimmer CK, Josephs SG, et al. Multidetector CT angiography of infrainguinal arterial bypass. Radiographics 2008; 28:529-548; discussion 549.

McCaslin JE, Macdonald S, Stansby G. Cryoplasty for peripheral vascular disease. Cochrane Database Syst Rev 2007; 4:CD005507.

Nelson PR, Anthony Lee W. Endovascular treatment of popliteal artery aneurysms. Vascular 2006; 14:297-304.

Perera GB, Lyden SP. Current trends in lower extremity revascularization. Surg Clin North Am 2007; 87:1135-1147, x.

Ramaiah V. Endovascular infrainguinal revascularization: technical tips for atherectomy device selection and procedural success. Semin Vasc Surg 2008; 21:41-49.

Rogers JH, Laird JR. Overview of new technologies for lower extremity revascularization. Circulation 2007; 116:2072-2085.

Silvers LW, Royster TS, Mulcare RJ. Peripheral arterial emboli and factors in their recurrence rate. Ann Surg 1980; 192:232-236.

Wain RA, Hines G. A contemporary review of popliteal artery aneurysms. Cardiol Rev 2007; 15:102-107.

REFERENCES

1. Haider SN, Kavanaugh EG, Forlee M, et al. Two-year outcome with preferential use of infrainguinal angioplasty for critical ischemia. J Vasc Surg 2006; 43:504-512.
2. Schillinger M, Sabeti S, Loewe C, et al. Balloon angioplasty versus implantation of nitinol stents in the superficial femoral artery. N Engl J Med 2006; 354:1879-1888.
3. BASIL trial participants. Bypass versus angioplasty in severe ischemia of the leg (BASIL): multicenter randomized controlled trial. Lancet 2005; 366:1925-1934.
4. Schillinger M, Sabeti S, Loewe C, et al. Sustained benefit at 2 years of primary femoropopliteal stenting compared with balloon angioplasty with optional stenting. Circulation 2007; 115:2745-2749.
5. Saxon RR, Coffman JM, Gooding JM, et al. Long-term results of ePTFE stent-graft versus angioplasty in the femoropopliteal artery: single center experience from a prospective randomized study. Circulation 2000; 102:2694-2699.
6. Kedora J, Hohmann S, Garrett W, et al. Randomized comparison or percutaneous Viabahn stent graft vs. prosthetic femoral-popliteal bypass in the treatment of superficial femoral arterial occlusive disease. J Vasc Surg 2007; 45:10-16.
7. Tolva V, Bertoni GB, Trimarchi S, et al. Unreliability of depopulated bovine ureteric xenograft for infrainguinal bypass surgery: mid-term results from two vascular centres. Eur J Endovasc Surg 2007; 33:214-216.
8. Patel A, Taylor SM, Langan EM 3rd, et al. Obturator bypass: a classic approach for the treatment of contemporary groin infection. Am Surg 2002; 68:653-659.
9. Laird JR, Biamino G, McNamara T, et al. Cryoplasty for the treatment of femoropopliteal arterial disease: extended follow-up results. J Endovasc Ther 2006; 13(Suppl 2):II52-II59.
10. Laird J, Jaff MR, Biamino G, et al. Cryoplasty for the treatment of femoropopliteal arterial disease: results of a prospective, multicenter registry. J Vasc Interv Radiol 2005; 16:1067-1073.
11. Bittl JA, Chew DP, Topol EJ, et al. Meta-analysis of randomized trials of percutaneous transluminal coronary angioplasty versus atherectomy, cutting balloon atherotomy, or laser angioplasty. J Am Coll Cardiol 2004; 43:936-942.
12. Dormandy JA, Rutherford RB. Management of peripheral arterial disease (PAD) TASC Working Group. TransAtlantic Inter-Society Consensus (TASC). J Vasc Surg 2000; 331(pt 2):S1-S296.
13. Norgren L, Hiatt WR, Dormandy JA, et al; TASC II Working Group. Inter-Society Consensus for the Management of Peripheral Arterial Disease (TASC II). J Vasc Surg 2007; 45(Suppl S):S5-S67.
14. Levy F, Butcher HR. Arterial emboli: an analysis of 125 patients. Surgery 1970; 68:968-973.
15. Eriksson I, Holmberg T. Analysis of factors affecting limb salvage and mortality after embolectomy. Acta Chir Scand 1977; 143:237-240.
16. Galbraith K, Collin J, Morris PJ, Wood RFM. Recent experience with arterial embolism of the limbs in a vascular unit. Ann R Coll Surg Engl 1985; 67:30-33.
17. Thompson JE, Staler L, Raut PS, et al. Arterial embolectomy: a 20 year experience with 163 cases. Surgery 1970; 67:212-220.

18. Atiani B, Evans WE. Immediate prognosis and five year survival after arterial embolectomy following myocardial infarction. Surg Gynecol Obstet 1980; 150:41-44.
19. Balas P, Bonatsos G, Xeromeritas N, et al. Early surgical results on acute arterial occlusion of the extremities. J Cardiovasc Surg 1985; 26:262-269.
20. Kairaluoma, K, Larmi TK. Surgical treatment of arterial embolism. Ann Chir Gyn 1976; 65:163-167.
21. Kendrick J, Thompson BW, Campbell GS, et al. Arterial embolectomy in the leg. Am J Surg 1981; 142:739-743.
22. Szczepanski KP. Results of surgical treatment of arterial embolism. Scand J Thorac Cardiovasc Surg 1979; 13:71-75.
23. Dryksjim M, Swedenborg J. Acute thrombosis and embolism of the extremities: factors influencing the result of treatment. Acta Chir Scand 1982; 148:135-139.
24. Webber GW, Jang J, Gustavson S, Olin JW. Contemporary management of postcatheterization pseudoaneurysms. Circulation 2007; 115:2666-2674.
25. Curi MA, Geraghty PJ, Merino OA, et al. Mid-term outcomes of endovascular popliteal artery aneurysm repair. J Vasc Surg. 2007; 45:505-510.
26. Davies RS, Wall M, Rai S, et al. Long-term results of surgical repair of popliteal artery aneurysm. Eur J Endovasc Surg 2007; 34:714.
27. Rajasinghe HA, Tzilinis A, Keller T, et al. Endovascular exclusion of popliteal artery aneurysms with expanded polytetrafluoroethylene stent-grafts: early results. Vasc Endovascular Surg 2006; 40:460-466.
28. Laganà D, Carrafiello G, Mangini M, et al. Endovascular treatment of femoropopliteal aneurysms: a five-year experience. Cardiovasc Intervent Radiol 2006; 29:819-825.
29. Mohan IV, Bray PJ, Harris JP, et al. Endovascular popliteal aneurysm repair: are the results comparable to open surgery? Eur J Vasc Endovasc Surg 2006; 32:149-154.
30. Tielliu IF, Verhoeven EL, Zeebregts CJ, et al. Endovascular treatment of popliteal artery aneurysms: results of a prospective cohort study. J Vasc Surg 2005; 41:561-567.
31. Antonello M, Frigatti P, Battocchio P, et al. Open repair versus endovascular treatment for asymptomatic popliteal artery aneurysm: results of a prospective randomized study. J Vasc Surg 2005; 42:185-193.

CHAPTER 115

Computed Tomographic Angiography of the Lower Extremities

Saurabh Jha and Harold Litt

Computed tomographic angiography (CTA) is at the forefront of noninvasive assessment of the peripheral arteries (CTA runoff).[1] The advantage of CTA over catheter angiography is the absence of complications attributed to its more invasive predecessor, such as pseudoaneurysm and arteriovenous fistula.[2] In addition, CTA requires a shorter stay for the patient, is less costly than catheter angiography, and has the potential to be more cost-effective than magnetic resonance angiography (MRA).[3]

CTA can assess the entire arterial tree from the aortic arch to the toes, if required, potentially making it a "one-stop" examination for extended field of view arterial illustration. With multidetector CT, large volume of coverage and high spatial resolution can be dually achieved, and the speed of acquisition allows reduction in the volume of iodinated contrast agent. CT can assess the arterial wall and the arterial lumen, making it an invaluable evaluator of atherosclerotic plaque burden and aneurysm morphology; this yields information beyond the lumen of the artery that can assist preoperative determination of suitability of vessels for grafting.

With the aid of postprocessing tools now available, CTA is able to provide the interpreting physician and vascular surgeon with information concerning the site of obstruction, extent of vascular disease, and strategy for the appropriate type of vascular intervention.[4]

The availability of CTA and the relative simplicity of its operation in comparison to MRI have led to the rapid adoption of CTA for noninvasive imaging for peripheral vascular disease. However, CTA has limitations and hazards. It involves the use of ionizing radiation and iodinated contrast agent, which are not appropriate in certain populations. In addition, there are inherent limitations to the examination itself; in such situations, MRA or catheter angiography is required to provide the clinical information.

TECHNICAL REQUIREMENTS

An appropriate CTA protocol must provide both large field of view coverage and spatial resolution optimized for maximal contrast agent bolus enhancement of the arterial tree while minimizing ionizing radiation exposure and contrast agent dose.[1]

The individual requirements are as follows:

- Multidetector CT (4 channels or more)
- Contrast agent with appropriate concentration of iodine and a dual injector. Typically, the concentrations used are 320 to 370 mg of iodine per milliliter.
- Software that allows optimal timing of the acquisition with respect to the contrast agent injection
- Postprocessing workstation
- Storage such as PACS (picture archiving and communication system)

Preparation of the patient involves appropriate hydration, and local policies with respect to prevention of contrast-induced nephropathy should be followed. Intravenous access must be of sufficient diameter (usually 20-gauge intravenous catheter) to allow rapid injection of iodinated contrast agent, typically around 4 mL/sec. Peripheral intravenous access is encouraged; the use of central catheters should strictly adhere to the manufacturer's guidelines with respect to the pressure limitations and maximum injection rates.

CHAPTER 115 • Computed Tomographic Angiography of the Lower Extremities

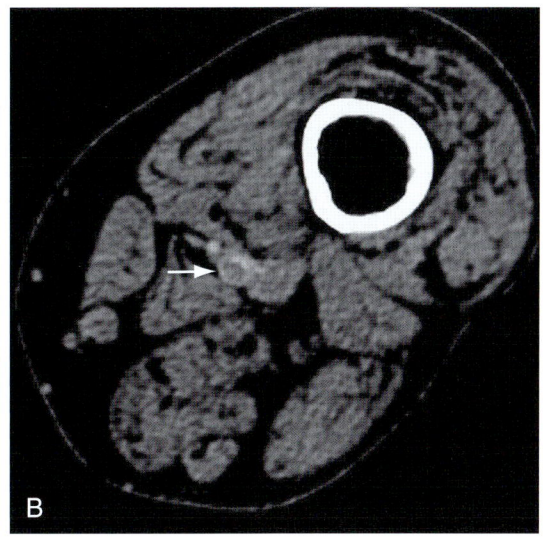

FIGURE 115-1 Sagittal (**A**) and axial (**B**) images show occlusion of the left superficial femoral artery (**A** and **B**, *arrows*), the superior aspect of which has a meniscal appearance (**A**, *arrowhead*), suggesting an acute or an acute on chronic event. CTA runoff is useful in the evaluation of patients with acute and chronic ischemic symptoms.

TECHNIQUES

Indications

- Systemic arterial disease due to atherosclerosis (Figs. 115-1 and 115-2)
- Nonatherosclerotic arterial disease (Buerger disease, vasospastic disease)
- Fibular graft vascular assessment[5]
- Trauma (Fig. 115-3)[6]
- Vascular masses and malformations[7]
  - Congenital
  - Acquired: aneurysm and pseudoaneurysm, arteriovenous fistula
- Compression of artery
  - Vascular invasion by musculoskeletal tumors (Fig. 115-4)[8]
  - Cystic adventitial disease[9]
  - Popliteal entrapment syndrome[10]
- Venous disease (Fig. 115-5)

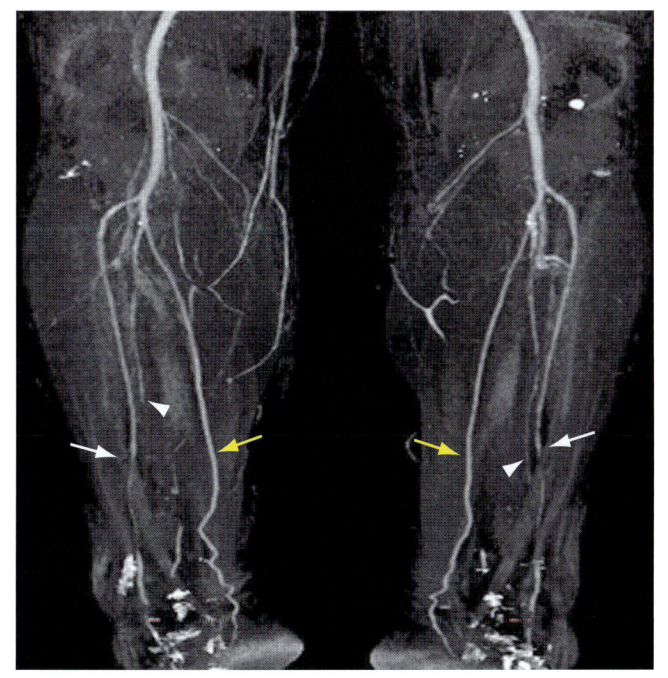

FIGURE 115-2 CTA runoff in patient with atherosclerotic peripheral vascular occlusive disease. Reformatted coronal maximum intensity projection (MIP) image of the calves shows segmental high-grade narrowing or occlusion in the mid and distal anterior tibial arteries (*white arrows*) and peroneal arteries (*arrowheads*) with relatively disease free posterior tibial arteries (*yellow arrow*). In this patient, the posterior tibial arteries were patent in their entirety and thus would be the preferred choice for distal attachment of a bypass procedure for a mid superficial femoral artery occlusion.

By far, the most common indication is peripheral arterial disease (also known as peripheral arterial occlusive disease) in both the acute and chronic setting and in patients for follow-up and surveillance after surgical or percutaneous revascularization (Figs. 115-6 and 115-7).

Trauma is an increasing indication for imaging, and CTA is readily accessible. CTA is able to assess coexisting injuries of neighboring and distant organs, making it preferable to conventional angiography in this setting. Notably, CTA is able to detect a host of vascular complications, such as hematoma, pseudoaneurysm, vascular compression, intimal tear, and vasospasm.

Assessment of the crural vessels for vascular variants is of importance in patients who may require fibular transfer, such as in complex craniofacial surgery, and thus recruitment of the peroneal artery.

Because of its limited ability to provide dynamic vascular information and soft tissue contrast, it may not be the best modality for the assessment of a vascular mass or popliteal entrapment syndrome. MRA and ultrasonography are more appropriate in these circumstances. Ultrasonography is more appropriate for the assessment of venous disease, which nonetheless may be encountered in surprisingly high frequency among those referred because of peripheral ischemia.

Contraindications

Renal Impairment

The ultimate decision to administer an intravenous contrast agent is a shared one between the interpreting

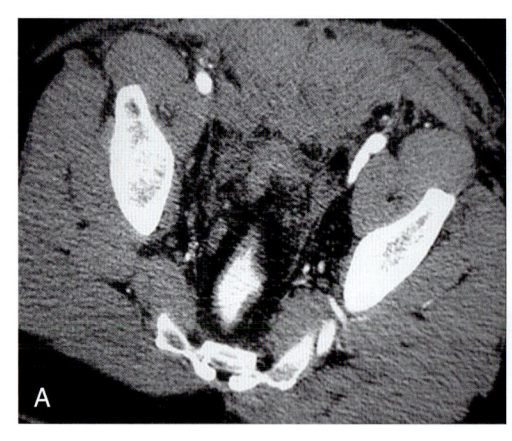

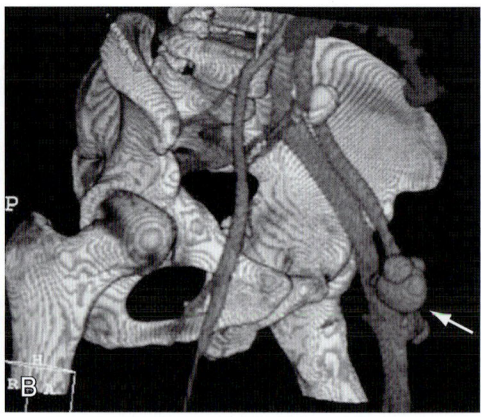

FIGURE 115-3 **A,** Pelvic CTA. Note the bright contrast in the left common iliac vein. **B,** Volume rendering of the pelvis demonstrates a large arteriovenous fistula system (*arrow*) between the femoral artery and femoral vein. *(From Fleiter TR, Mervis S. The role of 3D-CTA in the assessment of peripheral vascular lesions in trauma patients. Eur J Radiol 2007; 64:92-102.)*

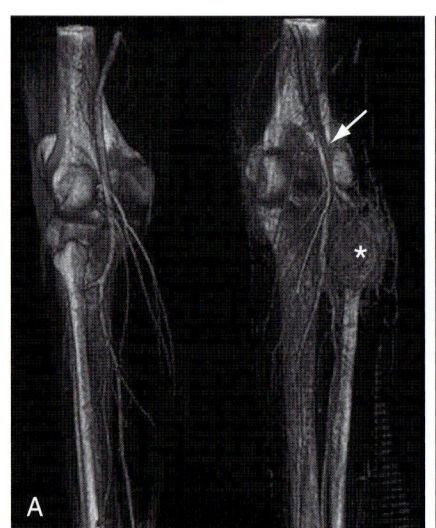

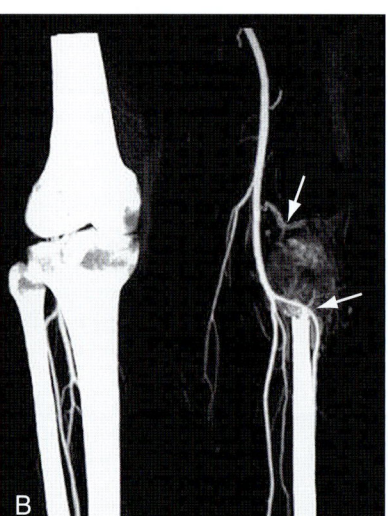

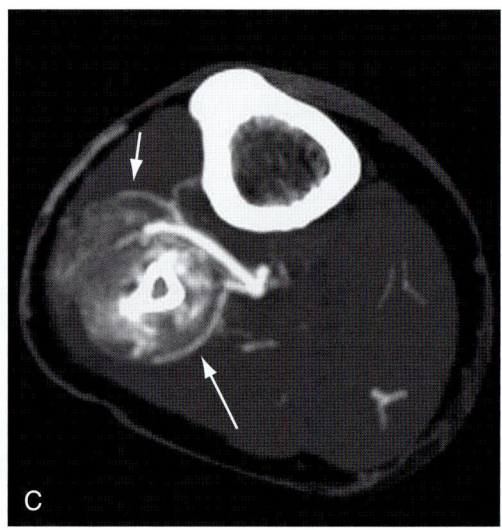

FIGURE 115-4 Extremity CTA of a 30-year-old man with a left fibular giant cell tumor. **A,** Three-dimensional volume rendered image demonstrates vascular supply of the proximal fibular mass (*asterisk*). Note early venous filling as a result of hypervascularity of the malignant giant cell tumor (*arrow*). Bones are removed on the side of the giant cell tumor. **B,** Coronal MIP image demonstrates vascular supply of the mass from the popliteal and anterior tibial arteries (*arrows*). **C,** Axial MIP image shows arterial supply of the mass from the popliteal (*long arrow*) and anterior tibial (*short arrow*) arteries. *(From Karcaaltincaba M, Aydingoz U, Akata D, et al. Combination of extremity computed tomography angiography and abdominal imaging in patients with musculoskeletal tumors. J Comput Assist Tomogr 2004; 28:273-277.)*

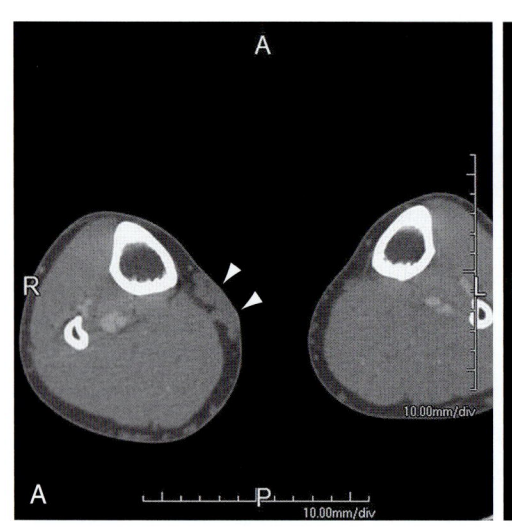

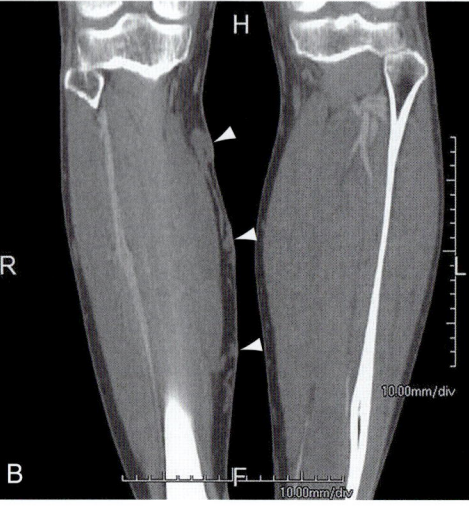

FIGURE 115-5 Axial (**A**) and coronal (**B**) images of the calf show dilated subcutaneous veins (*arrowheads*) in this patient with varicose veins. Venous disease is frequently discovered in patients imaged for peripheral ischemia.

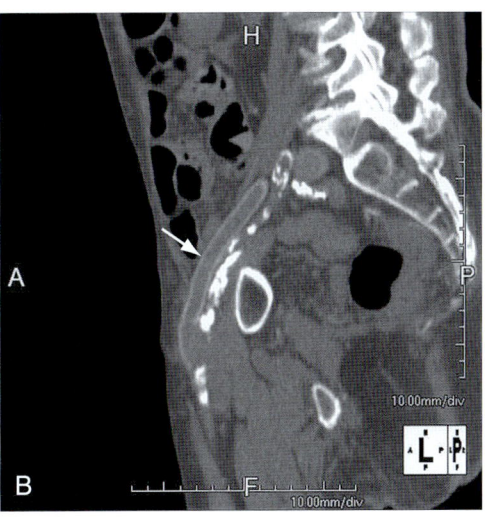

CHAPTER 115 • *Computed Tomographic Angiography of the Lower Extremities* 1613

FIGURE 115-6 Axial (**A**) and reformatted sagittal (**B**) images show an occluded left limb of the aortobifemoral graft (*arrows*). CTA is a useful modality for postoperative surveillance.

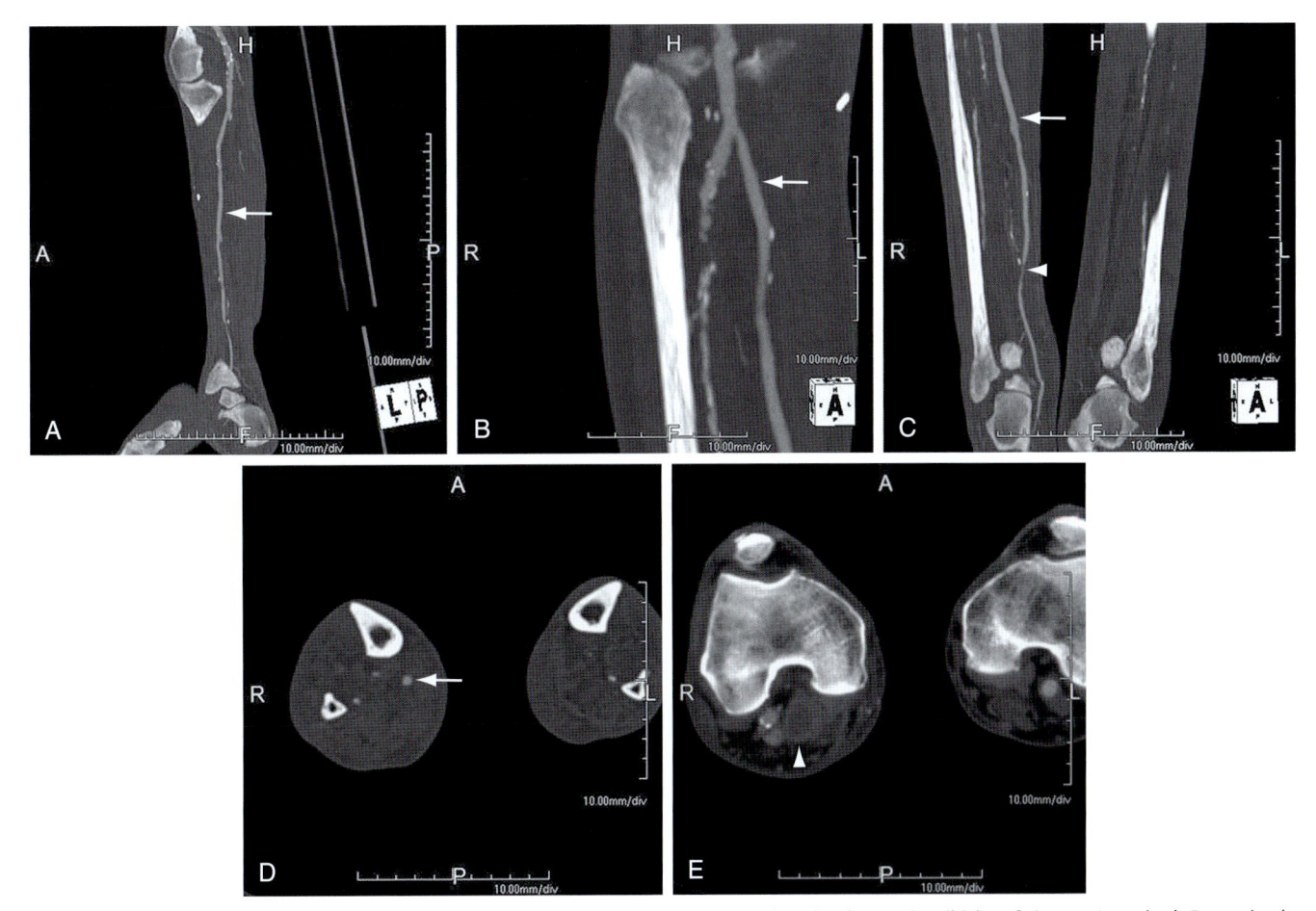

FIGURE 115-7 Multiplanar reformatted images in this patient with a right popliteal to distal posterior tibial graft (*arrow*; **A**, sagittal; **B**, proximal coronal; **C**, distal coronal; **D**, axial). The graft is patent, other than narrowing in its distal aspect (**C**, *arrowhead*). The right calf is edematous. The native posterior tibial artery is occluded. A rim-enhancing collection (**E**, *arrowhead,* axial view) posterior to the knee joint in the vicinity of the proximal anastomosis is suggestive of a graft infection.

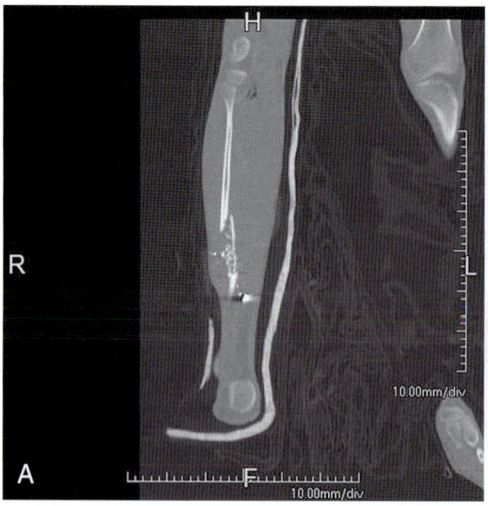

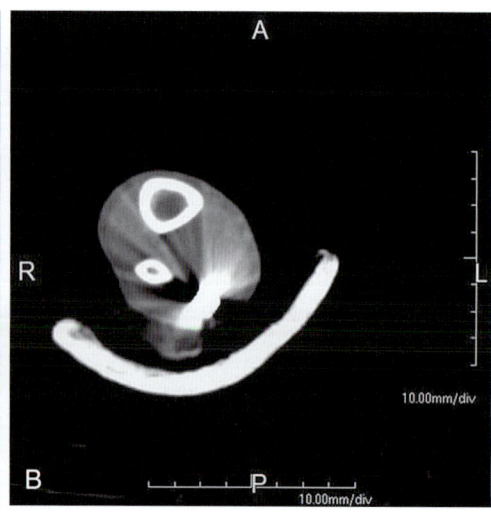

FIGURE 115-8 Reformatted coronal (**A**) and axial (**B**) images of the right calf in this patient with a gunshot wound, comminuted tibial-fibular fracture, and suspicion of a vascular injury. The CT images are degraded by high-attenuation artifact from the ballistic fragments, which is causing considerable streak artifacts. Under these circumstances, catheter angiography may be more appropriate.

physician and the referring physician after informed consent of the patient in the event of renal impairment. The timing of dialysis in relation to the time of the scan is of importance. MRA is an option and may have to be performed without intravenous gadolinium-chelate contrast agent if the patient is at risk for development of nephrogenic systemic fibrosis (e.g., glomerular filtration rate less than 30 mL/min/1.73 m^2).[11]

Contrast Allergy

It is important to determine if there is a true allergy to nonionic iodinated contrast agent and the nature of the allergic reaction. Steroid preparation can be given for those with documented history of mild to moderate contrast agent reactions.

Orthopedic Hardware or High-Attenuation Object

Although it is not technically a contraindication, the artifact resulting from a high-attenuation object[12] may obscure the artery of interest and limit the utility of the examination. Catheter angiography may be required because MRI may also be inflicted with significant artifact in such situations (Fig. 115-8).

Radiation-Sensitive Population

The risk of radiation-induced carcinogenesis must not be forgotten, and the principles of ALARA (as low as is reasonably achievable) should be respected in terms of radiation dose. The risk/benefit of CTA in the younger patient should be evaluated carefully.

Technique Description

Technique involves image acquisition and contrast agent administration.

Image Acquisition

Field of View

The field of view must answer the clinical question and provide information about associated vascular pathologic changes that would affect management. In the case of peripheral arterial occlusive disease, such as in patients with claudication, this involves the assessment of the abdominal aorta to assess the inflow and to exclude coexisting abdominal aortic aneurysm (Fig. 115-9).

An initial image through the abdomen and pelvis before the administration of the contrast agent is followed by arterial phase images from the celiac artery origin to the toes in a single acquisition. An immediate second acquisition is prudent through the calves, particularly with the newer scanners, in which outrunning of the contrast bolus can be a problem. Venous phase images are not routine and are obtained as clinically necessary. Breath-hold is required for the acquisition through the abdomen and pelvis.[1,13]

It is important to keep the patient's knees and legs together, close to the isocenter. Excessive plantar flexion can erroneously depict occlusion of the dorsalis pedis and should be avoided.[14]

Scanning Protocols

The acquisition parameters depend on the number of detectors and are vendor specific (Tables 115-1 and 115-2). Regardless, the scan time should be such that the entire arterial tree of interest is covered in a reasonable time during which the arteries remain maximally opacified (i.e., in the first and single pass of contrast bolus). With the latest multidetector CT scanners, this does not involve a tradeoff between spatial resolution and z-axis coverage. With the 4-detector CT, a choice usually needs to be made, as will be explained.

Background Principles

Further discussion of this area involves recapitulation of some concepts.

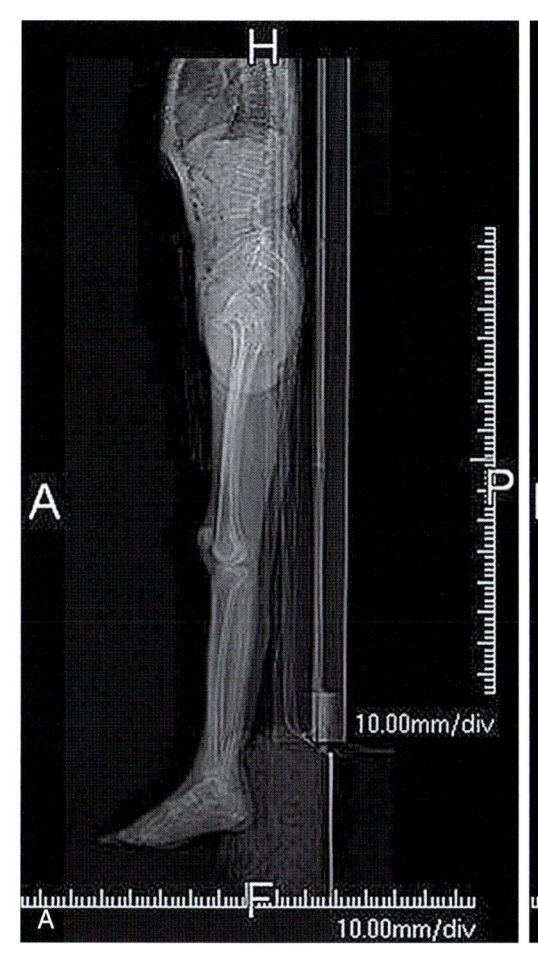

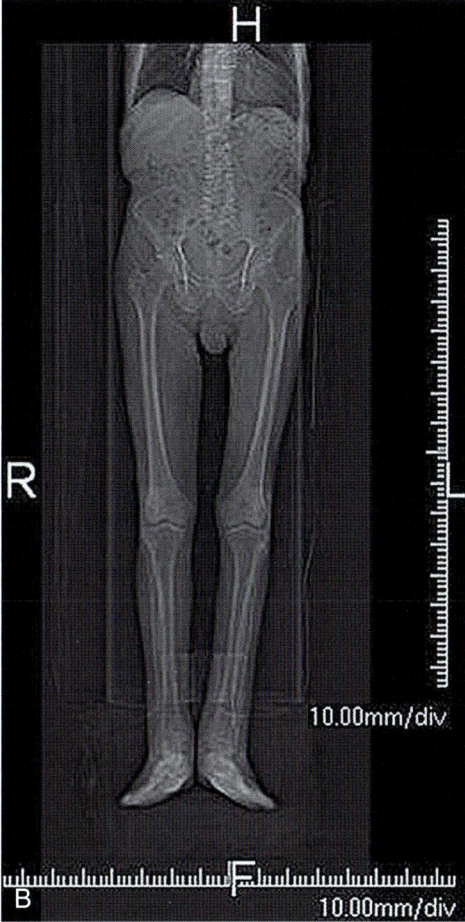

■ **FIGURE 115-9** Frontal and lateral scout topograms show the extended field of view in a typical CTA runoff study that is able to visualize the vasculature from the celiac artery to the toes. The lateral topogram ensures that the feet are included.

TABLE 115-1	CT Runoff: Typical Protocol for 16-Detector Scanner		
Patient preparation: 18- to 20-gauge angiographic catheter in antecubital vein			
Anteroposterior and lateral topograms to ensure that feet are in field of view			
	Before Administration of Contrast Agent	Angiography	Delay Calf
kVp	120	120	120
mAs	90	180	130
Slice collimation	0.75 mm	0.75 mm	0.75 mm
Slice width	5 mm	2 mm/1.5 mm	1.5 mm
Feed/rotation	15 mm	14.7 mm	13.0 mm
Rotation time	0.5 sec	0.5 sec	0.5 sec
Reconstruction kernel	B31f	B31f/B41f	B41f
Increment	5 mm	1.5 mm/1 mm	1 mm
Direction	Cranial-caudal	Cranial-caudal	Cranial-caudal
Coverage	Abdomen and pelvis	Above celiac to toes	Above knees to toes
Oral contrast agent	None		
Intravenous contrast agent	No	Yes	
Intravenous contrast agent injection rate		60 mL at 4 mL/sec, 60 mL at 2 mL/sec + 40 mL saline at 2 mL/sec	
Scanning delay		Aorta at celiac = 120 HU + 8 sec	Immediate
Reconstructions:			
Angiographic imaging: subtract bones, if needed, in abdomen and pelvis; must subtract bones in thighs and calves; can also subtract calcified plaques if needed, but save images before and after			
Coronal MIP of aorta and iliacs			
Oblique coronal MIPs of renal artery origins			
Sagittal MIP of celiac and superior mesenteric artery origins			
Oblique coronal MIPs of iliac and femoral bifurcations			
Coronal and sagittal MIPs of superficial femoral and popliteal arteries			
Coronal and oblique MIPs of calf vessels			
Coronal and sagittal MIPs of each foot—may need to rotate view for coronal view of feet			

TABLE 115-2   CT Runoff: Typical Protocol for 64-Detector Scanner

Patient preparation: 18- to 20-gauge angiographic catheter in antecubital vein
Anteroposterior and lateral topograms to ensure that feet are in field of view

	Before Administration of Contrast Agent	Angiography	Delay Calf
kVp	120	120	120
mAs	90	180	130
Slice collimation	0.6 mm	0.6 mm	0.6 mm
Slice width	5 mm	2 mm/1.5 mm	2 mm
Pitch	1.3	1.1	1.1
Rotation time	0.5 sec	0.5 sec	0.5 sec
Reconstruction kernel	B31f	B30f/B41f	B41f
Increment	5 mm	1.2 mm/1.0 mm	1.2 mm
Direction	Cranial-caudal	Cranial-caudal	Cranial-caudal
Coverage	Abdomen and pelvis	Above celiac to toes	Above knees to toes
Oral contrast agent	None		
Intravenous contrast agent	No	Yes	
Intravenous contrast agent injection rate		60 mL at 4 mL/sec, 60 mL at 2 mL/sec + 40 mL saline at 2 mL/sec	
Scanning delay		Aorta at celiac = 120 HU + 10 sec	Immediate

Reconstructions:
Angiographic imaging to toes: subtract bones, if needed, in abdomen and pelvis; must subtract bones in thighs and calves; can also subtract calcified plaques if needed, but save images before and after
Coronal MIP of aorta and iliacs
Oblique coronal MIPs of renal artery origins
Sagittal MIP of celiac and superior mesenteric artery origins
Oblique coronal MIPs of iliac and femoral bifurcations
Coronal and sagittal MIPs of superficial femoral and popliteal arteries
Coronal and oblique MIPs of calf vessels
Coronal and sagittal MIPs of each foot—may need to rotate view for coronal view of feet

- Table feed is equal to table speed multiplied by gantry rotation time.
- Collimation is equal to number of detectors multiplied by detector width.
- In-plane spatial resolution is inversely proportional to the field of view and directly proportional to the matrix and to the limit of the focal spot size (generally ~0.3 mm). Through-plane spatial resolution is determined by the slice thickness.
- Isotropic images are obtained when the spatial resolutions in all three planes are equal.
- Pitch is the proportion of the detector collimation that is covered in one gantry rotation (pitch = table feed in one gantry rotation/collimation).

Increasing the pitch results in the following:

- Reduced scan time for a constant z-axis coverage
- Increased z-axis coverage for a constant scan time
- Thinner slices for a constant z-axis coverage and scan time

A pitch greater than 1 broadens the slice sensitivity profile and in essence increases the effective section thickness.[12]

The z-axis is along the long axis of the body (i.e., in the direction the images are obtained). Clearly, the greater the number of detectors in the CT scanner, the greater the z-axis coverage in one gantry rotation. For example, if there are 64 detectors, each of width 0.625 mm, the area coverage is 4 cm in one rotation. If the pitch is 1.5 and the gantry rotation time is 500 ms, then 120 cm will be covered in 10 seconds. Assume the same parameters with 256 detectors; the scan time will be 2.5 seconds, which means that the acquisition will almost certainly outpace the contrast agent delivery to the lower extremity arteries. Thus, more detectors are not necessarily more beneficial in CTA runoff and after a certain number can actually be detrimental.

Consider this situation with a 4-detector scanner and a 1-mm individual detector width. It will take 100 seconds to cover 120 cm. This is too long and will result in one or more of the following: increased radiation dose, tube heating effects, increased contrast agent requirement, lower contrast agent administration rate, reduced arterial enhancement, and greater chance of venous enhancement. A choice must be made between the section thickness and the field of view, that is, one might have the entire field of view scanned for the thicker slices (e.g., 2.5-mm slices, which would mean a scan time of 40 seconds) or a smaller field of view scanned for thinner slices.

The optimal number of detectors that can provide submillimeter isotropic spatial resolution and coverage in a reasonable time without outrunning the bolus or incurring venous enhancement is 16 detectors. For proper visualization of the suprageniculate arteries in the absence of heavy calcification, a 4-detector scanner with 2.5-mm detector width can suffice. As a general rule, the larger the detector configuration, the lower the scanning pitch and the slower the gantry rotation speed.[1]

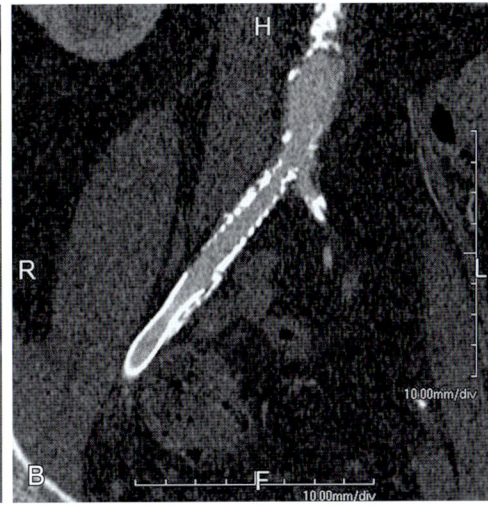

■ FIGURE 115-10 Slice thickness of 2 mm with a medium kernel (A) is compared with a slice thickness of 0.6 mm and a sharp kernel (B). Note that in B, the edges of the right iliac stents are crisper. The caveat to the increased edge definition in B is the increased image noise and reduced low-contrast resolution.

Scanning Parameters

A peak kilovoltage of 120 kVp is most frequently used for both the initial arterial phase CTA and the second delayed phase CTA, with the option to reduce to 100 kVp for thin patients and to increase to 140 kVp for the second delayed phase CTA acquisition through the calf if heavily calcified arteries are encountered. Noteworthy is that any change in peak kilovoltage settings has a disproportionate effect on the ionizing radiation dose (which is proportional to the square of the peak kilovoltage). The peak kilovoltage also affects image contrast, and lower peak kilovoltage settings will increase the attenuation of the arteries for a given dose of iodine.

Reconstruction Parameters

The major parameters in reconstruction are section thickness, overlap, and kernel.

The section thickness determines the through-plane spatial resolution (i.e., z-axis spatial resolution). Of course, having a thinner section (within the limits of the detector size) would mean a higher spatial resolution, but with the attendant increase in noise that may detrimentally affect both the signal-to-noise and contrast-to-noise ratios (Fig. 115-10). Thus, an optimal spatial resolution, which depends on the diameter of the smallest vessel that needs to be resolved, must be sought.

As a general rule, 2-mm thickness for the torso and thighs and 1.5-mm section thickness for the calf vessels suffice for most circumstances. The thinner section used for the calf vessels is necessary to compensate for the smaller size of vessels but also for their spatial proximity to bones. The bones cause high-attenuation artifact that can obscure the lumen of the neighboring artery. Thin sections reduce this artifact by reducing partial volume averaging.

Note that it is usual to acquire thinner slices (e.g., 0.6 mm) than are used for slice reconstruction (2 mm). This allows reconstruction of thinner slices if it is deemed necessary, if not as a matter of routine. This strategy reduces the number of images that need to be stored (because only the reconstructed slices, not acquired slices, are routinely stored) and also reduces the dose that one might be tempted to use to overcome the noise inherent in smaller voxels—thus the maxim "acquire thin and reconstruct thick."

Some degree of overlap of the reconstructed images is beneficial because it allows smoother three-dimensional reformats with minimal stair-step artifacts on oblique imaging views (Fig. 115-11).

The reconstruction kernel is essentially a tradeoff between low contrast resolution and spatial resolution. The sharper the kernel (higher numerical value), the higher the spatial resolution at the expense of increased noise and decreased low-contrast resolution. In general, calf and foot vessels (to reduce streak artifact from neighboring bone) and calcified arteries will benefit from a sharper kernel.

Summary of Acquisitions

- Scout topogram
- Non–contrast-enhanced scan (usually through the abdomen or pelvis or, in the context of trauma, through the affected limb part)
- Test bolus or bolus tracking scan
- Arterial phase CTA through the toes
- Delayed phase CTA through the calves (above knees to toes)

See Tables 115-1 and 115-2 for sample protocols.

Contrast Bolus Considerations

The aim of the injection protocol is to provide maximal enhancement of the peripheral arteries for the entire duration of the scan, with minimal enhancement of nonarterial structures. The exact contrast bolus protocol is scanner dependent and varies with the clinical question and the patient's factors. Therefore, rather than attempt to provide a specific protocol, the subsequent section emphasizes the principles.

1. The concept of iodine flux is important to understand.[15]
  The peak maximal enhancement of an artery depends

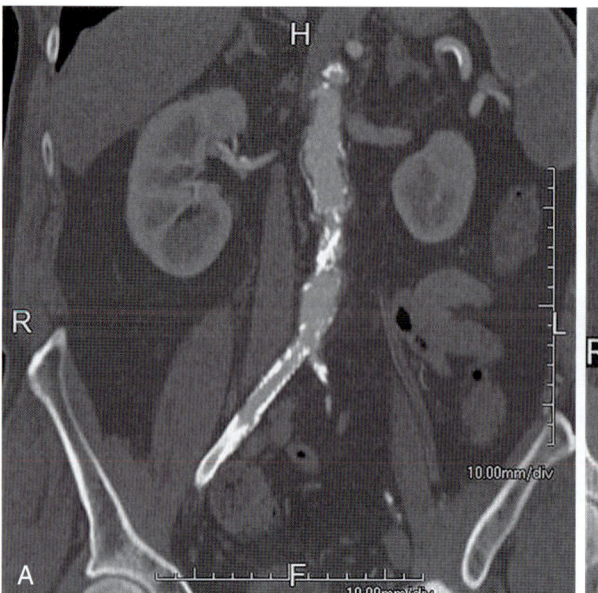

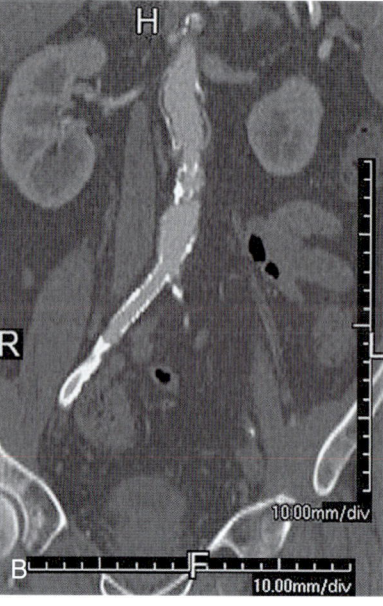

FIGURE 115-11 Reconstructed 2-mm slice thickness is compared with 1.2-mm overlap (**A**) and no overlap (**B**). A subtle difference lies in the quality of the reformatted images. Note that the edge of the innominate bone in **B** is more "streaky" than in **A**.

on both the rate of injection and the iodine concentration of the contrast agent (i.e., iodine delivery per unit time or iodine flux). In addition, the peak maximal enhancement increases with increasing volume of the contrast agent, which also increases the time to peak maximal enhancement.

2. A biphasic injection (i.e., two different injection rates) can be used to prolong the bolus duration and the resultant time of arterial contrast enhancement. Typically, this is used to lengthen the plateau phase of the bolus and prevents the sudden drop-off that occurs with a monophasic injection.[15,16]
3. Saline "tightens the bolus" by pushing it out of the peripheral veins into the central systemic circulation. This increases the duration of the arterial enhancement and has the potential to reduce the dose of contrast agent required.[15]
4. The contrast agent dose requirements increase with the patient's weight; however, at present, there are no formulas that can accurately predict the required amount.
5. Faster scanning speed (i.e., shorter scan time) requires a longer delay from the time of administration of the contrast bolus.[1]

Preferably, the contrast agent is administered through a 20-gauge antecubital peripheral venous catheter by means of a dual-chamber injector. The trick is to time the CT image acquisition with the peak contrast agent concentration in the target arteries. Of note, the acquisition does not follow the real-time first pass of the contrast agent through the arterial tree because such a task would require coordination of unattainable precision. Rather, the acquisition images the arteries during the period that the arteries are enhanced ("the contrast hangs around"). There are two approaches to ensure accurate timing[1]: bolus tracking and test bolus.

Bolus Tracking Technique

In bolus tracking (Figs. 115-12 and 115-13), a tracker (i.e., monitoring region) is set at an operator-determined location in the target arterial tree. This technique is automated; the scanner performs serial imaging of that tracker location, and the density within the tracker location is monitored. When the density of the tracker region of interest exceeds a predetermined threshold (e.g., 130 HU), CT scanning begins, typically after an operator-determined delay period (e.g., 5 seconds). The advantage

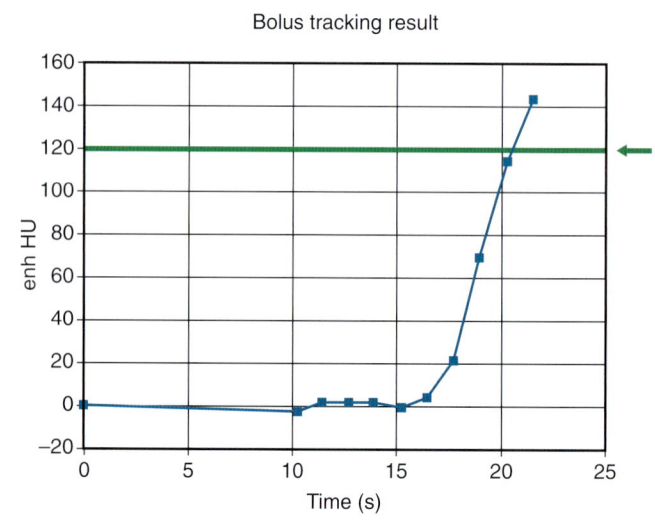

FIGURE 115-12 A typical bolus tracking graph. The operator has control of threshold Hounsfield units (HU) and the time delay of the start of the scan after the region of interest reaches the threshold HU. In this example, the threshold chosen is 120 HU (*arrow*). The time delay should take into consideration the volume of contrast agent, iodine concentration, and injection rate and factor a minimum delay that also allows the breath-hold instruction to be given and followed. enh, enhancement.

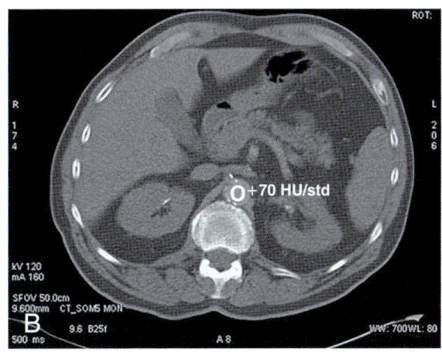

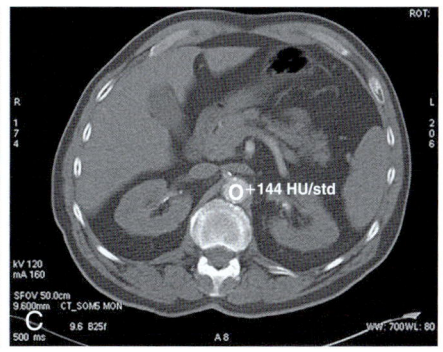

■ **FIGURE 115-13** Early (A), mid (B), and late (C) scans of the abdominal aorta after administration of an intravenous contrast agent bolus. During bolus tracking, a region of interest is placed in an artery, typically for a CTA runoff examination in the abdominal aorta as shown in these images. The tracker density is measured sequentially and in this case was increased from approximately 0 HU baseline density (A) to 70 HU (B) and 144 HU (C). With repetitive low-dose axial scans, the density within the tracker can be monitored for proper timing and initiation of the CTA scanning sequence. The density within the tracker region of interest, in this case the abdominal aorta, provides an automated method for detection of the contrast bolus arrival and for initiation of the CTA. This technique, however, provides timing only for the arrival of the contrast bolus, and should the patient have a slow circulatory time (e.g., heart failure patient), the resultant CTA may still outrun the contrast bolus arrival, especially at distal segments (i.e., below the knee).

of bolus tracking is its automated nature and resulting ease of operation. The disadvantage is its generalization and therefore inability to adapt to a patient's circulatory time. This may be important in patients with poor circulatory times, such as patients with heart failure or large aortic aneurysms.

Test Bolus Technique

The test bolus technique allows individualized timing for a patient's circulatory time. An area of the arterial tree is chosen and a region of interest is drawn. A certain volume of contrast agent (much less than the intended volume of injection, typically 15 to 20 mL) is injected at a rate equivalent to the intended rate of injection for the CTA, and serial CT images are performed of that location. For example, if the peripheral CTA bolus is intended to be 100 mL of contrast agent injected at a rate of 4.5 mL/sec, the test bolus will comprise an injection of 20 mL of contrast agent at 4.5 mL/sec followed by an equivalent volume (i.e., 20 mL) of saline at the same rate. The resulting Hounsfield unit measurements of the region of interest are plotted against time, and the time to peak maximal enhancement is noted. An adjustment factor is added to this time to factor in the extra volume of contrast agent (recall that both the peak maximal enhancement and the time to peak maximal enhancement increase with increasing volume of the contrast agent). The advantage of the test bolus is that it approximates to individual variation in the circulatory time, a fact of greater importance in those with cardiac impairment or slow arterial flow. The method also tests the patency of the intravenous access and thus potentially can reduce the frequency of extravasations.

The test bolus method has disadvantages. The test bolus is cumbersome to use. It requires an estimate of the adjustment factor because of the increased volume of contrast agent with the real injection, and this is, at best, a guess and certainly not based on an exact science. The test bolus also typically involves the administration of more iodinated contrast agent.

Pitfalls and Solutions

The pitfalls discussed are the ones specific to a peripheral CTA (runoff) examination. These can be categorized as acquisition considerations, interpretation considerations, and inherent CT limitations.

Acquisition Considerations

Poor image quality can result from poor synchronization of the peak maximal enhancement of arteries and image acquisition. Basically, the acquisition may have occurred too early or too late.[1]

Too early an acquisition may be due to scan parameters or patient factors. The scan parameters that predispose to premature acquisition include large detector collimation, fast gantry rotation, and high scanning pitch, essentially translating into faster anatomic coverage (i.e., scanning speed). The important patient factors to be appreciated are reduced cardiac function, increased volume of distribution resulting in contrast bolus dilution (e.g., aortic aneurysm), and steno-occlusive disease that delays contrast transit and can be strikingly asymmetric (Fig. 115-14).

The solutions are as follows:

1. Use a lower pitch, slower table speed, or slower gantry rotation time when using a large detector configuration (e.g., 64-detector CT scanner).
2. Increase the volume of the contrast bolus, slow the injection rate, or increase the delay time before the beginning of CT scanning.
3. Perform a second delayed phase CTA scan (i.e., a second "run") through the distal arteries in the calves to compensate for potential outrunning of the bolus during the initial arterial phase CTA.
4. Use a test bolus to individualize scan timing for the patient's circulatory time.

Alternatively, the acquisition may have been timed too late with respect to the peak maximal enhancement. It is

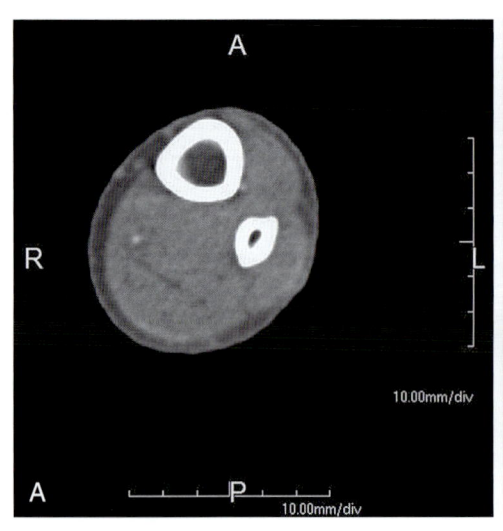

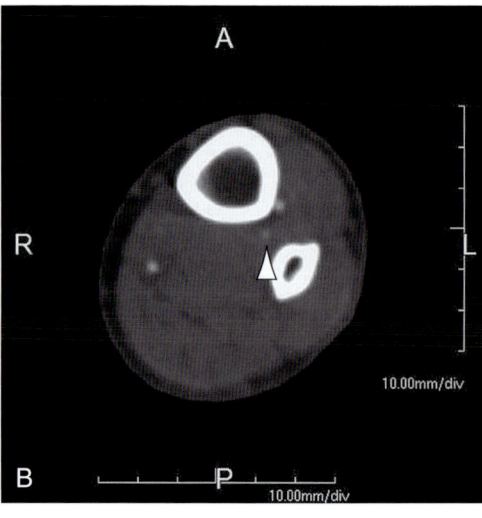

■ **FIGURE 115-14** Opacification of the left distal peroneal artery is noted in the second delayed phase CTA (**B**, *arrowhead*), not the first arterial phase CTA (**A**). The vessel is occluded proximally but filled by collaterals distally. Outrunning of the bolus may asymmetrically affect one side because of vascular disease, or it may affect both sides because of fast scan time. In either case, a second delayed phase CTA through the calf is prudent.

important to check the state of the aortic segment on which the tracker is placed for bolus tracking or test bolus. In the presence of disease, such as an atherosclerotic plaque or a dissection (which may not be apparent on the images obtained before the administration of the contrast agent), the tracker may be placed on the diseased part of the artery, such that the tracker attenuation values will not accurately reflect arterial luminal enhancement, thereby erroneously delaying the beginning of scanning.

The major problem with late acquisition is venous enhancement (or venous contamination). Patient factors that lead to venous contamination include (1) rapid venous filling due to regional hyperemia from inflammation, such as from an infected foot ulcer (a common situation in arteriopaths; Fig. 115-15), and (2) arteriovenous communication, such as an arteriovenous fistula or arteriovenous shunts, in the setting of severe occlusive disease.[17]

The point to be emphasized is that venous contamination can often be due to vascular pathologic processes and should not lead to a knee-jerk criticism of the technique or technologist. Appreciation of lower extremity vascular anatomy with cognizance of the fact that deep veins travel in pairs (venae comitantes) should allow distinction between veins and arteries in the cruropedal region by the experienced interpreter (Fig. 115-16). In addition, unlike MRA, CTA images generally have sub-millimeter resolution in the axial plane, where the arteries and veins can be viewed without overlap.

Interpretation Considerations

The most important problem in interpretation is the overestimation of stenoses due to calcification.[12] Calcium or any high-attenuation structure leads to the following:

- Blooming artifact because of spread of the point spread function (i.e., the structure looks bigger than it actually is)
- Beam hardening artifact
- Partial volume averaging leading to streak artifact

Overcalling of stenoses and occlusion can affect patient management. The strategies to overcome this pitfall are as follows:

- During acquisition
  - Use a higher peak kilovoltage. This reduces the beam hardening effect, although it also changes image contrast, reduces the attenuation of iodinated contrast material, and increases radiation dose.
  - Dual-energy CT. The concept of characterizing tissues by use of different energies has been

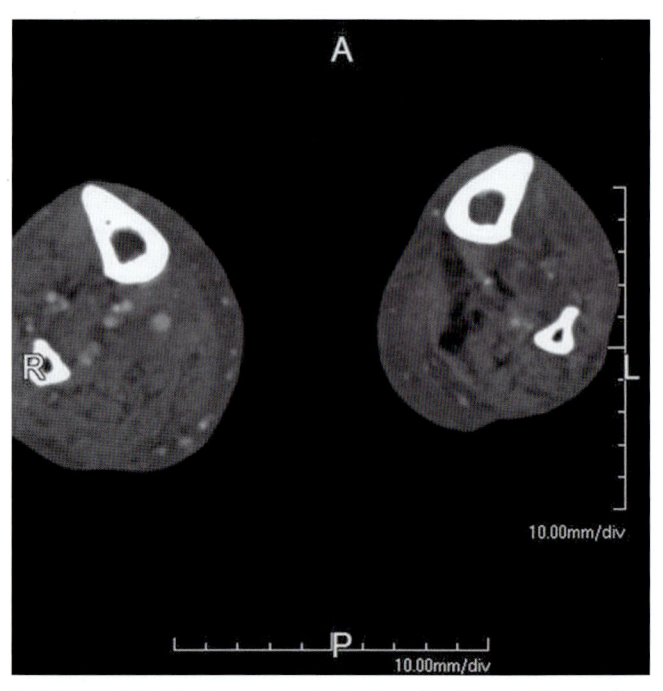

■ **FIGURE 115-15** Venous contamination of peripheral CTA runoff examination. Opacification of the leg veins can make the assessment of the arteries difficult. With current CT scanners, this is rarely due to slow scan speed. An inflammatory process has resulted in crural vein filling in the right leg. Severe arterial occlusive disease and resulting arteriovenous shunts can also lead to venous contamination.

receiving attention recently, almost 30 years after its first description. One method of dual-energy evaluation is to obtain simultaneous acquisitions with use of two source tubes operating at different kilovoltages (e.g., at 80 and 140 kVp). This allows separation of calcium from iodine and, theoretically, the ability to reduce the blooming associated with calcium and to facilitate more efficient bone subtraction algorithms.[18]

- During reconstruction
  - Use thinner slices. The partial volume averaging is reduced and edge definition is improved but at the expense of increased noise, which, if it is countered by increased milliamperes or kilovoltage, results in increased radiation dose.
- During interpretation
  - Use a wider window setting. Typical angiographic windows are centered at 150 HU with a width of 250 HU. For viewing of calcified vessels, the window can be centered to 200 HU with a width of 1000 HU (Fig. 115-17).
- Consider MRA or catheter angiography.

Inherent CT Limitations

See the section on contraindications.

Lack of Temporal and Flow Direction Information

The opacification of a vessel means that the contrast bolus has arrived, but in what temporal sequence is not dynamically captured by CTA. For example, opacification of the distal third of the posterior tibial may be due to retrograde flow through the plantar arch or antegrade flow through the proximal vessel. Single-station multiphase acquisitions (also known as time-resolved images) are required to answer this question. Although CT theoretically can do this, limited only by the gantry rotation time, the large radiation dose involved for the sequential assessment of flow dynamics makes it clinically untenable. However, time-resolved MRA with rapid temporal imaging may be an option in those in whom this information is critical before operative intervention.

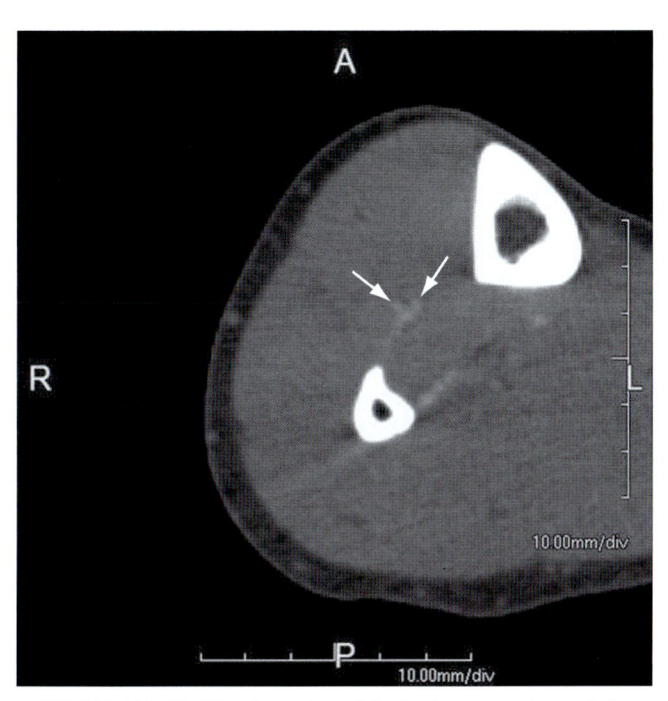

■ **FIGURE 115-16** The deep veins of the leg (venae comitantes) that accompany the tibioperoneal arteries travel in pairs, and this anatomic fact can aid in the identification of arteries when there is venous contamination. Note that the paired vascular structures surrounding the anterior tibial artery are the deep veins (*arrows*).

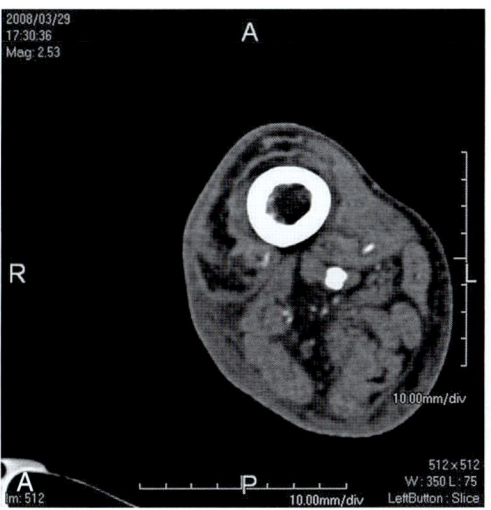

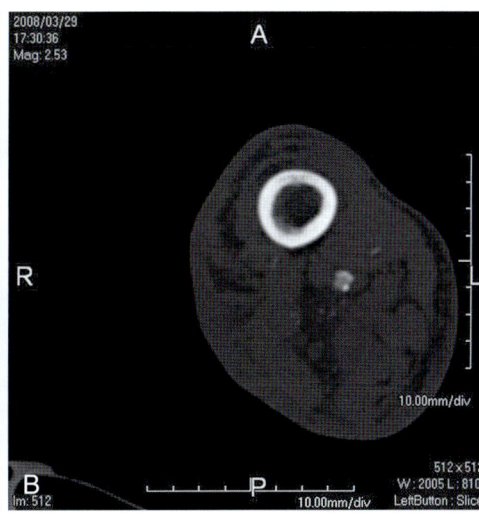

■ **FIGURE 115-17** Widening the window width and increasing the window level (**A,** narrow window; **B,** wide window) is a useful strategy at the workstation in dealing with the overestimation of stenosis in calcified vessels that is greater at narrower windows (**A**).

No Flow Quantification Information

CTA does not provide information about blood flow velocity, volume, or pressure gradients through areas of narrowing. If this information is necessary, catheter angiography and velocity-encoded phase contrast MRI are appropriate modalities for peripheral imaging, although MR will probably suffer from artifact if the vessel has a stent.

Image Interpretation

Postprocessing

The progress in three-dimensional image processing has created a worthy discipline in its own right and has revolutionized the handling of the extremely large data sets that accompany high-resolution and large field of view study, such as a peripheral CTA runoff examination.[1,19]

The following are basic principles to be appreciated.

- Stenoses should be quantified with referral to the axial source images.
- Interactive three-dimensional imaging permits the best approach to interpretation—a mechanism that is also often referred to as volume imaging.
- Visualization tools such as maximum intensity projection (MIP) and volume rendering are excellent for an overview (or a "road map") of the arterial tree, but their generation is typically operator dependent.
- Follow the "acquire thin and reconstruct thick" maxim. Assess nonvascular structures on the thicker reconstructions (e.g., 5 mm), then the vascular structures. Store the vascular images at a slice thickness thicker than the detector collimation (e.g., 2 mm).

Multiplanar Reformation

Multiplanar reformation, performed on standard operator or three-dimensional image workstations, consists of the processing of an image data set for viewing in a plane other than the one in which it is acquired. CT images are acquired helically and interpolated coaxially. Thus, rendition of CT data in a coronal, sagittal, or oblique plane is multiplanar reformation.

An underlying premise and fact of simple geometry is that when a structure runs in a plane that is off axis to the traditional cartesian planes, then to represent an accurate cross section of the structure, one must cut perpendicular to the plane of traversal or cut in a plane that is itself noncartesian. Put simply, to represent the cross-sectional area of a vessel accurately, one must be perpendicular to the centerline of the vessel. The generation of a predefined vascular centerline, curved multiplanar reformation, can be done by automated and partially automated software. The resulting cross section can thus be easily assessed for area and diameter change between diseased and nondiseased segments. The generation of these centerlines is arbitrary and may be erroneous in the presence of eccentric plaque, severe calcification, and extreme vessel tortuosity. As stated previously, the interpreter must rely on the axial source images when any ambiguity is encountered.

Curved multiplanar reformation lacks spatial perception, a problem that can be somewhat circumvented by the use of multipath curved planar reformation (Fig. 115-18).[20]

Maximum Intensity Projection

MIP processing will produce images similar to those of conventional angiography. MIP algorithms choose the highest attenuation voxels for projectional display in a prespecified volume, which would mean an accurate outline of arteries except that voxels from bone (necessitating bone editing) and other high-attenuation structures such as metal are often featured with disproportionate contribution. MIP provides an overview that is essential in conveying a large amount of clinical information in a single picture, including the presence of collaterals and the status of branch vessels. However, the technique can be misleading in terms of the degree of narrowing if there is extensive calcified atherosclerotic plaque, which is common at ostial segments in patients with atherosclerosis. MIP viewing may result in difficult interpretation in regions of calcified atherosclerotic plaque and in regions in which vessels travel in and out of the prescribed volume. Another pitfall of MIP is that it does not provide depth perception (Figs. 115-19 to 115-21).

Volume Rendering

As the name suggests, volume rendering uses the entire imaging volume (Fig. 115-22). Automated or manual assignment gives a tissue with a certain attenuation range a color and a level of transparency. For example, to visualize arteries separate from neighboring bone, volume rendering processing can be performed to designate that the tissue is red with no transparency between 200 and 500 HU and that the tissue is white with 100% transparency above 1000 HU. However, tissue attenuation values are a continuum with overlap of CT densities of plaque, iodinated contrast agent, and bone. Thus, accurate angiographic display of CTA data may still require a fair amount of manual and automatic editing of unwanted structures, making the process quite time-consuming even for the seasoned three-dimensional postprocessing operator.

Volume rendering is ideal for "snapshot" views of arterial segments. Depth perception is not lost when volume rendering is used. However, calcification and stents can obscure the lumen in much the same manner as in MIP images.

Thin Slab or Thick Slab

Basically, any three-dimensional postprocessing technique can be applied to the volume or less than the volume (subvolume, thin slab, thick slab). These terminologies merely emphasize the interactive nature of three-dimensional image processing in which the viewing direction and slab thickness are changed on the fly to incorporate as much or as little of the volume of interest according to the location and spacing of pathologic changes. Facility

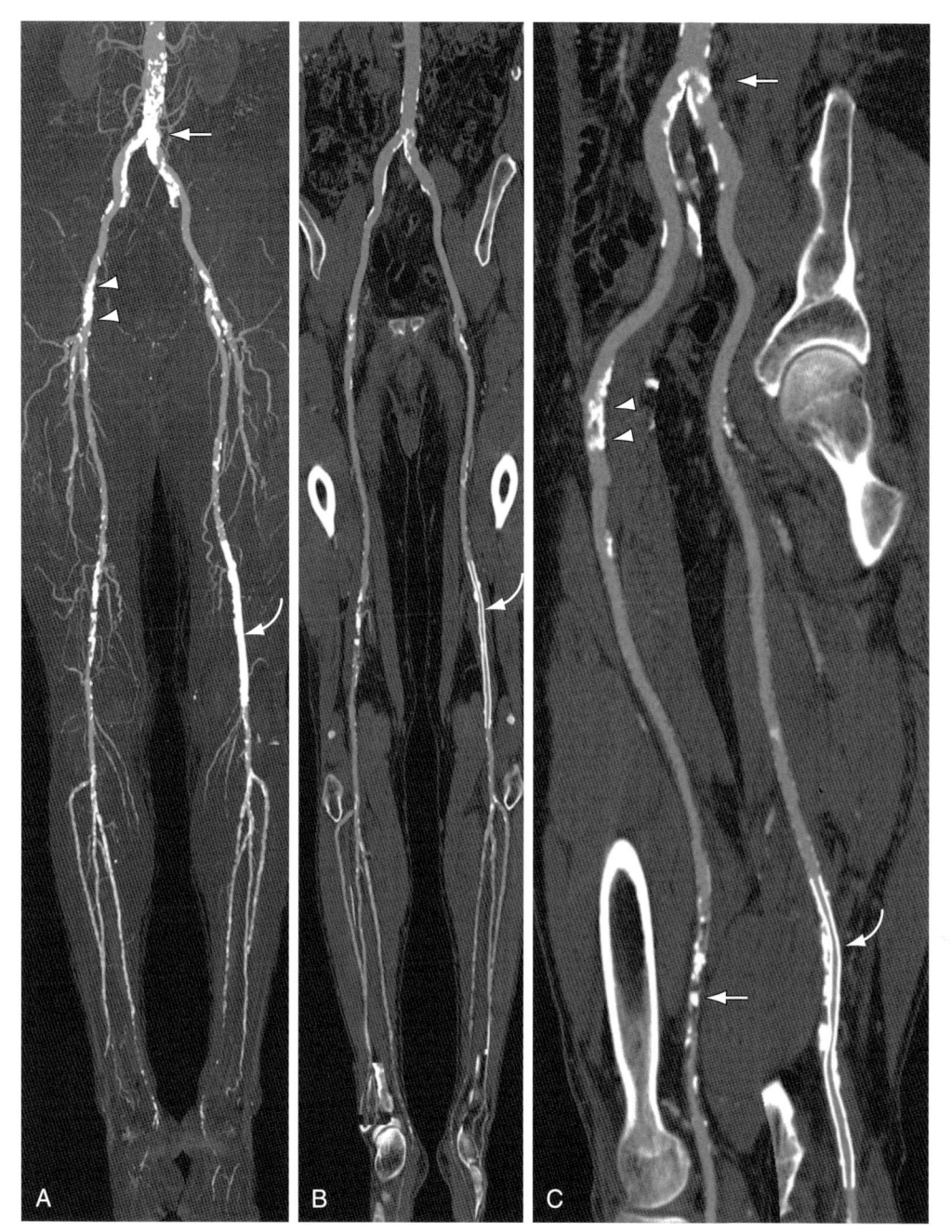

CHAPTER 115 • Computed Tomographic Angiography of the Lower Extremities

FIGURE 115-18 Peripheral CT angiography (16 × 0.75 mm, 2.0 mm/1.0 mm) of a diabetic male patient with bilateral claudication. MIP (**A**) shows arterial calcifications near the aortic bifurcation (*arrow*) as well as in the right (*arrowheads*) and left common femoral arteries, in the right femoropopliteal region, and in the crural vessels. A long stent is seen in the left femoropopliteal segment (*curved arrow*). Frontal view (**B**) and magnified 45-degree left anterior oblique (**C**) multipath CPR images provide simultaneous CPRs through the aorta and bilateral iliac through crural arteries. Note that prominent calcifications cause luminal narrowing in the proximal left common iliac artery (*arrow*) and in the right common femoral artery (*arrowheads*). The left common femoral artery is normal; the long femoropopliteal stent is patent (*curved arrow*). Mixed calcified and noncalcified occlusion of the right distal femoral artery is also seen (*open arrow*). (From Fleischmann D, Hallett RL, Rubin GD: CT angiography of peripheral arterial disease. J Vasc Interv Radiol 2006; 17:3-26.)

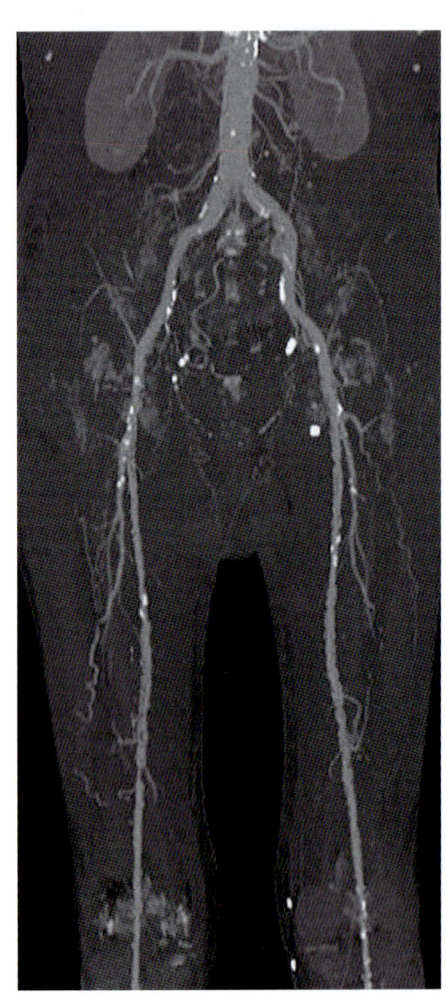

■ **FIGURE 115-19** MIP images provide a snapshot of the vasculature, giving information on the amount and extent of disease in the main vessels and the branches and also on the presence of collateral vessels. This is well demonstrated in this coronal MIP image with diffuse atherosclerosis that is shown by the diffuse calcified plaque and diffusely irregular arterial margins.

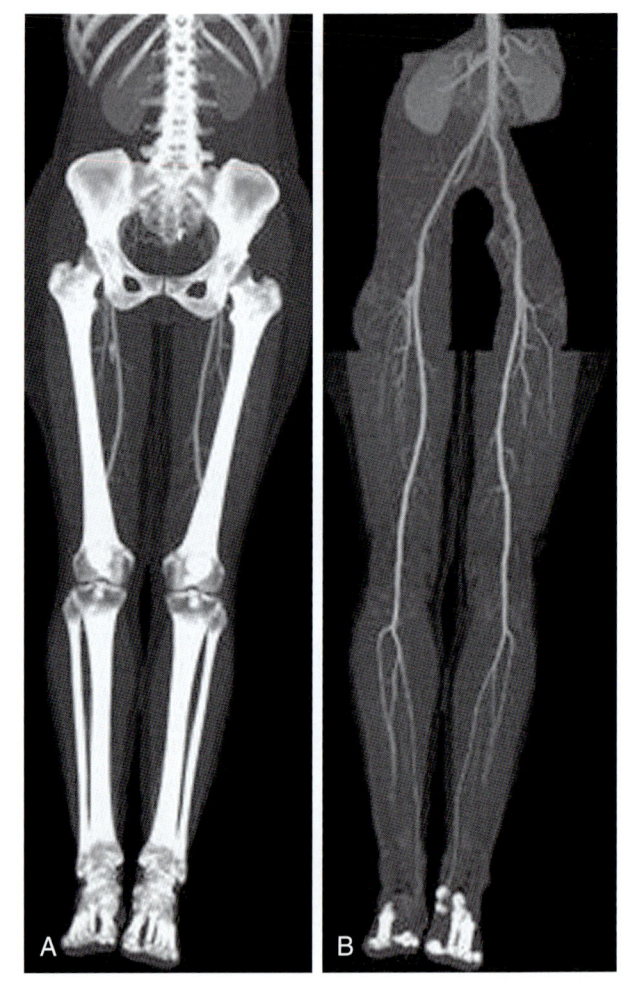

■ **FIGURE 115-20** MIP pitfall. Any high-attenuation structure is manifested on MIP images; the most problematic is bone (**A**), which therefore requires editing (**B**).

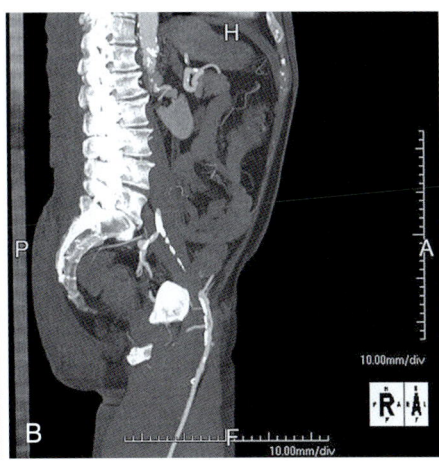

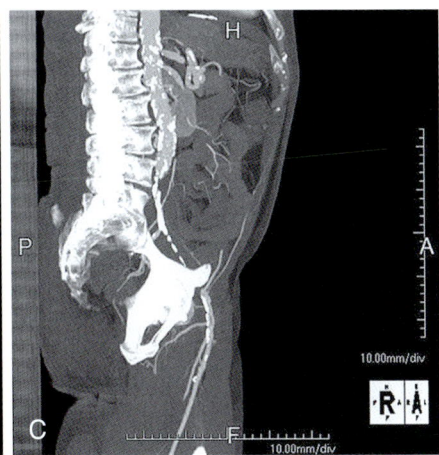

FIGURE 115-21 Increasing the thickness of the slab on which the MIP is extracted from 1 mm (**A**) to 30 mm (**B**) clearly results in more of the arterial tree visualized. However, this is at the expense of superimposition of bone and, eventually, at 60-mm slab thickness (**C**), obscuration of the arterial structure by bone.

with these techniques has the potential to dramatically speed up interpretation time, which is a common rate-limiting step in peripheral CTA interpretation.

Reporting

Reporting of imaging findings must convey to the referring physician information that aids in diagnosis, prognosis, and treatment planning. Interpreters of peripheral CTA examinations should be familiar with the recommendations of the TransAtlantic Inter-Society Consensus.[21] The Consensus document provides recommendations on the nature of intervention based on the location and length of the obstruction, among other factors, such as the status of the distal runoff and of the proximal inflow vasculature, and the presence and eccentricity of calcified

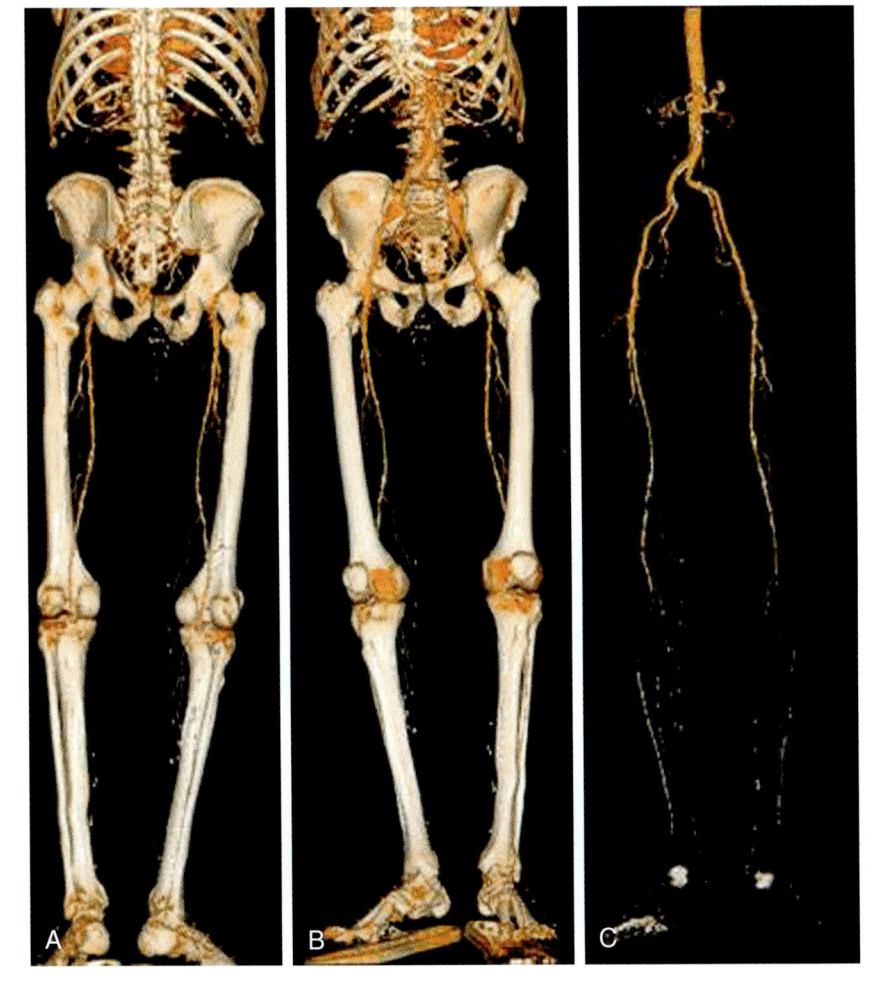

FIGURE 115-22 Volume rendered images without (**A** and **B**) and with (**C**) bone editing. Volume rendering affords more depth perception than MIP does, but it still requires bone editing. This is difficult to achieve in the foot because of both the shared CT attenuation values between contrast-enhanced arteries and bone and their proximity.

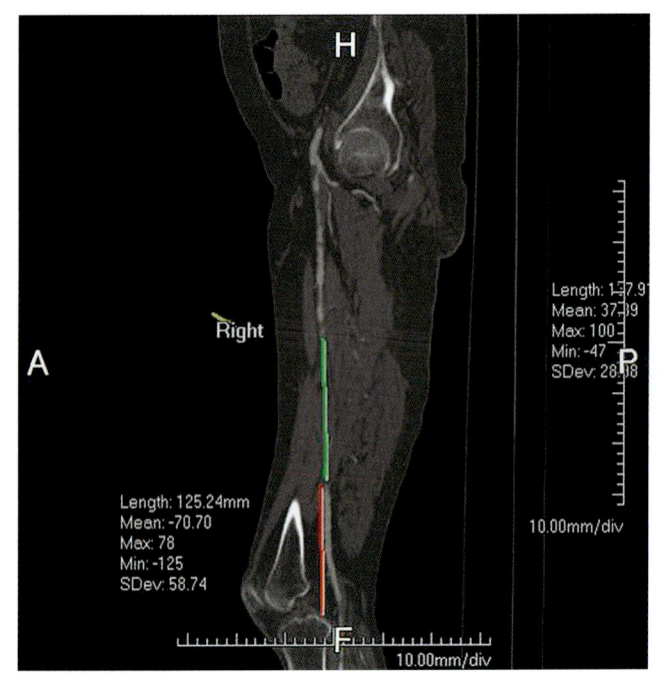

FIGURE 115-23 The report of a CTA runoff must contain information that assists the vascular surgeon with both diagnosis and treatment planning. The length of an occluded segment and the distance of the reconstituted segment from a bone landmark must be included, as should the status of the runoff. In the patient shown in Figure 115-2, for example, the posterior tibial arteries were patent in their entirety and would be the choice of distal attachment for a bypass of the mid superficial femoral artery occlusion. The anterior tibial and peroneal arteries were severely narrowed or occluded for most of their course.

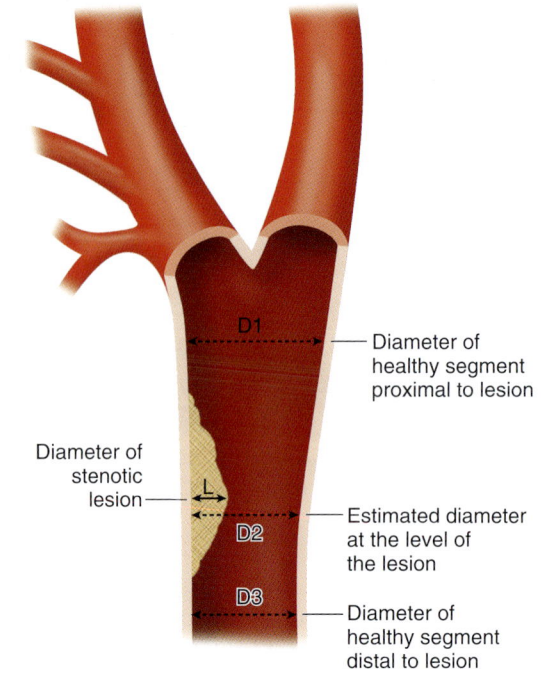

FIGURE 115-24 The key to calculating the percentage stenosis using the diameter or area is in choosing the reference segment, which may be either proximal (D1), at (D2), or distal to (D3) the stenotic segment. The degree of stenosis, for example, is L/D2.

plaque. The interpreter should avoid merely providing a litany of stenoses but attempt to think like a vascular surgeon in reporting peripheral CTA results (Fig. 115-23).

The report can be broadly divided into the following categories:

- Extent of vascular disease
- Patency of vessels and collaterals
- Nonvascular findings

The arterial tree is best subdivided into the following:

- Inflow (aortoiliac segment)
- Outflow (femoropopliteal segment)
- Runoff (calf and pedal vessels)

Patency can be described in the following manner:

- Occlusion—no flow or enhancement
- Critical stenosis (>70% narrowing)
- Moderate stenosis (30% to 70% narrowing)
- Mild stenosis (<30% narrowing)
- No stenosis but atherosclerotic plaque causing positive vessel remodeling
- Normal (no atherosclerotic plaque or stenosis)

When a vessel is occluded or has critical stenosis, it is important to state the following:

- Length of segment: Is the lesion focal or segmental?
- Is the lesion focal, multifocal, or multisegmental?
- What is the distance of the lesion to a bone landmark (e.g., knee or ankle)?
- If the vessel occludes, does it reconstitute, and which vessel provides the collateral supply? Distance should be measured from the point of reconstitution to a bone landmark.
- Is the lesion calcified or noncalcified? If it is calcified, what is the eccentricity of the calcification?

If there is diffuse atherosclerotic disease distal to an occlusion or critical stenosis, the length of the most disease free distal segment is described.

For the quantification of the degree of stenosis, the diameter or area of the artery in the diseased segment (L) is compared with the diameter or area of the artery in the healthy arterial segment (R). Percentage stenosis is calculated as $(1 - L/R) \times 100$ (Fig. 115-24). Although measurement of area stenosis is more accurate than measurement of diameter stenosis, it is the consistency of measurement that is more important.[22]

KEY POINTS

- CTA can provide an assessment of the arterial tree from the aortic arch to the toes in a single arterial phase scan.
- CTA provides the vascular surgeon essential information for determination of proper diagnosis, treatment, and operative strategy.
- Peripheral CTA does not require a 64-detector or above scanner.
- The presence of atherosclerotic calcifications may result in the overestimation of an arterial stenosis.
- Interpretation of large data sets requires a combination of two-dimensional and three-dimensional techniques.
- Axial source images must be used for interpretation to avoid interpretation mistakes that may result from three-dimensional postprocessing.

SUGGESTED READINGS

Fleischmann D, Hallett RL, Rubin GD. CT angiography of peripheral arterial disease. J Vasc Interv Radiol 2006; 17:3-26.

Ota H, Takase K, Rikimaru H, et al. Quantitative vascular measurements in arterial occlusive disease. Radiographics 2005; 25:1141-1158.

Roditi GH, Harold G. Magnetic resonance angiography and computed tomography angiography for peripheral arterial disease. Imaging 2004; 16:205-229.

REFERENCES

1. Fleischmann D, Hallett RL, Rubin GD. CT angiography of peripheral arterial disease. J Vasc Interv Radiol 2006; 17:3-26.
2. Waugh JR, Sacharias N. Arteriographic complications in the DSA era. Radiology 1992; 182:243-246.
3. Visser K, Kock MC, Kuntz KM, et al. Cost-effectiveness targets for multi-detector row CT angiography in the work-up of patients with intermittent claudication. Radiology 2003; 227:647-656.
4. Schernthaner R, Fleischmann D, Lomoschitz F, et al. Effect of MDCT angiographic findings on the management of intermittent claudication. AJR Am J Roentgenol 2007; 189:1215-1222.
5. Chow LC, Napoli A, Klein MB, et al. Vascular mapping of the leg with multi-detector row CT angiography prior to free-flap transplantation. Radiology 2005; 237:353-360.
6. Fleiter TR, Mervis S. The role of 3D-CTA in the assessment of peripheral vascular lesions in trauma patients. Eur J Radiol 2007; 64:92-102.
7. Hyodoh H, Hori M, Akiba H, et al. Peripheral vascular malformations: imaging, treatment approaches, and therapeutic issues. Radiographics 2005; 25:S159-S171.
8. Karcaaltincaba M, Aydingoz U, Akata D, et al. Combination of extremity computed tomography angiography and abdominal imaging in patients with musculoskeletal tumors. J Comput Assist Tomogr 2004; 28:273-277.
9. Chew FS, Bui-Mansfield LT. Imaging popliteal artery disease in young adults with claudication: self-assessment module. AJR Am J Roentgenol 2007; 189(Suppl):S13-S16.
10. Takase K, Imakita S, Kuribayashi S, et al. Popliteal artery entrapment syndrome: aberrant origin of gastrocnemius muscle shown by 3D CT. J Comput Assist Tomogr 1997; 21:523-528.
11. http://www.fda.gov/CDER/drug/InfoSheets/HCP/gccaHCP.htm. Accessed May 13, 2008.
12. Knollman F, Coakley FV (eds). Multidetector CT—Principles and Protocols. Philadelphia, Elsevier, 2005.
13. Rubin GD, Schmidt AJ, Logan LJ, Sofilos MC. Multi-detector row CT angiography of lower extremity arterial inflow and runoff: initial experience. Radiology 2001; 221:146-158.
14. Hartnell GG. Contrast angiography and MR angiography: still not optimum. J Vasc Interv Radiol 1999; 10:99-100.
15. Fleischmann D. Use of high-concentration contrast media in multiple-detector-row CT: principles and rationale. Eur Radiol 2003; 13(Suppl 5):M14-M20.
16. Fleischmann D, Rubin GD, Bankier AA, Hittmair K. Improved uniformity of aortic enhancement with customized contrast medium injection protocols at CT angiography. Radiology 2000; 214:363-371.
17. Milne EN. The significance of early venous filling during femoral arteriography. Radiology 1967; 88:513-518.
18. Johnson TR, Krauss B, Sedlmair M, et al. Material differentiation by dual energy CT: initial experience. Eur Radiol 2007; 17:1510-1517.
19. Fishman EK, Ney DR, Heath DG, et al. Volume rendering versus maximum intensity projection in CT angiography: what works best, when, and why. Radiographics 2006; 26:905-922.
20. Roos JE, Fleischmann D, Koechl A, et al. Multipath curved planar reformation of the peripheral arterial tree in CT angiography. Radiology 2007; 244:281-290.
21. Norgren L, Hiatt WR, Dormandy JA, et al; TASC II Working Group. Inter-Society Consensus for the Management of Peripheral Arterial Disease (TASC II). J Vasc Surg 2007; 45(Suppl S):S5-S67.
22. Ota H, Takase K, Rikimaru H, et al. Quantitative vascular measurements in arterial occlusive disease. Radiographics 2005; 25:1141-1158.

CHAPTER 116

Peripheral Magnetic Resonance Angiography

Tim Leiner

MR angiography (MRA) is a highly reliable technique that is widely used for imaging large and medium-sized arteries of the pelvis and lower extremities. In many hospitals worldwide, this technique has become an important adjunct to duplex ultrasonography (DUS) and x-ray catheter angiography, specifically intra-arterial digital subtraction angiography (IA DSA), in the workup of suspected peripheral artery disease (PAD). MRA, in many cases, is replacing diagnostic x-ray catheter angiography because it can provide similar diagnostic vascular road maps (Fig. 116-1) without the associated clinical concerns and risks related to invasive catheterization, ionizing radiation exposure, and use of iodinated contrast agents.

In this chapter, different MRA techniques that can be used for imaging the peripheral arteries are discussed. Currently, contrast-enhanced MR angiography (CE MRA), typically in conjunction with a bolus chase or multistation method, is the most widely used and validated technique for peripheral MRA and remains the standard of reference against which all other MRA methods are typically compared. Recently, there has been renewed interest in non-contrast-enhanced MR angiography techniques, mainly as an alternative to CE MRA in patients with severely compromised renal function. Although these techniques are elegant, their validity and clinical utility remain to be established.

PAD (also called peripheral arterial occlusive disease or peripheral vascular occlusive disease) is almost invariably the result of advanced atherosclerosis of the pelvic and lower extremity arteries. With increasing age, atherosclerotic plaque develops in the walls of the lower extremity arteries, leading to luminal narrowing and often arterial occlusion. This progression of events results in a recognizable clinical constellation of signs and symptoms that typically begins as intermittent claudication and progresses to lower extremity pain at rest and even nonhealing skin ulceration. The diagnosis of PAD is typically initially made on the basis of a single measurement of the ankle-brachial index (ABI) below 0.9.[1]

PREVALENCE AND EPIDEMIOLOGY

Atherosclerotic PAD is an important health care problem in Western society, with an estimated prevalence of about 3% of the general population in those older than 50 years. The prevalence rises to about 15% to 20% of the general population in those older than 70 years.[1]

ETIOLOGY AND PATHOPHYSIOLOGY

Patients with PAD typically present with a history of intermittent claudication. This term is derived from the Latin *claudicatio*, which means to limp. Claudication typically consists of cramping and pain in the buttocks, thighs, and lower legs that occurs with exercise (e.g. walking or climbing stairs). In these symptomatic patients with PAD, peripheral arterial blood flow is unable to augment to meet the increased metabolic demands of the lower extremity muscles during exercise. On cessation of exercise, these complaints typically disappear rapidly because arterial flow at rest is typically sufficient to meet the patient's basal metabolic needs.

In a minority of patients with intermittent claudication, the PAD will subsequently progress to critical ischemia, whereby even at rest the lower extremity arterial flow is insufficient to meet basal resting metabolic needs (i.e., oxygen and nutrient demand) of the lower extremity. Clinically, this is manifested by pain at rest and, in more severe cases, as nonhealing ulcers, cellulitis, and even gangrene. See Chapter 113 for an extensive discussion of the clinical aspects of PAD.

MANIFESTATIONS OF DISEASE

Clinical Presentation

The diagnosis of PAD is made on the basis of the typical history, physical examination (palpation of arterial pulsations), and measurement of the ABI. When a patient

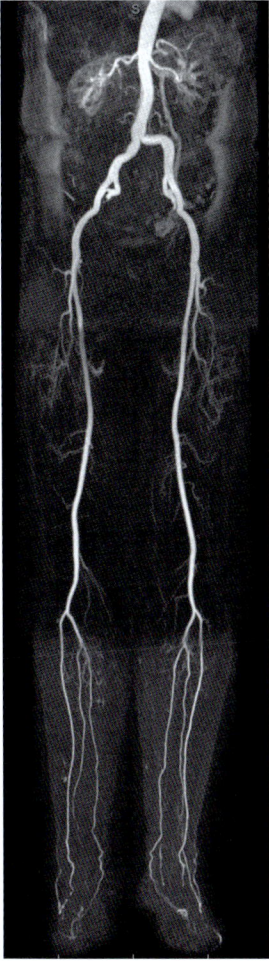

FIGURE 116-1 50-year-old patient suffering from complaints of intermittent claudication. Apart from iliac artery elongation, no abnormalities are present. Note the high-quality depiction of the peripheral vascular tree down to the pedal arteries.

presents to the general practitioner or vascular surgeon with complaints of PAD, first-line treatment consists of modification of and/or treatment for atherosclerotic risk factors, such as smoking, hypertension, hypercholesterolemia, and the institution of (supervised) exercise training.[2,3] Only when the patient's complaints become too limiting to pursue regular activities will invasive interventional treatments be considered. For patients with intermittent claudication, the decision to intervene is largely dependent on relative criteria (patient and surgeon preference), but for patients with chronic critical ischemia, the need to intervene is more urgent because tissue perfusion does not meet basic metabolic demands, even at rest. Of 100 patients presenting with PAD, 5 eventually undergo percutaneous or surgical treatment.[1] Although this is only a small minority of patients with PAD, the estimated annual number of percutaneous and surgical procedures performed for PAD in the United States alone was well over 200,000 in 2000, with sharp increases expected.[4]

Imaging Indications and Algorithm

Because the diagnosis of PAD is usually made from the typical history, physical examination, and ABI measurements, the need for imaging of the peripheral arteries only arises when a percutaneous or surgical intervention is considered. Imaging is needed to explore the extent of the disease process (e.g., number, location, and severity of atherosclerotic lesions) and to plan the correct approach for therapy.[5]

Traditionally, the standard of reference for imaging PAD has been x-ray catheter angiography, which initially had been through a translumbar aortic approach. In 1953, the transfemoral approach was developed by Seldinger, in which arterial access is gained through the superficial or common femoral artery.[6] Having been refined and technically optimized, this is the procedure most widely used in state of the art angiography today, and is still considered the standard of reference. When combined with digital subtraction techniques, high-resolution projection arteriograms of the peripheral arterial circulation can be obtained in a routine fashion. However, substantial rates of local and systemic procedure-related complications have sparked the search for noninvasive alternatives to IA DSA.

Patients with PAD are best served when they undergo as little testing as possible to establish a diagnosis and plan the appropriate therapy. The key clinical question is whether patients are candidates for a simple local procedure (e.g., percutaneous transluminal angioplasty or local endarterectomy) to treat focal disease or, alternatively, whether the disease is too diffuse and long segmented so that it requires a more extensive or complex procedure such as aortofemoral bypass surgery. CE MRA is well-suited for this purpose and can serve as the primary imaging modality for patients with PAD because it provides the necessary information for proper diagnosis and procedural decision making.

Imaging Techniques and Findings

Radiography

Conventional radiographs may demonstrate calcific deposits in the vessel wall but, in general, there is no role for dedicated radiography in the assessment of suspected peripheral arterial disease.

Ultrasound

DUS is widely used to determine the location, length, and severity of aortoiliac and femoropopliteal stenoses and obstructions. Duplex ultrasound was developed in the 1980s as an alternative to invasive angiography to avoid the inherent complications associated with the latter procedure. With DUS, the severity of a stenosis can be determined by using peak systolic velocity (PSV) measurements in arteries with reduced luminal diameter, PSV ratio at the site of stenosis and adjacent normal artery, end-diastolic velocity, and other less firmly established criteria. The sensitivity and specificity of DUS are generally moderate to high, ranging from 70% to 90%.[7] However, a relatively recent meta-analysis,[8] as well as a large prospective comparison study between CE MRA and DUS in 295 patients,[9] has found that CE MRA is more sensitive and specific compared with DUS for the detection of PAD.

Computed Tomography

Recent advances in CT technology have enabled fast and robust CT angiography (CTA) of the peripheral vascular tree. Although there are fewer reports comparing CTA with conventional angiography for the detection of PAD as compared with CE MRA, it is widely believed that CTA is a valid and reliable method.[10] The drawback of CTA is the enormous number of data sets that it generates—up to several thousand images per patient—and that heavily calcified arteries demand extensive user interaction to assess the underlying degree of stenosis adequately. In addition, the newest generation of multidetector row CT scanners is so fast that the contrast bolus may progress more slowly down the leg than the CT acquisition, leading to suboptimal opacification of the distal lower extremity arteries. For an in-depth discussion of CTA of the peripheral arteries, including these issues, see Chapter 115.

Magnetic Resonance Angiography

Although there are a variety of different MR angiography techniques, CE MRA is the most widely used method. Phase contrast (PC) and time of flight (TOF) MRA[11] were the subjects of intense investigation about a decade ago, but the intrinsic drawbacks associated with these methods, such as long imaging times and their propensity to overestimate the degree and length of arterial stenoses, have led to the abandonment of these techniques in favor of CE MRA. The superiority of CE MRA over other MRA methods for peripheral artery imaging has been confirmed in several meta-analyses.[12,13]

Recent concerns related to nephrogenic systemic fibrosis (NSF) have resulted in an increased interest in non-contrast-enhanced balanced steady-state free precession (bSSFP)–based techniques as alternatives for CE MRA. Although these techniques are promising, there are very limited data with regard to their diagnostic accuracy and clinical utility for imaging patients with PAD. Preliminary data have indicated that the value of these techniques lies in their high negative predictive value.

Contrast-Enhanced Magnetic Resonance Angiography of the Peripheral Arteries

The challenge for imaging patients with PAD is the need for imaging over an extended field of view (FOV) that begins at least from the level of the aortic bifurcation to the distal runoff vessels (ankles, feet), a region that typically requires imaging over three overlapping FOVs (abdomen-pelvis, thighs, and calves-feet). Current CE MRA techniques using some combination of bolus chase or stepping table CE MRA can usually cover the peripheral arterial tree within 15 minutes. However, adequate planning of peripheral CE MRA is essential. Operators must not only ensure proper anatomic coverage of the overlapping three-dimensional MRA volumes but also adjust the various imaging parameters to provide high image quality and spatial resolution for optimal benefit of the arterial phase of the contrast medium bolus. The exact spatial location of the three-dimensional CE MRA imaging volumes that cover the vascular tree of interest is determined on scout or localizer images. Scout scans are usually axial, thick-slice, low-resolution two-dimensional TOF scans or, more recently, steady-state free precession (SSFP) acquisitions. Acquisition of scout views in a sagittal or coronal orientation can also be useful. The advantage of using two-dimensional TOF images is that the vascular anatomy can be selectively viewed on postprocessed maximum intensity projections (MIPs). When the three-dimensional CE MRA volumes are prescribed, transverse source images should *always* be reviewed to ensure that all relevant vascular structures are included in the imaging volume. Failure to do so can result in the exclusion of relevant anatomy from the imaging volume.

Vascular Anatomy Considerations

In most patients, the anteroposterior coverage needed is usually less than 10 cm. When imaging in the presence of an aortic aneurysm, iliac arterial elongation, collateral bridging iliac or superficial femoral arterial obstructions, or femorofemoral crossover bypass graft, the anteroposterior (AP) coverage needed to depict these vessels may be markedly increased (up to 15 to 20 cm). Review of the transverse localizer images ensures that these structures are not excluded from the three-dimensional CE MRA imaging volume. This is particularly important if a patient has a femorofemoral crossover bypass graft because these grafts are usually not seen on axial TOF MIPs because of in-plane saturation artifacts. Particular attention should be paid to prescription of the MRA imaging volumes in patients with extra-anatomic bypass grafts because the grafts often extend beyond the traditional boundaries of a routine peripheral CE MRA and the scan volumes will need to be modified to include the grafts. Other patients that demand special attention are those with (thoraco-)abdominal aortic aneurysms in whom flow may be markedly slower compared with patients without an aortic aneurysm. If the scan delay (i.e., time period between the initiation of the contrast bolus injection and the beginning of MRI) is too short, there will be incomplete opacification of the abdominal aorta and its branches. This problem can be solved by use of a longer scan delay or a multiphase MRA acquisition technique (i.e., time-resolved MRA).

Synchronization of Three-Dimensional Contrast-Enhanced Magnetic Resonance Angiography Acquisition with Contrast Arrival

For successful CE MRA, care must be taken to synchronize peak arterial enhancement with image data acquisition, specifically acquisition of the central k-space data. The time of peak arterial enhancement is a function of many variables, the most important of which are injection rate and volume, amount and rate of saline flush,[14] and cardiac output.[15] Because the time of peak arterial enhancement can vary substantially among patients, the CE MRA examination needs to be tailored to the individual contrast arrival time. This is important for two main reasons: (1) to prevent "ringing" image artifacts and poor arterial opacification, which may occur if imaging is performed too early; and (2) to prevent suboptimal arterial enhancement and excessive venous and/or background enhancement, which occurs if imaging is performed too late.

To ensure acquisition of central k-space views during peak arterial enhancement, a two-dimensional time-resolved test bolus technique can be used. More recently, real-time bolus monitoring software packages have been introduced by all major MRI system vendors, and these are now considered the state of the art for CE MRA (e.g., BolusTrak, Philips Medical Systems, Best, The Netherlands; CareBolus, Siemens Medical Solutions, Erlangen, Germany; and Fluoro Trigger, General Electric Healthcare, Waukesha, Wisc). Instead of injecting a small amount of contrast material in a separate test bolus scan, real-time bolus monitoring allows the operator to time the imaging for the CE MRA in real time using a single contrast injection of the total volume of contrast material. Using real-time bolus monitoring, the operator monitors the contrast bolus progression and initiates MRA scanning when the desired signal enhancement in the target arterial bed has been reached. Automated bolus detection algorithms that do not require operator initiation of scanning are also available and are equally successful for achieving proper CE MRA timing.

Strategies to Optimize Vessel to Background Contrast

For multistation peripheral CE MRA (i.e., bolus chase CE MRA), the arterial T1 shortening associated with the sustained injection of a 0.1- to 0.3-mmol/kg dose of a standard (0.5 M) gadolinium-chelate contrast agent is generally insufficient to view the arteries preferentially over the extended FOVs over that of background tissue, especially in distal infrapopliteal arteries. The elimination of signal from background tissues, especially fat, because it has the shortest T1, is typically necessary for successful multistation peripheral CE MRA. The most commonly used technique to suppress background signal is image subtraction of nonenhanced mask three-dimensional MRA images from those of similarly acquired contrast-enhanced three-dimensional CE MRA. Although image subtraction decreases the signal-to-noise ratio by a factor of about 1.4 (√2 when the number of signals acquired is 1), vessel to background contrast improves to the extent that whole-volume MIPs become clinically useful, especially when using injection rates below 1.0 mL/sec.[16] A disadvantage of using mask scans is that patients may move in between acquisition of the mask and contrast-enhanced parts of the scan, which can lead to subtraction misregistration artifacts. Subtraction misregistration artifacts may also occur if table positioning between the precontrast mask and postcontrast CE MRA is not accurate, on the order of 1 mm or less.

Because the T1 of fat is close to that of contrast-enhanced arterial blood, another way to suppress background tissue is by spectral saturation of signal from protons in fat. Although a fat saturation prepulse can be integrated into the three-dimensional CE MRA sequence, this takes a significant amount of time, which in turn must be offset by decreasing spatial resolution to achieve the same desired overall acquisition duration. Results of using fat saturation pulses are mixed and their use can, therefore, not be universally recommended.[17,18]

A dedicated peripheral vascular surface coil is mandatory for high-quality imaging of the pelvic and lower leg arteries. Image quality and anatomic coverage are vastly improved when compared with imaging without these dedicated lower extremity coils.[19]

Strategies to Decrease Venous Enhancement

Venous contamination is an important problem for CE MRA. This problem is particularly prevalent in patients with cellulitis or arteriovenous fistulas or malformations.[20] Venous and background soft tissue contamination of arterial illustration are particularly prevalent in patients with diabetes mellitus.[21] Diabetic patients, furthermore, are more likely to have limb-threatening ischemia and to require peripheral distal bypass surgery, making them prime candidates for preoperative peripheral artery imaging using CE MRA.

The most straightforward way of preventing venous enhancement is by shortening the MRA acquisition duration. This should be done, first of all, by lowering the repetition time (TR) and echo time (TE) to the shortest possible value, without excessively increasing bandwidth. In addition, partial Fourier or fractional echo imaging can be used. When doing peripheral CE MRA (i.e., bolus chase CE MRA using three consecutive overlapping stations), it is particularly important to image the proximal two stations (aortoiliac and upper legs) as fast as possible. This affords a relatively longer scan period for high spatial resolution imaging of the smaller distal lower extremity (infrapopliteal) arteries. Use of centric or elliptical centric k-space filling schemes for this third and terminal station minimizes venous enhancement, despite the lateness of imaging relative to the overall contrast bolus duration. With the introduction of multielement surface coils, whereby multiple reception coils are used simultaneously to collect data, acquisition speed can be increased further by applying parallel imaging algorithms.

To avoid the limitations of imaging three consecutive stations, an alternative approach is to use two separate injections for peripheral CE MRA. In this approach, the distal lower legs (calves-feet or infrapopliteal region) are imaged during the first contrast medium bolus, and then a second contrast medium injection is administered to image the remaining two more proximal stations (the aortoiliac region and upper legs) using a two-station bolus chase CE MRA method. A benefit of this hybrid approach[22] is that it can provide more reliable high spatial resolution three-dimensional MRA of the distal lower leg station, because timing of imaging is specific for contrast arrival to the distal lower extremities versus arbitrary timing based on progression of the stepping table during a standard three-station multistation peripheral CE MRA. The initial acquisition of the lower legs is typically done using up to 15 to 20 mL of a standard 0.5 M Gd-chelate contrast agent; it can be performed as a single arterial phase or multiphase (arterial and delayed phase) acquisition. Because this first acquisition is a dedicated single-station MRA of the infrapopliteal region, synchronization of central k-space lines is optimized for peak contrast enhancement in the lower leg arteries, and venous enhancement is almost eliminated. After imaging the infrapopliteal region, a moving table acquisition is performed to image the proximal two stations (aortoiliac region and upper legs) using the remaining dose of 20 to 40 mL Gd-chelate contrast medium. Note that it is *not* recommended that any cumulative Gd-chelate contrast medium dose exceed an agent's approved dose levels, which in some cases is up to 0.3 mmol/kg dose for an adult patient. The greatest benefit of using the hybrid approach can be expected in patients with fast or highly variable arterial flow velocities, such as patients with chronic critical ischemia, arteriovenous fistulas, diabetes mellitus, and/or cellulitis.

In addition to the two-injection hybrid approach, there is also the technique in which separate injections are used for each imaging station (e.g., three separate injections, each for a different station). Although this approach can be used in the absence of dedicated multistation software and/or hardware, a disadvantage of the multiple injection technique is that the total dose of Gd-chelate contrast agent has to be divided into three or more separate injections, resulting in lower amounts of contrast agent available to image each station. This may lead to diminished vessel to background contrast with each subsequent injection secondary to increased background signal contamination with each contrast medium injection. Although escalating doses per injection can offset this issue, safety limitations of overall Gd-chelate contrast medium doses make this option not practical.

Over the past few years, all major MR vendors have implemented dedicated centric k-space filling algorithms. Centric k-space filling is useful for CE MRA because the time between arterial and venous opacification is usually shorter than the duration of a high spatial resolution three-dimensional CE MRA acquisition. The underlying principle is to collect central k-space data, which primarily determine image contrast, during peak contrast enhancement of the target arterial territory and before significant venous enhancement has taken place.[23,24] Peripheral k-space data primarily provide information related to edge detail of the image and can be acquired later during the bolus progression, with nominal impact on overall image quality. Therefore, use of centric k-space filling schemes for CE MRA timed for arterial phase of a bolus will result in preferential arterial images, with minimal venous contamination in most cases, even if the period between arterial and venous enhancement is shorter than the total duration of image acquisition.

Centric k-space filling is primarily useful for single-station abdominal and upper and lower leg acquisitions. However, centric k-space filling can also assist in optimization of multistation peripheral MRA. In the case of multistation peripheral MRA, centric k-space filling will advance central k-space sampling to the beginning of MRA data acquisition, which is preferred for imaging the second and third stations in the imaging progression to advance the sampling relative to the contrast medium bolus progression. That is to say, later imaging of central k-space data during a long bolus administration will increase the likelihood for venous contamination. When centric k-space filling is combined with parallel imaging, the chances of venous enhancement decrease even further.

Preferential arterial imaging can also be provided using time-resolved CE MRA, but it is crucial that temporal sampling be sufficient to image the arterial phase of the contrast medium bolus prior to significant venous enhancement. One popular time-resolved CE MRA technique uses repetitive centric k-space filling to obtain high spatial resolution MR angiograms with high temporal frame rate (i.e., time-resolved imaging at several seconds per frame). Korosec and colleagues[25] were first to describe this concept, which they termed *time-resolved imaging of contrast kinetics* (TRICKS). With TRICKS, the contrast-sensitive central part of k-space is oversampled (i.e., more often) than the peripheral resolution-sensitive views. After the acquisition is finished, central k-space lines are combined with peripheral lines through a process of temporal interpolation so that a series of time-resolved three-dimensional images of the vasculature are obtained. More recently, keyhole contrast-enhanced timing robust angiography (CENTRA) was described. With keyhole CENTRA, temporal resolution is increased by repetitive acquisition of the central part of k-space *only*. This information is later combined with a data set containing the peripheral part of k-space, which is acquired as part of the last frame of the time-resolved series.[26] Subsequently, these hybrid k-spaces can be reconstructed as a series of time-resolved three-dimensional CE MR angiograms. Combining keyhole imaging with parallel imaging can further increase temporal resolution. Time-resolved three-dimensional CE MRA is well suited for the initial dedicated distal lower leg (infrapopliteal) three-dimensional CE MRA of a hybrid peripheral MRA method.

Another final method to reduce venous contamination is by using midfemoral or infragenual venous compression with infrasystolic pressures of 50 to 60 mm Hg.[27,28] It remains to be determined whether patients with critical ischemia and/or ulcers, in which high-quality lower leg images are most important, can tolerate this type of compression.

All techniques discussed here can be combined to reduce the risk of disturbing venous enhancement even further.

Resolution Requirements

To describe the degree of stenosis accurately, it is paramount that the resolution of the three-dimensional data set meet minimal standards. For example, it is known from studies by Hoogeveen and associates[29] and Westenberg and coworkers[30] that at least three pixels are needed across the lumen of an artery to quantify the degree of stenosis with an error of less than 10%. When this constraint is kept in mind, it is rather obvious that a higher spatial resolution is needed to characterize stenoses in the hepatic or renal arteries accurately, which are smaller in diameter than the abdominal aorta or iliac arteries. In general, voxel dimensions should be kept as close to isotropic (equal length in all dimensions) as possible; otherwise, vessels become blurred when they are viewed on postprocessed oblique projections. Recommended voxel sizes resolution are about 4 to 5 mm^3 in the aortoiliac arteries, 3 to 4 mm³ in the upper legs, and 1 mm³ or more for hepatic, renal, or lower leg arteries.

Contrast Media and Injection Protocols

CE MRA relies on synchronizing maximum T1 shortening with acquisition of central k-space information. However, injection of gadolinium-chelate contrast medium only leads to transient T1 shortening of the blood pool. After having briefly enhanced the intravascular space, these contrast agents rapidly diffuse into the extracellular space. The intravascular half-life of commercially approved agents is about 90 seconds.[31] Enough contrast must be injected to decrease the T1 of blood to values smaller than those of stationary background tissues. To depict the vasculature selectively, this means that the T1 of blood must be reduced to a value well below that of fat (T1 at 1.5 T = 270 ms). The rate of gadolinium injection is dictated by the following equation:

$$\frac{1}{T_1} = \frac{1}{1200} + R_1 \times [Gd]$$

where T1 denotes the T1 of arterial blood at a given gadolinium concentration, 1200 is the T1 of arterial blood at 1.5 T, R1 is the T1 relaxivity of the contrast medium, and [Gd] is the arterial concentration of the gadolinium chelate. The rate of contrast injection should be such that an arterial T1 of about 50 ms or less is achieved. For example, when injecting a double dose (0.2 mmol/kg) of a 0.5 mmol/mL Gd-chelate contrast medium at 1.0 mL/sec in a 75-kg patient (i.e., 30 mL of contrast medium), assuming a relaxivity of 3.9 mmol⁻¹ · s⁻¹ and a cardiac output of 5 L/min, the lowest achievable T1 in arterial blood under first-pass conditions will be about 41 ms.

In almost all reported peripheral CE MRA studies, conventional 0.5 M extracellular contrast agents were used. Typically, between 0.1 and 0.3 mmol/kg of a Gd-chelate contrast agent is injected (e.g., from 15 to 45 mL for a 75-kg patient), followed by 15 to 30 mL saline injection to flush contrast from injection tubing and veins into the central venous and arterial circulations. When a time-resolved two-dimensional test bolus approach is used to image the lower legs and pedal arteries first, usually around 5 to 7 mL of contrast is used, followed by a slightly larger saline flush volume, to make sure that the contrast medium is flushed from the tubing and veins into the central circulation. When a hybrid approach is used, the lower legs are usually imaged with 15 to 20 mL of Gd-chelate contrast medium, and the aortoiliac and upper leg arteries with 20 to 25 mL of Gd-chelate contrast medium. Newer systems and systems capable of time-resolved imaging enable substantial reductions in the amount of contrast dose used; my experience is that peripheral CE MRA can be performed with Gd-chelate contrast medium doses as low as 20 mL.

At present, there is no single preferred injection protocol, although an empiric strategy that works well in clinical practice is that the contrast injection duration should be about 40% to 60% of the acquisition duration. The rationale for this strategy is twofold. First, because of contrast dilution at the leading and trailing edges of the contrast medium bolus, as well as variable transit times through different portions of the pulmonary circulation, contrast bolus duration will increase in the body (usually to about 5 to 7 seconds).[32] The second reason is that contrast injected after about half of the typical scan duration (on the order of 10 to 20 seconds) will not arrive in the arterial bed of interest before k-space lines contributing to contrast enhancement in the image are acquired.

The amount of Gd-chelate contrast medium to be injected, as well as injection speed and amount of saline flush, are dependent on other variables, such as the scan duration and technique used (i.e., single vs. multiple injection). Boos and colleagues[15] have found that increasing the amount of contrast injected, as well as saline flush volume, increases bolus length and improves small vessel conspicuity, but does not necessarily result in higher vessel to background contrast.

Novel Contrast Media

Vessel to background signal can also be improved by using other contrast agents than the standard 0.5 M gadolinium chelate contrast agents. Recently, the first 1.0-M agent (Gadobutrol, Schering AG, Berlin) was approved for clinical use in Europe for CE MRA. Gadobutrol is formulated at a higher Gd concentration of 1.0 mol/L and has about 20% higher relaxivity (T1 relaxivity in blood, 5.2 mmol⁻¹ · s⁻¹ at 37° C and 1.5 T) than traditional 0.5-M Gd-chelate contrast agents, generating lower blood T1 values compared with traditional contrast agents and thus offering an attractive method to increase intravascular signal.[33] In direct head to head comparisons between 1.0- and 0.5-M Gd-chelate contrast agents for pelvic MRA, Goyen and associates[34] found that the use of the 1.0-M agent led to significantly higher signal- and contrast-to-noise ratios and better delineation of especially small pelvic arteries.

Other promising agents for peripheral arterial imaging are gadobenate dimeglumine (Gd-BOPTA; MultiHance, Bracco Diagnostics, Milan, Italy) and gadofosveset trisodium (Ablavar; Lantheus Medical Imaging, Billerica, Mass). Both these agents exhibit reversible albumin binding (5% of injected dose for gadobenate dimeglumine and 85% of injected dose for gadofosveset trisodium), which leads to high-contrast images at lower doses compared with the conventional extracellular agents. Because of the high fraction that is protein-bound, gadofosveset trisodium is excreted much slower than extracellular agents, as evidenced by a mean intravascular half-life of about 30 minutes.[35] This leads to the possibility of not only acquiring images during the first pass, but also during the so-called steady state or equilibrium phase of the contrast bolus, a period during which the contrast agent has opacified both the arterial and venous systems. Because of the contrast agents' prolonged intravascular circulation time, images can be acquired with much higher spatial resolution compared with first-pass imaging, thus promising to increase the sensitivity and specificity of the resultant images for arterial disease detection and grading.[36]

Nonenhanced Magnetic Resonance Angiography of the Peripheral Arteries

Improvements in MR hardware and software, coupled with concerns about the safety of gadolinium-based contrast agents, have contributed to a renaissance of interest in nonenhanced MRA. An excellent and very comprehensive overview of the different nonenhanced techniques has recently been published by Miyazaki and Lee,[37] and the reader is referred to this article for further information about the technical details of these techniques.

However, despite the promising initial results, there is a paucity of studies in the literature in which noncontrast medium–enhanced techniques are compared with CE MRA or IA DSA. As of mid-2009, only a single study in 36 patients has been published[38] in which three-dimensional noncontrast medium–enhanced electrocardiograam (ECG)-gated MRA of the distal lower extremities was compared with CE MRA. Although the noncontrast medium–enhanced technique demonstrates a high negative predictive value 92.3%, the overall accuracy of 79.4% can be considered poor compared with CE MRA techniques.

Nuclear Medicine/Positron Emission Tomography

There is no role for nuclear medicine techniques in the diagnostic or preinterventional workup of PAD.

Angiography

Conventional IA DSA is still considered the standard of reference for the exact quantification of stenoses and occlusions of the peripheral vascular tree, although there is almost universal consensus that both MRA and CTA are as good as IA DSA for providing the clinically relevant information about the aorta and larger named arteries down to the ankle that is needed by the referring clinician. It is clear that a large fraction of the diagnostic IA DSA examinations can reliably be replaced by MRA or CTA, given the availability of the necessary imaging equipment and expertise. However, because of the superior spatial resolution of IA DSA, both MRA and CTA are presently not considered adequate alternatives for the characterization of lesions in smaller caliber arteries with a diameter smaller than 1 mm (e.g., small branch vessels and pedal arteries).

Classic Signs

The typical appearance of an atherosclerotic lesion is a focal excentric arterial narrowing, that may be relatively smooth or more serrated in appearance (Fig. 116-2). Lesions can be very short (several millimeters) or may extend over the entire vessel length. Long-standing high-grade stenoses and occlusions may be bridged by collateral vessels with a typical corkscrew appearance. Acute or very recent occlusions tend not to be very well collateralized.

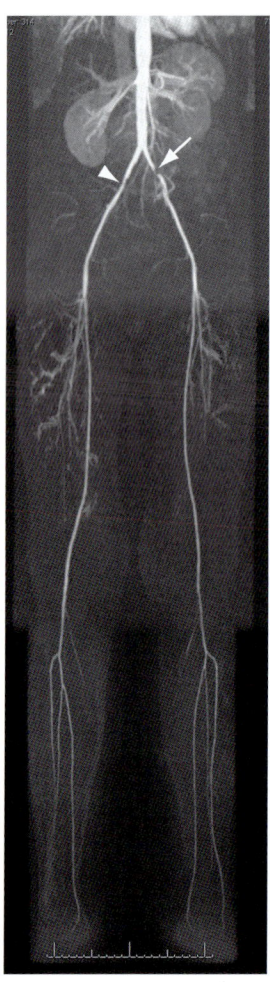

■ **FIGURE 116-2** Bilateral focal iliac stenoses in 55-year-old male patient suffering from left-sided intermittent claudication. The stenosis on the left (*arrowhead*) is a high-grade lesion; the stenosis on the right (*arrow*) is a mild nonsignificant lesion.

DIFFERENTIAL DIAGNOSIS

From Clinical Presentation

Although PAD in the lower extremities is almost invariably caused by atherosclerosis, there are well-known nonatherosclerotic diseases that may present with intermittent claudication or critical ischemia. An atypical history or clinical characteristics incongruent with those typically seen in atherosclerotic PAD should prompt consideration of alternative causes. There is an extensive list of differential diagnostic considerations. Some of the more frequently seen diseases are vasculitis, Buerger's disease, popliteal entrapment, cystic adventitial disease, and radiation-induced arteritis.[11]

From Imaging Findings

If a lesion in the peripheral vascular tree does not have the typical atherosclerotic appearance as described earlier, one should consider other diseases. Concentric smooth luminal narrowing is atypical in atherosclerosis and is generally suggestive of more uncommon causes of PAD,

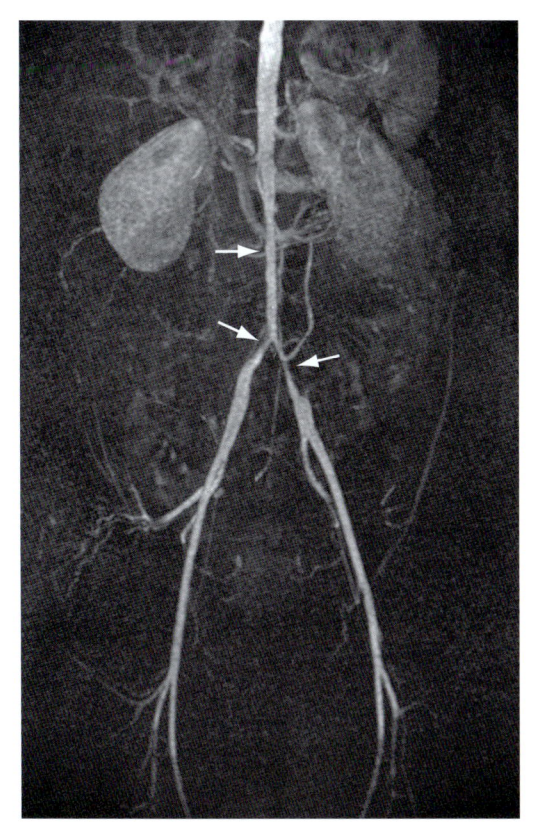

■ **FIGURE 116-3** A 29-year-old woman with long-standing complaints of intermittent claudication caused by Takayasu disease. Note the multiple smooth, segmental stenoses (*arrows*), which are characteristic of circumferential vessel wall thickening caused by inflammation.

such as vasculitis (Fig. 116-3) or cystic adventitial disease (Fig. 116-4). Evaluation of the soft tissues surrounding the artery of interest may reveal additional clues about other causes, such as aberrant insertion of the medial head of the gastrocnemius muscle in popliteal entrapment syndrome or the presence of high-signal intensity proteinaceous material in the popliteal artery wall in cystic adventitial disease.

SYNOPSIS OF TREATMENT OPTIONS

See Chapters 113 and 114 for an overview of treatment options for PAD.

REPORTING: INFORMATION FOR THE REFERRING PHYSICIAN

Aorta and Iliac Arteries

The aorta and iliac arteries are also referred to as inflow arteries in the context of peripheral arterial disease of the lower extremities. When evaluating the peripheral vasculature, it is important to describe the morphologic pattern of occlusive disease.

For lesions involving the aortic bifurcation and proximal iliac artery (Fig. 116-5), involvement of the contralateral iliac artery should also be noted, because this will change the preferred interventional treatment strategy. In case of aortic occlusion (Leriche syndrome; Fig. 116-6) or unilateral iliac artery occlusion, the site of distal reconstitution should be noted, because this will determine the

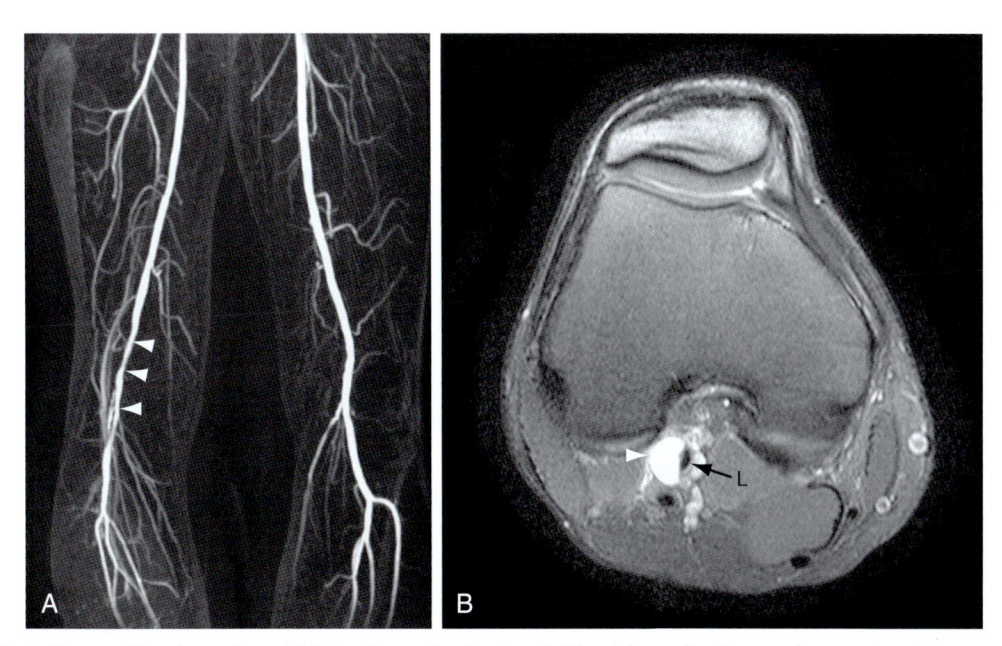

■ **FIGURE 116-4** A 40-year-old male smoker with intermittent claudication. **A,** The right popliteal artery shows a smooth segmental stenosis (*arrowheads*). **B,** Subsequent T2-weighted imaging in the transverse orientation demonstrates a cystic mass in the popliteal vessel wall (*arrowhead*) compressing the popliteal artery lumen (L).

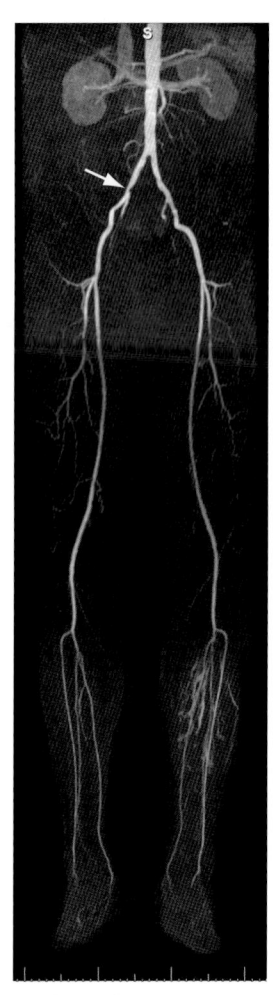

FIGURE 116-5 A 63-year-old male patient with mild intermittent claudication caused by a borderline significant stenosis in the right common iliac artery (*arrow*). Note slight venous contamination of the left lower leg.

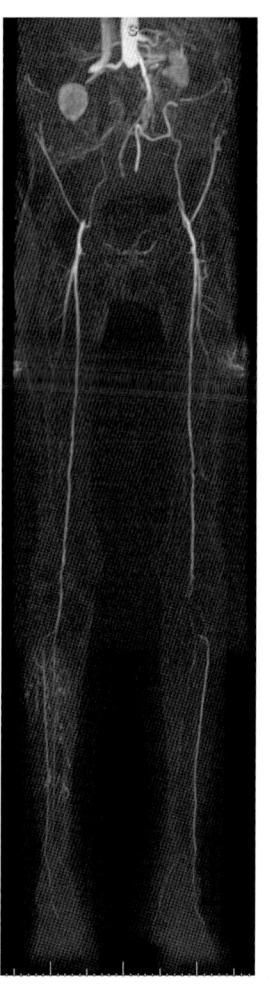

FIGURE 116-6 A 70-year-old male patient with characteristic infrarenal and bilateral iliac artery occlusions. These findings are diagnostic for the Leriche syndrome. Also note the severe distal PAD.

surgical approach. The easiest and most widely used way of measuring diameter reduction is simply to measure the maximum degree of luminal reduction on MIP images, analogous to how stenoses are measured on IA DSA images. A stenosis is generally considered to be hemodynamically significant when reduction of the luminal diameter exceeds 50%.

Femoropopliteal Arteries

CE MRA is an excellent modality to image infrainguinal disease, because inflow and outflow arteries can be imaged in a single examination. The key differentiation that must be made when evaluating the upper leg vasculature is whether there is a relatively short focal stenosis (see Fig. 116-2) or complete occlusion over a long segment (Fig. 116-7). This differentiation is particularly important in the setting of intermittent claudication, because patients and their vascular surgeons may only be interested in invasive treatment in case endovascular options can be considered.

The most common site of stenoses or occlusions is where the superficial femoral artery courses through the adductor (Hunter) canal. Current best clinical practice is to attempt endovascular treatment in patients in whom lesion length does not exceed 3 cm. Available evidence indicates that surgery is still the best treatment option when lesion length exceeds 5 cm.[1]

Lower Leg and Pedal Arteries

Although depiction of the infragenicular arterial system in patients with intermittent claudication is important, it is usually not the location of the lesions that causes symptoms, nor the target for invasive intervention, except in patients with diabetes mellitus.[39] This is opposed to the group of patients with chronic critical ischemia, those with rest pain and/or tissue loss. The angiographic hallmark of chronic critical ischemia is bilateral multiple stenoses and occlusions at different levels in the peripheral arterial tree. Patients with diabetes are a well-recognized

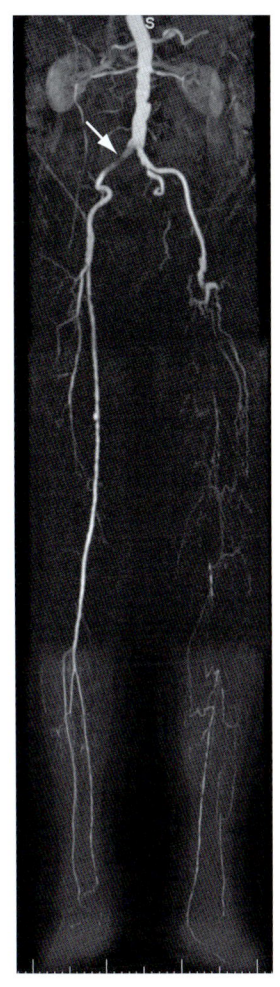

■ **FIGURE 116-7** A 67-year-old male patient with severe intermittent claudication caused by extensive occlusive disease of the left superficial femoral and popliteal arteries as well as the proximal lower leg arteries. MRA can confidently inform the vascular surgeon that bypass surgery is the preferred treatment option in this patient. Also note signal loss in the right common iliac artery (*arrow*) caused by prior stent placement.

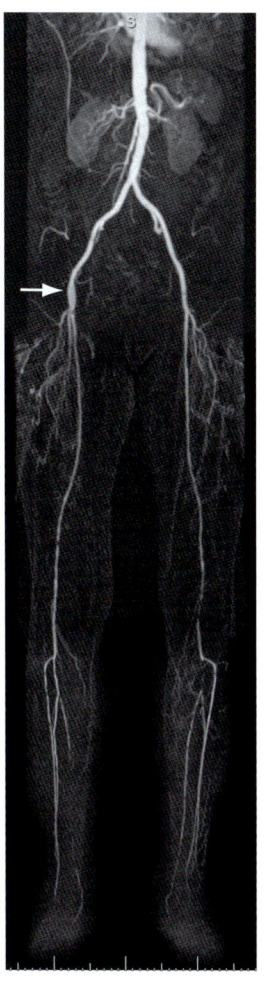

■ **FIGURE 116-8** A 54-year-old diabetic patient with complaints of intermittent claudication. The MRA scan shows relative preservation of the proximal inflow arteries and clinically relevant lesions in both popliteal arteries and lower legs. This pattern of PAD is characteristic for diabetes mellitus. Note the prior right common femoral endarterectomy (*arrow*).

subgroup, with primarily distal atherosclerotic occlusive disease and preservation of normal inflow (Fig. 116-8). Obtaining a full anatomic study from the infrarenal aorta down to the lower leg and pedal arteries is essential for the preinterventional workup of distal peripheral artery disease.

The guiding principle behind vascular surgical reconstruction in the lower legs of patients with chronic critical ischemia has evolved from conservative treatment, with eventual amputation, to restoration of pulsatile flow to the distal lower leg to end rest pain and achieve wound healing.[40,41] Distal bypass grafting has a much better limb salvage rate than conservative treatment.[42] Consequently, the vascular surgeon will bypass into the best available outflow vessel, regardless of anatomic level, provided that inflow into the artery and the origin of the graft are uncompromised. To determine the best possible treatment plan, it is essential for the vascular surgeon to obtain adequate anatomic information about lower leg arteries and the pedal arteries in addition to functional information from other tests, such as transcutaneous oxygen measurements and targeted high-resolution duplex ultrasonography.[1]

A thorough knowledge of below-knee and pedal vasculature and their anatomic variations is mandatory when reporting lower leg MRA studies. The most frequently encountered variations are high origins of the anterior and posterior tibial arteries. From a vascular surgical perspective, it is important to recognize variations in the dorsal pedal artery and medial and lateral plantar branches of the posterior tibial artery because nonfilling of one of the named segments does not necessarily mean that the vessel is occluded.[43] The crucial distinction to make in a report is whether the anterior circulation of the foot (most often the dorsalis pedis artery) anastomoses to the posterior circulation (posterior tibial, lateral and medial plantar arteries) via the deep plantar artery to constitute the pedal arch. Occlusion of the entire pedal arch is prognostic for a poor outcome of below-knee bypass grafting.[44]

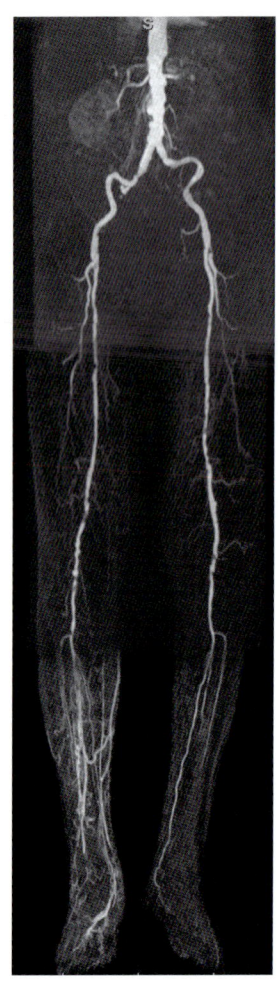

FIGURE 116-9 Disturbing venous enhancement in the right calf in a 60-year-old diabetic patient with bilateral intermittent claudication. There are multiple high-grade stenoses in both femoral arteries.

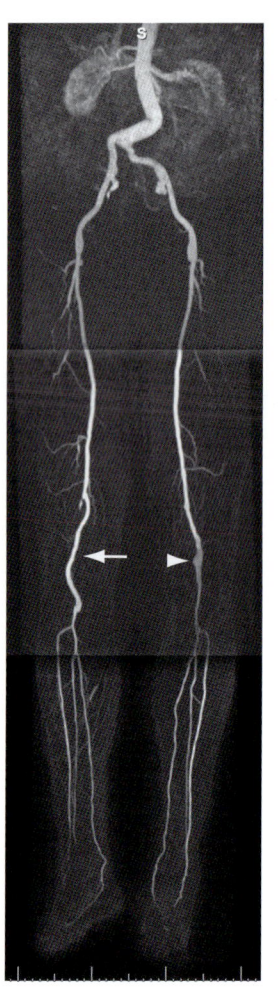

FIGURE 116-10 Short femoropopliteal bypass graft (*arrow*) repair in a 68-year-old man with a prior right popliteal artery aneurysm. Note that the patient also has a left popliteal artery aneurysm (*arrowhead*).

The most important pitfall for CE MRA is venous enhancement and contamination of arterial images, which occurs primarily in patients with cellulitis and diabetes (Fig. 116-9). A priori identification of these conditions helps determine the optimal imaging approach.[45] Exclusion of pedal arterial anatomy because of too small an imaging volume is a common mistake that can be avoided by meticulous review of localizer original partitions. Stenosis of the dorsalis pedis artery can be induced artifactually by tight straps and when the foot is imaged in plantar flexion. The cause of this latter so-called *ballerina sign artifact* is compression of the dorsal pedal artery by the distal part of the retinaculum extensorum.[46]

Postinterventional Imaging and Evaluation of Peripheral Arterial Bypass Grafts

Considering the chronic nature of the atherosclerotic disease process, many patients will ultimately present with renewed complaints after having been treated successfully for intermittent claudication or chronic critical ischemia (Figs. 116-10 and 116-11). Consequently, a substantial number of patients undergoing peripheral vascular imaging will have metallic implants such as vascular stent grafts, endoprostheses, and vascular surgical ligating clips. These implants are sometimes known to cause serious artifacts with MRI and MRA as a result of differences in susceptibility between the metal of which they are manufactured and human tissue. Susceptibility artifacts are highly variable but can be recognized by local or regional distortions or complete signal voids. In addition, artifacts may also be present after hip and knee joint replacement surgery. It is important to realize that artifact severity not only depends on the stent graft material, but also on the diameter of the stent graft or size of the ligating clip, field strength, echo time, angle to the main magnetic field, and orientation to the readout gradient.[47,48] Stents made of Nitinol suffer least from artifactual signal loss and stainless steel stents have the most signal loss. The proximal and distal anastomoses of the graft should be assessed carefully for the presence of stenoses. Clips may also be found in the vicinity of renal transplants, on side branches of venous grafts, and at sites of vein harvesting.

KEY POINTS

- Peripheral artery disease is prevalent, particulary in older patients. Up to 20% of the general population older than 70 years have signs of PAD.
- Technical advances, such as parallel imaging, centric k-space sampling, k-space view sharing, and dedicated multielement peripheral vascular coils enable the acquisition of high spatial resolution arterial images of the peripheral vascular tree in routine clinical practice.
- Contrast-enhanced MRA remains the standard of reference for the workup of PAD because this method has been shown to be highly reliable in comparison to IA DSA.
- Newer noncontrast medium–enhanced MRA methods remain to be validated against both CE MRA and IA DSA for peripheral artery visualization.
- More than 95% of all patients presenting with intermittent claudication or chronic critical ischemia suffer from atherosclerotic PAD. A history or imaging appearance incongruent with typical atherosclerotic PAD should prompt consideration of alternative causes of the complaints.

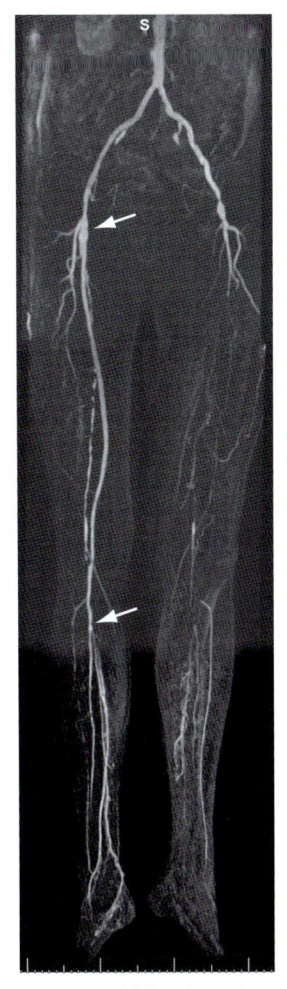

FIGURE 116-11 A 63-year-old female patient with rest pain in the left leg caused by chronic critical ischemia. There is a femorocrural bypass graft on the right side (*arrows*) originating in the proximal common femoral artery, with the distal anastomosis on the right tibioperoneal trunk. The left superficial femoral and popliteal arteries are almost completely occluded. There is poor runoff in the left lower leg because of relative lack of collateral formation.

SUGGESTED READINGS

Collins R, Burch J, Cranny G, et al. Duplex ultrasonography, magnetic resonance angiography, and computed tomography angiography for diagnosis and assessment of symptomatic, lower limb peripheral arterial disease: systematic review. BMJ 2007; 334:1257.

Kaufman JA. Lower extremity arteries. In Thrall JA (ed). Vascular and Interventional Radiology: The Requisites. Philadelphia, Mosby, 2004, pp 407-444.

Leiner T. Magnetic resonance angiography of abdominal and lower extremity vasculature. Top Magn Reson Imaging 2005; 16:21-66.

Miyazaki M, Lee VS. Nonenhanced MR angiography. Radiology 2008; 248:20-43.

Norgren L, Hiatt WR, Dormandy JA, et al. Inter-Society Consensus for the Management of Peripheral Arterial Disease (TASC II). J Vasc Surg 2007; 45(Suppl):S5-S67.

Rofsky NM, Adelman MA. MR angiography in the evaluation of atherosclerotic peripheral vascular disease. Radiology 2000; 214:325-338.

REFERENCES

1. Norgren L, Hiatt WR, Dormandy JA, et al. Inter-Society Consensus for the Management of Peripheral Arterial Disease (TASC II). J Vasc Surg 2007; 45(Suppl):S5-S67.
2. Beebe HG. Intermittent claudication: effective medical management of a common circulatory problem. Am J Cardiol 2001; 87:14D-18D.
3. Gardner AW, Poehlman ET. Exercise rehabilitation programs for the treatment of claudication pain. A meta-analysis. JAMA 1995; 274:975-980.
4. Krajcer Z, Howell MH. Update on endovascular treatment of peripheral vascular disease: new tools, techniques, and indications. Tex Heart Inst J 2000; 27:369-385.

5. Rofsky NM, Adelman MA. MR angiography in the evaluation of atherosclerotic peripheral vascular disease. Radiology 2000; 214:325-338.
6. Seldinger SI. Catheter replacement of the needle in percutaneous arteriography. Acta Radiol 1953; 39:368-375.
7. Koelemay MJ, den Hartog D, Prins MH, et al. Diagnosis of arterial disease of the lower extremities with duplex ultrasonography. Br J Surg 1996; 83:404-409.
8. Visser K, Hunink MG. Peripheral arterial disease: gadolinium-enhanced MR angiography versus color-guided duplex US—a meta-analysis. Radiology 2000; 216:67-77.
9. Leiner T, Kessels AG, Nelemans PJ, et al. Peripheral arterial disease: comparison of color duplex US and contrast-enhanced MR angiography for diagnosis. Radiology 2005; 235:699-708.
10. Collins R, Burch J, Cranny G, et al. Duplex ultrasonography, magnetic resonance angiography, and computed tomography angiography for diagnosis and assessment of symptomatic, lower limb peripheral arterial disease: systematic review. BMJ 2007; 334:1257.
11. Leiner T. Magnetic resonance angiography of abdominal and lower extremity vasculature. Top Magn Reson Imaging 2005; 16:21-66.
12. Koelemay MJ, Lijmer JG, Stoker J, et al. Magnetic resonance angiography for the evaluation of lower extremity arterial disease: a meta-analysis. JAMA 2001; 285:1338-1345.
13. Nelemans PJ, Leiner T, de Vet HC, van Engelshoven JM. Peripheral arterial disease: meta-analysis of the diagnostic performance of MR angiography. Radiology 2000; 217:105-114.
14. Schoenberg SO, Londy FJ, Licato P, et al. Multiphase-multistep gadolinium-enhanced MR angiography of the abdominal aorta and runoff vessels. Invest Radiol 2001; 36:283-291.
15. Boos M, Scheffler K, Haselhorst R, et al. Arterial first pass gadolinium-CM dynamics as a function of several intravenous saline flush and Gd volumes. J Magn Reson Imaging 2001; 13:568-576.
16. Ho KY, de Haan MW, Kessels AG, et al. Peripheral vascular tree stenoses: detection with subtracted and nonsubtracted MR angiography. Radiology 1998; 206:673-681.
17. Ruehm SG, Nanz D, Baumann A, et al. Three-dimensional contrast-enhanced MR angiography of the run-off vessels: value of image subtraction. J Magn Reson Imaging 2001; 13:402-411.
18. Leiner T, de Weert TT, Nijenhuis RJ, et al. Need for background suppression in contrast-enhanced peripheral magnetic resonance angiography. J Magn Reson Imaging 2001; 14:724-733.
19. Leiner T, Nijenhuis RJ, Maki JH, et al. Use of a three-station phased array coil to improve peripheral contrast-enhanced magnetic resonance angiography. J Magn Reson Imaging 2004; 20:417-425.
20. Wang Y, Chen CZ, Chabra SG, et al. Bolus arterial-venous transit in the lower extremity and venous contamination in bolus chase three-dimensional magnetic resonance angiography. Invest Radiol 2002; 37:458-463.
21. Zhang HL, Kent KC, Bush HL, et al. Soft tissue enhancement on time-resolved peripheral magnetic resonance angiography. J Magn Reson Imaging 2004; 19:590-597.
22. Morasch MD, Collins J, Pereles FS, et al. Lower extremity stepping-table magnetic resonance angiography with multilevel contrast timing and segmented contrast infusion. J Vasc Surg 2003; 37:62-71.
23. Wilman AH, Riederer SJ. Improved centric phase encoding orders for three-dimensional magnetization-prepared MR angiography. Magn Reson Med 1996; 36:384-392.
24. Willinek WA, Gieseke J, Conrad R, et al. Randomly segmented central k-space ordering in high-spatial-resolution contrast-enhanced MR angiography of the supraaortic arteries: initial experience. Radiology 2002; 225:583-588.
25. Korosec FR, Frayne R, Grist TM, Mistretta CA. Time-resolved contrast-enhanced three-dimensional MR angiography. Magn Reson Med 1996; 36:345-351.
26. Hoogeveen RM, von Falkenhausen M, Gieseke J. Fast, dynamic high resolution contrast-enhanced MR angiography with CENTRA keyhole and SENSE. Twelfth Scientific Meeting of the International Society for Magnetic Resonance in Medicine. Kyoto, Japan, May 2004.
27. Herborn CU, Ajaj W, Goyen M, et al. Peripheral vasculature: whole-body MR angiography with midfemoral venous compression—initial experience. Radiology 2004; 230:872-878.
28. Bilecen D, Schulte AC, Aschwanden M, et al. MR angiography with venous compression. Radiology 2004; 233:617-618.
29. Hoogeveen RM, Bakker CJ, Viergever MA. Limits to the accuracy of vessel diameter measurement in MR angiography. J Magn Reson Imaging 1998; 8:1228-1235.
30. Westenberg JJ, van der Geest RJ, Wasser MN, et al. Vessel diameter measurements in gadolinium contrast-enhanced three-dimensional MRA of peripheral arteries. Magn Reson Imaging 2000; 18:13-22.
31. Schmiedl U, Moseley ME, Ogan MD, et al. Comparison of initial biodistribution patterns of Gd-DTPA and albumin-(Gd-DTPA) using rapid spin echo MR imaging. J Comput Assist Tomogr 1987; 11:306-313.
32. Prince MR, Grist TM, Debatin JF. Three-dimensional Contrast MR Angiography. Berlin, Springer, 2003.
33. Hentsch A, Aschauer MA, Balzer JO, et al. Gadobutrol-enhanced moving-table magnetic resonance angiography in patients with peripheral vascular disease: a prospective, multi-centre blinded comparison with digital subtraction angiography. Eur Radiol 2003; 13:2103-2114.
34. Goyen M, Lauenstein TC, Herborn CU, et al. 0.5 M Gd chelate (Magnevist) versus 1.0 M Gd chelate (Gadovist): dose-independent effect on image quality of pelvic three-dimensional MR-angiography. J Magn Reson Imaging 2001; 14:602-607.
35. Perreault P, Edelman MA, Baum RA, et al. MR angiography with gadofosveset trisodium for peripheral vascular disease: phase II trial. Radiology 2003; 229:811-820.
36. Hadizadeh DR, Gieseke J, Lohmaier SH, et al. Peripheral MR angiography with blood pool contrast agent: prospective intraindividual comparative study of high-spatial-resolution steady-state MR angiography versus standard-resolution first-pass MR angiography and DSA. Radiology 2008; 249:701-711.
37. Miyazaki M, Lee VS. Nonenhanced MR angiography. Radiology 2008; 248:20-43.
38. Lim RP, Hecht EM, Xu J, et al. Three-dimensional nongadolinium-enhanced ECG-gated MRA of the distal lower extremities: preliminary clinical experience. J Magn Reson Imaging 2008; 28:181-189.
39. Menzoian JO, LaMorte WW, Paniszyn CC, et al. Symptomatology and anatomic patterns of peripheral vascular disease: differing impact of smoking and diabetes. Ann Vasc Surg 1989; 3:224-228.
40. Hughes K, Domenig CM, Hamdan AD, et al. Bypass to plantar and tarsal arteries: an acceptable approach to limb salvage. J Vasc Surg 2004; 40:1149-1157.
41. Pomposelli FB, Kansal N, Hamdan AD, et al. A decade of experience with dorsalis pedis artery bypass: analysis of outcome in more than 1000 cases. J Vasc Surg 2003; 37:307-315.
42. Holstein PE, Sorensen S. Limb salvage experience in a multidisciplinary diabetic foot unit. Diabetes Care 1999; 22(Suppl 2):B97-B103.
43. Alson MD, Lang EV, Kaufman JA. Pedal arterial imaging. J Vasc Interv Radiol 1997; 8:9-18.
44. Rutherford RB, Baker JD, Ernst C, et al. Recommended standards for reports dealing with lower extremity ischemia: revised version. J Vasc Surg 1997; 26:517-538.
45. Maki JH, Wilson GJ, Eubank WB, Hoogeveen RM. Predicting venous enhancement in peripheral MRA using a two-station timing bolus. Eleventh Scientific Meeting of the International Society for Magnetic Resonance in Medicine. Toronto, Ontario, May 2003.
46. Kaufman JA. Lower extremity arteries. In Thrall JA (ed). Vascular and Interventional Radiology: The Requisites. Philadelphia, Mosby, 2004, pp 407-444.
47. Weishaupt D, Quick HH, Nanz D, et al. Ligating clips for three-dimensional MR angiography at 1.5 T: in vitro evaluation. Radiology 2000; 214:902-907.
48. Meissner OA, Verrel F, Tato F, et al. Magnetic resonance angiography in the follow-up of distal lower-extremity bypass surgery: comparison with duplex ultrasound and digital subtraction angiography. J Vasc Interv Radiol 2004; 15:1269-1277.

PART
NINETEEN

The Upper Extremity Vessels

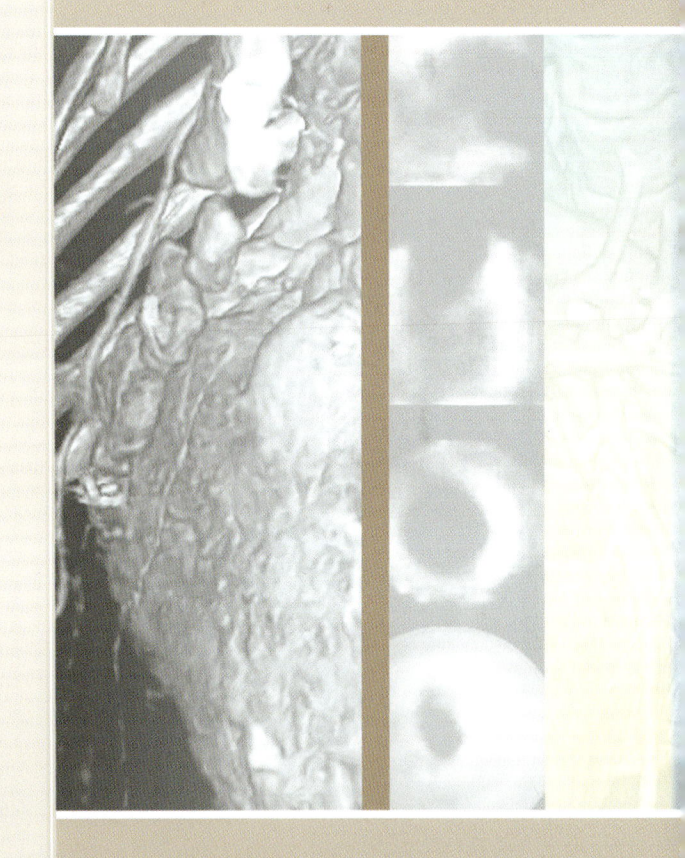

CHAPTER 117

Vascular Diseases of the Upper Extremities

Tim Leiner and Marc Kock

Symptomatic arterial occlusive disease of the upper extremity occurs much less frequently compared with arterial occlusive disease of the lower extremities. The spectrum of pathology that one is likely to encounter is also somewhat different. Whereas almost all lower extremity occlusive disease is the result of long-standing atherosclerosis, nonatherosclerotic disease and uncommon causes make up a substantial part of the case mix of clinicians dealing with patients suffering from upper extremity arterial disease. Furthermore, apart from intrinsic vascular disease, there are other well-recognized extrinsic entities that may compromise the arterial supply of the upper extremity.

There are several main reasons why examinations of the upper extremity arterial tree account for a minority of all vascular examinations in the average radiologic practice. The abundant collateral supply in the lower neck, shoulder, and upper arm regions provide a robust means for the reconstitution of distal perfusion, thus delaying symptoms. Also, a large fraction of patients suffer from small vessel disease, which is primarily managed medically instead of with percutaneous or surgical techniques. When the clinical history and laboratory information suggest small vessel disease, many patients are not even referred for vascular imaging because the information obtained does not necessarily influence treatment.

In this chapter, different vascular diseases affecting the upper extremity are discussed, as well as the relative merits and shortcomings of different techniques for imaging the upper extremity vasculature in the context of the most frequent diseases one is likely to encounter.

LARGE VESSEL DISEASE OF THE UPPER EXTREMITY

Large vessel occlusive disease of the upper extremity encompasses several well-recognized disease entities. The most frequently encountered disease underlying upper extremity ischemia is atherosclerosis. Other entities one is likely to encounter are thoracic outlet syndrome, autoimmune vasculitis, thromboembolism, and vascular damage caused by trauma, sports injuries, and radiation therapy.

Patients with atherosclerotic occlusive disease typically present with upper extremity claudication or steal phenomenon. The most common locations for upper extremity large vessel involvement include the brachiocephalic and subclavian arteries. However, atherosclerosis can also cause small vessel obstruction by atheromatous embolization or thromboembolism. A particularly helpful clinical clue in establishing the correct cause is the age of the patient. Atherosclerotic disease of the upper extremity tends to affect older adult patients, whereas nonatherosclerotic upper extremity arterial occlusive disease affects younger patients.[1]

The upper extremity is a frequent site for autoimmune vasculitis. Vasculitis is usually defined as a sterile inflammation of the vessel wall. In contrast to patients suffering from atherosclerosis, patients with vasculitis are often younger and have elevated erythrocyte sedimentation rates, antineutrophilic cytoplasmic antibodies (ANCA), and antiendothelial cell antibodies.[2] In addition to the local symptoms caused by vessel narrowing, many patients also suffer from concomitant constitutional symptoms such as fever, malaise, myalgia, and arthralgia. The upper extremity is most often affected by Takayasu disease and giant cell arteritis (GCA). These are histologically similar diseases but Takayasu disease tends to affect any of the aortic arch vessels as well as the arch itself, and sometimes the pulmonary and coronary arteries, whereas GCA tends to affect the subclavian arteries in a typical symmetrical pattern.[3] A specific clinical constellation associated with GCA is polymyalgia rheumatica. In polymyalgia rheumatica, the vasculitis is located more distally in the cervicocranial arteries. Up to 50% of patients suffer from intermittent claudication of the jaw, tongue, or throat, and up to 33% of patients present with visual complaints such as amaurosis fugax or even blindness.[4]

The group of neurovascular disorders caused by extrinsic compression of the subclavian and axillary arteries and veins as well as the brachial plexus is called cervicoaxillary compression syndrome. The more popular name for this disorder is the thoracic outlet syndrome (TOS). Symptoms are caused by compression at the interscalene triangle, costoclavicular space, or retropectoralis minor space.[5] Compression can be caused by a variety of causes such as a fibrous band, supernumerary cervical ribs, or excessive callus formation subsequent to a clavicular fracture. A large majority of cases (70% to 90%) is caused by involvement of the brachial plexus. In less than one third of cases, arteries and veins are involved.

Blunt and penetrating trauma to the chest and upper extremity may compromise the vascular supply as well. Other causes of injury to the upper extremity vessels are radiation therapy for malignancies of the breast, head, and neck and repetitive injury in athletes such as baseball pitchers, volleyball players, butterfly swimmers, and weight lifters.

Prevalence and Epidemiology

The incidence and prevalence of upper extremity atherosclerotic disease are not known. However, it is important to realize that the prevalence of atherosclerotic lesions in the upper extremity in absolute terms is much lower compared with the aortoiliac arteries and lower extremities. The reasons for this relative paucity of symptomatic atherosclerosis in upper extremity arteries remain unknown at present. Possible explanations include better collateral circulation, reduced muscle mass, and less vigorous use of the upper extremity compared with the lower extremity.

The estimated incidence of Takayasu arteritis is 2.6 cases per million in the United States, with higher incidences reported in young women and patients of Asian origin. Women in their second and third decades of life account for the vast majority of patients because they tend to be affected about eight to nine times more often than men. Conversely, GCA tends to affect older patients, peaking in the age group between 70 and 80 years. The estimated incidence of GCA is 2 to 20/million, with women being affected about two to four times more often than men.[6]

The incidence of thoracic outlet syndrome (TOS) is not well established. Although it is generally accepted that TOS is caused by compression of brachial plexus elements or subclavian vessels in their passage from the cervical area toward the axilla and proximal upper arm, there is much disagreement among clinicians regarding its diagnostic criteria and optimal treatment. Because there is no objective confirmatory test for TOS, the true prevalence of the disease remains elusive. Reported prevalence ranges from 3 to 80 cases/1000 population.[7] TOS is mostly considered a diagnosis of exclusion.

It is estimated that vascular injuries to the upper extremity represent approximately 30% to 50% of all peripheral vascular injuries. Usually, the brachial artery is involved and most injuries are caused by penetrating trauma.[8] Blunt injuries such as motor vehicle accidents account for 6% to 10% of upper extremity vascular trauma and are often associated with musculoskeletal injuries and neural injuries.[9] The functional impact of the trauma is often related to concomitant injury to peripheral nerves. The extent of the vascular compromise following radiation therapy is directly proportional to the amount of radiation given, but symptoms may present only decades after therapy.

Cause and Pathophysiology

Atherosclerosis is considered to be a chronic inflammatory disease of the large arteries.[10] The disease starts at an early age and remains clinically silent for decades. For a detailed discussion of the pathophysiology of atherosclerosis, see Chapters 51 and 88. It is important to note that imaging of the vascular lumen alone may underestimate the burden of disease related to atherosclerosis.

Takayasu arteritis is a classic vasculitis of unknown cause involving the upper extremity arteries. Infection, in particular tuberculosis, has been implicated in the pathogenesis of Takayasu arteritis, but a definitive link between the two diseases remains elusive at present.[3,11] The disease can be divided into two stages, with an acute period of large vessel vasculitis, followed by fibrosis and scarring. In the acute stage, the adventitial vessels of the arterial walls become inflamed as a result of unknown causes. This leads to a generalized, smooth, circumferential thickening of the affected segment, including the media. In the chronic stage, elastic tissue is replaced by fibrosis, with thickening of all three layers of the vessel wall, leading to irreversible segmental smooth luminal narrowing. Other vasculitides that affect the upper extremities are thought to be of similar pathogenesis, although the clinical manifestations may vary (see earlier).

Cervicoaxillary compression syndrome can be the result of a heterogeneous set of activities or trauma, as noted. The exact clinical symptoms depend on which anatomic structures are involved. Local vascular injury is often typified by intimal damage, with subsequent aneurysm formation. This, in turn, may lead to mural thrombus and potentially distal embolization.

Manifestations of Disease

Clinical Presentation

The most common presentations of chronic large vessel upper extremity occlusive disease are arm claudication, or steal phenomena. Clinical clues are helpful to elucidate the underlying disease process and a thorough medical, surgical, occupational and sports history should be obtained in every patient. Symptoms of upper extremity occlusive disease that suggest nonatherosclerotic causes are young age, long-standing fatigue and malaise, high erythrocyte sedimentation rate, and vigorous occupational or sports activities involving repetitive strain to the shoulder and hand, such as frequent baseball pitching, mountain biking, and using the hand to pound structures (e.g., carpenters). Patients with vasculitis typically report having had vague complaints for months or even years prior to consulting a physician. A possible explanation for the relative rarity of arm claudication symptoms is the reduced muscle mass, less vigorous use, and abundance of numerous and well-developed collateral pathways compared with the lower extremity.[12]

Patients with steal syndromes present with upper extremity weakness, dizziness, and sometimes angina. The most well-known steal syndrome is subclavian steal, or reversal of antegrade flow in the vertebral artery caused by the presence of ipsilateral significant subclavian artery stenosis or occlusion, proximal to the origin of the vertebral artery. Another well-known steal phenomenon can be seen in the coronary artery circulation after coronary artery bypass grafting using the internal thoracic artery. In the presence of a subclavian artery stenosis, flow may reverse in the internal thoracic artery to supply the upper extremity arterial bed instead of augmenting flow in the coronary arteries. It is important to realize that an angiographic steal phenomenon does not necessarily imply symptoms. In fact, only about one third of all patients with angiographically proven steal syndromes suffer from characteristic complaints.[13-15]

Acute injuries to the upper extremity often involve vascular structures and should be managed according to the presumed cause. In many cases, conventional angiography is the diagnostic modality of first choice because it allows for immediate intervention. This is also the case with suspected arterial embolism, for which catheter-based therapies can be used to perform thrombosuction and delivery of clot-lysing agents.

Imaging Indications and Algorithm

The noninvasive nature of Doppler ultrasonography (DUS), magnetic resonance imaging (MRI), and computed tomography (CT) has lowered the threshold for ordering imaging tests in patients with suspected upper extremity vascular involvement. Apart from the arguments in favor of safety and patient comfort, there is another major reason to use modern cross-sectional imaging techniques. DUS, CT, and MRI not only enable visualization of the arterial lumen but also of the arterial wall and surrounding bony and soft tissue structures. Because of this capability, DUS, MRI, and CT can identify lesions amenable to percutaneous transluminal angioplasty (PTA) and surgery, and can inform the surgeon about the best surgical approach.

When a patient presents with clinical symptoms suggestive of vascular involvement in the arteries of the upper arm, forearm, or hand, it is important to evaluate the entire upper extremity vascular tree from the aortic root to the digital arteries so as not to miss relevant lesions in the vascular tree. Suspected peripheral arterial or venous thrombosis is often evaluated with ultrasonography as the first-line imaging modality because it is a rapid, reliable, and less expensive imaging test, with high sensitivity and specificity. In cases of suspected arterial or venous lesions in the chest itself or in the parts of vessels that pass underneath the clavicle, CT and MRI are preferred, because the visualization of vascular structures in these locations is often poor with DUS. The choice of whether to use CT or MRI largely depends on local skill and preference. Both imaging modalities are capable of high-fidelity depiction of the vascular lumen and wall, as well as of the surrounding structures.

For diagnostic purposes, intra-arterial digital subtraction angiography (IA-DSA) has been relegated to a secondary role because the risks associated with the procedure outweigh the benefits for most patients. An exception is the evaluation of patients with suspected arterial thrombosis or embolization. These patients are vascular emergencies that should be treated without unnecessary delay. IA-DSA is the modality of first choice for this condition because it allows for an unequivocal diagnosis and concomitant treatment, if needed.

MEDIUM AND SMALL VESSEL DISEASE OF THE UPPER EXTREMITY

Atherosclerotic lesions in the forearm and hand arteries are rarely the cause of ischemic symptoms. Other diseases predominate in the list of differential diagnoses when distal upper extremity vascular disease is suspected.

The prototypical disease affecting the medium-sized arteries (and veins) of the upper limb is thromboangiitis obliterans, or Buerger disease (or Winiwarter-Buerger's disease). Although the lower extremity is involved far more often, Buerger disease may affect the radial and ulnar arteries and palmar arch. There are numerous other diseases that affect the distal forearm, hand, and digital arteries of the upper extremity. A full review of all conditions associated with distal upper extremity arterial disease is beyond the scope of this chapter but can be found in the excellent review by Greenfield and colleagues.[16] In many patients, arterial disease of the distal forearm and hand is not isolated but is associated with underlying systemic connective tissue disease such as scleroderma and CREST syndrome (*c*alcinosis cutis, *R*aynaud syndrome, *e*sophageal motility disorder, *s*clerodactyly, and *t*elangiectasia) or rheumatologic disorders such as rheumatoid arthritis, mixed connective tissue disease, systemic lupus erythematosus, antiphospholipid syndrome, polymyositis, and dermatomyositis.[17-19]

Occupational, recreational, and iatrogenic trauma are important sources of distal upper extremity ischemic symptoms. Repetitive pounding with the ulnar side of the hand or fist may result in aneurysm formation and digital artery occlusion. This condition is known as hypothenar hammer syndrome. A similar complex of symptoms can sometimes be encountered in patients with a history of long-standing pneumatic tool use or in mountain bikers, baseball catchers, volleyball players, or practitioners of karate. Arterial occlusion may also be a consequence of traumatic catheterization of the radial or ulnar arteries.

Raynaud phenomenon is a common ancillary finding in patients suffering from upper extremity vascular disease and may be the presenting symptom. It is defined as a reversible spasm of the small and medium-sized arteries, resulting in a characteristic triphasic white-blue-red color response. First, cessation of digital artery flow produces well-demarcated finger pallor. This is followed by vasorelaxation and return of arterial flow and subsequent postcapillary venule constriction, resulting in desaturated blood and producing cyanosis. Finally, postischemic hyperemia replaces cyanosis with rubor.[16,20,21] A distinction is made between primary Raynaud phenomenon (formerly Raynaud disease), if there is no underlying illness, and secondary Raynaud phenomenon (formerly Raynaud syndrome) if there is an associated disorder detected on assessment. In approximately one third of cases, Raynaud phenomenon is an isolated and benign condition not associated with underlying disease. In cases of inflammatory arteritis, Raynaud phenomenon is common.

Prevalence and Epidemiology

Atherosclerotic occlusive disease of the medium and small arteries of the upper extremity is uncommon and comprises a minority of patients presenting with symptoms of forearm and hand ischemia. The exact prevalence is unknown, because many patients may never come to medical attention.

The incidence of Buerger disease is estimated at 8 to 12.6/100,000.[22] Patients with Buerger disease are almost always young (younger than 45 years), use large amounts of tobacco, and characteristically show segmental occlusions in the radial, ulnar, palmar, and digital arteries, with typical bridging corkscrew collaterals. The disease is increasingly seen in women, commensurate with the increase in the proportion of female smokers.

Small vessel disease of the upper extremity is relatively common, especially as manifested as Raynaud disease and in the presence of systemic connective tissue disease. For example, over 90% of patients with scleroderma exhibit Raynaud-like symptoms (see later).

Hypothenar hammer syndrome (HHS) is an infrequent condition and its true prevalence is not known. Marie and associates[23] have found HHS to be the cause of symptoms in 47 of 4148 patients (1.1%) referred for evaluation of Raynaud phenomenon. Serious complications, defined as requiring surgical intervention, caused by iatrogenic injury of the upper extremity arteries are also relatively rare. Myers and coworkers[24] have reported 11 patients over 4 years, whereas Deguara and colleagues[25] have reported 6 patients over 20 years. The incidence of serious iatrogenic upper extremity injury depends largely on the case mix of patients seen in the hospital and on the types of procedures performed.

Raynaud's complex of symptoms is very common. Various studies that have been conducted in the general population in several different countries found the prevalence to range from 3% to 6% up to 30%. In these studies, between 70% and 90% of all reported patients were women. In a large United States registry of 1137 patients presenting with Raynaud, 356 (31.3%) suffered from pure vasospasm with no associated disease, 391 patients (34.4%) had associated connective tissue disease, and 389 patients (34.3%) suffered from other underlying diseases.[26]

Etiology and Pathophysiology

For a detailed discussion of the pathophysiology of atherosclerosis, see Chapters 51 and 88.

Although the cause of Buerger disease is not known, there is a strong association between the use of tobacco and Buerger disease. Most patients are heavy smokers, but Buerger disease has also been reported in users of smokeless tobacco such as chewing tobacco and snuff. Tobacco use plays a central role in the pathogenesis, initiation, and continuation of the disease and is an absolute requirement for diagnosis. Buerger disease is characterized pathologically by highly cellular thrombus with relative sparing of the blood vessel walls. Multinucleated giant cells can even be observed within the clot in Buerger disease.

Involvement of the small arteries of the upper extremity is frequently encountered in rheumatic diseases. Szekanecz and Koch[27] have recently reviewed the vascular biology underlying this process. Vascular injury is caused primarily by activated neutrophils and inflammatory mediators released by these cells. Rheumatic diseases are associated with accelerated atherosclerosis and increased cardiovascular morbidity and mortality.

Repetitive occupational or recreational trauma may damage the ulnar artery when it enters the hand through Guyon's canal. The type of arterial abnormality often depends on the nature of the damage to the vessel. Intimal damage favors thrombotic occlusion, whereas injury to the media favors palmar aneurysms.[28,29] Thrombosis and aneurysm are common features seen angiographically with HHS.[30]

In primary Raynaud phenomenon, patients have an abnormally strong vasospastic response to cold or emotional stimuli, with anatomically normal arteries. Primary Raynaud typically occurs in young women, is bilateral and not associated with ischemic ulcerations, has a benign course, and requires only symptomatic treatment. Secondary Raynaud is suggested by the following findings: an age of onset older than 30 years; episodes that are intense, painful, asymmetrical, or associated with skin lesions; clinical features suggestive of a connective tissue disease (e.g. arthritis and abnormal lung function); specific autoantibodies and evidence of microvascular disease on microscopy of nail fold capillaries.[21,31,32]

Manifestations of Disease

Clinical Presentation

Atherosclerosis of the distal upper extremity, although relatively rare, typically presents with classic symptoms of ischemia. Patients suffering from Buerger disease are mostly young tobacco smokers who present with complaints of distal extremity ischemia such as claudication and secondary Raynaud phenomenon of the hand, ischemic ulcers, or gangrene of the fingertips. The prevalence of disease has declined in the West over the last 30 years, which can be attributed to the decline in smoking. The disease is more prevalent in areas with a high proportion of smokers such as the Mediterranean, Middle East, and Asia. Because of the proclivity to involve more than one limb, arteriography of the upper and lower extremities should be performed in patients who present clinically with involvement of only one limb. It is common to see angiographic abnormalities consistent with Buerger disease in limbs that are not yet clinically involved.

Raynaud phenomenon is the classic presenting symptom of small vessel disease of the hand. As noted,

Raynaud phenomenon is not specific, because it is associated with a variety of conditions. As is the case with large vessel disease of the upper extremity, a thorough medical and surgical history should be obtained in every patient and will provide additional clues about the underlying disease. Occupational and recreational trauma to the small distal vessels of the hand may also present with Raynaud phenomenon.

Traumatic injury can also involve small and medium-sized vessels. Occupational exposure can lead to vibration or impact-induced small vessel vasospasm in the hand, followed by intimal injury, aneurysm formation, thrombosis, occlusion, and/or distal embolization. Blunt and penetrating hand trauma can lead to ischemia if the palmar arch is incomplete.

Imaging Indications and Algorithm

Imaging of the distal forearm and hand arteries is usually performed with CT angiography or MR angiography, or most often with IA-DSA. The latter modality remains the gold standard for depiction of the small vessels of the palmar arch and the digits. However, because of progressively better noninvasive imaging, such as 64-row (or more) multidetector computed CT angiography, or high spatial resolution (blood pool) contrast-enhanced MR angiography catheter angiography may not always be necessary. Although duplex ultrasonography allows real-time evaluation of arterial patency, interobserver variability limits its use to highly specialized centers with dedicated and experienced technicians.

In general, indications for imaging of the distal forearm and hand vessels may include arterial mapping prior to plastic surgery or radial or ulnar artery bypass grafting, HHS, suspected emboli from cardiac disease or atherosclerotic stenoses, or aneurysms in the subclavian artery, Raynaud syndrome, Buerger disease, scleroderma, rheumatoid arthritis, vasculitis, and repetitive trauma. Another indication is the presurgical evaluation of soft tissue tumors of the hand and fingers. Both CT and MR angiography can be combined with additional cross-sectional imaging to evaluate the surrounding soft tissue and bony structures. Raynaud syndrome or suspected distal emboli are particularly good indications for noninvasive vascular imaging techniques such as CTA and MRA; IA-DSA is generally not preferred because of the risk for embolic complications. In a small minority of patients suffering from Buerger disease, the disorder is exclusively located in the upper extremity; thus, when the disease is suspected, the lower extremities should be imaged as well.

Imaging Techniques and Findings

Radiography

When there is clinical suspicion of proximal upper extremity arterial disease, conventional radiographs of the thoracic outlet should be ordered. This will allow identification of supernumerary ribs, elongated transverse processes, or excessive callus formation in close proximity to vascular structures (Fig. 117-1). In patients with upper extremity trauma, conventional radiographs enable identification of

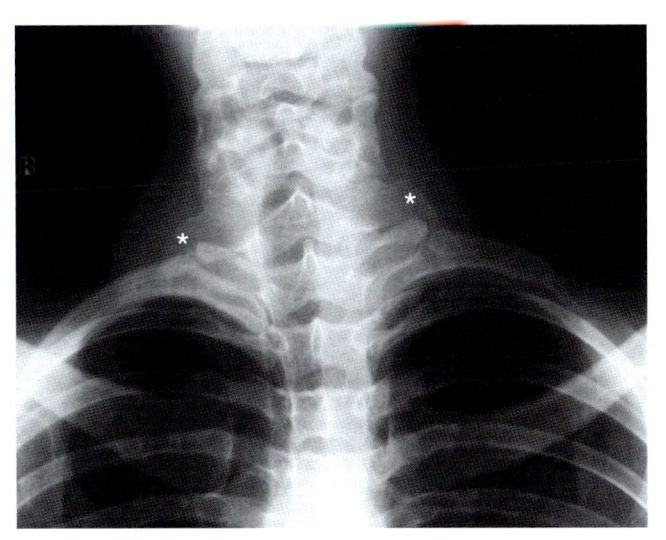

■ **FIGURE 117-1** Conventional x-ray of the lower cervical and upper thoracic spine showing bilateral cervical ribs (*asterisks*) in a 29-year-old woman with long-standing complaints of numbness and tingling in both arms.

fracture sites and the subsequent apposition of bone fragments and presence of radiopaque foreign material.

Ultrasound

Ultrasonography is a powerful first-line screening technique for evaluation of extrathoracic upper extremity arteries and veins. In contrast to the central large arteries and veins close to the heart or underneath the clavicle, the arteries of the upper extremity are easily accessible for ultrasonographic evaluation. There are enough imaging windows available so that the transducer can be placed over the artery of interest, without the presence of overlying bone. High-frequency transducers (more than 5 MHz) can normally be used because arteries and veins lie close to the skin, usually at a depth of several centimeters at most. Gray-scale imaging is useful for evaluating vascular diameter and the presence of atherosclerotic plaque or thrombotic material. Color Doppler flow imaging enables characterization of blood flow patterns and vascular patency. Because it is a noninvasive technique, ultrasonography is well suited for serial examinations. Arteries and veins can be evaluated reliably with ultrasonography from the axillary artery down to the distal radial and ulnar arteries, as well as the palmar arch and smaller digital branches. The normal flow pattern is triphasic. Expert ultrasonographers may be able to evaluate the subclavian artery for the presence of wall thickening associated with GCA or the presence of aneurysm formation and mural thrombus in patients with suspected TOS (Fig. 117-2).

A particularly powerful application of color Doppler ultrasonography is the evaluation of forearm arteries with regard to suitability for coronary artery bypass grafting as well as suspected pseudoaneurysms. Blood flow signals within a mass contiguous to an artery suggest the diagnosis of pseudoaneurysm, which is a complication that sometimes develops following arterial catheterization or penetrating trauma (Fig. 117-3). With an iatrogenic pseudoaneurysm of a native artery (e.g., after catheterization,

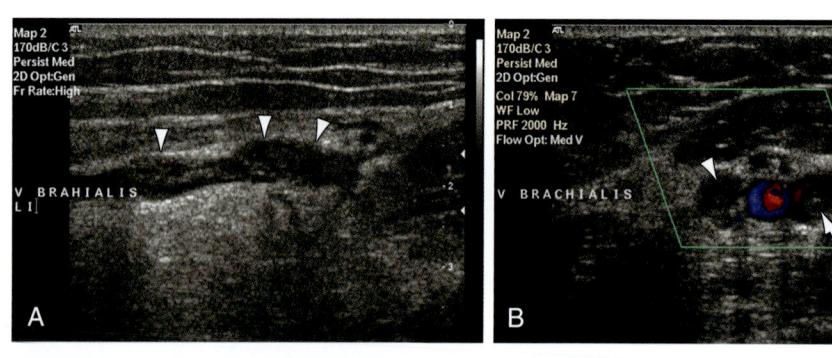

■ **FIGURE 117-2** Upper extremity deep venous thrombosis in 29-year-old male patient with recurrent non-Hodgkin lymphoma presenting with upper extremity swelling. Over the course of almost the entire left upper extremity, the radial and brachial veins could not be compressed at ultrasonography. **A,** Note the irregular shape of the brachial vein (*arrowheads*). **B,** There was normal flow in the brachial artery and thrombus material was in both accompanying veins (*arrow* and *arrowhead*).

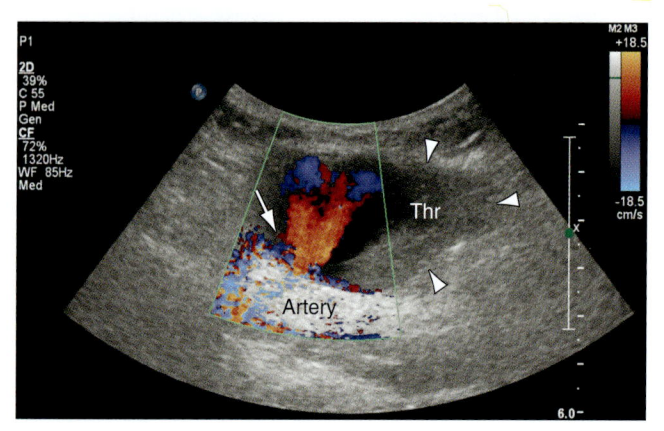

■ **FIGURE 117-3** Color Doppler ultrasonography in 55-year-old male patient presenting with a hypoechoic pulsatile mass in the left upper extremity after removal of an indwelling arterial catheter. Color Doppler analysis reveals a characteristic jet of blood directed into the false aneurysm (*arrow*; *arrowheads* demarcate the boundaries of the aneurysm). Thr, thrombus material.

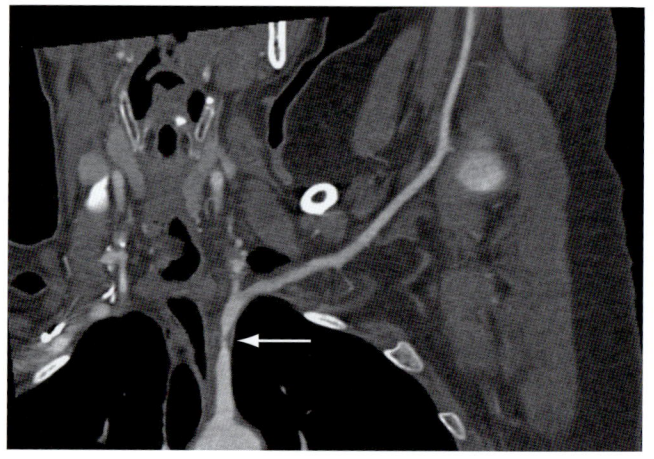

■ **FIGURE 117-4** Curved multiplanar reformation of 64-slice multidetector (MD) CT examination in a 67-year-old male patient with upper extremity intermittent claudication. There is a relatively short stenosis in the proximal left subclavian artery (*arrow*). Note the jagged appearance of the lesion. Also, there is no vessel wall thickening, suggesting that this lesion is of atherosclerotic origin.

unsuccessful arterial puncture, or placement or removal of indwelling arterial catheters), there is usually a small-diameter channel communicating with a larger contained collection of (partially thrombosed) blood. Color Doppler imaging shows blood flow signals and the pseudoaneurysm cavity. A jet and/or swirling motion or color yin yang sign is typically seen within the collection itself.[33] Color DUS is also well suited for the emergency evaluation of the upper extremity arteries in cases of suspected acute arterial embolus—for example, in patients with atrial fibrillation.

Computed Tomography

The main strength of cross-sectional imaging modalities such as CT and MRI is that the central thoracic vessels, which are often involved in upper extremity arterial disease, are much better accessible compared with color DUS. The resolution of current equipment allows high spatial resolution depiction of the arterial lumen and arterial wall. The capability for rapid image acquisition over a large field of view further increases the attractiveness of these techniques.

In general, three different CT angiography (CTA) protocols can be distinguished. For evaluation of the central thoracic vessels, one should use an aortic arch or proximal upper extremity protocol. For imaging the distal forearm and hands, a distal upper extremity runoff protocol should be used. Distinguishing these two indications allows for increased spatial resolution for imaging the distal arteries, which allows better depiction of subtle abnormalities such as those seen in small palmar and digital vessels. Upper extremity venous structures are usually imaged using indirect venographic protocols. Indirect imaging refers to the acquisition of a late-phase dataset after the injection of contrast medium (i.e., after the initial arterial first pass of contrast bolus) to avoid streak artifacts caused by undiluted iodinated contrast agents in the first pass. Delayed acquisitions may be useful in the setting of suspected vasculitis, vascular masses, and hemorrhage.

Properly executed, CTA allows recognition of arterial stenoses (Fig. 117-4) and aneurysm formation (Fig. 117-5) as seen in atherosclerosis, and the typical circumferential wall thickening as seen in vasculitis. An added benefit of CT over MRI is the improved ability to recognize and

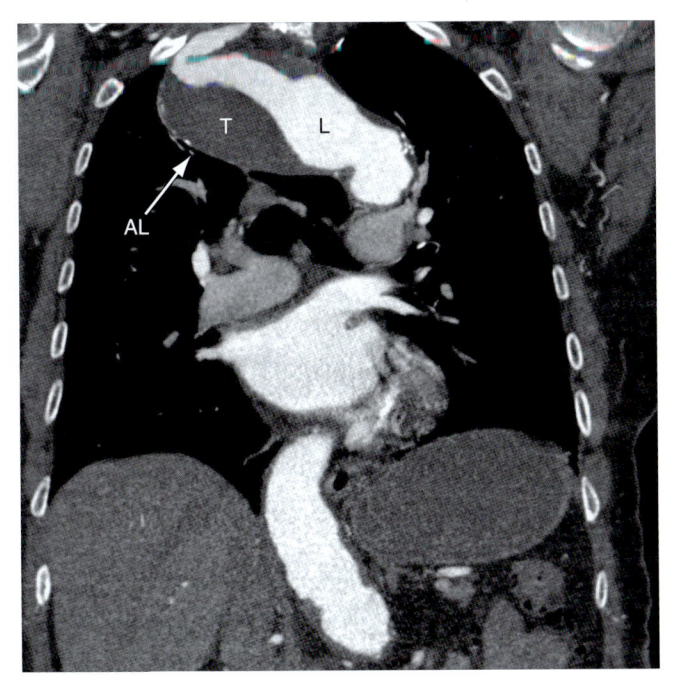

FIGURE 117-5 Curved multiplanar reformation of 64-slice MDCT examination in a 60-year old male patient presenting with acute chest pain. There is a giant aneurysm in the aberrant right subclavian artery. AL, arteria lusoria; L, arterial lumen; T, thrombus.

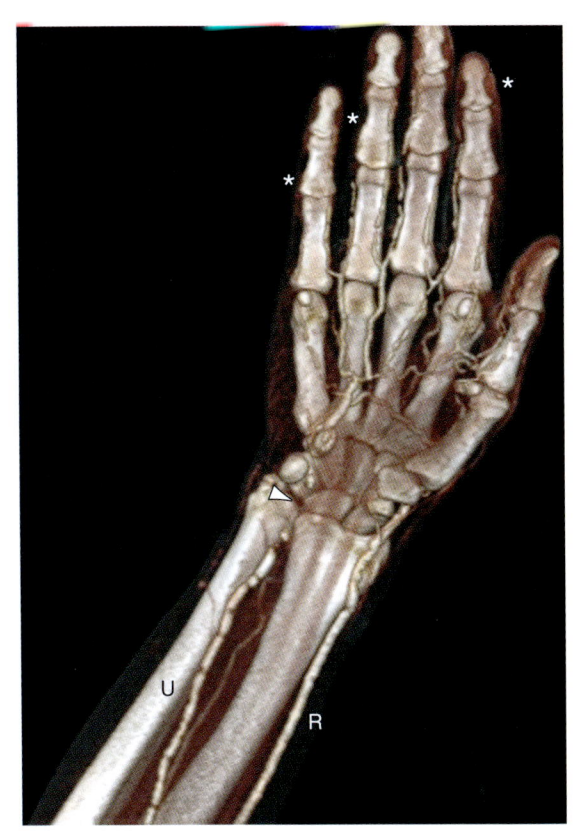

FIGURE 117-6 Color volume rendering of the distal upper extremity and hand arteries in a 75-year-old male patient presenting with intermittent claudication of the upper extremity. Image shows poor filling of the ulnar artery with an occlusion of the part of the ulnar artery (U) at the level of the wrist that connects to the palmar arch (*arrowhead*). Also note lack of filling of the proper digital arteries of the fingers (*asterisks*) and kinked radial artery (R).

display bony abnormalities. However, in most cases, these have already been detected with conventional radiography, which remains the first-line imaging study in patients with upper extremity complaints. With the current generation of 64-detector row CT scanners, care should be taken not to outrun the arrival of the contrast bolus—because incomplete vascular filling may erroneously suggest embolic occlusion of the vessel—as a result of the extremely fast acquisition speeds of these machines. Submillimeter collimation, a low pitch, and slower gantry speed are options to avoid this problem. Arterial embolism is usually characterized by an acute filling defect in the affected vessel, and is sometimes accompanied by increased density of contrast medium proximal to the occlusion, which often shows a typical meniscus sign.

When imaging the distal upper extremity, best image quality is achieved with the patient in the supine position, with the forearm and hand raised above the head. In patients with Buerger disease, arterial (and sometimes venous) occlusion can be seen, with typical bridging corkscrew collaterals that reconstitute distal flow. Key findings in small vessel disease are generally diminished enhancement in the radial, ulnar, and interosseous arteries and poor enhancement of the palmar and digital arteries in the hand (Fig. 117-6). Sometimes, narrowing and tapering of digital vessels can be seen.

In cases of suspected trauma, it is important to review the scout images for the presence of foreign material, such as bullets or shrapnel (Fig. 117-7).

Magnetic Resonance Imaging

Because of the wide array of different soft tissue contrasts and angiographic techniques, MRI has become one of the preferred modalities in the work-up of suspected upper extremity arterial disease. Although contrast-enhanced MRA (CE MRA) remains the standard of reference for evaluation of the vasculature, recent developments in nonenhanced pulse sequences for vascular imaging, combined with clinical concerns for potential risks of nephrogenic systemic fibrosis, have rekindled interest in these techniques.

There is a paucity of literature on the efficacy and diagnostic accuracy of nonenhanced techniques, so this section will focus on contrast-enhanced techniques. The limited maximum field of view (FOV) of 40 to 50 cm in commercially available MR scanners necessitates dedicated protocols for the central vessels in the chest and forearm and hand vessels, analogous to the dedicated protocols as described earlier for CT. An important pitfall of MRI is susceptibility-induced pseudostenosis in the subclavian artery ipsilateral to the site where the gadolinium (Gd) chelate contrast medium is injected. Because of the high concentration of Gd in the subclavian vein during the initial intravenous injection, it is possible to encounter signal drop-off (also known as T2* susceptibility artifact), which obscures visualization of the subclavian vein but also of the adjacent subclavian artery (Fig. 117-8). To avoid this artifact, it is necessary to acquire early and late arterial

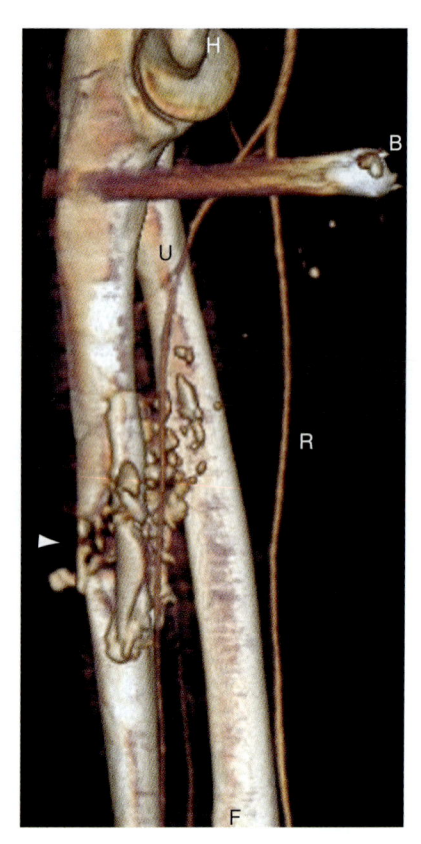

FIGURE 117-7 Color volume rendering of 64-slice CTA image of the left upper extremity of a 25-year-old male with a gunshot trauma. There is a comminuted fracture of the ulna (*arrowhead*). Both the radial (R) and ulnar artery (U) are patent and intact. The ulnar artery is slightly deviated because of soft tissue damage but is also intact and patent. B, bullet with streak artifacts.

phase images; the signal drop-off will disappear on the later phase images because of the natural reduction in the concentration of Gd over time, with hemodilution of the contrast agent.

Atherosclerotic lesions present as stenoses or occlusions in the aortic arch and brachial vessels over a relative short length and can be recognized by their typical serrated or jagged appearance (Fig. 117-9). This is opposed to the smooth, longer segmented stenoses with concomitant circumferential arterial wall thickening, which may be seen with vasculitis (i.e., arteritis). In cases of stenoses in one of the arch vessels, it is useful to supplement the MRI examination with phase contrast imaging of the cervical vessels to detect the presence of retrograde flow, or steal, in the vertebral artery.

Bilateral symmetrical smooth stenoses in the subclavian arteries are highly suggestive of GCA (Fig. 117-10). In patients with clinically suspected temporal arteritis, it is also useful to evaluate the superficial temporal artery with a dedicated high spatial resolution imaging protocol. The degree of arterial wall enhancement in this vessel has been found to correlate well with the amount of inflammatory activity at histology. Conversely, a return to lower degrees of enhancement and normal wall thickness detected by MRI after the institution of therapy reliably signifies a reduction of clinical disease activity.[34,35]

Aneurysmal widening of the subclavian artery can be seen in vasculitis but is more often encountered in patients with TOS. It is important to identify the presence of luminal thrombus in the artery, because this may pose a risk for distal embolization. It is often useful to image patients in the neutral anatomic position and with the arm(s) elevated above the head to assess the effect of postural changes on vascular patency (Fig. 117-11). Sagittal T1- and T2-weighted images in the neutral and elevated positions may also be of use to identify nonosseous compression of vascular structures such as fibrous bands. In patients with Buerger disease, arterial (and sometimes venous) occlusion can be seen, with typical bridging corkscrew collaterals (see later, "Angiography").

As is the case with CT, the best image quality is achieved with the patient in the supine position, with the forearm and hand raised above the head when imaging the distal upper extremity. Key findings in small vessel disease are slow and generally diminished enhancement of the forearm arteries and poor enhancement of the palmar and digital arteries in the hand (Fig. 117-12). The ability to perform time-resolved MR imaging is particularly helpful in this regard because it can readily demonstrate differential filling between both upper extremities or globally slowed arterial opacification. The introduction of the blood pool agent gadofosveset trisodium (Lantheus Medical Imaging; North Billerica, Mass) has facilitated ultrahigh spatial resolution equilibrium phase imaging of the vascular system in the hand and fingers, with voxel sizes as small as 64 µm. Narrowing and tapering of digital vessels can easily be appreciated on these images (Fig. 117-13).

MRI is not the preferred modality in cases of trauma. Patients are best imaged with CT or IA-DSA in these cases.

Nuclear Medicine and Positron Emission Tomography

The introduction of scanners capable of combined ^{18}fluorodeoxyglucose (^{18}FDG) positron emission tomography (PET) and CT imaging is potentially attractive for imaging inflammatory large vessel disease. Although no large-scale studies have been performed to date, there is anecdotal evidence that the combination of CT with PET (PET-CT) is of use for the evaluation of patients with large vessel vasculitis. A recent study by Henes and associates[36] in 13 patients who were newly diagnosed or re-evaluated for large vessel vasculitis has found that PET-CT could provide additional information over conventional serologic markers, such as erythrocyte sedimentation rate and C-reactive protein levels in blood. Stenotic lesions at CT were found in only 8 of 13 patients, whereas all patients with clinically active disease ($N = 12$) demonstrated uptake of ^{18}FDG in the aortic arch and branch vessels, indicating that PET imaging may be more sensitive in the early phases of the disease, when angiographic evaluation does not yet show luminal abnormalities (Fig. 117-14). Whether nuclear medicine techniques will still be used in the future remains to be determined because of the very high radiation doses involved (10 to 20 mSv/examination). No large comparative studies between MRI and PET-CT have been published so it is unclear to what extent these imaging modalities are complementary. Because of the

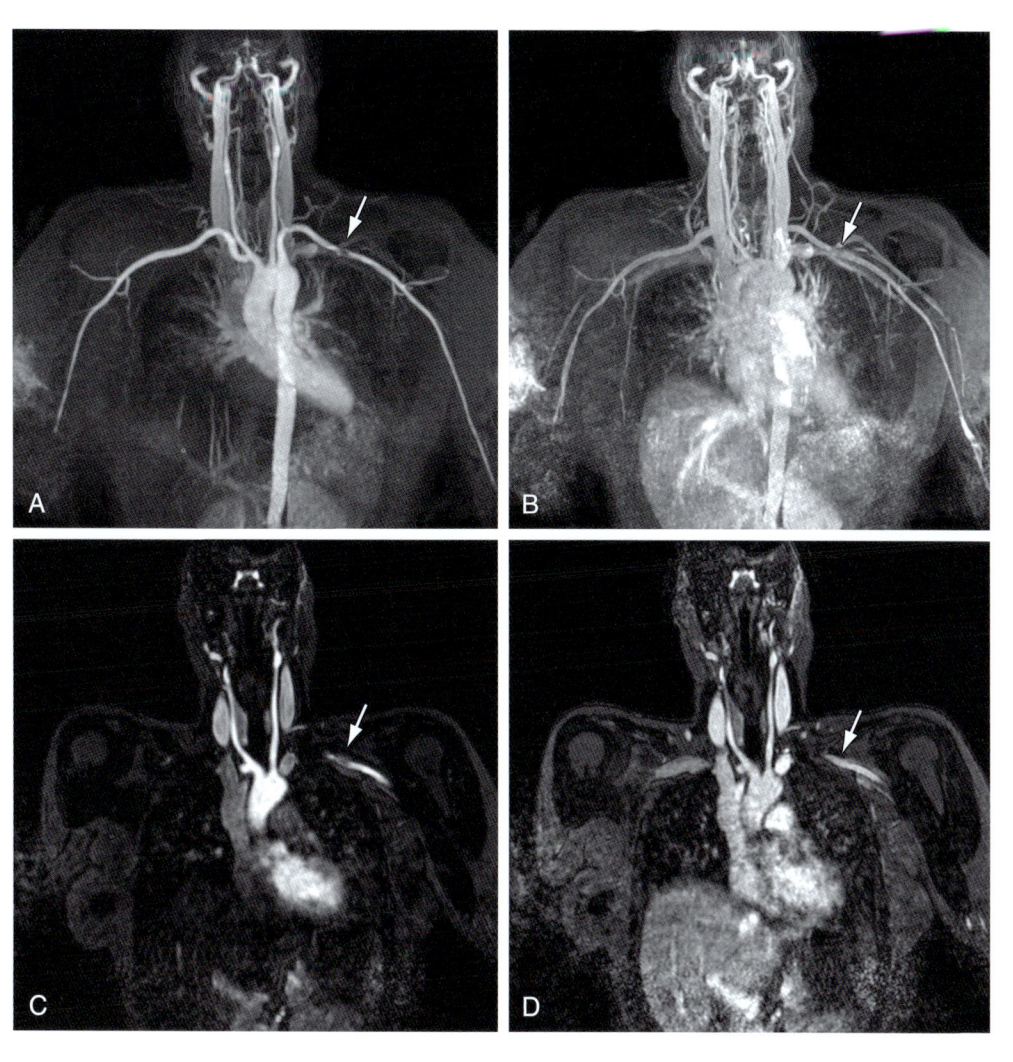

FIGURE 117-8 Whole-volume maximum intensity projection (MIP) by proximal upper extremity MRA in a 40-year-old male patient with complaints of bilateral upper extremity claudication. The physical examination was unremarkable and there was no blood pressure difference between both arms. Following a left antecubital venous injection of a Gd chelate contrast agent during CE MRA, the arterial phase MIP image suggests a stenosis in the left subclavian artery (*arrow*, **A**), which is confirmed on the accompanying source images (*arrow*, **C**). In the late arterial–early venous phase, the stenosis has disappeared on the MIP and source images (*arrows*, **B** and **D**). The stenosis is caused by T2* susceptibility-induced signal loss because of the highly concentrated gadolinium in the left subclavian vein. Note that this vessel exhibits far lower signal intensity compared with the jugular veins in **A**.

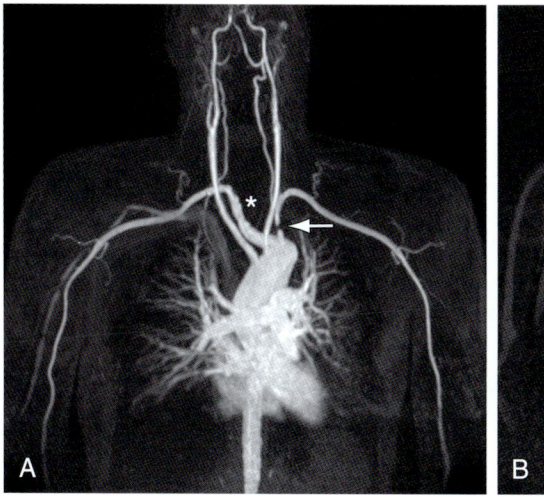

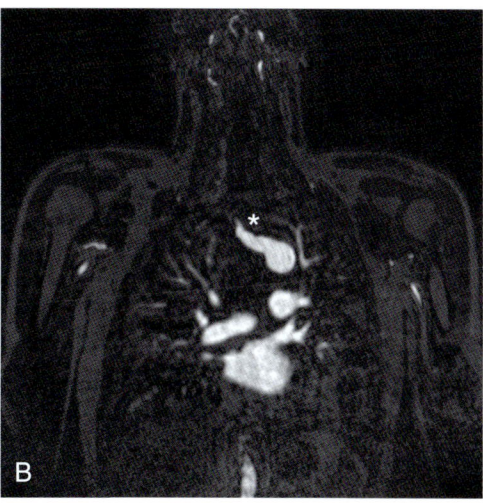

FIGURE 117-9 Whole-volume maximum intensity projection of proximal upper extremity MRA in 61-year-old male patient with complaints of bilateral upper extremity claudication. **A,** There is a short high-grade stenosis in the proximal left subclavian artery (*arrow*) and low-grade narrowing of the aberrant right subclavian artery. Note the serrated appearance of the lesion (*asterisks* in **A** and **B**). The absence of vessel wall thickening suggests that this lesion is of atherosclerotic origin.

high radiation burden and because many patients with vasculitis are young women, PET-CT is not a very attractive technique for repetitive imaging, as is often needed in the follow-up of vasculitis. In the foreseeable future, MRI remains the modality of first choice for these patients.

Angiography

Although CTA and MRA have largely overtaken DSA for the evaluation of the central thoracic arteries and veins, IA-DSA with the administration of vasodilators remains the

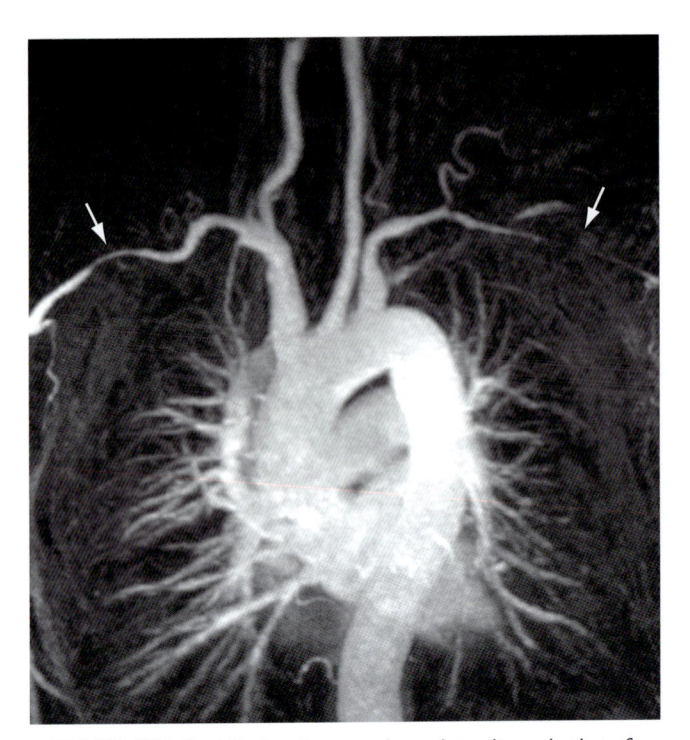

■ **FIGURE 117-10** Whole-volume maximum intensity projection of the aortic arch and branch vessels in a 67-year-old female patient with histologically proven giant cell arteritis. Note bilateral high-grade smooth subclavian artery stenoses (*arrows*). This finding is highly suggestive of arterial involvement caused by caused by giant cell arteritis. (*Courtesy of Dr. Thorsten Bley, Klinik und Poliklinik für Diagnostische und Interventionelle Radiologie, Universitätsklinikum Hamburg-Eppendorf, Hamburg, Germany.*)

standard for evaluation of digital arteries in most centers because of its unparalleled spatial and temporal resolution (Fig. 117-15). The major drawback, however, is the invasiveness and discomfort of the procedure, especially when vasodilators are used. Typical findings with regard to atherosclerotic or aneurysmal arterial disease, as well as findings suggestive of vasculitis or Buerger disease, are identical to those described earlier for CTA and MRA (Fig. 117-16). A limitation of IA-DSA is its inability to image the vessel wall. In clinical practice, IA-DSA of the central vessels is primarily performed in the context of endovascular treatment.

Classic Signs

The classic signs of atherosclerosis, vasculitis, Buerger disease, and small vessel disease have been discussed. It is important to note that many different diseases are associated with large or small vessel disease, and imaging findings are rarely specific for a certain disease. In suspected upper extremity vascular disease, imaging findings should always be considered in combination with the clinical picture.

DIFFERENTIAL DIAGNOSIS
From Clinical Presentation

As noted, a thorough medical, surgical, occupational, and sports history, including information about drug and alcohol use, remains the cornerstone of the workup of upper extremity vascular disease. This information should be supplemented with bilateral measurement of blood pressure, biochemical testing for hypercholesterolemia, and inflammatory marker screening. In selected cases, it is also useful to search for clotting disorders. The most important step to reach the correct diagnosis and subsequent treatment is to consider alternative diagnoses when the history and other demographic characteristics are incongruent with the most common cause of upper extremity arterial symptoms, atherosclerosis. The presence of a Raynaud complex of symptoms should prompt consideration of underlying systemic or connective tissue disease when this is the presenting complaint in patients. In about one third of the cases, however, Raynaud syndrome is a benign isolated finding, without serious implications.

From Imaging Findings

The main differentiation one can make on the basis of imaging appearance in the large thoracic and proximal upper extremity arteries is between a vasculitis and other diseases. As noted, vasculitis tends to present with longer, segmented, and smooth circumferential wall thickening and luminal narrowing. Small vessel abnormalities in the palmar arch and digital arteries are not specific for any given disease and are associated with many different conditions.

SYNOPSIS OF TREATMENT OPTIONS
Medical Treatment

Medical treatment is highly dependent on the underlying disease that causes the symptoms. As has become clear, imaging plays an important role to establish the nature and extent of underlying disease in many cases. Older patients will often be on anticoagulation and/or statin therapy. The only universally accepted treatment to stop progression of Buerger disease is complete cessation of tobacco use. This includes cessation of the use of tobacco variants such as snuff and chewing tobacco. In patients with small vessel disease, corticosteroids can be helpful.

Surgical and Interventional Treatment

In general, interventional radiologic and surgical techniques are used only in cases of obstructive symptomatic atherosclerosis of the central thoracic and proximal upper extremity arteries. Exact delineation of the site of occlusive disease is important from a therapeutic point of view, because many vascular surgeons prefer extrathoracic procedures to intrathoracic endarterectomy or bypass procedures, except in the management of complex occlusive disease of two or more major vessels. Modern interventional radiologic techniques allow for the successful repair of brachiocephalic, proximal carotid, and subclavian artery lesions, including stenting, when needed. PTA and

Text continued on p. 1658

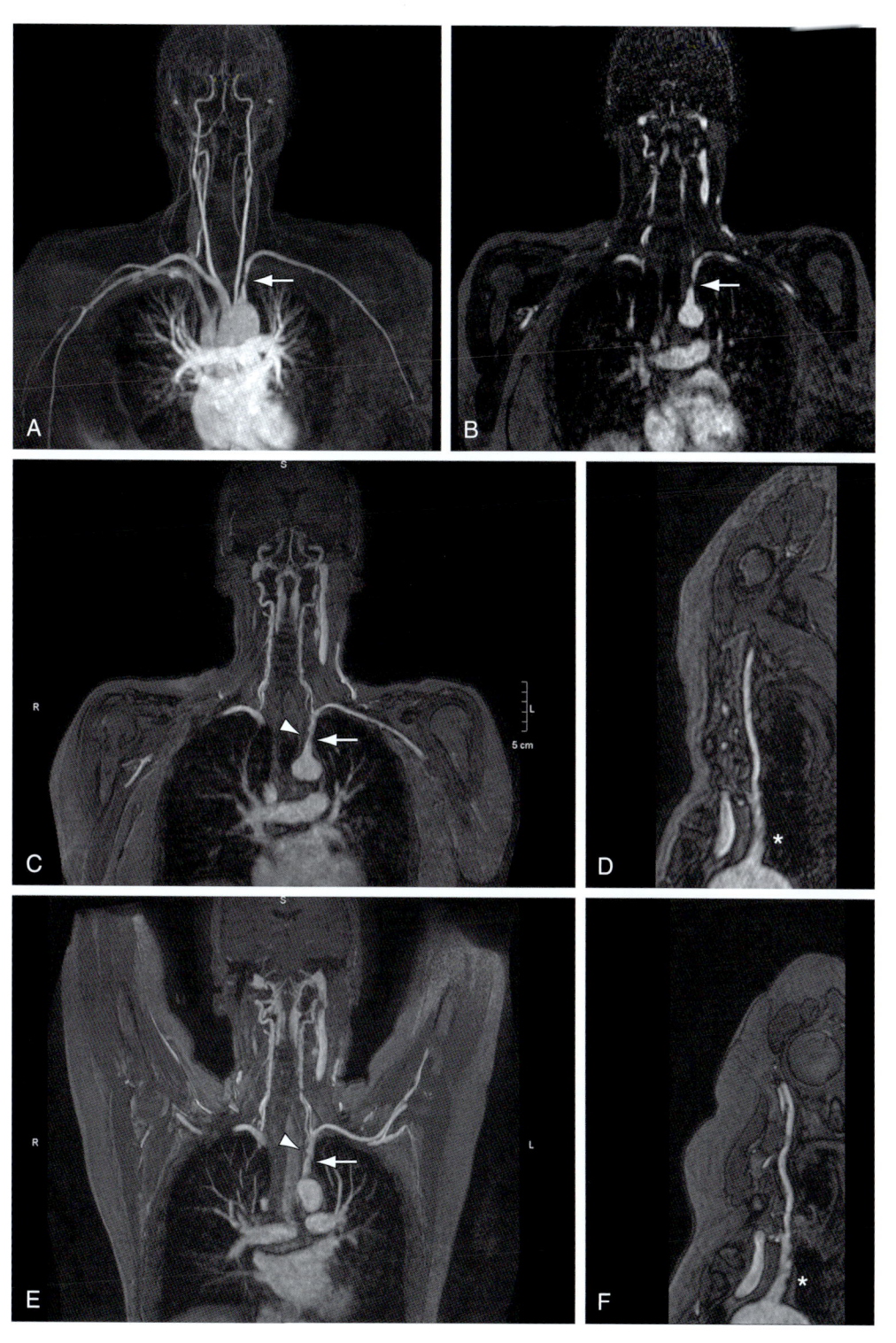

CHAPTER 117 • *Vascular Diseases of the Upper Extremities* 1653

FIGURE 117-11 Whole-volume maximum intensity projection (**A**) and corresponding source image (**B**) of proximal upper extremities in 57-year-old female patient with complaints of pain in the left shoulder and proximal upper extremity when lifting her arm above her head. The referring clinician wanted to rule out thoracic outlet syndrome. First-pass images were acquired in the anatomic position. Subsequent steady-state images were acquired in the anatomic position (**C**) and with the arms elevated above the head (**E**). There is a short 70% stenosis in the proximal left subclavian artery (*arrows*). Curved multiplanar reformations of the left subclavian artery reveal the stenosis in the proximal part (*asterisks* in **D** and **F**), but no compression or aneurysm formation was seen of the subclavicular portion of the subclavian artery. Gadofosveset, 10 mL, was used for the examination.

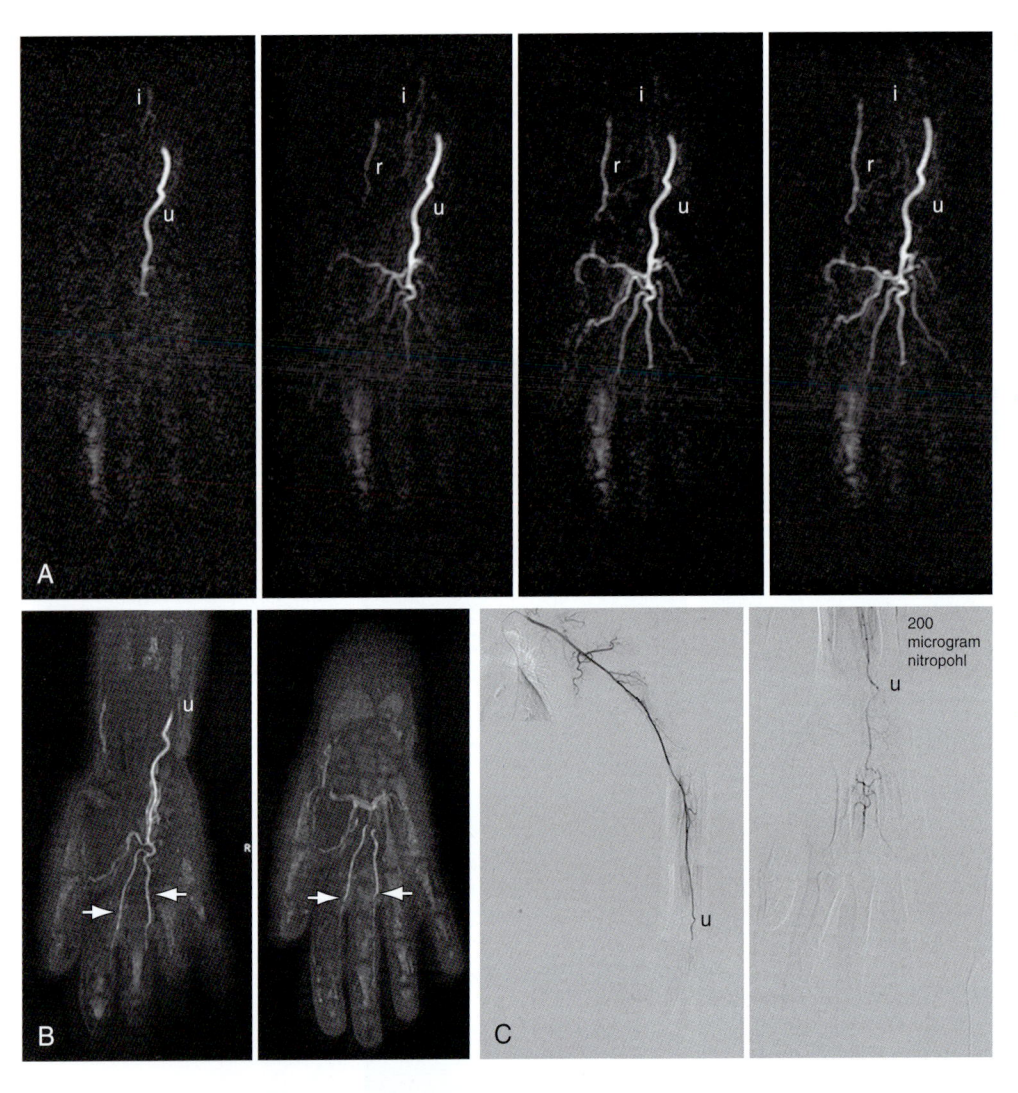

FIGURE 117-12 Time-resolved MR angiogram with subsequent steady-state acquisition in 47-year-old female patient with long-standing antiphospholipid syndrome. The patient presented with a cold hand that would not resolve. **A,** Four subsequent arterial phase images show very slow filling of the distal forearm and hand arteries. Note the absence of opacification of the digital arteries. **B,** Images acquired in the steady state (after distribution of contrast material in both the arterial and venous systems) show two digital arteries (*arrows*) in the proximal part of the hand (*left*) as well as the fingers (*right*). **C,** Intra-arterial digital subtraction angiography (DSA) was performed to ensure that MRA did not miss any arteries. As can be seen, even with vasodilation, DSA was not able to show any digital arteries, most likely because of the extremely slow flow in combination with the higher viscosity of the iodinated contrast agent. i, interosseous artery; r, radial artery; u, ulnar artery.

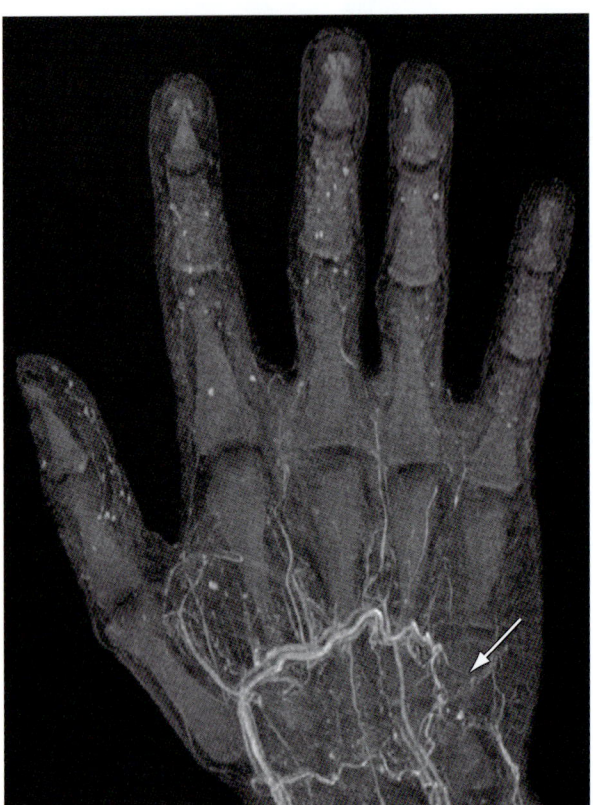

FIGURE 117-13 Whole-volume maximum intensity projection in 63-year-old female patient with gangrenous fingertips caused by steal after dialysis access creation in the proximal forearm. There is an almost complete lack of digital vessels, as well as a short occlusion of the palmar arch. Images were acquired in the steady state with an isotropic resolution of $0.4 \times 0.4 \times 0.4$ mm^3 (64 mµ) voxel size.

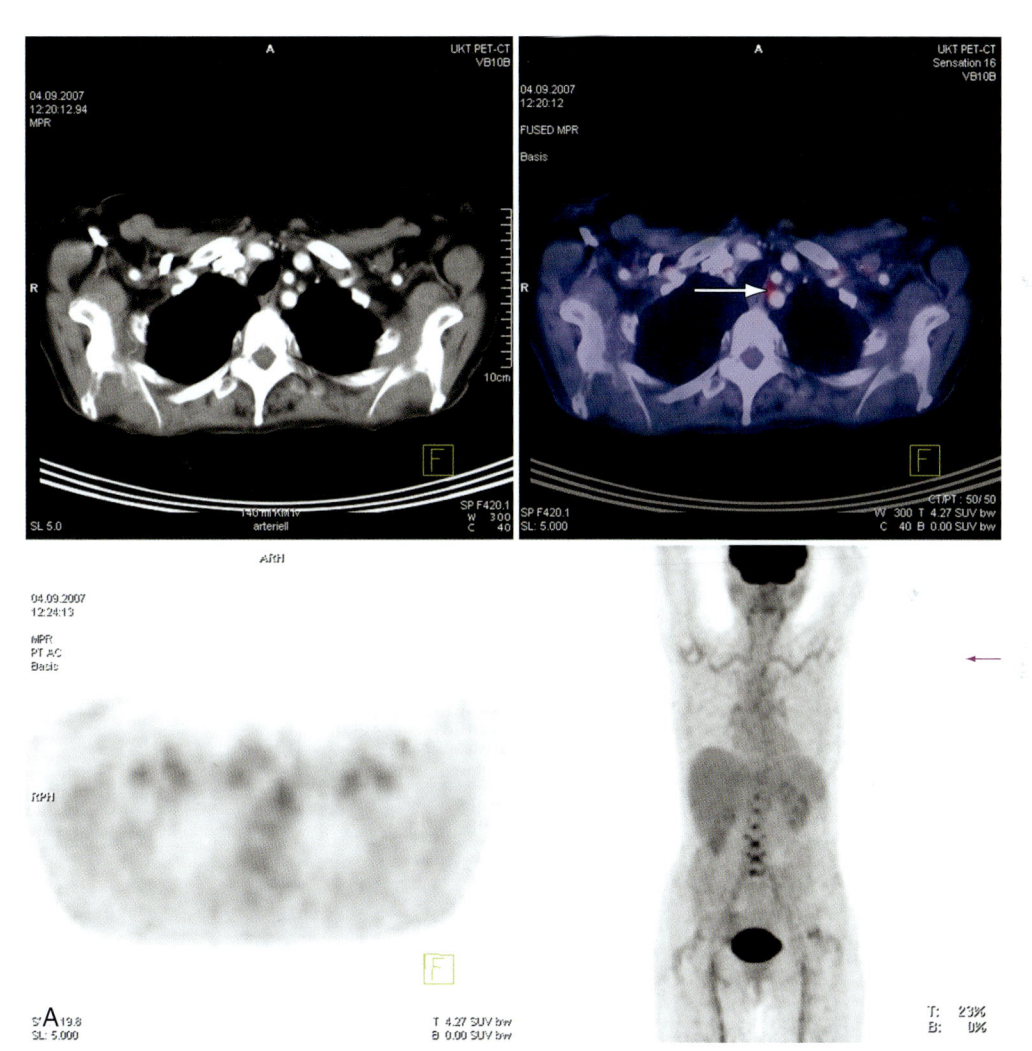

CHAPTER 117 • Vascular Diseases of the Upper Extremities 1655

■ **FIGURE 117-14** Whole-body PET-CT studies showing CT findings (*upper left panels*), PET findings (*lower panels*), and fused axial PET-CT images (*upper right panels*) at the upper chest level in three patients with minor (**A**), moderate (**B**), and extensive (**C**) vasculitis involving the subclavian arteries. **A,** The patient with minor disease was a 69-year-old woman suffering from weight loss, polymyalgia, and inadequate response to steroids. There is moderately increased uptake of ^{18}FDG in the left subclavian artery (*arrow*).

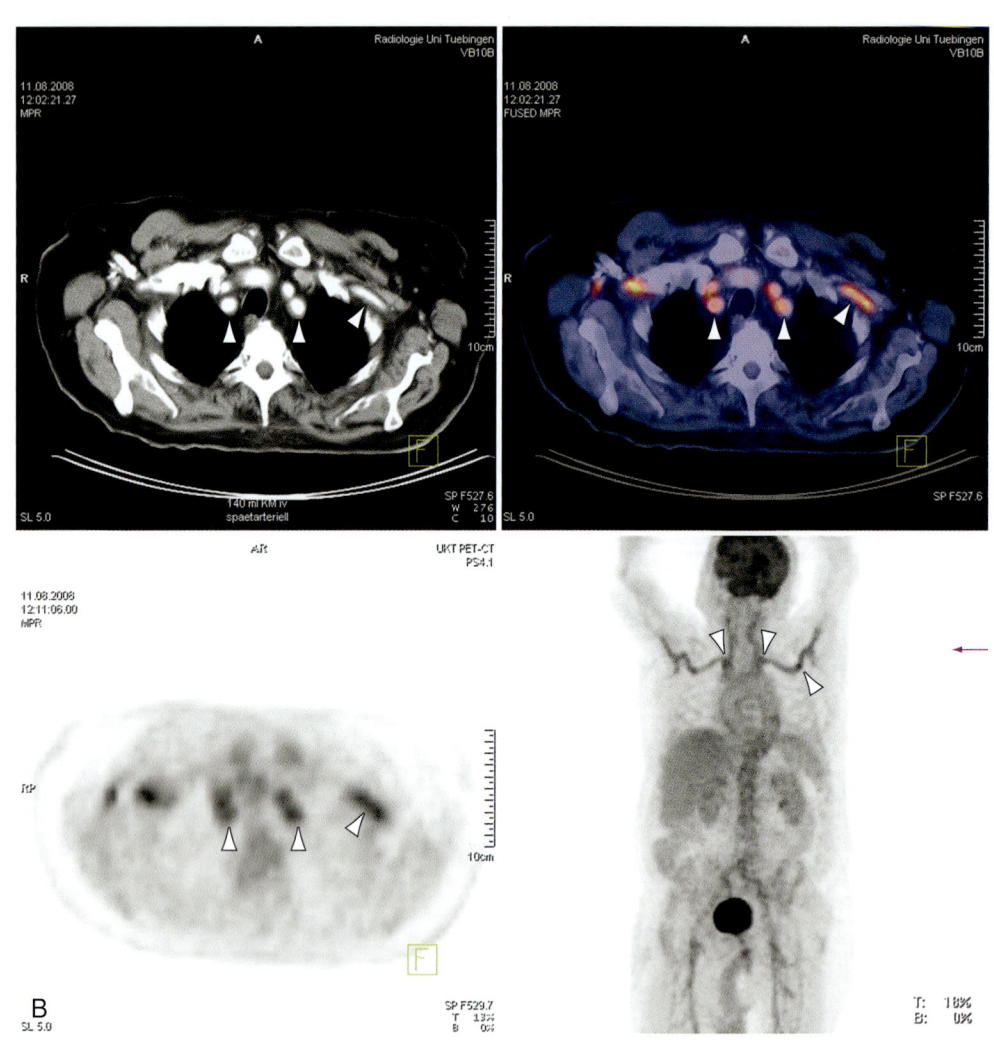

FIGURE 117-14, cont'd **B,** The patient with moderate disease was a 75-year-old man with initial complaints of polymyalgia, fever, visual impairment, jaw claudication, and inadequate response to steroid therapy as well. The CT, PET, and fusion images show mild thickening of both subclavian artery walls, with corresponding increased ^{18}FDG uptake (*arrowheads*).

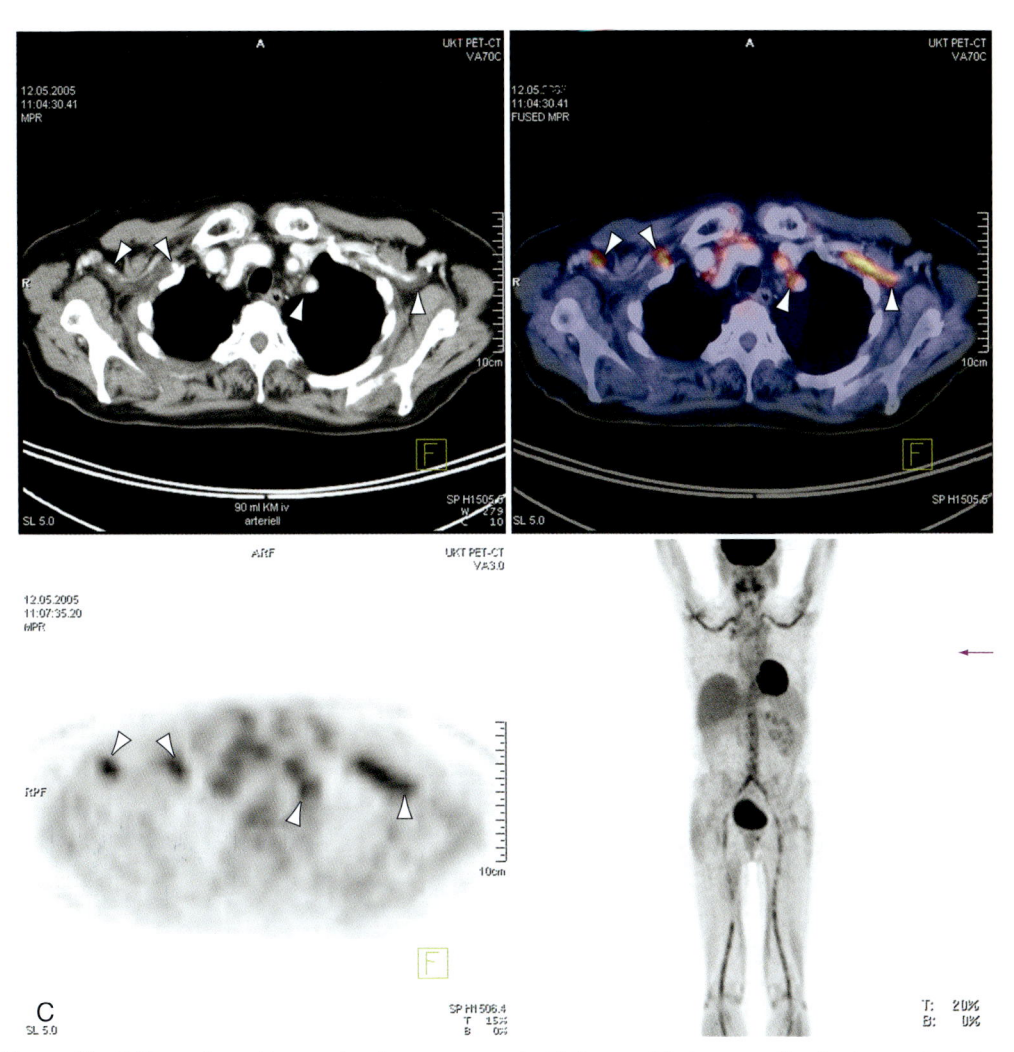

CHAPTER 117 • Vascular Diseases of the Upper Extremities 1657

■ **FIGURE 117-14, cont'd** C, The patient with extensive disease presented with fever, weight loss, arm claudication, and pulselessness of the left arm. There is extensive patchy arterial wall thickening with corresponding increased uptake of ^{18}FDG in the aortic arch and branch vessels (*arrowheads*). Also note the strong vascular wall enhancement throughout the entire peripheral vascular tree in the lower right image. *(Courtesy of Dr. Christina Pfannenberg and Dr. Jörg Henes, Erberhard Karls University Hospital, Tübingen, Germany.)*

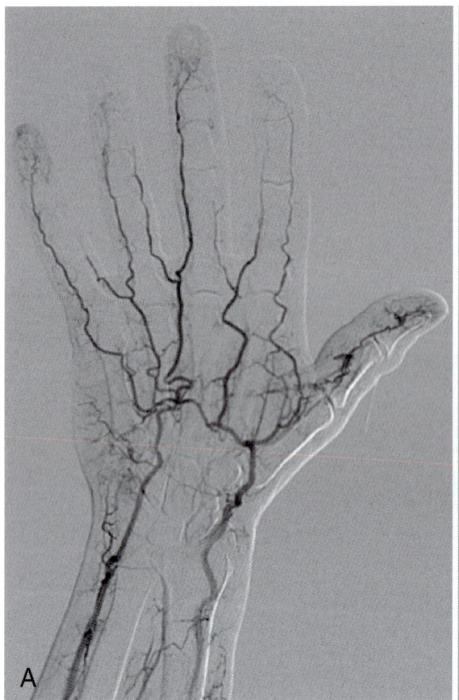

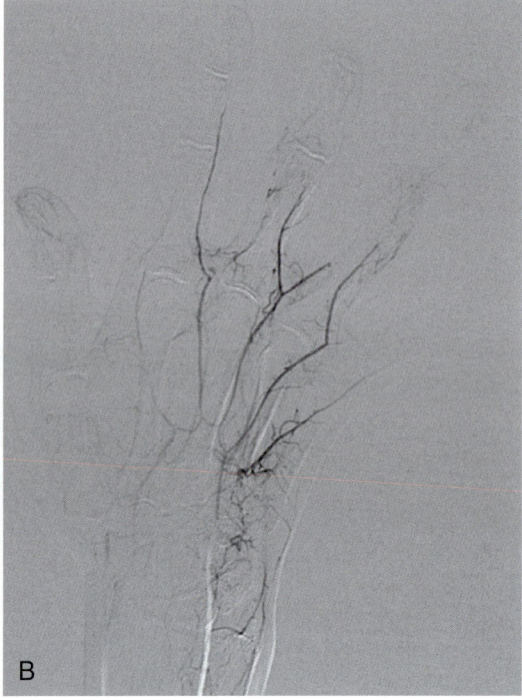

FIGURE 117-15 A, B, Intra-arterial digital subtraction angiograms of both hands in a 50-year-old female patient with the CREST syndrome presenting with Raynaud phenomenon. There is very slow flow in both hands, with extremely sparse vascularization of the right hand (B).

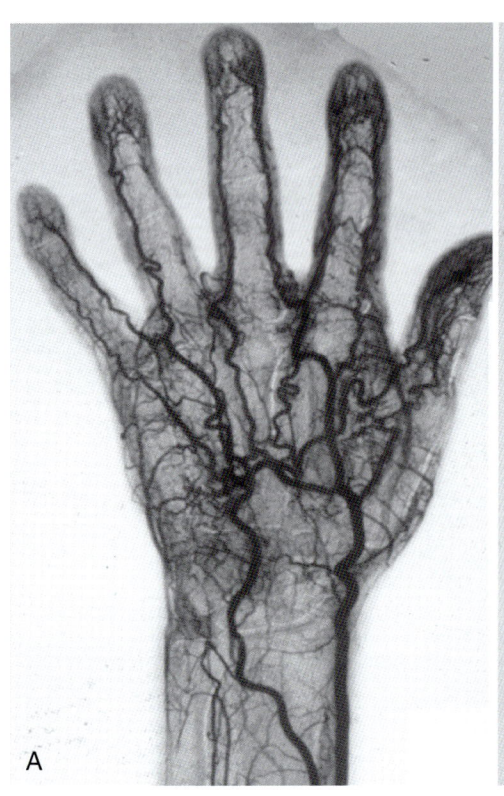

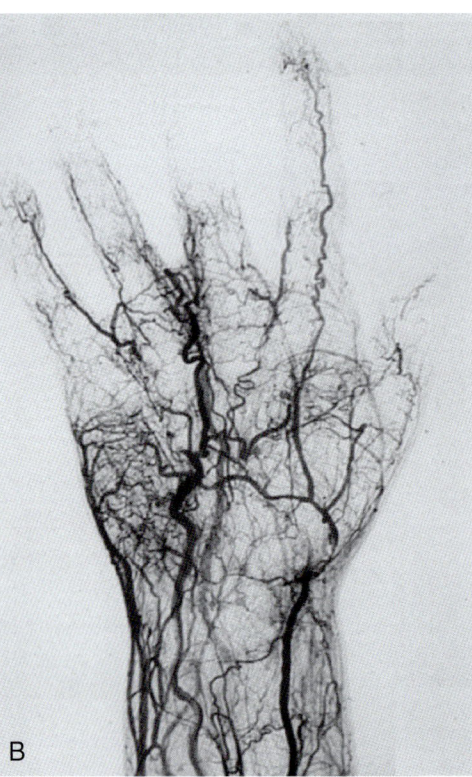

FIGURE 117-16 38-year-old male smoker presenting with painful and cold fingertips of the left hand. A, Image at presentation. At baseline, there were segmental occlusions of the fourth and fifth proper digital arteries with characteristic corkscrew collaterals, confirming the diagnosis of Buerger disease. The patient continued smoking. B, Two years later, there is significant advancement of the disease, with almost no digital arteries enhancing any more.

surgery have good long-term success rates. At present, PTA will often be attempted first. A key consideration for management options is the presence of concomitant carotid and coronary artery disease. In patients suffering from vasculitis, the usefulness of PTA with or without stenting has not been established.

REPORTING: INFORMATION FOR THE REFERRING PHYSICIAN

Key information that the interpreting physician should provide in the report of patients evaluated for suspected upper extremity vascular disease includes the location of the abnormality, whether it is symmetrical or bilateral, and the exact appearance of any stenotic lesion. Also, the presence or absence of steal phenomena should be documented. In addition to evaluation of the arterial tree, one should also comment on the appearance of the bony structures, including the presence of any supernumerary ribs or excessively large transverse processes. When evaluating small and distal arteries, the rate of arterial opacification should be noted and, in cases of occlusion, the presence of any corkscrew-like bridging collaterals.

KEY POINTS

- Symptoms of upper extremity vascular disease are the result of a heterogeneous set of conditions that affect the arteries and/or veins primarily, secondarily (associated with underlying systemic conditions), or by extrinsic compression or other trauma.
- A thorough medical, surgical, occupational, and sports history, including any habitual drug and/or alcohol use, is crucial to elucidate the source of the complaints; this often yields important information to complement imaging findings.
- Large artery disease of the upper extremity most often presents as intermittent claudication of the upper extremity, neck, tongue, or jaw. Alternatively, steal phenomena may be in the foreground.
- Suspected arterial occlusion of the forearm and hand arteries can be caused by distal embolization of thrombus fragments from the heart or from mural thrombus present in a proximal aneurysm.
- Medium-sized and small artery vascular disease in the upper extremity is almost never caused by atherosclerosis.
- Arterial disease of the hand often presents with Raynaud syndrome. In about one third of cases, this is a benign condition without clinical consequences. There is underlying connective tissue or systemic disease in about two thirds of patients.

SUGGESTED READINGS

Block JA, Sequeira W. Raynaud's phenomenon. Lancet 2001; 357: 2042-2048.

Demondion X, Herbinet P, Van Sint Jan S, et al. Imaging assessment of thoracic outlet syndrome. Radiographics 2006; 26:1735-1750.

Greenfield LJ, Rajagopalan S, Olin JW. Upper extremity arterial disease. Cardiol Clin 2002; 20:623-631.

Huang JH, Zager EL. Thoracic outlet syndrome. Neurosurgery 2004; 55:897-902.

Jennette JC, Falk RJ. Small-vessel vasculitis. N Engl J Med 1997; 337: 1512-1523.

Mills JL, Sr. Buerger's disease in the 21st century: diagnosis, clinical features, and therapy. Semin Vasc Surg 2003; 16:179-189.

Nastri MV, Baptista LP, Baroni RH, et al. Gadolinium-enhanced three-dimensional MR angiography of Takayasu arteritis. Radiographics 2004; 24:773-786.

Tann OR, Tulloh RM, Hamilton MC. Takayasu's disease: a review. Cardiol Young 2008; 18:250-259.

REFERENCES

1. Azakie A, McElhinney DB, Higashima R, et al. Innominate artery reconstruction: over 3 decades of experience. Ann Surg 1998; 228:402-410.
2. Jennette JC, Falk RJ. Small-vessel vasculitis. N Engl J Med 1997; 337:1512-1523.
3. Nastri MV, Baptista LP, Baroni RH, et al. Gadolinium-enhanced three-dimensional MR angiography of Takayasu arteritis. Radiographics 2004; 24:773-786.
4. Michet CJ, Matteson EL. Polymyalgia rheumatica. BMJ 2008; 336:765-769.
5. Demondion X, Herbinet P, Van Sint Jan S, et al. Imaging assessment of thoracic outlet syndrome. Radiographics 2006; 26:1735-1750.
6. Caselli RJ, Hunder GG. Giant cell (temporal) arteritis. Neurol Clin 1997; 15:893-902.
7. Huang JH, Zager EL. Thoracic outlet syndrome. Neurosurgery 2004; 55:897-902.
8. Andreev A, Kavrakov T, Karakolev J, Penkov P. Management of acute arterial trauma of the upper extremity. Eur J Vasc Surg 1992; 6:593-598.
9. Fitridge RA, Raptis S, Miller JH, Faris I. Upper extremity arterial injuries: experience at the Royal Adelaide Hospital, 1969 to 1991. J Vasc Surg 1994; 20:941-946.
10. Libby P. Vascular biology of atherosclerosis: overview and state of the art. Am J Cardiol 2003; 91:3A-6A.
11. Tann OR, Tulloh RM, Hamilton MC. Takayasu's disease: a review. Cardiol Young 2008; 18:250-259.
12. Kaufman JA. Upper-extremity arteries. In Kaufman JA, Lee MJ (eds). Vascular and Interventional Radiology: The Requisites. Philadelphia, Mosby, 2004, pp 142-162.
13. Cherry KJ Jr, McCullough JL, Hallett JW Jr, et al. Technical principles of direct innominate artery revascularization: a comparison of endarterectomy and bypass grafts. J Vasc Surg 1989; 9:718-723.
14. Kieffer E, Sabatier J, Koskas F, Bahnini A. Atherosclerotic innominate artery occlusive disease: early and long-term results of surgical reconstruction. J Vasc Surg 1995; 21:326-336.
15. Reul GJ, Jacobs MJ, Gregoric ID, et al. Innominate artery occlusive disease: surgical approach and long-term results. J Vasc Surg 1991; 14:405-412.
16. Greenfield LJ, Rajagopalan S, Olin JW. Upper extremity arterial disease. Cardiol Clin 2002; 20:623-631.
17. McLafferty RB, Edwards JM, Taylor LM Jr, Porter JM. Diagnosis and long-term clinical outcome in patients diagnosed with hand ischemia. J Vasc Surg 1995; 22:361-367.
18. Mills JL, Friedman EI, Taylor LM Jr., Porter JM. Upper extremity ischemia caused by small artery disease. Ann Surg 1987; 206:521-528.
19. Seibold JR. Critical tissue ischaemia in scleroderma: a note of caution. Ann Rheum Dis 1994; 53:289-290.

20. Block JA, Sequeira W. Raynaud's phenomenon. Lancet 2001; 357:2042-2048.
21. Wigley FM. Clinical practice. Raynaud's Phenomenon. N Engl J Med 2002; 347:1001-1008.
22. Mills JL Sr. Buerger's disease in the 21st century: diagnosis, clinical features, and therapy. Semin Vasc Surg 2003; 16:179-189.
23. Marie I, Herve F, Primard E, et al. Long-term follow-up of hypothenar hammer syndrome: a series of 47 patients. Medicine (Baltimore) 2007; 86:334-343.
24. Myers SI, Harward TR, Maher DP, et al. Complex upper extremity vascular trauma in an urban population. J Vasc Surg 1990; 12:305-309.
25. Deguara J, Ali T, Modarai B, Burnand KG. Upper limb ischemia: 20 years experience from a single center. Vascular 2005; 13:84-91.
26. Porter JM, Edwards JM. Occlusive and vasospastic diseases involving distal upper extremity arteries—Raynaud's syndrome. In Rutherford RB (ed). Vascular Surgery, 5th ed. Philadelphia, WB. Saunders, 2000, pp 1170-1183.
27. Szekanecz Z, Koch AE. Vascular involvement in rheumatic diseases: 'vascular rheumatology'. Arthritis Res Ther 2008; 10:224.
28. Kleinert HE, Volianitis GJ. Thrombosis of the palmar arterial arch and its tributaries: etiology and newer concepts in treatment. J Trauma 1965; 83:447-457.
29. Kleinert HE, Burget GC, Morgan JA, et al. Aneurysms of the hand. Arch Surg 1973; 106:554-557.
30. Vayssairat M, Debure C, Cormier JM, et al. Hypothenar hammer syndrome: seventeen cases with long-term follow-up. J Vasc Surg 1987; 5:838-843.
31. Kallenberg CG. Early detection of connective tissue disease in patients with Raynaud's phenomenon. Rheum Dis Clin North Am 1990; 16:11-30.
32. Kallenberg CG, Wouda AA, Hoet MH, van Venrooij WJ. Development of connective tissue disease in patients presenting with Raynaud's phenomenon: a six-year follow-up with emphasis on the predictive value of antinuclear antibodies as detected by immunoblotting. Ann Rheum Dis 1988; 47:634-641.
33. Polak JF, Donaldson MC, Whittemore AD, et al. Pulsatile masses surrounding vascular prostheses: real-time US color flow imaging. Radiology 1989; 170:363-366.
34. Bley TA, Ness T, Warnatz K, et al. Influence of corticosteroid treatment on MRI findings in giant cell arteritis. Clin Rheumatol 2006.
35. Bley TA, Wieben O, Vaith P, et al. Magnetic resonance imaging depicts mural inflammation of the temporal artery in giant cell arteritis. Arthritis Rheum 2004; 51:1062-1063.
36. Henes JC, Muller M, Krieger J, et al. [18F] FDG-PET/CT as a new and sensitive imaging method for the diagnosis of large vessel vasculitis. Clin Exp Rheumatol 2008; 26:S47-S52.

CHAPTER 118

Venous Sonography of the Upper Extremities and Thoracic Outlet

Jonathan D. Kirsch, Ulrike Hamper, and Leslie M. Scoutt

Upper extremity deep venous thrombosis (DVT) was historically considered an uncommon, benign, and self-limited condition.[1] As such, thrombi involving the upper extremities were thought to be of little clinical significance and often undertreated because the risk of propagation was also believed to be low. More recent studies have found this not to be the case. The incidence of upper extremity DVT is far more common than previously thought, especially with the increased use of central venous catheters and placement of cardiac pacemakers, and in patients with cancer and hypercoagulable states. Upper extremity DVT is also seen to be associated with significant complications, including pulmonary embolism, superior vena cava syndrome, postthrombotic venous insufficiency, and loss of venous access.

This chapter will review the anatomy of the upper extremity veins and thoracic outlet in addition to the prevalence, causes, clinical characteristics, complications, and diagnostic imaging of upper extremity deep venous thrombosis and thoracic outlet syndrome.

VENOUS ANATOMY

The relevant venous anatomy of the upper extremities and thoracic inlet includes the deep venous system composed of the internal jugular, brachiocephalic (or innominate), subclavian, axillary, and paired brachial veins. The superficial basilic and cephalic veins are also usually included in the examination (Fig. 118-1).

In the neck, the internal jugular vein courses from the jugular foramen at the base of the skull lateral to the carotid arteries within the carotid sheath. The internal jugular vein collects blood from the skull, brain, face, and neck. It joins the subclavian vein posterior to the medial clavicle, where it forms the brachiocephalic or innominate vein. A pair of valves is present in its caudal end near the confluence.

The right brachiocephalic vein is approximately 2.5 cm in length and courses in a caudal direction. The left brachiocephalic vein is approximately 6 cm in length, has a more horizontal course, and joins the right brachiocephalic vein to form the superior vena cava.

In the upper arm, the usually paired brachial veins flank the brachial artery. They may join with the basilic vein before forming the axillary vein. The axillary vein begins at the inferior border of the teres major muscle and continues through the axilla to the lateral border of the first rib, where it becomes the subclavian vein. The subclavian vein continues medially, deep to the clavicle, until it joins the internal jugular vein, forming the brachiocephalic vein. Valves may be seen in the subclavian vein near this confluence.

The axillary vein lies medial and inferior to the axillary artery. The subclavian vein is anterior and inferior to the subclavian artery (Fig. 118-2). Knowing these relationships will aid in identification of these vessels and help in distinguishing possible large collaterals from the native vessels.

PREVALENCE, ETIOLOGY, AND RISK FACTORS

Upper extremity deep venous thrombosis can be divided into primary and secondary thrombosis based on pathogenesis. Primary upper extremity DVT includes Paget-Schroetter Syndrome (effort thrombosis) and idiopathic upper extremity DVT. Secondary upper extremity DVT is found in patients with known inciting causes such as central venous catheters, pacemakers, and malignancy.

FIGURE 118-1 Venous anatomy of the upper extremity.

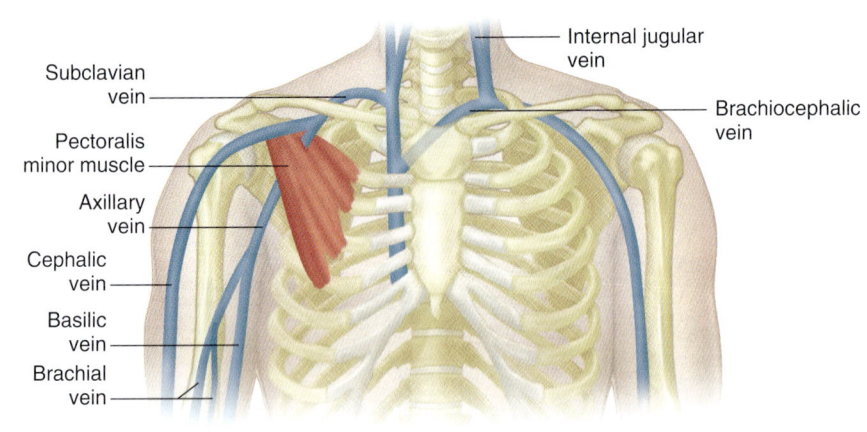

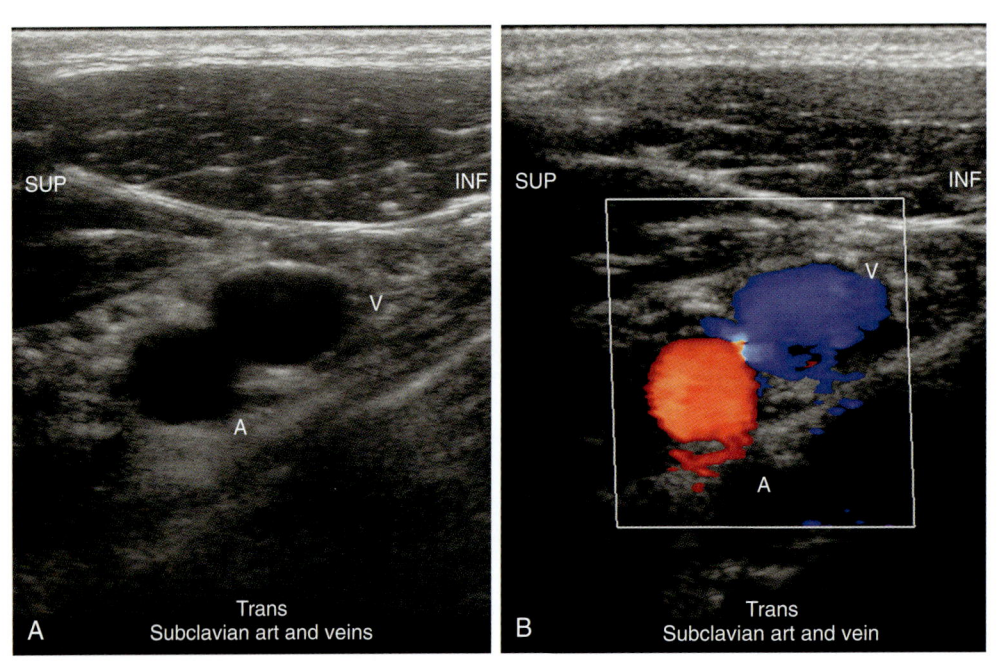

FIGURE 118-2 Transverse gray-scale (**A**) and color Doppler (**B**) images demonstrating the normal anatomic relationship of the subclavian vein (V) anterior and inferior (INF) to the subclavian artery (A). SUP, superior.

The exact prevalence of symptomatic upper extremity DVT in the general population is unknown but is estimated to be approximately 0.2%.[2] In patients with deep venous thrombosis, approximately 90% involve the lower extremity and the remaining 10% involve the upper extremity.[3]

With the increasing use of central venous catheters, the prevalence of upper extremity DVT has increased (Fig. 118-3). Earlier studies documented thrombosis in 2% to 12% of patients with central venous catheters.[4] In more recent studies, upper extremity DVT has been documented in 50% to 60% of patients with central venous catheters. The most powerful independent predictor of upper extremity DVT was the presence of a catheter, with the risk factor increasing sevenfold in these patients.[5,6] The position of the catheter tip has been found to correlate with the incidence of upper extremity DVT. Catheters at the junction of the right atrium and the superior vena cava and those in the mid superior vena cava (SVC) have the lowest incidence of associated thrombosis and those with the catheter tip in the brachiocephalic vein have a higher incidence.[4] The ideal position for the catheter tip is at the cavoatrial junction. Catheter material and diameter have also been found to affect the incidence of thrombus. The lowest rates have been for polyurethane and silicone catheters and for those with an external diameter less than 2.8 mm.[7,8] In the pediatric population, two thirds of DVT cases occur in the upper extremity, in contrast to adults, and are usually secondary to catheter placement.[6]

Cancer is a significant risk factor for upper extremity DVT secondary to alterations in coagulability factors, low-grade disseminated intravascular coagulation, and stasis secondary to tumor compression.[9] Bilateral upper extremity DVT was found to be more common in patients with malignancy. The risk of thrombosis increases signifi-

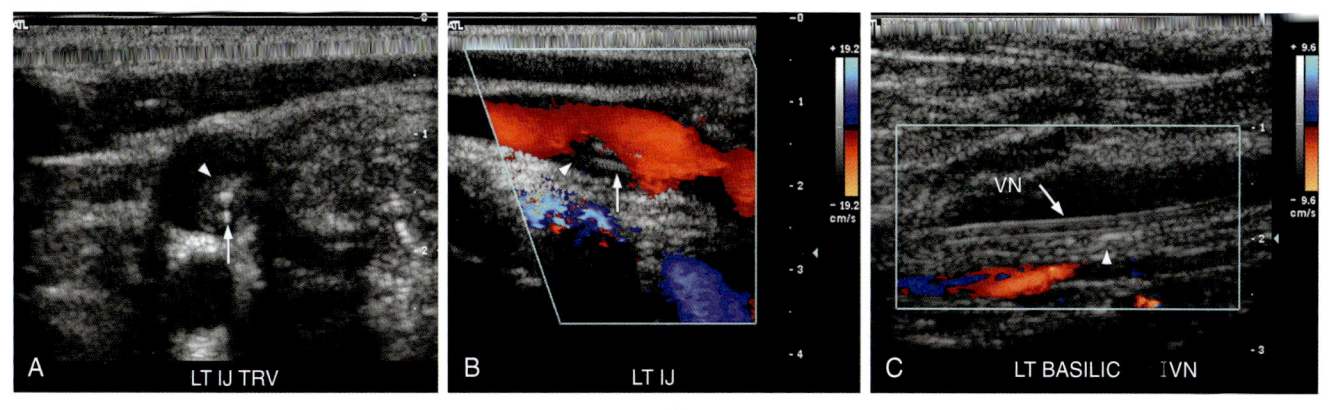

FIGURE 118-3 Transverse **(A)** and longitudinal **(B)** images show thrombus (*arrowhead*) around central venous line (*arrow*) in the internal jugular (IJ) vein. **C,** Longitudinal image shows echogenic thrombus (*arrowhead*) around peripherally inserted central catheter line (*arrow*) in the basilic vein (VN).

cantly in patients with both cancer and central venous catheters.[11]

Hypercoagulability (e.g., antithrombin, protein C, and protein S deficiencies; presence of antiphospholipid antibodies) is found to be prevalent in idiopathic upper extremity DVT in which no obvious associated disease or triggering factor is present. In patients with idiopathic upper extremity DVT, 42% to 56% of patients have been found to have clotting abnormalities in recent studies.[6,13,14] Transient causes of hypercoagulability such as estrogen use, pregnancy, and ovarian hyperstimulation have also been observed in women with idiopathic upper extremity DVT.[11,12]

Additional predisposing factors for upper extremity DVT include venous stasis, trauma, surgery, sepsis, and thoracic outlet obstruction secondary to anatomic anomalies. Interestingly, conventional risk factors associated with lower extremity DVT, including obesity, advanced age, and surgery were not significant risk factors for patients with non–catheter-related upper extremity DVT.[3] Patients with upper extremity DVT were found to be more often male, younger, leaner, and more likely to smoke than those with lower extremity DVT. Recent immobility and prior venous thromboembolism also play less of role in patients with upper extremity DVT; however, cancer was more common.[13]

COMPLICATIONS

The most serious complication of upper extremity deep venous thrombosis is pulmonary embolism (PE). Once thought to be uncommon, PE is now reported to have a prevalence of 7% to 36% in patients with upper extremity DVT.[2,13,14] Clinically, the prevalence of symptomatic PE at presentation has been reported to be fourfold less common in patients with upper extremity DVT when compared with patients with lower extremity DVT. However, after 3-month follow-up, the incidence of major or fatal bleeding, recurrent DVT, recurrent PE, or fatal PE was the same. Not surprisingly, patients with cancer were found to have the worst prognosis. Mortality from PE ranged from 11% to 34%.[13]

Other less common complications of upper extremity DVT include post-thrombotic venous insufficiency, loss of vascular access, superior vena cava syndrome, septic thrombophlebitis and, rarely, venous gangrene.

CLINICAL PRESENTATION

Clinically, the most common presentation of upper extremity DVT is upper extremity and face swelling and pain. The edema is typically nonpitting. Less common signs and symptoms include skin discoloration, a sense of coldness in the hand and forearm, tenderness over the affected vein, paresthesia, and numbness. Malfunction of a central venous catheter may also be an indication of thrombosis. Collateral veins can develop over the shoulder and chest wall. A tender cord may be palpable, especially in the axillary region. These signs and symptoms, however, are nonspecific and confirmation of the diagnosis by objective testing is necessary.[14] In addition, many cases of upper extremity DVT are asymptomatic, especially when related to catheter placement.[4]

IMAGING TECHNIQUE

Traditional x-ray venography, once considered the gold standard for imaging of upper extremity DVT, is a highly accurate examination. However, it is an invasive procedure that must be performed in the radiology department. It is uncomfortable for the patient and venous catheterization may be technically difficult secondary to arm swelling. Moreover, intravenous iodinated contrast administration carries the risk of nephrotoxicity and allergic reaction, in addition to predisposing to the development of thrombus. Venography may also fail to demonstrate the status of the internal jugular or brachiocephalic veins when more peripheral occlusive thrombus is present.

Color Doppler duplex ultrasonography with compression technique has become the imaging modality of choice for the diagnosis of upper extremity DVT and is highly accurate for making this diagnosis.[15] Sonography has the advantage of being noninvasive, requiring no venipuncture, ionizing radiation, or contrast agent. It is a potentially portable examination and can be performed at the bedside for critically ill patients. It can be performed regardless of renal function and serial

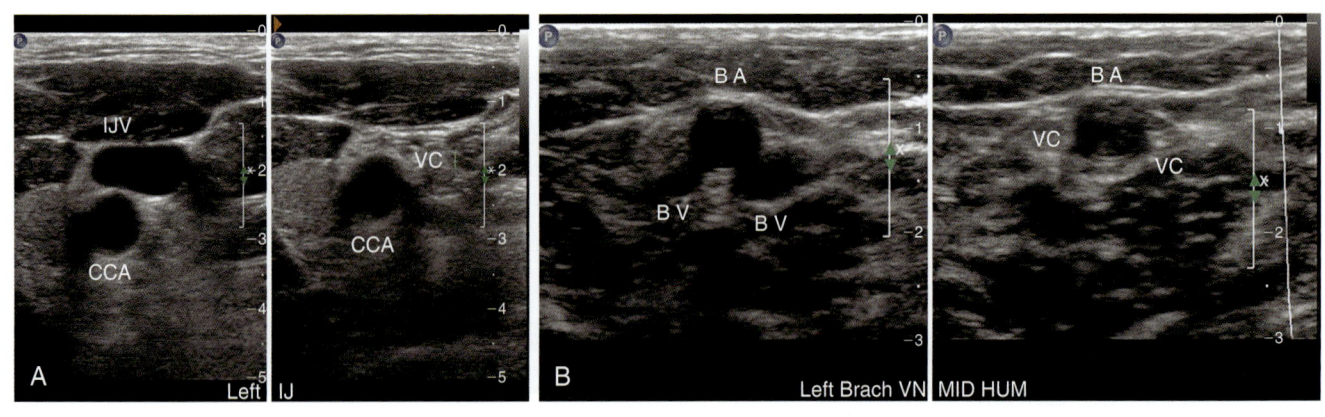

FIGURE 118-4 Transverse gray-scale split screen ultrasound images show complete compressibility of the normal (**A**) internal jugular vein and (**B**) paired brachial veins. BA, brachial artery; BV, brachial vein; CCA, common carotid artery; IJV, internal jugular vein; VC, vein compressed.

follow-up examinations are easily done. Unlike venography, the internal jugular and peripheral brachiocephalic veins can be evaluated, despite the presence of thrombus in the more peripheral vessels. Limitations of duplex sonography include inability to visualize the superior vena cava and more central portions of the brachiocephalic veins. In addition, small nonocclusive thrombus may be missed in the subclavian vein secondary to the inability to compress this vessel because of the overlying clavicle.[16] Furthermore, differentiation of a large collateral from the native vein may be difficult in patients with chronic deep venous thrombosis.

The reported sensitivity of color Doppler sonography for the diagnosis of upper extremity DVT has ranged from 78% to 100%, with a specificity of 82% to 100%.[17,18] False-positive examination results are thought to be rare. False-negative results can occur secondary to limitations in the ability to compress vessels (see earlier).

Variations exist in the recommended techniques and protocols for an ultrasound examination of the upper extremity venous system. At our institution, the internal jugular, subclavian, axillary, and brachial veins are imaged, in addition to the superficial basilic and cephalic veins to the level of the antecubital fossa.

The patient is placed supine, with the arm extended but not hyperabducted. The neck is turned slightly away from the side to be examined. Linear 12-5 or 7-4 MHz transducers are used. A curved 5-2 MHz transducer may be required for larger patients to obtain greater depth of penetration and obtain a larger field of view. A compression technique is used, starting with the internal jugular vein. Compression is always performed in the transverse plane because compression in the longitudinal plane may result in sliding off the vessel, potentially causing a false-negative result. All vessels are compressed except where limited by the clavicle.

The vessels are visualized with gray-scale and color Doppler imaging. The internal jugular vein is imaged in the sagittal and transverse planes. The subclavian vein is followed in its entirety and can be imaged from a supraclavicular approach medially and an infraclavicular approach laterally. It should be remembered that the subclavian vein lies anterior and caudal to the subclavian artery. The subclavian vein and artery should be visualized in the transverse plane to ensure the vein's correct location and proximity to the artery, allowing its differentiation from a large collateral, which will not run adjacent to the artery and will likely have a more tortuous course. The axillary and brachial veins are imaged in a similar manner. The axillary vein lies inferior and medial to the axillary artery. The brachial veins are usually paired and run adjacent to the brachial artery. The basilic vein is single, taking a more superficial and medial course in the upper arm. The cephalic vein courses more laterally. The basilic and cephalic veins run in the subcutaneous tissue, above the muscles of the arm, and do not course adjacent to an artery.

The medial subclavian vein and other centrally situated veins, including the brachiocephalic veins, can be difficult if not impossible to visualize. Use of a square phased-array transducer and a suprasternal-supraclavicular approach may aid in imaging these regions.

Spectral Doppler waveforms are obtained initially in the contralateral internal jugular and medial subclavian veins. These waveforms serve as an internal reference to evaluate for asymmetry, which may be indicative of more centrally located thrombosis not directly visualized by ultrasound examination. Waveforms are then obtained in the ipsilateral internal jugular vein and in the medial, mid, and distal portions of the subclavian vein. If possible, waveforms can also be obtained from the brachiocephalic veins.

ULTRASOUND FINDINGS

Ultrasound imaging of normal venous structures demonstrates complete apposition of the vessel walls with compression (Fig. 118-4). The vessel walls are thin and the lumens are generally anechoic, unless slow flow is present. Normal venous valves are easily visualized as thin leaf-like mobile structures and should not be mistaken for wall-adherent thrombus or sequelae from prior thrombosis.

Diagnostic criteria for upper extremity venous thrombosis by ultrasound are similar to those described for lower extremity deep venous thrombosis.[19] The principal criterion for the diagnosis of thrombus is noncompressibility of the vessel lumen. Acute thrombus usually fills and

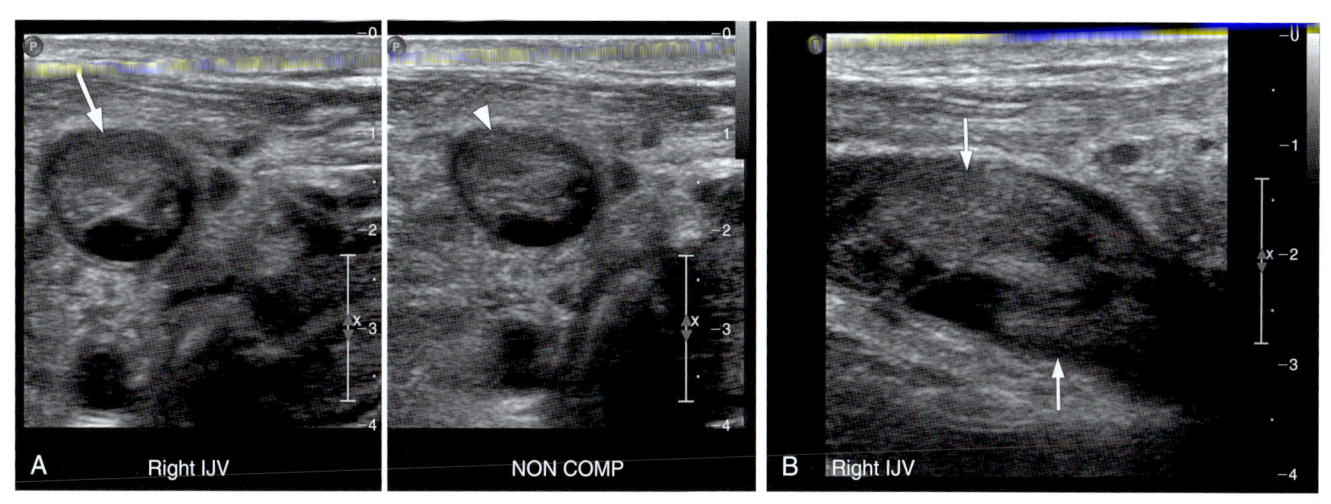

CHAPTER 118 • Venous Sonography of the Upper Extremities and Thoracic Outlet

FIGURE 118-5 A, Split-screen transverse image shows thrombus filling the internal jugular vein (IJV; *arrow*) which is noncompressible (*arrowhead*). B, Sagittal image demonstrates the same thrombus (*arrows*) filling and distending the vessel.

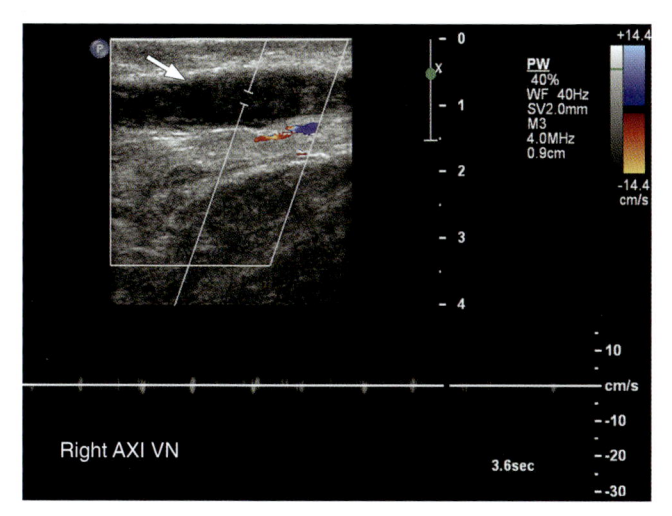

FIGURE 118-6 Longitudinal duplex Doppler image of the axillary vein (*arrow*) shows absence of flow on color Doppler flow imaging and spectral analysis.

distends the involved vessel and is typically anechoic to hypoechoic (Fig. 118-5). Color Doppler flow imaging makes visualization of anechoic and nonocclusive thrombus easier because it permits direct visualization of blood flow dynamics.[20] Spectral and color Doppler flow imaging demonstrate absence of flow in the presence of occlusive thrombus (Fig. 118-6). Nonocclusive thrombus will generally be outlined by color and demonstrate some evidence of flow in the vessel (Fig. 118-7).

The appearance and echogenicity of thrombus will evolve over time (Fig. 118-8). Generally, as thrombus becomes more chronic, its echogenicity increases and the clot retracts, with resultant decrease in the distention of the vessel. The visualized thrombus may be more eccentric and focal in location within the vessel lumen, with skip areas present. The wall may thicken and be incompletely compressible (Fig. 118-9). Although some veins may regain a normal appearance and compressibility over time, other vessels may demonstrate sequelae of chronic venous disease, such as frozen valve leaflets, synechia, and partial recanalization of the vessel. The affected native vessel may collapse and fibrose, with resulting collateral formation. In vessels in which thrombus has resolved, venous insufficiency or reflux may later be present.

The diagnosis of recurrent thrombosis or acute thrombosis superimposed on chronic thrombosis is problematic by ultrasound. Demonstration of new areas of thrombus not identified on the initial examination and/or considerable enlargement (>2 mm) of the compressed vein diameter between the two examinations have been used as criteria in clinical studies for recurrent lower extremity DVT.[21] Traditional x-ray or contrast-enhanced MR venography may be necessary for patients with clinically suspected recurrent DVT.

The normal spectral Doppler waveform of the upper extremity and neck veins are characterized by two phasic variations. Right atrial contraction results in a sawtooth pattern to the waveform, which is synchronized to the pulse rate. Superimposed on this cardiac pulsatility is a phasic change in amplitude caused by the respiratory cycle.[22] An increase in amplitude and venous return is seen during inspiration and a decrease is noted during expiration (Fig. 118-10). Luminal diameter will also vary with respiration. Sniffing can cause momentary collapse of a normal vessel; a Valsalva maneuver will cause the vessel to distend and velocity of venous flow to decrease.[15]

Although direct visualization of thrombus in the brachiocephalic veins and superior vena cava is difficult, if not impossible, it has been shown that loss or dampening of respiratory and cardiac phasicity in the subclavian and internal jugular veins is a very sensitive predictor of more centrally located thrombus in the brachiocephalic veins or SVC (Fig. 118-11). Loss of cardiac pulsatility has been reported as a more sensitive predictor than loss of respiratory phasicity alone. Conversely, the demonstration of normal cardiac and respiratory phasicity is highly predictive of the absence of thrombus in these vessels.[22] Comparison should be made to the waveform in the contralateral subclavian and internal jugular veins to confirm that the abnormal waveform is only present on the affected symp-

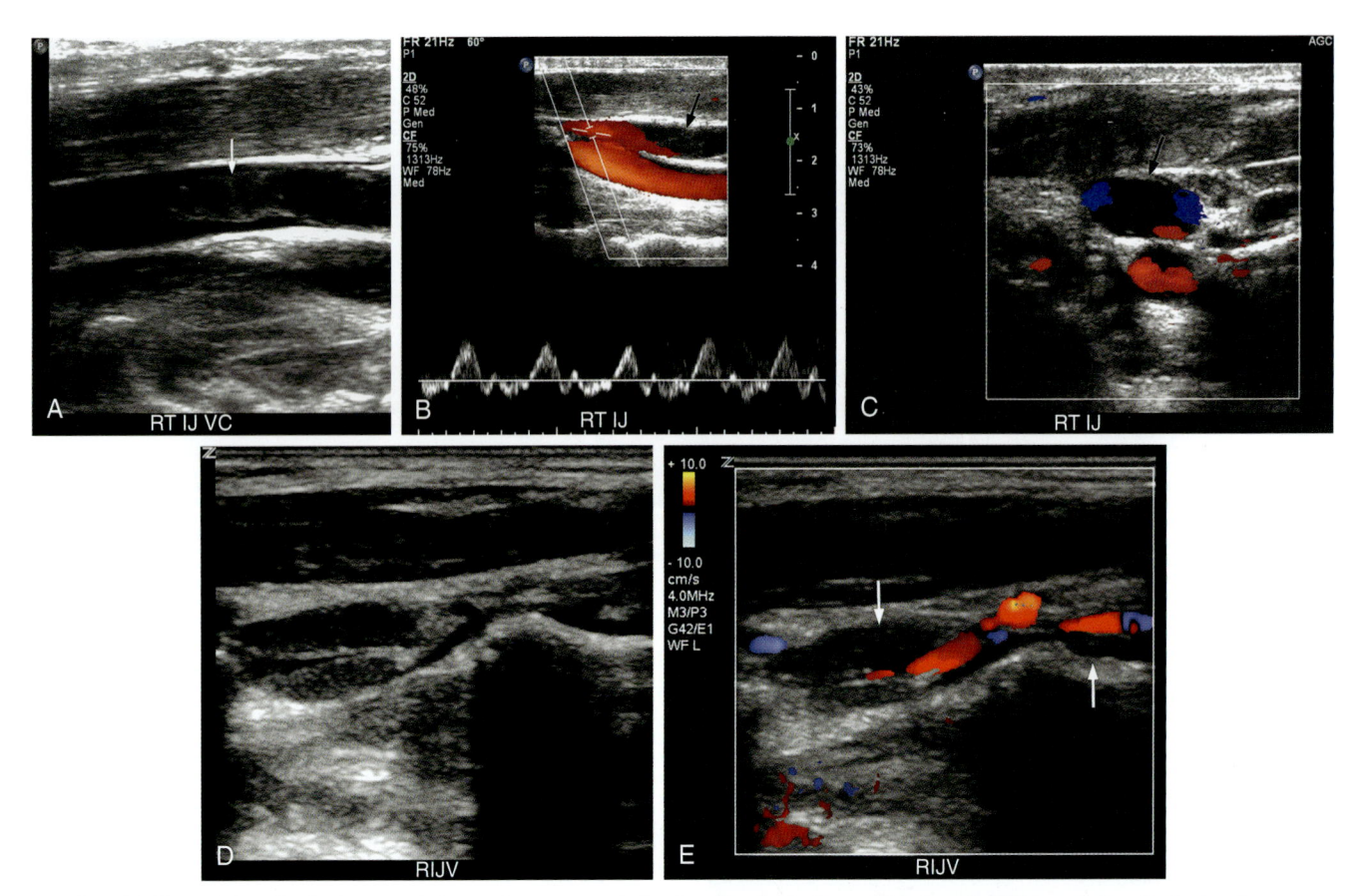

FIGURE 118-7 A, Longitudinal gray-scale image shows nonocclusive thrombus in the internal jugular vein (IJV; *arrow*). Longitudinal and transverse color Doppler flow images (**B, C**) demonstrate thrombus outlined by color (*arrows*). Longitudinal gray-scale (**D**) and color (**E**) images of the IJV demonstrate nonocclusive thrombus (*arrows*), with flow visualized around the thrombus on color Doppler flow images.

tomatic side. Bilateral dampening, however, can occur with thrombosis of the superior vena cava.

PITFALLS

There are limitations in duplex ultrasound imaging of the upper extremity and thoracic inlet venous structures. As noted, considerable constraint is placed by the normal anatomy of the region, with the clavicle, manubrium, and sternum limiting visualization and compressibility of the veins, especially centrally. Compression may also be limited by body habitus, overlying bandages, or indwelling catheters. Nonocclusive thrombus in regions that cannot be compressed may be missed. Color Doppler imaging may aid in the detection of nonocclusive thrombus, but care must be taken not to oversaturate the images with color, which can obscure thrombus (Fig. 118-12).

Slow-flowing blood can appear echogenic and mimic thrombus (Fig. 118-13). One should look carefully for swirling or slow-moving particles on real-time imaging, the presence of which will distinguish slow-flowing blood from true thrombus. Compressibility of the vessel will also confirm absence of thrombus.

Large collaterals can be mistaken for the native vessels, especially in the subclavian region. Proximity to the accompanying artery and the correct anatomic relationship between artery and vein should be looked for in the transverse plane.

SYNDROMES

Thoracic Outlet Syndrome

Thoracic outlet syndrome (TOS) can be defined as a set of symptoms caused by compression of the brachial plexus structures or vascular structures (subclavian artery and vein) as they pass from the lower cervical region or thoracic outlet to the axilla. It is more common in women than in men and occurs most commonly in the 20- to 50-year-old age range. An understanding of the anatomy of this region is helpful in understanding the pathophysiology of this syndrome.

The anatomy of the thoracic outlet region can functionally be thought of as composed of three areas of narrowing: (1) the interscalene triangle; (2) the costoclavicular space; and (3) the subcoracoid or retropectoralis minor space (Fig. 118-14). The interscalene triangle is bounded by the anterior and middle scalene muscles and the first rib to which they are attached. The three trunks of the brachial plexus and subclavian artery pass through this region. The subclavian vein passes anterior to the anterior scalene muscle. The divisions of the brachial plexus and

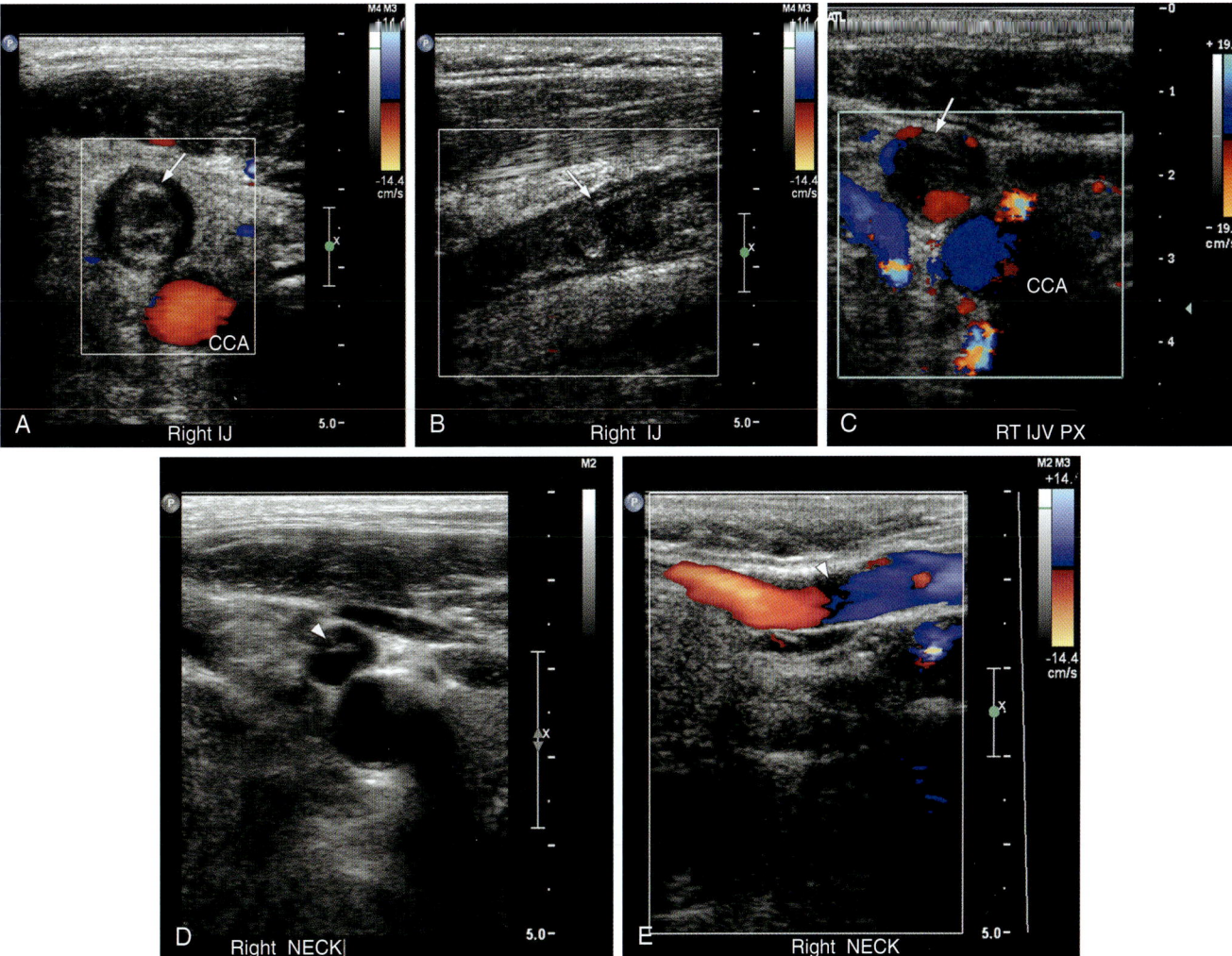

FIGURE 118-8 Transverse (**A**) and longitudinal (**B**) images of the internal jugular vein in 47-year-old man with neck pain and edema demonstrate occlusive thrombus (*arrows*). No flow is demonstrated on color Doppler flow imaging (CDFI). **C,** Follow-up imaging 3 weeks later demonstrates retraction of the clot (*arrow*), with partial recanalization of the IJV on CDFI. **D, E,** Follow-up imaging 4 months later demonstrates only a small amount of focal, eccentric, residual thrombus (*arrowhead*). Note that the IJV has decreased in size. CCA, common carotid artery.

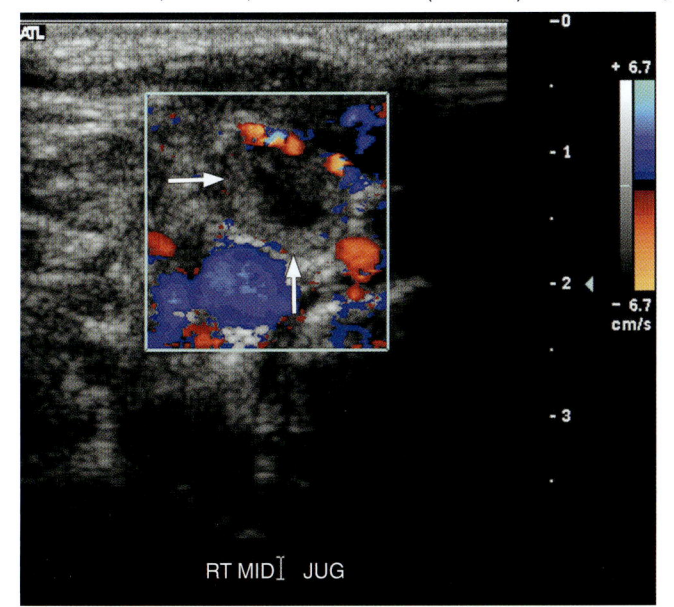

FIGURE 118-9 Transverse color Doppler flow image of the right internal jugular vein shows wall thickening and eccentric thrombus (*arrows*) consistent with chronic thrombus.

subclavian artery and vein then travel under the clavicle into the costoclavicular space, which lies between the clavicle and underlying first rib and is bounded anteriorly by the subclavius muscle. These structures enter the axilla through the subcoracoid (retropectoralis minor) space, bounded by the coracoid process and insertion of the pectoralis minor muscle superiorly and anteriorly and by the ribs posteriorly.

Compression and irritation of neural and vascular structures by repetitive movement and/or arm elevation can occur in these regions of narrowing. The interscalene triangle is the most common site of entrapment. The subclavian vein and artery are most often compressed at the costoclavicular space.[23] Anatomic variants such as cervical ribs, hypertrophy of the C7 transverse processes, and cervical bands can also result in entrapment.[24]

Clinically, the symptoms of thoracic outlet syndrome can be neurologic or vascular. Neurologic symptoms include pain (especially in an ulnar distribution), paresthesia, numbness, loss of dexterity, weakness, and occipital headache. Venous symptoms include upper extremity

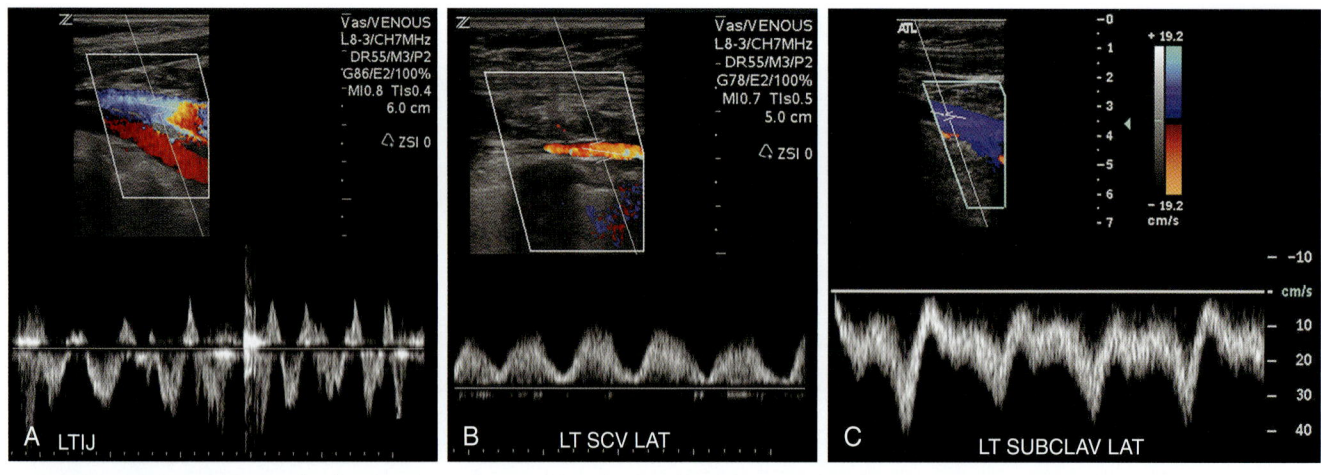

1668 PART NINETEEN ● *The Upper Extremity Vessels*

FIGURE 118-10 Color Doppler flow imaging and spectral Doppler imaging show normal cardiac and respiratory variability in the internal jugular (A) and subclavian (B, C) veins.

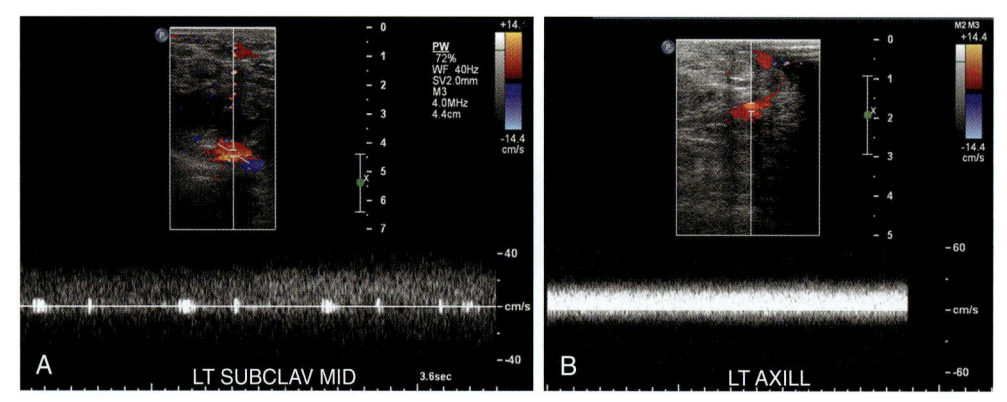

FIGURE 118-11 Duplex Doppler imaging in a 66-year-old man with central thrombus in the left brachiocephalic vein. A dampened waveform without respiratory or cardiac phasicity is seen in the mid left subclavian (A) and axillary (B) veins.

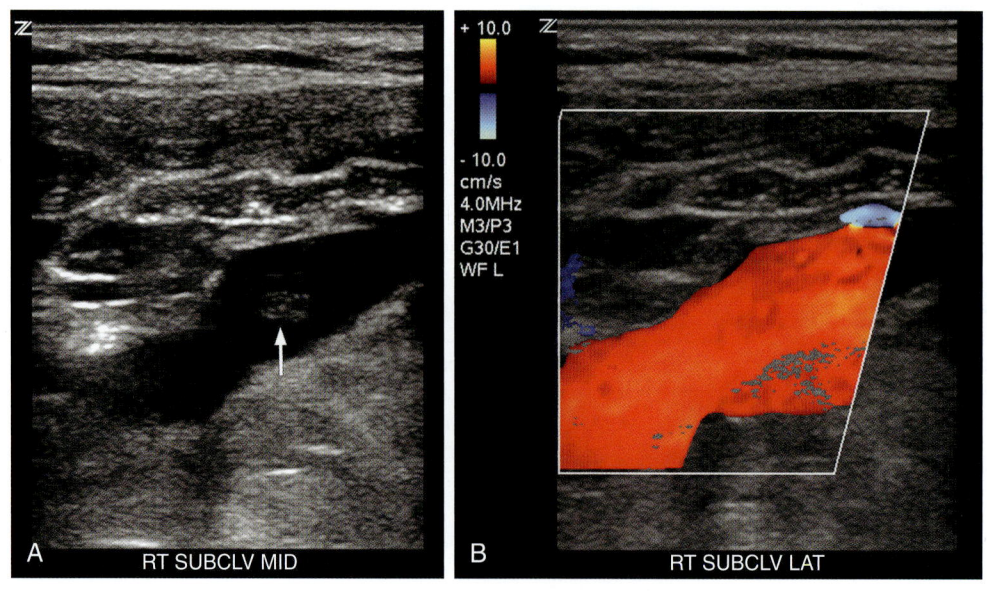

FIGURE 118-12 A, Longitudinal gray-scale imaging of the right subclavian vein shows nonocclusive thrombus (*arrow*). B, Oversaturation on color Doppler flow imaging obscures the thrombus.

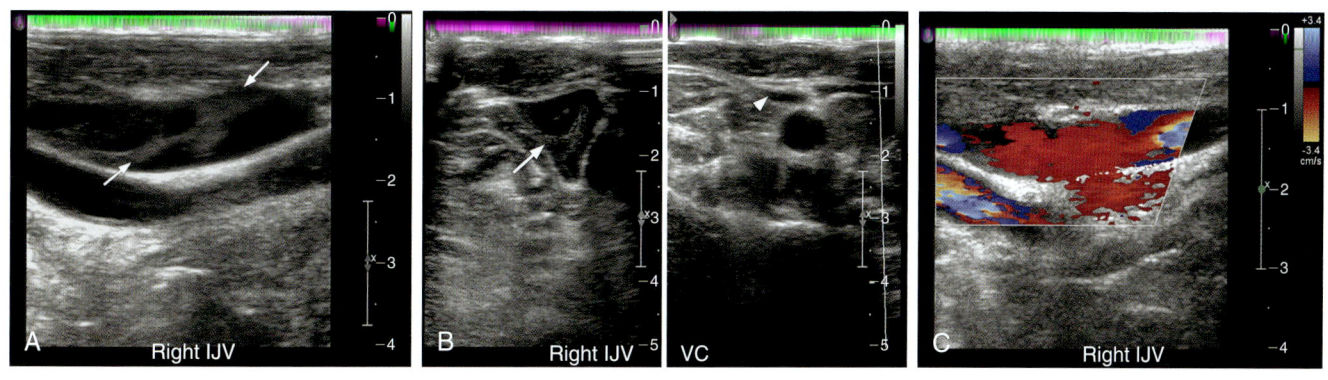

FIGURE 118-13 Echogenic material is seen on longitudinal (**A**) and transverse (**B**) images of the right internal jugular vein (IJV), which mimics thrombus (*arrows*). The echogenic material was seen to swirl on real-time imaging. **B,** Axial imaging demonstrates the vessel compressing completely (*arrowhead*). **C,** Longitudinal color Doppler imaging shows no evidence of flow void in the IJV. CCA, common carotid artery.

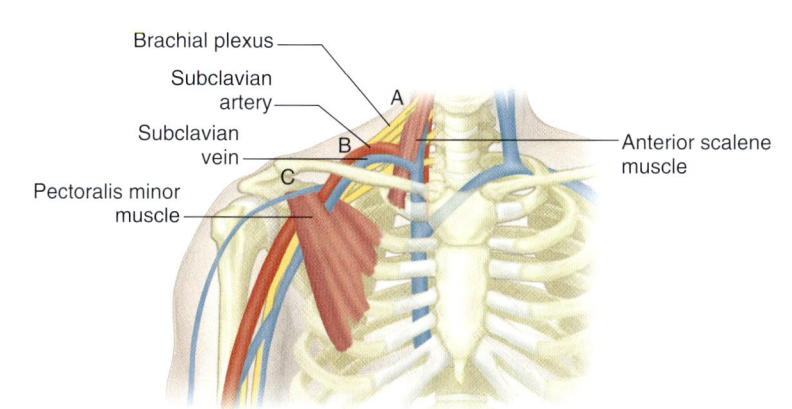

FIGURE 118-14 Anatomy of the thoracic outlet. A, interscalene triangle; B, costoclavicular space; C, subcoracoid (retropectoralis minor) space.

swelling and cyanosis. Claudication, pallor, and coldness can result from arterial compromise.

Provocative tests such as Adson's maneuver—checking the radial pulse with the shoulders depressed downward, head hyperextended and turned toward the affected side—and arm hyperabduction may aid in the diagnosis but demonstrate overlap in positive findings (variation in strength of the radial pulse during positional changes) with asymptomatic individuals.

Color Doppler sonography has been found to be a useful aid for the diagnosis of TOS because it allows direct visualization of the vessels in conjunction with spectral Doppler waveforms during maneuvers designed to result in vascular compression.[24] Longley and colleagues[23] have found that in symptomatic patients with thrombosis or significant compression of the subclavian vein during arm abduction (90 to 180 degrees), color Doppler sonography has a sensitivity of 92% and a specificity of 95% for the detection of thoracic outlet syndrome. Criteria used in this study for a positive result were detection of thrombus or change in the Doppler waveform, from a normal subclavian waveform to one showing complete loss of cardiac and respiratory pulsatility or cessation of flow. Evaluation of the subclavian artery yielded less helpful results, with 20% of asymptomatic individuals demonstrating changes in Doppler waveform on hyperabduction.

Venous imaging using CT angiography (CTA) or MR angiography (MRA) of TOS may also be useful, with imaging performed with the patient's arms alongside the body and then elevated over the head. Comparison of vascular patency using multiplanar and three-dimensional reformations of CTA or MRA can provide evidence for TOS. With CT or MRI, evidence of bony or soft tissue impingement on the brachial plexus can also be assessed. This technique has been found to be useful in evaluating the arterial structures but is less helpful in evaluating venous compression secondary to overlap of findings with asymptomatic individuals.[25]

Ultrasound offers the advantage of allowing visualization of the vessels during dynamically induced symptoms. Ultrasound also allows for imaging the patient in an upright or seated position, similar to a clinical examination, as opposed to CT or MRI, which have to be performed with the patient supine. Disadvantages include limited evaluation of the surrounding soft tissue and bony structures, especially in the region of the pulmonary apex.[25]

Paget-Schroetter Syndrome

James Paget and Leopold von Schroetter, independently, first described Paget-Schroetter syndrome, a primary form

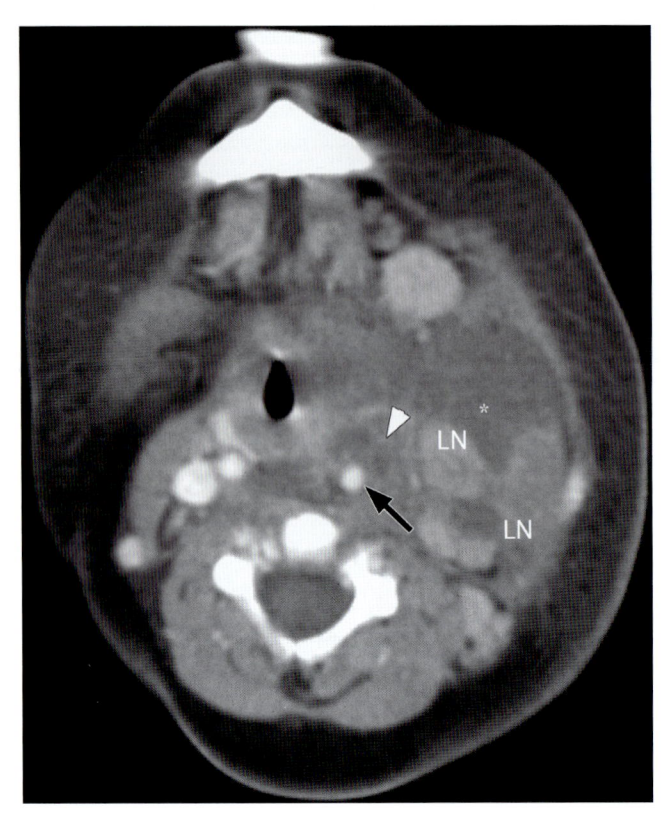

FIGURE 118-15 Transverse contrast-enhanced CT image through the mid neck demonstrates edema and inflammation (*) involving the left parapharyngeal region. The left internal jugular vein (*arrowhead*) is occluded. The *arrow* indicates the common carotid artery. LN, enlarged lymph nodes.

of cases was described by Lemierre in 1936. In the preantibiotic era, the mortality rate for the condition was 90%.[29]

Generally more common in young healthy adults, clinical signs and symptoms can be nonspecific. Patients typically present with pharyngitis but this may be absent in some cases. Fever, rigors, cervical adenopathy, and malaise are common accompanying symptoms. Because of their proximity to the carotid sheath, cranial nerves IX to XII may be affected, with associated neurologic signs and symptoms. In later stages, symptomatology is related to the location of the septic emboli.[28,30]

Ultrasound or CT imaging demonstrates thrombus within the internal jugular vein (Fig. 118-15). Surrounding inflammatory changes in the parapharyngeal region are best demonstrated by CT, as are septic emboli in the chest.

CONCLUSION

Although initially thought to be an uncommon, benign, and self-limited entity, upper extremity deep venous thrombosis is now known to be a fairly frequent condition, with significant resulting morbidity and mortality. The increased use of central venous lines and catheters, especially in patients with associated malignancies, has resulted in a dramatic increase in the occurrence of upper extremity DVT. Color Doppler sonography has proven to be a highly accurate imaging modality for screening, diagnosis, and follow-up of this entity, effectively replacing the traditional gold standard of invasive venography. Spectral and color Doppler sonography have also been found to be of benefit in the diagnosis of thoracic outlet syndrome. They can complement MRI and CT imaging, especially in the diagnosis of possible venous involvement.

of upper extremity DVT—also known as effort-induced thrombosis—in the mid to late 19th century. It is usually seen in young, otherwise healthy, individuals. Development of thrombus is usually seen in the dominant arm after strenuous activities such as weight lifting, pitching, or rowing. Damage to the intima is believed to occur from heavy exertion, resulting in activation of the coagulation cascade.[26] These patients are usually treated more aggressively with thrombolytic therapy because the risk for developing long-term sequelae such as post-thrombotic syndrome is higher.[27]

Lemierre's Syndrome

Lemierre's syndrome is a septic thrombophlebitis of the internal jugular vein usually caused by the anaerobic gram-negative rod *Fusobacterium necrophorum*, although other strains of fusobacterium have been implicated.[28] *F. necrophorum* makes up part of the normal flora of the mouth. Lemierre's syndrome is an uncommon sequela of acute pharyngotonsillitis that can be potentially life-threatening. Infection from the oropharynx may spread by direct extension to the parapharyngeal space or through venous or lymphatic dissemination. Thrombophlebitis of the internal jugular vein results from the surrounding inflammation and acts as a nidus for further septic embolization and septicemia. The lungs and joints are common locations for septic emboli and abscesses.[28] The first series

KEY POINTS

- Upper extremity deep venous thrombosis (DVT) has a much higher prevalence than originally thought, especially in the patient population with central venous catheters, underlying malignancy, and hypercoagulability states.
- Pulmonary embolism is the most serious complication of upper extremity DVT and has been reported in up to 35% of patients with upper extremity DVT.
- Color Doppler duplex sonography with compression technique is the imaging modality of choice for the diagnosis of upper extremity DVT.
- Loss of phasicity in the spectral Doppler waveforms in the internal jugular or subclavian veins can be indicative of more central thrombosis.
- Color and spectral Doppler imaging, along with CT and MRI, can aid in the diagnosis of thoracic outlet syndrome.
- Patients with Paget-Schroetter syndrome need to be treated more aggressively with thrombolytic therapy because the risk for developing long-term sequelae, such as post-thrombotic syndrome, is higher.

SUGGESTED READINGS

Chin, EE, Zimmerman PT, Grant EG. Sonographic evaluation of upper extremity deep venous thrombosis. J Ultrasound Med 2005; 24:829-838.

Demondion X, Herbinet P, et al. Imaging assessment of thoracic outlet syndrome. Radiographics 2006; 26:1735-1750.

Fraser JD, Anderson DR. Deep venous thrombosis: Recent advances and optimal investigation with US. Radiology 1999; 211:9-24.

Nazarian GK, Foshager MC. Color Doppler sonography of the thoracic inlet veins. Radiographics 1995; 15:1357-1371.

REFERENCES

1. Tilney NL, Griffiths HJG, Edwards EA. Natural history of major venous thrombosis of the upper extremity. Arch Surg 1970; 101:792-796.
2. Hingorani A, Ascher E. Upper extremity deep venous thrombosis. Perspect Vasc Surg Endovasc Ther 1999; 110:47-57.
3. Joffe HV, Kucher N, Tapson VF, Goldhaber SZ. Upper-extremity deep venous thrombosis: a prospective registry of 592 patients. Circulation 2004; 110:1605-1611.
4. Luciani A, Clement O, Halimi P, et al. Catheter-related upper extremity deep venous thrombosis in cancer patients: a prospective study based on Doppler US. Radiology 2001; 220:655-660.
5. Mustafa S, Stein PD, Patel KC, et al. Upper extremity deep venous thrombosis. Chest 2003; 123:1953-1956.
6. Gaitini D, Beck-Razi N, Haim N, Brenner B. Prevalence of upper extremity deep venous thrombosis diagnosed by color Doppler duplex sonography in cancer patients with central venous catheters. J Ultrasound Med 2006; 25:1297-1303.
7. Boswald M, Lugauer S, Bechert T, et al. Thrombogenicity testing of central venous catheters in vitro. Infection 1999; 27(Suppl 1): S30-S33.
8. Lokich JJ, Becker B. Subclavian vein thrombosis in patients treated with infusion chemotherapy for advanced malignancy. Cancer 1983; 52:1586-1589.
9. Chin EE, Zimmerman PT, Grant EG. Sonographic evaluation of upper extremity deep venous thrombosis. J Ultrasound Med 2005; 24:829-838.
10. Verso M, Agnelli G. Venous thromboembolism associated with long-term use of central venous catheters in cancer patients. J Clin Oncol 2003; 21:3665-3675.
11. Héron E, Lozinguez O, Alhenc-Gelas M, et al. Hypercoagulable states in primary upper extremity deep venous thrombosis. Arch Intern Med 2000; 160:382-386.
12. Prandoni P, Polistena P, Bernardi E, et al. Upper-extremity deep vein thrombosis. Risk factors, diagnosis, and complications. Arch Intern Med 1997; 157:57-62.
13. Munoz FJ, Mismetti P, Poggio R, et al. Clinical outcome of patients with upper-extremity deep vein thrombosis. Results from the REITE registry. Chest 2008; 133:143-148.
14. Longley DG, Finlay DE, Letourneau JG. Sonography of the upper extremity and jugular veins. AJR Am J Roentgenol 1993; 160: 957-962.
15. Sheikh MA, Topoulos AP, Deitcher SR. Isolated internal jugular vein thrombosis: risk factors and natural history. Vasc Med 2002; 7:177-179.
16. Falk RL, Smith DF. Thrombosis of upper extremity thoracic inlet veins: diagnosis with Duplex sonography. AJR Am J Roentgenol 1987; 149:677-682.
17. Mustafa BO, Rathbun SW, Whitsett TL, Raskob GE. Sensitivity and specificity of ultrasonography in the diagnosis of upper extremity deep vein thrombosis. Arch Intern Med 2002; 162:401-404.
18. Baarslag HJ, van Beek EJR, et al. Prospective study of color duplex ultrasonography compared with contrast venography in patients suspected of having deep venous thrombosis of the upper extremities. Ann Intern Med 2002; 136:865-872.
19. Fraser JD, Anderson DR. Deep venous thrombosis: recent advances and optimal investigation with US. Radiology 1999; 211:9-24.
20. Knudson GJ, Wiedmeyer DA, et al. Color Doppler sonographic imaging in the assessment of upper-extremity deep venous thrombosis. AJR Am J Roentgenol 1990; 154:399-403.
21. Simonneau G, Sors H, Charbonnier B, et al. A comparison of low-molecular-weight heparin with unfractionated heparin for acute pulmonary embolism. The THESEE Study Group. Tinzaparine ou Heparine Standard: Evaluations dans l'Embolie Pulmonaire. N Engl J Med 1997; 337:663-669.
22. Patel MC, Berman LH, Moss HA, McPherson SJ. Subclavian and internal jugular veins at Doppler US: abnormal cardiac pulsatility and respiratory phasicity as a predictor of complete central occlusion. Radiology 1999; 211:579-583.
23. Longley DG, Yedlicka JW, Molina EJ, et al. Thoracic outlet syndrome: evaluation of the subclavian vessels by color duplex sonography. AJR Am J Roentgenol 1992; 158:623-630.
24. Dubuisson AS. The thoracic outlet syndrome, 2008. Available at: http://www.medschool.lsuhsc.edu/Neurosurgery/nervecenter/TOS.html. Accessed October 6, 2009.
25. Demondion X, Herbinet P, Van Sint Jan S, et al. Imaging assessment of thoracic outlet syndrome. Radiographics 2006; 26:1735-1750.
26. Vijaysadan V, Zimmerman AM, Pajaro RE. Paget-Schroetter syndrome in the young and active. J Am Board Fam Pract 2005; 18:314-319.
27. Urchel HC, Razzuk MA. Paget-Schroetter syndrome: what is the best management? Ann Thorac Surg 2000; 69:1663-1669.
28. Screaton NJ, Ravenel JG, et al. Lemierre syndrome: forgotten but not extinct—report of four cases. Radiology 1999; 213:369-374.
29. Lemierre A. On certain septicemias due to anaerobic organisms. Lancet 1936; 1:701-703.
30. Hope A, Bleach N, Ghiacy S. Lemierre's syndrome as a consequence of acute supraglottitis. J Laryngol Otol 2002; 116:216-218.

CHAPTER 119

Hemodialysis Fistulas

Tim Leiner

INTRODUCTION

Chronic kidney disease (CKD) is a worldwide public health problem. Commensurate with the global epidemic of obesity and diabetes mellitus in the Western World, the incidence and prevalence of kidney failure are rising, and the costs are high. CKD remains underdiagnosed, which is unfortunate because adverse outcomes such as progression to kidney failure and advanced cardiovascular disease can often be prevented or delayed through early treatment. Although renal transplant is the treatment of choice for severe CKD, the supply of compatible renal donors lags the demand and many patients are not suitable candidates for renal transplantation. In these instances, renal dialysis is often the sole therapeutic option.

Hemodialysis, and to a lesser extent peritoneal dialysis, remains the mainstay of treatment of patients with CKD. In acute situations, such as in patients requiring immediate, short-term (less than 6 months) dialysis access, double-lumen catheters are often used. These catheters are inserted in the femoral, internal jugular, or subclavian vein. Long-term hemodialysis requires regular vascular access (e.g., two to five times a week), necessitating the surgical creation of an arteriovenous fistula for more robust vascular access, typically in an upper extremity. This can be performed using the patient's native artery and vein (arteriovenous fistula or AVF; Fig. 119-1) or with use of prosthetic graft material (arteriovenous graft or AVG; also called a prosthetic AVF; see Fig. 119-1).

Hemodialysis access fistulas are literally the lifelines of patients on hemodialysis and imaging is critical for proper preprocedural planning and management of hemodialysis patients. Preoperative imaging is particularly important prior to creation of a hemodialysis fistula (i.e., AVF or AVG) because patients typically have undergone numerous prior venous catheter placements, which predispose for development of venous stenoses that may jeopardize the success of the proposed dialysis fistula.

The main concern for a dialysis fistula is its patency and duration of patency. In general, a native AVF is believed to have longer problem-free patency rates than a prosthetic AVG and AVF has been the recommended first choice for long-term hemodialysis access by the National Kidney Foundation that was recommended in its 2000 Dialysis Outcomes Quality Initiative Clinical Practical Guidelines for Vascular Access (NKF/DOQI).[1] Most often, a hemodialysis fistula is created in the upper extremity by anastomosis of the cephalic vein to the radial artery, close to or in the *tabatière anatomique* or the anatomical snuffbox, or just proximal to the wrist. This latter type of hemodialysis fistula is also known as the radiocephalic or Brescia-Cimino (BC) fistula or shunt (see Fig. 119-1A). In patients in whom a BC shunt, an AVF, cannot be created, transposition of the basilic vein of the forearm to a ventral position with end-to-side radial-basilic anastomosis is a viable alternative option.[2] In patients in whom it is not possible to use autologous arteries and veins, a prosthetic AVG can be placed between an antecubital vein and the brachial artery (see Fig. 119-1B). The AVG is not the hemodialysis fistula of first choice, because the AVGs typically require more frequent (up to five times more frequent) therapeutic intervention compared with native AVFs to maintain their proper function.[3] The most common cause of AVG failure is development of stenosis at the arterial and venous anastomoses, which can cause critical flow decline and subsequent thrombosis of the graft. Alternatively, although the AVF fistula has a better patency rate compared to the AVG, an AVF requires much longer period of time to 'mature,' typically approximately 6 to 8 weeks. Maturation of the fistula is necessary for enlargement of the draining vein to accommodate its use for hemodialysis. This process of maturation is not successful in all patients and, therefore, AVF fistulas have a higher rate of early failure, sometimes necessitating catheter insertion to provide adequate dialysis. Maturation of AVGs is generally quicker, allowing their earlier use for hemodialysis.

The use of AVF, although greater than that of AVG, for dialysis initiation has been far from universal, a fact that may be attributable to a variety of factors to include practice differences and lack of timely access to specialty care.[4] There also remains a lack of sufficient evidence to

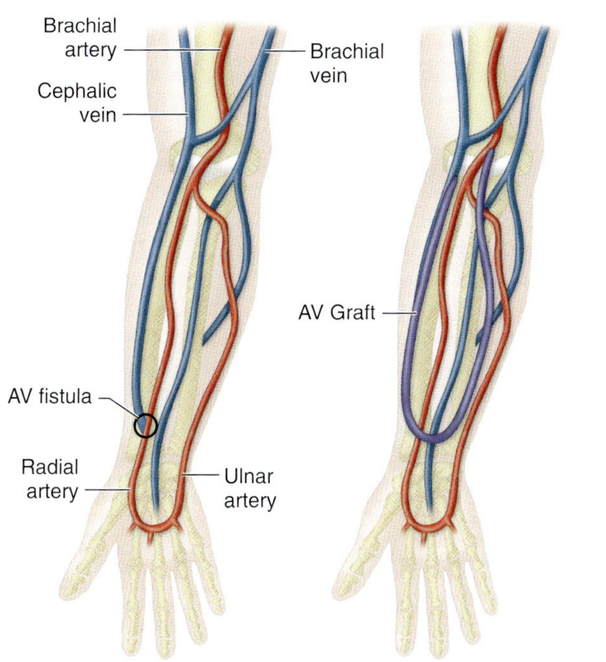

FIGURE 119-1 Schematic overview of a radial-cephalic wrist arteriovenous fistula (AVF; left) and a forearm loop arteriovenous graft (AVG; right). The graft anastomosed to the brachial artery and cephalic vein at the antecubital crease in an end (graft)-to-side (vessel) fashion. The loop has been tunneled underneath the skin to enable easy cannulation for dialysis sessions.

TABLE 119-1	Chronic Kidney Disease	
Stage	Description	GFR (mL/min per 1.73 m^2)
1	Kidney damage with normal or increased GFR	≥90
2	Kidney damage with mild decreased GFR	60-89
3	Moderately decreased GFR	30-59
4	Severely decreased GFR	15-29
5	Kidney failure	<15 or dialysis

GFR, glomerular filtration rate.

support the long-held notion of the supremacy of AVF to AVG.[5]

There are several special roles for imaging in the management of patients with hemodialysis fistulas. First, cross-sectional imaging techniques such as duplex ultrasonography (DUS), computed tomography (CT), and magnetic resonance angiography (MRA) can provide valuable preoperative information on arterial and venous diameters as well as identify stenotic vascular segments and anatomic variants that may influence the choice of hemodialysis fistula type and location. Second, imaging is essential for surveillance of vascular complications, notably stenosis of the hemodialysis fistula. The creation of hemodialysis fistula results in an unnatural or nonphysiologic flow situation in the upper extremity, which combined with a tendency for accelerated development of atherosclerotic stenoses and obstructions in this specific population, increases the likelihood for occlusion in affected segments, which may require endovascular intervention to maintain graft patency.[6]

Depending on the vitality, age, comorbid conditions, and social network, patients may also choose to undergo peritoneal dialysis (PD) when they are in need of long-term dialysis. The major advantage of PD is that patients can treat themselves or can be treated by others at home. Also, PD requires less medication and a less restrictive diet. Contraindications for PD are a history of major abdominal surgery, or diseases of the peritoneum. PD is also favored when the patient is unable to tolerate large fluctuations of vascular volume.

A very important consideration when choosing the optimal imaging strategy in patients who are candidates for or who already have a hemodialysis fistula is the presence of residual renal function. Residual renal function is a strong predictor of survival in patients with CKD,[7,8] illustrating the important fact that *dialysis clearance is not equivalent to renal clearance*. Residual function in the native kidneys retains a role in sodium and water removal, and dialysis (both hemodialysis and peritoneal dialysis) remains inefficient for removing larger and protein-bound uremic toxins. Thus, the preservation of even small amounts of residual renal function in patients on HD is of major clinical importance.[9] In general, residual kidney function is better preserved in patients who undergo PD versus HD. Care should be taken to avoid further reduction in residual renal function by use of large volumes of iodinated contrast agents. However, whereas MRA would seem a good alternative, the choice between different imaging modalities is becoming increasingly difficult because of the recent discovery of nephrogenic systemic fibrosis (NSF). NSF is a rare but potentially serious condition, almost exclusively seen in patients with severe CKD and renal failure, which has been linked to the administration of gadolinium-based contrast agents (GBCA) for MRA, and will be discussed in more detail in the section on MRI later. NSF has rekindled interest in nonenhanced MRA techniques, but at present these is no published data on the feasibility and accuracy of noncontrast media enhanced MRA in the preoperative workup of patients due to receive a hemodialysis fistula, nor in patients with hemodialysis fistula dysfunction due to suspected arterial or venous stenoses, although studies are underway to investigate these techniques for this purpose.

DISEASE

Definition

CKD is defined as either kidney damage or decreased kidney function for 3 or more months. The level of kidney function, regardless of diagnosis, determines the stage of CKD according to the National Kidney Foundation's Kidney Disease Outcomes Quality Initiative (K/DOQI) CKD classification into five stages (Table 119-1). It is important to realize that the prevalence of earlier stages of disease is more than 100 times greater than the prevalence of kidney failure. Kidney failure, also known as CKD stage 5, is defined as a patient with glomerular filtration rate (GFR) of less than 15 mL/kg/1.73 m^2, or in practical terms, a patient requiring renal dialysis therapy. It is important to note that kidney failure is not actually synonymous with the term "end-stage renal disease (ESRD)." *End-stage renal disease* is an administrative term used in the United States to indicate that a patient is undergoing renal dialysis in anticipation of renal transplantation, and is a condition for payment by the Medicare ESRD program.[10]

Prevalence and Epidemiology

CKD is highly prevalent and affects approximately 8.5% of the United States adult population (26 million adults in 2008). The number of persons with kidney failure in the United States who are treated with HD and transplantation is rising rapidly and projected to increase from 340,000 in 1999 to 651,000 in 2010.[10] Worldwide, an estimated 1.22 million patients were on HD in 2004, representing a 20% increase over 2001.[11,12] Because of a shortage in kidney donors, the majority of CKD patients are treated by renal dialysis therapy. With the steady growth of the aging population, the number of CKD patients continues to increase, especially in patients older than 65 years of age. The fraction of patients receiving a renal transplant decreases with age. Conversely, the percentage of patients being treated by HD increases with age. Over the next few years, the number of CKD patients in need of dialysis is expected to increase by approximately 5% per year, reaching over 3 million worldwide by 2010. Because of the chronic nature of the disease, CKD is accompanied by a large increase in healthcare-related costs. In 2008, the annual costs of the Medicare ESRD program were $20 billion, and $42 billion was the amount spent on treating patients with CKD.[13]

Etiology and Pathophysiology

Up to 10% to 20% of all newly created hemodialysis fistulas thrombose within the first week after creation due to insufficient flow.[14] Nonmaturation is defined as a hemodialysis fistula being inadequate for hemodialysis due to insufficient flow or insufficient venous distention within 6 weeks after creation. Causes of hemodialysis fistula nonmaturation are thought to include the use of small-diameter vessels (<1.6 mm in diameter),[15] and presence of stenoses or occlusions in arterial inflow and/or venous outflow segments.[16] The presence of large caliber side branches may also jeopardize hemodialysis fistula maturation due to altered flow distribution. Hemodialysis fistula nonmaturation rates within the first months after creation range from 5% up to 54%.[17]

Manifestations of Disease

Clinical Presentation

Patients in need of a hemodialysis fistula usually have a long medical history of renal disease. In fact, because almost all patients with stage 5 CKD are known to have this condition, the creation of a hemodialysis fistula can be anticipated, and sufficient time can be taken to allow for DAG maturation. The K/DOQI guidelines recommend that patients be referred for surgical evaluation when the creatinine clearance falls below 25 mL/min, or a serum creatinine >4 mg/dL (354 micromoles/L), or when creation of a hemodialysis fistula is anticipated within 1 year.[18]

Patients with functioning hemodialysis fistula should be under continuous surveillance for failure (i.e., stenosis or thrombosis). The K/DOQI guidelines recommend monthly flow measurements using an ultrasound-based dilution technique in every patient on HD. If absolute hemodialysis fistula flow at any time falls below 600 mL/min, or if the patient exhibits a decline >25% between two consecutive measurements in combination with an absolute flow of less than 1000 mL/min, the hemodialysis fistula is considered at risk for thrombosis.[18] If this is the case, imaging is indicated to investigate the presence of inflow and/or outflow stenoses.

Imaging Indications and Algorithm

Imaging is indicated (1) prior to creation of a hemodialysis fistula, and (2) in patients with a hemodialysis fistula who are suspected of having a stenosis or occlusion anywhere in the vascular system of the upper extremity within the vascular pathway between the left ventricle and right atrium.

Any presurgical workup should start with a thorough history and physical examination. Women, elderly patients, and patients suffering from diabetes mellitus, obesity, cardiovascular morbidity, and patients with a history of previous vascular access procedures as well as previous limb and thoracic surgery or radiation therapy are at increased risk for hemodialysis fistula nonmaturation.[19] Physical examination is an important and valuable tool in the workup of patients awaiting access surgery. Skin lesions, local infections, generalized dermatological problems and scars may indicate poor chance of successful hemodialysis fistula creation at standard locations and should be addressed. All patients should undergo bilateral blood pressure measurements of the upper extremity. A difference of more than 20 mm Hg or an arm-to-arm index of <0.9 are indicative for the presence of arterial pathology.

The anatomy of the venous system is also important to determine because it can be highly variable. The presence of small caliber veins, venous obstructions, low compliance segments, and large accessory veins is associated with higher hemodialysis fistula nonmaturation rates.[18] Physical examination is useful to identify factors influencing hemodialysis fistula maturation, but it is typically not sufficient to rely on by itself. For instance, Malovrh and colleagues examined 116 patients due to undergo access creation and found that physical examination failed to identify suitable vessels for hemodialysis fistula creation in more than half of the patients.[20] Venous imaging is critical for preprocedural planning for hemodialysis fistula placement.

In patients with a DAG already in place, continuous surveillance is mandated, as discussed earlier. In cases of suspected stenosis or occlusion, the patient should be referred for imaging and subsequent intervention without delay.

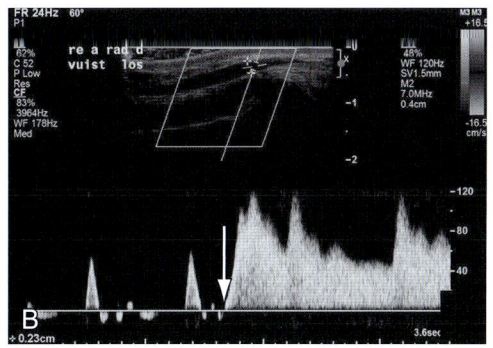

FIGURE 119-2 Duplex ultrasound assessment of radial artery flows at rest (**A**), during fist clenching (**B**), and during hyperemia after the fist clench has been released in a healthy volunteer. The *arrow* indicates the moment of fist clench release. Absence or diminished change in radial artery flow is associated with a higher risk of vascular access, early failure, and nonmaturation.

Imaging Techniques and Findings

Ultrasound

Duplex ultrasonography (DUS) is the imaging modality of first choice in patients due to undergo graft creation as well as in patients with a failing DAG. DUS enables assessment of vessel patency, diameter, flow volume and velocities. The application of DUS enables proper depiction and determination of suitable vessels for hemodialysis fistula creation that may not be detected by physical examination, especially in obese patients.[21-24]

Preoperative DUS examination should include assessment of the arteries and veins from the subclavian artery down to the radial and ulnar vessels at the wrist. The exact course and continuity as well as the presence of stenoses should be addressed because patients with arterial stenosis are thought to be at increased risk for developing hand and finger ischemia after AVF creation due to steal phenomena. For detection of relevant stenoses (defined as >50% luminal reduction) in the upper extremity arterial system, DUS has a sensitivity and specificity of 90.9% and 100% for the subclavian artery, 93.3% and 100% for upper arm arteries, 88.6% and 98.7% for forearm arteries, and for the arteries of the hand 70% and 100%, respectively.[25,26]

Another important morphologic parameter apart from the presence of arterial stenosis is arterial diameter. Arteries with diameters smaller than 1.5 to 3.0 mm have been associated with increased AVF nonmaturation rates.[14] Additional parameters such as radial artery flow volume and peak systolic velocities before or during reactive hyperemia have also been reported to be predictors of AVF maturation. In Figure 119-2 radial artery flow velocity changes due to fist clenching and reactive hyperemia are shown. Lockhart and associates, in contrast, found that arterial diameters, resistance indices, and peak systolic velocities had little if any predictive value for AVF outcome.[16]

The superficial venous system of the upper extremity is also easily assessable by DUS and—not surprisingly—results in detection of more veins compared to physical examination alone. DUS also allows for assessment of local hemodynamics, such as the determination of subclavian venous flow. A typical example of Doppler signal changes

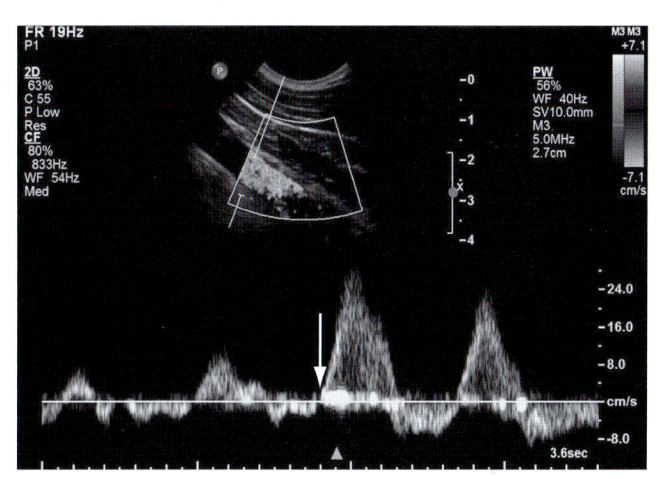

FIGURE 119-3 The effect of deep inspiration on subclavian vein flow assessed with duplex ultrasound. The *arrow* indicates the start of deep inspiration. Absence or diminished subclavian vein flow or change flow due to deep inspiration is indicated for central venous stenosis or occlusion.

of the subclavian vein during deep inspiration in a healthy volunteer is shown in Figure 119-3. The absence of changes in venous Doppler signal due to deep inspiration or loss of venous compressibility suggests the presence of a local venous stenosis or occlusion. Preoperative detection of stenoses and obstructions is important to avoid unsuccessful hemodialysis access surgeries. Nack and colleagues reported a DUS sensitivity, specificity, positive predictive value, and negative predictive value of 81%, 90%, 90%, and 78%, respectively, for detection of venous stenosis, thrombi, and occlusions when compared to DSA.[27] The clinical value of upper extremity DUS for detection of venous abnormalities is lower for proximal compared to distal veins. Nack and colleagues also reported progressively decreasing DUS sensitivities for detection of abnormalities in the subclavian vein (79%), innominate vein (75%), and superior vena cava (33%), when compared to DSA.[27] This can be explained by the fact that these veins course beneath bony structures such as the clavicle and ribs over a substantial length and/or are relatively distant from the skin surface and inaccessible by DUS.

As is the case for arteries, DUS-derived venous diameter is an important parameter for prediction of vascular access outcome. For assessment of venous diameter, a proximally applied cuff should be used to induce venous dilation for better appreciation of maximum or true venous diameter.[28] Reported venous cut-off diameters for successful hemodialysis fistula creation range from 1.6 to 2.6 mm.[6,28] This range may be partially explained by differences in vein mapping protocols because only few authors reported the measurement conditions and methods to achieve venous dilation. DUS venous diameter measurements, furthermore, are observer-dependent with an interobserver variation reported to be 0.5 mm.[29] Recently, Planken and associates have demonstrated that superficial forearm vein diameter measurements vary over time with a coefficient of variation of 27%.[28] Forearm superficial venous diameter measurement reproducibility also depends on the applied venous congestion pressure and best reproducibility is achieved at venous congestion pressures >40 mm Hg.[30]

The preoperative length of nondiseased contiguous vein >10 cm used for AVF in addition to venous diameter was predictive for the success of AVF creation.[31,32] Apart from venous diameter, some authors have found an association between the presence and size of venous side branches and AVF nonmaturation. Wong and colleagues suggested that a side branch <5 cm away from the planned anastomosis may impair AVF function, whereas Beathard and associates have stressed the importance of the size of the venous side branches. In the aforementioned studies nonmaturation was more likely in the event of a large venous side branch.[33,34] Turmel-Rodrigues and colleagues, in contrast, state that venous side branches are of no importance and come into play only in the presence of a venous outflow stenosis.[35]

Dynamic parameters to characterize upper extremity veins include flow volume and velocity measurements as well as assessment of flow wave changes due to respiratory maneuvers.[36] The capacity of superficial veins to dilate due to venous congestion (also known as venous compliance) has been reported to be higher in patients with successful AVF creation compared to patients with AVF failure or nonmaturation with venous diameter increase 48% and 11.8%, respectively, at a congestion pressure of 50 mm Hg.[24] Forearm superficial venous compliance measurements, however, have been reported to be poorly reproducible due to great variations in venous diameters at low venous congestion pressures.[30] The clinical value of forearm superficial venous compliance measurements is, therefore, considered of little if any use.

Multiple studies have shown the value of DUS in preoperative assessment of patients undergoing hemodialysis fistula creation. The performance of DUS prior to hemodialysis access fistula creation has been shown to result in changes in surgical procedure (31%), changes in site of exploration (9.6%), a decrease in unsuccessful explorations (11% to 0%), an increase in the relative number of AVFs created (as opposed to other types of access; 64% vs. 34%), and a decrease in AVF nonmaturation rates (e.g., 38% to 8.3%; and 66% to 46%), when compared to the use of physical examination alone.[14,19,20,23,37] However, the recommended threshold values of various DUS-derived parameters (i.e., diameter, flow-volume, velocities, compliance and resistive index) vary and no single parameter appears to be superior as a sole predictor for AVF success.[16,38] It remains to be established which combination of parameters might enable better prediction of vascular access function and minimize early failure and nonmaturation rates.

In patients with failing hemodialysis fistulas, DUS is highly sensitive and highly specific for the detection of stenoses and occlusions in the supplying arteries, as well as the draining veins, up to the shoulder region.[39] DUS is not reliable for imaging central to the subclavian region, and other techniques should be used instead. However, although regular hemodialysis fistula surveillance has been associated with a much lower rate of graft thrombosis, a randomized controlled trial in 101 patients with AVGs by Sam and coworkers found that 2-year graft survival was similar in patients when they were referred for intervention on the basis of clinical criteria, ultrasound dilution measurements, or DUS stenosis measurements.[40]

DUS is also highly sensitive for the detection of anastomotic problems such as aneurysm formation, which tend to have a wide neck if the aneurysm arises at the anastomosis of an autologous or synthetic graft. A drawback of DUS is the relatively long examination time, especially if the entire upper extremity needs to be evaluated.

CT

There are only a few studies[41-44] that have reported the use of computed tomography angiography (CTA) for both the preoperative workup of patients with CKD scheduled for hemodialysis access fistula surgery and for patients with dysfunctional hemodialysis fistulas. The largest study evaluated only 30 patients.[42] Not surprisingly, CTA was found capable of detecting vascular pathology in the hemodialysis fistula and the supplying as well as draining vessels with high accuracy (Figs. 119-4, 119-5, and 119-6).

The lack of studies on CTA underscores the tremendous usefulness and wide acceptance of DUS for hemodialysis fistula evaluation in clinical practice. On the other hand, it reflects the cautionary stance of the medical community toward the use of iodinated contrast agents in patients with severely compromised kidney function. However, with the advent of NSF concerns related to contrast-enhanced MRA, it is likely that physicians dealing with patients with CKD may revisit CTA evaluation of hemodialysis fistula patients in the future.

One of the most important issues standing in the way of universal acceptance of CTA for the assessment of the upper extremity vasculature is the lack of large prospective studies that address the long-term effects of iodinated contrast agents on residual renal function in the CKD patient population. Iodinated contrast agents have long been known to have nephrotoxic effects.[45] In any case, measures to prevent contrast-induced nephropathy such as adequate prehydration, use of N-acetylcysteine and or bicarbonate should be taken when patients with a preexisting decline in renal function are sent for contrast-enhanced CT examinations.

Most of the studies on residual renal function in HD patients are older, and were not performed using both modern generation low- or iso-osmolar contrast agents,

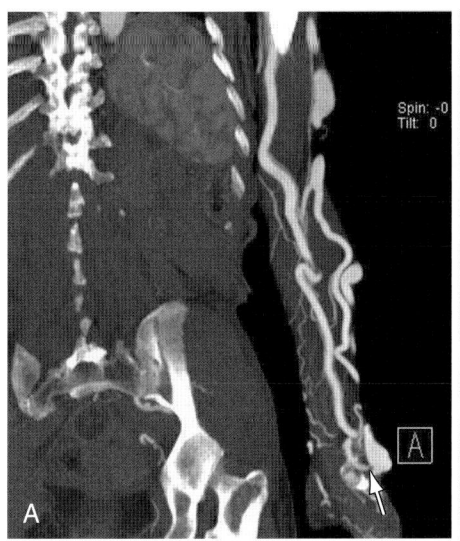

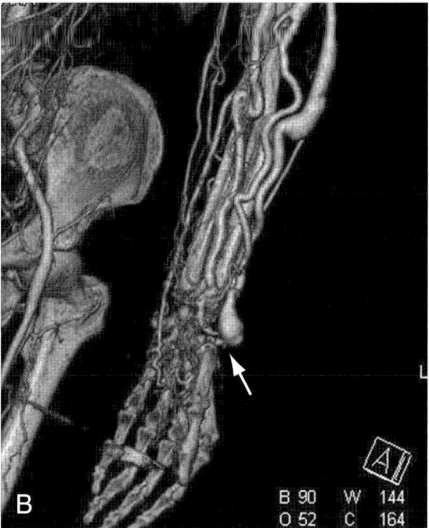

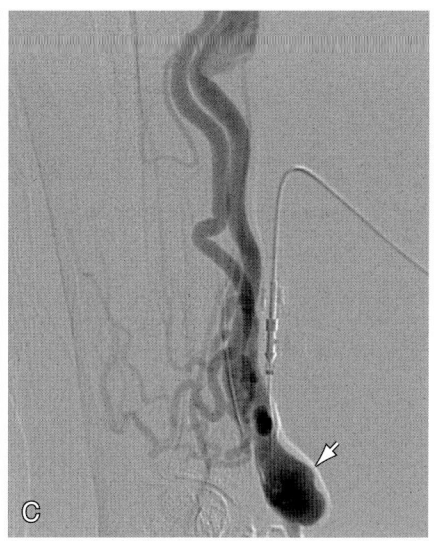

FIGURE 119-4 A 68-year-old woman with a left radial-cephalic AVF. Coronal subvolume maximum intensity projection (MIP, **A**) and volume rendered (VR, **B**) image from a CTA reveal a stenosis (*arrow*) at the radial artery anastomosis and an aneurysm in the draining vein with collateral formation. On the conventional x-ray fistulagram (**C**), the aneurysm (*small arrow*) was seen but the stenosis was obscured by overlying opacified vascular structures and not well seen. *(From E, Tarhan NC, Kayahan Ulu EM, et al. Evaluation of failing hemodialysis fistulas with multidetector CT angiography: comparison of different 3D planes. Eur J Radiol 2009; 69:184-192.)*

and the newest generation of biocompatible dialysis membranes, which are known to have a positive effect on contrast agent clearance and to ameliorate contrast nephrotoxicity. It is already known that residual renal function is conserved to a greater extent in patients on PD versus patients on HD, and two recent—but very small—studies have found that despite a limited transient decline in renal function, there was no accelerated decline after 2 weeks to 1 month after administration of iodinated contrast agent in PD patients when they were adequately prehydrated, and small volumes of contrast media (around 100 mL) were used.[46,47]

In conclusion, although CTA is likely to be accurate for the detection of vascular pathology in and around a hemodialysis fistula, there is a general lack of knowledge about the safety of iodinated contrast agent use in these patients. Nevertheless, preliminary evidence shows that at least some patients can probably be imaged safely. In patients who do not have residual renal function, it would be justifiable to use CTA as an imaging tool.

MRA

The enthusiasm for contrast-enhanced MRA (CE-MRA) for the depiction of upper extremity vasculature in patients due to undergo hemodialysis fistula creation, and in patients with failing grafts has waned acutely following the reported association of GBCA and NSF in 2006.[48] The safety of GBCA in patients with stage 4 and 5 CKD is a hotly contested issue and in continuous flux. An emerging consensus is that macrocyclic Gd-chelate contrast agents, which have not been unequivocally associated with NSF in even a single case, may indeed be safe when administered in small volumes (up to 0.1 mmol/kg) in patients with stage 4 and 5 CKD. Indeed, even the class of linear Gd-chelate contrast agents seem to have a much lower risk for NSF when used in low doses.[49] As with CTA, however, the risks of administration of the contrast agents for MRA should be carefully weighed against the diagnostic benefits that will be obtained.

Some widely used Gd-chelate contrast agents for CE-MRA purposes are gadopentetate dimeglumine (Magnevist, Schering, Berlin, Germany), gadoterate dimeglumine (Dotarem, Guerbet, Aulnay, France), gadodiamide (Omniscan, GE Health, Oslo, Norway), gadoversetamide (OptiMARK; Mallinckrodt, St Louis, Mo) and gadoteridol (ProHance, Bracco Diagnostics, Milan, Italy). The total incidence of adverse events related to gadolinium use for CE-MRA appears to be less than 5%. The incidence of any single adverse event is approximately 1%, or lower. By far the most common events are nausea, headache, and emesis.[50] When used intravenously, no detectable nephrotoxicity has been reported and the rates of adverse events are extremely low at the usual recommended doses.[51]

During the last decade, approximately 350 cases of nephrogenic systemic fibrosis (NSF), previously known as nephrogenic fibrosing dermopathy, have been reported worldwide. NSF is thought to be a chronic inflammatory reaction in response to the accumulation of free gadolinium in patients with severe renal failure. The reported clinical signs and symptoms of NSF are subacute progressive swelling of extremities followed by more proximal involvement and severe skin induration, pain, muscle restlessness, and loss of skin flexibility. NSF can lead to serious physical disability and wheelchair requirement, and even death.[52] The incidence of NSF is low—especially when low doses of GBCA are used—and the actual pathophysiology remains unknown.[49,52] To date, all linear Gd-chelate contrast agents, notably gadodiamide (Omniscan), are believed to be associated with NSF.[53,54] Because of these reported adverse events and the suspected causative relationship, many experts discourage the use of GBCA in CKD stage 4 and 5 patients until more data on safety are available.[53,54] A recent study by Chrysochou addressed the positive reporting bias regarding the link between gadolinium exposure and NSF and found that no patients with

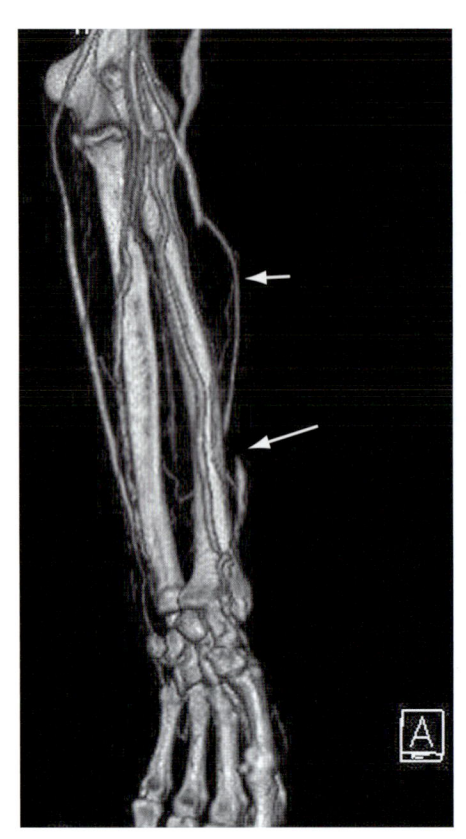

FIGURE 119-5 A 56-year-old man with left radial-cephalic AVF. Volume renedered image from a CTA reveals occlusion of the cephalic vein (*long arrow*) but filling of a venous collateral (*short arrow*). (From E, Tarhan NC, Kayahan Ulu EM, et al. Evaluation of failing hemodialysis fistulas with multidetector CT angiography: comparison of different 3D planes. Eur J Radiol 2009; 69:184-192.)

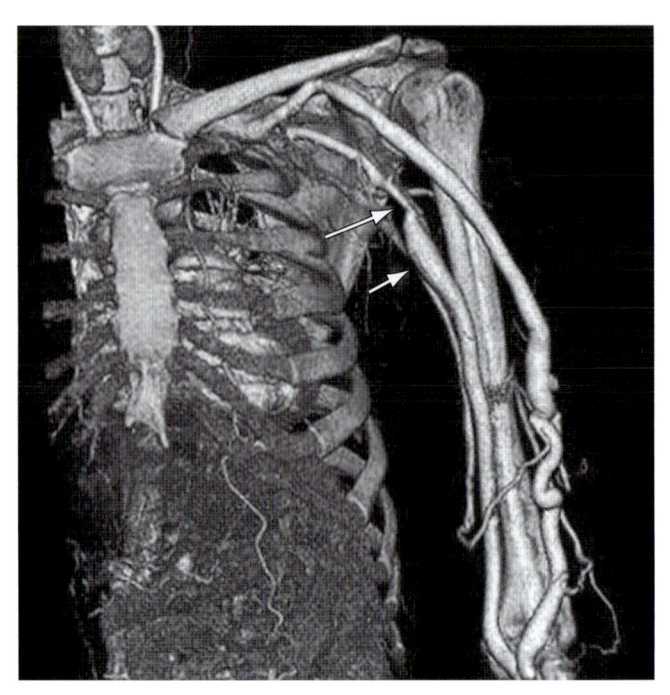

FIGURE 119-6 A 38-year-old woman with shoulder pain and patent left antecubital fossa AVF. Volume rendered image from a CTA reveals a brachial artery stenosis (*long arrow*) with poststenostic aneurysmal dilation (*short arrow*). (From E, Tarhan NC, Kayahan Ulu EM, et al. Evaluation of failing hemodialysis fistulas with multidetector CT angiography: comparison of different 3D planes. Eur J Radiol 2009; 69:184-192.)

CKD stage 4 developed NSF, regardless of the agent used.[55] Because there are no data published on the feasibility and accuracy of the newer, nonenhanced MRA techniques for evaluation of patients with hemodialysis fistulas, the subsequent discussion will focus on CE-MRA.

CE-MRA protocols enable image acquisition with high spatial (submillimeter voxel size) and temporal resolutions (<20 seconds per dynamic scan) with good to excellent image quality. For arterial imaging, a GBCA is injected in a contralateral antecubital or dorsal hand vein and imaging is timed for the return of the contrast bolus through the target arterial tree. Using this technique, further delayed imaging can reveal venous anatomy. An additional method for venous imaging is to use a direct method whereby MR imaging occurs during the initial injection of a diluted (1:15) contrast media bolus into an ipsilateral dorsal hand vein.

Because intrathoracic vessels are prone to movement during respiration, patients should hold their breath for about 15 to 20 seconds depending on scan protocol and technical factors related to system performance. Contrast medium is injected at speeds up to 3.0 mL/sec, followed by 25 mL of saline flush. Spatial resolution in recent reports is typically on the order of $1.0 \times 1.0 \times 1.2$ mm^3 (craniocaudal/frequency direction × left-right/phase-encoding directions × anteroposterior/slice direction).[6] Using this approach for imaging, upper extremity arteries and veins can be visualized with high accuracy (Fig. 119-7). Because upper extremity length of an adult is about 70 to 80 cm, depicting the entire upper extremity requires imaging of at least two fields of view because of the limited MR-bore length. An example of a preoperative contrast-enhanced MR arteriogram and venogram of an ESRD-patient is shown in Figure 119-8.

Synchronization of peak arterial and venous contrast concentration with sampling of central k-space profiles is very important in order to obtain selective imaging of arteries or veins, respectively. Currently, this is typically done by using either time-resolved sequences or real-time bolus monitoring software, followed by a high spatial-resolution 3D acquisition. If possible, parallel imaging techniques should be used to improve temporal resolution.

Planken and colleagues reported a multiphase approach using multiple dynamic scans that resulted in good to excellent subjective image quality images of upper extremity arteries down to the wrist.[56] Assessment of the arterial palmar arch and digital arteries remains cumbersome, however, with the currently acquired spatial resolutions, except when using timed arterial compression.[57] An important advance in this regard is the recent clinical introduction of blood pool contrast media, which enable ultra-high spatial resolution scans for assessment of the palmar arch and digital arteries (Fig. 119-9). Although CE-MRA is believed to be highly accurate for detection of arterial stenoses and obstructions, there are only limited studies about the accuracy and reproducibility for detection of thoracic and upper extremity arterial stenoses in patients with CKD. A typical example of a subclavian artery stenosis depicted by both CE-MRA and DSA is shown in Fig. 119-10.

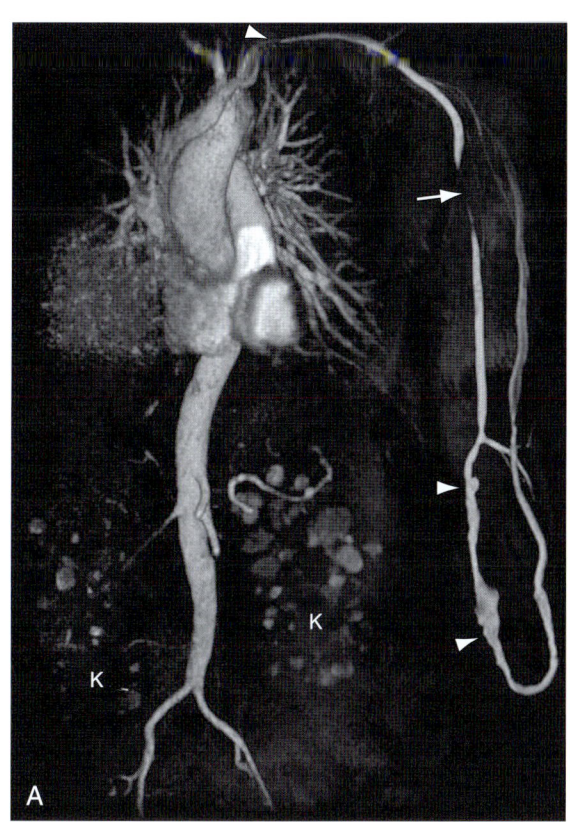

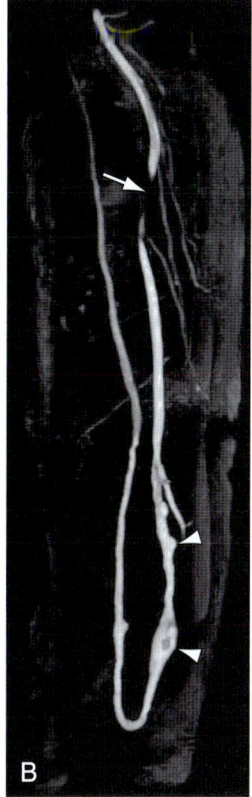

■ **FIGURE 119-7** A 67-year-old patient with polycystic kidney disease and flow declined hemodialysis access fistula in the left forearm (**A**). There are high-grade stenoses in the subclavian (*top arrowhead*) and brachial artery supplying the shunt (*arrow*). In addition, there are multiple aneurysmal dilations in the loop graft (**A**, *lower arrowheads*). Note enhancement of residual kidney parenchyma.
B, Zoomed subvolume maximum intensity projection of the left forearm and antecubital region more clearly shows high-grade stenosis (*arrow*) and aneurysms (*arrowheads*). K: kidney (TR/TE/SENSE factor: 4.0/1.5/2×).

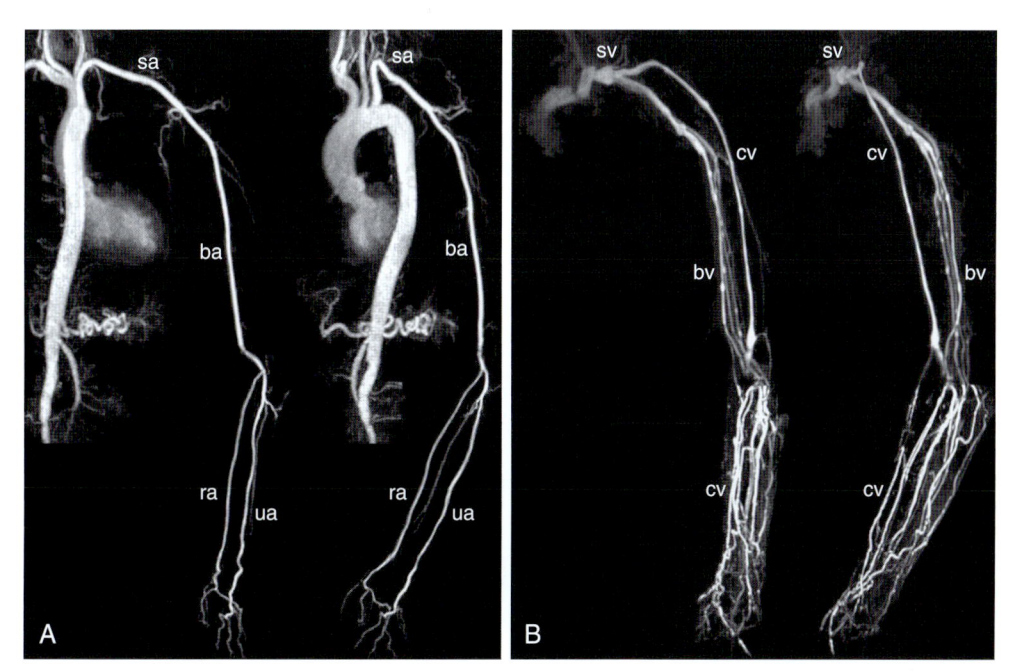

■ **FIGURE 119-8** Example of selective CE-MRA of upper extremity arteries (**A**) and veins (**B**), by contralateral and ipsilateral injection of contrast media, respectively. Images of the entire upper extremity vasculature were acquired in four consecutive phases. First distal arteries (forearm), second proximal arteries (upper arm and thorax), third proximal veins (upper arm and thorax) and fourth distal veins (forearm). sa, subclavian artery; ba, brachial artery; ra, radial artery; ua, ulnar artery; sv, subclavian vein; cv, cephalic vein; bv, basilic vein.

Reported contrast-enhanced MR venography techniques use either direct injection of diluted contrast-media (1:15 to 1:25 mL of gadolinium chelate in saline solution) in the ipsilateral extremity or contralateral intravenous injection of nondiluted contrast media, and acquisition during delayed venous enhancement after initial arterial first pass. Both techniques have their strengths and weaknesses. Direct venography with application of a proximal blood pressure cuff inflated to 60 mm Hg yields better vessel opacification with lower contrast dose as compared to the contralateral injection approach. Of course, this is very helpful in the context of concerns related to NSF risk. Examples of a central venous stenosis and obstruction by direct contrast-enhanced MR venography are shown in Figs. 119-11 and 119-12. Indirect contrast-enhanced MR venography using delayed venous enhancement techniques (i.e., after the first pass arterial phase) show relatively poor performance for detection of central venous stenosis and occlusions and are not recommended. Furthermore, on direct contrast-enhanced MR venography, diameter measurements have been shown to be more accurate compared to duplex ultrasonography when using surgical measurements as the standard of reference.[58] Because of the lower contrast dose, better vessel opacification and accuracy, direct contrast-enhanced MR venography seems to be the method of first choice for venous imaging.

Although CE-MRA is a promising and attractive modality for imaging the upper extremity arteries and veins, there are only sparse data about its clinical value for hemodialysis fistula planning or surveillance and future studies are needed. Recently, several new techniques for non-contrast enhanced MRA have been introduced. These promising techniques may prove to be important for hemodialysis fistula imaging and noninvasive vascular imaging of CKD patients in general but at present evidence is anecdotal (Fig. 119-13).

Angiography

Intra-arterial digital subtraction angiography (IA-DSA), using x-ray techniques and iodinated contrast media is considered the standard of reference for assessment of upper extremity arteries and veins. The major advantage of IA-DSA is that flow-limiting lesions can immediately be

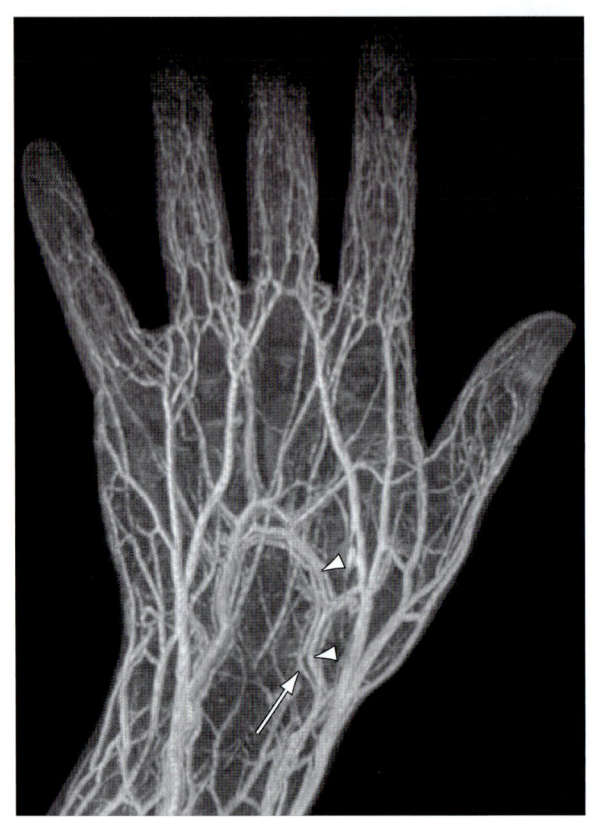

■ **FIGURE 119-9** Ultra high resolution (acquired voxel size: 0.4 × 0.4 × 0.4 mm³) steady-state CE-MRA of the arterial palmar arch and the proximal digital arteries, 45 sec after injection of a blood pool agent. Although both arteries and veins are equally opacified during steady state and separation of arteries and veins can be difficult, the arterial palmar arch (*arrowheads*) can be identified as well as accompanying veins (*arrow*).

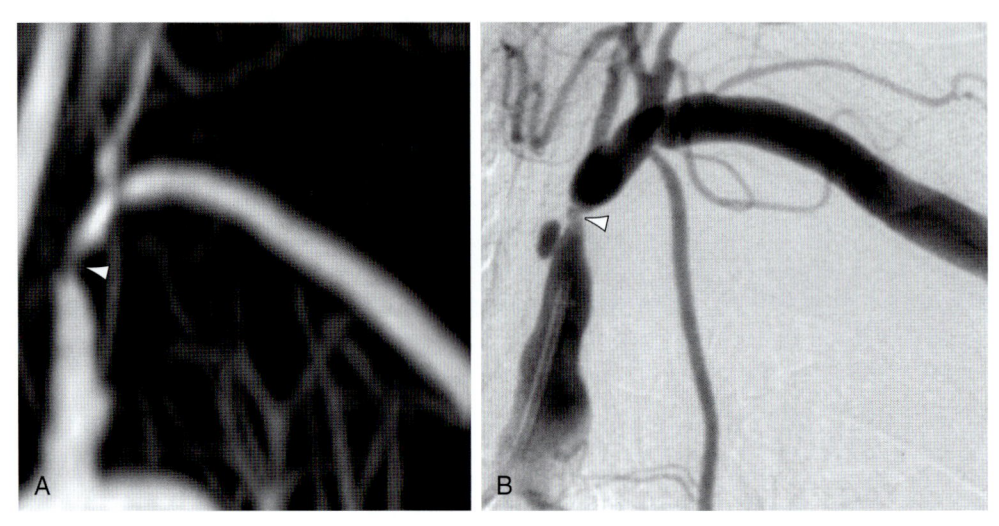

■ **FIGURE 119-10** Typical example of a subclavian artery stenosis (*arrowhead*), initially detected by CE-MRA (**A**) and confirmed by DSA (**B**, *arrowhead*).

CHAPTER 119 • Hemodialysis Fistulas   1681

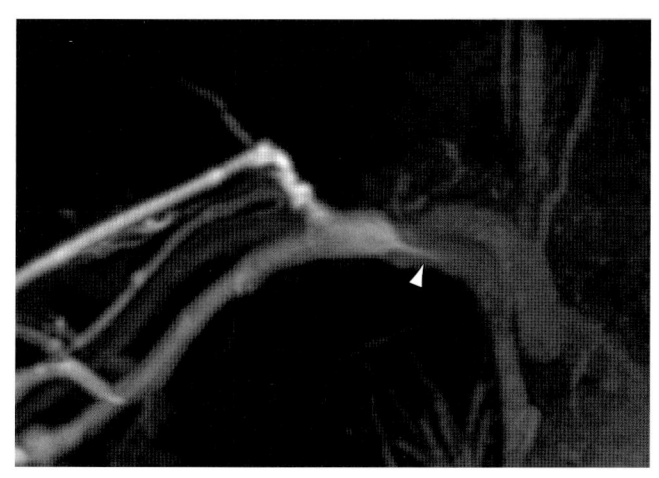

■ **FIGURE 119-11** Example of a direct MR venogram of a patient with a central venous stenosis (*arrowhead*).

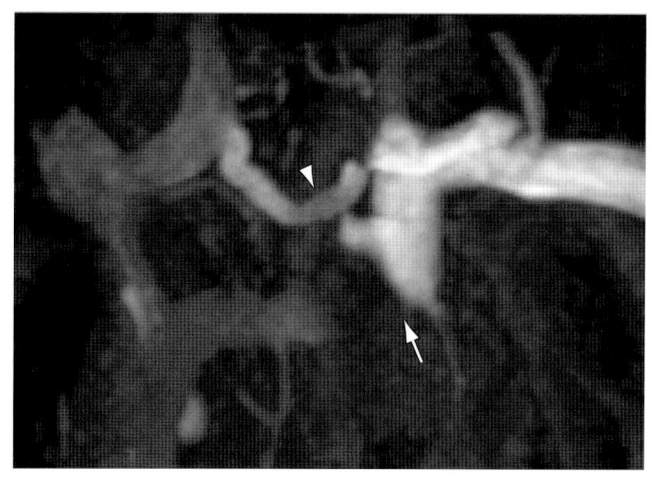

■ **FIGURE 119-12** Brachiocephalic vein occlusion (*arrow*) in a patient who had a history of multiple central venous catheters. The *arrowhead* indicates a draining collateral vein to the contralateral side.

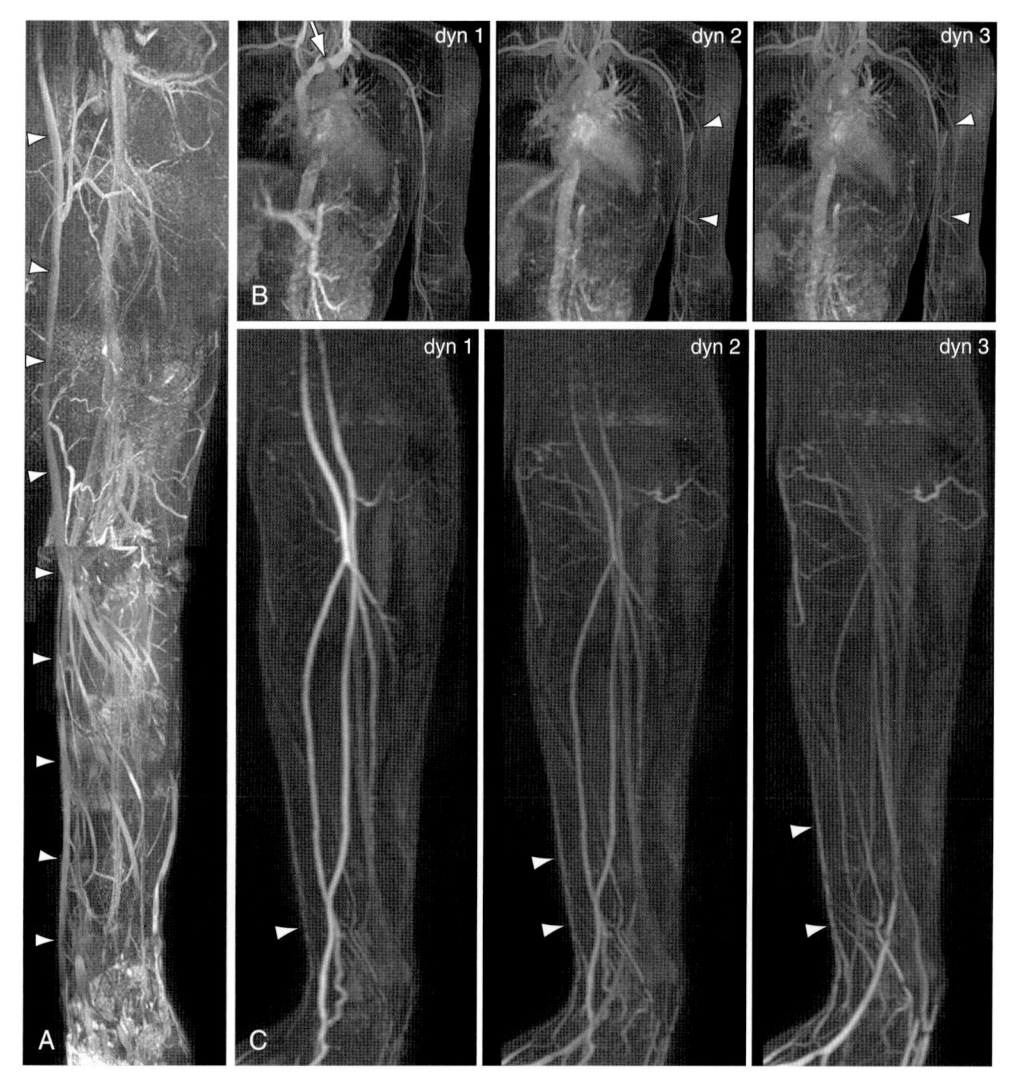

■ **FIGURE 119-13** Example of noncontrast-enhanced fat-saturated balanced turbo field echo acquisition of the upper arm and forearm vasculature in a 49-year-old male patient due to undergo dialysis access construction in the forearm (**A**). Note excellent depiction of both arteries and veins in a single image. Because of the high spatial resolution, arteries and veins can easily be differentiated in the source images. For comparison purposes the corresponding multiphase CE-MRA images of the upper arm (**B**) and forearm (**C**) are shown. Note how many more veins are depicted using the nonenhanced technique, and how much better the cephalic vein is depicted compared to the CE-MRA technique (*arrowheads* in **A-C**). CE-MRA images were acquired without venous compression, which leads to selective opacification of the dominant veins draining the arm only. Dyn, dynamic phase.

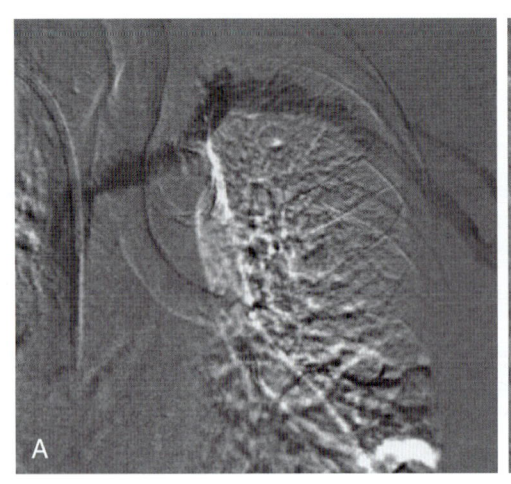

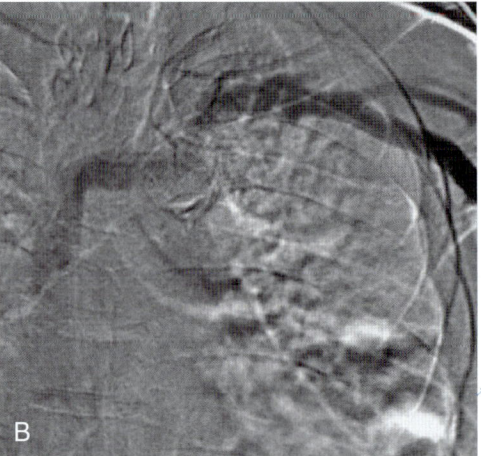

FIGURE 119-14 Example of venograms obtained in a single patient by CO_2 venography (**A**) and by conventional venography using iodinated contrast media (**B**). *(Images were kindly provided by Dr. S. Heye from the Department of Radiology, University Hospitals Gasthuisberg, Leuven, Belgium.)*

treated using endovascular therapies at the time of the study. The major drawback of IA-DSA is, of course, the use of iodinated contrast media, the issues of which have been discussed in the section on CTA above. In light of NSF concerns, IA-DSA should not be performed with GBCA.

Another alternative to iodinated contrast media and GBCA is carbon dioxide (CO_2) gas injection. Heye and colleagues have demonstrated that CO_2 venography is an acceptable alternative (sensitivity, 97%; specificity, 85%; accuracy, 95%) for assessment of upper-extremity and central veins in patients with contraindications to iodinated contrast material.[59] In Figure 119-14 a CO_2 venogram and corresponding conventional venogram using iodinated contrast media are shown. However, CO_2 injections may cause pain and the CO_2 contrast technique can lead to an overestimation of the degree of stenosis. The use of CO_2 contrast may furthermore lead to serious complications such as brain gas embolism, pulmonary embolism, or acute cardiac arrest.[59]

Upper extremity IA-DSA is traditionally performed by intra-arterial injection of contrast media. Arterial access can be achieved by femoral or brachial puncture. In patients with CKD, the brachial artery approach is generally avoided because it can be painful, it may jeopardize distal perfusion and thereby maturation and function of a (future) hemodialysis fistula created distal to the puncture site. Thrombosis of the brachial artery is a serious complication due to brachial punctures for catheter access in up to 7%.[60] The contralateral venous injection of contrast media is a less invasive alternative with fewer complications. However, in order to achieve sufficient arterial enhancement, this technique requires a high contrast dose, which is unacceptable in CKD patients due to the potential further deterioration of residual renal function. A recently described alternative by Duijm and colleagues is to insert the catheter through the access itself or the draining vein. This strategy enabled full depiction of both the outflow (venous) trajectory, as well as the inflow (arterial) trajectory by retrograde catheterization of the arterial inflow in 162/166 (97.7%) of patients.[61] The authors concluded, however, that hemodialysis fistula evaluation by noninvasive imaging such as DUS is sufficient in the majority of patients as isolated proximal arterial inflow stenoses were seen in only 4.8% of patients.

Central venous stenosis and obstruction occur frequently after central venous catheter insertion or placement of pacemaker wires; however, often patients remain asymptomatic until after the hemodialysis fistula is created. Imaging of the subclavian and innominate veins and the superior vena cava prior to hemodialysis fistula creation is important because CKD patients typically have had central venous catheters and up to 40% of patients with a history of central venous catheters have central venous stenosis or obstruction.[62] Examples of central venous obstructions due to pacemaker wires and central venous catheter use are shown in Figures 119-15 and 119-16. Venography by cannulation of an ipsilateral dorsal hand vein allows imaging of the entire cephalic or basilic veins from the hand up to the confluence of the basilic and brachial veins into the subclavian vein. Although the superficial veins of the upper extremity are connected to each other at multiple levels, the puncture site will limit venous opacification to the draining vein of the puncture site only. It is important to avoid puncturing veins proximal to the distal radius in order to preserve draining veins for future access use. It is the experience of this author that the use of a proximal tourniquet inflated to 60 mm Hg enables depiction of collateral veins and improves assessment of venous diameter because of dilation.

Classic Signs

The classic sign associated with a dysfunctioning hemodialysis fistula is a stenosis at the arteriovenous anastomosis, or in the venous outflow trajectory proximal to the hemodialysis fistula. Less frequently, the artery supplying the hemodialysis fistula is stenotic. An arterial stenosis should always be searched for when imaging of the hemodialysis fistula is negative for flow-limiting lesions.

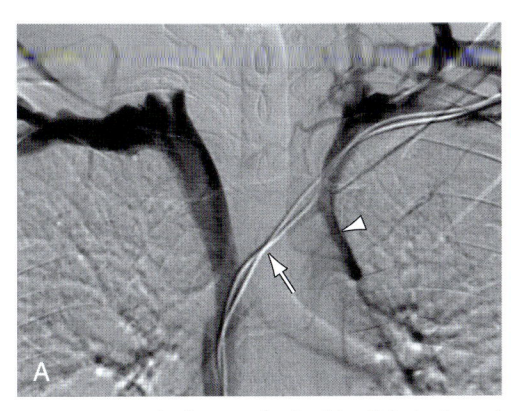

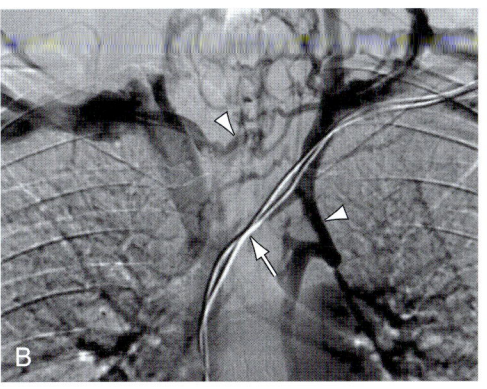

■ **FIGURE 119-15** Two consecutive images obtained by digital subtraction angiography of a central venous obstruction (*arrow*) due to pacemaker wires. *Arrowheads* point at collateral draining veins.

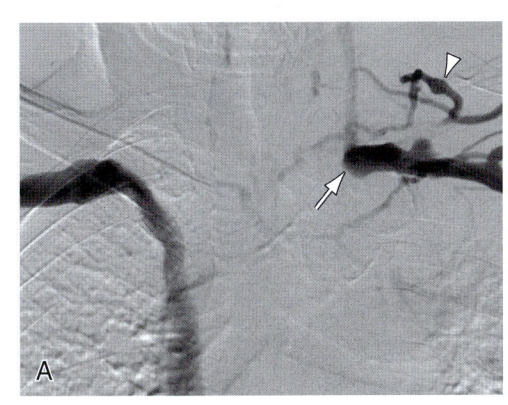

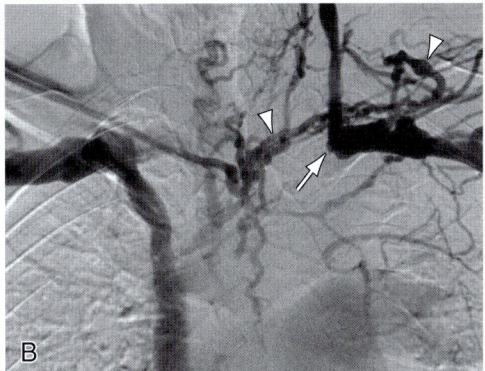

■ **FIGURE 119-16** Two consecutive images obtained by digital subtraction angiography of a central venous obstruction (*arrow*) due to central venous catheter use. *Arrowheads* point at collateral draining veins.

DIFFERENTIAL DIAGNOSIS

From Clinical Presentation

The cause of flow decline in an existing hemodialysis fistula is almost always the presence of a stenosis somewhere in the vascular pathway between the left ventricle and the right atrium. At first, imaging should focus on the hemodialysis fistula itself and the venous outflow as most stenoses will form in these locations. If imaging of this trajectory does not yield evidence of flow-limiting lesions, the arterial inflow should be imaged.

From Imaging Findings

Stenoses in the hemodialysis fistula itself and the draining vein are mainly caused by intimal hyperplasia, which is thought to be secondary to the altered flow conditions after creation of the arteriovenous fistula. Stenoses in feeding arteries to a hemodialysis fistula can also be attributable to accelerated atherosclerosis which is common in patients with CKD.

SYNOPSIS OF TREATMENT OPTIONS

Medical

There is no adequate medical treatment for a failing AVF or AVG.

Surgical/Interventional

Percutaneous transluminal angioplasty with direct insertion of the catheter and balloon through the AVF or AVG is the treatment of first choice in case of suspected hemodialysis fistula dysfunction due to a flow-limiting stenosis or graft thrombosis. In cases of nonmaturation, the treatment of first choice is also endovascular intervention of the flow limiting lesions. However, if no lesions are found, treatment is ligation of large side-branches of the draining vein. Nonetheless, it is best always to investigate the vasculature of the upper extremity in detail prior to creation of a hemodialysis fistula, in order to avoid the problem of nonmaturation in the first place.

REPORTING: INFORMATION FOR THE REFERRING PHYSICIAN

When describing the findings of vascular imaging of the upper extremity, one must state exactly what part of the upper extremity was imaged, keeping in mind that an examination is not complete if the central thoracic arteries and veins are not depicted. If stenoses are found, it is important to describe their exact location (inflow, in the graft, or in the outflow trajectory) and degree of luminal narrowing. With regard to MRI, it is important to comment on any artifacts associated with surgical clips, as these may obscure an underlying stenosis or occlusion.

KEY POINTS

- Long-term hemodialysis requires vascular access and the surgical creation of a hemodialysis fistula, typically in the patient's distal forearm. Hemodialysis fistulas can be created using the patient's native arteries and veins (arterial venous fistula or AVF), or by using a prosthetic graft (arteriovenous graft or AVG). Generally, AVF is the preferred type of hemodialysis fistula. Imaging plays a key role for the preoperative planning and postoperative surveillance of patients with hemodialysis fistulas. Residual renal function is a key predictor of survival in patients with chronic kidney disease. The preservation of even small amounts of residual renal function in patients on dialysis is of major clinical importance.
- Duplex ultrasonography is the imaging test of first choice in patients due to undergo hemodialysis fistula creation, as well as in patients with dysfunctional hemodialysis fistulas.
- Although CTA is capable of demonstrating vascular stenoses with high accuracy, there is limited data on the effect of iodinated contrast media administration on residual renal function.
- Because of concern for nephrogenic systemic fibrosis (NSF), contrast-enhanced MR angiography probably should not be performed with linear gadolinium (Gd)-chelate contrast agents in patients with stage 4 and 5 chronic kidney disease. However, preliminary evidence suggests that macrocyclic Gd-chelate contrast agents at a dose of 0.1 mmol/kg or less may be safely used in these patients
- Intra-arterial DSA with direct puncture of the vascular access allows comprehensive imaging and endovascular therapy in almost all patients with stenoses in the arterial inflow, the access itself, and the venous outflow.

SUGGESTED READINGS

Clinical practice guidelines for hemodialysis adequacy, update 2006. Am J Kidney Dis 2006; 48 Suppl 1:S2-90.

Levey AS, Coresh J, Balk E, et al. National Kidney Foundation practice guidelines for chronic kidney disease: evaluation, classification, and stratification. Ann Intern Med 2003; 139:137-147.

Persson PB, Hansell P, Liss P. Pathophysiology of contrast medium-induced nephropathy. Kidney Int 2005; 68:14-22.

Planken RN, Tordoir JH, Duijm LE, et al. Current techniques for assessment of upper extremity vasculature prior to hemodialysis vascular access creation. Eur Radiol 2007; 17:3001-3011.

Tordoir JH, Mickley V. European guidelines for vascular access: clinical algorithms on vascular access for haemodialysis. Edtna Erca J 2003; 29:131-136.

United States Renal Data System. USRDS Annual data report. Minneapolis, MN: USRDS Coordinating Center, 2008 [http://www.usrds.org/adr.htm] Accessed August 1, 2009.

REFERENCES

1. National Kidney foundation, K/DOQI Clinical Practice Guidelines for Vascular Access, 2000. Am J Kidney Dis 2001; 37:S137-S181.
2. Sidawy AN. Strategies of arteriovenous dialysis access. In Rutherford RB, ed. Vascular Surgery, 6th ed. Philadelphia, Saunders, 2005.
3. Staramos DN, Lazarides MK, Tzilalis VD, et al. Patency of autologous and prosthetic arteriovenous fistulas in elderly patients. Eur J Surg 2000; 166:777-781.
4. Foley RN, Chen SC, Collins AJ. Hemodialysis access at initiation in the United States, 2005-2007: Still "catheter first." Hemodial Int 2009; 13(4):533-542.
5. Huber TS, Buhler AG, Seegar JM. Evidence-based data for the hemodialysis access surgeon. Semin Dial 2004;17(3), 217-223.
6. Planken RN, Tordoir JH, Duijm LE, et al. Current techniques for assessment of upper extremity vasculature prior to hemodialysis vascular access creation. Eur Radiol 2007; 17:3001-3011.
7. Termorshuizen F, Dekker FW, van Manen JG, et al. Relative contribution of residual renal function and different measures of adequacy to survival in hemodialysis patients: an analysis of the Netherlands Cooperative Study on the Adequacy of Dialysis (NECOSAD)-2. J Am Soc Nephrol 2004; 15:1061-1070.
8. Perl J, Bargman JM. The importance of residual kidney function for patients on dialysis: a critical review. Am J Kidney Dis 2009; 53:1068-1081.
9. Marron B, Remon C, Perez-Fontan M, et al. Benefits of preserving residual renal function in peritoneal dialysis. Kidney Int Suppl 2008:S42-S51.
10. Levey AS, Coresh J, Balk E, et al. National Kidney Foundation practice guidelines for chronic kidney disease: evaluation, classification, and stratification. Ann Intern Med 2003; 139:137-147.
11. Moeller S, Gioberge S, Brown G. ESRD patients in 2001: global overview of patients, treatment modalities and development trends. Nephrol Dial Transplant 2002; 17:2071-2076.
12. Grassmann A, Gioberge S, Moeller S, Brown G. ESRD patients in 2004: global overview of patient numbers, treatment modalities and associated trends. Nephrol Dial Transplant 2005; 20:2587-2593.
13. United States Renal Data System. USRDS Annual data report. Minneapolis, Minn: USRDS Coordinating Center, 2008 [http://www.usrds.org/adr.htm] Accessed August 1, 2009.
14. Robbin ML, Gallichio MH, Deierhoi MH, et al. US vascular mapping before hemodialysis access placement. Radiology 2000; 217:83-88.
15. Lauvao LS, Ihnat DM, Goshima KR, et al. Vein diameter is the major predictor of fistula maturation. J Vasc Surg 2009; 49:1499-1504.
16. Lockhart ME, Robbin ML, Allon M. Preoperative sonographic radial artery evaluation and correlation with subsequent radiocephalic fistula outcome. J Ultrasound Med 2004; 23:161-168; quiz 169-171.
17. Leblanc M, Saint-Sauveur E, Pichette V. Native arterio-venous fistula for hemodialysis: what to expect early after creation? J Vasc Access 2003; 4:39-44.
18. Clinical practice guidelines for hemodialysis adequacy, update 2006. Am J Kidney Dis 2006; 48 Suppl 1:S2-90.
19. Allon M, Bailey R, Ballard R, et al. A multidisciplinary approach to hemodialysis access: prospective evaluation. Kidney Int 1998; 53:473-479.
20. Silva MB, Jr., Hobson RW, 2nd, Pappas PJ, et al. A strategy for increasing use of autogenous hemodialysis access procedures: impact of preoperative noninvasive evaluation. J Vasc Surg 1998; 27:302-307; discussion 307-308.

21. Katz ML, Comerota AJ, DeRojas J, et al. B-mode imaging to determine the suitability of arm veins for primary arteriovenous fistulae. J Vasc Technol 1987; 11:172-174.
22. Vassalotti JA, Falk A, Cohl ED, et al. Obese and non-obese hemodialysis patients have a similar prevalence of functioning arteriovenous fistula using pre-operative vein mapping. Clin Nephrol 2002; 58:211-214.
23. Mihmanli I, Besirli K, Kurugoglu S, et al. Cephalic vein and hemodialysis fistula: surgeon's observation versus color Doppler ultrasonographic findings. J Ultrasound Med 2001; 20:217-222.
24. Malovrh M. Native arteriovenous fistula: preoperative evaluation. Am J Kidney Dis 2002; 39:1218-1225.
25. Wittenberg G, Landwehr P, Moll R, et al. [Interobserver variability of dialysis shunt flow measurements using color coated duplex sonography]. Rofo 1993; 159:375-378.
26. Wittenberg G, Schindler T, Tschammler A, et al. [Value of color-coded duplex ultrasound in evaluating arm blood vessels—arteries and hemodialysis shunts]. Ultraschall Med 1998; 19:22-27.
27. Nack TL, Needleman L. Comparison of duplex ultrasound and contrast venography for evaluation of upper extremity venous disease. J Vasc Technol 1992; 16:69-73.
28. Planken RN, Keuter XH, Hoeks AP, et al. Diameter measurements of the forearm cephalic vein prior to vascular access creation in end-stage renal disease patients: graduated pressure cuff versus tourniquet vessel dilatation. Nephrol Dial Transplant 2006; 21:802-806.
29. Lees TA, Manzo R, Strandness DE, Appleton D. Observer variation in the measurement of venous diameters using duplex scanning. J Vasc Technol 1994; 18:177-180.
30. Planken RN, Keuter XH, Kessels AG, et al. Forearm cephalic vein cross-sectional area changes at incremental congestion pressures: towards a standardized and reproducible vein mapping protocol. J Vasc Surg 2006; 44:353-358.
31. Lemson MS, Leunissen KM, Tordoir JH. Does pre-operative duplex examination improve patency rates of Brescia-Cimino fistulas? Nephrol Dial Transplant 1998; 13:1360-1361.
32. Allon M, Lockhart ME, Lilly RZ, et al. Effect of preoperative sonographic mapping on vascular access outcomes in hemodialysis patients. Kidney Int 2001; 60:2013-2020.
33. Beathard GA, Arnold P, Jackson J, Litchfield T. Aggressive treatment of early fistula failure. Kidney Int 2003; 64:1487-1494.
34. Wong V, Ward R, Taylor J, et al. Factors associated with early failure of arteriovenous fistulae for haemodialysis access. Eur J Vasc Endovasc Surg 1996; 12:207-213.
35. Turmel-Rodrigues L, Mouton A, Birmele B, et al. Salvage of immature forearm fistulas for haemodialysis by interventional radiology. Nephrol Dial Transplant 2001; 16:2365-2371.
36. Tordoir JH, Mickley V. European guidelines for vascular access: clinical algorithms on vascular access for haemodialysis. Edtna Erca J 2003; 29:131-136.
37. Allon M, Robbin ML. Increasing arteriovenous fistulas in hemodialysis patients: problems and solutions. Kidney Int 2002; 62:1109-1124.
38. Robbin ML, Chamberlain NE, Lockhart ME, et al. Hemodialysis arteriovenous fistula maturity: US evaluation. Radiology 2002; 225:59-64.
39. Tordoir JH, de Bruin HG, Hoeneveld H, et al. Duplex ultrasound scanning in the assessment of arteriovenous fistulas created for hemodialysis access: comparison with digital subtraction angiography. J Vasc Surg 1989; 10:122-128.
40. Ram SJ, Work J, Caldito GC, et al. A randomized controlled trial of blood flow and stenosis surveillance of hemodialysis grafts. Kidney Int 2003; 64:272-280.
41. Rooijens PP, Serafino GP, Vroegindeweij D, et al. Multi-slice computed tomographic angiography for stenosis detection in forearm hemodialysis arteriovenous fistulas. J Vasc Access 2008; 9:278-284.
42. Karadeli E, Tarhan NC, Ulu EM, et al. Evaluation of failing hemodialysis fistulas with multidetector CT angiography: comparison of different 3D planes. Eur J Radiol 2009; 69:184-192.
43. Ye C, Mao Z, Rong S, et al. Multislice computed tomographic angiography in evaluating dysfunction of the vascular access in hemodialysis patients. Nephron Clin Pract 2006; 104:c94-100.
44. Lin YP, Wu MH, Ng YY, et al. Spiral computed tomographic angiography—a new technique for evaluation of vascular access in hemodialysis patients. Am J Nephrol 1998; 18:117-122.
45. Persson PB, Hansell P, Liss P. Pathophysiology of contrast medium-induced nephropathy. Kidney Int 2005; 68:14-22.
46. Dittrich E, Puttinger H, Schillinger M, et al. Effect of radio contrast media on residual renal function in peritoneal dialysis patients—a prospective study. Nephrol Dial Transplant 2006; 21:1334-1339.
47. Moranne O, Willoteaux S, Pagniez D, et al. Effect of iodinated contrast agents on residual renal function in PD patients. Nephrol Dial Transplant 2006; 21:1040-1045.
48. Grobner T. Gadolinium—a specific trigger for the development of nephrogenic fibrosing dermopathy and nephrogenic systemic fibrosis? Nephrol Dial Transplant 2006; 21:1104-1108.
49. Prince MR, Zhang H, Morris M, et al. Incidence of nephrogenic systemic fibrosis at two large medical centers. Radiology 2008; 248:807-816.
50. Shellock FG, Kanal E. Safety of magnetic resonance imaging contrast agents. J Magn Reson Imaging 1999; 10:477-484.
51. Cochran ST, Bomyea K, Sayre JW. Trends in adverse events after IV administration of contrast media. AJR Am J Roentgenol 2001; 176:1385-1388.
52. Thomsen HS. Nephrogenic systemic fibrosis: A serious late adverse reaction to gadodiamide. Eur Radiol 2006; 16:2619-2621.
53. Marckmann P, Skov L, Rossen K, et al. Nephrogenic systemic fibrosis: suspected causative role of gadodiamide used for contrast-enhanced magnetic resonance imaging. J Am Soc Nephrol 2006; 17:2359-2362.
54. Kuo PH, Kanal E, Abu-Alfa AK, Cowper SE. Gadolinium-based MR contrast agents and nephrogenic systemic fibrosis. Radiology 2007; 242:647-649.
55. Chrysochou C, Buckley DL, Dark P, et al. Gadolinium-enhanced magnetic resonance imaging for renovascular disease and nephrogenic systemic fibrosis: critical review of the literature and UK experience. J Magn Reson Imaging 2009; 29:887-894.
56. Planken RN, Leiner T, Nijenhuis RJ, et al. Contrast-enhanced magnetic resonance angiography findings prior to hemodialysis vascular access creation: a prospective analysis. J Vasc Access 2008; 9:269-277.
57. Wentz KU, Frohlich JM, von Weymarn C, et al. High-resolution magnetic resonance angiography of hands with timed arterial compression (tac-MRA). Lancet 2003; 361:49-50.
58. Planken RN, Tordoir JHM, de Haan MW, et al. Contrast enhanced-MR angiography of upper extremity arteries and veins prior to vascular access surgery. Blood Purif 2005; 23:227-261.
59. Heye S, Maleux G, Marchal GJ. Upper-extremity venography: CO_2 versus iodinated contrast material. Radiology 2006; 241:291-297.
60. Heenan SD, Grubnic S, Buckenham TM, Belli AM. Transbrachial arteriography: indications and complications. Clin Radiol 1996; 51:205-209.
61. Duijm LE, Overbosch EH, Liem YS, et al. Retrograde catheterization of haemodialysis fistulae and grafts: angiographic depiction of the entire vascular access tree and stenosis treatment. Nephrol Dial Transplant 2009; 24:539-547.
62. Surratt RS, Picus D, Hicks ME, et al. The importance of preoperative evaluation of the subclavian vein in dialysis access planning. AJR Am J Roentgenol 1991; 156:623-625.

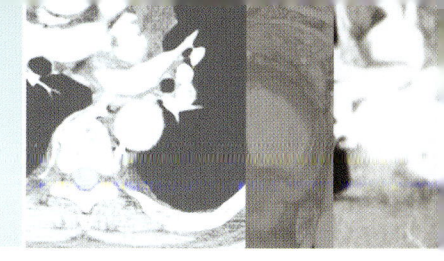

Index

A

A number, 270, 271t
Abdomen
  arterial anatomy of, 969-977. *See also named artery, e.g.*, Abdominal aorta.
  CT angiography of, 1061t, 1065-1068
    aorta in, 1065-1066, 1067f
    hepatic vasculature in, 1066, 1068f
    mesenteric vasculature in, 1066-1068, 1069f
    pancreas in, 1066, 1067f
    renal vasculature in, 1066, 1067f-1068f
  vascular disorders of, MR imaging of, 1451-1470. *See also under specific disorder.*
    gadolinium use and safety in, 1453
    methodology in, 1451
    of arteries, 1451-1452
    of veins and soft tissue, 1452-1453
  venous anatomy of
    portal circulation in, 1005-1009, 1006f-1007f
      differential considerations of, 1008-1009, 1008f, 1008t
      variants of, 1008
    systemic circulation in, 1009-1012, 1009f-1010f
      differential considerations of, 1011-1012, 1011f-1012f
      variants of, 1010-1011
Abdominal aorta, 969-976
  acute occlusion of, 1410-1411, 1411f-1413f
  anatomy of
    descriptions in, 969, 970f
    differential considerations of, 975, 976f
    normal variants in, 970-975
    pertinent imaging considerations and, 975-976
    specific areas in, 970-976
  aneurysm of. *See* Abdominal aortic aneurysm.
  aortography of, 1158-1159
  descending, 955-956
  dissection of, 1416-1417, 1416f
  imaging of
    contrast media in, 1398-1399
      dosage of, 1399
    CT angiography in, 1065-1066, 1067f
      protocol parameters for, 1061t
    CT scans in, technique of, 1397
    Doppler ultrasound in, anatomic considerations in, 1508, 1508f-1509f
    MR scans in
      coil choice for, 1398
      patient position for, 1397-1398
      pulse sequences in, 1398, 1398f
      technique of, 1397-1398
    techniques of, 1397-1398

Abdominal aorta *(Continued)*
  major branches of, 971t, 973f
  traumatic injury of, 1409-1410, 1410f
Abdominal aortic aneurysm, 1399-1404
  atherosclerotic disease causing, 1194, 1199
  clinical manifestations of, 1400
  differential diagnosis of, 1207t, 1402
  endovascular repair of, 1420, 1421f
    aneurysm sac (endoleak) after, 1426, 1428t
    clinical presentation after, 1426
    complication(s) of
      arterial dissection as, 1436
      colon necrosis as, 1435-1436
      endoleaks as, 1431-1434, 1431f-1434f
      graft infection as, 1434
      graft kinking as, 1434
      graft occlusion as, 1434-1435
      graft thrombosis as, 1434, 1434f-1436f
      hematoma at arteriotomy site as, 1436
      shower embolism as, 1435
    death during, 1426
    goal of, 1420
    graft placement in, 1422-1423, 1424f-1426f
      surgical conversion after, 1423-1424, 1427f, 1440, 1441t
    imaging of
      indications and algorithm for, 1426-1429
      techniques and findings in, 1429-1436, 1429f-1430f, 1430t
    postoperative assessment of, 1420-1436, 1423f-1428f
    postoperative management after, 1436-1437
    preprocedural interventions and, 1422-1423, 1423f
    success of, 1422
      anatomic appearance after, 1426, 1428f
    vs. open surgical repair, 1424-1426
  etiology and pathophysiology of, 1399-1400
  hybrid repair procedures in, 1181-1182, 1183f-1184f
  imaging of
    FDG-PET, 1402
    indications and algorithm for, 1400, 1400t
    MRA scan in, 1205-1206, 1401, 1402f
    radiography in, 1400, 1400f
    ultrasound in, 1400-1401, 1401f
  prevalence and epidemiology of, 1399
  rupture of, 1420
    signs of, 1401-1402, 1402f-1404f
  screening for, 1200
  surgical repair of, 1179-1180, 1211
    clinical presentation after, 1440-1441
      anastomotic pseudoaneurysms, 1441, 1447, 1449f
        postoperative management of, 1449

Abdominal aortic aneurysm *(Continued)*
      aortic graft infection, 1441, 1443-1447, 1446f-1447f
        postoperative management of, 1449
      aortocaval fistula, 1441, 1443
      aortoenteric fistula, 1441, 1445-1447, 1448f
        postoperative management of, 1447
      aortoiliac occlusive disease, 1441, 1447, 1448f
      renal infarction, 1447, 1449f
    complications of
      early postoperative, 1439-1440
      late postoperative, 1440
    contraindications to, 1180
    conversion from endovascular repair to, 1440, 1441t
    imaging after
      indications and algorithm for, 1441-1442
      techniques and findings in, 1442-1443, 1443f-1445f
    imaging findings in, 1180-1181, 1181f-1182f
    indications for, 1180
    mortality and survival after, 1440
    outcomes and complications of, 1176f, 1180
    postoperative assessment of, 1439-1447
    postoperative management of, 1447-1449
    vs. endovascular repair, 1424-1426
  treatment options for, 1402-1404
Abdominal trauma, vascular, 1468-1469, 1469f
AbiRahma criteria, in diagnosis of carotid stenosis, 1173, 1174t
Ablation procedures
  for arrhythmogenic right ventricular dysplasia, 894
  for atrial fibrillation, 445-446, 446f
  for left ventricular outflow tract obstruction, 881-882
Above-knee amputation, for chronic limb ischemia, 1583-1584
Above-knee femoropopliteal graft, patency of, 1590, 1590t
Abscess, embolization and, 1170
Acceleration index (AI), in Doppler imaging, 1045, 1513
Acceleration time (AT), in Doppler imaging, 1045, 1513
Acipimox, in ^{18}FDG imaging, 332-333
Acoustic noise, of MRI scanners, 267
Acoustic power, in Doppler ultrasonography, 1040

Acquisition protocols, for myocardial
    perfusion imaging with SPECT, 745-746
  dual isotope, 746
  same-day rest-stress Tc 99m radiotracer
    protocol, 746
  stress-redistribution thallium 201 protocol,
    746
  two-day rest-stress Tc 99m radiotracer
    protocol, 746
Acute aortic syndrome, 1288-1305
  dissection as, 1288-1296
  intramural hematoma as, 1296-1299
  penetrating atherosclerotic ulcer as,
    1299-1302
  ruptured aneurysm as, 1302-1303, 1303f
Acute coronary syndrome, 715-725
  angiography of, 722
  classic signs of, 722
  clinical presentation of, 716
  CT imaging of, 717-721, 718f-720f
    protocol parameters for, 720t
    University of Maryland triage studies in,
      721t
  definition of, 715
  differential diagnosis of, 723
  etiology and pathophysiology of, 715-716
  imaging of
    indications and algorithm for, 716
    technique and findings in, 716-722
  MR imaging of, 721, 721f
  myocardial perfusion imaging of, 742
  nuclear imaging of, 722, 722f
  percutaneous coronary interventions for,
    402, 723
  plaque rupture and, 61
  prevalence and epidemiology of, 715
  radiography of, 716, 717f
  reporting of, 723
  treatment options for, 723
  ultrasonography of, 716-717
Acute limb ischemia. See Limb ischemia, acute.
Acute lung injury, 1376
Acyanotic congenital heart disease. See
    Congenital heart disease (CHD),
    acyanotic.
Adaptive detector, in multislice CT, 1053-
    1054, 1053f
Adenocarcinoma, pancreatic. See Pancreatic
    adenocarcinoma.
Adenosine, 353
  chemical structure of, 284f
  in cardiac MRI stress testing, 267
  infusion of, in MR imaging, 733-734
  mechanism of action of, 354f
  perfusion imaging protocol with, 353, 355f
    contraindications to, 205, 206t
    exercise and, 357
    in PET, 316
    in SPECT, 284-285, 744-745
  side effects of, 353, 354t
Adrenal artery, 973
Adrenocortical carcinoma, inferior vena cava
    invasion by, 1530
Adson's maneuver, for thoracic outlet
    syndrome, 1669
Adult, congenital heart disease in, radiographic
    studies of, 89, 91f-92f
Adult respiratory distress syndrome (ARDS),
    1376-1377
  causes of, 1377b
  histopathologic abnormalities in, 1376-1377
  imaging findings in
    during exudative phase, 1377-1378, 1378f
    during proliferative phase, 1378, 1378f
  stages of, 1377b

Adventitial cystic disease, 987, 1600
  imaging of, 1604, 1605f
Agatson score, 459
Age, advanced, atherosclerosis and, 1196
Air accumulation, in ischemic heart disease,
    813
Air space (alveolar) edema, 1375f, 1376
Akinesia, definition of, 232
Alcohol, as embolic agent, 1168
Alcohol septal myocardial ablation, for left
    ventricular outflow tract obstruction,
    881-882
Aliasing, in Doppler ultrasonography, 1041,
    1041t
Allergy, contrast, as contraindication to CT
    angiography, 1614
Allograft(s), kidney
  Doppler ultrasonography of, 1519,
    1519f-1520f
  segmental infarction in, 1520, 1521f
Allograft rejection
  after cardiac transplantation, 812
  aortic, 820
  diagnosis of, 818
  postoperative management of, 821-823,
    822f
  renal, 1519, 1520f
Allograft renal vessels
  parameters in, normal values of, 1519b
  stenosis of, criteria for, 1519b
  thrombosis of, pitfalls in sonography of,
    1513
Alpha particles, 272, 272t
Alveolar damage, diffuse
  permeability edema with, 1376-1378. See
    also Pulmonary edema, permeability.
  permeability edema without, 1379
Alveolar (air space) edema, 85-87, 1375f, 1376
Alveolar hemorrhage, diffuse, 1383-1384, 1391
Ambiguity, directional, in Doppler
    ultrasonography, 1042, 1042f
American College of Rheumatology
    classification, of Takayasu arteritis, 1315t
American College of Rheumatology criteria,
    for giant cell arteritis, 1320t
American Heart Association (AHA)
    recommendations, for coronary artery
    bypass graft surgery, 416t
Ammonia N 13
  in PET imaging
    for identifying myocardial viability,
      799-800
    myocardial perfusion imaging with,
      749-750
  in PET/CT imaging, 325-326, 339-340, 340f,
    340t
Ampere-Maxwell law, 263
Amplatz vascular plug, as embolic agent, 1168
Amplitude, in Doppler imaging, 1043
Amputations, for chronic limb ischemia,
    1583-1584
Amyloid deposits, 861
  characteristics of, 861
Amyloidosis
  clinical presentation of, 862
  definition of, 861
  etiology and pathophysiology of, 861-862
  imaging of
    echocardiographic, 115-116, 116f
    indications and algorithm for, 862
    technique and findings in, 862-864,
      862f-864f, 872t
  prevalence and epidemiology of, 861
Analgesia, intravenous, for acute coronary
    syndrome, 723

Anastomosis
  microvascular, in coronary artery bypass
    graft surgery, 413, 415f-416f
  piggy-back technique of, in hepatic
    transplantation, 1534-1535, 1534f-1535f
Anastomotic pseudoaneurysm, 1441, 1447,
    1449f
  after abdominal aortic aneurysm repair,
    1180
  postoperative management of, 1449
Aneurysm
  aortic. See Aortic aneurysm.
  arterial, lower extremity. See Lower
    extremity aneurysm.
  bypass graft, after CABG surgery, 525
  coronary artery. See Coronary artery
    aneurysm.
  Doppler imaging of, 1044
  ductus, vs. patent ductus arteriosus,
    590-591, 591f
  false, 1271, 1277, 1277f. See also
    Pseudoaneurysm.
    delayed hyperenhancement MR imaging
      of, 209-210
  formation of, after surgical repair of
    coarctation of aorta, 539-540, 540f
  iliac artery. See Iliac artery aneurysm.
  nontraumatic, vs. patent ductus arteriosus,
    592-594, 594f
  popliteal artery. See Popliteal artery
    aneurysm.
  post–myocardial infarction, 94
  renal artery, Doppler ultrasound diagnosis
    of, 1515
  splanchnic artery, 1462-1463, 1463f-1464f
  true, 1271, 1277
  venous, after liver transplantation, 1551,
    1554f
Aneurysm sac, opacification of, after stent
    graft insertion. See Endoleak(s).
Angina
  stable, 715-716
    percutaneous coronary interventions for,
      402
  typical, definition of, 61-62
  unstable, percutaneous coronary
    interventions for, 402
Angiography, 1157-1161
  cerebral, 1159
  cine, of arrhythmogenic right ventricular
    dysplasia, 887, 887t
  computed tomographic. See Computed
    tomographic angiography (CTA).
  contraindications to, 1160
  contrast agents in, choice of, 1158
  digital subtraction. See Digital subtraction
    angiography (DSA).
  first-pass radionuclide, of ventricular
    function
    data acquisition in, 776-778, 779f
    image interpretation in, 778-779
    indications for, 775-776
  hepatic, 1159
  indications for, 1159-1160
  mesenteric, 1159
  multiple overlapping thin slab, 1094, 1094f
  of abdominal aorta, 1158-1159
  of acute coronary syndrome, 722
  of amyloidosis, 864
  of aortic aneurysm
    abdominal, 1442
    thoracic, 1282
  of aortic arch, 1158, 1158f
  of aortic dissection, 1294, 1294f
  of aortic trauma, thoracic, 1310-1311

Index

Angiography (Continued)
  of arteriovenous fistula failure, 1680-1682, 1682f-1683f
  of atherosclerosis, 1206-1207, 1207f
  of atrial septal defect, 568-569
  of cardiomyopathy
    dilated, 858
    hypertrophic, 882
    siderotic, 868
  of carotid arteries, 1159
  of carotid stenosis, 1219-1220, 1219f-1220f
  of chronic thromboembolic pulmonary hypertension, 1349-1350, 1367
    differential diagnosis in, 1350, 1351f
  of coarctation of aorta, 537
    during and after repair, 373, 376f
  of cor triatriatum, 633
  of coronary arteries, 412, 413f
  of coronary atherosclerosis, 708
  of double-outlet right ventricle, 684
  of eosinophilic endomyocardial disease, 866
  of giant cell arteritis, 1321, 1322f, 1414
  of inferior vena cava anomalies, 1529
  of inferior vena cava stenosis, after hepatic transplantation, 1535, 1536f-1537f
  of inferior vena cava tumors, 1531-1532
  of intramural hematoma of aorta, 1297-1298
  of ischemic heart disease, postoperative, 815
  of limb ischemia
    acute, 1577
    chronic, 1583
  of mycotic aortic aneurysm, 1407
  of myocarditis, 899
  of patent ductus arteriosus
    postoperative, 370, 374f
    preoperative, 370, 371f-374f
  of penetrating atherosclerotic ulcer, 1300-1301
  of peripheral artery disease, 1634
  of pulmonary artery stenosis, 375-377, 377f
    postoperative, 377, 379f
  of pulmonary hypertension
    chronic thromboembolic, 1349-1350, 1367
    differential diagnosis in, 1350, 1351f
    idiopathic, 1359
    with unclear multifactorial mechanisms, 1371
  of pulmonary insufficiency, 380-381, 380f-381f
  of pulmonary venous connections
    partial anomalous, 628
    total anomalous, 636, 637f
  of renal artery stenosis, 1502f, 1505
    in transplant recipient, 1564
  of renal vasculature, in living kidney donor, 1568
  of sarcoidosis, 870-871
  of single ventricle, 677, 678f
  of subclavian steal syndrome, 1329, 1330f
  of Takayasu arteritis, 1319f, 1389-1390, 1389f, 1414
  of tetralogy of Fallot, 646-647, 662
  of transposition of great arteries, 660
  of truncus arteriosus, 666
  of upper limb, 1159, 1159f
  of upper limb medium and small vessel disease, 1651-1652, 1658f
  of ventricular septal defect, 577-579, 580f
  outcomes and complications of, 1160
  pelvic, 1159
  postprocedural surveillance after, 1161
  preprocedural planning in, 1160-1161

Angiography (Continued)
  pulmonary, 1159f, 1336
    contraindications to, 1337b
  renal, 1159, 1160f
  specific regions of interest in, 1158-1159, 1158f-1160f
  three-dimensional
    optimal, 1131-1133, 1134f-1135f
    simulating, 1133, 1135f
  vascular access for, 1157-1158
Angiomyolipoma, renal, 1533, 1533f
Angioplasty, 1161-1163, 1161f
  and stent placement, in lower extremity revascularization, 1591-1592, 1592f-1593f
  for mesenteric atherosclerotic disease, 1212
  for Takayasu arteritis, 1318
  imaging findings in, 1162-1163
  indications for and contraindications to, 1162, 1163f
  outcomes and complications of, 1162
  percutaneous balloon, for coarctation of aorta, 539
  percutaneous transluminal, for peripheral artery disease, 1210-1211, 1210t
  percutaneous transluminal coronary. See Percutaneous transluminal coronary angioplasty (PTCA).
  special considerations in, 1162
Angiosarcoma
  definition of, 925
  differential diagnosis of, 926-927
  echocardiography of, 116
  manifestations of disease in, 925-926, 926f-927f
  pathology of, 925, 926f
  prevalence of, 925
  treatment options for, 927
Angiotensin-converting enzyme (ACE) inhibitor(s)
  for cerebrovascular atherosclerotic disease, 1208
  for peripheral artery disease, 1208-1209
  radiolabeled, 805, 806f
Angiotensin-converting enzyme inhibitor (ACEI) scintigraphy, of renal arteries
  captopril administration in, 1493
  contraindications to, 1492-1493
  enalaprilat administration in, 1493
  indications for, 1492
  pitfalls and solutions in, 1494
  postprocessing of, 1494
  procedure in, 1493-1494
  protocol for
    1-day, 1493
    2-day, 1493-1494
  reporting of, 1492, 1495f
  ^{99m}Tc-DTPA in, 1494
  ^{99m}Tc-MAG3 in, 1494
  technical requirements for, 1492
Angle of correction, in Doppler ultrasonography, 1040
Angle of insonation, in Doppler ultrasonography, 1039-1040, 1040f
  plaque evaluation and, 1229-1231, 1231f
Ankle-brachial index (ABI)
  in intermittent claudication, 1580-1581
  in peripheral artery disease, 1194
  ultrasound measurement of, 1202
Anomalous origin of left coronary artery from pulmonary artery (ALCAPA), 470, 606-607
  myocardial ischemia in, 470-471
  surgical treatment for, 471

Anomalous pulmonary venous connections, 18
  partial, 625-628. See also Partial anomalous pulmonary venous connections (PAPVC).
  total, 634-638. See also Total anomalous pulmonary venous connections (TAPVC).
Antecubital vein, median, 1020
Anterior interventricular vein (AIV), 51, 54f
Anticoagulants, for inferior vena cava thrombosis, 1539
Antihypertensive agents
  for cerebrovascular atherosclerotic disease, 1208
  for peripheral artery disease, 1208-1209
Antiplatelet therapy
  for cerebrovascular atherosclerotic disease, 1208
  for ischemic stroke or transient ischemic attack, 1222
  for peripheral artery disease, 1209
  preprocedural, for carotid artery stenting, 1224
Aorta
  abdominal. See Abdominal aorta.
  anatomy of, 549, 556, 556f
  aneurysm of. See Aortic aneurysm.
  ascending, post-stenotic dilation of, 1275, 1276f
  calcification of, 89, 90f
  coarctation of. See Coarctation of aorta.
  descending, mild bulging of, 1273, 1275f
  dissection of. See Aortic dissection.
  elastic lamina of, 549, 550f
  elasticity of
    MR imaging of, 556, 557f-558f
    reduced, 550
  in Marfan syndrome, 550-551, 551f
  intramural hematoma of, 1296-1299. See also Intramural hematoma, aortic.
  malposition of, 18, 20f
  MR imaging of, technique and protocol in, 555-556, 555t, 556f-558f
  occlusion of, balloon catheter embolectomy for, 1578
  penetrating atherosclerotic ulcer of
    definition of, 1299
    differential diagnosis of, 1301
    etiology and pathophysiology of, 1299
    manifestations of, 1299-1301, 1299f-1301f
    prevalence and epidemiology of, 1299
    reporting of, 1302
    treatment options for, 1301-1302
  post-traumatic pseudoaneurysm of, 592, 593f
  pseudocoarctation of, 539, 539f
  thoracic
    ascending. See Thoracic aorta, ascending.
    descending, 955-956
  traumatic injury of, vs. patent ductus arteriosus, 592, 593f
  wall of, intrinsic abnormalities of, 549
Aortic aneurysm, 434
  abdominal. See Abdominal aortic aneurysm.
  ascending, 1276
  endovascular repair of, endoleaks after, 1407-1409
    etiology and pathophysiology of, 1408, 1408f, 1408t
    imaging of
      indications and algorithm for, 1408
      techniques and findings in, 1408-1409, 1409f
    prevalence and epidemiology of, 1407
    treatment options for, 1409

Aortic aneurysm (Continued)
  inflammatory, 1404-1406
    clinical manifestations of, 1404
    definition of, 1404
    differential diagnosis of, 1405
    etiology and pathophysiology of, 1404
    imaging of, 1405, 1405f-1406f
    prevalence and epidemiology of, 1404
    treatment options for, 1405-1406
  mycotic (infectious), 594, 594f, 1406-1407, 1407f
  rupture of
    definition of, 1302
    etiology and pathophysiology of, 1302
    manifestations of, 1302-1303, 1303f
    treatment options for, 1303
  thoracic. See Thoracic aortic aneurysm.
  thoracoabdominal
    Crawford classification of, 1176-1177, 1177f, 1276, 1277f
    repair of, 1176-1178
Aortic arch
  anatomy of, 955, 957f-958f
  anomalous position of, 960-961, 961f
  aortography of, 1158, 1158f
  defined, 955
  development of, 10-11, 12f
    pathology in, 11
  double, 11, 544, 544f-545f, 958, 959f
  embryonic development of, 957, 958f
  interruption of
    vs. coarctation of aorta, 537-538, 539f
    vs. patent ductus arteriosus, 595, 595f
  left, with aberrant right subclavian artery, 544, 546f, 959-960, 960f
  radiography of, 72-73, 73f
  right
    subtypes of, 959, 959f
    with aberrant left subclavian artery, 11, 72, 73f, 544, 545f-546f, 959, 960f
    with mirror image branching, 11
Aortic atherosclerotic disease. See also Atherosclerosis.
  medical treatment of, 1209
  presenting findings in, 1198t
  prevalence and epidemiology of, 1194
  surgical/interventional treatment of, 1211
Aortic balloon valvotomy, 407f, 408-409
Aortic bifurcation, lesions involving, MR angiography of, 1635-1636
Aortic border, radiography of, ascending aorta in, 75-76
Aortic bypass graft, for Takayasu arteritis, 1318-1319, 1319f
Aortic dissection, 433-434, 434f
  abdominal, 1416-1417, 1416f
  aneurysmal, 1273, 1275f
  angiography of, 1294, 1294f
  chest radiography of, 1290, 1290f
  classic signs of, 1294, 1294f-1295f
  classification of, 434, 434f, 1289, 1289f
  clinical presentation of, 1289, 1289f
  CT imaging of, 1291, 1292f-1293f
  differential diagnosis of, 1294
  echocardiography of, 117, 118f
  etiology and pathophysiology of, 1288-1289, 1289f
  imaging of, indications and algorithm for, 1289-1290
  medical treatment of, 1295
  MR imaging of, 1291-1294, 1293f
  prevalence and epidemiology of, 1288
  repair of, surveillance studies after, 420f, 437
  reporting of, 1296

Aortic dissection (Continued)
  risk factors for, 433-434, 434t
  surgical/interventional treatment of
    for type A (ascending) dissection, 1295
    for type B (descending) dissection, 1295-1296, 1296f
  ultrasonography of, 1290-1291, 1290f
Aortic graft infection, 1441, 1443-1447, 1446f-1447f
  postoperative management of, 1449
Aortic isthmus
  other vascular entities at, vs. patent ductus arteriosus, 588-595, 590f
  traumatic injury to, 1306, 1308f
Aortic neck dilation, after abdominal aortic aneurysm repair, 1440
Aortic root
  anatomy of, 955, 956f
  dilation and regurgitation of, in tetralogy of Fallot, 641
Aortic root-to-right heart shunt, in acyanotic congenital heart disease, 384, 385t
Aortic sac, 3-4
Aortic spindle, vs. patent ductus arteriosus, 588, 590f
Aortic valve
  anatomy of, 35-36, 36f, 417, 417f
  bicuspid, 7
    MR imaging of, 66f, 552, 552f
    pathophysiology of, 551-552
    prevalence and epidemiology of, 551
  calcifications in, 87, 88f
    patterns of, 87
  prosthetic
    mechanical bileaflet, 420, 420f
    tissue, 420, 421f
    advantage of, 421
  replacement of, 418-419, 418f-419f
  velocity-encoded MR imaging of, 556
Aortic valve disease, surgery for, 417-422
  anatomic considerations in, 417-419, 417f-419f
  contraindications to, 420
  indications for, 419-420, 419t-420t
  outcomes and complications of, 418f, 420-421, 420f-421f
  postoperative surveillance after, 416
  preoperative imaging in, 421-422, 422f-423f
Aortic valve insufficiency
  severity of, classification of, 419t
  surgical intervention for, 389
Aortic valve regurgitation
  after arterial switch operation, 555
  clinical presentation of, 832
  definition of, 831
  etiology of, 831-832
  imaging of
    echocardiographic, 110, 832-833
    indications for, 832
    radiographic, 92-93
    techniques of, 832-833, 832f-833f
  medical treatment of, 833
  pathophysiology of, 418, 831-832
  prevalence of, 831
  quantification of, 241, 243f
  surgical treatment of, 833-834
    indications for, 420t
Aortic valve stenosis, 65
  catheter-based intervention for, 389
  clinical presentation of, 827-828
  critical, vs. coarctation of aorta, 538-539
  definition of, 827
  etiology of, 827

Aortic valve stenosis (Continued)
  imaging of
    echocardiographic, 109, 828
    indications for, 828
    radiographic, 92
    techniques of, 828-829, 828f-831f
  medical treatment of, 830
  pathophysiology of, 417-418, 827
  prevalence of, 827
  severity of, classification of, 419t
  surgical treatment of, 830, 832f. See also Prosthetic aortic valve.
    indications for, 419t
    success of, 421, 422f
Aorticopulmonary window, 72-73
Aortitis, 1314-1325. See also Giant cell arteritis; Takayasu arteritis.
  classification of, 1314, 1315t
  infected, 1275
  syphilitic, 1322-1324, 1322t, 1323f
  thoracic, differential diagnosis of, 1323-1324, 1324f
Aortobifemoral bypass, 1182
  contraindications to, 1182-1184
  imaging findings in, 1184-1185, 1184f-1185f
  indications for, 1182
  outcomes and complications of, 1184
Aortocaval fistula, 1441, 1443
Aortoduodenal fistula, after abdominal aortic aneurysm repair, 1180
Aortoenteric fistula, 1415-1416, 1416f, 1441, 1445-1447, 1448f
  postoperative management of, 1447
Aortography
  abdominal, 1158-1159
  arch, 1158, 1158f
Aortoiliac occlusive disease, 1441, 1447, 1448f
  hybrid procedures for, 1188-1189, 1188f
Aortoplasty, for aortic coarctation, 539
Aortopulmonary window, vs. patent ductus arteriosus, 588
Aortopulmonary-level shunt, in acyanotic congenital heart disease, 384, 385t
Apical thinning, myocardial perfusion imaging and, 748
Apolipoprotein E (APOE) gene, lipid abnormalities associated with, 1196
Apoptosis, 792
  targeting, 805
Arc of Buehler, 975
Arc of Riolan, 975, 976f
Arcuate artery, Doppler ultrasonography of, anatomic considerations in, 1507
Area-length method, of global left ventricular function, 231
Arrhythmias. See also specific arrhythmia.
  in arrhythmogenic right ventricular dysplasia, 885-886
Arrhythmogenic right ventricular cardiomyopathy (ARVC), 113, 237, 237f
Arrhythmogenic right ventricular dysplasia (ARVD), 884-895
  chest radiography of, 887
  cine angiography of, 887, 887t
  clinical presentation of, 885-892, 888f-889f
  CT imaging of, 888, 888f
  definition of, 884
  diagnosis of, 886, 886t
  differential diagnosis of, 890f, 892-893, 892t
  echocardiographic evaluation of, 113, 887-888, 888t
  electrocardiographic evaluation of, 886-887, 887t
  etiology and pathophysiology of, 884-885, 885f

Arrhythmogenic right ventricular dysplasia
  future directions for, 894
  genetics of, 885, 885t
  MR imaging of, 888-892, 889f-892f, 891t
  nuclear ventriculoscintigraphy of, 887
  patterns of disease in, 884
  prevalence and epidemiology of, 884
  reporting of, 894
  treatment options for, 893-894
Arterial dynamics, contrast media–enhanced, 160-161, 160f
  basic rules of, 161
Arterial embolic occlusion. See also Embolus (embolism).
  site of, in acute limb ischemia, 1574-1575, 1574f
Arterial mapping, left, contrast media injection protocol for, 164t-165t
Arterial stenosis, Doppler imaging of, 1044
Arterial switch procedure
  aortic regurgitation after, 555
  for transposition of great arteries, 554-555, 608, 608f-609f
    cardiac-gated CTA after, 612, 612f
    surgical outcome of, 608-609, 609f
Arterial thrombosis. See Thrombosis, arterial.
Arteriography. See Angiography.
Arterioles, pulmonary, 1353
Arterioportal shunting, MR imaging of, 1455-1456, 1456f
Arteriotomy site, hematoma at, after endovascular aneurysm repair, 1436
Arteriovenous fistula, 1600-1601, 1601f, 1672-1685
  after renal transplantation, 1520-1521, 1521f
  dysfunction of
    classic signs in, 1682
    differential diagnosis of, 1683
    treatment options for, 1683
  in hemodialysis patient
    creation of, 1672, 1673f
    role of imaging of, 1673
    use of, 1672-1673
    vascular evaluation of
      angiography in, 1680-1682, 1682f-1683f
      CT angiography in, 1676-1677, 1677f-1678f
      indications and algorithm for, 1674
      MR angiography in, 1677-1680, 1679f-1681f
      ultrasound in, 1675-1676, 1675f
  in renal transplant recipient, 1520-1521, 1521f
  vascular evaluation of, 1564-1566
    clinical presentation of, 1565
    etiology and pathophysiology of, 1564-1565
    imaging of
      indications and algorithm for, 1565
      technique and findings in, 1565, 1565f-1566f
    prevalence and epidemiology of, 1564
    treatment options for, 1565-1566, 1566f
  involving carotid arteries, Doppler imaging of, 1244, 1246f
  management of, 1601
    endovascular exclusion procedures in, 1603
Arteriovenous graft, 1672
Arteriovenous malformations
  hepatic, 1468
  splenic, 1468
Arteriovenous shunts, Doppler imaging of, 1044

Arteritis
  giant cell. See Giant cell arteritis.
  Takayasu. See Takayasu arteritis.
Artery(ies). See named artery.
Artifact(s). See also specific artifact.
  in cardiac CT imaging, 147, 147f-148f
  in coronary CT angiography, 495-500, 495t, 496f
  in Doppler ultrasonography, 1041-1043, 1041t
Aspirin
  for acute coronary syndrome, 723
  for cerebrovascular atherosclerotic disease, 1208
  for ischemic stroke or transient ischemic attack, 1222
  preprocedural, for carotid artery stenting, 1224
Asplenia complex, 18
ASTRAL trial, 1480
Asymmetric septal hypertrophy, in cardiomyopathy, MR imaging of, 875, 876f-877f
Asymptomatic Carotid Atherosclerosis Study (ACST), 1172, 1210
Atherectomy, 1156-1157, 1167
  devices for, 1156-1157
  in lower extremity revascularization, 1592, 1593f-1594f
  percutaneous transluminal coronary rotational, 400, 401f
Atheroembolus, 1575. See also Embolus (embolism).
Atheroma, 705
  thin cap, and vulnerable plaque, 706
Atherosclerosis
  aortic, 1194
    medical treatment of, 1209
    presenting findings in, 1198t
    prevalence and epidemiology of, 1194
    surgical/interventional treatment of, 1211
  cerebrovascular, 1194
    medical treatment of, 1208
    surgical/interventional treatment of, 1210
  clinical presentation of, 1198-1199, 1198t
  coronary, 59-62, 60f-61f. See also Coronary artery disease (CAD), atherosclerotic.
    calcium associated with, 457. See also Coronary artery calcium (CAC).
  definition of, 1193
  differential diagnosis of, 1207-1208, 1207t
  etiology and pathophysiology of, 1195-1196
  extracellular matrix formation in, 1195
  fibrous cap in, 1195, 1196f
  Glagov phenomenon in, 1195, 1195f
  imaging of
    angiographic, 1206-1207, 1207f
    CT angiography of, 1203-1204, 1203f
    indications and algorithm for, 1199-1200, 1200f
    MR angiography of, 1204-1206, 1205f
    PET scan, 1206
    radiographic, 1201
    technique and findings in, 1201-1207, 1201t
    ultrasound, 1201-1203, 1202f
  injury hypothesis of, response to, 1195
  mesenteric, 1194
    medical treatment of, 1210
    surgical/interventional treatment of, 1212
  oxidation hypothesis of, 1195
  peripheral, 1194. See also Peripheral arterial disease.

Atherosclerosis (Continued)
  medical treatment of, 1208-1210
  surgical/interventional treatment of, 1210-1211, 1210t
  physical examination of, 1199
  plaque in. See Plaque, atherosclerotic.
  prevalence and epidemiology of, 1193-1194
  primary stages of, 1195
  progression of, to clinical significance, 1195-1196, 1195f-1196f
  renal. See Renal atherosclerotic disease.
  reporting of, 1212
  risk factors for, 1196-1198, 1197t
    modifiable, 1196-1198, 1197f
    non-modifiable, 1196
    novel, 1198
  thoracic aortic aneurysm caused by, 1271, 1272f
  treatment options for
    medical, 1208-1210
    surgical/interventional, 1210-1212, 1210t
  vascular biology of, 60-61, 60f-61f
Atherosclerotic ulcer, penetrating
  definition of, 1299
  differential diagnosis of, 1301
  etiology and pathophysiology of, 1299
  manifestations of, 1299-1301, 1299f-1301f
  prevalence and epidemiology of, 1299
  reporting of, 1302
  treatment options for, 1301-1302
Atoll sign, in Wegener's granulomatosis, 1385, 1386f
Atom, structure of, 270, 271f
Atresia, premature, of pulmonary vein, 1001-1002
Atrial amyloidosis, isolated, 861. See also Amyloidosis.
Atrial baffle leak, after atrial switch procedure, 612
Atrial border, left, radiography of, 74, 74f-75f
  in lateral projection, 77
Atrial fibrillation
  clinical presentation of, 443
  clinically relevant anatomy in, 443-444, 443f-445f
  definition of, 442
  epidemiology of, 442
  lone, 442
  pathophysiology of, 442-443
  prevalence of, 442
  reporting of, 451-452
  treatment of, 444-451
    ablation procedure in, 445-446, 446f
    imaging techniques in, 446-450
      image fusion, 449-450, 450f
      MRI scans, 449, 450f
      multidetector CT, 447-449, 447f-449f
    postprocedural imaging after, 450-451
      atrioesophageal fistula in, 451, 451f
      pulmonary venous stenosis in, 450-451, 451f
      recurrent atrial fibrillation in, 451
    Wolf mini-Maze procedure in, 445, 446f
Atrial isthmus, left, implication of, in recurrent atrial fibrillation, 451
Atrial kick, 57, 59
Atrial myxoma, 906. See also Myxoma.
Atrial septal defect (ASD), 363-366
  angiography of, 568-569
  clinical presentation of, 564
  considerations regarding, 383, 385t
  coronary sinus, 563, 567f
  CT imaging of, 566, 568f
  definition of, 563

Atrial septal defect (ASD) (Continued)
    device closure for, 363
        contraindications to, 363-364
        indications for, 363
        outcomes and complications of, 364
        postoperative surveillance after, 365-366, 367f-368f
        preoperative imaging and, 364-365, 364f-366f
    differential diagnosis of, 570
    etiology and pathophysiology of, 563-564
    imaging of
        indications and algorithm for, 564
        technique and findings in, 564-569
    medical treatment of, 570
    MR imaging of, 566-567, 568f-569f
    nuclear imaging of, 567-568, 569f
    ostium primum, 8, 563, 566f
    ostium secundum, 8, 363, 563-564
        radiography of, 90, 91f
    prevalence and epidemiology of, 563
    radiography of, 564-565, 565f-566f
    reporting of, 570
    sinus venosus, 563, 567f
    surgical/interventional treatment of, 570
    types of, 563
    ultrasonography of, 117-118, 565-566, 566f-567f
    vs. partial anomalous pulmonary venous connections, 628
Atrial septum
    anatomy of, 33
    anomalies associated with, evaluation of, 24, 26f
    developmental pathology of, 8
    formation of, 7-8, 9f
Atrial situs ambiguous, 16, 17f
Atrial switch procedure
    atrial baffle leak after, 612
    for transposition of great arteries, 389, 609-610, 609f-610f
    imaging after, 612
Atrial tumors
    left, 432, 433f
    right, 432, 433f
Atrial-level shunt, in acyanotic congenital heart disease, 383, 385t
Atrioesophageal fistula, after ablation for atrial fibrillation, 451, 451f
Atrioventricular canal, developmental pathology of, 5
Atrioventricular connection(s)
    biventricular, types of, 19-20, 22f
    twisted, 20, 24f
    univentricular, 119, 119f
        types of, 20, 23f
Atrioventricular groove, 39-40, 40f
Atrioventricular junction
    first connecting segment of, 19-20, 22f-24f
    second connecting segment of, 22-24, 25f
Atrioventricular node
    abnormal development in, congenitally corrected transposition of great arteries, 606
    in cardiac electrophysiology, 57
Atrioventricular septal defect
    multiple-level shunts in, 386
    surgical treatment of, 386, 387f
Atrioventricular sulcus, 3-4
Atrium (atria). See also Atrial entries.
    identification of, 13-14, 14f
    left
        accessory appendage of, 32-33, 32f, 443, 443f. See also Left atrial appendage.

Atrium (atria) (Continued)
    anatomy of, 32-33, 32f, 443-444, 443f
    diastolic filling patterns in, 103, 106f
    echocardiographic imaging of, 103, 104f-105f
    formation of, 10, 11f
    morphologic, features of, 14, 14f
    oblique vein of, 53-55
    venous component of, 443-444, 444f-445f
    vestibular component of, 443
    primitive, paired, 3-4
    right
        anatomy of, 30-31, 32f
        formation of, 8-10, 10f
        morphologic, features of, 13-14, 14f
    third, 632. See also Cor triatriatum.
Attenuation, in photon-matter interactions, 276
Attenuation correction, in PET imaging, 308
    protocols for, 311-312
    placement of, 312
Attenuation event, in PET imaging, 306, 306f-307f
Attenuation maps, in PET imaging, and conversion to CT images, 308-309, 309f
Attenuation mismatch, in PET imaging, 309-311
    patient motion causing, 309, 310f
    respiratory and contractile cardiac motion causing, 309-310, 311f
    thoracic cavity drift causing, 310-311, 311f
Auger electron, 271-272, 272f
Autocorrelation, in Doppler ultrasonography, 1035-1036
Autonomic innervation, targeting, 805-807, 806f
Autoregulation, of coronary blood flow, 352
Autosomal dilated cardiomyopathy, 851-852. See also Cardiomyopathy, dilated.
Autosomal dominant inheritance, of arrhythmogenic right ventricular dysplasia, 884-885, 885t
Autosomal dominant myxoma, 905. See also Myxoma.
Autosomal recessive inheritance, of arrhythmogenic right ventricular dysplasia, 884-885, 885t
Axial images
    in cardiac CT imaging, 168-169
    in coronary CT angiography, 500
    in phase contrast MR angiography, 1096, 1097f
Axial resolution, in CT angiography, 1056
Axillary artery, 989-990, 990f
Axillary vein, 1661, 1662f
Axillary-femoral bypass graft, 981-982, 982f
Axillofemoral bypass graft, 1586-1588, 1587f
Azygos vein
    anatomy of, 1000, 1000f-1001f
    variations in, 1000, 1002f
    continuation of, in inferior vena cava anomaly, 1525, 1526f
    radiography of, 76-77

B

Back pain, postoperative new-onset, ischemic heart disease and, 813
Balloon(s)
    as embolic agent, 1168
    compliant and noncompliant, 1156
    in percutaneous vascular interventions, 1156

Balloon angioplasty
    cryoplasty, 1156
    cutting, 1156
        in lower extremity revascularization, 1593
    percutaneous, for coarctation of aorta, 539
Balloon catheter embolectomy, for saddle embolus, 1578
Balloon dilation, for pulmonary artery stenosis, 375. See also Pulmonary artery stenosis, balloon dilation for.
Balloon pump placement, intra-aortic, carotid Doppler waveform pattern after, 1244-1245, 1247f
Balloon thrombectomy, for iliac occlusion, 1578, 1578f
Balloon valvotomy
    aortic, 407f, 408-409, 830
    mitral, 407f, 408, 836
    pulmonic, 408f, 409
Balloon valvuloplasty, mitral, percutaneous, 427, 428t
Balloon-mounted stents, 1157
Banding artifacts, in CT angiography, 1070
Bare metal stent, 515, 516f
    risk of thrombosis in, 516, 517f
Baseline shift, in Doppler ultrasonography, 1041
Basilic vein, in upper extremity, 1020-1022, 1021f-1022f
Bat-wing appearance, of pulmonary edema, 86
Beak sign, in type B aortic dissection, 1294, 1294f
Beam(s), ultrasound, 1033, 1034f
Beam filtration, increased, to reduce radiation in CT imaging, 153-154
Beam hardening artifacts, in coronary CT angiography, 495-496, 495t, 496f
Beam pitch, increased, to reduce radiation in CT imaging, 153
Beam-hardening artifact, in CT angiography, 1070
Beer's law, 1047
Behçet syndrome, 1387, 1388f
Below-knee amputation, for chronic limb ischemia, 1583-1584
Below-knee femoropopliteal graft, patency of, 1590, 1590t
Bernoulli equation, modified, estimation of pressure gradients by, 99, 240, 241f
Beta particle emission, 272, 272t, 273f
Beta-blockers
    for aortic dissection, 1295
    for peripheral artery disease, 1208-1209
    used in cardiac imaging, 156
        contraindications to, 158t
        effects mediated by, 157t
        protocols for, 143-144, 156-157, 158t
B-flow image, in ultrasonography, 1034, 1037
Bidirectional superior cavopulmonary connection (BSCC), in single ventricle repair, 671-672
    MR imaging after, 674-675
Bile duct injury, 1468
Binding energy, 271
Bipolar gradients, in phase contrast MR angiography, 1095, 1096f
Black blood imaging, 1099-1100, 1100f
    of cardiac anatomy, 182-184
        acquisition parameters in, 183-184, 184f
        blood suppression achievement in, 183, 183f
Blalock-Taussig shunt
    for decreased pulmonary blood flow, 391
    modified, for tetralogy of Fallot, 648

Bleed localization scan, GI. *See* Gastrointestinal bleed localization scan.
Bleeding. *See* Hemorrhage.
Blood flow
  in Doppler imaging
    quantification of, 1045
    turbulent, 1043, 1043t
  MR evaluation of, 239-250
    flow-encoding axes in, 239-240, 241f
    indications for, 240
    limitations and pitfalls in, 240, 242f
    phase contrast imaging in, 239-240, 240f
    technical requirements for, 239-240, 240f-242f
    techniques for, 240-249
      in coarctation of aorta, 242-243, 244f
      in pulmonary flow evaluation, 244-249, 246f-248f
      in shunting, 243-244, 245f
      in valvular heart disease, 241-242, 243f
    velocity encoding in, 240, 242f
  pulmonary, anatomy and physiology of, 1353
Blood vessels. *See also named artery or vein.*
  in three-dimensional image
    automated extraction of, 1129
    automated pathline detection of, 1135-1136, 1136f
      validation of, 1136, 1136t
    bifurcation of, projection overlap in, 1133, 1135f
    lumen analysis of, 1134
    presegmentation of, 1129, 1130f
    segmentation of, 1131-1132, 1133f
      lumen, 1136-1137, 1137f-1138f
      validation of, 1137, 1139f, 1139t
    stenosis of, quantification of, 1131
    wall morphology of, assessment of, 1137-1138, 1139f-1140f
  wall of
    CT angiography of, 488-489, 489f-490f
    layers of, 60, 60f
Blooming artifact
  in coronary CT angiography, 495t, 496, 496f-497f
  in Doppler evaluation of plaque, 1228-1229, 1230f
Blunt trauma
  aortic, 1306, 1307f. *See also* Thoracic aortic trauma.
    acute injury due to, 592, 593f
    with deceleration mechanism injury, 1273
  upper extremity, 1644
Blurring artifacts, in coronary CT angiography, 495t, 496-499, 498f-499f
B-mode ultrasonography, 1034. *See also* Ultrasonography.
  image in, 1034, 1037
Bohr atom, 270, 271f
Bolus
  in contrast-enhanced CT angiography
    testing of, 1059-1060, 1062, 1399
    tracking of, 1058-1060, 1062
  in contrast-enhanced MR angiography, timing of, 1086-1087, 1088f, 1399
Bolus-triggering technique, of contrast media injection, 161-162, 1399
Bony pelvis. *See also* Pelvis.
  venous origin outside, 1012, 1013f-1014f
Bovine arch, 957, 958f
Bovine jugular venous valve, in pulmonary insufficiency repair, 379, 379f
Bovine xenograft, in vascular bypass surgery, 1586, 1587f

Brachial artery
  anatomy of
    normal, 991-994, 992f-993f
    variants of, 994
  angiographic access via, 1158
Brachial artery reactivity testing, 1202
Brachial vein, anatomy of, 1023, 1023f, 1661, 1662f
Brachiocephalic vein, anatomy of, 1023, 1023f, 1661, 1662f
  variant, 999
Brain perfusion tomography
  image interpretation of, 1149-1150, 1150f
  indications and contraindications to, 1148, 1149f
  pitfalls and solutions in, 1148-1149
Breath-hold technique
  used in cardiac CT imaging, 144
  used in MR imaging, 1398, 1398f
    cardiac, 202
Breathing, sleep-disordered, 1365-1366
Bremsstrahlung, 274-275
Bronchial artery, 965
Brugada syndrome, vs. arrhythmogenic right ventricular dysplasia, 893
Bruit, in carotid stenosis, 1218-1219
Budd-Chiari syndrome, 1011, 1011f, 1529
  clinical presentation of, 1461
  definition of, 1461
  differential diagnosis of, 1462
  etiology and pathophysiology of, 1461
  MR imaging of, 1461, 1462f
  treatment options for, 1462
Buerger disease (thromboangiitis obliterans), 1645, 1651-1652, 1658f. *See also* Upper extremity, medium and small vessel disease of.
  etiology and pathophysiology of, 1646
  incidence of, 1646
Bulboventricular looping, of primitive heart tube, 4, 5f
Bulbus cordis, 3-4
Bundle of His, in cardiac electrophysiology, 57-58
Butterfly appearance, of pulmonary edema, 86
N-Butyl cyanoacrylate, as embolic agent, 1168
Bypass graft(s)
  aneurysm of, after CABG surgery, 525
  arterial, 981-982. *See also specific bypass graft, e.g.,* Coronary artery bypass graft (CABG) *entries.*
  choice of conduit for, 522
  extra-anatomic, in vascular bypass surgery, 1586-1588, 1587f-1589f
  thrombosis and occlusion of, after CABG surgery, 524-525, 527f-529f
  thrombosis of, 1573

C

^{11}C-acetate, in PET imaging, 343-344
Cadaveric hepatic transplantation. *See also* Hepatic transplantation.
  surgical anatomy of, 1546-1547, 1547f
Calcification(s)
  aortic aneurysm, 1279
  atherosclerosis associated with, 60-61, 457, 707. *See also* Plaque, atherosclerotic.
  coronary. *See* Coronary artery calcium (CAC).
  femoral artery, 1188, 1188f
  great vessel, 89, 90f

Calcification(s) *(Continued)*
  heavy, in coronary CT angiography, 479-481, 483f-484f
  myocardial, 87, 87f
  pericardial, 82, 82f
  valvular, 87, 88f
Calcified amorphous cardiac tumor, 919-920, 919f-920f
Calcified stenosis, angioplasty and, 1162
Calcium channel blockers, used in cardiac imaging, 157, 158t
  contraindications to, 158t
Camera
  gamma
    components of, 276, 276f
    used in SPECT, 739
  PET, 304-305
Cancer. *See at anatomic site; specific neoplasm.*
Captopril, oral administration of, in ACEI renal scintigraphy, 1493
^{15}O-Carbon monoxide, 340
Cardiac. *See also* Heart *entries.*
Cardiac amyloidosis. *See* Amyloidosis.
Cardiac anomalies. *See specific anomaly.*
Cardiac catheterization
  for hypertrophic cardiomyopathy, 882
  in diagnosis and treatment of heart defects, 383
  standard projection views for, 416t
Cardiac cycle, abnormal Doppler waveform patterns involving, 1242-1245
  arteriovenous fistula, 1244, 1246f
  carotid dissection, 1243, 1245f
  carotid pseudoaneurysm, 1243, 1246f
  intra-aortic balloon pump, 1244-1245, 1247f
Cardiac devices, as MRI safety issue, 264-266
Cardiac electrophysiology, 57-58, 58f
Cardiac embryology, 3-25, 4f-27f. *See also specific components of heart.*
Cardiac events, coronary artery calcium as predictor of, 461-462
Cardiac function analysis, in hypertrophic cardiomyopathy, MR imaging of, 876-877, 879f-880f
Cardiac myocytes. *See* Myocytes.
Cardiac pacemakers, as MRI safety issue, 264-265
Cardiac resynchronization therapy (CRT), for dilated cardiomyopathy, 858
Cardiac rupture, post-myocardial, 94
Cardiac sarcoidosis. *See* Sarcoidosis.
Cardiac segment(s), major
  first: viscerotrial situs, 16-18, 17f-19f
  second: ventricular loop, 18, 19f
  third: great arterial relationship, 18, 20f
  analysis of, 16-18
  identification of, 13-16
Cardiac surgery, coronary CT angiography in, 486-487, 488f
Cardiac tamponade. *See* Tamponade.
Cardiac tumors, 905-937
  benign, 905-920. *See also named tumor, e.g.,* Myxoma.
  differential diagnosis of, 935t
  in hypertrophic cardiomyopathy, MR imaging of, 876, 878f
  malignant, 920-934. *See also named tumor, e.g.,* Angiosarcoma.
  metastatic, 921-922
  summary of, 934-935
Cardiac vein(s)
  anatomy of, 36
  anterior, 55
  great, 51-52, 54f

Cardiac vein(s) (Continued)
  middle, 52-53, 54f
  small, 53, 54f
Cardiac wall motion
  abnormalities of, 216-217
    during dobutamine infusion, 218, 220f
  MR assessment of, 188-190, 189f-190f
Cardiac wall thickness, end-diastolic, 782
Cardiomegaly
  in Ebstein anomaly, 653, 654f
  with decreased pulmonary vascularity, 651-653, 652f
Cardiomyopathy
  arrhythmogenic right ventricular, 237, 237f
  dilated
    clinical presentation of, 852
    definition of, 851
    differential diagnosis of, 858
    etiology and pathophysiology of, 851-852
    imaging of
      angiographic, 858
      CT scans in, 853-855, 854f
      indications and algorithm for, 852
      MR scans in, 855-857, 856f-857f
      nuclear medicine, 857-858, 857f
      radiographic, 852
      ultrasound, 110, 852-853, 853f
    medical treatment of, 858
    prevalence and epidemiology of, 851
    reporting of, 859
    surgical/interventional treatment of, 858
    vs. arrhythmogenic right ventricular dysplasia, 893
  hypertrophic, 63, 874-883
    asymmetric septal, MR imaging of, 875, 876f-877f
    cardiac function analysis in, MR imaging of, 876-877, 879f-880f
    cardiac neoplasms in, MR imaging of, 876, 878f
    clinical presentation of, 874
    coronary reserve flow in, MR imaging of, 879
    etiology and pathophysiology of, 874
    imaging of
      angiographic, 882
      CT, 874-875, 875f
      MRI scans in, 875-882
        morphology in, 875-876, 875t, 876f-878f
        radiographic, 94
        ultrasound, 110-113, 874
    impaired myocardial perfusion in, MR imaging of, 877
    left ventricular outflow tract obstruction in
      MR imaging of, 879-882, 881f
      treatment of, 881-882
    myocardial viability in, MR imaging of, 877-879, 880f
    prevalence and epidemiology of, 874
    surgical/interventional treatment of, 882
    ventricular mass in, MR imaging of, 875-876, 878f
  ischemic, 62
  noncompaction, echocardiography of, 113, 114f-115f
  restrictive, 861
    additional causes of, 871
    amyloidosis associated with, 861-864
    differential diagnosis of, 871
    eosinophilic endomyocardial disease associated with, 864-866

Cardiomyopathy (Continued)
    imaging features of, 872t
      echocardiographic, 113
      radiographic, 94
    reporting of, 871
    sarcoidosis associated with, 868-871
    treatment options for, 871
  siderotic
    clinical presentation of, 867
    definition of, 866
    etiology and pathophysiology of, 866-867
    imaging of
      indications and algorithm for, 867
      technique and findings in, 867-868, 868f, 872t
    medical treatment of, 871
    prevalence and epidemiology of, 866
  tako-tsubo, 107
Cardiopulmonary bypass, in coronary artery bypass graft surgery, 412-413, 414f
Cardiovascular disease, syphilitic manifestations in, 1322t
Cardioverter-defibrillators, implantable
  as MRI safety issue, 264-265
  as PET image artifact, 321-322, 322f
  for arrhythmogenic right ventricular dysplasia, 894
Carney complex, 905
Carotid artery
  anatomy of, 961-963, 961f-963f
    variations in, 962-963, 963f-964f
  angiography of, 1159
  bifurcation of, 961-962, 961f
    disease at, risk factors for, 1227
    variability of, 962
  common
    division of, 961
    normal Doppler tracing of, 1231-1232, 1232f. See also Doppler ultrasonography, of carotid arteries.
  CT angiography of, 1060, 1062f, 1260-1267. See also Computed tomographic angiography (CTA), carotid.
    protocol parameters for, 1061t
  dissection of, 1242-1243
    CT angiography of, 1262, 1263f
    Doppler imaging of, 1243, 1245f
  external, 961, 961f-962f
    normal Doppler tracing of, 1231-1232, 1232f. See also Doppler ultrasonography, of carotid arteries.
    variations of, 963, 963f
    vs. internal carotid artery, 1232, 1233f
  internal, 961-962, 961f-962f
    normal Doppler tracing of, 1231-1232, 1232f. See also Doppler ultrasonography, of carotid arteries.
    stenosis of. See also Carotid artery stenosis.
      caliper measurements of
        direct, 1258, 1259f
        multiplanar reformations in, 1258, 1259f
      grading of, 1227, 1228f, 1233, 1234f-1235f
      in contralateral side, 1236-1237, 1238f
      measuring and reporting of, 1258-1259
      vs. external carotid artery, 1232, 1233f
    MR angiography of, 1252-1259. See also Magnetic resonance angiography (MRA), contrast-enhanced, of carotid arteries.

Carotid artery (Continued)
  occlusive disease of, 1217-1226. See also Carotid artery stenosis.
  pseudoaneurysm of, Doppler imaging of, 1243, 1246f
  stenting of, status and patency in, CT angiographic evaluation of, 1261-1262, 1262f
  tortuous, peak systolic velocity in, 1235, 1236f
  ulceration of, CTA detection of, 1266-1267
  ultrasound evaluation of, 1227-1250. See also Doppler ultrasonography, of carotid arteries.
Carotid artery stenosis, 1217-1225. See also Stroke.
  asymptomatic, treatment of, 1222
  clinical presentation of, 1218-1219
  definition of, 1217
  differential diagnosis of, 1221
  etiology of, 1218
  imaging of
    angiographic, 1219-1220, 1219f-1220f
    CT angiography in, 1220
    indications and algorithm for, 1219
    MR angiography in, 1220
    ultrasound, 1220, 1220f
  internal
    caliper measurements of
      direct, 1258, 1259f
      multiplanar reformations in, 1258, 1259f
    grading of, 1227, 1228f, 1233, 1234f-1235f
    in contralateral side, 1236-1237, 1238f
    measuring and reporting of, 1258-1259
  pathophysiology of, 1218, 1218f
  plaque in, morphology of, 1220-1221, 1221f
  prevalence and epidemiology of, 1217-1218
  reporting of, 1224-1225
  symptomatic, treatment of, 1222
  treatment option(s) for
    carotid artery stenting as, 1222-1224
      procedure for, 1224, 1224f
    carotid endarterectomy as, 1222, 1223f. See also Carotid endarterectomy.
    current indications in, 1224
    for asymptomatic carotid stenosis, 1222
    for symptomatic carotid stenosis, 1222
    medical, 1222
    synopsis of, 1221-1224
Carotid artery stenting, 1222-1224
  procedure for, 1224, 1224f
  recommendations for, 1224
  status and patency in, CT angiographic evaluation of, 1261-1262, 1262f
Carotid coils, dedicated, in contrast-enhanced MR angiography, 1253-1254
Carotid endarterectomy, 1172-1175, 1222, 1223f
  contraindications to, 1172-1173
  for cerebrovascular atherosclerotic disease, 1210
  imaging findings in
    postoperative surveillance and, 1174-1175
    preoperative assessment and, 1173-1174, 1173f-1175f, 1174t
    preoperative planning and, 1174
  indications for, 1172
  outcomes and complications of, 1173
Carotid intimal-medial thickness (CIMT), ultrasound measurement of, 1199-1202, 1202f
Carotid Revascularization Endarterectomy versus Stent Trial (CREST), 1222-1223

Carotid triangle, 961-962, 963f
Carotid-subclavian bypass, 1175
 contraindications to, 1175
 imaging findings in, 1175-1176, 1175f-1176f
 indications for, 1175
Carrel patch, 1546
Catecholamines, radiolabeled, in PET/SPECT imaging, 806, 806f
Catheter(s), 1155-1156
 central venous, deep vein thrombosis associated with, 1662, 1663f
 Fogarty embolectomy, 1577-1578, 1577f
Catheter ablation, for arrhythmogenic right ventricular dysplasia, 894
Caudate lobe vein, 1010
Celiac stenosis, CT angiography of, 1066-1068
Celiac trunk, branches of, 970-972, 971f, 973f
Cell death
 after myocardial ischemia, 792
 programmed, 792
 targeting, 805
Cell survival, programmed, 792
Central venous catheter, deep vein thrombosis associated with, 1662, 1663f
Cephalic vein, in upper extremity, 1020-1022, 1021f-1022f
Cerebral angiography, 1159
Cerebral artery, fetal origin of, 963, 964f
Cerebral embolism, in infective endocarditis, 429, 429f
Cerebrovascular atherosclerotic disease. *See also* Atherosclerosis.
 differential diagnosis of, 1207t
 medical treatment of, 1208
 presenting findings in, 1198t
 prevalence and epidemiology of, 1194
 surgical/interventional treatment of, 1210
Cervicoaxillary compression syndrome, 1644
CHARGE syndrome, 640
Chelation therapy, for peripheral artery disease, 1209
Chest pain
 acute, 715. *See also* Acute coronary syndrome.
 clinical classification of, 482t
 in emergency department setting
  coronary artery calcium assessment and, 462
  CT angiographic evaluation of, 485-486, 487f
 sudden-onset, postoperative, ischemic heart disease and, 813
Chest radiography. *See also* Radiography.
 in intensive care, 94-96, 95f, 95t
 of acute coronary syndrome, 716, 717f
 of amyloidosis, 862
 of angiosarcoma, 926
 of aortic aneurysm
  ruptured, 1302
  thoracic, 1279-1280, 1280f
 of aortic dissection, 1290, 1290f
 of aortic regurgitation, 92-93, 832, 832f
 of aortic stenosis, 92, 828, 828f
 of aortic trauma, thoracic, 1306-1307, 1308f
 of aortitis, syphilitic, 1323, 1323f
 of arrhythmogenic right ventricular dysplasia, 887
 of atherosclerotic ulcer, penetrating, 1300
 of atrial septal defect, 564-565, 565f-566f
  ostium secundum, 90, 91f
  postoperative, 365-366, 368f
 of Behçet syndrome, 1387, 1388f
 of cardiac borders, 71-97
  aortic arch and, 72-73, 73f
  aortic border in, ascending, 75-76

Chest radiography *(Continued)*
 atrial border in, left, 74, 74f-75f
  in lateral projection, 77
 azygos vein and, 76-77
 in left anterior oblique projection, 77-78, 80f
 in right anterior oblique projection, 77, 79f
 left ventricle in, lateral projection of, 77
 measurement of heart size by, 78-80
 mediastinal border in
  left, 72, 72f-73f
  right, 75, 76f
 normal and abnormal, 71-78
 pulmonary artery border in, 74, 74f
 ventricular border in
  left, 74-75, 75f-76f
  right, 75
 of cardiac metastases, 923, 923f
 of cardiac tumor, calcified amorphous, 919, 920f
 of cardiomyopathy
  dilated, 852
  hypertrophic, 94
  restrictive, 94
  siderotic, 867
 of Churg-Strauss syndrome, 1390, 1390f
 of coarctation of aorta, 536
  classic signs in, 537, 537f
  thoracic, 89-90, 91f
 of congenital heart disease, in adult, 89, 91f-92f
 of cor triatriatum, 632, 633f
 of coronary artery calcification, 88, 89f
 of diffuse alveolar hemorrhage, 1384
 of double-outlet right ventricle, 682, 682f
 of Ebstein anomaly, 653, 654f
 of eosinophilic endomyocardial disease, 865
 of fibroma, 912
 of Goodpasture syndrome, 1393
 of great vessel calcification, 89, 90f
 of intramural hematoma of aorta, 1296-1297
 of ischemic heart disease, postoperative, 813
 of leiomyosarcoma, 928
 of lipoma, 915
 of mitral regurgitation, 93-94, 837
 of mitral stenosis, 93, 93f, 834-835, 834f
 of myocardial calcification, 87, 87f
 of myocarditis, 897, 897f
 of myxoma, 907, 907f
 of nonthrombotic embolization, 1369
 of osteosarcoma, 929
 of papillary fibroelastoma, 910
 of paraganglioma, 918
 of patent ductus arteriosus, 585, 586f
 of pericardial calcification, 82, 82f
 of pericardial constriction, 80-82
 of pericardial cyst, 82, 83f
 of pericardial effusion, 80, 81f, 942, 943f
 of pericarditis
  acute, 946
  constrictive, 949-950
 of pericardium, 80-82
  normal, 80, 81f
 of pneumothorax, postoperative, 96
 of primary cardiac lymphoma, 932, 933f
 of pulmonary capillary hemangiomatosis, 1363
 of pulmonary edema, 85-87, 86f
  hydrostatic, 1373-1374, 1374b, 1375f
  neurogenic, 1379, 1379f
  permeability, 86-87, 1377-1378
  postoperative, 96
  re-expansion, 1380, 1380f

Chest radiography *(Continued)*
 of pulmonary embolism, 1333-1334, 1333f-1334f
 of pulmonary hemosiderosis, idiopathic, 1392
 of pulmonary hypertension, 1356, 1357f
  arterial, 84-87, 85f
  caused by lung disease/hypoxia, 1366
  chronic thromboembolic, 1345, 1346f-1348f, 1367
  idiopathic, 1358
  related to associated conditions, 1360, 1361f
  venous, 85
  with left heart disease (venous), 1364, 1364f
  with unclear multifactorial mechanisms, 1371
 of pulmonary valve regurgitation, 846
 of pulmonary valve stenosis, 92, 92f, 846
 of pulmonary vasculature, 82-89
  abnormal blood flow in, 84, 84f-85f
  normal anatomy in, 82-84, 83f-84f
 of pulmonary veno-occlusive disease, 1362, 1362f
 of pulmonary venous connections
  partial anomalous, 626, 627f
  total anomalous, 635, 635f
 of rhabdomyoma, 913
 of rhabdomyosarcoma, 930
 of sarcoid granulomatosis, necrotizing, 1392
 of sarcoidosis, 869, 870f
 of single ventricle, 672, 673f
 of sinus venous defect, 629, 630f
 of subaortic stenosis, 92-94
 of Takayasu arteritis, 1316
 of tetralogy of Fallot, 641-647, 641f-642f, 660, 661f
 of thorax, lateral view in, 77, 78f
 of transposition of great arteries, 657, 658f
  complete, 611-612, 612f
 of tricuspid valve regurgitation, 845
 of truncus arteriosus, 664
 of valvular calcification, 87, 88f
 of vascular rings, 543
 of ventricular septal defect, 574, 574f-575f
 of Wegener's granulomatosis, 1385, 1385f
 postoperative, early, 96
Chest trauma, blunt, aortic, 1306, 1307f. *See also* Thoracic aortic trauma.
 acute injury due to, 592, 593f
 with deceleration mechanism injury, 1273
Chest wall
 arteries of, 964-965
 venous drainage of, 999, 1000f
Child-Turcotte-Pugh score, 1453
Cholangiocarcinoma, intrahepatic, 1458-1459
Cholesterol ester transfer protein *(CETP)* gene, lipid abnormalities associated with, 1196
Chronic kidney disease (CKD), 403
 classification of, 1673t
 clinical presentation of, 1674
 definition of, 1673-1674
 etiology and pathophysiology of, 1674
 hemodialysis for, 1672. *See also* Arteriovenous fistula, in hemodialysis patient; Arteriovenous graft.
 in patients with coronary artery disease, 403
 prevalence and epidemiology of, 1674

Chronic kidney disease (CKD) *(Continued)*
  vascular imaging in
    angiography in, 1680-1682, 1682f-1683f
    CT angiography in, 1676-1677, 1677f-1678f
    indications and algorithm for, 1674
    MR angiography in, 1677-1680, 1679f-1681f
    ultrasound in, 1675-1676, 1675f
Chronic limb ischemia. *See* Limb ischemia, chronic.
Chronic obstructive pulmonary disease (COPD)
  definition of, 1365
  etiology and pathophysiology of, 1365
  manifestations of, 1366-1367
  prevalence and epidemiology of, 1365
  pulmonary hypertension caused by, 1365
Chronic thromboembolic pulmonary hypertension (CTPH), 1344-1351, 1366-1368. *See also* Pulmonary hypertension.
  classic signs of, 1350
  clinical presentation of, 1345, 1366-1367
  definition of, 1366
  differential diagnosis of, 1350, 1351f
  etiology and pathophysiology of, 1344, 1366
  imaging of
    indications and algorithm for, 1345
    technique and findings in, 1345-1350, 1346f-1350f, 1367
  medical treatment of, 1350-1351, 1367-1368
  prevalence and epidemiology of, 1344
  reporting of, 1351
  surgical/interventional treatment of, 1351, 1368
Churg-Strauss syndrome, 1390, 1390f
  diagnostic criteria for, 1391b
Cilostazol, for peripheral artery disease, 1209
Circle of Willis, 1217
Circulation. *See* Blood flow.
Circumferential-longitudinal shear angle, of left ventricle, 234-235
Cirrhosis
  clinical presentation of, 1453
  definition of, 1453
  differential diagnosis of, 1456-1457
  etiology and pathophysiology of, 1453
  imaging of
    indications and algorithm for, 1454, 1454f
    technique and findings in, 1454-1456
  treatment options for, 1457
Claudication, intermittent, 1578-1581, 1579f
  differential diagnosis of, 1583
  in peripheral artery disease, 1628. *See also* Peripheral arterial disease (PAD).
Clopidogrel
  for ischemic stroke or transient ischemic attack, 1222
  for peripheral artery disease, 1209
  preprocedural, for carotid artery stenting, 1224
Clopidogrel versus Aspirin in Patients at Risk of Ischemic Events (CAPRIE) trials, 1208
Clubbing, in Eisenmenger syndrome, 585
Coarctation of aorta, 371-373, 535, 536f
  blood flow in
    abnormal, 248f
    MR evaluation of, 242-243, 244f
  classic signs of, 537, 537f-538f
  clinical manifestations of, 535-537
  definition of, 535
  differential diagnosis of
    from clinical presentation, 537-539, 539f
    from imaging findings, 539, 539f

Coarctation of aorta *(Continued)*
  etiology and pathophysiology of, 535
  imaging studies of, 535
    in pediatric patients, 536
    postoperative, 697-698, 698f-699f
  medical treatment of, 539
  pathophysiology of, 552-553
  prevalence and epidemiology of, 535, 552
  surgical repair of, 371-372, 539-540, 540f
    abnormal circular-type flow after, 248f
    considerations regarding, 373, 388, 388t
    contraindications to, 373
    indications for, 372-373
    mortality rate from, 539-540
    outcomes and complications of, 373
    postoperative management after, 698, 698f-699f
    postoperative surveillance after, 373, 376f-377f, 552-553, 553f
    preoperative imaging in, 373, 375f-376f
  thoracic, radiography of, 89-90, 91f
  vs. patent ductus arteriosus, 594, 594f
Cobweb sign, in type B aortic dissection, 1294, 1295f
Coeur en sabot sign, in tetralogy of Fallot, 647
Coils. *See* Gradient coils.
COL3A1 gene, in Ehlers-Danlos syndrome, 1273
Colchicine, for pericarditis, 947
Colic vein, 1006, 1006f-1007f
Collateral pathways, of lower extremity arteries, 985-986, 986f-987f
Collett and Edwards classification, of truncus arteriosus, 616, 617f
Collimator(s)
  in SPECT, 276-277, 277f-278f
  low-energy all purpose, 277
Colon necrosis, after endovascular aneurysm repair, 1435-1436
Color and spectrum invert, in Doppler ultrasonography, 1041
Color Doppler ultrasonography, 1036. *See also* Doppler ultrasonography.
Color flash artifact, in Doppler ultrasonography, 1043
Color flow imaging, in Doppler ultrasonography, 98-100, 101f
Color gain
  in Doppler ultrasonography, 1040, 1040f
  setting of, 1042
  incorrect, in carotid artery Doppler ultrasonography, 1234
Commissurotomy, open, for mitral stenosis, 836
Compartment pressure, measurement of, 1575-1576
Complementary *s*patial *m*odulation of *m*agnetization (C-SPAMM) technique, for quantifying myocardial motion, 230
Complete transposition of great arteries, 601. *See also* Transposition of great arteries (TGA), complete.
Compliance index, 1512
Compliant balloons, in vascular interventions, 1156
Compression syndrome, cervicoaxillary, 1644
Compton scatter
  in PET imaging, 306
  in photon-matter interactions, 275, 275f, 1047
Computed tomographic angiography (CTA), 1055-1077
  abdominal, 1065-1068
    of aorta, 1065-1066, 1067f
    of hepatic vasculature, 1066, 1068f

Computed tomographic angiography (CTA) *(Continued)*
    of mesenteric vasculature, 1066-1068, 1069f
    of pancreas, 1066, 1067f
    of renal vasculature, 1066, 1067f-1068f
  advantages of, 1055-1056, 1064f-1065f
  carotid, 1060, 1062f, 1260-1267
    contraindications to, 1262-1263
    detection of ulceration in, 1266-1267
    image interpretation of, 1264-1267
    imaging parameters for, 1263-1264, 1264t
    indications for, 1260-1262, 1260f-1263f
    pitfalls and solutions in, 1264
    postprocessing of, 1264-1266, 1265f
    reporting of, 1266f, 1267
    technical requirements for, 1260
    technique of, 1263-1264, 1264t
  cerebral, 1060, 1061f
  contrast media in
    administration of, 145
    bolus tracking of, 1058-1059
    concentration of, 1059
    detection and administration of, 1058-1060
    dual-head power injectors for, 1059-1060
    fixed scan delay and, 1058
    test bolus of, 1059
  coronary, 123-132
    after arterial switch procedure, 612, 612f
    after pulmonary artery banding, 611f, 612
    after Rastelli procedure, 612-613, 613f
    angiographic views in, 124-126, 124f-127f
    artifact(s) in, 495-500, 495t, 496f
      beam hardening, 495-496, 496f
      blooming (partial volume), 496, 496f-497f
      blurring (patient motion), 496-499, 498f-499f
      incomplete coverage, 499-500
      noise-induced, 499
      poor vessel enhancement, 499
      stair-step, 499, 500f-501f
      streaks (metallic materials), 496, 497f-498f
    contraindications to, 123, 494
    contrast media in, injection protocol for, 164t-165t
    emerging applications of, 485-489
      in cardiac surgery, 486-487, 488f
      in chest pain evaluation, 485-486, 487f
      in noncardiac surgery, 486
      in vessel wall imaging, 488-489, 489f-490f
    estimation of cardiovascular risk and pretest probability for CAD with, 482t-483t
    image interpretation of, 127-131, 127f-131f, 500-504
      plaque characterization in, 503-504
      postprocessing, 500-502
        axial images in, 500
        maximum intensity projection in, 502
        multiplanar reformation in, 500, 502f
        volume rendering in, 502
      stenosis assessment in, 502-503, 503f
    indications for, 123, 478, 479f-482f, 494
      in asymptomatic patients, 478
    of aneurysms, 510f-513f, 513
    overview of evidence and trends in, 477-478

Computed tomographic angiography (CTA) (*Continued*)
   patient-related consideration(s) in, 479-485
      heart rate and heart rate variability as, 481-482, 485f
      heavy calcifications as, 479-481, 483f-484f
      obesity as, 484-485, 485f-486f
      renal insufficiency as, 485
   pitfalls and solutions in, 126
   procedure-related risks associated with, 489-490
   radiation exposure associated with, 346-347, 346f
      dose reduction in, 348-350, 349f-350f
   reporting of, 504-507, 504f-506f, 506t
   role of, in context of other noninvasive tests, 479
   segment-based and patient-based analysis in, 478-485
   technical requirements in, 123, 493-494
   technique of, 123-124, 494-507, 1061t, 1063-1064
  detectors in, 1056-1057
  dual-energy mode of, 1057
  ECG dose modulation in, 1058
  image acquisition in, 1057-1058
  image interpretation in, 1073-1075
  image quality in, 1056
  of aortic aneurysm
    abdominal, 1181, 1181f, 1441-1442
    thoracic, 1178-1179, 1178f-1179f
  of aortic occlusion, 1411, 1412f-1413f
  of arteriovenous fistula failure, 1676-1677, 1677f-1678f
  of atherosclerosis, 1203-1204, 1203f
  of atherosclerotic ulcer, penetrating, 1299-1300, 1299f, 1301f
  of carotid stenosis, 1220
  of celiac artery thrombosis, 1548-1549, 1549f
  of chronic thromboembolic pulmonary hypertension, 1348, 1348f
  of coarctation of aorta, 536
  of cor triatriatum, 632-633
  of graft infection, after lower extremity bypass, 1185-1186, 1186f
  of hepatic artery stenosis, 1550, 1552f-1553f
  of hepatic artery thrombosis, 1548-1549, 1549f-1551f
  of inferior vena cava stenosis, 1553-1554, 1555f-1556f
  of limb ischemia
    acute, 1576
    chronic, 1582-1583
  of lower extremities, 1610-1627
   contraindications to, 1611-1614, 1614f
   contrast bolus considerations in, 1617-1619
     bolus tracking technique, 1618-1619, 1618f-1619f
     test bolus technique, 1619
   image acquisition in, 1614-1617
     field of view and, 1614, 1615f
     reconstruction parameters and, 1617, 1617f-1618f
     scanning protocols and, 1614-1617, 1615t-1616t
   image interpretation in, 1622-1627
     maximum intensity projection, 1622, 1624f-1625f
     multiplanar reformation, 1622, 1623f
     reporting of, 1625-1627, 1626f
     thin slab or thick slab, 1622-1625
     volume rendering, 1622, 1625f

Computed tomographic angiography (CTA) (*Continued*)
   indications for, 1611, 1611f-1613f
   pitfalls and considerations in, 1619-1622
     acquisition considerations, 1619-1620, 1620f-1621f
     inherent limitations, 1621-1622
     interpretation considerations, 1620-1621, 1621f
   technical requirements for, 1610
  of lower extremity vasculature, 1068-1069, 1069f-1072f
  of portal vein thrombosis, 1551, 1553f-1554f
  of pulmonary venous connections
   partial anomalous, 627
   total anomalous, 636, 636f
  of renal arteries, 1066, 1067f-1068f
   contraindications to, 1485
   image interpretation in, 1488-1490, 1489f-1490f
   pitfalls and solutions in, 1488
   reporting of, 1490
   technique of, 1485-1486, 1485t, 1486f
  of renal artery stenosis, 1475, 1475f-1476f
  of subclavian artery occlusion, 1176, 1176f
  of thoracic outlet syndrome, 1669
  of thoracic vasculature, 1060-1062, 1063f-1064f
  pitfalls and solutions in, 1069-1073
  postprocessing in, 1073-1074
   limits of, 1074-1075
  preoperative
   of carotid artery stenosis, 1174, 1174f
   of thoracoabdominal aortic aneurysm, 1177-1178
  prestent and poststent protocol for, 1429, 1430t
  prospective gating in, 1057-1058
  pulmonary, 1062-1063, 1064f-1065f
  radiation and dosage in, 1070-1073
  reconstruction techniques in, 1058
  retrospective gating in, 1057
  scanner design in, 1056
  scanner noise in, 1056
  technical components and design in, 1056-1057
  techniques of, 1060-1075, 1061t
  three-dimensional postprocessing in, basic, 1120-1127. *See also* Three-dimensional postprocessing, in CTA and MRA.
Computed tomographic venography (CTV), of pulmonary embolism, 1340
Computed tomography (CT). *See also* CT *entries;* PET/CT imaging systems.
  after surgical repair of truncus arteriosus, 622-623, 622f
  cardiac
   artifacts in, 147, 147f-148f
   clinical techniques of, 143-149
   contrast media in, 159
    administration of, 145-146, 145f
    early arterial dynamics of, 160-161, 160f
    injection of, 161
     clinical protocols for, 163-165, 164t-165t
     timing of, 161-162, 162f
    safety issues of, 159-160
    saline flushing and, 163, 163f
   dual-source, 140
   ECG-synchronized, 134, 135f
   goals of, definition of, 133

Computed tomography (CT) (*Continued*)
   imaging processing in, 167-179, 168f-171f
    axial images in, 168-169
    coronal and sagittal images in, 170-171, 172f
    curved planar reconstruction in, 171-173, 173f-175f
    maximum intensity projection in, 173-176
    technical requirements for, 167-168
    volume rendering technique of, 176-178, 177f
   imaging reconstruction techniques in, 134
   imaging requirements in, 133
   in myocardial perfusion studies, 326
   medications for, 156-159, 157f, 157t-158t. *See also specific medication.*
   new developments in, 140-141
   patient preparation for, 143-144, 144f
   physics of, 133-142
   postprocedural considerations in, 146-147
    pitfalls and solutions in, 147, 147f-148f
   radiation dose reduction in, 348-350, 349f-350f
    increased beam filtration technique for, 153-154
    increased beam pitch technique for, 153
    increased reconstructed slice thickness technique for, 154, 154f
    reduced tube current technique for, 150-152, 151f
    reduced tube voltage technique for, 152-153
    shortened scan length technique for, 153
    technical requirements for, 150
    tubal modulation for, 146
   radiation exposure associated with, 346-347, 346f, 347t
   scanning technique of, 144-146
    contrast administration in, 145-146, 145f
    image quality in, 144-145
    minimizing radiation dose in, tubal modulation to, 146
   technical principle(s) of, 134-140
    ECG tube current modulation, 138-140, 139f
    multisegment image reconstruction, 136-137, 138f-139f
    optimal reconstruction phase, 137
    prospective triggering, 134-136, 135f
    retrospective gating, 136, 137f
   with volume detectors, 140-141
  dual-source, technology of, 1057
  electron-beam
   of coronary artery calcium, vs. multidetector CT imaging, 460
   technology of, 1056
  high-resolution
   of ARDS during exudative phase, 1377, 1378f
   of ARDS during proliferative phase, 1378, 1378f
  multidetector, 1055
   of atrial fibrillation, 447-449, 447f-449f
   of coronary artery calcium, 459
    vs. electron-beam CT imaging, 460
   of pulmonary embolism, 1339-1340, 1339t
    limitations of, 1339-1340
   of thoracic aortic trauma, 1307-1308

Computed tomography (CT) *(Continued)*
  of acute coronary syndrome, 717-721, 718f-720f
    protocol parameters for, 720t
    University of Maryland triage studies in, 721t
  of amyloidosis, 863, 863f
  of angiosarcoma, 926, 926f-927f
  of aortic aneurysm
    abdominal, 1441-1442
    inflammatory, 1405, 1405f-1406f
    mycotic, 1407, 1407f
    ruptured, 1302-1303, 1303f
    thoracic, 1280-1281, 1281f
  of aortic dissection, 1291, 1292f-1293f
  of aortic regurgitation, 833
  of aortic stenosis, 828-829, 829f-831f
  of aortic trauma
    abdominal, 1410, 1410f
    thoracic, 1307-1309
      aortic pseudoaneurysm in, 1308, 1309f
      contour abnormality in, 1308
      contrast agent extravasation in, 1309
      intimal flap in, 1308
      multidetector technique of, 1307-1308
      periaortic mediastinal hemorrhage in, 1309, 1309f
  of aortitis, syphilitic, 1323, 1323f
  of aortoenteric fistula, 1415-1416, 1416f
  of arrhythmogenic right ventricular dysplasia, 888, 888f
  of atherosclerotic plaque, ulcerated, 1299-1300, 1300f
  of atrial septal defect, 566, 568f
  of atrium
    left, 32-33, 32f
    right, 30-31, 32f
  of Behçet syndrome, 1387, 1388f
  of cardiac function, 758, 759f
    during stress, 769
    left ventricular, 761
    regional, 766-767
    right ventricular, 762-763
  of cardiac lymphoma, primary, 933, 933f-934f
  of cardiac metastases, 921f-924f, 924
  of cardiac tumor, calcified amorphous, 919
  of cardiomyopathy
    dilated, 853-855, 854f
    hypertrophic, 874-875, 875f
    sideritic, 867
  of chronic thromboembolic pulmonary hypertension, 1345-1349, 1346f-1349f, 1367
  of coarctation of aorta, 536
    classic signs in, 537, 538f
    repaired, 373, 377f
  of coronary anomalies, congenital, 467
  of coronary artery bypass graft, 523, 523f
  of coronary atherosclerosis, 710, 710f-711f
  of diffuse alveolar hemorrhage, 1384, 1384f, 1391
  of double-outlet right ventricle, 683-684
  of endoleaks, 1409
  of eosinophilic endomyocardial disease, 865, 866f
  of fibroma, 912-913, 912f
  of giant cell arteritis, 1320-1321, 1321f, 1391, 1391f, 1414, 1415f
  of Goodpasture syndrome, 1393-1394, 1393f
  of inferior vena cava anomalies, 1528
  of inferior vena cava thrombosis, 1537, 1538f
  of inferior vena cava tumors, 1530
    findings in, 1530-1531, 1531f-1533f

Computed tomography (CT) *(Continued)*
  of in-stent restenosis and thrombosis, 518-519, 519f
  of intramural hematoma, 1297, 1297f
  of ischemic heart disease, 755, 756t
    postoperative, 814
  of leiomyosarcoma, 928
  of lipoma, 915, 915f
  of lipomatous hypertrophy of interatrial septum, 916, 916f
  of liposarcoma, 931, 932f
  of mitral regurgitation, 837
  of mitral stenosis, 835, 835f
  of myocardial perfusion, 326, 730-733
    animal studies in, 730-731, 731t
    contraindications to, 733
    human studies in, 731-733, 732t
    image interpretation in, 735
    indications for, 733
    pitfalls and solutions in, 734
    reporting of, 735-736
    stress multidetector, 733
    technique of, 734
  of myocardial viability, 784-787, 787f
    limitations of, 787-788
  of myocarditis, 897-899, 898f
  of myxoma, 907-908, 907f-908f
  of nonthrombotic embolization, 1369, 1369f-1370f
  of osteosarcoma, 929, 929f
  of papillary fibroelastoma, 910, 911f
  of paraganglioma, 918
  of patent ductus arteriosus, 585-586, 587f
  of pericardial effusion, 942
  of pericarditis
    acute, 946, 947f
    constrictive, 950, 950f
  of peripheral artery disease, 1630
  of pulmonary capillary hemangiomatosis, 1363, 1363f
  of pulmonary edema, hydrostatic, 1374, 1374b, 1375f
  of pulmonary embolism, 1337-1339
    benefits and accuracy of, 1338
    classic findings in, 1337-1338, 1338f
    limitations of, 1338-1339
    multidetector, 1339-1340, 1339t
      limitations of, 1339-1340
    technical considerations in, 1337
  of pulmonary hemosiderosis, idiopathic, 1392, 1393f
  of pulmonary hypertension, 1356-1357, 1357f
    caused by lung disease/hypoxia, 1366
    chronic thromboembolic, 1345-1349, 1346f-1349f, 1367
    idiopathic, 1358, 1358f-1359f
    related to associated conditions, 1360
    with left heart disease (venous), 1364, 1365f
    with unclear multifactorial mechanisms, 1371
  of pulmonary veno-occlusive disease, 1362
  of renal vasculature, in living kidney donor, 1568
  of rhabdomyoma, 913
  of rhabdomyosarcoma, 930
  of sarcoidosis, 869, 870f
  of single ventricle, 673
  of sinus venous defect, 630
  of subclavian steal syndrome, 1328, 1328f
  of Takayasu arteritis, 1316, 1316f, 1388-1389, 1389f
  of tetralogy of Fallot, 643, 644f

Computed tomography (CT) *(Continued)*
  of transposition of great arteries, 658
    levo-, 679-680
  of truncus arteriosus, 664-665, 665f-666f
  of upper extremity medium and small vessel disease, 1648-1649, 1648f-1650f
  of vascular anatomy, in pancreas transplant recipient, 1569
  of vascular rings, 544
  of ventricular septal defect, 574-575, 577f-578f
  of Wegener's granulomatosis, 1385-1386, 1386f
  postoperative, of occluded aortobifemoral bypass limb, 1185, 1185f
  radionuclides in, 325-326. *See also* Radionuclide(s).
  x-ray
    fundamentals of, 1047, 1048f
    important performance parameters in, 1047-1051, 1048f-1051f
    multislice, 1053-1054, 1053f
    physics of, 1047-1054
    step-and-shoot vs. helical (spiral), 1051-1053, 1051f-1052f
Conal septum, in double-outlet right ventricle physiology, 682
Conduction system, of heart, 57-58, 58f
Conduit(s), in vascular bypass surgery
  autogenous saphenous vein as, 1585-1586
  definition of, 1585
  extra-anatomic bypass grafts as, 1586-1588, 1587f-1589f
  prosthetic, 1586
  xenografts as, 1586, 1587f
Congenital heart disease (CHD). *See also specific cardiac defect, e.g.*, Tetralogy of Fallot.
  acyanotic
    with shunt, 383-387, 385f, 385t
      surgery for
        contraindications to, 386
        indications for, 386, 387f
        outcomes and complications of, 386
        postoperative surveillance after, 387
        preoperative imaging in, 386-387
    without shunt, 387-389, 388t
      surgery for
        indications for and contraindications to, 388-389
        postoperative surveillance after, 389
  adult, in general population, 383, 384t
  complex, 656
  cyanotic
    evaluation of patient with, 651-653, 652f
    with decreased pulmonary blood flow, 390-392, 391t
      surgery for, 391-392
    with increased pulmonary blood flow, 389-390, 389t
      surgery for, 390
  diagnosis and management of, segmental approach to, 12-13, 13f
  echocardiography of, 117-118
  in adult, 89, 91f-92f
  incidence of, 651
  postoperative evaluation of
    coronary artery imaging, perfusion imaging, and myocardial viability in, 693-694, 693f-694f
    gadolinium-enhanced three-dimensional MR angiography in, 693, 693f
    MR imaging of, 689-701
      cine imaging, 690-691, 690f-691f
      clinical presentation indicating, 694

Congenital heart disease (CHD) *(Continued)*
    indications and algorithm for, 694
    spin-echo imaging, 691, 691f
    technique and findings in, 694-700, 695f-699f
    velocity-encoded cine sequences, 691-693, 692f
  relative frequency of, 383, 384t
Congenital venolobar syndrome, 625, 626f-627f
  repair of, baffle obstruction after, 628, 629f
Congenitally corrected transposition of great arteries, 601. *See also* Transposition of great arteries (TGA), congenitally corrected.
Connective tissue disease, 1391
  pulmonary hypertension associated with, 1359
Conotruncus, development of, 22-24, 25f
Constrictive pericarditis. *See* Pericarditis, constrictive.
Continuous wave Doppler ultrasonography, 98-99, 1036-1037. *See also* Doppler ultrasonography.
Contour abnormality(ies), in thoracic aortic trauma, 1308
Contractile cardiac motion, causing attenuation mismatch, in PET imaging, 309-310, 311f
Contrast agents, 1398-1399. *See also specific agent entries, e.g.*, Gadolinium.
  allergy to, as contraindication to CT angiography, 1614
  clinical injection protocols for, 163-165, 164t-165t
  dosage of, 1399
  extravasation of, in thoracic aortic trauma, 1309
  in angiography, choice of, 1158
  in contrast-enhanced MR angiography. *See also* Magnetic resonance angiography (MRA), contrast-enhanced.
    injection protocols for, 1633
    novel, 1633
  in CT angiography
    administration of, 145
    bolus tracking of, 1058-1059
    concentration of, 1059
    detection and administration of, 1058-1060
    dual-head power injectors for, 1059-1060
    fixed scan delay and, 1058
    test bolus of, 1059
  in CT imaging, 159
    administration of, 145-146, 145f
    early arterial dynamics of, 160-161, 160f
    injection of, 161
      clinical protocols for, 163-165, 164t-165t
      timing of, 161-162, 162f
    safety issues of, 159-160
    saline flushing and, 163, 163f
  in MR imaging, 251-260
    classification of, 255-259, 255f, 257t-258t
    cost of, 255
    development of, 251
    pharmacovigilance of, 253
    regulatory label of, 251-252
    safety issues of, 252-253, 266
  in perfusion imaging, dosing range of, 206
Contrast bolus, in CT angiography
  of abdominal aorta
    detection/triggering methods of, 1399
    timing techniques of, 1399

Contrast bolus, in CT angiography *(Continued)*
  of lower extremities, 1617-1619
    bolus tracking technique and, 1618-1619, 1618f-1619f
    test bolus technique and, 1619
Contrast-enhanced harmonic imaging, in ultrasonography, 1037
Contrast-induced nephropathy (CIN), 159
Contrast-to-noise ratio, in contrast-enhanced MR angiography, 1258
Conus branch, of right coronary artery, 40, 42f
Conus cordis, 3-4
Cor adiposum, vs. arrhythmogenic right ventricular dysplasia, 893
Cor triatriatum
  clinical presentation of, 632
  definition of, 632
  differential diagnosis of, 633
  etiology and pathophysiology of, 632
  imaging technique and findings in, 632-633, 633f
  incidence of, 632
  reporting of, 634
  treatment options for, 634
CORAL trial, 1480
Coronal images, in cardiac CT imaging, 170-171, 172f
Coronary allograft vasculopathy, after cardiac transplantation, 813
  angiography of, 815
Coronary angioplasty, percutaneous transluminal. *See* Percutaneous transluminal coronary angioplasty (PTCA).
Coronary artery(ies), 38-56
  anatomy of
    normal, 39-48, 39f
    segmental, 48f, 49-50
  calcium in. *See* Coronary artery calcium (CAC).
  congenital anomalies of
    classification of, 467t
    CT imaging of, 467
    definition of, 466
    differential diagnosis of, 468-473
    etiology and pathophysiology of, 466-467
    manifestation of disease in, 467
    MR imaging of, 467
    of intrinsic anatomy, 472-473, 473f-474f
    of origin and course, 468-472, 468f-473f
      duplication in, 48-49, 471-472, 472f
      from noncoronary sinus, 471, 471f
      from opposite sinus of Valsalva, 468-469, 468f-470f
      from pulmonary artery, 470-471
      high arterial origin, 471, 471f
      multiple ostia in, 471, 472f
      single artery, 472, 473f
    of termination: fistula, 473, 474f
    prevalence and epidemiology of, 466
  diagnostic computed angiography of, 123-132. *See also* Computed tomographic angiography (CTA), coronary.
  diseased, evaluation of collateral flow to, 129-131, 130f-131f, 130t
  dissection of, 129, 129f
  duplication of, 48-49, 471-472
  intramuscular, prevalence of, 49
  left, anatomy of, 43-44, 43f-44f, 413f
  left anomalous, diagnosis of, 386

Coronary artery(ies) *(Continued)*
  left anterior descending, 44-46, 44f-45f, 412, 413f
    aneurysm of, 509, 510f
    duplication of, 471-472, 472f
  left circumflex, 46, 46f-47f, 413f
    aneurysm of, 509, 510f
  MR imaging of, 190-191, 191f
    in postoperative congenital heart disease patients, 693-694, 693f-694f
    respiratory-navigator techniques of, 190-191, 191f
    short breath-hold three-dimensional techniques of, 190
  narrowing of
    diffuse, 128, 128f
    discreet, 127-128, 128f
  network of, 38
  percutaneous transluminal coronary angioplasty of. *See* Coronary artery disease (CAD), percutaneous coronary intervention for.
  ramus intermedius, 46, 47f
  right
    aneurysm of, 509, 510f, 513f
    branches of, 39-41, 40f-42f, 413f
    dominance of, 46-48, 48f
    single, anomalous, 472, 473f
  stenosis of
    calcification as indicator of, 461, 461t
    CT assessment of, 502-503, 503f
  stenting of. *See* Coronary stents.
  thrombus in, during angioplasty intervention, 129, 129f
  variations in
    definitions of, 38-39
    normal, 48-49, 48f-50f
Coronary artery aneurysm, 128-129, 128f-129f
  angiography of, 513
  atherosclerotic, 509
  clinical presentation of, 509-512
  congenital, 472, 473f
  CT angiography of, 510f-513f, 513
  definition of, 509
  differential diagnosis of, 513
  epidemiology of, 509, 510f-513f
  etiology and pathophysiology of, 509
  incidence of, 509
  medical treatment of, 513
  radiographic imaging of, 512-513
  surgical treatment of, 513, 514f
Coronary artery bypass graft (CABG), computed angiography of, contrast media injection protocol for, 164t-165t
Coronary artery bypass graft (CABG) surgery, 412-417
  anatomic considerations in, 412-413, 413f
  arterial grafts in, 522
  assessment of, 522-530
    background in, 522
    CT imaging in, 523, 523f
    MR imaging in, 523-524
  cardiopulmonary bypass in, 412-413, 414f
  choice of conduits in, 522
  complication(s) of, 524-525
    graft aneurysm as, 525
    graft thrombosis and occlusion as, 524-525, 527f-529f
  contraindications to, 413-414, 416t
  for coronary atherosclerosis, 713
  goals of, 412, 413f
  indications for, 413, 416t
  internal mammary artery grafts in, 522
  microvascular anastomoses in, 413, 415f-416f

Coronary artery bypass graft (CABG) surgery *(Continued)*
 outcomes and complications of, 414-415
 postoperative evaluation of, 524, 525f-526f
 postoperative surveillance after, 417
 preoperative imaging for, 413, 416f, 416t
 preoperative planning in, 524
 preoperative risk factors for, 416t
 saphenous vein grafts in, 522
 technique of, 412
Coronary artery calcium (CAC)
 as indicator of stenosis, 461, 461t
 as predictor of cardiac events, 461-462
 assessment of, in elderly populations, 462-463
 imaging of, 458-460, 458f
  clinical importance of, 461-462
  electron-beam CT in, 458-459
  interscan reproducibility in, 460
  multidetector CT in, 459
   vs. electron-beam CT imaging, 460
  radiation dosage in, 460
  radiographic, 88, 89f
  standardization of, 459-460, 460f
 in asymptomatic individuals, risk assessment of, 462
 in patients with chest pain, presenting to emergency departments, 462
 in plaque formation, 457-458. *See also* Plaque, atherosclerotic.
 in specialized populations, 462-463
 pathophysiology of, 457-458
 prevalence of, in renal failure, 463
 screening for
  in diabetic patients, 463
  with treadmill and nuclear stress imaging, 463
Coronary artery calcium (CAC) score, 331, 331f
 progression of, 463
  effect of statins on, 463-464
 relationship between race and, 462
 reporting of, 459
 zero, value of, 461
Coronary artery disease (CAD)
 atherosclerotic. *See also* Atherosclerosis; Plaque, atherosclerotic.
  angiography of, 708
  biology of, 60-61, 60f-61f
  calcium associated with, 457. *See also* Coronary artery calcium (CAC).
  clinical presentation of, 708
  CT imaging of, 710, 710f-711f
  definition of, 705
  differential diagnosis of, 712-713
  etiology and pathophysiology of, 705-707, 706f-707f
  imaging of
   indications and algorithm for, 708
   investigational catheter-based techniques, 712, 712f
   technique and findings in, 708-712
  MR imaging of, 710-711
  nuclear imaging of, 711-712
  prevalence and epidemiology of, 705
  treatment options for, 713
  ultrasonography of, 107, 708-709, 709f
 chronic, 61-62
 CT angiography of, 1063
  protocol parameters for, 1061t
 evaluation of, prognostic approach to, 281, 282f
 lifetime risk of, 790
 multivessel, evaluation of, 329, 329f-330f

Coronary artery disease (CAD) *(Continued)*
 obstructive
  CT angiography of. *See also* Computed tomographic angiography (CTA), coronary.
   image interpretation of, 127-131, 127f-131f, 500-504
    plaque characterization in, 503-504
    postprocessing, 500-502
     axial images in, 500
     maximum intensity projection in, 502
     multiplanar reformation in, 500, 502f
     volume rendering in, 502
    stenosis assessment in, 502-503, 503f
   reporting of, 504-507, 504f-506f, 506t
  definition of, 477
 percutaneous coronary intervention for, 394-403
  adverse periprocedural events in, 405, 405f-406f
  after saphenous vein bypass graft, 394-395, 396f
  chronic total occlusion and, 395-397, 398f
  contraindications to, 402
  in stent era, 403-405, 404f
   restenosis and, 404, 405f
  indications for, 401-402
  of bifurcation-type lesions, 394, 395f
  of complex, angulated, and lesions distal to proximal vessel tortuosity, 395, 396f-397f, 397
  of left main artery stenosis, 397, 398f-399f
  of long lesions and diffuse disease, 397, 398f
  of specific lesion subsets, catheter modification in, 400, 401f
  outcomes and complications of, 402-403
  ST segment elevation myocardial infarction and, 399, 400f
  stent thrombosis and, 399, 400f
 perfusion imaging of
  diagnostic accuracy of, 342t
  myocardial, 739, 741f-743f
   accuracy of, 749
   pharmacologic stress agents in, 356-357
  pretest probability of, according to age and sex, 483t
 surgery for, 412-417. *See also* Coronary artery bypass graft (CABG) surgery.
 ultrasonography of, 107, 108f-109f
Coronary artery fistula, 473, 474f
Coronary blood flow, 352-353
 at rest vs. hyperemia, 354f
Coronary collateral pathways, common, 130t
Coronary flow reserve, 352-353, 353f
 and radiotracer uptake, 353, 354f
Coronary ostia
 congenital stenosis of, 472, 473f
 location of, 39, 39f
 multiple, anomalous origin of coronary artery from, 471, 472f
 number of, 39
Coronary reserve flow, in hypertrophic cardiomyopathy, MR imaging of, 879
Coronary reverse flow, 61-62
Coronary sinus, 50-51, 53f
 formation of, 8-10, 10f
 tributaries of, 51-52

Coronary stents, 403-405
 for atherosclerosis, 713
 in-stent restenosis and thrombosis
  clinical presentation of, 516-517
  etiology, prevalence, and pathophysiology of, 515-516, 516f-517f
  imaging of, 517-522
   analysis of, 519-520, 520f-521f
   CT scans in, 518-519, 519f
   MR scans in, 518
   radiography in, 517
   ultrasound in, 517-518
  percutaneous coronary intervention for, 399, 400f, 520
  reporting of, 520
  treatment options for, 520
 noninvasive evaluation of, 515-522, 516f
Coronary syndrome, acute. *See* Acute coronary syndrome.
Coronary vein(s)
 anatomy of, 50-55, 53f-54f
 mapping of, contrast media injection protocol for, 164t-165t
Corticosteroids, for Takayasu arteritis, 1318
Costocervical trunk, 989, 990f
Count density, in PET/CT imaging, 327-328
Cox Maze procedure, for atrial fibrillation, 445
^{11}C-palmitate, in PET imaging, 343-344
Crawford classification, of thoracoabdominal aortic aneurysm, 1176-1177, 1177f, 1276, 1277f
C-reactive protein, increased levels of, 1197-1198
Crescent sign, in intramural hematoma of aorta, 1298
CREST syndrome, 1645, 1658f
 pulmonary hypertension associated with, 1359
Crista terminalis, 8-10
Critical limb ischemia, 1579, 1580f-1582f, 1581. *See also* Limb ischemia.
 differential diagnosis of, 1583
Cryogens, as MRI safety issue, 264
Cryoplasty, in lower extremity revascularization, 1592, 1595f
Cryoplasty balloons, 1156
Crystals, scintillation, in SPECT, 277, 278t
CT. *See also* Computed tomography (CT).
CT number
 accuracy of, CT scanner and, 1049-1050
 equation defining, 1049
 in water phantom, 1049, 1050f
CT scanner
 320-slice, 1057
 CT number accuracy of, 1049-1050
Current, x-ray tube, in computed tomography, reduction of, 150-152, 151f
Curved multiplanar reformatted (CMPR) image, 1129, 1130f
 contour detection of, 1129-1131, 1131f-1132f
Curved planar reconstruction (CPR)
 in cardiac CT imaging, 171-173, 173f-175f
 in carotid CT angiography, 1265
Cutting balloon(s), 1156
Cutting balloon angioplasty, in lower extremity revascularization, 1593
Cyanosis, in Eisenmenger syndrome, 585
Cyanotic congenital heart disease. *See* Congenital heart disease (CHD), cyanotic.
Cyst(s), pericardial, radiography of, 82, 83f
Cystic disease, adventitial, 987, 1600
 imaging of, 1604

Cystic medial necrosis, thoracic aortic aneurysm caused by, 1272-1273, 1273f-1274f
Cystic vein, 1008

D

Damus-Kaye-Stansel procedure
  for single-ventricle defects, 390
  for transposition of great arteries, 611, 611f
Dana Point classification, of pulmonary hypertension, 1354-1356, 1356b
Data
  acquisition of, in MR angiography, 1078-1081
  reconstruction and display of, in PET imaging, 318-319
Data processing, three-dimensional, in CTA and MRA, 1120-1127. *See also* Three-dimensional postprocessing, in CT and MRA.
David's and Yacoub's surgical technique, for type A aortic dissection, 1295
D-Dimer assay, sensitivity and specificity of, 1333t
D-Dimer levels, in pulmonary embolism, 1333
Death
  during endovascular aneurysm repair, 1426
  sudden, arrhythmogenic right ventricular dysplasia and, 884
DeBakey classification, of aortic dissection, 434, 434f, 1289, 1289f
Decay constant, of radionuclide, 273-274
Deep vein(s). *See also named vein.*
  of lower extremity, 1027-1029
  of upper extremity, 1022-1023, 1023f
Deep vein thrombosis (DVT)
  ultrasound detection of, 1334-1335
  upper extremity, 1661
    clinical presentation of, 1663
    complications of, 1663
    etiology of, 1661
    imaging of, 1663-1664
      findings in, 1664-1666, 1664f-1668f
      pitfalls in, 1666, 1668f-1669f
      ultrasound, 1647, 1648f
    prevalence, etiology, and risk factors for, 1661-1663, 1663f
Delayed hyperenhancement magnetic resonance imaging (DE-MRI)
  description of, 210-211, 211f
  indications for, 207-210, 208f-210f
  pitfalls and solutions in, 212, 212f
  reporting of, 212-213, 213f
Detector(s)
  in CT angiography, 1056-1057
  in PET, material properties of, 306-308, 308t
Dextrotransposition of great arteries, 601. *See also* Transposition of great arteries (TGA).
Diabetes mellitus
  atherosclerosis associated with, 1197, 1197f
  coronary artery calcium screening in, 463
  in patients with coronary artery disease, 403
  peripheral artery disease associated with, 1197
  restrictive cardiomyopathy associated with, 871
Diastole
  MRI in assessment of, 218, 219f
  physiology of, 63
  ventricular, 59
Diastolic filling ration, early-to-late, 754

Diastolic flow abnormalities, waveform analysis of, in carotid arteries, 1241-1242, 1241f-1244f
Diastolic function
  echocardiography of, 103, 104f-106f
  left ventricular, image interpretation of, 235, 235f
  right ventricular, image interpretation of, 237
Dietary restriction protocols, for PET imaging, 316
Diffuse alveolar hemorrhage, 1383-1384, 1391
Digital subtraction angiography (DSA), 1055, 1060
  of aortic occlusion, 1184, 1184f
  of aortitis, syphilitic, 1323, 1323f
  of arteriovenous fistula failure, 1680-1682, 1683f
  of carotid artery stenosis, 1251
  of femoral artery calcifications, 1188, 1188f
  of graft thrombosis, after lower extremity bypass, 1185-1186, 1186f
  of peripheral artery disease, 1206, 1207f
  of renal artery stenosis, 1478, 1479f-1480f
  of stenosis, after vascular bypass surgery, 1589, 1590f
  of subclavian artery occlusion, 1176, 1176f
  preoperative
    of carotid artery stenosis, 1174, 1175f
    to assessment of inflow, outflow, and runoff, before bypass, 1186-1187, 1188f
Digital vein(s), dorsal
  of lower extremity, 1024-1026, 1026f
  of upper extremity, 1019, 1020f
Dilated cardiomyopathy, 851-860. *See also* Cardiomyopathy, dilated.
Dilators, vascular, 1156
Dipyridamole, 353-355
  chemical structure of, 284f
  mechanism of action of, 354f
  perfusion imaging protocol with, 355, 355f
  in PET, 316
  in SPECT, 284-285, 745
  side effects of, 354t, 355
Directional ambiguity, in Doppler ultrasonography, 1042, 1042f
Displacement encoding with stimulated echoes (DENSE), for quantifying myocardial motion, 230-231, 230t, 765, 765f
Dissection(s)
  aortic. *See* Aortic dissection.
  arterial, after endovascular aneurysm repair, 1436
  carotid artery, 1242-1243
    CT angiography of, 1262, 1263f
    Doppler imaging of, 1243, 1245f
  coronary artery, 129, 129f
  during angioplasty, 1162
Diverticulum of Kommerell, vs. patent ductus arteriosus, 591-592, 591f-592f
Dobutamine, 356
  chemical structure of, 285f
  for MR stress imaging, 267-268
  MR assessment of cardiac function with, 218-223, 767-768
    diagnostic criteria and, 768, 769f
    myocardial ischemia and, 218-221, 220t, 221f
    myocardial viability and, 221-222, 222f, 782
    patient prognosis and, 222-223, 223f
    physiology and safety profile of, 218, 220f

Dobutamine *(Continued)*
  protocols for, 768
  sensitivity and specificity of, 220t
  myocardial viability assessment with, 358
  perfusion imaging protocol with, 355f, 356
    contraindications to, 205, 206t
    in SPECT, 285, 745
    vs. echocardiography, 357-358, 357f
  side effects of, 354t, 356
Dobutamine stress echocardiography (DSE). *See also* Echocardiography.
  vs. dobutamine MR imaging, 218-219
Döhle-Heller syndrome, 1323
Doppler angle, incorrect choice of, in carotid artery ultrasonography, 1233-1234, 1235f
Doppler frequency shift, 1034-1035, 1035f, 1039-1040
  choice of, 1038
  formula for, 1035
Doppler indices, 1045, 1045t
Doppler signal, 1041, 1041t
Doppler spectrum, 1043, 1043f
Doppler ultrasonography. *See also* Echocardiography; Ultrasonography.
  artifacts, pitfalls, and solutions in, 1041-1043, 1041t
  color, 1036
  color flow imaging in, 98-100, 101f
  continuous wave, 98-99, 1036-1037
  contraindications to, 1038
  historical perspective on, 1034-1036, 1035f
  image interpretation in, 1043-1044, 1043f-1044f
  indications for, 1037
  of amyloidosis, 862
  of carotid arteries, 1227-1250
    assessment of plaque in, 1237-1240, 1238f-1239f
    complex waveform pattern in, 1248f, 1249
    components of, 1228
    contraindications to, 1228
    grading of stenosis in, 1233, 1234f-1235f
    indications for, 1228
    normal findings in, 1231-1232, 1232f-1233f
    pitfalls in
      pathological, 1235-1237, 1236f-1238f
      technical, 1233-1234, 1235f
    protocol for, 1231
    technical requirements in, 1227-1237
    technique of, 1228-1231, 1229f-1231f
    waveform analysis in, 1240-1245
      abnormal patterns involving cardiac cycle and, 1242-1245
      arteriovenous fistula, 1244, 1246f
      carotid dissection, 1243, 1245f
      carotid pseudoaneurysm, 1243, 1246f
      intra-aortic balloon pump, 1244-1245, 1247f
      diastolic flow abnormalities in, 1241-1242, 1241f-1244f
      systolic peak abnormality(ies) in, 1240-1241
        parvus tardus waveform, 1240, 1240f
        pulsus alternans waveform, 1241, 1241f
        pulsus bisferiens waveform, 1241, 1241f
  of dilated cardiomyopathy, 852
    anatomic considerations in, 1505-1509
    functional assessment in, 1509, 1510f
    of abdominal aorta, 1508, 1508f-1509f

Vol. I: pages 1-952; Vol. II: pages 953-1686

Doppler ultrasonography *(Continued)*
  of renal arteries, 1505-1507, 1507f-1508f
  of renal veins, 1507-1508, 1508f
  of segmental, interlobar, and arcuate arteries, 1507, 1508f
  fibromuscular dysplasia and, 1498, 1503f
  image interpretation in, 1513-1522
    diagnosis of renal artery aneurysm, 1515
    diagnosis of renal artery stenosis, 1513
      direct criteria for, 1513, 1513b, 1514f
      indirect criteria for, 1513, 1513b, 1515f
    diagnosis of renal artery thrombosis, 1515
    diagnosis of renal vein thrombosis, 1515-1519, 1518f
    diagnostic accuracy of, 1513
    postangioplasty renal artery assessment and, 1514-1515, 1516f-1518f
    renal transplants and, vascular evaluation of, 1519-1522, 1519b, 1519f-1522f
  indications for, 1498b
  pitfalls and solutions in, 1512-1513
    allograft renal vein thrombosis and, 1513
    renal artery stenosis and, 1497-1498
      atherosclerotic, 1497-1498, 1499f-1502f
    renal artery thrombosis and, 1498-1505, 1505f
    renal transplant assessment in, 1505
    renal vein thrombosis and, 1505, 1506f
    Takayasu arteritis and, 1498, 1503f-1504f
  technical considerations in, 1509-1512
    of intrarenal arteries, 1511, 1512f
    of renal arteries, 1509-1511, 1510f-1511f
    of renal morphology, 1511-1512
  technical requirements for, 1497
  techniques of, 1497-1505
    description of, 1505-1512
  of subclavian steal syndrome, 1247-1249, 1247f-1248f
  of thoracic outlet syndrome, 1669
  of upper extremity arteries, 1647-1648, 1648f
  of upper extremity deep vein thrombosis, 1663-1664
    findings in, 1664-1666, 1664f-1668f
    limitations of, 1666, 1668f-1669f
  of vertebral artery, 1246-1249
  postprocessing in, 1044-1045, 1045t
  power, 1036-1037
  pulsed wave, 1036-1037
  reporting of, 1045
  spectral, 1037
  technique of, 1037-1045
    acoustic power in, 1040
    angle of correction in, 1040
    angle of insonation in, 1039-1040, 1040f
    baseline shift in, 1041
    choice of instrumentation in, 1038
    choice of probe and frequency in, 1038
    choice of pulse repetition frequency/velocity scale in, 1038, 1039f
    color and spectrum invert in, 1041
    dwell time in, 1041
    focal zone in, 1041
    gain in, 1040, 1040f
    high-pass filter in, 1040-1041
    sample volume in, 1038, 1039f

Dor procedure, for ischemic heart disease, 811
  postoperative appearance of, 817, 818f
  postoperative complications of, 812
  imaging of, 817-818
Dorsal veins
  digital
    of lower extremity, 1024-1026, 1026f
    of upper extremity, 1019, 1020f
  of penis, 1014
Dorsal venous plexus, upper extremity, 1019-1020, 1021f
Dorsalis pedis artery, 984-985, 985f
Dose modulation, radiation, in CT angiography, 1058
Dosimetry, PET, 319
Double aortic arch, 544, 544f-545f, 958, 959f. *See also* Aortic arch.
Double-outlet right ventricle (DORV), 680-684
  clinical presentation of, 682-684
  definition of, 680
  differential diagnosis of, 607, 608f, 684-685
  etiology and pathophysiology of, 682
  imaging of
    indications and algorithm for, 682
    technique and findings in, 682, 682f-685f
  incidence and epidemiology of, 680-682
  medical treatment of, 685-686
  pathology of, 7
  surgical/interventional treatment of, 686-687
DRASTIC trial, 1480
Dressler syndrome, 94
Drug(s). *See also named drug or drug group;* Pharmacologic stress agent(s).
  as risk factor for pulmonary hypertension, 1359b
  illicit, ventricular septal defect risk associated with, 572-573
  in cardiac MRI stress testing, 267-268
  in CT imaging, 156-159, 157f, 157t-158t
Drug-eluting stents, 515, 517f, 1157
  effectiveness of, 515-516
  repeat stenting with, 520
  risk of thrombosis in, 516, 517f
Dual-energy mode
  in CT angiography, 1057
  of CT angiography, 1057
Dual-head power injectors, of contrast, in CT angiography, 1059-1060
Dual-isotope imaging protocols, with thallium 201 and Tc 99m, for SPECT, 282-283, 746
Ductus aneurysm
  definition of, 590-591
  vs. patent ductus arteriosus, 590-591, 591f
Ductus arteriosus
  patent. *See* Patent ductus arteriosus (PDA).
  physiologic closure of, 583, 584f
    mechanism of, 583
    schematic of, 584f
Ductus bump, vs. patent ductus arteriosus, 588, 590f
Ductus diverticulum
  definition of, 588-590
  vs. patent ductus arteriosus, 588-590, 590f
  vs. traumatic aortic pseudoaneurysm, 1311, 1311f
Duplex ultrasonography. *See also* Ultrasonography.
  of atherosclerotic carotid plaque, 1220-1221, 1221f
  of atherosclerotic disease, 1202-1203
  of carotid and vertebral arteries, in subclavian steal syndrome, 1175, 1175f
  of carotid stenosis, 1220, 1220f

Duplex ultrasonography *(Continued)*
  of limb ischemia
    acute, 1576
    chronic, 1582
  of lower extremity bypass, 1187, 1188f
  of peripheral artery disease, 1629
  of renal artery stenosis, 1473-1475, 1474f
  preoperative, of carotid artery stenosis, 1173-1174, 1173f, 1174t
Duplication(s)
  coronary artery, 48-49
  inferior vena cava, 1525, 1525f
    with retroaortic left renal vein and azygos continuation, 1527
    with retroaortic right renal vein and hemiazygos continuation, 1526-1527
  superior vena cava, 998, 998f
Dwell time, in Doppler ultrasonography, 1041
Dynamic (multiframe) imaging protocol, in emission scanning, 326-327
Dyskinesia, definition of, 232

E

Ebstein anomaly, 653-654, 654f
  considerations regarding, 388, 388t, 391, 391t
  echocardiography of, 119, 653-654
ECG. *See also* Electrocardiography (ECG).
ECG dose modulation, in CT angiography, 1058
ECG gated imaging protocol, in emission scanning, 326-327
ECG gating, in MR angiography, 1103
ECG triggering, prospective, in CT imaging, 134-136, 135f
ECG tube current modulation, in CT imaging, 138-140, 139f
ECG-based reduction, in x-ray tube current, 151
  pitfalls and solutions for, 151-152
ECG-gated reconstruction, retrospective, in CT imaging, 136, 137f
Echocardiography, 98-122. *See also* Ultrasonography.
  contrast, 107
  dobutamine stress, vs. dobutamine MR imaging, 218-219
  Doppler. *See* Doppler ultrasonography.
  fundamental image in, 98
  harmonic image in, 98
  intracardiac, 101-110
    indications for, 101-110
  M mode, 98, 99f
  of amyloidosis, 115-116, 116f
  of aortic aneurysms, thoracic, 1280
  of aortic dissection, 117, 118f
  of aortic regurgitation, 110, 832-833
  of aortic stenosis, 109, 828
  of arrhythmogenic right ventricular dysplasia, 113, 887-888, 888t
  of atrial septal defect, 117-118
  of cardiomyopathy, 110-113
    dilated, 110
    hypertrophic, 110-113
    noncompaction, 113, 114f-115f
    restrictive, 113
  of congenital heart disease, 117-118
  of coronary artery disease, 107, 108f-109f
  of cyanotic heart lesions, 651
  of diastolic function, 103, 104f-106f
  of Ebstein anomaly, 119, 653-654
  of endocarditis, 110, 113f

Echocardiography (Continued)
of fibroma, 116
of ischemic heart disease, postoperative, 813-814
of malignant tumors, 116
of mitral regurgitation, 110, 837
of mitral stenosis, 109-110, 111f-112f, 835, 835f
of myxoma, 116, 117f
of papillary fibroelastoma, 116
of patent ductus arteriosus, 118
of pericardial diseases, 113-115
of pericarditis, constrictive, 115, 116f
of prosthetic valves, 110
of pulmonary hypertension, 105, 106f, 1356
chronic thromboembolic, 1345
with left heart disease (venous), 1364
of pulmonary insufficiency, 381, 381f
of pulmonary valve stenosis, 846
of pulmonary venous connections, anomalous, 118
of rhabdomyoma, 116
of systemic veins, anomalous, 118
of systolic function and quantification, 103, 104f-105f
of tamponade, 113
of tetralogy of Fallot, 119, 642
postnatal, 642-643, 643f
of transposition of great arteries
complete, 119, 611-612
after atrial switch procedure, 612
congenitally corrected, 119
of tricuspid valve regurgitation, 845
of univentricular atrioventricular connection, 119, 119f
of valvular heart disease, 65-66, 107
of ventricular outflow tract obstruction, 118
of ventricular septal defect, 118
stress
of acute coronary syndrome, 717
of coronary artery disease, 107
of dilated cardiomyopathy, 853
technical requirements in, 98-110
three-dimensional, 101
tissue velocities and strain imaging in, 119-122, 120f-121f
transesophageal. See Transesophageal echocardiography (TEE).
transtracheal. See Transtracheal echocardiography (TTE).
two-dimensional, 98, 100f
vs. dobutamine stress perfusion imaging, 357-358, 357f
Echo-planar imaging (EPI) technique, of MR imaging, 228-229, 228t
Edema, pulmonary. See Pulmonary edema.
Edge artifact, in Doppler ultrasonography, 1043
Edwards hypothetical double aortic arch, 542, 543f
Effective orifice area (EOA), patient-prosthetic mismatch due to, 421
Effective orifice area (EOA) index, 421
Effusion
pericardial. See Pericardial effusion.
pleural, postoperative, radiographic features of, 96
Effusive pericarditis, 438, 438f. See also Pericarditis.
Ehlers-Danlos syndrome, 1601, 1603f
vascular, 1273
Eisenmenger syndrome, 573, 577, 584, 1359
cyanosis and clubbing in, 585

Ejection fraction (EF), 3A
left ventricular
^{99m}Tc-sestamibi imaging of, 286f
calculation of, 103, 106f
change in, after revascularization, 335t
coronary artery disease and, 329, 329f-330f
MR assessment of, 216
Simpson's rule in, 215
Elastic recoil
contributing to coronary restenosis, 515, 516f
in angioplasty, 1162
Elbow, brachial artery at, 993, 993f
Elderly populations, coronary artery calcium assessment in, 462-463
Electrical impulse, conduction of, 57
Electricity, as MRI safety issue, 263
Electrocardiography (ECG). See also ECG entries.
abnormal, in arrhythmogenic right ventricular dysplasia, 886-887, 887t
during gated MPI acquisition, in ventricular function assessment, 772
monitoring of, during exercise or pharmacologic stress imaging, 358-359
normal appearance of, 57, 58f
synchronization of, with computed tomography, 134, 135f
Electromagnetic energy, in radiation, 270
Electron(s)
Auger, 271-272, 272f
physics of, 270, 271f
recoil, 275
Electron capture, 272-273, 272t, 273f
Electron shells, 270, 271f
Electron transition, mechanisms of, 271-272, 272f
Embolectomy, balloon catheter, for saddle embolus, 1578
Embolic agents, 1167-1169
liquid, 1168-1169
particulate, 1167-1168
Embolization, 1167-1170
for arteriovenous fistula and pseudoaneurysm, in renal transplant recipient, 1565-1566, 1566f
imaging findings in, 1170
indications for and contraindications to, 1170
liquid agents for, 1168-1169, 1169f
mechanical occlusion devices for, 1168
nontarget, 1170
nonthrombotic, 1368-1370
clinical presentation of, 1369
etiology and pathophysiology of, 1368
imaging technique and findings in, 1369-1370, 1369f-1370f
outcomes and complications of, 1170
particulate agents for, 1167-1168
principles of, 1169-1170
Embolus (embolism)
cerebral, in infective endocarditis, 429, 429f
coronary artery, 129
in myxomas, 906-907
pulmonary. See Pulmonary embolism.
shower, after endovascular aneurysm repair, 1435
sites of, in acute limb ischemia, 1574-1575, 1574f
Embryogenesis, of inferior vena cava, 1527
Emission scans, in myocardial perfusion studies, 326-327
Enalaprilat, IV administration of, in ACEI renal scintigraphy, 1493

Endarterectomy, carotid. See Carotid endarterectomy.
Endarterectomy versus Angioplasty in patients with Symptomatic Severe Carotid Stenosis (EVA-3S) trial, 1223
End-diastolic velocity (EDV), effect of heart rate on, 1235-1236
Endocardial cushion defect, 5
Endocarditis
infective. See Infective endocarditis.
Löffler, 864-866. See also Eosinophilic endomyocardial disease.
Endograft(s). See also Stent(s).
aneurysm repair with, 1420, 1421f
clinical presentation after, 1426
complication(s) of
arterial dissection as, 1436
colon necrosis as, 1435-1436
endoleaks as, 1431-1434, 1431f-1434f
graft infection as, 1434
graft kinking as, 1434
graft occlusion as, 1434-1435
graft thrombosis as, 1434, 1434f-1436f
hematoma at arteriotomy site as, 1436
shower embolism as, 1435
death during, 1426
endoleak after, 1426, 1428t
goal of, 1420
graft placement in, 1422-1423, 1424f-1426f
surgical conversion after, 1423-1424, 1427f, 1440, 1443f
imaging of
indications and algorithm for, 1426-1429
techniques and findings in, 1429-1436, 1429f-1430f, 1430t
postoperative assessment of, 1420-1436, 1423f-1428f
postoperative management after, 1436-1437
preprocedural interventions and, 1422-1423, 1423f
success of, 1422
anatomic appearance after, 1426, 1428f
vs. open surgical repair, 1424-1426
classification of, 1408t
percutaneous placement of, for aortic atherosclerotic disease, 1195-1196
Endoleak(s)
after endovascular aneurysm repair, 1407-1409, 1431-1434
classification of, 1426, 1428t
etiology and pathophysiology of, 1408, 1408f, 1408t
imaging of
indications and algorithm for, 1408
techniques and findings in, 1408-1409, 1409f
prevalence and epidemiology of, 1407
treatment options for, 1409
Type I, 1431-1434, 1431f-1432f, 1436
Type II, 1431-1434, 1432f-1433f, 1436-1437
Type III, 1431-1434, 1434f, 1437
Type IV, 1437
definition of, 1436
postoperative management of, 1436-1437
primary and secondary, 1436
recurrent, 1436
Endomyocardial fibrosis, 864-866. See also Eosinophilic endomyocardial disease.
radiation-induced, 871

Endovascular aortic aneurysm repair (EVAR), 1181-1182, 1183f-1184f
  complications of, 1407-1409. *See also* Endoleak(s).
Endovascular Aortic Aneurysm Repair (EVAR) trial, 1420-1422
Endovascular procedure(s)
  exclusion or occlusion, for lower extremity aneurysm, 1604-1608. *See also* Lower extremity aneurysm, endovascular exclusion procedures for.
  for abdominal aortic aneurysm. *See* Abdominal aortic aneurysm, endovascular repair of.
  for penetrating atherosclerotic ulcer, 1301-1302
  for thoracic aortic trauma, 1312-1313, 1312f
  for type B aortic dissection, 1295-1296, 1296f
  lower extremity, 1591-1598
    anatomic considerations in, 1591-1594, 1592f-1595f
    angioplasty and stent placement as, 1591-1592, 1592f-1593f
    atherectomy as, 1592, 1593f-1594f
    contraindications to, 1596
    cryoplasty as, 1592, 1595f
    cutting balloon angioplasty as, 1593
    imaging findings in, 1597-1598, 1597f
    indications for, 1594-1596, 1595t, 1596f
    outcomes and complications of, 1596-1597
Endovascular stents, 1157
End-stage renal disease, 1673-1674
Energy discrimination, in SPECT, 278
Energy metabolism, alterations of, in hibernating myocardium, 792
Enzyme-linked immunosorbent assay (ELISA), sensitivity and specificity of, 1333, 1333t
Eosinophilic endomyocardial disease
  clinical presentation of, 865
  definition of, 864
  etiology and pathophysiology of, 864-865
  imaging of
    indications and algorithm for, 865
    technique and findings in, 865-866, 865f-866f, 872t
  medical treatment of, 871
  prevalence and epidemiology of, 864
Epigastric artery
  inferior, 978, 979f
  thoracoabdominal arterial anastomosis through, 985, 986f
Equilibrium gated blood pool imaging, of ventricular function
  indications for, 773
  technique of, 773-775, 774f-778f
Esophageal varices, from portal hypertension, 1008-1009, 1008f
  MR imaging of, 1454-1455, 1455f
Esophagus, CT imaging of, 447-448, 448f
Ethylene-vinyl alcohol copolymer, as embolic agent, 1168-1169, 1169f
EUROSTAR registry, of endoleaks, 1407
Evian classification, of pulmonary hypertension, 1354, 1354b
Excitation, of transferred energy, 271
Exclusion procedure(s), lower extremity
  endovascular methods as, 1604-1608
  surgical excision and vascular bypass as, 1600-1604
Exercise
  for peripheral artery disease, 1209
  MR assessment of cardiac function with, 223-224, 223f, 767

Exercise stress protocols
  in SPECT, 283, 283t, 744
  vs. pharmacologic stress protocols, 358-359, 359t, 744
Extracellular matrix formation, in atherosclerosis, 1195
Extremity
  lower. *See* Lower extremity.
  upper. *See* Upper extremity.

F

False aneurysm, 1271, 1277, 1277f. *See also* Pseudoaneurysm.
  delayed hyperenhancement MR imaging of, 209-210
Faraday's law, 263
Fast low-angle shot (FLASH) technique
  comparison of left ventricular volume by, vs. steady-state free precession, 231-232
  of MR imaging, 227, 228t
Fast pulse sequences, in accelerated MR imaging, 194-195, 194f
Fast-field echo (FFE) technique, of MR imaging, 227, 228t
Fat pad sign, epicardial, in pericardial effusion, 942
Fatty acid radiotracers, in PET/SPECT imaging, 800-801, 801f-802f
Fatty streaks, in atherosclerosis, 60
FBN1 gene, in Marfan syndrome, 550
Femoral artery
  calcifications in, digital subtraction angiography of, 1188, 1188f
  common, 978, 979f, 983
    angiographic access via, 1157-1158
  superficial, 983, 983f, 987f
Femoral vein, deep, 1028
Femoral-femoral bypass graft, 981-982, 982f
  right-to-left, 1586-1588, 1588f
Femoral-popliteal bypass graft, 981-982, 982f
Femoropopliteal artery(ies), occlusion of, MR angiography of, 1636, 1637f
Femoropopliteal bypass graft
  above-knee, 1590, 1590t
  below-knee, 1590, 1590t
Ferucarbotran (SHU555), 258t, 259
Feruglose (NC100150), 258t, 259
Ferumoxide (AMI 25), 258t, 259
Ferumoxtran (AMI 227), 258t, 259
Fever, postoperative, ischemic heart disease and, 813
Fibrillation, atrial. *See* Atrial fibrillation.
Fibroatheroma, 457-458
Fibroelastoma, papillary, 116, 909-910, 910f-911f
Fibroma
  differential diagnosis of, 913
  echocardiography of, 116
  manifestations of disease in, 911-913, 912f
  pathology of, 911, 911f
  prevalence of, 911
  treatment options for, 913
Fibromuscular dysplasia
  arterial narrowing or aneurysm caused by, 975, 976f
  Doppler ultrasonography of, 1498, 1503f
  renal artery stenosis caused by, 1471
    prevalence and epidemiology of, 1471-1472
Fibrosing mediastinitis
  clinical presentation of, 1371
  etiology and pathophysiology of, 1370-1371
  imaging of, 1371

Fibrosis, nephrogenic systemic, 253-255
  as contraindication to contrast-enhanced MR angiography, 1255-1257
  causes of, 254
  in chronic kidney disease, 1673
  risk of, gadolinium-containing contrast agents and, 254, 1453
Fibrous cap, in atherosclerosis, 1195, 1196f
Field of view
  in contrast-enhanced MR angiography, 1254-1255, 1255f-1256f
  in CT angiography of lower extremities, 1614, 1615f
Field strength, in MR angiography, 1102
Filter
  in Doppler ultrasonography
    high-pass, 1040-1041
    wall, setting of, 1041-1042
  inferior vena caval, 1540, 1540f
Filtered back projection (FBP) approach
  to PET reconstruction, 313
  to SPECT reconstruction, 279
Fistula
  aortocaval, 1441, 1443
  aortoduodenal, after abdominal aortic aneurysm repair, 1180
  aortoenteric, 1415-1416, 1416f, 1441, 1445-1447, 1448f
    postoperative management of, 1447
  arteriovenous. *See* Arteriovenous fistula.
  atrioesophageal, after ablation for atrial fibrillation, 451, 451f
  coronary artery, 473, 474f
  hemodialysis, 1672-1685. *See also* Arteriovenous fistula, in hemodialyis patient; Arteriovenous graft.
Fixed scan delay, in CT angiography, 1058
Fleischner lines, 1334
Flow direction artifact, in Doppler ultrasonography, 1042, 1042f
Flow-encoding axes, in MR evaluation of blood flow, 239-240, 241f
Fluorodeoxyglucose (FDG)
  in PET imaging, 801
    protocol(s) in, 801-803
      hyperinsulinemic-euglycemic clamping, 803
      intravenous glucose loading, 803
      nicotinic acid derivative, 803
      oral glucose loading, 802-803
  in PET/CT imaging, 326, 342-343, 342f-343f
    of myocardial perfusion, 333-334, 333f-334f
    patient preparation for, 332-333, 333f
  in SPECT imaging, 805
  kinetics of, 315
Focal neurologic deficits, postoperative, ischemic heart disease and, 813
Focal zone, in Doppler ultrasonography, 1041
Fogarty embolectomy catheter, 1577-1578, 1577f
Fontaine stages, of peripheral artery disease, of limbs, 1578, 1579t
Fontan procedure
  MR imaging after, 675-676, 676f-677f, 699-700
  variant of, for single-ventricle defects, 390
  postoperative management after, 699-700
Food and Drug Administration (FDA)
  regulatory approval, of contrast agents, 251-252
Foot amputation, for chronic limb ischemia, 1583-1584

Foramen ovale
  anatomy of, 443
  patent. See Patent foramen ovale.
Fourier transform scanning, two-dimensional, 1080, 1080f-1081f
  gradient pulse echo sequence for, 1080, 1080f
Fracture, rib, 1306-1307
Frequency shift, Doppler, 1034-1035, 1035f, 1039-1040
  choice of, 1038
  formula for, 1035
Frequency-encoding gradient, in MR angiography, 1080
Friction rub, in pericarditis, 945-946
Fusobacterium necrophorum, in Lemierre's syndrome, 1670

G

Gadobenate, 256, 257t
Gadobuterol, 256, 257t
Gadodiamide, 256, 257t
Gadolinium agents
  pharmacovigilance of, 253
  physiochemical characteristics of, 257t
  standard nonprotein interacting, 256
  use and safety of, in MR imaging of abdominal vascular disorders, 1453
  with macromolecular structures, 253-254
  with strong protein interaction, 256-258
  with weak protein interaction, 256
Gadopentate dimeglumine, 256, 257t
Gadotexetate disodium, 256, 257t
Gadoversetamide, 256, 257t
Gamma camera
  components of, 276, 276f
  used in SPECT, 739
Gamma ray(s), 270
  emission of, 272t, 273
Gangrene
  lower limb, 1581
  wet, 1581
Gastric artery, 970, 973f
Gastric vein, 1006f-1007f, 1007-1008
Gastroduodenal artery, 972, 973f
Gastroduodenal pseudoaneurysm, 1463, 1464f, 1469f
Gastroepiploic vein
  left, 1006-1007, 1006f-1007f
  right, 1006, 1006f-1007f
Gastrointestinal bleed localization scan
  image interpretation of, 1146
  indications and contraindications to, 1144-1146
  pitfalls and solutions in, 1146, 1147t
Gated blood pool (GBP) imaging, of ventricular function
  indications for, 773
  technique of, 773-775, 774f-778f
Gating
  in cardiac MR imaging, 201-202
    electrocardiographic, 201-202
    navigator echo technique of, 202, 203f
  in CT angiography
    prospective, 1057-1058
    retrospective, 1057
Gauss' law, 263
Gelfoam, as embolic agent, 1167
Gender, role of, in atherosclerosis, 1196
Generalized autocalibrating partially parallel acquisitions (GRAPPA), in parallel imaging, 195

Genetic mutations, in arrhythmogenic right ventricular dysplasia, 884-885, 885t
Genetic predisposition, to atherosclerosis, 1196
Genetic screening
  for dilated cardiomyopathy, 851
  for truncus arteriosus, 618
Giant cell arteritis, 1390-1391, 1414-1415
  aneurysm dilation due to, 1275
  clinical presentation of, 1320, 1391
  definition of, 1320
  diagnosis of, American College of Rheumatology criteria for, 1320t
  differential diagnosis of, 1414
  etiology and pathophysiology of, 1320, 1414
  imaging of
    indications and algorithm for, 1320, 1414
    technique and findings in, 1320-1321, 1321f-1322f, 1391, 1391f, 1414, 1415f
  incidence of, 1644
  prevalence and epidemiology of, 1320, 1414
  treatment options for, 1322, 1415
  upper extremity affected by, 1643-1644
  vs. Takayasu arteritis, 1319t
Glagov phenomenon, in atherosclerosis, 1195, 1195f
Glucocorticoids, for giant cell arteritis, 1322
Glucose loading
  in ^{18}FDG-PET imaging, 332-333
    intravenous, 803
    oral, 802-803
    principle of, 316
Gluteal artery, inferior, 978-981, 980f
Gluteal vein, 1012, 1013f-1014f
Gonadal artery, 975, 981
Goodpasture syndrome, 1393-1394, 1393f
Gorlin syndrome, fibromas associated with, 911
Gradient coils
  as embolic agents, 1168
  in MR angiography, 1084, 1084f
    birdcage, 1083
    contrast-enhanced, dedicated, 1253-1254
    gradient, 1102
    phased-array surface, 1102-1103
    RF field detection by, 1083
Gradient system, magnetic field
  as MRI safety issue, 263
  in MR angiography, 1083
Gradient-recalled-echo (GRE) techniques, of MR imaging, 181
  three-dimensional, 1452
Graft(s). See also Allograft(s); Bypass graft(s); Prosthetic graft(s); Xenograft(s).
  arteriovenous, 1672
  failure of, focal lesion causing, 1591
  placement of, in endovascular aneurysm repair, 1422-1423, 1424f-1426f
  success of, 1423-1424, 1427f
Graft aneurysm, after CABG surgery, 525
Graft infection
  after abdominal aortic aneurysm repair, 1180, 1180f
  after endovascular aneurysm repair, 1434
  after lower extremity bypass, 1185-1186, 1186f
  after vascular bypass surgery, 1589
  aortic, 1441, 1443-1447, 1446f-1447f
  postoperative management of, 1449
Graft kinking, after aneurysm repair, 1434
  endovascular, 1434

Graft occlusion
  after CABG surgery, 524-525, 527f-529f
  after endovascular aneurysm repair, 1434-1435
Graft patency
  femoropopliteal
    above-knee, 1590, 1590t
    below-knee, 1590, 1590t
  in revascularization procedures, 1589
  infrapopliteal, 1590, 1591t
Graft thrombosis
  after endovascular aneurysm repair, 1434, 1434f-1436f
  after lower extremity bypass, 1185-1186, 1186f
Granulomatosis
  necrotizing sarcoid, 1392
  Wegener's. See Wegener's granulomatosis.
Grating artifact, in Doppler ultrasonography, 1042
Great arteries. See also Aorta; Pulmonary artery(ies).
  identification of, 16, 16f
  relationship of, 18, 20f
  transposition of. See Transposition of great arteries (TGA).
Grey-Turner sign, in abdominal aortic aneurysm, 1440
Ground-glass opacity
  in Wegener's granulomatosis, 1385, 1386f
  of lung, 1376
Guide wires, 1156

H

Half-Fourier acquisition single-shot turbo spin-echo (HASTE) imaging, 204
Hampton hump sign, in pulmonary embolism, 1334, 1334f
Hand
  arch variations in, 994f
  arterial anatomy of, 993f
  superficial veins of, 1019-1020, 1020f-1021f
Harmonic imaging, contrast-enhanced, in ultrasonography, 1037
Hazards, associated with MR imaging, 261-262
Head and neck
  arterial blood supply to, 1217
  venous drainage of, 999
Hearing protection, for MR imaging, 267
Heart. See also Cardiac; Cardio-; Myocardial *entries*.
  anatomy of, 30-37, 31f-36f
  boot-shaped, in tetralogy of Fallot, 641-642, 642f
  chambers of. See also Atrial *entries*; Atrium (atria); Ventricle(s); Ventricular *entries*.
    anatomy of, 30, 31f
    blood flow through, 58-59, 59f
    contraction of, 57
    identification of, 13
  conduction system of, 57-58, 58f
  coronary arteries of, 412, 413f. See also Coronary artery(ies).
  CT imaging of, 133-142. See also Computed tomography (CT), cardiac.
  echocardiography of, 98-122. See also under Echocardiography.
  hypertrophy of, 63
  left-sided lesions of, extreme forms of, 388, 388t

Heart (Continued)
  MR imaging of, 180-200, 215-226. See also Magnetic resonance imaging (MRI), cardiac.
  physiology of, 57-68
  radiology of, 71-97. See also Chest radiography.
    normal and abnormal cardiac borders in, 71-78. See also Chest radiography, of cardiac borders.
    right-sided lesions of, 388, 388t
    size of, radiographic measurement of, 78-80
    types of, different, 19-25, 21f
Heart disease
  congenital. See Congenital heart disease (CHD).
  ischemic. See Ischemic heart disease (IHD).
  segmental approach to, 3
    case study in, 27f, 28
    embryologic basis for, 11-12
    evaluation of function in, 24-25, 27f
  valvular
    catheter-based management of, 405-409, 407f-408f
    MR evaluation of blood flow in, 241-242, 243f
    radiographic studies of, 92-94, 93f
Heart failure
  congestive, 810
  hyperadrenergic state of, 805
  mortality rates associated with, 790
Heart murmur, holosystolic, in ventricular septal defect, 573
Heart rate
  effect of, on peak systolic velocity and end-diastolic velocity, 1235-1236, 1236f
  in three-dimensional steady-state free precession MR angiography, 1107
  variability of, in coronary CT angiography, 481-482, 485f
Heart rhythm, in three-dimensional steady-state free precession MR angiography, 1107
Heart sounds, S_2, in atrial septal defect, 564
Heart transplantation
  for arrhythmogenic right ventricular dysplasia, 894
  for ischemic heart disease, 811-812
    postoperative appearance of, 818, 819f-820f
    postoperative complications of, 812-813
      imaging of, 818-820, 821f
Heart tube
  components of, 3-4, 4f
  formation of, 3-13
Heart valves. See also named valve.
  anatomy of, 34-36, 35f-36f
  function of, 58-59
  insufficiency or stenosis of, 64-66. See also under specific valve.
    imaging assessment of, 65-66, 66f
  prosthetic. See Prosthetic heart valve.
Heart-to-blood pool count ratio, in PET/CT imaging, 327-328
Heath-Edwards grading system, of pulmonary hypertension, 1359-1360
Helical (spiral) computed tomography. See also Computed tomography (CT).
  vs. step-and-shoot CT, 1051-1053, 1051f-1052f
Helical pitch (h)
  definition of, 1051-1052
  increased helical artifacts with, 1052, 1052f
  selection of, 1053
Helium, liquid, used in MRI scanners, 264

Hemangiomatosis, pulmonary capillary, 1362-1363, 1363f
Hematoma
  at arteriotomy site, after endovascular aneurysm repair, 1436
  intramural
    CT imaging of, 816-817, 817f
    of aorta, 1296-1299. See also Intramural hematoma, aortic.
Hemiazygos vein, anatomy of, 1000, 1001f
Hemitruncus, 621
Hemodialysis, for chronic kidney disease, 1672
  access fistulas in, 1672, 1673f. See also Arteriovenous fistula, in hemodialysis patient; Arteriovenous graft.
Hemodialysis-associated amyloidosis, 861. See also Amyloidosis.
Hemolytic anemia, chronic, pulmonary hypertension associated with, 1360
Hemorrhage
  after vascular bypass surgery, 1589
  diffuse alveolar, 1383-1384, 1391
  mediastinal, postoperative, radiographic features of, 96
  periaortic mediastinal, in thoracic aortic trauma, 1309, 1309f
  perioperative
    in operative field, 816, 817f
    ischemic heart disease and, 813
  pulmonary, differential diagnosis of, 1384t
Hemorrhagic telangiectasia, hereditary, 1468
Hemosiderosis, idiopathic pulmonary, 1392-1393, 1393f
Heparin
  for inferior vena cava thrombosis, 1539
  preprocedural, for carotid artery stenting, 1224
Hepatic. See also Liver entries.
Hepatic angiography, 1159
Hepatic arteriovenous malformations, 1468
Hepatic artery, 971-972, 972f
  anatomy of
    CT angiography of, 1545, 1545f-1546f
    Michel classification of, 1545, 1546t
    variant donor, 1546, 1546f
Hepatic artery pseudoaneurysm, after liver transplantation, 1551, 1553f
Hepatic artery stenosis, after liver transplantation, 1550, 1552f-1553f
Hepatic artery thrombosis
  after liver transplantation, 1548-1551, 1548f-1552f
  MR imaging of, 1460-1461, 1460f
Hepatic transplantation, 1544-1558
  cadaveric, surgical anatomy of, 1546-1547, 1547f
  complication(s) after, 1547-1554
    hepatic artery pseudoaneurysm as, 1551, 1553f
    hepatic artery stenosis as, 1550, 1552f-1553f
    hepatic artery thrombosis as, 1548-1551, 1548f-1552f
    inferior vena cava stenosis as, 1534-1535, 1553-1554, 1555f-1556f
      clinical presentation of, 1534
      definition of, 1534
      differential diagnosis of, 1535
      imaging of, 1534-1535, 1534f-1537f
      prevalence and epidemiology of, 1534
      treatment options for, 1535
    portal vein stenosis as, 1551-1553, 1554f-1555f

Hepatic transplantation (Continued)
    portal vein thrombosis as, 1551, 1553f-1554f
    venous aneurysms as, 1551, 1554f
  contraindications to, 1544
  imaging prior to
    indications and algorithm for, 1459-1460
    technique and findings in, 1460-1461, 1460f-1461f
  indications for, 1544
  manifestations of disease prior to, 1459
  pretransplant work-up for, 1544-1546
    imaging of liver transplant recipients in, 1544-1545
    imaging of potential living donors for, 1545-1546, 1545f-1546f, 1546t
  prevalence and epidemiology of, 1459
Hepatic vasculature, CT angiography of, 1066, 1068f
Hepatic vein, anatomy of, 1010, 1010f, 1545-1546
  variations of, 1010-1011
Hepatic veno-occlusive disease, vs. Budd-Chiari syndrome, 1461, 1462f
Hepatocellular carcinoma
  inferior vena cava invasion by, 1530-1531, 1533f
  MR imaging of, 1458-1459, 1459f
  vs. arterioportal shunts, 1457
Hereditary amyloidosis, 861. See also Amyloidosis.
Hereditary hemorrhagic telangiectasia, 1468
Heterotaxy
  definition of, 16-18
  syndromic approach to, 18, 18f-19f
High-altitude pulmonary edema, 1381-1382
High-attenuation object, as contraindication to CT angiography, 1614, 1614f
High-pass filter, in Doppler ultrasonography, 1040-1041
Holosystolic murmur, in ventricular septal defect, 573
Human herpes virus 6, in myocarditis, 898-899
Human immunodeficiency virus (HIV) infection, pulmonary hypertension associated with, 1359-1360
Hunter's canal, 983
Hybrid devices, for valvular heart disease, 409
Hybrid procedures
  for aortoiliac and lower extremity occlusive disease, 1188-1189, 1188f
  in abdominal aortic aneurysm repair, 1181-1182, 1183f-1184f
  in thoracic aortic aneurysm repair, 1178-1179, 1178f-1179f
Hypercoagulability, in deep vein thrombosis, 1663
Hyperenhancement
  delayed, in cardiac MR imaging
    description of, 210-211, 211f
    indications for, 207-210, 208f-210f
    pitfalls and solutions in, 212, 212f
    reporting of, 212-213, 213f
  of myocardial viability, MR imaging of, 782-784, 783f-786f
Hyperinsulinemic-euglycemic clamping, 332-333
  in ^{18}FDG-PET imaging, 803
Hyperperfusion syndrome, after carotid endarterectomy, 1173

Hypertension
   atherosclerosis associated with, 1196-1197
   portal. *See also* Portal hypertension.
   pulmonary, 1353-1358. *See also* Pulmonary hypertension.
   renovascular
      ACEI scintigraphy of. *See* Angiotensin-converting enzyme inhibitor (ACEI) scintigraphy, of renal arteries.
      secondary to renal artery stenosis, 1471, 1492
Hypertrophic cardiomyopathy, 63, 874-883. *See also* Cardiomyopathy, hypertrophic.
Hypoplastic left heart syndrome (HLHS), 8
   etiology and pathophysiology of, 671-672
   Norwood procedure for, 389, 672
   prevalence and epidemiology of, 671
   vs. coarctation of aorta, 538
Hypothenar hammer syndrome, 1645
   incidence of, 1646
Hypoxia, pulmonary hypertension caused by, 1365-1366

I

Ibuprofen, for pericarditis, 947
Idiopathic hypereosinophilic syndrome (IHES), 864-866. *See also* Eosinophilic endomyocardial disease.
Idiopathic pulmonary hemosiderosis, 1392-1393, 1393f
Idiopathic pulmonary hypertension, 1358-1359, 1358f-1359f. *See also* Pulmonary hypertension.
   definition of, 1358
Ileal vein, anatomy of, 1005, 1006f
Ileocolic vein, anatomy of, 1006, 1006f
Iliac artery
   circumflex, deep and superficial, 978, 979f
   common, 975, 978, 979f, 1028-1029
   external, 978, 979f, 1028-1029
   internal, 978
      anterior division of, 978-981, 980f
      posterior division of, 978, 980f
      variations of, 981
   lesions involving, MR angiography of, 1635-1636, 1636f
Iliac artery aneurysm
   definition of, 1019
   endovascular repair of, 1420, 1422f. *See also* Endograft(s), aneurysm repair with.
   goal of, 1420
Iliac occlusion, balloon thrombectomy for, 1578, 1578f
Iliac vein
   common, 1012
   external, 1012, 1013f
   internal, 1012-1014, 1013f-1014f
Iliac vein compression syndrome (IVCS), 1015, 1015f, 1535
Iliolumbar artery, 978, 980f
Illicit drug use, ventricular septal defect risk associated with, 572-573
Image acquisition
   in CT angiography, 1057-1058
   in MR imaging, 227-229
Image aliasing artifact, in MR imaging, 1397
Image encoding, in MR angiography, 1079-1081, 1080f-1082f
Image generation, in SPECT, 279

Image interpretation
   of brain perfusion tomography, 1148-1150
   of CT angiography, 1073-1075
      coronary, 127-131, 127f-131f, 500-504
   of GI bleed localization scan, 1146
   of Meckel diverticulum scan, 1148
   of SPECT, 285-296, 286f-296f
   of three-dimensional contrast-enhanced MR angiography, 1116-1118
   of three-dimensional steady-state free precession MR angiography, 1108-1109, 1108f
   of time-of-flight MR angiography, 1105
   of TR MR angiography, 1112
Image quality
   in cardiac CT imaging, 144-145
   in CT angiography, 1056
   in PET/CT systems, 320-322
      elevated activity in inferior wall at stress and, 322, 323f
      metal implants and, 321-322, 322f
      prompt gamma correction and, 321, 321f
      streaking and lateral wall overcorrection and, 321, 321f
      truncation and, 322, 323f
Image reconstruction
   in MR angiography, 1078-1081
   in PET imaging, 313-314, 314f
Imaging modalities. *See specific modality*.
Imaging processing, in computed tomography, 168-171, 172f
Imaging times, prolonged, in time-of-flight MR angiography, 1105
Implantable cardioverter-defibrillators (ICDs)
   as MRI safety issue, 264-265
   as PET image artifact, 321-322, 322f
   for arrhythmogenic right ventricular dysplasia, 894
Implants, metallic, as contraindication to contrast-enhanced MR angiography, 1257
Infarction
   myocardial. *See* Myocardial infarction.
   renal, 1447, 1449f
   segmental, in renal allograft, 1520, 1521f
   splenic, 1466-1467, 1467f
Infection
   after cardiac transplantation
      imaging of, 818-819, 821f
      mediastinal, 812-813, 819-820
      postoperative management of, 821-823
   aortic aneurysm after, 594, 594f
      thoracic, 1275, 1276f
   aortic graft, 1441, 1443-1447, 1446f-1447f
      postoperative management of, 1449
   graft
      after endovascular aneurysm repair, 1434
      after lower extremity bypass, 1185-1186, 1186f
   prosthetic graft, 1284-1285
Infectious agents
   causing acute pericarditis, 945, 946t
   causing myocarditis, 896
Infective endocarditis, 429-432
   clinical manifestations of, 429, 429f-430f, 430t
   echocardiography of, 110, 113f
   surgery for
      contraindications to, 430-431
      goals of, 430, 430f
      indications for, 430, 430t-431t
      outcomes and complications of, 431
      postoperative surveillance after, 431-432, 432f
      preoperative imaging in, 431-432, 432f-433f

Inferior vena cava
   anastomosis of, 1547, 1547f
   anatomy of, 998-999
      normal, 1524, 1525f
      variations in, 998-999, 999f, 1014-1015
   azygos continuation of, 1525, 1526f
   circumaortic left renal vein anomaly of, 1525, 1527f
   circumcaval ureter anomaly of, 1526
   congenital anomalies of, 1524-1527, 1525f-1527f
      clinical presentation of, 1527-1528
      etiology and pathophysiology of, 1527
      imaging of
         indications and algorithm for, 1528
         technique and findings in, 1528-1529
      prevalence and epidemiology of, 1527
      reporting of, 1529
   duplicated right renal vein anomaly of, 1526
   duplication of, 1525, 1525f
      with retroaortic left renal vein and azygos continuation, 1527
      with retroaortic right renal vein and hemiazygos continuation, 1526-1527
   embryogenesis of, 1527
   formation of, 1009, 1009f
   inflow to, 1009-1010, 1010f
   left-sided anomaly of, 1525
   partial/complete absence of, 1526
   retroaortic left renal vein anomaly of, 1525
   tumors of, 1529-1532
      clinical presentation of, 1529
      differential diagnosis of, 1532-1533, 1533f
      etiology and pathophysiology of, 1529
      imaging of
         indications and algorithm for, 1529-1530
         technique and findings in, 1530-1532, 1531f-1533f
      prevalence and epidemiology of, 1529
      reporting of, 1533
      treatment options for, 1533
Inferior vena cava interventions
   definition of, 1540
   filters, 1540, 1540f
   shunts, 1540-1541, 1541f
   stents, 1541-1542, 1541f
Inferior vena cava obstruction syndrome, 1529
Inferior vena cava stenosis, after liver transplantation, 1534-1535, 1553-1554, 1555f-1556f
   clinical presentation of, 1534
   definition of, 1534
   differential diagnosis of, 1535
   imaging of, 1534-1535, 1534f-1537f
   prevalence and epidemiology of, 1534
   treatment options for, 1535
Inferior vena cava thrombosis, 1535-1540
   clinical presentation of, 1536-1539
   definition of, 1535
   differential diagnosis of, 1539-1540
   etiology and pathophysiology of, 1536, 1537t
   imaging of
      CT scan in, 1537, 1538f
      indications and algorithm for, 1536
      MR scan in, 1537-1539, 1539f
      nuclear medicine, 1539
      ultrasound, 1536
   prevalence and epidemiology of, 1536
   reporting of, 1540
   treatment options for, 1539
Infrapopliteal bypass graft, 1590, 1591t

Injection, of contrast media, 161
  clinical protocols for, 163-165, 164t-165t
  MR power-controlled, 1085, 1086f
  timing of, 161-162, 162f
Injection duration (ID), of contrast media, 160-161
Injury hypothesis, of atherosclerosis, response to, 1195
Innominate artery, tracheal compression of, 544, 547f
Inotropic agents, 355-356
  mechanism of action of, 355-356, 355f
  perfusion imaging protocol for, in SPECT, 285, 285f
Insertable loop recorders (ILRs), as MRI safety issue, 265
Instrumentation
  in Doppler ultrasonography, choice of, 1038
  in positron emission tomography, 319-320
  in single-photon emission computed tomography, 276-279, 276f. See also Single-photon emission computed tomography (SPECT), instrumentation in.
Integrins, 58
Intensive care unit (ICU), chest radiography in, 94-96, 95f, 95t
Interatrial septum
  developmental pathology of, 8
  formation of, 7-8, 9f
  lipomatous hypertrophy of, 916-917, 916f-917f
Interlobar artery, Doppler ultrasonography of, anatomic considerations in, 1507
Interlobular septal thickening, from hydrostatic pulmonary edema, 1374-1375, 1375f
Intermittent claudication, 1578-1581, 1579f
  differential diagnosis of, 1583
  in peripheral artery disease, 1628. See also Peripheral arterial disease (PAD).
Intermuscular veins, of lower extremity, 1028
Internal conversion, radioactive, 272t, 273, 273f
Internal mammary artery bypass graft, 522
  postoperative evaluation of, 524
Interpolation, in image reconstruction, 1120-1121, 1123f
Interposition graft, for penetrating atherosclerotic ulcer, 1301-1302
Interstitial edema, 85-87, 1374
Interventricular septum
  anatomy of, 34, 34f
  developmental pathology of, 4
  formation of, 4, 5f-6f
Interventricular sulcus, 3-4
Intima, of blood vessels, 60, 60f
Intimal flap, in thoracic aortic trauma, 1311
  CT imaging of, 1308
Intimal tear, with pseudoaneurysm, 1311, 1311f
Intra-aortic balloon pump, placement of, carotid Doppler waveform pattern after, 1244-1245, 1247f
Intracranial vascular disease, CT angiography of, 1060, 1061f
  protocol parameters for, 1061t
Intramural hematoma, aortic
  classic signs of, 1298
  definition of, 1296
  differential diagnosis of, 1298
  etiology and pathophysiology of, 1296
  imaging of
    indications and algorithm for, 1296
    technique and findings in, 1296-1298, 1297f-1298f

Intramural hematoma, aortic (Continued)
  medical treatment of, 1298
  prevalence and epidemiology of, 1296
  reporting of, 1299
  surgical/interventional treatment of, 1298-1299
Intramuscular veins, of lower extremity, 1028
Intrarenal artery(ies), Doppler ultrasonography of
  anatomic considerations in, 1507, 1508f
  technical considerations in, 1511, 1512f
Intravenous glucose loading protocol, in ^{18}FDG-PET imaging, 803
Intravoxal dephasing, in time-of-flight MR angiography, 1105
Inversion-recovery turbo field-echo (IF-TFE) sequences, in cardiac MR imaging, 211
Ionization, 271
Iron oxide contrast agents
  physiochemical characteristics of, 258t
  superparamagnetic, 254
Ischemic cardiomyopathy, 62. See also Cardiomyopathy.
Ischemic heart disease (IHD), 726. See also specific ischemic process.
  algorithm for management of, 726-727, 727f
  cardiac transplantation for, 811-812
    postoperative appearance of, 818, 819f-820f
    postoperative complications of, 812-813
      imaging of, 818-820, 821f
    clinical presentation of, postoperative, 813
  evaluation of
    CT imaging in, 755, 756t
    MRI scans in, 755, 755t
  postoperative assessment of, 812-813
    angiography in, 815
    CT imaging in, 814
    echocardiography in, 813-814
    MRI scans in, 814
    nuclear imaging in, 814-815
    PET scans in, 814-815
    radiography in, 813
    specific, 812-813
    surgery-related complications in, 812
  postoperative management of, 821-823, 822f
  prevalence, epidemiology, and background of, 810-812
  surgical ventricular restoration for: Dor procedure, 811
    postoperative appearance of, 817, 818f
    postoperative complications of, 812
      imaging of, 817-818
  ventricular assist device for, 810-811
    postoperative appearance of, 815, 816f
    postoperative complications of, 812
      imaging of, 816-817, 817f
    preoperative and perioperative assessment of, 815
Isobar, 271t
Isomer, 271t
Isometric transition, 273
Isotone, 271t
Isotope, 271t
Iterative reconstruction, of SPECT images, 279
Iterative reconstruction method, of PET image reconstruction, 313-314, 314f

J

Jejunal vein, 1005, 1006f
Judkins' technique, of coronary angiography, 123-124

Jugular vein(s)
  head and neck drainage via, 999
  internal, anatomy of, 1661, 1662f
Jugular venous valve, bovine, in pulmonary insufficiency repair, 379, 379f

K

Kawasaki's disease, aneurysm dilation in, 509, 511f-512f
Kerley A lines, 1374-1375
Kerley B lines, 1374-1375
Kidney. See Nephro-; Renal entries.
Kinetic energy, in radiation, 270
Kinetics, tracer, 314-315
Knee, arteries in
  collateral pathways of, 985-986, 987f
  pathologies of, 986
Knuckle sign, in pulmonary embolism, 1334
K-space, in contrast-enhanced MR angiography, 1088-1089, 1089f, 1399
K-space filling, triggering of
  in three-dimensional contrast-enhanced MR angiography, 1115-1116
  in three-dimensional steady-state free precession MR angiography, 1107
K-t methods, of accelerated MR imaging, 195-197
Kussmaul sign, in constrictive pericarditis, 949

L

Large vessel occlusive disease, of upper extremity, 1643-1645
  cause and pathophysiology of, 1644
  clinical presentation of, 1644-1645
  imaging indications and algorithm for, 1645
  prevalence and epidemiology of, 1644
Larmor equation, 1078-1079
LDL receptor gene, mutations of, 1196
Lecompte maneuver, for tetralogy of Fallot with absent pulmonary valve, 648, 649f
Left anterior descending (LAD) artery
  anatomy of, 44-46, 44f-45f
  segmental, 49
  aneurysm of, 509, 510f
  duplication of, 471-472, 472f
  subtypes of, 48-49, 48f
Left anterior oblique (LAO) projection, in chest radiography, 77-78, 80f
Left atrial appendage, 32-33, 32f, 443. See also Atrial entries.
  thrombus in, 443, 443f
    CT imaging of, 447, 447f-448f
Left bundle branch block (LBBB), 58
  myocardial perfusion imaging and, 358, 748
Left circumflex (LCX) artery
  anatomy of, 46, 46f-47f
  segmental, 49
  aneurysm of, 509, 510f
Left ventricle. See Ventricle(s), left.
Left ventricular assist device (LVAD), temporary percutaneous, 811
Left ventricular border, radiography of, 74-75, 75f-76f
Left ventricular function. See also Ventricular function.
  CT assessment of, 761
  diastolic, 235, 235f
Left ventricular mass, image interpretation of, 232

Left ventricular outflow tract (LVOT) obstruction, in hypertrophic cardiomyopathy
  MR imaging of, 879-882, 881f
  treatment of, 881-882
Left-to-right shunt
  in acyanotic heart defects, surgical intervention for, 386
  in patent ductus arteriosus, 584
  in ventricular septal defect, 573, 577-579
  quantification of, 243-244, 245f
Leiomyosarcoma, 927-928
  inferior vena cava invasion by
    extraluminal, 1530
    intraluminal, 1530, 1531f
Lemierre's syndrome, 1670, 1670f
Lenz effect, 265
Leriche syndrome, 1635-1636, 1636f
Lethargy, postoperative, ischemic heart disease and, 813
Levotransposition of great arteries, 602, 677-680. *See also* Transposition of great arteries (TGA).
  clinical presentation of, 678-680
  definition of, 677
  etiology and pathophysiology of, 678
  imaging of
    indications and algorithm for, 678
    technique and findings in, 678-680, 679f-681f
  incidence and epidemiology of, 677-678
Life cycling, of atherosclerotic plaque, 707
Lifestyle changes, for peripheral artery disease, 1209
Limb ischemia
  acute, 1573-1578
    clinical presentation of, 1573-1577, 1574f
    critical categorization of, 1575-1576, 1575t, 1576f, 1598, 1598t
    definition of, 1573
    differential diagnosis of, 1577
    etiology and pathophysiology of, 1573, 1574t
    imaging of
      indications and algorithm for, 1576
      technique and findings in, 1576-1577
    medical treatment of, 1577
    prevalence and epidemiology of, 1573, 1574t
    surgical/interventional treatment of, 1577-1578, 1577f-1578f
  chronic, 1578-1584
    clinical presentation of, 1580-1581
    critical, 1579, 1580f-1582f, 1581
    definition of, 1578, 1579t
    differential diagnosis of, 1583
    etiology and pathophysiology of, 1579-1580
    imaging of
      indications and algorithm for, 1581-1582
      technique and findings in, 1582-1583
    intermittent claudication in, 1578-1581, 1579f
    medical treatment of, 1583
    prevalence and epidemiology of, 1578-1579, 1579f-1580f
    Rutherford categorization of, 1578, 1579t, 1588, 1589t
    surgical/interventional treatment of, 1583-1584
Linear attenuation coefficient (μ), 276
Linear interpolation, in image reconstruction, 1121

Lipid abnormalities
  genes promoting, 1196
  in atherosclerotic process, 1197
Lipid-lowering therapy
  for cerebrovascular atherosclerotic disease, 1208
  for peripheral artery disease, 1209
Lipomatous hypertrophy, 916
Lipomatous hypertrophy of interatrial septum (LHIS), 916-917, 916f-917f
Liposarcoma, 931-932, 932f
Liquid embolic agents, 1168-1169
Liquid helium, used in MRI scanners, 264
List mode imaging protocol, in emission scanning, 326-327
Liver. *See also* Hepatic *entries.*
Liver cancer, 1458-1459. *See also* Cholangiocarcinoma; Hepatocellular carcinoma.
  endovascular treatment of, 975-976
Liver disease
  cirrhotic. *See* Cirrhosis.
  pulmonary hypertension associated with, 1360
Liver transplant recipients. *See also* Hepatic transplantation.
  manifestations of disease in, 1459
  pretransplant imaging of, 1544-1545
    indications and algorithm for, 1459-1460
    MR scans in, 1460
Living donors
  for hepatic transplantation
    pretransplant imaging of, 1545-1546, 1545f-1546f, 1546t
    split-liver, 1534
  for renal transplantation, vascular evaluation of, 1567-1568
Loeys-Dietz syndrome, 1273, 1274f
Löffler endocarditis, 864-866. *See also* Eosinophilic endomyocardial disease.
Long-segment stenosis, of carotid arteries, Doppler ultrasonography of, 1236, 1237f
Low contrast detectability (LCD), in CT systems, 1050, 1050f-1051f
Low-density lipoprotein (LDL), oxidation of, 1195
Lower extremity
  arterial anatomy of, 983-988. *See also* named artery, e.g., Femoral artery.
    collateral pathways in, 985-986, 986f-987f
    differential considerations in, 986-987
    general description of, 983-985, 983f-985f
    normal variants of, 985-986
    pertinent imaging considerations in, 987-988
  CT angiography of, 1610-1627. *See also* Computed tomographic angiography (CTA), of lower extremities.
  exclusion procedure(s) for. *See also specific procedure.*
    endovascular methods, 1604-1608
    surgical excision and vascular bypass, 1600-1604
  occlusive disease of
    bypass procedures for. *See* Lower extremity bypass.
    hybrid procedures for, 1188-1189, 1188f
    pulse volume recordings identifying, 1186, 1187f
    revascularization procedure(s) for. *See also specific procedure.*
    catheter-directed or pharmacomechanical thrombolysis, 1597f, 1599-1600
    endovascular methods, 1591-1598

Lower extremity (Continued)
    surgical thromboembolectomy, 1598-1599, 1598t
    vascular bypass surgery, 1585-1591
  thrombosis in, ultrasound detection of, 1334-1335
  vasculature of, CT angiography of, 1068-1069, 1069f-1072f
    protocol parameters for, 1061t
  venous anatomy of, 1023-1029, 1024f-1025f. *See also named vein.*
    deep veins in, 1027-1029
    perforator veins in, 1029
    superficial veins in, 1024-1027, 1026f-1028f
Lower extremity aneurysm
  endovascular exclusion procedures for, 1604-1608
    anatomic considerations in, 1604
    contraindications to, 1605
    imaging findings in, 1606-1608, 1606f-1607f
    indications for, 1605
    outcomes and complications of, 1605-1606
  surgical excision and vascular bypass of
    anatomic considerations in, 1600-1601, 1601f
    contraindications to, 1601-1602
    imaging findings in, 1603-1604, 1604f-1605f
    indications for, 1601, 1602f-1603f
    outcomes and complications of, 1602-1603
Lower extremity bypass, 1185
  contraindications to, 1185
  imaging findings in
    postoperative surveillance and, 1187, 1188f
    preoperative assessment and, 1186, 1186t-1187t, 1187f
    preoperative planning and, 1186-1187, 1188f
  indications for, 1185
  outcomes and complications of, 1185-1186, 1186f, 1186t
Lumber artery, 975
Lumber vein, 1009, 1010f
Lung(s). *See also* Pulmonary; Respiratory *entries.*
  ground-glass opacity of, 1376
Lung disease
  chronic obstructive. *See* Chronic obstructive pulmonary disease (COPD).
  pulmonary hypertension caused by, 1365-1366
  thromboembolic, 1332-1343. *See also* Pulmonary embolism.
    definition of, 1332
Lung injury
  acute, 1376
  direct and indirect, 1377b
Lymphoma
  metastatic to heart, 922
  primary cardiac
    definition of, 932
    manifestations of disease in, 932-933, 933f-934f
    pathology of, 932
    prevalence of, 932

M

M mode, in echocardiography, 98, 99f
Macrophages, lipid-laden, 60, 60f

Magnetic fields
  as MRI safety issue
    gradient, 263
    static, 263, 263t
  in MR angiography, gradient, 1083
Magnetic resonance angiography (MRA)
  after surgical repair of truncus arteriosus, 622-623, 623f
  black blood, 1099-1100, 1100f
  contrast-enhanced, 1086-1091, 1087f, 1398-1399
    agent dosage in, 1399
    k-space view ordering in, 1088-1089, 1089f, 1399
    mask mode subtraction in, 1091, 1091f
  of carotid arteries, 1252-1255, 1253f
    contraindication(s) to
      metallic implants as, 1257
      nephrogenic systemic fibrosis as, 1255-1257
    dedicated carotid coils in, 1253-1254
    field of view in, 1254-1255, 1255f-1256f
    image interpretation of, 1258-1259, 1259f
    imaging parameters for, 1257, 1257t
    indications for, 1252
    parallel imaging in, 1253, 1254f
    pitfalls and solutions in, 1258
    spatial resolution in, 1252-1253
    technical requirement for, 1252
    technique of, 1257-1258, 1257t
  of coarctation of aorta, 373, 375f, 536-537
  of coronary atherosclerosis, 711
  of penetrating atherosclerotic ulcer, 1300, 1301f
  of peripheral artery disease, 1630-1634
    contrast media and injection protocols in, 1633
    novel contrast media in, 1633
    resolution requirements in, 1632-1633
    strategies to decrease venous enhancement in, 1631-1632
    strategies to optimize vessel to background contrast in, 1631
    three-dimensional, with contrast arrival, 1630-1631
    vascular anatomy considerations in, 1630
  of renal arteries, 1487-1488
  of tetralogy of Fallot, 643-645, 645f-646f
  overall scan time in, 1087-1088, 1089f
  preoperative, of carotid artery stenosis, 1174
  techniques of, 1086-1100, 1087f
  three-dimensional, 1112-1118
    contraindications to, 1115
    indications for, 1113-1115, 1113f-1118f
    of arterial system, 1451
    of venous system and soft tissue, 1452
    pitfalls and solutions in, 1115-1116
    postprocessing of, 1116-1117
    reporting of, 1117-1118
    time-resolved, 1089-1091, 1090f-1091f
  data acquisition in, 1078-1081
  ECG gating in, 1103
  field strength in, 1102
  gadolinium-enhanced three-dimensional, of postoperative congenital heart disease patients, 693, 693f
  gradient coils in, 1102
  image encoding in, 1078, 1080f-1082f
  image reconstruction in, 1078-1081, 1079f
  new developments in, 1487-1488
  nonenhanced, of peripheral artery disease, 1634

Magnetic resonance angiography (MRA) (Continued)
  of abdominal aortic aneurysm, 1205-1206, 1401, 1402f, 1442
  of aortic dissection, 1292, 1293f
  of arteriovenous fistula and pseudoaneurysm, in renal transplant recipient, 1565, 1566f
  of arteriovenous fistula failure, 1677-1680, 1679f-1681f
  of atrium, right, 30-31, 32f
  of carotid stenosis, 1220
  of cyanotic heart lesions, 652
  of heart valves, 34-36, 35f-36f
  of inferior vena cava stenosis, 1553-1554, 1556f
  of interventricular septum, 34, 34f
  of limb ischemia
    acute, 1576
    chronic, 1583
  of pericardium, 30, 31f
  of portal vein stenosis, 1551-1553, 1554f-1555f
  of pulmonary hypertension, related to associated conditions, 1361, 1361f
  of renal arteries, 1485, 1487-1488
    contraindications to, 1485
    contrast-enhanced, 1487-1488
    image interpretation in, 1488-1490, 1488f
    indications for, 1483-1485, 1484f
    pitfalls and solutions in, 1488
    reporting of, 1490
    technical requirements for, 1483
    technique of, 1486-1487, 1486t
  of renal artery stenosis, 1475-1477, 1477f-1478f, 1483-1484, 1484f
    in transplant recipient, 1561-1564, 1563f
    accuracy of, 1562t
  of renal artery thrombosis, in transplant recipient, 1567
  of renal donor, 1484-1485, 1484f
  of renal vasculature, in living kidney donor, 1568
  of renal vein thrombosis, in transplant recipient, 1567
  of subclavian steal syndrome, 1328-1329, 1328f-1330f
  of thoracic outlet syndrome, 1669
  of vascular anatomy, in pancreas transplant recipient, 1569
  of ventricle
    left, 33-34, 34f
    right, 33, 33f
  parallel imaging techniques in, 1102-1103
  patient preparation for, 1103
  phase contrast, 1094-1098, 1095f-1097f, 1105-1106
    intravoxel dephasing in, 1096
    postprocessing in, 1096-1098, 1097f-1098f
  phased-array surface coils in, 1102-1103
  steady-state free precession, 1098-1099, 1099f
    three-dimensional, 1106-1109, 1107f-1108f
    contraindications to, 1106
    image interpretation in, 1108-1109, 1108f
    indications for, 1106
    pitfalls and solutions in, 1107-1108
  technical requirements in, 1081-1085, 1102-1103
    gradient system and, 1083
    magnetic resonance scanner and, 1082-1083, 1082f

Magnetic resonance angiography (MRA) (Continued)
  parallel imaging and, 1084, 1085f
  patient monitoring and, 1084-1085
  power injector and, 1085, 1086f
  radiofrequency system and, 1083-1084, 1083f-1084f
  three-dimensional postprocessing in, basic, 1120-1127. See also Three-dimensional postprocessing, in CTA and MRA.
  time-of-flight, 1091-1094, 1092f, 1103-1105, 1104f
    contraindications to, 1103-1105
    image interpretation in, 1105
    indications for, 1103
    of carotid artery stenosis, 1252
    pitfalls and solutions in, 1105
    three-dimensional, 1093
    sequential, 1094, 1094f
    two-dimensional, 1092-1093, 1092f-1093f
  time-resolved, 1109-1112, 1109f
    contraindications to, 1110-1111
    contrast-enhanced, 1089-1091, 1090f-1091f
    image interpretation in, 1112
    indications for, 1109-1110, 1110f-1111f, 1112t
    pitfalls and solutions in, 1111
Magnetic resonance imaging (MRI). See also MRI entries.
  cardiac, 180-200, 215-226
    accelerated, 192-198
      fast pulse sequences in, 194-195, 194f
      k-t methods of, 195-197
      parallel imaging in, 195, 196f
      real-time, 197-198
    anatomic overview in, 203-205, 204f
    application-specific methods of, 181-192
    black blood imaging used in, 182-184, 183f-184f
    cardiovascular protocol for, 555t
    clinical applications of, 180
    clinical techniques of, 201-214
    delayed hyperenhancement in
      description of, 210-211, 211f
      indications for, 207-210, 208f-210f
      pitfalls and solutions in, 212, 212f
      reporting of, 212-213, 213f
    determining global measures in, 215-216
    diastolic function and, 218, 219f
    dynamic left ventricular function and
      with dobutamine, 218-223, 220f-223f, 220t
      with exercise, 223-224, 223f
    image acquisition technique(s) for, 227-229
      echo-planar imaging, 228-229, 228t
      in assessing quantitative analysis of myocardial motion, 229-231, 229f, 230t
      sensitivity encoding parallel imaging, 228t, 229
      spoiled gradient echo, 227, 228t
    interpretation of, 231-237
      left ventricular volume and function and, 231-235, 231f-232f, 233t, 234f-235f
      right ventricular volume and function and, 235-237, 236t, 237f
    motion compensation in, 201-203, 202f-203f
    perfusion in
      contraindications to, 205, 206t
      description of, 205-207

Magnetic resonance imaging (MRI) (Continued)
    indications for, 205, 205f
    pitfalls and solutions in, 207
    reporting of, 207
    phase contrast images in, 192, 192f-194f
    resting regional wall motion abnormalities and, 216-217
    right ventricular function and, 217, 217f
    spatial resolution in, 180-181
    technical requirements for, 215
    temporal resolution in, 180-181
  contrast agents in, 251-260, 1398-1399
    classification of, 255-259, 255f, 257t-258t
    cost of, 255
    development of, 251
    dosage of, 1399
    pharmacovigilance of, 253
    regulatory label of, 251-252
    safety of, 252-253, 266
  of acute coronary syndrome, 721, 721f
  of amyloidosis, 863, 863f-864f
  of angiosarcoma, 926, 927f
  of aorta, 555-556, 555t, 556f-558f
  of aortic aneurysm
    abdominal, 1442
    inflammatory, 1405, 1406f
    ruptured, 1303
    thoracic, 1281-1282
  of aortic dissection, 1291-1294, 1293f
  of aortic regurgitation, 833, 833f
  of aortic stenosis, 829, 831f
  of aortic trauma, thoracic, 1309-1310, 1310f
  of arrhythmogenic right ventricular dysplasia, 888-892, 889f-892f, 891t
    black blood breath-hold fast spin-echo, 890-891
    bright blood cine gradient, 890
    functional abnormalities in, 889, 890f-891f, 891t
    morphologic abnormalities in, 889, 889f-890f, 891t
    right ventricular intramyocardial fat on, 891
    screening role of, 892
  of atherosclerosis, 1204-1206, 1205f
  of atherosclerotic carotid plaque, 1220-1221, 1221f
  of atrial fibrillation, 449, 450f
  of atrial septal defect, 566-567, 568f-569f
    postoperative, 365-366, 368f
    preoperative, 364, 365f-366f
  of blood flow, 239-250
    flow-encoding axes in, 239-240, 241f
    indications for, 240
    limitations and pitfalls in, 240, 242f
    phase contrast, 239-240, 240f
    technical requirements in, 239-240, 240f-242f
    techniques for, 240-249
      in coarctation of aorta, 242-243, 244f
      in pulmonary flow evaluation, 244-249, 246f-248f
      in shunting, 243-244, 245f
      in valvular disease, 241-242, 243f
    velocity encoding in, 240, 242f
  of Budd-Chiari syndrome, 1461, 1462f
  of cardiac function, 756-757
    anatomic planning and standard views in, 756
    during stress, 218-223, 767-768
      diagnostic criteria and, 768, 769f
      exercise, 223-224, 223f, 767

Magnetic resonance imaging (MRI) (Continued)
    pharmacologic agents in, 767-768. See also specific agent. e.g., Dobutamine.
    protocols for, 768
  image analysis in, 757, 758f
  left ventricular, 556, 733-734, 758-759, 760t-761t
  regional, 764-766, 765f-767f
    image interpretation of, 232-235, 233t, 234f-235f, 237, 237f
  right ventricular, 217, 217f, 761-762, 762t-763t
  sequences in, 756-757
  of cardiac lymphoma, primary, 933, 934f
  of cardiac metastases, 921f, 923f, 924, 925f
  of cardiac tumor, calcified amorphous, 919, 920f
  of cardiomyopathy
    dilated, 855-857, 856f-857f
    hypertrophic, 875-882
      morphology in, 875-876, 875t, 876f-878f
      siderotic, 867-868, 868f
  of coarctation of aorta, 373, 376f, 536-537
    classic signs in, 537, 538f
  of congenital heart disease, postoperative evaluation in, 689-701
    cine imaging, 690-691, 690f-691f
    clinical presentation indicating, 694
    indications and algorithm for, 694
    spin-echo imaging, 691, 691f
    technique and findings in, 694-700, 695f-699f
    velocity-encoded cine sequences, 691-693, 692f
  of cor triatriatum, 633
  of coronary anomalies, congenital, 467
  of coronary arteries, 190-191, 191f
  of coronary artery bypass graft, 523-524
  of coronary atherosclerosis, 710-711
  of cyanotic heart lesions, 652
  of double-outlet right ventricle, 684, 685f
  of endoleaks, 1409, 1409f
  of eosinophilic endomyocardial disease, 865, 866f
  of fibroma, 912f, 913
  of giant cell arteritis, 1321, 1321f-1322f
  of hereditary hemorrhagic telangiectasia, 1468
  of inferior vena cava anomalies, 1528-1529
  of inferior vena cava thrombosis, 1537-1539, 1539f
  of inferior vena cava tumors, 1531
  of in-stent restenosis and thrombosis, 518
  of intramural hematoma of aorta, 1297, 1298f
  of ischemic heart disease
    advantages and disadvantages of, 756t
    indications for and applications of, 755, 755t
    postoperative, 814
  of leiomyosarcoma, 928
  of lipoma, 915
  of lipomatous hypertrophy of interatrial septum, 916, 917f
  of liposarcoma, 931
  of mitral regurgitation, 837, 837f
  of mitral stenosis, 835
  of myocardial perfusion, 184-185, 185f-187f, 728-730
    contraindications to, 733
    image interpretation in, 734-735, 735f
    indications for, 733

Magnetic resonance imaging (MRI) (Continued)
    pitfalls and solutions in, 734
    preclinical and clinical evaluation in, 728-730, 728f-729f, 730t
    reporting of, 735-736
    technique of, 733-734
  of myocardial viability, 185-188, 187f-189f
    contraindications to, 787
    hyperenhancement on, 782-784, 783f-786f
    in postoperative congenital heart disease patients, 693-694, 693f-694f
    wall thickness in, 782
    with dobutamine, 221-222, 222f, 782
  of myocarditis, 897-899, 898f
  of myxoma, 908, 908f-909f
  of osteosarcoma, 929, 929f
  of pancreatic adenocarcinoma, 1465-1466, 1465f-1466f
  of papillary fibroelastoma, 910
  of paraganglioma, 918, 918f
  of patent ductus arteriosus, 586-588, 587f-589f
  of pericardial effusion, 943
  of pericarditis
    acute, 946
    constrictive, 950-951, 951f
  of polyarteritis nodosa, 1468
  of pulmonary artery stenosis, 377, 378f
  of pulmonary embolism, 1340
  of pulmonary hypertension, 1357-1358
    chronic thromboembolic, 1349, 1367
    with left heart disease (venous), 1364
    with unclear multifactorial mechanisms, 1371
  of pulmonary insufficiency, 380-381, 380f
  of pulmonary valve regurgitation, 846-847
  of pulmonary valve stenosis, 846
  of pulmonary venous connections
    partial anomalous, 627
    total anomalous, 636, 637f
  of rhabdomyoma, 913-914, 914f
  of rhabdomyosarcoma, 930, 931f
  of sarcoidosis, 869-870, 870f
  of single ventricle, 673-676
    after bidirectional superior cavopulmonary connection, 674-675
    after Fontan procedure, 675-676, 676f-677f
    after stage I, 674
    in native state, 674
  of sinus venosus defect, 630, 631f
  of splanchnic artery aneurysm, 1463, 1464f
  of splenic infarcts, 1467, 1467f
  of tagging and wall motion, 188-190, 189f-190f, 764-765, 765f
  of Takayasu arteritis, 1316-1317, 1317f-1318f, 1389, 1389f
  of tetralogy of Fallot, 643-646, 645f-647f, 661, 662f-663f
  of transposition of great arteries, 658-660, 659f
  of tricuspid valve regurgitation, 845
  of truncus arteriosus, 665-666, 667f-670f
  of upper extremity medium and small vessel disease, 1649-1650, 1651f-1654f
  of valvular disease, 66, 66f
  of vascular rings, 544
  of ventricular function, 181-182, 181f-182f
    left, 556, 733-734, 758-759, 760t-761t
    right, 217, 217f, 761-762, 762t-763t
  of ventricular septal defect, 575-577, 578f-579f

Magnetic resonance imaging (MRI) *(Continued)*
  repetition time in, 181-182
  safety of, 261-269, 262b
    acoustic noise and, 267
    future issues in, 268
    general concerns regarding, 261-264
      cryogens and, 264
      electricity and magnetism and, 263
      gradient magnetic fields and, 263
      hazards and, 261-262
      MRI clinic and, 262-263, 262f
      radiofrequency fields and, 263-264
      static magnetic field strength and, 263, 263t
    hearing protection and, 267
    insertable loop recorders and, 265
    pacemakers, implantable cardioverter-defibrillators, other devices and, 264-265
    prosthetic heart valves and, 265
    sedation and, 266-267, 266t
    stents and, 265-266
    stress testing and, 267-268
    terminology issues and, 264, 264t-265t
  steady-state free precession, 181, 228, 228t, 1398, 1398f
  dilated cardiomyopathy diagnosis with, 855, 856f
  evaluation of cardiac function in, 756-757
  image acquisition techniques for, 228, 228t
  localization of heart in, 733-734
Magnetic resonance scanner, in MR angiography, 1082-1083, 1082f
Magnetism, as MRI safety issue, 263
Malignancy. *See also* Metastases; *specific neoplasm.*
  as risk factor in deep vein thrombosis, 1662-1663
  renal vein thrombosis associated with, 1518-1519, 1518f
Marfan syndrome, cystic medial necrosis in, 1272-1273, 1273f-1274f
  pathophysiology and follow-up of, 550-551, 551f
  prevalence and epidemiology of, 550
Marginal artery of Drummond, 975
Marginal veins
  cardiac, 52
  lower extremity, 1024-1026, 1027f
Mask mode subtraction, in contrast-enhanced MR angiography, 1091, 1091f
Matrix detector, in multislice CT, 1053-1054, 1053f
Matter, radiation interactions with, 274-276, 275f-276f
Maximum intensity projection (MIP)
  in CT angiography, 1074, 1121-1123, 1123f-1124f
    carotid, 1265-1266
    coronary, 502
    lower extremity, 1622, 1624f-1625f
    renal, 1489, 1489f
  in CT imaging, cardiac, 173-176
  in MR angiography, 1488, 1488f
    contrast-enhanced, 1258, 1259f
    time-of-flight, 1105
  sliding, 173-176
May-Thurner syndrome, 1015, 1015f, 1535
Mechanical occlusion devices, as embolic agents, 1168
Meckel diverticulum scan, 1146-1148

Mediastinal border, radiography of
  left, 72, 72f-73f
  right, 75, 76f
Mediastinal hemorrhage
  periaortic, in thoracic aortic trauma, 1309, 1309f
  postoperative, radiographic features of, 96
Mediastinal infection, after cardiac transplantation, 812-813, 819-820
Mediastinal widening, in thoracic aortic trauma, 1311
Mediastinitis
  fibrosing
    clinical presentation of, 1371
    etiology and pathophysiology of, 1370-1371
    imaging of, 1371
  postoperative, ischemic heart disease and, 813
Medium vessel disease, of upper extremity, 1645-1652. *See also* Upper extremity, medium and small vessel disease of.
Melanoma, metastatic, to heart, 922
Mesenteric angiography, 1159
Mesenteric artery
  inferior, 972, 973f-974f
  superior, 972, 973f-974f
Mesenteric atherosclerotic disease. *See also* Atherosclerosis.
  clinical presentation of, 1198t, 1199
  CT angiography of, 1203-1204
  differential diagnosis of, 1207t
  medical treatment of, 1210
  prevalence and epidemiology of, 1194
  screening for, 1200
  surgical/interventional treatment of, 1212
Mesenteric ischemia
  angiography of, 1207
  MR angiography of, 1205
Mesenteric vasculature, CT angiography of, 1066-1068, 1069f
Mesenteric vein
  inferior, 1006f-1007f, 1007
    variations of, 1008
  superior, 1005-1006, 1006f-1007f
    variations of, 1008
  thrombosis of, 1457-1458
Mesocaval shunt, inferior vena cava, 1541
Metabolic agents, radionuclide. *See also specific radionuclide.*
  in PET imaging, 342-344, 342f-343f
Metabolic storage diseases, restrictive cardiomyopathy associated with, 871
Metacarpal veins, 1024-1026, 1026f
123-Metaiodobenzylguanidine, radiolabeled, in PET/SPECT imaging, 806, 806f
Metallic components, implantable, as PET image artifact, 321-322, 322f
Metallic implants, as contraindication to contrast-enhanced MR angiography, 1257
Metallic material artifacts, in coronary CT angiography, 496, 497f-498f
Metastases
  cardiac
    clinical presentation of, 922-923
    definition of, 921-922, 921f-922f
    differential diagnosis of, 924-925
    imaging technique and findings in, 923-924, 923f-925f
    pathology of, 922
    prevalence of, 922-925
    treatment options for, 925

Metastases *(Continued)*
    myocardial, 922
    pericardial, 922
    pericardial effusion in, 941
Metoprolol
  used in cardiac imaging, 144
  used in CTA examination, 1064
Michel classification, of hepatic artery anatomy, 1545, 1546t
Microscopic polyangiitis, 1386-1387
Mirror image artifact, in Doppler ultrasonography, 1042
Mitral annulus velocities, 103
Mitral balloon valvotomy, 407f, 408, 836
Mitral balloon valvuloplasty, percutaneous, indications for, 427, 428t
Mitral inflow velocities, 103
Mitral valve
  anatomy of, 34, 35f, 422-424, 423f-424f
  calcifications in, 87, 88f
  formation of, 5
Mitral valve disease, surgery for, 417-429
  anatomic considerations in, 422-426, 423f-427f
  contraindications to, 427-428
  indications for, 426-427, 427t-428t
  outcomes and complications of, 424f, 426f, 428
  postoperative surveillance after, 415
  preoperative imaging in, 428-429
Mitral valve insufficiency, 64-65
Mitral valve regurgitation
  clinical presentation of, 837
  definition of, 836
  etiology of, 836
  imaging of
    echocardiographic, 110, 837
    indications for, 837
    radiographic, 93-94
    techniques of, 837, 837f
  medical treatment of, 837
  pathophysiology of, 424, 425f, 836
  prevalence of, 836
  quantification of, 241-242
  surgical treatment of, 837-838
    considerations regarding, 387-388, 388t
    indications for, 426-427, 427t
Mitral valve stenosis, 65
  clinical presentation of, 834
  definition of, 834
  etiology of, 834
  imaging of
    echocardiographic, 109-110, 111f-112f, 835, 835f
    indications for, 834
    radiographic, 93, 93f
    techniques of, 834-835, 834f-835f
  medical treatment of, 424-425, 836
  pathophysiology of, 424, 834
  percutaneous balloon valvuloplasty for, indications for, 427, 428t
  prevalence and epidemiology of, 834
  surgical treatment of, 426f-427f, 836
    indications for, 427, 428t
Mitral valve vegetation, in infective endocarditis, 429f-430f
Mixed edema, 1379, 1379b
Modulation transfer function (MTF), of CT systems, 1048-1049
Morphine, intravenous, for acute coronary syndrome, 723
Mortality rate
  for abdominal aortic aneurysm repair, 1440
  for heart failure, 790
  for infective endocarditis, 431

Mortality rate (Continued)
  for mitral valve repair, 429
  for thoracic aortic repair, 136
MRI. See also Magnetic resonance imaging (MRI).
MRI clinic, zones of, 262-263, 262f
MRI compatible, definition of, 263t-264t, 264
MRI safe, definition of, 263t-264t, 264
MRI scanners, acoustic noise of, 267
MRI suite, rapid evacuation of, emergency procedures for, 267
MRI unsafe, definition of, 264, 264t
MR-IMPACT trial, 730
Multi-Ethnic Study of Atherosclerosis (MESA) trial, 460
Multiframe (dynamic) imaging protocol, in emission scanning, 326-327
Multiplanar (reconstruction) reformation (MPR)
  in contrast-enhanced MR angiography, 1258, 1259f
  in CT angiography, 1073-1074, 1120-1121, 1121f-1122f
    carotid, 1264-1265
    coronary, 500, 502f
    lower extremity, 1622, 1623f
  in steady-state free precession MR angiography, 1108
  interpolation in, 1120-1121, 1123f
  linear interpolation in, 1121
Multiple overlapping thin slab angiography (MOTSA), 1094, 1094f
Multiple-level shunt, in acyanotic congenital heart disease, 385t, 386
Multisegment image reconstruction, in CT imaging, 136-137, 138f-139f
Muscle tissue deficits, in acute limb ischemia, 1574
Muscular septum, long/short, myocardial perfusion imaging and, 748
Mustard and Stenning procedure, for transposition of great arteries, 389
Mycotic aortic aneurysm, 594, 594f, 1406-1407, 1407f
Myectomy, for left ventricular outflow tract obstruction, 881
Myocardial bridging, of coronary arteries, 49, 49f-50f, 472-473, 474f
Myocardial calcification, radiography of, 87, 87f
Myocardial contractility, evaluation of, MRI scans in, 757
Myocardial delayed enhancement (MDE) imaging, 734
  hyperenhancement on, 782-784, 783f-786f
Myocardial function
  assessment of, 756-767
    CT imaging in, 758, 759f
      during stress, 769
      of left ventricle, 761
      of right ventricle, 762-763
    MR imaging in, 756-757
      anatomic planning and standard views in, 756
      during stress, 218-223, 767-768
        diagnostic criteria and, 768, 769f
        exercise, 223-224, 223f, 767
        pharmacologic agents for, 767-768. See also specific agent, e.g., Dobutamine.
        protocols for, 768
      image analysis in, 757, 758f
      of left ventricle, 758-759, 760t-761t
      of right ventricle, 761-762, 762t-763t
      sequences in, 756-757
  disorders of, systolic, 62

Myocardial function (Continued)
  regional
    CT assessment of, 766-767
    MRI assessment of, 764-766, 765f-767f
    nomenclature for, 763, 764f
Myocardial hibernation, 62, 331
  definition of, 781, 790
  energy metabolism alterations in, 792
  phenomenon of, 792, 792f
  schematic of, 791f
Myocardial infarction
  chronic coronary artery disease and, 62
  complications of, 94
  definition of, 61
  imaging after, 357-358
    delayed hyperenhancement MR, 208, 209f
  non–ST segment elevation, 715
    percutaneous coronary interventions for, 402, 723
  pericardial effusion in, 941
  prognosis after, 754
  ST segment elevation, 715
    percutaneous coronary interventions for, 399, 400f, 723
Myocardial ischemia
  causes of, 726
  definition of, 792, 792f
  dobutamine MRI and, 218-221, 220t, 221f
  identification of, stress multidetector CT in, 733
  injury resulting from, categorization of, 792, 793f
Myocardial metabolism, 800-805
  ^{18}FDG PET imaging of, 801
    protocol(s) in, 801-803
      hyperinsulinemic-euglycemic clamping, 803
      intravenous glucose loading, 803
      nicotinic acid derivative, 803
      oral glucose loading, 802-803
  fatty acid radiotracer PET/SPECT imaging of, 800-801, 801f-802f
Myocardial metastases, 922
Myocardial motion
  causing attenuation mismatch, in PET imaging, 309-310, 311f
  compensation for, during MR imaging, 201-203, 202f-203f
  MRI quantitative analysis of, 229-231
    displacement encoding with stimulated echoes in, 230-231, 230t
    phase-contrast velocity mapping in, 230, 230t
    tagged imaging in, 229-230, 229f, 230t
Myocardial perfusion
  assessment of, 326-331, 727-728
    CT imaging in, 326, 730-733
      animal studies of, 730-731, 731t
      contraindications to, 733
      human studies of, 731-733, 732t
      image interpretation of, 735
      indications for, 733
      pitfalls and solutions in, 734
      reporting of, 735-736
      stress multidetector, 733
      technique of, 734
    emission scans in, 326-327
    MR imaging in, 184-185, 185f-187f, 205-207, 728-730
      contraindications to, 205, 206t, 733
      image interpretation of, 734-735, 735f
      indications for, 205, 205f, 733
      pitfalls and solutions in, 207, 734
      preclinical and clinical evaluation of, 728-730, 728f-729f, 730t

Myocardial perfusion (Continued)
    reporting of, 207, 735-736
    technique of, 733-734
    PET/CT imaging in, 326-331
      diagnostic accuracy of, 328-329, 329t
      evaluation of coronary artery disease and, 329, 329f-330f
      glucose-loaded ^{18}FDG patterns in, 333-334, 333f-334f
      imaging protocols for, 326-327, 327f
      quality assurance for, 327-328, 328f
      risk stratification and, 329-331, 331f
  defects in, ^{99m}Tc-sestamibi imaging of, 285-296, 287f-296f
  functional recovery of, after revascularization, 334-335, 335t
  impaired, in hypertrophic cardiomyopathy, MR imaging of, 877
Myocardial perfusion imaging (MPI)
  with gated SPECT, of ventricular function, 771-773
    data processing, reconstruction, and analysis of, 772-773
    electrogram gated acquisition in, 772
    pitfalls and solutions in, 773
    technique(s) of, 773-779
      equilibrium gated blood pool imaging, 773-775, 774f-778f
      first-pass radionuclide angiography, 775-779, 779f
  with PET, 749-751
    clinical indications for, 749, 750f
    future directions of, 751-752
    image acquisition data in, 750-751
    myocardial viability and, 751, 752f
    pitfalls and solutions in, 751
    radiotracers in, 749-750
    stress protocols for, 750
    technical aspects of, 749-750
    technique and protocols for, 750-751, 750f
  with SPECT, 738-749. See also under Single-photon emission computed tomography (SPECT).
    description of technique and protocols in, 744-746
    image interpretation of, 746-749, 747f-748f
    technical aspects of, 738-739
    techniques of, 739-744, 741f-743f
Myocardial scarring, 331
Myocardial strain, 764
Myocardial stunning, 62, 331, 721
  definition of, 781, 790
  phenomenon of, 792, 792f
  schematic of, 791f
Myocardial tagging, MR imaging of, 188-190, 189f-190f, 764-765, 765f
Myocardial torsion, 764
Myocardial twist, 764
Myocardial viability, 62-63
  assessment of, 331-336
    CT imaging in, 784-787, 787f
      limitations of, 787-788
    hibernation vs. stunning in, 331-332
    impact of, on patient outcomes, 335-336, 336f, 336t
    PET/CT imaging protocols in, 332-333, 332f
      accuracy of, predicting functional recovery, 334-335, 335t
      myocardial perfusion and glucose-loaded ^{18}FDG patterns in, 333-334, 333f-334f
      patient preparation for, 332-333, 333f
      with dobutamine, 358

Myocardial viability (Continued)
  definitions of, 781-782, 790-794
  identification of, nuclear imaging
      technique(s) in, 794-800. See also
      under specific imaging modality.
    fatty acid radiotracers in, 800-801,
        801f-802f
    ^{18}FDG, 801
    ^{18}FDG-PET mismatch and match patterns,
        803-804
      functional recovery in, 803, 804f
      prognosis of, 803-804, 804f
    ^{18}FDG-PET protocols, 801-803
    ^{18}FDG-SPECT, 805
    future opportunities for, 805-807, 806f
    PET, 799-800, 799f-800f
    SPECT, 794-797, 795f-798f
  in hypertrophic cardiomyopathy, MR
      imaging of, 877-879, 880f
  MR imaging of, 185-188, 187f-189f, 782-784
    contraindications to, 787
    hyperenhancement on, 208, 209f,
        782-784, 783f-786f
    in postoperative congenital heart disease
        patients, 693-694, 693f-694f
    wall thickness in, 782
    with dobutamine, 221-222, 222f, 782
  studies of, end points used in, 792-794,
      794f
  ^{201}Tl-labeled SPECT imaging showing,
      299-300, 300f
    accuracy of, 749
Myocarditis, 896-901
  classic signs in, 899
  clinical presentation of, 896
  definition of, 896
  differential diagnosis of, 899
  etiology and pathophysiology of, 896
  imaging of
    indications and algorithm for, 896-897
    technique and findings in, 897, 897f-898f
  isolated, vs. arrhythmogenic right
      ventricular dysplasia, 893
  prevalence and epidemiology of, 896
  reporting of, 900
  treatment options for, 900
Myocytes
  contraction of, 58, 59f
  glucose and fatty acid pathways in, 342,
      342f
  necrosis of, 61
Myopericarditis, 945-946
Myotomy, for left ventricular outflow tract
    obstruction, 881
Myxoma
  clinical presentation of, 906-907
  definition of, 905
  differential diagnosis of, 908-909
  imaging of
    echocardiographic, 116, 117f
    technique and findings in, 907-908,
        907f-909f
  pathology of, 905-906, 906f
  prevalence of, 905
  surgery for, 432-433, 432f-433f, 909
Myxoma cells, 905-906, 906f

N

Naked aorta sign, 1207
National Electronic Manufacturers Association
    (NEMA) procedures, 319
Native artery thrombosis, 1573
Navier-Stokes equations, 245-249

Navigator band location, in three-dimensional
    steady-state free precession MR
    angiography, 1107
Navigator echo gating, motion compensation
    with, in cardiac MR imaging, 202, 203f
Near-infrared spectroscopy (NIRS), of coronary
    arteries, 712, 712f
Necrosis, colon, after endovascular aneurysm
    repair, 1435-1436
Necrotizing sarcoid granulomatosis, 1392
Negative remodeling mechanism, contributing
    to coronary restenosis, 515, 516f
Neointimal proliferation, contributing to
    coronary restenosis, 515, 516f
Neonate, respiratory distress in, cyanotic heart
    lesions causing, 652, 652f
Nephrogenic systemic fibrosis, 253-255
  as contraindication to contrast-enhanced MR
      angiography, 1255-1257
  causes of, 254
  in chronic kidney disease, 1673
  risk of, gadolinium-containing contrast
      agents and, 254, 1453
Nephropathy, contrast-induced, 159
Nerve tissue deficits, in acute limb ischemia,
    1574
Neurohormonal agents, radiotracer, in PET
    imaging, 344, 344t
Neutron(s), physics of, 270
New York University Renal CTA Protocol,
    1485t
New York University Renal MRA Protocol,
    1486t
Nicotinic acid derivative protocol, ^{18}FDG-PET
    imaging, 803
Nitroglycerin
  sublingual, for acute coronary syndrome,
      723
  used in cardiac imaging, 144, 157-159, 158t
    contraindications to, 158t, 159
Noise
  acoustic, of MRI scanners, 267
  of CTA scanners, 1056
Noise-induced artifacts, in coronary CT
    angiography, 499
Noncardiac surgery, coronary CT angiography
    in, 486
Noncompliant balloons, in vascular
    interventions, 1156
Non–ST segment elevation myocardial
    infarction (NSTEMI), 715
  percutaneous coronary interventions for,
      402, 723
Nonthrombotic embolization, 1368-1370
  clinical presentation of, 1369
  etiology and pathophysiology of, 1368
  imaging technique and findings in,
      1369-1370, 1369f-1370f
North American Symptomatic Carotid
    Endarterectomy Trial (NASCET), 1172,
    1210, 1227
Norwood procedure, for hypoplastic left heart
    syndrome, 389, 672
Nubbin sign, in graft occlusion, 524-525, 528f
Nuclear medicine imaging
  extrathoracic, 1144-1151
    bleeding studies in, 1144, 1145f
    brain perfusion tomography, 1148-1150,
        1149f-1150f
    gastrointestinal bleed localization scan,
        1144-1146, 1147t
    Meckel diverticulum scan, 1146-1148
    technical requirements in, 1144
  of acute coronary syndrome, 722, 722f
  of amyloidosis, 864

Nuclear medicine imaging (Continued)
  of aortic aneurysm
    mycotic, 1407
    thoracic, 1282
  of arrhythmogenic right ventricular
      dysplasia, 887
  of atrial septal defect, 567-568, 569f
  of coronary atherosclerosis, 711-712
  of dilated cardiomyopathy, 857-858, 857f
  of double-outlet right ventricle, 684
  of inferior vena cava thrombosis, 1539
  of inferior vena cava tumors, 1531
  of ischemic heart disease, postoperative,
      814-815
  of myocarditis, 899
  of paraganglioma, 918
  of pulmonary capillary hemangiomatosis,
      1363
  of pulmonary venous connections, partial
      anomalous, 628
  of renal artery stenosis, 1477-1478, 1479f
    in transplant patient, 1564
  of sarcoidosis, 870
  of single ventricle, 677
  of tetralogy of Fallot, 661
  of transposition of great arteries, 660
  of truncus arteriosus, 666
  of ventricular septal defect, 577
  stress, coronary artery calcium screening
      with, 463
  technique(s) of, for identifying myocardial
      viability, 794-800
    fatty acid radiotracers in, 800-801,
        801f-802f
    ^{18}FDG, 801
    ^{18}FDG-PET mismatch and match patterns,
        803-804
      functional recovery in, 803, 804f
      prognosis of, 803-804, 804f
    ^{18}FDG-PET protocols, 801-803
    ^{18}FDG-SPECT, 805
    future opportunities for, 805-807, 806f
    PET, 799-800, 799f-800f
    SPECT, 794-797, 795f-798f
  ventilation-perfusion (V/Q)
    of pulmonary embolism, 1335,
        1335f-1336f
    of pulmonary hypertension
      chronic thromboembolic, 1349, 1350f,
          1367
      idiopathic, 1358-1359
      with unclear multifactorial mechanisms,
          1371
    of pulmonary veno-occlusive disease,
        1362
    of tumor embolization, 1370
Nuclear nomenclature, 270, 271t
Nuclear pulmonary flow scan, of stenosis,
    before and after repair, 375-377,
    378f
Nuclear transformation, 272
Nucleus
  electrons orbiting, 270, 271f
  proton:neutron ratio in, 270, 271f
Nuclide, 271t. See also Radionuclide(s).
Nutcracker syndrome, 1011-1012, 1012f

O

Obesity
  and accuracy of coronary CT angiography,
      484-485, 485f-486f
  definition of, 484-485
Oblique vein of Marshall, 53-55

Obturator artery, 978-981, 980f
Obturator lymphnode, 1506-1509, 1509f
Obturator vein, 1012, 1013f
Occlusion. *See also at anatomic site.*
  bypass graft, after CABG surgery, 524-525, 527f-529f
  chronic, angioplasty and, 1162
Occlusion devices, mechanical, as embolic agents, 1168
Oculostenotic reflex, 127
One-day ^{99m}Tc labeled imaging protocol, for SPECT, 282
Optical coherence tomography (OCT), of coronary arteries, 712
Oral glucose loading protocol, in ^{18}FDG-PET imaging, 802-803
Orthopedic hardware, as contraindication to CT angiography, 1614
Osler-Weber-Rendu disease, 1468
Osteosarcoma, 928-930, 929f
  echocardiography of, 116
Ostial stenosis, congenital, in coronary arteries, 472, 473f
Ostium (ostia), coronary
  location of, 39, 39f
  multiple, anomalous origin of coronary artery from, 471, 472f
  number of, 39
Ostium primum, in atrial septal defect, 8, 563, 566f
Ostium secundum, in atrial septal defect, 8, 363, 563-564
  radiography of, 90, 91f
Ovarian vein, 1010, 1010f
Oxidation, of low-density lipoprotein, 1195
Oxidation hypothesis, of atherosclerosis, 1195
Oxygen 15–carbon monoxide, 340
Oxygen 15–water, in PET imaging, 340, 340t
  of myocardial viability, 800, 800f
Oxygen tension measurements, transcutaneous, in wound healing, 1186, 1187t
Oxygen therapy, for acute coronary syndrome, 723

P

Pacemaker(s), as MRI safety issue, 264-265
Pacemaker leads, as MRI safety issue, 265
PAD Awareness, Risk, and Treatment: New Resources for Survival (PARTNERS) study, 1194
Pain
  back, 813
  chest. *See* Chest pain.
Pair production, in photon-matter interactions, 275, 275f
Palmar arch, 1022
  variants of, 994f-995f, 995
Palmar vein, 1020
Pancreas, CT angiography of, 1066, 1067f
Pancreas transplant recipients, vascular evaluation of, 1568-1569
Pancreatic adenocarcinoma
  clinical presentation of, 1464
  definition of, 1464
  differential diagnosis of, 1466
  etiology and pathophysiology of, 1464
  imaging of
    indications and algorithm for, 1464-1465
    technique and findings in, 1465-1466, 1465f-1466f

Pancreatic adenocarcinoma (Continued)
    staging of, multiphasic CT in, 1066
  treatment options for, 1466
Pancreatic vein, 1007
Pancreaticoduodenal artery, 972, 973f
Pancreaticoduodenal vein, 1006, 1006f-1007f
Papillary fibroelastoma, 116, 909-910, 910f-911f
Papillary muscle rupture, post-myocardial, 94
Paraesophageal varices, from portal hypertension, MR imaging of, 1454-1455, 1455f
Paraganglioma
  differential diagnosis of, 918-919
  manifestations of disease in, 917-918, 918f
  pathology of, 917, 917f
  prevalence of, 917
  treatment options for, 919
Parallel imaging
  in accelerated MR imaging, 195, 196f
  in MR angiography, 1084, 1085f, 1102-1103
    contrast-enhanced, 1253, 1254f
Paraplegia
  after aortic aneurysm rupture repair, 1303
  after thoracic aortic aneurysm repair, with prosthetic graft, 1285, 1285f
Parasitic embolization
  clinical presentation of, 1369
  etiology and pathophysiology of, 1368
  imaging technique and findings in, 1369
Paraumbilical vein, 1005
PARR-2 study, 336
Partial anomalous pulmonary venous connections (PAPVC), 625-628
  classic signs of, 628
  clinical presentation of, 625-626
  definition of, 625
  differential diagnosis of, 628
  etiology and pathophysiology of, 625, 626f
  imaging of
    indications and algorithm for, 626
    technique and findings in, 626-628, 627f
  medical treatment of, 628
  prevalence and epidemiology of, 625
  reporting of, 625
  surgical/interventional treatment of, 628, 629f
Partial anomalous pulmonary venous return, 1001-1002, 1003f
Particulate embolic agents, 1167-1168
Particulate embolization
  etiology and pathophysiology of, 1368
  imaging technique and findings in, 1369
Parvovirus B19, in myocarditis, 898-899
Parvus tardus waveform, 1240, 1240f
Patch aortoplasty, for aortic coarctation, 539
Patent ductus arteriosus (PDA), 366-369
  clinical presentation of, 585-588
  complications of, 585
  CT imaging of, 585-586, 587f
  definition of, 583
  device closure for, 369-370
    contraindications to, 370
    indications for, 370
    outcomes and complications of, 370-371
    postoperative surveillance after, 370-371, 374f
    preoperative imaging for, 370, 371f-374f
  differential diagnosis of, 588-595
  echocardiography of, 118
  etiology and pathophysiology of, 584-585
  grading of, 585
  imaging of, technique and findings in, 585-588
  medical treatment of, 596

Patent ductus arteriosus (PDA) (Continued)
  MR imaging of, 586-588, 587f-589f
  prevalence and epidemiology of, 583-584
  radiography of, 585, 586f
  surgical/interventional treatment of, 596-597, 596f. *See also* Patent ductus arteriosus, device closure of.
  ultrasonography of, 585, 586f
  vs. aortic spindle or ductus bump, 588, 590f
  vs. aortopulmonary window, 588
  vs. coarctation of aorta, 594, 594f
  vs. diverticulum of Kommerell, 591-592, 591f-592f
  vs. ductus aneurysm, 590-591, 591f
  vs. ductus diverticulum, 588-590, 590f
  vs. interrupted aortic arch, 595, 595f
  vs. nontraumatic aneurysm and pseudoaneurysm, 592-594, 594f
  vs. other vascular entities at aortic isthmus, 588-595, 590f
  vs. traumatic aortic injury, 592, 593f
Patent foramen ovale, 366-369, 368f
  CT imaging of, 447, 448f
  device closure of, 366
    contraindications to, 368
    indications for, 367-368
    outcomes and complications of, 368
    postoperative surveillance after, 369
    preoperative imaging for, 369, 369f
Patient monitoring, in MR angiography, 1084-1085
Patient motion
  causing attenuation mismatch, in PET imaging, 309, 310f
  in three-dimensional steady-state free precession MR angiography, 1107-1108
Patient positioning
  in MR imaging, 1397-1398
  in PET protocols, 316
Patient preparation
  for cardiac computed tomography, 143-144, 144f
  for MR angiography, 1103
  PET protocols of, 316
Patient prognosis, dobutamine MRI and, 222-223, 223f
Patient-prosthetic mismatch, in aortic valve surgery, 421
Pauli exclusion principle, 270
Peak filling rate (PFR), 754
Peak systolic velocity (PSV)
  effect of Doppler angle on, 1233-1234, 1235f
  effect of heart rate on, 1235-1236, 1236f
  in carotid artery stenosis, 1233, 1234f-1235f
    effect of contralateral occlusion on, 1236-1237, 1238f
  in renal artery stenosis, 1513
  in tortuous carotid arteries, 1235, 1236f
  increased, in vertebral artery, 1246
Pedal artery(ies), occlusion of, MR angiography of, 1636-1638, 1637f-1638f
Pediatric cardiology. *See also* Congenital heart disease (CHD).
  impact of prostaglandins on, 383
  milestones in, 383, 384t
Pelvic angiography, 1159
Pelvic congestion syndrome, 1015-1016, 1016f
Pelvis
  arterial anatomy of, 978-983
    differential considerations in, 981-983, 982f
    general descriptions of, 978-981, 979f-980f

Index

Pelvis *(Continued)*
  normal variants in, 981, 981f
  pertinent imaging considerations in, 983
  venous anatomy of, 1012-1016
    differential considerations in, 1015-1016, 1015f-1016f
    of specific veins, 1012-1014, 1013f-1014f
    pertinent imaging considerations in, 1016, 1017f
    variants in, 1014-1015
Penetrating atherosclerotic ulcer, of aorta. *See* Aorta, penetrating atherosclerotic ulcer of.
Penetrating trauma, upper extremity, 1644
Penicillin, for syphilitic aortitis, 1323
Penis, dorsal veins of, 1014
Pentoxifylline, for peripheral artery disease, 1209
Percutaneous coronary intervention (PCI), for coronary artery disease. *See* Coronary artery disease (CAD), percutaneous intervention for.
Percutaneous transluminal angioplasty (PTA)
  for peripheral artery disease, 1210-1211, 1210t
  for transplant renal artery stenosis, 1564
Percutaneous transluminal coronary angioplasty (PTCA)
  historical aspects of, 393, 394f, 515
  of coronary arteries. *See also* Coronary artery disease (CAD), percutaneous coronary intervention for.
    anatomic considerations regarding, 394-400, 395f-401f
    contraindications to, 402
    in stent area, 403-405, 404f-406f, 520
    indications for, 401-402
    outcomes and complications of, 402-403
Percutaneous transluminal coronary rotational atherectomy, 400, 401f
Percutaneous vascular interventions, 1155-1171. *See also specific intervention, e.g.,* Angiography.
  equipment and tools used in, 1155-1157
Perforator veins, of lower extremity, 1029
Perfusion, myocardial. *See* Myocardial perfusion.
Perfusion agents
  contraindications to, 206t
  radiotracer. *See also specific radionuclide.*
    diagnostic accuracy of, 342, 342t
    in PET imaging, 339-342, 340f-341f, 340t
Perfusion imaging protocols
  for MR imaging, 205-207, 206t
  for PET, 317-318, 317f-318f
Periaortic mediastinal hemorrhage, in thoracic aortic trauma, 1309, 1309f
Peribronchial cuffing, 1375, 1375f
Pericardial calcification, radiography of, 82, 82f
Pericardial constriction, radiography of, 80-82
Pericardial cyst, radiography of, 82, 83f
Pericardial disease, 63-64, 437-440
  disorders associated with, 438t
  echocardiography of, 113-115
  rheumatoid, 941
Pericardial effusion
  clinical presentation of, 941
  definition of, 941, 942f
  differential diagnosis of, 943
  etiology and pathophysiology of, 941
  imaging of
    indications and algorithm for, 941
    radiographic, 80, 81f, 439, 440f
    technique and findings in, 942-943, 943f

Pericardial effusion *(Continued)*
  prevalence and epidemiology of, 941
  reporting of, 943
  treatment options for, 943
  with tamponade, 941
  without tamponade, 64f
Pericardial metastases, 922
Pericardiectomy
  radical, for constrictive pericarditis, 951
  technique of, 438, 439f
Pericardiotomy
  for pericardial effusion, 943
  for pericarditis, 947
Pericarditis
  acute
    classic signs of, 946
    clinical presentation of, 945-946
    definition of, 945
    differential diagnosis of, 946-947
    etiology and pathophysiology of, 945, 946t
    imaging of
      indications and algorithm for, 946
      technique and findings in, 946, 947f
    medical treatment of, 947
    prevalence and epidemiology of, 945
    reporting of, 948
    surgical treatment of, 438-439, 947, 947f
  chronic, surgical treatment of, 438-439
  constrictive, 64, 65f, 65t, 437-438, 438t
    causes of, 64t
    classic signs of, 951
    clinical presentation of, 949
    definition of, 949
    differential diagnosis of, 951
    etiology and pathophysiology of, 949, 950t
    imaging of
      echocardiographic, 115, 116f
      indications and algorithm for, 949
      technique and findings in, 949-951, 950f-951f
    medical treatment of, 951
    prevalence and epidemiology of, 949
    reporting of, 952
    surgical treatment of, 438-439, 439f, 951
      indications for and contraindications to, 439
      outcomes and complications of, 439
      postoperative surveillance after, 439-440
      preoperative imaging in, 439, 440f
  effusive, 438, 438f
Pericardium
  anatomy of, 30, 31f, 63, 63f, 437, 437f
  normal, radiography of, 80, 81f
Perihilar haze, 1375, 1375f
Peripheral arterial bypass grafts, imaging and evaluation of, postinterventional, 1638-1639, 1638f-1639f
Peripheral artery disease (PAD), 1573-1584. *See also specific disorder, e.g.,* Limb ischemia.
  classic signs of, 1634, 1634f
  clinical presentation of, 1198t, 1199, 1628-1634
  diagnostic algorithm for, 1200f
  differential diagnosis of, 1207t, 1634-1635, 1635f
  etiology and pathophysiology of, 1628
  imaging of
    angiography in, 1634
    CT angiography in, 1203
    CT scans in, 1630

Peripheral artery disease (PAD) *(Continued)*
    digital subtraction angiography in, 1206, 1207f
    indications and algorithm for, 1629
    MR angiography in, 1206, 1630-1634. *See also* Magnetic resonance angiography (MRA), contrast-enhanced, of peripheral artery disease.
    radiography in, 1629
    technique and findings in, 1629-1634
    ultrasound in, 1629
  increased risk of, pathologic mechanisms for, 1197
  medical treatment of, 1208-1209
  prevalence and epidemiology of, 1194, 1628
  reporting of, 1635-1639
    in aorta and iliac arteries, 1635-1636, 1636f
    in femoropopliteal arteries, 1636, 1637f
    in lower leg and pedal arteries, 1636-1638, 1637f-1638f
  screening for, 1200
  surgical/interventional treatment of, 1210-1211, 1210t
Peripheral vascular ischemia, sudden-onset, postoperative, ischemic heart disease and, 813
Peritoneal dialysis, for chronic kidney disease, 1673
Peroneal artery, 984, 984f
  occluded, 987f
Peroneal vein, 1028
Persistent truncus arteriosus, 618. *See also* Truncus arteriosus.
PET/CT imaging systems. *See also* Computed tomography (CT); Positron emission tomography (PET).
  cardiac
    accuracy of, 334-335, 335t
      diagnostic, 328-329, 329t
    future directions of, 336-337
    imaging protocols for, 332-333, 333f
    quality assurance for, 327-328, 328f
    risk stratification in, 330
  of upper extremity medium and small vessel disease, 1650-1651, 1655f-1657f
Pharmacologic stress agent(s), 352-360. *See also specific agent.*
  in MR imaging, 767-768
  in PET imaging, 316-317
  in SPECT
    protocols for, 283-285, 284f-285f, 744-745
    vs. echocardiography, 357-358, 357f
  inotropic, 355-356
    mechanism of action of, 355-356, 355f
    utility of, in coronary artery disease, 356-357
  vasodilator, 352-355
    side effects of, 354t
  vs. exercise stress protocols, 358-359, 359t
Pharmacomechanical thrombolysis, 1599-1600
Pharmacovigilance, of MR contrast agents, 253
Phase contrast images, in cardiac MR imaging, 192, 192f-194f
Phase contrast magnetic resonance angiography, 1094-1098, 1095f-1097f, 1105-1106. *See also* Magnetic resonance angiography (MRA).
  postprocessing in, 1096-1098, 1097f-1098f
Phase shift, in Doppler ultrasonography, 1035-1036
Phase-contrast velocity mapping, for quantifying myocardial motion, 230, 230t

Phased array surface coils, in MR angiography, 1102-1103
Phase-encoding gradient, in MR angiography, 1080, 1080f
Photoelectric effect, in photon-matter interactions, 275, 275f, 1047
Photomultiplier tubes, in SPECT, 277-278, 279f
Photon(s)
  energy transmitted by, 271
  matter interactions with, 274-276, 275f
    probability of, 275-276, 276f
  physics of, 270
  x-ray, 1047
Photon attenuation, in PET imaging, 306, 307f
Phrenic artery, inferior, 973-975, 975t
Phrenic vein, inferior, 1009, 1010f
Picture archiving and communication system (PACS), 1128
Pink tetralogy, 641
Pixels, ultrasound, 1033
Plantar artery, 984, 985f
Plantar vein
  deep, 1027-1028
  superficial, 1026
Plaque, atherosclerotic
  accumulation of, 60, 61f
  calcification in, 60-61, 707
  CTA image interpretation of, 503-504
  development of, 457-458
  Doppler ultrasound assessment of, 1228-1229, 1230f, 1237-1240, 1238f-1239f
  echotexture of, 1228, 1229f
  erosion of, 707, 707f
  fibrointimal thickening and, 1237-1240, 1239f
  histologic evaluation of, 1218, 1218f
  hypoechoic, 1237, 1238f
  irregular, 1237, 1239f
  life cycling of, 707
  morphology of, 1220-1221, 1221f
  progression of
    atheromatous, 706, 706f
    nonatheromatous, 707, 707f
  stages of, 706
  rupture of, 61, 458
    and acute coronary syndromes, 61
  surface contour of, 1228, 1230f
  three-dimensional image assessment of, 1140-1142, 1140f-1141f, 1140t
  ulcerated, 1237, 1239f
    CT imaging of, 1299-1300, 1300f
    vs. penetrating atherosclerotic ulcer, 1299-1300, 1299f
  vulnerable, thin cap atheroma and, 706
Pleural effusion, postoperative, radiographic features of, 96
Plexogenic pulmonary arteriopathy, 1354
Pneumothorax, radiography of, 96
Point spread function (PSF), in contrast-enhanced MR angiography, 1254-1255
PolarCath angioplasty system, 1156
Polyangiitis, microscopic, 1386-1387
Polyarteritis nodosa, 1467-1468
Polysplenia complex, 18
Polyvinyl alcohol, as embolic agent, 1167-1168
Poor vessel enhancement artifact, in coronary CT angiography, 495t, 499
Popliteal artery, 983, 984f
  adventitial cystic disease of, 987
  angiographic access via, 1158
  division of, 985

Popliteal artery aneurysm, 987
  repair of, indications for, 1601, 1602f
  with limb ischemia, 1578
Popliteal artery entrapment syndrome (PAES), 986, 1600
  classification of, 986-987
  surgical treatment of, 1601
Popliteal vein, 1028
Porta hepatis, 971-972
Portal hypertension, 1008-1009, 1008f, 1008t
  clinical presentation of, 1453
  definition of, 1453
  differential diagnosis of, 1456-1457
  etiology and pathophysiology of, 1453, 1454f
  imaging of
    indications and algorithm for, 1454, 1454f
    technique and findings in, 1454-1456, 1455f-1456f
  treatment options for, 1457
Portal vein
  anastomosis of, 1546
  anatomy of, 1005, 1006f-1007f
    imaging of, 1545, 1546f
    variations in, 1008
Portal vein stenosis, after liver transplantation, 1551-1553, 1554f-1555f
Portal vein thrombosis, 1457-1458, 1457f
  after liver transplantation, 1551, 1553f-1554f
Portal venous circulation
  anatomy of, 1005-1008
    in specific veins, 1005-1008, 1006f-1007f
    variants of, 1008
  differential considerations of, 1008-1009, 1008f, 1008t
Portosystemic gradient (PSG), 1008
Portosystemic shunting, intrahepatic, MR imaging of, 1454-1455, 1456f
Positron emission, 272, 272t, 273f
Positron emission tomography (PET). See also PET/CT imaging systems.
  and CT coregistration, 312
  attenuation correction in, 308
    protocols for, 311-312
      placement of, 312
  attenuation event in, 306, 306f-307f
  attenuation maps in, conversion of CT images to, 308-309, 309f
  attenuation mismatch in, 309-311
    patient motion causing, 309, 310f
    respiratory and contractile cardiac motion causing, 309-310, 311f
    thoracic cavity drift causing, 310-311, 311f
  detectors in, 306-308, 308t
  dilated cardiomyopathy assessment with, 858
  dosimetry in, 319
  fatty acid radiotracers in, of myocardial metabolism, 800-801, 801f-802f
  FDG-labeled
    mismatch and match patterns in, 803-804, 804f, 806f
    of abdominal aortic aneurysm, 1402
    of giant cell arteritis, 1414
    of lipomatous hypertrophy of interatrial septum, 916
    of myocardial metabolism, 801
      protocol(s) in, 801-803
        hyperinsulinemic-euglycemic clamping, 803
        intravenous glucose loading, 803
        nicotinic acid derivative, 803
        oral glucose loading, 802-803

Positron emission tomography (PET) (Continued)
    of sarcoidosis, 870
    of Takayasu arteritis, 1317, 1318f, 1414
  for identifying myocardial viability, 799-800, 799f-800f
    ammonia N 13 as radiotracer in, 799-800
    rubidium 82 as radiotracer in, 799, 799f
  image reconstruction in, 313-314, 314f
  myocardial perfusion imaging with, 749-751
    clinical indications for, 749, 750f
    future directions of, 751-752
    image acquisition data in, 750-751
    myocardial viability and, 751, 752f
    pitfalls and solutions in, 751
    radiotracers in, 749-750
    stress protocols for, 750
    technical aspects of, 749-750
    technique and protocols for, 750-751, 750f
  myocardial perfusion studies with, 326-331
    coronary artery disease evaluation in, 329, 329f-330f
    diagnostic accuracy of, 328-329, 329t
    imaging protocols for, 326-327, 327f
    quality assurance for, 327-328, 328f
    risk stratification and, 329-331, 331f
  myocardial viability assessment with, 331-336
    accuracy of, 328f-329f, 334-335, 751
    hibernation vs. stunning and, 331-332
    imaging protocols for, 332-333, 332f-333f
    impact of, on patient outcome, 330f, 335-336, 336f
    perfusion and glucose-loaded ^{18}FDG patterns in, 333-334, 333f-334f
  of atherosclerosis, 1206
    coronary, 712
  of giant cell arteritis, 1321
  of ischemic heart disease, postoperative, 814-815
  of myocarditis, 899
  of thoracic aortic aneurysms, 1282
  prompt gamma event in, 306, 307f
  protocol(s) in, 315-319
    data reconstruction and display, 318-319
    dietary restriction, 316
    patient preparation and positioning, 316
    pharmacologic stress, 316-317
    rest-stress, 317-318, 317f-318f
    viability, 318, 318f
  quality control in, 319-322
    image, 320-322, 321f-323f
    PET/CT systems, 319-320
    ^{82}Rb generator, 320
  radiation exposure associated with, 347-348, 348f
    dose reduction in, 348-350, 349f
  radionuclides in, 325-326, 339-344. See also Radionuclide(s).
    metabolic agents, 342-344, 342f-343f
    neurohormonal agents, 344, 344t
    perfusion agents, 339-342, 340f-341f, 340t
    diagnostic accuracy of, 342, 342t
  scanner physics in, 304-314, 305f
  scatter correction in, 312-313
  scatter event in, 306, 307f
  tracer kinetics in, 314-315
    fluorodeoxyglucose, 315
    rubidium 82, 314-315
  vs. SPECT, 328-329
Postembolization syndrome, 1170
Posterior descending artery, coronary, 39-41, 41f-42f
Posterior lateral ventricular vein, 52, 54f

Posterolateral ventricular branch, of coronary artery, 39-41, 41f-42f
Post-infarct imaging, 357-358
Post-stenotic dilation, of ascending aorta, 1275, 1276f
Potential energy, 271
Potts shunt, for decreased pulmonary blood flow, 391
Power Doppler ultrasonography, 1036-1037. See also Doppler ultrasonography.
Power injector
  dual-head, in CT angiography, 1059-1060
  in MR angiography, 1085, 1086f
Pravastatin, for cerebrovascular atherosclerotic disease, 1208
Precapillary vs. postcapillary etiology classification, of pulmonary hypertension, 1354, 1355b
Premature atresia, of pulmonary vein, 1001-1002
Pressure gradients, estimation of, modified Bernoulli equation in, 99, 240, 241f
Pressure overload, 63
Primary amyloidosis, 861. See also Amyloidosis.
Primary cardiac lymphoma
  definition of, 932
  manifestations of disease in, 932-933, 933f-934f
  pathology of, 932
  prevalence of, 932
Probe, in Doppler ultrasonography, choice of, 1038
Profunda femoral artery, 983, 983f
  variants of, 985
Programmed cell death, 792
  targeting, 805
Programmed cell survival, 792
Prompt gamma event, in PET imaging, 306, 307f
  failure to correct, 321, 321f
Prospective gating, in CT angiography, 1057-1058
Prospective Investigation of Pulmonary Embolism Disorders (PIOPED) I study, 1333-1334
  V/Q scan in, 1335
Prospective Investigation of Pulmonary Embolism Disorders (PIOPED) II study, 1339
  diagnostic reference standard for, 1339t
  limitations of, 1339
Prostacyclin, and patent ductus arteriosus, 583
Prostaglandin(s), impact of, on pediatric cardiology, 383
Prostaglandin E_2, and patent ductus arteriosus, 583
Prosthetic graft(s)
  complications of, 1284-1285, 1285f
  for thoracic aortic aneurysm, 1284, 1284f
  used in vascular bypass surgery, 1586
Prosthetic heart valve
  as MRI safety issue, 265
  echocardiography of, 110
  for aortic regurgitation, 833-834
    indications for, 420t
  for aortic stenosis, 830, 832f
    indications for, 419t
    success of, 421, 422f
  mechanical bileaflet, 420, 420f
  tissue, 420, 421f
    advantage of, 421
Prosthetic valve endocarditis, 429. See also Infective endocarditis.
  surgery for, indications for, 431t

Proton, 270
Pseudoaneurysm, 1271, 1277, 1277f. See also Aneurysm.
  anastomotic, 1441, 1447, 1449f
    after abdominal aortic aneurysm repair, 1180
    postoperative management of, 1449
  aortic, post-traumatic, 592, 593f
  carotid artery
    Doppler imaging of, 1243, 1246f
    traumatic dissection with, 1262, 1263f
  chronic calcified, 1312, 1312f
  Doppler imaging of, 1044
  gastroduodenal, 1463, 1464f, 1469f
  hepatic artery, after transplantation, 1551, 1553f
  in renal transplant recipient, vascular evaluation of, 1564-1566
    clinical presentation of, 1565
    etiology and pathophysiology of, 1564-1565
    imaging of
      indications and algorithm for, 1565
      technique and findings in, 1565, 1565f-1566f
    prevalence and epidemiology of, 1564
    treatment options for, 1565-1566, 1566f
  in thoracic aortic trauma, 1311
    CT imaging of, 1308, 1309f
  lower extremity
    post-catheterization, imaging of, 1603-1604, 1604f
    repair of, 1600
      contraindications to, 1601-1602
      indications for, 1601
  nontraumatic, vs. patent ductus arteriosus, 592-594, 594f
Pseudoartifact, in Doppler ultrasonography, 1043
Pseudocoarctation of aorta, 539, 539f. See also Coarctation of aorta.
Pseudofilling defects, in three-dimensional contrast-enhanced MR angiography, 1115-1116
Pseudohypocalcemia, after gadolinium-enhanced MR angiography, 252-253
Pseudothrombus artifact, 1537
Pseudotruncus, 621
Pudendal artery, internal, 978-981, 980f
Pudendal plexus, 1014
Pudendal vein, 1012, 1013f-1014f
Pulmonary. See also Lung entries.
Pulmonary angiography, 1159, 1336
  contraindications to, 1337b
  CT, 1337-1340
    single-detector helical, 1337
      accuracy of, 1337
Pulmonary arterioles, 1353
Pulmonary arteriopathy, plexogenic, 1354
Pulmonary artery(ies)
  anatomy of, 965-966, 965f
    variations in, 966, 967f
  anomalous origin of coronary artery from, 470-471
  calcification of, 89
  flow in
    decreased, radiographic evaluation of, 84, 85f
    increased, radiographic evaluation of, 84, 84f
    MR evaluation of, 244-249, 246f
      secondary parameters in, 245-249
      time-resolved, three-dimensional phase contrast, 244-249, 247f-248f
  involvement of, in Takayasu arteritis, 1315

Pulmonary artery(ies) (Continued)
  left, 965, 965f
    anomalous, 545, 547f
    lower lobe, 966, 967f
    radiography of, 74
    upper lobe, 966, 967f
  main, radiography of, 74, 74f
  right, 965, 965f
    lower lobe, 966, 967f
    upper lobe, 966, 966f
  segmental, 966
Pulmonary artery banding, CT angiography of, 611f
Pulmonary artery pressure, increased, pulmonary embolism and, 1332
Pulmonary artery sling, 545, 547f, 966
Pulmonary artery stenosis, 375-377
  balloon dilation for, 375
    contraindications to, 375
    indications for, 375
    outcomes and complications of, 375
    postoperative surveillance after, 377, 378f-379f
  preoperative imaging for, 375-377, 377f-378f
Pulmonary balloon valvotomy, 408f, 409
Pulmonary blood flow
  decreased, cyanotic congenital heart disease with, 390-392, 391t, 651-653, 652f
    surgery for, 391-392
  increased, cyanotic congenital heart disease with, 389-390, 389t
    surgery for, 390
Pulmonary capillary hemangiomatosis, 1362-1363, 1363f
Pulmonary circulation, anatomy and physiology of, 1353
Pulmonary edema, 1373-1382
  air space (alveolar), 85-87, 1376
  high-altitude, 1381-1382
  hydrostatic, 1373-1376
    classic signs of, 1374-1376
    course and clearing of, 1373
    CT imaging of, 1374, 1375f
    distribution of, 1376, 1376b
    etiology and pathophysiology of, 1373
    radiographic findings in, 1373-1374, 1374b, 1375f
  interstitial, 85-87, 1374
  mixed, 1379, 1379b
  neurogenic, 1379, 1379f
  permeability, 86-87, 1376-1378
    clinical presentation of, 1376-1377, 1377b
    differential diagnosis of, 1379, 1379b
    etiology and pathophysiology of, 1376
    imaging findings in
      during ARDS exudative phase, 1377-1378, 1378f
      during ARDS proliferative phase, 1378, 1378f
  postoperative, radiography of, 96
  re-expansion, 1379-1381, 1380f
  subpleural, 1375-1376
  types of, radiographic differentiation of, 1381-1382, 1381b
Pulmonary embolism
  angiography of, 1336, 1337b
  chest radiography of, 1333-1334, 1333f-1334f
  chronic, 1344-1351. See also Chronic thromboembolic pulmonary hypertension (CTPH).
  definition of, 1344
  clinical presentation of, 1333, 1333t
  consequences of, 1332

Pulmonary embolism (Continued)
 CT imaging of, 1337-1339
  benefits and accuracy of, 1338
  classic findings in, 1337-1338, 1338f
  limitations of, 1338-1339
  multidetector, 1339-1340, 1339t
   limitations of, 1339-1340
  technical considerations in, 1337
 CT venography of, 1340
 definition of, 1332
 differential diagnosis of, 1340-1341
 etiology and pathophysiology of, 1332
 imaging techniques and findings in, 1333-1340
 inferior vena cava tumors causing, 1529
 MR imaging of, 1340
 prevalence and epidemiology of, 1332
 treatment options for, 1341
 ultrasonography of, in lower and upper extremity, 1334-1335
 upper extremity DVT associated with, 1663
 V/Q scintigraphy of, 1335, 1335f-1336f
 V/Q SPECT of, 1335-1336, 1336f
 Wells clinical decision rule for, 1333t
Pulmonary hemorrhage, differential diagnosis of, 1384t
Pulmonary hemosiderosis, idiopathic, 1392-1393, 1393f
Pulmonary hypertension, 1353-1358. See also Chronic thromboembolic pulmonary hypertension (CTPH).
 arterial, radiographic evaluation of, 84-87, 85f
 caused by lung disease/hypoxia, 1365-1366
 classification of, 1354-1356
  Dana Point, 1354-1356, 1356b
  Evian, 1354, 1354b
  precapillary vs. postcapillary etiologies in, 1354, 1355b
  Venice-revised WHO, 1354, 1355b
 definition of, 1344, 1353
 etiology and pathophysiology of, 1353
 idiopathic, 1358-1359, 1358f-1359f
  definition of, 1358
  manifestations of
   echocardiographic, 105, 106f, 1356
   imaging technique and findings in, 1356-1358, 1357f
  pathogenesis of, 1353
  primary, 1358
  related to associated conditions, 1359-1361, 1359b
   clinical presentation of, 1360
   definition of, 1359
   etiology and pathophysiology of, 1359-1360
   imaging technique and findings in, 1360-1361, 1361f
  secondary, 1358
  venous, radiographic evaluation of, 85, 86f
  with left heart disease (venous)
   definition of, 1363
   etiology and pathophysiology of, 1364
   manifestations of, 1364, 1364f-1365f
   treatment options for, 1355
  with unclear multifactorial mechanisms
   definition of, 1370
   etiology and pathophysiology of, 1370-1371
   manifestations of, 1371
Pulmonary infundibulum spasm, in tetralogy of Fallot, 641
Pulmonary thromboembolism. See also Pulmonary embolism.
 definition of, 1332

Pulmonary valve
 anatomy of, 26, 26f, 836
 failure of, disease causing, 839, 840f, 842f-844f
 normal function of, 845
Pulmonary valve atresia, 840f
Pulmonary valve insufficiency, 375-381, 842f-844f
 valve implantation for, 377
  contraindications to, 379, 379f
  indications for, 379
  outcomes and complications of, 379
  postoperative surveillance after, 381, 381f
  preoperative imaging for, 380-381, 380f-381f
Pulmonary valve regurgitation
 clinical presentation of, 846
 imaging of, 846
 quantification of, 241
 treatment options for, 847, 847f
Pulmonary valve stenosis, 843f-844f
 clinical presentation of, 845
 imaging of
  indications and algorithm for, 845-846
  radiographic, 92, 92f
  technique and findings in, 846
 interventional catheterization for, 389
 treatment options for, 846
Pulmonary vasculature. See also Pulmonary artery(ies); Pulmonary vein(s).
 CT angiography of, 1062-1063, 1064f-1065f
  protocol parameters for, 1061t
 radiography of, 82-89
  abnormal blood flow in, 84, 84f-85f
  normal anatomy in, 82-84, 83f-84f
Pulmonary vasculitis, 1384, 1385t
Pulmonary vein(s)
 anatomy of, 1001, 1002f
  variations in, 1001-1004, 1003f
 developmental pathology of, 10
 flow velocities in, 103
 formation of, 10, 11f
Pulmonary veno-occlusive disease
 definition of, 1361
 etiology and pathophysiology of, 1361
 manifestations of, 1362, 1362f
Pulmonary venous connections, anomalous, 10
 echocardiography of, 118
 partial, 625-628. See also Partial anomalous pulmonary venous connections (PAPVC).
 total, 634-638. See also Total anomalous pulmonary venous connections (TAPVC).
Pulmonary venous return, anomalous, 10
 partial, 1001-1002, 1003f
 total, 1002-1004, 1003f
  infracardiac, 1008
Pulmonary venous stenosis, after ablation for atrial fibrillation, 450-451, 451f
Pulsatility index (PI), in Doppler imaging, 1513
Pulsation artifacts, in CT angiography, 1070
Pulse repetition frequency, in Doppler ultrasonography, 1036
 choice of, 1038, 1039f
Pulse sequences, MR, 1398
Pulse volume recordings, in location of arterial occlusive disease, 1581, 1582f
Pulse wave velocity, calculation of, for aortic arch and descending aorta, 556, 558f
Pulsed wave Doppler ultrasonography, 1036-1037. See also Doppler ultrasonography.

Pulsus alternans waveform, 1241, 1241f
Pulsus bisferiens waveform, 1241, 1241f
Pulsus paradoxus, 63-64

Q

Qp:Qs ratio, 243
 in atrial septal defect, 565, 568-569
 in partial anomalous pulmonary venous connections, 628
 measurement of, 243-244, 245f
 in single ventricle, 674-675
Quadrilateral space syndrome, 991, 991f
Quality assurance (QA) program
 for gamma camera SPECT operation, 743-744
 for PET/CT systems, 327-328, 328f
Quality control
 image. See Image quality.
 of CT instrumentation, 320
 of PET instrumentation, 319-320
 of PET/CT systems, 319-320
 of SPECT instrumentation, 279

R

Race, CAC score and, 462
Radial artery
 anatomy of, 994-995
 angiographic access via, 1158
 branches of, 993-994
Radial vein, 1022-1023, 1023f
Radiation
 exposure to, ^{201}Tl-labeled SPECT imaging and, 300-301, 300t, 301f
 interactions of, with matter, 274-276, 275f-276f
 ionizing
  in CT angiography, 1070-1073
   dose modulation of, 1058
  in PET/CT systems, 344-345, 345f, 345t
   dose reduction in, 348-350, 349f-350f
   for CT portion of examination, 346-347, 346f, 347t
   for PET portion of examination, 347-348, 348f
 physics of, 270-271
Radiation dose, effective, in CT imaging of coronary calcium, 460
Radiation reduction strategy(ies), 1073
 in computed tomography, 150-155
  increased beam filtration technique, 153-154
  increased beam pitch technique, 153
  increased reconstructed slice thickness technique, 154, 154f
  reduced tube current technique, 150-152, 151f
  reduced tube voltage technique, 152-153
  shortened scan length technique, 153
  technical requirements for, 150
  tubal modulation, 146
Radiation-sensitive population, as contraindication to CT angiography, 1614
Radioactive decay, 273-274
 types of, 272t
Radioactivity, 270-273, 272f-273f
Radioembolization, using yttrium 90, 975-976
Radiofrequency system, in MR angiography, 1083-1084, 1083f-1084f
Radiofrequency ablation, for atrial fibrillation, 445-446

Radiofrequency coils, in carotid MR angiography, 1252
Radiofrequency excitations, in MR angiography, 1079
Radiofrequency fields
 as MRI safety issue, 263-264
 in MR angiography, 1078-1079
Radiography
 chest. See Chest radiography.
 of abdominal aortic aneurysm, 1400, 1400f
 of calcifications, in atherosclerosis, 1201
 of endoleaks, 1408-1409
 of inferior vena cava anomalies, 1528
 of inferior vena cava tumors, 1530
 of in-stent restenosis and thrombosis, 517
 of peripheral artery disease, 1629
 of transplant renal artery stenosis, 1560
 of ulcer or gangrenous wounds, in limb ischemia, 1582
 of upper extremity medium and small vessel disease, 1647, 1647f
Radionuclide(s). See also specific radionuclide.
 half-life of, 273-274
 in PET imaging, 325-326, 339-344
  metabolic agents, 342-344, 342f-343f
  neurohormonal agents, 344, 344t
  perfusion agents, 339-342, 340f-341f, 340t
   diagnostic accuracy of, 342, 342t
 in PET/CT imaging, 325-326
  ammonia N 13, 325-326
  fluorodeoxyglucose 18, 326
  rubidium 82, 325
 in SPECT imaging, 298-303
  technetium 99m labeled, 301
  technetium 99m-N-NOET, 302
  technetium 99m-sestamibi, 301, 739, 740f-741f
  technetium 99m-teboroxime, 302
  technetium 99m-tetrofosmin, 301-302, 739
  thallium 201, 298-301, 299f-301f, 738-739
 manufacture of, 274
 photons released from, 271
 specific activity of, 274
Radionuclide angiography, first-pass, of ventricular function
 data acquisition in, 776-778, 779f
 image interpretation in, 778-779
 indications for, 775-776
Radionuclide medicine imaging. See Nuclear medicine imaging.
Radiotracer(s). See Radionuclide(s).
Ramipril, for peripheral artery disease, 1208-1209
Ramus intermedius (RI) artery, anatomy of, 46, 47f
Rastelli procedure, 390
 for complete transposition of great arteries, 610-611, 610f
 imaging after, 612-613, 613f
Rayleigh scattering, 1047
Raynaud's complex, 1646
Raynaud's phenomenon, 1645-1647. See also Upper extremity, medium and small vessel disease of.
Recoil electron, 275
Reconstruction parameters, for CT angiography of lower extremities, 1617, 1617f-1618f
Reconstruction phase, optimal, in CT imaging, 137
Rectal venous plexus, 1013, 1014f
Redistribution phenomenon, in ^{201}Tl cardiac imaging, 796

Reflex, oculostenotic, 127
Regadenoson protocol, for PET imaging, 317
Relative velocity, in Doppler ultrasonography, 1034, 1035f
Renal allograft
 Doppler ultrasonography of, 1519, 1519f-1520f
 rejection of, 1519, 1520f
 segmental infarction in, 1520, 1521f
Renal angiography, 1159, 1160f
Renal angiomyolipoma, 1533, 1533f
Renal artery(ies), 972-973, 1483-1491
 ACEI scintigraphy of
  captopril administration in, 1493
  contraindications to, 1492-1493
  1-day protocol for, 1493
  2-day protocol for, 1493-1494
  enalaprilat administration in, 1493
  indications for, 1492
  pitfalls and solutions in, 1494
  postprocessing of, 1494
  procedure in, 1493-1494
  reporting of, 1492, 1495f
  ^{99m}Tc-DTPA in, 1494
  ^{99m}Tc-MAG3 in, 1494
  technical requirements for, 1492
 aneurysm of, Doppler ultrasound diagnosis of, 1515
 CT angiography of, 1066, 1067f-1068f
  contraindications to, 1485
  image interpretation in, 1488-1490, 1489f-1490f
  pitfalls and solutions in, 1488
  reporting of, 1490
  technique of, 1485-1486, 1485t, 1486f
 Doppler ultrasonography of
  anatomic considerations in, 1505-1507, 1507f-1508f
  technical considerations in, 1509-1511, 1510f-1511f
 fibromuscular disease affecting, 975, 976f, 1471
  Doppler ultrasonography of, 1498, 1503f
  prevalence and epidemiology of, 1471-1472
 MR angiography of
  contraindications to, 1485
  contrast-enhanced, 1487-1488
  image interpretation in, 1488-1490, 1488f
  indications for, 1483-1485, 1484f
  pitfalls and solutions in, 1488
  reporting of, 1490
  technical requirements for, 1483
  technique of, 1486-1487, 1486t
 postangioplasty, Doppler assessment of, 1514-1515, 1516f-1518f
Renal artery stenosis, 1471
 atherosclerotic. See Renal atherosclerotic disease.
 classic signs of, 1478
 clinical presentation of, 1472
 differential diagnosis of, 1478-1480
 Doppler ultrasonography of, 1497-1498
  image interpretation in, 1513
   direct criteria for, 1513, 1513b, 1514f
   indirect criteria for, 1513, 1513b, 1515f
 etiology and pathophysiology of, 1472
 imaging of
  indications and algorithm for, 1472, 1473f
  technique and findings in, 1473-1478, 1474f-1480f
 in allograft vessels, criteria for, 1519b
 in transplant patient, 1519-1520, 1520f
 MR angiography of, 1483-1484, 1484f
 prevalence and epidemiology of, 1471-1472

Renal artery stenosis (Continued)
 renovascular hypertension caused by, 1471, 1492
 reporting of, 1480-1481
 transplant, 1559-1564. See also Transplant renal artery stenosis (TRAS).
 treatment options for, 1480
Renal artery thrombosis
 Doppler ultrasonography of, 1498-1505, 1505f
 image interpretation in, 1515
 in renal allograft, 1520, 1521f, 1566-1567
Renal atherosclerotic disease, 1471. See also Atherosclerosis.
 conventional angiography of, 1206
 differential diagnosis of, 1207t
 Doppler ultrasonography of, 1497-1498, 1499f-1502f
 medical treatment of, 1209
 MR angiographic assessment of, 1205, 1205f
 presenting findings in, 1198t
 prevalence and epidemiology of, 1194, 1471
 screening for, 1200
 surgical/interventional treatment of, 1211-1212
Renal cell carcinoma, inferior vena cava invasion by, 1530, 1532f
Renal disease
 chronic. See Chronic kidney disease (CKD).
 end-stage, 1673-1674
Renal donor, evaluation of, MR angiography in, 1484-1485, 1484f
Renal failure
 after ruptured aortic aneurysm repair, 1303
 as contraindication to CT angiography, 1262-1263
 coronary artery calcium and, 463
Renal impairment, as contraindication to CT angiography, 1611-1614
Renal infarction, 1447, 1449f
Renal insufficiency, CT angiography and, 485
Renal morphology, Doppler ultrasonography of, technical considerations in, 1511-1512
Renal transplantation
 Doppler ultrasound assessment of, 1505
 living donor for, vascular evaluation of, 1567-1568
 vascular evaluation of, 1559-1568
  arteriovenous fistula and pseudoaneurysm in, 1564-1566
   clinical presentation of, 1565
   etiology and pathophysiology of, 1564-1565
   imaging of
    indications and algorithm for, 1565
    technique and findings in, 1565, 1565f-1566f
   prevalence and epidemiology of, 1564
   treatment options for, 1565-1566, 1566f
  Doppler ultrasound assessment in, 1519-1522, 1519b, 1519f-1522f
  transplant renal artery and vein thrombosis in, 1566-1567
  transplant renal artery stenosis in, 1559-1564. See also Transplant renal artery stenosis (TRAS).
Renal tumor, imaging evaluation of, 1485
Renal vein(s), 1009, 1010f
 Doppler ultrasonography of, anatomic considerations in, 1507-1508, 1508f
 left
  circumaortic, 1525, 1527f
  retroaortic, 1525

Renal vein(s) (Continued)
  right, duplicated, 1528
  variants of, 1011
    reporting of, 1529
Renal vein thrombosis
  Doppler ultrasonography of, 1505, 1506f
    image interpretation in, 1515-1519, 1518f
  in renal allograft, 1521, 1522f, 1566-1567
  pitfalls of sonography of, 1513
Renal-aortic ratio (RAR)
  calculation of, 1509
  in renal artery stenosis, 1513
Renin-angiotensin system, targeting, 805, 806f
Renovascular hypertension
  ACEI scintigraphy of. See Angiotensin-converting enzyme inhibitor (ACEI) scintigraphy, of renal arteries.
  secondary to renal artery stenosis, 1471, 1492
Resistive index (RI), in Doppler imaging, 1512-1513
Resolution phantoms, of CT systems, 1048, 1048f
Resolution testing patterns, of CT systems, 1048, 1048f
Respiratory acceptance window, in three-dimensional steady-state free precession MR angiography, 1107
Respiratory artifacts, in cardiac CT imaging, 147, 147f
Respiratory distress, neonatal, cyanotic heart lesions causing, 652, 652f
Respiratory distress syndrome. See Adult respiratory distress syndrome (ARDS).
Respiratory rhythm, in three-dimensional steady-state free precession MR angiography, 1107
Rest and stress perfusion, multidetector CT
  animal studies of, 730-731, 731f
  human studies of, 731-733, 732t
Rest pain, ischemic, 1581
Restenosis
  after angioplasty, 1162
  in-stent. See Coronary stents, in-stent restenosis and thrombosis.
  recurrent, after carotid endarterectomy, 1173
Resting perfusion
  CT sequence of, 734
  MRI sequence of, 733-734
  PET sequence of, 750
Restrictive cardiomyopathy, 861-873. See also Cardiomyopathy, restrictive.
Rest-stress protocols
  for PET imaging, 317-318, 317f-318f
  for SPECT
    same-day Tc 99m radiotracer, 746
    two-day Tc 99m radiotracer, 746
Retrospective gating, in CT angiography, 1057
Revascularization procedure(s). See also specific procedure, e.g., Coronary artery bypass graft (CABG) surgery.
  for peripheral artery disease, 1210-1211, 1210t
  for renal atherosclerotic disease, 1211-1212
  lower extremity
    catheter-directed or pharmacomechanical thrombolysis, 1597f, 1599-1600
    endovascular methods, 1591-1598
    surgical thromboembolectomy, 1598-1599, 1598t
    vascular bypass surgery, 1585-1591
    with stents, 1163-1164, 1164f
Rhabdomyolysis, in acute limb ischemia, 1576
Rhabdomyoma, 116, 913-914, 914f

Rhabdomyosarcoma, 930-931, 931f
  echocardiography of, 116
Rheumatoid arthritis, atherosclerosis associated with, 1196
Rib fracture, 1306-1307
Rib notching, bilateral symmetrical, 89
Right anterior oblique (RAO) projection, in chest radiography, 77, 79f
Right ventricle. See also Ventricle(s); Ventricular entries.
  double-outlet. See Double-outlet right ventricle (DORV).
  normal values of, 65t
Right ventricular border, radiography of, 75
Right ventricular cardiomyopathy, arrhythmogenic, 237, 237f
Right ventricular dysplasia, arrhythmogenic, 884-895. See also Arrhythmogenic right ventricular dysplasia (ARVD).
Right ventricular function. See Ventricular function, right.
Right ventricular outflow tract (RVOT), vs. arrhythmogenic right ventricular dysplasia, 893t
Roger disease, 580
Roof ablation line, 446
Ross procedure, for aortic valve disease, 389
Rubidium 82 (^{82}Rb)
  decay of, in prompt gamma, 306, 307f
  generator activity of, 320
  in myocardial perfusion imaging with PET, 750
  in PET imaging, 799, 799f
  in PET/CT imaging, 325, 340t, 341-342, 341f
  kinetics of, 314-315
  manufacture of, 274
Rutherford categorization
  of acute limb ischemia, 1575, 1575t
  of chronic limb ischemia, 1578, 1579t, 1588, 1589t

S

S_2 heart sounds, in atrial septal defect, 564
Saccular aneurysm. See Pseudoaneurysm.
Sacral artery
  lateral, 978, 980f
  median, 975
Sacral vein, lateral, 1012
Saddle embolus, 1575. See also Embolus (embolism).
  balloon catheter embolectomy for, 1578
Safety
  of contrast agents, 159-160, 252-253
  of MR imaging, 261-269, 262b. See also Magnetic resonance imaging (MRI), safety issues of.
Safety profile, of dobutamine MRI, 218, 220f
Sagittal images, in cardiac CT imaging, 170-171, 172f
Saline flushing, contrast media and, 163, 163f
Same-day ^{99m}Tc radiotracer protocol, for SPECT, 746
Sample volume, in Doppler ultrasonography, 1038, 1039f
Saperstein principle, 298
Saphenous vein
  great, 1024-1027, 1026f, 1028f
    in vascular bypass surgery, 1585-1586
  small, 1027, 1027f
Saphenous vein bypass graft, 522
  aneurysm of, 509, 511f
Sarcoid granulomatosis, necrotizing, 1392

Sarcoidosis
  cardiac involvement in, delayed hyperenhancement MR imaging of, 209, 210f
  clinical presentation of, 869
  definition of, 868
  etiology and pathophysiology of, 868-869
  imaging of
    indications and algorithm for, 869
    technique and findings in, 869-871, 870f, 872t
  medical treatment of, 871
  prevalence and epidemiology of, 868
  vs. arrhythmogenic right ventricular dysplasia, 892-893
Sarcomas, echocardiography of, 116
Saturation, in time-of-flight MR angiography, 1105
Scan delay, fixed, in CT angiography, 1058
Scan length, shortened, to reduce radiation in CT imaging, 153
Scan time, in MR angiography, 1087-1088, 1089f
Scanner
  CTA
    16-detector, protocol for, 1615t-1616t
    design of, 1056
  PET, 304-314, 305f
    events recorded in
      multiple, 306, 306f
      types of, 305, 305f
Scanning protocols
  for cardiac computed tomography, 144-146, 145f
  for CT angiography of lower extremities, 1614-1617, 1615t-1616t
Scatter correction, in PET imaging, 312-313
Scatter event, in PET imaging, 306, 307f
Schistosomiasis, pulmonary, 1368
  hypertension associated with, 1360
Sciatic artery, persistent, 981, 981f
  clinical importance of, 982
Scimitar sign, in partial anomalous pulmonary venous connections, 628
Scimitar syndrome, 625, 626f-627f
  repair of, baffle obstruction after, 628, 629f
Scintigraphy. See Nuclear medicine imaging.
  ACEI. See Angiotensin-converting enzyme inhibitor (ACEI) scintigraphy.
Scintillation crystals, in SPECT, 277, 278t
Scintillation detector, in PET scanners, 304, 305f
Scintillation event, 277
  localization of, in SPECT, 278
Secondary amyloidosis, 861. See also Amyloidosis.
Sedation
  depth of, four levels of, 266, 266t
  in MR imaging, safety issues of, 266-267
Segmental artery(ies), Doppler ultrasonography of, anatomic considerations in, 1507, 1508f
Self-expanding stents, 1157
Senile systemic amyloidosis, 861. See also Amyloidosis.
Sensitivity encoding (SENSE)
  in parallel MR angiography, 1084, 1085f
  in parallel MR imaging, 195, 228t, 229
Septal defect(s)
  asymmetric, in hypertrophic cardiomyopathy, MR imaging of, 875, 876f-877f
  atrial. See Atrial septal defect (ASD).
  atrioventricular
    multiple-level shunts in, 386
    surgical treatment of, 386, 387f

Septal defect(s) (Continued)
  ventricular. See Ventricular septal defect (VSD).
Septal thickening, interlobular, from hydrostatic pulmonary edema, 1374-1375, 1375f
Septum primum, 7-8, 9f
Septum secundum, 7-8, 9f
Shaded surface display, in CT angiography, 1074
Sheaths, vascular, 1156
Shower embolism, after endovascular aneurysm repair, 1435
Shunt(s). See also specific type of shunt.
  acyanotic congenital heart disease with, surgery for, 383-387, 385f, 385t, 387f
  acyanotic congenital heart disease without, surgery for, 387-389, 388t
  arterioportal, MR imaging of, 1455-1456, 1456f
  arteriovenous, Doppler imaging of, 1044
  inferior vena cava, 1540-1541
    mesocaval, 1541
    side-to-side portacaval, 1541, 1541f
  veno-venous (intrahepatic), MR imaging of, 1454-1455, 1456f
Sickle cell disease, pulmonary hypertension associated with, 1360
Side-lobe artifact, in Doppler ultrasonography, 1042
Siderotic cardiomyopathy, 866-868. See also Cardiomyopathy, siderotic.
Side-to-side portacaval shunt, inferior vena cava, 1541, 1541f
Signal-to-noise ratio
  in MR angiography, 1081, 1102, 1252-1253
    contrast-enhanced, 1258
  in MR imaging, 1398
Simpson's rule
  in MRI assessment of ejection fraction, 215
  in MRI determinants of left ventricular volume, 215
  multislice, of global left ventricular function, 231, 231f-232f
Simultaneous acquisition of spatial harmonics (SMASH), in parallel imaging, 195, 1084
Simvastatin, for cerebrovascular atherosclerotic disease, 1208
Single-detector helical CT pulmonary angiography, 1337
  accuracy of, 1337
Single-photon emission computed tomography (SPECT)
  fatty acid radiotracers in, of myocardial metabolism, 800-801, 801f-802f
  ^{18}FDG-labeled, 805
  for identifying myocardial viability, 794-797
    Tc 99m labeled radiotracers in, 794-795, 795f
    Tc 99m labeled radiotracers with nitrate administration in, 795-796, 796f
    thallium 201 in, 796-797
      protocols for, 797, 797f-798f
  gated, 283
  image interpretation in, 285-296, 286f-296f
  instrumentation in, 276-279, 276f
    advances in, 279
    collimators, 276-277, 277f-278f
    energy discrimination and, 278
    image generation and, 279
    photomultiplier tubes, 277-278, 279f
    quality control of, 279
    scintillation crystals, 277, 278t
    scintillation event localization and, 278

Single-photon emission computed tomography (SPECT) (Continued)
  myocardial perfusion imaging with, 738-749
    acquisition protocols for, 745-746
      dual isotope, 746
      same-day rest-stress Tc 99m radiotracer protocol, 746
      stress-redistribution thallium 201 protocol, 746
      two-day rest-stress Tc 99m radiotracer protocol, 746
    artifacts and normal variants in, 748-749
    contraindications to, 743
    exercise protocols for, 744
    image interpretation in, 747-748, 747f-748f
    indications for, 739-743, 741f-743f
    instrumentation in, 739
    pharmacologic protocols for
      adenosine, 744-745
      dipyridamole, 745
      dobutamine, 745
    pitfalls and solutions in, 743-744
    postprocessing in, 746-747
    quality assurance of, 743-744
    radionuclide imaging protocols for, 744-745
    radiotracer in, 738-739, 740f-741f
      characteristics of, 298
      technetium 99m labeled, 301, 739, 740f-741f
      thallium 201 labeled, 298-301, 738-739
    stress protocols for, 744
    technical aspects of, 738-739
    techniques of, 739-744
    test accuracy of, 749
  of acute coronary syndrome, 722
  of coronary atherosclerosis, 712
  of dilated cardiomyopathy, 857-858, 857f
  physics of, 270-276
    anatomic structure in, 270, 271f, 271t
    interactions of matter in, 274-276, 275f-276f
    radioactive decay in, 273-274
    radioactivity and, 270-273, 272f-273f, 272t
    radionuclide manufacture and, 274, 274f
  radiotracer imaging agent(s) in. See also specific radionuclide.
    technetium 99m labeled, 301
    technetium 99m–N-NOET, 302
    technetium 99m–sestamibi, 301
    technetium 99m–teboroxime, 302
    technetium 99m–tetrofosmin, 301-302
    thallium 201, 298-301, 299f-301f
  stress protocols for, 283-285
    exercise, 283, 283t
    pharmacologic, 283-285, 284f-285f
  ^{99m}Tc-labeled imaging protocol(s) for, 282-283
    dual-isotope protocol, 282-283
    one-day protocol, 282
    two-day protocol, 282
  technical requirements for, 281-283
    description of, 298-302
  ^{201}Tl imaging protocols for, 281-282
  ventilation-perfusion (V/Q), of pulmonary embolism, 1335-1336, 1336f
  vs. PET imaging, 328-329
Sinoatrial nodal artery, 40-41, 42f
Sinoatrial node
  anatomy of, 444, 445f
  depolarization initiated by, 57, 58f
  electrical impulses originating in, 57

Sinus of Valsalva
  aneurysms of, imaging of, 1279-1280
  coronary arteries arising from, 39, 39f-40f, 956f, 957-961
  noncoronary cusp of, 39
  opposite, anomalous origin of coronary arteries from, 468-469, 468f-470f
Sinus venarum, 8-10
Sinus venosus, formation of, 3-4
Sinus venous defect
  clinical presentation of, 629
  definition of, 628-629
  differential diagnosis of, 631
  etiology and pathophysiology of, 629
  imaging of, technique and findings in, 629-631, 630f-631f
  prevalence and epidemiology of, 629
  reporting of, 632
  surgical/interventional treatment of, 631-632
Situs invertus, visceral, 16, 17f
Situs solitus, visceral, 16, 17f
  in Ebstein anomaly, 653
Sized-based reduction, in x-ray tube current, 151, 151f
  pitfalls and solutions for, 152
Sleep-disordered breathing, 1365-1366
Slice thickness, increased, CT radiation reduction and, 154, 154f
Small vessel disease, of upper extremity, 1645-1652. See also Upper extremity, medium and small vessel disease of.
Snowman sign, in pulmonary venous connections
  partial anomalous, 628
  total anomalous, 636
Sodium tetradecyl, as embolic agent, 1168
Soft tissue, abdominal, MR imaging of, 1452-1453
Sones' technique, of coronary angiography, 123-124
Spasm, pulmonary infundibulum, in tetralogy of Fallot, 641
Spatial encoding, in MR angiography, 1079-1080
Spatial modulation of magnetization (SPAMM) technique, for quantifying myocardial motion, 229-230
Spatial resolution
  in cardiac MR imaging, 180-181
  in contrast-enhanced MR angiography, 1252-1253
    while minimizing imaging time and motion artifact, 1258
  in CT angiography, 1049, 1049f, 1056
Specialized populations, coronary artery calcium in, 462-463
Specific absorption rate (SAR), of MRI scanners, FDA recommendations for, 263-264
Specific activity, of nuclide, 274
Spectral broadening artifact, in Doppler ultrasonography, 1042
Spectral Doppler ultrasonography, 1037. See also Doppler ultrasonography.
Spectral gain
  in Doppler ultrasonography, 1040, 1040f
  incorrect, in carotid artery Doppler ultrasonography, 1234
Spectral window, in Doppler imaging, 1043, 1043t
Splanchnic artery aneurysm, 1462-1463, 1463f-1464f
Splenic arteriovenous malformations, 1468
Splenic artery, 970-971, 973f

Splenic infarction, 1466-1467, 1467f
Splenic trauma, 1468
Splenic vein, 1006-1007, 1006f-1007f
Spoiled gradient echo technique, of MR imaging, 227, 228t
ST segment elevation myocardial infarction (STEMI), 715
  percutaneous coronary interventions for, 399, 400f, 723
Stable coronary disease, percutaneous coronary interventions for, 402
Stair-step artifact
  in CT angiography, 1070
    coronary, 495t, 499, 500f-501f
  in CT imaging, cardiac, 147, 147f
Stanford classification, of aortic dissection, 434, 434f, 1289, 1289f
Stanford protocol, for medications used in cardiac imaging, 156-157, 158t
Static magnetic field strength, as MRI safety issue, 263, 263t
Statins
  effect of, on progression of CAC score, 463-464
  for coronary atherosclerosis, 713
Steady-state free precession (SSFP) technique
  comparison of left ventricular volume by, vs. FLASH, 231-232
  of MR angiography, 1098-1099, 1099f
    three-dimensional, 1106-1109, 1107f-1108f
      contraindications to, 1106
      image interpretation in, 1108-1109, 1108f
      indications for, 1106
      pitfalls and solutions in, 1107-1108
  of MR imaging, 181, 228, 228t, 1398, 1398f
    dilated cardiomyopathy diagnosis with, 855, 856f
    evaluation of cardiac function in, 756-757
    localization of heart in, 733-734
Steal phenomenon, Doppler imaging of, 1044
Stenosis. *See under* anatomy.
Stent(s). *See also* Endograft(s).
  as MRI safety issue, 265-266
  balloon-mounted, 1157
  bare metal, 515, 516f
    risk of thrombosis in, 516, 517f
  carotid, 1222-1224
    procedure for, 1224, 1224f
    recommendations for, 1224
    status and patency of, CT angiographic evaluation of, 1261-1262, 1262f
  coronary, 403-405. *See also* Coronary stents.
  drug-eluting, 515, 517f, 1157
    effectiveness of, 515-516
    repeat stenting with, 520
    risk of thrombosis in, 516, 517f
  endovascular, 1157
    for thoracic aortic aneurysm, 1283, 1284f
    for thoracic aortic injury, 1312-1313, 1312f
    for type B aortic dissection, 1295-1296, 1296f
  inferior vena caval, 1541-1542, 1541f
  placement of, angioplasty and, in lower extremity revascularization, 1591-1592, 1592f-1593f
  revascularization with, 1163-1164, 1164f
  self-expanding, 1157
Stent graft(s), 1157
  revascularization with, 1163-1164, 1164f
Stent-Protected Angioplasty versus Carotid Endarterectomy (SPACE) trial, 1223

Step-and-shoot computed tomography. *See also* Computed tomography (CT).
  vs. helical (spiral) CT, 1051-1053, 1051f-1052f
Storage diseases, metabolic, restrictive cardiomyopathy associated with, 871
Strain, in Doppler imaging, 119-122
Strain rate, 120
Strandness criteria, in diagnosis of carotid stenosis, 1173, 1174t
Streak artifacts, in CT angiography, 1069
  coronary, 496, 497f-498f
Streptokinase, for inferior vena cava thrombosis, 1539
Stress, evaluation of cardiac function during, 767-769
  CT imaging in, 769
  MR imaging in, 767-768
    diagnostic criteria in, 768, 769f
    dobutamine stress protocol and, 768
    pharmacologic stress agents and, 767-768
Stress perfusion, CT, 322, 323f, 734
Stress protocols
  for MR imaging, dobutamine, 768
  for PET imaging, 750
  for SPECT, 283-285, 744
    exercise, 283, 283t, 744
    pharmacologic, 283-285, 284f-285f, 744-745. *See also* Pharmacologic stress agent(s).
Stress test(ing)
  in MRI setting, 267-268
  selection of, 359t
Stress-perfusion MRI studies, diagnostic accuracy of, 729, 730t
Stress-redistribution thallium 201 protocol, in SPECT, 746
Stroke
  antiplatelet therapy for, 1222
  causes of, 1227
  CT angiography of, 1060
  etiology of, 1217
  prevalence of, 1217
  probability of, noninvasive testing and, sensitivity and specificity of, 1251, 1252f
  risk factors for, 1218
  risk reduction of, carotid endarterectomy in, 1172
Stroke volume, definition of, 58
Subaortic conus, development of, 22-24, 25f
Subaortic stenosis, radiography of, 92-94
Subclavian artery
  aberrant
    associated with tetralogy of Fallot, 640
    left, right aortic arch with, 11, 72, 73f, 544, 545f-546f, 959, 960f
    right
      aneurysmal origin of, 591-592. *See also* Diverticulum of Kommerell.
      left aortic arch with, 544, 546f, 959-960, 960f
  anatomy of
    normal, 989-991, 990f
    variants of, 990-991
  aneurysm of, CT imaging of, 1648-1649, 1649f
  differential considerations of, 991, 991f
  involvement of, in Takayasu arteritis, 1315
  stenosis of, 1326. *See also* Subclavian steal syndrome.
    carotid-subclavian bypass for, 1175-1176, 1175f-1176f
    MR imaging of, 1650, 1651f-1653f

Subclavian flap aortoplasty, for aortic coarctation, 549
Subclavian steal syndrome, 1326-1331
  carotid-subclavian bypass for, 1175, 1175f-1176f
  clinical presentation of, 1326-1327, 1645
  definition of, 1326
  differential diagnosis of, 1329
  etiology and pathophysiology of, 1326
  imaging of
    angiographic, 1329, 1330f
    CT scans in, 1328, 1328f
    indications and algorithm for, 1327
    MR scans in, 1328-1329, 1328f-1330f
    ultrasound, 1327-1328, 1327f
      Doppler, 1247-1249, 1247f-1248f
  prevalence and epidemiology of, 1326
  treatment options for, 1329-1330
    surgical and interventional, 1330
Subclavian vein
  anatomy of, 1661, 1662f
  upper extremity drainage via, 999
Subpleural edema, 1375-1376
Subpulmonary conus, development of, 22-24, 25f
Sudden death, arrhythmogenic right ventricular dysplasia and, 884
Superficial veins
  of lower extremity, 1024-1027, 1026f-1028f
  of upper extremity, 1019-1022, 1020f-1022f. *See also* named vein.
Superior vena cava, anatomy of, 996-998, 997f
  variations in, 997-998, 997f-998f
Supraduodenal artery, 972
Suprarenal vein, 1010, 1010f
Surgical excision, of lower extremity aneurysm
  anatomic considerations in, 1600-1601, 1601f
  contraindications to, 1601-1602
  imaging findings in, 1603-1604, 1604f-1605f
  indications for, 1601, 1602f-1603f
  outcomes and complications of, 1602-1603
Surgical ligation, for patent ductus arteriosus, 596-597
Surgical thrombolectomy, lower extremity, 1598-1599, 1598t
Surgical ventricular restoration (Dor procedure), for ischemic heart disease, 811
  postoperative appearance of, 817, 818f
  postoperative complications of, 812
  imaging of, 817-818
Sympathetic nervous system, neurohormonal PET imaging of, 344, 344t
Syphilitic aortitis, 1322-1324, 1322t, 1323f
Systemic fibrosis, nephrogenic, as contraindication to contrast-enhanced MR angiography, 1255-1257
Systemic lupus erythematosus, 1391
  atherosclerosis associated with, 1196
Systemic veins
  anomalous, echocardiography of, 118
  formation of, 8-10, 10f
Systolic function
  disorders of, etiologies of, 790
  echocardiography of, 103, 104f-105f
  global, 756-758
  left ventricular, image interpretation of, 232-235, 233t, 234f
Systolic peak, abnormality(ies) of, carotid vessel stenosis causing, 1240-1241
  parvus tardus waveform, 1240, 1240f
  pulsus alternans waveform, 1241, 1241f
  pulsus bisferiens waveform, 1241, 1241f

T

T lymphocytes, activation of, in atherosclerosis, 1195-1196
Tagged imaging, for quantifying myocardial motion, 229-230, 229f, 230t
Takayasu arteritis, 1411-1414
  aneurysm dilation in, 509, 511f, 1275
  arteriography of, 1414
  classification of, 1315t
  clinical presentation of, 1314-1315, 1315f, 1388
  CT and MR scans of, 1413, 1413f
  definition of, 1314
  diagnostic criteria for, 1388t
  differential diagnosis of, 1390, 1413
  Doppler ultrasonography of, 1498, 1503f-1504f
  etiology and pathophysiology of, 1314, 1388, 1411, 1644
  FDG-PET scan of, 1414
  imaging of
    indications and algorithm for, 1315-1316, 1413-1414
    technique and findings in, 1316-1318, 1316f-1319f, 1388-1390, 1389f
  incidence of, 1644
  prevalence and epidemiology of, 1314, 1388
  treatment options for, 1318-1319, 1319f, 1414
  upper extremity affected by, 1643-1644
  vs. giant cell arteritis, 1319f
Tako-tsubo cardiomyopathy, 107
Tamponade, 63-64, 64f
  causes of, 64t
  echocardiography of, 113
  pericardial effusion with, 941
Technetium 99m (^{99m}Tc), manufacture of, 274
Technetium 99m (^{99m}Tc) erythrocyte scan
  of gastrointestinal bleed, 1144-1146
  pitfall of, 1146
  report of, 1146
Technetium 99m (^{99m}Tc) labeled radiotracer, 301
  in ACEI renal scintigraphy, 1494
  in SPECT
    for identifying myocardial viability, 794-795, 795f
      with nitrate administration, 795-796, 796f
    imaging protocol(s) of, 282-283
      dual-isotope, 282-283
        with thallium 201 and, 282-283, 746
      one-day, 282
      two-day protocol, 282
Technetium 99m (^{99m}Tc)-pertechnetate scan, of Meckel diverticulum, 1146-1148
Technetium 99m (^{99m}Tc) radiotracer protocol(s), rest-stress
  same-day, 282, 746
  two-day, 282, 746
Technetium 99m–N-NOET radiotracer, in SPECT, 302
Technetium 99m–sestamibi radiotracer, in SPECT, 301, 739, 740f-741f, 750f
Technetium 99m–teboroxime radiotracer, in SPECT, 302
Technetium 99m–tetrofosmin radiotracer, in SPECT, 301-302, 739
Telangiectasia, hereditary hemorrhagic, 1468
Temporal artery biopsy, for giant cell arteritis, 1322
Temporal resolution, in cardiac MR imaging, 180-181
Terminology issues, in MRI safety, 264, 264t-265t
Test bolus, in contrast CT angiography, 1059-1060, 1062
Test bolus injection, of contrast media, 161-162
Testicular vein, 1010, 1010f
Tet spells, treatment of, 648
Tetralogy, pink, 641
Tetralogy of Fallot, 640-650
  angiography of, 646-647, 662
  classic signs of, 647
  clinical presentation of, 641, 660
  considerations regarding, 390, 391t
  coronary artery anomalies associated with, 640
  CT imaging of, 643, 644f, 661
  definition of, 640, 660
  differential diagnosis of, 647-648
  etiology and pathophysiology of, 640-641, 660
  imaging of
    indications and algorithm for, 641, 660
    technique and findings in, 641-647, 660-662
  medical treatment of, 648
  MR imaging of, 643-646, 645f-647f, 661, 662f-663f
  postoperative, 694-695, 695f
  nuclear imaging of, 661
  pathology of, 7
  pathophysiology and follow-up of, 554, 554f
  prevalence and epidemiology of, 553-554, 640, 660
  radiography of, 641-647, 641f-642f, 660, 661f
  reporting of, 648-649
  surgical repair of, 391, 648, 649f
    postoperative management after, 694-695, 695f
  ultrasonography of, 119, 642-643, 643f, 660-661, 661f-662f
  postnatal, 642-643, 643f
  vs. double-outlet right ventricle, 684
Thallium 201 (^{201}Tl)
  in SPECT, 298-301, 738-739
    dosage and image quality of, 301
    dual-isotope imaging protocol with Tc 99m and, 282-283, 746
    extraction and biodistribution of, 299, 299f
    for identifying myocardial viability, 796-797
      protocols for, 797, 797f-798f
    imaging protocols for, 281-282, 746
    radiation exposure to, 300-301, 300t, 301f
    redistribution of, 299, 299f
    showing myocardial viability, 299-300, 300f
  manufacture of, 274
  physical properties of, 298
  washout of, necrotic myocardial tissue and, 796
Thienopyridines, for cerebrovascular atherosclerotic disease, 1208
Thigh arteries, collateral pathways of, 985
Thoracic aorta. See also Aorta; Aortic entries.
  anatomy of
    normal, 955-961, 956f-958f
    variant, 957-961, 958f-961f
  ascending
    anatomy of, 955, 956f
    pathologic conditions of, 433. See also Aortic aneurysm; Aortic dissection.

Thoracic aorta (Continued)
  surgical repair of, 433-437
    anatomic considerations in, 435, 435f
    contraindications to, 436
    indications for, 436
    outcomes and complications of, 436
    postoperative surveillance after, 437, 437t
    preoperative imaging in, 436-437, 436f
  descending, 955-956
  injury to. See Thoracic aortic trauma.
Thoracic aortic aneurysm, 1271-1286
  asymptomatic, 1277
  causes of, 1271
  clinical presentation of, 1277-1278
  definition of, 1271
  differential diagnosis of, 1282
  etiology and pathophysiology of, 1271-1277
    atherosclerosis in, 1271, 1272f
    cystic medial necrosis in, 1272-1273, 1273f-1274f
    dissection in, 1273, 1275f
    increased aortic flow in, 1276
    infection and inflammation in, 1275, 1276f
    post-stenotic dilation in, 1275, 1276f
    trauma in, 1273, 1275f
  false, 1277, 1277f
  imaging of
    echocardiographic, 1280
    indications and algorithm for, 1278-1279, 1278f
    technique and findings in, 1279-1282, 1280f-1281f
  prevalence and epidemiology of, 1271, 1272f
  reporting of, 1285-1286
  rupture of, 1278
  symptomatic, 1278
  treatment option(s) for, 1282-1285
    hybrid procedures in, 1178-1179, 1178f-1179f
    medical, 1282-1283
    prosthetic graft as, 1284, 1284f
      complications of, 1284-1285, 1285f
    stent graft as, 1283, 1284f
  true, 1277
Thoracic aortic trauma
  angiography of, 1310-1311
  classic signs of, 1311
  clinical presentation of, 1306
  CT imaging of, 1307-1309
    aortic pseudoaneurysm in, 1308, 1309f
    contour abnormality in, 1308
    contrast agent extravasation in, 1309
    intimal flap in, 1308
    periaortic mediastinal hemorrhage in, 1309, 1309f
    technique of, 1307-1308
  differential diagnosis of, 1311, 1311f
  etiology and pathophysiology of, 1306-1313, 1307f-1308f
  imaging of, indications and algorithm for, 1306
  medical treatment of, 1312, 1312f
  MR imaging of, 1309-1310, 1310f
  radiography of, 1306-1307, 1308f
  reporting of, 1313
  surgical/interventional treatment of, 1312-1313, 1312f
  ultrasonography of, 1307
Thoracic aortitis, 1314-1325. See also Giant cell arteritis; Takayasu arteritis.
  differential diagnosis of, 1323-1324, 1324f
Thoracic artery, internal, 964-965, 989, 990f

Thoracic cavity drift, causing attenuation mismatch, in PET imaging, 310-311, 311f
Thoracic outlet, anatomy of, 1666-1667, 1669f
Thoracic outlet syndrome, 991, 991f, 1644, 1666-1669
  definition of, 1666
  imaging of, 1669
  incidence of, 1644
  tests for, 1669
Thoracic vasculature, CT angiography of, 1060-1062, 1063f-1064f
  protocol parameters for, 1061t
Thoracic vein, 996
Thoracoabdominal aortic aneurysm
  Crawford classification of, 1176-1177, 1177f, 1276, 1277f
  repair of, 1176-1178
Thoracotomy, for thoracic aortic injury, 1312
Thorax
  arterial anatomy of, 955-968. *See also* named artery, e.g., Thoracic aorta.
  radiography of. *See also* Chest radiography.
    lateral view of, 77, 78f
  venous anatomy of, 996-1004. *See also* named vein, e.g., Superior vena cava.
    azygos and hemiazygos systems in, 1000
    chest wall drainage via, 999, 1000f
    normal, 996
    pulmonary veins and, 1001-1004
    upper extremity and head drainage via, 999
    venae cavae and, 996-999
Three-dimensional echocardiography, 101. *See also* Echocardiography.
Three-dimensional postprocessing, in CTA and MRA
  advanced, 1128-1143
    accurate assessment of, 1133-1134
    application of x-ray angiographic planning purposes in, 1131
    automated vessel extraction in, 1129
    automated vessel lumen analysis from, 1134
    automated vessel lumen segmentation in, 1136-1137, 1137f-1138f
      validation of, 1137, 1139f, 1139t
    automated vessel pathline detection in, 1135-1136, 1136f
      validation of, 1136, 1136t
    centerline detection in, 1129, 1130f
    contour detection in, 1129-1131, 1131f-1132f
    coronary vessel presegmentation in, 1129
    curved multiplanar reformatting in, 1129, 1130f
    introduction to, 1128-1142
    optimal angiographic view in, 1133, 1135f
    plaque assessment in, 1140-1142, 1140f-1141f, 1140t
    projection overlap in, 1133, 1134f
    region of interest in, 1132, 1134f
    segmentation steps in, 1131-1132, 1133f
    simulating angiographic views in, 1133, 1135f
    stenosis quantification in, 1131
    technical requirements for, 1129-1131
    user interaction in, 1134-1135
    vessel wall morphology in, automated assessment of, 1137-1138, 1139f-1140f
  basic, 1120-1127
    maximum intensity projection in, 1121-1123, 1123f-1124f

Three-dimensional postprocessing, in CTA and MRA (Continued)
    multiplanar reformation in, 1120-1121, 1121f-1122f
    interpolation in, 1120-1121, 1123f
    linear interpolation in, 1121
  of arterial system, 1451
  of venous system and soft tissue, 1452
  volume rendering in, 1122f, 1123-1125, 1124f-1126f
Thrombectomy
  balloon, for iliac occlusion, 1578, 1578f
  mechanical, 1599
Thrombin, as embolic agent, 1169
Thromboangiitis obliterans (Buerger disease), 1645, 1651-1652, 1658f. *See also* Upper extremity, medium and small vessel disease of.
  etiology and pathophysiology of, 1646
  incidence of, 1646
Thrombolectomy, surgical, lower extremity, 1598-1599, 1598t
Thrombolysis, 1164-1167
  agents in, 1599
  catheter-directed, 1597f, 1599-1600
    for acute limb ischemia, 1577
  contraindications to, 1166
  for acute coronary syndrome, 723
  for inferior vena cava thrombosis, 1539
  for mesenteric atherosclerotic disease, 1210
  imaging findings in, 1166-1167
  indications for, 1165-1166
  outcomes and complications of, 1166
  pharmacomechanical, 1599-1600
  special considerations in, 1165, 1166f
Thrombosis
  arterial
    coronary, during angioplasty intervention, 129, 129f
    hepatic
      after liver transplantation, 1548-1551, 1548f-1552f
      MR imaging of, 1460-1461, 1460f
    native, 1573
    renal. *See* Renal artery thrombosis.
  during angioplasty, 1162
  extremity, ultrasound detection of, 1334-1335
  graft, 1573
    after CABG surgery, 524-525, 527f-529f
    after endovascular aneurysm repair, 1434, 1434f-1436f
    after lower extremity bypass, 1185-1186, 1186f
  in- stent. *See* Coronary stents, in-stent restenosis and thrombosis.
  venous
    deep. *See* Deep vein thrombosis (DVT).
    Doppler imaging of, 1044
    inferior vena cava, 1535-1540, 1537t, 1538f-1539f
    mesenteric, 1457-1458
    portal, 1457-1458, 1457f
      after liver transplantation, 1551, 1553f-1554f
    renal. *See* Renal vein thrombosis.
Thrombus
  in left atrial appendage, 443, 443f
    CT imaging of, 447, 447f-448f
  intracardiac, delayed hyperenhancement MR imaging of, 210, 210f
  tricuspid valve, 841f
  tumor, 1458
Thyrocervical trunk, 989, 990f

Tibial artery
  anterior, 983, 984f
  posterior, 984, 984f
Tibial vein
  anterior, 1028
  posterior, 1028
Ticlopidine Aspirin Stroke Study (TASS), 1208
Time to peak filling rate to R-R interval (tPFR/RR), 754
Time-of-flight (TOF) magnetic resonance angiography, 1091-1094, 1092f, 1103-1105, 1104f. *See also* Magnetic resonance angiography (MRA).
  contraindications to, 1103-1105
  image interpretation in, 1105
  indications for, 1103
  of carotid artery stenosis, 1252
  pitfalls and solutions in, 1105
  three-dimensional, 1093
  sequential, 1094, 1094f
  two-dimensional, 1092-1093, 1092f-1093f
Time-resolved imaging of contrast kinetics (TRICKS), three-dimensional, 1090-1091
Time-resolved (TR) magnetic resonance angiography, 1109-1112, 1109f. *See also* Magnetic resonance imaging (MRA).
  contraindications to, 1110-1111
  contrast-enhanced, 1089-1091, 1090f-1091f
  image interpretation in, 1112
  indications for, 1109-1110, 1110f-1111f, 1112t
  pitfalls and solutions in, 1111
Tissue Doppler imaging (TDI), 119-122, 120f-121f, 230
  of amyloidosis, 862-863
Tissue phase mapping (TPM), for quantifying myocardial motion, 230, 230t
Tissue plasminogen activator (tPA), for inferior vena cava thrombosis, 1539
Tissue-weighting factors, in irradiation, 1070-1071
Tobacco use
  atherosclerosis associated with, 1197, 1197f
  Buerger disease associated with, 1646
Toe amputation, for chronic limb ischemia, 1583-1584
Torsion, renal transplant, 1521-1522
Total anomalous pulmonary venous connections (TAPVC)
  classic signs of, 636
  clinical presentation of, 635-636
  definition of, 634
  differential diagnosis of, 636-637
  etiology and pathophysiology of, 634-635
  imaging of
    indications and algorithm for, 635
    technique and findings in, 635-636, 635f
  medical treatment of, 637
  prevalence and epidemiology of, 634
  reporting of, 638
  surgical/interventional treatment of, 638
Total anomalous pulmonary venous return (TAPVR), 1002-1004, 1003f
  infracardiac, 1008
Toxin(s), as risk factor for pulmonary hypertension, 1359b
Tracer kinetics, 314-315
  fluorodeoxyglucose 18, 315
  rubidium 82, 314-315
Tracheal compression, of innominate artery, 544, 547f

TransAtlantic Inter-Society Consensus (TASC) Working Group classification, of aortoiliac and infrainguinal occlusive disease, 1594, 1595t
Transcatheter intravascular ultrasonography, of in-stent restenosis and thrombosis, 517-518
Transcatheter occlusion, for patent ductus arteriosus, 596, 596f
Transcutaneous oxygen tension measurements, in wound healing, 1186, 1187t
Transducers, ultrasound, 1033
  types of, 1034f
Transesophageal echocardiography (TEE), 101, 102f. *See also* Echocardiography.
  contraindications to, 120
  dobutamine, vs. dobutamine MRI, 221-222
  of aortic dissection, 1290-1291, 1290f
  of atrial septal defect, 564-565, 566f-567f
    postoperative, 365-366, 367f
    preoperative, 364, 364f-365f
  of intramural hematoma of aorta, 1297
  of patent foramen ovale, 369, 369f
  of penetrating atherosclerotic ulcer, 1300
  of thoracic aortic trauma, 1307
  of ventricular septal defect, 576f
  pitfalls and solutions in, 120-122
Transient ischemic attack (TIA). *See also* Stroke.
  antiplatelet therapy for, 1222
Transient ischemic dilation (TID), 359
Transit time (TT), of contrast media, 160
Transmission-emission misalignment, in PET/CT imaging, 327-328, 328f
Transplant renal artery stenosis (TRAS), 1559-1564
  clinical presentation of, 1559-1560
  differential diagnosis of, 1564
  etiology and pathophysiology of, 1559, 1560f
  imaging of
    angiographic, 1564
    indications and algorithm for, 1560
    MR angiographic, 1561-1564, 1562t, 1563f
    nuclear medicine, 1564
    radiographic, 1560
    ultrasound, 1560-1561, 1560f-1561f
  prevalence and epidemiology of, 1559
  treatment options for, 1564
Transplantation
  heart. *See* Heart transplantation.
  liver. *See* Hepatic transplantation.
  pancreas, vascular evaluation of recipient of, 1568-1569
  renal. *See* Renal transplantation.
Transposition of great arteries (TGA), 389t, 601-615
  cardiac anomalies associated with, 604-605, 604f-605f
  classifications of, 601-602, 602f
  clinical manifestations of, 605-606, 606f, 657
  complete, 601
    cardiac anomalies associated with, 604, 604f-605f
    clinical presentation of, 603
    definition of, 601
    embryology of, 603-604
    imaging of, 611-612
      echocardiographic, 119

Transposition of great arteries (TGA) *(Continued)*
    surgery for, 607-611, 608f-611f. *See also specific procedure, e.g.,* Arterial switch procedure.
      imaging after, 611-613, 612f-613f
    vs. double-outlet right ventricle, 607, 608f
  congenitally corrected, 601
    abnormal AV node development in, 606
    cardiac anomalies associated with, 604-605, 605f
    definition of, 602
    embryology of, 604
    imaging of, 613-614
      echocardiographic, 119
    late complications of, 606, 606f
    physiology and natural history of, 606
    surgery for, 611
  definition of, 601-602, 656
  dextro-, 601, 656-657
  differential diagnosis of, 606-607, 607f-608f
  epidemiology of, 603
  etiology and pathophysiology of, 603-605, 604f-605f, 657
  genetics of, 603
  imaging of
    indications and algorithm for, 611-613, 657
    postoperative, 695-697, 696f-697f
    technique and findings in, 657-660, 658f-659f
  levo-, 602, 677-680. *See also* Levotransposition of great arteries.
  medical treatment of, 607
  pathology of, 7
  pathophysiology of, 555
  prevalence and epidemiology of, 554-555, 656-657
  surgical treatment of, 389-390, 607-611, 608f-610f
    follow-up after, 555, 555f
    postoperative management after, 696-697, 696f-697f
  three-letter scheme categorizing, 602, 603f
  vs. double-outlet right ventricle, 684
Transthoracic echocardiography (TTE). *See also* Echocardiography.
  of atrial septal defect, 564, 566f-567f
  of cardiac metastases, 923-924
  of ventricular septal defect, 574, 576f
Trauma. *See at specific anatomic site.*
Treadmill stress testing, coronary artery calcium screening with, 463
Triangle of dysplasia, in arrhythmogenic right ventricular dysplasia, 884-885, 885f
Tricuspid valve
  anatomy of, 839-844
  anomalies of, 388, 388t
  failure of, disease causing, 839, 840f-841f
  formation of, 5
  normal function of, 839-844
Tricuspid valve atresia, 840f
  single-ventricle palliation pathway for, 391-392
Tricuspid valve insufficiency, 841f
Tricuspid valve regurgitation
  clinical presentation of, 844
  echocardiography of, 845
  imaging of
    indications and algorithm for, 844-845
    technique and findings in, 845
Tricuspid valve thrombus, 841f
Trigeminal artery, persistent, 963, 964f
Trigger delay, in cardiac MR imaging, 201, 202f

Trig window, in MR imaging, 181-182
Trisacryl gelatin microspheres, as embolic agent, 1168
True aneurysm, 1271, 1277. *See also* Aneurysm.
Truncal valve
  tricuspid, 619, 619f
  ventricular septal defect and, 618-619, 618f
Truncation, of CT image, 322, 323f
Truncus arteriosus, 3-4, 616-624
  angiography of, 666
  cardiac anomalies associated with, 618-620, 618f-619f
  classification of, 616-618, 617f, 662-663
  clinical presentation of, 620, 620f, 664
  CT imaging of, 664-665, 665f-666f
  definition of, 616, 662-663
  differential diagnosis of, 621
  embryology of, 618
  epidemiology of, 618
  etiology and pathophysiology of, 618-620, 663-664
  genetic screening for, 618
  imaging of
    indications and algorithm for, 664
    technique and findings in, 664-666, 665f-670f
  MR imaging of, 665-666, 667f-670f
  nuclear imaging of, 666
  pathology of, 7
  persistent, 618
  radiography of, 664
  septation of, 6-7, 7f-8f
  surgical treatment of, 621, 621f
    imaging after, 622-623, 622f-623f
    prognosis after, 621-622
  ultrasonography of, 664, 665f
  vs. double-outlet right ventricle, 684-685
Tubal modulation, radiation dose minimization with, in cardiac CT imaging, 146
Tumor(s). *See named tumor; at anatomic site.*
Tumor embolization
  clinical presentation of, 1369
  etiology and pathophysiology of, 1368
  imaging technique and findings in, 1369-1370
Tumor thrombus, 1458
Tunica adventia, of blood vessels, 60, 60f
Tunica media, of blood vessels, 60, 60f
Turbo spin-echo (TSE) sequences, in cardiac MR imaging, 204, 204f
Turbulent flow, in Doppler imaging, 1043, 1043f
Twinkle artifact, in Doppler ultrasonography, 1043
Two-day ^{99m}Tc radiotracer protocol, for SPECT, 282, 746
Two-dimensional echocardiography, 98. *See also* Echocardiography.

U

Uhl anomaly, vs. arrhythmogenic right ventricular dysplasia, 893
Ulcer (ulceration)
  atherosclerotic, penetrating. *See* Atherosclerotic ulcer, penetrating.
  carotid artery, detection of, 1266-1267
  lower limb, 1581, 1581f
Ulnar artery
  anatomy of, 994-995
  at elbow, 993f, 994
  branches of, 994
  CT angiography of, 1648-1649, 1649f-1650f

Ulnar vein, 1022-1023, 1023f
Ultrasonography, See also Echocardiography.
  aortic trauma, thoracic, 1307
  B mode, 1033-1034
    image in, 1034, 1037
  contrast-enhanced harmonic imaging in, 1037
  Doppler. See Doppler ultrasonography.
  duplex. See Duplex ultrasonography.
  lower and upper extremity, for pulmonary embolism, 1334-1335
  of acute coronary syndrome, 716-717
  of amyloidosis, 862-863, 862f
  of angiosarcoma, 926
  of aortic aneurysm
    abdominal, 1180, 1400-1401, 1401f, 1441
    inflammatory, 1405
    thoracic, 1280
  of aortic dissection, 1290-1291, 1290f
  of aortic occlusion, acute, 1411, 1411f
  of arteriovenous fistula and pseudoaneurysm, in renal transplant recipient, 1565, 1565f
  of arteriovenous fistula failure, 1675-1676, 1675f
  of atherosclerosis, 1201-1203, 1202f
  of atrial septal defect, 565-566, 566f-567f
  of cardiomyopathy
    dilated, 852-853, 853f
    hypertrophic, 874
    siderotic, 867
  of carotid stenosis, 1220, 1220f
  of chronic thromboembolic pulmonary hypertension, 1345
  of coarctation of aorta, 536
  of cor triatriatum, 632, 633f
  of coronary atherosclerosis, 708-709, 709f
  of double-outlet right ventricle, 682, 683f-684f
  of endoleaks, 1409
  of eosinophilic endomyocardial disease, 865, 865f
  of fibroma, 912
  of giant cell arteritis, 1320
  of inferior vena cava anomalies, 1528
  of inferior vena cava stenosis, after hepatic transplantation, 1534-1535, 1534f-1535f
  of inferior vena cava thrombosis, 1536
  of inferior vena cava tumors, 1530
  of in-stent restenosis and thrombosis, 517-518
  of intramural hematoma of aorta, 1297
  of lipoma, 915
  of lipomatous hypertrophy of interatrial septum, 916
  of liposarcoma, 931
  of myocarditis, 897
  of myxoma, 907, 907f
  of papillary fibroelastoma, 910
  of paraganglioma, 918
  of patent ductus arteriosus, 585, 586f
  of penetrating atherosclerotic ulcer, 1300
  of pericardial effusion, 942
  of pericarditis
    acute, 946
    constrictive, 950
  of primary cardiac lymphoma, 933
  of pulmonary valve regurgitation, 846
  of pulmonary venous connections
    partial anomalous, 626-627
    total anomalous, 635-636
  of renal artery and vein thrombosis, in transplant recipient, 1567

Ultrasonography (Continued)
  of renal artery stenosis, in transplant recipient, 1560-1561, 1560f-1561f
  of rhabdomyoma, 913
  of rhabdomyosarcoma, 930
  of sarcoidosis, 869
  of single ventricle, 672, 674f-675f
  of sinus venous defect, 629-630, 630f
  of subclavian steal syndrome, 1327-1328, 1327f
  of Takayasu arteritis, 1316, 1316f
  of tetralogy of Fallot, 642-643, 643f, 660-661, 661f-662f
  of transposition of great arteries, 657-658, 658f
  of truncus arteriosus, 664, 665f
  of upper extremity medium and small vessel disease, 1647-1648, 1648f
  of vascular anatomy, in pancreas transplant recipient, 1569
  of vascular rings, 543
  of ventricular septal defect, 574, 576f
  vascular
    physical principles and instrumentation in, 1033-1037, 1034f-1035f
    techniques of, 1037-1045. See also Doppler ultrasonography.
Unaliasing by Fournier-encoding overlaps using temporal dimension (UNFOLD), in parallel imaging, 197
University of Maryland triage, for cardiac multidetector CT studies, 721t
Unstable angina/non–ST segment elevation myocardial infarction, percutaneous coronary interventions for, 402
Upper extremity
  angiography of, 1159, 1159f
  arterial anatomy of, 989-995. See also named artery, e.g., Subclavian artery.
  large vessel disease of, 1643-1645
    cause and pathophysiology of, 1644
    clinical presentation of, 1644-1645
    imaging indications and algorithm for, 1645
    prevalence and epidemiology of, 1644
  medium and small vessel disease of, 1645-1652
    classic signs in, 1652
    clinical presentation of, 1646-1647
    differential diagnosis of, 1652
    etiology and pathophysiology of, 1646
    imaging of
      angiographic, 1651-1652, 1658f
      CT scan in, 1648-1649, 1648f-1650f
      indications and algorithm for, 1647
      MR scan in, 1649-1650, 1651f-1654f
      PET-CT, 1650-1651, 1655f-1657f
      radiographic, 1647, 1647f
      ultrasound, 1647-1648, 1648f
    prevalence and epidemiology of, 1646
    reporting of, 1658-1659
    treatment options for, 1652-1658
  thrombosis in
    deep vein. See Deep vein thrombosis (DVT), upper extremity.
    ultrasound detection of, 1334-1335
  venous anatomy of, 1019-1023, 1661, 1662f
    deep veins in, 1022-1023, 1023f
    superficial veins in, 1019-1022, 1020f-1022f
  venous drainage of, 999
Ureter(s), circumcaval (retrocaval), 1526
Urokinase, for inferior vena cava thrombosis, 1539

Uterine artery, 980f, 981
Uterine plexus, 1014

V

VACTERL syndrome, 640
Vaginal artery, 981
Valve implantation, for pulmonary insufficiency, 377. See also Pulmonary insufficiency, valve implantation for.
Valve replacement
  for aortic regurgitation, 833-834
    indications for, 420t
  for aortic stenosis, 830, 832f
    indications for, 419t
  for mitral stenosis, 836
Valvotomy, balloon. See Balloon valvotomy.
Valvular calcification, radiography of, 87, 88f
Valvular heart disease
  catheter-based management of, 405-409, 407f-408f
  echocardiography of, 65-66, 107
  MR evaluation of blood flow in, 241-242, 243f
  radiographic studies of, 92-94, 93f
Valvuloplasty, balloon. See Balloon valvuloplasty.
Van Praagh and Van Praagh classification, of truncus arteriosus, 616, 617f, 662-663
Van Praagh's types, of human heart, 19, 21f
Varices, esophageal, from portal hypertension, 1008-1009, 1008f
  MR imaging of, 1454-1455, 1455f
Vascular access, in angiography, 1157-1158
Vascular bypass surgery, lower extremity, 1585-1591
  anatomic considerations in, 1585-1588, 1586f-1589f
  conduits in
    autogenous saphenous vein as, 1585-1586
    definition of, 1585
    extra-anatomic bypass grafts as, 1586-1588, 1587f-1589f
    prosthetic, 1586
    xenografts as, 1586, 1587f
  contraindications to, 1588-1589
  imaging of
    postoperative surveillance with, 1591
    preoperative planning with, 1591
  indications for, 1588, 1589t
Vascular dilators, 1156
Vascular disorders, of abdomen, MR imaging of, 1451-1470. See also under specific disorder.
  gadolinium use and safety in, 1453
  methodology in, 1451
  of arteries, 1451-1452
  of veins and soft tissue, 1452-1453
Vascular indistinctness, in pulmonary edema, 1375
Vascular interventions, percutaneous, 1155-1171. See also specific intervention, e.g., Angiography.
  equipment and tools used in, 1155-1157
Vascular plug, Amplatz, as embolic agent, 1168
Vascular rings, 542
  classic sign(s) of, 544-545
    anomalous left pulmonary artery, 545, 547f
    double aortic arch, 544, 544f-545f
    innominate artery compression, 544, 547f

I-42 *Index*

Vascular rings *(Continued)*
    left aortic arch with aberrant right
        subclavian artery, 544, 546f
    right aortic arch with aberrant left
        subclavian artery, 544, 545f-546f
  clinical presentation of, 542-543
  complete, 542
  definition of, 542
  differential diagnosis of, 545-546
  etiology and pathophysiology of, 542, 543f
  formation of, 11
  imaging studies of, 543-544
  incomplete, 542
  prevalence and epidemiology of, 542
  surgical/interventional treatment of, 546-547
Vascular sheaths, 1156
Vascular slings, 542
Vascular trauma, abdominal, 1468-1469, 1469f
Vasculitis. *See also specific type, e.g.*, Takayasu arteritis.
  definition of, 1643-1644
  pulmonary, 1384, 1385t
  upper extremity, 1643-1644
Vasodilator agents, 352-355. *See also specific vasodilator.*
  in SPECT
    contraindications to, 745
    protocol for, 284-285, 284f
Vein(s), abdominal, MR imaging of, 1452-1453
Velocity encoding (VENC)
  in MR evaluation of blood flow, 240, 242f
  in phase contrast MR angiography, 1094-1095, 1095f-1096f, 1105
Velocity scale, in Doppler ultrasonography, choice of, 1038, 1039f
Vena cava. *See* Inferior vena cava; Superior vena cava.
Vena cordia parva, 53, 54f
Venice-revised WHO classification, of pulmonary hypertension, 1354, 1355b
Venography
  CO_2, of arteriovenous fistula failure, 1682, 1682f
  CT, of pulmonary embolism, 1340
  x-ray, of upper extremity deep vein thrombosis, 1663
Veno-occlusive disease, hepatic, vs. Budd-Chiari syndrome, 1461, 1462f
Venous aneurysms, after liver transplantation, 1551, 1554f
Venous flow, in Doppler imaging, 1043-1044
Venous obstruction, Doppler imaging of, 1044
Venous plexus, dorsal, upper extremity, 1019-1020, 1021f
Venous thrombosis. *See* Thrombosis, venous.
  deep. *See* Deep vein thrombosis (DVT).
Veno-venous shunt, intrahepatic, MR imaging of, 1454-1455, 1456f
Ventilation-perfusion (V/Q) scintigraphy. *See* Nuclear medicine imaging, ventilation-perfusion (V/Q).
Ventricle(s)
  developmental pathology of, 4
  formation of, 4, 5f-6f
  identification of, 15-16, 15f-16f
  left
    anatomy of, 33-34, 34f
    circumferential-longitudinal shear angle of, 234-235
    dysfunction of
      associated with coronary artery disease, 403
      management of, 62
    ejection fraction of. *See* Ejection fraction, left ventricular.

Ventricle(s) *(Continued)*
    normal values of, 65t
    pressure-volume relationships in, 58-59, 59f
    radiography of, of cardiac borders, in lateral projection, 77
    segmentation of, 49-50, 51f-52f
    ^{99m}Tc-sestamibi imaging of, 286f
    two-dimensional echocardiographic imaging of, 103
  primitive, 3-4
  right
    anatomy of, 33, 33f
    double-outlet. *See* Double-outlet right ventricle (DORV).
    echocardiographic imaging of, 103
    normal values of, 65t
  single, 671-677
    angiography of, 677, 678f
    clinical presentation of, 672
    CT imaging of, 673
    defects of, 389-390, 389t
      repair of, 390
    definition of, 671
    etiology of, 671
    imaging of
      indications and algorithm for, 672
      technique and findings in, 672-677
    MR imaging of, 673-676
      after bidirectional superior cavopulmonary connection, 674-675
      after Fontan procedure, 675-676, 676f-677f, 699-700
      after stage I, 674
      in native state, 674
    nuclear imaging of, 677
    pathophysiology of, 671-672
    prevalence and epidemiology of, 671
    radiography of, 672, 673f
    ultrasonography of, 672, 674f-675f
Ventricular assist device (VAD)
  for ischemic heart disease, 810-811
  postoperative appearance of, 815, 816f
  postoperative complications of, 812
    imaging of, 816-817, 817f
  preoperative and perioperative assessment of, 815
  long-term, 811
  temporary percutaneous, 811
Ventricular border, radiography of
  left, 74-75, 75f-76f
  right, 75
Ventricular cardiomyopathy, right, arrhythmogenic, 237, 237f
Ventricular dysplasia, right, arrhythmogenic, 884-895. *See also* Arrhythmogenic right ventricular dysplasia (ARVD).
Ventricular function
  gated MPI assessment of, 771-773
    data processing, reconstruction, and analysis of, 772-773
    electrogram gated acquisition in, 772
    pitfalls and solutions in, 773
    technique(s) of, 773-779
      equilibrium gated blood pool imaging, 773-775, 774f-778f
      first-pass radionuclide angiography, 775-779, 779f
  global, image interpretation of, 231-232, 231f-232f
  left
    CT assessment of, 761
    diastolic, 235, 235f

Ventricular function *(Continued)*
    MRI assessment of, 181-182, 181f-182f, 556, 733-734, 758-759, 760f-761t
      using dobutamine, 218-223
        contraindications to, 223
        image interpretation in, 223
        indications and clinical utility for, 218-223, 220f-223f, 220t
        pitfalls and solutions in, 223
      using exercise, 223-224, 223f
    normal values of, in healthy persons, 233t
    regional, image interpretation of, 232-235, 233t, 234f-235f
  right
    CT assessment of, 762-763
    diastolic, 237
    global, image interpretation of, 235, 236t
    MRI assessment of, 217, 217f, 761-762, 762t-763t
    normal values of, in healthy persons, 236t
    regional, image interpretation of, 237, 237f
    systolic, 232-235, 233t, 234f
Ventricular loop, analysis of, 18, 19f
Ventricular mass
  in hypertrophic cardiomyopathy, MR imaging of, 875-876, 878f
  left, image interpretation of, 232
Ventricular myxoma, 906. *See also* Myxoma.
Ventricular outflow tract(s)
  developmental pathology of, 7, 8f
  formation of, 6-7, 7f-8f
  right, vs. arrhythmogenic right ventricular dysplasia, 893t
Ventricular outflow tract obstruction
  echocardiography of, 118
  left, in hypertrophic cardiomyopathy
    MR imaging of, 879-882, 881f
    treatment of, 881-882
Ventricular septal defect (VSD)
  angiography of, 577-579, 580f
  associated with d-TGA, 657
  clinical presentation of, 573
  considerations regarding, 383, 385f, 385t
  CT imaging of, 574-575, 577f-578f
  definition of, 572
  developmental pathology of, 4
  differential diagnosis of, 579-580
  etiology and pathophysiology of, 572-573
  imaging of
    indications and algorithm for, 573
    technique and findings in, 574
  medical treatment of, 580
  MR imaging of, 575-577, 578f-579f
  nuclear imaging of, 577
  prevalence and epidemiology of, 572
  radiography of, 574, 574f-575f
  reporting of, 581
  subtruncal, 618-619, 618f
  surgical repair of, 621, 621f
  surgical/interventional treatment of, 386, 580-581
  type I, 572
  type II, 572
  type III, 572
  type IV, 572
  ultrasonography of, 118, 574, 576f
Ventricular septum
  anatomy of, 34, 34f
  anomalies associated with, evaluation of, 24, 26f
  developmental pathology of, 4
  formation of, 4, 5f-6f
Ventricular strain, left, 234-235, 235f

Ventricular volume
　left
　　MRI determinants of, Simpson's rule in, 415
　　quantification of, FLASH vs. steady-state free precession in, 231-232
　　right, image interpretation of, 235-237
Ventricular-level shunt, in acyanotic congenital heart disease, 383, 385t
Ventriculoarterial (VA) discordance, in levotransposition of great arteries, 677
Ventriculoscintigraphy, of arrhythmogenic right ventricular dysplasia, 887
Vertebral artery, 989, 990f
　Doppler ultrasonography of, 1246-1249
　　normal tracing in, 1231-1232, 1232f
　　pre-steal waveform of, 1247-1249, 1247f
Vesical artery, inferior, 981
Vesical venous plexus, 1014
Viability protocols, for PET imaging, 318, 318f
Visceral plexus(es), venous origin in, 1013-1014, 1014f
Visceral situs solitus, in Ebstein anomaly, 653
Visceroatrial situs, analysis of, 16-18, 17f-19f
Voltage, x-ray tube, in computed tomography, reduction of, 152-153
Volume detectors, in CT imaging, 140-141
Volume overload, 63
Volume rendering technique (VRT)
　equation for, 1124
　of CT angiography, 1074, 1122f, 1123-1125, 1124f-1126f
　　carotid, 1266
　　coronary, 502
　　lower extremity, 1622, 1625f
　　renal, 1489, 1490f
　of CT imaging, cardiac, 176-178, 177f
Voxel, volume flow rate through, calculation of, 1097

W

Walking adenosine protocol, 357. *See also* Adenosine.
Warfarin, for inferior vena cava thrombosis, 1539
　of myocardial viability, 800, 800f
Water flask silhouette, in pericardial effusion, 942
Water phantom, in CT systems, 1049, 1050f
Waterston shunt, for decreased pulmonary blood flow, 391
Waveform, in Doppler imaging, 1043
Waveform analysis, Doppler, of carotid arteries, 1240-1245
　abnormal patterns involving cardiac cycle, 1242-1245
　　arteriovenous fistula, 1244, 1246f
　　carotid dissection, 1243, 1245f
　　carotid pseudoaneurysm, 1243, 1246f
　　intra-aortic balloon pump, 1244-1245, 1247f
　diastolic flow abnormalities in, 1241-1242, 1241f-1244f
　systolic peak abnormality(ies) in, 1240-1241
　　parvus tardus waveform, 1240, 1240f
　　pulsus alternans waveform, 1241, 1241f
　　pulsus bisferiens waveform, 1241, 1241f
WaveProp algorithm, 1129
Wegener's granulomatosis, 1384-1386
　clinical manifestations of, 1385
　differential diagnosis of, 1386
　imaging of, 1385-1386, 1385f-1386f
　limited, 1386
　prevalence and epidemiology of, 1385
Wells clinical decision rule, for pulmonary embolism, 1333t
Westermark sign, in pulmonary embolism, 1333f, 1334
Wet gangrene, 1581
Whitwater-Buerger disease, 1043
Wires, guide, 1156
Wolf mini-Maze procedure, for atrial fibrillation, 445, 446f
Wolff-Parkinson-White syndrome, 606
Wooden shoe sign, in tetralogy of Fallot, 647

X

Xenograft(s), bovine, in vascular bypass surgery, 1586, 1587f
X-linked dilated cardiomyopathy, 852. *See also* Cardiomyopathy, dilated.
X-ray(s), 270
　characteristic, 271, 272f
X-ray photons, 1047
X-ray physics, fundamentals of, 1047, 1048f
X-ray tube current, in CT imaging
　ECG-based reduction of, 151
　　pitfalls and solutions for, 151-152
　size-based reduction of, 151, 151f
　　pitfalls and solutions for, 152
X-ray tube voltage, in CT imaging, reduction of, 152-153

Y

Yttrium 90, radioembolization using, 975-976

Z

Z number, 270, 271t
Zellaballen, 917, 917f